TEXTBOOK OF PEDIATRIC EMERGENCY PROCEDURES

TEXTBOOK OF PEDIATRIC EMERGENCY PROCEDURES

Editors

Fred M. Henretig, M.D., F.A.A.P.
Associate Professor of Pediatrics
University of Pennsylvania School of Medicine
Director, Section of Clinical Toxicology
Division of Emergency Medicine
The Children's Hospital of Philadelphia
Medical Director, The Poison Control Center
Philadelphia, Pennsylvania

Christopher King, M.D., F.A.C.E.P.
Assistant Professor of Emergency Medicine and
Pediatrics
University of Pittsburgh School of Medicine
Attending Physician, Emergency Medicine
University of Pittsburgh Medical Center
Children's Hospital of Pittsburgh
Pittsburgh, Pennsylvania

Associate Editors
Mark D. Joffe, M.D.
Brent R. King, M.D.
John Loiselle, M.D.
Richard M. Ruddy, M.D.
James F. Wiley II, M.D.

Illustrator
Christine D. Young, A.M.I.

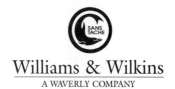

Williams & Wilkins
A WAVERLY COMPANY

BALTIMORE • PHILADELPHIA • LONDON • PARIS • BANGKOK
BUENOS AIRES • HONG KONG • MUNICH • SYDNEY • TOKYO • WROCLAW

Editor: Kathleen Courtney Millet
Managing Editors: Karen K. Gulliver, Joyce A. Murphy
Production Coordinator: Marette D. Magargle-Smith
Copy Editor: Carey Lange
Designer: Rita Baker-Schmidt
Typesetter: Maryland Composition Co., Inc.
Printer & Binder: Quebecor Printing

Copyright © 1997, Williams & Wilkins

351 West Camden Street
Baltimore, Maryland 21201-2436 USA

Rose Tree Corporate Center
1400 North Providence Road
Building II, Suite 5025
Media, Pennsylvania 19063-2043 USA

Accurate indications, adverse reactions, and dosage schedules for drugs are provided in this book, but it is possible that they may change. The reader is urged to review the package information data of the manufacturers of the medications mentioned.

Printed in the United States of America

Library of Congress Cataloging-in-Publication Data

Textbook of pediatric emergency procedures / editors, Fred M.
  Henretig, Christopher King ; associate editors, Mark D. Joffe . . .
  [et al.] ; illustrator, Christine D. Young.
     p.   cm.
  Includes index.
  ISBN 0–683–03971–7
  1. Pediatric emergencies.   2. Pediatric intensive care.
I. Henretig, Fred M.   II. King, Christopher, 1959– .
  [DNLM: 1. Emergencies—in infancy & childhood. 2. Emergency
Medicine—methods.   WS 205 P371 1996]
RJ370.P456   1996
618.92′0025—dc20
DNLM/DLC
for Library of Congress   96–661
                               CIP

The publishers have made every effort to trace the copyright holders for borrowed material. If they have inadvertently overlooked any, they will be pleased to make the necessary arrangements at the first opportunity.

To purchase additional copies of this book, call our customer service department at **(800) 638-0672** or fax orders to **(800) 447-8438.** For other book services, including chapter reprints and large quantity sales, ask for the Special Sales department.

Canadian customers should call **(800) 268-4178,** or fax **(905) 470-6780.** For all other calls originating outside of the United States, please call **(410) 528-4223** or fax us at **(410) 528-8550.**

Visit Williams & Wilkins on the Internet: **http://www.wwilkins.com** or contact our customer service department at **custserv@wwilkins.com.** Williams & Wilkins customer service representatives are available from 8:30 am to 6:00 pm, EST, Monday through Friday, for telephone access.

98 99 00
3 4 5 6 7 8 9 10

For Marnie, Jon and Jeff, and Elizabeth and Max

–FMH

For Tammy and Jordan

–CK

FOREWORD

In a small conference room on the second floor of the Children's Hospital of Philadelphia, Fred Henretig introduced us to the vivid writing of William Carlos Williams. It was a routine emergency medicine morning conference in 1982. Somehow, of all of the conferences given on all the mornings, this one is remembered. Fred's topic was "How to Perform Procedures on Pediatric Patients." He began by reading from Williams' essay entitled "The Use of Force." The words were magic. They described young Dr. Williams encountering a flushed and febrile little girl who he suspected of having diphtheria at a time when diphtheria was killing children in his practice. It was imperative that he perform the procedure of examining the child's throat in order to make the diagnosis and provide the correct therapy. The treatment room was the family's kitchen, for this was in the time of the three-dollar house call.

"Well I said, suppose we take a look at the throat first. I smiled in my best professional manner and asking for the child's first name I said, come on, Mathilda, open your mouth and let's take a look at your throat.

Nothing doing."

We had all been in that very same situation. Anyone who has worked with children has faced the same awful dilemma. Those of us who had dedicated our careers to pediatric emergency medicine had faced a similar predicament on a daily basis. The conference room was filled with staff, residents, and students, who listened on.

"Aw, come on, I coaxed, just open your mouth wide and let me take a look. Look, I said opening both hands wide. I haven't anything in my hands. Just open up and let me see."

Fred read on, and we smiled as we listened to the common scenario. But soon the coaxing turned more serious. As Dr. Williams became more aggressive the child parried with even more determined resistance. The parents tried to coax her as well, but the child's mouth remained tightly clenched and resolute.

"As I moved my chair a little nearer, suddenly with one cat like movement both her hands clawed instinctively for my eyes and she almost reached them too. In fact she knocked my glasses flying and they fell, though unbroken, several feet away from me on the kitchen floor."

The conference room fell silent. Now this was getting serious. I think we all began to reflect on similar moments of confrontation in our past. I need to get the job done and the child will not let me. Do I push on? Do I try another technique? And through it all, perhaps a bit of anger is starting to infiltrate my professional demeanor. It is an uncomfortable feeling. I am there to help my young patients, not to be angry with them—they are only kids. Yes, but sometimes they are provoking. Yes, but always they seem to be so fragile, so dependent. Around the room, some smiles were gone, some heads were downed. As the story continued Dr. Williams saw that the child was breathing fast and appearing more ill. He decided to do what we had often done, appeal to the parents.

"I had to have a throat culture for her own protection. But first I told the parents that it was entirely up to them. I explained the danger but said that I would not insist on a throat examination so long as they would take responsibility."

This too was an all too familiar vignette. Shift the responsibility to the parents. Force them into action. Make them sign out against medical advice when we have failed. But it often works and the parents may put on the pressure, as they did in the case of Mathilda.

"If you don't do what the doctor says you'll have to go to the hospital the mother admonished her severely."

And then finally, it had to be done, the way no one prefers to perform a procedure, by the use of force. The father was asked to hold the child. The child started shrieking.

"Stop it! You're killing me!"

Williams grew furious. He tried first with a wooden tongue blade, but she splintered it. Determined to go through with the procedure, he asked the mother for a spoon. The child's tongue was cut and bleeding. She shrieked. Our conference room was spellbound by Fred and his choice of reading and by our own remembering.

"The damned little brat must be protected against her own idiocy, one says to oneself at such times. Others must be protected against her. It is a social necessity. And all these things are true. But a blind fury, a feeling of adult shame, bred of a longing for muscular release are the operatives. One goes to the end.

In the final unreasoning assault I overpowered the child's neck and jaws. I forced the heavy silver spoon back of her teeth and down her throat until she gagged. And there it was—both tonsils covered with membranes. She had fought valiantly to keep me from knowing her secret. She had been hiding the sore throat for three days at least and lying to her parents in order to escape such an outcome as this."

Dr. Henretig now confronted an audience as involved as an audience could be in the difficult role we have in performing procedures on children. As a master teacher he had recognized the components needed to perform any procedure: the knowledge, the equipment, and, most importantly, the attitude. He had given us a profound lesson in the latter. The emotion in the room was heavy. People began to speak of their experiences—their victories and their defeats. Most of all they began to talk about their feelings and how difficult it was to have to hurt in order to heal.

We were then ready to learn about the specifics that Fred had to teach us. It was one of those teaching/learning experiences that you never forget. William Carlos Williams, a University of Pennsylvania medical student who graduated in 1906, and Fred Henretig, a University of Pennsylvania faculty member in 1982, had teamed up to teach us something about pediatric procedures and how to perform them.

In later years Chris King was to join us from the Medical College of Pennsylvania. He too focused us on procedures and brought the world of general emergency medicine to our pediatric hospital setting. Chris also proved to be an excellent teacher and highly skilled clinician.

Both Dr. Henretig and Dr. King taught us that performing procedures takes more than the correct psychological mindset and caution in working with children. It takes information about the indications and contraindications for performing the task. It takes the proper equipment. It takes a step-by-step approach. These elements are all important, whether the procedure is the removal of a wayward fishhook or the placement of a central venous catheter. In these times, correct procedural technique also includes gaining the appropriate, informed parental consent and protecting oneself and staff colleagues from possible hazardous exposures.

Dr. Williams wrote more than 40 volumes of poems, fiction, essays, and plays. Dr. Henretig and Dr. King, along with our other colleagues, have prepared this excellent volume on pediatric procedures. It embodies all the strong teaching principles and dedication to the needs of our young patients that characterized that single emergency medicine conference described above. The authors have not been theorists working in their laboratories; they have all been front-line combatants in the battle to improve the lives of ill and injured children. Each has spent countless hours tending to his or her patients whenever the need was felt. Each has also been a master educator in training students, residents, fellows, and colleagues in the science and in the art of medical practice. This book reflects their knowledge and their spirit. It is comprehensive in scope, meticulous in detail, and presented with the beautiful illustrations of Christine Young as well as with many photographs. We are proud that Henretig and King's *Textbook of Pediatric Emergency Procedures* follows the *Textbook of Pediatric Emergency Medicine* as part of a series of books published by Williams & Wilkins. We salute the editors, illustrator, and authors, and thank them for their magnificent accomplishment.

Stephen Ludwig, M.D.
Gary Fleisher, M.D.

PREFACE

This book is intended for physicians who care for children with acute illness or injury. Virtually all of these patients will require some type of procedural intervention, whether it is as simple as an otoscopic examination or as complex as endotracheal intubation. We have attempted to codify both the experience of clinicians and the medical literature relating to the various hands-on techniques used in treating pediatric patients. In deciding what constitutes an "emergency" procedure, we have used as a general criterion procedures that are performed routinely in a hospital emergency department (ED). This obviously includes the more invasive techniques involved in the emergency management of life-threatening processes. Yet since a great deal of primary care takes place in every ED, this definition also encompasses most procedures performed in other acute care settings as well as office-based practice. Our hope is that this book will therefore be an equally useful resource for the emergency physician, pediatrician, and family practitioner.

One might well ask why produce an entire textbook devoted to pediatric emergency procedures? Why now? The answer reflects in part the evolution of our respective background disciplines (pediatrics for FH, emergency medicine for CK) and, more specifically, the recent growth and development of our chosen hybrid subspecialty of pediatric emergency medicine (PEM). The past 15 years has witnessed the publication of several authoritative texts in PEM and emergency medicine. In 1983, the appearance of Fleisher and Ludwig's *Textbook of Pediatric Emergency Medicine* served as a milestone in the recognition of PEM as a legitimate subspecialty. The Fleisher and Ludwig book is now in its third edition. Over this same period, a proliferation of titles in emergency medicine has kept pace with the rapid development and subspecialization of that field, including procedural titles covering the encyclopedic approach to a previously under-represented aspect of emergency medicine. We consider these pioneering texts as landmarks in the evolution of their respective disciplines, and believe that the *Textbook of Pediatric Emergency Procedures* owes a debt of ancestry to these foundational works.

In 1992, the American Board of Pediatrics and the American Board of Emergency Medicine jointly offered the first examination for certification in the newly recognized subspecialty of PEM. We believe that with this recognition will come a further expansion in the PEM body of literature, serving as the infrastructure in building this new discipline. The scope of PEM is broad, spanning the entire pediatric age range and the gamut of medical and surgical conditions of every organ system. It provides the opportunity for critical life support interventions as well as a full range of diagnostic and therapeutic ambulatory care challenges. Furthermore, the procedural nature of PEM is an innate part of its appeal. Achieving technical proficiency is an essential component of its practice, and striving for mastery in this realm is an ongoing quest for all its practitioners. A textbook focused on this aspect of the discipline therefore seems appropriate at this time, and we hope that the publication of this effort will be a timely contribution toward expanding the academic foundation of the field.

One of our primary aims for this book was to achieve a balance between the dual roles of a comprehensive reference and a

Acknowledgments

"user-friendly," clinically useful procedural guide. On the one hand, we have endeavored to produce an authoritative, well-referenced text, with sufficient detail for the reader to fully appreciate relevant basic science, indications, equipment requirements, comparative approaches, and potential complications for each procedure described. We believe the novice practitioner will find all the depth needed to provide a complete resource for learning about a given procedure de novo, while the more experienced clinician can also find enough information to enhance one's knowledge or skill. At the same time, each chapter affords the senior physician a quick and easy review of the key points of a procedure just prior to performing it (for those who want a brief reminder about a technique not done in some time, or who wish to cast a few "pearls" while teaching a resident, etc.). A lengthy reading of the text should not be necessary in this situation. The format of this book was designed to meet this need through the liberal use of step-by-step illustrations combined with highlighted tables containing a distillation of the important information in the chapter. A quickly directed review of the figures and tables for each procedure should allow the practitioner to "just do it."

We feel especially fortunate in having had the privilege of working from the inception of this endeavor with a talented and experienced medical illustrator. Christine Young has illustrated all three editions of Fleisher's and Ludwig's book, as well as several titles in pediatric surgery. We believe her ability to "see" how procedures are done and to convey this in her artwork is masterful and will be immediately obvious to the reader perusing the illustrations in each chapter.

The contents of this book are organized into chapters covering one or more techniques and procedures relevant to specific clinical situations. The chapters are in turn grouped into sections, which have overlapping areas of focus. Each chapter is structured similarly in order to provide a familiar format for the reader, allowing information to be retrieved quickly and efficiently. The background anatomy, physiology, and other relevant science is briefly reviewed. Issues regarding the likely setting for the procedure are addressed, as are specific indications and contraindications. Available equipment options are listed and compared. The procedure is then detailed in a step-by-step fashion, linked closely with illustrations to provide an "at-the-bedside" view of the methods involved. Where appropriate, various approaches for performing the procedure are presented and contrasted, with the authors indicating their prioritization of choices. Potential complications are described, along with suggestions for minimizing their likelihood of occurrence. Summary tables and tables providing "clinical tips" (i.e., focused suggestions for optimizing technique) are included to facilitate a rapid review of the key points. Finally, each chapter is fully referenced, so that the interested reader can critically pursue the scientific basis of the procedural recommendations.

The first section includes chapters related to the general care of the pediatric patient in the emergency and acute care settings. Sections two and three provide in-depth discussions of medical and trauma life support procedures. Section four focuses on methods of sedation and anesthesia. Section five describes procedures relevant to managing neonatal emergencies that may require intervention in the ED. Sections six through fourteen detail procedures classified by disorders of the various major organ systems. The last several sections are devoted to more generic emergency procedures, including those related to minor outpatient procedures, bedside laboratory investigations, toxicologic and environmental exposures, the use of ultrasonography in the ED, and pediatric transport procedures.

This textbook is respectfully offered to our fellow practitioners with the hope that it will enhance the capabilities—and, ideally, the resultant professional satisfaction experienced—of those who care for pediatric patients. Ultimately, it will be the sick and injured children who stand to benefit the most from skillfully and compassionately performed procedures. To the extent that this book makes even a small contribution to this end, we would consider that the most gratifying accomplishment.

Fred M. Henretig, M.D.
Christopher King, M.D.

ACKNOWLEDGMENTS

We wish to thank all those who participated in the development and preparation of the *Textbook of Pediatric Emergency Procedures*. As with any first-edition medical text, much of the work required in completing this task involved defining a particular area of practice and attempting to organize information into a clinically relevant and useful format. The opportunity to collaborate in this endeavor with many talented experts from around the country has truly been a rewarding experience.

We would also like to acknowledge the support of friends and coworkers in the emergency department. We owe a special thanks to Evi Allessandrini, M.D., Bill Angelos, M.D., Doug Baker, M.D., Lou Bell, M.D., Mananda Bhende, M.D., Vidya Chande, M.D., Mike Decker, M.D., Dennis Durbin, M.D., Joel Fein, M.D., Susan Fuchs, M.D., Marc Gorelick, M.D., Bob Hickey, M.D., Ray Karasic, M.D., Jane Lavelle, M.D., Mary Pierce, M.D., Steve Selbst, M.D., Kathy Shaw, M.D., Abby Wolfson, M.D., Tony Woodward, M.D., and Don Yealy, M.D. These superb clinicians, educators, and scientists have, like us, chosen to pursue the ongoing journey of exploration and discovery that our still relatively young field represents. We are privileged to have them as colleagues, and we greatly appreciate their help and encouragement during this undertaking.

We gratefully acknowledge the devotion and hard work of the secretarial staff who assisted in preparing this textbook: Sandee Skversky, Janice Basich, Rose Beato, and Tracey Sampson. Their logistical efforts during this process were invaluable. In addition, photographs by Margi Ide and Jon Henretig are greatly appreciated. We also wish to recognize those individuals at Williams & Wilkins who were instrumental in fostering the development of this text. Specifically, we thank Katey Millet, David Retford, Karen Gulliver, Joyce Murphy, and Marette Magargle-Smith. Their continuing support and dedication to this project are sincerely appreciated.

Finally, we thank our current and former chiefs and mentors, who have provided advice and guidance throughout the preparation of this text: Holly Davis, M.D., Gary Fleisher, M.D., Steve Ludwig, M.D., Paul Paris, M.D., and David Wagner, M.D.

CONTRIBUTORS

BARBARA J. ABRAMS, M.D., F.A.C.E.P.
ASSISTANT PROFESSOR
DIRECTOR OF ULTRASOUND EDUCATION
DEPARTMENT OF EMERGENCY MEDICINE
ERIE COUNTY MEDICAL CENTER
BUFFALO, NEW YORK

WILLIAM AHRENS, M.D.
ASSISTANT PROFESSOR OF PEDIATRICS AND
    EMERGENCY MEDICINE
DIRECTOR, PEDIATRIC EMERGENCY
    MEDICINE
UNIVERSITY OF ILLINOIS COLLEGE OF
    MEDICINE
CHICAGO, ILLINOIS

PETER J. ALDERSON, M.A., M.B.A., M.B.
STAFF ANAESTHETIST, DEPARTMENT OF
    ANAESTHESIA
CALDERDALE HEALTHCARE NMS TRUST
HALIFAX, ENGLAND

EVALINE A. ALESSANDRINI, M.D., F.A.A.P.
ASSISTANT PROFESSOR OF PEDIATRICS
DIVISION OF EMERGENCY MEDICINE
THE CHILDREN'S HOSPITAL OF PHILADELPHIA
PHILADELPHIA, PENNSYLVANIA

MICHAEL F. ALTIERI, M.D., F.A.A.P.
ASSOCIATE CLINICAL PROFESSOR OF
    PEDIATRICS AND EMERGENCY MEDICINE
GEORGE WASHINGTON UNIVERSITY
    SCHOOL OF MEDICINE
GEORGETOWN UNIVERSITY SCHOOL OF
    MEDICINE
WASHINGTON, D.C.
CHIEF OF PEDIATRIC EMERGENCY MEDICINE
FAIRFAX HOSPITAL
FALLS CHURCH, VIRGINIA

ANGELA C. ANDERSON, M.D.
ASSISTANT PROFESSOR OF PEDIATRICS
BROWN UNIVERSITY SCHOOL OF MEDICINE
ATTENDING PHYSICIAN, PEDIATRIC
    EMERGENCY MEDICINE
RHODE ISLAND HOSPITAL
HASBRO CHILDREN'S HOSPITAL
PROVIDENCE, RHODE ISLAND

JEFFREY R. AVNER, M.D., F.A.A.P.
ASSOCIATE PROFESSOR OF PEDIATRICS
ALBERT EINSTEIN COLLEGE OF MEDICINE
ASSOCIATE DIRECTOR, PEDIATRIC
    EMERGENCY SERVICE
JACOBI MEDICAL CENTER
BRONX, NEW YORK

DAVID T. BACHMAN, M.D., F.A.A.P.
DIRECTOR, PEDIATRIC EMERGENCY
    SERVICES
MAINE MEDICAL CENTER
PORTLAND, MAINE

M. DOUGLAS BAKER, M.D., F.A.A.P.
ASSOCIATE PROFESSOR OF PEDIATRICS
UNIVERSITY OF PENNSYLVANIA SCHOOL OF
    MEDICINE
ASSOCIATE DIRECTOR OF EMERGENCY
    MEDICINE
CHILDREN'S HOSPITAL OF PHILADELPHIA
PHILADELPHIA, PENNSYLVANIA

BRENT BARNES, M.D.
DEPARTMENT OF EMERGENCY MEDICINE
UNIVERSITY OF OKLAHOMA COLLEGE OF
    MEDICINE
OKLAHOMA CITY, OKLAHOMA

JUDITH C. BAUSHER, M.D., F.A.A.P.
ASSOCIATE PROFESSOR OF PEDIATRICS AND
EMERGENCY MEDICINE
UNIVERSITY OF CINCINNATI COLLEGE OF
MEDICINE
ATTENDING PHYSICIAN, DIVISION OF
EMERGENCY MEDICINE
CHILDREN'S HOSPITAL MEDICAL CENTER
CINCINNATI, OHIO

LOUIS M. BELL, M.D., F.A.A.P.
ASSOCIATE PROFESSOR OF PEDIATRICS
UNIVERSITY OF PENNSYLVANIA SCHOOL OF
MEDICINE
ATTENDING PHYSICIAN, INFECTIOUS
DISEASES AND EMERGENCY MEDICINE
CHILDREN'S HOSPITAL OF PHILADELPHIA
PHILADELPHIA, PENNSYLVANIA

**COURTNEY A. BETHEL, M.D., M.P.H.,
F.A.C.E.P**
ASSISTANT PROFESSOR OF EMERGENCY
MEDICINE
MCP ◆ HAHNEMANN SCHOOL OF
MEDICINE OF ALLEGHENY
UNIVERSITY OF THE HEALTH SCIENCES
PHILADELPHIA, PENNSYLVANIA

**MANANDA S. BHENDE, M.D., F.A.A.P,
F.A.C.E.P.**
ASSOCIATE PROFESSOR OF PEDIATRICS
UNIVERSITY OF PITTSBURGH SCHOOL OF
MEDICINE
ATTENDING PHYSICIAN, CHILDREN'S
HOSPITAL OF PITTSBURGH
PITTSBURGH, PENNSYLVANIA

JEFREY BIEHLER, M.D.
DEPARTMENT OF PEDIATRIC EMERGENCY
MEDICINE
MIAMI CHILDREN'S HOSPITAL
MIAMI, FLORIDA

A. FELIPE BLANCO, M.D.
INSTRUCTOR IN PEDIATRICS
UNIVERSITY OF COSTA RICA SCHOOL OF
MEDICINE
DIVISION OF EMERGENCY MEDICINE
HOSPITAL NACIONAL DE NIÑOS
SAN JOSÉ, COSTA RICA

DOUGLAS A. BOENNING, M.D.
ASSOCIATE PROFESSOR OF PEDIATRICS
GEORGE WASHINGTON UNIVERSITY
SCHOOL OF MEDICINE
ASSOCIATE DIRECTOR FOR RESEARCH
EMERGENCY MEDICAL TRAUMA CENTER
CHILDREN'S NATIONAL MEDICAL CENTER
WASHINGTON, D.C.

G. RANDALL BOND, M.D., F.A.A.P.
ASSISTANT PROFESSOR OF PEDIATRICS AND
INTERNAL MEDICINE
UNIVERSITY OF VIRGINIA
CHARLOTTESVILLE, VIRGINIA

**GREGORY S. BUCHERT, M.D., M.P.H.,
F.A.A.P.**
MEDICAL DIRECTOR, DEPARTMENT OF
AMBULATORY CARE SERVICES
CHILDREN'S HOSPITAL OF ORANGE
COUNTY
ORANGE, CALIFORNIA

JOHN H. BURTON, M.D.
ATTENDING PHYSICIAN, DEPARTMENT OF
EMERGENCY MEDICINE
MAINE MEDICAL CENTER
PORTLAND, MAINE

JAMES M. CALLAHAN, M.D., F.A.A.P.
CLINICAL ASSISTANT PROFESSOR OF
PEDIATRICS
UNIVERSITY OF PENNSYLVANIA SCHOOL OF
MEDICINE
ATTENDING PHYSICIAN, EMERGENCY
DEPARTMENT
THE CHILDREN'S HOSPITAL OF PHILADELPHIA
PHILADELPHIA, PENNSYLVANIA

**RICHARD M. CANTOR, M.D., F.A.A.P.,
F.A.C.E.P.**
ASSOCIATE PROFESSOR OF EMERGENCY
MEDICINE AND PEDIATRICS
STATE UNIVERSITY OF NEW YORK HEALTH
SCIENCE CENTER AT SYRACUSE
SYRACUSE, NEW YORK

CAROLYN M. CAREY, M.D.
ASSISTANT PROFESSOR OF NEUROSURGERY
ASSISTANT PROFESSOR OF PEDIATRICS
DEPARTMENT OF NEUROSURGERY, DIVISION
OF PEDIATRIC NEUROSURGERY
UNIVERSITY OF UTAH SCHOOL OF
MEDICINE
PRIMARY CHILDREN'S MEDICAL CENTER
SALT LAKE CITY, UTAH

VIDYA T. CHANDE, M.D., F.A.A.P.
ASSISTANT PROFESSOR OF PEDIATRICS
UNIVERSITY OF PITTSBURGH SCHOOL OF
MEDICINE
ATTENDING PHYSICIAN, PEDIATRIC
EMERGENCY DEPARTMENT
CHILDREN'S HOSPITAL OF PITTSBURGH
PITTSBURGH, PENNSYLVANIA

Contributors

JENNIFER PRATT CHENEY, M.D., F.A.A.P.
ASSISTANT PROFESSOR OF PEDIATRICS
GEORGE WASHINGTON UNIVERSITY
  SCHOOL OF MEDICINE
ATTENDING PHYSICIAN, EMERGENCY
  MEDICAL TRAUMA CENTER
CHILDREN'S NATIONAL MEDICAL CENTER
WASHINGTON, D.C.

CINDY W. CHRISTIAN, M.D., F.A.A.P.
ASSISTANT PROFESSOR OF PEDIATRICS
UNIVERSITY OF PENNSYLVANIA SCHOOL OF
  MEDICINE
MEDICAL DIRECTOR, CHILD ABUSE
  SERVICES
THE CHILDREN'S HOSPITAL OF
  PHILADELPHIA
PHILADELPHIA, PENNSYLVANIA

MARK C. CLARK, M.D., F.A.C.E.P.
CLINICAL ASSISTANT PROFESSOR OF
  SURGERY
UNIVERSITY OF FLORIDA COLLEGE OF
  MEDICINE
ASSISTANT MEDICAL DIRECTOR,
  DEPARTMENTS OF EMERGENCY
  MEDICINE AND PEDIATRICS
ORLANDO REGIONAL MEDICAL CENTER
ORLANDO, FLORIDA

KATHLEEN M. CONNORS, M.D.
ASSISTANT PROFESSOR OF EMERGENCY
  MEDICINE
STATE UNIVERSITY OF NEW YORK HEALTH
  SCIENCE CENTER AT SYRACUSE
SYRACUSE, NEW YORK

RICHARD T. COOK, JR., M.D.
ATTENDING PHYSICIAN, EMERGENCY
  DEPARTMENT
LEHIGH VALLEY MEDICAL CENTER
ALLENTOWN, PENNSYLVANIA

ANDREW T. COSTARINO, JR., M.D., F.A.A.P.
ASSOCIATE PROFESSOR OF
  ANESTHESIOLOGY AND PEDIATRICS
THE UNIVERSITY OF PENNSYLVANIA SCHOOL
  OF MEDICINE
ATTENDING PHYSICIAN, CRITICAL CARE
  MEDICINE
THE CHILDREN'S HOSPITAL OF
  PHILADELPHIA
PHILADELPHIA, PENNSYLVANIA

ELLEN F. CRAIN, M.D., PH.D., F.A.A.P.
PROFESSOR OF PEDIATRICS
ALBERT EINSTEIN COLLEGE OF
  MEDICINE
DIRECTOR, PEDIATRIC EMERGENCY
  MEDICINE
JACOBI MEDICAL CENTER
BRONX, NEW YORK

KATHLEEN M. CRONAN, M.D., F.A.A.P.
CLINICAL ASSISTANT PROFESSOR OF
  PEDIATRICS
THOMAS JEFFERSON MEDICAL COLLEGE
DIRECTOR, EMERGENCY SERVICES
ALFRED I. DUPONT INSTITUTE, CHILDREN'S
  HOSPITAL
WILMINGTON, DELAWARE

SANDRA J. CUNNINGHAM, M.D.
ASSISTANT PROFESSOR OF PEDIATRICS
ALBERT EINSTEIN COLLEGE OF
  MEDICINE
ASSISTANT DIRECTOR, PEDIATRIC
  EMERGENCY MEDICINE
JACOBI MEDICAL CENTER
BRONX, NEW YORK

JAMES D'AGOSTINO, M.D.
ASSISTANT PROFESSOR OF EMERGENCY
  MEDICINE AND PEDIATRICS
ATTENDING PHYSICIAN, PEDIATRIC
  EMERGENCY MEDICINE
DEPARTMENT OF EMERGENCY MEDICINE
STATE UNIVERSITY OF NEW YORK
SYRACUSE, NEW YORK

HOLLY W. DAVIS, M.D., F.A.A.P.
ASSOCIATE PROFESSOR OF PEDIATRICS
UNIVERSITY OF PITTSBURGH SCHOOL OF
  MEDICINE
DIRECTOR, PEDIATRIC EMERGENCY
  MEDICINE
CHILDREN'S HOSPITAL OF PITTSBURGH
PITTSBURGH, PENNSYLVANIA

JOANNE M. DECKER, M.D.
ASSISTANT PROFESSOR OF EMERGENCY
  MEDICINE AND PEDIATRICS
ALLEGHENY UNIVERSITY OF THE HEALTH
  SCIENCES
ATTENDING PHYSICIAN, EMERGENCY
  MEDICINE
ST. CHRISTOPHER'S HOSPITAL FOR
  CHILDREN
PHILADELPHIA, PENNSYLVANIA

Contributors

DOUGLAS S. DIEKEMA, M.D., M.P.H., F.A.A.P.
ASSISTANT PROFESSOR OF PEDIATRICS
UNIVERSITY OF WASHINGTON SCHOOL OF
  MEDICINE
ATTENDING PHYSICIAN, DEPARTMENT OF
  EMERGENCY SERVICES
CHILDREN'S HOSPITAL MEDICAL CENTER
SEATTLE, WASHINGTON

GREGG A. DiGIULIO, M.D., F.A.A.P.
ASSISTANT PROFESSOR OF PEDIATRICS
UNIVERSITY OF CINCINNATI COLLEGE OF
  MEDICINE
ATTENDING PHYSICIAN, DIVISION OF
  EMERGENCY MEDICINE
CHILDREN'S HOSPITAL MEDICAL CENTER
CINCINNATI, OHIO

E. HOWARD DIXON III, M.D., F.A.A.P.
ASSISTANT PROFESSOR OF EMERGENCY
  MEDICINE
UNIVERSITY HOSPITAL OF JACKSONVILLE
JACKSONVILLE, FLORIDA

ALFRED T. DORSEY, M.D., F.A.A.P.
ASSISTANT PROFESSOR OF ANESTHESIOLOGY
TEMPLE UNIVERSITY SCHOOL OF MEDICINE
ST. CHRISTOPHER'S HOSPITAL FOR CHILDREN
PHILADELPHIA, PENNSYLVANIA

SUSAN DUFFY, M.D.
CLINICAL ASSISTANT PROFESSOR OF PEDIATRICS
BROWN UNIVERSITY SCHOOL OF MEDICINE
ATTENDING PHYSICIAN, PEDIATRIC
  EMERGENCY MEDICINE
RHODE ISLAND HOSPITAL
PROVIDENCE, RHODE ISLAND

ANN-CHRISTINE DUHAIME, M.D.
DEPARTMENT OF NEUROSURGERY
UNIVERSITY OF PENNSYLVANIA SCHOOL OF
  MEDICINE
THE CHILDREN'S HOSPITAL OF PHILADELPHIA
PHILADELPHIA, PENNSYLVANIA

DENNIS R. DURBIN, M.D., F.A.A.P.
ASSISTANT PROFESSOR OF PEDIATRICS
UNIVERSITY OF PENNSYLVANIA SCHOOL OF
  MEDICINE
SENIOR SCHOLAR, CENTER FOR CLINICAL
  EPIDEMIOLOGY AND BIOSTATISTICS
THE CHILDREN'S HOSPITAL OF PHILADELPHIA
PHILADELPHIA, PENNSYLVANIA

ROBERT EBERLEIN, M.D.
CLINICAL INSTRUCTOR
NORTHEASTERN OHIO UNIVERSITIES
  COLLEGE OF MEDICINE
ROOTSTOWN, OHIO
ATTENDING PHYSICIAN, DEPARTMENT OF
  EMERGENCY MEDICINE
ROBINSON MEMORIAL HOSPITAL
RAVENNA, OHIO

JOEL A. FEIN, M.D., F.A.A.P.
ASSISTANT PROFESSOR OF PEDIATRICS
UNIVERSITY OF PENNSYLVANIA SCHOOL OF
  MEDICINE
ATTENDING PHYSICIAN, EMERGENCY
  DEPARTMENT
THE CHILDREN'S HOSPITAL OF
  PHILADELPHIA
PHILADELPHIA, PENNSYLVANIA

GEORGE L. FOLTIN, M.D., F.A.A.P., F.A.C.E.P.
ASSISTANT PROFESSOR OF CLINICAL
  PEDIATRICS
NEW YORK UNIVERSITY SCHOOL OF
  MEDICINE
DIRECTOR OF PEDIATRIC EMERGENCY
  MEDICINE
BELLEVUE HOSPITAL CENTER
NEW YORK UNIVERSITY SCHOOL OF
  MEDICINE
NEW YORK, NEW YORK

SCOTT H. FREEDMAN, M.D.
ASSISTANT PROFESSOR OF PEDIATRICS
ATTENDING PHYSICIAN, PEDIATRIC
  EMERGENCY DEPARTMENT
UNIVERSITY OF MARYLAND SCHOOL OF
  MEDICINE
BALTIMORE, MARYLAND

JANET H. FRIDAY, M.D.
DIVISION OF EMERGENCY MEDICINE
CONNECTICUT CHILDREN'S MEDICAL
  CENTER
HARTFORD, CONNECTICUT

LEONARD R. FRIEDLAND, M.D., F.A.A.P.
ASSISTANT PROFESSOR OF PEDIATRICS AND
  MEDICINE
TEMPLE UNIVERSITY SCHOOL OF
  MEDICINE
DIRECTOR, PEDIATRIC EMERGENCY
  MEDICINE
TEMPLE UNIVERSITY HOSPITAL
PHILADELPHIA, PENNSYLVANIA

SUSAN M. FUCHS, M.D., F.A.A.P.
  ASSOCIATE PROFESSOR OF PEDIATRICS
  NORTHWESTERN UNIVERSITY SCHOOL OF
    MEDICINE
  ASSOCIATE DIRECTOR, DIVISION OF
    EMERGENCY MEDICINE
  CHILDREN'S MEMORIAL HOSPITAL
  CHICAGO, ILLINOIS

RONNIE S. FUERST, M.D., F.A.A.P.
  MEDICAL DIRECTOR, CHILDREN'S
    EMERGENCY CENTER
  CHILDREN'S HOSPITAL OF RICHLAND
    MEMORIAL HOSPITAL
  ATTENDING PHYSICIAN, EMERGENCY
    MEDICINE
  RICHLAND MEMORIAL HOSPITAL
  COLUMBIA, SOUTH CAROLINA

ANGELO P. GIARDINO, M.D., M.S.E.D.,
F.A.A.P.
  CLINICAL ASSISTANT PROFESSOR OF
    PEDIATRICS
  DIVISION OF CHILD DEVELOPMENT AND
    REHABILITATION
  UNIVERSITY OF PENNSYLVANIA SCHOOL OF
    MEDICINE
  ASSISTANT PHYSICIAN-IN-CHIEF
  CHILDREN'S SEASHORE HOUSE
  PHILADELPHIA, PENNSYLVANIA

TIMOTHY G. GIVENS, M.D., F.A.A.P.
  ASSISTANT PROFESSOR OF PEDIATRICS
  DIRECTOR, PEDIATRIC EMERGENCY
    MEDICINE FELLOWSHIP PROGRAM
  UNIVERSITY OF LOUISVILLE
  ATTENDING PHYSICIAN, ASSOCIATE
    MEDICAL DIRECTOR, EMERGENCY
    DEPARTMENT
  KOSAIR CHILDREN'S HOSPITAL
  LOUISVILLE, KENTUCKY

ROBERT F. GOCHMAN, M.D., F.A.A.P.
  ASSISTANT PROFESSOR OF PEDIATRICS
  ALBERT EINSTEIN COLLEGE OF MEDICINE
  BRONX, NEW YORK
  DIRECTOR, PEDIATRIC EMERGENCY
    MEDICINE FELLOWSHIP PROGRAM
  SCHNEIDER CHILDREN'S HOSPITAL/LONG
    ISLAND
  JEWISH MEDICAL CENTER
  NEW HYDE PARK, NEW YORK

JULIUS G.K. GOEPP, M.D., F.A.A.P.
  ASSISTANT DIRECTOR, PEDIATRIC
    EMERGENCY MEDICINE
  DEPARTMENT OF PEDIATRICS
  THE JOHNS HOPKINS SCHOOL OF
    MEDICINE
  BALTIMORE, MARYLAND

JAVIER A. GONZALEZ DEL REY, M.D.,
F.A.A.P.
  ASSISTANT PROFESSOR OF PEDIATRICS
  DIVISION OF EMERGENCY MEDICINE
  DEPARTMENT OF PEDIATRICS
  CHILDREN'S HOSPITAL MEDICAL CENTER
  CINCINNATI, OHIO

MARC H. GORELICK, M.D.
  ASSISTANT PROFESSOR OF PEDIATRICS AND
    EPIDEMIOLOGY
  UNIVERSITY OF PENNSYLVANIA SCHOOL OF
    MEDICINE
  ATTENDING PHYSICIAN, DIVISION OF
    PEDIATRIC EMERGENCY MEDICINE
  THE CHILDREN'S HOSPITAL OF
    PHILADELPHIA
  PHILADELPHIA, PENNSYLVANIA

JOHN W. GRANETO, D.O., M.ED.
  ATTENDING PHYSICIAN, DIVISION OF
    PEDIATRIC EMERGENCY MEDICINE
  DEPARTMENTS OF EMERGENCY MEDICINE
    AND PEDIATRICS
  LUTHERAN GENERAL CHILDREN'S HOSPITAL
  PARK RIDGE, ILLINOIS

MICHAEL GREEN, M.D.
  DEPARTMENT OF EMERGENCY MEDICINE
  MERCY HOSPITAL
  CHICAGO, ILLINOIS

RUSSELL H. GREENFIELD, M.D., F.A.C.E.P.
  DIRECTOR, EMERGENCY DEPARTMENT
  PRESBYTERIAN MATTHEWS HOSPITAL
  MATTHEWS, NORTH CAROLINA

ELLIOTT M. HARRIS, M.D., F.A.A.P.
  ASSISTANT PROFESSOR OF EMERGENCY
    MEDICINE AND PEDIATRICS
  STATE UNIVERSITY OF NEW YORK HEALTH
    SCIENCE CENTER
  SYRACUSE, NEW YORK

Contributors

MARY A. HEGENBARTH, M.D., F.A.A.P.
Assistant Professor of Pediatrics
University of Missouri–Kansas City
School of Medicine
Attending Physician, Division of
Emergency Medicine
Children's Mercy Hospital
Kansas City, Missouri

MARK L. HELPIN, D.M.D.
Chairman and Associate Professor,
Pediatric Dentistry
University of Pennsylvania School of
Dental Medicine
Chief, Division of Dentistry
The Children's Hospital of
Philadelphia
Philadelphia, Pennsylvania

FRED M. HENRETIG, M.D., F.A.A.P.
Associate Professor of Pediatrics
University of Pennsylvania School of
Medicine
Director, Section of Clinical
Toxicology
Division of Emergency Medicine
The Children's Hospital of
Philadelphia
Medical Director, The Poison
Control Center
Philadelphia, Pennsylvania

DEE HODGE III, M.D., F.A.A.P., F.A.C.E.P.
Assistant Clinical Professor of
Pediatrics
University of California, San
Francisco
Director, Emergency Medicine
Children's Hospital Oakland
Oakland, California

CYNTHIA HOECKER, M.D., F.A.A.P.
Assistant Clinical Professor of
Pediatrics
University of California, San Diego
School of Medicine
Attending Physician, Division of
Pediatric Emergency Medicine
Children's Hospital and Health
Center
San Diego, California

SONIA O. IMAIZUMI, M.D., F.A.A.P.
Associate Professor of Clinical
Pediatrics
Robert Wood Johnson Medical
School
Associate Director of Neonatal
Services
Children's Regional Hospital at
Cooper
Camden, New Jersey

DANIEL J. ISAACMAN, M.D., F.A.A.P.
Associate Professor of Pediatrics
Eastern Virginia Medical School
Chief, Division of Pediatric Emergency
Medicine
Children's Hospital of The King's
Daughters
Norfolk, Virginia

DIETRICH JEHLE, M.D., F.A.C.E.P.
Associate Professor of Emergency
Medicine
State University of New York at
Buffalo School of Medicine
Director, Department of Emergency
Medicine
Erie County Medical Center
Buffalo, New York

MARK D. JOFFE, M.D., F.A.A.P.
Associate Professor of Pediatrics
Temple University School of Medicine
Director, Emergency Medicine
St. Christopher's Hospital for
Children
Philadelphia, Pennsylvania

JEAN MARIE KALLIS M.D.
Assistant Professor of Pediatrics
Division of Emergency Medicine
Kosair Children's Hospital
Louisville, Kentucky

ZACH KASSUTTO, M.D.
Assistant Professor of Emergency
Medicine and Pediatrics
MCP ◆ Hahnemann School of
Medicine of Allegheny University of
the Health Sciences
Attending Physician
St. Christopher's Hospital for
Children
Philadelphia, Pennsylvania

Contributors

xviii

JOHN J. KELLY, D.O., F.A.C.E.P.
ASSOCIATE PROFESSOR OF MEDICINE
TEMPLE UNIVERSITY SCHOOL OF
   MEDICINE
ADJUNCT ASSOCIATE PROFESSOR OF
   EMERGENCY MEDICINE
MEDICAL COLLEGE OF PENNSYLVANIA
ASSOCIATE CHAIRMAN, DEPARTMENT OF
   EMERGENCY MEDICINE
ALBERT EINSTEIN MEDICAL CENTER
PHILADELPHIA, PENNSYLVANIA

KATHLEEN P. KELLY, M.D., F.A.C.E.P.
ASSISTANT PROFESSOR OF EMERGENCY
   MEDICINE
GEORGETOWN UNIVERSITY SCHOOL OF
   MEDICINE
WASHINGTON, D.C.
ATTENDING PHYSICIAN
FAIRFAX HOSPITAL
FALLS CHURCH, VIRGINIA

SIGMUND J. KHARASCH, M.D., F.A.A.P.
ASSISTANT PROFESSOR
DEPARTMENT OF PEDIATRICS
BOSTON UNIVERSITY SCHOOL OF
   MEDICINE
CLINICAL DIRECTOR
PEDIATRIC EMERGENCY DEPARTMENT
BOSTON CITY HOSPITAL
BOSTON, MASSACHUSETTS

HNIN KHINE, M.D., F.A.A.P.
ASSISTANT PROFESSOR
DEPARTMENT OF PEDIATRICS
ALBERT EINSTEIN COLLEGE OF MEDICINE
ATTENDING PHYSICIAN, PEDIATRIC
   EMERGENCY SERVICES
JACOBI MEDICAL CENTER
BRONX, NEW YORK

BRENT R. KING, M.D., F.A.A.P.
ASSOCIATE PROFESSOR OF EMERGENCY
   MEDICINE AND PEDIATRICS
CHIEF, DIVISION OF PEDIATRIC EMERGENCY
   MEDICINE
MCP ◆ HAHNEMANN SCHOOL OF
   MEDICINE OF ALLEGHENY UNIVERSITY OF
   THE HEALTH SCIENCES
MEDICAL DIRECTOR, PEDIATRIC TRANSPORT
   TEAM
ST. CHRISTOPHER'S HOSPITAL FOR
   CHILDREN
PHILADELPHIA, PENNSYLVANIA

CHRISTOPHER KING, M.D., F.A.C.E.P.
ASSISTANT PROFESSOR OF EMERGENCY
   MEDICINE AND PEDIATRICS
DEPARTMENT OF EMERGENCY MEDICINE
UNIVERSITY OF PITTSBURGH SCHOOL OF
   MEDICINE
ATTENDING PHYSICIAN, EMERGENCY MEDICINE
UNIVERSITY OF PITTSBURGH MEDICAL CENTER
CHILDREN'S HOSPITAL OF PITTSBURGH
PITTSBURGH, PENNSYLVANIA

**NIRANJAN KISSOON, M.D., F.A.A.P.,
F.C.C.M.**
PROFESSOR OF PEDIATRICS
UNIVERSITY OF FLORIDA HEALTH SCIENCE
   CENTER
DIRECTOR, PEDIATRIC CRITICAL CARE UNIT
WOLFSON CHILDREN'S HOSPITAL
JACKSONVILLE, FLORIDA

BRUCE L. KLEIN, M.D., F.A.A.P.
ASSOCIATE PROFESSOR OF PEDIATRICS AND
   EMERGENCY MEDICINE
THE GEORGE WASHINGTON UNIVERSITY
   SCHOOL OF MEDICINE AND HEALTH
   SCIENCES
ASSOCIATE MEDICAL DIRECTOR,
   EMERGENCY MEDICAL TRAUMA CENTER
CHILDREN'S NATIONAL MEDICAL CENTER
WASHINGTON, D.C.

JEAN E. KLIG, M.D., F.A.A.P.
ASSISTANT PROFESSOR OF PEDIATRICS
YALE UNIVERSITY SCHOOL OF MEDICINE
ATTENDING PHYSICIAN, PEDIATRIC
   EMERGENCY DEPARTMENT
YALE-NEW HAVEN HOSPITAL
NEW HAVEN, CONNECTICUT

SUSANNE KOST, M.D., F.A.A.P.
CLINICAL ASSISTANT PROFESSOR OF
   PEDIATRICS
JEFFERSON MEDICAL COLLEGE
ATTENDING PHYSICIAN, PEDIATRIC
   EMERGENCY MEDICINE
A.I. DUPONT INSTITUTE CHILDREN'S
   HOSPITAL
WILMINGTON, DELAWARE

ROY M. KULICK, M.D., M.S., F.A.A.P.
ASSOCIATE PROFESSOR
DEPARTMENT OF PEDIATRICS
UNIVERSITY OF CINCINNATI COLLEGE OF
   MEDICINE
ASSOCIATE DIRECTOR
DIVISION OF EMERGENCY MEDICINE
CHILDREN'S HOSPITAL MEDICAL CENTER
CINCINNATI, OHIO

Contributors

Nanette C. Kunkel, M.D., F.A.A.P.
Assistant Professor of Pediatrics
University of Utah School of
Medicine
Attending Physician, Pediatric
Emergency Medicine
Primary Children's Medical Center
Salt Lake City, Utah

Mary E. Lacher, M.D., F.A.A.P.
Assistant Professor of Pediatrics
University of Cincinnati College of
Medicine
Division of Emergency Medicine
Children's Hospital Medical Center
Cincinnati, Ohio

Natalie E. Lane, M.D.
Assistant Professor of Pediatrics
University of Louisville
Attending Physician, Division of
Pediatric Emergency Medicine
Kosair Children's Hospital
Louisville, Kentucky

Bernard J. Larson, D.D.S.
Resident, Department of Pediatric
Dentistry
Children's National Medical Center
Washington, D.C.

Jane Lavelle, M.D., F.A.A.P.
Assistant Professor of Pediatrics
The University of Pennsylvania School
of Medicine
Associate Director, Emergency
Medicine
Division of Pediatric Emergency
Medicine
The Children's Hospital of
Philadelphia
Philadelphia, Pennsylvania

David C. Lee, M.D., F.A.A.E.M., D.A.C.M.T.
Assistant Professor of Emergency
Medicine
Department of Emergency Medicine
MCP ◆ Hahnemann University School
of Medicine of Allegheny University
of the Health Sciences
Philadelphia, Pennsylvania

Alex V. Levin, M.D., F.A.A.P., F.R.C.S.C.
Assistant Professor of
Ophthalmology, Pediatrics, and
Genetics
University of Toronto
Pediatric Ophthalmology Staff
The Hospital for Sick Children
Toronto, Ontario
Canada

William J. Lewander, M.D.
Director, Pediatric Emergency
Medicine
Departments of Pediatrics and
Emergency Medicine
Brown University School of Medicine
Hasbro Children's Hospital of Rhode
Island Hospital
Providence, Rhode Island

Lisa S. Lewis, M.D., F.A.A.P.
Assistant Professor of Pediatrics
Adjunct Assistant Professor of
Emergency Medicine
University of Cincinnati College of
Medicine
Attending Physician
Division of Emergency Medicine
Children's Hospital Medical Center
Cincinnati, Ohio

Kathleen A. Lillis, M.D., F.A.A.P.
Assistant Professor of Pediatrics and
Emergency Medicine
State University of New York at
Buffalo School of Medicine
Chief, Division of Emergency Medicine
Children's Hospital of Buffalo
Buffalo, New York

James G. Linakis, Ph.D., M.D., F.A.A.P.
Assistant Professor of Pediatrics
Brown University
Associate Director, Pediatric
Emergency Medicine
Hasbro Children's Hospital
Rhode Island Hospital
Providence, Rhode Island

Jordan D. Lipton, M.D., FACEP
Attending Physician,
Department of Emergency Medicine
Mercy Hospital South
Charlotte, North Carolina

Contributors

xx

JOHN LOISELLE, M.D., F.A.A.P.
ASSISTANT PROFESSOR OF EMERGENCY
MEDICINE AND PEDIATRICS
MCP ◆ HAHNEMANN SCHOOL OF
MEDICINE OF ALLEGHENY UNIVERSITY OF
THE HEALTH SCIENCES
ATTENDING PHYSICIAN
ST. CHRISTOPHER'S HOSPITAL FOR
CHILDREN
PHILADELPHIA, PENNSYLVANIA

DAVID A. LOWE, M.D., F.C.C.M., F.A.A.P.
ASSOCIATE PROFESSOR OF
ANESTHESIOLOGY
TEMPLE UNIVERSITY SCHOOL OF
MEDICINE
DIRECTOR, DEPARTMENT OF ANESTHESIA
AND CRITICAL CARE
ST. CHRISTOPHER'S HOSPITAL FOR
CHILDREN
PHILADELPHIA, PENNSYLVANIA

JOSEPH W. LURIA, M.D.
ASSISTANT PROFESSOR OF PEDIATRICS
THE OHIO STATE UNIVERSITY
SECTION OF EMERGENCY MEDICINE
CHILDREN'S HOSPITAL
COLUMBUS, OHIO

**ROBERT C. LUTEN, M.D., F.A.A.P.,
F.A.C.E.P.**
PROFESSOR OF EMERGENCY MEDICINE
UNIVERSITY OF FLORIDA HEALTH SCIENCE
CENTER
DIRECTOR, PEDIATRIC EMERGENCY
SERVICES
UNIVERSITY MEDICAL CENTER
JACKSONVILLE, FLORIDA

JACALYN S. MALLER, M.D., F.A.A.P.
CLINICAL ASSISTANT PROFESSOR OF
PEDIATRICS
UNIVERSITY OF PENNSYLVANIA SCHOOL OF
MEDICINE
ASSISTANT PHYSICIAN, DIVISIONS OF
EMERGENCY MEDICINE AND GENERAL
PEDIATRICS
PRIMARY CARE CENTER
THE CHILDREN'S HOSPITAL OF
PHILADELPHIA
PHILADELPHIA, PENNSYLVANIA

STEVE MARCINAK, M.D.
DEPARTMENT OF EMERGENCY MEDICINE
COLLEGE OF MEDICINE WEST
CHICAGO, ILLINOIS

JAMES R. MATEER, M.D., F.A.C.E.P.
ASSOCIATE PROFESSOR OF EMERGENCY
MEDICINE
DIRECTOR, EMERGENCY MEDICINE
ULTRASONOGRAPHY FELLOWSHIP
MEDICAL COLLEGE OF WISCONSIN
MILWAUKEE, WISCONSIN

CONSTANCE M. McANENEY, M.D., F.A.A.P.
ASSISTANT PROFESSOR OF PEDIATRICS
UNIVERSITY OF CINCINNATI COLLEGE OF
MEDICINE
ATTENDING PHYSICIAN, DIVISION OF
EMERGENCY MEDICINE
CHILDREN'S HOSPITAL MEDICAL CENTER
CINCINNATI, OHIO

**ROBERT M. McNAMARA, M.D.,
F.A.C.E.P.**
PROFESSOR OF EMERGENCY MEDICINE
DIRECTOR, RESIDENCY PROGRAM
MCP ◆ HAHNEMANN SCHOOL OF
MEDICINE OF ALLEGHENY UNIVERSITY OF
THE HEALTH SCIENCES
PHILADELPHIA, PENNSYLVANIA

**LEO G. NIEDERMAN, M.D., M.P.H.,
F.A.A.P.**
CLINICAL ASSOCIATE PROFESSOR OF
PEDIATRICS
UNIVERSITY OF ILLINOIS AT CHICAGO
HEAD, GENERAL AND EMERGENCY
PEDIATRICS
DEPARTMENT OF PEDIATRICS
UNIVERSITY OF ILLINOIS HOSPITAL AND
CLINICS AND MICHAEL REESE
HOSPITAL
CHICAGO, ILLINOIS

RONALD I. PAUL, M.D., F.A.A.P.
ASSOCIATE PROFESSOR OF PEDIATRICS
PEDIATRIC EMERGENCY MEDICINE
UNIVERSITY OF LOUISVILLE SCHOOL OF
MEDICINE
MEDICAL DIRECTOR, EMERGENCY
DEPARTMENT
KOSAIR CHILDREN'S HOSPITAL
LOUISVILLE, KENTUCKY

MARY CLYDE PIERCE, M.D.
Assistant Professor of Pediatrics
University of Pittsburgh School of
Medicine
Attending Physician
Children's Hospital of Pittsburgh
Pittsburgh, Pennsylvania

SHARI L. PLATT, M.D., F.A.A.P.
Clinical Instructor in Pediatrics
Pediatric Emergency Service
Bellevue Hospital
Department of Pediatrics
Bellevue Hospital Center/New York
University Medical Center
New York, New York

META PODRAZIK, M.D.
Assistant Professor of Emergency
Medicine
Allegheny University of the Health
Sciences
Attending Physician, Pediatric
Emergency Medicine
St. Christopher's Hospital for
Children
Philadelphia, Pennsylvania

MICHAEL P. POIRIER, M.D.
Assistant Professor of Pediatrics
Eastern Virginia Medical School
Division of Pediatric Emergency
Medicine
Children's Hospital of The King's
Daughters
Norfolk, Virginia

J. CHRISTOPHER POST, M.D.
Assistant Professor of
Otolaryngology
University of Pittsburgh School of
Medicine
Co-director, Department of Pediatric
Otolaryngology
Children's Hospital of Pittsburgh
Pittsburgh, Pennsylvania

LINDA QUAN, M.D., F.A.A.P.
Associate Professor of Pediatrics
University of Washington School of
Medicine
Chief, Emergency Services
Children's Hospital and Medical
Center
Seattle, Washington

PETER D. QUINN, D.M.D., M.D.
Chairman, Oral and Maxillofacial
Surgery
University of Pennsylvania Medical
Center
Philadelphia, Pennsylvania

SCOTT REEVES, M.D.
Assistant Professor of Pediatrics
Baylor College of Medicine
Division of Emergency Medicine
Texas Children's Hospital
Houston, Texas

CLARK A. ROSEN, M.D.
Assistant Professor of
Otolaryngology
University of Pittsburgh School of
Medicine
Director, University of Pittsburgh
Voice Center
Pittsburgh, Pennsylvania

STEVEN G. ROTHROCK, M.D., F.A.C.E.P.
Research Director, Department of
Emergency Medicine
Orlando Regional Medical Center
Orlando, Florida

RICHARD M. RUDDY, M.D., F.A.A.P.
Professor of Clinical Pediatrics
University of Cincinnati College of
Medicine
Director, Division of Emergency
Medicine
Department of Pediatrics
Children's Hospital Medical Center
Cincinnati, Ohio

GAIL RUDNITSKY, M.D., F.A.A.P., F.A.C.E.P.
Assistant Professor of Emergency
Medicine
MCP ◆ Hahnemann School of
Medicine of Allegheny University of
the Health Sciences
Philadelphia, Pennsylvania

SEEMA SACHDEVA, M.D., F.A.A.P.
Director, Physicians for Children and
Adolescents
Pikeville Methodist Hospital
Pikeville, Kentucky

Contributors

xxii

RICHARD A. SALADINO, M.D.
Assistant Professor of Pediatrics
Department of Medicine
Harvard Medical School
Attending Physician, Emergency
Department
Children's Hospital
Boston, Massachusetts

MORTON E. SALOMON, M.D., F.A.A.P.,
F.A.C.E.P.
Associate Professor of Pediatrics and
Emergency Medicine
Albert Einstein College of Medicine
Director of Emergency Services and
Vice-Chairman
Montefiore Medical Center and
North Central Bronx Hospital
Bronx, New York

RICHARD J. SCARFONE, M.D.
Assistant Professor of Pediatrics
Temple University School of Medicine
Associate Director and Fellowship
Director, Section of Pediatric
Emergency Medicine
St. Christopher's Hospital for
Children
Philadelphia, Pennsylvania

ROBERT W. SCHAFERMEYER, M.D., F.A.A.P.,
F.A.C.E.P
Clinical Professor of Pediatrics and
Emergency Medicine
University of North Carolina School
of Medicine
Chapel Hill, North Carolina
Associate Chairman, Department of
Emergency Medicine
Carolinas Medical Center
Charlotte, North Carolina

CHARLES J. SCHUBERT, M.D., F.A.A.P.
Assistant Professor of Pediatrics
University of Cincinnati
Division of Emergency Medicine
Children's Hospital Medical Center
Cincinnati, Ohio

JEFF E. SCHUNK, M.D., F.A.A.P.
Department of Pediatrics
University of Utah
Primary Children's Medical Center
Salt Lake City, Utah

GARY SCHWARTZ, M.D., F.A.A.P.
Assistant Professor of Emergency
Medicine
Vanderbilt University Medical Center
Nashville, Tennessee

PHILIP V. SCRIBANO, D.O.
Assistant Professor of Pediatric
Emergency Medicine
University of Connecticut
Farmington, Connecticut

MICHAEL SHANNON, M.D., M.P.H.,
F.A.A.P., F.A.C.E.P.
Associate Professor of Pediatrics
Harvard Medical School
Assistant Director, Pediatric
Emergency Medicine
Children's Hospital
Boston, Massachusetts

ROBERT ALLAN SHAPIRO, M.D., F.A.A.P.
Associate Professor of Clinical
Pediatrics
University of Cincinnati
Director, Child Abuse Program
Department of Emergency Medicine
Children's Hospital Medical Center
Cincinnati, Ohio

KATHY N. SHAW, M.D., F.A.A.P.
Associate Professor of Pediatrics
University of Pennsylvania School of
Medicine
Acting Director, Division of
Emergency Medicine
The Children's Hospital of Philadelphia
Philadelphia, Pennsylvania

BENJAMIN K. SILVERMAN, M.D., F.A.A.P.
Staff, Pediatric Emergency Medicine
Children's Hospital of Orange
County
Orange, California

HAROLD K. SIMON, M.D.
ASSISTANT PROFESSOR OF PEDIATRICS
EMORY UNIVERSITY SCHOOL OF MEDICINE
ATTENDING PHYSICIAN, EMERGENCY
DEPARTMENT
EGLESTON CHILDREN'S HOSPITAL AND
HUGHES SPALDING CHILDREN'S HOSPITAL
ATLANTA, GEORGIA

STEPHEN A. STAYER, M.D., F.C.C.M.
ASSISTANT PROFESSOR OF ANESTHESIA AND
PEDIATRICS
TEMPLE UNIVERSITY SCHOOL OF MEDICINE
DEPARTMENT OF ANESTHESIA AND CRITICAL
CARE
ST. CHRISTOPHER'S HOSPITAL FOR
CHILDREN
PHILADELPHIA, PENNSYLVANIA

DALE STEELE, M.D., F.A.A.P.
ASSISTANT PROFESSOR OF PEDIATRICS
BROWN UNIVERSITY SCHOOL OF MEDICINE
ATTENDING PHYSICIAN, PEDIATRIC
EMERGENCY MEDICINE
RHODE ISLAND HOSPITAL
PROVIDENCE, RHODE ISLAND

MARIA STEPHAN, M.D., F.A.A.P.
ASSOCIATE PROFESSOR OF PEDIATRICS
UNIVERSITY OF CINCINNATI COLLEGE OF
MEDICINE
ATTENDING PHYSICIAN, DIVISION OF
EMERGENCY MEDICINE
CHILDREN'S HOSPITAL MEDICAL CENTER
CINCINNATI, OHIO

RICHARD T. STRAIT, M.D., F.A.A.P.
ASSISTANT PROFESSOR OF PEDIATRICS
MEDICAL COLLEGE OF WISCONSIN
DEPARTMENT OF PEDIATRICS
SECTION OF EMERGENCY MEDICINE
ATTENDING PHYSICIAN, EMERGENCY
MEDICINE
CHILDREN'S HOSPITAL OF WISCONSIN
MILWAUKEE, WISCONSIN

GARY R. STRANGE, M.D.
ASSOCIATE PROFESSOR AND HEAD,
DEPARTMENT OF EMERGENCY MEDICINE
CHIEF, EMERGENCY SERVICES
THE UNIVERSITY OF ILLINOIS AT CHICAGO
CHICAGO, ILLINOIS

**MILTON TENENBEIN, M.D., F.A.A.P.,
F.A.A.C.T., F.R.C.P.C.**
PROFESSOR OF PEDIATRICS AND
PHARMACOLOGY
UNIVERSITY OF MANITOBA
DIRECTOR, EMERGENCY SERVICES
CHILDREN'S HOSPITAL
WINNIPEG, MANITOBA
CANADA

THOMAS E. TERNDRUP, M.D., F.A.C.E.P.
ASSOCIATE PROFESSOR OF EMERGENCY
MEDICINE AND PEDIATRICS
DIRECTOR, PEDIATRIC EMERGENCY
DEPARTMENT
STATE UNIVERSITY OF NEW YORK HEALTH
SCIENCE CENTER
SYRACUSE, NEW YORK

SUSAN B. TORREY, M.D., F.A.A.P.
INSTRUCTOR OF PEDIATRICS
HARVARD MEDICAL SCHOOL
ASSISTANT IN MEDICINE
CHILDREN'S HOSPITAL
BOSTON, MASSACHUSETTS

NICHOLAS TSAROUHAS, M.D., F.A.A.P.
ASSISTANT PROFESSOR OF CLINICAL
PEDIATRICS AND SURGERY
ROBERT WOOD JOHNSON MEDICAL
SCHOOL
DIRECTOR, PEDIATRIC EMERGENCY
MEDICINE
DEPARTMENT OF EMERGENCY MEDICINE
COOPER HOSPITAL/UNIVERSITY MEDICAL
CENTER
CAMDEN, NEW JERSEY

VERENA T. VALLEY, M.D.
EMERGENCY MEDICINE ULTRASONOGRAPHY
FELLOW
MEDICAL COLLEGE OF WISCONSIN
DEPARTMENT OF EMERGENCY MEDICINE
MILWAUKEE, WISCONSIN

PATRICIA L. VANDEVANDER, M.D.
ASSISTANT PROFESSOR OF SURGERY
DIVISION OF EMERGENCY MEDICINE
UNIVERSITY OF COLORADO HEALTH
SCIENCES CENTER
DENVER, COLORADO

Contributors

xxiv

JULIE LANGE VARGA, M.D., F.A.C.E.P.
DEPARTMENT OF EMERGENCY MEDICINE
ILLINOIS MASONIC MEDICAL CENTER
CHICAGO, ILLINOIS

ROBERT J. VINCI, M.D., F.A.A.P.
ASSOCIATE PROFESSOR OF PEDIATRICS
BOSTON UNIVERSITY SCHOOL OF MEDICINE
DIRECTOR, PEDIATRIC EMERGENCY
DEPARTMENT
BOSTON CITY HOSPITAL
BOSTON, MASSACHUSETTS

MICHELE R. WADSWORTH, M.D.
ASSISTANT PROFESSOR OF PEDIATRICS
DIVISION OF EMERGENCY MEDICINE
EASTERN VIRGINIA MEDICAL SCHOOL
CHILDREN'S HOSPITAL OF THE KING'S
DAUGHTERS
NORFOLK, VIRGINIA

DAVID K. WAGNER, M.D., F.A.C.E.P.
PROFESSOR AND CHAIR, DEPARTMENT OF
EMERGENCY MEDICINE
MCP ◆ HAHNEMANN SCHOOL OF
MEDICINE OF THE ALLEGHENY
UNIVERSITY OF THE HEALTH SCIENCES
PHILADELPHIA, PENNSYLVANIA

GARY SETH WASSERMAN, D.O., F.A.A.P.
PROFESSOR OF PEDIATRICS
UNIVERSITY OF MISSOURI–KANSAS CITY
SCHOOL OF MEDICINE
PEDIATRICIAN IN EMERGENCY MEDICINE
CHIEF, SECTION OF CLINICAL TOXICOLOGY
DIRECTOR, POISON CONTROL CENTER
THE CHILDREN'S MERCY HOSPITAL
KANSAS CITY, MISSOURI

JAMES F. WILEY II, M.D., F.A.A.P.
ASSOCIATE PROFESSOR OF PEDIATRICS
THE SCHOOL OF MEDICINE AT THE
UNIVERSITY OF CONNECTICUT HEALTH
CENTER
FARMINGTON, CONNECTICUT
DIRECTOR, EMERGENCY MEDICAL SERVICES
CONNECTICUT CHILDREN'S MEDICAL
CENTER
HARTFORD, CONNECTICUT

GEORGE ANTHONY WOODWARD, M.D., F.A.A.P.
ASSISTANT PROFESSOR OF PEDIATRICS
THE UNIVERSITY OF PENNSYLVANIA SCHOOL
OF MEDICINE
DIVISION OF EMERGENCY MEDICINE AND
TRANSPORT
MEDICAL DIRECTOR, TRANSPORT SERVICE
THE CHILDREN'S HOSPITAL OF PHILADELPHIA
PHILADELPHIA, PENNSYLVANIA

GRACE M. YOUNG, M.D., F.A.A.P., F.A.C.E.P.
ASSOCIATE PROFESSOR OF PEDIATRICS
UNIVERSITY OF MARYLAND SCHOOL OF
MEDICINE
ATTENDING PHYSICIAN, PEDIATRIC
EMERGENCY DEPARTMENT
UNIVERSITY OF MARYLAND MEDICAL
CENTER
BALTIMORE, MARYLAND

STEPHEN ZDERIC, M.D.
ASSISTANT PROFESSOR OF UROLOGY
UNIVERSITY OF PENNSYLVANIA SCHOOL OF
MEDICINE
ATTENDING UROLOGIST
CHILDREN'S HOSPITAL OF PHILADELPHIA
PHILADELPHIA, PENNSYLVANIA

CONTENTS

Section One:
General Concepts
Editor: Fred M. Henretig

Section Two:
Cardiopulmonary Life
Support Procedures
Editor: Christopher King

Section Three:
Trauma Life Support
Procedures
Editor: Brent R. King

Section Four:
Anesthesia and
Sedation Procedures
Editor: Mark D. Joffe

Section Five:
Special Procedures for
Neonates
Editor: John Loiselle

Section Six:
Neurologic and
Neurosurgical
Procedures
Editor: James F. Wiley II

Section Eleven:
Pulmonary
Procedures
Editor: Richard M. Ruddy

Section Twelve:
Gastrointestinal
Procedures
Editor: James F. Wiley II

Section Thirteen:
Genitourinary
Procedures
Editor: Mark D. Joffe

General Concepts

Section Editor: Fred H. Henretig

CHAPTER 1

PATIENT AND FAMILY ISSUES

Fred M. Henretig

INTRODUCTION

A child is rushed to the emergency department (ED) by anxious parents. This scenario unfolds tens of millions of times per year in the United States, but remains a uniquely compelling event for all the persons involved: patient, family, and medical staff. In the most dramatic of cases, the child's life depends on the skill of the ED staff in rapidly diagnosing the injury or illness, instituting life support, and initiating definitive treatment as a prelude to hospitalization. Unfortunately, some of these visits end tragically with the death of a child in the ED, despite a technically optimal resuscitation effort. In the vast majority of visits, the family returns home within a few hours, the child sporting some new sutures, or a new cast, or an antibiotic prescription for that unbearable middle-of-the-night ear infection. In every case, the child and/or family bears a lasting impression of their experience, even if the pathophysiologic aberration is readily corrected. Their pain and fear of the ED visit, and how it was addressed by the ED staff, may be remembered long after the physical wounds heal. Conversely, even an otherwise forgettable pediatric walk-in visit, perhaps one of dozens experienced during a busy shift, can be a residual source of frustration to the ED physician who battled to examine a screaming child or tried five times to "get the i.v." The general approach to these psychosocial stresses on child, parent, and medical staff are the focus of this chapter.

All patients are potentially traumatized by an ED experience, but some factors pertain uniquely to the pediatric visit (1, 2). Children vary enormously in age and developmental status, but as a group they have an innate fear of needles and procedures. The younger child in particular fears strangers (and especially physicians, who are often perceived as sources of pain). Parents are the natural protectors and sources of comfort for their children during a physical or emotional crisis. When their child is sick, parents feel an obligation to serve in a helping role. They may also feel some share of responsibility for having "allowed" the illness or injury to occur. Thus, parents are functioning in dual roles when their child visits the ED. On the one hand they wish to be composed and to function as a member of the helping team. At the same time, they are stressed and anxious, and may feel some guilt over their child's illness. In essence, they too are patients. Medical staff often diminish both of these parental roles in their zeal to get things done efficiently. This is generally a mistake. Parents, in most situations, are able to function as considerable sources of comfort and support to their children in the ED setting, and belong at the bedside during the vast majority of interventions that might occur. This chapter explores background issues related to parental involvement in pediatric ED procedures. It offers an approach to take maximal advantage of parents as allies in the effort to accomplish such procedures successfully from both the child and the family and the staff perspective.

DEVELOPMENTAL AND PSYCHOLOGIC ISSUES

Psychologists consider the first year of life to be a period when children experience their world as an extension of their parents. Although toddlers aged 1 to 3 years begin to understand themselves as individuals, there is still a very close bond to parents that requires a nearly constant sense of parental presence within the immediate environment for maximal sense of security. Infants beyond 6 to 9 months of age have intense stranger anxiety, often lasting to the age of 3 years. Maintaining close contact with parents is crucial to optimizing psychological support during a stressful event in this age group (see also Chapter 2, p. 9, and Table 2.1, p. 10).

Although older preschool and school-aged children are obviously able to tolerate brief separations from parents, they still derive a strong sense of comfort from ready access to them. Dental literature has reported that children aged 41 to 49 months of age are less fearful and more cooperative when their parents stay with them (3). Other researchers observed that behavioral manifestations of discomfort may actually increase if parents are present (4); this may reflect the child's perception that parental presence gives them permission to verbalize their discomfort. However, the goal of pain management during procedures is obviously not to produce a cooperative child who bravely suffers in silence. When surveyed, more than 90% of children 9 to 12 years old reported that the "thing that helped most" during a painful procedure was to have parents present (5). Also, parental anxiety about the procedure may influence the child's experience (6), and obviously individual parental differences in this regard need to be taken into account. As a corollary, parental preparation for the procedure may be as important as preparing the child.

Parents were surveyed regarding their preferences about being present during procedures on their children. In one study performed in a Boston pediatric ED (7), 78% of parents surveyed indicated they would want to be present when their child had blood drawn or an i.v. started. Of this group, 80% said it would make them personally feel better, 91% thought it would make their child feel better, and 73% felt it would help the physician. A follow-up study by the same authors (8) reported on actual observations of 50 venipunctures or intravenous cannulations. Parents remained with their children during 62% of the procedures. Many of the parents who did not stay indicated they would have preferred to, but were either directly asked to leave or given nonverbal cues strongly suggesting that they should. Overall, only 10% of this group of parents stated they had not wanted to be with their child during the procedure.

Physicians and nurses, along with parents, have also been surveyed about their attitudes and practice regarding parental presence during pediatric procedures. In a 1990 report, 212 pediatricians, 59 nurses, and 77 parents were surveyed in the Salt Lake City area (9). The procedures included in the survey were immunizations, venipunctures, laceration suturing, intravenous cannulation, lumbar puncture, radiologic tests, and trauma evaluations in both conscious and unconscious patients. Of physicians, 58% reported they usually encouraged parents to remain with their child. The likelihood of asking parents to leave varied with the perceived invasiveness of the procedure. Nurses' responses were similar. Parents confirmed that they were present during the majority of procedures, including more than 90% of the time for immunizations, sutures, and venipunctures, and 75% for i.v. access and lumbar puncture. Only 2% of the parents in this survey felt they would be too upset to help their child, though many felt that physicians might exclude them out of fear that they would overreact or interfere with the procedure. The majority of parents believed an explanation of the procedure to both them and their child would be the most helpful coping strategy for the child.

Intuitively, it may strike many clinicians that the more traumatic the circumstances, the less appropriate it would be for parents to remain with their child during emergency procedures, such as those associated with significant anatomical disfigurement or potential death. In many such situations, the child will be unconscious and unlikely to be objectively comforted by parental presence. Whether parents would feel a measure of comfort in having participated and helped all they could is another matter. Little research has actually been done in this area. Some case reports have indicated that parents express gratitude and appreciation for having been allowed to be with their child and speak to him or her during an unsuccessful trauma resuscitation (10). A survey of families of cardiac arrest victims, who had been allowed into the resuscitation room, also tended to indicate a sense that participation had been beneficial to the grieving process and was comforting to the dying relative (11). In these reports, endotracheal intubation and other invasive procedures had usually been accomplished before bringing the family into the room, and ED staff were assigned to accompany the family members during the remainder of the resuscitation effort.

Anecdotal evidence suggests that physicians may believe they are more anxious and perform procedures less effectively when parents are present (12). This has not been studied to date, but even if true, it seems likely that increased experience with parental participation would obviate such differences. Medical students and resident physicians are often nervous about their pediatric physical examination skills, but are expected to become comfortable with these procedures done in the presence of the family, and most manage to do so. Some physicians also believe that children will suffer less psychic trauma after a painful or frightening procedure if parents leave the treatment room and then return as the rescuers at the completion of the procedure. This also is an unstudied phenomenon. It seems likely that the parental role of providing comfort to their child during procedures would also be enhanced by physician-directed preparation and guidance in this situation. Bauchner and colleagues studied the impact of such a brief educational effort for parents whose children less than 3 years old required procedures in the ED (13, 14). The procedures included venipuncture, intravenous cannulation, and urethral catheterization. The educational intervention included instructions for the parents to situate themselves near the head of the bed, and to talk with and touch their child soothingly. They were not expected to help in restraint. They were also warned that their child might cry, and they were asked not to tell the child that the procedure would not

hurt. Parents were randomized into three groups—those who stayed with their child and received the educational intervention (group 1), those who stayed for the procedure but did not receive the intervention (group 2), and those who did not stay (group 3). The groups were equivalent for a number of sociodemographic factors. Of the 101 parents in the intervention group, 89% were effective in following the instructions and 93% stated the instructions were helpful. Only 46% of the 101 parents who stayed, but did not receive the specific guidelines, used similar strategies in comforting their child. Of the parents in group 1, 95% were satisfied with their child's care versus 81% in group 2. Among both groups who stayed, the vast majority reported they would be likely to stay with their child for a future procedure (93% of group 1, 95% of group 2) versus only 53% of those who did not stay (group 3).

Some procedures exist for which the inherent aversiveness to parents may be overwhelming, and there may be some parents who simply can not cope with any procedure being performed. A common example of the former context might be the actual reduction of a displaced forearm fracture. The combination of visual and auditory sensations, as well as the nearly unavoidable though very transient pain to the child, makes this an exceedingly difficult moment for most parents. The family could easily remain with their child during the initial evaluation, intravenous line placement, and initiation of conscious sedation. One method is to gently suggest to the parents that the reduction per se will be very brief, and the appropriately sedated and narcotized child would be unlikely to miss their transient absence. The family might briefly leave, or at least stand away from the bedside, and then return immediately at the completion of the reduction, during the casting and subsequent reevaluation. Some parents may still choose to stay, and such a decision should be supported with appropriate forewarnings of what they will see and hear. For the vast majority of procedures, if emergency physicians and pediatricians attempt to foster the parents' role as ally and partner in their child's treatment, such occasions necessitating the parents leaving the bedside would likely be the exception.

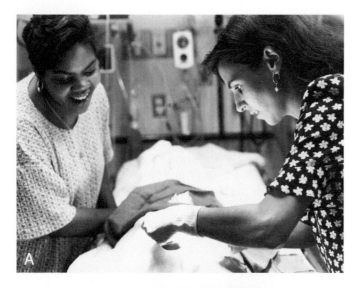

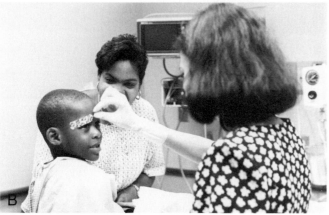

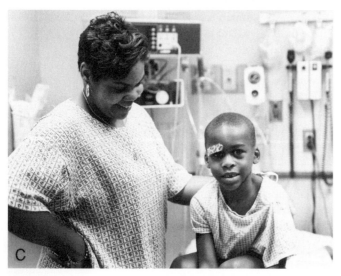

Figure 1.1.
A. Mother is holding child's hand and comforting him during facial laceration repair.
B. Procedure completed; this child is not terrified of physician.
C. Both child and parent can take pride in "their accomplishment."

APPROACH TO INVOLVING THE PARENTS

The first step in engaging parents is to offer them the opportunity to be with and to help their child during the procedure. It should be made clear that they are not being asked to take on a medical or nursing role; rather, they are being asked to remain as comforters and empathizers to their child. Many parents who might faint during their own venipunctures can nurture their child through a complex and bloody laceration repair, if they (*a*) know what to expect, (*b*) trust their physicians's competence and sense of caring for their child, and (*c*) understand that everything possible will be done medically to relieve their child's pain. If, after such an offer, parents continue to appear hesitant or express discomfort with remaining present, they should certainly not be made to feel inadequate. Such parents may remain with the child during the preparations for the procedure, be separated as short a time as possible, and be immediately ushered in as comforters at the procedure's completion.

Both parents and child need some preparation involving information about the technical and sensory aspects of the procedure. They need to know what the steps of the procedure will be, approximately how long it will take, an honest estimation of the degree of discomfort the child may encounter, and how that discomfort will be mitigated by the physician. Sensory input includes describing the sights, sounds, smells, and physical sensations the child will experience during the procedure, and allowing the child, when appropriate, to see and feel the equipment. For those parents who have chosen to stay, their role should be made more explicit. They will be asked to position themselves so that their child may see them, if possible. Their job will be to talk soothingly and touch their child as much as possible. Suggestions may be offered regarding the content of the parents' comforting words, such as telling a favorite adventure story, particularly one that might engage the child in a fantasy. Parents should not tell their child that the procedure will not hurt, but rather reaffirm the physician's assurances that significant pain will be avoided and/or treated pharmacologically as necessary. They will not be expected to participate in the medical or surgical aspects of the procedure or to help with restraint (other than in the briefest, pain-free situations such as an otoscopic examination). Parents are not expected to be critically observing the procedure itself, but rather to be fully engaged with comforting their child.

As the procedure begins, parents may need continued guidance and reinforcement of these points. The ED staff should help to position the parents at the head of the bed, or as appropriate for the particular procedure. They need to be continuously updated and reassured about the procedure's steps toward completion, and the child's condition. If parents become anxious and falter, a second or two of directed interaction with them may suffice to help them back into their role. There may be some cases where it will be obvious that everyone would be better off if the parents left the room momentarily. Again, they should be supported in this decision and returned to the child as soon as feasible to resume their comforter role.

The issue of exactly which procedures are appropriate for parental presence is a complex one, and no arbitrary rules are offered here. Conditions vary for any given procedure; physician experience, parental experience with previous emergency interventions, and the medical circumstances of the particular context in which the procedure is necessary all contribute to making such a determination of appropriateness. The reader is urged to seriously consider the value of parental presence in virtually any pediatric emergency procedure.

SUMMARY

Parents should be encouraged and guided in remaining with their child through most pediatric emergency procedures. Their presence will be comforting not only to the child, but also will play a therapeutic role for the parents themselves, and will often facilitate the successful completion of the procedure. Emergency department staff should offer parents the option of remaining, prepare them for their comforter role, and provide continuing guidance to them during the procedure.

REFERENCES

1. Zeltzer LK, Jay SM, Fisher DM. The management of pain associated with pediatric procedures. Pediatr Clin North Am 1989;36: 941–964.
2. Selbst SM, Henretig FM. The treatment of pain in the emergency department. Pediatr Clin North Am 1989;36:965–978.
3. Frankl S, Shiere F, Fogels H. Should the parent remain with the child in the dental operatory? J Dent Child 1962;29:152–163.
4. Shaw EG, Routh DK. Effect of mother presence on children's reduction of aversive procedures. J Pediatr Psychol 1982;7:33–44.
5. Ross DM, Ross SA. The importance of type of question, psychological climate and subject set in interviewing children about pain. Pain 1984;19:71–79.
6. Jay SM, Ozolins M, Elliot CH, et al. Assessment of children's distress during painful medical procedures. Health Psychol 1983;2: 133–147.
7. Bauchner H, Vinci R, Waring C. Pediatric procedures: do parents want to watch? Pediatrics 1989;84:907–909.
8. Bauchner H, Waring C, Vinci R. Parental presence during procedures in an emergency room: results from 50 observations. Pediatrics 1991;87:544–548.
9. Merrit KA, Sargent JR, Osborn LM. Attitudes regarding parental presence during medical procedures. Am J Dis Child 1990;144: 277–271.
10. Eichhorn DJ, Meyers TA, Guzzetta CE. Family presence during resuscitation: it is time to open the door. Capsules and Comments in Critical Care Nursing 1995;3:8–13.
11. Doyle CJ, Post H, Burney RE, et al. Family participation during resuscitation: an option. Ann Emerg Med 1987;16:673–675.
12. Bauchner H. Procedures, pain and parents. Pediatrics 1991;87:563–565.
13. Bauchner H, Vinci R, Pearson C. Parental presence during procedures: satisfaction with care. Am J Dis Child 1993;147:426–427.
14. Bauchner H, Vinci R, May A. Teaching parents how to comfort their children during common medical procedures. Arch Dis Child 1994;70:548–550.

SUMMARY
1. Offer parents the option of staying with their child.
2. Explain that their presence, if calm and supportive, will help the child.
3. Prepare them for role as providers of emotional support, not technical assistants.
4. Position them, if possible, within the child's sight.
5. Ask them to speak soothingly and touch their child throughout the procedure.
6. Update and reassure them on procedural steps and child's condition.
7. Indicate how supportive their presence has been to their child.

TECHNIQUES FOR EXAMINING THE FEARFUL CHILD

Janet H. Friday and Fred M. Henretig

INTRODUCTION

In caring for children in the outpatient setting, most of us have been humbled at some time by the difficulty of examining an uncooperative child. Although no single, fail-proof technique exists to avoid this problem, a calm and relaxed approach that incorporates a knowledge of developmental stages can smooth the interaction (1-4). This method should not significantly increase the time spent on the examination. Instead, it will help to establish a relationship with the family, provide a basis for future interventions, and allow an optimal diagnostic evaluation in a timely manner. The related subject of minimizing fear and anxiety during procedures is approached in Chapter 35.

PHYSIOLOGY—NORMAL DEVELOPMENTAL STAGES

Recognition of childhood developmental stages and their accompanying issues will help the examining physician to interact with the child in a way that optimizes patient comfort and acceptance of the examination (Table 2.1).

Infants (Birth to 1 Year)

Until the appearance of stranger anxiety around 8 to 9 months of age, the infant exam-ination is not constrained by fear; however, infants are quite sensitive to their immediate environment. After stranger anxiety appears, the infant may be threatened by the physician's presence, and will remain most cooperative in the parent's arms.

Toddlers (1 to 3 Years)

Although the young toddler may appear relatively nonverbal, the child's receptive language skills develop sooner than the expressive ones. Therefore, the physician must be careful of what is said in the child's presence. The toddler is most cognizant of his or her developing individuality and independence. Negativism of the "terrible two's" is prevalent. The child fears separation from the parents, and will be best examined in the parent's lap.

Preschool Age (3 to 5 Years)

The preschooler has developed expressive skills and a strong concept of self. Magical thinking and fantasy play become important during preschool years, and can be incorporated into the examination.

School Age (5 to 10 Years)

Development of logic and reason, and a good grasp of language allows the older child to co-

Table 2.1.
Developmental Approach to Pediatric Emergency Care Patients

Age (yr)	Important Development Issues	Fears	Useful Techniques
Infancy: 0–1	Minimal language Feel an extension of parents Sensitive to physical environment	Stranger anxiety	Keep parents in sight and touch Avoid hunger Use warm hands Keep room warm
Toddler: 1–3	Receptive language more advanced than expressive See themselves as individuals Assertive will	Brief separation Pain	Maintain verbal communication Examine in parent's lap Allow some choices when possible
Preschool: 3–5	Excellent expressive skills for thoughts and feelings Rich fantasy life Magical thinking Strong concept of self	Long separation Pain Disfigurement	Allow expression Encourage fantasy and play Encourage participation in care
School age: 5–10	Fully developed language Understanding of body structure and function Able to reason and compromise Experience with self-control Incomplete understanding of death	Disfigurement Loss of function Death	Explain procedures Explain pathophysiology and treatment Project positive outcome Stress child's ability to master situation Respect physical modesty
Adolescence: 10–19	Self-determination Decision making Peer group important Realistic view of death	Loss of autonomy Loss of peer acceptance Death	Allow choices and control Stress acceptance by peers Respect autonomy Stress confidentiality

From Fleisher G, Ludwig S (eds). Textbook of Pediatric Emergency Medicine. 3rd ed. Baltimore: Williams & Wilkins, 1993, with permission.

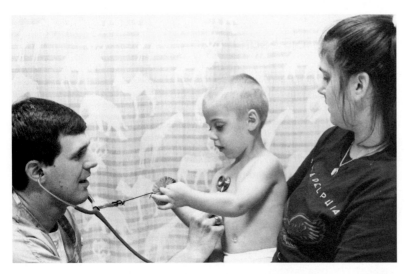

Figure 2.1.
A simple toy may engage the toddler.

operate with the examination. An understanding of body function and structure can be incorporated during these years. Even before the development of sexual maturation, modesty will emerge and should be anticipated.

Adolescence (10 to 19 Years)

In general, cooperation with the physical examination is not an issue with the adolescent.

However, appreciation for the importance of his or her particular issues with autonomy, peer group importance, self-determination, and control will certainly ease the interaction.

INDICATIONS

Every encounter with the child who is not critically ill will be enhanced by a few efforts to gain trust and cooperation. The ability to detect subtle but important physical findings (e.g., a heart murmur or friction rub, the presence of pulmonary rales or asymmetric air entry, or abdominal tenderness or mass) will certainly be optimized by examining a child who is cooperative (or at least not screaming and resisting).

In certain circumstances, the examiner may anticipate that a difficult situation will arise even before entering the examination room. This will allow him or her to take special care not to rush the interaction and to carefully apply the appropriate techniques. Such situations include children with chronic diseases, irritable toddlers, and any child who already has had difficult interactions with other members of the health care team. The obvious contraindication to using the following approaches would be a seriously ill or injured child where attention to immediate resuscitation or stabilization takes precedence over all else.

EQUIPMENT

Every experienced pediatric specialist has a few tricks of the trade which he or she uses to put a child at ease. For infants, this will often be offering a pacifier or bottle during the examination. At around 3 months of age, babies will become enamored with simple noises such as lip-smacking or jingling keys. In toddlers, any toy may work wonders in engaging the child (Fig. 2.1). Many examination tools can be incorporated into a game which will transition nicely into the actual examination. Part of the ascertainment of a child's well-being will be seeing him or her doing normal activities, so therefore giving out crayons and paper during a waiting period is helpful in this regard.

For actual examination equipment, many pediatricians prefer long stethoscope tubing so the examination may be accomplished at some distance from the anxious child (Fig. 2.1). It has become dogma that children are afraid of the "white coat," which may be somewhat true. However, children are not easily fooled; and if afraid of doctors, will notice the scrub suits, beepers, and stethoscopes that characterize them. In general, an unfamiliar examiner will be challenged to gain a child's trust no matter how he or she is attired.

PROCEDURE

Ensuring a warm, quiet environment and offering a bottle when appropriate will provide a good milieu for the physical examination in most infants. Speaking to the parent in a soft, friendly voice and establishing a rapport with him or her before approaching the child will make the examination more accepted. Much of the examination can be accomplished while the parent is holding the infant in his or her lap (Fig. 2.2). Washing with hot water will warm the examiner's hands and thus

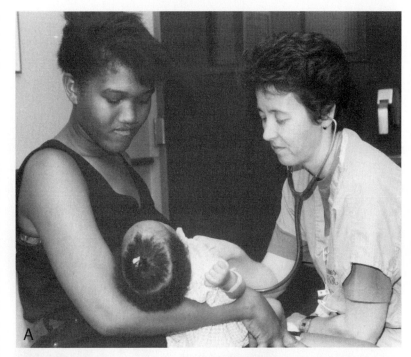

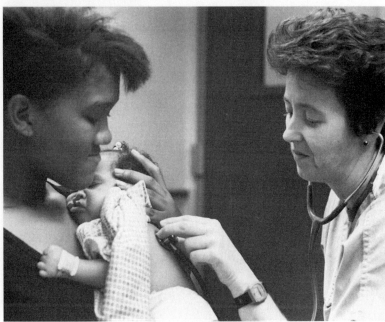

Figure 2.2.
The infant examination is often begun on mother's lap or against her chest.

avoid startling the infant, in addition to its antimicrobial benefit. Instruments, especially the stethoscope, can be "rubbed up" to warm them as well. The examination should be ordered so that auscultation of the heart, lungs, and abdomen occur first, followed by palpation of the abdomen. Any disruptive or painful procedure (e.g., removing the diaper

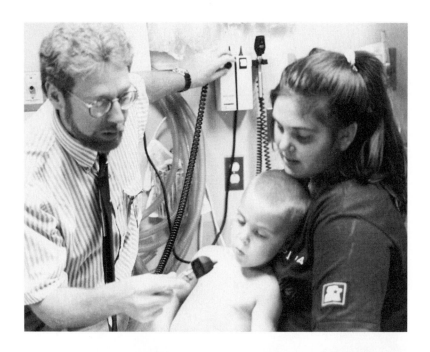

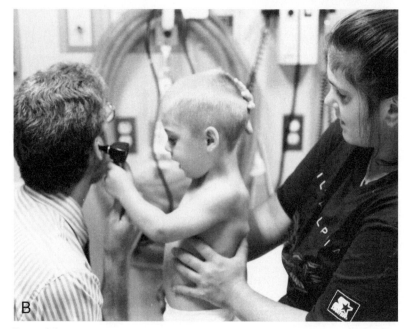

Figure 2.3.
A. Toddler "blows out" the light prior to otoscopic examination.
B. Toddler "examines" physician's ears.

Chapter 2
Techniques for
Examining the Fearful
Child

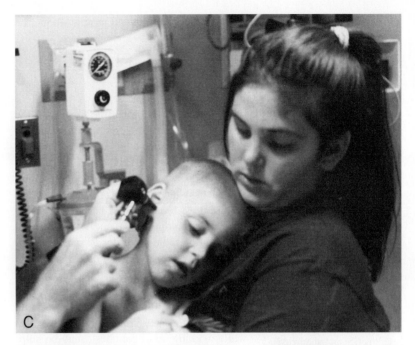

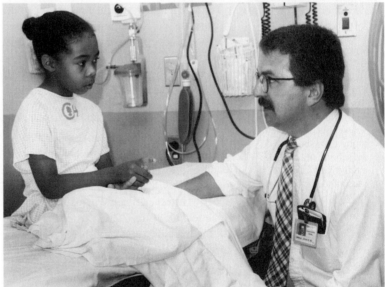

Figure 2.3. (continued)
C. Toddler now allows ear examination with minimal restraint from mother.
D. Respect for modesty is crucial in school age children.

SUMMARY
1. Age-related approach
2. Applicable to all encounters except critically ill patients
3. Wash (and warm) hands
4. Infants and toddlers: utilize parents as much as possible
5. Preschool: encourage fantasy, play, and participation in the examination
6. School age: explain actions, respect modesty
7. Adolescence: stress confidentiality, respect modesty and autonomy

CLINICAL TIPS
1. Practice an "unhurried" demeanor
2. Handwashing reassures parents and patients, warms hands
3. Infants: use props (pacifier, bottle, jingling keys)
4. Toddlers: play games (blowing out the otoscope light, and auscultating their shoes)
5. Preschool: utilize magical thinking and fantasy (auscultate or palpate favorite foods in the abdominal examination, look for animals or cartoon characters in the ears)
6. School age: explain each step
7. Adolescence: allow choices, control as possible

or examining the ears and mouth) should be done last.

Toddlers

In most cases, it is preferable to discuss the history with the parents first keeping in mind that the child understands much of the conversation. For the fearful toddler, this discussion should occur prior to any threatening approach. When it comes time for the examination, most toddlers will be comforted by the parents holding them, and will prefer not to sit on the table. In order to gain the toddler's trust, the examiner should begin with examining the feet or hands. The subsequent order should be the same as for infants (see previous section). Playing some simple games, such as auscultating the extremities while working up to the chest, may be helpful. The examiner should not offer choices when none exist and, similarly, not ask any question unless prepared to hear the response "no" (e.g., not "Would you like to roll on your tummy now?" when it is preferable to say, "Roll over now, please."). When undergoing ear and mouth examination, the toddler should be given a chance to cooperate, but noncompliance should be anticipated. Games such as blowing out the otoscope light or pretending to examine the doctor's ears can be attempted with older toddlers (Fig. 2.3.A, 2.3.B). However, they will usually require some restraint (Fig. 2.3.C, Chapter 4). Overall, the examiner must seek assistance when necessary and move fast!

Preschool Age

At the preschool age, the examination begins to become less difficult. A more direct interaction with the child is appropriate and accepted. For example, greeting the child and complementing their attire will no longer be a threat (Hi! How are you today? I like those Mickey Mouse sneakers!). Allowing the child to express fears or desires and participate will often lend to a better examination. Some of the magical thinking and fantasy can be incorporated into the examination (e.g., listening for french fries in the tummy or looking for monkeys in the ears). Again it is preferable to leave any intrusive part until last.

School Age

For the most part, examination of the school-age child does not need to differ greatly in content from that of an adult. At this age, children become extraordinarily inquisitive and are interested in what the examiner is really doing and why. Explaining the examination as one precedes may be helpful. Appreciation for modesty at this age is an absolute necessity (Fig. 2.4).

Adolescence

Again, the examination of an adolescent is usually not different from that of an adult. Appreciation of autonomy and confidentiality, and respect for modesty and decision making should be used. Allowing for choices and control, when appropriate, may be helpful.

SUMMARY

In conclusion, it can be difficult to ease the fears of an uncooperative young child. The approach and techniques detailed here are no substitute for years of experience (and mistakes). However, used judiciously, while adapting to unique situations, they will maximize the information which can only be obtained by a thorough examination. The trust established with the child and family will serve as a foundation for further care.

REFERENCES

1. Selbst SM, Henretig FM. The treatment of pain in the emergency department. Pediatr Clin North Am (36)4:965–978.
2. Hughes WT, Buescher ES. Preparation of the patient. In: Pediatric procedures. 2nd ed. Philadelphia: WB Saunders, 1980, pp. 1–25.
3. Fleisher GR, Ludwig S. Textbook of pediatric emergency medicine. Baltimore: Williams and Wilkins, 1993, pp. xxxvii–xi.
4. Hoekelman RA. The physical examination of infants and children. In: Bates B, ed. A guide to physical examination and history taking. 5th ed. Philadelphia: JB Lippincott, 1991, pp. 561–635.

CHAPTER 3

RESTRAINT TECHNIQUES

Joel A. Fein and M. Douglas Baker

INTRODUCTION

In the course of managing patients in an acute care setting, we sometimes find it necessary to restrain the violent or uncooperative patient. Approximately 50% of human service providers are victims of violence (1). Twenty-five percent of adult emergency departments restrain at least one patient per day (2). In the absence of psychiatric illness, intoxication, or organic brain syndromes, the most common person requiring restraint for procedures is the uncooperative child. It is therefore important that both the equipment and the overall approach used are age appropriate. Since restraint procedures are also used in the prehospital, inpatient, or intensive care unit settings, EMTs, nurses, physicians, and security personnel should be familiar with the risks and benefits of these techniques. The techniques involved are temporizing, and frequent reassessment of the need and method of restraint is the rule. Although the actual application of physical or chemical restraints is straightforward, the ethical and legal issues surrounding these procedures are more complex.

ANATOMY AND PHYSIOLOGY

One must recognize the developmental level of the child in need of a potentially painful procedure (see also Table 2.1, p. 10). Whereas the 5- or 6-year-old child might be adept at the art of negotiation, he or she is not as adept at keeping his or her end of the bargain when faced with a noxious stimulus. Ten- or 11-year-old children may have the ability to understand the necessity for a procedure in the abstract, but will often require some help in immobilization during the procedure itself.

In contrast, the older patient who is noncompliant with emergency medical care may have some physiologic disturbance that can alter judgment, self-control, or ability to assess pain. These patients may suffer from a variety of conditions, including organic brain syndrome, intoxication, functional psychosis, or personality disorder. In these cases one must recognize that the patient may not stop struggling while tissue injury is occurring. A striking example of this problem is seen in adolescent patients with exposure to phencyclidine (PCP), which is discussed in the following sections.

INDICATIONS

Two situations exist in which health care professionals must consider the use of physical or chemical restraints on a patient. The first scenario is one in which the patient will not or cannot cooperate with the performance of a medically necessary emergent procedure. The patient may be a developmentally appropriate child or an older individual with some alteration of mental status. A psychiatric consultant is helpful in the diagnosis and treatment of patients with psychosis or personality disorders.

The second situation in which physical restraint may be required occurs when someone's actions are assessed as being either personally harmful or harmful to others. The person requiring restraint may be a patient, or may be a visitor to the health care facility. In this case, the goal of the hospital personnel is to use verbal, physical, and chemical coercion to eliminate the risk of injury to the person and those around him or her.

There are few absolute contraindications to restraining patients in need of acute care. However, alternative methods should be considered if the use of chemical or physical restraints would exacerbate a medical condition and render the patient medically unstable, or would inhibit continuous monitoring required by a critically ill patient. In addition, one should not attempt to restrain a patient if there are not enough personnel or equipment to perform the technique safely and efficiently.

A special case in which physical restraint may be harmful to the patient is after PCP ingestion. PCP users can be unpredictable and are not aware of their behavior. These patients should be allowed to remain in a quiet, dark room with as little stimulation as possible. One should not attempt to talk to the patient (3). Physical restraint should be applied only if the patient becomes a danger to others. Because the patient is not aware of the tissue damage occurring as a result of fighting against the restraints, severe physical injury can occur.

Table 3.1.
List of Equipment Necessary for Patient Restraint

- Papoose boards of various sizes (Fig. 3.1)
  Canvas flaps and Velcro® fasteners
  (Olympic Medical, Seattle, WA)
- Leather four-point restraint bracelets with leather straps
  (Stuarts Drug and Surgical Supply, Greensburg, PA)
- Philadelphia collar
- Monitoring equipment
  CR monitor
  Pulse oximeter

EQUIPMENT

The equipment necessary for restraining patients appropriately is listed in Table 3.1. Equipment used for restraint should be easy to apply, and padded and contoured to minimize damage to patient. Papoose boards should have a portion for head immobilization that is integral to the unit. In order to minimize the risk of the patient getting free during a procedure, it is better to overestimate than to underestimate board size. Leather restraints should be padded internally, and have adjustable ring clips.

Appropriate monitoring equipment is necessary to supplement the continuous observation of the restrained patient. This includes frequent assessment of vital signs in potentially unstable patients, as well as the potential measurement of oxygenation by pulse oximetry. Further details regarding monitoring devices are reviewed in Chapter 5 of this text.

RESTRAINT PROCEDURES

As mentioned, patients require restraint for a variety of reasons. The approach to the uncooperative pediatric patient depends on the size and strength of the child. In addition, the overtly violent patient is more likely to require a systematic approach toward the protection of hospital or office personnel.

Consent Issues

Obtaining consent in order to restrain a patient seems to be a contradiction in terms. However, in the absence of an emergency, one needs the consent of the patient or the parents before any treatment can be initiated. This consent need not be written, and may be implied in the explanation of the procedure. In the event of a life-threatening emergency, consent is usually considered to be implied. When in doubt, the patient should be restrained and treated. The damages incurred by not treating are usually greater than those incurred from restraining the patient (4). Simply informing the patient of the method and timing of how he or she is going to be restrained is a helpful and necessary part of the restraint procedure. Adolescent or adult patients with organic brain syndromes or psychiatric illness might not be considered competent to make an intelligent choice regarding their treatment. A more detailed discussion of consent and competence issues is reviewed in Chapter 9.

Techniques

The Violent Patient

During an interaction with a violent or potentially violent patient, the goals are to prevent injury to the patient and the health care team and to provide the appropriate medical treatments as necessary. In order to prevent personal injury, the best positioning would allow both the patient and the interviewer to have access to the door; however, if this is not possible, then it is best to position the interviewer between the patient and the door. Speak calmly but definitively, and first request the patient's cooperation in a nonthreatening manner. Explain that violence is unacceptable, and in a noncondescending tone, explain the consequences of the patient's actions. As these negotiations proceed, it may be helpful to provide a show of force, using the restraint team, security, and local police if available. This often provides the patient with an excuse that he or she was outnumbered, and could not possibly win. Once the decision to physically restrain a patient is made, there is no further negotiation. At this point, the restraint team should use the five-point restraint technique described below. A thorough weapons search should be conducted as soon as the patient is immobilized (see Table 3.2).

Papoose

For the uncooperative but otherwise nonviolent patient, monitoring systems should be placed before the restraint procedure. Infants or small children may only require immobilization of the body part on which the procedure is being performed. This is usually the case during intravenous catheter placement, when the person performing the procedure might provide his or her own immobilization,

or might only need the help of a colleague. For longer or more complex procedures, immobilization of the whole body can be accomplished using a papoose board, as shown in Figs. 3.1 and 3.2. For this procedure, the board is placed on the stretcher or bed, and a sheet is folded and placed on top of the padded backing inside the canvas straps. The child is then placed supine on top of the sheet, which prevents abrasions from developing after the canvas straps envelop the patient and connect with velcro. The child is initially restrained across the midabdomen, followed by trunk and arms, and then by legs, as necessary. Papoose boards come in a variety of sizes. If the board is appropriately sized, then holes in the fabric allow one or both arms to extrude from the papoose if necessary. Some brands of papoose boards contain additional straps for head immobilization. If a papoose board is not available, a folded sheet may be used to immobilize the child's arms and body, as shown in Fig. 3.3. First, the child stands on the stretcher. Next, the sheet is

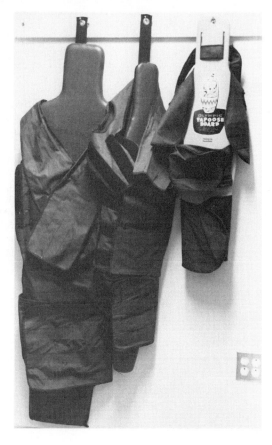

Table 3.2.
Approach to the Violent Patient

- Universal access to door
- Speak calmly but definitively request cooperation explain consequences
- Show of force
- Five-point restraint technique
- Weapons search

Figure 3.1.
Papoose boards should be available in several sizes.

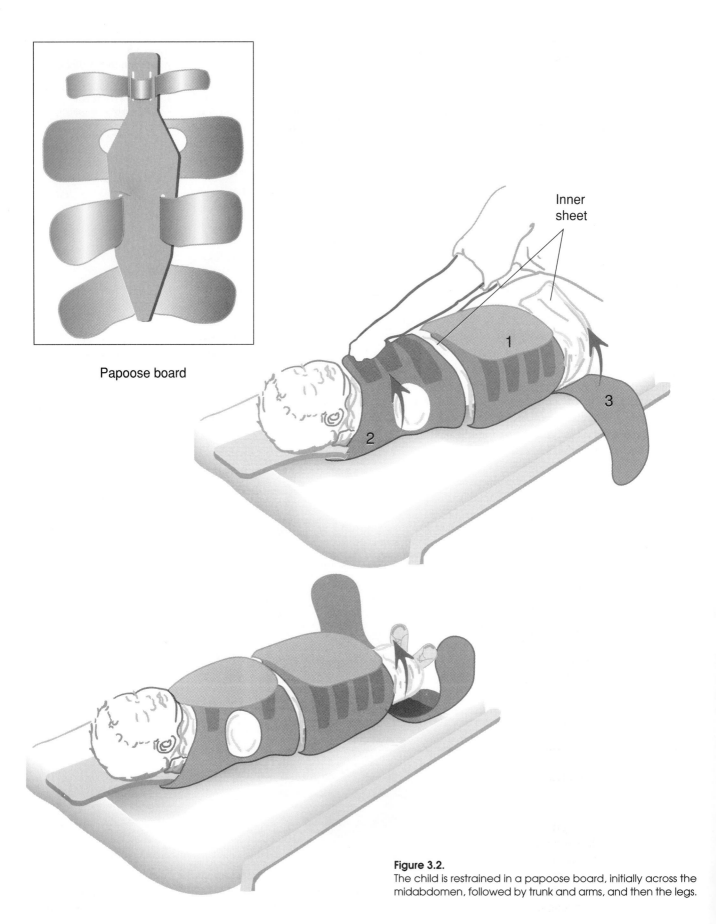

Papoose board

Inner sheet

Figure 3.2.
The child is restrained in a papoose board, initially across the midabdomen, followed by trunk and arms, and then the legs.

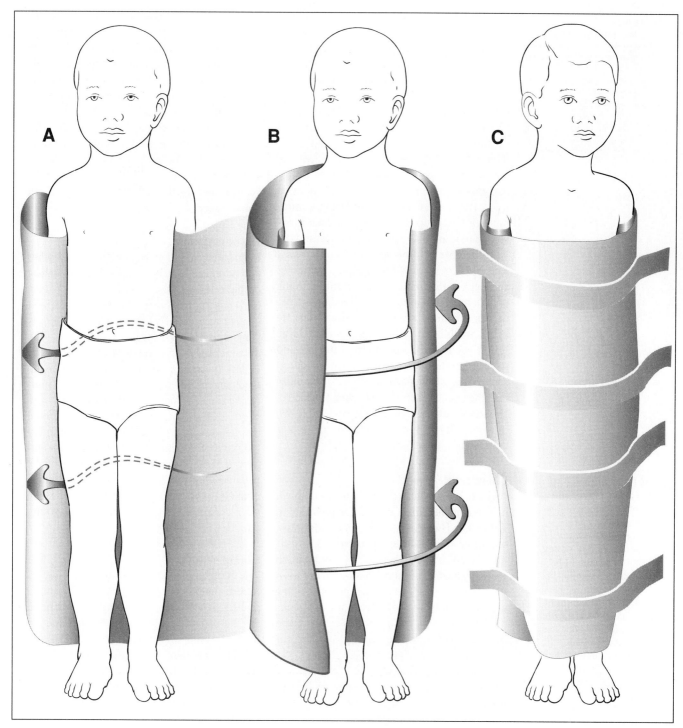

Figure 3.3.
Folded sheet immobilization (see text this page).

folded on itself along its length to a width that covers the child's trunk and legs. It is then initially placed behind the back, with the short end tucked under the right axilla and folded around the right arm, ending behind the back (**A**). The long end is tucked under the left axilla, wrapped around the left arm, then behind the back and around the chest to behind the back again (**B**). Now the child can be placed prone or supine, as desired, and secured with several strips of wide adhesive tape to the sides of the stretcher (**C**).

Five-Point Restraint

Older children or adolescents will usually comply with painful procedures if the reasons and methods are described to them beforehand. If the patient requires immobilization for an emergency procedure, or is a danger to himself or herself or others, then a five-point restraint system should be enacted (Table 3.3). In a similar fashion to other medical emergencies, the most successful approach to this procedure involves a predesignated restraint team with well-defined roles, directed by one person. Using a minimum of five people, one team member is assigned to immobilize each extremity, and the fifth member controls the head and airway. The placement of a Philadelphia collar or soft neck collar helps to prevent injury to the patient or team members sustained by the patient's thrashing or biting. Extremities are best immobilized by holding down the large joints such as the shoulders, elbows, and knees. Leather restraints are first secured around the distal portion of each extremity and then secured to the stretcher. These restraints should be tight enough to hold down the extremity without causing neurovascular compromise (Fig. 3.4).

Chemical Restraint

A list of the medications used to accomplish or supplement patient restraint is provided in Table 3.4. The dosage, indications, and most common side effects are provided. Anxiolytic medications, when used in conjunction with physical restraint procedures, can lessen the force necessary to restrain patients. They are commonly used before painful procedures in children. Various forms can be given intravenously, intramuscularly, rectally, or intranasally (see also Chapters 34 and 35). Neuroleptic medications may obviate the need for prolonged physical restraint. Barbiturates or antihistamines are infrequently used as adjuncts to patient restraint.

Maintenance and Removal of Restraints

While physical restraints are in place, serial monitoring of vital signs and physical examination should occur every 30 minutes. Restraints should be removed one extremity at a time if signs of neurovascular compromise appear. Patients who require pharmacologic interventions such as anxiolytics or neuroleptics need to be monitored more continuously. The sedative and anticholinergic effects of these medications can act alone or in conjunction with drugs of abuse to cause respiratory depression, neurologic depression, or extrapyramidal reactions.

The same criteria used to apply physical restraints should be used to remove them. If the threat that the patient had originally responded to is removed, such as a painful procedure, then further restraint is most likely unnecessary.

Documentation

Restraining a patient is similar to any other procedure, in that it requires documentation of the technique (see also Chapter 11). In certain cases, this procedure is performed against the patient's wishes, and therefore is subject to potential legal complications. The documentation should therefore speak to the events preceding the restraint, the decision mechanisms, the type of restraint used, application times, removal times, the patient's reaction to restraint, and the patient's eventual disposition. Preprinted forms can facilitate this kind of documentation. The documentation of these events need not be as comprehensive when implied or expressed consent is obtained from the patient's guardian, as is the case during a laceration repair in a young child.

Complications

The complications that may occur secondary to restraint procedures range from psychological to physiologic. It is admittedly difficult for the patient, parents, and medical staff to avoid an emotional response toward the restraint of a patient against his or her will. It is therefore important for the medical staff to understand the risks and benefits of performing the procedure, and to communicate this information to the patient, parents, and each other. In addition, all alternative methods of achieving the medical goals should be explored before restraining the patient.

Of general emergency departments, 13% report physically injuring patients during restraint procedures (2). The most serious physical injury that can occur involves respiratory compromise from poor airway positioning.

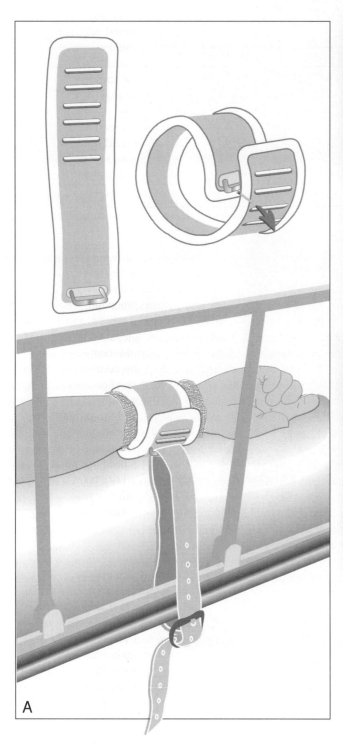

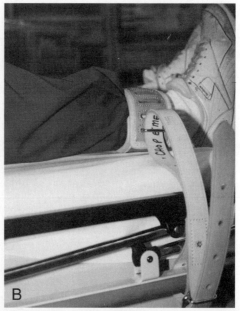

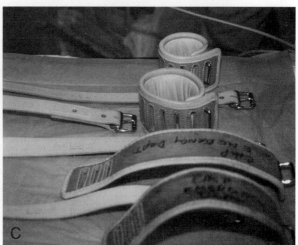

Figure 3.4.
A. Leather restraints are first fastened to distal extremity, then tied down.
B. Restraints should be snug enough to hold down extremity, without causing neuroavscular compromise.
C. A set of leather restraints.

Table 3.4.
Medications Used During Restraint Procedures

Drug Class	Examples	Dose/Route*	Indications	Side Effects
Anxiolytics	Diazepam (Valium®) Lorazepam (Ativan®) Midazolam (Versed®)	0.05–0.1 mg/kg or 1–2 mg IV/IM q1–4 hr 0.05–0.1 mg/kg IV 0.2–0.4 mg/kg IN***	Ethanol withdrawal Drug intoxication/withdrawal** Anger/aggression	Sedation Respiratory depression
Neuroleptics High potency	Haloperidol (Haldol®)	0.1 mg/kg or 5–10 mg IM, PO q 30–60 min	Hallucinations Delusions Violence	Extrapyramidal symptoms Sedation
Low potency	Chlorpromazine (Thorazine®)	1–2 mg/kg or 100–200 mg q 1hr IM/IV		Sedation α-Adrenergic blockade Anticholinergic

* Dose suggested as mg/kg (for young children) or total mg (for adolescent/young adult). Route as indicated: note diazepam is not well absorbed IM, and many practitioners advocate use of IV haloperidol, though such use is not FDA-approved.
** May need large doses for severe symptoms of acute toxicity due to amphetamine, phencyclidine, cocaine, etc.
*** IN = intranasal (maximum dose 6 mg).

This complication can be minimized by dedicating one member of the restraint team to control and monitor the airway. In addition, noninvasive monitoring by cardiorespiratory monitor or pulse oximeter will supplement the information achieved through physical examination. Cardiopulmonary compromise occurs more often in intoxicated patients, small children, or patients with underlying medical illness.

Neurovascular injury can occur if the restraint materials are placed too tightly around an extremity, or if the patient is struggling violently against the restraints. Frequent monitoring of the general appearance, pulses, capillary refill, the range of motion of restrained extremities can prevent permanent injury. In addition, one should use only the force necessary to immobilize a patient quickly. As mentioned previously, this force may be reduced by the judicious use of anxiolytic or neuroleptic medications.

Legal complications of restraint procedures may be avoided or lessened by following the consent methods as delineated in this chapter, and documenting the thought processes and techniques used from beginning to end.

SUMMARY

The restraint of patients for procedures or protection is, unfortunately, at times a necessary part of providing the best care for our patients and families. One must, however, determine beforehand the indications, equipment, techniques, and personnel that will be used for restraint procedures in any given clinical setting. A stepwise approach toward the violent or uncooperative patient is useful, beginning with verbal intervention and progressing to physical restraint and chemical adjuncts if necessary. Careful monitoring and documentation is paramount in these situations and can be facilitated by preprinted forms. The proper technique for patient restraint involves a multidisciplinary approach, which may involve medical, security, and law enforcement personnel. In order to provide safe and effective care, all individuals involved should be aware of the psychological, physiologic, and legal issues surrounding restraint procedures.

REFERENCES

1. Rice MM, Moore GP. Management of the violent patient: therapeutic and legal considerations. Emerg Med Clin North Am 1991;9(1): 13–30.
2. Lavoie FW, Carter GL, Danzl DE, et al. Emergency department violence in United States teaching hospitals. Ann Emerg Med 1988; 17(11):143–138.
3. Neinstein LS, Scott DI. Hallucinogens. In: Adolescent health care: a practical guide. 2nd ed., Baltimore: Urban & Schwarzenberg, 1991.
4. George JE, Quattrone MS. Law and the emergency nurse: restraining patients: can you be sued? Part II. J Emerg Nurs 1993:19:57.

SUMMARY
1. Assess potential for danger to patient or emergency department staff.
2. Use verbal intervention first.
3. Papoose for younger children, five-point restraint for others.
4. Form a standard restraint team with specific roles.
5. Chemical restraint when indicated and safe.
6. Monitor frequently: cardiopulmonary, neurovascular, and mental status.
7. Remove as soon as patient proves to be in control.
8. Document decisions, times, and monitoring.

EVALUATION OF VITAL SIGNS

Jefrey Biehler and Brent Barnes

INTRODUCTION

Initial physical assessment of emergency department (ED) patients includes evaluation of the vital signs. The systematic evaluation of respiratory status, heart rate, systemic blood pressure, and body temperature, as well as peripheral capillary refill, contributes to a rapid estimation of the severity of illness. Intermittent, repeat determination of vital signs allows medical care providers to evaluate the patient's ongoing status and responses to therapy. Continuous monitoring of certain parameters is also frequently employed, and the use of electronic devices for this purpose is discussed in Chapter 5. Because the physiology and procedural aspects of blood pressure and tympanic thermometry monitoring are detailed there, these topics are only briefly alluded to in this chapter. The measurement and assessment of vital signs in children may present special problems given the wide range of sizes and physiologic development spanning the pediatric age range.

ANATOMY AND PATHOPHYSIOLOGY

Consideration of several patient factors is important in the measurement and evaluation of pediatric vital signs. Factors such as patient's emotional status, age, weight, and methods used in obtaining measurements play an important role in the proper interpretation of pediatric vital signs. Anxiety, anger, and pain may each influence the measurement of vital signs. The interpretation of measured vital signs must include consideration of these influences. Large variations in normal values exist among the age groups of pediatric patients. Emergency physicians who do not frequently administer care to children should have references providing pediatric normal values immediately available for review. Failure to recognize the importance of patient age in the interpretation of vital signs may result in the erroneous assumption that a critical condition exists. The misinterpretation of normal vital signs as abnormal may result in unnecessary or perhaps even dangerous medical intervention.

INDICATION

The measurement of vital signs may be used to provide an initial insight into the severity of patient illness. In apparently ill patients these measurements may reflect alterations in physiologic status. These measurements help the physician estimate the seriousness of current illness and assist in determining the need for various forms of medical intervention. Vital sign determination in the apparently well patient may also serve as a screening tool, occasionally identifying patients with unsuspected pathologic conditions.

The most serious problem encountered in any medical setting is a patient with cardiac arrest. Unlike adult patients, cardiac arrests among children are rarely the result of sudden cardiac dysrhythmia or infarction. Cardiac arrests occurring in pediatric patients are more likely the result of a compromised airway or failure of pulmonary ventilation. Recognition of the early signs of cardiorespiratory compromise allows for therapeutic intervention and possible prevention of further clinical deterioration. The propensity of pediatric patients to suffer from respiratory compromise requires that physicians approach ill children with a systematic schema of evaluating physical findings and vital signs. One system, currently advocated in the American Heart Association's Pediatric Advanced Life Support course (1), utilizes the "ABC" mnemonic approach. This system emphasizes the early recognition of airway (**A**) related problems, determination of the adequacy of breathing (**B**), and the status of patient circulation (**C**). This chapter will use a similar approach in the determination and interpretation of pediatric vital signs.

COMPLICATIONS

Although vital signs are an important component of the initial ED evaluation, medical staff should not permit the precise measurement of vital signs to delay the establishment of an unobstructed airway or adequate respirations. The temptation to measure patient vital signs at the expense of necessary emergency interventions can have disastrous consequences. A rapid survey of the ABCs and interventions necessary to correct any problems should always take precedence over detailed measurement of routine vital signs.

PROCEDURES

Vital Impression

Evaluation of a patient begins with a general assessment. This rapid survey or vital impression includes an assessment of airway patency, appraisal of the adequacy of respirations, quality of cry, skin color, and a general visual assessment of the degree of patient illness. Level of consciousness, eye contact and visual tracking (especially in the young infant), and age-appropriate interactiveness all contribute to this global assessment. This vital impression is helpful as a rapid first screen in determining the need for emergency interventions.

Respiration

After establishing the patency of the airway, ensuring the adequacy of ventilation must take priority over all other medical interventions. The evaluation of respirations should include the rate, effectiveness, pattern of breathing, and work of breathing. A patient's respiratory rate is the number of breaths taken in 1 minute. The effectiveness of respiration is clinically estimated by determining the adequacy of air movement, the presence or absence of cyanosis, and any changes in patient mental status.

Equipment and Procedure
Respiratory rates are routinely measured and recorded during the course of most ED evaluations. Respiratory rates should be measured while the patient is relaxed (asleep, if possible, in infants) and breathing at a rate unaffected by the process of evaluation. Attempts to calm or distract anxious or uncooperative patients may result in measured rates more accurately reflecting the patient's true clinical status. Respiratory rates may be measured directly by auscultation of breath sounds during a measured length of time. In the young or uncooperative patient, respiratory rate may sometimes be determined more accurately by simply counting chest or abdominal movements over a determined period. The accuracy of respiratory rates improves when the period of time for determination is lengthened. Counting respirations for 1 minute helps to ensure accurate results. Respiratory rates may also be determined by respiratory inductive plethysmography. By measuring changes in thoracic impedance between two cardiac chest leads, the number of chest wall movements over a set time can be determined.

However, one must not rely on electronic measurement of respirations as the sole method in determining the respiratory rate of patients. Electronic measurement of chest wall movements may not accurately correlate with the number of effective respirations. Electronic measurement of respiratory rates may further be erroneously influenced by voluntary or involuntary patient movements, precordial cardiac activity, improper application/standardization of equipment, or equipment failure. Chest wall movement does not ensure the presence of an unobstructed airway or the adequacy of air exchange. Emergency department personnel should not rely solely on electronic monitors for the ongoing observation of severely ill children (see also Chapter 5). Failing to detect the presence of a respiratory emergency because of electronic monitor malfunction may have serious medical and legal ramifications.

Interpretation

The interpretation of respiratory rates among children requires consideration of patient age and emotional status at the time of measurement (Table 4.1). Normal resting respiratory rates vary between pediatric age groups (2). Respiratory rates of patients who are emotionally upset, in pain, or feel threatened by the interventions of medical personnel should be interpreted in the context of these stresses. Fever will elevate respiratory rate. The respiratory rate taken in a crying child does not accurately reflect the child's respiratory status. The ED record should reflect the presence of factors that may affect the measurement of respiratory rates.

Aberrant respiratory rates or patterns may be the result of abnormalities in the patient's airway, pulmonary ventilation, oxygen exchange, acid-base status, central nervous system abnormalities due to metabolic or toxicologic derangement, various brain or spinal cord lesions, seizures, patient emotional status, or patient cooperation.

Heart Rate

As with respiratory rates, the measurement and interpretation of heart rate in pediatric patients requires that clinicians consider patient age, clinical condition, and emotional state. Clinical evaluation of heart rate may also provide the first indication of cardiac rhythm disturbances.

Equipment and Procedure

Heart rate may be determined by several different methods. Palpation of pulses, auscultation of heart sounds, observation or palpation of apical chest wall movement, and electronic ECG monitors may be used to determine heart rates and the regularity of rhythm. The latter technique is detailed in Chapter 5. Palpation of pulses provides additional informa-

tion concerning pulse volume, and has a time-honored mystique which may confer some significant advantages in older children, adolescent, and adult patients (3). If possible, the patient's heart rate should be determined while the patient is relaxed and unaffected by the process of evaluation, though this is typically difficult in the ED setting. Counting the number of heart beats over a defined period determines the beats per minute heart rate. It has been found that counting the beats for 1 minute helps to ensure accurate results. Measuring the rate for shorter periods of time may increase the chances of erroneous results and misguided clinical intervention.

Interpretation

Interpretation of heart rate and rhythm, like that of respiratory rate, depends on numerous physiologic and pathologic variables. Age-appropriate heart rates are listed in Table 4.2. Assuming an accurate measurement in a resting state, a heart rate significantly elevated for age may reflect numerous conditions including fever, hyperthyroidism, hypovolemia, hypoxia, hypoglycemia, acidosis, anemia, decreased cardiac function, tachyarrhythmia, vasodilatation, increased sympathomimetic activity via any of a variety of exogenous or endogenous causes, or anticholinergic agents. Bradycardia may be seen with increased intracranial pressure, hypothermia, hypothyroidism, bradyarrhythmia, excess vagal tone, as a response to hypoxia (early in newborns, later in older infants and children), and with several drugs, particularly digoxin, β-blockers, and calcium channel blockers.

Pulse volume may be increased in patent ductus arteriosus, aortic insufficiency, hyperthyroidism, fever, and anemia. Decreased pulse volume is noted in shock and aortic stenosis.

The approach to diagnosis of an irregular pulse is beyond the scope of this chapter, and has been summarized elsewhere (4). However, a common cause of concern to the physician less experienced with children is the observation of sinus arrhythmia. In this physiologic rhythm the pulse rate increases with inspiration and decreases during expiration. Young children may have very impressive sinus arrhythmia, with the heart seeming to pause perceptibly after a deep breath. If the

Table 4.1.*
Age-Adjusted Respiratory Rates

Term infant	30–50
1 to 6 months	20–40
6 months to 2 years	20–30
2 to 12 years	16–24
Adolescent	12–20

* Adapted from Silverman B, 1993.

Table 4.2.*
Age-Adjusted Heart Rates

Age	Heart Rate (per minute)
Neonate	80–180
1 week to 1 month	80–160
3 months to 2 years	80–150
2 to 10 years	75–110
10 years to adult	50–100

* Adapted from Silverman B, 1993.

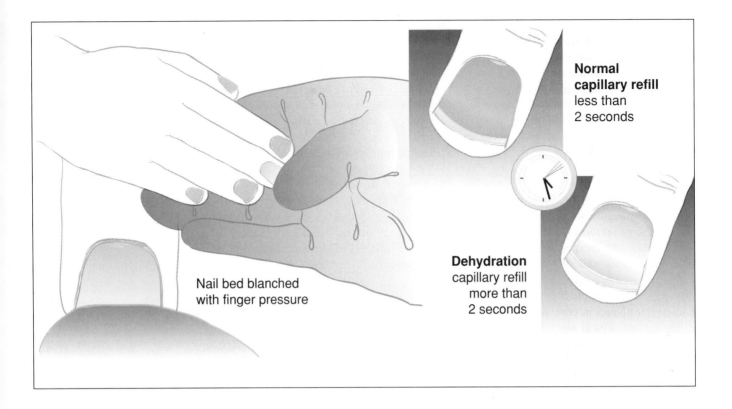

Normal capillary refill less than 2 seconds

Dehydration capillary refill more than 2 seconds

Nail bed blanched with finger pressure

Figure 4.1.
The assessment of capillary refill time at the fingernail bed.

relation to respiration is not easily apparent clinically, and convincing, a quick electrocardiographic rhythm strip will establish the diagnosis.

Capillary Refill

The measurement of capillary refill time as an indicator of the adequacy of peripheral perfusion, although not classically included in the vital signs, per se, is a useful tool in the initial assessment of all ill children. Changes in capillary refill time may reflect decreased vascular volume or alteration in systemic vascular resistance and vascular shunting. The capillary refill time is considered by many to be the earliest measurable clinical indicator of inadequate peripheral circulation (5, 6).

Procedure
The determination of capillary refill time is simple, reliable, and takes only a few seconds. Capillary refill time is best determined by gently pressing the fingernail bed. The time required for the blanched nailbed to return to the normal color is determined (Fig. 4.1). When utilizing capillary refill time to

measure the response to medical therapy it is recommended that serial determinations are measured at the same anatomic location.

Interpretation
Normal capillary refill time for the pediatric patient is usually considered to be less than 2.0 seconds. The upper limit of normal for capillary refill time is slightly higher in adults. Schriger reported an upper limit of normal for adult men of 2.0 seconds and 2.9 seconds for women (5). Skin temperature also plays a role in determining capillary refill time. Capillary refill time may vary significantly with changes in skin temperature, including changes due to a cool environment such as that encountered in an air-conditioned ED (7).

A delay in capillary refill of greater than 2.0 to 3.0 seconds may reflect inadequacy of peripheral perfusion. Saavedra reported a correlation between the degree of dehydration in pediatric patients and prolongation of capillary refill time (6). In patients admitted to the hospital for diarrhea, a refill time of 1.5 to 3.0 seconds suggested a fluid deficit of greater than 100 mL/kg.

Other conditions that may result in a prolongation of capillary refill time include heart failure, hypothermia, electrolyte abnormalities, hypotension resulting from any clinical condition, and conditions resulting in alterations of circulatory regulation.

Blood Pressure

Routine measurement of blood pressure is occasionally omitted in pediatric patients attending EDs, which is most likely a consequence of inexperience and impatience, and often a lack of appropriate equipment. However, the blood pressure is a valuable adjunct in pediatric assessment, as it is at any age. Although hypotension is usually heralded by obvious changes in sensorium, heart rate, pulse volume, skin color, and capillary refill, mild to moderate hypertension may be more occult and yet be an important early warning of serious systemic (especially renal) disease.

Several types of instruments to measure blood pressure are available, including mercury or aneroid sphygmomanometers using stethoscope- or ultrasound-based (Doppler) determinations of blood flow, and oscillometric-based instruments such as the Dinamap. Chapter 5 (pp. 34–36) discusses the latter in some detail, with an overview of the physiologic basis of blood pressure measurement in general, and proper Dinamap technique in particular. The primary emphasis here is that cuff size is of crucial importance to all forms of blood pressure determination. Whereas most authors focus on cuff width in relation to arm length (e.g., the former should be at least two-thirds of the latter), it is probably more accurate, especially in obese

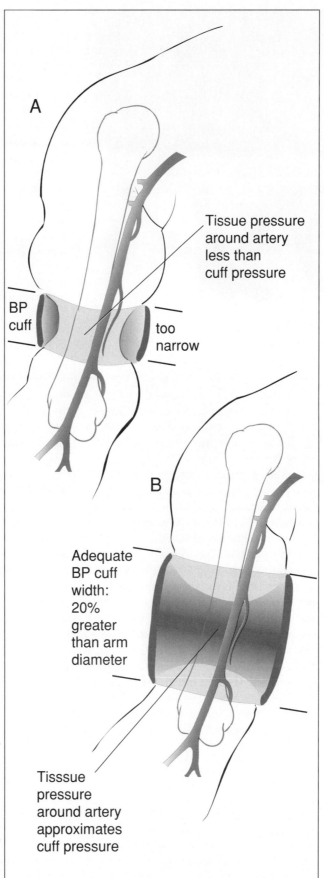

A.

Tissue pressure around artery less than cuff pressure

BP cuff

too narrow

B.

Adequate BP cuff width: 20% greater than arm diameter

Tisssue pressure around artery approximates cuff pressure

Figure 4.2.
A. Cuff pressure is transmitted through the arm in a diminishing band.
B. An appropriate cuff width in relation to arm diameter is necessary for adequate transmission of cuff pressure to tissue pressure surrounding the brachial artery, and thus accurate blood pressure measurement. (Adapted from Park et al., 1976, and Kirkendall WM et al., Circulation 1967;36:980.)

Chapter 4
Evaluation of Vital
Signs

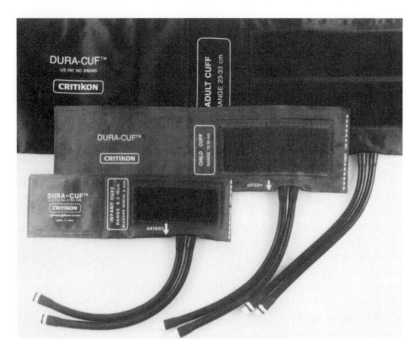

Figure 4.3.
The pediatric ED should stock several different cuff sizes.

patients, to relate cuff width to arm *diameter* (8). Park and colleagues have shown that a cuff width 20% greater than arm diameter, which allows proper transmission of cuff bladder pressure to the level of the brachial artery in most patients, will accurately measure a blood pressure that correlates closely with pressure measured from an intraarterial catheter (Fig. 4.2). Cuff widths significantly narrower (e.g., less than 10% wider than arm diameter) will falsely elevate measured pressure by a range of 10 to 15 mm Hg, and cuffs too large (e.g., 30 to 45% wider than arm diameter), will falsely lower pressure 3 to 6 mm Hg. The cuff length is also a consideration, and most authors favor a cuff length that completely encircles the arm. The ED should have cuffs in widths of 3, 5, 8, 12, and 18 cm for all sizes of pediatric patients (Fig. 4.3). If the proper sized cuff is not available, folding down a larger cuff will suffice. When choice is very limited, a cuff larger than optimal is probably preferable, because the discrepancy with overly wide cuffs is less than with those that are too narrow.

Procedure

The patient should be relatively calm, in a supine position or with arm held at level of the heart (Fig. 4.4). The proper sized cuff is wrapped snugly around the patient's arm (or leg), and the cuff inflated. It is often recom-

mended to first estimate systolic pressure by palpation of the distal pulse. The cuff is reinflated to 10 to 20 mm Hg above the point of pulse disappearance, and then deflated slowly, no more than 2 to 4 mm Hg per second. Auscultation of the first Korotkoff sound indicates systolic pressure; muffling of sounds indicates diastolic pressure, although in some children distinct onset of muffling is difficult to ascertain and disappearance of sounds is accepted as the diastolic pressure. In busy and noisy EDs, the Dinamap approach is favored for accuracy of measurement, and because when left in place the anxious child is more likely to become relaxed without the nurse's or physician's close proximity.

Interpretation

Numerous pathophysiologic states alter blood pressure. Hypotension is classically associated with hypovolemia, cardiac (pump) failure, or profound vasodilatation from any of innumerable causes. Hypovolemia in children is most commonly secondary to dehydration from gastroenteritis, but of course may be secondary to traumatic blood loss, plasma deficit as occurs in burns, and other fluid losses as might occur in adrenal insufficiency or diabetic ketoacidosis. Distributive shock (vasodilatation) is most frequently caused by sepsis in the pediatric population; other causes include anaphylaxis, drug overdoses, and spinal injury. Cardiogenic shock in children may be due to congenital cardiac defects, particularly those such as hypoplastic left heart syndrome that are dependent on a patent ductus for systemic circulation, and which present in fulminant heart failure when the ductus closes. Other causes of cardiogenic shock in children include viral myocarditis, certain drug overdoses, and dysrhythmias.

Hypertension is being increasingly recognized as a pediatric problem. Generally a blood pressure above the 95th percentile for age is considered to be hypertensive, and pressures greater than the 99th percentile represent severe hypertension. Common pediatric causes include renal parenchymal and renovascular disease and aortic coarctation in infancy and early childhood, and essential hypertension, renal and renovascular disorders in school-age and adolescent children. Age-appropriate blood pressures are summarized in Table 4.3. A good rule of thumb to approximate the 50th percentile systolic pressures by age, in mm Hg, is: neonate = 70; infant to 1 year = 80; > 2 years = 90+ (2 × age in years) (1).

Temperature

The measurement of body temperature is an essential vital sign assessment. Alterations of body temperature, including hyperthermia and hypothermia, can be an indication of benign or potentially life-threatening pathologic processes. Though changes in body temperature are most often the result of infection, other etiologies should be considered. Intoxication, malignancies, collagen vascular disease, thyroid disorders, nutritional insufficiency, and exposure to environmental temperature extremes are all important causes of changes in body temperature.

The evaluation of body temperature in the pediatric population is a common task facing health care providers. Indeed, febrile illnesses in children account for over 20% of ED visits. Inaccurate measurement of body temperature can result in serious errors in diagnosis and treatment.

The ideal thermometer should be easy to use, accurately reflect core body temperature, minimize the spread of contagious diseases, provide rapid results, and cause no patient discomfort or embarrassment. At present, a number of body sites and thermometer types are utilized to measure body temperature. These include oral, axillary, rectal, and tympanic membrane sites, and the use of glass mercury and electronic digital thermometers, tympanic membrane digital thermometers, esophageal and bladder probes, and pulmonary artery catheter probes. Recent attempts to measure temperature noninvasively have included temperature-sensitive pacifiers and forehead strips, but these have not been found reliable in young children. Obviously, not all of these methods are convenient for the ambulatory setting, and none fit the aforementioned definition of an ideal thermometer. Presently, the most popular methods of measuring body temperature in the ED include oral, rectal, axillary, and tympanic membrane sites with glass mercury or electronic devices. An understanding of the proper use and limitations of each method of

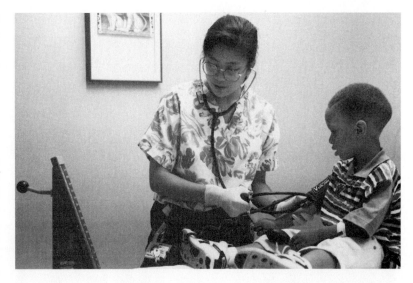

measuring body temperature is important in preventing errors in diagnosis.

Oral Temperature Measurements

Oral temperatures are commonly used in older children and adolescents. Oral temperatures are obtained easily and quickly by glass mercury or electronic thermometers. Inaccuracies may result from recent ingestion of hot or cold oral liquids, respiratory distress or tachypnea, and an inability to cooperate. Patients with these conditions should have their temperature measured by another method.

The measurement of oral temperature with a glass mercury thermometer should begin with ensuring the thermometer has been adequately cleaned and sterilized before use. The mercury level should be well below normal body temperature (accomplished by shaking down the thermometer) and then placed under the tongue, slightly off midline in the sublingual pocket. The child's mouth should then be closed. Temperature can be read after 2 to 3 minutes. Oral electronic thermometers should be calibrated regularly (usually on a weekly or monthly basis) and the disposable plastic probe should be changed between use to minimize the spread of disease. The probe is placed under the tongue, and measurement is completed within a few seconds with an audible tone indicating equilibration with body temperature.

Axillary Temperature Measurement

Axillary temperatures are commonly used in infants, especially in the first month of life.

Figure 4.4.
The blood pressure is taken with the arm held at the level of the heart with a (hopefully) relaxed and cooperative child.

Table 4.3.*
Age-Adjusted Blood Pressure

Age	Pressure (systolic/diastolic in mm Hg)	
Neonate	Range 40–80/20–55	
	Percentile	
	50th	95th
2 years	96/60	112/78
6 years	98/64	116/80
9 years	106/68	126/84
12 years	114/74	136/88

* Adapted from Silverman B, 1993.

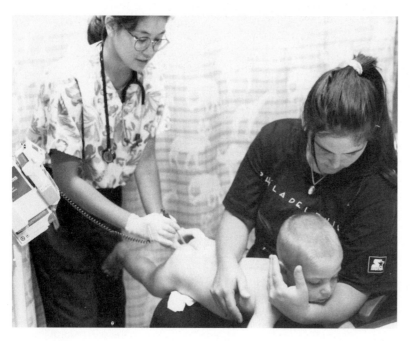

and the temperature read after 2 to 3 minutes. Obtaining axillary temperatures by electronic thermometers is done easily and quickly. Again, the digital thermometer should be calibrated regularly, and the probe placed in the axillary region. Temperature will reach equilibrium and can be read in a few seconds.

Rectal Temperature Measurement

Rectal temperature has long been considered the gold standard of temperature measurement. It has generally been the temperature measurement of choice in studies involving correlations between bacteremia and temperature in infants and young children. Despite the fact that rectal temperature has been the standard of temperature measurement, recent studies have indicated that rectal temperature may lag behind and poorly reflect rapid changes in body temperature (9, 10). It has been found that rectal temperature is slow to reflect changes in body temperature due to vascular insulation from the relatively poor blood flow to the rectum (11). Rectal temperatures are easily obtained, but the procedure is uncomfortable and brings about patient embarrassment in older children. Therefore rectal temperature is most commonly used in infants. Rectal temperatures are considered contraindicated in patients with recent rectal surgery or neutropenia.

Rectal temperatures can be obtained via glass or digital thermometers. With the patient in a supine, prone, or on-the-side position and the hips flexed, the glass thermometer should be placed 2 to 3 centimeters into the rectal vault, with the nurse or parent securing the infant (Fig. 4.5). The temperature may be read in 2 to 3 minutes. With a digital thermometer, the rectal probe should be similarly inserted into the rectum and temperature equilibration will be reached within a few seconds. In either case, care should be taken so the thermometer is not placed directly into a mass of fecal matter, which may falsely lower the temperature reading.

Figure 4.5.
The rectal temperature being taken with the infant secured on mother's lap in the prone position, with hips flexed.

Figure 4.6.
Using the tympanic thermometer. (Photograph courtesy of Thermoscan, Inc., San Diego, CA)

This method of temperature measurement is done quickly and easily in patients unable to cooperate. Though axillary temperature correlates fairly well with rectal temperature, axillary temperature is easily affected by skin perfusion and environmental temperature variations and by bundling of an infant. Obtaining an axillary temperature with a mercury glass thermometer is similar to obtaining a temperature orally. The thermometer should be placed snugly in the axillary region

Tympanic Temperature Measurement

The first tympanic membrane thermometers used thermistor probes in direct contact with the eardrum, but this method was painful and not practical. Recently, tympanic membrane thermometers have been developed that use an infrared sensor probe oriented toward, but

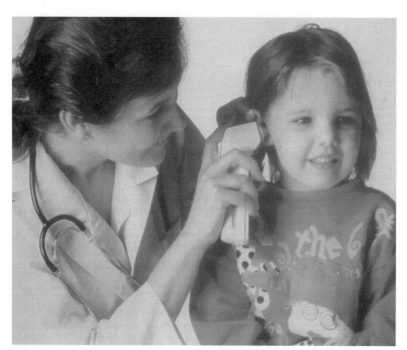

not in contact with, the membrane, which senses the temperature of the tympanic membrane (Fig. 4.6). These thermometers have become widely used because temperature can be taken within seconds without removal of clothing or concern about recent oral fluids, mouth breathing, or tachypnea. Though the initial tympanic membrane thermometers were shown to lack sensitivity in comparison to rectal thermometers, recent advancements in the development of the tympanic thermometer have led to measurements that are quite accurate in comparison with the traditional oral and rectal methods. Theoretically, the tympanic membrane thermometer most closely parallels the true core body temperature, as the hypothalamus and the tympanic membrane both receive their blood supply from the internal carotid artery. As an electronic device used to monitor temperature, the discussion of tympanic thermometry is detailed further in Chapter 5 (p. 36).

Interpretation

Fever is an elevation of body temperature in response to a pathologic stimulus. It is difficult to ascertain the least elevation of temperature which is abnormal for all children under all circumstances. Temperature varies with environment, clothing, activity, digestion, and diurnal rhythms (12). Most children have a peak temperature in early evening, between 5:00 PM and 7:00 PM. For a child at rest who has been appropriately dressed for the ambient temperature, we define fever as a rectal or tympanic temperature of 38° C (100.4° F). Oral temperatures are usually 0.6° C (1.0° F), and axillary temperatures 1.1° C (2° F) lower than rectal, respectively. The evaluation of febrile children in regard to the diagnosis of infectious diseases is a complex issue and will not be detailed here. Briefly, several factors play an important role in the evaluation of fever, including the age of the patient, overall clinical appearance, host defense status, evidence of focal infection on clinical evaluation, and degree of temperature elevation beyond normal (12). Infants under 8 to 12 weeks of age may have serious infections with normal or low grade temperatures. In children 3 to 36 months of age, the likelihood of severe illness and bacteremia increases with the degree of temperature elevation.

Fever can also be a prominent symptom in many important noninfectious processes. Malignancies, collagen vascular disease, endocrinologic abnormalities, drug intoxications, and environmental exposure are examples of these processes.

Hypothermia, defined as a temperature of less than 35° C, is also an important sign of disease. In infants less than 8 weeks old and in immunocompromised patients, hypothermia can be the result of overwhelming sepsis and warrants aggressive investigation. Other causes of hypothermia include endocrinologic failure, nutritional insufficiency, erythrodermas, and environmental exposure. Hypothermia is also frequently seen in major resuscitations, especially trauma victims. Patients suffering severe trauma often have prolonged cold exposure and aggressive fluid and blood replacement which can lead to hypothermia if fluids and blood are not warmed. Hypothermia in trauma victims may lead to profound coagulopathy and poor outcome. Hypothermia is particularly compelling in small infants undergoing resuscitation from any cause, and must be carefully guarded against. The appropriately equipped ED should have access to delivery room type overhead warmers, heated bedding, and/or blankets as necessary for pediatric resuscitations.

SUMMARY
1. Careful evaluation of vital signs is crucial to every emergency department encounter.
2. Pediatric vital signs include rapid global assessment and capillary refill time as well as heart rate, respiratory rate, blood pressure, and temperature.
3. Heart rate, respiratory rate, and blood pressure vary considerably by age and by the child's anxiety level, so therefore the most accurate reflection of physiologic status is gained in the calm, resting child.
4. Capillary refill is an excellent pediatric technique to estimate intravascular volume status.
5. Appropriate blood pressure cuff size is critical to an accurate determination.
6. Tympanic temperature measurement is quick, accurate, and relatively noninvasive for the child over 3 months of age.

REFERENCES

1. American Heart Association. Textbook of pediatric advanced life support, 1988.
2. Silverman BK. Practical information. In: Fleisher GR, Ludwig S, eds. Textbook of pediatric emergency medicine. 3rd ed. Baltimore: Williams & Wilkins, 1993.
3. Athreya B, Silverman BK. Pediatric physical diagnosis, East Norwalk, CT: Appleton-Century-Crofts, 1985.
4. Gewitz MH, Vetter VL. Cardiac emergencies. In: Fleisher GR, Ludwig S, eds. Textbook of pediatric emergency medicine. 3rd ed. Baltimore: Williams & Wilkins, 1993.
5. Schriger DL, Baraff LJ. Defining normal capillary refill: variation with age, sex and temperature. Ann Emerg Med 1988;17:932–935.
6. Saavedra JM, Harris GD, Li S, Finberg L. Capillary filling (skin turgor) in the assessment of dehydration. Am J Dis Child 1991; 145:296–298.
7. Gorelick MH, Shaw KN, Baker MD. Effect of ambient temperature on capillary refill in healthy children. Pediatrics 1993;62: 699–702.

8. Park MK, Kawabori I, Guntheroth WG. Need for an improved standard for blood pressure cuff size. Clin Pediatr 1976;15:784–787.

9. Terndrup T, Milewski A. The performance of two tympanic thermometers in a pediatric emergency department. Clin Pediatr 1991: (Suppl):18–22.

10. Brennan D, Falk J, et al. Reliability of infrared tympanic thermometry in the detection of rectal fever in children. Ann Emerg Med 1995;25:21–29.

11. Chamberlain J, Grandner J, et al. Comparison of a tympanic thermometer to rectal and oral thermometers in a pediatric emergency department. Clin Pediatr 1991; (Suppl): 24–28.

12. Henretig FM. Fever. In: Fleisher GR, Ludwig S, eds. Textbook of pediatric emergency medicine. 3rd ed. Baltimore: Williams & Wilkins, 1993.

CHAPTER 5

USE OF MONITORING DEVICES

Jacalyn S. Maller, and Marc H. Gorelick

INTRODUCTION

Monitoring is the process of observing the clinical condition of a patient, typically by repeated measurement of vital signs. Although such monitoring may be done by human observers, the task is frequently performed by automated devices. In this section, methods and equipment for several of the most commonly monitored parameters in pediatric emergency medicine—heart rate and rhythm, blood pressure, and temperature—are discussed. First, pulse oximetry is mentioned briefly here, since it is the subject of a separate chapter (Chapter 77).

PULSE OXIMETRY

The use of pulse oximetry, a noninvasive method of measuring the oxygen saturation of blood, has expanded rapidly since its introduction into clinical practice in the early 1980s. The pulse oximeter uses the differential light absorption spectra of various hemoglobin species to measure transcutaneously the relative amount of oxygenated hemoglobin in arterial blood. Because of its ease of use, painlessness, and availability of appropriate sized equipment, pulse oximetry is particularly suited to use in pediatrics.

Indications for pulse oximetry include screening for the presence or development of hypoxemia, as well as continuous monitoring to measure response to therapy. It is commonly used in the assessment of children with acute respiratory illness such as pneu-

monia, asthma, or upper airway obstruction. It is also recommended in monitoring patients undergoing conscious sedation (2). The anatomy, physiology, and technology underlying pulse oximetry are detailed in Chapter 77, as well as a discussion of proper technique and interpretation of findings.

ELECTROCARDIOGRAPHIC MONITORING

Physiology

Electrocardiographic (ECG) monitors measure and display heart rate and rhythm by detecting the electrical activity of cardiac muscle. The device consists of a sensing component, the electrode, which when placed on the skin surface can detect changes in electrical potential (i.e., depolarization and repolarization) originating in the heart. Two electrodes comprising a lead are required to detect cardiac activity by measuring the difference in electrical potential between two sites. Standard limb leads are placed on the left arm, right arm, and left leg. A right leg electrode serves as a ground. Each lead detects a different view of the heart and when viewed as a whole gives a complete picture of cardiac activity. A 12-lead ECG involves both limb and chest leads, placed in a standard configuration, and allows a look at the activity of a specific lead. Routine monitoring in the ED usually involves only three electrodes, placed at the base and apex of the heart with a reference electrode at the upper

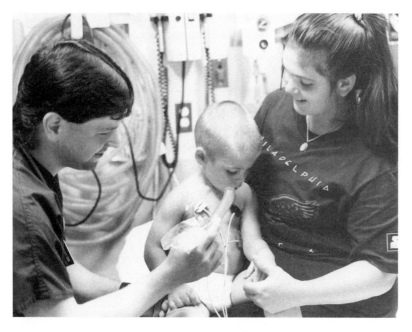

movement, involuntary shivering, seizure activity, or interference by nearby electronic devices can produce artifact. Good contact must occur between the skin and the electrode to produce an accurate tracing. The machine must be standardized so a given voltage of activity produces a consistent deflection and both patient and machine should be properly grounded.

As with all monitoring devices, the ECG must not replace frequent clinical assessment of the patient. The results of the ECG can be normal with organic heart disease or abnormal in a healthy individual. As with any laboratory test, ECG findings must be interpreted in conjunction with the clinical status of the patient.

BLOOD PRESSURE

Monitoring of blood pressure in the emergency department is used as a screen to (*a*) assess the level of cardiovascular stability for patient triage, (*b*) follow clinical response or adverse reactions to therapy, and (*c*) follow clinical course in a potentially unstable condition. In the majority of cases this can be done noninvasively with a blood pressure cuff and stethoscope, or with an automated oscillometric device such as the Dinamap. Invasive blood pressure monitoring is reserved for those critically ill patients requiring intensive care unit admission, multiple repeated measurements of arterial blood gases, and continuous monitoring.

Physiology

The principle of noninvasive blood pressure monitoring involves the use of a compression cuff applied to the limb and inflated with air to a pressure above systolic blood pressure, thereby terminating distal flow. Blood pressure is determined by detecting the pressure at which blood flow resumes as the cuff is deflated. Auscultatory methods include using a stethoscope to detect Korotkoff's sounds, which is the result of turbulent blood flow as cuff pressure falls below arterial systolic pressure. The first sound auscultated approximates systolic blood pressure. Diastolic blood pressure is the pressure at which muffling of sounds occurs. If auscultation is dif-

Figure 5.1.
Electrocardiograph monitoring leads are placed at the three usual sites: base and apex of the heart, and upper left chest.

left chest wall to reduce electrical interference (3).

Electrical potentials detected by the leads require amplification to detect the low voltage signal. The amplifier also has a filtration system to reduce electrical "noise." Cardiac activity can be displayed continuously on an oscilloscope and/or recorded on ECG graph paper as a plot of voltage versus time. Most monitors also have the capacity to freeze and record a tracing in the last few seconds before an abnormality activates the monitor alarm (4). Monitor alarms, both auditory and visual, indicate equipment problems including loose or defective electrodes, heart rate parameters which have exceeded the programmed limits, or abnormal cardiac rhythms.

Procedure

Intended electrode sites are cleansed with alcohol. Conductive gel is used at each area of contact between the electrode surface and skin to stabilize the electrode. Most disposable electrodes are pre-gelled. The electrode and lead wire should be firmly applied to dry skin. As previously noted, for routine continuous ED monitoring, three thoracic sites (base and apex of the heart, and upper left chest) are usually chosen (Fig. 5.1).

Potential sources of difficulty can be patient or equipment related. Any voluntary

ficult because of noise level or a low flow state, the arterial pulse can be palpated as the cuff is deflated or an ultrasonic flow detector can detect when flow resumes. These two latter methods cannot be used to determine diastolic pressures.

An alternative method of blood pressure detection is the oscillometric method utilized in the Dinamap machine. This method is based on the principle that pulsatile blood flow through a blood vessel produces arterial wall oscillations which are transmitted to a blood pressure cuff (5). The machine operates with a pressure transducer and a microcomputer both of which sense cuff pressure, initiate cuff inflation and deflation, control for motion artifact, and record points of changing amplitude of oscillations. At systolic blood pressure, a rapid increase occurs in the amplitude of oscillations. Diastolic pressure is the point at which a sudden decrease occurs in oscillations. The mean arterial pressure is the point at which the amplitude of oscillations reaches a maximum. These three independently measured values are digitally displayed at the completion of each inflation/deflation cycle.

Procedure

Errors in blood pressure measurement can be cuff or patient related (6). The most common error is incorrect cuff size—in particular, a cuff that is too small—which falsely elevates the blood pressure. The cuff should cover two-thirds of the upper arm length, fully encircling the arm with a snug fit. In obese children, a cuff width 20% greater than area diameter will provide a more accurate reading (Fig. 4.2). Rapid deflation rate is another source of measurement error, creating falsely low blood pressure measurements. Cuff deflation rate should be no more than 2 to 3 mm Hg per second. Before cuff application and in between determinations, ensure that all residual air is eliminated.

Patient-related sources of error include having a crying or anxious child and placing the extremity above or below heart level during measurement.

Use of the Dinamap machine begins with placing the proper sized cuff on the selected limb, which in most cases is the upper arm. Other sites including the forearm and ankle

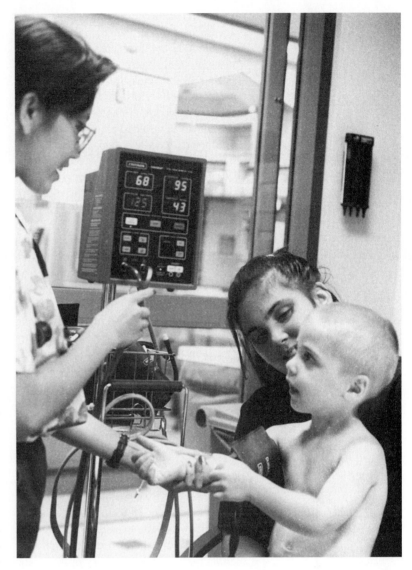

are more comfortable for prolonged periods of monitoring in the conscious patient, but are less helpful when dealing with the patient with shock or peripheral vasoconstriction. Before applying the cuff, all residual air must be squeezed out and the cuff applied snugly, but not so tight as to cause venous congestion. If residual air remains in the cuff or the cuff is not snug, blood pressure readings will be falsely elevated. The cuff and the patient's heart must be at the same level to avoid the effect of hydrostatic pressure on the reading, which is falsely high when the cuff is below the heart and falsely low when the cuff is above the heart. The conscious, cooperative patient must be told to remain quiet and avoid movement (Fig. 5.2).

Problems with noninvasive blood pres-

Chapter 5
Use of Monitoring
Devices

sure monitoring occur with shock and peripheral vasoconstriction. Palpation and auscultatory methods are insensitive in low flow states. The Dinamap is more useful during shock because it measures pressure oscillations instead of sounds. In severe cases only mean arterial pressure may be measurable, if at all, and invasive blood pressure monitoring is warranted. Other situations in which accurate noninvasive monitoring is compromised occur in patients with frequent arrhythmias or on mechanical ventilation, when large variability in systolic blood pressures exists.

Accuracy of the Dinamap is superior to auscultation when compared with an arterial catheter, with a mean error of less than 5 mm Hg (5, 6) and standard deviation of less than 8 mm Hg. Because of its accuracy, lack of interobserver variability, improved patient cooperation, usefulness in a noisy environment, and improved BP detection over auscultatory methods in low flow states, the Dinamap is the method of choice for monitoring blood pressure in the pediatric ED. It is crucial to remember that use of automated devices must not preclude direct clinical examination of the patient.

TYMPANIC THERMOMETRY

Measurement of body temperature is essential in the evaluation of acutely ill children. The traditional method of temperature measurement uses a glass mercury or electronic thermometer at one of several sites: rectal, oral, or axillary. More recently, devices have been developed that measure body temperature by infrared emission detection from the tympanic membrane. These tympanic thermometers are gaining widespread use in pediatrics because of relative ease of operation, greater parent and child acceptability, and concerns about infection control with other types of thermometers.

Physiology

Tympanic thermometers measure infrared emissions from the tympanic membrane, which correlates closely with core body temperature (hypothalamic or pulmonic artery temperature) (7, 8, 9). Because core temperature is lower than rectal temperature, with

which clinicians are most familiar, most ear thermometers use a microprocessor to add an "offset" to the tympanic temperature, yielding a rectal or oral equivalent. The algorithm for this offset is different for each of the six different ear thermometers currently marketed in the United States.

Procedure

To use the tympanic thermometer, a disposable cover is placed over the otoscope-like probe. This probe is then inserted in the auditory canal (Fig. 4.6). Care should be taken to aim the probe at the tympanic membrane for the most accurate results. An ear tug is recommended to straighten the canal as much as possible—posteriorly for infants, and posteriorly and superiorly for older children (10). A reading is available in 1 to 3 seconds. Neither cerumen nor concomitant otitis media has a significant effect on the accuracy of tympanic temperature measurement (11, 12, 13). Extremes of ambient temperature will distort the results, particularly in infants with shallow ear canals (14).

A large number of studies of tympanic thermometry have been performed in adults and children, with varying results (8, 11, 15-19). Much of the discrepancy is the result of differences in technique, choice of different gold standards for comparison, and differences in offsets between devices. Based on current literature, tympanic temperature is not recommended in infants less than 3 months of age. In older children, careful attention to technique as described previously is essential. In addition, because of the use of varying correction offsets, the interpretation of tympanic temperature can be problematic when treatment decisions are based on equivalent rectal temperature. Thus, familiarity with the particular device being used is also helpful.

REFERENCES

1. Alexander CM, Teller LE, Gross JB. Principles of pulse oximetry: theoretical and practical considerations. Anaesth Analg 1989;68: 368–376.
2. Sacchetti A, Schafermeyer R, Gerardi M, et al. Pediatric analgesia sedation. Ann Emerg Med 1994;23(2):237–250.

SUMMARY
1. Electronic monitoring is not a substitute for careful clinical surveillance.
2. All monitoring techniques have both patient- and device-related sources of error.
3. For ECG: minimize motion artifact, ensure good skin-lead contact.
4. For BP: choose correct cuff size, extremity at level of heart, slow deflation, Dinamap more accurate than auscultation in low flow states.
5. For tympanic temperature: aim probe at TM; not recommended for infants under 3 months of age.

Chapter 5
Use of Monitoring
Devices

3. Morriss FC, Mast CP. Electrocardiographic and respiratory monitors. In Levin DL, ed. A practical guide to pediatric intensive care. St. Louis: CV Mosby, 1984, pp. 474–478.
4. Nobel JJ. ECG monitors. Ped Emerg Care 1993;9(1):52.
5. Park MK, Menard SM. Accuracy of blood pressure measurement by the Dinamap monitor in infants and children. Pediatrics 1987;79:907–914.
6. Ramsey M. Knowing your monitoring equipment. Blood pressure monitoring: automated oscillometric devices. J Clin Monit 1991;7:56
7. Nobel JJ. Infrared ear thermometry. Ped Emerg Care 1992;8(1):54–58.
8. Terndrup TE. An appraisal of temperature assessment by infrared emission detection tympanic thermometry. Ann Emerg Med 1992;21(12):1483–1492.
9. Milewski A, Ferguson KL, Terndrup TE. Comparison of pulmonary artery, rectal, and tympanic membrane temperatures in adult intensive care unit patients. Clin Pediatr 1991;30(4):13–16.
10. Pransky SM. The impact of technique and conditions of the tympanic membrane on infrared tympanic thermometry. Clin Pediatr 1991;30(4):50–52.
11. Chamberlain JM, Grandner J, Rubinoff JL, Klein BL, Waisman Y, Huey M. Comparison of a tympanic thermometer to rectal and oral thermometers in a pediatric emergency department. Clin Pediatr 1991;30(4):24–29.
12. Terndrup TE, Wong A. Influence of otitis media on the correlation between rectal and auditory canal temperatures. AJDC 1991;145:75–78.
13. Kelly B, Alexander D. Effect of otitis media on infrared tympanic thermometry. Clin Pediatr 1991;30(4):46–48.
14. Zehner WJ, Terndrup TE. The impact of moderate ambient temperature variance on the relationship between oral, rectal, and tympanic membrane temperatures. Clin Pediatr 1991;30(4):61–64.
15. Talo H, Macknin ML, Medendorp SV. Tympanic membrane temperatures compared with rectal and oral temperatures. Clin Pediatr 1991;30(4):30–33.
16. Terndrup TE, Milewski A. The performance of two tympanic thermometers in a pediatric emergency department. Clin Pediatr 1991;30(4):18–23.
17. Rhoads FA, Grandner J. Assessment of an aural infrared sensor for body temperature measurement in children. Clin Pediatr 1990;29(2):112–115.
18. Muma BK, Treloar DJ, Wurmlinger K, Peterson E, Vitae A. Comparison of rectal, axillary, and tympanic membrane temperatures in infants and young children. Ann Emerg Med 1991;20(1):41–44.
19. Kenney RD, Fortenberry JD, Surratt SS, Ribbeck BM, Thomas WJ. Evaluation of an infrared tympanic membrane thermometer in pediatric patients. Pediatrics 1990;85(5):854–857.

EMERGENT DRUG DOSING AND EQUIPMENT SELECTION

Robert C. Luten

INTRODUCTION

Most procedures performed in the emergency department (ED) do not require rapid selection of drugs and equipment. Although the majority of ED procedures are of an urgent or nonelective nature, the clinician usually has adequate time for measurement of a patient's weight, selection of equipment, and calculation of drug dosages required before performing a procedure. Examples include the suturing of lacerations, reduction of fractures, or suprapubic aspirations.

Some procedures, however, do not afford the clinician this luxury. These procedures must be done immediately. Failure to do so can cause loss of life or limb. There is no time to obtain an accurate weight on a patient. Efforts spent in equipment selection and drug dosage calculation only exacerbate this problem. Anxiety produced when faced with this dilemma, as well as error from inaccurate drug dosage calculation and equipment selection also compound the problem. An example is endotracheal intubation which requires correct sized laryngoscopes, ET tubes, and suction catheters, as well as medications for rapid sequence induction of anesthesia.

The advent of organized, educational, resuscitative efforts for adults, Advanced Cardiac Life Support (ACLS), and children, Pediatric Advanced Life Support (PALS), brought about attempts to solve drug dosage and equipment selection problems as it became clear that this area of resuscitation was fraught with error and delays in the resuscitative process (1).

Drug dosing in children requires several steps:
1. Knowledge of the correct dose
2. Knowledge of a patient's weight, which can only be estimated in emergent situations because weight measurements are impractical (weight estimation by clinicians has been shown to be fraught with error) (2)
3. Error-free calculation
4. Error-free delivery

Equipment selection also frequently depends on estimation of an accurate weight or age.

Other than memory, clinicians' early efforts to solve this problem relied on cards or charts that contained the drug dose. These efforts were also full of error and anxiety because the clinician had to rely on an estimated weight and also because calculations were frequently erroneous—especially 1/10 or 10X the correct dose. The next advance utilized precalculated handbooks, cards, and computer printouts (3). Though an improvement, the clinician still had to rely on estimations of weight and/or age.

Recently, the patient's length has been used to estimate weight (3, 4) and to determine certain equipment sizes. (Table 6.1). A patient's length not only estimates weight better than experienced clinicians, but also

Figure 6.1.
A. The Broselow tape, with 25 color-coded weight spaces.
B. The child is measured in the recumbent position, from crown to heel.

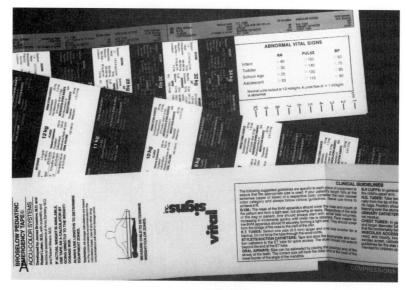

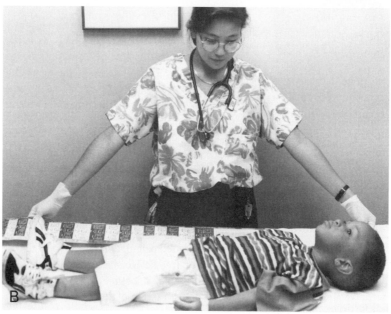

predicts certain equipment more accurately than existing, commonly used methods. Using length has been shown to be the most accurate method of endotracheal tube selection in children, more accurate than existing formulas (5), and also more accurate than existing anthropomorphic methods (e.g., the little finger or the nares) (6).

ANATOMY

Length is related to several biologic phenomena, such as intestinal absorption and renal function. It is a stronger determinant of body surface area than weight. Length is also a more important variable than body habitus or age in estimating body weight (3).

The National Center for Health Statistics studied 20,000 U.S. children between 1963 and 1975, and published a widely used set of percentile curves for height and weight by age in 1979 (7). The 50th percentile weight for many heights spanning the pediatric spectrum were used by James Broselow to develop a measuring tape marked by weight categories (4). Each space was labeled with appropriate drug doses and equipment sizes for that weight bracket (Fig. 6.1.A). This tape has been validated on studies in large numbers of children and is very accurate, particularly for children of less than 25 kg. In direct comparison to clinicians' estimates of weight based on knowledge of patient age and direct observation, the tape correctly predicted weight within 10% error in 85% of test scenarios versus 47% for the clinicians' estimates (4).

Procedure

The child is measured in the recumbent position, the likely posture during critical care interventions (Fig. 6.1.B). The tape is stretched from the crown of the head to the heel. It is not crucial to measure to the nearest millimeter, nor to obsess over perfect straightening of the child. There are only 25 "weight spaces", which vary from approximately 2.5 to 5 cm in length, and which increase from 3 kg to 20 kg by one-kg increments, and then from 20 kg to 34 kg by 2 kg increments. A child's length being "off" by one space would thus be quite unlikely to result in a clinically significant error in drug dosing. Drugs and other modalities incorporated into the Broselow tape are shown in Figure 6.2.

DRUGS
Paralytic Agents
  Succinylcholine
  Pancuronium
  Vecuronium
Defasciculating
  Agents
  Pancuronium
  Vecuronium
Infusions
  Isoproterenol
  Epinephrine
  Norepinephrine
  Dopamine
  Dobutamine
  Lidocaine
  PGE
  Nitroprusside
  Nitroglycerine
  Amrinone
ICP Agents
  Mannitol
  Furosemide
Overdose
  D25W
  Naloxone

EQUIPMENT
  BVM's
  ET Tubes
  Stylets
  Suction Catheters
  Oral Airway
  O2 Masks
  NG Tubes
  Urinary Catheters
  Chest tubes
  Vascular Access
    Modalities

Seizure
  Diazepam (IV & PR)
  Phenobarbital
  Phenytoin
  Lorazepam
Resuscitation
  Epinephrine
  Atropine
  Sodium Bicarbonate
  Calcium Choride
  Lidocaine
Defibrillation Doses
Cardioversion Doses

FLUIDS
  Volume Expansion
  Maintenance Fluids

**OTHER
  INFORMATION**
  Ventilator Settings
  Pediatric Trauma
    Score
  Abnormal Vital
    Signs

Figure 6.2.
Drugs, equipment, and other emergency modalities contained in the Broselow tape.

Table 6.1.
Evaluation of Methods for Selection of Pediatric Equipment and Drug Dosages

	Weight-Based Methods			Length-Based Methods		
Memory	Drug/Equipment Cards	Precalculated Equipment Cards and Computer Printouts	Length-Based Chart (Table 6.2)	First 5 Minutes	Broselow System
3 steps	2 steps	1 step	2 steps	2+ steps	1 step
1. Recollection of dose 2. Weight estimation 3. Calculation 4. Associated with anxiety and error	Associated with anxiety and error Require calculation in crisis situation Associated with error, 1/10 or 10X common	Associated with anxiety and error	Measure, access chart Minimal anxiety and error	Measurement, determination of habitus, then reference to a book Minimal anxiety and error	Measure and read directly from tape. Minimal anxiety and error

Legend: Progressing from left to right increases accuracy and decreases anxiety, error, and time lost. All weight-based methods are only as accurate as the clinicians weight estimation. The same is true for formulas used to predict equipment size, which are based on age or weight.

Table 6.2.
Length-Based Equipment Chart*

Item	Length (cm)						
	58–70	70–85	85–95	95–107	107–124	124–138	138–155
ET tube size (mm)	3.5	4.0	4.5	5.0	5.5	6.0	6.5
Lip–tip length (mm)	10.5	12.0	13.5	15.0	16.5	18.0	19.5
Laryngoscope	1 straight	1 straight	2 straight	2 straight or curved	2 straight or curved	2–3 straight or curved	3 straight or curved
Suction catheter	8 F	8–10 F	10 F	10 F	10 F	10 F	12 F
Stylet	6 F	6 F	6 F	6 F	14 F	14 F	14 F
Oral airway	Infant/small child	Small child	Child	Child	Child/small adult	Child/small adult	Medium adult
Bag-valve-mask	Infant	Child	Child	Child	Child	Child/adult	Adult
O₂ mask	Newborn	Pediatric	Pediatric	Pediatric	Adult	Adult	Adult
Vascular access catheter/butterfly	22–24/23–25, intraosseous	20–22/23–25, intraosseous	18–22/21–23, intraosseous	18–22/21–23, intraosseous	18–20/21–23	18–20/21–22	16–20/18–21
Nasogastric tube	5–8 F	8–10 F	10 F	10–12 F	12–14 F	14–18 F	18 F
Urinary catheter	5–8 F	8–10 F	10 F	10–12 F	10–12 F	12 F	12 F
Chest tube	10–12 F	16–20 F	20–24 F	20–24 F	24–32 F	28–32 F	32–40 F
Blood pressure cuff	Newborn, infant	Infant, child	Child	Child	Child	Child/adult	Adult

Legend: Directions for use:

1. Measure patient length with centimeter tape.

2. Using measured length in centimeters, access appropriate equipment column.

* Adapted from Luten RC, Wears RL, Broselow J, et al. Length-based endotracheal tube sizing for pediatric resuscitation. Ann Emerg Med 1992;21:900–904.

Table 6.3.
Average Weight for Age in Childhood

Approximate 50th percentile

Age	Weight (kg)
NB	3.5
6 mos	7
12 mos	10
2 yrs	12
3 yrs	14
4 yrs	16
5 yrs	18
6 yrs	20
7 yrs	22
8 yrs	25
9 yrs	28
10 yrs	32
11 yrs	36
12 yrs	40
13 yrs	45
14 yrs	50
15 yrs	55
16 yrs	60
17 yrs	66 M
	56 F
18 yrs	69 M
	57 F

Adapted from Hamil et al[7]

SUMMARY

1. Access the Broselow tape, if available, and use it as noted.
2. In lieu of the Broselow tape, measure patient and access the length-based chart (Table 6.2) for appropriate selection of resuscitation equipment.
3. Weight by age-based estimates should be used only as a last choice in the absence of length-based resources.

SUMMARY

Table 6.2 may be used as an adjunct for equipment selection. Using a single length measurement in centimeters, the clinician can access pediatric equipment using this chart.

The Broselow tape permits immediate access to precalculated drug doses as well as to equipment directly from the tape by a single length measurement. As emphasized in this chapter, estimates based on assumed (or known) age and/or clinical appearance are less accurate than length-derived estimates. In the event that no measuring tape or Broselow tape is available, Table 6.3 provides, as a rough guideline, the average weights for age.

REFERENCES

1. Oakley PA. Inaccuracy and delay in decision-making in pediatric resuscitation and a proposed reference chart to reduce error. Br Med J 1988;297:817–819.
2. Luten RC. Pediatric resuscitation chart and equipment shelf: aids to mastering age-related problems. J Emerg Med 1986;4:9–14.
3. Garland JS, Kishaba RG, Nelson DB, et al. A rapid and accurate method of estimating body weight. Am J Emerg Med 1986; 4(5):390–393.
4. Lubitz DS, Seidel JA, Chameides L, et al. A rapid method for estimating weight and resuscitation drug dosages for length in the pediatric age group. Ann Emerg Med 1988;17:576.
5. Luten RC, Wears RL, Broselow J, et al. Length-based endotracheal tube sizing for pediatric resuscitation. Ann Emerg Med 1992;21: 900–4.
6. Hinkle AJ. A rapid and reliable method for selecting endotracheal tube size in children (abstract). Anaesth Analg 1988;67:S92.
7. Hamill PVV, Drizd TA, Johnson CL, et al. Physical growth: National Center for Health Statistics Percentiles. Am J Clin Nutr 1979;32: 607–629.

Chapter 6
Emergent Drug Dosing
and Equipment
Selection

CHAPTER 7

ASEPTIC TECHNIQUE

Evaline A. Alessandrini and Jacalyn S. Maller

INTRODUCTION

Aseptic technique is the process utilized to prevent the access of microorganisms to a sterile field where a procedure or operation is being performed. The word "antisepsis" translates from the Greek, "against putrefaction." The concept of antisepsis was recognized in the mid-19th century by Oliver Wendell Holmes when he observed that a physician performing an autopsy was infected and subsequently killed by the same disease as the patient being autopsied. This resulted in improved handwashing and changing of clothing during such procedures. In 1867, Lister published his first description of "antiseptic principles" when the discovery of bacteria and their role in wound infection was realized.

Aseptic technique employs several methods: the use of sterile instruments, antiseptic hand scrubs, the wearing of sterile gowns, gloves, and masks by personnel, and also cleansing of the patient's skin with antiseptics. Other modalities are included in aseptic technique. *Sterilization* is the ultimate in disinfection for it is defined as the process of killing all microorganisms by either physical or chemical agents. Steam under pressure is the most commonly used method of sterilizing instruments for pediatric procedures. An *antiseptic* is a chemical agent applied to the body that kills or inhibits the growth of pathogenic organisms. A *disinfectant* is a chemical substance used on inanimate objects, such as floors and countertops, to eliminate bacteria.

Aseptic technique is an important prelude to many of the other procedures described in this text. Proper aseptic technique should be used by physicians, nurses, and other health professionals performing pediatric procedures to eliminate potentially serious infectious complications.

ANATOMY AND PHYSIOLOGY

The anatomy of the skin and its microbial inhabitants must be understood in order to properly perform aseptic technique. Two types of microorganisms are causative in both skin and wound infections and have been termed resident flora and transient flora. Resident flora are those bacteria that live and grow in the skin and can be repetitively cultured from it. These microorganisms live in the cracks and dead cells of the horny layer of the skin. Most organisms are of low virulence and include *Staphylococcus epidermidis*, micrococcus, and diphtheroids such as *Propionibacterium acnes*. Transient skin flora coexist with the resident flora in the horny skin layer and are barred from deeper skin invasion by the cells of the tightly packed stratum corneum. The transient organisms are acquired by contact with colonized or infected materials, often in the hospital environment. Subsequently these organisms are more likely to be resistant to many antibiotics and responsible for nosocomial infections. *Staphylococcus aureus* and Gram-negative enterobacteria are frequently identified as transient flora. The goal of cleansing and preparation of the skin with antiseptics is to remove the transient bacteria and reduce the levels of resident flora to a low level.

These potentially infectious microorganisms must be removed from both the patient and the health care provider. Subsequently it is important to understand the bacterial load of various areas of the body, for it has been determined that organism counts exceeding 10^5 per square centimeter are more likely to become infected (1). Organisms are actually sparse on the palms and dorsum of the hands. However, most hand flora are harbored under the nails and around the lateral nail folds, achieving counts of 10^4 to 10^6 per square centimeter. Most of the body surface, including the trunk, arms and legs, are colonized with only a few thousand organisms per square centimeter. Other moist places such as the perineum, axilla, and intertriginous areas harbor millions of bacteria per square centimeter. These bacterial counts must be considered in preparation of a field during aseptic technique.

The physiology of the body and its relation to aseptic technique have been reviewed. The physical characteristics of barriers used in aseptic techniques are also important. Various barrier methods are used in aseptic technique to eliminate passage of microorganisms onto the sterile field, including masks, gloves, and gowns worn by the health care provider as well as sterile drapes to define and preserve the boundaries of the sterile field. Masks should be worn, especially by those with upper respiratory tract infections, to decrease transmission of respiratory flora to the sterile field. Speaking while wearing a mask promotes leaking of respiratory flora from the sides of the mask and so should be kept at a minimum during the procedure. Gowns and gloves are worn to provide a barrier to transfer of the physician's bacterial flora to the patient. Gowns impermeable to moisture prevent the wicklike effect of transferring bacteria from one side of the gown to the other. Latex gloves, and to a lesser extent vinyl gloves, serve as protective barriers to health care workers' hands. However, bacteria multiply under moist gloves and hand contamination can occur even when gloves are worn, so handwashing is recommended routinely after gloves are removed (2).

INDICATIONS

Aseptic technique is indicated to minimize the risk of infectious complications from various invasive procedures. These procedures include lumbar puncture, urine catheterization, suprapubic bladder aspiration, central venous access procedures, thoracentesis, chest tube placement, paracentesis, joint aspiration, wound repair, and tapping of a ventriculoperitoneal shunt.

Good judgment, as well as specific institutional guidelines, should be used in determining the level of aseptic technique necessary for a given procedure. The following list details what level of aseptic technique is recommended for various procedures:

Full aseptic technique (mask, gown, gloves, drapes, and skin preparation)
   Central venous access procedures
   Thoracentesis
   Paracentesis
   Chest tube placement
Aseptic technique including skin preparation, draping, and sterile gloves
   Lumbar puncture
   Wound repair
   Tapping a ventriculoperitoneal shunt
Partial aseptic technique (skin preparation and sterile gloves)
   Suprapubic bladder aspiration
   Urine catheterization
   Joint aspiration

There are no true contraindications to aseptic technique. Latex sensitivity must be considered in patients at risk, especially those with spina bifida. Although allergies to the various antiseptic solutions are rare, history of sensitivity to povidine-iodine or other antiseptics must be elicited.

EQUIPMENT

Disposable mask
Sterile gown
Sterile gloves
Antiseptic solution
Disposable sponges or gauze pads with hemostats
Sterile drapes

Sterile gowns and drapes may be purchased in disposable, single-use types which

Table 7.1.
Table of Skin Antiseptics

Antiseptic	Uses	Antibacterial Spectrum	Benefits	Drawbacks
Povidine-iodine scrub "Betadine scrub"	Handwashing	Highly bactericidal against Gram-positive and negative organisms	Nontoxic	Minimally toxic to wound tissues
Povidine-iodine solution "Betadine solution"	Skin preparation	As above	Can be used for large body surface areas	Iodism rare. Stains skin temporarily
Chlorhexidine "Hibiclens"	Handwashing Alternative skin preparation	Highly bactericidal against Gram-positive organisms, less bactericidal against Gram-negative organisms	Persistent protective residue after single handwashing. Rarely causes dermatitis	Ototoxicity if instilled in middle ear
Hexachlorophene "phisoHex"	Handwashing	Good activity against Gram-positive organisms, poor against Gram-negative organisms	Persistent protective residue after handwashings	Teratogenic, CNS toxicity with repeated usage
Benzalkonium chloride "Zephiran"	Skin preparation	Effective against Gram-positive and Gram-negative organisms	None. Use not often recommended	Storage prone to contamination. Inactivated by soaps and detergents
Alcohols	Skin preparation	Effective against Gram-positive and Gram-negative organisms	Organic solvent, removes oil and debris	Requires 2 minutes of moist application to achieve good antisepsis

are often made of waterproof material that is nonwoven and therefore not likely to be penetrated by bacteria. More traditional woven cloth can also be used. These cloths may be reused after laundering, but should be washed no more than 75 times to maintain their barrier integrity (3).

If disposable sponges are not available, fine-pore (90 pores per inch) 4 × 4 gauze pads may be soaked in a disinfectant and used to cleanse the field.

Any type of sterile glove may be used, though studies have shown that latex gloves are more protective and resistant to organism penetration than vinyl gloves (2).

Several types of antiseptic solutions are available for preparation of the sterile field and handwashing. The most commonly used antiseptics are summarized in Table 7.1. Povidine-iodine solution is most often used for skin preparation because of its highly bactericidal effects against both Gram-positive and Gram-negative organisms (4, 5). Chlorhexidine may also be used for skin preparation in the event that a hypersensitivity to povidine-iodine exists. Chlorhexidine is the antiseptic of choice for handwashing because it leaves a protective bactericidal residue on the skin after cleansing. Chlorhexidine does not stain or cause dermatitis, reactions which are often encountered when povidine-iodine scrub is used for handwashing (4, 5). Hexachlorophene, benzalkonium chloride, and alcohols are infrequently used for reasons listed in Table 7.1.

PROCEDURE

Operator Preparation

An orderly approach to aseptic technique will ensure the best results. First, a mask is placed snugly over the mouth and nose and tied securely behind the head. An appropriate method of handwashing is next. Friction with soap and water is adequate to remove transient flora for procedures such as urinary catheterizations and lumbar punctures. However, a several-minute scrub with an antiseptic such as an iodophor with broad antibacterial activity or hexachlorophene with its sustained suppressant action on the skin flora is beneficial in more invasive procedures such as chest tube placement (1). Special attention to the lateral nail folds and nail tips are necessary to eliminate the majority of organisms. At this point, a sterile gown is donned.

Two methods of gloving are used for aseptic procedures. The first is the *closed method* which is utilized in the operating room and will not be described further. The *open method* (6) is more commonly used in the ED and will be described here (Fig. 7.1). Before scrubbing or washing the hands, the outer wrapper of the gloves is opened. If the procedure requires gowning it is done before glove placement, with the cuffs of the gown pulled over the hands from inside the sleeve by an assistant.

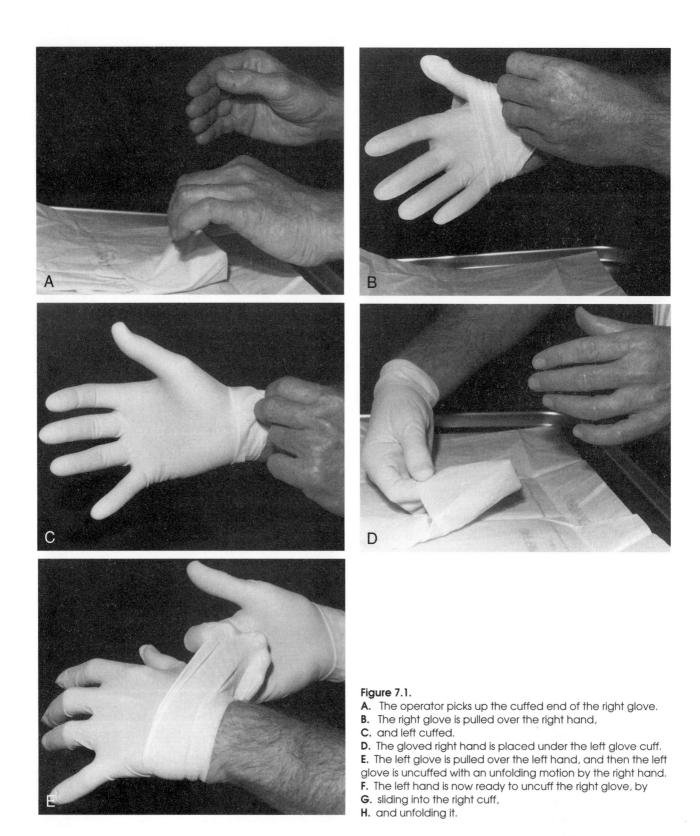

Figure 7.1.
A. The operator picks up the cuffed end of the right glove.
B. The right glove is pulled over the right hand,
C. and left cuffed.
D. The gloved right hand is placed under the left glove cuff.
E. The left glove is pulled over the left hand, and then the left glove is uncuffed with an unfolding motion by the right hand.
F. The left hand is now ready to uncuff the right glove, by
G. sliding into the right cuff,
H. and unfolding it.

Placement of the Right Glove

First the inner glove cover is opened. By convention, the right glove is placed first. The right glove is grasped by the left fingers at the folded cuff end and lifted up. The right hand is then placed inside the right glove while the left hand continues to pull out the glove cuff until it hits the cuff of the gown. Avoid contamination of the gown with the unsterile left hand.

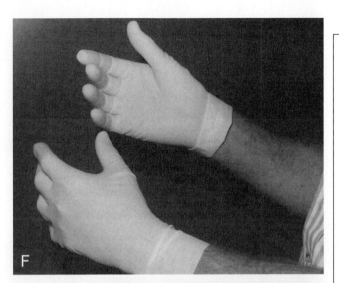

F

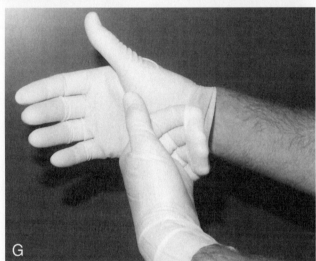

G

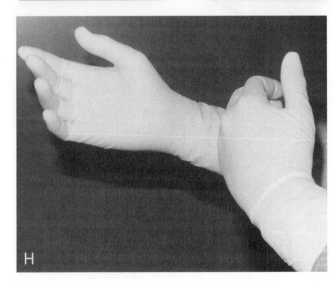

H

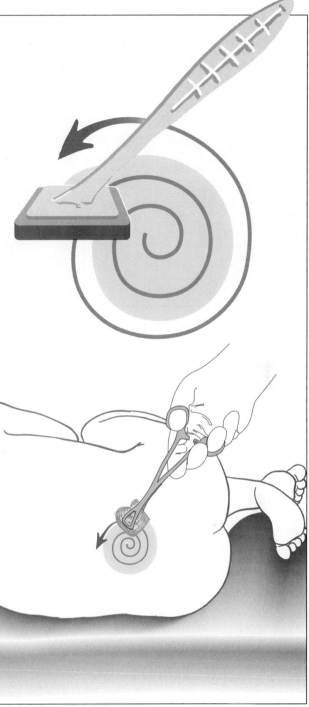

Figure 7.2.
Skin preparation for a
"clean" procedure such as
lumbar puncture.

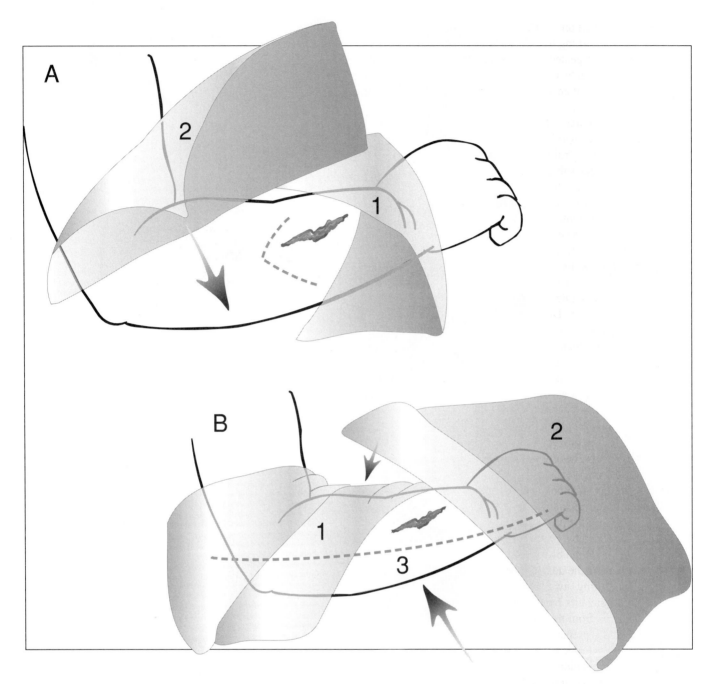

Figure 7.3.
Sterile draping to prepare the procedural field
A. Using a two-towel technique to create a "diamond-shaped" field.
B. Using three towels to create a "triangle-shaped" field.

Placement of the Left Glove

The left glove is then picked up with the right fingers by the folded cuff. The right gloved fingers are then placed under the left glove cuff and the glove is pulled onto the left hand until it hits the gown cuff. The cuff of the left glove is unfolded by the right hand which is still slid under the left glove cuff. Finally, the right glove cuff is turned by sliding the left gloved fingers under the right glove cuff and unfolding it over the right gown cuff.

Field Preparation

It is important to change gloves if they break or touch any unsterile objects. Gloves should be kept at waist level or above and should always be easily visible to prevent any inadvertent contamination. Skin preparation is performed next (Fig. 7.2), which is begun at the incision or procedure site, using a concentric motion starting centrally and moving peripherally. The antiseptic is placed on a sterile sponge and rubbed on firmly. A new sponge is used when returning to the central site and the procedure is repeated four times. Preparation of a dirty or infected area, such as incision and drainage of an abscess, is performed differently. Skin preparation is begun at the outer boundaries and continued toward the incision site (peripheral to central) to avoid spreading bacteria from a dirty site onto a clean surface. Each subsequent preparation is begun approximately 0.5 centimeters inside the outer boundaries of the first wash (6). Draping is done immediately after the antiseptic preparation is completed.

Sterile drapes are used to establish a sterile field around the area in which a procedure is performed. They provide a barrier to minimize the passage of microorganisms from unsterile to sterile sites. Drapes should be held higher than the level of the physician's waist and the bed on which the procedure is performed. Draping is done from the operative or "clean" site to the periphery, using either two or three drapes as illustrated in Figure 7.3.A and 7.3.B. The draping material is cuffed back over the gloved hands to preserve the sterility of the gloves. Once a drape is in place, it should not be moved. Excessive handling, which may generate air currents and spread droplets or other particles, must be avoided. The physician should always face the sterile area. If the physician must face the unsterile area for any reason, a distance of a least 12 inches should be maintained between the physician and the unsterile objects (6).

When turning away from the sterile field, the physician's back should again remain 12 inches from the sterile area. At this point, the field is prepared for the initiation of the procedure. Aseptic technique may be violated by contamination or tear of a glove or other objects on the sterile field. At the moment this is recognized, all contaminated items must be replaced.

COMPLICATIONS

Performing aseptic technique may potentially be complicated by allergic reactions to either latex gloves or an antiseptic solution. This complication may be minimized by taking a good history before initiation of aseptic technique.

The most unfavorable outcome of improperly performed aseptic technique is an infection at the site of the procedure. This may range from a urinary tract infection as the result of an improperly performed urethral catheterization to a bacteremic illness as the result of an infection from central line placement. Clinicians may avoid complications by strict adherence to aseptic technique and rapid correction of any recognized violations.

REFERENCES

1. Steere AC, Mallison GF. Handwashing practices for the prevention of nosocomial infections. Ann Intern Med. 1975;83:683–690.
2. Olsen RJ, Lynch P, Coyle MB, Cummings J, Bokete T, Stamm WE. Examination gloves as barriers to hand contamination in clinical practice. JAMA. 1993;270(3):350–353.
3. Beck WC. Aseptic barriers in surgery: their present status. Arch Surg. 1981;116:240–244.
4. Kaul AF, Jewett JF. Agents and techniques for disinfection of the skin. Surg Gynecol Obstetr 1981;152:677–685.
5. Sebben JE. Surgical antiseptics. J Am Acad Derm. 1983;9(5):759–765.
6. Brooks SM. Fundamentals of operating room nursing. St. Louis; CV Mosby, 1975, pp. 65–69, 96–99. 100–102.

SUMMARY
1. Elicit history of relevant allergy: latex, antiseptics, etc.
2. Gauge level of aseptic technique to invasiveness of procedure.
3. Handwashing with emphasis on nail tips and lateral nail folds.
4. Proper order: mask, handwashing, gown, gloves, skin preparation, draping.
5. Prepare skin from procedure site to periphery for "clean" procedures, and from periphery to procedure site for "dirty" procedures.

Protecting the Health Professional Against Hazardous Exposures

Leonard R. Friedland and Louis M. Bell

Introduction

Health care workers (HCWs) practice medicine in a potentially dangerous environment. Occupational health hazards include infectious disease and chemical and radioactive exposures. The high volume, high acuity, and unscheduled nature of emergency medicine practice make emergency health professionals unique in their potential for such exposures. This is particularly important in the practice of pediatric emergency medicine when infectious disease and accidental poisoning are commonly encountered. HCWs need to be aware of and continually educated about their risks from hazardous exposures. This chapter provides an overview of the risks associated with occupational exposure to infectious, chemical, and radioactive agents. Guidelines for exposure prevention and control are discussed.

Infectious Disease Exposures

Microbiologic Considerations

HCWs are at risk of acquiring many different infectious diseases which can be transmitted via blood and respiratory and other body fluids. Routes of exposure to infectious agents include percutaneous inoculation of, and contact with, nonintact skin or mucous membranes by contaminated blood or body fluids. More than 20 different infectious diseases can be transmitted via blood- or body fluid-contaminated needlestick injuries. Of particular importance among these agents are human immunodeficiency virus (HIV) and hepatitis B virus (HBV). Exposure by aerosol droplets from the respiratory tract of infected patients and direct contact with infected secretions can place the HCW at risk of acquiring many serious illnesses. These include tuberculosis, measles, varicella, pertussis, cytomegalovirus, meningococcus, *Haemophilus influenzae,* and adenovirus infections.

Indications

The care of pediatric emergency department patients is highly procedure oriented and is the subject of this textbook. Medical and trauma resuscitations are particularly high-risk situations that place the HCW in close contact with blood and other body fluid secretions. Close patient contact makes occupational exposure to infectious diseases common for emergency medicine HCWs in their everyday practice. This is particularly true for pediatric emergency medicine HCWs because children do not routinely have good hygienic practices and, in comparison to adults, have an increased incidence of infections. Precautions to limit HCW exposure and prevent occupational acquisition of infectious diseases are indicated in virtually every ED encounter and rest on two fundamental principles: most infectious diseases are contagious before the patient and HCW are aware of the diagnosis, and following infection control guidelines will help prevent exposure.

PROCEDURES

Guidelines for Infection Control

Hospital employee health services should provide for HCWs annual or biannual screening with Mantoux skin testing for tuberculosis, annual influenza vaccination, and for those regularly exposed to blood, vaccination against HBV if the HCW is without HBV immunity. In addition, HCWs immunity should be documented, either by history of disease or by immunization, to varicella, rubella, measles, mumps, pertussis, and polio. If immunity is lacking, the appropriate vaccine should be administered. For infections that are not preventable by vaccination, for example adenovirus conjunctivitis and varicella, the HCW should be counseled about the risks of exposure. Some infections pose increased risk for pregnant HCWs, and will be discussed later in this chapter.

Needlestick Injuries

Health care workers gave little concern to the frequency of needlestick injuries in the ED before the AIDS epidemic. This was despite the well-known 6 to 30% risk of infection with HBV to a hepatitis B surface antibody-negative HCW following a needlestick exposure from a hepatitis B surface antigen-positive patient. The difference in the current era is that infection with HIV is likely to prove fatal. The risk of occupational HIV transmission is small but real. One percutaneous exposure to the blood of an HIV-infected patient places the HCW at an approximate 0.3% risk of acquiring HIV infection (1, 2). Nonparenteral (mucous membrane and nonintact skin) exposure to the blood of an HIV-infected patient is associated with a decreased rate of acquisition. The risk of acquisition following percutaneous exposure to certain other body fluids of an HIV-infected patient

is unknown. The likelihood of a HCW becoming infected at work with HIV or other bloodborne pathogen depends on the rate of parenteral or nonparenteral exposure to the blood of an infected patient and the prevalence of the infection. Mucous membrane and skin exposure to blood is a commonplace event in the practice of pediatric emergency medicine (3). Virtually all hospital-related blood contacts involve the hand (3, 4). Needlestick injury is less common but does occur. As the prevalence of HIV infection continues to rise so does the rate of recognized and unrecognized HIV-infected patients presenting for emergency care. Several reports out of inner-city and non-inner-city EDs have focused attention on the high prevalence rates of HIV infection in adult patients (5–11). Published data on the prevalence rate of HIV among children presenting to the ED are limited (12). With adolescent heterosexuals and reproductive-age women representing ever-increasing groups of HIV-infected individuals, these numbers are likely to rise and not be restricted to certain geographic inner-city EDs.

Universal Precautions

Recognizing the risks of occupational exposure to HIV and other bloodborne pathogens in health care settings, the Centers for Disease Control and Prevention (CDCP) published in 1985 recommendations for preventing HIV transmission in the workplace (13). The CDCP referred to this approach as "universal blood and body fluid precautions" or "universal precautions." The CDCP has subsequently consolidated and updated their recommendations (14–17).

Universal precautions are a method of barrier precautions based on infection control principles designed to prevent parenteral, nonintact skin, and mucous membrane exposures to bloodborne pathogens (18). The tenets of universal precautions include routine use of gloves, masks, protective eyewear, impervious gowns, and precautions to prevent injuries when handling needles and sharp instruments. Table 8.1 reviews infection control requirements for exposure to body fluids and procedures performed in the ED.

Table 8.1.
Infection Control Requirements for Exposure to Body Fluids and Procedures Performed in the Emergency Department

	Gloves	Mask and Protective Eyewear	Gown	No Precautions Required
Body Fluids				
stool	Yes	No	No	
urine	Yes	No	No	
vomitus	Yes	No	No	
blood	Yes	Optional	Optional	
oral secretions	Yes	No	No	
tears				Yes
Procedures				
venipuncture	Yes	No	No	
intravenous line	Yes	No	No	
control of minor bleeding	Yes	No	No	
control of profuse bleeding	Yes	Yes	Yes	
endotracheal intubation	Yes	Yes	No	
naso/orogastric tube placement	Yes	Yes	No	
tracheostomy care	Yes	Yes	No	
oral examination	Yes	No	No	
wound irrigation	Yes	Yes	Optional	
diaper changing	Yes	No	No	

Universal precautions are currently our best strategy to prevent occupational exposure to blood and body fluids. Currently no established efficacious postexposure HIV prophylaxis regimen exists. Studies of postexposure zidovudine use are ongoing and preliminary reports suggest that efficacy is not absolute (1).

Gloves should be worn during all vascular access procedures (e.g., phlebotomy, arterial blood sampling, intravenous line placement), during examination of nonintact skin and mucous membranes, and when touching blood and body fluids. Wearing gloves may provide some protection against needlestick injuries (19). Gloves should be changed and hands washed thoroughly after contact with each patient. Handwashing, and when appropriate, glove and gown use, are very important procedures in preventing nosocomial infections (20).

Masks and protective eyewear (a face shield will work as both) should be worn to protect the mucous membranes of the face when procedures are performed that could generate a spray of blood or blood-containing body fluids (e.g., wound irrigation, endotracheal intubation, naso/orogastric tube placement). Impervious gowns should be worn when there is profuse bleeding or procedures are performed that could create splashes of blood or blood containing body fluids (e.g., arterial line placement, central line place-

ment, cutdown, thoracostomy tube placement) (Fig. 8.1). Mouth-to-mouth resuscitation should be avoided and alternative ventilation devices should be used (e.g., bag-valve mask-ventilation).

Needles should never be recapped, bent, or broken by hand. All sharp objects should be handled with exceptional care. Puncture-resistant containers should be used for needle and sharp instrument disposal. These containers should be readily accessible and if possible within arm's reach of the working area (Figs. 8.2.A and 8.2.B).

Figure 8.1.
The pediatric trauma team prepares for patient arrival with gown, mask, goggles, and gloves.

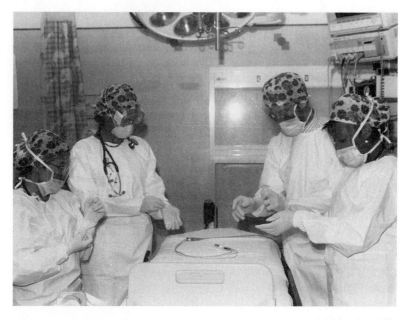

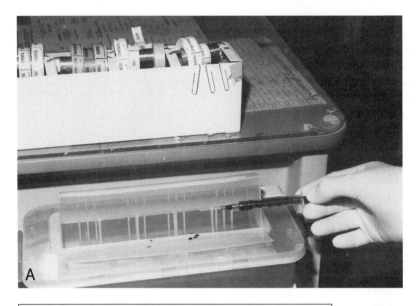

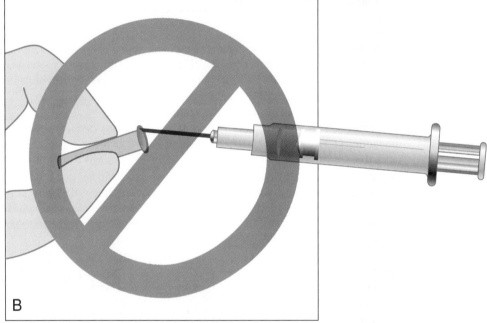

Figure 8.2.
A. The proper disposal of contaminated needles.
B. Needles should never be recapped before disposal.

Universal precautions will be useful in preventing the occupational transmission of bloodborne and other pathogens only if HCWs adhere to them. Studies from EDs and other health care settings have demonstrated that glove use and other barrier precautions by HCWs are far from universal (21–25). Educational interventions have been somewhat successful in improving HCW compliance with universal precautions (26–28). The Occupational Safety and Health Administration (OSHA) issued regulations that mandate HCWs to wear gloves for all phlebotomy procedures in hospitals, and that

hospital personnel train their employees annually regarding the reasons and need to wear gloves during all phlebotomy procedures (29). HCWs can be fined for infractions.

Reasons for poor compliance by HCWs with universal precautions are numerous. They include lack of time to put on protective materials, uncomfortable protective materials, failure to remember, judging the patient not high risk, and interference with proficient performance of procedures. In particular, HCWs often complain that they cannot perform vascular access procedures when wearing gloves. However, investigators from Philadelphia reported no difference in the success rate on the first attempt at vascular access with and without wearing gloves by nurses and residents in a pediatric ED (26). HCWs should be advised that retraining can be easily accomplished through practice and patience.

Universal precautions are very effective barrier protectors against cutaneous and mucous membrane exposures to blood and body fluids. However, percutaneous exposure from needlestick and sharp instrument injuries account for the vast majority of occupational HIV and HBV transmission. In a study of 1201 HCWs exposed to blood or body fluids of HIV-infected patients, needlestick injuries accounted for 80% of the exposures, and sharp instruments 8% (30). Exposure causes included manipulating needles (36%), recapping needles (17%), and improper disposal of sharp objects (14%). Two exposures that resulted in HIV seroconversion were from needlestick injuries inflicted by coworkers during resuscitation procedures (Fig. 8.3).

Training and educating HCWs to take extraordinary precautions while handling sharp items is not sufficient. In addition to implementing universal precautions, hospitals must continue to create a safer working environment for HCWs, government bureaus must continue to enact safety regulation guidelines, and industry must create safer devices (31).

"Safe" needle devices are being developed and marketed (18, 32, 33). As of August 1992, over 340 patents for sharp safety devices had been issued, and the Food and Drug Administration has approved for marketing at least 88 needlestick prevention devices (34). Examples of devices to perform procedures with fewer sharp instruments include compressed-air injection systems (Fig. 8.4), needleless i.v. and vial access systems (Figure 8.5), and needles that can be used and disposed with no risk of injury (Figs. 8.6.A and 8.6.B).

The vast majority of blood contacts by HCWs are cutaneous. Latex gloves are a reliable protection against cutaneous exposure to blood and body fluids; however, they will not preclude needlestick or sharp instrument injuries. Wearing two pair of gloves can decrease the risk of inner glove perforation (19).

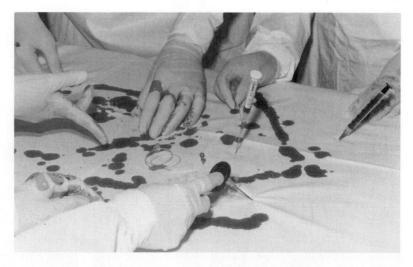

Cut-resistant glove liners designed to be worn under latex gloves are available.

In many EDs a simple, needleless device is used to irrigate wounds, which prevents splash of blood-contaminated irrigation fluid (Figs. 8.7.A and 8.7.B). This product is a clear plastic, parabolic cup which attaches to the tip of a Luer-Lok or slip-tip syringe. Its self-contained nozzle creates a high-pressure stream for irrigation, while the shield protects against contaminated splashback.

Disposable gloves, masks, protective eyewear, impervious gowns, sharp containers, and the newly developed safe needles and other safe devices are expensive, (35); however, they are currently our best protection

Figure 8.3.
Improper, careless scattering of used needles and sharps, including their insertion into a mattress, creates a hazardous environment for health care workers.

Figure 8.4.
The Biojector® 2000, an advanced needle-free system for intramuscular and subcutaneous injections, was engineered by Bioject inc. of Portland, Oregon.

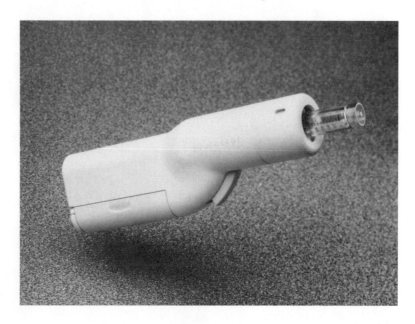

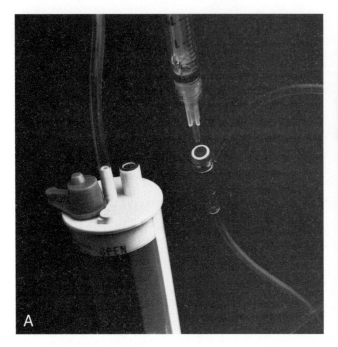

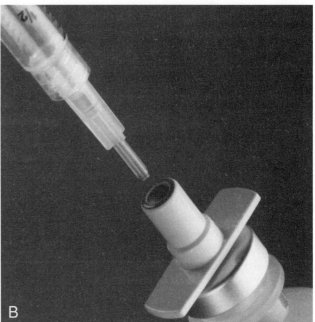

Figure 8.5.
A. Representative needle-less i.v. tubing and
B. Needleless vial access systems.

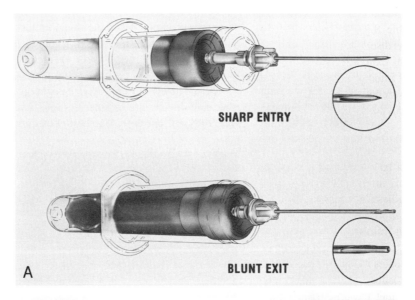

SHARP ENTRY

BLUNT EXIT

A

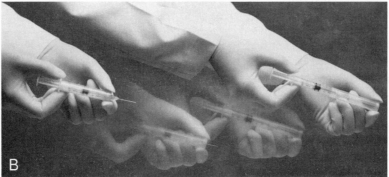

B

Figure 8.6.
A. A "blunt" needle system.
B. A safety syringe with a protective shield.

against occupational acquisition of blood-borne and other pathogens. The benefit of possibly preventing cases of occupationally acquired HIV, HBV, or other infections far outweighs the costs of barrier protective materials and the newer safer devices.

SELECTED INFECTIONS THAT OCCUR FOLLOWING EXPOSURE TO BLOOD OR SECRETIONS

Although universal precautions as previously described are the recommended approach in caring for all patients, it is prudent to review some of the more common infections that could affect HCWs. Despite careful adherence to Infection Control Procedures and Policy during the management of acutely ill or injured patients, exposures will occur. In evaluating the risk of exposure and infection after exposure, the HCW should consider the infectious agent, the mode of transmission, individual susceptibility, type of contact exposure, and recognition of high-risk patients or situations. Table 8.2 outlines the more common infectious diseases in terms of most common source of exposure, transmission, incubation, risk of infection following exposures, high-risk patients and situations, and postexposure prophylaxis.

HIV

HCWs exposed to HIV-containing blood or secretions are rarely infected. The risk of infection after a needlestick exposure to HIV-infected blood is approximately 0.3% (1, 2, 36). HIV infection following mucous membrane exposure is even less. Proper handling and disposal of needles will prevent a majority of these exposures (37). If exposed, HCWs should contact the employee health department in their institution for counseling and testing. Table 8.3 outlines the steps to follow after accidental exposure.

The use of zidovudine for postexposure prophylaxis is unproven (1, 38, 39). Despite this, many institutions offer it to HCWs with needlestick injuries. If given, zidovudine should be started as soon as possible after exposure at a dose of 200 mg every 4 hours for 4 to 6 weeks. Zidovudine is usually not recommended more than 48 hours after the ex-

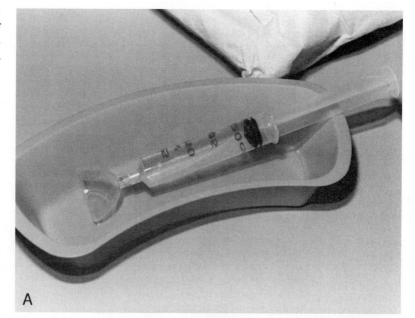

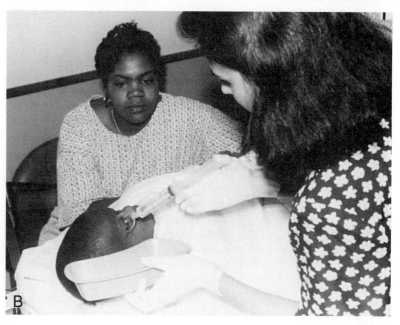

posure, if the exposure was superficial (not bleeding), or was a mucous membrane exposure (38, 39). HCWs of child-bearing age should have a negative pregnancy test.

Hepatitis B

Hepatitis B infection is a major cause of acute and chronic hepatitis, cirrhosis, and primary hepato-cellular carcinoma. The reported incidence of acute hepatitis B in the United States increased by 37% from 1979 to 1989 with an estimated 200,000 to 300,000 new infections occurring from 1980 to 1991 (40).

Figure 8.7.
A. A clear, plastic splash guard attached to an irrigation syringe.
B. Irrigation of a laceration using the syringe-splash guard technique.

**Chapter 8
Protecting the Health Professional Against Hazardous Exposures**

Table 8.2.
Summary of Potential Infectious Diseases Following Exposure to Blood and Secretion

Infectious Agent	Source	Transmission and Incubation	Risk of Infection After Exposures (Needlestick) to Contaminated Blood	High-Risk Patients[a]	High-Risk Situations[b]	Postexposure Prophylaxis
Human immunodeficiency virus (HIV)	• Blood, bloody secretions, genital secretions of infected persons	• Intravenous inoculations • Splash accidents (most seroconverted within 1st 12 weeks)	0.3%	• Intravenous drug use in caretakers • Transfusions before 1985 in mother or child	• Recapping needles • Medical or trauma ''code'' situations	• Zidovudine 200 mg every 4 hr for 4–6 wk[c]
Hepatitis B	• Blood or bloody secretions of a person infected or carrier	• Intravenous innoculations • Close and sexual contact (45 to 160 days)	26%	• Intravenous drug use in caretakers • Sexually active adolescents	• As above	• See Table 8.4
Hepatitis C	• Blood or bloody secretions of an infected person	• Intravenous innoculations • Sexual contact	Unknown	• Intravenous drug use • Transfusions	• As above	• None[d]

[a] Reference 42.
[b] References 5 and 7.
[c] Efficacy is unproven.
[d] Consider immunoglobin (0.06 mL/kg) given i.m. if hepatitis B prophylaxis is not indicated.

All HCWs who work in EDs should be immunized with hepatitis B vaccine. The chance of infection following percutaneous exposure from blood contaminated with hepatitis B is approximately 85 times more likely than the same exposure with HIV-contaminated blood (40). Table 8.4 outlines the recommendations for postexposure prophylaxis.

Protective antibody levels of 10 or more multi-international units develop in 85 to 96% of those receiving vaccine. The vaccine should be given in the deltoid muscle in adults—this site has the highest response rate. Vaccination with either Recombivax HB (Merck & Co.) or Energix B (Smith Kline Beecham) is recommended. Adults over 20 years of age should be given 10 mg (1.0 mL) of hepatitis B surface antigen protein of the Recombivax HB or 20 mg (1.0 mL) of the Energix B intramuscularly at 0, 1, and 6 months (40).

After the series of immunizations, postvaccinate testing should also be considered for persons at risk for exposures such as ED HCWs. Such testing should be performed 1 to 6 months after completion of the series. For persons who do not respond, two to three additional doses will produce adequate antibody levels in up to 50% of adults (40).

Hepatitis C

The transmission of hepatitis C virus (HCV) occurs by exposure to parenteral blood or blood products that contain the virus. Although most cases of transfusion-related non-A, non-B hepatitis are due to HCV, infection by transfusion accounts for only 5 to 10% of the total number of clinical infections (38). Infection during i.v. drug use and sexual transmission are thought to play major roles in the spread of HCV. The risks for HCWs following a needlestick or mucous membrane exposure is unknown.

Tuberculosis

Unlike HIV or hepatitis B and C, tuberculosis (TB) in HCWs occurs following exposure to the aerosolized secretions of infected patients or coworkers. Control of tuberculosis within

Table 8.3.
Management of Exposed HCW to Blood or Bloody Secretions from an HIV-Positive Patient*

• Confirmation that the patient is HIV positive
• Evaluation of the HCW clinically and serologically for HIV infection immediately after exposure
• If seronegative, retesting at 6 weeks, 3 months, 6 months, and 12 months after exposure
• Offer zidovudine for chemoprophylaxis[+]
• Counseling about risk from exposure

* Adapted from Centers for Disease Control, 1989.
[+] The data on the use of zidovudine for postexposure prophylaxis is inconclusive for both efficacy and safety. Consult the infectious diseases expert in your hospital.

Table 8.4.
Recommendations for Hepatitis B Prophylaxis After Percutaneous Exposure to Blood That Contains (OR Might Contain) HBsAg*

Exposed Person	Treatment when source is found to be		
	HBsAg-Positive	HBsAg-Negative	Unknown or Not Tested
Unvaccinated	Administer HBIG × 1† and initiate hepatitis B vaccine‡	Initiate hepatitis B vaccine‡	Initiate hepatitis B vaccine
Previously vaccinated Known responder	Test exposed person for anti HBs§ 1. If adequate, no treatment 2. If inadequate, hepatitis B vaccine booster dose‡	No treatment	No treatment
Known nonresponder	HBIG × 2 or HBIG × 1 plus 1 dose of hepatitis B vaccine‡	No treatment	If known high-risk source, may treat as if source were HBsAg-positive
Person for whom response is unknown	Test exposed person for anti HBs§ 1. If inadequate, HBIG × 1, plus hepatitis B vaccine booster dose‡ 2. If adequate, no treatment	No treatment	Test exposed person for anti HBs§ 1. If inadequate, hepatitis B vaccine booster dose‡ 2. If adequate, no treatment

* Reproduced from Centers for Disease Control and Prevention. MMWR 1991:40(RR-13):22.
† Hepatitis B immune globulin (HBIG) dose 0.06 ml/kg, intramuscularly.
‡ See Recommendations American Academy of Pediatrics. In: Peter G, ed. 1994 Red Book: report of the Committee on Infectious Diseases. 23rd ed. Elk Grove Village, IL. American Academy of Pediatrics 1994:229, Table 3.12.
§ Adequate anti-HBs is ≥10 milli-international units.

a hospital setting depends on early identification and treatment of persons with TB, on proper function and use of isolation rooms, and on an aggressive surveillance program to identify transmission of TB to HCWs (41).

TB surveillance is especially important for the HCWs in the ED. Because of the nature of emergency medicine as the front line or interface with the community, exposure to TB may be frequent. Screening using the Mantoux technique (the intradermal injection of five tuberculin units of purified protein derivative) should be done at least yearly and perhaps every 6 months, depending on the prevalence of TB in the population served.

Control of TB in the ED also depends on engineering concerns both in ventilation (number of air exchanges within a defined space) and direction of air flow (negative or low into the isolation room). The best movement and housing of the patient and family within the ED should be determined with these factors in mind (41).

CHEMICAL EXPOSURES

Certain chemical materials may pose a hazard to patients via continuing contamination, and to HCWs via cross contamination. Cross contamination may occur if hazardous chemicals gather on HCWs clothes or skin, or ED equipment, during the process of caring for patients involved in chemical incidents (e.g., chemical spills, explosions, gas leaks, fires, accidental poisonings, suicide attempts). Preferably, a receiving ED will be notified by prehospital care providers before the arrival of any patients involved in chemical incidents. The ED team's preparation will be improved with prior knowledge about the chemical involved and details of the incident. On notification, the ED team should contact both the hospital's safety officer, and the regional poison control center. The poison control center can help determine the extent of acute or chronic medical problems that may arise from the chemical involved, and if decontamination is necessary. This information also will assist the safety officer in readying possible special decontamination materials. Effective decontamination begins in the field and continues in the hospital.

Toxicologic Considerations

Occupational exposure to hazardous chemicals may occur via three main routes: inhalation, ingestion, and skin absorption. Inhalation exposure occurs through introduction of toxic compounds into the respiratory system.

Examples include gases or vapors of volatile liquids, although solids and liquids can be inhaled as dusts or aerosols. Inhalation exposure usually results in a rapid systemic dosage because of the lung's large surface area and high vascularity. Ingestion exposure is an uncommon source of exposure. One route is the incidental transfer of chemical materials when a HCW wipes his or her mouth with his or her hand or sleeve. Skin contamination is a common route of occupational exposure. It is estimated that hazards exist for skin absorption from one in four industrial chemicals (43). Skin exposure can cause local effects, as well as systemic. Systemic effects are usually not as rapid as with inhalation exposure, although some chemicals are rapidly absorbed. In addition, some chemicals that come in contact with the eye can also be absorbed.

PROCEDURES

Guidelines for Chemical Control

Decontamination is the process that removes or neutralizes hazardous chemicals collected on HCWs clothes or skin, or ED equipment, during the process of caring for patients involved in chemical incidents (44–46). Decontamination is important to HCW safety, and we recommend that ED health care workers regularly familiarize themselves with the decontamination process. Along with decontamination, the patient's medical needs also must be assessed, and appropriate resuscitative measures and antidotes initiated.

Avoiding contact with the hazardous chemical is the most effective method; however, HCW contamination is often unavoidable. Steps to limit this include wearing impermeable gowns, rubber gloves and eye shields when handling contaminated patients, and completely removing and placing in closed plastic bags all the patient's clothing, including diapers. Patients who are able and cooperative may assist with their own decontamination. In an effort to limit continuing contamination to the patient and cross contamination to the HCW, the entire body (including hair, nails, skin folds, and groin) of a stable victim of a skin chemical exposure should be copiously lavaged with water and a mild soap. This process should be repeated two more times. If available, tincture of green soap, which is 30% alcohol, is effective in removing fat-soluble compounds. Only a saline irrigation should be used over vesiculated skin, and victims of an eye chemical exposure should have their eyes copiously lavaged with saline for 20 minutes (see also Chapter 51). Afterward, if exposed to the hazardous chemical, HCWs should remove their contaminated clothes and wash as just described.

Residues of the decontamination process must be considered hazardous wastes. The assistance of the hospital's safety officer will be needed for proper disposal. Some hospitals have special ED decontamination rooms equipped with a shower and a self-contained water disposal system (Fig. 8.8). In the case of a hospital hazardous chemical spill, the hospital's safety officer must be contacted to direct the containment and disposal process.

Special Considerations

Health care workers are at particular risk of developing toxicity via skin cross contamination from patients exposed to organophosphates, hydrocarbons, caustics, and via inhalation cross contamination from the clothes of patients exposed to lacrimators (used as riot-control agents).

Organophosphate occupational exposure is of specific importance to the pediatric HCW because these compounds are commonly used as interior house and garden insecticides, often stored in garages, and are highly contaminating. Organophosphates represent an estimated 2 to 3% of ingestions by children less than 5 years old, and up to 50% of fatal poisonings in young children. The route of accidental exposure in children is oral. Its unexpected taste and garliclike or petroleum odor is likely to cause the child to stop drinking and to throw down the bottle, thereby spilling the chemical on their clothes and skin. Contamination to the child, and cross contamination to the HCW, is secondary to its high lipid solubility, leading to easy skin, ocular, pulmonary, and gastrointestinal absorption. These factors along with inattention to the principles of chemical decontamination may lead to HCW toxicity while caring for these victims. Symptoms of acute toxicity are primarily systemic secondary to excess cholinergic effects, but can also include dermal irritation. Management principles, in addition to thorough skin and ocular decontamination, include cardiorespiratory support, gastrointestinal decontamination, and administration of antidotes (atropine and pralidoxime). When treating a victim of an organophosphate exposure, HCWs should wear rubber gloves, protective eyewear, and impermeable gowns. If cross contaminated, HCWs should remove their contaminated clothes and copiously irrigate their exposed skin and eyes with saline.

Occupational skin exposure to hydrocarbons (e.g., gasoline, kerosene, phenol), acids (e.g., hydrogen chloride), and alkalis (e.g., sodium hydroxide) via cross contamination can lead to dermal erythema, blistering, and deeper burns. When handling patients with these chemical exposures, HCWs should wear rubber gloves, protective eyewear, and impermeable gowns. If cross contaminated, HCWs should remove their contaminated clothes and copiously irrigate their exposed skin and eyes with saline. Ocular alkali exposure requires immediate ophthalmologic consultation in addition to irrigation.

RADIOACTIVE EXPOSURES

Radiation exposure in the ED is another potential health hazard facing HCWs. Exposure is almost exclusively related to diagnostic radiographs or roentgenograms taken during resuscitation efforts. Although rare, radiation accidents do occur and may contaminate health care workers if proper procedures are not followed. From 1944 until October 1990, 331 radiation accidents occurred worldwide (47). Most of these were in the United States.

Radiation Biology

Radiation denotes energy released from a source and comes in two forms—nonionizing (light, microwaves, radiowave, ultraviolet, etc.) and ionizing. Ionizing radiation is the most damaging to tissue and can be either nonparticulate (x-rays, gamma rays) or particulate. Particulate ionizing radiation is fur-

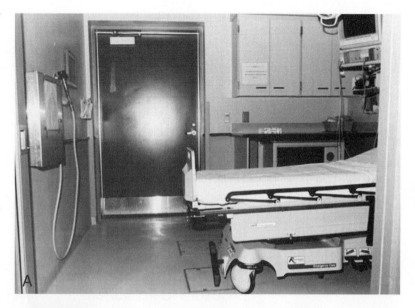

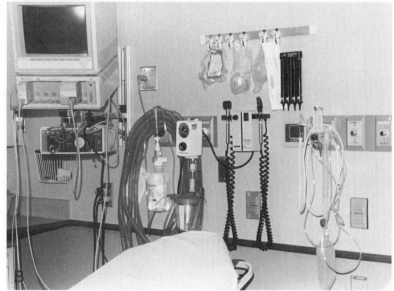

ther subdivided into uncharged (neutrons) and charged (α and β rays).

Because of tissue penetration, radiation exposures can result in somatic and hereditary effects. Tissues most at risk following exposure are bone marrow, breast, thyroid, and gonadal tissues. The dose equivalent of radiation is a rem. One rad is approximately equal to 1 rem. For example, the maximum permissible occupational dose equivalent for the whole body is 5 rems per year. However, pregnant women are allowed only 0.5 rem during the gestational period. The hands can be exposed to 75 rems per year, but no more than 25 rems in each quarter (48).

Figure 8.8.
A. A decontamination room has wall-mounted shower head, floor drain, and external entry door, in addition to
B. Usual monitoring and resuscitation capability.

In a United Kingdom study from 1992, 143 patients required emergency radiographs during resuscitation (49). A total of 790 radiographs were taken, and 4% were repeated. Seven physicians and one nurse were monitored for the cumulative exposure to their hands. Although none received radiation exceeding the acceptable limits, shield gloves were used infrequently. In only 5 of 85 occasions were lead gloves worn by the doctor during cross-table, lateral cervical radiographs.

PROCEDURES

Guidelines to Control the Exposure to Radiation

All hospitals are required to have an ED plan for handling radiation accidents. Main components of a plan are outlined in Table 8.5. Of

Table 8.5.
Hospital Plan for Emergency Treatment of Patient Contaminated with Radioactive Materials

Goal
    Hospital is prepared to provide care of patients contaminated with radioactive material in a manner that will minimize risk to staff and other patients.
Components:
    Notification:
        • Related injuries, type of exposure, number of patients?
        • Instruct ambulance crews to wait in ambulance on arrival
        • Notify hospital radiation safety officer
        • Notify other HCWs
    Emergency Department Area Preparation:
        • Assign a buffer zone nurse
        • Ensure that the ED decontamination room is prepared
        • Secure the area
    Health Care Worker Preparation:
        • Protective clothing and dosimeters are dispensed
        • Caps, surgical masks, water repellent gown, shoe covers, and gloves
    Patient arrival:
        • Meet patient at ambulance if condition permits. Remove and treat clothing as contaminated. Wrap clothing in sheet and transport with patient to decontamination room
        • Radiation officer measures radiation of patient and ambulance
        • Transport patient immediately to decontamination room by shortest route possible
        • Hold ambulance until determined free of radioactive contamination
    Patient Treatment (see also Table 129.2)
        • Proceed with medical needs
        • Internal and external decontamination
    HCW Decontamination
        • All HCWs should be carefully checked for contamination before leaving area and decontaminated if necessary

Table 8.6.
Rules to Protect the Health Care Worker from Radiation Exposure in the Emergency Department

The radiology technician should:
• set proper collination of the x-ray beam
• minimize retakes
The other health care workers should:
• use mechanical means of immobilization or adequate shielding
• maintain distance during procedure
• not order radiographs unless indicated

course, each hospital will design individualized plans based on staffing and the physical plant. Care of life-threatening conditions must always take priority over containment of contamination. Because radiation accidents are rare, drills should be conducted periodically in order to evaluate and familiarize HCWs with the protocol.

Furthermore, adherence to a few simple rules will reduce risk of radiation exposure when diagnostic radiographs are required (Table 8.6). The amount of exposure to x-rays is governed by time, distance, and shielding. Time is not often a factor in the ED. Having distance between the clinician and the radiation source (i.e., the radiographic machine) is frequently the best course. X-rays are governed by the "inverse square law," meaning that by doubling the distance from a source of radiation, the amount of exposure is reduced to 25%. Tripling the distance will reduce the exposure to 1% (47).

However, following this "distance" rule requires having mechanical methods to immobilize the child during the radiographic procedure rather than relying on parents or HCWs as "holders." If the HCW or parent is required to restrain the patient, proper shielding is important. Finally, quality improvement programs to reduce the number of repeat or unnecessary radiographs will reduce exposures in the ED.

SUMMARY

This chapter has provided an overview to protecting the NCW from occupational exposures. Procedural details are summarized in Tables 8.1 to 8.6 and Figs. 8.1 to 8.10.

REFERENCES

1. Tokars JI, Marcus R, Culver DH, et al. Surveillance of HIV and zidovudine use among health care workers after occupational exposure to HIV-infected blood. Ann Intern Med 1993;118:913–919.
2. Henderson DK, Fahey BJ, Willy M. Risk of occupational transmission of human immunodeficiency virus type 1 (HIV-1) associated with clinical exposures. Ann Intern Med 1990;113:740–746.
3. Marcus R, Bell D, Srivastava P, et al. Contact with HIV-infected blood among emergency care providers. Presented at the Third International Conference on Nosocomial Infections. Atlanta, GA: July 31–August 3, 1990.
4. Wong ES, Stotka JL, Chinchilli VM, et al. Are universal precautions effective in reducing the number of occupational exposures among health care workers? a prospective study of physicians on a medical service. JAMA 1991;265:1123–1128.
5. Baker JL, Kelen GD, Sivertson KT, Quinn TC. Unsuspected human immunodeficiency virus in critically ill emergency patients. JAMA 1987;257:2609–2611.
6. Kelen GD, Fritz S, Qaquish B, et al. Unrecognized human immunodeficiency virus infection in emergency department patients. N Engl J Med 1988;318:1645–1650.
7. Kelen GD, Fritz S, Qaquish B, et al. Substantial increase in human immunodeficiency virus (HIV-1) infection in critically ill emergency patients: 1986 and 1987 compared. Ann Emerg Med 1989;18:378–382.
8. Lewandowski C, Ognjan A, Rivers E, et al. Health care worker exposure to HIV-1 and HTLV I-II in critically ill, resuscitated emergency department patients. Ann Emerg Med 1992;21:1353–1359.
9. Baraff LJ, Talan DA, Torres M. Prevalence of HIV antibody in a non-inner-city university hospital emergency department. Ann Emerg Med 1991;20:782–786.
10. Rhee KJ, Albertson TE, Kizer KW, Hughes MJ, Ascher MS. The HIV-1 seroprevalence rate of injured patients admitted through California emergency departments. Ann Emerg Med 1991;20:969–972.
11. Sturm JT. HIV prevalence in a midwestern emergency department. Ann Emerg Med 1991;20:276–278.
12. Schweich PJ, Fosarelli PD, Duggan AK, et al. Prevalence of human immunodeficiency virus seropositivity in pediatric emergency room patients undergoing phlebotomy. Pediatrics 1990;86:660–665.
13. Centers for Disease Control and Prevention. Recommendations for preventing transmission of infection with human T-lymphotropic virus type III/ lymphadenopathy-associated virus in the workplace. MMWR 1985;34:681–686,691–695.
14. Centers for Disease Control and Prevention. Recommendations for the prevention of HIV transmission in health care settings. MMWR 1987;36(suppl 2S):1–18.
15. Centers for Disease Control and Prevention. Update: universal precautions for prevention of transmission of human immunodeficiency virus, hepatitis B virus, and other bloodborne pathogens in health care settings. MMWR 1988;37:377–382,387–388.
16. Centers for Disease Control and Prevention. Guidelines for prevention of transmission of human immunodeficiency virus and hepatitis B virus to health care and public safety workers. MMWR 1989;38(suppl 6S):1–37.
17. Centers for Disease Control and Prevention. Recommendations for preventing transmission of human immunodeficiency virus and hepatitis B virus to patients during exposure-prone invasive procedures. MMWR 1991;40(RR-8):1–9.
18. Friedland LR. Universal precautions and safety devices which reduce the risk of occupational exposure to bloodborne pathogens: a review for emergency health care workers. Pediatr Emerg Care 1991;7:356–362.
19. Mast ST, Gerberding JL. Factors predicting infectivity following needlestick exposure to HIV: an in vitro model. Clin Res 1991;39:58A.
20. Leclair JM, Freeman J, Sullivan BF, Crowley CM, Goldman DA. Prevention of nosocomial respiratory syncytial virus infections through compliance with glove and gown isolation precautions. N Engl J Med 1987;317:329–334.
21. Kelen GD, DiGiovanna TA, Celentano DD, et al. Adherence to universal (barrier) precautions during interventions on critically ill and injured emergency department patients. J Acquir Immune Defic Syndr 1990;3:987–994.
22. Baraff LJ, Talan DA. Compliance with universal precautions in a university hospital emergency department. Ann Emerg Med 1989;18:654–657.
23. Hammond JS, Eckes JM, Gomez GA, et al. HIV, trauma, and infection control: universal precautions are universally ignored. J Trauma 1990;30:555–558.
24. Courington KR, Patterson SL, Howard RJ. Universal precautions are not universally followed. Arch Surg 1991;126:93–96.
25. Henry K, Campbell S, Maki M. A comparison of observed and self-reported compliance with universal precautions among emergency department personnel at a Minnesota public teaching hospital: implications for assessing infection control programs. Ann Emerg Med 1991;21:940–946.
26. Friedland LR, Joffe M, Wiley JF, Schapire A, Moore DF. Effect of educational program on compliance with glove use in a pediatric emergency department. Am J Dis Child 1992;146:1355–1358.
27. Kelen GD, Green GB, Hexter DA, et al. Substantial improvement in compliance with universal precautions in an emergency depart-

ment following institution of policy. Arch Intern Med. 1991;151:2051–2056.

28. Talan DA, Baraff LJ. Effect of education on the use of universal precautions in a university hospital emergency department. Ann Emerg Med 1990;19:1322–1326.

29. Occupational Safety and Health Administration. Occupational exposure to bloodborne pathogens: final rule. Federal Register. 1991;56:64,175–64,182.

30. Marcus R, and the CDC Cooperative Needlestick Surveillance Group. Surveillance of health care workers exposed to blood from patients infected with the human immunodeficiency virus. N Engl J Med 1988;319:1118–1123.

31. Jagger J, Hunt EH, Brand-Elnaggar J, Pearson RD. Rates of needlestick injury caused by various devices in a university hospital. N Engl J Med 1988;319:284–288.

32. Emergency Care Research Institute. Needlestick prevention devices. Health Devices. 1991 May;20:154–180.

33. Schuman AJ. Preventing needlesticks and their consequences. Contemp Peds 1992 June;9:76–106.

34. Owens-Schwab E, Fraser VJ. Needleless and needle protection devices: a second look at efficacy and selection. Infect Control Hosp Epidemiol 1993;14:657–660.

35. Doebbeling BN, Wenzel RP. The direct costs of universal precautions in a teaching hospital. JAMA 1990;264:2083–2087.

36. American Academy of Pediatrics. In: Peter G, ed. 1994 Red Book: report of the Committee on Infectious Diseases. 23rd ed. Elk Grove Village, IL: American Academy of Pediatrics; 1994:254.

37. Klontz KC, Gunn RA, Caldwell JS. Needlestick injuries and hepatitis B immunization in Florida paramedics: a statewide survey. Ann Emerg Med 1991 December;20:1310–1313.

38. Go GW, Baraff LJ, Schriger DL. Management guidelines for health care workers exposed to blood and body fluids. Ann Emerg Med 1991;20:1341–1350.

39. Callaham ML. Prophylaxis with zidovudine (AZT) after exposure to human immunodefi-

ciency virus: a brief discussion of the issues for emergency physicians. Ann Emerg Med 1991;20:1351–1354.

40. Centers for Disease Control and Prevention. Hepatitis B virus: a comprehensive strategy for eliminating transmission in the US through universal childhood vaccinations, recommendations of the ACIP. MMWR 1991;40(RR-13)1.

41. Guidelines for preventing the transmission of tuberculosis in health care settings, with special focus on HIV-related issues. MMWR 1990;39(RR-17):1–29.

42. Fein JA, Friedland LR, Rutstein R, Bell LM. Children with unrecognized human immunodeficiency virus infection: an emergency department perspective. Am J Dis Child 1993;147:1104–1108.

43. Kay MM, Henschel AF, Butler J, et al., eds. Occupational diseases. A guide to their recognition. Washington, DC: HEW, 1977, p. 16.

44. Agency for Toxic Substances and Disease Registry. Managing hazardous materials incidents. Volume 2: Hospital emergency departments—a planning guide for the management of contaminated patients. Atlanta, GA, 1992.

45. Ellenhorn MJ, Barceloux DG. Introduction and initial evaluation. In: Medical toxicology, Elsevier, New York: 1988.

46. Hartnett L. Environmental contamination. In: Goldfrank LR et al., eds, Toxicologic Emergencies. Norwalk, CT: Appleton and Lange, 1990.

47. Mettler FA, Royal HD, Drum DE. Environmental emergencies (radiation accidents). In: Fleisher GL, Ludwig S, eds. Textbook of pediatric emergency medicine. Baltimore, MD: Williams & Wilkins, 1993, 824–837.

48. National Institutes of Health. Report of the National Institutes of Health ad hoc Working Group to Develop Radioepidemiological Tables. NIH Publication 85-2748. Washington DC: US Department of Health and Human Services, 1985.

49. Evans RJ, Cusack S, Parkek T. Exposure of the hands to ionizing radiation in the resuscitation room of an accident and emergency department. Arch Emerg Med 1992;9:220–224.

CHAPTER 9

INFORMED CONSENT

Richard T. Strait and Richard M. Ruddy

INTRODUCTION

Every person has the right to be informed regarding their medical care and then consent or dissent to the proposed treatments. A person's age and mental capacity may impact on the degree of self-determination exercised in receiving medical care. In this chapter, the concept of informed consent is developed in relation to the pediatric emergency physician, the patient, and the parent or guardian. This chapter will discuss the legal principles of informed consent and provide definitions of the concept of informed consent, minor consent, dissent and leaving against medical advice. It will conclude with some illustrative examples of common problems of informed consent in the pediatric emergency department (ED) and options for solution. References are provided for the reader seeking further in-depth discussion of informed consent.

LEGAL PRINCIPLES

Consent for medical treatment is a fairly recent notion. As late as 1847, the American Medical Association Code of Ethics stated, "The obedience of a patient to the prescriptions of his physician should be prompt and implicit. He should never permit his own crude opinions as to their fitness to influence his attention to them." (1) In 1914 Justice Cordozzo (*Schloendorff v. New York Hospital*) made his statement that began the ideal of consent, "Every human being of adult years and sound mind has a right to determine what shall be done with his own body . . . ." Later

came not just an interest in consent, but also in its quality (1, 2). In 1957, the case of *Salvo v. Leland Stanford Jr. University Board of Trustees* offered a legal decision which is believed to be the birth of informed consent. The court stated that it is the physician's duty to disclose "any facts which are necessary to form the basis of intelligent consent by the patient to the proposed treatment" (1). This simply means that for consent to be valid the patient must be given sufficient information to understand the nature of the decision. This decision marked the beginning of the shift of medicolegal cases based on assault, battery, and tort law to ones based on negligence or malpractice (Table 9.1).

In the early 1970s, another shift occurred characterized by the emphasis that disclosure of information regarding medical therapy fit the patient's needs. The 1972 *Canterbury v. Spence* decision stated "the scope of the physician's communication to the patient . . . must be measured by the patient's need, and that need is the information material to the decision" (3). The American Medical Association endorsed this theory at that time asserting "the patient's right of self-decision can be effectively exercised only if the patient possesses enough information to enable an intelligent choice" (3).

The concept of informed consent is somewhat more complex and often imprecise when applied to consent for minors. Two centuries ago, English common law held that the father's right of custody of his children took precedence over the mother's and all other's (4). In colonial times, children had no constitutional rights so parents had absolute control

Table 9.1.
Legal Terminology

Assault—unlawful placing of an individual in fear of immediate
 bodily harm
Battery—intentional touching of another person's body without
 authorization
Tort—intentional wrong
Negligence—omission of reasonable care or action

over them. This is known as "parental sovereignty" and is still held highly by the courts today. In 1912, in the case of *Luka v. Lowrie,* the court decided that in an emergency any child may be treated without parental consent, which was a break from the traditional ideal of parental sovereignty (4). However, in 1933 in the case of *Zuman v. Schultz,* it was decided that nonemergency treatment of a child without the consent of a parent gives rise to assault and battery charges against the physician rendering care (4). This decision reinforced the ideal of parental control. In 1967, the Supreme Court ruled that a child may be treated differently from an adult by a government entity (referring to a government-funded hospital) only if the difference accrues to the child's benefit (4). This means that lack of consent should not keep a minor from receiving the proper medical care equivalent to that of an adult. This has been interpreted to include treatment at all medical facilities, not just at ones that are federally funded. In 1971, voting age dropped from 21 to 18 years old and subsequently the age of majority in each state has dropped to 18.

DEFINITIONS OF INFORMED CONSENT

According to Holder, *informed consent* is "the duty (of the physician) to warn a patient of the hazards, possible complications and expected and unexpected results of a proposed treatment" (4). Informed consent should contain the following five basic elements (5, 6, 7) (*a*) the patient and/or parent should be told in lay terms the diagnosis and prognosis; (*b*) the nature and purpose of the proposed treatment should be explained in detail; (*c*) the significant risks and consequences of the proposed treatment need to be discussed. *Significant risk* is best interpreted

to mean any consequent event of treatment with a high probability of occurring or with a devastating enough result that a person would want to know; (*d*) the probability and degree of success of the proposed treatment are communicated; and (*e*) all feasible alternative treatments and their benefits, risks, and success rates are discussed. The last four elements are referred to as the "reasonable patient standard" (6) which is the information that any reasonable patient and/or parent would need in order to make an informed decision about the treatment (Table 9.2).

Variation can exist in content of communicated information according to geographic location and individual situation. This difference in content from area to area is referred to as "*local practice standards.*" Recently the court system has shifted away from local to more national standards for informed consent (4). Given the "information highway" that exists now and access to information to most people, this direction for the courts is not surprising. The specifics of the information rendered should be adapted to the ability of the patient or parent to understand.

A key aspect of consent is the patient's or the parent or guardian's ability to understand the information and have the capacity to make decisions. Capacity is a person's decision-making ability. Health care providers assess whether patients or parents understand options for treatment, the consequences of options for treatment, and the personal cost and benefits of the treatment (1, 7). They also attempt to consider the apparent level of intelligence of the patient or guardian and his or her ability to express choice. Evidence of patient and parent understanding should be communicated back to the health care provider by the patient or the parent or guardian. The physician also seeks to understand the reasonableness of the choice that is made when obtaining consent. Strictly speaking, if the patient lacks capacity to give con-

Table 9.2.
Components of Informed Consent

1. Diagnosis and condition of the patient
2. "Reasonable patient standard":
   - Nature and purpose of the proposed treatment
   - Risks and consequences of the proposed treatment
   - Probability of success
   - Feasible alternatives with benefits, risks, and success rates

sent, the physician must obtain consent from a third party. The physician, absent a serious emergency, must have a patient or guardian's consent before initiating treatment. However, the physician should not allow the lack of consent to unduly affect the patient's health.

In an emergency setting, other types of consent are important to understand for anyone providing care to children. Whenever a patient enters a hospital ED to be treated, he or she is asked to sign a *general consent* form (3). This usually involves signing the ED record and agreeing to evaluation and treatment. It usually takes place at registration and little or no information on medical care is exchanged before this consent. The general consent form should be thought of as a statement of a willingness to be examined and have minor treatment done. It is not informed consent and all significant interventions unless immediately life-saving will require further consent by the patient or parent. In *expressed consent,* the patient or parent is aware of the proposed care, agrees to such, and in some manner demonstrates a willingness to proceed (3). This is common when the physician wants to obtain a blood sample and the parent approves of the test being done. An additional subtype is *implied consent,* (2, 5) which is consent inferred by the actions of the patient without specific agreement. An example is when a patient rolls up a sleeve to receive an injection. A further subtype of *implied consent* is implied parental consent. For example, parents send their child to the ED for care of a laceration and phone approval is obtained. It is implied that the parent would want care to be definitive at that visit. Physicians may treat any minor seeking emergency care if they believe that any reasonable parent would agree to treatment. The legal term for this implied parental consent is "in loco parentis." *Deferred consent* is consent after the fact. An example is treatment with epinephrine for severe bronchospasm given to an obtunded patient and getting consent after the patient has improved (3). There is legitimate debate as to whether this is informed consent or deferred support or assent to what already was done.

An important subtype of consent for an ED physician is *emergency consent* (3, 5) It applies in situations when "immediate treatment is deemed necessary to prevent loss of life or permanent disability and the patient lacks the capacity to make independent decisions." The physician is allowed and expected to act in the patient's best interests. Most states have broadened this to include those conditions that require prompt treatment such as alleviating pain, suturing, or fracture reduction (5). The physician does not have to be certain as to the actual eventuality of harm, but only that harm or injury is a reasonable possibility. These laws are deliberately broad to encourage treatment without fear of liability. States such as South Carolina, North Carolina, and Oklahoma require a second opinion if surgery is contemplated (5). Although a second opinion is not required by law elsewhere, it may often be prudent to obtain one if the process will not greatly increase risk of less than optimal outcome.

ISSUES AND DEFINITIONS IN CONSENT FOR MINORS

A *minor* is defined by law to be a person who has not yet reached the age of 18 years. Minors are legally incapable of giving consent (6). Therefore a parent or guardian must consent for them. However, there are no reported legal decisions that hold a physician liable for treating a minor for his or her own benefit in a nonelective situation without consent. Also, in most states, *minor treatment statutes* allow for older minors to consent to "ordinary medical treatment" (4). Ordinary medical treatment in this setting refers to treatment with only minimal risk.

Additional confusion exists as to when minors are able to consent for themselves. These exceptions are based on the minors themselves and on specific medical problems. Exceptions based on minors fall under two categories—*emancipated minor* and *mature minor*. The precise definitions of each vary from state to state, but the following holds for most states. A minor is considered emancipated and able to give consent if he or she is living alone and/or financially independent, a high school graduate, serving in the military, or married, pregnant, or a parent (Table 9.3) (3–6, 8).

A minor can be considered mature and therefore able to give consent if he or she is 15 years old and understands the nature and

Table 9.3.
Minor Issues Definitions

Minor—any person under the age of 18 years
Emancipated minor—living alone and/or financially independent such as:
- high school graduate
- serving in the military
- married, pregnant, or parent

Mature minor—15 years old *and* understands nature and risks of the treatment and physician believes all of the following:
- the patient can make an informed decision
- treatment is in the minor's best interest
- treatment does not involve serious risks

risks of the treatment and the physician believes the following three items are true. First, the minor can make an informed decision. Secondly, treatment is in the minor's best interest. Lastly, treatment does not involve serious risks (Table 9.3) (3–6, 8).

Exceptions to minor consent based on medical problems are in place in many states. These exceptions are based on the belief that the need to be treated outweighs the parents' right to consent in some medical situations when it is in the minor's or society's best interest. An example is a sexually transmitted disease. The minor and society both benefit from treatment. These are known as *minor treatment statutes*. In order to encourage minors to seek medical care for these problems, the statutes allow for immediate and confidential treatment for the minor. Some states go so far as to forbid informing the parents unless it puts the minor at undo risk not to inform the parents. Common medical problems covered under the majority of state statutes are mental illness, substance abuse, pregnancy, sexually transmitted diseases, emergencies, suspected child abuse, and victims of crime (4–6, 8).

In some circumstances, consent for treatment for minors can seem confusing and troublesome, especially when deciding which adult parent can give consent for the minor. A physician may treat a minor with consent of only one parent as long as there is no reason to believe the other parent would object (4, 5) No cases are found of a physician being successfully sued under these circumstances. In divorce the custodial parent retains the duty to provide care and give consent. However, the parent with actual physical control at the time the health need arises may give consent (4, 5, 8). In foster care, the foster parents or the institution or agency may give consent for

routine health care. However, for elective or major treatment the person empowered to give consent depends on whether the placement was voluntary or involuntary. If placement was voluntary the parents must give consent, and if involuntary then the social agency gives consent and the foster parents may not (5, 8). In detention facilities the parents maintain custody and therefore right to consent (5, 8). When a child is away from the care of his or her parents such as at school or camp there is often a blanket consent form that the parents sign, which gives consent for treatment. These consents do not cover nonemergency care. Because there is support for true emergency care implied from the law, these forms do not add additional support for treatment of a non-emergency without consent (4, 5, 8). When runaways are involved, the parent maintains custody and right of consent unless the child can be considered mature or emancipated (4, 8). Lastly, if the parent is a minor then the courts tend to view this parent like any other parent. The minor then may give his or her own consent if he or she has the capacity to understand (4, 5, 6).

DISSENT

Dissent or refusal of treatment can be very troubling to ED staff. However, the reality is that if a patient has a right to consent, there exists a right to dissent. The decision to dissent must be accepted just as readily as that of consent. Numerous reasons exist why people dissent for treatment. One of the most frequent is for religious beliefs. Patients and/or parents may refuse medical treatment on religious grounds as long as there is no threat to the health of others (6). An example when dissent is disallowed would be treatment for tuberculosis. Additionally, parents do not have the right to deny emergency medical care to their child (*State v. Perricone,* 1962) (8). However, at the same time, states will provide immunity from prosecution for medical neglect to parents who withhold consent for religious reasons (5).

Another difficult situation arises about consent when it is refused by the adolescent. Even if the parents consent, there are some circumstances where the minor's dissent takes priority. An adolescent's dissent must be accepted if he or she can be considered a mature minor, an emancipated minor, or if the situation falls under specific treatment statutes (4).

Arguably the most difficult situation occurs when the parent refuses consent. Courts generally support parental control over the child's health care. Still, a child's health cannot be seriously jeopardized because of the parent's limitations or convictions (6, 8). Additionally, parents do not have the authority to deny life-saving treatment for their child. The physician and states depend on the child abuse statutes for help in obtaining custody and rendering treatment (8).

The physician's role in refused treatment varies according to the type of patient and the degree to which treatment is needed and beneficial. The more serious the illness and the more beneficial the treatment, the greater the physician's involvement and efforts should be. With the *mature or emancipated minors*, the physician must first decide on the capacity of the patient. If the patient appears competent, then the physician should try to discover the reason(s) for the dissent. Often it is related to anger and/or anxiety. The anger can come from a perception and frustration of a long wait, a rude staff member, the feeling of being used in an experiment, or a misunderstanding of the disease and its treatment. Anxiety can come from lack of understanding about the disease or treatment, from observing other occurrences in the ED, or from a sense of a loss of control.

Once the reason for dissent is known, addressing that reason may be all that is necessary to obtain consent. If discussion with the patient does not work, then involving another individual that the patient trusts such as the primary caregiver, a friend, a family member, or a religious leader may assist in obtaining consent.

If the physician fails to obtain consent, then the refusal of treatment should be thoroughly documented as follows. A careful history and physical examination should be noted, assuming the patient allowed such a clinical evaluation. The reasons for considering the patient to be competent should be clearly stated. The patient must be competent for refusal to be accepted. The risks and benefits of the proposed treatment and any alternative treatments including no treatment should be included. A brief explanation of why the physician feels the proposed treat-

Table 9.4.
Documentation of Dissent

- History and physical examination if obtained
- Reasons for considering the patient and/or guardian competent
- Risks and benefits of the proposed treatment
- Risks and benefits of alternative treatment including no treatment
- Why the proposed treatment was refused
- That an offer was made to provide treatment at any future time if the patient and/or parent changes their mind
- Witness of refusal

ment was refused is noted. The patient should understand that if he or she has a change of mind at any time, treatment will be available, and the offer is further documented. Lastly, the refusal and the documentation of the refusal should be witnessed. It is worthwhile to have the patient and a third party read and sign the documented refusal if possible (Table 9.4).

The physician's role in the refusal of treatment involving an *immature or unemancipated minor* differs from refusal of an adult. Again the physician must decide on competency, but in this case it is both of the minor and of the parents. The physician should try to define exactly why the treatment is being refused and address those issues. If refusal remains, then the physician should involve a trusted individual of the patient's or parents'. If despite good efforts refusal of care persists, the physician must decide on the degree to which intervention is required. If the condition is life threatening then the physician has four options. The best option depends on the urgency of the situation. The physician can (*a*) take temporary protective custody based on the child neglect statutes; (*b*) report to the hospital administrator and attorney; (*c*) contact the local child protective agency; or (*d*) obtain a court order to render care (5).

Taking custody is the quickest option, but the physician is usually treading in unfamiliar territory. If possible it is best to engage someone who is more familiar with the legal system. Relying on the hospital attorney and/or administrator to settle the issue can take time. Regardless of the option chosen, hospital staff should be informed of the situation in a timely manner. The best option, if there is little time, is to involve the hospital social worker and the local child protective agency. They know the system and can work

Figure 9.1.
Parents who refuse consent
for their child's lumbar
puncture.

A 5-month-old infant presents to the ED with fever, irritability and vomiting. After evaluation, the ED physician recommends lumbar puncture to exclude the diagnosis of meningitis. The parents initially refuse consent.

- The physician notes the child's ill appearance and abnormal examination findings, and emphasizes that these are suggestive of meningitis.
- The physician explains the potential serious consequences of delayed diagnosis and treatment of meningitis.
- The relatively low risk and frequent experience in performing lumbar puncture are detailed.

The parents listen attentively, and are assessed as competent to give informed consent, but continue to refuse.

- The parents are asked to discuss their reluctance. It is revealed that in the father's family a relative had been ill, underwent lumbar puncture and subsequently suffered paralysis. This event had occurred more than 50 years ago, and the story had been passed down through several generations.
- The physician attempts to put this family history into context, pointing out that the illness occurred during the poliomyelitis era, and at a time when treatment for bacterial meningitis was not available. The likely relationship between the disease itself and the paralysis is noted. The rarity of neurologic complications from lumbar puncture in febrile infants is re-emphasized.

The parents now give consent.	The parents continue to refuse.

- Under these circumstances, it would be advisable to document the discussion in the medical record, and obtain written consent.

- Options to the ED physician include:
- Consider empiric antibiotic therapy, without preceding lumbar puncture. This course may be more acceptable to this family, without unduly delaying treatment. However, definitive diagnosis is delayed or lost, and hospitalization may be prolonged, or have been unnecessary. Detailed documentation is necessary.
- Initiate emergency assumption of protective custody, with hospital security assistance as necessary. Simultaneously, notify hospital attorney, social worker, child protective agency or courts, as per community protocols. Perform lumbar puncture, and start antibiotic treatment as indicated. Detailed documentation is necessary.

in a very efficient manner if need be. The last option of obtaining a court order can be very time consuming. The reality is that all of these people and agencies may become involved eventually in difficult cases.

Most courts tend to prefer that the child protective agencies seek the court order for treatment. If there is no time to involve the child protective services then physicians should seek the court order themselves. Historically, the courts have supported the parents' right to refuse care in nonserious and nonlife-threatening conditions. When the courts do get involved they use a case-by-case analysis. Factors that are taken into account include whether the treatment will restore the patient to a normal life, whether refusal has suicidal or homicidal motives, the competence of the patient and parent, the age of the patient (i.e., could the decision

wait until the child can be considered mature, emancipated, or an adult), and whether the patient has dependent children. Conflicting medical opinions on the proposed treatment or alternative treatments can be an important factor in the court denying or maintaining the parent or guardian's right to decide on medical care. Figure 9.1 illustrates an example of an approach to parents who refuse consent for lumbar puncture on their infant with likely meningitis.

LEAVING AGAINST MEDICAL ADVICE

Another difficult situation for the emergency physician is when the patient or parent wants to leave against medical advice. This can and should be handled in much the same manner as dissent. The physician needs to decide on the competence of the patient and/or parent. If they are felt to be competent then the reason for wanting to leave needs to be discovered and specifically addressed. The approach to the family and patient needs to be one of compassion, sensitivity, and diplomacy. Involvement of a trusted family member can be very helpful. If the physician fails to persuade the patient to stay, then the decision on just how imperative it is that the patient stay to be evaluated and treated must be made. **Parents may not leave with a child if a life-threatening condition exists, if there is suspected child abuse, or if the parent is incompetent** (6, 7, 8). The same actions and documentation should occur as for the patient or parent who refuses treatment.

OBTAINING AND DOCUMENTING INFORMED CONSENT

Ideally the physician performing the procedure should obtain the consent, but there may be a designee to do this. It would be wise to first have the performing physician obtain the consent while the future designee observes this interaction. Then when comfortable and knowledgeable about the procedure, the designated physicians should be allowed to obtain consent while the performing physician observes the process. This sequence allows education of the designees about the purpose and significant risks of the procedure, allows them to be mentored, and provides the performing physicians an opportunity to assess that future informed consent is complete and accurate even in their absence. When discussing the proposed procedure and obtaining the informed consent from the parent or patient, the physician should address the five elements discussed in Table 9.2. The consent process should also be witnessed by a third party and documented in writing when appropriate.

Documentation should ideally record exactly what was discussed. The more risky the treatment the more detailed the documentation should be. Common and low risk treatments, as many routine ED procedures are, need minimal informed consent and little or no written consent. This does not mean that consent should be overlooked in this situation, only that it can be abbreviated. Additionally, physicians need to decide for themselves how comfortable they are with the amount of written documentation they obtain (see also Chapter 11, pp. 79–82).

In uncommon, controversial, and high risk treatments more comprehensive written documentation should be obtained. The patient or the guardian should read and sign a consent form, which includes all risks and benefits. Remember that written consent does not substitute for the informed consent discussion between the physician and the patient. A well-informed patient or parent averts future legal cases more than a signed consent form.

WHEN INFORMED CONSENT IS NOT NECESSARY

Five different instances occur when full, informed consent is not necessary. The first is when patients or parents state they do not want to know the risks and will proceed with the treatment (1,5). It is still optimal for physicians to attempt informed consent, but they are not obligated in this circumstance. A second instance when informed consent can be waived is known as "therapeutic privilege." The physician believes that disclosure of the risks would substantially or adversely affect the patient's health. It does not apply to minors since the parents are the ones who must consent, and disclosure of the risk only to the parents may avoid the patient being placed at risk by the discussion of the issues (1, 4, 5). The third instance is when the risk of the treatment is considered common knowledge (5). Examples include an injection or placement of an intravenous line. In this instance, the patient and family should be informed as part of the procedure, but it may not require the detail indicated for more complex problems. The fourth instance is when the situation does not allow informed consent, such as a patient in cardiac arrest (1). Last is the setting in which the physician assesses patients and/or parents as lacking the capacity to understand their plight and/or the proposed treatment (1). In this instance, the physician needs to fully document the assessment in the record.

SUMMARY

Informed consent is a key element in the proper delivery of quality health care in the ED. As outlined, the components of good consent generally follow common sense, but are predicated on the principle that patients or their guardians have the right to understand and concur with the therapies the children are to receive. In true emergencies, the need to provide timely care can and should preclude the detailed explanation of treatment to maximize the likelihood of good outcomes. Though documentation is important, thorough and easy to understand explanations to patients and parents are the most important components of informed consent.

REFERENCES

1. Botkin JR. Informed consent for lumbar puncture. Am J Dis Child 1989;143:899–904.
2. Iserson KV. Bioethics. In: Rosen P, Barkin RM, Braen GR et al. eds. Emergency medicine: concepts and clinical practice. St. Louis: CV Mosby, 1992, 37–48.
3. Seigel DM. Consent and refusal of treatment. Emerg Med Clin North Am 1993;11:833–840.
4. Holder AR. Legal issues in pediatrics and adolescent medicine. New Haven, CT: Yale University Press, 1985, chapter 5.
5. Morrissey JM, Hofmann AD, Thorpe JC. Consent and confidentiality in the health care of children and adolescents: a legal guide. New York: Free Press, 1986.
6. Korin JB, Selbst SM. Legal aspects of emergency department pediatrics. In: Fleisher GR and Ludwig S, eds. Textbook of pediatric emergency medicine. Baltimore: Williams & Wilkins, 1993, 1559–1564.
7. Rice MM. Emergency department patients leaving against medical advice. Foresight 1994;29:1–8.
8. Sullivan DJ. Minors and emergency medicine. Emerg Med Clin North Am 1993;11:841–851.

CHAPTER 10

TEACHING PROCEDURES

Roy M. Kulick

INTRODUCTION

Teaching procedures is an integral, yet challenging aspect of pediatric emergency medicine practice. The challenge stems from the complexity of psychomotor skills, the hectic, unpredictable emergency department (ED) setting, uncooperative patients, and frantic parents. In addition, opportunities to perform potentially life-saving emergency procedures are rare and when they do occur, it is often not the appropriate time for student practice.

"See one, do one, teach one." This familiar saying describes the traditional approach to teaching procedures to medical students, residents and fellows. Perry Klass' less generous version—"See three, try four, miss them all" reflects the problems with this approach (1). The purpose of this chapter is to move beyond this haphazard teaching tradition to describe a structured, systematic approach to teaching procedures based on principles of psychomotor skill learning.

Teaching a psychomotor skill can be thought of as a procedure in and of itself. To illustrate this point, this chapter will, to the extent possible, follow the textbook's general chapter outline for procedures. In "Anatomy and Physiology" we will discuss the theoretical framework for understanding how adults learn psychomotor skills, in "Equipment" the advantages and disadvantages of available teaching resources, in "Procedure" a step-by-step approach to teaching procedures, and in "Complications" special considerations when teaching procedures at the bedside. Finally the section "Other Issues" is added,

which is a brief discussion on documenting competency, credentialing, and maintaining skills.

ANATOMY AND PHYSIOLOGY

Three phases of psychomotor learning have been described (2). During the *cognitive phase* the student intellectually analyzes the skill and develops a mental image. This is followed by the *fixation phase* during which motor patterns are practiced until correct behaviors are well established. Finally, during the *autonomous phase* the student becomes more "expert" in developing increasing speed and precision. The student moves from initially performing the procedure awkwardly under total conscious control to performing the procedure smoothly under total or near-total automatic control.

Three important conditions exist that influence the acquisition of new skills (2). *Contiguity* is the proper sequence and appropriate timing of motor responses. *Practice* is second and involves rehearsal and fixation of the skill. The amount of practice required will vary depending on the ability of the student and the complexity of the task. *Feedback* is the third and possibly most important condition that influences the learning of psychomotor skills. Feedback provides the learner with immediate evaluation of his or her current performance to improve future performance. Without feedback, accurate performance is not reinforced, and errors remain uncorrected and persist. Red Auerbach, the legendary Boston Celtic coach, eloquently summarized this point in basketball when he said "Practice does not make perfect, ... *perfect* practice makes perfect" (3).

EQUIPMENT

Many resources are currently available to facilitate teaching procedures, each with advantages and disadvantages (3–6)

Mannequins such as the familiar Resusianne and other man-made models are used widely. They are available for a variety of procedures including CPR, intubation, and venipuncture. Because they can be used multiple times, mannequins are considerably less expensive than live animal models. Although their quality continues to improve, their major disadvantage is limited reality.

Pig's feet or ears for wound care and chicken legs for intraosseous infusion are useful models. These animal parts are readily available and inexpensive.

Live animals such as pigs or dogs treated compassionately under approved protocols are effective models for invasive procedures such as cricothyroidotomy, thoracostomy, peritoneal lavage, and central venous access (4). Using animals for this purpose has become increasingly controversial as animal rights groups have become more vocal and influential. In addition, live animals are expensive.

Human volunteers, both paid and unpaid, are useful for relatively noninvasive procedures such as casting, splinting, intravenous catheter placement, and nasogastric tube placement. Students can also practice many of these procedures on each other.

Human cadavers may also be used to practice procedures. There are few procedures that cannot be done nearly as well on a fresh cadaver as on a live human being and the experience is generally highly rated by students (6). Cadavers, however, are expensive.

Using the "newly dead" for learning procedures is practiced in some training programs. The debate related to the ethics of this practice and whether family consent is necessary has recently resurfaced. Of recently surveyed U.S. training programs in adult and pediatric critical care and emergency medicine, 39% described using newly deceased patients for teaching resuscitation procedures (7). The highest proportion was among emergency medicine residency programs (68%), and tracheal intubation was by far the most common procedure. Among the 39% who use the newly dead, only 10% attempted to get verbal or written consent from the family. As difficult as getting consent may seem, in a recent prospective study, 59% of 46 families gave consent to perform wire-guided retrograde intubation on their newly deceased adult relatives in the ED (8).

Most recently, computer virtual reality systems, similar to that used to train airline pilots, have been developed to simulate the human body. Prototype systems for practicing surgical procedures are under development. "Using a head-mounted display and DataGlove,™ a person can learn anatomy from a new perspective by 'flying' inside and around organs, or can practice surgical procedures with a scalpel and clamps" (9). Although not yet readily available, this technology is likely to become more commonplace over the next several years.

Resources for teaching the cognitive component of procedures (indications, equipment, anatomy, etc.) include textbooks, videotapes (commercial and locally produced), and computer technology such as videodisks and CD-ROM. These resources allow students to study the material at their own convenience and to stop and review critical parts of the procedure. Computer-based systems may, in addition, allow the student to interact with the material and receive instant feedback on their responses (3, 5, 9, 10).

Finally, physician colleagues in related specialties are valuable teaching resources. For example, airway skills may be taught and practiced in the operating room under the supervision of anesthesiologists. Similarly, colleagues from other specialties such as surgery, plastic surgery, and ophthalmology may be available. In addition, nurses and allied health professionals may be adept at teaching the procedures they routinely perform such as splinting and wound care.

PROCEDURE

The cognitive component of a procedure includes relevant anatomy and physiology, indications, contraindications, complications, and equipment. The correct performance of

Table 10.1.
Basic Steps of Orotracheal Intubation in Adults and Older Children

1. Put on gloves and goggles	19. Insert blade into mouth
2. Check patient ventilation	20. Lift at 45° angle
3. Select correct size of ET tube	21. Gently advance blade, observing landmarks
4. Check cuff for leaks	22. Suction as needed
5. Leave syringe attached	23. Apply cricoid pressure as needed
6. Insert stylet into tube	24. Expose tracheal opening
7. Recess stylet 1 cm from end of tube	25. Place tube between cords
8. Bend tube appropriately	26. Advance tube to position
9. Lubricate tube	27. Remove stylet
10. Attach blade to handle	28. Inflate cuff and remove syringe
11. Ensure that light is working	29. Ventilate patient
12. Turn on suction device	30. Observe for chest rise
13. Instruct assistant for time counts, handing over suction or tube	31. Auscultate for breath sounds and air entering stomach
14. Position patient	32. Secure tube in position
15. Hyperventilate with mask	33. Recheck for proper tube position
16. Grasp laryngoscope	34. Document breath sounds heard and any complication
17. Open patient's mouth	35. Clean or dispose of contaminated equipment
18. Begin timing	

Adapted with permission from Thomas H. Teaching procedural skill: beyond "see one—do one." Acad Emerg Med 1994;1:399.

each step of the procedure is then described. These concepts should be reviewed and understood before actually performing the psychomotor skill.

The key to teaching the psychomotor component of a procedure is to divide it into small discrete steps (2, 3, 5, 11). The appropriate level of detail in each step will vary depending on the degree of exactness the students will need to learn the skill. An example of the discrete, component steps used to teach paramedics orotracheal intubation is illustrated in Table 10.1 (3, 12).

The process of teaching a procedure itself may be similarly divided into three broad phases corresponding to the phases of psychomotor learning already discussed (2). The introductory (cognitive) phase allows the student to develop a mental plan for the procedure. During the practice (fixation) phase the student is supervised while rehearsing the skill and is given feedback to reduce errors and strengthen correct responses. Finally, the perfecting (autonomous) phase is generally a more extended period during which the student performs the skill under realistic clinical conditions and improves speed and precision. A fourth phase that many would add is the teaching phase, which provides students the opportunity to demonstrate their mastery of the skill by successfully teaching it to a new student (3). Table 10.2 lists the first three phases divided into their component steps as they would be presented in, for example, the setting of a procedure workshop (2).

Many times procedures are taught and practiced at the bedside in the less controlled ED setting. Teaching a procedure on patients in the ED requires modification of the sequence outlined above (11). The instructor should initiate a brief, focused, preprocedure discussion as outlined in Table 10.3. Using a diagram and/or model will facilitate this discussion. Often a brief review of the surface anatomy of the student or instructor will suffice. Ideally, this brief teaching interaction should be conducted out of sight and hearing of the patient and family. The family should, however, be informed of the student-instructor relationship. This will make it more comfortable for the instructor

Table 10.2.
Phases of Teaching a Procedure*

Introductory (Cognitive) Phase
1. Explicitly describe the objective of the session and the expected performance outcome.
2. Describe the relevant anatomy and physiology, indications, contraindications, and potential complications.
3. Familiarize the student with the required equipment.
4. Demonstrate and simultaneously articulate how each sequential step of the procedure is correctly performed.

Practice (Fixation) Phase
1. Both verbally and physically guide the first attempt of each student to perform the procedure.
2. Provide immediate feedback by instructor and/or peers.
3. Allow time for independent practice.
4. Document that the student is able to correctly perform the procedure in the practice setting.

Perfecting (Autonomous) Phase
1. Provide the opportunity for students to practice and receive feedback under realistic clinical conditions.

* Adapted from Whitman N, Lawrence P, 1991.

Table 10.3.
Bedside Preprocedure Focused Discussion*

1. Relevant anatomy and physiology
2. Indications
3. Contraindications
4. Equipment
5. Patient information (informed consent)
6. Step-by-step procedure demonstration
7. Complications

* Adapted from Hedges JR, 1994.

to coach the student during the actual procedure. Still, it is often useful to surreptitiously guide the student through the procedure while "explaining" the procedure step-by-step to the patient.

Another principle of an effective procedure demonstration in any setting is to have the student observe the procedure from the appropriate position (11). This position is the one from which the student will actually perform the procedure and often requires standing behind the instructor and viewing over the instructor's shoulder (Fig. 10.1). This method facilitates a better understanding of spatial orientation and handedness. Understanding what each hand does and the direction of hand movements in relation to the operator are important to the learning process.

Importantly, the instructor that is the most expert at performing a procedure is not always the most effective teacher. The "expert" often performs the skill under total automatic control and may have difficulty

Figure 10.1
A., B. The student gains correct spatial orientation and an appreciation of each hand's movements during the procedure by observing over the instructor's shoulder.

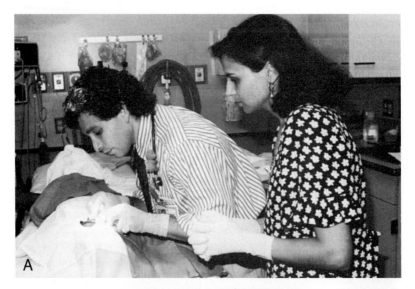

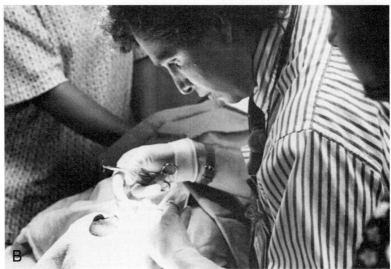

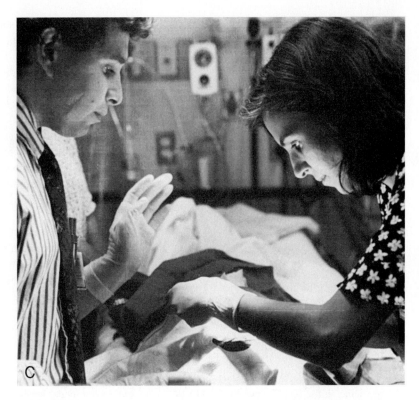

SUMMARY
1. The three phases of psychomotor learning are cognitive, fixation, and autonomous.
2. The three critical conditions that influence procedural learning are contiguity, practice and feedback.
3. Divide the procedure into small discrete steps (Table 10.1).
4. Teach the procedure in three phases that correspond to the three phases of psychomotor learning: introductory (cognitive), practice (fixation), and perfecting (autonomous) (Table 10.2).
5. If possible, allow the student to observe the procedure from the position in which the student will actually perform the procedure (i.e., from over the instructor's shoulder). This facilitates a better understanding of spatial orientation and handedness (Fig. 10.1).
6. Bedside teaching of procedures in the ED requires a preprocedure discussion (Table 10.3) and demonstration, if possible. Explaining each step to the patient and/or family may further serve as additional guidance to the student.

demonstrating and articulating separate component steps to a trainee. In addition, the role of enthusiasm coupled with patience cannot be underestimated.

COMPLICATIONS/PRECAUTIONS

Teaching procedures on actual patients in the ED requires the instructor to weigh the benefit to the student against the risk and discomfort of the patient (11). Factors that must be considered include the acuity of the patient's condition and the urgency of the procedure, the risks of the procedure, the ability of the patient to cooperate, the skill level and experience of both the student and instructor, other simultaneous clinical and administrative demands on the instructor, and the wishes of the family. Although instructors should strive to facilitate every opportunity for students to practice procedures, many situations will require the student to observe or assist only. Although it is difficult to give general guidelines, the patient should never be exposed to undue risk or discomfort.

OTHER ISSUES

Virtually every medical specialty requires their physicians to be competent in certain procedures; however, the process for determining competency and credentialing physicians is generally poorly defined (13). Although the number of procedures performed is often taken as a proxy for competency, this has never been demonstrated in the literature. A recent study found that neither thoracotomy experience nor cognitive knowledge of the procedure content adequately predicts thoracotomy competency (14).

A related problem is the maintenance of procedural skills while in practice. This may be particularly problematic for academic physicians who may have less clinical time and must often allow trainees to perform procedures. It is not clear to what extent teaching and supervising procedures without actually performing them prevents deterioration of psychomotor skills. Some potential solutions include computer-based cognitive review and assessment, live animal workshops, "mini rotations" in focused clinical areas (e.g., anesthesia), or arranging additional clinical shifts allowing greater exposure to direct patient care.

REFERENCES

1. Klass P. A not entirely benign procedure: four years as a medical student. New York: New American Library, 1987.
2. Whitman N, Lawrence P. Teaching procedures. In: Surgical teaching: practice makes perfect. Salt Lake City: University of Utah School of Medicine, 1991:65–80.
3. Thomas H. Teaching procedural skills: beyond "see one—do one." Acad Emerg Med 1994;1 398–401.
4. Homan CS, Viccellio P, Thode HC, Fisher W. Evaluation of an emergency-procedure teaching laboratory for the development of proficiency in tube thoracostomy. Acad Emerg Med 1994;1:382–387.
5. Foley RP. Smilanksy J. Skill lessons. In: Teaching techniques. A handbook for health professionals. New York: McGraw-Hill, 1980:71–91.
6. Nelson MS. Models for teaching emergency medicine skills. Ann Emerg Med 1990;19: 333–335.
7. Burns JP, Reardon FE, Troug RD. Using newly deceased patients to teach resuscitation procedures. N Engl J Med 1994;331: 1652–1655.
8. McNamara RM, Monti S, Kelly JJ. Requesting consent for an invasive procedure in newly deceased adults. JAMA 1995;273: 310–312.
9. Satava RM. Emergency medical applications of virtual reality: a surgeon's perspective. Artificial Intelligence in Med 1994;6:281–288.
10. Chapman DM. Use of computer-based technologies in teaching emergency procedural skills. Acad Emerg Med 1994;1:404–407.
11. Hedges JR. Pearls for the teaching of procedural skills at the bedside. Acad Emerg Med 1994;1:401–404.
12. Stratton SJ, Kane G, Gunter CS, et al. Prospective study of mannequin only versus mannequin and human subject endotracheal intubation training of paramedics. Ann Emerg Med 1991;20:1314–1318.
13. Brain GR, Munges BS. Evaluation of procedural skills. Acad Emerg Med 1994;1:325.
14. Chapman DM, Marx JA, Honigman B, Rosen P, Cavanaugh SH. Emergency thoracotomy: comparison of medical student, resident, and faculty performances on written, computer, and animal-model assessments. Acad Emerg Med 1994;1:373–381.

CHAPTER 11

DOCUMENTATION

Philip V. Scribano

INTRODUCTION

When encountering the pediatric patient in the emergency department (ED) who requires a diagnostic or therapeutic procedure, the practitioner must be vigilant in the documentation of that procedure, keeping in mind medicolegal and medical care aspects of this encounter (1–6). The Joint Commission on Accreditation of Healthcare Organizations (JCAHO) requirement for the ED record at minimum requires a report of any procedure including tests sent and results documented appropriately on the ED chart. An important component of the medicolegal aspect is that related to informed consent, which is detailed in Chapter 9.

Discussion of this topic here will therefore focus on other medicolegal issues and particularly medical care issues. These will be elaborated by reviewing the appropriate documentation of surgical procedures such as laceration repair, and of medical procedures such as lumbar puncture and thoracentesis.

Briefly, informed consent in the pediatric patient evokes some unique issues in comparison to the otherwise competent adult patient. The law views the pediatric patient as incompetent to consent to treatment or procedures, and is clear in providing that legal right to natural parents or legal guardians on behalf of the child. Although the competent adult patient has the legal and moral right to refuse consent to a procedure and or treatment, parents are not given this absolute right to refuse treatment or to have a procedure performed

on behalf of their child under the conditions of an emergency.

An *emergency* has been defined as "any condition that requires prompt medical intervention, but is not restricted to a condition that may cause death or disability. If the life or health of the child would be adversely affected by a delay caused by the parents' refusal, the situation is deemed an emergency (6). Limitations on parental authority have been supported by the Committee on Bioethics of the American Academy of Pediatrics and the President's Commission for the Study of Ethical Problems in Medicine and Biomedical and Behavioral Research. Further discussion of informed consent and refusal may be found in Chapter 9.

THE DOCUMENTATION PROCESS

The purposes of documentation of procedures in the ED are many. First, any encounter with a patient should generate a record of that encounter and events surrounding that interaction, especially when an action has the potential to cause an untoward result to the patient's well-being. This record serves to protect both the patient and the physician. Second, to maintain optimal communication with other health care professionals that may be caring for the patient, a description of the procedure and results maximize that communication, especially if verbal communication is not possible. Third, from an academic standpoint, the well-documented procedure note provides education to other health care professionals regarding the approach to a particular procedure and the associated issues such as anesthesia and/or use of conscious sedation, use of specific equipment, and positioning of the patient. It also affords researchers the opportunity to critically review certain aspects of a given technique and provides the ability to suggest improvements in how the procedure may be performed in the future.

The approach to documentation of the procedure itself should focus on several key features. First, the practitioner should describe in detail the area of interest. For instance, a laceration requiring repair should be described regarding its length, the depth of the wound (i.e., through the dermis, through the fascia), unique shape (i.e., curvilinear, jagged), body area of involvement, presence of active bleeding, and the overall integrity of the soft tissues (i.e., avulsed or intact). Second, documentation of the preparation of the wound area should be included. Irrigation with saline and/or providine-iodine solution to the area and debridement of devitalized skin or underlying soft tissue should be discussed. Third, the use and type of anesthesia must be noted. Particular features including concentration and volume of anesthetic (i.e., 3 ml of 1% lidocaine without epinephrine) and route of administration (i.e., topical using preparations such as TAC—tetracaine, adrenaline, cocaine—or LET—lidocaine, epinephrine, tetracaine), or simple infiltration with lidocaine by needle should be documented. If conscious sedation is required, documentation of the type of sedative used, the amount given, and its route of administration (i.e., oral, rectal, intranasal, or intravenous) as well as the use of appropriate monitoring such as pulse oximetry and cardiac monitoring is suggested. Fourth, the repair itself should be recorded including materials used, type and number of sutures (i.e., 4-5.0 nylon, interrupted sutures, 2-4.0 nylon vertical mattress sutures or 3-4.0 chromic,

Figure 11.1.
Example of laceration repair procedure note.

> "Consent issues regarding repair and conscious sedation discussed with parent/guardian; risks and benefits of repair and sedation were explained and informed consent was obtained. Midazolam, 3 mg PO was given and continuous pulse oximetry and cardiac monitoring was used. In the supine position, under sterile conditions, a 2.5 linear laceration along the lateral aspect of the right thigh was irrigated with 200 ml NSS, followed by preparation of the site with povidine; topical anesthetic 3 ml (lidocaine 4%, epinephrine 0.05%, tetracaine 0.5%) was applied to the wound over 20 minutes. Three- 4.0 chromic, interrupted sutures were placed subcuticular to approximate the wound margins; 6- 4.0 interrupted nylon sutures were placed with good approximation of wound margins. Antibiotic ointment was applied with a sterile dressing. The patient tolerated the procedure well. No evidence of lasting sedative effects noted and the patient was stable for discharge from the E.D."

subcuticular, interrupted sutures). A comment on the overall approximation of the repair should be made (i.e., good approximation of the wound margins is observed). Lastly, wound dressing including the use of antibiotic ointment, the type of sterile dressing applied, and the use and type of splints should be documented in the chart.

Documentation of a medical procedure such as a lumbar puncture, thoracentesis, or arthrocentesis requires some additional details that are less crucial in most minor surgical procedures. More emphasis is on the position of the patient, a description of the approach to the procedure, and the actual findings related to the procedure.

For example, when performing a lumbar puncture, it should be documented whether the patient was placed in a lateral recumbent or seated upright position for the procedure. This is especially important if opening and closing pressures will be assessed. As previously mentioned for surgical procedures, preparation of the needle entry site and use and type of anesthesia should be documented. Again, special mention should be made if conscious sedation is being used with a comment on the monitoring employed. A description of the cerebrospinal fluid specimen as it is being obtained also should be commented on (i.e., CSF was noted to be clear or bloody). If multiple attempts have been made, this too should be documented. The description of the approach should include details such as the size gauge needle used and site of penetration (i.e., L3-L4 interspace). A comment on the

patient's condition after the lumbar puncture has been performed should be included (i.e., the child tolerated the procedure well). Any adverse events related to or occurring at the time of the procedure should be recorded. After the appropriate studies have been sent, recording these laboratory findings on the chart is required.

Similarly, if an arthrocentesis is being performed, a description of the position of the patient (i.e., supine or prone) and the extremity (i.e., extension, flexion) is important. Description of the approach should include details such as the size gauge needle used and the site of penetration (i.e., inferolateral to the patella). A description of the synovial fluid specimen (i.e., straw-colored, turbid, sanguinous) should be made. As previously mentioned for surgical procedures, preparation of the site, and use and type of anesthesia should be documented. Again, special mention should be made if conscious sedation is being used with a comment on the monitoring employed.

Documentation of a procedure such as thoracentesis requires slightly more vigilance than those procedures previously described for several reasons. First, because of the upright positioning required, immobilization of the anxious pediatric patient may be less than optimal and may therefore lessen the overall success of the procedure. Second, some patients may have immediate life-threatening disease putting them at higher risk, especially if a complication results. Third, the complications of a thoracentesis have a higher morbid-

"Consent issues discussed with parent/guardian; risks and benefits of lumbar puncture explained and informed consent was obtained. In the lateral recumbent position and under sterile conditions, the child was prepped with povidine and 1 ml of 1% lidocaine without epinephrine was injected at the L3-4 interspace followed by a $2\frac{1}{2}$ inch spinal needle in the usual fashion. Six ml of clear CSF fluid was obtained without difficulty. A sterile dressing was applied to the puncture site and the patient tolerated the procedure well."

Figure 11.2.
Example of lumbar puncture procedure note.

SUMMARY
Key Features of a Well-Documented Medical or Surgical Procedure
1. Position of the patient
2. Preparation of the body area
3. Use of anesthetic/conscious sedation
4. General technique
5. Specimen/gross findings
6. General condition of patient
7. Results of laboratory tests on specimens obtained
8. Potential complications

ity than those procedures previously discussed and may not be immediately apparent (i.e., pulmonary contusion, hepatic or splenic trauma).

Documentation of the child's position (i.e., in the sitting position with the arms and head supported on a pillow) should be made. A brief description of the approach including the preparation of the area, the use of anesthetics and conscious sedation, and the location of needle insertion (i.e., at the 7th intercostal space along the posterior axillary line) and needle size should be recorded. Mention of the thoracentesis specimen findings such as volume of pleural fluid obtained and color (i.e., serous, serosanguinous, sanguinous) should be made. A comment on the patient's condition, after the procedure, is recommended. Lastly, after successful completion of the procedure, the results of laboratory tests as well as an upright chest radiograph should be recorded to document any presence of iatrogenic complications.

SUMMARY

Good documentation of medical or surgical procedures will provide the information necessary to maintain optimal communication to those caring for the patient after the procedure has been performed, and can be helpful and instructional to those reviewing the medical record in the future. The basic elements in this documentation should provide the reader with a clear understanding of the patient at the time of the procedure, the actual procedure performed, the results of the procedure, and any untoward events resulting from or temporally related to the procedure. These features are summarized in the Summary Table.

REFERENCES

1. Botkin J. Informed consent for lumbar puncture. AJDC 1989;143:899–903.
2. Bukata WR. Emergency department medical record. In: Henry GL, ed. Emergency medicine risk management. Dallas: American College of Emergency Physicians, 1991, p. 235.
3. Fosarelli P, Baker MD. What you don't record can hurt you: documentation in the emergency department. Pediatr Emerg Care 1985;1:223–227.
4. Korin J, Selbst, S. Legal aspects of emergency department pediatrics. In: Fleisher G, Ludwig S, et al., eds. Textbook of pediatric emergency medicine. Baltimore: Williams & Wilkins, 1993, p. 1544.
5. Selbst S. Medicolegal considerations. In: Diekmann RA, et al., eds. Pediatric emergency care systems. Baltimore, 1992, p. 421.
6. Wilde J, Pedroni A. My boy doesn't need an iv. Contemp Pediatr 1990 December; pp. 15–24.

CARDIOPULMONARY LIFE SUPPORT PROCEDURES

Editor: Christopher King

BASIC LIFE SUPPORT

Judith C. Bausher and Constance M. McAneney

INTRODUCTION

Basic life support (BLS) encompasses early recognition and intervention for respiratory and cardiopulmonary arrest. The goal of BLS is to artificially supply oxygen to the body, most importantly to the brain and heart, through the use of rescue breathing and chest compressions. BLS can represent a definitive intervention, since spontaneous respirations and normal cardiac activity will sometimes resume, or as in most cases, a temporizing measure until advanced life support (ALS) can be administered. BLS is a crucial component of the overall emergency medical system for children, which includes bystander cardiopulmonary resuscitation (CPR), rapid response by appropriately trained prehospital personnel, and transport to a hospital emergency department (ED). Prompt initiation of BLS is critical for a good outcome. Consequently, all individuals responsible for the care of children including parents and other caregivers, emergency medical personnel, nurses, and physicians should have training in this procedure.

Cardiopulmonary arrest in the pediatric population is an uncommon event. In fact, only 10 to 15% of all arrest victims are younger than 19 years of age (1). The age range most commonly affected is children under 1 year, representing approximately half of all pediatric arrests. Among the remaining patients, children between the ages of 1 and 4 years account for 15 to 30% of pediatric arrests, school-age children (5 to 12 years) 15

to 20%, and teenagers 10 to 15% (1–4). With children younger than 4 years of age, the causative event is most likely to occur in or around the home, including apparent life-threatening events (formerly called "near miss" sudden infant death syndrome), household injuries, respiratory illnesses, drownings, and neurologic diseases. For school-age children, the streets and recreational areas are more common sites, with injuries and drownings representing the most common causes (2, 5, 6, 7).

Asystole is by far the most common arrest rhythm seen among pediatric patients, accounting for 75 to 90% of documented cases (1, 6, 8, 9). Unlike the common scenario with adults, fewer than 10% of children experiencing a pulseless arrest have ventricular fibrillation (VF). Pediatric patients presenting with VF are likely to have a specific insult to the heart, such as accidental ingestion of a cardiotonic medication, metabolic abnormalities, or underlying cardiac disease (2, 6, 8, 9). Coronary artery insufficiency is a rare cause of pediatric arrest. As a result, whereas adults usually suffer a sudden, primary cardiac arrest, cardiopulmonary arrest in children generally represents a "final common pathway" after progressively worsening compromise as a result of other illnesses. Indeed, respiratory etiologies of arrest are far more likely among pediatric patients than are cardiac etiologies.

Most studies of out-of-hospital, normothermic cardiac arrest in children report survival averages of 10%, although most of these victims suffer permanent neurologic impairment (4, 7, 10, 11). Not surprisingly, the highest rate of intact survival is achieved with witnessed arrests when there has been prompt institution of BLS and ALS procedures (2, 3, 5, 8). Conversely, the intact survival rate for respiratory arrest alone may exceed 50% with rapid intervention (4, 9, 10). This relatively high rate of survival underscores the importance of early recognition and resuscitation for pediatric patients who suffer a primary respiratory arrest.

This chapter focuses exclusively on the CPR component of BLS for children. Although traditionally included with BLS procedures, the initial management of upper airway foreign bodies (i.e., back blows, Heimlich maneuver) is not discussed in this chapter. A complete description of both the basic and advanced techniques for managing upper airway foreign bodies is found in Chapter 54.

ANATOMY AND PHYSIOLOGY

Airway/Breathing

Various techniques for attempted resuscitation of the dead or near-dead have been described since ancient times (12). Proposed methods for reviving victims have included rolling on a barrel, bouncing on a galloping horse, and using bellows to blow air into the lungs. Manual methods of ventilation using either back pressure/arm lift or chest pressure/arm lift date back almost 150 years (13, 14). The Schafer "prone pressure method" was taught by the American Red Cross until the late 1950s, when mouth-to-mouth resuscitation was recognized as being more effective.

References to mouth-to-mouth ventilation date as far back as biblical times. In 1771, Tossach described inflating a person's lungs using the rescuer's expired air (15). Yet it was the pivotal studies by Safar and Gordon published in the 1950s that demonstrated that mouth-to-mouth ventilation was superior to other methods for all age groups in providing rescue breathing (16–18). This report, along with the landmark publication of Kouwenhoven et al. describing closed chest compression (19), began the modern era of CPR.

A number of important differences exist between pediatric patients and adults that are relevant to airway control and rescue breathing (20, 21) (Fig. 12.1). For example, the occiput of an infant is more prominent, which may cause a flexed airway when the infant is lying in the supine position. Furthermore, when compared with adults, infants and younger children have a larger tongue relative to the size of the hypopharynx and greater laxity of the pharyngeal soft tissues. These characteristics contribute to the fact that pediatric patients are prone to develop airway obstruction simply from lying supine. In addition, the neck is short and chubby, making appropriate positioning more difficult. The tracheal cartilage is soft and easily compressible; as a result, hyperextension of the infant's head and neck can produce airway obstruction. There is also greater airway resistance, caused by the narrower luminal diameter of the pediatric airway. According to Poiseuille's law, resistance to flow is inversely proportional to the 4th power of the radius (21). A pediatric airway one-half the diameter of an adult airway will therefore have a 16-fold greater resistance to flow. For this reason, even small changes in airway diameter (e.g., due to inflammation, edema, or improper positioning) may cause significant respiratory compromise. Further discussion of this concept and other aspects of pediatric airway anatomy can be found in Chapters 14 and 16.

Many aspects of the mechanics of breathing are also unique to infants and children. Because the pediatric rib cage is very pliable and more horizontally oriented, it does not provide the same degree of support as with an adult, and therefore the residual capacity of the lungs is decreased. If there is diminished air entry resulting from intrinsic lung disease or upper airway obstruction, the negative pressure created during inspiration causes paradoxical movement of the chest. In addition, infants and younger children are more dependent on diaphragmatic excursion for ventilation. Any conditions that hamper movement of the diaphragm (abdominal distension, masses, etc.) can therefore significantly impair gas exchange. Children also develop hypoxemia in response to respiratory insults more rapidly than adults due in part to differences in the work of breathing and alveolar surface area. Efficient respiratory effort takes place when a minimum of energy is ex-

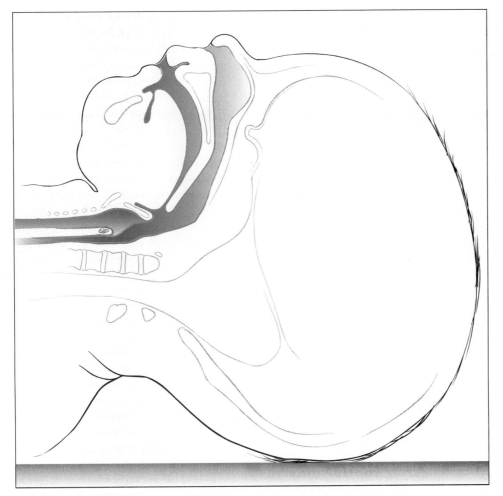

Figure 12.1.
Anatomy of the infant airway. The infant has a more prominent occiput than an adult, resulting in neck flexion and potential airway obstruction when the patient is lying supine on a flat surface. The tongue of an infant is also large in relation to the size of the oropharynx, as well as being more superiorly positioned. Both characteristics increase the likelihood of airway obstruction by the tongue.

pended to provide an adequate respiratory rate and tidal volume. Increased airway resistance and greater chest wall compliance cause children to achieve efficient breathing at higher relative rates than adults, disproportionately increasing the metabolic demands of respiration (21). Furthermore, the smaller alveolar surface area of a pediatric patient results in a diminished reserve for gas exchange. As a result, processes that cause mismatching of ventilation and perfusion in the lungs are more likely to produce significant hypoxemia in children.

As mentioned previously, respiratory failure is the primary cause of cardiopulmonary arrest among pediatric patients. Respiratory failure results from inadequate oxygenation of blood and/or inadequate ventilation. Inadequate oxygenation, which is usually caused by either intrinsic lung disease or upper airway obstruction, leads to a suc-cession of adverse effects including tissue hypoxia, lactic acid production, and metabolic acidosis. Initially the patient attempts to compensate by increasing the respiratory effort and rate; when this can no longer be sustained, the patient develops progressively worsening hypoxemia and acidosis, resulting eventually in full cardiopulmonary failure. By contrast, ventilatory dysfunction impairs excretion of CO_2 (hypercarbia) producing a respiratory acidosis. This is generally a more gradual process resulting from conditions that inhibit the normal function of the "respiratory pump" (i.e., those systems of the body responsible for producing effective ventilation) (see also Chapter 16). With progressively increasing levels of CO_2 in the blood, respiratory effort will wane and finally cease altogether. The patient then develops hypoxemia as well as hypercarbia, profound acidosis, and ultimately cardiac arrest.

Circulation

Although adults usually have abrupt cardiovascular collapse as a prelude to arrest, pediatric patients often develop gradually worsening circulatory compromise and shock. Simply stated, the shock state is characterized by delivery of oxygen and substrate to tissues that is insufficient to meet metabolic demands. This outcome depends on the circulating blood volume, cardiac output, and vasomotor tone, which are continually regulated to maintain tissue perfusion. Significant changes in any one of these variables result in altered function of the others as the body attempts to maintain an adequate blood pressure. For example, a drop in vasomotor tone (e.g., septic shock) is accompanied by an elevated cardiac output through increased heart rate and stroke volume; significant blood loss or dehydration causes both increased vasomotor tone and cardiac output. In addition, compensatory mechanisms, such as the release of endogenous catecholamines, also operate to maintain an adequate blood pressure despite compromise to one or more of these physiologic mechanisms. As shock progresses, however, these compensatory mechanisms become inadequate and the patient develops global deficits in oxygen and substrate delivery to vital organs, resulting in multiple organ system failure and eventually cardiopulmonary arrest.

For purposes of discussion, shock is divided into three general categories: hypovolemic, distributive, and cardiogenic. Hypovolemic shock, the most common type in the pediatric age group, is characterized by inadequate intravascular volume resulting in a diminished stroke volume and cardiac output. Dehydration and hemorrhage are by far the most common causes, but "third-spacing" of fluids (i.e., sequestering fluids within the body but outside the cardiovascular system) can also cause hypovolemic shock. Distributive shock is characterized by peripheral vasodilatation resulting in a drop in systemic blood pressure. The cardiac output may be normal or even elevated, but the maldistribution of blood flow causes inadequate perfusion of vital organs. This type of shock is seen in anaphylaxis, certain drug ingestions, and early sepsis. As septic shock progresses, significant intravascular fluid losses occur as well as myocardial dysfunction. Thus in the later phases of septic shock a low cardiac output state also develops. Cardiogenic shock is characterized by myocardial dysfunction. Even though the intravascular volume and heart rate are adequate or even increased, poor myocardial contractility results in a diminished stroke volume and cardiac output. Cardiogenic shock is usually seen in patients with underlying heart disease (congenital or acquired) and metabolic derangements such as acidosis, hypoxia, hypoglycemia, or hypocalcemia.

The first scientific reports of cardiac compression were published in the late 19th and early 20th centuries. The impetus of this work was the occurrence of sudden, unexpected death of patients receiving chloroform anesthesia. Open cardiac massage was initially advocated for treating arrest patients (22, 23), but this technique proved to be fraught with complications and required the expertise of highly trained physicians. The method of closed chest compression was initially described by Boehm in 1878 using laboratory animals (24). Further reports on this technique appeared sporadically over the next 70 years, but it was not until the work of Kouwenhoven et al., published in 1960, that closed chest cardiac compression was considered a potential intervention for arrest patients.

The exact mechanism by which cardiac compressions produce forward blood flow has been a point of controversy over the years (Fig. 12.2). In what has become known as the "cardiac pump theory," Kouwenhoven et al. postulated that the heart is directly compressed between the sternum and the thoracic spine, causing blood flow as the heart empties (19). Relaxation of the pressure on the chest allows the heart to refill with blood, and the cycle is continued. Although the myocardium no longer contracts, the heart nonetheless functions as a pump across which there is a pressure gradient. It was theorized that during compression, the aortic and pulmonic valves open, while retrograde flow is prevented by closure of the mitral and tricuspid valves. During the relaxation phase, the ventricles reexpand to their original size and are filled by suction effect, while arterial pressure was thought to close the aortic and pulmonic valves.

The cardiac pump theory was generally

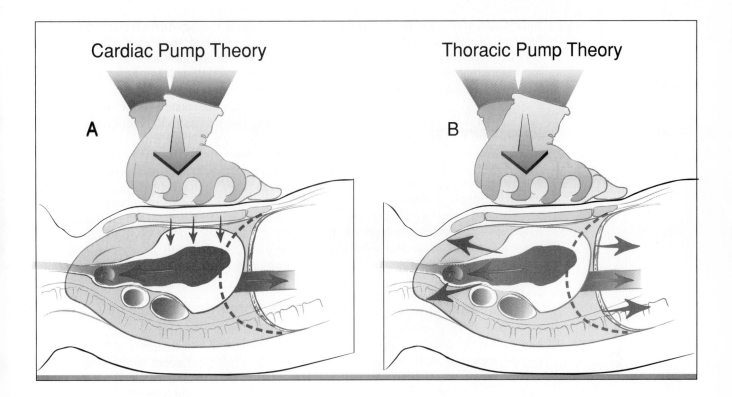

Cardiac Pump Theory

A

Thoracic Pump Theory

B

accepted until 1976, when Criley et al. (25) described a patient undergoing cardiac catheterization who developed VF. The patient began coughing in a rhythmic fashion and surprisingly remained conscious, raising questions about the mechanism of CPR. Changes in intrathoracic pressure, rather than any direct compressive effect on the heart, appeared to produce significant forward blood flow during coughing. This observation became the basis for the "thoracic pump theory." Experimental studies with large animals have shown that chest compressions produce an equal rise in pressure of all other intrathoracic structures as well as the heart (26). In other words, the heart does not function as a pump, but simply a passive conduit. During compression, an intrathoracic-to-extrathoracic pressure gradient causes forward flow through the arterial system; retrograde flow is prevented by venous valves and collapse of the veins. When the chest compression is released, the pressure gradient is reversed and blood flows from the extrathoracic to the intrathoracic venous system (Fig. 12.2).

As might be expected, the debate has not ended there, particularly with regard to pediatric patients. More recent studies in small animals using higher forces for chest compression have shown that intrathoracic vascular pressures are in fact much greater than pleural pressures (27). This higher than expected rise in vascular pressure would seem to be a consequence of direct cardiac compression, as originally proposed by Kouwenhoven. Although the exact mechanism has yet to be determined, it seems likely that *both* proposed theories are applicable in differing degrees with pediatric patients. Infants and younger children, who have a relatively small, compliant chest wall, probably depend more on direct cardiac compression for forward blood flow. With older children and adolescents, overall changes in intrathoracic pressure are likely to predominate. The most recent recommendations of the American Heart Association for the rate and duration of chest compressions are designed to have maximal effectiveness irrespective of the mechanism of flow (28).

INDICATIONS

The purpose of BLS is to provide circulation of oxygenated blood to vital organs, most importantly to the heart and brain. The outcome of resuscitation depends not only on the underlying condition but also on the timeliness

Figure 12.2.
Cardiac pump theory versus thoracic pump theory. These two theories have been proposed to explain the effects of chest compressions during CPR. The cardiac pump theory postulates that direct compression of the heart causes forward flow of blood. The heart serves as a pump. The thoracic pump theory postulates that pressure generated in the entire thoracic cavity causes forward blood flow, while the heart functions more as a passive conduit. It is likely that both mechanisms play a role for infants and younger children.

and effectiveness of the resuscitation effort. The most common clinical scenarios requiring BLS procedures for pediatric patients are respiratory failure and arrest, cardiopulmonary failure, and cardiopulmonary arrest.

Respiratory Failure

Respiratory failure should be suspected in any patient with significant respiratory distress manifested by increased work of breathing. The most common causes of respiratory failure among pediatric patients are lower airway diseases (e.g., pneumonia, asthma, bronchiolitis, and aspiration) and processes affecting upper airway patency (e.g., croup syndromes, foreign bodies, intrinsic mass, epiglottitis, and laryngospasm). Ventilatory dysfunction usually occurs in patients with lung disease who can no longer sustain the increased respiratory effort necessary to adequately excrete CO_2. Pulmonary muscle fatigue leads to progressively worsening hypercarbia. Ventilatory dysfunction also can occur in patients with central nervous system depression as a result of drug overdose, head trauma, and seizures. Hypoxemia in early respiratory failure causes a child to be agitated and difficult to console. The patient may also develop cyanosis and bradycardia. Hypercarbia generally causes lethargy, and in more severe instances, unconsciousness. As respiratory failure progresses, the resulting acidosis leads to worsening cardiac output, hypotension, and poor tissue perfusion (mottling, cool extremities, prolonged capillary refill). With cases of isolated respiratory failure, prompt institution of ventilatory support with either rescue breathing or positive pressure ventilation will prevent this progression of symptoms.

Respiratory Arrest

Untreated respiratory failure eventually leads to respiratory arrest. When an abrupt primary respiratory arrest occurs, circulation of oxygenated blood may continue for a few minutes. Because cardiac activity is still present, the brain and other vital organs receive oxygen and substrate, albeit in a progressively abnormal and inadequate manner, and these patients have a pulse. After several minutes, however, profound hypoxemia occurs depressing brain and cardiac function. Clinically, this is manifested by a depressed level of consciousness, as well as a weak, slow pulse and signs of poor perfusion such as delayed capillary refill, pallor or cyanosis, and cool extremities. This relatively brief interval of time when respirations have ceased and a pulse is still present is a critical period. Intervention at this point usually produces a good clinical outcome whereas failure to intervene almost certainly results in progression to cardiopulmonary arrest. Once the patient develops a significant cardiac arrhythmia in this situation, the prognosis is much worse.

Cardiopulmonary Failure

Cardiopulmonary failure may occur in the patient with progressive respiratory failure, when hypoxemia and acidosis cause myocardial dysfunction resulting in decreased heart contractility and rate. It may also be seen with the patient in shock when inadequate oxygen and substrate delivery to tissue has a similar effect on the heart. The patient in early or compensated shock maintains a systolic blood pressure within normal range, although other signs of circulatory compromise are present. The patient commonly presents with diminished peripheral pulses, cool distal extremities, delayed capillary refill, increased pulse rate, and widened pulse pressures. The patient may appear anxious or agitated as a result of high circulating levels of endogenous catecholamines. As the shock state progresses, compensatory mechanisms become inadequate and hypotension ensues. Peripheral pulses are absent and central pulses are weak. The skin is mottled or cyanotic and the patient may be diaphoretic. The coolness of the distal extremities progresses proximally. The patient becomes lethargic and difficult to arouse.

If untreated, both respiratory and circulatory failure will lead to progressive cardiopulmonary failure as a result of global deficits in oxygen and substrate delivery to vital organs. The patient in impending cardiopulmonary failure will be minimally responsive or unresponsive with central pulses that are weak and slow. The patient may also exhibit gasping or agonal respirations. Because respiratory failure is by far the most common cause of cardiopulmonary failure, establishing an airway and performing rescue breathing will often reverse this cascade of events. However, if the heart rate of a child remains below 60 bpm despite adequate airway control and ventilation, chest compressions should be initiated to provide circulatory support.

Cardiopulmonary Arrest

Untreated cardiopulmonary failure will eventually result in complete cessation of breathing and circulation. Patients will be unresponsive, apneic, cyanotic, and have no palpable central pulse. The electrocardiogram may show profound sinus bradycardia, an idioventricular rhythm, asystole, or rarely VF. Although there may be some cardiac output with an organized rhythm (e.g., sinus bradycardia), this will not be enough to perfuse vital organs or produce a palpable pulse (pulseless electrical activity). BLS must be started immediately in this situation. As soon as appropriate personnel and equipment are available, further assessment and treatment of the underlying condition that caused the arrest can then be initiated.

PROCEDURE

Basic life support requires no equipment and can be accomplished in almost any location. Outcome largely depends on the timely initiation of CPR, the skill with which the procedures are performed, and the rapidity of instituting ALS interventions.

Determining Responsiveness

The initial step in any resuscitation is a general assessment of the patient. This should always be performed in a systematic way so that no pertinent clinical data which may influence necessary actions is omitted. The child's state of consciousness, ability to breathe, and extent of any injuries should be quickly determined. Gently shaking the child (assuming there is no risk of cervical spine injury) and speaking in a loud voice are helpful in assessing the level of responsiveness. Respiratory effort and effectiveness, as well as attempts to speak, should be noted. If a head or neck injury is suspected, the cervical spine should be immobilized. The presence of significant injuries can be quickly established by looking for any deformities, bleeding, or environmental clues that indicate trauma.

Once these three quick assessments are performed, a verbal call for help is made. If there is a lone rescuer and CPR is necessary, it should be performed for 1 minute before notifying EMS. Although not the protocol for adults, this is done for children because a primary respiratory insult, the most likely etiology of a pediatric arrest, may be completely reversible with initial BLS interventions. If there are two rescuers, one can initiate CPR while the other notifies EMS.

Airway Control

Next the airway should be assessed for patency. Using the "look, listen, feel" approach, the operator observes the patient for airway compromise, listens over the patient's nose and mouth for breathing, and/or places a hand or cheek close to the patient's face to feel any air movement (Fig. 12.3). If obstruction is suspected, the operator must act immediately to establish a patent airway. For medical arrests, the head tilt-chin lift maneuver is preferred. Any child who suffers a traumatic arrest should have full immobilization of the head and neck, and airway patency is established using the jaw thrust maneuver. With either method, the child is first placed supine on a firm, flat surface, minimizing any movement of the neck as necessary. To perform the head tilt-chin lift maneuver, the operator places one hand on the patient's forehead and one or two fingers of the other hand just lateral to the chin. The neck is then extended slightly by gently pushing the forehead while pulling upward on the mandible (Fig. 12.4). Care must be taken not to close the mouth or inadvertently compress the soft tissue under the chin, because these actions may obstruct the airway. The jaw thrust maneuver allows the operator to open the airway without significantly moving the neck. The third and/or fourth fingers of both hands are "hooked" under the angle of the mandible as both thumbs

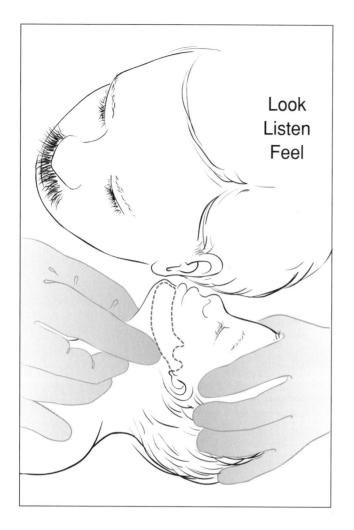

Look
Listen
Feel

are used to provide countertraction by pressing against the forehead. The mandible is lifted upward and outward with moderate force to open the mouth and displace the tongue anteriorly (Fig. 12.5). This maneuver is most comfortably performed with the operator's elbows resting on the surface just above the patient's head. The child with airway difficulty who is conscious should then be transported by experienced prehospital personnel to a facility where ALS and airway management can be provided.

Breathing

After airway patency has been established, the operator should assess the child's respirations. Once again, the standard "look, listen, feel" method is used. If the child is apneic or has inadequate respirations despite a patent airway, rescue breathing should be performed. With an infant, the operator places his or her mouth over the nose and mouth of the patient creating a tight seal (Fig. 12.6). For the older child, the operator places his or her mouth over the mouth of the patient while pinching the patient's nose closed to prevent air escape (Fig. 12.7). If not already performed, the head tilt-chin lift maneuver is used to keep the airway open, as long as there is no risk of cervical spine injury.

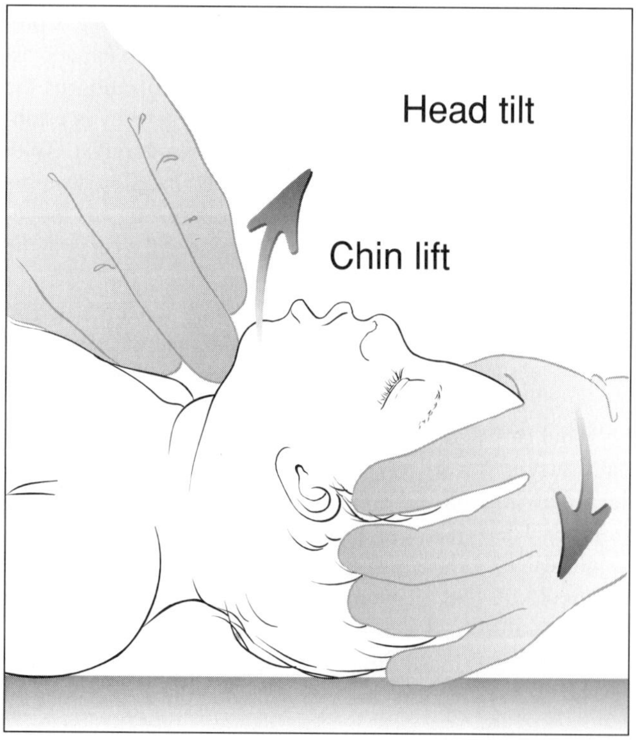

Figure 12.3.
"Look, listen, feel" method of assessing air movement.

Head tilt

Chin lift

Figure 12.4.
Head tilt-chin lift maneuver. Note that the fingers should not extend over the submental area as this may produce airway obstruction.

Chapter 12
Basic Life Support

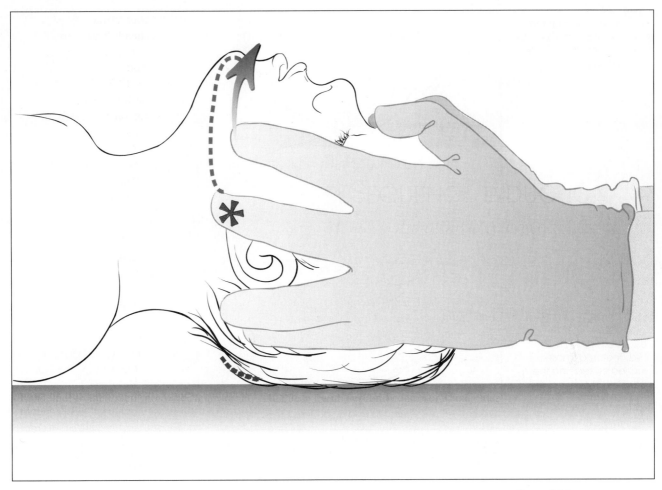

Figure 12.5.
Jaw thrust maneuver with
stabilization of the cervical
spine.

Two breaths should be delivered slowly (over approximately 1 to 2 seconds) with a pause between breaths. Delivering the breaths slowly will minimize the pressure required to provide adequate ventilation and decrease the likelihood of gastric distension. The pause between these initial rescue breaths allows the operator to also take a breath, replenishing the operator's "dead space" gas. Because approximately the first third of a normal exhalation is not involved in gas exchange (i.e., CO_2 excretion), this "dead space" gas is essentially atmospheric air and therefore has a higher oxygen concentration. The optimal delivered inspiratory pressures and volume of the rescue breaths depend primarily on the patient. The small airways of an infant have greater resistance and are prone to turbulent flow, necessitating relatively slow breaths. In order to reduce confusion, the most recent American Heart Association guidelines recommend a ventilatory rate of 20 per minute for both infants and children (also refer to the following section). Rescue breaths that produce chest excursions which are similar to normal deep respirations ensure an appropriate tidal volume. If the chest fails to rise, then the volume of the rescue breath is inadequate or the child has an obstructed airway. In the latter case, the patient's head and neck are first repositioned, because failure to open the airway initially is the most common cause of obstruction. If unsuccessful, the patient may have an airway foreign body; maneuvers to identify and alleviate this type of obstruction should then be performed (see Chapter 54).

Circulation

Checking the Pulse

After the airway has been positioned and two rescue breaths have been administered, the need for chest compressions is determined by

Figure 12.6.
Rescue breathing for the infant. The operator's mouth covers the infant's nose and mouth.

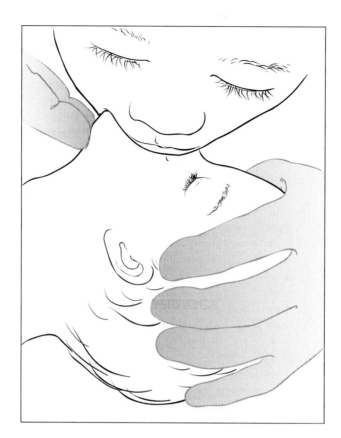

Figure 12.7.
Rescue breathing for the child. The child's nose is pinched closed and the operator's mouth covers the child's mouth.

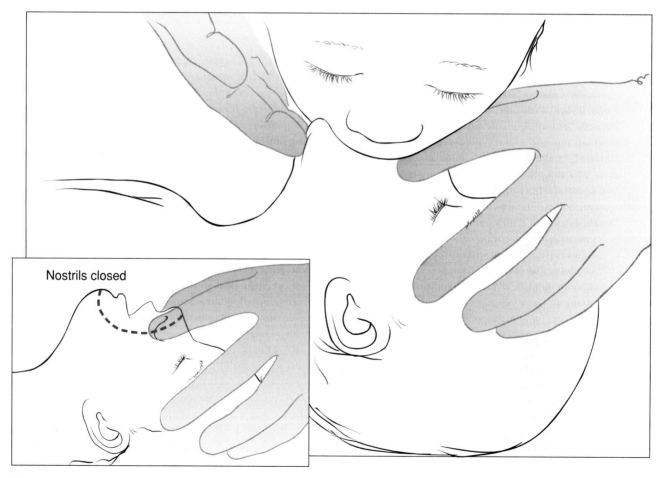

Nostrils closed

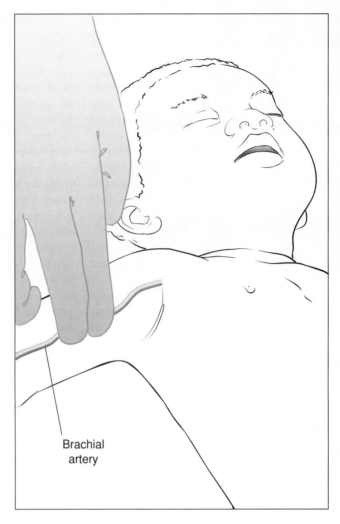

Figure 12.8.
Palpating the pulse. Because infants have a short, chubby neck, palpating the brachial pulse is a more reliable method.

Brachial
artery

SUMMARY
Determine responsiveness
  Gently shake infant or
    child if no injury
    suspected
  Speak loudly
Call out for help
Position infant or child
  Place supine on firm
    surface
  Keep neck immobilized
    if injury suspected
Assess airway patency
  Head tilt-chin lift
  Jaw thrust (if neck injury
    suspected)
Assess breathing
  Watch for chest
    movement
  Listen, feel for breaths
Ventilate twice
  Give two slow breaths
  Watch for chest to rise
  If no air movement,
    reposition and repeat
  If still no air movement
    despite repositioning,
    perform airway
    obstruction maneuvers
Check pulse
  Use brachial or femoral
    in infant (<1 yr)
  Use carotid in child (> 1
    yr)
  Check for 3–5 seconds
*Perform chest
  compressions*
Infant (< 1 yr)
  Position: one
    fingerbreath below
    intermammary line
  Technique: 3rd and 4th
    fingers on sternum
  Depth: 1/3–1/2 depth of
    chest (0.5–1.0 inch)
  Rate: at least 100 times
    per minute
  Ratio: 5 compressions to
    1 ventilation
      (continued)

palpating for a central pulse. In children older than 1 year, the carotid artery is the most accessible central artery for palpation. Because infants have short, chubby necks, the carotid pulse may be difficult to locate; consequently, palpating the brachial artery on the medial aspect of the upper arm is a more reliable method for checking the pulse with these patients (Fig. 12.8). Alternatively, the femoral pulse may also be used. The apical impulse of the heart should not be used to verify pulselessness, because the absence of a palpable peripheral pulse does not necessarily preclude the presence of cardiac activity. If a pulse is present and the rate is greater than 60 bpm, then rescue breathing alone should be continued. If no pulse is palpable or the heart rate is less than 60 bpm with signs of poor systemic perfusion, then chest compressions should be initiated and coordinated with ventilation.

Chest Compressions

The victim should be supine on a hard, flat surface in order to achieve optimal compressions. If an infant must be carried during CPR, the operator's forearm is used as a support for the infant's torso, while the head and neck are supported by the operator's hand. The other hand is used to perform compressions. The head should not be higher than the rest of the body. The compressions should be smooth and rhythmic, with equal time for compression and relaxation. The area of compression for both infants and children is the lower third of the sternum (29, 30).

Infant chest compressions are performed using an imaginary line between the nipples (intermammary line) as a landmark. With the operator at the patient's side, the index finger is placed on the sternum just below the intermammary line. Sternal compressions are

SUMMARY *(Continued)*
Child (1 to 8 yr)
  Position: one
    fingerbreath above
    xyphoid-sternal margin
  Technique: heel of hand
  Depth: 1.0–1.5 inches
  Rate: 100 times per
    minute
  Ratio: 5 compressions to
    1 ventilation
Child (> 8 yr)
  Position: lower third of
    sternum
  Technique: two hands
  Depth: 1.5–2.0 inches
  Rate: 80–100 times per
    minute
  Ratio: 5 compressions to
    1 ventilation for one
    rescuer; 15
    compressions to 2
    ventilations for two
    rescuers
Activate EMS
  Call EMS after 1
    minute of CPR
Continue CPR
*Reassess airway,
  breathing, circulation*

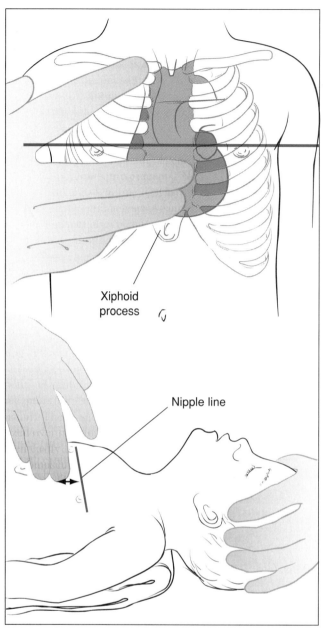

Xiphoid process

Nipple line

sion rate of approximately 80 per minute. This 5:1 compression to ventilation ratio produces a rescue breathing rate of 20 per minute or greater and is maintained whether there is one or two rescuers. With one rescuer, the hand not performing chest compressions stays on the victim's forehead to maintain a patent airway. In this way, no time is lost repositioning the head each time a rescue breath is delivered. If the airway cannot be maintained with the head tilt alone, then the operator uses both hands to perform the head tilt-chin lift maneuver for each rescue breath.

For children 1 to 8 years of age, chest compressions are performed using the heel of the hand on the lower sternum. The area of compression is located at the midline of the sternum two fingerbreadths superior to the xiphoid process (Fig. 12.10). The fingers are held away from the ribs during compressions to avoid injury to the ribs. Compressions should be one-third to one-half the total anteroposterior diameter of the chest, which for the child corresponds to a compression depth of approximately 1 to 1½ inches. The rate of compressions should be 100 times per minute; with pauses for ventilation after five compressions, the effective rescue breathing rate is 20 per minute and the compression rate is 80 per minute. As with the infant, the 5:1 compression to ventilation ratio is maintained whether there is one or two rescuers. The recommendations for ventilatory and compression rates for infants and children have been simplified by the American Heart Association in an effort to eliminate confusion about various memorized protocols. With one rescuer, the hand not performing compressions remains on the forehead to perform the head tilt. However, with children, unlike infants, head tilt alone usually does not maintain a

performed with the third and fourth fingers positioned one fingerbreadth below the intermammary line (Fig. 12.9). The depth of compression is one-third to one-half the total anteroposterior diameter of the chest, which corresponds to a compression depth of approximately ½ to 1 inch in the infant. The fingers should not be removed from the chest when pressure is released at the end of each compression, so that abrupt movements are avoided. The compression rate should be at least 100 times per minute. There should be a 1 to 2 second pause for ventilation after five compressions, producing an overall compres-

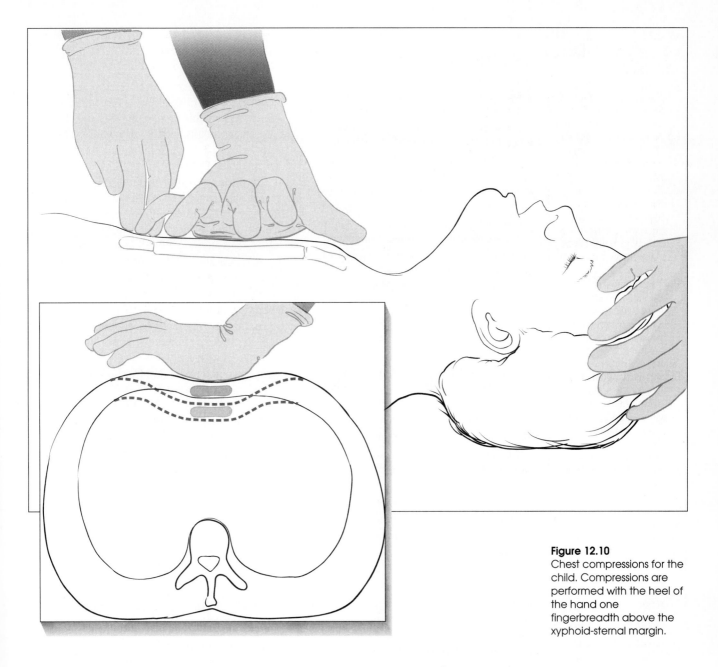

Figure 12.10
Chest compressions for the child. Compressions are performed with the heel of the hand one fingerbreadth above the xyphoid-sternal margin.

patent airway. Therefore the hand performing chest compressions must be removed each time to provide a chin lift during the ventilation phase. So that valuable time is not lost with this movement, relocating the landmarks on the chest for compressions can be done visually. For children older than 8 years of age, adult guidelines for rescue breathing and chest compressions are used.

COMPLICATIONS

Complications from BLS are relatively few and usually result from improper technique.

For example, failure to adequately immobilize the neck with a trauma victim may result in cervical cord injury. In such cases, the jaw thrust maneuver combined with in-line immobilization should be used to maintain airway patency. In addition, the patient should be fully immobilized before any transport.

Improper positioning of the patient can also prevent effective rescue breathing. If the head tilt-chin lift maneuver is performed and adequate chest excursions are not produced, the rescuer should reposition the head until a more favorable alignment of the airway is achieved and then reattempt rescue breathing. If this occurs when the jaw thrust maneuver is performed, the operator should exert greater force in displacing the mandible anteriorly, maintaining immobilization of the cervical spine as necessary. The operator can actually cause airway obstruction by pressing too firmly on the soft tissues of the submental area so that the tongue is pushed against the palate. In addition, overly aggressive extension of the neck can cause "kinking" of the airway and resulting obstruction. Maintaining a patent airway is often a matter of trial and error until the optimal position of the head and neck are established.

Failure to deliver adequate rescue breaths may be caused by leakage from an improper seal between the operator's mouth and the patient's mouth or nose and mouth. This also can occur when an inadequate tidal volume is delivered. In such cases, the patient may receive minimal oxygenation, increasing the risk of a poor outcome. Conversely, administering excessively high volumes or inspiratory pressures during rescue breathing will often cause gastric distension, which may lead to vomiting and aspiration. In extreme cases, pneumothorax can occur. These complications generally can be avoided if the operator delivers slow breaths and is careful to observe the patient's chest excursions.

Failure to deliver chest compressions at the recommended rate and depth will compromise blood flow to vital organs. Compressions that are too slow or too shallow must be avoided. The operator should concentrate on performing compressions in a smooth and rhythmic fashion, avoiding any abrupt or jerky movements. To maximize forward blood flow, the ratio of compression to relaxation should be roughly 1:1 (i.e., 50% of the time in compression and 50% of the time in relaxation). Although a common concern about performing chest compressions, fracturing ribs is in fact a relatively uncommon complication. A study by Feldman and Brewer (31) failed to demonstrate rib fractures even after prolonged CPR done by health providers with variable levels of skill. Excessive force should obviously be avoided, but the pliability of the infant's and child's rib cage makes fractures unlikely.

SUMMARY

Although sudden respiratory and cardiac arrest are less common among infants and children than adults, BLS procedures are nonetheless commonly indicated for pediatric patients. By far the most frequent cause of a pediatric arrest is respiratory compromise. Consequently, rescue breathing is often the only initial intervention required. The overall outcome from such a respiratory insult is generally good with appropriate management. Cardiovascular compromise requiring chest compressions is usually the result of a more gradual process in the pediatric population. Primary heart disease is rare. Prevention of this progression to cardiovascular collapse is therefore imperative. For children who present with arrest as a result of a cardiac event, the outcome is poor. Cardiopulmonary resuscitation can be performed without additional equipment by both health professionals and lay persons. All practitioners who care for children should be knowledgeable about the indications for CPR and skillful at performing the necessary procedures.

REFERENCES

1. Eisenberg M, Bergner L, Hallstrom A. Epidemiology of cardiac arrest and resuscitation in children. Ann Emerg Med 1983;12: 672–674.
2. Torphy DE, Minter MG, Thompson BM. Cardiorespiratory arrest and resuscitation of children. AJDC 1984;138:1099–1102.
3. Rosenberg NM. Pediatric cardiopulmonary arrest in the emergency department. Am J Emerg Med 1984;2:497–499.
4. Zaritsky A, Nadkarni V, Getson P, Kuehl K. CPR in children. Ann Emerg Med 1987; 16:1107–1111.
5. Friesen RM, Duncan P, Tweed WA, Bristow G. Appraisal of pediatric cardiopulmonary resuscitation. Can Med Assoc J 1982;126: 1055–1058.
6. Barzilay Z, Somekh E, Sagy M, Boichis H. Pediatric cardiopulmonary resuscitation outcome. J Med 1988;19:229–241.
7. Schoenfeld PS, Baker MD. Management of cardiopulmonary and trauma resuscitation in the pediatric emergency department. Pediatrics 1993;91:726–729.
8. Gillis J, Dickson D, Reider D, Steward D, Edmonds J. Results of inpatient pediatric resuscitation. Crit Care Med 1986;14:469–471.

9. Walsh CK, Krongrad E. Terminal cardiac activity in pediatric patients. Am J Cardiol 1983;51:557.

10. Lewis JK, Minter MG, Eshekman SJ, Witte MK. Outcome of pediatric resuscitation. Ann Emerg Med 1983;12:297–299.

11. O'Rourke PP. Outcome of children who are apneic and pulseless in the emergency room. Crit Care Med 1986;14:466–468.

12. Safar P. History of cardiopulmonary-cerebral resuscitation. In: Kaye W, Bircher N, eds. Cardiopulmonary resuscitation. New York: Churchill Livingstone, 1989.

13. Silvester HR. A new method of resuscitating stillborn children and of restoring persons apparently dead or drowned. Br Med J 1858;2:576.

14. Schafer EA. Description of a simple and efficient method of performing artificial respirations in the human subject. Transactions of the Royal Medical and Chiurgical Society 1904;87:609.

15. Tossach W. Man dead in appearance recovered by distending lungs with air. In: Medical essays and observations. 5th ed. London: T. Cadell and J. Balfour, 1771, vol 5 part 2, pp. 108–111.

16. Safar P, Escarraga L, Elam JO. A comparison of mouth-to-mouth and mouth-to-airway methods of artificial respiration with the chest-pressure arm-lift method. N Engl J Med 1958;671–677.

17. Gordon AS, Frye CE, Gittleson L, et al. Mouth-to-mouth verses manual artificial respiration for children and adults. JAMA 1958;167:320–328.

18. Elam JO, Brown ES, Elder JD. Artificial respiration by mouth-to-mask method: study of respiratory gas exchange of paralyzed patients ventilated by operator's expired air. N Engl J Med 1954;250:749–754.

19. Kouwenhoven WB, Jude JR, Knickerbocker GC. Closed chest cardiac massage. JAMA 1960;173:1064–1067.

20. Steward DJ, ed. Manual of pediatric anesthesia. New York: Churchill Livingstone, 1985, pp. 10–17.

21. Nichols DG, Rogers MC. Developmental physiology of the respiratory system. In: Rogers MC, ed. Textbook of pediatric intensive care. Baltimore: Williams & Wilkins, 1987, pp. 83–111.

22. Keen WW. A case of total laryngectomy (unsuccessful) and a case of abdominal hysterectomy (successful) in both of which massage of the heart for chloroform collapse was employed. With notes of 25 other cases of cardiac massage. Therap GAZ 1904;28:217.

23. Stephenson HE, Reid LC, Hinton JW. Some common denominators in 1200 cases of cardiac arrest. Ann Surg 1953;137:731–744.

24. Boehm R. Uber weiderbelelung nach vergiftunger und asphyxie. Arch Exp Pathol Pharmakol 1878;8:68.

25. Criley JM, Blaufuss AN, Kissel GC. Cough-induced cardiac compression. JAMA 1976;236:1246–1250.

26. Rudikoff MT, Maughan WL, Effron M, Freund P, Weisfeldt ML. Mechanisms of blood flow during cardiopulmonary resuscitation. Circulation 1980;61:345–351.

27. Maier GW, Tyson GS Jr, Olsen CO, Kernstein KH, et al. The physiology of external cardiac massage: high impulse cardiopulmonary resuscitation. Circulation 1984;70:86–101.

28. Emergency Cardiac Care Committee and Subcommittee, American Heart Association. Guidelines for cardiopulmonary resuscitation and emergency care: Pediatric basic life support. JAMA 1992;268:2251–2261.

29. Orlowski JP. Optimum position for external cardiac compression in infants and young children. Ann Emerg Med 1986;15:667–673.

30. Finholt DA, Kettrick RG, Wagner HR, Swedlow DB. The heart is under the lower third of the sternum: implications for external cardiac massage. AJDC 1986:646–649.

31. Feldman KW, Brewer DK. Child abuse, cardiopulmonary resuscitation, and rib fractures. Pediatrics 1984;339–342.

Airway Adjuncts, Oxygen Delivery, and Suctioning the Upper Airway

Richard J. Scarfone

Introduction

Adults typically suffer sudden death as a result of primary cardiac events such as myocardial infarction or dysrhythmias. In contrast, most pediatric cardiac arrests occur secondary to respiratory failure leading to hypoxemia and acidosis (1). One series of hospitalized children experiencing cardiopulmonary arrest demonstrated that 27% were resuscitated with airway and ventilatory interventions alone (2). Status asthmaticus, bronchiolitis, pneumonia, and laryngotracheobronchitis are among the many pulmonary diseases commonly seen in children which may lead to respiratory failure. In addition, status epilepticus, sedative or narcotic overdose, and overwhelming sepsis may lead to hypoventilation or apnea. Furthermore, unlike pediatric arrests resulting primarily from cardiac disease, which are generally associated with significant morbidity and mortality despite aggressive management, compromise resulting from a respiratory insult is often readily reversible. For these reasons skillful management of respiratory dysfunction is especially important in pediatric resuscitation.

The first step in the assessment of any seriously ill or injured child is the evaluation of the patency of the airway and the adequacy of ventilation. For the child with mild to moderate respiratory distress who has a patent airway, simple delivery of oxygen may be the only method of support necessary. If the patient has airway obstruction, suctioning and/or the introduction of a pharyngeal airway may serve as definitive treatment or as a temporizing measure before endotracheal intubation. This chapter describes the proper methods of performing these adjunctive airway procedures for the infant or child with respiratory distress.

Anatomy and Physiology

Airway Anatomy

Beginning at the nose and lips and proceeding down the airway of the infant or young child, several important anatomic differences are encountered as compared to the adult (Fig. 13.1). Many of these differences predispose the child to airway obstruction; for example, the tongue of the infant or young child is relatively large in proportion to the oral cavity. In addition, since the larynx has a more superior position in the neck of a pediatric patient compared with an adult, the tongue has a more rostral location in the hypopharynx (3). Consequently, a child lying supine will often develop airway obstruction due solely to posterior displacement of the tongue, a problem that can be alleviated with a pharyngeal airway. Infants are also obligate nasal breathers until approximately 3 to 5

Chapter 13
Airway Adjuncts,
Oxygen Delivery,
and Suctioning
the Upper Airway

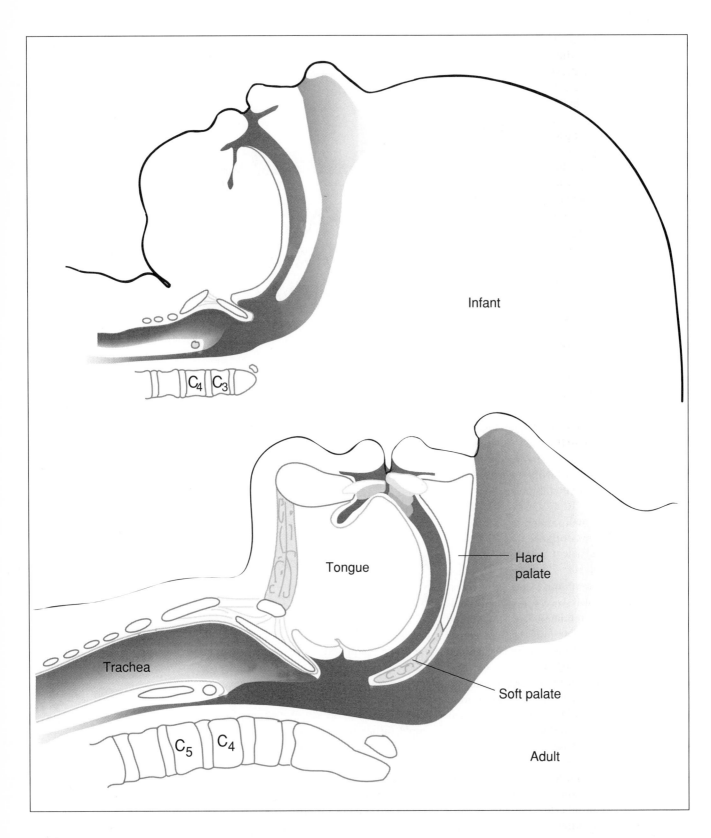

Infant

Tongue

Hard palate

Trachea

Soft palate

Adult

C_4 C_3

C_5 C_4

**Chapter 13
Airway Adjuncts,
Oxygen Delivery,
and Suctioning
the Upper Airway**

Figure 13.1.
Infant vs. adult airway anatomy. Characteristics of the airway of an infant
include a large tongue relative to the overall size of the oropharynx and a more superior
location of the tongue and larynx (opposite C3-C4) compared with the adult (opposite C4-C5).
These factors produce an increased tendency for airway obstruction in the infant.

months of age (3). As a result, swelling of the nasal mucosa, thick rhinorrhea, nasal foreign bodies, or choanal atresia may cause significant respiratory distress in the young infant. Perhaps the most obvious and important difference from the adult patient is children have smaller corresponding airway luminal diameters. Because the resistance to air flow is inversely related to the 4th power of the radius, disease states which cause further narrowing of the airways (edema, secretions, etc.) disproportionately increase the work of breathing and resulting oxygen demand in children compared with adults (Fig. 13.2). Further discussion of pediatric airway anatomy can be found in Chapters 14 and 16.

Physiology of Oxygen Utilization and Delivery

The oxygen consumption index of an infant is roughly twice that of an adult, due primarily to a higher rate of metabolism. As a result, pediatric patients develop hypoxemia more rapidly in response to inadequate oxygen delivery. Most practitioners have witnessed the precipitous decline in the oxygen saturation reading of a pulse oximeter which can occur when oxygen flow to a child in respiratory distress is interrupted.

In general, the rate of oxygen flow delivered should be sufficient to maintain an oxygen saturation of 100% whenever possible. Although the concentration of oxygen delivered to the patient (F_iO_2) corresponds to the rate of flow, a linear relationship does not exist. A number of other important variables also contribute to the F_iO_2. These include the patient's nasal and oropharyngeal resistance, inspiratory flow rate, tidal volume, and entrainment of atmospheric gases into the oxygen delivery system. The greater the patient's inspiratory flow rate and minute ventilation, the lower the F_iO_2 for any given oxygen flow rate. For example, assuming a constant oxygen flow of 3 L/min, a patient with minute ventilation of 12 L/min will breathe more oxygen-poor atmospheric air than a patient with a minute ventilation of 9 L/min. Although the rate of oxygen flow is the same, F_iO_2 is greater for the patient with a lower minute ventilation. Similarly, an older child with a greater tidal volume will need a higher oxygen flow to achieve the same F_iO_2 as a younger child. In addition, the delivery system used will influence oxygen concentration delivered to the patient. At a given oxygen flow, a nonrebreathing mask will provide a higher F_iO_2 than a simple face mask, because the latter system allows for greater contamination with room air.

OXYGEN DELIVERY

Indications

There are several diseases affecting children that may result in hypoxemia and for which the administration of oxygen is indicated. The most common of these is reactive airway disease (i.e., asthma and bronchiolitis). With reactive airway disease, bronchoconstriction and airway inflammation increase lower airway resistance, contribute to atelectasis and ventilation/perfusion mismatching, and increase the patient's work of breathing and

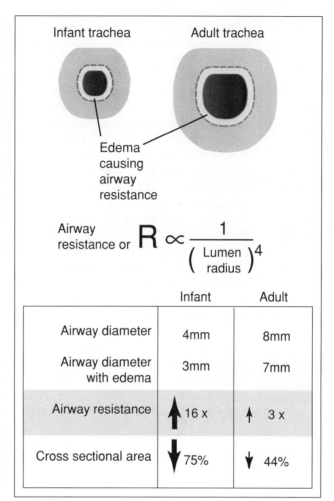

Figure 13.2.
Effects of airway narrowing for infants vs. adults. Airway diameter of an infant is significantly smaller than that of an adult at comparable anatomic levels. Because the resistance to gas flow is inversely proportional to the 4th power of the radius, small decreases in luminal diameter result in large increases in resistance for both infants and adults. However, this also means that with a given decrease in luminal diameter (e.g., 1 mm), the smaller lumen of the infant airway experiences a much greater increase in resistance compared with the adult.

Modified with permission from Cote CJ, Todres ID: The Pediatric Airway. In: Cote CJ, Ryan JF, Todres ID, et al. (eds) A Practice of Anesthesia for Infants and Children. 2nd ed. Philadelphia, Saunders, 1993.

oxygen consumption. The degree of hypoxemia may be exacerbated if the child has underlying chronic lung disease such as bronchopulmonary dysplasia or cystic fibrosis. Pneumonia and laryngotracheobronchitis (croup) also commonly affect children and may necessitate the administration of oxygen. In addition to primary pulmonary processes, other common indications for oxygen administration include status epilepticus and hypoventilation secondary to an overdose of a sedative or narcotic. Hypercarbia and acidosis may be relatively well tolerated by a child, but even a short period of oxygen deprivation can lead to bradycardia or cardiac arrest (2). Once it is determined that the spontaneously breathing child with respiratory distress has a patent airway, oxygen should be administered empirically.

The most important physical finding indicating hypoxemia in a child is cyanosis. Typically, the perioral region and distal extremities are the first areas of the body to become cyanotic. Other signs include agitation, lethargy, and bradycardia. Determination of

oxygen saturation by pulse oximetry provides a means of quantifying the degree of hypoxemia (see Chapter 77). Unless adequacy of ventilation is a concern, there is usually little need to perform a painful and time-consuming arterial puncture for blood gas analysis. Pulse oximetry offers a noninvasive, "real-time" modality which rapidly gives an indirect but generally reliable indication of the PaO_2. In interpreting the pulse oximeter reading, it is important to remember that the patient will maintain an oxygen saturation over 90% as long as the PaO_2 is above 60 mm Hg, even if the PaO_2 is decreasing. Physiologically, this corresponds to the initial "flat" segment of the oxyhemoglobin dissociation curve (Fig. 13.3) Once the PaO_2 falls below 60 mm Hg, however, oxygen saturation will drop dramatically as the patient reaches the "steep" segment of the curve. Therefore, oxygen saturation of 90% is only minimally acceptable in most clinical situations. If an oxygen saturation of at least 90% cannot be maintained with a given method of delivery, a system capable of administering a higher concentration should be employed. In such cases, controlled or assisted ventilation may also prove necessary.

Equipment

When administering oxygen, the clinician first determines the concentration that must be delivered and, based on this assessment, selects an appropriate delivery system. These decisions are affected by a number of patient variables including age, degree of cooperation, respiratory effort, and extent of hypoxemia. For example, a child in mild to moderate respiratory distress and minimal hypoxia may receive oxygen via a low flow system such as a nasal cannula or simple face mask. However, many younger children become extremely agitated and uncooperative when such devices are used, increasing oxygen consumption and potentially exacerbating hypoxemia. In such cases, it may be more effective to use a less efficient but better tolerated delivery method, such as a hollow plastic tube held close to the child's face. For the child in greater distress, a nonrebreathing face mask may be necessary to maintain an adequate oxygen saturation. The clinician should be knowledgeable about the charac-

Figure 13.3.
Oxyhemoglobin dissociation curve. The oxygen saturation stays relatively constant at approximately 90% along the initial "flat" segment of the curve. However, when the PaO_2 falls below 60 mm Hg, the "steep" segment of the curve is reached, and the oxygen saturation falls rapidly.

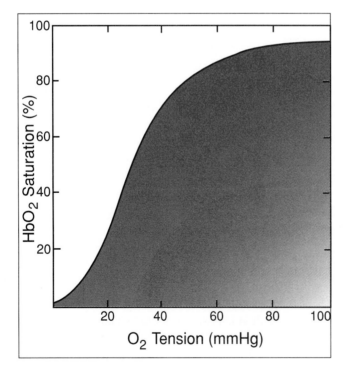

Chapter 13
Airway Adjuncts,
Oxygen Delivery,
and Suctioning
the Upper Airway

teristics of each delivery system, the manner in which they are best used, and the advantages and disadvantages of each.

Nasal Cannula

This simple, low flow, oxygen delivery system consists essentially of a small diameter, hollow plastic tube. One end of the tube is connected to the oxygen source via an adapter, with two short prongs at the other end which are placed into the anterior nares, delivering oxygen into the nasopharynx (Fig. 13.4). This system is most useful when a low oxygen flow (3 L/min or less) is adequate to maintain an acceptable oxygen saturation. Its principal advantage is that the light plastic tubing is less bulky and bothersome than a face mask. A nasal cannula device is particularly useful for young infants who are obligate nasal breathers and for whom a properly sized face mask may not be available or is poorly tolerated.

The main disadvantage of the nasal cannula system is that it is difficult to deliver oxygen in excess of 3 L/min. Higher flow rates cause irritation of the nasopharynx and are therefore not well accepted by most children. In addition, this is obviously not a "closed" system, and the F_iO_2 may vary widely if the child is mouth breathing or crying. Consequently, a nasal cannula may not meet the oxygen demands of a patient requiring consistent delivery of a higher F_iO_2.

Simple Oxygen Mask

This delivery system consists of a clear plastic or rubber mask that fits snugly over the nose and mouth (Fig. 13.5). Centers caring for children should have a wide range of sizes available. Transparent masks allow for the visualization of vomitus, blood, or other secretions. Each side of the mask has openings which serve as exhalation ports. These openings also permit inhalation of room air if the oxygen flow rate does not match the patient's tidal volume or if the oxygen source becomes disconnected. The simple mask may be used when a relatively low oxygen flow is adequate to maintain an appropriate oxygen saturation. This system can be expected to deliver a higher F_iO_2 than can be achieved with a nasal cannula, but it may not be as well tolerated. At an oxygen flow rate of 6 to 10 L/min, a simple oxygen mask will deliver an

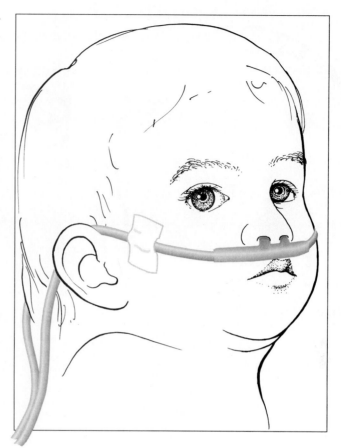

oxygen concentration of between 35 and 60%, depending on the patient's respiratory rate (1). The principal disadvantage of this system is that the F_iO_2 is lowered by entrainment of room air through the exhalation ports. A minimum oxygen flow rate of 6 L/min must be used to maintain a higher oxygen concentration and prevent rebreathing of exhaled carbon dioxide (1).

Partial Rebreathing and Nonrebreathing Masks

A partial rebreathing mask consists of a simple face mask with a reservoir bag attached. With the simple face mask, the patient's inspired air is contaminated by the inhalation of room air through the exhalation ports and the rebreathing of oxygen-poor exhaled gases. The purpose of the reservoir bag is to reduce rebreathing. Roughly the first third of exhaled gas enters the reservoir bag, and because the source of this gas is primarily the airway rather than the lungs, it is not significantly involved with gas exchange and is therefore relatively oxygen-rich (1). Remain-

Figure 13.4.
Nasal cannula for oxygen administration.

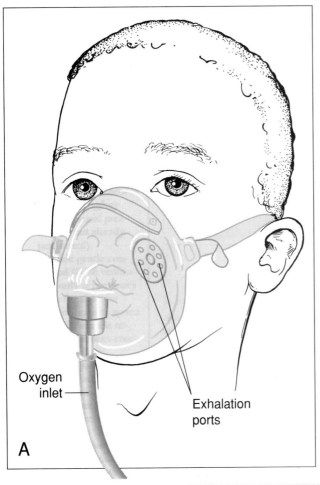

Oxygen inlet

Exhalation ports

A

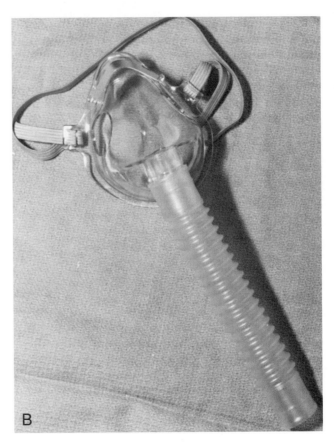

B

Figure 13.5.
A. Simple oxygen face mask.
B. Oxygen mask with corrugated tube reservoir.

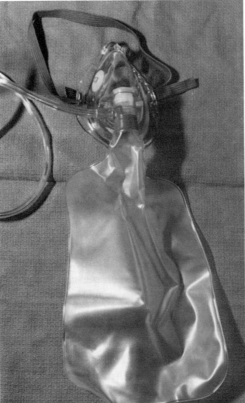

Figure 13.6.
Nonrebreathing face mask.

**Chapter 13
Airway Adjuncts,
Oxygen Delivery,
and Suctioning
the Upper Airway**

ing expired gases are vented through the exhalation ports. Assuming adequate oxygen flow into the reservoir bag (the bag should not fully deflate during inspiration), it should contain close to 100% oxygen which is inspired by the patient. Although the rebreathing of exhaled gases is reduced, room air is still entrained through the exhalation ports. With a flow rate of 10 to 12 L/min, an oxygen concentration of 50 to 60% can normally be achieved.

A nonrebreathing face mask also contains a reservoir bag and functions in much the same manner as a simple face mask but with a few important modifications. The nonrebreathing mask contains rubber seals serving as one-way valves over the exhalation ports (Fig. 13.6). This allows egress of exhaled gases while preventing entrainment of room air into the mask during inhalation. In addition, a second one-way valve is located between the bag and mask. This valve diverts oxygen-poor, exhaled gases away from the bag and thereby further reduces rebreathing.

Assuming that oxygen flow is sufficient to prevent collapse of the reservoir bag on inspiration (10 to 12 L/min) and that the face mask fits properly, an inspired oxygen concentration of over 95% can usually be achieved. ANSI standards mandate that only one of the two exhalation ports be sealed so that the patient can breathe room air should the oxygen source become disconnected from the reservoir bag. If both ports were sealed, the interruption of oxygen flow would result in the equivalent of complete airway obstruction. Although this safety measure is absolutely necessary, it reduces the F_iO_2 slightly because atmospheric gases are inspired through the open exhalation port. Nonrebreathing delivery systems are also available for infants, with the only modification being

that a small plastic tube, rather than a bag, serves as the reservoir.

Oxygen Hood

An oxygen hood is most useful for infants who require prolonged administration of oxygen, when a face mask or nasal cannula might be poorly tolerated. It consists of either a clear, soft plastic enclosure or a hard Plexiglas dome placed over the patient's head (Fig. 13.7). Because medical personnel have access to the infant's trunk and extremities while the hood is in use, general nursing care

Figure 13.7.
Oxygen hood.

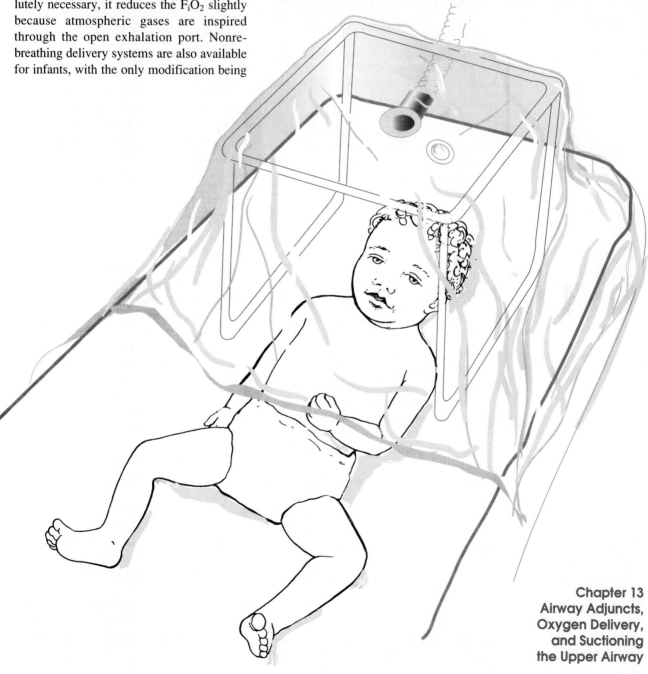

can be performed without lowering the F_iO_2. In addition, administration of cool or warm humidified oxygen will not significantly affect the patient's body temperature. It is possible to deliver oxygen concentrations of 80 to 90% with an oxygen hood.

The principal disadvantages of an oxygen hood are that it is cumbersome to use and often impractical in an emergency setting. The hood also restricts access to the infant's head and neck. Furthermore, it is not recommended for patients over 1 year of age, because their mobility will allow them to easily separate themselves from the oxygen source.

Oxygen Tent

An oxygen tent is similar in concept to a hood except that it is designed to encircle the entire trunk and head of an older child (Fig. 13.8). As with a hood, it is most useful for prolonged oxygen administration to a child who needs a higher oxygen concentration than is provided by a nasal cannula and who will not tolerate prolonged use of a face mask. Most tents allow control of oxygen concentration, temperature, and humidity.

Oxygen concentration maintained within the tent depends on the rate of flow, the tent volume, the adequacy of the seal between the tent walls and bed, and the frequency with which this seal is broken to tend to the patient. Minimal oxygen flows needed to provide oxygen concentrations of 50% have been established for various tent designs (4).

This system is effective for delivering humidity to the patient but is inefficient for delivering high concentrations of oxygen reliably. The tent must be displaced frequently to administer routine nursing care to the patient, allowing oxygen-poor room air to mix with the gases within the tent. Maintaining a consistent seal between the tent and the bed can also be difficult with a moving child, although placing blankets or small sand bags at the base of the tent walls may help in this regard. With adequate oxygen inflow, it is generally possible to maintain a reliable F_iO_2 of at least 50% within the tent.

Procedure

The nasal cannula is easily applied by inserting each short prong into the nares and draping the plastic tubing behind each ear. Taping the tubing to each cheek may help to prevent dislodgment. The child should be assessed periodically to ensure that the prongs have not become displaced. A face mask is attached to the oxygen source via a clear plastic tube and is held on the face with an adjustable strap placed around the occiput. It should fit snugly over the nose and mouth to decrease the amount of room air that is inspired.

When using either a nasal cannula or a face mask to deliver oxygen, the child should be allowed to assume a position of comfort. If the child is forced into the supine position, he or she may become frightened or agitated and increase oxygen consumption while struggling to remove the device. It may be more prudent in these cases to allow the child to sit on a parent's lap.

A child may be in either the prone or the supine position when placed within an oxygen hood or tent. The older child may choose to sit upright in an oxygen tent. Care should be taken to ensure that the base of the tent walls forms an adequate seal with the mattress of the bed to prevent mixing of room air within the system.

Complications

For many adults with chronic respiratory disease, high concentrations of oxygen can cause a suppressed respiratory drive. For the large majority of children, however, high F_iO_2 can be delivered safely without fear of causing respiratory depression. Exceptions include children with chronic respiratory diseases such as cystic fibrosis or bronchopulmonary dysplasia, who may sometimes experience hypoventilation with the administration of high concentrations of oxygen. For these children, respiratory effort must be monitored closely during oxygen administration and the physician must be prepared to assist ventilation if this becomes necessary. In general, oxygen may be safely delivered to children with congenital cardiac disease, although one notable exception is the child with hypoplastic left heart syndrome. Here, oxygen will serve to dilate the pulmonary vasculature which will increase left-to-right shunting of blood across a patent ductus arteriosus and impair peripheral perfusion.

Chapter 13
Airway Adjuncts,
Oxygen Delivery,
and Suctioning
the Upper Airway

108

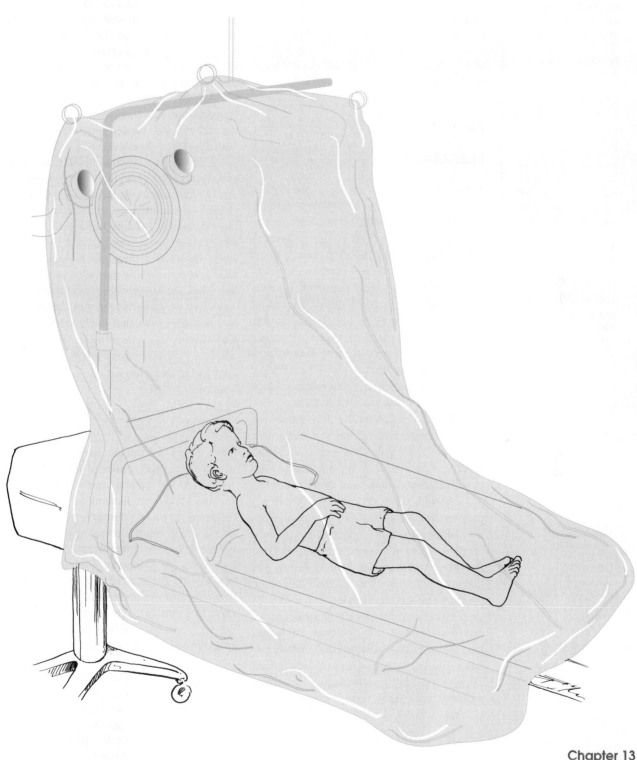

Figure 13.8.
Oxygen tent.

Chapter 13
Airway Adjuncts,
Oxygen Delivery,
and Suctioning
the Upper Airway

109

SUMMARY:
OXYGEN DELIVERY
1. Administer heated, humidified oxygen empirically once it has been established that the spontaneously breathing child with moderate respiratory distress has a patent airway.
2. Use pulse oximetry to assess oxygen saturation.
3. Maintain minimally acceptable oxygen saturation of 90% and, in most cases, near 100%.
4. Use nasal cannula device or simple face mask for patients requiring only low flow oxygen.
5. Use partial rebreathing or nonrebreathing mask for patients requiring higher concentrations of oxygen.
6. Consider using oxygen hood or oxygen tent for infants or younger children requiring prolonged administration of oxygen and humidity.

Chapter 13
Airway Adjuncts,
Oxygen Delivery,
and Suctioning
the Upper Airway

110

All patients receiving supplemental oxygen should undergo serial examinations. The clinician must ensure that the delivery system has not become dislodged from the oxygen source and that the patient has not experienced a clinical deterioration requiring a change to a different oxygen delivery system, or in more severe cases, assisted or controlled ventilation.

SUCTIONING

Indications

As stated earlier, the first step in the assessment of any child who is in respiratory distress is to ensure patency of the airway. Signs of airway obstruction in a child include tachypnea, stridor, snoring, poor aeration despite good chest wall movement, and cyanosis. In many cases, simple suctioning of the mouth and nose may provide prompt and complete alleviation of obstruction. One example is the patient who develops respiratory distress after sustaining oral trauma for whom suctioning of blood and teeth from the oropharynx may be necessary. A child who experiences significant blunt head trauma or who receives conscious sedation may have an altered level of consciousness followed by emesis. Here suctioning may be required to aid in the clearance of liquid and particulate material from the oropharynx. Alternatively, suctioning may be used in conjunction with other maneuvers to provide a patent airway. For example, airway obstruction following a seizure may be due to a combination of excessive secretions and laxity of the pharyngeal musculature, causing the tongue to fall against the posterior wall of the pharynx. In this case, manual methods of opening the airway together with suctioning of secretions, mucus, or blood from the mouth may be necessary to reestablish airway patency. Finally, suctioning is often an important step in facilitating visualization of the airway anatomy during direct laryngoscopy.

Equipment

Three commonly available types of suctioning devices are catheter tip, dental tip, and tonsil tip (Yankauer) devices (Fig. 13.9). The operator should be familiar with the features that make each of these useful in distinct clinical situations.

Catheter Tip Suction Devices

A catheter tip suction device is simply a narrow tube made of a soft, flexible plastic. It is connected via an adapter to a longer, hard plastic tube which is attached to wall suction. The catheter should be inserted gently into the patient's nasopharynx or oropharynx. Negative pressure is applied when the operator occludes the side opening on the catheter with a finger or thumb.

Catheter tip suction devices are best suited for gentle suctioning of the nasopharynx, which can often greatly improve gas exchange and resulting oxygenation, particularly for infants. In addition, these devices are well suited for suctioning thin secretions from the trachea through an endotracheal tube or tracheostomy cannula (see Chapter 81). They are not useful for suctioning thick secretions or particulate matter, because the narrow catheter lumen is likely to become occluded.

Dental Tip and Tonsil Tip Suction Devices

In most cases, airway obstruction secondary to secretions or particulate matter will most readily be alleviated with either a dental tip or tonsil tip suction device. Each consists of a wide bore catheter made of hard plastic or stainless steel. Each is attached to the wall vacuum via a hard plastic tube. Of the two, the dental tip suction device is more effective for removing vomitus from the pharynx, as it is less likely to become occluded by particulate matter (5). The end of the tonsil tip suction device is rounded and therefore less likely to cause injury to the pharyngeal tissues. It is primarily recommended for suctioning blood, because its design prevents obstruction of the tip by tissue or clot (5).

Procedure

Most devices require the operator to occlude a side hole to apply negative pressure through the lumen. In general, suctioning should be performed under direct visualization to avoid injury to the pharynx. It should also be done in brief intervals not exceeding 30 seconds to avoid prolonged hypoxemia. Supplemental

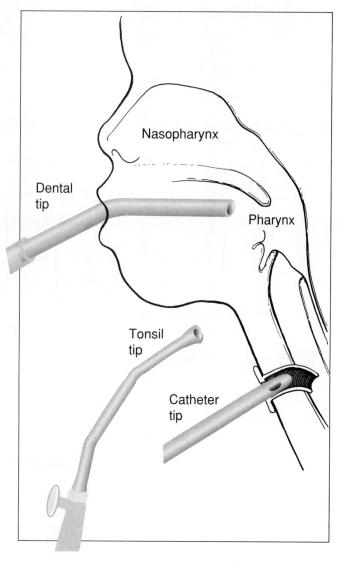

Figure 13.9.
Suction devices.

Nasopharynx

Dental tip

Pharynx

Tonsil tip

Catheter tip

SUMMARY:
SUCTIONING THE AIRWAY
1. Perform suctioning under direct visualization in brief intervals not exceeding 30 seconds.
2. Provide supplemental oxygen during intervals between suctioning.
3. Use catheter tip suction device for suctioning nasopharynx or for suctioning through an endotracheal tube or tracheostomy cannula.
4. Use dental tip suction device for removing vomitus or particulate matter from pharynx.
5. Use tonsil tip suction device for removing blood and blood clots from pharynx.

oxygen should be provided in the intervals between suctioning. The heart rate should be monitored, because vagal stimulation resulting in bradycardia may occur from catheter stimulation of the posterior pharynx (1).

Complications

Suctioning is normally a safe and well-tolerated procedure in pediatric patients. Excessively deep suctioning of any patient should be avoided to minimize the risk of vomiting with subsequent aspiration or laryngospasm. Should vomiting occur, the child's head is first turned to one side, and suctioning is continued with a dental tip device until the emesis is cleared. This obviously assumes that the child is not at risk for possible cervical cord

injury from movement of the neck. If such a risk exists, the child's neck should be immobilized (manually or with a cervical collar), and the entire body should be rolled to one side, preferably on a spine immobilization board (Fig. 13.10). In this way, suctioning can be effectively performed, and the child's head turned to one side without movement of the neck.

Nasal suctioning may cause mild epistaxis, although this is not generally a significant problem if the clinician avoids excessive force. In addition, there have been several reports of nasogastric tubes and nasopharyngeal airways being inadvertently introduced into the cranium of patients with an injury to the cribiform plate (6–8). Although this complication is rare, it underscores the need for caution when inserting a suction catheter into

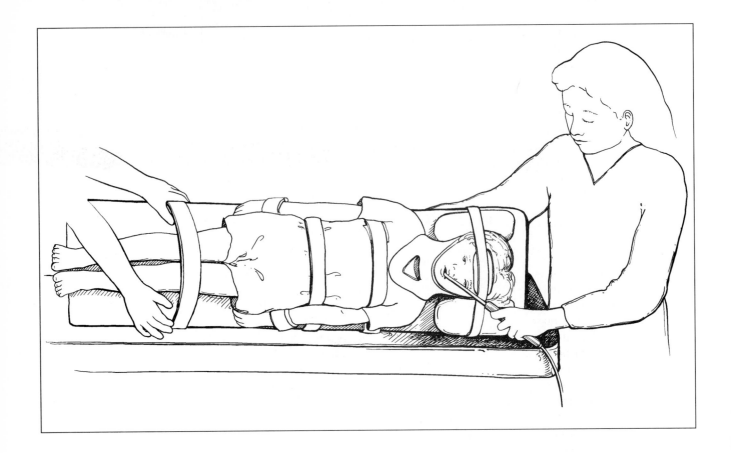

Figure 13.10.
Preferred method for suctioning the oropharynx of a child with possible cervical spine injury. The patient's head is turned to the side without moving the neck.

the nasopharynx of a patient with head or facial injuries.

USE OF ARTIFICIAL AIRWAYS

Inflammation and disease involving the soft tissues of the pharynx and supraglottic area are important causes of airway obstruction in children. In addition, the relatively large tongue and lax airway characteristic of pediatric patients result in a greater tendency for obstruction owing to causes such as mental status depression or simply lying in a supine position. Occlusion of the airway as a result of these "fixed" processes is obviously not amenable to suctioning, but both types of conditions may be easy to reverse with insertion of an artificial airway. An oropharyngeal or nasopharyngeal airway will often bypass the obstructing tissue, allowing either the patient to resume spontaneous respirations or the operator to effectively assist ventilation with a BVM circuit. In such cases, proper use of an artificial airway may therefore obviate the need for endotracheal intubation or at least provide a temporizing measure until intubation can be performed.

Indications

The optimal situation for using an oropharyngeal airway is with an unconscious child who has an intact gag reflex and readily reversible airway obstruction resulting from laxity of the tongue and pharyngeal soft tissues. If the underlying process is transient (e.g., iatrogenic overdose with a short-acting sedative), an oral airway can often be used to maintain patency until the child regains consciousness. If the process is more serious (overwhelming sepsis, head injury, etc.), an oral airway can be used to facilitate BVM ventilation before endotracheal intubation. It can also be used as a bite block after the patient has been intubated. Because an oropharyngeal airway directly contacts the tongue and supraglottic structures, it may induce vomiting. It is for this reason that the child with an impaired gag reflex is not a good candidate for insertion of an oral airway, as vomiting may lead to aspiration pneumonitis. With such patients, an oropharyngeal airway should be used only for brief periods and only when necessary. A nasal airway should be used in this situation whenever possible. If the child is fully awake, an oropharyngeal airway is likely to cause gagging, vomiting, soft tissue injury, or laryngospasm and should therefore not be used (9).

A nasopharyngeal airway provides an alternative means for overcoming obstruction of the airway not alleviated with simple suctioning. It is particularly useful for a child who is conscious and not likely to tolerate an oropharyngeal airway. For example, a child who has had a prolonged seizure and is postictal may experience relaxation of the muscles of the floor of the mouth, allowing the base of the tongue to occlude the larynx. In such cases, a nasopharyngeal airway will often prevent obstruction until the child is more alert, while being much less likely than an oropharyngeal airway to induce emesis. A nasopharyngeal airway may also be useful for the patient with partial airway obstruction as a result of oral or mandibular trauma, when limited mouth opening or injury to the teeth makes use of an oropharyngeal airway inadvisable. A child with infectious mononucleosis or bacterial pharyngitis may have significant tonsillar hypertrophy causing partial airway obstruction. For these patients, a nasopharyngeal airway will often provide an effective conduit for gas exchange, bypassing the obstructing tissues. Such children may also have enlarged adenoids; therefore, special care must be exercised in inserting a nasopharyngeal airway to avoid mucosal injury and bleeding.

Equipment

An oropharyngeal airway is a molded piece of hard plastic consisting of a curved body (stent), a short bite block, and a flange (Fig. 13.11) The flange serves as a site for taping the airway into place as well as preventing the airway from being advanced too far into the pharynx. The bite block fits between the teeth causing the mouth to remain slightly open. A central air channel is contained within the stent, providing a passage for air exchange and allowing insertion of a suction catheter. The curved stent is designed to fit over the posterior aspect of the tongue to prevent it from contacting the pharyngeal wall. A variety of pediatric oropharyngeal airway sizes are available, ranging from 4 to 10 cm in length.

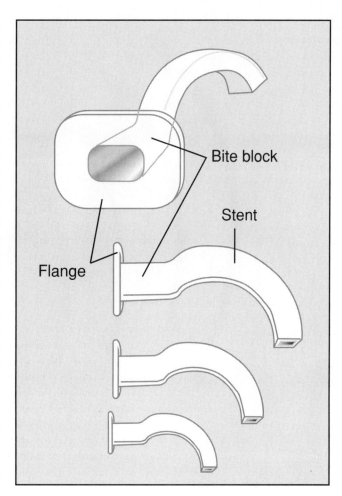

Bite block

Stent

Flange

Figure 13.11.
Oropharyngeal airway.

Standard nasopharyngeal airways (Leyland) are simply red rubber tubes which are narrow and flexible (Fig. 13.12). The distal end is angled to facilitate passage of the tube over the nasal turbinates. As with an oropharyngeal airway, a flange at the proximal end prevents further passage into the nose. Nasopharyngeal airways range in size from 12 to 36 French and are progressively longer as the diameter of the lumen increases. The proper size for most infants is 12 French, which is approximately the caliber of a 3 mm ID endotracheal tube.

More recent designs of nasopharyngeal airways have been successfully used with adult patients. A cuffed airway has been demonstrated as effective for anesthetized, spontaneously breathing adults (14). The tip of this airway is positioned just above the epiglottis and the inflated cuff contacts the soft palate, securing it in place. This device is not recommended for use during prolonged periods of assisted ventilation, because the

Figure 13.12.
Nasopharyngeal airways.

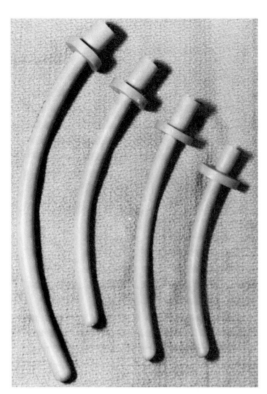

airway is not protected. Another design, the Linder airway, is made of soft plastic and has an introducer with a smooth, rounded tip designed to minimize the likelihood of bleeding. In a study of 85 adult patients, the Linder airway was found to have a lower incidence of nasal bleeding on insertion than other commonly used airways (15). It is likely that such modifications of the standard nasopharyngeal airway soon will be available for use with pediatric patients.

Procedure

Oropharyngeal Airway Insertion

An oropharyngeal airway of proper size is estimated by first placing it adjacent to the patient's face, with the flange at the level of the central incisors and the bite block parallel to the hard palate. Held in this position, the tip of a properly sized airway should reach the angle of the mandible (1, 10). All centers caring for children should have an array of sizes of oropharyngeal airways available.

Before inserting an oropharyngeal airway, the operator should ensure that the patient is appropriately monitored and receiving supplemental oxygen. A suction device and a

Figure 13.13.
Insertion of an oropharyngeal airway using a tongue blade.

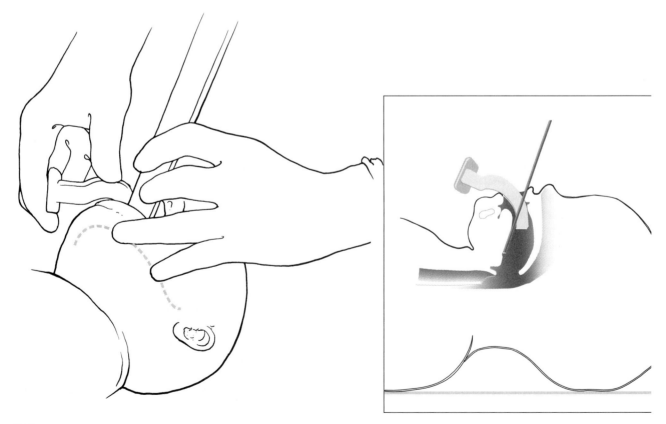

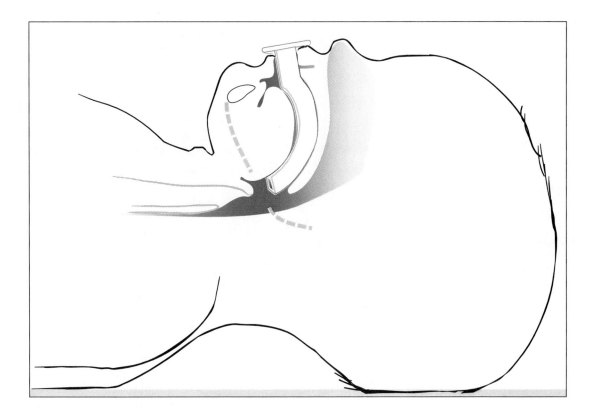

BVM circuit should be available in case of vomiting or airway compromise. The child should be lying in the supine position. Using a tongue depressor to displace the tongue, the operator first inserts the airway into the mouth with the concave side pointing posteriorly (Fig. 13.13). The airway is then gently guided under direct visualization along the length of the soft palate until the tip is located in the posterior hypopharynx. The curved portion of the airway separates the tongue from the posterior pharyngeal wall and pulls the epiglottis slightly forward (11) (Fig. 13.14). An alternative method of placement involves inserting the airway with the concave side pointing superiorly and then rotating it 180°. This technique is not recommended for pediatric patients, because it is more likely to cause posterior displacement of the tongue and injury to the soft palate, tonsils, or teeth (12).

Once the airway is in place, it may be secured to the face with tape. Assuming the obstruction was caused by occlusion of the airway by the tongue or other pharyngeal soft tissues, a properly placed oropharyngeal airway should result in prompt alleviation of the obstruction. The clinician should appreciate decreased work of breathing and improved gas exchange and oxygenation. If the child's condition fails to improve, this may indicate that an improperly sized airway has been inserted or that a problem exists which is not readily reversible. When this occurs, the airway should be quickly withdrawn and rechecked to ensure it is the appropriate size for the patient. If the obstruction cannot be alleviated with an oropharyngeal airway and proper positioning, preparations should be made for securing a definitive airway.

Nasopharyngeal Airway Insertion

The same preparatory steps described for oropharyngeal airway insertion should be performed before inserting a nasopharyngeal airway. As with the previous procedure, it is important to select a nasopharyngeal airway that is appropriately sized for the patient. In general, the proper length is equal to the distance between the nostril and the lobule of the ear, as measured by holding the airway next to the child's face (Fig. 13.15). This length allows the tip of the airway to reside just above the epiglottis.

The use of a topical vasoconstrictor such as neosynephrine is recommended 1 to 2 minutes before insertion in order to minimize the risk of bleeding. Each nostril can be occluded

Figure 13.14.
Proper position for an oropharyngeal airway.

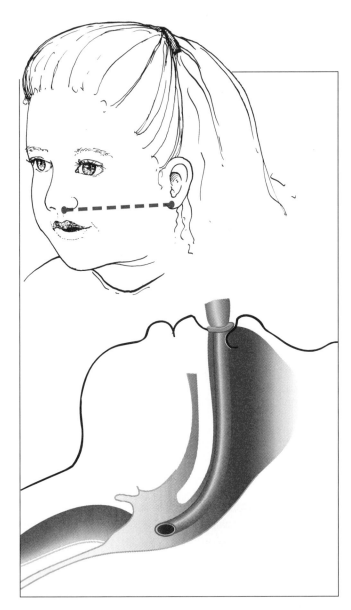

Figure 13.15.
Insertion of a
nasopharyngeal airway.
The airway can be sized
properly by placing it
adjacent to the child's
face. The correct size will
match the distance from
the lobule of the ear to the
nostril. After insertion, the tip
of the airway should be
positioned at the
supraglottic region.

Chapter 13
Airway Adjuncts,
Oxygen Delivery,
and Suctioning
the Upper Airway

116

in turn to determine which is more patent. The nasal airway should be liberally lubricated and inserted into the nare so the angled side faces the nasal septum. This decreases the likelihood of injuring the turbinates. If resistance is met on one side, then insertion should be attempted on the other. It may be necessary to rotate the airway 180° (i.e., the concave side faces superiorly) in order to have the angled side of the tip facing the septum. When this is done, the airway can then be rotated back into its proper orientation after the tip reaches the posterior pharynx.

The patient should be reassessed following nasopharyngeal airway insertion. Hopefully the clinician will see a decrease in the patient's respiratory effort and improved air flow and oxygenation if the airway has been inserted properly. As with the oropharyngeal airway, if adequate airway patency is not established more definitive measures will likely be necessary.

Complications

Use of an oropharyngeal airway that is either too small or too large can exacerbate airway obstruction. An airway that is too small can push the base of the tongue against the posterior pharyngeal wall, whereas an airway that is too large can displace the epiglottis inferi-

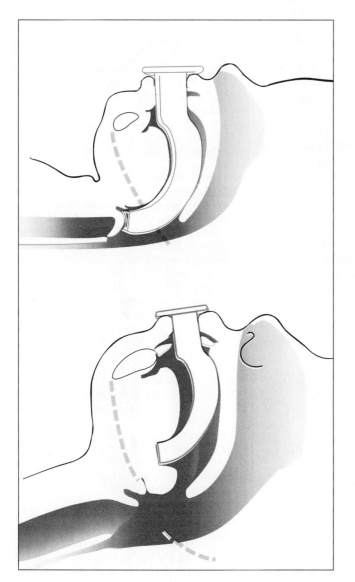

Figure 13.16.
Improperly sized oropharyngeal airways. An oropharyngeal airway that is too large will displace the epiglottis inferiorly over the glottic opening. An airway that is too small will impinge on the tongue displacing it posteriorly into the hypopharynx.

orly over the glottic opening (Fig. 13.16). In addition, an oropharyngeal airway may induce vomiting, which can in turn cause aspiration pneumonitis in the patient with depressed airway reflexes. If the child is fully awake, insertion of an oral airway can cause laryngospasm or injury of the pharyngeal soft tissues due to coughing and gagging. Such complications can usually be avoided by using an appropriately sized airway and proper patient selection. As stated previously, the most appropriate patient for use of an oral airway is an unconscious child with an intact gag reflex.

Few significant complications are associated with using a nasopharyngeal airway. Occasionally the airway may cause injury to nasal mucosa or adenoidal tissue resulting in

epistaxis. If the patient has a coagulopathy, such bleeding can be profuse and may cause problems with maintaining airway patency. In such cases, intervention by an otolaryngologist may be required. Clearly, caution in inserting a nasal airway must be exercised with all patients. Prolonged use of a nasopharyngeal airway has been associated with ulceration of the nasal mucosa, otitis media, and sinusitis, although these complications are not a concern during an emergent resuscitation. If the patient has a basilar skull fracture, a nasal airway may be inserted through a disruption in the cribiform plate into the anterior cranial fossa (6–8). Although this is a rare complication, a nasopharyngeal airway should not be used for any child suspected of having this injury.

Chapter 13
Airway Adjuncts,
Oxygen Delivery,
and Suctioning
the Upper Airway

117

SUMMARY

Respiratory difficulties are an important cause of pediatric cardiopulmonary arrest. Medical personnel must be adept at providing supplemental oxygen, achieving and maintaining a patent airway, and assisting the ventilation of any critically ill child. Once it has been established that a spontaneously breathing child in respiratory distress has a patent airway, oxygen should always be provided. The clinician must be familiar with various oxygen delivery devices and select an appropriate system based on the patient's needs. In all but a few exceptional situations, an oxygen concentration should be delivered that is adequate to maintain an oxyhemoglobin saturation of 100%.

For a child with evidence of airway obstruction, suctioning of the nasopharynx or oropharynx is often beneficial. In addition, airway maneuvers may be effective in establishing patency. If these measures are unsuccessful, insertion of an artificial airway may be necessary. A nasopharyngeal airway is best suited for an alert child whereas an oropharyngeal airway is most effective for the obtunded patient who has an intact gag reflex. Depending on the clinical situation, insertion of an artificial airway may serve as a definitive procedure or as a temporizing measure before endotracheal intubation. Familiarity with these adjunctive procedures and mastery of the necessary manual skills are essential for all medical personnel who care for critically ill or injured children.

REFERENCES

1. Chameides L. Pediatric airway management. In: American Heart Association textbook of pediatric advanced life support, 1988.

2. Ludwig S, Kettrick RG, Parker M. Pediatric cardiopulmonary resuscitation. Clin Ped 1984;23:71–75.

3. Cote CJ, Todres DI. The pediatric airway. In: Ryan JF, Cote CJ, eds. A practice of anesthesia for infants and children. Philadelphia: WB Saunders, 1986.

4. Gas regulation, administration, and controlling devices. In: McPhearson SP, ed. Respiratory therapy equipment. St. Louis: CV Mosby, 1990.

5. Clinton JE, Ruiz E. Respiratory procedures. In: Roberts JR, Hedges J, eds. Clinical procedures in emergency medicine. Philadelphia: WB Saunders, 1991.

6. Muzzi DA, Losasso TJ, Cucchiara RF. Complication from a nasopharyngeal airway in a patient with a basilar skull fracture. Anesthesiology 1991;74:366–368.

7. Fremstad JD, Martin SH. Lethal complication from insertion of nasogastric tube after severe basilar skull fracture. J Trauma 1978;18:820–822.

8. Fletcher SA, Henderson LT, Minor ME, Jones JM. The successful surgical removal of intracranial nasogastric tubes. J Trauma 1987;27:948–952.

9. American Heart Association. Pediatric advanced life support. JAMA 1986;255:2961–2968.

10. Kettrick R, Ludwig S. Resuscitation—Pediatric basic and advanced life support. In: Fleisher G, Ludwigs S, eds. Textbook of Pediatric Emergency Medicine. Baltimore: Williams & Wilkins, 1988.

11. Face Masks and Airways. In: Dorsch JA, Dorsch SE, eds. Understanding anesthesia equipment—construction, care and complications. Baltimore: Williams & Wilkins, 1984.

12. American College of Surgeons. Advanced trauma life support. Upper Airway Management, pp. 23–29.

13. Hwang CL, et al. Estimation of the length of nasopharyngeal airway in Chinese adults. Anaesth Sinica 1990;28:49–54.

14. Feldman SA, Fauvel NJ, Ooi R. The cuffed pharyngeal airway. Eur J Anesthes 1991;8:291–295.

15. Gallagher WJ, Pearce AC, Power SJ. Assessment of a new nasopharyngeal airway. Brit J Anesthes 1982;66:112–115.

BAG-VALVE-MASK VENTILATION

Christopher King and Alfred T. Dorsey

INTRODUCTION

The first steps in most pediatric resuscitations are to establish a patent airway and to provide adequate ventilatory support. Although definitive management of a respiratory emergency normally involves endotracheal intubation, this may not be possible initially if the appropriate equipment is unavailable or properly trained personnel are not present. Even in settings where intubation can be performed rapidly, the patient may require respiratory support before the procedure. It is in such situations that bag-valve-mask (BVM) ventilation is indicated. Patients requiring assisted or controlled ventilation may be managed on an immediate basis with minimal preparation using this procedure. In most cases, BVM ventilation serves as a temporizing measure to be used before intubation and during intervals between intubation attempts. It is often possible, however, to support a patient through a brief apneic episode (e.g., oversedation) with BVM ventilation alone.

BVM ventilation is a skill that many health care providers—including physicians, nurses, respiratory therapists, and paramedics—are called on to perform. It is undoubtedly the procedure most commonly used by medical personnel in the initial management of pediatric respiratory emergencies. But this should by no means indicate that BVM ventilation is a simple procedure. Most practitioners who care for critically ill children can relate experiences during which performing manual ventilation proved far more difficult

than endotracheal intubation. In addition, published studies have questioned the effectiveness of BVM ventilation in the hands of less experienced operators. For these reasons, as with any airway intervention, the attention of the team leader in a pediatric resuscitation should never be far from the proficiency with which BVM ventilation is being performed.

ANATOMY AND PHYSIOLOGY

A number of anatomic differences exist between pediatric and adult patients which have important clinical implications regarding the use of BVM ventilation (Fig. 14.1). Not surprisingly, these differences are most apparent among infants and become less pronounced as the patient matures through older childhood and adolescence. One such characteristic is that the tongue of an infant or younger child is larger relative to the oral cavity when compared with an adult. In addition, the tongue has a more rostral (superior) location in relation to the roof of the mouth. The larger size and "higher" position of the tongue greatly increase the likelihood of airway obstruction when the patient is lying supine. Using an artificial airway is therefore often necessary when performing BVM ventilation with a pediatric patient (see Chapter 13). Infants also exhibit obligate nasal breathing until about 3 to 5 months of age as a result of obstruction of the oropharyngeal airway as the tongue rests against the roof of the mouth. Occlusion of the nares because of stenosis or choanal atresia, as well as transient causes

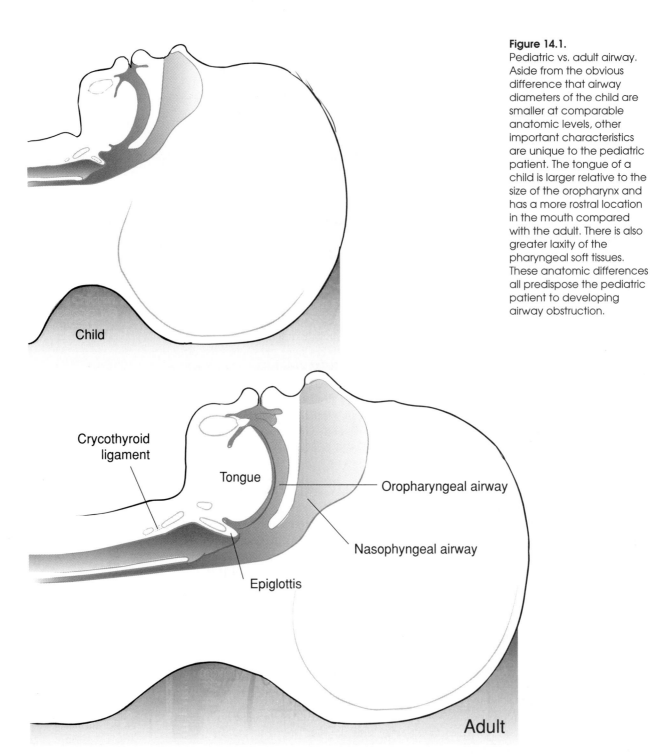

Figure 14.1.
Pediatric vs. adult airway. Aside from the obvious difference that airway diameters of the child are smaller at comparable anatomic levels, other important characteristics are unique to the pediatric patient. The tongue of a child is larger relative to the size of the oropharynx and has a more rostral location in the mouth compared with the adult. There is also greater laxity of the pharyngeal soft tissues. These anatomic differences all predispose the pediatric patient to developing airway obstruction.

Child

Crycothyroid ligament

Tongue

Oropharyngeal airway

Nasophyngeal airway

Epiglottis

Adult

such as blood, vomitus, or secretions, can produce profound respiratory distress and even asphyxia in an infant (1, 2). In such cases, BVM ventilation is an effective means of bypassing the obstruction and providing gas exchange via the oropharynx.

The immature laryngeal cartilages of the pediatric airway are more compliant, allowing wider variation in the airway diameter in response to compressive or distending forces (3, 4). As a result, pediatric patients with partial airway obstruction are more prone to develop dynamic collapse of the extrathoracic airway as a result of high negative intraluminal pressures, increasing the work of breathing. Manual ventilation is often effective in such situations, because this negative pressure is reduced or eliminated (see below). Infants and children also have greater laxity of the cervical spine and neck musculature (5–7). This can lead to excessive rotation of the head during attempts to establish a patent airway, which can result in complete airway obstruction (Fig. 14.2).

As described in Chapter 16, the optimal position of the head and neck for airway patency is the so-called "sniffing position." The neck is slightly flexed while the head is rotated into extension. This is said to be the position assumed when one is "sniffing the air," and it results in the most favorable alignment of the oral, pharyngeal, and tracheal axes (8) (Fig. 14.3). With adolescents and adults, it is generally necessary to place a small towel roll or pad under the head to achieve the proper degree of neck flexion. However, because infants and younger children have a relatively large occiput, such measures are not usually required (Fig. 14.4).

The relative immaturity of the pediatric diaphragm, intercostal muscles, and ribs can also impact on the use of BVM ventilation. The chest wall of an infant or child is significantly more compliant than that of an adolescent or adult (9). As a result, there is less "protective" resistance provided by the chest wall, which results in a higher incidence of barotrauma during BVM ventilation. In addition, pediatric patients have a greater tendency to develop early respiratory muscle fatigue, potentially leading to respiratory arrest. This is primarily the result of the immature diaphragm having a lower content of Type I muscle fibers (slow twitch, high oxidative capacity) which confer fatigue resistance (10). The infant's diaphragm is also more horizontal and therefore less efficient in expanding the lungs. One clinical consequence of these characteristics relates to pediatric patients with processes causing significant upper airway obstruction such as epiglottitis. For many years, respiratory arrest due to epiglottitis was believed to be the result of complete obstruction of the airway which could only be relieved with endotracheal intubation or a surgical airway. More recent experience has shown that arrest results primarily due to diaphragmatic muscle fatigue (i.e., the child simply tires after prolonged breathing against a "tight" partial airway obstruction, and respiration eventually ceases). This in part accounts for the more benign clinical course of adult epiglottitis. As a result, BVM ventilation can often be used very effectively to ven-

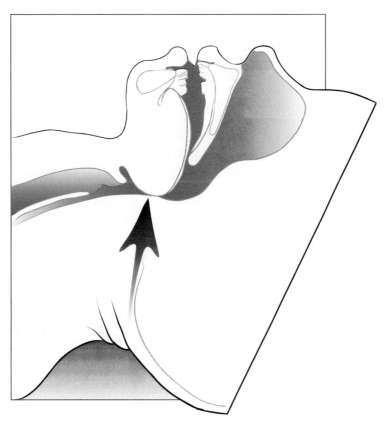

Figure 14.2.
Excessive extension of the neck in an attempt to establish airway patency can actually cause or worsen obstruction.

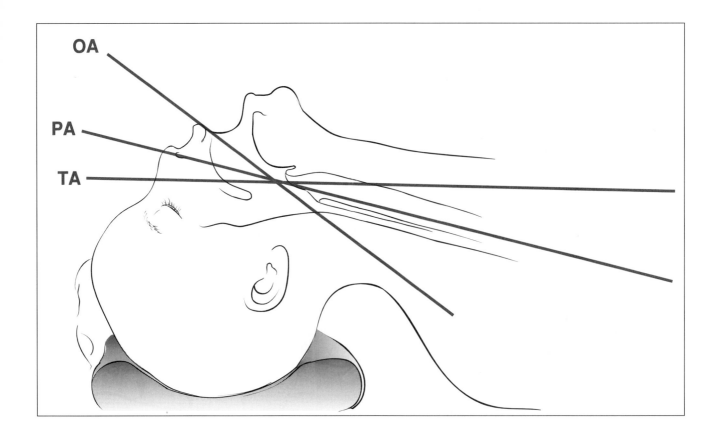

Figure 14.3.
The sniffing position results in the most favorable alignment of the oral, pharyngeal, and tracheal axes for airway patency. Note that a small pad may be necessary to achieve the necessary flexion of the neck for an older child or adolescent (see also Fig. 16.3).

Chapter 14
Bag-Valve-Mask
Ventilation

tilate a patient whose respiratory musculature can no longer overcome the increased airway resistance caused by epiglottitis (11, 12).

Certain congenital abnormalities of the face and airway can make BVM ventilation difficult or impossible to perform. For example, achieving an adequate mask seal may not be possible if the child has micrognathia or other midfacial anomalies. This is also true for patients with severe trauma to the face or mandible. In addition, administering manual ventilation may be problematic for children with macroglossia due to difficulty maintaining a patent airway. In such cases, providing positive pressure ventilation (PPV) to treat respiratory failure may require immediate endotracheal intubation.

Use of BVM ventilation may be affected by several characteristics of pediatric respiratory physiology. As with endotracheal intubation, BVM ventilation is a useful means of providing respiratory support because it offers a method of delivering PPV. Although normal spontaneous ventilation and PPV both result in oxygen delivery to the body, in many ways these two processes have opposing physiologic effects. Spontaneous respiration occurs when the negative intrathoracic

pressure generated by contraction of the respiratory muscles (primarily the diaphragm) causes expansion on the lungs and passive movement of air into the upper airway. As the term implies, positive pressure ventilation with a BVM circuit involves forced air entry through the upper airway and into the lungs, which is produced by an externally applied pressure. One clinically important result of this difference is the contrasting effects these two modes of ventilation have on the extrathoracic airway (Fig. 14.5). With spontaneous respiration, the extrathoracic airway experiences negative intraluminal pressures (relative to atmospheric pressure) during inspiration. As mentioned previously, this negative pressure may be significantly increased with partial airway obstruction and can result in dynamic collapse of the airway proximal to the obstruction (3), which can worsen the patient's respiratory distress and increase the work of breathing. Controlled ventilation with a BVM circuit tends to "stent" the extrathoracic airway open, even when partial obstruction is present, as the airway experiences positive intraluminal pressures throughout inspiration (Fig. 14.6).

Physiologic differences between sponta-

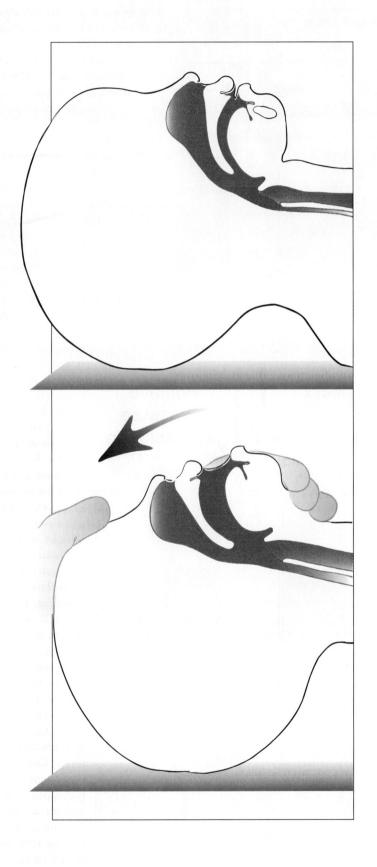

Figure 14.4.
Infants and younger children have a relatively large occiput which displaces the neck anteriorly when the patient is lying supine on a flat surface, so that placing a pad under the head is unnecessary. The only maneuver needed to achieve the sniffing position is extension (rotation) of the head.

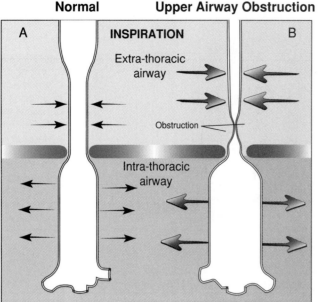

A INSPIRATION B

Extra-thoracic
airway

Obstruction

Intra-thoracic
airway

Figure 14.5.
A. During spontaneous respiration, the extrathoracic airway experiences negative intraluminal pressure on inspiration.
B. With airway obstruction, this negative pressure increases greatly and may produce collapse of the extrathoracic airway proximal to the obstruction.

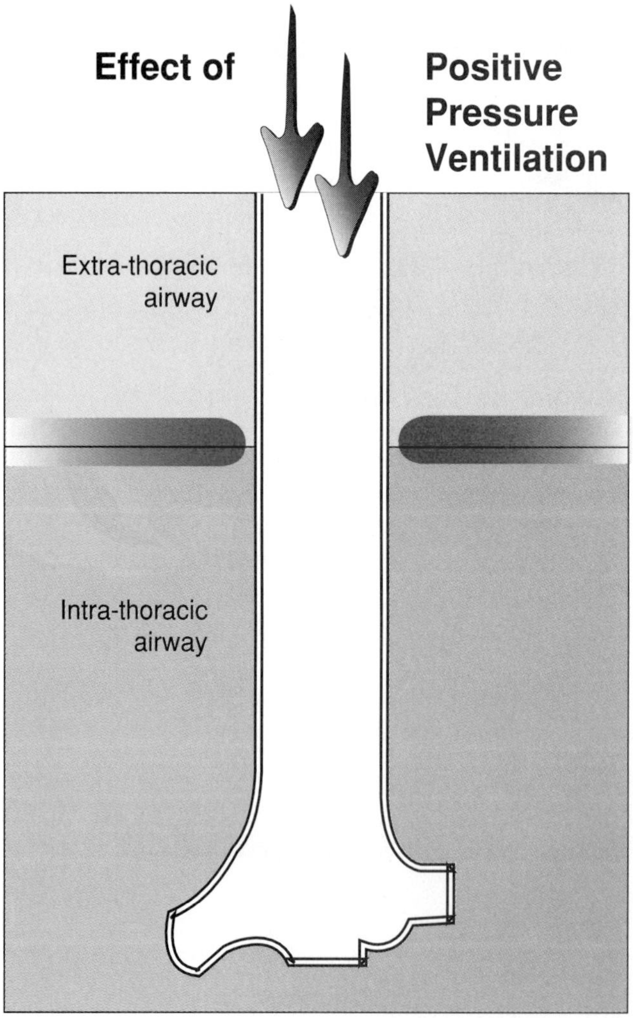

Effect of **Positive Pressure Ventilation**

Extra-thoracic
airway

Intra-thoracic
airway

Figure 14.6.
During BVM ventilation, the extrathoracic airway is "stented" open by the effect of positive intraluminal pressure throughout the respiratory cycle.

**Chapter 14
Bag-Valve-Mask
Ventilation**

neous ventilation and PPV may also play a role in some adverse consequences associated with BVM ventilation. For example, the elevated intrathoracic pressure that occurs with PPV reduces venous return to the heart and can cause a decrease in cardiac output (13), although interestingly, this may be less pronounced in children than adults (14). This effect normally has clinical significance only for patients with hypovolemia or borderline cardiac function. Consequently, such patients who receive BVM ventilation may require increased intravenous fluid administration to maintain stable hemodynamics. In addition, BVM ventilation can exacerbate ventilation-perfusion (VQ) mismatching (15, 16). With spontaneous ventilation, the lung bases receive the majority of both air entry and blood flow during inspiration; ventilation and perfusion are therefore well matched. When a patient receives BVM ventilation, the distribution of air entry is determined primarily by compliance of the lung parenchyma, which is greatest in the apices. As a result, while blood continues to flow preferentially to the bases, the majority of air entry now goes to the apices, resulting in VQ mismatch. This accounts for the spontaneously breathing patient who may have a decrease in oxygen saturation when assisted ventilation with a BVM circuit is initiated. For this reason, the delivered oxygen concentration should be maximized whenever manual ventilation is performed.

One of the more unwelcome events during BVM ventilation of a pediatric patient is the sudden, dramatic decline in oxygen saturation that results when oxygen delivery is inadequate, which is also related to a unique characteristic of pediatric physiology. Compared with adults, the rate of oxygen consumption among infants and children is significantly higher; the baseline oxygen consumption of a neonate is approximately twice that of an adult

(17). As a result, if the concentration of oxygen delivered by manual ventilation is insufficient for any reason (e.g., unrecognized mask leak, rebreathing of expired gases), the pO_2 of a pediatric patient will drop more rapidly as compared with an adult (18). This appears to be even more pronounced among children with upper respiratory infections (19). Because the oxygen dissociation curve has an initial flat segment, the oxygen saturation reading of the pulse oximeter remains relatively stable despite the fact that the pO_2 is falling (Fig. 14.7). If this problem is not recognized, oxygen saturation will suddenly decline precipitously when the pO_2 reaches the steep segment of the curve. This diminished margin for error makes the timely recognition of problems leading to inadequate oxygen delivery an important priority with pediatric patients.

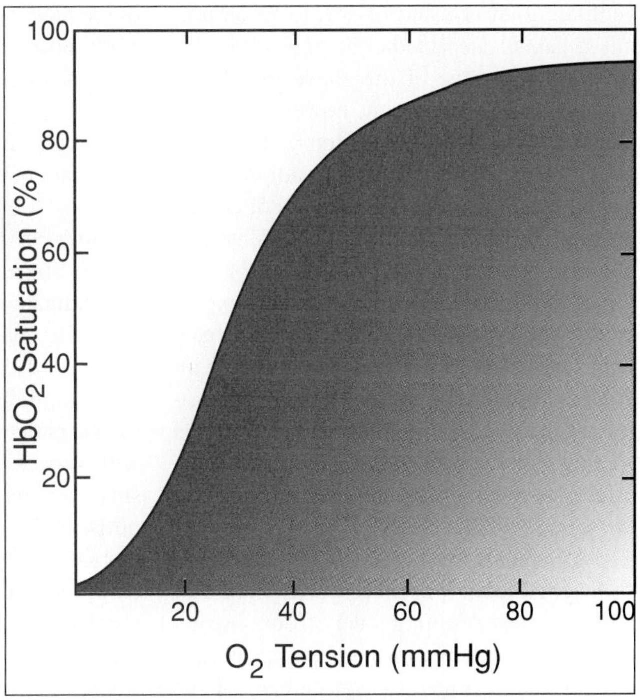

Figure 14.7.
Oxyhemoglobin dissociation curve.

INDICATIONS

The primary indication for the use of BVM ventilation is to provide temporary ventilatory support until definitive management can be undertaken or the patient resumes spontaneous respiration. There are few contraindications to BVM ventilation. Relative contraindications include any problems that significantly undermine the effectiveness of the procedure, such as congenital or traumatic facial deformities so severe that a mask seal is impossible to maintain, or a high-grade airway obstruction that prevents delivery of adequate ventilatory support. If such a process becomes apparent when BVM ventilation is attempted, an alternate procedure (e.g., immediate endotracheal intubation, percutaneous transtracheal ventilation, or a surgical airway) should be performed. In addition, BVM ventilation should not be used for any significant length of time with a patient who is suspected of having a tension pneumothorax before the appropriate interventions for this process. Continued delivery of PPV can further increase the elevated intrathoracic pressure. BVM ventilation can be used for immediate stabilization if such a patient is apneic, but needle thoracostomy and/or chest tube insertion (Chapter 30) should be performed as soon as possible. The only situations that represent absolute contraindications to the use of this procedure are the initial management of a thick meconium delivery (Chapter 39) and the presence of a diaphragmatic hernia (Chapter 41), both of which require immediate endotracheal intubation.

Indications for the use of BVM ventilation can be divided into two general categories—problems of the airway and problems with ventilation. Airway indications for BVM ventilation include the various causes of upper airway obstruction affecting pediatric patients that can lead to significant respiratory compromise. For example, partial airway obstruction resulting from bacterial and viral infections such as croup, epiglottitis, and retropharyngeal abscess may serve as an indication for BVM ventilation. As discussed previously, pediatric patients may develop respiratory arrest as a result of airway obstruction long before BVM ventilation would be difficult to administer. In other words, the obstruction is rarely "complete." Thus the operator should not be dissuaded from making an initial attempt at manually ventilating an arrested or severely compromised patient suspected of having airway obstruction from one of the above mentioned processes. It is important, however, to emphasize that assisted ventilation with a BVM circuit is *not* indicated for a child with suspected epiglottitis or another cause of airway obstruction who is stable and breathing adequately. Such a patient should not be disturbed, but should instead be managed expectantly with airway equipment close at hand until surgical and anesthesia personnel are involved. Fortunately, the incidence of epiglottitis in the pediatric population has declined sharply with the widespread availability of an effective vaccine against *Haemophilus influenzae* (20–22).

As mentioned above, infants and younger children may present with frank respiratory arrest resulting solely from obstruction caused by laxity of the pharyngeal musculature and posterior displacement of the tongue. Such patients normally have other medical problems (e.g., sepsis or toxic ingestion), causing a profoundly depressed mental status. In this situation, the use of BVM ventilation, combined with proper positioning and insertion of an artificial airway, offers an effective approach to managing the respiratory component of the overall presentation. Other obstructive processes that can be initially managed using BVM ventilation include hematoma, supraglottic edema, and upper airway foreign body. For the patient with a rapidly expanding hematoma of the upper airway, BVM ventilation can be used in the early stage of management, but tracheal intubation should be performed as soon as the patient is stabilized. In addition, foreign bodies should normally be removed from the airway whenever possible before initiating BVM ventilation, because smaller objects may be propelled distally by the force of ventilations (see Chapter 54).

The ventilatory indications for the initial use of BVM ventilation include (*a*) nonobstructive causes of hypoventilation and respiratory arrest, (*b*) processes that lead to ineffective ventilation, and (*c*) insults to the lungs that cause impaired gas exchange. Hypoventilation and respiratory arrest in the pediatric population can result from a wide variety of neurologic, infectious, toxicologic, and metabolic disorders. In the ED, overwhelming sepsis and traumatic brain injury are two of the most common causes. Infants are especially prone to develop apnea as the first significant manifestation of an underlying illness. BVM ventilation should be initiated during a neonatal resuscitation whenever the heart rate is below 100 or the patient has apneic spells lasting 30 seconds or longer (see Chapter 38). Transient hypoventilation resulting from iatrogenic drug overdose (e.g., benzodiazapines for status epilepticus) can often be managed with BVM ventilation alone until the patient resumes spontaneous respiration. Ineffective ventilation among pediatric patients is most frequently associated with processes which affect patency of the small airways, such as asthma and bronchiolitis. Fatigue leading to hypoxia and hypercarbia usually accounts for the child's worsening condition. With these patients, BVM ventilation can be used to temporarily reduce the work of breathing, although in such situations, endotracheal intubation will usually prove necessary. The decision to initiate manual ventilation is based primarily on the clinician's assessment of the severity of the patient's respiratory compromise. Impaired alveolar gas exchange results from diverse etiologies, such as lung infection, near-drowning, and pulmonary contusion. With more severe and diffuse involvement of the lungs, the patient may manifest clinical findings consistent with adult respiratory distress syndrome. These children may develop profound hypoxemia and frequently require endotracheal intubation. When BVM ventilation is used in the initial management of such patients, the circuit should be configured to reliably deliver a concentration of oxygen near 100%, and if necessary, to administer positive end expiratory pressure (PEEP).

EQUIPMENT

Equipment and materials used to perform BVM ventilation are listed in Table 14.1. Figure 14.8 shows a typical self-inflating BVM circuit. Appropriate sizes should be selected carefully, as use of the proper equipment will often determine the success or failure of the procedure. As this is often a process of trial and error, the operator should not be reluctant to change equipment during BVM ventilation should this prove necessary. As with most pediatric procedures, an array of equipment

Table 14.1.
Equipment for BVM Ventilation

Array of face masks
Infant, pediatric, and adult resuscitation bags
Pressure manometer (when available)
Suction devices
Oxygen source
Oropharyngeal and nasopharyngeal airways
Monitors (pulse oximetry, cardiac monitor, capnography)

sizes should be available for all age groups (Fig. 14.9). In selecting the proper face mask, the operator should choose the smallest size that completely covers the patient's nose and mouth (Fig. 14.10). A mask that is too large may extend below the mandible, so that a good seal will be difficult or impossible to establish. A large mask may also be inadvertently positioned over the eyes. Compression of the eyes can produce bradycardia as a result of vagal stimulation or ocular injury. Conversely, a small mask will not cover the entire mouth, causing an air leak when PPV is administered. As stated above, it is often necessary to try more than one mask size before finding the proper fit.

The most important consideration in selecting a resuscitation bag is that delivery of an adequate tidal volume must be ensured. As a general rule, a resuscitation bag one size too large will produce better results than one that is too small, as long as the operator is careful not to deliver an excessive tidal volume. For example, a bag that would be suitable for an adolescent can normally be used effectively to administer BVM ventilation to a child. This may be particularly relevant to neonatal resuscitations. Investigators have demonstrated that apneic newborns require initial sustained ventilatory pressures in the range of 20 to 40 cm H_2O to produce adequate lung expansion (23–25). Field et al. found that a pediatric bag was actually superior to a neonatal bag for use during resuscitation of asphyxiated newborn infants, since only the pediatric bag would deliver the higher sus-

Figure 14.8.
Typical self-inflating BVM circuit.

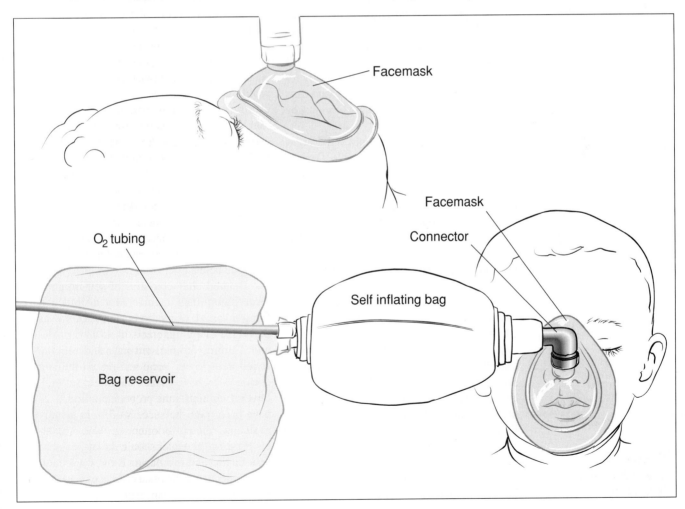

Facemask

Facemask

Connector

O_2 tubing

Self inflating bag

Bag reservoir

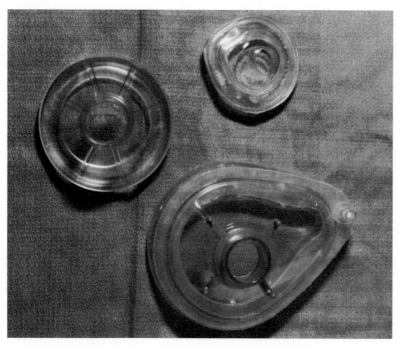

Figure 14.9.
Face masks of various sizes and shapes. Premature infant through adult sizes should be available.

circular Laerdal infant mask was found to be superior among several available models in a comparison of the quality of construction, methods for cleaning and sterilization, and the occurrence of mask leak (28). For children and adolescents, various sizes of the traditional triangular masks are generally appropriate. The Laerdal pocket mask, which is often carried by prehospital personnel, is not recommended for infants, because it was found to give unacceptable results due to poor fit (27).

BVM ventilation can be performed with two types of resuscitation bags—self-inflating and conventional anesthesia bags. Of the two, self-inflating bag systems are more widely employed in the emergent management of pediatric patients primarily because they are easier to use. As the name implies, the bag is designed to reinflate when released, without requiring any additional maneuvers or adjustment of the equipment. This characteristic, however, also represents one of the primary limitations of these systems, because the bag will refill regardless of the quality of the mask seal or the rate of oxygen flow. The operator may be unaware that a significant mask leak is present or that the oxygen source is malfunctioning or depleted. In addition, the rapid reexpansion of a self-inflating bag causes entrainment of room air (21% oxygen) into the system, reducing the delivered concentration of oxygen. Even when connected to a standard oxygen inflow of 10 to 15 L/min, a self-inflating BVM unit with no oxygen reservoir delivers an inconsistent oxygen concentration, ranging from 30 to 80% (29, 33). Fortunately, the widespread use of reservoir devices in the design of pediatric BVM systems has largely overcome this disadvantage (see below).

Desired characteristics of self-inflating resuscitation bags include easy disinfection using a variety of methods; non-stick valves that resist clogging; standard 15 mm (male) and 22 mm (female) fittings; and reliable function at lower temperatures so the bag does not freeze (e.g., in a cold field setting). Several comparisons of resuscitation bags have been published (26, 30–33). In a study evaluating the performance of various models used for neonates, the Laerdal pediatric resuscitator and the Ambu baby resuscitator were found to be the most effective in a series of 45 resuscitations (26). For infants and chil-

tained pressures required (26). Overall, mask fit appears to be a more important factor in ensuring adequate ventilation than bag size (27). Clearly, the use of a resuscitation bag that is far too large for the patient increases the risk of administering excessive tidal volume and ventilatory pressures, potentially resulting in gastric distension and barotrauma. In all cases, the chest wall excursions must be closely monitored.

A variety of different shapes and designs of pediatric face masks are available. Desired characteristics for masks include (*a*) one-piece construction, so the mask does not come apart during the procedure; (*b*) transparent materials, so emesis or perioral cyanosis can be readily seen; (*c*) easy cleaning and disinfection with a wide range of methods (gas sterilization, cold sterilization, steam autoclaving, etc.); (*d*) small "dead space" to minimize the amount of gas in the system not delivered to the patient; (*e*) nonirritating materials; and (*f*) a low pressure, high volume air-filled silicone seal. Hard rubber seals cause a higher incidence of air leak and facial nerve injury. The seal of some masks are designed with a valve that allows the operator to increase or decrease inflation, although this feature is normally useful only during changes in ambient pressure as with air transports. The optimal shape of the mask depends on the size and age of the patient. For premature infants and full-term neonates, the

dren, Finer et al. have recommended the Laerdal pediatric resuscitator based on laboratory tests using an artificial lung model (33).

The quality of the materials and design of self-inflating BVM units have improved significantly over the last several years. As mentioned previously, some of the more recent designs can be configured to deliver PEEP when necessary. In addition, many currently available models are disposable, eliminating the risk of disease transmission. Other enhancements that have been incorporated into most popular systems include nonstick one-way valves that are less susceptible to clogging with secretions, various methods for increasing the F_iO_2 delivered, in-line pressure monitors, and a "pop-off" pressure valve. The purpose of a pop-off valve is to limit the ventilatory pressures generated within the circuit to a designated level (generally between 35 and 45 cm H_2O), a feature that reduces the risk of barotrauma. However, when airway resistance is high or pulmonary compliance is low, the presence of a functioning pop-off valve has been shown to significantly diminish the F_iO_2 delivered and/or prevent administration of an adequate tidal volume (33). Any BVM unit equipped with a pop-off valve should therefore have a simple mechanism for disabling this device when necessary (34). In such cases, an in-line manometer should be used when available to prevent excessive peak inspiratory pressures and possible barotrauma (35).

In contrast to self-inflating resuscitation bags, conventional anesthesia bag circuits offer the advantage of providing a more reliable means of delivering high concentrations of oxygen. Proposed designs for a variety of these systems were originally described by Mapleson (36). The configurations most widely used for pediatric patients today are the Mapleson D circuit and two modifications of this system—the modified Mapleson D (Bain circuit) (36) and the Mapleson F (Jackson Rees circuit) (37). A schematic diagram of each of these systems is shown in Figure 14.11. All three circuits share the common elements of (a) a conventional anesthesia bag, (b) an oxygen outlet, and (c) a venting mechanism. They differ with regard to where these features are positioned on the unit. The Mapleson D circuit has the oxygen inlet positioned close to the patient and the

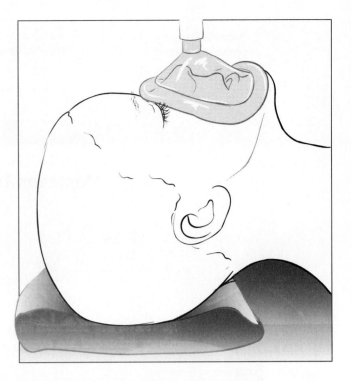

Figure 14.10.
The smallest mask that completely covers the nose and mouth should be selected.

venting mechanism close to the anesthesia bag, an arrangement that minimizes rebreathing of expired gases by the patient. The Bain circuit has both the oxygen inlet and the venting mechanism close to the anesthesia bag, with a narrow inner tube that extends from the oxygen inlet to a point near the patient. This facilitates warming and humidification of oxygen as it flows into the system. With the Jackson Rees circuit, the venting mechanism (which is often simply an opening to the atmosphere) is incorporated into the resuscitation bag. This circuit is especially popular for use in the operating room because of its light weight and simple design, although it has the disadvantage of requiring a higher rate of oxygen inflow to minimize rebreathing (38, 39).

Several important differences are found in both design and function between conventional anesthesia circuits and self-inflating BVM units. For one, anesthesia circuits do not require a reservoir system to deliver a high oxygen concentration. The bag itself serves as both the oxygen reservoir and the means of administering PPV. In addition, anesthesia circuits have some type of venting mechanism, consisting normally of an adjustable pressure limiting (APL) valve which opens to the atmosphere. The resistance of the valve is increased or decreased by the operator as needed. The purpose of the APL

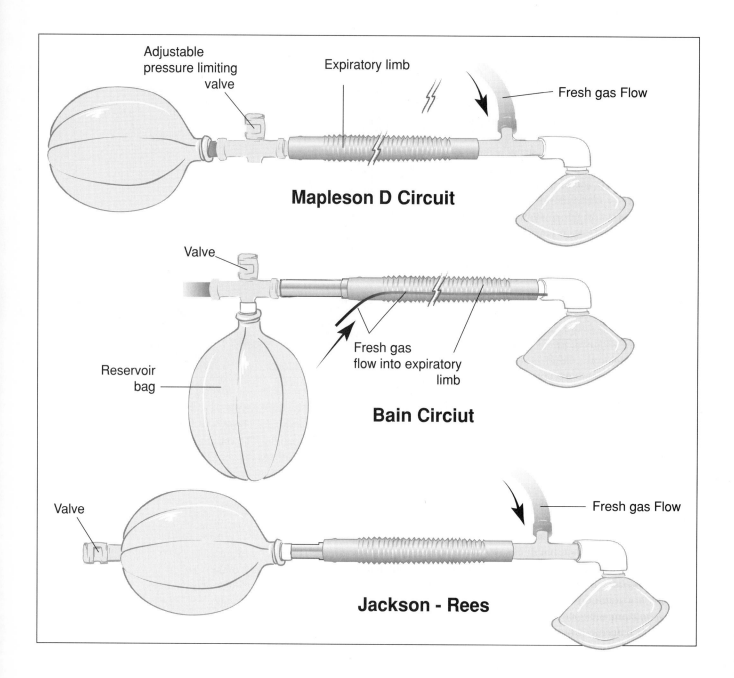

Adjustable
pressure limiting
valve

Expiratory limb

Fresh gas Flow

Mapleson D Circuit

Valve

Fresh gas
flow into expiratory
limb

Reservoir
bag

Bain Circiut

Valve

Fresh gas Flow

Jackson - Rees

Figure 14.11.
Commonly used
conventional anesthesia
bag circuits (see text for
description).

**Chapter 14
Bag-Valve-Mask
Ventilation**

valve is to vent gases exhaled by the patient while at the same time limiting the pressure within the circuit, much like a pop-off valve. Unlike self-inflating BVM units, anesthesia circuits have no one-way valves, which increases the possibility of the patient rebreathing expired gases. However, this potential drawback is more than offset by the fact that anesthesia circuits do not share the primary disadvantage of self-inflating BVM units (i.e., refilling with some fraction of atmospheric gases). As described previously, a significant percentage of the gas that enters a self-inflating bag when it reinflates is ambi-

ent air, whereas the only gas entrained into an anesthesia circuit is 100% oxygen. Furthermore, with the use of an appropriate oxygen flow rate and proper adjustment of the APL valve, the degree of rebreathing that occurs with an anesthesia bag circuit is generally minimal (38).

Several innovations in oxygen supplementation have been developed to increase the delivered F_iO_2 of self-inflating BVM units. The most commonly used device for this purpose is the oxygen reservoir system. Generally consisting of a length of corrugated tubing or a small plastic bag, a reservoir

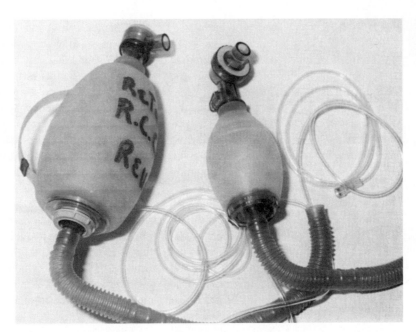

system allows oxygen to accumulate within the circuit during the interval between ventilations, substantially increasing the delivered F_iO_2. Importantly corrugated tube reservoirs (Fig. 14.12) have been found to provide an inconsistent and often inadequate F_iO_2, as their function depends on such variables as the length of the tube, bag refill time, and the rate of ventilation (29). These systems can be used for low level oxygen supplementation but are not recommended for patients requiring a consistently high concentration of oxygen. Bag reservoir systems (Fig. 14.8) deliver a higher F_iO_2 and offer the additional advantage of alerting the operator to a malfunctioning oxygen source, since most do not inflate if oxygen flow is interrupted. In general, a minimum oxygen flow of 10 to 15 L/min is necessary to maintain an adequate oxygen volume in the reservoir of a pediatric self-inflating BVM unit (33). Table 14.2 shows the various oxygen enrichment devices currently available and the range of oxygen concentrations each delivers. Oxygen supplementation for patients who receive BVM ventilation in the field is generally provided through an oxygen tank. Specific issues relating to the use of an oxygen tank are discussed in Chapter 13.

Even with the addition of a reservoir system, self-inflating resuscitation bags will optimally deliver only about 95% oxygen at the higher ventilatory rates used for children, and the F_iO_2 drops significantly if the oxygen inflow is not maintained at an appropriate level. A "low tech" method of increasing the delivered F_iO_2 of a self-inflating unit is to increase the refilling time (40). Normally, a self-inflating bag will reexpand immediately when released. The operator then waits a few seconds before delivering the next breath. If the refilling time is intentionally increased to about 4 seconds, a greater percentage of oxygen relative to ambient air will be entrained into the system. The operator accomplishes this by releasing the bag slowly, causing it to gradually reinflate over the entire interval between ventilations. This has been shown to increase the delivered F_iO_2 by as much as 40% over the traditional method. Unfortunately, this technique is only applicable to older children and adolescents, because the gradual refilling required cannot be performed effectively with ventilatory rates greater than 20 per minute (29).

Table 14.2.
Oxygen Enrichment for BVM Ventilation[a]

Device	Oxygen Concentration Delivered[a]
Oxygen line connected to bag	0.41
Corrugated tube reservoir	0.51–0.53[b]
2.5 liter bag reservoir	0.95–1.0

[a] Assumes an oxygen inflow rate of 15 l/min with self-inflating resuscitation bag. When used properly, a conventional anesthesia bag system reliably delivers an oxygen concentration of 1.0.

PROCEDURE

Management of the patient who requires BVM ventilation first involves standard basic life support (BLS) assessment and intervention. A detailed discussion of this initial approach is provided in Chapter 12. The primary operator takes a position above the head of the patient at the start of the resuscitation. When possible, the height of the bed should be adjusted to an appropriate level to both improve effectiveness and reduce fatigue. As described previously, airway patency is maximized when the patient is placed in the "sniffing" position, i.e., slight flexion of the neck with extension (rotation) of the head (Figs. 14.3 and 14.4). The airway is established using either the chin lift or jaw thrust maneuvers, and the operator then assesses the patient using the "look, listen, feel" method (see Chapter 12). A useful sign indicating success in opening the airway is an audible "sighing" sound that may be heard as the patient exhales. In fact, when obstruction is solely the result of posterior displacement of the tongue, the patient may resume spontaneous respirations. If patency is not initially established, the operator should attempt to achieve a more favorable alignment of the airway by repositioning the head and neck. For example, as previously mentioned, excessive rotation of the head can actually cause airway obstruction, and it may therefore be necessary to reduce slightly the degree of force used in performing the chin lift maneuver. Similarly, when performing the jaw thrust maneuver, it may be necessary to apply greater force in anteriorly displacing the mandible if the child has a large tongue.

Once a patent airway has been estab-

Figure 14.13.
Chin lift maneuver to maintain airway patency and secure the mask. This method enhances control of the mask if the patient is moving. In other cases, most clinicians prefer to hold the mask in place with the index finger and thumb positioned over the air-filled seal.

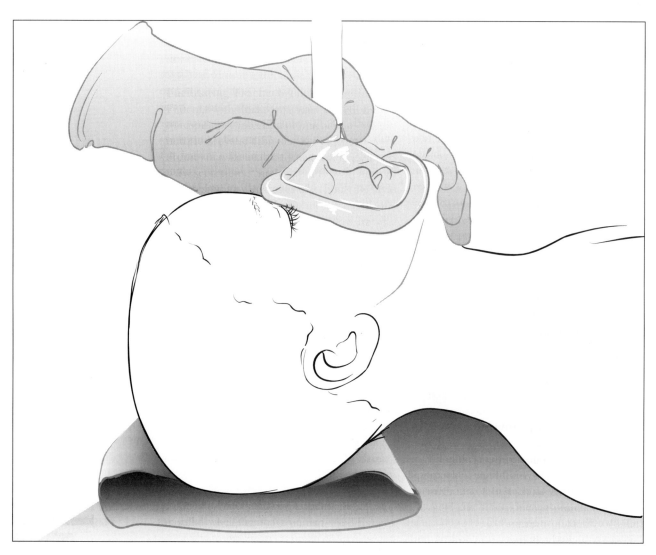

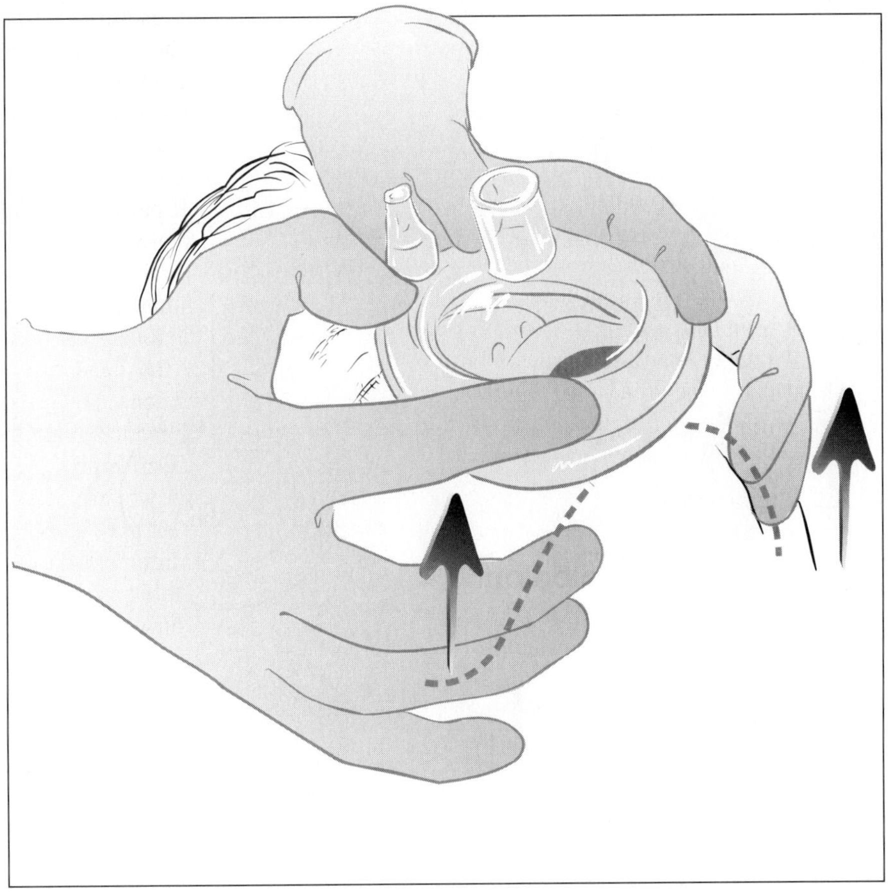

Figure 14.14.
Jaw thrust maneuver to
maintain airway patency
and secure the mask.

lished, the operator is ready to begin performing BVM ventilation. Selection of a proper face mask and resuscitation bag is based on guidelines described previously (see Equipment). When the chin lift maneuver is used to maintain the airway and apply the mask, this should be performed with the non-dominant hand, so the dominant hand is free to compress the resuscitation bag. The mask is held in place with the thumb and index finger (Fig. 14.13). If the jaw thrust maneuver is used, the mask is secured by the thumb and index finger of both hands (Fig. 14.14). Downward pressure on the mask also provides countertraction to facilitate displacement of the mandible anteriorly. If the patient is an infant or younger child, the fifth finger can sometimes be used to simultaneously apply cricoid pressure (Sellick's maneuver). Cricoid pressure reduces the incidence of aspiration during BVM ventilation by (a) preventing regurgitation of stomach contents into the oropharynx, and (b) limiting air entry into the stomach, preventing the accumulation of an excessively high intragastric pres-

sure which may cause vomiting (41, 42). This maneuver is performed by pressing firmly downward over the cricoid cartilage (Fig. 14.15). With an older child or adolescent, an assistant can be enlisted to perform Sellick's maneuver. Whatever maneuver is used to maintain the airway and secure the mask, the operator must take care to avoid pressing on the tissues of the submental area as this will often result in airway obstruction, particularly with younger patients.

It is important to ensure that the mask fits snugly on the face so that no air leak can occur. The fit should be checked frequently throughout the procedure by listening and feeling around the rim of the mask. Detection of a mask leak is especially important with a self-inflating resuscitation bag, because reexpansion occurs even when there is a significant mask leak. As mentioned previously, maintaining a good mask seal may be difficult if the child has a facial anomaly (e.g., micrognathia), trauma to the face (mandibular or midfacial fractures, burns, etc.) or when a nasogastric tube has been inserted. In such

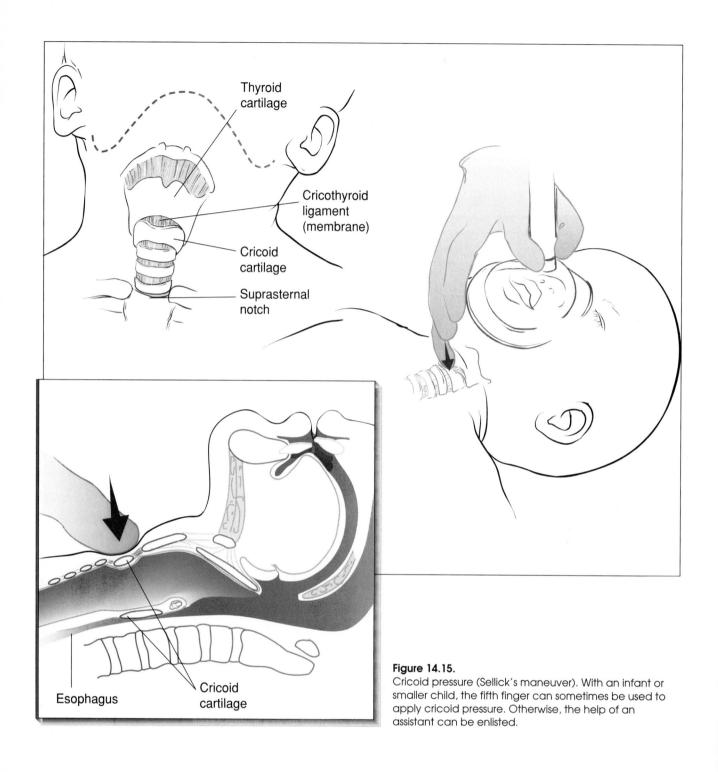

Figure 14.15.
Cricoid pressure (Sellick's maneuver). With an infant or smaller child, the fifth finger can sometimes be used to apply cricoid pressure. Otherwise, the help of an assistant can be enlisted.

Labels in figure:
- Thyroid cartilage
- Cricothyroid ligament (membrane)
- Cricoid cartilage
- Suprasternal notch
- Esophagus
- Cricoid cartilage

cases, a better fit may be achieved by placing gauze pads around the rim of the mask (43). Integrity of the seal is also affected by the strength of the operator's hand and the size of the mask. Although a perfect seal may not be obtainable—and in fact may not be necessary to adequately ventilate the patient—the success or failure of the procedure will often de-pend on the degree to which mask leaks are minimized.

After the mask is properly applied, the operator administers PPV by compressing the resuscitation bag. The dominant hand is used to ensure delivery of an adequate tidal vol-ume. Appropriate ventilatory rates for pedi-atric age groups are shown in Table 14.3.

When a patient is simultaneously receiving chest compressions, one ventilation should be given after every five compressions. Since measurement of delivered gases during BVM ventilation is usually impractical in an emergent situation, estimation of the patient's weight is not generally useful in determining the appropriate tidal volume. The operator should instead rely on careful observation of the patient's chest excursions during ventilation. Compression of the resuscitation bag should produce chest wall movement similar to normal deep inspirations. As mentioned previously, patients with partial airway obstruction or diminished lung compliance may require higher ventilatory pressures to overcome the increased resistance. The operator accomplishes this by disabling the pop-off valve, performing more forceful compressions of the resuscitation bag, and ensuring that the mask is held tightly in place to prevent air leaks. Here again, observation of the chest excursions serves as the primary indicator in determining the necessary force of ventilation.

Using a conventional anesthesia bag system differs from using a self-inflating BVM unit in several important respects. Unlike a self-inflating bag, the resuscitation bag in an anesthesia circuit will inflate properly only if the following conditions are met: (*a*) the oxygen inflow is adequate, (*b*) no significant mask leak occurs, and (*c*) the APL valve is properly set. This is why using such a system can sometimes seem like juggling three balls at once. First, the rate at which oxygen flows into the system must be maintained at an appropriate level to reinflate the bag and minimize rebreathing of exhaled gases. For pediatric patients, this is generally 2 to 3 times the minute ventilation of the patient, depending on the circuit used (38, 39). Second, the operator must at all times maintain a closed system. If there is any significant mask leak, the resuscitation bag will not reinflate properly and administration of adequate PPV will be impossible. Finally, the APL valve must be adjusted so an appropriate pressure is maintained within the system. In determining the correct setting for this valve, the operator must take into account such variables as pulmonary compliance, oxygen inflow, and tidal volume. The APL valve often proves to be one of the more problematic features of an anesthesia circuit for less experienced operators. If the resistance of the valve is set too high, the bag will progressively overinflate like a balloon as the pressure in the system increases. If the resistance is too low, the outflow of gas will be greater than the oxygen inflow, and the bag will not inflate sufficiently. When all these tasks are combined with the additional responsibility of maintaining a patent airway, the high failure rate demonstrated by novice practitioners with this procedure is easy to understand (44). Nevertheless, in the hands of an experienced operator, an anesthesia bag circuit is the preferred system when the patient requires 100% oxygen.

If the operator has difficulty administering ventilations, this may be the result of one of several problems. For example, it may sometimes prove impossible to adequately compress the resuscitation bag while maintaining airway patency. This can occur if the patient requires higher ventilatory pressures, the operator has small hands, or managing the airway is particularly troublesome. In such situations, employing the two-person technique of BVM ventilation usually provides an effective solution (see below). Assuming the airway is patent, one of the most frequent causes of inadequate ventilation is a significant air leak caused by an improper mask fit and/or poor technique. These problems can normally be avoided with careful selection of an appropriate mask size and ongoing vigilance in assessing the seal. Using a resuscitation bag that is too small for the patient can also lead to ineffective ventilation, because the tidal volume delivered will be inadequate. Poor chest wall excursions should indicate that a larger bag is needed. It is noteworthy that a progressive increase in the amount of force necessary to deliver ventilations over a short period of time can be an ominous sign. The patient may simply have gastric distension that has reached a point of restricting expansion of the lungs, which can normally be relieved by inserting a nasogastric tube. However, if ventilations do not become significantly easier to administer after nasogastric tube placement, this may indicate that the patient has a tension pneumothorax. The approach to this especially dangerous problem is discussed below (see Complications).

During the procedure, the operator should frequently reevaluate the patient to ascertain whether BVM ventilation is having the desired effects. Several clinical indicators

Table 14.3.
Ventilatory Rates for Pediatric Patients

Infant	20–24 breaths/min
Child	16–20 breaths/min
Adolescent	12–16 breaths/min

Chapter 14
Bag-Valve-Mask
Ventilation

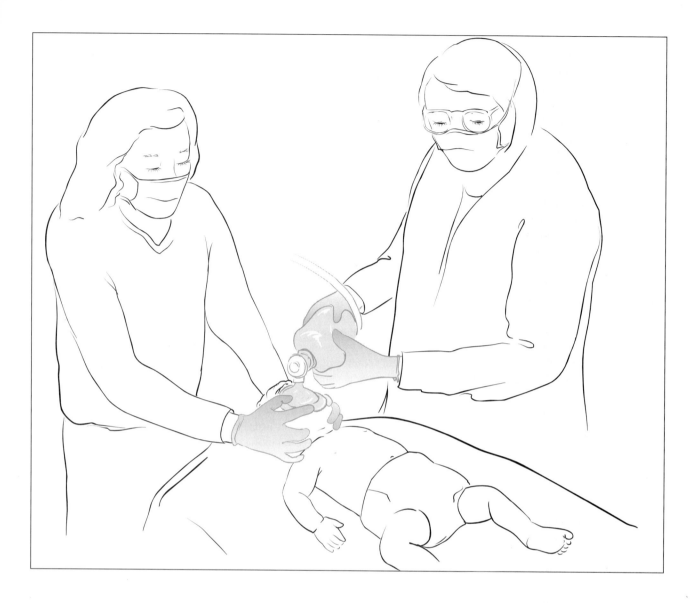

Figure 14.16.
Two-person technique for BVM ventilation.

and monitoring methods can be used in this assessment. The skin color should progressively change from dusky or cyanotic to pink with adequate PPV. The heart rate of a patient with bradycardia as a result of hypoxemia should also return to normal. For the patient with a depressed mental status, the level of consciousness will often improve and the child may open his or her eyes or begin to cry. Pulse oximetry (Chapter 77) provides a noninvasive, "real-time" reading of the blood oxygen saturation and therefore serves as an indirect indicator of how effectively oxygen is being delivered. However, the pulse oximeter gives no information about the ventilatory state of the patient, because the level of CO_2 in the blood is not measured. Capnography may be used for this purpose when available (Chapter 78). The gold standard for

evaluating the effect of BVM ventilation is determination of arterial blood gases, but this involves a successful arterial puncture and the results are delayed by transport and laboratory analysis. In all cases, information obtained from the laboratory and monitoring devices must be carefully considered, but the operator should rely primarily on changes in the patient's clinical condition in judging the effectiveness of BVM ventilation.

A number of published studies have demonstrated that simultaneously performing all the skills involved with BVM ventilation can be a difficult task for one person to accomplish, particularly when the operator has less experience with this procedure (27, 44–48). Based on the results of a manikin trial, Jesudian and colleagues were the first to recommend that a two-person technique for

BVM ventilation (Fig. 14.16) should be used whenever feasible (49). This recommendation has been adopted by the American Heart Association (50). The two-person technique allows one operator to use both hands to position the patient, maintain a patent airway, and hold the mask securely in place. The second operator can then use both hands if necessary to compress the resuscitation bag. This method more reliably accomplishes the two primary goals of (a) minimizing the occurrence of mask leak and problems with airway obstruction, and (b) increasing the likelihood that an adequate tidal volume will be delivered. It is particularly useful with the more complicated apparatus of an anesthesia circuit. When the number of available medical personnel is limited (e.g., prehospital settings), the two-person technique may not be a practical alternative. Furthermore, the experienced practitioner may be capable of performing the procedure without assistance. However, for many pediatric resuscitations initial use of the two-person technique will enhance the effectiveness with which BVM ventilation is performed.

COMPLICATIONS

In general, BVM ventilation is a safe procedure. A number of relatively minor problems can occur and only a few specific complications can be more serious. Minor complications are primarily related to the mechanical forces involved in performing the procedure. For example, neuropraxia of the facial or trigeminal nerves can occur when excessive or prolonged pressure is applied while holding the face mask in place. During the limited course of an emergent resuscitation, this is not usually a problem. If the mask extends too high on the face, the patient may sustain injury to the eyes or periorbital area, possibly resulting in a corneal abrasion or periorbital edema. Pressure on the eyes can also cause vagal stimulation in younger patients, producing bradycardia if unrecognized. Selection of an appropriate mask size and careful adherence to proper technique will reduce the likelihood of these complications. Finally, patients who are allergic to material in the mask, or to chemicals used for sterilization, may develop a mild dermatitis of the face. These complications are generally self-limited, and in most cases, can be easily treated if necessary after the patient is stabilized.

A potentially serious complication of BVM ventilation is causing damage to the cervical cord in the patient with an unstable cervical spine injury. Although rare among pediatric patients (5–7, 51), unstable cervical spine injuries should be suspected with any significant trauma (falls, motor vehicle accidents, etc.). In all instances, the possibility of cervical spine instability requires extreme caution when manipulating the head and neck to control the airway. The cervical spine should be completely immobilized during BVM ventilation until radiographic and clinical assessments can be performed to exclude the possibility of cervical spine injury (see Chapter 23). To limit extension of the neck, airway patency is established using the jaw thrust maneuver. The two-person technique for BVM ventilation should be employed in this situation. This allows one operator to concentrate solely on maintaining the airway and securing the face mask, while at the same time minimizing any movement of the cervical spine. Immobilization of the cervical spine, although important, should not be given such a high priority that airway obstruction and impaired ventilation are not appropriately addressed. Published studies have indicated that morbidity in such cases is more likely to result from cerebral hypoxia, as a result of delayed or inadequate intervention for respiratory compromise, than from exacerbating a cervical spine injury (52–54).

Another significant complication of BVM ventilation is aspiration pneumonitis. Patients requiring this procedure are likely to have a combination of characteristics which predispose to vomiting and aspiration (i.e., an impaired mental status, a diminished or absent gag reflex, and a full stomach) (55). Aspiration pneumonitis as a result of BVM ventilation usually results from the following sequence of events: (a) positive pressure ventilation exceeds the opening pressure of the esophagus, resulting in air entry into the stomach; (b) the progressive increase in intragastric pressure eventually results in vomiting; and (c) regurgitated stomach contents enter the trachea and lungs due to impaired airway reflexes. Excessively elevated intragastric pressure can also impede delivery of an adequate tidal volume, as the stomach

SUMMARY
1. Assess patient—airway, breathing, circulation
2. Establish airway patency
   a. Chin lift (if no danger of cervical spine injury)
   b. Jaw thrust
3. Select appropriate equipment sizes
   a. Face mask should be the smallest size that completely covers the nose and mouth
   b. Resuscitation bag should be large enough to ensure delivery of an adequate tidal volume
4. Apply mask to face with nondominant hand (or with both hands when two-person technique is used)
5. Compress resuscitation bag at appropriate rate with dominant hand (or with both hands as necessary when two-person technique is used)
6. If anesthesia BVM circuit is used, adjust oxygen inflow and APL valve setting as necessary to maintain appropriate pressure within system
7. Assess for mask leak
8. Observe chest excursions and modify delivered tidal volume as needed
9. Monitor patient response

Chapter 14
Bag-Valve-Mask
Ventilation

presses upward against the diaphragm and limits expansion of the lungs. The severity of the resulting pneumonitis depends on the volume and acidity of the aspirated material, as well as the amount of particulate matter in the stomach contents (56). The operator can take several steps to prevent this complication. For one, the operator or an assistant can perform Sellick's maneuver to prevent air entry into the stomach. This is particularly important when higher ventilatory pressures are necessary because of diminished lung compliance. In addition, any patient who receives BVM ventilation for longer than 2 minutes should have a gastric tube inserted. This reduces the likelihood of significant aspiration by removing air and undigested food from the stomach. Finally, the operator should carefully monitor the chest wall excursions during BVM ventilation. Using the minimum force necessary to deliver an adequate tidal volume is one of the most effective means of reducing air entry into the stomach.

A final potentially serious complication of BVM ventilation is pneumothorax (57–59). As described previously, pediatric patients are more at risk for this complication than adults because of greater chest wall compliance. The risk is further increased for children with an underlying lung disease such as cystic fibrosis or congenital lobar emphysema (60). This complication can be largely prevented if the operator is careful in observing the chest wall excursions to ensure that overinflation of the lungs does not occur. If a pneumothorax is unrecognized during BVM ventilation, gases escaping from the lung into the thoracic cavity may lead to the development of a tension pneumothorax. Should this occur, the operator will notice that increasing force is necessary to compress the resuscitation bag despite insertion of a gastric tube. The patient will have diminished breath sounds and a tympanitic hemithorax on the affected side. Tracheal deviation may occur, although this is often difficult to detect in children. Eventually, the vena cava is "kinked" as the mediastinum shifts away from the tension pneumothorax, resulting in decreased venous return to the heart and a precipitous drop in systemic blood pressure. Early placement of a chest tube in any patient receiving prolonged PPV who develops a pneumothorax will prevent this complication. As a result of the potentially rapid progres-

sion of this process, the operator who suspects the presence of a tension pneumothorax should immediately perform a needle thoracostomy and/or chest tube insertion rather than waiting to confirm the diagnosis with a chest radiograph. A complete discussion of the techniques used in the management of pneumothorax can be found in Chapter 30.

SUMMARY

BVM ventilation is an effective method for delivering PPV to pediatric patients with respiratory compromise. Although a few potential complications are associated with this procedure, they can usually be avoided with careful use of proper technique. Although similar to the methods used for adult patients, BVM ventilation for infants and children requires certain specific modifications based on unique characteristics of pediatric airway anatomy and respiratory physiology. Equipment selection is an especially important aspect of this procedure, because the use of a face mask or resuscitation bag that is inappropriate for the size of the patient may result in complications or failure to provide adequate ventilatory support. BVM ventilation of a pediatric patient can sometimes challenge the abilities of even the most skillful practitioner, particularly when performed by a single operator. For this reason, the two-person technique is recommended whenever the procedure proves more difficult. In addition, the use of a conventional anesthesia circuit should only be undertaken by an experienced operator because of the complexity of the apparatus. The advantages of immediate availability, low incidence of complications, and wide clinical utility make BVM ventilation one of the most valuable tools for the health professional who provides emergent care for pediatric patients.

REFERENCES

1. Passy V, Newcron S, Snyder S. Rhinorrhea with airway obstruction. Laryngoscope 1975; 85:888–895.
2. Maniglia AJ, Goodwin WJ Jr. Congenital choanal atresia. Otolaryngol Clin North Am 1981; 14:167–173.
3. Wittenborg MH, Gyepes MT, Crocker D. Tracheal dynamics in infants with respiratory dis-

tress, stridor, and collapsing trachea. Radiology 1967; 88:653–662.

4. Polgar G, Kong GP. Nasal resistance in newborn infants. J Pediatr 1961; 67:557–567.

5. Bohn D, Armstrong D, Becker L, Humphreys R. Cervical spine injuries in children. J Trauma 1990; 30:463–469.

6. Rachesky I, Boyce T, Duncan B, Bjelland J, Sibley B. Clinical prediction of cervical spine injuries in children. Arch Dis Child 1987; 141:199–201.

7. Stauffer ES, Mazur JM. Cervical spine injuries in children. Pediatr Ann 1982; 11: 502–511.

8. Morikawa S, Safar P, DeCarlo J. Influence of the head-jaw position on upper airway patency. Anesthesiology 1961; 22:265–279.

9. Papastamelos C, Panitch HB, England SE, Allen JL. Developmental changes in chest wall compliance in infancy and early childhood. J Appl Physiol 1995; 78(1):179–184.

10. Keens TG, Ianuzzo CD. Development of fatigue-resistant muscle fibers in human ventilatory muscles. Am Rev Respir Dis 1979; 2 (Suppl 119):139–141.

11. Glicklich M, Cohen R, Jona J. Steroids and bag and mask ventilation in the treatment of acute epiglottis. J Pediatr Surg 1979; 14: 247–251.

12. Szold P, Glicklich M. Children with epiglottis can be bagged. Clin Pediatr 1976; 15: 792–793.

13. Cournand A, Motley HL, Wesko L, et al. Physiologic studies of the effects of intermittent positive pressure breathing on cardiac output in man. Am J Physiol 1948; 152: 162–174.

14. Clough JB, Duncan AW, Sly PD. The effect of sustained positive airway pressure on derived cardiac output in children. Anaesth Intensive Car 1994; 22(1):30–34.

15. Watson WE. Observations of physiologic deadspace during intermittent positive pressure ventilation. Br J Anaesth 1962; 35: 502–506.

16. Kerr JH. Pulmonary oxygen transfer during IPPV in man. Br J Anaesth 1975; 47(6): 695–705.

17. Cross KW, Tizard JPM, Trythall DAH. The gaseous metabolism of the newborn infant. Acta Paediatr 1957; 46:265–285.

18. Patel R, Lenczyk M, Hannallah RS, McGill WA. Age and the onset of desaturation in apnoeic children. Can J Anaesth 1994; 41(9): 771–774.

19. Kinouchi K, Tanigami H, Tashiro C, et al. Duration of apnea in anesthetized infants and children required for desaturation of hemoglobin to 95%. The influence of upper respiratory infection. Anesthesiology 1992; 77(6):1105–1107.

20. Alho OP, Jokinen K, Pirila T, et al. Acute epiglottis and infant conjugate Haemophilus influenzae type B vaccination in northern Finland. Arch Otolaryngol Head Neck Surg 1995; 121(8):898–902.

21. Wurtele P. Acute epiglottis in children: results of a large-scale antiHaemophilus type B immunization program. J Otolaryngol 1995; 24(2):92–97.

22. Keyser JS, Derkay CS. Haemophilus influenzae type B epiglottis after immunization with HbOC conjugate vaccine. Am J Otolaryngol 1994; 15(6):436–443.

23. Boon AW, Milner AD, Hopkin IE. Physiologic responses of the newborn infant to resuscitation. Arch Dis Child 1979; 54: 492–498.

24. Milner AD, Boon AW, Hopkin IE. Lung expansion, tidal exchange and formation of the functional residual capacity during resuscitation of asphyxiated infants. J Pediatr 1979; 6:1031–1036.

25. Vyas H, Milner AD, Hopkin IE. Physiologic response to prolonged and slow rise inflation. J Pediatr 1981; 99:635–638.

26. Field D, Milner AD, Hopkin IE. Efficiency of manual resuscitators at birth. Arch Dis Child 1985; 61:300–302.

27. Terndrup TE, Kanter RK, Cherry RA. A comparison of infant ventilation methods performed by prehospital personnel. Ann Emerg Med 1989; 18(6):607–611.

28. Palme C, Nystrom N, Tunell R. An evaluation of the efficiency of face masks in the resuscitation of newborn infants. Lancet 1985; 1:207–210.

29. Campbell TP, Stewart RD, Kaplan RM, et al. Oxygen enrichment of bag-valve-mask units during positive-pressure ventilation: a comparison of various techniques. Ann Emerg Med 1988; 17(3):232–235.

30. Carden E, Hughes T. An evaluation of manually operated self-inflating resuscitation bags. Anaesth Analg 1975; 54:133–138.

31. Carden E, Bernstein M. Investigation of the nine most commonly used resuscitator bags. JAMA 1970; 212(4):589–592.

32. Carden E, Freidman D. Further studies of manually operated self-inflating resuscitation bags. Anaesth Analg 1977; 56:202–206.

33. Finer NN, Barrington KJ, Al-Fadley F, Peters K. Limitations of self-inflating resuscitators. Pediatrics 1986; 77(3):417–420.

34. Kauffman GW. A simple PEEP system for the Laerdal resuscitation bag. Resp Ther 1981; 11: 3–4.

35. Kauffman GW, Hess DR. Modification of the infant Laerdal resuscitation bag to monitor airway pressure. Crit Care Med 1982; 10(2): 112–113.

36. Bain JA, Speorel WE. A streamlined anaesthetic system. Can Anaesth Soc J 1972; 19(4)426–435.

37. Rees GJ. Anaesthesia in the newborn. Brit Med J 1950; 2:1419–1422.

38. Bain JA, Spoerel WE. Flow requirements for a modified Mapleson D system during controlled ventilation. Can Anaesth Soc J 1973; 20(5):629–636.

39. Willis BA, Pender JW, Mapleson WW. Rebreathing in a T-piece: volunteer and theoret-

Chapter 14
Bag-Valve-Mask
Ventilation

ical studies of the Jackson-Rees modification of Ayre's T-piece during spontaneous respiration. Br J Anaesth 1975; 47:1239–1245.

40. Priano LL, Ham J. A simple method to increase the F_DO_2 of resuscitator bags. Crit Care Med 1978; 6(1):48–49.

41. Vyas H, Milner AD, Hopkin IE. Face mask resuscitation: does it lead to gastric distension? Arch Dis Child 1983; 58:373–375.

42. Salem MR, Wong AY, Mani M, Sellick MB. Efficacy of cricoid pressure in preventing gastric inflation during bag-mask ventilation in pediatric patients. Anesthesiology 1974; 40(1):96–98.

43. Backofen JE, Rogers MC. Emergency management of the airway. In: Rogers MC, ed. Textbook of pediatric intensive care. 2nd ed. Williams & Wilkins, Baltimore, 1992.

44. Kanter RK. Evaluation of mask-bag ventilation in resuscitation of infants. Arch Dis Child 1987; 141:761–763.

45. Harrison RR, Maull KI, Keenan RL, Boyan PC. Mouth-to-mouth ventilation: a superior method of rescue breathing. Ann Emerg Med 1982; 11(2):39–41.

46. Elling BA, Politis J. An evaluation of emergency medical technicians' ability to use manual ventilation devices. Ann Emerg Med 1983; 12(12):53–56.

47. Hess D, Baran C. Ventilatory volumes using mouth-to-mouth, mouth-to-mask, and bag-valve-mask techniques. Am J Emerg Med 1985; 3(4):292–296.

48. Lawrence PJ, Navaratnam S. Ventilation during cardiopulmonary resuscitation: which method? Med J Aust 1985; 143:443–445.

49. Jesudian MCS, Harrison RR, Leenan RL, Maull KI. Bag-valve-mask ventilation; two

rescuers are better than one: preliminary report. Crit Care Med 1985; 13(2):122–123.

50. Pediatric advance life support. JAMA 1992; 268(16):2262–2275.

51. Lally KP, Senac M, Hardin WD Jr, et al. Utility of the cervical spine radiograph in pediatric trauma. Am J Surg 1989; 158:540–542.

52. Rhee KJ, Green W, Holcroft JW, et al. Oral intubation in the multiple injured patient: the risk of exacerbating cervical spine damage. Ann Emerg Med 1990; 19(5)45–48.

53. Holley J, Jorden R. Airway management in patients with unstable cervical spine fractures. Ann Emerg Med 1989; 18(11):151–153.

54. Grande CM, Barton CR. Appropriate techniques for airway management of emergency patients with suspected spinal cord injury [letter]. Anaesth Analg 1988; 67:710–718.

55. Hupp JR, Peterson LJ. Aspiration pneumonitis: etiology, therapy, and prevention. J Oral Surg 1981; 39(6):430–435.

56. Sladen A, Zanca P, Hadnott WH. Aspiration pneumonitis—the sequelae. Chest 1971; 59(4):448–450.

57. Miller RD, Hamilton WK. Pneumothorax during infant resuscitation. JAMA 1969; 210:1090–1092.

58. Hirschman AM, Kravath RE. Venting vs ventilating. A danger of manual resuscitation bags. Chest 1982; 82(3):369–370.

59. Dwyer ME. Pneumothorax. Aust Paediatr J 1975; 11(4):195–200.

60. Luck SR, Raffensperger JG, Sullivan HJ, Gibson LE. Management of pneumothorax in children with chronic pulmonary disease. J Thorac Cardiovasc Surg 1977; 74(6): 834–839.

RAPID SEQUENCE INDUCTION

Joanne M. Decker and David A. Lowe

INTRODUCTION

A detailed discussion of the various methods for performing emergent endotracheal intubation can be found in Chapter 16. The purpose of this chapter is to review the techniques of pharmacologic facilitation of intubation. The standard procedure of providing sedation and inducing neuromuscular paralysis in preparation for intubation is called rapid sequence induction (RSI). Its purpose is to allow a safe, expedient intubation while reducing the likelihood of aspiration pneumonitis. RSI minimizes or prevents many of the patient's responses to the noxious stimuli of intubation, including vomiting, coughing, breathholding, and laryngospasm. This procedure and its modifications can also limit adverse physiologic effects of intubation, such as increased intracranial pressure (ICP), systemic hypertension and hypotension, cardiac arrhythmias, and elevated intraocular pressure. In addition, RSI facilitates laryngoscopic visualization of the airway in situations when this might otherwise be impossible (i.e., with patients who are seizing, unable to cooperate, or combative as a result of mental status changes).

Certain clinical situations require using one of several modifications of the standard RSI procedure. For example, muscle relaxants should not be administered if bag-valve-mask (BVM) ventilation and/or intubation is anticipated to be difficult. With such patients, paralysis followed by an unsuccessful intubation produces apnea without a patent airway and therefore may be lethal. In this situation, sedation alone is indicated to facilitate intubation without eliminating respiratory function. Other modifications of RSI involve the use of alternative agents for sedation and neuromuscular blockade to prevent increases in ICP (e.g., with cerebral edema or a space-occupying intracranial lesion) or circulatory collapse for the patient with hypovolemia or a low cardiac output state. Agents with vasodilating or myocardial depressant effects which can exacerbate preexisting physiologic derangements must obviously be titrated carefully or avoided. Medications are substituted which may increase systemic blood pressure or decrease ICP, depending on the clinical situation. In its classic form, RSI involves pre-oxygenating the patient by providing 100% mask O_2 during spontaneous respiration. BVM ventilation is not performed following administration of the induction agents to avoid filling the stomach with gas and thereby reduce the likelihood of vomiting before intubation. However, patients with preexisting respiratory compromise and hypoxemia may not tolerate even a brief period of apnea despite preoxygenation. These patients therefore require skilled BVM ventilation with cricoid pressure for 45 to 90 seconds with 100% O_2 until the peak effect of the muscle relaxant has been achieved and endotracheal intubation can be attempted. These and other modifications of RSI are described in this chapter.

Depending on the availability and experience of medical personnel, RSI is generally performed by either an emergency physician or anesthesiologist. Because the potential for morbidity is high with this procedure, the physician performing RSI must be skillful with pediatric endotracheal intubation and thoroughly familiar with the risks and benefits of the medications and techniques used. Optimal settings for this procedure are the emergency department (ED), intensive care unit (ICU) or operating room. Above all, practitioners must keep in mind that RSI suppresses all respiratory effort and eliminates the ability of the patient to protect and maintain the airway. Consequently, this procedure should be performed with the highest degree of caution and only when indicated.

ANATOMY AND PHYSIOLOGY

Clinically important features of pediatric airway anatomy and physiologic effects of endotracheal intubation are described in Chapter 16. However, additional factors specifically related to the use of pharmacologic agents for facilitating intubation merit further discussion. For one, the child with a "difficult airway" represents a major concern for the operator performing RSI, because the suppression of spontaneous respirations before obtaining a secure airway is particularly dangerous with such patients. In addition, the physiology of the normal protective airway reflexes and the "full stomach" state have important consequences with regard to preventing aspiration pneumonitis, one of the primary purposes of this procedure. Finally, the operator should fully understand the pharmacologic properties and physiologic effects of the agents used in performing RSI.

In most instances, the patient with a difficult airway can be identified before attempted intubation. Unfortunately, this is not always possible, even when an intubation is performed on an elective basis. In the limited time available before an urgent or emergent intubation, the operator must make a rapid assessment of the patient and, to the extent possible, ascertain that BVM ventilation and endotracheal intubation will not be difficult. If time permits, obtaining historical information from the parent or caretaker may be helpful in making this judgment. A known congenital abnormality, previous problems with intubation, or a history of difficulty breathing (e.g., while asleep or feeding, with upper res-

piratory infections) can all indicate a potentially difficult airway. A wide diversity of congenital anomalies has been associated with difficult intubation. Examples include Klippel-Fiel syndrome, Down's syndrome, achondroplasia, the Pierre-Robin sequence, Treacher-Collins syndrome, Marfan's syndrome, Cornelia de Lange syndrome, Moebius syndrome, and familial osseous dysplasia (cherubism). The approach to such patients can only be properly tailored to the specific challenges posed by each syndrome when time is not a concern, as with an elective intubation. A complete discussion of these issues is therefore beyond the scope of this chapter. Readers interested in more information on this subject are referred to standard pediatric and anesthesiology texts. More importantly in the emergent setting, physical examination will usually reveal anatomic characteristics that would make laryngoscopy and/or manual ventilation problematic, such as micrognathia (best evaluated while viewing the patient's profile), macroglossia, cleft or high arched palate, protruding upper incisors, small mouth, limited temporomandibular joint mobility, or limited cervical spine mobility (Table 15.1). Difficult laryngoscopy should also be anticipated when the patient has any of the following acquired abnormalities: hoarsness, stridor, drooling, a preferred posture, facial burns, blunt or penetrating injury to the neck, facial bone fractures, oral trauma, epiglottitis, retropharyngeal abscess, and a foreign body in the extrathoracic airway (Table 15.2). For the patient with a potentially unstable cervical spine, laryngoscopy and intubation may be hindered by inline stabilization and use of a cervical collar, which limit neck flexion and extension as well as mouth opening.

Normal protective effects of airway reflexes can also be a significant obstacle to performing endotracheal intubation. Instrumentation of the airway may stimulate gagging, coughing, jaw clenching, increased production of secretions, and possible laryngospasm. These reflexes must often be suppressed for the intubation to be atraumatic and successful. The physiology of the various mechanisms that mediate the airway reflexes is complex. To briefly summarize, irritation of upper airway and digestive tract mucosa stimulates the glossopharyngeal (9th) and vagus (10th) nerves, which project to the nucleus of the solitary tract (NTS) in the medulla (1). Gagging and coughing are produced by nerve impulses relayed from the NTS back to the motor efferents of the upper airway, diaphragm, and intercostal and abdominal muscles. In addition, nerve tracts from the NTS to the medulla activate a "vomiting center," which induces emesis by coordinating such responses as contraction of the abdominal musculature, closure of the glottis, opening of the lower esophageal sphincter, and increased salivation. This medullary vomiting response can also be stimulated by the area postrema of the brainstem, which is sensitive to noxious substances circulating in the bloodstream (1). Sympathetic outflow resulting from stimulation of the NTS can cause an increase in heart rate and blood pressure, which in turn can lead to dysrhythmias and increased ICP. However, the most pronounced response to oropharyngeal manipulation in children is generally transmission from the NTS to the dorsal vagal nucleus, producing marked bradycardia. Because cardiac output in infants and younger children depends more on heart rate than changes in stroke volume, bradycardia can have a significant deleterious effect on systemic blood pressure.

Any patient undergoing emergent intubation is presumed to have a "full stomach," defined as recent ingestion of food (within the past 8 hours) or liquid (within the past 2 hours) or delayed gastric emptying as a result of intestinal obstruction, trauma, pain, pregnancy, elevated ICP, or shock. Presumption of a full stomach state means the patient is at risk for emesis or regurgitation and subsequent aspiration of gastric contents. Factors increasing this risk include agitation, persistent gagging or coughing, and elevated intragastric pressure as a result of gas entry into the stomach during BVM ventilation or swallowing of air and/or blood. The normal gag response provoked by stimulation of the pharynx can be suppressed with pharmacologic agents, thereby decreasing the likelihood of vomiting. However, these agents also reduce or eliminate the patient's ability to protect his or her airway should any vomiting or regurgitation of stomach contents occur.

The ideal pharmacologic properties of medications used in RSI are rapid onset and short duration of effect. Anatomic and physiologic characteristics of pediatric patients can have important clinical effects on these prop-

erties. Onset and duration time depend on the total body compartments of fat, muscle, and water. Total body water is 75 to 80% of body composition in a newborn, decreasing to the adult proportion of 60% at about 6 months of age. This explains why infants may require a larger initial dose of water soluble drugs than adults. In addition, agents that depend on redistribution to fat and muscle for termination of effect will have a longer duration of action in younger patients, because they have lower body fat and muscle content. With older children, the half-life of a medication will generally be shorter, because a larger proportion of the cardiac output is delivered to the liver and kidneys causing more rapid metabolism of the drug. As a general rule, drugs have a more rapid onset of effect and a shorter duration of action in children as compared with adults, and a larger dose (based on body weight) will be required to achieve the same anesthetic effect.

The primary desired effects of pharmacologic facilitation of intubation are sedation, analgesia, and muscle relaxation. Sedation is generally provided by barbiturates, benzodiazepines and/or opioids. Barbiturates have several actions in the central nervous system (CNS) that produce sedation. Most importantly, they potentiate the neuroinhibitory actions of gamma-aminobutyric acid (GABA), which is accomplished by increasing chloride conductance and decreasing depolarization induced by glutamate. Evidence also exists of depression of the calcium-dependent action potential (2). Benzodiazepines potentiate GABA-mediated inhibition as well, but little is known about their direct actions. Neurologic inhibition by the opiates is more complex. There are three known major categories of opioid receptors in the CNS. Analgesia is produced by endogenous and exogenous peptides that bind to the μ receptors in the brain, κ receptors in the spinal cord, and δ receptors distributed in both the brain and spinal cord. Inhibition at these sites is accomplished by a reduction in the release of neurotransmitters and inhibition of adenyl cyclase at μ and δ receptors. Evidence also exists of inhibition of calcium channels at κ receptors (2). Activation of opioid receptors causes a decrease in the sensation of pain, as well as modification of the perception of a stimulus as painful. For example, the periaqueductal grey matter in the midbrain contains δ and μ receptors, and

Table 15.2.
Acquired Abnormalities Indicating a Potentially Difficult Airway

Hoarseness
Stridor
Drooling
A preferred posture
Facial burns
Blunt or penetrating injury to the neck
Facial bone fractures
Oral trauma
Epiglottitis
Retropharyngeal abscess
Foreign body in the extrathoracic airway

agonists at these sites inhibit the processing of nociceptive information from the spinal cord. In addition, an abundance of μ receptors are found in the locus ceruleus, which is responsible for feelings of alarm, panic, fear, and anxiety (2). Inhibition at these receptors increases the tolerance for pain and the associated psychological stress.

Muscle relaxation is produced at the motor end plate by depolarizing agents or nondepolarizing competitive agents. Normally, release of acetylcholine (ACh) from the presynaptic membrane causes summation of electrical potentials which form an action potential that stimulates muscle contraction. Depolarizing agents mimic ACh and bind directly to the postsynaptic ACh receptor, causing all skeletal muscles to depolarize. This is evident as muscle fasciculations followed by flaccid paralysis, which remains until postsynaptic receptors again regain their ability to transmit an electrical stimulus (2). Nondepolarizing neuromuscular blocking agents competitively inhibit the nicotinic postsynaptic receptors for ACh so depolarization cannot occur. These agents are normally metabolized over time to less active forms which are then easily displaced by ACh. Both types of neuromuscular blockers have no direct CNS effects and do not decrease awareness. Using these agents alone without sedation therefore leaves a patient in the terrorized state of being awake but unable to move or breathe.

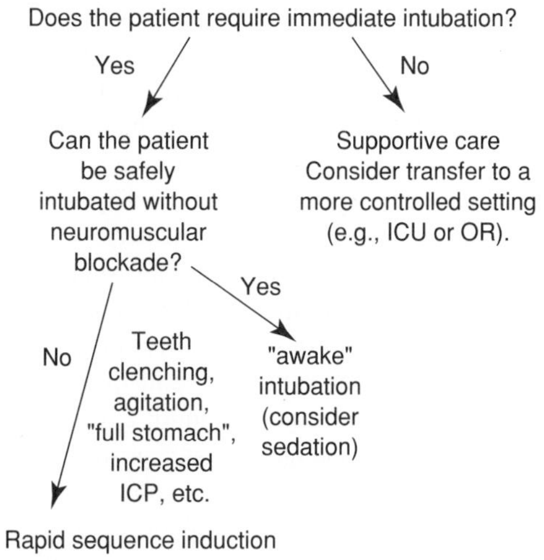

INDICATIONS

Rapid sequence induction is performed to facilitate endotracheal intubation. Consequently, the indications for RSI in the acute care setting are in part determined by the indications for emergent intubation. Yet only a minority of patients who require intubation on an emergent basis are appropriate candidates for RSI. An algorithm illustrating the assessments and decisions involved with determining the subset of patients who should undergo RSI is presented in Figure 15.1. In general, RSI is indicated for patients with airway or ventilatory compromise who cannot be intubated without using sedatives and neuromuscular blocking agents or who would be at increased risk for complications without these drugs and techniques. Indications for one of the modifications of RSI depend on the

Rapid sequence induction

Figure 15.1.
Determining indications for rapid sequence induction.

specific clinical circumstances (see below). As mentioned previously, even in the best of situations RSI is a challenging and potentially dangerous procedure. It should be performed only when the operator presumes with reasonable certainty that the trachea can be intubated promptly. If intubation is delayed or impossible, subsequent positive pressure ventilation (PPV) with a BVM circuit may increase intragastric pressure, causing decreased total lung compliance and a greater likelihood of aspiration. In the worst case scenario, BVM ventilation may be ineffective, and therefore adequate respiratory support cannot be provided. For these reasons, RSI should be performed only after the airway has been evaluated as thoroughly as possible under the circumstances and a judgment made that endotracheal intubation, or at a minimum BVM ventilation with cricoid pressure, can be successfully accomplished.

The first question asked in determining whether a standard RSI is indicated should be "Does the child require immediate intubation?" As described in Chapter 16, there are seven primary indications for emergent intubation: (1) maintenance of the airway, (2) protection of the airway (e.g., before gastric lavage for the obtunded patient), (3) administration of positive pressure ventilation, (4) oxygen administration, (5) delivery of resuscitation drugs through the endotracheal tube, (6) access to the trachea for suctioning, and (7) respiratory support when other systems are failing in the unstable patient. Numerous disease processes and injuries can cause sufficient respiratory compromise in pediatric patients to require emergent endotracheal intubation. However, in certain instances intubation will be necessary, but not immediately. Patients with impending respiratory failure may be stable enough to transfer to a more controlled setting such as the operating room or ICU. In such cases, temporary respiratory support is provided by assisted or controlled ventilation using a BVM circuit.

If intubation is necessary and cannot be delayed, the second question that must be asked is "Can the patient be safely intubated without neuromuscular blockade?" Many intubations in the ED are performed on patients who are moribund, and therefore drugs are not needed to facilitate intubation and prevent undesirable autonomic responses. Furthermore, many physicians prefer to make one attempt at an "awake" intubation (i.e., no muscle relaxant but possibly some degree of sedation) whenever this can be performed without additional risk to the patient. But many situations exist in which either an awake intubation is hazardous and/or the likelihood of success with this method is clearly low from the outset. For example, when the patient is struggling forcefully and restraint is necessary or the patient's jaw is firmly clenched (e.g., during seizure activity), an awake intubation is likely to be impossible. In such cases, attempted intubation without neuromuscular blockade may cause trauma and bleeding, which make subsequent attempts more difficult, while increasing the likelihood of aspiration. Thus for the patient who requires immediate intubation, but for whom this cannot be accomplished safely without sedation and muscle relaxation, a standard RSI is indicated.

As discussed previously, coughing, gagging, and vomiting as a result of airway manipulation are all known to cause an increase in ICP. For this reason, a modification of the RSI procedure often called a "neurologic induction" (or "neurologic intubation") should be considered with any patient, including infants, who may have elevated ICP. A neurologic induction simply refers to special measures taken to avoid further increases in ICP which can produce cerebral hypoperfusion, cerebral swelling, and possible herniation. These patients present with such conditions as head trauma, meningitis, acute en-

cephalopathy, ventriculoperitoneal (VP) shunt dysfunction, or CNS tumors. For a neurologic induction, thiopental is usually used as the sedating agent, because it is reliable in protecting the brain by preventing a rise in ICP during noxious stimulation. In addition, intravenous lidocaine can be administered, because it also may attenuate the rise in ICP. Neuromuscular blockade should be provided to suppress the airway and autonomic reflexes, although the agent of choice in this situation is somewhat controversial (see Procedure). Prolonged apnea after administration of the muscle relaxant must be carefully avoided, as cerebral hypercarbia will exacerbate an elevated ICP. It should be noted that thiopental has a potent myocardial depressant effect and therefore must be avoided or administered in small, frequent doses to patients with hypovolemia or a low cardiac output state. If the patient suspected of having increased ICP is also in cardiovascular shock, another sedative (e.g., midazolam and/or fentanyl) should be used.

Other indications that require special consideration relate to specific clinical presentations. For example, the patient with a possible open globe injury should not receive succinylcholine or ketamine, because both of these agents increase intraocular pressure and may cause extrusion of the vitreous. In addition, any patient with either a low cardiac output or significant hypovolemia should not receive any medications that may induce or exacerbate hypotension. For the patient with severe asthma who requires intubation, ketamine may be substituted as the sedation agent, because it both supports the systemic circulation and acts as a bronchodilator. A more detailed approach to patients with these conditions is described later in this chapter.

Many physicians prefer to intubate young infants without paralysis and often without sedation. This is usually more appropriate in the delivery room, where the degree of urgency and lack of intravenous access often do not permit a controlled intubation procedure. Although paralysis may seem unnecessary because an infant is more easily and effectively restrained, rapid sequence intubation is recommended when indicated in the ED. At the least, a sedating agent should be considered even in young infants.

There are a few important contraindications to RSI. For example, any child who is

Table 15.3.
Equipment for Rapid
Sequence Induction

Standard equipment for endotracheal
  intubation (see Chapter 16)
Cardiac monitor
Blood pressure monitor
Pulse oximetry
Capnography (if available)
Intravenous catheters
Tape
Benzoin
Medications:
  Atropine
  Lidocaine
Sedating agents:
  thiopental
  midazolam
  ketamine
  fentanyl
Paralytic agents:
  succinylcholine
  vecuronium
  pancuronium
  rocuronium

apneic and pulseless at presentation should undergo endotracheal intubation early in the resuscitation without undue delay. Pharmacologic agents are unnecessary in this situation. Similarly, a patient who is moribund as a result of an overwhelming disease process (e.g., sepsis) may gain no benefit from undergoing RSI. In such situations, performing RSI would add needless complexity to the management of the patient, potentially prolonging the period of inadequate oxygenation and ventilation, without enhancing the safety of intubation. As mentioned previously, standard RSI is relatively contraindicated when the patient has one or more conditions associated with a potentially difficult airway and is breathing spontaneously or requires only 100% oxygen, continuous positive airway pressure, or minimal assistance with BVM ventilation. Should endotracheal intubation become necessary, an awake procedure (with judicious sedation as needed) should be attempted. In such cases, muscle relaxants should be withheld at least until effective BVM ventilation can be ensured. This is done after careful titration of sedative agents permits first assisted, then controlled, BVM ventilation without eliminating protective airway reflexes. Nondepolarizing muscle relaxants should generally be avoided when the patient has a neuromuscular disease (e.g., Werdnig-Hoffman, myasthenia gravis, or Duchenne's muscular dystrophy), because paralysis can persist for an excessively long period of time. In such cases, benzodiazepines may be used exclusively or in conjunction with an opiate. Succinylcholine, a depolarizing muscle relaxant, is absolutely contraindicated in patients with preexisting hyperkalemia, susceptibility to malignant hyperthermia, and denervating neuromuscular diseases. Finally, RSI is contraindicated for any spontaneously breathing patient suspected of having a tension pneumothorax, pericardial tamponade, or a mediastinal mass compressing the heart, great vessels, or large airways. In these patents, sedative agents may directly or indirectly cause vasodilation and myocardial depression that could precipitate circulatory collapse. In patients with mediastinal masses, neuromuscular blocking agents will also remove muscle tone which helps to maintain intrathoracic airway patency. In general, such children should be intubated only when necessary, optimally with the patient awake, sitting in a partially upright position, using a topical anesthetic as the only medication.

EQUIPMENT

The equipment necessary for performing RSI is shown in Table 15.3. Patients should have at least one reliable peripheral or central access site verified as intravenous. The appropriate pharmacologic agents should be drawn in labeled syringes. The general classifications of medications used to perform RSI are described below, with particular attention given to the most commonly used agent in each category.

Sedatives

Barbiturates (Thiopental)

Barbiturates are potent sedatives. From this class of drugs, thiopental is used most frequently in performing RSI. It is a rapidly acting agent, producing its peak transient effect in 10 to 20 seconds (3, 4). The duration of effect depends on the rate of redistribution to fat and muscle (3, 5) but is generally between 5 and 30 minutes (4, 6). Thiopental decreases the metabolic demands of the brain, thereby decreasing cerebral blood flow. It is therefore an excellent agent to use when the patient has a known or presumed elevated ICP (4, 6).

Precautions

Thiopental is both a myocardial depressant and a peripheral vasodilator. It can cause hypoperfusion associated with hypotension in patients with preexisting myocardial depression or hypovolemia. Normally, baroreceptors detect a low blood pressure and compensate by producing a reflex tachycardia. However, hypovolemic patients with tachycardia may be incapable of mounting any further increase in heart rate and are therefore likely to become hypotensive. Patients with underlying cardiovascular disease may not produce adequate coronary perfusion under these conditions (3, 4, 5). Consequently, any patient suspected of hypovolemia or cardiovascular disease should not receive thiopental or, if no appropriate substitute is available, should only receive it in small (1 to 3 mg/kg), frequent doses as tolerated based on blood pressure (3, 4).

The physician choosing thiopental should also be aware that it is a poor analgesic. Patients given thiopental may have laryngospasm or cough in response to airway manipulation as a result of inadequate anesthetic effect (7). "Light" anesthesia may also allow a catecholamine response leading to systemic or intracranial hypertension in response to intubation or other noxious interventions. For these reasons, it is often beneficial for thiopental to be administered in conjunction with an analgesic, particularly when the patient is at risk for elevated ICP. In addition, extravasation or intraarterial injection of thiopental can cause severe tissue necrosis (3). Extra care must therefore be taken to inject into an access site that recently has been verified as intravenous. It is also important to use only a dilute solution (2.5%) for injection.

Other precautions relate to the respiratory effects of this agent. Thiopental has minimal direct effects on bronchomotor tone, but bronchospasm may occur due to light anesthesia during noxious airway manipulation, particularly in asthmatic patients. It also depresses the respiratory center in the brainstem. Patients may have precipitous onset of apnea, particularly if there is associated hypovolemia or head trauma (3). The respiratory depressant effect is related to the dose and rate of administration (3, 5).

How Supplied

Thiopental comes in kits stored at room temperature to be prepared at the time of injection. The most common is called Pentothal which comes in a three-piece kit (Fig. 15.2). The pieces are put together with matching colors at the ends. As the diluent is drawn up it simultaneously mixes with the powder yielding 20 mL of a 25 mg/mL (2.5%) solution.

Dose

For normotensive patients with a normal or elevated cardiac output, the recommended dose is 5 to 7 mg/kg given rapidly as a bolus. If the patient is hypotensive but has increased ICP, a lower dose of 1 to 3 mg/kg may be used at frequent intervals if blood pressure remains acceptable.

Benzodiazepines (Diazepam, Midazolam)

The benzodiazepines produce sedation, amnesia, and hypnosis. They also have anxiolytic and anticonvulsant effects. Diazepam normally has an onset of action within 1 to 3 minutes (although this can be variable) (3, 4) and a duration of 10 to 30 minutes (4). Diazepam is oil-based and causes pain and occasionally phlebitis with intravenous administration (3, 5, 6). Midazolam is a newer benzodiazepine that has several advantages over diazepam. Midazolam has a more rapid and consistent rate of onset (approximately 80 seconds) (3) and a shorter duration (5 to 20 minutes) (3, 6). Because it is water soluble, midazolam does not cause pain with injection. ICP is not affected by benzodiazepines but midazolam does lower intraocular pressure (3). Most authorities recommend using midazolam and not diazepam for performing RSI.

Precautions

Although the benzodiazepines produce fewer cardiovascular side effects than the barbiturates, they are associated with a slight transient decrease in systemic blood pressure because of a decrease in systemic vascular resistance. Evidence suggests that an increase in venous capacitance caused by midazolam is offset by a shift of blood volume out of the splanchnic circulation and a transient in-

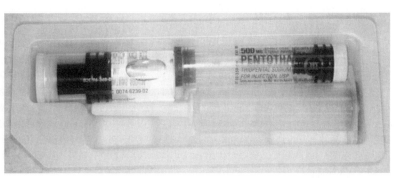

Figure 15.2.
Pentothal (thiopental) kit.

crease in heart rate (8). For some patients, a small decrease in blood pressure can be beneficial in attenuating both the pressor response and the rise in ICP that can occur with laryngoscopy (9). However, the patient whose increased sympathetic activity is compensating for significant hypovolemia is most susceptible to the hypotensive effects of midazolam (10). In most patients with cardiovascular disease, cardiac output and coronary blood flow are not adversely affected by midazolam.

Similar to barbiturates, benzodiazepines have a respiratory depressant effect which may induce apnea. This is potentiated by both rapid rate of administration and concomitant use of narcotics (3). Benzodiazepines do not provide analgesia, nor will they enhance the analgesic effects of other drugs. Consequently, when used for induction, midazolam is normally paired with an agent that has analgesic properties such as fentanyl or ketamine (see below).

How Supplied

Midazolam (Versed) is an injectable solution supplied in concentrations of 1 mg/ml and 5 mg/mL, and is stored at room temperature.

Dose

The recommended dosage range of midazolam for pediatric patients is 0.1 to 0.3 mg/kg. The lower end of the range is often chosen for use in conjunction with potent analgesics and the higher end for use of midazolam alone.

Narcotics (Morphine and Fentanyl)

Narcotics produce sedation and analgesia. Morphine produces varying degrees of histamine release which can cause hypotension, although this is less common among pediatric patients than adults (11). This effect is not inhibited or reversed by naloxone (11). Fentanyl does not cause histamine release and has minimal cardiovascular effects; it is therefore a superior choice for sedation and analgesia when the patient is hemodynamically unstable (11, 12). Because fentanyl is more highly lipid soluble than morphine, it crosses the blood-brain barrier more rapidly and has a more rapid redistribution time. As a result, fentanyl has a faster onset of action (about 1 to 2 minutes to peak effect) (4, 6) and a shorter duration (30 to 40 minutes) (2).

At higher doses, termination of the effect of fentanyl depends not on redistribution, but on hepatic clearance as the drug accumulates in the body. A more prolonged effect of fentanyl can therefore be obtained at higher doses. A second peak can also occur as a result of release from pulmonary or skeletal muscle stores (6, 11). Fentanyl has been shown to inhibit muscle fasciculations caused by succinylcholine (13) and to blunt the hemodynamic effects of laryngoscopy (14).

Precautions

All opiates produce respiratory depression. This effect is dose dependent and can be reversed with naloxone. Another significant adverse effect of both morphine and fentanyl is chest wall rigidity, which can interfere with spontaneous, assisted, or controlled ventilation (4, 15). Chest wall rigidity is normally prevented by the concomitant use of muscle relaxants or by administering the narcotic slowly (11, 15). This also may be reversible with naloxone (3).

Fentanyl has minimal cardiovascular effects, but it can cause a transient reduction in heart rate (5, 11). A vagolytic (e.g., atropine) therefore should be used in conjunction with fentanyl when this would be undesirable. Case reports of generalized tonic-clonic seizures after fentanyl administration have appeared in the literature (16, 17). However, these patients did not have simultaneous EEG recordings during the apparent seizure activity. It has been suggested that the seizurelike episodes may have instead been myoclonus or severe muscular rigidity (18, 19).

Although fentanyl has been generally considered to have little or no effect on ICP, some controversy does exist on this subject. A recent case report was published which described transient but significant increases in ICP noted immediately following administration of two separate 5 μg/kg doses of fentanyl to an 11-year-old boy with closed head injury (20). The child's ICP increased from a baseline of 12 to 18 mm Hg up to 42 mm Hg after the first dose and 38 mm Hg after the second dose. Both increases were managed easily without complications using hyperventilation and administration of 2 mg/kg of thiopental. Cuillerier et al. (21) studied the effects of fentanyl in 40 adult patients undergoing surgery for CNS aneurysms and arterial-venous malformations. The researchers found an increase in CSF pressure resulting in a reduction in cerebral perfusion pressure. In an investigation of adults with head trauma, Sperry et al. (22) found an average increase in ICP of 8 mm Hg after a dose of 3 μg/kg of fentanyl. To date no formal studies of the effect of fentanyl on ICP during emergent intubation of pediatric patients have been done. Fentanyl is known to blunt the pressor response during intubation, which contributes to the rise in ICP. However, it also appears that through a separate mechanism fentanyl may cause a direct increase in ICP. The clinical significance of this effect is currently unknown, although widespread experience supports the safety of fentanyl for patients with elevated ICP. Despite these isolated reports, fentanyl continues to be recommended for use during neurologic induction by most authorities. In practice, fentanyl is used routinely for RSI with pediatric patients suspected of having elevated ICP. Further study is therefore warranted on this subject, particularly as it relates to infants and children.

How Supplied
Fentanyl (Sublimaze) is supplied as a 50 μg/mL injectable solution. It should be stored at room temperature away from light.

Dose
The recommended dosage range of fentanyl for use in RSI is 2 to 10 μg/kg.

Ketamine
Ketamine is a dissociative anesthetic that rapidly provides sedation, anesthesia, analgesia, and amnesia. Within seconds of intravenous administration, the patient is sedated and unresponsive to pain (6, 11, 23). However, the patient may appear awake because ketamine does not affect the reticular activating system; instead, it acts to interrupt the connection between thalamoneocortical tracts and the limbic system (6, 23). Termination of the sedating effects depends on redistribution and usually occurs after 10 to 20 minutes (3, 5, 6). Termination of the analgesic effect is somewhat longer (40 to 45 minutes) (3).

Ketamine has important properties that make it a particularly valuable agent for fa-

cilitating intubation of the asthmatic patient. It causes the release of endogenous catecholamines, dilating bronchial smooth muscle, and stimulating β receptors in the lungs, which can increase pulmonary compliance and relieve bronchospasm (3, 23). Ketamine also increases oropharyngeal and tracheobronchial secretions, which in some instances can reduce mucus plugging (6). Excessive production of secretions may interfere with visualization of the larynx during direct laryngoscope and can be controlled when administration of ketamine is preceded by atropine (see below).

The sympathomimetic effects of ketamine also affect the cardiovascular system. Primarily through a centrally mediated mechanism, ketamine causes an increase in heart rate, blood pressure, and cardiac output (3, 23). This pressor response tends to mask its mild inherent myocardial depressant effect found in vitro (3, 23). Consequently, ketamine is often a good choice for a patient with hypotension, particularly when caused by early endotoxic shock, severe dehydration, acute hemorrhage, cardiac tamponade, or restrictive pericarditis (3, 23).

Precautions
The stimulatory effects of ketamine on the cardiovascular system are detrimental to the patient with hypertension, unstable angina, or a recent myocardial infarction, although all of these are rare in children. In addition, any patient with an intracranial, thoracic, or abdominal aneurysm should not receive ketamine because of the deleterious effects of increased blood pressure on these conditions. Although ketamine has beneficial effects on cardiac output in some acutely hypotensive or hypovolemic patients, some evidence shows that it may worsen hypotension in patients who have been in shock for more prolonged periods, whose chronic low cardiac output state has been supported by endogenous catecholamines that have become depleted (23).

Ketamine produces an increase in ICP by causing cerebral vasodilation and increasing systemic blood pressure (23). Therefore, it is contraindicated for any patient with possible head injury, intracranial mass, hemorrhage, or VP shunt obstruction. It may also cause a slight increase in intraocular pressure (3) and thus should be avoided in patients with an open globe injury.

A potential complication when ketamine is used as the only sedative is the occurrence of postemergence reactions, which have an overall reported incidence ranging from 3 to 50% (3). In children under 16 years of age, the incidence is less than 10% (24). These reactions range from mild floating sensations and dizziness to vivid, unpleasant dreams, auditory and visual hallucinations, and frank delirium (3, 23). Most of the reactions resolve once the patient is fully awake, but some have symptoms for weeks (25, 26). Preceding ketamine with midazolam (at least 0.1 mg/kg) will normally prevent these postemergence problems without prolonging the recovery from anesthesia (26).

Ketamine does not generally cause respiratory depression. However, apnea does occur in a small percentage of cases and therefore should be anticipated whenever this agent is used (3, 23, 27). Laryngeal reflexes are usually maintained with ketamine, making it advisable to use a muscle relaxant concomitantly to avoid vomiting or laryngospasm during airway manipulation. In addition, increased production of saliva and tracheal secretions occurring with administration of ketamine may cause gagging or difficulty in visualizing the airway during laryngoscopy. For this reason, an antisialagogue (either glycopyrrolate or atropine) also should be routinely administered (25, 28). Since atropine may increase the incidence of post-emergence dreams, glycopyrolate should be used when available for older children and adolescents.

How Supplied
Ketamine (Ketaject, Ketalar) is supplied as an injectable solution in 10 mg/mL, 50 mg/mL, and 100 mg/mL concentrations and is stored at room temperature.

Dose
The intravenous dose of ketamine is 1 to 2 mg/kg. When intravenous access is unobtainable making RSI impossible, ketamine may be given as an intramuscular injection at a dose of 2 to 10 mg/kg. The onset of action and peak effect of the drug will obviously be less reliable in this situation.

Neuromuscular Blockade

Depolarizing Agents (Succinylcholine)
Succinylcholine acts by directly binding to the ACh receptor site at the motor end plate, causing prolonged depolarization of the muscle (often evidenced by fasciculations) and subsequent paralysis. Although succinylcholine is rapidly hydrolyzed by plasma pseudocholinesterase, the muscle remains refractory to further contraction until the membrane returns to the resting state.

Succinylcholine is water soluble and rapidly distributed to the extracellular space (5). It has a rapid onset (20 to 60 seconds) and a short duration of effect (5 to 10 minutes) (3, 29, 30–34). In general, an intravenous dose of 1.5 mg/kg will reliably produce rapid onset of profound muscle paralysis in any child over 1 year of age (3, 29, 32, 33). Infants have a higher body composition of extracellular fluid and therefore require a higher dosage range for succinylcholine compared to that for older children and adolescents. Intraosseous administration of succinylcholine has been shown to be equally effective and to have a comparable rate of onset to intravenous injection (35). Succinylcholine may be given via intramuscular injection at a dose of 4 mg/kg, although the onset time is much longer (2 to 4 minutes) (5, 37). The intraosseous route is therefore preferred over the intramuscular route for RSI when timely intravenous access cannot be established.

Precautions
Many experts believe that the rapid onset and short duration of this agent make it the muscle relaxant of choice for most standard RSI intubations. However, succinylcholine does have several side effects, as well as relative and absolute contraindications. Because of its similarity to acetylcholine, succinylcholine produces varying degrees of vagal stimulation, ranging from mild to profound bradycardia and even asystole. Infants and young children are most susceptible (3, 29). For this reason, atropine should be routinely given before succinylcholine when performing RSI. Administration of atropine after bradycardia is already present may be ineffective in reversing this effect.

Because of its depolarizing action, succinylcholine may produce muscle fasciculations before paralysis. The contraction of the diaphragm and abdominal muscles can cause an increase in intragastric pressure which theoretically could lead to regurgitation. However, reflux is normally prevented by the greater rise in lower esophageal sphincter pressure. In addition, since children younger than 4 years have a relatively small muscle mass, significant fasciculations are unlikely in these patients (29, 32, 34, 37, 38). Regurgitation of stomach contents can generally be avoided if cricoid pressure is applied and overzealous BVM ventilation is avoided. A "defasciculating dose" of vecuronium or pancuronium (0.01 mg/kg) given 1 to 2 minutes before administering succinylcholine is often advocated to prevent fasciculations (37). However, this dosing is not routine practice because it is believed unnecessary for most pediatric intubations; it is a potential distraction from more important interventions; it can produce weakness (causing dysphoria and decreasing the patient's ability to protect the airway); and it eliminates a valuable sign (fasciculations) of the onset of profound paralysis when laryngoscopy can begin. One important exception involves the patient with an open globe injury. Intraocular pressure is increased by succinylcholine as a direct result of extraocular muscle contractions during the fasciculation phase (3, 29). This drug is therefore contraindicated for any patient with a penetrating eye injury unless preceded by a defasciculating dose of a nondepolarizing muscle relaxant.

Succinylcholine can cause a transient increase in serum potassium levels of approximately 0.5 mEq/L (29, 34, 38). In certain patient groups, this increase may be as high as 5 to 11 mEq/L (29, 34), potentially leading to ventricular arrhythmias and asystole (3). Patients at increased risk for this complication are those with massive tissue destruction (e.g., extensive burns or crush injuries) or muscular wasting secondary to denervating neuromuscular disorders (e.g., spinal cord injury, recent onset of multiple sclerosis, or stroke) (3, 29). In patients with these conditions, risk of life-threatening hyperkalemia does not begin until days after the injury or onset of symptoms (3, 6). The vulnerable period for patients with burns, for example, is 5

to 120 days after the injury (3) and perhaps longer after the wounds have healed. Succinylcholine is therefore not contraindicated for burn or crush injury patients immediately following their injury.

Use of succinylcholine for patients with increased ICP is controversial. Some investigators have found that it causes a transient rise in ICP (39), whereas others have found no change in ICP with this agent. In fact, succinylcholine has actually been shown to eliminate the increase in ICP that occurs with endotracheal suctioning, probably by suppressing the cough reflex (7). Initial use of 0.01 mg/kg of vecuronium or pancuronium prevents fasciculations caused by succinylcholine, which may contribute to any theoretical increase in ICP. However, our practice is to administer succinylcholine as the only paralytic agent during RSI to patients with elevated ICP unless otherwise contraindicated. We do not use a defasciculating dose of a nondepolarizing agent for reasons mentioned previously. Succinylcholine has a rapid onset, is highly potent, and has a short duration of effect. These properties combine to decrease the likelihood of hypoxemia and hypercarbia, which have significant detrimental effects on cerebral blood flow and metabolism. They also decrease the likelihood of aspiration, which would require higher airway pressures and a resulting rise in ICP. These demonstrable advantages are believed by many to outweigh any theoretical risks associated with succinylcholine. Other rare adverse effects include malignant hyperthermia, which occurs in approximately 1 in 15,000 children (40), masseter spasm, and myoglobinuria, which is a more common complication among children than adults (3).

How Supplied
Succinylcholine (Anectine, Quelicin, Sucostrin) is supplied as an injectable solution in concentrations of 20 mg/mL (preferred), 50 mg/mL, and 100 mg/mL. It should be kept refrigerated to preserve potency.

Dose
For children and adolescents, the standard dose for succinylcholine is 1 to 1.5 mg/kg. For infants, the dose is 1.5 to 2 mg/kg.

Nondepolarizing agents (Pancuronium, Vecuronium, Rocuronium).
Nondepolarizing agents block neuromuscular transmission by competitive inhibition of ACh at the motor end plate receptor sites. Unlike depolarizing agents, they have no neurotransmitter capability. Instead, they prevent the muscle from contracting.

Pancuronium is a long-acting agent. The onset time for good intubating conditions following a dose of 0.1 mg/kg is about 90 seconds in infants and about 3 minutes in older children and adolescents (3, 32). Its duration of action (generally 40 to 90 minutes) initially depends on redistribution and then subsequently on renal and hepatic excretion (6, 30, 32). The relatively long onset and duration times have limited the use of pancuronium for RSI as newer agents have been developed.

Vecuronium is an intermediate-acting nondepolarizing agent. At a dose of 0.1 mg/kg (the standard dose used for elective intubation), vecuronium has an onset of 1 to 3 minutes (6, 32) and a duration of about 75 minutes in infants and 35 to 55 minutes in older children and adolescents (29, 32). Increasing the dose to 0.3 mg/kg has been shown to shorten the onset time to 40 to 60 seconds (30, 31), which decreases the risk of aspiration during RSI. However, at this higher dose the duration of effect is at least 75 minutes in children.

Rocuronium is a new nondepolarizing muscle relaxant with a fast onset and relatively short duration of effect compared with vecuronium and pancuronium. Several studies in adults have shown that rocuronium produces good to excellent intubating conditions in 60 to 90 seconds (41–43). Duration of action has been reported at between 24 and 37 minutes (42–44). Although currently used primarily by anesthesiologists, rocuronium will undoubtedly gain wider application for pediatric patients in the ED as greater clinical experience is obtained, particularly for situations in which succinylcholine is contraindicated.

How Supplied
Pancuronium (Pavulon) is supplied in injectable solutions of 1 mg/mL and 2 mg/mL that must be refrigerated. Vecuronium (Norcuron) is supplied as a powder in 10 mg vials that do not require refrigeration. It must be mixed at the time of injection by adding 5 mL of normal saline to each vial to produce a 2 mg/mL solution. Rocuronium (Zemuron) is supplied as a 10 mg/mL injectable solution in 5 and 10 mL vials which must be refrigerated.

Dose
The routine dose for pancuronium and vecuronium for elective intubations is 0.1 mg/kg. The dose for RSI is 0.15 mg/kg for pancuronium and 0.3 mg/kg for vecuronium. At these higher doses, the onset time is 90 seconds for pancuronium and 60 seconds for vecuronium. As mentioned previously, a defasciculating dose of 0.01 mg/kg of either pancuronium or vecuronium may be given as indicated 1 to 2 minutes before administering succinylcholine to suppress fasciculations.

Rocuronium has been only minimally studied in pediatric patients at present. In one series (6), a dose of 0.6 mg/kg was used in children between ages 1 and 5 years with profound paralysis induced after approximately 60 seconds. For RSI, our practice is to use a higher dose (1 mg/kg) to achieve a more rapid onset of effect. Evidence also indicates that infants may require a higher dose than older children to achieve acceptable onset times (45, 46). In adults, the duration of action of rocuronium at a dose of 1.2 mg/kg has been reported at between 67 and 73 minutes (44, 47).

Ancillary Agents

Atropine
Except in rare cases (e.g., mitral stenosis, coronary artery disease, or preexisting tachyarrhythmia) atropine should always be used during RSI for infants and younger children. Atropine is a rapid-onset acetylcholine receptor antagonist which increases the heart rate for a duration of approximately 30 minutes (3). This vagolytic effect also blocks the bradycardia caused by airway manipulation or succinylcholine administration. In contrast to adults, children are more likely to respond with profound bradycardia and even asystole when an anticholinergic agent has not been administered. Atropine also reduces salivary and airway secretions, thereby facilitating laryngoscopy.

How Supplied

Atropine is supplied in ampules with concentrations ranging from .05 mg/mL to 1 mg/mL solutions. We prefer the 0.4 mg/mL solution supplied in 1 mL vials for pediatric patients. Atropine can be stored at room temperature.

Dose

The dose for premedication before intubation is 0.02 mg/kg, with a minimum dose of 0.15 mg (about 0.4 mL of the 0.4 mg/mL solution) and a maximum dose of 0.4 mg.

Lidocaine

Lidocaine is an antiarrhythmic and local anesthetic agent which has been advocated for use to blunt the rise in ICP that occurs during laryngoscopy and other noxious stimuli. Intravenous and intratracheal lidocaine have been extensively studied in patients with elevated ICP (7, 35, 48–50). It is intended to decrease the rise in systemic blood pressure that occurs with instrumentation without significantly decreasing myocardial contractility, as a large dose of thiopental might do. However, the usefulness of lidocaine in this context remains controversial. It has not been shown to effectively blunt the catecholamine response to intubation in children (49). Nonetheless, many practitioners routinely administer intravenous lidocaine 2 to 3 minutes before intubation for the patient presumed to have increased ICP (50). Intravenous and intratracheal lidocaine may also suppress the cough response. Percutaneous transtracheal administration of lidocaine is described in Chapter 16.

How Supplied

Lidocaine (Xylocaine) is supplied in either 10 mg/mL or 20 mg/mL solutions in preservative-free single-use 5 mL vials and is stored at room temperature.

Dose

For preintubation purposes, the intravenous dose of lidocaine is 1 to 2 mg/kg.

PROCEDURE

In this section, standard RSI for endotracheal intubation is described first, followed by modifications of the procedure which are indicated in specific clinical situations. The success of RSI intubation depends on the participation and skill of at least three qualified individuals: one person to provide 100% oxygen and perform the intubation, another to apply cricoid pressure, and a third to administer the medications. Ideally, a resuscitation team leader not involved with the procedure will have the sole task of monitoring the patient's clinical status and directing overall patient care. In this situation, individuals are assigned to perform specific duties while the team leader oversees and organizes treatment. In reality, the supervising physician will often have the responsibility of performing one or more aspects of RSI as well. When available, any additional personnel can assist by restraining the patient as necessary and documenting the procedure.

Oxygenation and ventilation are maintained by spontaneous, assisted, or controlled ventilation during setup for the procedure. Intravenous access is obtained and heart rate, blood pressure, and oxygen saturation monitoring are established. Preparation includes acquiring maximum access to the patient around the stretcher, clearly describing assignments to assistants, verifying intravenous access, and testing all necessary equipment (e.g., suction, laryngoscopes, endotracheal tubes).

As these preparations are finalized, the patient is preoxygenated by administering 100% F_iO_2 via face mask. In the optimal situation, this occurs as the patient spontaneously breathes oxygen from a nonrebreathing mask. Three minutes of spontaneous respirations at a consistent F_iO_2 of 100% has been shown to allow at least 2 minutes of apnea without desaturation in healthy children (52). When a rapid onset muscle relaxant is used, effective preoxygenation in this manner obviates the need for immediate BVM ventilation should the patient become apneic after administration of the sedative but before complete paralysis. Positive pressure ventilation can wait until after the endotracheal tube is in place and the airway is protected. This is believed to lower the risk of vomiting and aspiration by avoiding air entry into the stomach during BVM ventilation. Importantly, patients with reduced functional residual capacity (FRC) or underlying lung disease will desaturate more rapidly despite adequate preoxygenation.

SUMMARY: STANDARD RAPID SEQUENCE INDUCTION

(Note: this method is used when there is no risk of increased ICP. Patients suspected of having increased ICP should undergo the "neurologic induction" method.)

1. Establish appropriate monitoring (EKG, blood pressure cuff, pulse oximeter)
2. Establish intravenous access
3. Maintain a patent airway and an effective seal of the face mask
4. Pre-oxygenate with 100% FiO_2 for 2–3 minutes if FRC is normal, up to 5 minutes if FRC is very high or very low. If respiratory insufficiency exists, assist or control ventilation with a BVM circuit while applying cricoid pressure
5. Give atropine (0.02 mg/kg, minimum dose of 0.15 mg, maximum dose 0.4 mg)
6. Give sedation: Thiopental (3–7 mg/kg)

   If decreased systemic blood pressure, use midazolam (0.1–0.3 mg/kg), ketamine (1–2 mg/kg), or fentanyl (1–5 mg/kg)

   If patient has status asthmaticus, use ketamine (1–2 mg/kg).

   If patient has diminished sensorium, sedation may be unnecessary.

7. Give muscle relaxant (unless contra-indicated) Succinylcholine (1.5 mg/kg) If succinylcholine is contraindicated, use vecuronium (0.3 mg/kg) or rocuronium (1 mg/kg)
8. Apply cricoid pressure (if not already performed)
9. Provide gentle controlled BVM ventilation only if necessary from the time the sedative causes apnea until the muscle relaxant produces complete paralysis
10. Perform laryngoscopy, visualize the tube entering the trachea, and begin positive pressure ventilation
11. Auscultate both lung fields under each axilla to check tube placement
12. If available, use CO_2 detector to verify tracheal placement
13. Release cricoid pressure once the tube is verified to be in the trachea
14. Secure the tube at mid-tracheal position
15. Insert orogastric or nasogastric tube to suction gastric contents
16. Obtain chest radiograph to confirm tube position
17. Consider additional sedation with narcotics, which can be completely antagonized with naloxone if necessary

Chapter 15
Rapid Sequence
Induction

154

Table 15.4.
Medications and Dosages for Standard Rapid Sequence Induction

Vagolytic
  Atropine 0.02 mg/kg (minimum dose 0.15 mg, maximum dose 0.4 mg)
Sedation
  Thiopental 3–7 mg/kg
  If patient is hypotensive, use
    Ketamine 1–2 mg/kg
    OR
    Midazolam 0.1–0.3 mg/kg
Neuromuscular blockade
  Succinylcholine 1.5 mg/kg
  If succinylcholine contraindicated, use
    Vecuronium 0.3 mg/kg
    OR
    Rocuronium 1 mg/kg

For the spontaneously breathing patient, it is generally advisable to administer a few assisted ventilations using a BVM circuit during the preoxygenation phase (see Chapter 14). As mentioned previously, this provides reasonable assurance that adequate BVM ventilation can be provided should intubation prove unsuccessful after the neuromuscular blocking agent has been administered. Adequacy of the mask seal, patency of the airway, and any difficulty with delivering PPV should be carefully assessed. As mentioned previously, administration of a paralytic agent would be contraindicated if there is a concern that BVM ventilation may be impossible. In this situation, an awake intubation (with judicious use of sedating agents as necessary) should be attempted.

The medications and dosages used for standard pediatric RSI are shown in Table 15.4. Although the sedating and neuromuscular blocking agents are given in rapid sequence immediately before intubation, atropine (0.02 mg/kg) may be administered at any time during the preoxygenation phase. Sedation for a standard RSI is provided by thiopental (3 to 7 mg/kg). This allows for induction of anesthesia in 20 to 60 seconds. Immediately following administration of thiopental, succinylcholine (1.5 mg/kg) is given to produce profound paralysis within 20 to 60 seconds. Cricoid pressure may be performed at this point to prevent regurgitation of stomach contents (see below). Notably many practitioners use rocuronium (1 mg/kg) or vecuronium (0.3 mg/kg) to provide neuromuscular blockade. As mentioned previously, succinylcholine may be preferred for

RSI unless contraindicated due to its potency, faster onset, and shorter duration of effect. The rapid onset of succinylcholine normally allows the operator to safely avoid BVM ventilation after induction agents are administered, since the time to complete paralysis is brief. Whatever agent is selected, laryngoscopy should begin as soon as fasciculations occur or apnea and hypotonia are observed. These signs indicate the patient is sufficiently paralyzed to insert the endotracheal tube without eliciting coughing or gagging. When succinylcholine is used for neuromuscular blockade and preoxygenation is completed with no entrainment of room air, the operator generally has at least 2 minutes of "safe" time to insert the endotracheal tube (i.e., before desaturation occurs and before return of normal muscle tone). Once the endotracheal tube has been placed, the lung fields should be ascultated and capnography used when available to confirm proper tube position (see Chapter 16). Cricoid pressure should be maintained until tube placement is confirmed. The patient should be ventilated manually or by mechanical ventilation and the tube should be taped in place. A nasogastric tube should be placed and a chest radiograph obtained to verify tube position. The operator may consider giving longer-acting sedative and paralytic agents to facilitate mechanical ventilation and/or transport.

Modifications

The ideal circumstances for performing an endotracheal intubation using RSI are unfortunately not always present in an emergent situation. Often one or more problems require a modification of RSI. As previously described, the optimal method of preoxygenating the patient is to apply a nonrebreathing face mask delivering 100% oxygen for 2 to 5 minutes before intubation while the patient breathes spontaneously. When succinylcholine is used for RSI in this situation, its rapid effect often allows the operator to avoid performing BVM ventilation during the brief interval between the onset of apnea (caused by the sedative) and complete paralysis. However, the patient with significant respiratory compromise may require assisted or controlled ventilation with a BVM circuit and a modified preoxygenation phase. The risk of aspiration is already high when the patient is acutely ill and is likely to have a full stomach. Positive pressure ventilation before intubation adds to this risk to the extent that air enters the stomach and increases the intragastric pressure. When the patient is receiving BVM ventilation before intubation, the rapid onset of succinylcholine is less of an advantage. In addition, there is a theoretical possibility that regurgitation of stomach contents may be produced by fasciculations as a result of succinylcholine, further increasing the risk of aspiration. In this situation, a nondepolarizing agent such as rocuronium or vecuronium may therefore be preferred.

For the patient requiring ongoing assisted or controlled ventilation, cricoid pressure (Sellick's maneuver) should be performed by an assistant from the time BVM ventilation is initiated until the trachea is successfully intubated. This prevents the accumulation of excessive intragastric pressure and possible regurgitation of stomach contents or vomiting (53–58). The technique for performing Sellick's maneuver is shown in Figure 16.17 on page 191. The cricoid cartilage can be palpated inferior to the thyroid cartilage as a firm ring-shaped structure. With the patient supine, pressure is applied directly downward over the cricoid cartilage to compress the esophagus. Notably, excessive pressure that distorts the airway must be avoided, as this will make laryngoscopy and passage of the endotracheal tube more difficult. In addition, cricoid pressure should be discontinued if the patient vomits, because extreme pressures generated in this situation may result in gastric or esophageal rupture. Above all, the operator managing the airway must take particular care to administer "gentle" BVM ventilation, so that chest excursions are adequate to maintain good oxygenation but not so forceful that excessive inspiratory pressures cause air entry into the stomach. Positive pressure ventilation must obviously continue until the patient is fully paralyzed, at which point the operator may proceed with laryngoscopy. The remainder of the procedure is the same as with standard RSI.

Another modification of RSI is designed to prevent increases in ICP to protect the brain when the patient is suspected of having an elevated ICP. In this situation, it is particularly important to avoid hypoxemia, hypercarbia, systemic hypertension or hypoten-

Table 15.5.
Medications and Dosages for Neurologic Induction

Premedications
    Atropine 0.02 mg/kg (minimum dose 0.15 mg, maximum dose 0.4 mg)
    Fentanyl 1 μg/kg
    Vecuronium 0.01 mg/kg (may be given as a "defasciculating dose" if desired when succinylcholine is used for muscle relaxation)
    Lidocaine 1 mg/kg
Sedation
    Thiopental 3–7 mg/kg
    If patient is hypotensive, use
        Midazolam 0.2–0.3 mg/kg
        OR
        Fentanyl (1–5 μg/kg)
        OR
        Thiopental (1–3 mg/kg)
Neuromuscular blockade
    Succinylcholine 1.5 mg/kg
    If succinylcholine contraindicated, use
        Vecuronium 0.3 mg/kg
        OR
        Rocuronium 1 mg/kg

sion, excessive positive airway pressure, and noxious stimulation with inadequate anesthesia. Examples of the medications and dosages for pediatric neurologic induction are shown in Table 15.5. This method includes two additional agents in the premedication phase while the patient is receiving 100% oxygen. After the atropine has been given, intravenous fentanyl (1 μg/mg) can be administered. Fentanyl has been shown to decrease the pressor response and the rise in ICP that occurs with laryngoscopy among both children and adults (14). It should be given at least 30 to 60 seconds before intubation during the preoxygenation phase. Because it acts as a respiratory and CNS depressant, immediate elimination of soft tissue obstruction, initiation of PPV, and suctioning may become necessary. As an adjunct, intravenous lidocaine (1 to 1.5 mg/kg) can then be given immediately before administering the sedative. Lidocaine may attenuate the rise in ICP during intubation with little myocardial depressant effect. Thiopental (3 to 7 mg/kg) is the primary sedative agent in this situation because of its protective effect on the brain. As discussed previously, the patient at risk for increased ICP who has low cardiac output may be given small, frequent 1 to 3 mg/kg doses of thiopental every 20 to 60 seconds, titrated to sedative effect and hemodynamic stability. Alternatively, midazolam may be used (0.1 to 0.3 mg/kg).

SUMMARY: NEUROLOGIC INDUCTION
(Note: this method should be used for patients with head trauma, intracranial mass lesion, CNS infection, VP shunt dysfunction, or another CNS process causing potentially elevated ICP.)

1. Establish appropriate monitoring (ECG, blood pressure cuff, pulse oximeter)
2. Establish intravenous access
3. Maintain patent airway and effective seal of the face mask
4. Preoxygenate with 100% F_iO_2 for 2 to 3 minutes if FRC is normal, up to 5 minutes if FRC is very high or very low. If respiratory insufficiency exists, assist or control ventilation with BVM circuit while applying cricoid pressure.
5. Give premedication: Atropine (0.02 mg/kg, minimum dose 0.15 mg, maximum dose 0.4 mg) Fentanyl (1 μg/kg) (optional) Vecuronium (0.01 mg/kg) (optional) Lidocaine (1 mg/kg)
6. If necessary, remove front piece of cervical collar and provide inline stabilization
7. Give sedation: Thiopental (3 to 7 mg/kg) If decreased systemic blood pressure, use midazolam (0.1 to 0.3 mg/kg), fentanyl (1 to 5 μg/kg), or thiopental (1 to 3 mg/kg, titrate doses)

Chapter 15
Rapid Sequence
Induction

155

8. Give muscle relaxant (unless contraindicated):
   Succinylcholine (1.5 mg/kg)
   If succinylcholine is contraindicated, use vecuronium (0.3 mg/kg) or rocuronium (1 mg/kg)
9. Apply cricoid pressure (if not already performed)
10. Provide gentle controlled BVM ventilation only if necessary from time sedative causes apnea until muscle relaxant produces complete paralysis
11. Perform laryngoscopy, visualize tube entering trachea, and begin PPV
12. Auscultate both lung fields under each axilla to check tube placement
13. If available, verify tracheal placement with CO_2 detector
14. Release cricoid pressure once tube is verified to be in trachea
15. Secure tube at midtracheal position
16. Insert orogastric or nasogastric tube to suction gastric contents
17. Obtain chest radiograph to confirm tube position
18. Consider additional sedation with narcotics, which can be completely antagonized with naloxone if necessary

Either succinylcholine or a potent nondepolarizing drug in a high dose is acceptable as part of the neurologic RSI. Of the neuromuscular blockers, succinylcholine provides the fastest onset of paralysis, and many prefer it to minimize the likelihood of hypoxemia, hypercarbia, and aspiration. However, some animal evidence shows it can cause a transient increase in ICP, in part as a result of muscle fasciculations, although many practitioners consider this effect unimportant clinically. If desired, a defasciculating dose of vecuronium or pancuronium (0.01 mg/kg) can be given 2 to 3 minutes before the succinylcholine to prevent muscle fasciculations. As described previously, some experts believe this is unnecessary for pediatric patients and adds needless complexity and risk to the procedure. An alternative approach is to substitute a competitive blocker such as vecuronium (0.3 mg/kg) or rocuronium (1 mg/kg). At the higher doses used for RSI, the time to complete paralysis with these agents is closer to that of succinylcholine. However, it may be necessary to administer gentle PPV from the time the peak effect of thiopental occurs (about 15 to 40 seconds) until complete paralysis is observed (60 to 90 seconds with vecuronium or rocuronium) to prevent hypercarbia. Even with cricoid pressure, this approach may increase the likelihood of vomiting and aspiration due to air entry into the stomach during BVM ventilation. It should also be remembered that use of the higher doses of the nondepolarizing agents significantly prolongs the time that the patient will be paralyzed. As long as intubation is accomplished rapidly, this longer duration of effect poses no problem. In fact, it will often be desirable because paralysis will facilitate head imaging studies that require the patient to be motionless. But for the rare patient who proves unexpectedly difficult to both intubate and manually ventilate, such a prolonged period of paralysis can lead to significant morbidity or mortality. Many practitioners, primarily for these reasons, prefer succinylcholine in such emergency circumstances.

For the patient requiring RSI who is hypotensive but not at risk for increased ICP, ketamine (1 to 2 mg/kg) is preferred for sedation over thiopental. Ketamine causes the release of endogenous catecholamines which maintain or even raise the systemic blood pressure, unlike thiopental which has a potent myocardial depressant effect. A secondary option in this situation would be midazolam (0.1 to 0.3 mg/kg) which has minimal cardiovascular effects.

Ketamine is also an excellent choice for sedation of the asthmatic patient who requires intubation. Unlike thiopental and midazolam, ketamine is a bronchodilator. Ketamine also increases airway and salivary secretions. Although this may have some beneficial effect in relieving mucus plugging, it can significantly hinder laryngoscopy, and therefore ketamine should always be preceded by atropine or glycopyrrolate.

A final modification of RSI relates to patients with glaucoma or possible open globe injury. These patients should not receive succinylcholine for neuromuscular blockade unless preceded by a defasciculating dose of a nondepolarizing agent. Fasciculations caused by succinylcholine cause the intraocular pressure to rise, and in patients with an eye injury, extrusion of the ocular contents can occur. The preference in this situation is to use vecuronium (0.3 mg/kg) or rocuronium (1 mg/kg) to produce muscle relaxation.

COMPLICATIONS

Aspiration is a serious potential complication of RSI because the technique is performed with patients presumed to have a full stomach (59, 60). Cricoid pressure, avoidance of BVM ventilation, and proper use of pharmacologic agents will decrease the likelihood of aspiration. If BVM ventilation is required, it should be performed using the minimum necessary inspiratory pressures, so excessive air entry into the stomach is avoided. Complete elimination of soft tissue obstruction with an effective jaw thrust and avoidance of excessive tidal volumes, with peak inflating pressures ideally below 15 to 20 cm H_2O, will reduce the risk of elevated intragastric pressure.

Sympathetic stimulation associated with laryngoscopy and intubation can lead to cardiovascular collapse, particularly when the patient presents with hypoxemia, myocardial ischemia, or a low cardiac output state. In addition, vagotonic effects of laryngoscopy often predominate in infants and younger children (60, 61), potentially leading to significant bradycardia and asystole. Both complications can normally be avoided with careful selection of induction agents tailored to the patient's clinical status. Hypotensive patients should receive an agent that does not further depress myocardial function and systemic blood pressure. In many cases, there will be sufficient time to perform a volume resuscitation while temporizing with BVM ventilation. Many believe that atropine should always be given to children before intubation to both avoid bradycardia and reduce airway secretions.

Exacerbation of an elevated ICP may occur during intubation if an inappropriate or poorly executed RSI regimen is used (39). Most patients suspected of having increased ICP—such as those with space occupying lesions and/or cerebral edema—should undergo a neurologic induction. Although this modification of RSI will minimize the effect of laryngoscopy and endotracheal intubation on ICP, the most important priorities remain the prevention of hypoxemia and aspiration.

Inadequate sedation during RSI can lead to systemic hypertension, dysrhythmias, and myocardial ischemia. Furthermore, the patient can have the terrifying experience of being awake but paralyzed even before a painful stimulus is applied. Proper sedation, as a bolus or titrated in small frequent increments, can be safely achieved in almost all patients who require neuromuscular blocking agents.

If laryngoscopy is performed before complete sedation and paralysis, the patient may cough, vomit, or have adverse cardiovascular changes. Conversely, if the period of apnea before intubation is prolonged, profound hypoxemia may result. The operator must therefore wait an appropriate length of time before initiating intubation, but then act immediately once paralysis is complete. Clearly, timing is a critical element in the success of RSI.

Finally, failure to accomplish intubation in a paralyzed patient creates an immediate dependency on BVM ventilation as the lifesaving means of gas exchange. If intubation is unsuccessful after RSI has been performed, BVM ventilation should be administered with effective cricoid pressure until the effects of the neuromuscular blocking agent have subsided or another airway intervention can be performed. It cannot be overemphasized that before choosing to administer a muscle relaxant, the operator must ensure to the extent possible that both intubation and manual ventilation can be accomplished with minimal difficulty. Otherwise, spontaneous ventilation must be preserved with intubation performed using little or no sedation and no muscle relaxant.

CLINICAL TIPS

1. Materials and setup should be properly organized and assignments precisely communicated to assistants before any drug is administered.
2. A muscle relaxant should not be used unless both BVM ventilation and endotracheal intubation are very likely to be achieved without difficulty.
3. Intravenous placement of the peripheral access catheter should be verified and all tubing connections should be checked before administering medications.
4. An effective mask seal should be ensured at all times during preoxygenation.
5. Drugs should be administered through an access port close to the patient, preferably through a T-connector attached to the intravenous catheter.
6. Laryngoscopy should begin at the moment of full muscle relaxation. Premature instrumentation may cause trauma or vomiting. Delayed instrumentation reduces the time available for intubation before the onset of desaturation.
7. Cricoid pressure should not be released until correct tube position is confirmed unless the patient vomits. Continued cricoid pressure during vomiting can cause gastric or esophageal rupture.
8. For the hypotensive patient, thiopental should be avoided or administered in low doses of 1 to 3 mg/kg and titrated to adequate sedation and hemodynamic stability. Midazolam or fentanyl may be substituted.
9. Ketamine supports the circulation and acts as a bronchodilator, indications for its use in the asthmatic requiring intubation. Ketamine should not be used when the patient has an open globe injury or is at risk for increased ICP.
10. Succinylcholine should never be administered to patients with glaucoma or possible open globe injury unless preceded by a defasciculating dose of a nondepolarizing muscle relaxant. Succinylcholine is contraindicated in patients with denervating neuromuscular diseases, susceptibility to malignant hyperthermia, and thermal and crush injuries beginning days after the traumatic event.

Summary

The purpose of RSI is to facilitate a safe endotracheal intubation. It is intended to protect the patient from several potentially adverse effects of intubation. Patients presenting acutely who require emergent intubation are presumed to have a full stomach and are therefore at risk for aspiration of gastric contents. RSI is designed to minimize this risk. In addition, modifications of this procedure include methods that are intended to attenuate the rise in ICP associated with intubation, to avoid exacerbating systemic hypotension, and to facilitate intubation of the asthmatic patient. Familiarity with the necessary induction agents and muscle relaxants is essential to successful RSI. The operator must also understand the indications, limitations, and potential hazards of this procedure. When used appropriately, RSI significantly enhances the capabilities of those who provide emergency airway management for pediatric patients.

References

1. West JB, ed. Best and Taylor's physiological basis of medical practice. 12th ed. Baltimore, MD: Williams & Wilkins, 1991.
2. Gilman AG, Rall TW, Nies AS, Taylor P, eds. Goodman and Gilman's the pharmacological basis of therapeutics. 8th ed. New York: Pergamon Press, 1990.
3. AMA Drug Evaluations, 5th ed., Chicago: American Medical Association, 1983.
4. Yamamoto LG, Kim GK, Britten AG. Rapid sequence anesthesia induction for emergency intubation. Ped Emerg Care 1990;6:200–212.
5. Cotæ CJ. Pediatric anesthesia. In: Miller RD, ed. Anesthesia. 3rd ed. New York: Churchill Livingstone Inc., 1990:1897, 1924.
6. Dronen SC. Pharmacologic adjuncts to intubation. In: Roberts J, Hedges J, eds. Clinical procedures in emergency medicine. 2nd ed. Philadelphia: WB Saunders, 1991.
7. White PF, Schlobohm RM, Pitts LH, Lindauer JM. A randomized study of drugs for preventing increases in intracranial pressure during endotracheal suctioning. Anesthesiology 1982;57:242–244.
8. Gelman S, Reves JG, Harris D. Circulatory responses to midazolam anesthesia: emphasis on canine splanchnic circulation. Anesth Analg 1983;62:135–139.
9. Chraemnzer-Jorgensen B, Hertel S, Strom J, et al. Catecholamine response to laryngoscopy and intubation. Anesthesia 1992;47:750–756.
10. Adams P, Gelman S, Reves JG, et al. Midazolam pharmacodynamics and pharmacokinetics during acute hypovolemia. Anesthesiology 1985;63:140–146.
11. Fackler JC, Arnold JH. Anesthetic principles and operating room anesthesia regimens. In: Fuhrman BP, Zimmerman JS, eds. Pediatric critical care. St. Louis: Mosby-Year Book, Inc., 1992, pp. 1265–1273.
12. Chudnofsky DR, Wright SW, Dronen SC, et al. The safety of fentanyl use in the emergency department. Ann Emerg Med 1989;18:635–639.
13. Lindgren L, Saarnivaara L. Effect of competitive myoneural blockade and fentanyl on muscle fasciculations caused by suxamethonium in children. Br J Anaesth 1983;55:747–751.
14. Sims CH, Splinter WM. Fentanyl blunts the haemodynamic response of children to laryngoscopy. Can J Anaesth 1990;37:591.
15. Hill AB, Nahrwold ML, DeRosayro AM, et al. Prevention of rigidity during fentanyl-oxygen induction of anesthesia. Anesthesiology 1981;55:452–454.
16. Hoien AO. Another case of grand mal seizure after fentanyl administration. (Letter) Anesthesiology 1984;60:387–388.
17. Safwat AM, Daniel D. Grand mal seizure after fentanyl administration. (Letter) Anesthesiology 1983;59:78.
18. Scott JC, Sarnquist FH. Seizurelike movements during a fentanyl infusion with absence of seizure activity in a simultaneous EEG recording. Anaesthesia 1985;62:812–814.
19. Sebel PS, Bovill JG. Fentanyl and convulsions. (Letter) Anaesth Analg 1983;62:858–859.
20. Tobias JD. Increased intracranial pressure after fentanyl administration in a child with closed head trauma. Pediatr Emerg Care 1994;10:89–90.
21. Cuillerier DJ, Manninen PH, Gelb AW. Alfentanil, sufentanil and fentanyl: effect on cerebral perfusion pressure. Anaesth Analg 1990;70:S75.
22. Sperry RJ, Bailey PL, Reichman MV, et al. Fentanyl and sufentanil increase intracranial pressure in head trauma patients. Anaesthesia 1992;77:416–420.
23. White PF, Way WL, Trevor AJ. Ketamine—its pharmacology and therapeutic uses. Anaesthesia 1982;56:119–136.
24. Perel A, Davidson JT. Recurrent hallucinations following ketamine. Anaesthesia 1976;31:1081–1083.
25. Meyers EF, Charles P. Prolonged adverse reactions to ketamine in children. Anesthesiology 1978;49:39–40.
26. White PF. Pharmacologic interactions of midazolam and ketamine in surgical patients. Clin Pharmacol Ther 1982;31:280.
27. Berman W, Fripp RR, Rubler M, Alderele L. Hemodynamic effects of ketamine in children undergoing cardiac catheterization. Pediatr Cardiol 1990;11:72–76.

28. Morgan M, Loh L, Singer L. Ketamine as the sole anaesthetic agent for minor surgical procedures. Anaesthesia 1971;26:158–165.
29. Cook DR. Neuromuscular blocking agents. In: Fuhrman BP, Zimmerman JS, eds. Pediatric critical care. Philadelphia: Mosby-Year Book, Inc., 1992, pp. 1251–1263.
30. Sloan MH, Lerman J, Bissonnette B. Pharmacodynamics of high-dose vecuronium in children during balanced anesthesia. Anaesthesia 1991;74:656–659.
31. Koller ME, Husby P. High-dose vecuronium may be an alternative to suxamethonium for rapid sequence intubation. Acta Anaesthesiol Scand 1993;37:465–468.
32. Meretoja OA. Neuromuscular blocking agents in paediatric patients: influence of age on the response. Anaesth Intens Care 1990;18:440–448.
33. Brown TCK, Meretoja OA, Bell B, Clare D. Suxamethonium—electromyographic studies in children. Anaesth Intensive Care 1990;18:473–476.
34. DeGarmo BH, Dronen S. Pharmacology and clinical use of neuromuscular blocking agents. Ann Emerg Med 1983;12:48–55.
35. Tobias JD, Nichols DG. Intraosseous succinylcholine for orotracheal intubation. Pediatr Emerg Care 1990;6:108–109.
36. Lui LMP, De Cook TA, Goudsouzian et al.: Dose response to intramuscular succinylcholine in children. Anesthesiology 1981;55:599–602.
37. Nugent SK, Lavaruso R, Rogers MC. Pharmacology and use of muscle relaxants in infants and children. J Pediatr 1979;94:481–487.
38. Salem MR, Wong AY, Lind YH. The effect of suxamethonium on the intragastric pressure in infants and children. Br J Anaesth 1972;44:166.
39. Burney R, Winn HR. Increased cerebrospinal fluid pressure during laryngoscopy and intubation for induction of anesthesia. Anaesth Analg 1975;54:687.
40. Tsang HS, Schoenfeld FG. Malignant hyperthermia. IMJ 1976;471–473.
41. Tryba M, Zorn A, Thole H, Zenz M. Rapid sequence orotracheal intubation with rocuronium: a randomized double-blind comparison with suxamethonium—preliminary communication. Eur J Anaesth 1994; (supp) 9:44–48.
42. Huizinga AC, Vandenbrom RH, Wierda JM, Hommes FD. Intubating conditions and onset of neuromuscular block of rocuronium (Org 9426); a comparison with suxamethonium. Acta Anaesth Scand 1992;36(5):463–468.
43. Cooper R, Mirakhur RK, Clarke RS, Boules Z. Comparison of intubating conditions after administration of Org 9246 (rocuronium) and suxamethonium. Br J Anaesth 1992; 69(3):269–273.
44. Magorian T, Flannery KB, Miller RD. Comparison of rocuronium, succinylcholine, and vecuronium for rapid-sequence induction of anesthesia in adult patients. Anaesthesia 1993;79(5): 913–918.
45. Vuksanaj D, Fisher DM. Pharmacokinetics of rocuronium in children aged 4–11 years. Anaesthesia 1995;82(5):1104–1110.
46. Viby-Mogensen J. Dose-response relationship and time course of action of rocuronium bromide in perspective. Eur J Anaesth 1994; (supp) 9:28–32.
47. Wright PM, Caldwell JE, Miller RD. Onset and duration of rocuronium and succinylcholine at the adductor pollicis and laryngeal adductor muscles in anesthetized humans. Anaesthesia 1994;81(5):1110–1115.
48. Yano M, Nishiyama H, Yokota H, et al. Effect of lidocaine on ICP response to endotracheal suctioning. Anesthesiology 1986;64:651–653.
49. Splinter WM. Intravenous lidocaine does not attenuate the hemodynamic response of children to laryngoscopy and tracheal intubation. Can J Anaesth 1990;37:440–443.
50. Hamill JF, Bedford RF, Weaver DC, et al. Lidocaine before endotracheal intubation: intravenous or laryngotracheal? Anaesthesia 1981;55:578–581.
51. Videira RL, Neto PP, do Amaral RV, Freeman JA. Preoxygenation in children: for how long? Acta Anaesthesiol Scand 1992;36:109.
52. Sellick BA. Cricoid pressure to control regurgitation of stomach contents during induction of anaesthesia. [Preliminary Communication] Lancet 1961;2:404–406.
53. Salem MR, Wong AY, Mani M, Sellick BA. Efficacy of cricoid pressure in preventing gastric inflation during bag-mask ventilation in pediatric patients. Anesthesiology 1974;40:96.
54. Admani M, Yeh TF, Jain R, et al. Prevention of gastric inflation during mask ventilation in newborn infants. Crit Care Med 1985;13:592.
55. Moynihan RJ, Brock-Utne JG, Archer JH, et al. The effect of cricoid pressure on preventing gastric insufflation in infants and children. Anesthesiology 1993;78:652.
56. Fanning GL. The efficacy of cricoid pressure in preventing regurgitation of gastric contents. Anesthesiology 1970;32:553.
57. Salem MR, Wong AY, Fizzotti GF. Efficacy of cricoid pressure in preventing aspiration of gastric contents in paediatric patients. Br J Anaesth 1972;44:401.
58. Hupp JR, Peterson LJ. Aspiration pneumonitis: etiology, therapy, and prevention. J Oral Surg 1981;39(6):430–435.
59. Sladen A, Zanca P, Hadnott WH. Aspiration pneumonitis—the sequelae. Chest 1971;59(4):448–450.
60. Codero L Jr, Hon EH. Neonatal bradycardia following nasopharyngeal stimulation. J Ped 1971;78:441.
61. Marshall TA, Keeder R, Pai S, et al. Physiologic changes associated with endotracheal intubation of preterm infants. Crit Care Med 1984;12:501.

EMERGENT ENDOTRACHEAL INTUBATION

Christopher King and Stephen A. Stayer

INTRODUCTION

Few procedures have the same degree of potential impact on the care of a critically ill infant or child as endotracheal intubation. It represents one of the central elements of pediatric resuscitation. Yet the term obviously does not specify a single procedure. It encompasses a variety of techniques that, when successful, lead to the same outcome, i.e., insertion of a tube into the trachea for the purpose of delivering positive pressure ventilation to the lungs. By far the most commonly used approach for this procedure is conventional orotracheal intubation via direct laryngoscopy. Mastery of this technique is essential for any practitioner who provides emergency care to children. Blind nasotracheal intubation is a popular choice in the management of adult respiratory emergencies; however, for a variety of reasons discussed later in this chapter, its use is much more restricted among pediatric patients. Nontraditional intubation methods, such as retrograde intubation and tactile intubation, can be effective when used in appropriate clinical circumstances. In addition, improvements in fiberoptic technology have added lighted stylet intubation and flexible fiberoptic intubation to the options available for pediatric patients. Although the majority of endotracheal intubations are managed routinely with orotracheal intubation, proficiency with one or more of these alternative techniques can prove invaluable when dealing with the more challenging situations.

The focus of this chapter is emergent intubation, which differs in several respects from elective intubation. The most obvious difference is the importance of time as a constraint during an emergent intubation, because the patient's condition may be rapidly deteriorating. Furthermore, the patient must always be assumed to have a full stomach, which significantly increases the risk of vomiting and aspiration of gastric contents into the lungs. Depending on the presentation, sedative and paralytic medications may be contraindicated, adding the movements of a struggling child to the list of potential challenges. Finally, compromise due to trauma or an underlying disease process may make the patient more susceptible to adverse physiologic effects of the procedure. These and other factors combine to increase both the complexity and the potential morbidity of emergent endotracheal intubation.

Although it is a skill that requires considerable technical expertise, pediatric intubation is performed by a diverse group of health professionals, which includes emergency physicians, anesthesiologists, pediatricians, nurse anesthetists, and paramedics. The complexity of this procedure can vary greatly depending on the clinical circumstances. As discussed in Chapter 14, endotracheal intubation can at times prove to be less difficult than properly performed bag-valve-mask (BVM) ventilation. Although the prospect of intubating an apneic child can be a source of anxiety for those who primarily treat adults, certain aspects of pediatric anatomy (e.g., a supple neck, absence of teeth in infants) in fact may pose less of a challenge. However, all of this is not to say that emergent endotracheal intubation of a pediatric patient can ever be approached casually, because a host of potential hazards must be carefully avoided. This procedure is best approached with an appropriate mix of confidence and caution to ensure the greatest likelihood for success.

ANATOMY AND PHYSIOLOGY

The most obvious anatomic difference between the airway of an infant or child as compared with an adult is size. However, differences also are found in the shape, orientation, and relative positions of structures. These anatomic characteristics change progressively from infancy through adolescence as a result of growth and continuing maturation of the head and neck (Fig. 16.1). Proceeding along the airway from the nose and mouth, several unique features of pediatric anatomy can be identified which have clinical importance in performing endotracheal intubation. Adenoid hypertrophy is common among pediatric patients and may contribute to nasal airway obstruction during manual ventilation. Enlarged adenoids also are more likely to be injured when an endotracheal tube is passed through the nasopharynx, even when gentle pressure is used. Tooth eruption typically begins at between 4 and 6 months of age. The emerging teeth of a younger child can potentially be damaged from excessive force applied during direct laryngoscopy. Although infants lack dentition, injury to the alveolar ridge can occur in a similar manner, potentially resulting in abnormalities in subsequent dental development. Primary teeth are shed between 5 and 10 years of age. Accidental dislodgment of one or more primary teeth is not generally harmful to the developing dentition, but an avulsed tooth can be aspirated into the tracheobronchial tree (see Complications).

The tongue of a pediatric patient is large in proportion to the rest of the oral cavity (1). With most adults, the mouth will open wide enough to permit the operator to insert a large laryngoscope blade, making retraction of the tongue less difficult. For infants and children, the combination of a small mouth opening and a relatively large tongue frequently requires using a laryngoscope blade that may not easily displace the tongue. Although an often repeated axiom, the pediatric larynx is not anterior but is actually rostral (superior) when compared with an adult (2). For example, the larynx of an infant is opposite the C3-C4 interspace, while the larynx of an adult is opposite the C4-C5 interspace (Fig. 16.1). This more superior location of the larynx creates difficulty with direct visualization of airway landmarks as a result of the more acute angulation between the base of the tongue and the glottic opening. The vallecula is the space between the base of the tongue and the epiglottis. Anterior traction by a curved blade in the vallecula stretches the hyoepiglottic ligament which retracts the epiglottis from view. The epiglottis of an adult is broad and has a longitudinal axis that is essentially parallel to that of the trachea. The epiglottis of an infant or young child is relatively narrow, omega shaped, and has a more acute angle in relation to the axis of the trachea (Fig. 16.2) (3). This angled orientation causes the epiglottis to cover more of the glottic opening and makes retraction with a laryngoscope blade more difficult.

When considering the anatomical structures involved with direct laryngoscopy, it is useful to conceptualize the airway as forming 3 axes—the oral axis, the pharyngeal axis, and the tracheal axis (Fig. 16.3). Direct visualization of the anatomic landmarks is greatly facilitated by achieving the most favorable alignment possible of these axes. This is best accomplished by placing the child in the so-called sniffing position, i.e., slight anterior displacement of the neck and extension (rotation) of the head. This is said to be the position normally assumed when a person is "sniffing the air." With adolescents, achieving the necessary anterior displacement of the neck often requires placing a pad or small towel roll under the head. Because infants and younger children have a relatively large occiput, the neck is already displaced anteriorly when the patient is lying supine, making such additional measures unnecessary. With these younger patients, extension of the head is generally the only maneuver required to achieve the sniffing position.

The major cartilaginous skeleton of the larynx is formed by the thyroid cartilage anteriorly and by the arytenoid and cricoid car-

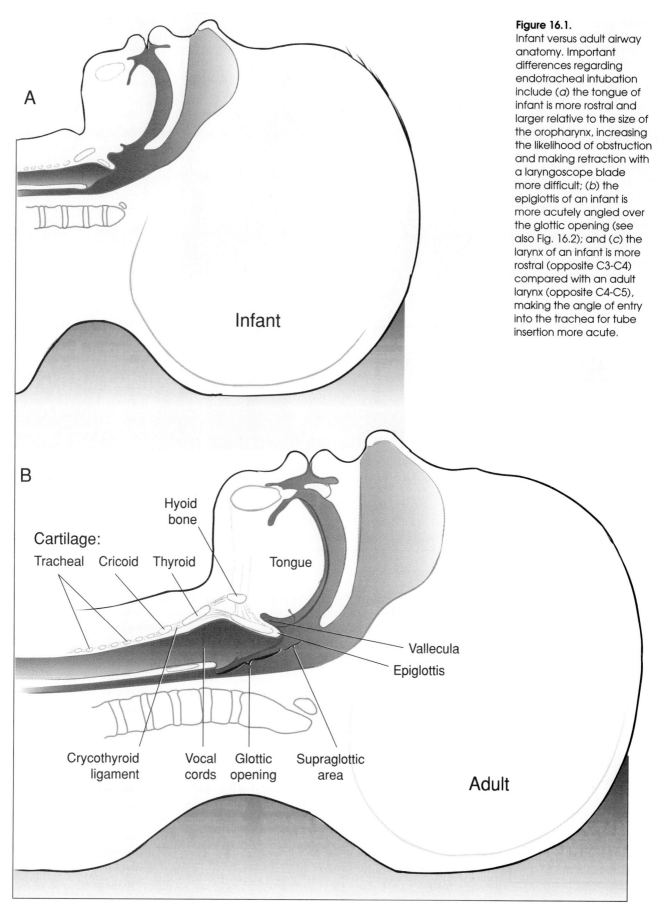

A

Infant

B

Cartilage:
Tracheal   Cricoid   Thyroid

Hyoid
bone

Tongue

Vallecula

Epiglottis

Crycothyroid
ligament

Vocal
cords

Glottic
opening

Supraglottic
area

Adult

Figure 16.1.
Infant versus adult airway anatomy. Important differences regarding endotracheal intubation include (*a*) the tongue of infant is more rostral and larger relative to the size of the oropharynx, increasing the likelihood of obstruction and making retraction with a laryngoscope blade more difficult; (*b*) the epiglottis of an infant is more acutely angled over the glottic opening (see also Fig. 16.2); and (*c*) the larynx of an infant is more rostral (opposite C3-C4) compared with an adult larynx (opposite C4-C5), making the angle of entry into the trachea for tube insertion more acute.

163

Figure 16.2.

The epiglottis of an infant has a greater angle relative to the axis of the trachea, so that it covers more of the glottic opening. The epiglottis of an adult has a more parallel orientation. In addition, an infant's vocal cords have a lower attachment anteriorly than posteriorly, whereas the vocal cords of an adult are perpendicular to the trachea. This "slanted" position of the cords increases the likelihood that an endotracheal tube will be caught in the anterior commissure. (Modified with permission from Cote CJ, Todres ID: The Pediatric Airway. In: Cote CJ, Ryan JF, Todres ID, et al. (eds). A Practice of Anesthesia for Infants and Children. 2nd ed. Philadelphia: WB Saunders, 1993.)

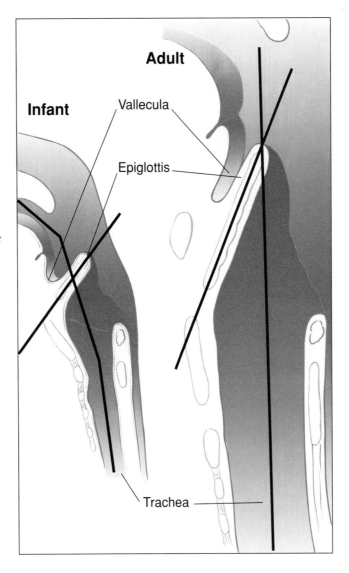

tilages posteriorly. The overall shape of the airway formed by these cartilages is different in infants as compared with adults. Because of an underdeveloped cricoid cartilage, the airway of an infant is shaped like a cone, whereas the airway of an adult has a more cylindrical shape (Fig. 16.4). The arytenoids are the cartilaginous attachments of the true vocal cords. During a difficult laryngoscopy, the arytenoids (which appear white compared with the surrounding tissues) may be the only structures of the larynx visualized. In such cases, the endotracheal tube can be guided into the larynx by directing it along the midline anterior to the arytenoid cartilages and thereby through the glottic opening. An infant's vocal cords have a lower attachment anteriorly than posteriorly, so that the cords slant "away from" the laryngoscopist, whereas the vocal cords of an adult are essentially perpendicular to the trachea (Fig. 16.2) (3). This angled orientation of the cords increases the likelihood that an endotracheal tube will be held up at the anterior commissure during nasal intubation of an infant or younger child.

The trachea of a newborn is 4 to 5 cm in length and grows to 7 cm by around 18 months of age. The adult trachea is approximately 12 cm long (4). Consequently, movement of the endotracheal tube of only 2 cm within the trachea of an infant may result in endobronchial intubation or tracheal extubation. It is therefore crucial to confirm midtracheal placement of the tube and to properly secure the tube so that minimal movement can occur. The narrowest segment of the larynx in an infant or younger child is at the level of the cricoid cartilage, whereas the adult extrathoracic airway is narrowest at the vocal cords (5). An endotracheal tube that passes through the glottis of an adult fits loosely in the trachea, because the airway beyond has a larger diameter. However, an endotracheal tube that passes easily through the vocal cords of a pediatric patient may fit tightly in the subglottic region, possibly leading to injury over time. By approximately 10 to 12 years of age the cricoid and thyroid cartilages have matured sufficiently that both the angulation of the vocal cords and the narrowed subglottic area are no longer present.

After birth, the number of alveoli in the lungs increases rapidly. Approximately 20 million alveolar saccules are present at birth (6), increasing to approximately 300 million alveoli by 8 years of age (7). The alveoli grow in both size and number as the child matures, which in turn increases gas exchanging surface area of the lung. Therefore, the alveolar surface area of an infant is only one-third to one-half that of an adult, even when normalized for body surface. The adult lung also contains small channels that allow ventilation distal to an obstructed bronchus; these pathways are not present in infancy, developing subsequently between the first and second year of life (8). The smaller size of the alveolus and the absence of channels for collateral ventilation combine to increase the risk for development of atelectasis among infants.

Anatomic features of the pediatric cervical spine also may have clinical importance with regard to performing endotracheal intubation, because many patients who require intubation present with head and neck trauma. Factors influencing the incidence and types of cervical spine injuries that characteristically occur among infants and children include (a) the cervical spine of a child is less rigid (more compliant) and therefore more likely to absorb the forces of flexion and extension without a fracture; (b) children have more cartilage relative to bone in the cervical spine than adults, also protecting against fracture; (c) the facet joints at C1 and C2 of a child are more horizontal and the ligaments more lax, leading to a greater incidence of high cervical cord injuries; (d) the relatively large head and short neck of a pediatric patient also contribute to the propensity for high cord injuries; and (e) the presence of an epiphysis at the base of the dens increases the probability of a dens fracture (9). The greater compliance of the cervical spine and lower likelihood of fracture also account in part for the higher incidence of spinal cord injury without radiographic abnormality, an entity that also is commonly referred to by its acronym SCIWORA (10, 11).

To understand pulmonary ventilation and the pathophysiologic processes that lead to respiratory failure in children, it is useful to review the functional subdivisions of the lungs (Fig. 16.5). The relative size of the lung compartments is approximately constant from infancy through adulthood. Total lung capacity (TLC) is the maximum lung volume allowed by the strength of the inspiratory muscles stretching the thorax and lungs. Residual volume (RV) is the amount of air remaining in the lung after maximum expiration and comprises approximately one-fourth of TLC. The functional residual capacity (FRC) is lung volume at the completion of normal, unforced exhalation. FRC is determined by the balance between the outward stretch of the thorax versus the inward recoil of the lung and normally comprises one-half of TLC. As gas is exhaled and lung volumes decrease, the terminal bronchioles are no longer supported by the elastic recoil of the lung and eventually collapse. Lung volume at which this occurs is the closing volume (CV). When CV is reached, alveolar units distal to the collapsed bronchioles do not participate in gas exchange. Lungs of infants and younger children are extremely compliant (i.e., have a low elastic recoil) probably because the elastic fibers are insufficiently developed. This characteristic resembles that of geriatric, emphysematous lungs in which the closing volume is greater than FRC. Consequently, some lung segments will not be ventilated during normal tidal breathing when younger patients lie supine (12, 13). This results in an intrapulmonary shunt which contributes to the rapid desaturation that occurs when ventilation is interrupted.

One of the most important physiologic concepts with regard to airway management of a pediatric patient is Poiseuille's law, which states that the resistance to gas flowing through an airway is inversely proportional to the 4th power of the radius of the airway. In other words, a small decrease in the diameter of an airway results in a large increase in resistance. This can have a profound impact on

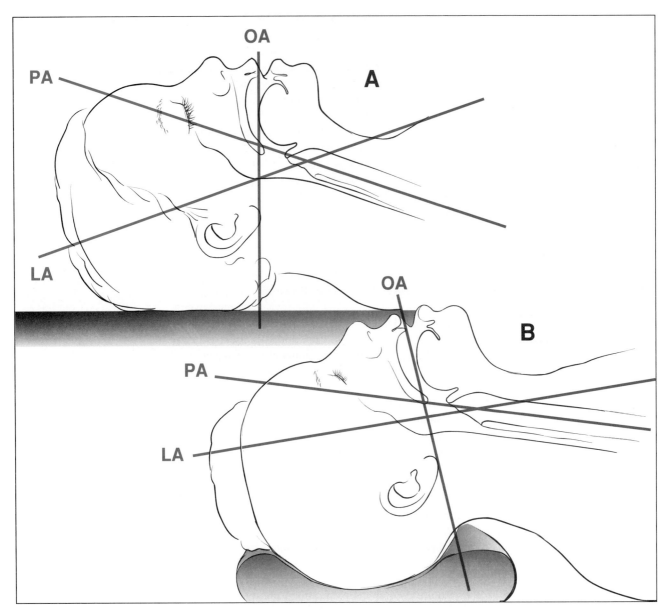

Figure 16.3.
"Sniffing position." The most favorable position for airway patency and insertion of an endotracheal tube is achieved when the oral axis (OA), pharyngeal axis (PA), and laryngeal axis (LA) are optimally aligned. This is the position naturally assumed by a child with airway compromise when sitting upright, because resistance to gas flow is minimized. **A.** When the patient is lying supine on a flat surface, the axes are poorly aligned. **B.** Placing a small pad or towel roll under the head better aligns the pharyngeal and tracheal axes.

the work of breathing. Because the airway of a child is smaller to begin with, a decrease in the internal diameter by a given amount (due to edema, obstruction, etc.) results in a greater increase in resistance for pediatric patients compared with adults (Fig. 16.6). Furthermore, disease processes that lead to narrowing of small airways disproportionately increase the work of breathing in infants and children, which accounts for the greater incidence of lower airway obstructive disease seen in this age group.

In both adults and children, the tracheal and bronchial walls are compliant and thus vary in diameter during the respiratory cycle

(14–16). The degree of variation that occurs is a function of (*a*) the elasticity of the supportive tissues and (*b*) the distending or compressive forces applied. The compliance of the larynx, trachea, and bronchi of an infant or younger child are significantly greater than that of an adult; as a result, the same force applied to an immature airway will produce a much greater variation in diameter. This exaggerated effect has particular clinical importance regarding airway obstruction. During normal inspiration, negative intrathoracic pressure dilates and stretches the intrathoracic airway (17). The extrathoracic trachea is slightly narrowed due to a pressure differ-

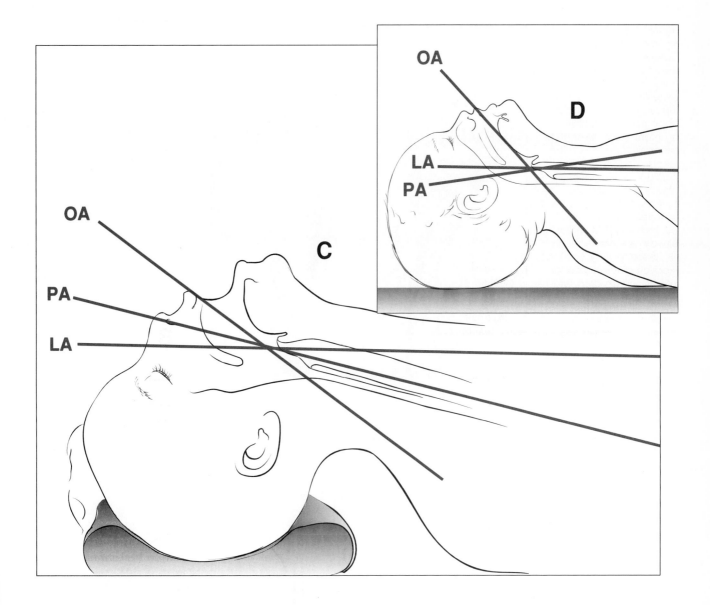

Figure 16.3 (Cont'd)
C. Extension of the neck then aligns all three axes.
D. Because infants have a relatively large occiput making the use of a towel roll unnecessary, extension of the neck is the only maneuver needed to achieve the sniffing position. (Modified with permission from Cote CJ, Todres ID: The Pediatric Airway. In: Cote CJ, Ryan JF, Todres ID, et al. (eds). A Practice of Anesthesia for Infants and Children. 2nd ed. Philadelphia: WB Saunders, 1993.)

ential between the intratracheal and atmospheric pressures. Inspiration against an upper airway obstruction results in the development of a more negative intrathoracic pressure, which dilates the intrathoracic airways and leads to collapse of the extrathoracic trachea proximal to the obstruction (Fig. 16.7). This periodic collapse produces inspiratory stridor (18–23). With a fixed intrathoracic tracheal obstruction (e.g., foreign body or vascular ring), stridor may occur during both inspiration and expiration (24, 25).

Because infants and younger children have a highly compliant chest wall and horizontally positioned ribs, thoracic ventilation is relatively inefficient. These patients therefore rely predominately on diaphragmatic breathing (26, 27). For this reason, increases in abdominal pressure will significantly compromise ventilation, because movement of the diaphragm is impeded. In addition, infants are predisposed to ventilatory muscle fatigue because they have a lower percentage of slow-twitch, fatigue-resistant muscle fibers in the diaphragm (28–30).

Although most physiologic mechanisms for controlling ventilation are functional by 3 to 4 weeks of age, this system remains immature for somewhat longer, particularly in preterm infants. As a result, premature infants exhibit periodic breathing, i.e., pauses of 10 to 15 seconds in the respiratory cycle (31). Apnea is defined as a respiratory pause of longer than 20 seconds; approxi-

Figure 16.4.
Airway cartilages. Compared with an adult, the infant's cricoid cartilage is relatively underdeveloped, so that the airway has a conical appearance. The airway of an infant is narrowest at the cricothyroid ligament. The relatively larger cricoid cartilage of the adult airway gives it a more cylindrical shape. (Modified with permission from Cote CJ, Todres ID: The Pediatric Airway. In: Cote CJ, Ryan JF, Todres ID, et al. (eds). A Practice of Anesthesia for Infants and Children. 2nd ed. Philadelphia: WB Saunders, 1993.)

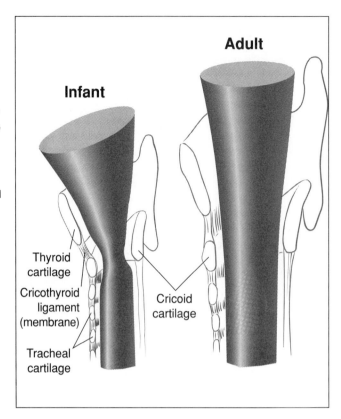

Figure 16.5.
Physiologic subdivisions of the lungs.

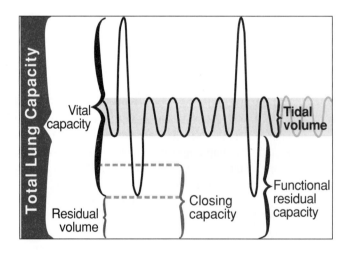

Chapter 16
Emergent
Endotracheal
Intubation

mately 25% of preterm infants will have at least one episode of apnea (32). The ventilatory response of an infant to hypercarbia and hypoxemia also differs from that of an adult. When challenged with increasing CO_2, a neonate will increase minute ventilation, but not to the same degree as an adult (33, 34). The newborn has a biphasic response to hypoxemia; transient hyperventilation is followed by ventilatory depression as oxygen tension decreases (35). Responses to hypercarbia and hypoxemia normally mature in the first few weeks of life, although again abnormal responses may persist longer in the premature infant (36). Poor respiratory control is probably a major factor in the occurrence of sudden infant death syndrome (SIDS), which is the second leading cause of infant loss between ages 3 and 9 months (37, 38).

Respiratory failure may be defined as the inability of the respiratory system to meet the metabolic demands of the body for the uptake of oxygen and CO_2 excretion. Respiratory failure is caused by one of two processes—either failure of the lungs to exchange gas or failure of the respiratory pump to ventilate the lungs. Gas exchange involves conduction of gas through airways, diffusion of gas across the alveoli, and distribution of gas from the pulmonary circulation to the body. Disease processes that affect any of these physiologic mechanisms will impair the gas-exchanging capability of the lungs. In the majority of patients, the primary disturbance is an alteration in the normal ventilation (V) and perfusion (Q) in the lung resulting in hypoxemia. The term "respiratory pump" is used when referring to those structures and mechanisms that control ventilation of the lungs (i.e., the nervous system, respiratory musculature, and

thoracic cage). In response to changes in pCO_2 and pO_2, respiratory centers in the brainstem send a signal via the phrenic and intercostal nerves to the respiratory muscles. The resulting contraction of these muscles causes expansion of the thorax and the development of negative pressure within the pleural space. The pressure gradient produced causes gas flow into the lungs. Exhalation occurs passively through elastic recoil of the lungs and chest wall. Failure of gas exchange,

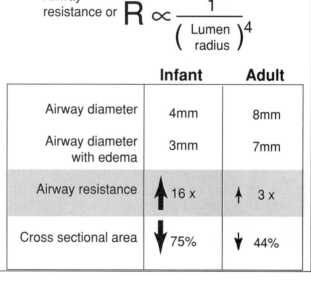

Airway

	Infant	Adult
Airway diameter	4mm	8mm
Airway diameter with edema	3mm	7mm
Airway resistance	16 x	3 x
Cross sectional area	75%	44%

Airway resistance or

$$R \propto \frac{1}{\left(\text{Lumen radius}\right)^4}$$

Figure 16.6.
Effects of airway narrowing. Resistance to gas flow is inversely proportional to the 4th power of the radius of the airway lumen, meaning that small decreases in luminal diameter result in large increases in airway resistance. Because infants and children have smaller airways than adults at comparable levels, the same amount of airway narrowing (e.g., 1 mm) results in a disproportionate increase in resistance for these patients. This problem is compounded by the fact that the immature respiratory musculature of a pediatric patient is less efficient, and therefore more prone to fatigue, than that of an adult. (Modified with permission from Cote CJ, Todres ID: The Pediatric Airway. In: Cote CJ, Ryan JF, Todres ID, et al. (eds). A Practice of Anesthesia for Infants and Children. 2nd ed. Philadelphia: WB Saunders, 1993.)

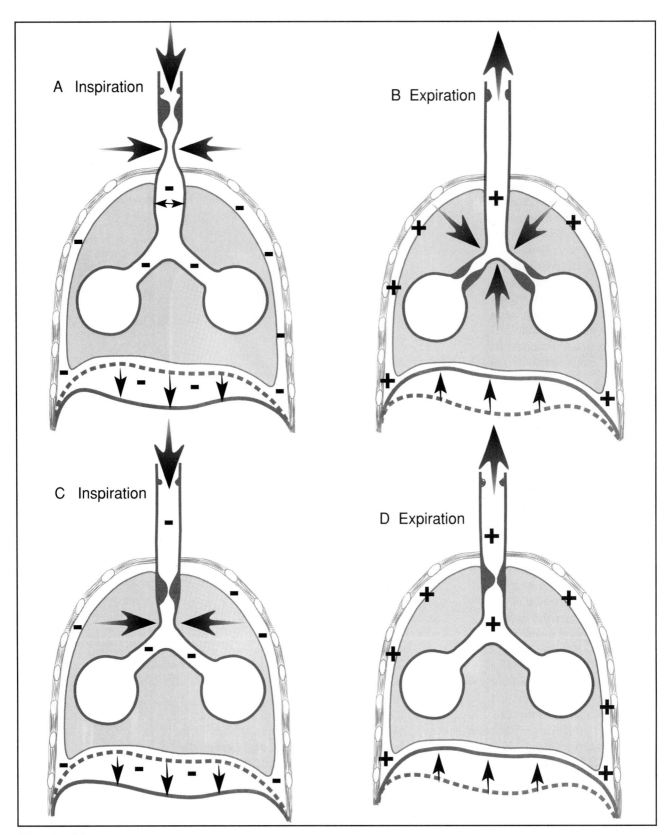

A Inspiration

B Expiration

C Inspiration

D Expiration

through VQ mismatch or intrapulmonary shunting, primarily impairs oxygenation. By contrast, disorders that affect ventilation manifest predominately with hypercarbia as a result of inadequate excretion of CO_2. Mild hypoxia also may be present with ventilatory insufficiency, because increased CO_2 in the alveolus dilutes available O_2.

Physiologic characteristics of the pediatric cardiovascular system also can have important clinical consequences during endotracheal intubation. For example, infants (and particularly neonates) have an exaggerated response to vagotonic stimuli, due primarily to a relative lack of sympathetic development in the heart (39, 40). Consequently, vagal stimulation can sometimes cause profound bradycardia in these patients (41, 42). Furthermore, neonatal lamb studies suggest that immature myocardium has a limited ability to increase stroke volume, and therefore cardiac output primarily depends on heart rate (43, 44). The combination of these two factors accounts for the fact that vagal stimuli have a much greater negative impact on cardiac output in younger patients, potentially resulting in significant hypotension. Laryngoscopy can have a wide range of physiologic effects on the cardiovascular system (Table 16.1). Catecholamine release during laryngoscopy can lead to an increase in heart rate and systemic blood pressure, although this is more common among adults; with pediatric patients, the vagal effects of upper airway instrumentation tend to predominate. Another potential adverse consequence of tracheal intubation relates to the institution of positive pressure ventilation, which may produce hypotension when venous return is diminished as a result of elevated intrathoracic pressure. During spontaneous ventilation, the negative intrathoracic pressure generated favors venous return to the heart. In a hypovolemic patient, a significant fall in cardiac output and blood pressure may occur when spontaneous ventilation is converted to controlled ventilation.

INDICATIONS

Disease processes and clinical situations that serve as indications for emergent endotracheal intubation are so numerous that it would be beyond the scope of this chapter to discuss all possibilities in detail. Instead, an overview of the most clinically important topics is given. Commonly encountered pediatric illnesses and conditions that may require intubation, as well as certain unusual but illustrative indications, are discussed first. Then several of the typical management scenarios involving emergent intubation are reviewed, along with issues regarding the use of specific approaches. Finally, contraindications to this procedure are discussed. Primary indications for emergent endotracheal intubation of the pediatric patient are listed in Table 16.2.

Airway Obstruction

Intubation is often indicated to ensure a patent airway in patients with large airway obstruction. The term "upper airway" is frequently used to describe the large airways; however, borders that delineate the upper airway are somewhat ambiguous. We prefer to define airways by their anatomic boundaries and to divide a large airway based on the

Table 16.1.
Physiologic Effects of Laryngoscopy

Pain
Anxiety
Hypertension
Tachycardia (catecholamine release)
Bradycardia (vagal stimulation)
Hypoxemia
Hypercarbia
Increased intracranial pressure
Increased intraocular pressure

Figure 16.7.
A. With extrathoracic airway obstruction, inspiration results in greatly increased negative intraluminal pressures, causing dynamic collapse of the extrathoracic airway proximal to the obstruction. The patient with this type of obstruction will often have inspiratory stridor. The intrathoracic airways are dilated as a result of the increased pressure generated in the chest during forced inspiration.
B. Processes that cause lower airway obstruction (e.g., asthma, bronchiolitis) produce narrowing of the intrathoracic airways during expiration (wheezing). Although the airways experience positive intraluminal pressures, this is offset by the pressure generated in the chest during forced expiration.
C, D. With a fixed intrathoracic obstruction, airway narrowing is not dependent on forced inspiration, and the patient will often have inspiratory and expiratory stridor.
(Modified with permission from Cote CJ, Todres ID: The Pediatric Airway. In: Cote CJ, Ryan JF, Todres ID, et al. (eds). A Practice of Anesthesia for Infants and Children. 2nd ed. Philadelphia: WB Saunders, 1993.)

Table 16.2.
Indications for Emergent Endotracheal Intubation of Pediatric Patients

Airway Obstruction
  Congenital anomalies
  Acquired airway lesions
    Infection
      Retropharyngeal abscess
      Ludwig's angina
      Peritonsillar abscess
      Laryngotracheal bronchitis (croup)
      Bacterial tracheitis
      Epiglottitis
    Airway trauma
    Burns (chemical or thermal)
    Foreign body aspiration
Respiratory Failure
  Impaired gas exchange
    Obstructive lung disease
      Bronchopulmonary dysplasia
      Bronchiolitis
      Asthma
    Pneumonitis and pneumonia
    Pulmonary edema (cardiogenic and ARDS)
    Thoracic trauma
    Near drowning
  Respiratory pump failure
    Apnea
    Spinal cord trauma
    Neuromuscular diseases
      Tetanus
      Poliomyelitis
      Guillain-Barre syndrome
      Myasthenia gravis
      Botulism
Common Clinical Scenarios
  Cardiopulmonary resuscitation
  Drug administration via endotracheal tube
  Facilitate hypocapnic ventilation
  Decrease intracranial pressure
  Eliminate work of breathing for patient in circulatory failure
  Suction tracheobronchial debris
  Protect lungs from aspiration pneumonitis in patient with absent protective airway reflexes

more physiologic designation of extrathoracic versus intrathoracic airway. The extrathoracic airway extends from the nose through the nasopharynx, oropharynx, and larynx to the thoracic inlet. The intrathoracic airway originates at the thoracic inlet and includes the intrathoracic portion of the trachea extending to the terminal bronchi.

When the airway is partially obstructed, airflow becomes turbulent and noisy respirations or stridor can be heard as gas passes through the narrowed portion of the airway. Observation of the timing of stridor can aid in diagnosing the location of airway obstruction (Fig. 16.7) (45). Inspiratory stridor is common when airway narrowing is located at the supraglottic or glottic airway. Negative pressure generated during inspiration will cause

further narrowing of the extrathoracic airway, increasing the turbulence of gas flow. On exhalation the extrathoracic airway dilates, eliminating turbulent flow and noise. Expiratory stridor is more often noted with airway compression below the level of the thoracic inlet. Both inspiratory and expiratory stridor will be heard with fixed lesions such as subglottic stenosis which do not change airway diameter with respirations (46). Pitch of stridor is also sometimes helpful in localizing obstructive lesions (45), and a coarse, low pitch noise is commonly observed with oropharyngeal or nasopharyngeal airway obstruction. A high pitch is noted with glottic lesions such as vocal cord paralysis. A barking cough is frequently described with subglottic narrowing, as with laryngotracheal bronchitis. With some etiologies of airway obstruction, stridor and respiratory distress may be altered by a change in position. Infants with laryngomalacia or a vascular anomaly compressing the airway frequently show improvement when placed prone with mild extension of the neck. Infants with micrognathia and airway obstruction from the tongue are improved by lying lateral or prone with the neck extended.

The extent of airway obstruction will determine which clinical signs are present. Children with mild obstruction may have stridor only with increased airflow, as with crying. Moderate airway obstruction usually causes retractions, tachypnea, tachycardia, restlessness, and confusion. As airway obstruction progresses, small children will manifest paradoxical chest wall movement—with attempted inspiration against the obstructed airway, the diaphragm distends as the abdomen protrudes, and the compliant chest wall retracts. Cyanosis is a late sign of airway obstruction and necessitates emergency intervention.

Appropriate treatment for the child with airway obstruction is based on diagnosis, rate of progression of symptoms, and initial response to therapy. Presence of fever suggests an infection. Patients with congenital anatomic abnormalities (e.g., vocal cord paralysis, laryngomalacia, vascular ring, congenital subglottic stenosis, laryngeal web, or laryngeal cyst) will usually manifest stridor at birth. The acute onset of stridor in a toddler is more likely caused by foreign body aspiration, croup, or epiglottitis. Children aged 2 to

8 years frequently develop enlarged tonsils and adenoids which may lead to airway obstruction (46).

The compliant cartilaginous airway of a child will exhibit further compromise when a child is crying. The operator must therefore make every effort to calm a child who has airway obstruction to prevent excessive crying. However, it should be emphasized that sedatives or narcotics should not be used for this purpose before securing a definitive airway. Using these drugs can lead to suppression of respiratory drive resulting in hypoventilation or apnea. Parents can be enlisted to distract and comfort the patient (3). The child should be maintained in a comfortable position, humidified oxygen delivered via face mask, and protective airway reflexes maintained until the diagnosis is made. For any child who presents with airway obstruction and severe respiratory distress, emergency preparations should be made to secure the airway. Because routine direct laryngoscopy may be difficult or impossible because of altered anatomy, assistance should be sought from a qualified anesthesiologist or otolaryngologist when available. The course of action should be carefully planned, including the primary approach (usually conventional orotracheal intubation) and one or more backup approaches (e.g., fiberoptic laryngoscopy or retrograde intubation). Preparations also should be made for emergency tracheotomy or cricothyroidotomy if personnel capable of performing these procedures are present. A variety of endotracheal tube sizes should be available in case the initially estimated size does not pass through the narrowed airway. Because a surgical procedure may become necessary in this situation, optimal management of the patient would take place in the operating room, assuming that the child's clinical condition allows sufficient time for transport.

Acquired Airway Lesions
Infection
Patients with retropharyngeal cellulitis or abscess typically present with one or more of the following: a history of preceding upper respiratory infection or sore throat, dysphasia, drooling, stridor, meningismus, and a toxic appearance. This process usually affects younger children. On lateral neck radiograph, a widening of the soft tissues between the air column and cervical vertebrae is evi-dent (46), and an air-fluid level associated with an abscess also may be seen. Caution must be exercised with intubation because the normal anatomy of the larynx may be distorted, and abscess rupture can occur.

Ludwig's angina is an infection of the sublingual, submandibular, and submaxillary spaces. Symptoms are caused by rapidly spreading inflammation resulting in an edematous tongue and induration of the suprahyoid area. The tongue is pushed upward and posteriorly, promoting airway obstruction (46). Presenting signs and symptoms include a remarkably firm, tender anterior neck, difficulty with talking and swallowing, trismus, limited neck mobility, drooling, dyspnea and stridor with significant airway obstruction. The usual source of infection is a dental abscess or caries. Difficulty with intubation should be anticipated.

Acute laryngotracheal bronchitis (croup) usually occurs between the ages 6 months and 3 years. It is characterized by a preceding upper respiratory tract infection, gradual onset of a hoarse, barking cough, stridor, and thin copious secretions (46). Diagnosis is generally made on clinical grounds, but can be confirmed by a funnel-shaped appearance of the glottic and subglottic area on frontal radiograph of the neck. Inhaled racemic epinephrine usually reverses airway obstruction. Indications for establishment of an artificial airway include cyanosis, fatigue, and frequent (more often than every 30 minutes) need for racemic epinephrine. This is best accomplished in the operating room where facilities for bronchoscopy and tracheostomy are readily available (46). Bacterial tracheitis occurs most commonly in infants and toddlers (47). Many patients will initially have croup followed by the acute onset of stridor, fever, hoarseness, dysphasia, and a brassy cough. The child generally appears quite ill. Suctioning through an artificial airway is frequently necessary because of significant obstruction from the purulent tracheal exudate (48).

Acute epiglottitis usually occurs in children between the ages of 2 and 6 years, although any age group may be affected including adults. Patients with epiglottitis typically present with the abrupt onset of fever, sore throat, stridor, and dysphasia, evolving rapidly to involve significant airway obstruction. The child appears anxious and characteristically assumes a "tripod" position, sitting upright braced on the outstretched arms with the head forward in an exaggerated sniffing position. Epiglottitis may be associated with varying degrees of respiratory distress, from mild discomfort to frank respiratory arrest. When the child is clinically stable, diagnosis can be made by lateral neck radiograph revealing an enlarged epiglottis. Direct examination of the airway is avoided because of the child's tenuous respiratory status. Agitation resulting from an examination of the pharynx may exacerbate airway obstruction as the swollen epiglottis is drawn over the laryngeal inlet by more extreme negative inspiratory effort. Similarly, blood drawing and intravenous catheterization generally should not be performed until after the child has a secure airway. The optimal setting for endotracheal intubation in this situation is the operating room, where the child can first receive inhalation induction of general anesthesia. An otolaryngologist also should be present and prepared to perform an emergency tracheotomy (46).

Blunt Trauma

Potential causes of airway obstruction resulting from orofacial trauma include (*a*) foreign body (e.g., dislodged teeth); (*b*) laryngeal or tracheal disruption, or (*c*) external compression of the airway by an enlarging hematoma. Mandibular fractures are commonly associated with trismus, which will impede mouth opening during intubation. Patients may present with hemoptysis, stridor, subcutaneous emphysema, pneumomediastinum, or pneumothorax when an airway injury has occurred (49–53). Restlessness and agitation may be the result of hypoxemia and therefore should not be treated with sedatives or analgesics until after the airway is secured. If the patient is stable, bronchoscopy and fiberoptic laryngoscopy can be used both to evaluate the extent of trauma to the airway and to secure an artificial airway. The patient who is spontaneously breathing, even with evidence of partial airway obstruction, should not be given muscle relaxants before intubation. The lighted stylet can be a useful alternative in this situation when other methods of intubation have failed. The lighted stylet facilitates tracheal intubation without head extension or visualization of the larynx. However, it should not be used when laryngeal trauma is suspected, because the endotracheal tube

may be blindly passed through a traumatic false passage. Evaluation and appropriate management of potential cervical spine injury must always be considered in patients who have significant orofacial trauma.

Burns

Thermal burns in the airway occur from direct flame injury, explosion products, hot gases, or steam. Patients who present with burns of the face or singed facial hair have been exposed to high temperature gas that should be assumed to have caused a respiratory burn. Thermal injury usually affects the nasopharynx and larynx, and infrequently leads to a burn injury below the vocal cords, because the temperature of dry gas decreases rapidly in the extrathoracic airway. Patients who have been exposed to high temperature gases should be observed for evidence of respiratory obstruction or distress (54, 55). If progressive respiratory distress develops, intubation is indicated to clear secretions and carbonaceous sputum, and to bypass an edematous larynx. It is important to have available smaller sized endotracheal tubes than the one estimated for age because of the possibility of airway narrowing as a result of laryngeal and tracheal edema. Fiberoptic bronchoscopy may be useful for removal of debris and evaluation of the airway below the larynx at the time of intubation.

Chemical burns of the airway usually occur in children after ingestion of caustic substances, particularly following emesis and aspiration. The glottis and subglottic regions are most commonly affected, typically exhibiting inflammation, ulceration, and edema. Because the areas of involvement may be discontinuous, any child with a history of caustic ingestion should undergo examination of the larynx. Tracheal intubation is indicated for patients presenting with respiratory distress (46).

Foreign Body Aspiration

Aspiration of a foreign body usually occurs in toddlers from 1 to 3 years of age. Although virtually any small household article may be aspirated (marbles, toys, etc.), the most commonly retrieved object is a peanut. The most likely cause of significant large airway obstruction in a child is a piece of hot dog (56, 57). If the patient is unable to speak or otherwise phonate, complete tracheal obstruction should be presumed, and emergent laryngoscopy is indicated for foreign body removal or possible intubation. A stable patient with partial airway obstruction should not undergo direct laryngoscopy in the emergency department (ED). A foreign body in a mainstem bronchus may produce a ball-valve effect with positive pressure ventilation. An already hyperinflated lung may become further distended, shifting the mediastinum and leading to cardiovascular collapse. Notably, endotracheal intubation may further advance a foreign body causing complete tracheal obstruction. The child with a partial airway obstruction from a foreign body should therefore be given supportive therapy until the object can be removed endoscopically in the operating room. Only when severe dyspnea and cyanosis occur as a result of airway obstruction and respiratory fatigue should immediate laryngoscopy for removal or intubation be attempted in the ED. A complete discussion of the management of airway foreign bodies can be found in Chapter 54.

Respiratory Failure

Respiratory failure is a common indication for endotracheal intubation and mechanical ventilation. As described previously, disease processes that lead to respiratory failure affect either gas exchange in the lungs or the normal function of the respiratory pump (see Anatomy and Physiology). Children with respiratory failure resulting from poor gas exchange demonstrate obvious signs of respiratory distress: tachypnea, nasal flaring, intercostal and suprasternal retractions, and use of accessory muscles of respiration. Arterial blood gases or pulse oximetry will reveal hypoxemia well before the onset of hypercarbia. Persistent hypoxemia causes the patient to be tachypneic and agitated. The decision to intubate is based on the presence of physical findings suggesting excessive work of breathing, hypoxemia that is unresponsive to supplemental oxygen, and the response of the patient to initial therapeutic interventions. By comparison, patients with respiratory pump failure commonly do not appear distressed. Arterial blood gas analysis will reveal CO_2 retention reflecting the degree of ventilatory insufficiency. For these patients, endotracheal intubation should be performed when it

is apparent that ventilatory efforts are inadequate or the clinical condition deteriorates.

Impaired Gas Exchange

Obstructive Lung Disease

Bronchiolitis, asthma, and bronchopulmonary dysplasia (BPD) primarily affect gas flow through the small airways in the lung and are common causes of respiratory failure in children. BPD results from unresolved neonatal lung injury. These children manifest diminished lung compliance as a result of widespread fibrosis and a decreased number of alveolar units. They also have increased small airway resistance which can often be partially corrected with bronchodilators (58, 59). Bronchiolitis is an acute inflammatory disease of the lower respiratory tract resulting in obstruction of small airways. Infants who develop bronchiolitis initially manifest symptoms of an upper respiratory tract infection (cough, sneeze, and rhinorrhea) which progresses to marked respiratory distress characterized by tachypnea, nasal flaring, chest wall retractions, audible wheezing, and irritability. A low-grade fever is typically present, and marked dyspnea interferes with feedings. Lungs are hyperinflated, and auscultation reveals wheezing, prolonged expiration, and rales (60). Asthma is a diffuse obstructive pulmonary disease associated with generalized narrowing of the lower airways from mucosal edema, pulmonary secretions, and constriction of bronchial smooth muscle. Asthma is characterized by airway obstruction that is intermittent and reversible. Patients with status asthmaticus (i.e., asthma that is unresponsive to standard therapy) present with persistent dyspnea, prolonged expiratory wheezing, tachycardia, use of accessory respiratory muscles, and eventually cyanosis. The only absolute indications for emergent intubation of patients with status asthmaticus, bronchiolitis, or respiratory failure from BPD are cardiopulmonary arrest and coma. Aggressive medical management is preferable to endotracheal intubation and mechanical ventilation when feasible, because such patients may be difficult to ventilate and are prone to problems from air trapping (e.g., pneumothorax).

Intubation, however, should be strongly considered whenever the patient has any of

**Table 16.3.
Conditions Predisposing
to a Reduction in
Functional Residual
Capacity**

Supine position
Abdominal distention
Thoracic or abdominal surgery
Atelectasis
Thoracic trauma
Pulmonary edema
ARDS
Near drowning
Diffuse pneumonitis
  Aspiration
  Idiopathic interstitial
  Bacterial
  Viral
  Opportunistic organisms
  Radiation

the following: (*a*) a decreased respiratory effort as a result of progressive exhaustion (61, 62), (*b*) deterioration in mental status (61, 63), (*c*) absence of both breath sounds and wheezing (suggesting minimal gas exchange) (64), (*d*) cyanosis despite receiving 40% oxygen (64), (*e*) hypoxemia with a pO_2 less than 60 while receiving six liters of O_2 per min (64, 65), (*f*) hypercapnia with a pCO_2 over 65 torr and increasing by more than 5 torr per hour (64). Even with successful intubation, patients may develop reflex bronchospasm, which can lead to worsened hypoxemia and cardiac arrest. The patient's blood pressure, cardiac rhythm, and oxygen saturation must be carefully monitored during this procedure.

Diffuse Pneumonitis

Pneumonitis is one of several conditions that can lead to a reduction in FRC causing impaired gas exchange (Table 16.3). These processes result in terminal closure of gas-exchanging units as alveoli collapse (or become fluid filled) producing a large intrapulmonary shunt. Shunting of desaturated blood through the lung causes the patient to manifest significant hypoxemia. Lung compliance also is reduced leading to an increase in the work of breathing. The decision to perform endotracheal intubation in this situation is based on the response to supplemental oxygen therapy and the degree of respiratory compromise. Patients receiving face mask oxygen of 60% or greater who have persistent cyanosis or an oxygen saturation of less than 90% require intubation and positive pressure ventilation. Intubation also should be performed when the patient has an altered mental status or shows signs suggesting excessive work of breathing (e.g., respiratory rate greater than twice normal or accessory respiratory muscle use).

Pneumonitis is characterized by inflammation of the lung parenchyma. It is a common cause of life-threatening lower respiratory disease observed in pediatric patients (66). In most cases the etiology is infectious, although pneumonitis can result from a wide diversity of causes. An initial insult to the lung parenchyma leads to the generation of toxic-free radicals, recruitment of inflammatory cells (primarily neutrophils), and the activation of complement and chemotactic factors (67). The resulting inflammatory response causes widespread pulmonary disease. With a chemical pneumonitis, initial lung injury may be caused by aspiration, inhalation, or ingestion of toxins. Aspiration of gastric contents rarely causes significant pneumonia in the patient with a normal sensorium. However, patients with preexisting central nervous system deficits have an increased incidence of gastroesophageal reflux and may be unable to adequately protect the lungs from soilage due to aspiration. Inhalation of noxious fumes, gases, or soot in smoke can result in chemical injury to the lung parenchyma. Ciliary function in impaired and mucosal edema develops, often leading to a diffuse pneumonitis (68, 69). Bacterial pneumonia is a form of pneumonitis involving a defined area of alveolar consolidation which occurs when the pulmonary defense mechanisms are disrupted. Bacteria then invade the respiratory system from aspiration or hematogenous spread. Patients present with tachypnea, fever, and/or hypoxemia. Viral interstitial pneumonitis is a common cause for hospitalization of young children. Patients typically have a gradual onset of low-grade fever, rhinorrhea, cough, and progressive tachypnea. Although differentiation of bacterial versus viral pneumonia cannot be made solely based on radiographic appearance, viral pneumonia normally reveals peribronchial thickening, patchy involvement of multiple areas of the lung, and areas of hyperinflation adjacent to areas of atelectasis (70). An opportunistic pulmonary infection such as fungal pneumonitis or Pneumocystis carinii pneumonia should be suspected when an immunocompromised host presents with fever, tachypnea, and an infiltrate on chest radiograph.

Pulmonary Edema

Pulmonary edema occurs when extravascular fluid accumulates in the lungs. Cardiogenic (hydrostatic) pulmonary edema occurs due to impaired left ventricular function as a result of congenital or acquired cardiac disease. When hydrostatic pressure in the pulmonary vasculature increases above 18 mm Hg, fluid is forced across the alveolar-capillary membrane. Therapy should be directed toward improving cardiac function with pharmacologic or surgical therapies. Noncardiogenic pulmonary edema or adult respiratory distress syndrome (ARDS) occurs following primary lung injury (pneumonia, hydrocarbon aspiration, smoke inhalation, near drowning) or an insult not directly involving the lungs (shock, trauma, sepsis). In this case, pulmonary edema develops from increased permeability of the alveolar-capillary membrane (71). Patients with pulmonary edema exhibit agitation, tachypnea, and hypoxemia from intrapulmonary shunting of venous blood. Hypoxemia may be particularly profound with patients who have noncardiogenic pulmonary edema. The need for endotracheal intubation is based on the patient's clinical condition and the response to initial therapy for the underlying disease.

Thoracic Trauma

The incidence of acute respiratory failure after chest trauma is approximately 10%, with motor vehicle accidents accounting for the majority of cases (72). Two primary causes of impaired gas exchange in this situation are pulmonary contusion and flail chest. Pulmonary contusion occurs when the lung experiences significant force from blunt trauma to the chest wall. Children are particularly susceptible to this injury because they have increased chest wall compliance and reduced protection from the ribs. Hypoxemia from a reduction in FRC occurs with pulmonary contusion when alveoli collapse and fill with fluid and/or blood. Flail chest is a less common injury among children that results from multiple rib fractures and causes a disruption in chest wall integrity. A free-floating portion of the chest wall (the flail segment) moves paradoxically with respiration (i.e., inward with inspiration and outward with expiration). This paradoxical movement leads to atelectasis and VQ mismatching of the underlying lung parenchyma which often results in significant hypoxemia. Patients with a flail chest frequently have a coexisting pulmonary contusion.

Respiratory Pump Failure

As described previously, the respiratory pump refers to the bellows function of the chest and muscles that move gas through the conducting airways (see Anatomy and Physiology). The pump is primarily controlled in the brainstem through the input of chemoreceptors sensitive to $PaCO_2$, PaO_2, and pH, and through input from the lung regarding airway irritation and stretch applied to the intercostal muscles. The brain, spinal cord, pe-

ripheral nerves, neuromuscular junction, and muscles make up the five anatomic components necessary for normal function of the respiratory pump. Respiratory pump failure may therefore result from muscle weakness or lack of respiratory drive. Endotracheal intubation should be considered whenever a patient manifests the following: (a) frequent episodes of apnea which resolve only with significant stimulation or which are associated with hypoxemia and/or bradycardia; (b) a pCO_2 increasing at greater than 5 torr per hour; (c) arterial pH less than 7.25; and (d) insufficient strength to generate a cough or gag. Inspiratory muscle strength may be evaluated by measuring the maximum negative inspiratory force, or forced vital capacity (FVC). Inspiratory pressure values less than –20 cm H_2O and FVC less than 2 times the predicted tidal volume are associated with severe respiratory compromise and impending respiratory failure (73).

Apnea

As mentioned, apnea is one of the most common forms of respiratory pump failure among pediatric patients. Risk factors include prematurity, cardiac or pulmonary disease, viral respiratory infection, brain injury, gastroesophageal reflux, sepsis, and drug ingestion (Table 16.4). Newborn or premature infants do not display the same increased ventilatory drive from hypoxemia or hypercarbia as adults (33–35), and they commonly develop apnea in response to an increased respiratory load (see Anatomy and Physiology). Viral infections—particularly respiratory syncytial virus—can cause central apnea in infants. Infants with cyanotic congenital heart disease have chronic hypoxemia and do not express the normal increased ventilatory drive in response to lower oxygen tension (74). Patients with underlying chronic pulmonary disease (e.g., bronchopulmonary dysplasia) may have chronic CO_2 retention and an abnormal sensitivity to increasing CO_2 (75). The brain-injured patient most often develops hyperventilation or abnormal respiratory patterns which lower arterial CO_2, such as Cheyne-Stokes respiration, although apnea also commonly occurs with injury to the brainstem. Indications for emergent intubation of these patients include (a) impairment or loss of protective airway reflexes; (b) prolonged seizures; and (c) progression of the

Table 16.4.
Differential Diagnosis of Apnea

	Neonate, Infant	Older Child
Central nervous system	Infection (meningitis, encephalitis)	Infection
	Seizures	Toxin
	Prematurity	Tumor
	Intraventricular hemorrhage	Seizure
	Increased ICP	Increase ICP (trauma, hydrocephalus)
	Congenital anomaly (Arnold Chiari)	Obstructive sleep apnea
	Breath-holding spell	
Upper airway	Laryngospasm (gastroesophageal reflux)	Infection (epiglottitis, croup)
	Infection (croup)	Foreign body
	Congenital anomaly (Down's syndrome)	
Lower airway	Infection (pneumonia, bronchiolitis)	Infection
	Infant botulism	Asthma
	Congenital anomaly	Guillain-Barré syndrome
	Spinal cord injury	
	Flail chest	
Other	Hypocalcemia, hypoglycemia	Arrhythmia
	Anemia	
	Sepsis	
	Arrhythmia	
	Sudden infant death syndrome	

brain injury leading to abrupt onset of hypoventilation or apnea.

Patients with systemic infection have stress-related release of catecholamines, glucagon, and cortisol which contribute to a hypermetabolic state. Normal response to infection is hyperventilation, although overwhelming sepsis usually leads to respiratory depression (76). When a child with sepsis fails to hyperventilate, incipient respiratory failure should be suspected. Temperature has a direct effect on ventilatory drive. Hyperventilation usually accompanies both heat and cold stress, but deep accidental hypothermia can profoundly depress ventilatory drive. Infants are particularly prone to develop apnea in response to hypothermia. Finally, numerous drugs administered therapeutically or ingested accidentally may suppress normal respiratory efforts. These include opioids and other analgesics, benzodiazepines, and barbiturates. When even small doses of these medications are administered to an acutely ill patient, the effects on respiratory drive may cause hypoventilation or apnea.

Spinal Cord Trauma
Respiratory motor deficits are directly related to the level of spinal injury. High cervical cord injuries (C1-C2), which children are especially prone to sustain, result in apnea and early death without respiratory support. Injury to the middle cervical cord (C3-C5) results in loss of diaphragmatic, intercostal, and

abdominal muscle function (77). Accessory muscles of inspiration in the neck and shoulders remain intact, but hypoventilation rapidly develops because these accessory muscles are inadequate to maintain gas exchange. Injury to the spinal cord below the level of C5 may lead to respiratory failure through the development of neurogenic pulmonary edema, but respiratory muscle function is usually adequate to maintain ventilation. Although spinal cord injuries are rare in children, a high index of suspicion should be maintained for all patients with severe head and neck trauma, especially those manifesting coma, flaccidity, hypotension, or hypoventilation. Patients who present with a spinal cord injury and associated decreased level of consciousness, diminished airway reflexes, inability to clear pulmonary or pharyngeal secretions, or frank hypoventilation should be immediately intubated. A complete discussion of the approach to the child with a potentially unstable cervical spine injury who requires emergent intubation is provided later in this chapter.

Neuromuscular Diseases
Several diseases that occur during childhood that may affect the nerves, neuromuscular junction, or the muscles of the respiratory pump include tetanus, poliomyelitis, Guillain-Barré syndrome, myasthenia gravis, botulism, and myopathies involving the skeletal muscles. Tetanus is now rare because of

widespread immunization. Cases of neonatal tetanus, which usually result from contamination and infection of the umbilicus, are still seen occasionally. Laryngospasm and/or spasm of the respiratory muscles may lead to inadequate ventilation (78, 79). Poliomyelitis is caused by an acute viral infection of the CNS which, in severe cases, results in muscle paralysis with associated respiratory failure. In the United States, sporadic cases are seen among immunocompromised patients exposed to live attenuated virus used for active immunization (80). Guillain-Barré syndrome is an acute inflammatory peripheral neuropathy of unknown etiology that affects both adults and children. Patients typically develop progressive muscle weakness which is most severe in the lower extremities. Approximately 20% of children with Guillain-Barré syndrome ultimately develop respiratory failure (81). Myasthenia gravis results from production of antibodies to the acetylcholine receptor leading to dysfunction of signal transmission at the neuromuscular junction. The disease takes several forms in the pediatric population, each with a unique pathogenesis and clinical picture. Weakness is apparent soon after birth with both the congenital and the neonatal forms of myasthenia and develops later in childhood with juvenile myasthenia (82). Botulism is an acute paralytic disorder caused by ingestion of neurotoxin released by *Clostridium botulinum*. The toxin is found in food contaminated with the organism which is processed under anaerobic conditions (83). Patients who ingest the toxin manifest generalized muscle weakness within 36 hours. Infant botulism is a form of the disease unique to children under 9 months of age. The organism is ingested in vivo and colonizes the gastrointestinal tract of the infant leading to a slow release of toxin. These patients most commonly present between 2 and 4 months of age and manifest poor feeding, constipation, lethargy, and generalized hypotonia. In severe cases, these infants may require emergent intubation and mechanical ventilation (84–86). Many peripheral neuromuscular diseases are complicated by respiratory failure, which most commonly develops from upper airway obstruction or aspiration pneumonitis. Muscle weakness results in glossopharyngeal hypotonia with associated airway obstruction that occurs when the tongue obstructs the posterior pharynx.

An impaired ability to swallow oropharyngeal secretions also may give rise to aspiration pneumonitis.

Common Clinical Scenarios

Cardiopulmonary Resuscitation

The most frequent cause of cardiac arrest in pediatric patients is a preceding respiratory arrest. In a review of the causes of cardiac arrest in 119 patients younger than 18 years of age, the most common presentation was SIDS (32%), followed by drowning (22%), other respiratory causes (9%), congenital cardiac problems (4%), cancer (3%), other cardiac causes (3%), drug overdose (3%), and smoke inhalation (2%) (87). Initial attempts to restore oxygenation and ventilation should first be performed with BVM ventilation. If no spontaneous respirations return, the practitioner should proceed with endotracheal intubation. During cardiopulmonary resuscitation, certain medications (atropine, epinephrine, lidocaine, and naloxone) may be delivered via the endotracheal tube and absorbed into the systemic circulation (88).

Airway Protection

Patients with a depressed mental status and absent cough and gag reflexes should undergo endotracheal intubation to prevent aspiration of oropharyngeal secretions and gastric contents. Potential causes for this type of presentation include drug ingestion, trauma, metabolic encephalopathy, or intracranial mass lesion. Intubation is particularly important for such patients if gastric lavage will be performed for a suspected ingestion.

Facilitating Hypocapnic Ventilation

Lowering the $PaCO_2$ will decrease cerebral arterial blood flow and lower intracranial pressure. Patients with head trauma who present with a Glasgow coma score less than 8 should undergo endotracheal intubation to protect the airway and reduce intracranial pressure before performing an imaging study. Using anesthetic agents and muscle relaxants is indicated to avoid the rise in intracranial pressure associated with endotracheal intubation (see Chapter 15). Lowering the $PaCO_2$ or raising the PaO_2 also will decrease pulmonary artery pressure. Patients who have right-to-left shunting from congenital heart disease (tetralogy of Fallot, Eisenmenger complex) may present with severe cyanosis, unresponsive to supplemental oxygen therapy. Emergent tracheal intubation and the institution of hypocapnic ventilation can reverse the shunt and improve oxygenation.

Ventilatory Support During Circulatory Failure

The child with circulatory failure may have compromised oxygen delivery from both poor circulation and respiratory dysfunction. In addition, decreased respiratory pump function may result from diminished respiratory muscle perfusion, acidosis, hypoxia, and electrolyte abnormalities (89). In this situation, endotracheal intubation and mechanical ventilatory support may improve cardiac output and oxygen delivery while decreasing the work of breathing. Cautious use of sedatives and preparation for rapid administration of intravenous fluids should be established before attempting intubation of patients in circulatory failure, because the procedure itself may precipitate hypotension.

Facilitating Tracheobronchial Suctioning

Patients with thick, tenacious secretions due to respiratory infection or mucociliary abnormalities (cystic fibrosis, Kartagener's syndrome) may be unable to adequately clear airway secretions. Such patients will present with respiratory distress and hypoxemia. Tracheal intubation will provide access to the airway below the vocal cords, allowing suctioning with saline lavage and improved pulmonary toilet (see Chapter 81). Neonatal patients delivered in the ED who have thick meconium-stained amniotic fluid should undergo immediate awake endotracheal intubation. Direct suction should be applied to the endotracheal tube as it is removed. If meconium-stained fluid is noted below the vocal cords, repeat endotracheal intubation should be performed to remove as much of this material as possible (see Chapter 39).

Use of Specific Approaches

Initial attempts to establish a patent airway should be via BVM ventilation. Adults are frequently intubated awake, either orally or nasally, when they have an increased risk for complications with the use of anesthetic agents or muscle relaxants. Awake intubations are usually performed after the application of topical anesthesia and administration of a sedative or analgesic. However, even with excellent topical anesthesia and sedation, it is frequently difficult to talk a child through an awake procedure. In children less than 4 to 6 months of age, awake intubation is frequently used to avoid both the risks associated with anesthetic agents and the loss of protective airway reflexes. Rarely does harm come from an attempt at awake intubation, and many authorities recommend this approach for their patients when appropriate. Indications for awake intubation include (a) known anatomic abnormality of the airway, (b) inexperience with pediatric intubation, (c) circulatory instability, and (d) severe hypoxemia. Even a short disruption in ventilation may significantly worsen preexisting hypoxemia, and the hemodynamically unstable patient often will not tolerate the circulatory effects of sedatives or analgesics.

By far the majority of emergent and urgent tracheal intubations in children will be performed via the oral route using direct laryngoscopy. Direct laryngoscopy for nasotracheal intubation requires prolonged laryngoscopy and is therefore not generally recommended in an emergent situation. Blind nasotracheal intubation is rarely successful in patients younger than 8 years of age for several reasons—it requires a substantial degree of patient cooperation, the larynx is in a more superior position, and the vocal cords are angled, resulting in poor alignment of the nasopharyngeal airway and glottic opening. Additionally, children commonly have enlarged adenoids that may be traumatized during passage of a nasotracheal tube, often causing significant bleeding. Consequently, nasal intubation should not be performed for urgent or emergent airway control for young children, although this approach may be considered for older children or adolescents.

Several techniques for tracheal intubation have been developed as alternatives to direct laryngoscopy. Although extremely useful in the appropriate circumstances, these approaches would only rarely be considered as methods of first choice. Included in this category are fiberoptic nasotracheal intubation, lighted stylet intubation, tactile (digital) intubation, and retrograde intubation. All these techniques require ongoing practice to master, and they are only useful when performed or supervised by an experienced operator. Primary indications for alternative intubation approaches are (*a*) the patient has a known unstable cervical spine injury, (*b*) the patient has an airway abnormality resulting from injury or congenital malformation that may significantly interfere with direct laryngoscopy, and (*c*) conventional orotracheal intubation is unsuccessful and the patient cannot be adequately ventilated using a BVM circuit. This last indication would be particularly relevant when the patient is a poor candidate for a surgical airway. In such situations, percutaneous transtracheal ventilation often represents an effective temporizing measure until other airway interventions can be performed (see Chapter 17). In addition, case reports in the literature indicate that insertion of a laryngeal mask airway also may be beneficial in the emergent "cannot intubate, cannot manually ventilate" situation. However, because of the lack of airway protection against aspiration, this application remains controversial at present. As a general rule, the route of intubation used should be the one that the operator has the greatest confidence in performing with the least likelihood of harming the patient, which in most cases will be direct laryngoscopy and orotracheal intubation.

Many practitioners would choose fiberoptic nasotracheal intubation as the preferred method for patients with the following conditions: (*a*) small or ankylosed mandible, (*b*) micrognathia (e.g., Robin sequence), (*c*) a mass lesion on the palate or pharynx, (*d*) a penetrating neck injury without damage to the trachea, or (*e*) patients with limited neck mobility. The primary disadvantage of fiberoptic intubation is that excessive secretions or bleeding can make visualization of the anatomy difficult or impossible. Tactile intubation might well be considered as a primary approach for an otherwise normal infant requiring intubation. Advantages of tactile intubation are that the larynx need not be visualized, no special equipment is required, and it is easily practiced so the operator can maintain the necessary skills. Similarly, retrograde intubation and lighted stylet intubation may be attempted initially when the patient has a known unstable cervical spine injury. Disadvantages to using the lighted stylet, however, also exist. The larynx is not directly visualized, so laryngeal anomalies may be missed. Depth of intubation is not verified at the vocal cord level, increasing the potential for endobronchial intubation. In addition, it may be necessary to dim the room lights and thus visual detection of cyanosis may not be possible. With neonates, the esophagus also may transilluminate brightly, making verification of endotracheal placement unreliable. Above all, it cannot be overemphasized that the most important consideration in using an alternative intubation technique is the individual operator's capabilities and expertise.

Contraindications

No absolute contraindications exist for securing the airway. Because inadequate oxygenation rapidly leads to brain injury and death, control of the airway takes precedence over other considerations in the severely compromised patient. However, one circumstance does exist in which endotracheal intubation should not be the primary method of securing the airway—an unstable patient with blunt or penetrating injury to the larynx should undergo emergency cricothyrotomy or tracheotomy without attempted direct laryngoscopy. When the larynx is fractured or disrupted, an endotracheal tube passed through the vocal cords may dissect into the soft tissues of the neck creating a traumatic false passage. When positive pressure ventilation is then attempted, gas will be forced into the soft tissues, further distorting the anatomic structures of the neck and thereby making attempted tracheotomy difficult or impossible.

In addition, situations occur in which endotracheal intubation should be delayed if possible until additional interventions can be performed or until the patient can be moved to a more controlled setting, such as the operating room or the intensive care unit (Table 16.5). This obviously depends on the degree of respiratory compromise and how rapidly the patient's clinical condition is deteriorating.

A problematic intubation should be anticipated whenever the patient has a prior history of either difficult intubation or episodes

**Table 16.5.
Situations in Which Increased Risk of Complications From Endotracheal Intubation Occur**

Anatomic abnormalities of the airway
Increased risk of aspiration
Unstable cervical spine
Elevated intracranial pressure
Hypovolemia or shock
Open globe injury
Preexisting hypoxemia

of airway obstruction that suggest an anatomic abnormality. Clearly, obtaining a detailed history in this regard may not be possible in the emergent situation. However, a brief physical examination will often reveal findings that may make both manual ventilation and visualization of the larynx difficult (e.g., macroglossia, micrognathia, facial clefts, midface hypoplasia, facial asymmetry, small mouth, or short neck). Limited mobility of the temporomandibular joint or cervical spine also increases the difficulty of visualizing the larynx by direct laryngoscopy. A vast array of congenital anomalies has been associated with potentially difficult intubation. Because this is most relevant for elective intubation, a detailed discussion of these abnormalities is beyond the scope of this chapter. Readers interested in further information on this subject are referred to standard pediatric and anesthesiology texts.

In addition, patients with head and neck trauma may have midfacial instability, airway bleeding, edema, masses, or foreign bodies that distort or obscure normal airway anatomy. The operator should carefully plan the approach to intubation for these patients, ideally having available the items necessary for at least one backup method as well as the standard intubation equipment. If the patient's clinical condition allows, it is generally prudent in these situations to delay intubation until the patient can be transferred to the operating room, because a surgical airway will often be necessary.

Contraindications to awake intubation with a pediatric patient include raised intracranial pressure and an unstable cervical spine. Rise in intracranial pressure associated with laryngoscopy and intubation should be suppressed using anesthetic agents in patients who have suspected head injury (see Chapter 15). In addition, head and neck movement by a struggling patient with an unstable cervical spine can potentially exacerbate a cord injury. Although awake blind nasotracheal intubation has been advocated for this situation, it is not common practice to use this approach for pediatric patients. Not only is this technique difficult to perform successfully with a child lying immobilized in a supine position, but pediatric patients are rarely if ever capable of providing the degree of cooperation required for an atraumatic intubation. When endotracheal intubation is immediately necessary in this situation, many authorities recommend that the clinician (a) immobilize the neck with in-line stabilization, (b) perform a rapid sequence induction, and (c) intubate the patient using the method least likely to produce movement of the neck which the operator is capable of performing. Alternative techniques such as lighted stylet intubation and tactile intubation can often be accomplished with minimal head and neck movement. However, if the clinician is confident only with conventional orotracheal intubation, then this approach should be used. Additional discussion of this subject is provided in the Complications section of this chapter.

In many cases, likelihood of complications as a result of an endotracheal intubation may be minimized if, instead of being performed immediately, the procedure is momentarily delayed until after intravenous access is obtained and medications or other therapy are given. For example, most patients who require emergent intubation are at increased risk for aspiration of gastric contents. When time allows, intravenous administration of the medications used for rapid sequence induction (see Chapter 15) can often significantly diminish this risk. Patients with preexisting hypovolemia or shock should ideally receive a bolus of intravenous fluid before intubation, because positive pressure ventilation can exacerbate hypotension. Endotracheal intubation of a patient with significant head injury should ideally be delayed until medications can be administered which will attenuate the rise in intracranial pressure during laryngoscopy. In addition, because intubation can cause an increase in intraocular pressure, the patient with an open globe injury should receive intravenous lidocaine before the procedure (see also Complications). However, it is important to remember that these are only relative contraindications to immediate intubation. Securing control of the airway is always the first priority, and the operator must not wait until fluids or medications can be administered if the patient is not being adequately oxygenated. Yet when the airway can be appropriately managed on a temporary basis using manual ventilation, such interventions can significantly reduce the incidence of morbidity associated with emergent intubation.

EQUIPMENT

An important goal that must be accomplished before endotracheal intubation is to ensure that all necessary equipment is readily available. Reaching a crucial step only to find that a needed piece of equipment is not at hand can force the operator to abort the procedure and start over from the beginning. In many instances, emergent intubation must be performed with little warning or time to prepare. Therefore, it is highly important that all equipment necessary for intubation be assembled and checked before a patient with respiratory failure arrives in the ED. Preparing a cart that contains all the items needed to intubate any patient from neonate to adult is one method of organizing the necessary materials. One drawer may contain all the endotracheal tubes, ranging in size from 2.5 to cuffed 8.0 mm tubes. Another drawer can be used to hold an array of laryngoscope blades and extra laryngoscope handles. A third drawer may contain useful adjuncts for BVM ventilation and endotracheal intubation, such as Yankauer and flexible suction catheters, stylets of different sizes, oral airways from size 50 to 100 mm, nasopharyngeal airways, tincture of benzoin, and tape. A lockable drawer can hold syringes and medications.

Other such systems can be devised based on the needs of each individual facility. Whatever method is used, adequate stocking with functional equipment should be checked at each shift, and materials must be cleaned and replaced immediately after they are used. A helpful memory aid in going through the mental checklist of equipment needed for an endotracheal intubation is SOAPIM (a variation on the "SOAP" mnemonic)—suction, oxygen, airway equipment, pharmacologic agents, intravenous access, and monitors (Table 16.6).

Suction

A large bore (14 French) flexible suction catheter is preferred when intubating children under 1 year of age. The catheter should be multiorifice and without a control port (i.e., providing continuous suction). These catheters are easily directed in the mouth of an infant and are less cumbersome than a Yankauer style suction device when mouth opening is limited. The vacuum source should always be on full (200 cm H_2O). For older children who consume solid foods, a Yankauer suction device is superior because of its large diameter suction orifice and rigid design, allowing the operator greater ease in removing particulate matter (see also Chapter 13).

Oxygen and Positive Pressure Delivery System

A wall oxygen source with flow meter that permits 10 L/min or greater flow should be used whenever possible. An oxygen tank is less desirable, because there is a risk of emptying the tank. Oxygen delivery systems are further discussed in Chapter 13. Two types of positive pressure resuscitation bags are available—self-inflating or conventional anesthesia systems. Self-inflating bags are used most commonly in the ED because of the simplicity of the apparatus. Primary drawbacks to self-inflating systems are that they generally deliver a lower concentration of oxygen and provide a lack of tactile feedback to the operator. Because the bag reinflates when released, a poor seal with the face mask may go unrecognized. Furthermore, when the bag reinflates room air may be entrained into the system, lowering the inspired oxygen concentration. Disadvantages of anesthesia delivery systems are that they are more difficult for a single person to operate, and they may lead to rebreathing of CO_2. When using such a system, the face mask must have a tight seal

---

Table 16.6.
Equipment Checklist: SOAPIM Mnemonic

Suction. Flexible catheter (for infants and children under 1 year) and/or Yankauer suction device (for older children and adolescents); suction tubing; functioning wall suction set on full (200 cm H_2O).

Oxygen and positive pressure delivery system. Face masks; oxygen tubing; high-flow oxygen source (wall mounted or tank oxygen); resuscitation bags.

Airway equipment. Laryngoscope handles and blades; endotracheal tubes; stylets; nasopharyngeal and oropharyngeal airways; equipment used for alternative approaches (e.g., fiberoptic laryngoscope, lighted stylet, extra-long guide wire for retrograde intubation).

Pharmacologic agents. Sedatives; analgesics; neuromuscular blocking agents; atropine.

Intravenous access. Peripheral and/or central venous catheters; intravenous tubing; intravenous fluids.

Monitors. Cardiac monitor; pulse oximetry; capnography.

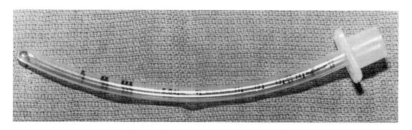

Figure 16.8.
Mallinckrodt® oral endotracheal tube.

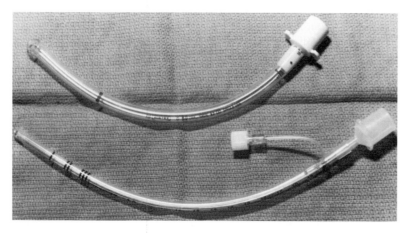

Figure 16.9.
Portex endotracheal tubes may be used for oral or nasal intubation.

Figure 16.10.
Styletted endotracheal tube molded into "hockey stick" configuration.

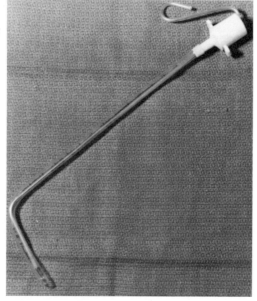

times; otherwise, exhaled CO_2 will be redelivered to the patient by the anesthesia bag (90). A low profile, clear mask with a high volume, low pressure cuff lining should be used during BVM ventilation before intubation. Such masks provide an optimal seal against the child's face, minimize dead space, and allow the operator to see perioral cyanosis or emesis in the mask. A detailed description of positive pressure delivery systems can be found in Chapter 14.

Airway Equipment

Airway equipment includes everything used in manipulating the airway during an intubation (i.e., endotracheal tubes, stylet, laryngoscope, and artificial airways). Any additional items necessary for performing an alternative intubation approach—such as a flexible fiberoptic laryngoscope, a lighted stylet, or equipment used for a retrograde intubation—also would be considered as part of the airway equipment.

Disposable, sterile implant-tested endotracheal tubes are used exclusively in the United States. Most endotracheal tubes designed for pediatric use have length markers starting at the tip to aid the operator in ensuring the proper depth of insertion. A Mallinckrodt® oral tube (Fig. 16.8) is relatively short and therefore cannot be used for nasal intubation. Endotracheal tubes manufactured by Portex® are slightly longer, allowing them to be used as either oral or nasal tubes (Fig. 16.9). Most tubes have single, double, and triple circumferential line markers at the distal tip approximately 1 cm apart. Positioning the double line marking at the glottis usually ensures the proper depth of insertion.

Many experts recommend using a stylet for all conventional orotracheal intubations. The stylet confers stiffness to an otherwise floppy endotracheal tube, allowing the operator to more precisely direct the tube in the confined space of a small airway. Furthermore, the tube and stylet can be molded into a so-called "hockey stick" configuration, so that an acute angle of entry into the trachea is more easily negotiated (Fig. 16.10). If intubation proves to be uncomplicated, the presence of a stylet in the tube does not hinder the procedure in any way, even though it may not

for the bag to refill. If a good seal is not obtained, administering adequate BVM ventilation will be difficult or impossible.

Once the endotracheal tube is in place, using an anesthesia circuit to deliver positive pressure ventilation is less difficult. Oxygen flow into the system must exceed the patient's minute ventilation by at least 2.5 to 3

Table 16.7.
Formulas for Calculating Endotracheal Tube Sizes in Children*

Internal diameter (mm) = [16 + age (yr)]/4
    OR
    = [age (yr)]/4 + 4
    OR
    = [height (cm)]/20

* The internal diameter is also approximately equal to the size of the patient's fifth finger.

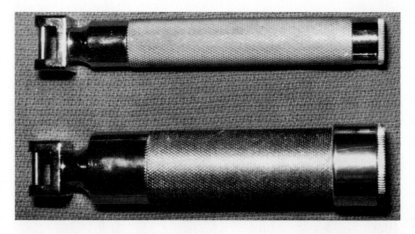

Figure 16.11.
Standard and pediatric laryngoscope handles.

have been needed. However, if the trachea has a particularly superior location and intubation is more difficult, no time will be lost removing the tube and inserting a stylet. To avoid injury to the airway soft tissues, the stylet should not extend beyond the tip of the endotracheal tube. In addition, the stylet should be lubricated with a water soluble jelly so that it can be easily removed after intubation without dislodging the tube.

As mentioned previously, the narrowest portion of the airway in most children younger than 8 years of age is at the cricoid cartilage, which is where the tip of the endotracheal tube will lie. Because the tip fits snugly within the airway at this level, inflating a cuff is unnecessary to achieve an adequate seal. An uncuffed tube is therefore recommended for these patients. Because a cuff adds about 0.5 mm to the outer diameter of an endotracheal tube, using an uncuffed tube also offers the advantage of allowing passage of a larger tube, which reduces airway resistance. If a cuffed tube is used, the cuff should be inflated before intubation and tested to ensure that there is no leak. After a cuffed tube is passed into the trachea, it should be inflated

to a "just seal" pressure, because excessive inflation pressure can result in injury to the subglottic region over time (91). The appropriate cuffed and uncuffed tube sizes can be estimated based on the patient's age (Tables 16.7 and 16.8). Unfortunately, as a result of the normal anatomic variation among pediatric patients, selection of the proper endotracheal tube is never an exact science. For this reason, it is generally advisable to have available at least two additional tubes (one 0.5 mm larger and one 0.5 mm smaller) in case the initial estimation proves incorrect.

Laryngoscope handles of standard length are suitable for pediatric use, although those of smaller diameter are much easier to manipulate and are recommended when available (Fig. 16.11). The operator should always have at least one backup laryngoscope handle available in case the first one fails during the procedure. A straight blade is generally more suitable than a curved blade for infants and young children, because it facilitates lifting the base of the tongue and exposing the glottic opening (see Conventional Orotracheal Intubation later in this chapter). The blade size and type selected depends on the size of the patient and the preference of the laryngoscopist (Table 16.9).

Table 16.8.
Pediatric Endotracheal Tube Sizes

Weight/Age	Internal Diameter (mm)*	Tube Marking at Lips (cm)
Under 1500 g	2.5 uncuffed	wt in kg + 6.0 cm
1500–5000 g	3.0 uncuffed	wt in kg + 6.0 cm
>5000 g–6 mo	3.5 uncuffed	12.0–13.0
6–18 mo	3.5–4.0 uncuffed	13.0–14.0
18 mo–3 yr	4.0–4.5 uncuffed	13.5–14.5
3–5 yr	4.5 uncuffed	14.5–15.5
5–6 yr	5.0 uncuffed	15.5–17.0
6–8 yr	5.5–6.0 uncuffed	17.0–19.0
8–10 yr	5.5–6.0 cuffed	19.0–20.0
10–12 yr	6.0–6.5 cuffed	20.0–21.0
12–14 yr	6.5–7.0 cuffed	21.0–22.0
14–16 yr	7.0–7.5 cuffed	22.0–23.0

* Two additional endotracheal tubes (one-half size larger and smaller) should also be readily available in case the initial estimation proves incorrect.

Table 16.9.
Pediatric Laryngoscope Blade Sizes

Age/Weight	Size (Type)
2.5 kg	0 (straight)
0–3 mo	1.0 (straight)
3 mo–3 yr	1.5 (straight)
3 yr–12 yr	2.0 (straight or curved)*
12 yr–18 yr	3.0 (straight or curved)

* A curved blade may be used for older children, but a straight blade is generally preferred.

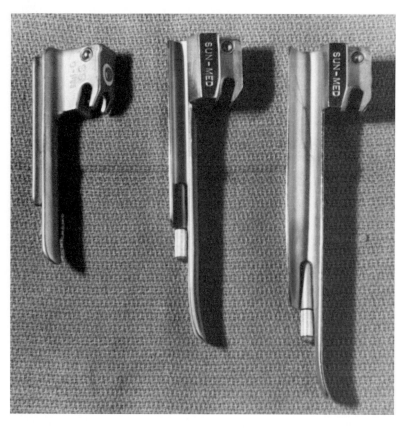

Figure 16.12.
Miller (straight) blades.

Figure 16.13.
Macintosh (curved) blades.

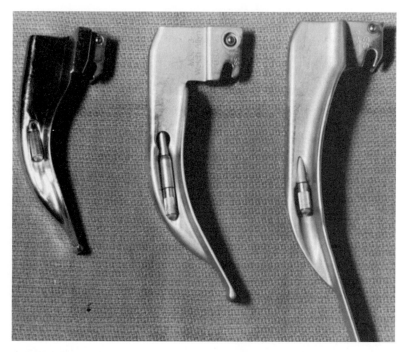

Several differences exist among the various straight laryngoscope blades available. The curved tip of the Miller straight blade (Fig. 16.12) makes it possible to retract the epiglottis indirectly by advancing the tip into the vallecula and applying pressure to the hyoepiglottic ligament. If the patient is an infant, the wider bore of the Wisconsin and Flagg blades generally give the operator a better view and allow easier passage of the endotracheal tube than does the flattened profile of a Miller blade. Children aged 2 to 4 years are commonly intubated with a Wis-Hipple 1.5 blade, which has a light source very near the tip and a low profile. For older children, the Miller blade is preferred since it is less likely to chip large new incisors. As mentioned previously, children older than 8 to 10 years are normally intubated with a cuffed tube. For these patients, a Macintosh (curved) blade (Fig. 16.13) may prove easier to use because it allows more room for passage of the bulky cuff, although many practitioners prefer to use a straight blade for all pediatric patients. Predicting which laryngoscope blade will work best before performing an intubation may not be possible, and therefore it is always advisable to have available an array of blades in various sizes and styles. When testing a laryngoscope blade, the clinician should first ensure that the lightbulb is functional by snapping the blade into the proper position on the handle. An acceptable bulb will produce a high intensity light. A dim, yellow light denotes a failing battery and may not provide adequate illumination of the airway. Newer laryngoscopes have a high intensity, gas-filled bulb housed in the handle rather than on the blade itself. They emit a cool, bright light through a fiberoptic glass filament that extends to the tip, eliminating the problems associated with electrical connections that can occur with traditional laryngoscopes.

An artificial airway is often an effective adjunct to manual ventilation before intubation. As mentioned previously, a child's tongue is relatively large in proportion to the oropharynx and is therefore prone to obstruct the airway. Pharyngeal hypotonia is also a relatively common cause of partial airway obstruction in the pediatric patient. Inserting an oral or nasopharyngeal airway will displace the tongue and airway soft tissues, thereby providing a passage for unobstructed gas exchange (see also Chapter 13).

Certain specialized items of airway equipment are needed to perform the alternative intubation approaches discussed later in this chapter. With advances in fiberoptic technology came the development of flexible fiberoptic laryngoscopes in sizes suitable for use with pediatric patients (Fig. 16.14). Currently, fiberoptic laryngoscopes with a diameter of 2.2 mm are available, a size that can easily accommodate a 3.0 ID endotracheal tube. The primary drawback of these smaller laryngoscopes is the lack of a suction port, which can make visualization of the airway anatomy more difficult. Ancillary equipment used to displace the tongue and maintain BVM ventilation during fiberoptic laryngoscopy also must be available. The features and characteristics of the fiberoptic laryngoscope, as well as proper maintenance procedures, are fully discussed in Chapter 64.

A lighted stylet (light wand) also uses fiberoptic technology, but in this case only the transmission of light and not actual visualization of an image occurs via the fiberoptic strand. The large size of commercially available lighted stylets has previously limited their usefulness for pediatric patients. However, smaller pediatric lighted stylets have recently been developed which will accommodate tracheal tubes with an internal diameter of 3.5 mm or greater (Fig. 16.15). A lighted stylet consists of a handle containing batteries, similar to a standard laryngoscope handle, attached to a stylet which is combined with a fiberoptic element. The fiberoptic strand transmits light to the tip of the stylet. An endotracheal tube is fitted over this stylet so that the tip is positioned just inside the distal end of the tube. We use pediatric fiberoptic lighted stylets manufactured by Anesthesia Medical Specialties, Inc. (Santa Fe Springs, CA) and Aaron Medical Industries (St. Petersburg, FL).

Airway equipment used to perform a retrograde intubation is shown in Table 16.10. The only item in this list not likely to be commonly available in an acute care facility is the extra-long (at least 125 cm), heavy gauge (at least 0.035 mm diameter) guide wire. A wire from a central line kit will not be adequate for this purpose. A suitable extra-long guide wire can be obtained from the angiography suite of most radiology departments or from the cardiac catheterization laboratory. If retrograde intubation is planned as an option for endotracheal intubation, it is recommended to

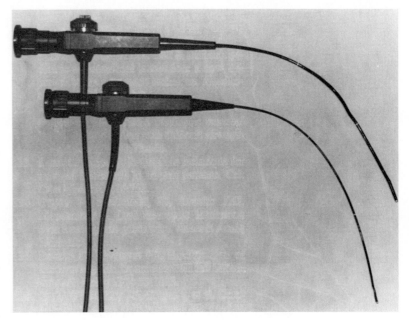

have all the necessary items available in a prepared tray.

Figure 16.14.
Pediatric fiberoptic laryngoscopes.

Pharmacologic Agents

Although drug-free intubation is certainly possible and sometimes even required, physiologic and psychological benefits associated with sedatives, analgesics, and paralytic agents often outweigh their potential disadvantages. However, excellent airway skills are an important prerequisite to using pharmacologic agents during an intubation, because

Figure 16.15.
Pediatric lighted stylets.

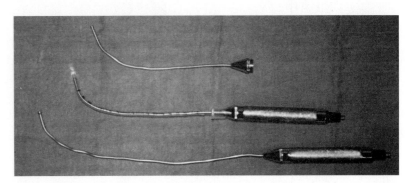

Table 16.10.
Equipment Used for Retrograde Intubation

Extra-long (at least 125 cm), heavy gauge (at least 0.035 mm diameter) guide wire 5 mL syringe
Intravenous catheter (18 gauge or 16 gauge)
Magill forceps
Endotracheal tubes

loss of airway control in this situation invites catastrophe. A thorough discussion of the use of medications to facilitate endotracheal intubation is presented in Chapter 15. An anticholinergic agent such as atropine or glycopyrrolate should generally be administered before intubation of younger pediatric patients, both to reduce oral secretions and to prevent bradycardia. Because of its availability, atropine (0.02 mg/kg, minimum dose 0.1 mg, maximum dose 0.4 mg) is usually the preferred agent. Atropine is safe, inexpensive, and rarely causes adverse effects. Whether this approach is necessary for all children is debatable, but most sources recommend routinely using an anticholinergic agent before intubation for any patient under 1 year of age. With older children and adolescents, pretreatment with atropine can be performed at the discretion of the practitioner.

Intravenous Access

An intravenous line, either central or peripheral, should be inserted before intubation whenever possible (see Chapters 18 and 75). Intravenous access allows the administration of medications and intravenous fluids both to facilitate intubation and to treat the hemodynamic effects of intubation and positive pressure ventilation. Antisialagogues, sedatives, hypnotics, or muscle relaxants can be administered intravenously when indicated. Obviously, if the patient requires immediate intubation as a result of severe airway or ventilatory compromise, establishing intravenous access becomes a secondary priority.

Monitors

Patients who undergo intubation generally have significant cardiovascular or respiratory dysfunction. Furthermore, profound physiologic changes often occur as a direct result of intubation or medications administered during the procedure. For these reasons, patients must be adequately monitored at all times. The minimum necessary monitors for any intubation in the ED include electrocardiogram (Chapter 5), blood pressure monitor, and pulse oximeter (Chapter 77). Capnography should also be used when available, because this modality is the most rapid and reliable method of avoiding inadvertent esophageal intubation (92, 94–96) (Chapter 78). Additional personnel should be enlisted to assess changes in heart rate, blood pressure, and oxygen saturation and to alert the laryngoscopist about the need to resume BVM ventilation.

Importantly the operator must understand the limitations of pulse oximetry to use this modality correctly during endotracheal intubation. The pulse oximeter measures oxygen saturation, not PaO_2. Oxygen saturation is maintained at greater than 90% as the PaO_2 falls from over 500 to approximately 60 along the flat portion of the oxyhemoglobin dissociation curve (Fig. 16.16). This decrease occurs especially rapidly in pediatric patients, because they have a higher metabolic rate and consequently a higher rate of oxygen consumption. Not until the PaO_2 falls below 60 will there be a similarly rapid decrease in oxygen saturation reflected by the pulse oximeter reading. Furthermore, a pulse oximetry transducer applied to the digit of an extremity has a delay of approximately 30 seconds in response time compared to measurements of arterial blood (93). For these reasons, efforts to intubate a patient should be

Figure 16.16. Oxyhemoglobin dissociation curve.

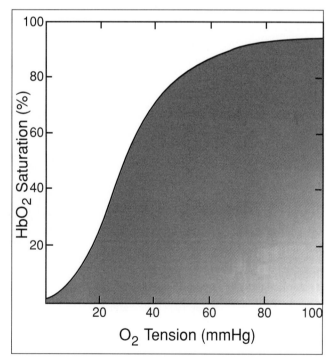

aborted as soon as the oxygen saturation reading reaches 90%, assuming that the patient had a normal saturation at the beginning of the procedure. Even with prompt restoration of ventilation at this point, true arterial saturation will frequently fall below 70%.

PROCEDURE

Overview

As with all technically complex tasks, one of the most important keys to performing a successful endotracheal intubation is to work in an unhurried, methodical manner. Sudden or rushed movements increase the likelihood of injuring the patient and do not generally result in accomplishing intubation more rapidly. The operator should proceed from one stage of the procedure to the next with deliberate and efficient actions. In addition, endotracheal intubation is greatly facilitated by focusing attention solely on the goal at hand and, to the extent possible, ignoring all distractions. Obviously, this can be difficult in the frequently loud and eventful setting of a pediatric resuscitation. Yet the skillful operator often appears virtually oblivious of the noisy surroundings while performing this procedure.

Although sometimes overlooked in the rush of events, the role of an experienced assistant who aids the primary operator can also be extremely important. This person may be a physician, nurse, or other health care professional. A good assistant will make the proper piece of equipment available at precisely the right moment, so that the operator's attention need not be diverted from the patient. The assistant also can perform other necessary maneuvers (e.g., neck extension or flexion, cricoid pressure, retraction of the cheek or lip) at critical points in the procedure. Finally, as mentioned previously, the assistant can make the operator aware of important information, such as rate or rhythm changes on the cardiac monitor, a declining oxygen saturation on the pulse oximeter, or the time interval since initiation of an intubation attempt. Such assistance can be invaluable in ensuring a smooth and successful intubation.

Steps Common to All Approaches

Certain actions performed during an endotracheal intubation are similar regardless of the method selected. Most of these steps will be a routine part of any intubation. More specific maneuvers are described later in the sections on each individual approach.

Monitoring

As discussed previously, monitoring modalities used during an endotracheal intubation will vary depending on the status of the patient and the setting for the procedure (see Equipment). When an intubation is performed outside the hospital (as with prehospital interventions or during an interhospital transport), cardiac monitoring may be the only available method. Patients who undergo emergent intubation in the hospital should have at least cardiac monitoring and pulse oximetry, although pulse oximetry is not likely to be useful initially for patients who arrive in full arrest. Capnography is also gaining widespread availability for emergent intubation. The value of these monitoring techniques is that the operator has continuous, "real time" information about the cardiovascular and respiratory status of the patient during the invasive and potentially compromising maneuvers of intubation.

Although it is certainly important to concentrate on the technical aspects of an endotracheal intubation, the operator should nevertheless maintain ongoing awareness of the monitor readings. Ideally, the team leader will be someone other than the person performing the intubation, so that the primary responsibility for following the monitor readings can be assumed by an individual not directly involved in the procedure. In reality, the person who leads the resuscitation will often be required to perform the intubation as well. When this is the case, the operator can continue to follow the readings while managing the airway by listening to the audible tones produced by the monitors. If pulse oximetry is not available, the heart rate can be used as a crude guide to the oxygenation status of the patient, because infants and children rapidly develop bradycardia as oxygen saturation decreases. When no monitoring modality is available, each intubation attempt should be continued for no longer than 30 to 45 seconds before the patient again receives positive pressure ventilation with a BVM circuit. As mentioned already, an assistant can be enlisted to call out appropriate time intervals during the procedure.

Preoxygenation

One primary factor contributing to the difficulty of an emergent endotracheal intubation is the time limitation. The patient's overall clinical status may be deteriorating to the extent that securing a definitive airway must take place rapidly. In addition, each intubation attempt involves a period of apnea or hypoventilation during which the procedure is performed, and the patient's oxygen saturation often begins to decline within a short period. This is a particular problem with younger patients, because a linear relationship exists between the onset of desaturation and age (97). However, one way to offset this limitation is to "pre-load" the patient with oxygen, which will significantly increase the time available to perform the procedure (98–100). Preoxygenation of the spontaneously breathing patient may be accomplished simply by administering 100% oxygen via face mask for 2 to 3 minutes before attempting intubation. It is essential that a tight mask seal is maintained so that oxygen delivery is optimized. If the child is struggling, one hand may be used to properly position the head while the other hand secures the mask. For the hemodynamically stable patient receiving assisted or controlled ventilation with a BVM circuit, adequate preoxygenation can be achieved by delivering 100% oxygen over approximately 2 minutes (see Chapter 14). For most children, this will provide at least 2 minutes of "safe" apnea during which direct laryngoscopy can be performed (100). When a rapid sequence induction is performed, preoxygenation should take place during spontaneous ventilation whenever possible (i.e., before the paralytic agent is administered) because positive pressure ventilation after paralysis greatly increases the risk of vomiting and aspiration (see Chapter 15). Preoxygenation is less effective for the patient in full arrest, because the benefits are greatly diminished in the low flow state that results with chest compressions. In this situation, intubation should be accomplished as rapidly as possible.

Selecting an Approach

Primary determinants in selecting an approach for endotracheal intubation have been discussed in detail (see Indications). In general, the clinical condition of the patient, the nature of the underlying illness, and the skill of the operator with a given technique should all be considered in making this decision. The need for sedatives or neuromuscular relaxants also will be an important factor in selecting an approach. Clearly, a procedure that the operator does not feel confident in performing should not be the method of choice, regardless of how appropriate it might otherwise be given the clinical situation. Above all, it is important to have a well-formulated plan of action in the event that intubation is initially unsuccessful. In addition to the primary approach selected, the operator must be prepared to perform one or more backup procedures for providing respiratory support should this become necessary. Secondary techniques include temporizing measures such as laryngeal mask airway insertion or percutaneous transtracheal ventilation (see Chapter 17), alternative methods of endotracheal intubation (e.g., retrograde or lighted stylet intubation), and a surgical airway (see Chapter 25). Equipment for these secondary methods should be readily accessible, ideally in a prepackaged kit.

Preparation and Testing of Equipment

Before initiating the procedure, the operator must ensure that all necessary equipment is functional and readily available. It is potentially dangerous to reach a critical step only to find that a piece of equipment does not work properly or is not at hand. The operator should develop a standard routine for gathering the appropriate equipment (such as the SOAPIM mnemonic described previously) and for performing necessary testing. This should be consistently practiced with every intubation. The equipment is logically arranged within easy reach, and medications are drawn up in the appropriate dosages with the syringes labeled. As mentioned previously, estimating the size of the tracheal diameter can sometimes be difficult with pediatric patients, and therefore at least three

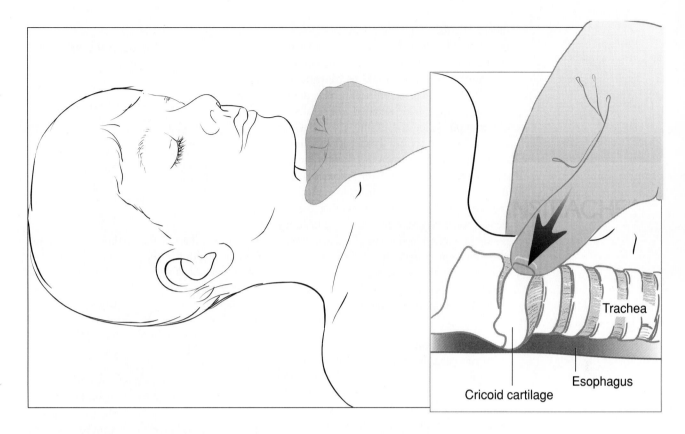

endotracheal tubes should be available—the size that will be used on the initial attempt as well as the next larger and smaller sizes. When an assistant is available, the operator should review specific points during the procedure when that person will be needed to provide a particular piece of equipment. Depending on the method of intubation used, testing the equipment will involve such actions as checking the laryngoscope blade for an adequate light source, inflating the endotracheal tube cuff to identify a possible air leak, assessing the quality of the image obtained with a fiberoptic laryngoscope, etc. Further information about testing individual pieces of equipment can be found in the Equipment section and in the sections on specific intubation approaches.

Gastric Tube Insertion and Cricoid Pressure

Regurgitation and aspiration of gastric contents during endotracheal intubation can result in pneumonitis and pulmonary edema (see Complications). Inserting a gastric tube and using cricoid pressure are two measures that may reduce the incidence of these complications. Primary factors that lead to aspiration pneumonitis are the presence of undigested food and gastric acid in the stomach,

lack of protective airway reflexes, and elevated intragastric pressure as a result of air swallowing and/or forced entry of gases into the stomach during manual ventilation (101, 102). When appropriate, insertion of a gastric tube before endotracheal intubation allows evacuation of stomach contents thereby reducing intragastric pressure (see also Chapter 86). Gastric tube placement should only be performed when the patient has an intact gag reflex, or after the airway is protected, because inserting the tube may itself induce vomiting.

Cricoid pressure (Sellick's maneuver) is a simple technique that can be highly beneficial both before and during an intubation. Before the procedure, cricoid pressure limits the amount of gas entering the stomach during BVM ventilation (103–105). During an intubation, cricoid pressure prevents reflux of gastric contents into the oropharynx (106, 107), reducing the likelihood of aspiration pneumonitis and facilitating intubation approaches which involve direct visualization of the larynx. The maneuver is performed by placing the thumb and index finger over the superior cricoid cartilage and applying downward pressure (Fig. 16.17). The stiff rings of cartilage maintain patency of the tracheal lumen while the more compliant esophagus is occluded. For older children and adolescents, firm pressure may be necessary to collapse the esophagus, but it should be remembered that with infants, even relatively gentle cricoid pressure may actually induce airway obstruction. Cricoid pressure also provides an effective method for displacing the glottic opening posteriorly when the view of the trachea appears to be anterior (superior). Although generally a safe maneuver, cricoid pressure should not be continued if the patient is forcefully vomiting, because this may result in excessive pressure in the stomach and esophagus potentially leading to rupture. Furthermore, excessive pressure may distort the airway, increasing the difficulty of visualizing the larynx or passing the endotracheal tube.

Confirming Proper Tube Position

After inserting the endotracheal tube, the operator must first ensure that the tip lies within the trachea. The traditional method for making this assessment is to auscultate the chest while positive pressure ventilation is delivered. The operator listens first over both lungs (in the axilla) to confirm that equal breath sounds are heard and then over the stomach for signs of air entry. Unequal breath sounds in the lungs indicate an endobronchial intubation, whereas transmitted sounds over the abdomen suggest that the tube is in the esophagus. Unfortunately, the small size of a pediatric thorax can make auscultation for this purpose difficult to interpret. Breath sounds may be heard equally well on both sides of the chest as well as over the abdomen. A more reliable method for assessing tube position is using capnography (94–96), because a high concentration of CO_2 in the exhaled gases confirms tracheal placement (see Chapter 78). Colorimetric devices indicate the presence of CO_2 with a change in color; if no color change is seen, the endotracheal tube is in the esophagus. Handheld infrared capnography units also are now avail-

Table 16.11.
Signs Indicating Tube Placement in the Trachea

Most reliable
  Capnography
  Direct visualization of tube insertion through vocal cords
Less reliable
  Equal breath sounds in both lungs
  No breath sounds over stomach
  Symmetric rise of chest wall
  ''Fogging'' of endotracheal tube with expiration
  No gastric distension
  Consistently high oxygen saturation by pulse oximetry

able. Regardless of the method used to confirm the position of the endotracheal tube, the importance of this step cannot be overstated, because an unrecognized esophageal intubation is associated with significant potential morbidity or mortality. Additional findings that may be useful in distinguishing tracheal versus esophageal intubation are listed in Table 16.11.

The operator must next position the tube at the proper depth of insertion within the trachea. The ideal location for the tip of the endotracheal tube is at the midpoint between the thoracic inlet and the carina. If the tip is too high (rostral) it may become dislodged from the trachea with any movement of the patient. If the tip is too low (caudal) it increases risk of endobronchial intubation with changes in head position. For infants and young children, proper position will normally be 1 to 2 cm above the carina. For children over the age of 5 to 6 years, this distance may be increased to 3 cm (108). With adults, positioning the endotracheal tube correctly can generally be ensured by placing a given external demarcation on the tube at the incisors. Unfortunately, no such single measurement applies to the various sizes of infants and children. Age- and weight-dependent formulas have been devised for this purpose, but these can be difficult to recall or calculate during a resuscitation. One favored method is shown in Figure 16.18. After the endotracheal tube

Figure 16.18.
Confirming proper depth of tube insertion.
A. While auscultating the left chest, the operator advances the endotracheal tube until breath sounds are diminished or absent (right mainstem intubation).
B. The tube is then withdrawn until breath sounds are first heard again normally on the left, indicating the tip is just proximal to the carina.
C. The tube is then withdrawn an additional 1 to 3 cm (depending on the age and size of the patient) to achieve proper midtracheal positioning of the tip.

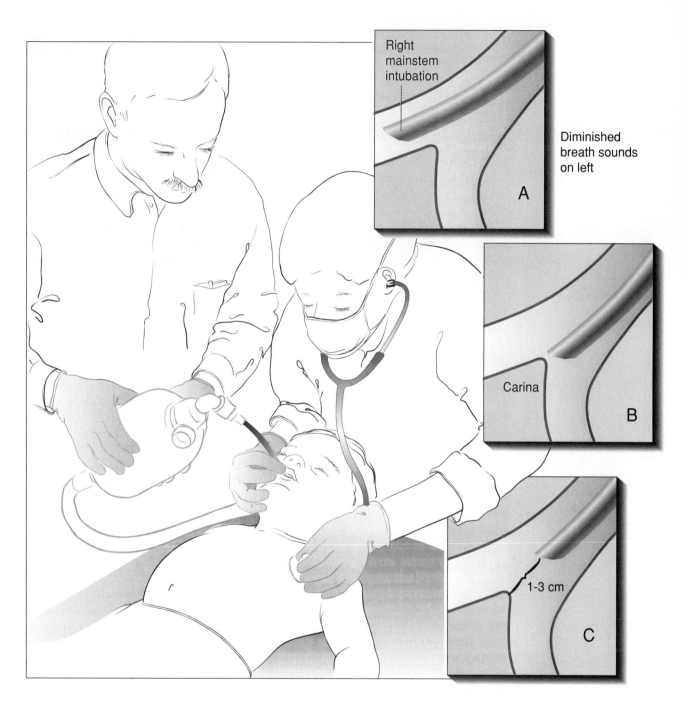

Right mainstem intubation

Diminished breath sounds on left

A

Carina

B

1-3 cm

C

is inserted into the trachea, the operator first confirms that equal breath sounds are heard on both sides of the chest as positive pressure ventilation is delivered. While listening continuously with the stethoscope to the left chest at the axilla, the operator then advances the tube until a decrease in the breath sounds is heard (right endobronchial intubation). Because the breath sounds are so well transmitted in the chest of a child, it is not necessary to advance the tube until breath sounds disappear entirely, as this usually indicates that the

tube has passed several branches in the airway. At this point, the tube is slowly withdrawn to the point that breath sounds are first well heard again on the left, indicating that the tip is at the level of the carina. Finally, the operator withdraws the tube an additional 1 to 3 cm, so that the tip is located at the midtracheal position. Aside from being relatively simple to perform, primary advantages of this method are that it is applicable to any age group, it provides consistently reliable results, and it does not involve memorized for-

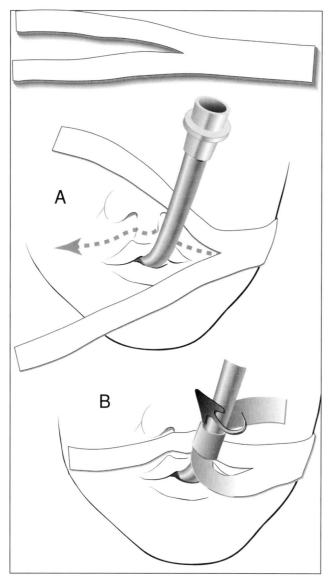

the bag with sufficient force to produce chest excursions similar to normal spontaneous respirations. Consistently inadequate tidal volumes will result in retention of CO_2, whereas excessive tidal volumes can cause a pneumothorax. Occasionally, the size of the endotracheal tube necessary for the patient is significantly underestimated, resulting in an excessive air leak around the tube during positive pressure ventilation. So much air may escape that delivering an adequate tidal volume is impossible. If this is the case, it will be necessary to remove the endotracheal tube and replace it with a larger size. Once the operator has established that the endotracheal tube is in the correct position and positive pressure ventilation can be properly administered, mechanical ventilation can then be safely initiated (see Chapter 84).

Securing the Tube

The final step of an intubation is to secure the endotracheal tube in such a way that it will not be accidentally dislodged from the trachea or further advanced into a mainstem bronchus. Before securing the tube, the operator should note mentally (and later document in the chart) the external centimeter marking on the tube that corresponds with the level of the central incisors or alveolar ridge. This should then be rechecked after the tube is secured to ensure that it has not been inadvertently advanced or withdrawn.

The most common method for securing an endotracheal tube is with standard adhesive tape as shown in Figure 16.19. Applying tincture of benzoin to the face and tube before taping enhances adhesion. It is important to remember that with patients who are not paralyzed, securing the tube may also involve appropriately restraining the hands. For increased stability (e.g., before transport), the tape may be extended around the back of the patient's head, and then the tube is taped on both sides. Tracheotomy tapes may be used in a similar manner. Synthetic straps using this same principle, which have attachment devices that hold the tube in place rather than adhesive, also are available commercially. The primary advantage of these methods is that the need for frequent retaping is eliminated, because there is no problem with decreased adhesion as a result of traction and contact with saliva. The disadvantage of tracheotomy tapes is that they must be tied

Figure 16.19.
Securing the endotracheal tube.
A. The tape is split into a *Y* and the base is applied to the cheek.
B. One strip of tape is then applied to the skin above or below the lips while the other secures the tube. A second piece of tape may be applied from the other side in a similar manner for greater stability. Tincture of benzoin also may be used to increase adhesion.

Chapter 16
Emergent
Endotracheal
Intubation

mulas (108). Definitive confirmation of proper tube position should always be obtained with a chest radiograph.

Positive Pressure Ventilation

Immediately after intubation, the patient should receive positive pressure ventilation delivered using a resuscitation bag attached to the endotracheal tube. A thorough description of the various features of self-inflating bags and conventional anesthesia circuits is given in Chapter 14. The patient should always initially receive the highest concentration of oxygen the circuit is capable of administering; this can later be adjusted as appropriate. Because the exact tidal volume delivered with a resuscitation bag cannot be easily measured, the operator should squeeze

tightly to limit movement of the tube to less than 1 cm. This can lead to pressure necrosis of the skin under the ties over time. Placing gauze padding under the ties reduces the likelihood of this complication.

Conventional Orotracheal Intubation

As discussed previously, this is by far the most commonly used method for emergent pediatric intubation. Practitioners who must care for critically ill children should be thoroughly familiar and skillful with this procedure. Gaining facility with the alternative approaches to be described later is a secondary priority after achieving mastery with conventional orotracheal intubation.

Positioning

While standing above the head of the bed, the operator places the patient in the sniffing position (Fig. 16.3). As described previously, this position results in the most favorable alignment of the pharyngeal and laryngeal axes for airway patency (see Anatomy and Physiology). The neck is extended by placing the palm of the right hand on the patient's forehead (with the fingers on the patient's scalp) and applying pressure posteriorly (Fig. 16.20). This maneuver also causes the patient's mouth to open, allowing insertion of the laryngoscope blade. It should be empha-

Figure 16.20.
Positioning the head and neck for insertion of the laryngoscope blade. Posterior pressure on the forehead extends the neck and usually causes the mouth to open.

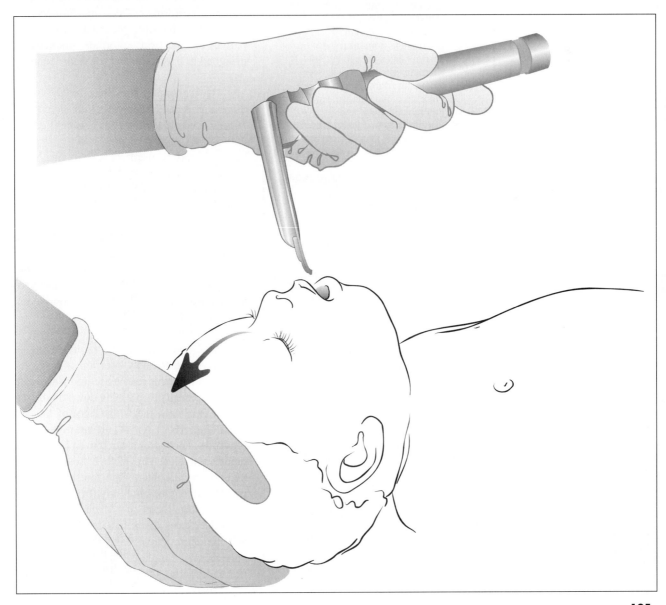

sized that excessive neck extension must be avoided with any patient who may have an unstable cervical spine injury. If conventional orotracheal intubation is the approach selected in this situation, in-line stabilization should be performed and movement of the neck must be minimized.

Direct Laryngoscopy

Perhaps the most important aspect of orotracheal intubation is obtaining an adequate view of the airway anatomy during direct laryngoscopy. Once this is accomplished, insertion of the endotracheal tube is relatively straightforward. As with any complex task, the likelihood of success with laryngoscopy is increased when a given series of actions is systematically reproduced each time the procedure is performed. If this standardized approach fails, the operator must then be prepared to perform alternate maneuvers designed to overcome any problems encountered.

The techniques for direct laryngoscopy differ significantly depending on the type of laryngoscope blade used (i.e., straight versus curved). As discussed previously, a straight blade should be used for infants and most children. A curved blade may be used for some older children and adolescents, although the method preferred by many is to use a straight blade for all pediatric patients. The handle of the laryngoscope is held in the left hand as shown in Figure 16.21, leaving the right hand free to position the patient and to insert the endotracheal tube. All laryngoscopes, except specially ordered equipment, are designed to be held in the left hand, regardless of whether the operator is right- or left-hand dominant. If the mouth must be opened further to allow insertion of the laryngoscope blade, this can be accomplished with younger patients by pressing down on the patient's chin with the fifth finger of the left hand (Fig. 16.21.A). When neuromuscular blockade is not administered to a child with a tendency to clench the teeth, a "scissor" technique using the thumb and forefinger of the right hand may be necessary (Fig. 16.21.B).

The large flange of a Macintosh (curved) blade facilitates displacement of the tongue, and the curve allows easy insertion into the vallecula. A straight blade has the advantage of not retracting the larynx into a more anterior (angulated) position, as well as allowing the operator to directly lift the epiglottis to expose the glottic opening. Although direct laryngoscopy with a straight blade additionally requires maneuvers not necessary with a curved blade, the ability to retract the epiglottis and thus provide a better view of the larynx offsets this difficulty. Traditionally, the novice practitioner is taught to insert a straight laryngoscope blade into the patient's mouth from the right side and "sweep" the tongue to the left (Fig. 16.22). However, inserting a straight blade just to the right of the midline is equally effective and generally a simpler technique. When inserting the blade, the operator must always make certain that the patient's lower lip is not caught against the teeth to avoid causing a laceration. An assistant can be enlisted to retract the lip if necessary.

As described previously, the operator should use the largest straight blade that will readily fit into the patient's mouth. A common mistake made with pediatric intubations is to select a blade that is inappropriately small for the patient, making adequate retraction of the tongue and soft tissues difficult or impossible. After the laryngoscope blade has been inserted into the vallecula the handle is then pulled upward at an angle of approximately 45° relative to the patient (Fig. 16.21.C). The operator must take care to avoid levering the laryngoscope blade on the maxillary teeth or alveolar ridge, as this may result in tooth avulsion or gingival injury. Moreover, even though levering the blade may sometimes marginally improve the view of the larynx, the patient's mouth opening will be compromised, making it more difficult to pass the endotracheal tube. These problems are best avoided by always pulling along the axis of the handle and minimizing any rotation of the wrist.

Once the tongue and soft tissues are retracted, the important structures of the extrathoracic airway must be identified. When using a straight blade, the next step is to elevate the epiglottis so that the glottic opening can be visualized. This can be accomplished using one of two methods. The technique used most commonly is to insert the tip of the blade below (or posterior to) the epiglottis and then lifting it directly (Fig. 16.21.D). Because the epiglottis is relatively large and floppy, and airway secretions make it prone

to slip off the blade, this is generally the most difficult aspect of direct laryngoscopy with a straight blade. A superior approach is to make one attempt to elevate the epiglottis by advancing the tip of the blade into the vallecula and lifting upward, much in the same way that a curved blade is used (see next paragraph). In addition to being easier to perform, this method has the advantage of minimizing trauma to the epiglottis, which is not directly instrumented. Unfortunately, the operator will not always obtain an adequate view of the glottic opening, because the relatively large floppy epiglottis of a child may not be sufficiently retracted. In such cases, the standard method of lifting the epiglottis with the tip of the blade is then performed.

As mentioned previously, a curved laryngoscope blade is inserted in the mouth just to the right of the midline following the contour of the tongue. The blade is advanced under direct visualization down the base of the tongue into the vallecula (Fig. 16.23). Estimating the proper size of a curved blade to be used for a pediatric patient is crucial to successful laryngoscopy. If the laryngoscope blade is too large, the tip will force the epiglottis down obscuring the glottic opening; if the blade is too small, the tongue and epiglottis may not be adequately retracted. Once the laryngoscope blade is inserted, the operator pulls upward on the handle at a 45° angle relative to the patient to retract the tongue. This is done in exactly the same manner performed when using a straight blade. However, in this case upward tension on the hyoepiglottic ligament displaces the epiglottis so that the glottic opening can be visualized. The additional step of directly lifting the epiglottis with the tip of the blade is unnecessary. Although this method is almost always effective for older adolescents and adults, the large epiglottis and lax airway soft tissues of infants and children frequently make it impossible to adequately elevate the epiglottis using a curved blade. Even when proper technique is used, the operator will often pull upward on the laryngoscope handle only to find the epiglottis completely covering the glottic opening. For this reason, attempting direct laryngoscopy using a curved blade is not recommended for younger patients.

Anatomic landmarks to be identified during direct laryngoscopy are shown in Figure 16.24. The epiglottis is a flat, elongated structure with an anterior attachment that drapes over the glottis like a hood. It appears omega shaped in infants and younger children. Perhaps the most easily recognizable landmarks are the arytenoid cartilages, which are white structures on either side of, and posterior to, the glottic opening. In some cases, the arytenoids may not be visible until the epiglottis is retracted. The vocal cords are upright, slightly tilted structures that are separated by the dark midline space of the glottis. They can often be seen to move rhythmically with respirations if the patient is breathing. The most posterior structure seen during direct laryngoscopy is the esophagus. Although the esophagus is sometimes confused with the glottic opening, certain features make it distinguishable. The margins of the glottic opening appear sharp and well defined, whereas the margin of the esophagus has a ridged or puckered appearance. The glottic opening also is surrounded by the characteristic geometric shapes of cartilaginous structures, whereas the area immediately adjacent to the esophagus is homogenous.

For the patient with a potentially unstable cervical spine injury who undergoes conventional orotracheal intubation, performing direct laryngoscopy requires certain modifications. For one, in-line stabilization of the neck should always be provided by assistants (Fig. 16.25) (109–111). Because it may impede displacement of the chin and mandible, the front piece of the cervical collar is normally removed (or a one-piece collar is opened) before direct laryngoscopy and then subsequently replaced. In-line stabilization should be performed during this entire time, both to prevent any voluntary movements by an awake patient and to limit movement of the neck during direct laryngoscopy. To perform in-line stabilization, the assistant places his or her hands firmly on either side of the patient's head and maintains the neck in a neutral position. To avoid interfering with the actions of the laryngoscopist, the assistant should kneel until his or her head is at or below the level of the patient. This technique must be explicitly distinguished from in-line traction, which involves pulling back on the patient's head along the axis of the body. Although previously recommended by many sources, in-line traction has been shown in cadaver models to increase subluxation of an unstable cervical spine and should not be performed (110). A second assistant should hold the patient's shoulders down against the stretcher to prevent movement of the upper torso (see also Fig. 23.7, p. 338). As mentioned previously, another modification is that the operator must attempt to perform direct laryngoscopy causing as little movement of the patient's head and neck as possible. Maneuvers that involve significant flexion or extension of the neck, although sometimes necessary during a standard intubation, should be avoided when the patient has a potentially unstable cervical spine. Such maneuvers could only be considered if immediate intubation is necessary to save the patient's life and no other airway intervention can be performed. In most cases, adequate oxygenation and ventilation can be achieved temporarily using a BVM circuit until an alternative method of securing the airway is possible.

A number of potential obstacles may be encountered during direct laryngoscopy that can limit the view of the larynx. Some of the more common problems include the presence of vomitus or secretions in the hypopharynx, difficulty in retracting the tongue and epiglottis, and anatomic variations or abnormalities.

Figure 16.21.
Direct laryngoscopy using a straight blade.
A. The head is positioned with the right hand and the mouth is opened using the fifth finger of the left hand (if necessary).
B. Alternatively, the mouth may be opened with the thumb and index finger of the right hand using a "scissor" technique.
C. The laryngoscope blade is inserted under direct vision over the tongue and into the vallecula. One attempt may be made at this point to elevate the epiglottis by lifting upward on the laryngoscope handle at a 45° angle.
D. If unsuccessful, the tip of the blade is used to directly retract the epiglottis, revealing the vocal cords and glottic opening.

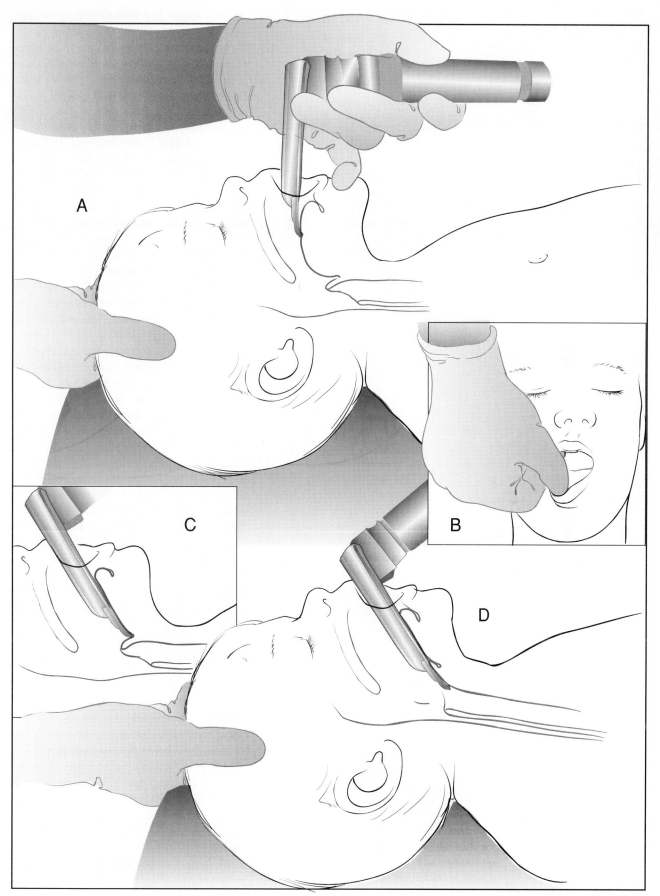

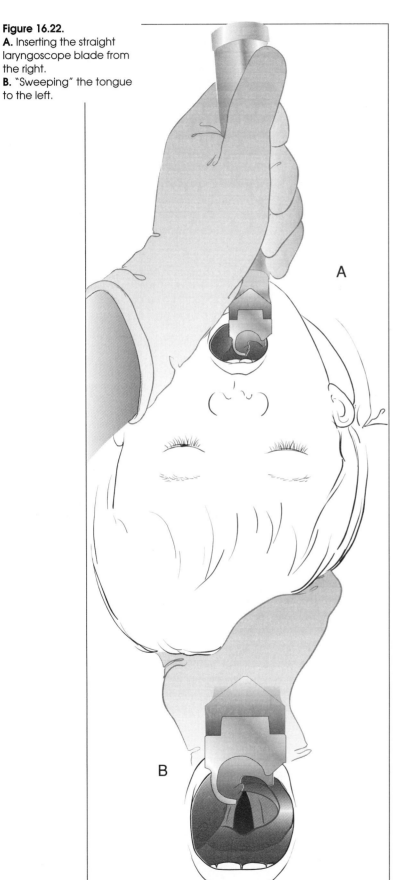

Figure 16.22.
A. Inserting the straight laryngoscope blade from the right.
B. "Sweeping" the tongue to the left.

When copious secretions impair visualization, properly suctioning the oropharynx can be an important key to successful laryngoscopy (see also Chapter 13). Taking the time to obtain a clear field in the posterior hypopharynx can greatly facilitate identification of anatomic landmarks. A Yankauer or tonsil-tip suction device is usually most effective for older children and adolescents, although with children under 2 years, these larger devices may be too bulky. A 14F multiorifice, flexible suction catheter without a control valve (i.e., providing continuous suction) is therefore recommended for younger patients. Whatever device is used, the vacuum should be set at the maximum level of 200 cm H_2O.

At times the tongue and epiglottis cannot be adequately retracted even though the laryngoscope blade has been inserted properly and the handle pulled upward with appropriate force. This is almost always because the blade selected is too small for the patient. If this becomes apparent, the operator should quickly abort the procedure, remove the laryngoscope, and replace the blade with a larger size. Distortion of the anatomy as a result of mucosal swelling (e.g., airway edema, trauma from prior intubation attempts) may make visualization of the larynx difficult despite adequate retraction of the tongue. In such cases, the operator must often rely on a thorough understanding of the relative positions of the anatomic structures. For example, even if the vocal cords are not visible, the bright reflection of the arytenoids can be recognized in most instances. Once these landmarks are located, the operator then looks anteriorly along the midline to find the darkened silhouette of the glottic opening. If the difficulty is in locating the epiglottis, it may be helpful to intentionally insert the laryngoscope blade into the esophagus and then slowly remove it. As the blade is withdrawn, the epiglottis will fall into view. Although often effective, this technique should only be used when other methods have failed, because abrasion of the epiglottis may cause swelling and make subsequent laryngoscopy attempts more difficult.

If the angle of entry into the trachea is especially severe, any attempts at visualizing the larynx may be obstructed by the base of the tongue. In this situation, further extension of the neck, well beyond the normal position achieved during laryngoscopy, may bring the

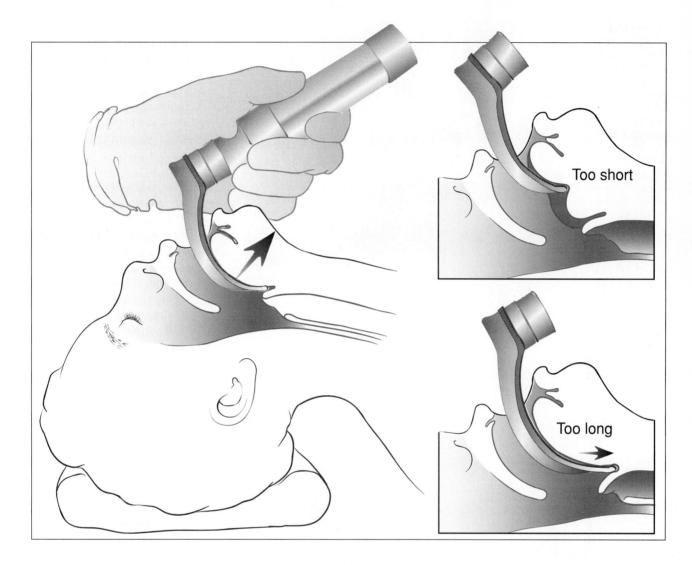

Too short

Too long

desired structures into view. Simultaneous cricoid pressure also may be effective in displacing the trachea posteriorly so that the glottic opening can be seen. If these measures fail, it may be necessary to use more resourceful methods. One favored approach is to insert the laryngoscope blade and retract the tongue in the normal fashion with the left hand, but in this case using the right hand to manipulate the anterior neck to achieve a favorable position of the larynx. The operator may apply cricoid pressure or shift the laryngeal structures to the right or left as necessary. Once the glottic opening is in view, an assistant can be instructed to position the larynx in the exact same manner while the operator continues to retract the patient's tongue with the laryngoscope. When the glottis is again visualized, the operator can then insert the endotracheal tube.

Inserting the Endotracheal Tube

After the operator has successfully performed direct laryngoscopy, the next task is to insert the endotracheal tube through the glottic opening and into the trachea. Ideally, once the anatomic landmarks are visualized the operator will not have to shift his or her gaze or concentration from these structures until the patient is intubated. Losing a clear view of the vocal cords because of a distraction requires the operator to readjust the laryngoscope and prolong the period of apnea. Once again, the aid of an assistant can be very helpful. When the glottis is visualized, the operator holds out his or her right hand, without diverting attention from the patient, and receives the endotracheal tube from the assistant. If no assistant is available, the tube should be placed in a nearby position where it can be easily retrieved "by feel."

Figure 16.23.
Direct laryngoscopy using a curved blade. The blade is inserted under direct vision until the tip is positioned in the vallecula. Pulling upward on the laryngoscope handle at 45° angle retracts the tongue and at the same time elevates the epiglottis, revealing the vocal cords and glottis. Selection of the appropriate laryngoscope blade is especially important with this technique. A blade that is too small will impinge on the midportion of the tongue potentially obscuring the landmarks, whereas a blade that is too large can displace the epiglottis posteriorly over the glottic opening.

201

Figure 16.24.
Anatomic landmarks for direct laryngoscopy.
A. After initial retraction of the tongue with a straight blade, the epiglottis may remain draped posteriorly, partially or completely covering the glottic opening.
B. Retraction of the epiglottis with the tip of the blade allows visualization of the glottis and surrounding structures.

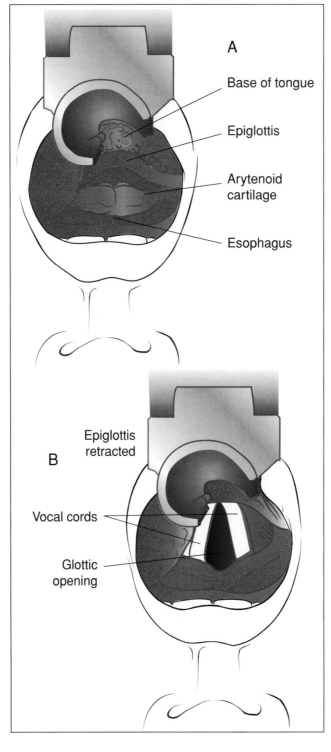

A
- Base of tongue
- Epiglottis
- Arytenoid cartilage
- Esophagus

B
Epiglottis retracted

Vocal cords

Glottic opening

the tube so that this plane is perfectly vertical (i.e., with the tube concave directly upward). In the small opening of a pediatric airway, this often results in having both the tube and the operator's hand obstruct the line of vision. A superior method is to insert the tube in a more horizontal plane, which allows the operator to keep the cords in constant view while watching the tip enter the glottic opening. The tube can then be rotated into the vertical plane after intubation is accomplished. Another technique that will aid the operator in maintaining visualization of the vocal cords is to introduce the endotracheal tube into the patient's mouth somewhat right of the midline. This also keeps the tip of the tube from blocking the operator's view. Although this may sometimes be difficult with a younger patient because of the small size of the mouth, enlisting the aid of an assistant to retract the cheek will generally provide the additional space needed.

While inserting the endotracheal tube, the operator should always stay far enough back from the patient that binocular vision is preserved. Getting so close that both eyes are not used (or closing one eye to "aim") causes the operator to lose valuable depth perception. As with threading a needle, inserting an endotracheal tube is greatly facilitated by using both eyes. Occasionally the angled tip of a styletted endotracheal tube will impinge on the anterior wall of the trachea after insertion, preventing further entry of the tube. If this happens, the tube should be advanced as the stylet is carefully removed, in much the same manner that an intravenous catheter is advanced off the needle into a vein.

Another potential problem occurs when

As mentioned previously, we recommend using a stylet for all conventional orotracheal intubations. The endotracheal tube is held between the thumb and first two fingers of the right hand (Fig. 16.26). If the natural arc of the tube is imagined as occupying a single plane, one common error is to insert

the vocal cords are tightly constricted during a prolonged cough or a mild episode of laryngospasm, temporarily making insertion of the endotracheal tube impossible. In most cases, the operator need only wait a few seconds until the patient takes a breath, at which time the vocal cords will abduct allowing the tube to

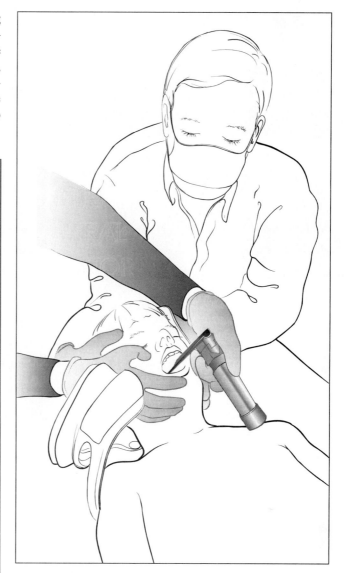

Figure 16.25.
In-line stabilization of the head and neck. A second assistant should hold the shoulders in place against the stretcher to prevent movement of the torso.

---

pass. If this does not happen after 15 to 20 seconds, the patient may be experiencing a more significant episode of laryngospasm that will not resolve spontaneously, requiring the administration of a rapid onset muscle relaxant (see Chapter 15).

Although relatively uncommon, occasional instances will occur in which the glottic opening cannot be identified despite appropriate laryngoscopy technique. In such cases, it may be necessary to insert the endotracheal tube without direct visualization. If the epiglottis is the only recognizable structure, the operator uses a styletted endotracheal tube that has a 90° angle 2 to 3 cm from the tip. The tube is slipped under the epiglottis and advanced in as anterior a trajectory as

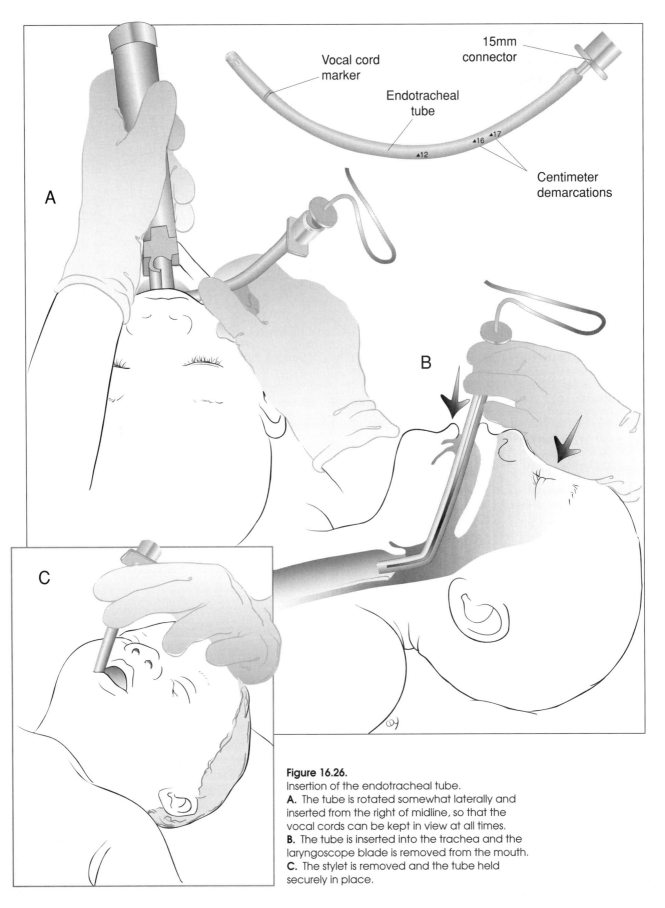

Figure 16.26.
Insertion of the endotracheal tube.
A. The tube is rotated somewhat laterally and inserted from the right of midline, so that the vocal cords can be kept in view at all times.
B. The tube is inserted into the trachea and the laryngoscope blade is removed from the mouth.
C. The stylet is removed and the tube held securely in place.

possible along the midline. This will normally result in successful intubation of the trachea. It should be emphasized that inserting an endotracheal tube in this manner without direct visualization significantly increases the likelihood of esophageal intubation. Confirmation of proper tube position using the methods described previously is therefore especially important. If no alternative technique of intubation can be immediatley performed, however, this method is worth a single attempt before undertaking an emergent surgical airway. Because of the risks associated with this method, it should only be performed by the most experienced available operator. In all cases, the most effective and reliable way of avoiding an esophageal intubation is to directly observe the tube as it passes between the vocal cords into the trachea.

Once the patient is intubated, the tube should be held securely in place at all times with the thumb and index finger, while the other three fingers rest against the patient's face (Fig. 16.26.C). Maintaining contact in this way ensures that the operator's hand will follow any unexpected movements of the patient's head so that the tube does not become accidentally dislodged. Confirmation of the appropriate depth of insertion and securing the tube in place are performed as described previously.

Blind Nasotracheal Intubation

As discussed in the Indications section, this approach is only rarely used with pediatric patients. The more cephalad position of the larynx in younger patients does not allow the glottic opening to align with the nasopharyngeal air passage. Consequently, blind passage of the tube is virtually impossible with infants and children. Furthermore, a significant degree of patient cooperation is required to perform this procedure successfully. A crying, struggling child is not a candidate for blind nasotracheal intubation. Finally, the likelihood of passing the tube through the vocal cords is substantially increased when the patient is making strong respiratory efforts. An adult patient with an exacerbation of emphysema or congestive heart failure normally has a deep, prolonged inspiratory

phase during which the vocal cords are widely abducted. This greatly facilitates blind insertion of the tube. Conditions requiring emergent intubation that cause a similar increased respiratory effort among children are relatively uncommon. Thus the most likely pediatric patient for whom blind nasotracheal intubation might prove useful would be a cooperative adolescent with status asthmaticus, or in rare cases, severe congestive heart failure or ARDS. Although this approach is often advocated for pediatric trauma patients requiring cervical spine immobilization, experience has shown that this is extremely difficult to perform successfully even in the most favorable circumstances. Blind nasotracheal intubation is contraindicated for the child with a bleeding tumor or abscess above the glottis due to the risk of hemorrhage and further encroachment of the airway (112).

With those caveats in mind, it is worth examining the potential benefits of blind nasotracheal intubation. The most important advantage is that the patient is awake and maintains spontaneous respirations and intact airway reflexes at all times, eliminating risks associated with administration of anesthetic agents or neuromuscular blockade. Aspiration of gastric contents is rare, and if the procedure is unsuccessful the patient is still conscious and breathing ("no bridges are burned"). An adolescent patient with airway anomalies who is suspected of having a potentially difficult airway, or for whom manual ventilation may be problematic, might well be considered for this approach. The second major advantage is that many of the potential complications associated with direct laryngoscopy are avoided. Used in the appropriate circumstances, blind nasotracheal intubation offers a highly safe, controlled method for securing the airway (113–116). Nasotracheal intubation under direct laryngoscopic visualization is rarely performed on an emergent basis and is therefore not discussed here. Readers interested in information on this approach are referred to standard pediatric anesthesiology texts.

Before performing a blind nasotracheal intubation, the operator should take steps to minimize any discomfort experienced by the patient. This not only makes the procedure as humane as possible, but because patient cooperation is so essential, it also increases the

1. If blind nasotracheal intubation is unsuccessful after three or four attempts, an alternative method should be used.
2. This procedure is best suited for adolescents. Children are rarely if ever good candidates for blind nasotracheal intubation.
3. If the tip of the endotracheal tube gets caught in one of the pyriform sinuses, the operator will appreciate a bulge lateral to the midline on either side of the neck. In such cases, the tube should be rotated back to a midline position before the next attempt at passage.
4. If the tip of the tube gets caught in the vallecula or anterior commissure of the vocal cords, the operator will appreciate a bulge in the submental region of the neck. In such cases, the patient's neck should be flexed somewhat before the next attempt at passage.
5. If the tube persistently enters the esophagus, the following may be effective: (a) using an Endotrol™ tube and pulling the ring to deflect the tip anteriorly, (b) applying cricoid pressure during insertion, and (c) extending the patient's neck.
6. If the ring of an Endotrol™ tube sits tightly against the nose after insertion, the ligature should be cut and the ring removed. Otherwise, tension on the ligature will cause the tube to exert continuous anterior pressure on the trachea.

Chapter 16
Emergent
Endotracheal
Intubation

mg/mL) lidocaine solution also can be performed to provide a greater degree of anesthesia (see Retrograde Intubation later in this chapter), although this is not generally required to successfully perform a blind nasotracheal intubation. Whatever methods are used, the operator must make certain that the maximum allowable dosage of lidocaine (approximately 5 to 7 mg/kg) is not exceeded. Another possible option for enhancing patient cooperation is to administer a small dose of an intravenous sedative such as midazolam (0.1 mg/kg). For the patient with severe asthma, ketamine (1 to 2 mg/kg, administered in increments of 0.5 mg/kg/dose) is also an excellent choice, because it produces bronchodilation as well as sedation and analgesia (see Chapter 15). Although judicious doses of these agents may facilitate the procedure, deep sedation is obviously not appropriate, because the primary aim with this approach is to maintain airway reflexes. With a mature adolescent who is fully cooperative, sedation is usually unnecessary.

Preparation of the nasal mucosa also includes application of a topical vasoconstrictor to decrease mucosal edema and limit potential bleeding. Significant epistaxis often will force the operator to abort this approach. Phenylephrine spray (0.25%) can be used if it is the only available agent, but oxymetazoline spray (0.05%) is preferred because it does not cause systemic hypertension. For adolescent patients, topical phenylephrine should be diluted to 0.1% and the total dose limited to 2 to 3 mL. As with application of the topical anesthesia, the vasoconstrictor should be applied 2 to 4 minutes before performing the procedure, so that the full effect is obtained.

Unfortunately no simple formulas are available for determining the proper tube size for a blind nasotracheal intubation. Because this procedure will rarely be performed with a child younger than 8 years, a cuffed tube will virtually always be necessary. In general, the internal diameter of the tube used with this approach should be 0.5 to 1 mm smaller than one that would be appropriate for a conventional orotracheal intubation. For example, if a patient is estimated to require a 7.0 ID tube for an oral intubation, a reasonable first choice for a nasal intubation would be a 6.5 or 6.0 ID tube. The tube must be large enough to adequately ventilate the patient without being so large that the nasal mucosa is injured dur-

likelihood of success. Enhancing patient tolerance is best provided by the application of topical anesthesia to the airway mucosa. Because a few minutes must pass before the full anesthetic effect is achieved, this should be one of the first steps performed. For most patients, spraying the hypopharynx with a topical anesthetic (e.g., cetacaine) and instilling a small amount of lidocaine jelly into the nares are sufficient to produce adequate anesthesia. Both nares are anesthetized so that if one side does not permit insertion of the tube, passage can be attempted on the other side without delay. Transtracheal instillation of 1% (10

ing insertion. In addition, pressure on the nasal mucosa from a tube that fits too tightly may cause ulceration and necrosis over time.

The child should be positioned sitting upright with the hands gently restrained as necessary to prevent grabbing at the tube. Before the endotracheal tube is inserted, patency of the nares should be assessed by occluding each one in turn and observing any obstruction to air flow. If both nares are equally patent, the tube is inserted on the right side so that the bevel faces the nasal septum, as this will decrease the chances of injuring the turbinates. The tube is held concave downward in the dominant hand and carefully inserted using a "straight in" approach, perpendicular to the plane of the patient's face (Fig. 16.27.A). A common error is to insert the tube in a superior (rostral) direction in the mistaken belief that the nasal passage initially follows an upward course. This is painful for the patient and increases the likelihood of injury. Should passage on the right side prove difficult, an attempt can be made on the left side by inverting the tube (i.e., rotating it 180°), so that again the bevel will face the septum (Fig. 16.28). Once the tip reaches the posterior pharynx, the tube is then rotated back to the normal orientation. If passage is unsuccessful on both sides, a smaller tube should be used. If this also fails, or if the tube must be so small that ventilating the patient will be difficult, orotracheal intubation will likely be necessary. It cannot be overemphasized that excessive force must never be used in inserting the tube through the nasal passage, because this greatly increases the likelihood of injury and bleeding.

Once the endotracheal tube is inserted into the nasopharynx, the angle at the posterior pharyngeal wall must be negotiated (Fig. 16.27.B). Here again, the tube should not be forced at any point, because tonsillar or adenoid tissue can be avulsed, or in rare instances, the tube can actually create a traumatic false passage into the posterior hypopharynx. Ideally, the endotracheal tube should be inserted in one easy, continuous motion from the nose to the supraglottic region. As the tip approaches the glottic opening, the operator will begin to see fogging of the tube with each expiration and hear breath sounds transmitted through the tube. Slowly advancing the endotracheal tube until these signs are lost and then withdrawing slightly ensures that the tip is positioned just superior to the glottic opening (Fig. 16.27.C). If breath sounds are difficult to appreciate through the tube because of a noisy environment or the patient's poor respiratory effort, using a BAAM (Beck airway airflow monitor) may assist the operator in positioning the tube (117, 118). This simple and inexpensive device, which fits the proximal opening of an endotracheal tube, has a small aperture that makes a distinctive whistling sound even when the patient has diminished respirations. Location of the tip of the endotracheal tube at the proper level is indicated when this whistling sound is most prominent.

At this point, the operator is ready to intubate the trachea. Passage of the tube must be carefully timed with the patient's respirations, so that the vocal cords will be fully abducted when the tube is inserted. A useful practice is to spend a few seconds listening to the respirations to get a good sense of their rhythm. At the moment the patient first begins inspiration, when exposure and patency of the glottic opening are greatest, the tube is briskly advanced into the trachea (Fig. 16.27.D). If the operator is successful, the patient will normally have a prolonged cough and will be unable to phonate. Any recognizable vocalization (speaking, moaning, etc.) indicates that the tube has been passed into the esophagus. If this happens, the tube should be withdrawn back to a point just superior to the glottic opening, and another attempt should be made using an appropriate corrective maneuver (to be described). After successful intubation, the balloon is inflated and the tube secured. If the procedure has not been accomplished after three to four attempts, the operator should consider performing a conventional orotracheal intubation or using one of the alternative approaches described later in this chapter.

Although blind nasotracheal intubation offers distinct advantages in the appropriate clinical circumstances, it can sometimes be difficult to perform successfully even for the experienced practitioner. Undoubtedly, this is another reason why this procedure is not commonly performed on an emergent basis. The primary problem is that the endotracheal tube can get "hung up" by various structures in the airway, and the operator obviously has no way of directly visualizing where this has occurred. However, several suggestive clinical findings can be used to determine the na-

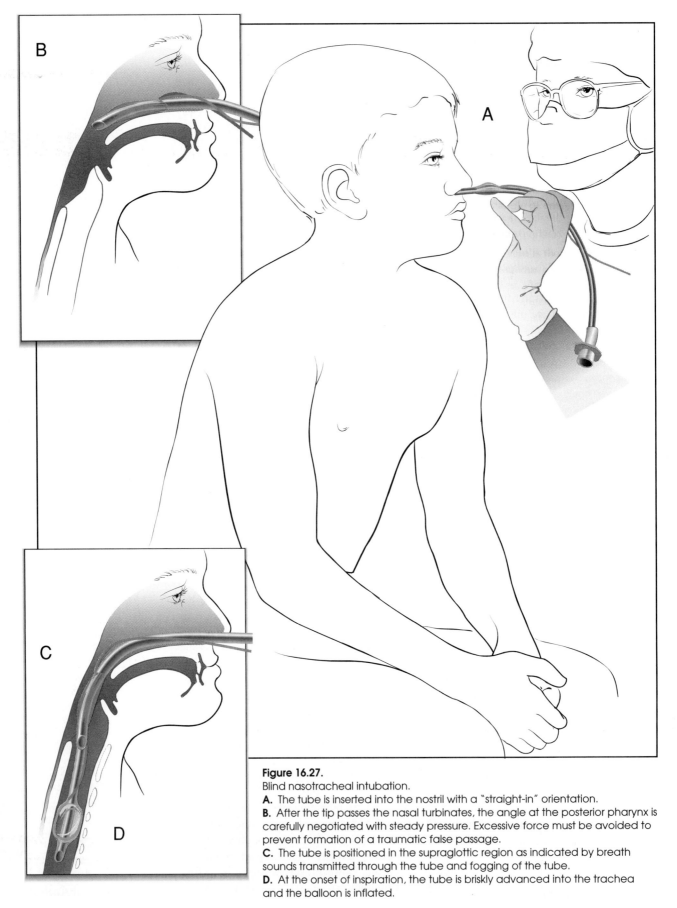

Figure 16.27.
Blind nasotracheal intubation.
A. The tube is inserted into the nostril with a "straight-in" orientation.
B. After the tip passes the nasal turbinates, the angle at the posterior pharynx is carefully negotiated with steady pressure. Excessive force must be avoided to prevent formation of a traumatic false passage.
C. The tube is positioned in the supraglottic region as indicated by breath sounds transmitted through the tube and fogging of the tube.
D. At the onset of inspiration, the tube is briskly advanced into the trachea and the balloon is inflated.

ture of such problems, along with corresponding corrective maneuvers that may overcome them. For example, the endotracheal tube may travel too far anteriorly during insertion, causing the tip to get caught in the vallecula or the anterior commissure of the vocal cords. This can normally be recognized without difficulty, because the operator will appreciate a prominent midline bulge in the anterior neck when the tube is advanced. If this happens, the tube should first be withdrawn far enough to remove the tip from the vallecula. The patient's neck is then flexed slightly, so that the tube follows a more posterior trajectory on reinsertion. Another potential problem occurs when the tube is inadvertently rotated during insertion causing the tip to get caught in one of the piriform sinuses. This also can be identified based on the presence of a bulge in the neck, although in this case it will be somewhat lateral to the midline on either side. To reposition the tip in the midline, the operator rotates the proximal end of the tube away from the involved piriform sinus. In other words, if the tip is caught in the left piriform sinus, the tube is rotated in a clockwise direction; if the tip is in the right piriform sinus, the tube is rotated counterclockwise.

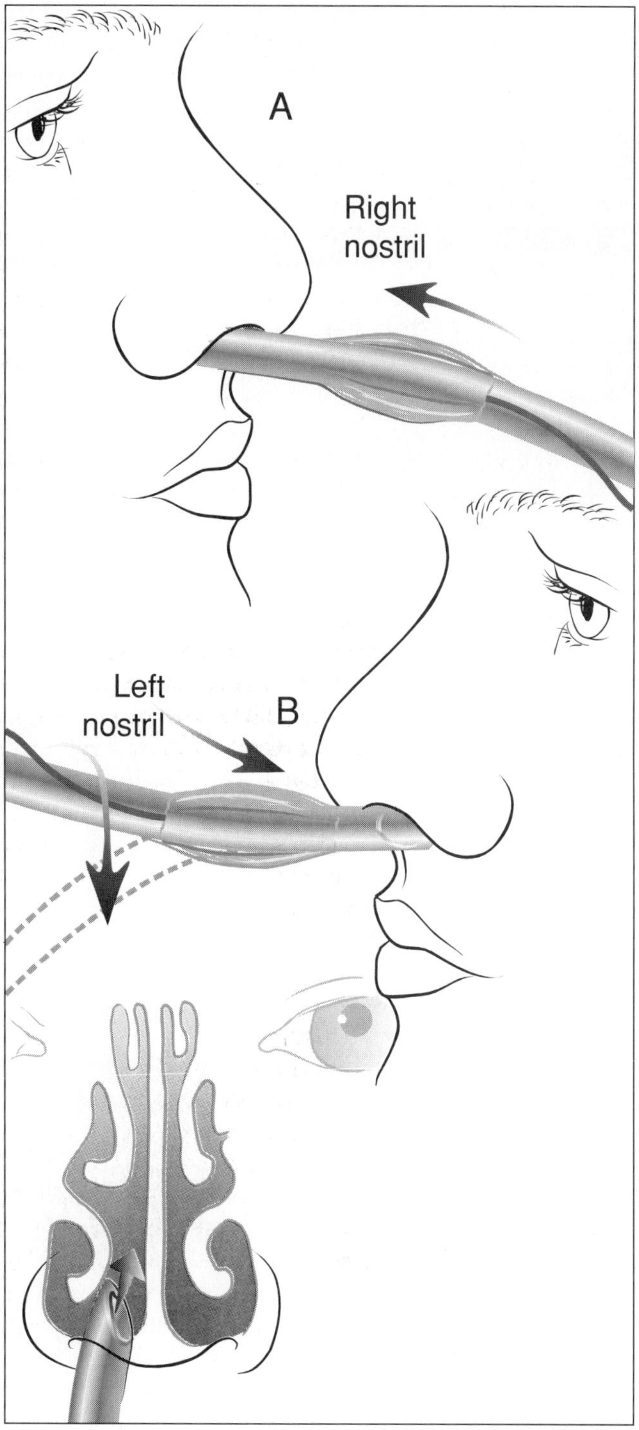

As mentioned, one of the most common problems with blind nasotracheal intubation occurs when the angle of entry into the trachea is so acute that the tube persistently passes into the esophagus. In most instances, this results from a particularly cephalad location of the trachea, which makes negotiating the turn at the base of the tongue more difficult than normal. One simple technique for overcoming this is to extend the patient's head some-what as the tube is inserted, so that the angle of entry into the glottis is not as severe. This often allows the normal curvature of the tube to project the tip far enough anteriorly that it will enter the glottic opening. Another method is to enlist the aid of an assistant to perform gentle cricoid pressure during the procedure. As with orotracheal intubation, the posterior displacement of the trachea

Figure 16.28.
During blind nasotracheal intubation, the bevel of the endotracheal tube should face the septum to minimize the risk of injury to the nasal turbinates.
A. With the tube concave downward (the standard initial approach), this necessitates insertion on the right side.
B. If the right nostril is not adequately patent, the tube may be inserted on the left side by inverting it 180°. The tube can then be rotated back to the normal position after the tip reaches the posterior pharynx.

**Chapter 16
Emergent
Endotracheal
Intubation**

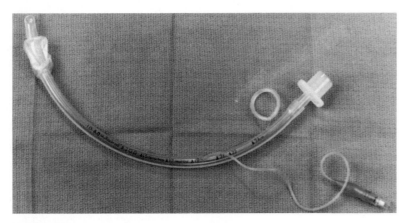

Figure 16.29.
Endotrol™ tube.

Figure 16.30.
Pulling the ring of an Endotrol™ tube exerts tension on the plastic ligature, which in turn increases the curvature of the tube. In this way, the operator can direct the tip to some extent during insertion. This facilitates passage of the tube at the posterior pharynx by deflecting the tip inferiorly. In addition, persistent passage of the tube into the esophagus when the patient has a more superiorly positioned trachea also may be overcome using this technique.

achieved with cricoid pressure makes the glottis more accessible for insertion of the tube. Perhaps the most effective technique in this situation involves using an Endotrol™ tube (Fig. 16.29). These tubes have a plastic ligature along the inner (concave) side that connects to a ring at the proximal end. By pulling this ring during insertion, the operator can increase the curvature of the tube as needed, which in turn projects the tip anteriorly or inferiorly depending on the position of the tube (Fig. 16.30). Ability to direct the tip of the endotracheal tube with some degree of precision can greatly facilitate the procedure and often make other measures unnecessary. Notably, if the ring is sitting firmly against the nares after intubation, the tip of the tube may exert continuous anterior pressure on the trachea. In such cases, the ligature should be cut and the ring removed.

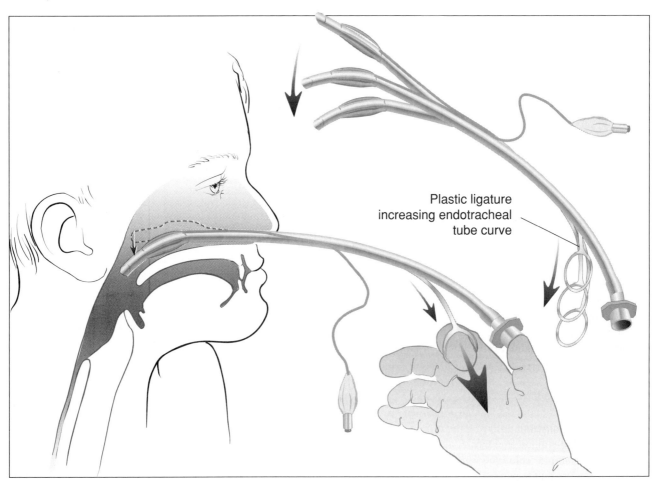

Plastic ligature increasing endotracheal tube curve

Alternative Intubation Techniques

From time to time, patients requiring emergent intubation will be encountered who are not candidates for blind nasotracheal intubation and for whom conventional orotracheal intubation either has potential undesirable effects or proves impossible to perform. As discussed previously, these patients may have airway anomalies (e.g., micrognathia, macroglossia), possible or known cervical spine injury, or severely restricted neck movement or mouth opening. Several techniques have been advocated to deal with such situations, but the ones most suitable for the emergent situation are lighted stylet intubation, tactile intubation, retrograde intubation, and fiberoptic nasotracheal intubation. Although the majority of pediatric endotracheal intubations will be performed using conventional orotracheal intubation, skill with one or more of these alternative approaches can be highly valuable in selected cases. Because the clinical indications for these techniques are rare, they are best performed in a controlled setting such as the operating room when possible.

Lighted Stylet (Light Wand) Intubation

When a focused light source is directed anteriorly within the trachea, transillumination through the skin of the neck occurs in a characteristic fashion. Lighted stylet intubation represents a practical application of this effect (119–122). As described previously, a light wand is essentially a stylet combined with a fiberoptic bundle attached to a handle containing a light source (Fig. 16.15). An endotracheal tube is placed over the stylet, and the light projected to the tip of the fiberoptic bundle provides a focused beam that is inserted into the trachea. The primary advantage of this technique is that direct laryngoscopy is unnecessary, eliminating the need to visualize the anatomic landmarks of a potentially difficult airway and possibly decreasing any movement of the patient's head and neck. Although formerly used only for adults, advances in fiberoptic technology have recently made lighted stylets suitable for pediatric patients widely available.

In preparing the equipment for this approach, the operator should first fully lubricate the stylet so that it can be easily removed

from the endotracheal tube when necessary. The tube is then threaded over the stylet. As with any stylet used for intubation, it should extend the entire length of the tube but should not protrude beyond the distal tip, to minimize the risk of injury to the patient while ensuring that the light source is properly positioned at the tip of the endotracheal tube. It is sometimes necessary to shorten a larger endotracheal tube to achieve the desired position of the stylet. This is done by removing the 15 mm connector and cutting off a segment of the tube from the proximal end. In addition, a smaller endotracheal tube may only just fit the stylet, requiring the 15 mm connector to be left off during the entire procedure and replaced subsequently. To facilitate insertion into the trachea, the styletted

SUMMARY: LIGHTED STYLET (LIGHT WAND) INTUBATION

1. Prepare patient
   a. Administer assisted or controlled BVM ventilation as needed
   b. Attach patient to monitoring devices
   c. Preoxygenate patient with 100% oxygen
   d. Insert gastric tube to evacuate stomach contents as necessary
2. Prepare and test necessary equipment
   a. Check intensity of light from fiberoptic element of lighted stylet
   b. Inflate balloon on cuffed endotracheal tube (if used) to ensure there are no leaks
   c. Lubricate stylet liberally and insert into tube; if necessary, cut segment from proximal end of tube and/ or remove 15 mm connector
   d. Bend styletted tube to 110° angle approximately 2 to 3 cm from distal end
3. Grasp tongue and mandibular block with nondominant hand and pull outward to open mouth
4. Dim room lights as necessary
5. Insert styletted endotracheal tube into patient's mouth along midline following contour of tongue
6. When tube reaches supraglottic region, direct it as far anteriorly as possible and continue to advance it until it passes through glottic opening into trachea
7. Observe anterior neck to see characteristic focused, cherry-red glow at suprasternal notch ("jack-o-lantern" effect)
8. Carefully remove stylet
9. Confirm tracheal placement (equal breath sounds, no sounds over stomach, capnography)
10. Position tube at midtracheal level
11. Secure endotracheal tube
12. Confirm proper tube position with chest radiograph

CLINICAL TIPS: LIGHTED STYLET (LIGHT WAND) INTUBATION

1. Lighted stylet intubation can often be performed with minimal movement of the patient's head and neck.
2. It may be necessary to dim the lights in a bright room to appreciate the appearance of the light from the lighted stylet on the patient's anterior neck. Whenever this is done, special attention must be given to the monitoring equipment during this time, because visual cues regarding the patient's clinical condition (e.g., cyanosis) will not be readily observed.
3. Esophageal intubation with a lighted stylet can be recognized by the characteristic dim, unfocused light seen on the anterior neck.
4. In the event of an esophageal intubation, the tube should be withdrawn to the hypopharynx before making another attempt. The operator will often appreciate a subtle "pop" as the tube flips out of the esophagus and into the supraglottic region.
5. Because of the sharp bend in the styletted endotracheal tube, removal of the stylet may result in buckling of the tube and inadvertent extubation. For this reason, the tube should be held firmly in place against the patient's tongue as the stylet is carefully withdrawn with firm, steady pressure
6. As with any stylet used during an endotracheal intubation, the tip should not extend beyond the distal end of the tube to avoid injury to the soft tissues.

endotracheal tube is bent to approximately 110° at a point 2 to 3 cm from the distal end.

Much of the literature regarding lighted stylet intubation suggests that the operator should stand to one side of the patient. Standing above the head of the bed, as with a conventional orotracheal intubation, is also an effective position, because this facilitates performing manual ventilation as necessary between attempts. Preoxygenation is performed before intubation as described previously. Unless the patient is deeply comatose or presents in full arrest, this procedure should normally be performed on a fully anesthetized, paralyzed patient (see Chapter 15). To begin the procedure, the operator first grasps the tongue and mandibular block with the nondominant hand and pulls them outward to open the mouth (Fig. 16.31.A). A small gauze pad may be placed over the tongue to aid in maintaining traction. Before insertion of the lighted stylet, it may be helpful to dim the room lights somewhat so that light can be better observed on the patient's anterior neck. However, it is not necessary or desirable to have a completely darkened room; in fact, as the operator gains experience with this approach, it may prove unnecessary to dim the lights at all. It should be emphasized that whenever the ambient light is decreased, the operator must maintain a heightened awareness of the monitor readings, because visual signs of the patient's condition (e.g., cyanosis) will be more difficult to discern. The styletted endotracheal tube is then inserted into the patient's mouth along the midline following the contour of the tongue (Fig. 16.31.B). The operator should attempt to insert the tube as anterior as possible, hugging the base of the tongue until the tube passes through the glottis or meets resistance at the vallecula.

When the endotracheal tube enters the trachea, a focused cherry-red glow will be observed in the midline superior to the suprasternal notch. This appearance has been referred to as a "jack-o-lantern" effect. A more diffuse light on either side of the midline indicates that the tip is in one of the pyriform sinuses. If this happens, the tube should be withdrawn somewhat, redirected toward the midline, and then reinserted until the desired light pattern is seen. A bright glow in the submental area indicates that the tip is in the vallecula, requiring the operator to rein-

sert the tube in a more posterior direction. An esophageal intubation can normally be recognized by a characteristic diffuse, unfocused light on the anterior neck. If this is seen, the tube should be withdrawn to the supraglottic region, redirected anteriorly, and reinserted as before. As the tube is withdrawn, the operator may feel it "give" slightly as the tip flips out of the esophagus and into the area proximal to the glottic opening. Infants and younger children will have a sharp red glow in the midline of the neck if the esophagus is intubated and then pulled anteriorly against the trachea. This makes recognition of esophageal intubation more difficult in this age group, although a recent investigation using this same technique with a fiberoptic strand incorporated into the endotracheal tube demonstrated a high success rate with intubation of young infants (123). Further study of lighted stylet techniques in this age group is warranted.

Once the trachea has been successfully intubated, the stylet should be carefully withdrawn while at the same time the tube is advanced to the appropriate depth of insertion. Because of the sharp bend in the styletted endotracheal tube, the tube may be prone to buckle as the stylet is removed, potentially resulting in inadvertent extubation. As a result, this step must be performed with slow, steady pressure rather than any rapid movements, and the operator should support the tube against the patient's tongue as the stylet is removed (Fig. 16.31.C). Proper midtracheal position of the tube should then be confirmed using methods described previously.

Tactile (Digital) Intubation

As mentioned previously, this is an old procedure that has gone in and out of favor multiple times over the years. More recently, it has been well documented as an effective method for adults (124–127). However, as pointed out by Hancock and Peterson (128), neonates and young infants may be the ideal candidates for this approach for two reasons: (a) they are edentulous, eliminating the risk of bite injuries to the operator and (b) they have a relatively small extrathoracic airway, making it easier to reach the supraglottic structures even for those not endowed with large hands. Tactile intubation has the additional advantages of potentially decreasing neck movement for the patient with a possible cervical spine injury as well as requiring a minimum of equipment to perform. Although not widely used for pediatric patients, the benefits offered by this technique for emergent intubation may increase its popularity once again.

Depending on individual preference, this procedure may be performed with or without using a stylet. Although sometimes recommended to facilitate insertion of the endotracheal tube, many practitioners who are experienced with tactile intubation do not find using a stylet to be necessary. If the operator elects to use a stylet, the endotracheal tube should be molded into a gentle arc rather than the "hockey stick" configuration used for orotracheal intubation (Fig. 16.32). As always, the tip of the stylet should not extend beyond the end of the tube to prevent injury to the airway soft tissues.

The tip of the endotracheal tube should be lightly lubricated or moistened with sterile water, so that it will slide more easily into the glottic opening. This procedure is best performed with the operator standing to one side of the patient (a right-handed operator to the patient's left). Following appropriate preoxygenation, the nondominant index finger is inserted into the mouth along the midline of the tongue until the epiglottis and arytenoid cartilages are felt (Fig. 16.32.A). If necessary, the epiglottis should be gently lifted so that the arytenoids can be palpated. The endotracheal tube is then inserted into the mouth with the dominant hand, while the index finger of the nondominant hand is used to direct the tube along the midline (Fig. 16.32.B). The thumb of the nondominant hand also may be used to apply cricoid pressure, which steadies the trachea and displaces it posteriorly to facilitate insertion of the tube. As the tube is advanced, the index finger of the nondominant hand guides the tip into the glottic opening. The tube is then further advanced to the appropriate depth of insertion, and the stylet (if used) is removed. Proper midtracheal position of the endotracheal tube is confirmed using the methods described previously.

Retrograde Intubation

Although somewhat unorthodox, this approach is well supported by the literature for application in both adults and children (129–133). Retrograde intubation is in many ways analogous to the Seldinger technique for central venous cannulation (Chapter 18), because a guide wire is used to facilitate insertion of an endotracheal tube into the trachea. However, in this case the wire is placed in a retrograde fashion, as the name of the procedure implies. Because the clinical indications for this procedure will be rare, it should be regularly practiced with cadaver or animal models if it is to be a viable option in the ED. A wide array of special adaptations has been developed for performing this procedure, but for the sake of clarity only the methods most suitable for the emergency setting are described here. The reader wishing more information on these modifications is referred to other sources (131, 132, 134, 135).

Initial steps of a retrograde intubation are exactly the same as those performed for percutaneous transtracheal ventilation (Chapter 17). As the patient continues to receive manual ventilation, the skin of the anterior neck overlying the trachea is thoroughly cleansed with an antiseptic solution and a sterile field is established. Standing to one side of the patient (a right-handed operator at the patient's right), the operator identifies the relevant external anatomic landmarks (Fig. 17.1). This is

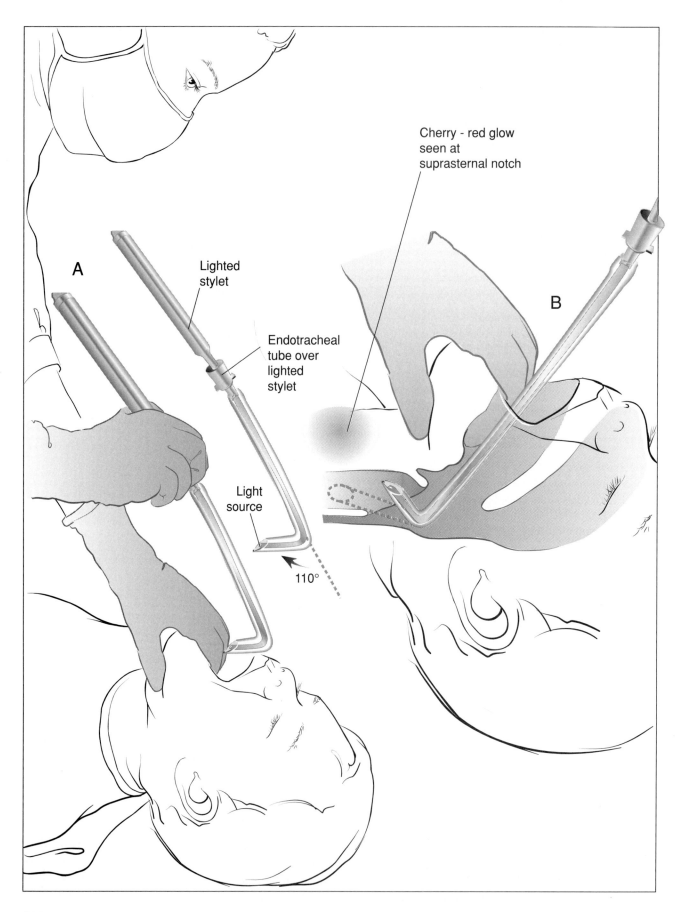

A

Lighted stylet

Endotracheal tube over lighted stylet

Light source

110°

Cherry - red glow seen at suprasternal notch

B

done by first palpating the laryngeal prominence (thyroid cartilage) and then moving down along the midline until a small "bump" is felt at the superior aspect of the cricoid cartilage. The cricothyroid membrane is just cephalad to this point. With younger patients who do not have a well-developed laryngeal prominence, it may be necessary to proceed upward from the tracheal rings until the bulge at the cricoid cartilage is appreciated. If the location of the cricothyroid membrane cannot be determined using these methods, a lower point of entry in the midline of the trachea through an intercartilaginous space may be used without added risk to the patient.

If the patient is conscious, a local anesthetic should be infiltrated into the subcutaneous tissue overlying the planned insertion site. Because this approach involves more aggressive manipulation of the extrathoracic airway, the operator also may elect to perform transtracheal instillation of lidocaine. This is done by first attaching a small-gauge needle to a syringe filled with 1 to 2 mL of 1% (10 mg/mL) lidocaine. The operator then inserts the needle through the cricothyroid membrane while applying negative pressure on the syringe (Fig. 16.33). The needle is gradually advanced until air bubbles are first detected in the lidocaine, indicating that the tip has entered the tracheal lumen. The lidocaine is rapidly instilled into the trachea and the needle is immediately removed to prevent injury to the vocal cords when the patient coughs. Although more invasive than other methods of airway anesthesia, insertion of a needle through the cricothyroid membrane in this manner has been shown to have minimal complications in large patient series (136–138). However, the operator should be aware that transtracheal anesthesia will suppress the patient's airway reflexes, increasing the possibility of aspiration of regurgitated stomach contents.

To perform retrograde–intubation, a second fluid-filled syringe is first attached to a standard 18-gauge intravenous catheter. Alternatively, the operator may choose to simply use an 18-gauge needle alone. The guide wire should be an extra-long, heavy duty wire as described previously (see Equipment). The thumb and index finger of the nondominant hand are used to stabilize the trachea as the needle is inserted with the dominant hand (Fig. 16.34.A). The needle should initially be inserted in a "straight in" (i.e., perpendicular) or slightly caudad direction to decrease the risk of injury to the vocal cords. As with the

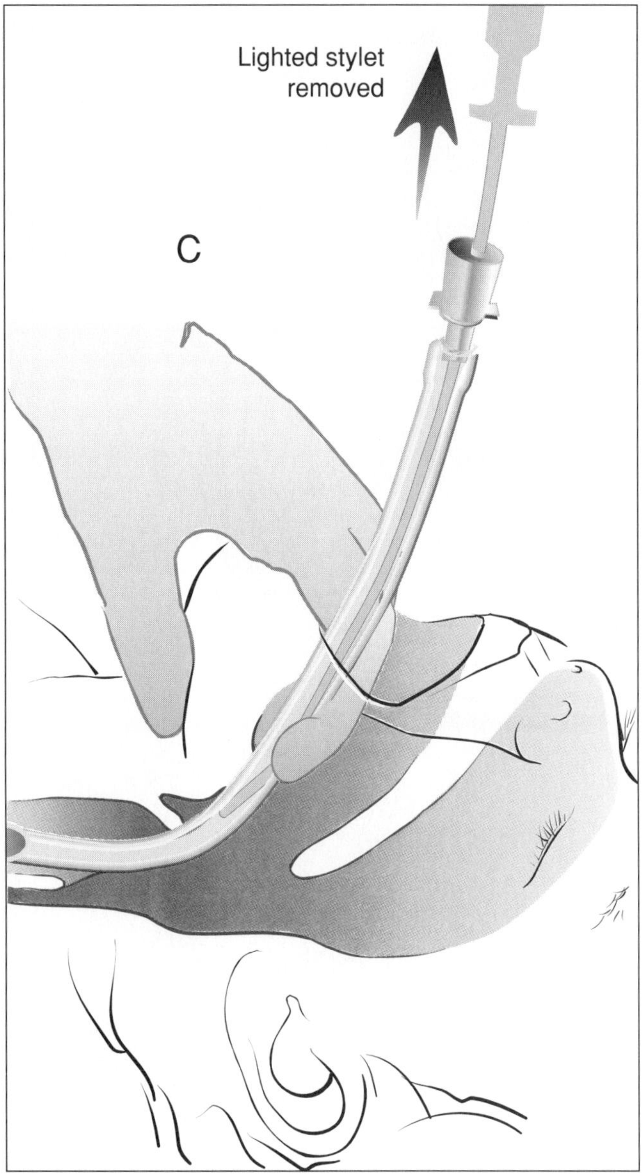

Lighted stylet removed

C

Figure 16.31.
Lighted stylet (light wand) intubation.
A. The mandibular block is grasped and pulled outward with the nondominant hand.
B. The styletted endotracheal tube is inserted over the tongue along the midline until a focused, cherry-red glow is seen at the anterior neck proximal to the suprasternal notch.
C. The tube is secured against the tongue with the index finger and the lighted stylet is carefully removed.

Figure 16.32.
Tactile (digital) intubation.
A. The index finger of the nondominant hand is used to palpate the arytenoids and retract the epiglottis.
B. The tube is inserted using the index finger to guide the tip into the trachea. The thumb may be used to apply simultaneous cricoid pressure.

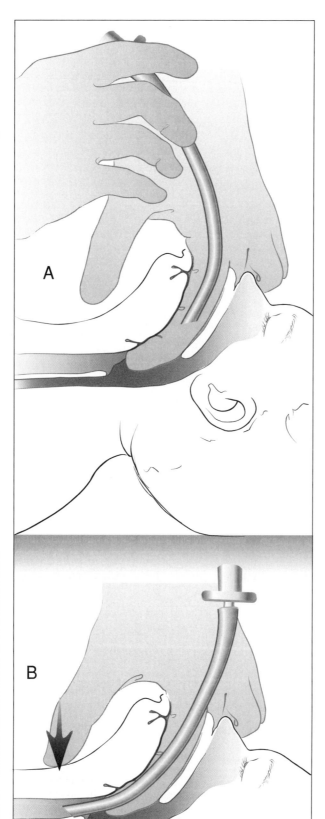

SUMMARY: RETROGRADE INTUBATION

1. Prepare patient
   a. Administer assisted or controlled BVM ventilation as needed
   b. Attach patient to monitoring devices
   c. Preoxygenate patient with 100% oxygen
   d. Insert gastric tube to evacuate stomach contents as necessary
   e. Prepare anterior neck aseptically and drape field

SUMMARY: RETROGRADE INTUBATION (CONTINUED)

   f. Infiltrate skin and subcutaneous tissues overlying planned insertion site with local anesthetic
   g. Perform transtracheal instillation of lidocaine (optional)
2. Prepare and test necessary equipment
   1. Attach standard 18-gauge intravenous catheter to fluid-filled syringe
   2. Use extra-long, heavy gauge wire
   3. Inflate balloon on cuffed endotracheal tube (if used) to ensure there are no leaks
3. Stabilize trachea with thumb and index finger of nondominant hand and locate cricothyroid membrane
4. Insert needle using "straight in" (or slightly caudad) approach; apply negative pressure on syringe so that entry into trachea is indicated by appearance of bubbles in fluid
5. As soon as needle enters trachea, rotate syringe so that needle points superiorly and advance catheter until hub rests against skin
6. Remove needle and syringe
7. Insert guide wire until a sufficient length extends out nose or mouth of patient and then clamp wire at anterior neck
8. Thread endotracheal tube over wire into nose or mouth of patient until tip of tube is in supraglottic region
9. Pull wire taut and pass tube into trachea
10. Remove clamp and withdraw tube through cephalad end of tube
11. Confirm tracheal placement (equal breath sounds, no sounds over stomach, capnography)
12. Position tube at midtracheal level (see Fig. 16.18)
13. Secure endotracheal tube
14. Confirm proper tube position with chest radiograph

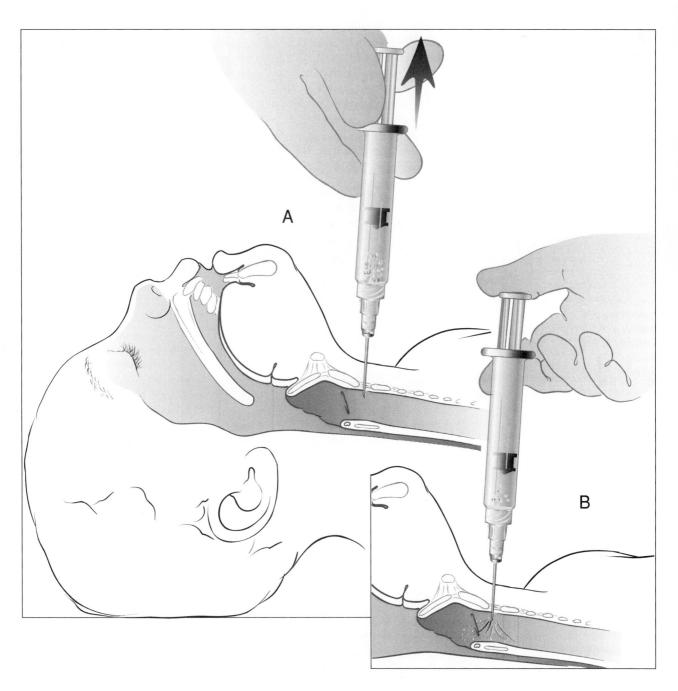

A

B

transtracheal block, negative pressure is applied to the syringe, so that entry into the trachea will be indicated by the appearance of bubbles in the fluid. When this occurs, the needle is advanced no further, and the syringe is rotated so that the needle now points cephalad. If an intravenous cannula is used, the catheter is advanced to its hub into the trachea, and the needle and syringe are removed (Fig. 16.34.B). The guide wire is then inserted through the catheter and threaded up the airway until it exits from the patient's nose or mouth. If necessary, blunt forceps can

be used to retrieve the wire from the posterior pharynx. At this point, BVM ventilation is discontinued.

After a sufficient length of wire has been withdrawn to accommodate the endotracheal tube, the caudal segment of the wire protruding from the catheter is clamped with a hemostat to secure it in place. The tube is passed over the guide wire and inserted until its tip lies in the supraglottic region (Fig. 16.34.C). The cephalad end of the wire is then pulled taut in order to provide a stable guide, and the tube is advanced into the trachea (Fig.

Figure 16.33.
Transtracheal anesthesia.
A. The needle is advanced through the cricothyroid membrane with negative pressure on the syringe. Entry into the trachea is indicated by the appearance of bubbles in the syringe.
B. Lidocaine is injected into the trachea and the needle is rapidly removed to avoid injury to the vocal cords when the patient coughs.

Figure 16.34.

Retrograde intubation.
A. The needle is inserted through the cricothyroid membrane with negative pressure on the fluid-filled syringe. Entry into the trachea is indicated by the appearance of bubbles in the fluid.
B. The needle is directed anteriorly and the needle and syringe are removed as the catheter is advanced to its hub. The guide wire is inserted through the catheter until it can be retrieved from the nose or mouth.
C. The endotracheal tube is threaded over the wire after the wire has been secured at the skin with a hemostat. The wire should be threaded through the Murphy side hole.
D. The wire is pulled taut and the tube is advanced into the trachea over the wire.
E. After successful intubation, the hemostat is removed, the wire is withdrawn through the proximal end of the tube, and the tube is advanced to the appropriate depth of insertion.

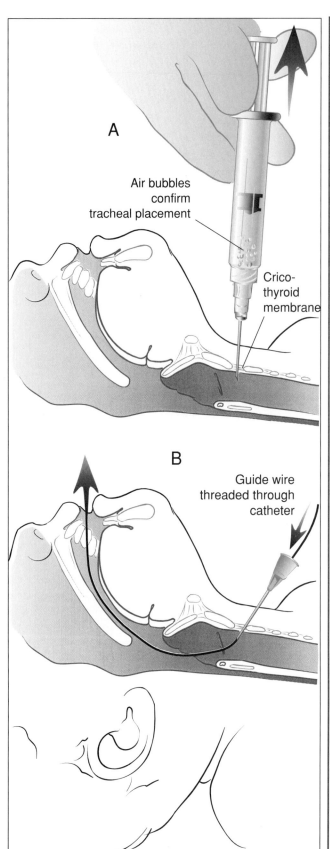

Air bubbles confirm tracheal placement

Crico-thyroid membrane

A

B

Guide wire threaded through catheter

CLINICAL TIPS: RETROGRADE INTUBATION

1. With adolescents and some older children, the laryngeal prominence (thyroid cartilage) is the first landmark used in locating the cricothyroid membrane. The operator palpates inferiorly from this point until the second "bump" of the superior margin of the cricoid cartilage is felt. The cricothyroid membrane is just cephalad to this point.

2. The laryngeal prominence is not well developed in infants and younger children and can therefore not be used as a landmark for locating the cricothyroid membrane. With these patients, it is necessary to palpate upward from the trachea until the more subtle prominence of the cricoid cartilage is located.

3. If the cricothyroid membrane cannot be located, a lower point of entry through an intercartilaginous space in the midline of the trachea can be used with additional risk to the patient.

4. The entry needle should be attached to a fluid-filled syringe so that entry into the trachea is indicated by the appearance of bubbles in the fluid.

5. It may be necessary to retrieve the guide wire from the hypopharynx using blunt forceps. If the wire is retrieved from the nose, a nasal intubation may be performed.

6. If the tube cannot be passed easily into the trachea over the wire, the tube should be withdrawn somewhat as the tension in the wire is diminished. The wire should then be pulled taut again and another attempt made. In such instances, it may also be helpful to rotate the tube 90° before reinsertion or to use a smaller tube.

7. Failure to intubate the trachea after two or three attempts with the retrograde technique indicates that another method should likely be used.

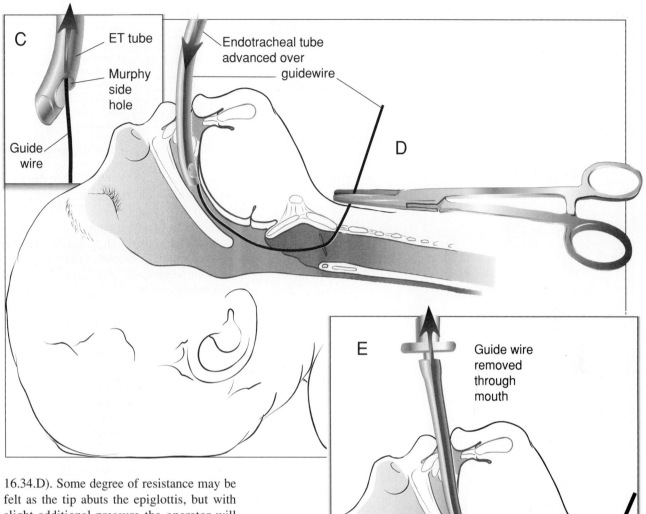

C ET tube

Murphy side hole

Guide wire

Endotracheal tube advanced over guidewire

D

E Guide wire removed through mouth

16.34.D). Some degree of resistance may be felt as the tip abuts the epiglottis, but with slight additional pressure the operator will normally feel a faint "pop" as the tube slips into the trachea. If this does not occur, it may be helpful to relax the tension on the guide wire, withdraw the endotracheal tube some-what, and then reattempt insertion. Additional maneuvers, such as rotating the tube 90° before insertion or using a smaller endotracheal tube, also may be effective. Although each attempt should normally require only a few seconds to perform, failure to intubate the trachea after two to three attempts indicates that another intubation technique should be considered.

Once the trachea is intubated, the operator releases the hemostat and then removes the guide wire by pulling it out through the cephalad end of the endotracheal tube, while taking care to maintain the position of the tube (Fig. 16.34.E). This method of removal theoretically decreases the likelihood of contaminating the airway structures with oral flora, although this has not been demonstrated in a controlled trial. Finally the endo-

tracheal tube is advanced to the appropriate depth of insertion and the catheter is removed from the skin. Proper midtracheal position of the tube is confirmed using methods described previously. As with all approaches, using excessive force to advance the tube greatly increases the risk of injury to the patient and should therefore be avoided.

Fiberoptic Nasotracheal Intubation
Improving fiberoptic technology has resulted in the manufacture of progressively smaller, flexible fiberoptic laryngoscopes, until cur-

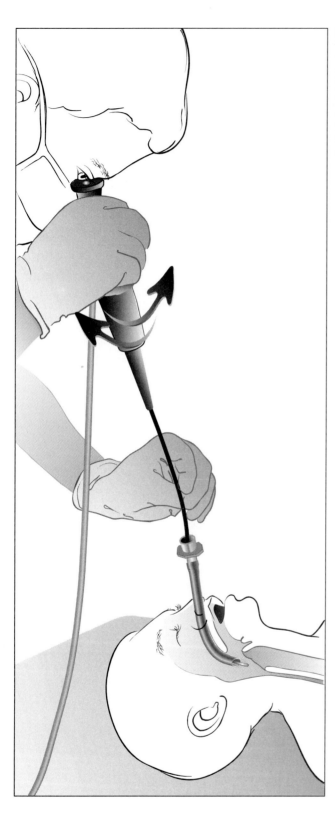

Figure 16.35.
Using this method, the endotracheal tube is first inserted until the tip reaches the supraglottic area. The fiberoptic laryngoscope is then inserted through the tube until the appropriate landmarks can be seen through the eyepiece. The trachea is then intubated as shown in Figure 16.36. This method should only be used when the nasal mucosa has been adequately prepared with a vasoconstrictor, because prior insertion of the tube will otherwise cause bleeding that may obscure visualization.

rently pediatric sizes are available that offer good illumination and high quality image resolution. The utility of this technique in the emergent setting has been demonstrated in several case series (132, 134, 139–144). Important general principles of fiberoptic laryngoscopy are described in detail in Chapter 64. Endotracheal intubation using this technique involves a few relatively straightforward modifications of these principles. Although fiberoptic intubation can be performed orally, the nasal approach greatly increases the likelihood of maintaining a midline position, which is crucial to success with this procedure (139, 140). For this reason, only the nasotracheal method is described here. It should be emphasized that fiberoptic intubation requires a high degree of skill to be used effectively and should therefore only be performed by practitioners with appropriate training and experience.

Perhaps more than any other intubation approach, fiberoptic nasotracheal intubation requires a high degree of cooperation from the patient. Proper patient selection is therefore especially important. In general, emergent fiberoptic nasotracheal intubation should be performed with a spontaneously breathing patient. A mild sedative may be administered to the awake patient to facilitate the procedure. Although it is possible to perform this procedure on an unconscious, apneic patient, this should only be attempted by a practitioner with extensive experience, since the time available to accomplish intubation is greatly diminished. Because of its effect on patient cooperation, adequate airway anesthesia is essential. As with blind nasotracheal intubation, lidocaine jelly should be instilled in both nares, so that if the laryngoscope cannot be passed on one side, an attempt can be made on the other side without waiting. The posterior pharynx should be sprayed with a topical anesthetic such as cetacaine. The operator also may choose to perform transtracheal anesthesia as described (see Retrograde Intubation). In addition, as with blind nasotracheal intubation, a topical vasoconstrictor should always be applied to the nasal mucosa 2 to 4 minutes before the procedure. Significant epistaxis is one of the most common causes of failure with fiberoptic nasotracheal intubation, because obtaining an adequate view of the larynx becomes impossible.

Next the operator should prepare the necessary equipment. The laryngoscope is tested to ensure that the tip can be easily manipulated throughout its full range of positions and that a good image is seen through the eyepiece. If the fiberoptic laryngoscope has a suction port, this should be connected to wall suction. Alternatively, many practitioners prefer using high flow oxygen through the suction port, because this can serve as an effective method for dispersing secretions or blood in the airway while at the same time delivering 100% oxygen. When adequate time is available, the operator also can immerse the tip of the endotracheal tube in warm water for a few minutes to soften it, which decreases the likelihood of injury to the nasal mucosa when the tube is inserted. If necessary, the 15 mm connector is removed so that the endotracheal tube can be passed as far as possible up the fiberoptic laryngoscope. The laryngoscope and endotracheal tube are then generously lubricated, both to facilitate passage and to allow easy removal of the laryngoscope at the appropriate time.

Depending on individual preference, the operator can stand to one side of the bed (facing superiorly toward the patient's head) or in the traditional position used for direct laryngoscopy above the head of the bed. It should be noted that the images seen through the eyepiece from one of these two positions will be inverted 180° when compared with those obtained in the other position. The patient's head and neck are maintained in a neutral position during fiberoptic laryngoscopy. One of two methods may be used for insertion of the laryngoscope and endotracheal tube. If a topical vasoconstrictor has been applied to the nasal mucosa for a sufficient length of time, the endotracheal tube may be first passed through the most patent nostril until it reaches the hypopharynx in a manner similar to a blind nasotracheal intubation. The fiberoptic laryngoscope is then inserted through the

tube and easily passed into the supraglottic region (Fig. 16.35). This method allows the endotracheal tube to serve as a guide for the laryngoscope and also to facilitate subsequent insertion of the tube into the trachea. However, if the topical vasoconstrictor has not been applied for a sufficient length of time, prior passage of the tube may cause bleeding that can greatly hinder laryngoscopy. In this situation, the narrow fiberoptic element of the laryngoscope, which is less likely to injure the nasal mucosa, is inserted into the trachea first and only then is the endotracheal tube passed. Using this method, a longer fiberoptic laryngoscope is required, because it must accommodate the endotracheal tube with sufficient length remaining to allow passage of the tip into the trachea. To perform this technique, the operator first slides the tube as far as possible up the entire length of the laryngoscope. The operator then inserts the fiberoptic element of the laryngoscope into the patient's nose until it reaches the posterior pharynx, taking care not to injure the turbinates or nasal mucosa (Fig. 16.36.A). It is important to emphasize that the laryngoscope should always be advanced under direct vision (through the eyepiece), because blind insertion will lead to mucosal

---

CLINICAL TIPS: FIBEROPTIC NASOTRACHEAL INTUBATION

1. The nasal mucosa should be prepared with a topical vasoconstrictor whenever possible 2 to 4 minutes before laryngoscopy. Epistaxis is one of the primary causes of failure for this procedure.
2. Mild sedation may be necessary to facilitate a fiberoptic nasotracheal intubation. However, spontaneous respirations and normal airway reflexes should be preserved.
3. The suction port of a fiberoptic laryngoscope may be connected to high flow oxygen. This port can then be used to "blow" secretions from the field of view while simultaneously delivering oxygen to the patient.
4. The laryngoscope should always be advanced under direct vision through the eyepiece, because blind insertion will lead to mucosal injury and bleeding.
5. If a patient has not been intubated within the first 3 minutes after initiating a fiberoptic nasotracheal intubation, the likelihood of success decreases significantly and another approach should be considered.

SUMMARY: FIBEROPTIC NASOTRACHEAL INTUBATION

1. Prepare patient
   a. Attach patient to monitoring devices
   b. Preoxygenate patient with 100% oxygen
   c. Insert gastric tube to evacuate stomach contents as necessary
   d. Apply topical anesthetic and topical vasoconstrictors to nares
   e. Perform transtracheal instillation of lidocaine (optional)
   f. Administer mild sedative as needed
2. Prepare and test the necessary equipment
   a. Check laryngoscope to see that fiberoptic tip can be manipulated through full range of positions
   b. Check eyepiece to assure good image resolution
   c. Attach laryngoscope to wall suction or high flow oxygen
   d. Generously lubricate fiberoptic strand of laryngoscope
   e. Select endotracheal tube and test balloon for any leaks
3. Check nares for patency by occluding each one in turn; if patency is equal in both nares, then right side should be used for intubation
4. Perform laryngoscopy
   a. If nasal mucosa are adequately prepared with topical vasoconstrictor, the following method may be used:
      1. Insert endotracheal tube until tip reaches posterior hypopharynx
      2. Pass fiberoptic filament of laryngoscope through endotracheal tube until it reaches supraglottic region
      3. Deflect tip of fiberoptic filament and rotate laryngoscope back and forth to obtain panoramic view of supraglottic structures
   b. If nasal mucosa cannot be adequately prepared, the following method must be used:
      1. Remove 15 mm connector from endotracheal tube if necessary
      2. Slide endotracheal tube up entire length of fiberoptic laryngoscope
      3. Insert fiberoptic filament through nose, around angle at posterior pharynx, and into supraglottic region
      4. Deflect tip of fiberoptic filament and rotate laryngoscope back and forth to obtain a panoramic view of supraglottic structures
5. Insert fiberoptic filament into tracheal to level of carina
6. Advance endotracheal tube into trachea
7. Remove laryngoscope
8. Confirm tracheal placement (equal breath sounds, no sounds over stomach, capnography)
9. Position tube at midtracheal level (see Fig. 16.18)
10. Secure endotracheal tube
11. Confirm proper tube position with chest radiograph

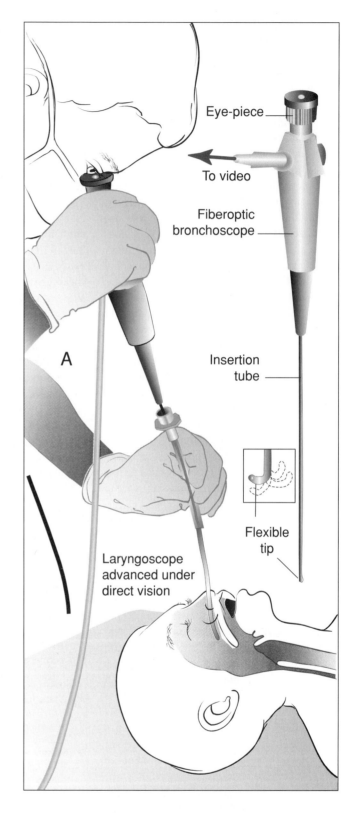

Figure 16.36.
Fiberoptic nasotracheal intubation.
A. Using this method, the endotracheal tube is first threaded up the entire length of the fiberoptic strand. The fiberoptic laryngoscope is then inserted into the nose under direct visualization through the eyepiece.

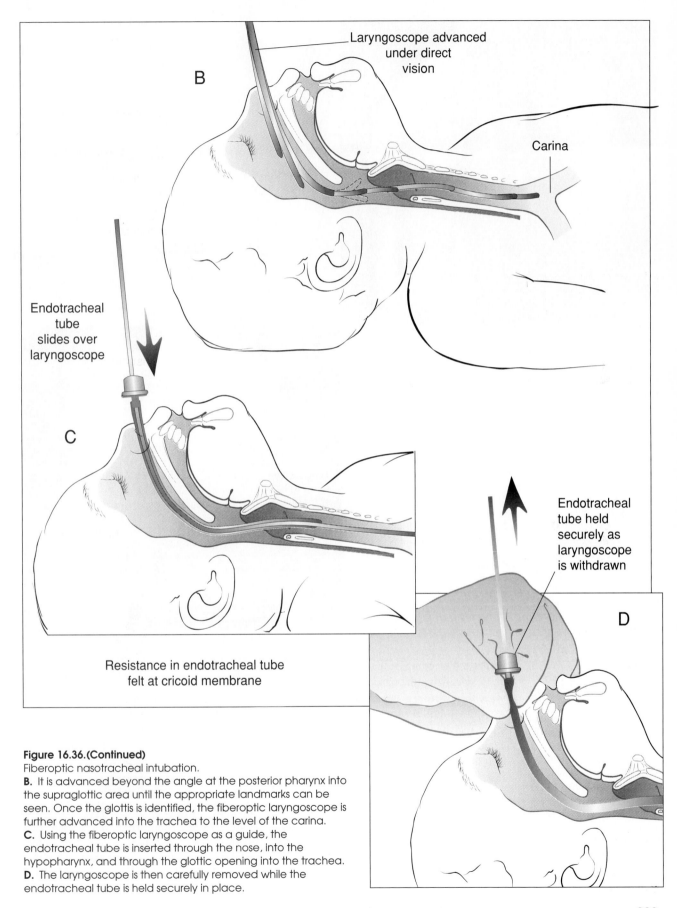

B Laryngoscope advanced under direct vision

Carina

Endotracheal tube slides over laryngoscope

C

Resistance in endotracheal tube felt at cricoid membrane

Endotracheal tube held securely as laryngoscope is withdrawn

D

Figure 16.36.(Continued)
Fiberoptic nasotracheal intubation.
B. It is advanced beyond the angle at the posterior pharynx into the supraglottic area until the appropriate landmarks can be seen. Once the glottis is identified, the fiberoptic laryngoscope is further advanced into the trachea to the level of the carina.
C. Using the fiberoptic laryngoscope as a guide, the endotracheal tube is inserted through the nose, into the hypopharynx, and through the glottic opening into the trachea.
D. The laryngoscope is then carefully removed while the endotracheal tube is held securely in place.

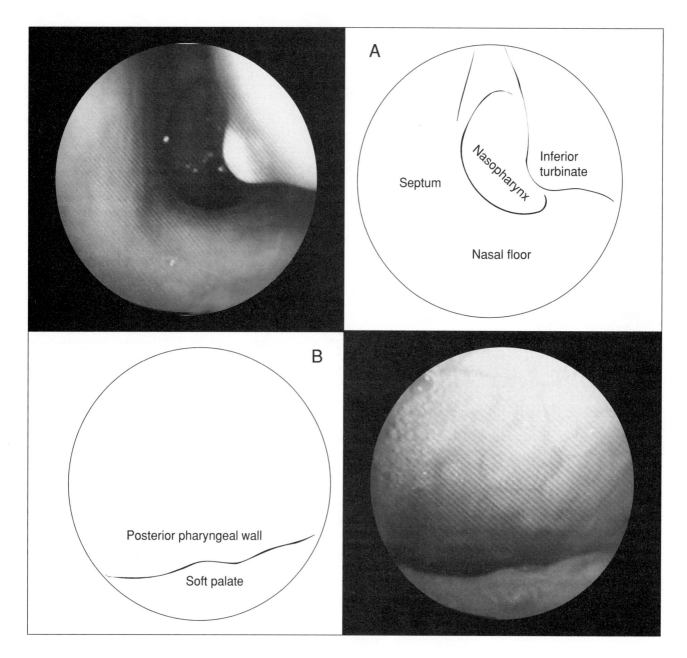

Figure 16.37.
Laryngoscopic views at various levels of the airway.
A. Nasal cavity.
B. Posterior nosopharynx.
C. Proximal oropharynx.
D. Supraglottic region.
(Photographs courtesy of Dr. Clark Rosen, University of Pittsburg School of Medicine.)

injury and bleeding. If the operator has difficulty visualizing the nasopharyngeal air passage, the fiberoptic laryngoscope should be withdrawn until a patent airway comes into view and then advanced again slowly. The angle at the posterior pharynx is then negotiated by deflecting the tip inferiorly and carefully advancing the laryngoscope into the supraglottic region.

With either of these two techniques, once the fiberoptic laryngoscope is positioned just proximal to the glottic opening, the operator should angle the tip and rotate the laryngoscope back and forth to obtain a panoramic view of the anatomic landmarks (Fig. 16.36.B). Although remarkably flexible, the fiberoptic insertion tube is designed to be stiff enough that rotation of the laryngoscope head along its axis will be translated into a similar movement of the distal tip. If the view is obscured by airway secretions or blood, the accessory portal can be used to clear the field of view by suctioning or "blowing" with high flow oxygen. Once the landmarks are identified, the tip of the fiberoptic laryngoscope is passed through the vocal cords into the trachea to the level of the carina. The trachea is recognized by its char-

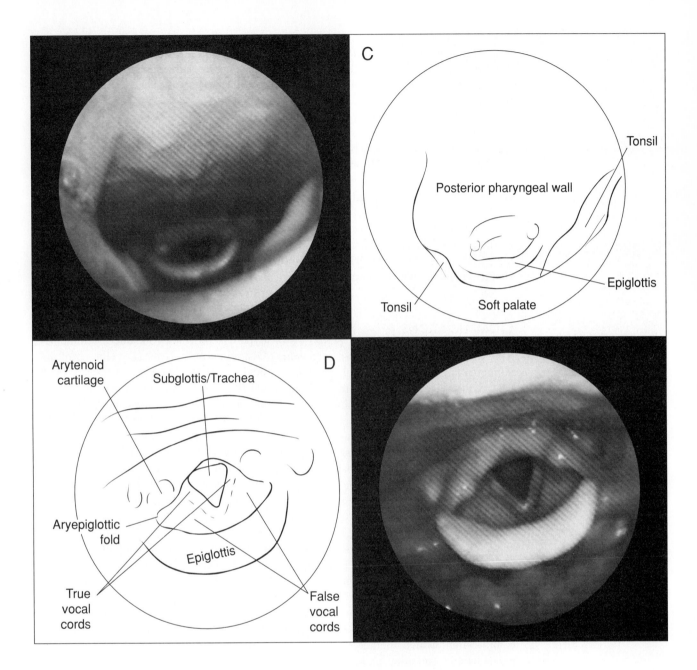

C

Tonsil

Posterior pharyngeal wall

Tonsil

Epiglottis

Soft palate

D

Arytenoid cartilage

Subglottis/Trachea

Aryepiglottic fold

Epiglottis

True vocal cords

False vocal cords

acteristic cartilaginous rings. While maintaining the position of the laryngoscope, the operator slides the endotracheal tube along the fiberoptic element through the glottic opening until resistance is felt at the cricothyroid ligament (Fig. 16.36.C). The fiberoptic laryngoscope is then carefully withdrawn as the tube is held securely in place (Fig. 16.36.D). Figure 16.37 shows the various levels of the airway as seen during fiberoptic laryngoscopy. These images were obtained during laryngoscopy performed at the patient's side, with the operator facing superiorly toward the patient's head. They are

therefore the standard anatomic views seen with an upright patient, rather than the "upside down" views of the airway seen during fiberoptic laryngoscopy performed with the operator standing above the head of the bed.

One of the greatest potential obstacles to successfully performing this procedure is inadequate patient cooperation. Even with optimal conditions, fiberoptic nasotracheal intubation requires considerable skill on the part of the primary operator; with a struggling child, it becomes virtually impossible. When necessary, intravenous sedation may be used to facilitate the procedure, although this must be done judiciously so that the patient continues to have normal respirations and airway reflexes (see Chapter 35). Another pitfall that may be encountered is difficulty in identifying the anatomic landmarks. This can be the result of bleeding from excessive secretions or vomitus, mucosal injury, or variants in airway anatomy (145). When such problems become apparent, it is generally prudent to abort the procedure rather than persist with an excessively prolonged attempt. In fact, investigators have recommended that if the patient is not intubated within the first 3 minutes after initiating a fiberoptic intubation, the likelihood of success decreases significantly and another approach should be used (141).

COMPLICATIONS

Several potential complications can occur during an emergent endotracheal intubation. Clearly the most effective way to avoid any possible risk of such complications is to refrain from attempting the procedure in the first place. This raises the question of when *not* to perform an emergent intubation. In a review of complications associated with endotracheal intubation of pediatric trauma patients, Nakayama et al. (146) contended that in over 30% of cases the procedure was not indicated on an emergent basis, because the patients had a Glasgow coma score of greater than 10 and no signs of airway compromise or apnea. The majority of these patients were intubated at the scene or in the ED of a referring hospital. Approximately one in three patients had what was considered a significant complication, which included vocal cord paralysis and aspiration pneumonitis. Certainly, an endotracheal intubation should be performed expeditiously when necessary, but if the procedure can be safely delayed until the patient is in a more controlled environment, this approach is generally advisable. Other factors that have been shown to increase the likelihood of complications include hemodynamic instability of the patient, difficult intubation, raised intracranial pressure, an unstable cervical spine, use of equipment that is inappropriate for the size of the patient, and inexperience on the part of the operator (147, 148). Because the subject of this chapter is emergent intubation, only the acute complications encountered in this clin-

ical situation are described here. Readers interested in information about long-term complications of endotracheal intubation are referred to standard pediatric anesthesiology texts.

Adverse Physiologic Effects

As described previously, primary effects of endotracheal intubation on cardiovascular physiology are the result of a combination of sympathetic discharge and vagal stimulation (see Anatomy and Physiology). These two processes have opposing physiologic effects, and the overall outcome largely depends on which reflex predominates (40, 41, 149). Patients who are not adequately anesthetized commonly experience tachyarrhythmias and hypertension from sympathetic stimulation. Occasionally patients develop profound bradycardia and hypotension because of vagal effects. Infants and younger children may be particularly susceptible to this response (40). Bradycardia also can be the result of hypoxemia during an excessively prolonged intubation attempt. The likelihood of significant bradycardia can be decreased by administering atropine before the procedure. As stated, the necessity of routinely administering atropine to all pediatric patients is somewhat controversial (150–152). However, because the bradyarrhythmias that can result are often resistant to therapy once they occur, many experts recommend pretreating all young patients who undergo intubation with atropine unless some overriding contraindication exists (e.g., mitral stenosis, coronary artery disease, or preexisting tachyarrhythmia).

Another immediate adverse physiologic effect of endotracheal intubation is increased intracranial pressure. Exactly why this occurs is not well understood, although it is likely due in part to a combination of elevated cerebral venous pressure (coughing, straining, changes in head position) and increased cerebral arterial pressure from the systemic hypertension that occurs during laryngoscopy (153–155). This effect normally has clinical significance only when preexisting elevated intracranial pressure is exacerbated (ruptured cerebral aneurysm, epidural hematoma, etc.). In extreme cases, development of a cerebral herniation syndrome is possible. When the patient is at risk for these complications, pharmacologic agents that blunt the rise in intracranial pressure should be administered (see Chapter 15). Patients also develop elevated intraocular pressure during endotracheal intubation (156–158). This effect is similar to what is observed with the use of intravenous succinylcholine, although more pronounced. For normal children, and even for those with glaucoma, the rise in intraocular pressure during intubation is normally inconsequential. However, serious damage to the eye can result if the patient has an open globe injury. In a study of 40 children undergoing eye surgery, Drenger et al. (158) found that intravenous lidocaine (2 mg/kg) significantly attenuated the rise in intraocular pressure that occurred during endotracheal intubation. For this reason, many authorities recommend routinely using lidocaine before intubation of patients at risk for this complication.

Inadequate Oxygenation

One of the most significant complications of endotracheal intubation is ischemic brain injury due to inadequate oxygenation. This can result from any of the following causes: (*a*) inability to provide adequate bag-valve-mask ventilatory support, (*b*) excessively prolonged laryngoscopy, (*c*) unrecognized esophageal intubation, (*d*) endobronchial intubation, (*e*) obstruction of the endotracheal tube, and (*f*) pneumothorax. While a persistent episode of laryngospasm also can prevent oxygenation during laryngoscopy, this complication is rare when anesthetic agents are not used. In most cases, laryngospasm is transient and subsides spontaneously after several seconds. Should prolonged laryngospasm occur, administration of intravenous succinylcholine (0.5 to 2 mg/kg) is universally effective in relaxing the vocal cords. Atropine (0.02 mg/kg, minimum dose 0.1 mg) should be routinely administered before succinylcholine to avoid potential bradyarrhythmias from this agent, which are more likely with preexisting hypoxemia. Esophageal intubation can result either from inadvertent insertion of the endotracheal tube into the esophagus or from subsequent movement of the patient's head which dislodges the tube from the trachea. This can normally be recognized before any injury to the patient occurs with the use of pulse oximetry (Chapter 77) and capnography (Chapter 78). Capnography is the superior modality for identifying esophageal intubation, because the capnograph will immediately display an abnormally low or absent CO_2 level (92, 94–96). By the time pulse oximetry indicates a drop in oxygen saturation, several ventilatory cycles have gone unattended, and the patient may have significant desaturation before the situation can be corrected. As mentioned previously, the most effective way to avoid an esophageal intubation is to directly observe the tube passing between the vocal cords and into the trachea whenever this is possible.

Another potential cause of inadequate oxygenation is insertion of the endotracheal tube into a mainstem bronchus. This can result from advancing the tube too far into the trachea during intubation, inadequately securing the tube, or from movement of the patient's head (159–162). Interestingly, although endobronchial intubation almost always occurs on the right side, inadvertent left mainstem intubation has been reported as a complication of tactile intubation in adults (163). After endotracheal intubation is performed, a chest radiograph should always be obtained to assess the location of the tube within the trachea. The tip of the endotracheal tube should lie halfway between the thoracic inlet and the carina. Should an endobronchial intubation occur, the patient will normally have a persistently low oxygen saturation measured by the pulse oximeter. A sudden rise in inspiratory pressures also may be necessary to expand the chest, as evidenced by greater difficulty performing manual ventilation or the necessity for higher peak inflating pressures from a mechanical ventilator. This complication is best avoided by performing serial auscultatory examinations of the chest to ensure that equal breath sounds are heard. This is particularly important when monitoring modalities are not available, as in field settings or during transport. Simple observation of the patient is not sufficient, because chest excursion may appear symmetric despite endobronchial intubation. If this problem is suspected, the patient's head should be repositioned or the endotracheal tube should be withdrawn until equal breath sounds are heard in both lungs.

Impaired oxygenation also occurs when

the endotracheal tube becomes partially obstructed. With infants, this may occur acutely when the tip of the tube abuts against the tracheal wall. Brasch et al. (164) found that the likelihood of this complication is increased when the infant's head is turned to one side and the bevel of the tube faces the opposite direction. Mean pulmonary resistance was found to be 4 times greater than normal in these patients. Thus when an infant shows signs suggesting the endotracheal tube is obstructed, the only measure necessary may be simply to reposition the head. Obstruction of the endotracheal tube from airway secretions is far more common, although this usually occurs after longer periods of intubation. Redding et al. (165) found in a consecutive series of endotracheal tubes removed from 81 pediatric patients that the incidence of partial obstruction from airway secretions was approximately 20%. Obstruction was not found to correlate with either duration of intubation, the presence of a Murphy side hole, or small tube size. The most important factor for avoiding obstruction was believed to be humidification of inspired gases. Suctioning the endotracheal tube is normally sufficient to relieve a partial obstruction resulting from airway secretions. Instillation of saline before suctioning also may be helpful. However, if the patient continues to have increased pulmonary resistance that cannot be explained by other factors, the endotracheal tube should be replaced.

Barotrauma

Pediatric patients are at greater risk than adults for sustaining barotrauma to the lungs from positive pressure ventilation (166–168), primarily because infants and children have greater compliance of the ribs and chest wall musculature. The relatively diminished protective effects of chest wall resistance result in a greater likelihood for pulmonary overinflation and lung injury. Risk is further increased for children with an underlying lung disease such as cystic fibrosis or congenital lobar emphysema (169). Complications from barotrauma which are normally minor include pneumomediastinum, subcutaneous emphysema, and pneumopericardium. These are usually self-limited processes that do not generally require intervention. In rare cases,

pneumopericardium can cause cardiac tamponade, necessitating emergent decompression. Complications from barotrauma more commonly associated with significant morbidity are pneumothorax and tension pneumothorax. When the peak pressure within the lungs reaches a sufficiently high level, the alveolar wall may rupture. Gas dissects along a perivascular sheath into the mediastinum and from there through the visceral pleura into the pleural space. Tube thoracostomy should be performed whenever a patient receiving positive pressure ventilations develops a pneumothorax. If a pneumothorax is not promptly recognized and treated appropriately in this setting, the patient is at increased risk for developing a tension pneumothorax, a potentially life-threatening complication. Positive pressure ventilation in the presence of a pneumothorax produces a ball-valve effect when air moving in a one-way direction out of the injured lung and into the thoracic cavity results in a progressive increase in pressure. The mediastinal structures are shifted away from the affected side, eventually causing a precipitous drop in blood pressure when venous return to heart is impaired as a result of deformation and compression of the vena cava. As mentioned previously, the characteristic findings of a tension pneumothorax include a tympanitic hemithorax with diminished breath sounds, hypotension, and deviation of the trachea. Management of pneumothorax and tension pneumothorax is described fully in Chapter 30.

Mechanical Trauma

The most common type of complication resulting from endotracheal intubation is mechanical trauma. Because the procedure involves relatively forceful manipulation and instrumentation of various structures of the head and neck, a wide array of injuries can occur, ranging from minor abrasions to potentially life-threatening hemorrhage. Although sometimes unavoidable, this type of complication can normally be minimized if the operator maintains a high degree of awareness and employs careful technique.

A relatively minor injury that can result during an intubation is corneal abrasion. Even such seemingly trivial actions as leaning a forearm against the patient's brow to steady the hand or inadvertently sweeping a sleeve over the patient's face can cause a corneal abrasion. Vigilance regarding the possibility of this complication is generally the most effective way of avoiding it. If the patient is unconscious, the eyelids should be taped shut after the airway is secured so that subsequent injury to the eyes does not occur.

The teeth of older children (or the alveolar ridge of infants) also may be injured during an intubation. This usually results when the laryngoscope blade is used to lever the mouth open, with the teeth or gingiva serving as a fulcrum. Obviously this practice must be carefully avoided. Significant trauma to the gingiva of an infant can lead to abnormal tooth eruption and/or dental development (170). If a tooth is accidentally avulsed during intubation, it should be immediately retrieved to prevent aspiration of the tooth into the trachea. A "lost" tooth may well be found later on chest radiograph in a bronchus.

A potentially serious complication resulting from mechanical forces is airway bleeding, which usually results from injury to the nasal turbinates, adenoids, or palatine tonsils (148). Mucosal surfaces of these structures may be abraded by the laryngoscope blade or endotracheal tube, and if subjected to sufficient force, adenoids and palatine tonsils can be partially or completely avulsed. Such tissue avulsions can result in airway obstruction and bleeding. Significant epistaxis may occur with blind nasotracheal intubation (113–115) and fiberoptic nasotracheal intubation (140, 141, 145). Direct laryngoscopy during an orotracheal intubation may result in injury to the tonsils. Percutaneous puncture of the cricothyroid membrane to perform transtracheal anesthesia or retrograde intubation also can cause bleeding in the airway (129). Although in most cases these are minor problems representing more of a temporary impediment to the procedure than a danger to the patient, a child with hemophilia or an acquired coagulopathy can develop extensive and potentially life-threatening airway bleeding or obstruction due to a hematoma (171, 172). Any child with a clinically significant bleeding disorder should obviously undergo intubation in the least traumatic manner possible. Approaches such as blind nasotracheal intubation and fiberoptic nasotracheal intubation would be inadvisable. If bleeding is extensive and persistent, the airway should be secured as rapidly as possible, and an otolaryngologist should be urgently consulted to evaluate the patient.

Other soft tissue injuries resulting from the mechanical effects of endotracheal intubation may involve the lips, tongue, retropharynx, epiglottis, arytenoids, trachea, and esophagus (148,175-178). Indeed, virtually any airway structure above the bronchi can be traumatized. Hematoma and subcutaneous emphysema of the anterior neck can occur with percutaneous puncture of the cricothyroid membrane during retrograde intubation. The epiglottis and arytenoid cartilages can be abraded by the laryngoscope blade, particularly if the blade is first inserted into the esophagus and then withdrawn. Insertion of the endotracheal tube has been associated with a wide variety of complications, including dislocation of the arytenoids and perforation of the retropharynx, trachea, and epiglottis. Laceration injuries are particularly common when the tip of a stylet improperly extends beyond the end of the tube. Although smaller than an endotracheal tube, a fiberoptic laryngoscope can cause similar injuries during insertion. Arytenoid subluxation and dislocation have been reported in adults during lighted stylet intubation (177). Once again, the overzealous use of force in performing laryngoscopy or advancing the tube is generally to blame for this type of complication.

Aspiration Pneumonitis

Pediatric patients who undergo emergent endotracheal intubation are likely to have one or more of the following primary risk factors for aspiration of gastric contents into the lungs: a decreased level of consciousness, a diminished or absent gag reflex, and/or a full stomach. A full stomach state exists when the patient has had a recent meal, has an intestinal obstruction, or has some process causing decreased gastric motility (increased intracranial pressure, extreme pain, pregnancy, etc.). The severity of resulting lung injury is related to the acidity and volume of the aspirate and the amount of particulate matter aspirated (101). Clinical consequences of aspiration can have a wide range of manifestations, including no detectable effect, a self-limited pneumonitis, significant hypoxemia, bacterial pneumonia, and in more severe cases, lung abscess formation and the development of ARDS (102). Although possible after intubation is successfully accomplished, aspiration is far more likely to occur during the actual procedure, when instrumentation causes vomiting before the airway is protected. In a prospective study of 50 infants and children, Goitein et al. (178) found that among patients who showed no signs of aspiration after intubation was initially performed, only three demonstrated evidence of a significant aspiration event before extubation. Several steps can be taken to reduce the incidence of aspiration during an emergent intubation. Prior insertion of a gastric tube evacuates much of the stomach contents, and therefore the likelihood that the patient will vomit during the procedure is decreased. If a rapid sequence induction is performed, the patient with spontaneous respirations patient should not receive manual ventilation until after successful intubation, so that vomiting is not induced by forced air entry into the stomach. Preoxygenation is performed by allowing the patient to breath 100% by mask before administration of neuromuscular blocking agents (see Chapter 15). Aspiration also is less likely to occur when cricoid pressure (Sellick's maneuver) is performed (103–107). Salem et al. (107) demonstrated in a study of postmortem infants that cricoid pressure was effective in preventing reflux of gastric contents even in the presence of elevated intragastric and intraesophageal pressures. Unless contraindicated, this technique is recommended for all children with an impaired or absent gag reflex who undergo emergent endotracheal intubation.

Pulmonary Edema

A relatively unusual but physiologically interesting complication of endotracheal intubation in pediatric patients is acute pulmonary edema that occurs after relief of extrathoracic airway obstruction (179–183). Children with severe croup, epiglottitis, or other causes of airway obstruction who undergo intubation may develop the typical clinical signs of pulmonary edema—frothy secretions, diffuse alveolar densities on chest radiograph, and hypoxemia. This complica-

tion also can occur when a child bites down on an endotracheal tube already in place, resulting in transient complete airway obstruction. The pathogenesis of this process remains poorly understood, although it is likely due in part to increased hydrostatic pressure in the lungs during labored respirations causing a rapid influx of interstitial fluid. If a child is intubated without using a paralytic agent, the operator should insert a bite block when appropriate to prevent occlusion of the endotracheal tube. Furthermore, any pediatric patient with a known cause of significant airway obstruction who requires intubation should be considered at risk for developing acute pulmonary edema. In most cases, manifestations of this complication are relatively mild, and basic supportive measures (e.g., increased supplemental oxygen delivery and positive end-expiratory pressure) are generally the only interventions necessary.

Cervical Cord Injury

Perhaps the most intensively studied complication of endotracheal intubation is exacerbation of spinal cord trauma in the patient with an unstable cervical spine (184–192). The best approach to airway management for these patients remains highly controversial. Some practitioners believe that orotracheal intubation has proven to be a safe procedure even in the presence of a cervical spine injury. They cite the experience with thousands of patients managed at major trauma centers who have shown no demonstrable evidence of worsened neurologic outcome among patients with cervical spine injuries after orotracheal intubation. Many authorities contend that the most important source of morbidity for such patients is ischemic brain injury as a result of inadequate airway intervention resulting from a misplaced overemphasis on protecting the cervical cord. Others believe that the maneuvers involved with an orotracheal intubation represent a significant risk for causing neurologic injury in the patient with a potentially unstable cervical spine. This view is based primarily on cadaver studies which show that even with in-line stabilization, distraction and subluxation at the site of injury can occur. Some practitioners recommend using airway interventions that minimize movement of the neck, such as blind nasotracheal intubation, awake fiberoptic intubation, digital intubation, retrograde intubation, or a surgical airway.

The possibility of exacerbating a cord injury during intubation is fortunately less of a concern with pediatric patients compared with adults, because the incidence of unstable cervical spine fractures among infants and children is low. In a retrospective study of 2133 pediatric patients who had cervical spine radiographs, Rachesky et al. (193) found that only 1.7% had a radiographic abnormality. Lally et al. (10) found that during a 36-month period at the Children's Hospital of Los Angeles only one child had a confirmed cervical spine fracture. Nevertheless, the relative rarity of cervical spine injuries among pediatric patients does not make the question of how best to manage this presentation an easy one. In the absence of any definitive case series on the safety of conventional orotracheal intubation for the patient with an unstable cervical spine injury, it would seem most prudent to intubate the patient using the least traumatic approach that the operator is capable of performing. If the operator is proficient with an alternative intubation technique that minimizes movement of the patient's neck, then making an attempt using that method would be a logical approach. Conversely, if a patient with a potentially unstable cervical spine requires immediate intubation, and the operator is competent only with conventional orotracheal intubation, then this method should be used with appropriate caution. In this case, an assistant should maintain in-line stabilization as described previously and movement of the neck must be minimized. Above all, the perceived threat of injury to the cervical cord in a pediatric trauma patient must not take precedence over the very real need to provide adequate airway and ventilatory support.

SUMMARY

Emergent endotracheal intubation of pediatric patients presents a unique set of challenges and rewards. Unlike adults, children are often unable to cooperate with the procedure out of fear or lack of understanding. The confined spaces, relatively large tongue, and small mandible can test the skill of even the most experienced practitioner. Furthermore,

an emergent intubation allows the operator much less time for preparation than an elective intubation, because respiratory decompensation (or for that matter, the arrival of the patient at the hospital) may occur with very little warning. This leads to a greater degree of urgency and more restrictive time constraints. However, despite these obstacles, few accomplishments are more gratifying in medical practice than a successful intubation that preserves the life of a child.

Emergent endotracheal intubation is an invasive procedure associated with several potential complications. The operator must be knowledgeable about appropriate indications for emergent intubation, because the best way to avoid complications is to perform the procedure only when truly necessary. Optimal management may involve transferring the patient to a more controlled environment before intubation is attempted. Unfortunately, relatively few easily defined rules are available for deciding when an emergent intubation should be performed. Laboratory tests and imaging techniques consume valuable time and seldom provide a definitive answer. The most important determining factor generally proves to be the experience and judgment of the practitioner in evaluating the condition of the patient. Considering the number and potential severity of the complications associated with this procedure, it is in fact surprising that they are not encountered more frequently in clinical practice. In reality, when endotracheal intubation is performed in an appropriate setting using proper technique, significant complications can normally be avoided.

Certainly the most dreaded circumstance occurs when the patient cannot be intubated and BVM ventilation is not adequately effective. This represents a worst case scenario in which a surgical airway, with all the attendant risks of that procedure, must then be attempted. The most effective way to avoid such an unwelcome situation is to develop skills in performing at least one other intubation technique, so that failure with one approach can be quickly followed by success with another. Although conventional orotracheal intubation is by far the most commonly used method, alternative approaches such as those described in this chapter may prove invaluable in a difficult situation. Although it is by no means necessary to become adept at all these additional techniques, the resourceful practitioner will always have another "arrow in the quiver" when orotracheal intubation is unsuccessful.

REFERENCES

1. Motoyama E. Endotracheal intubation. In: Motoyama EK, Davis PJ, eds. Smith's anesthesia for infants and children. 5th ed. St. Louis: Mosby, 1990, p. 276.
2. Sasaki CT, Levine PA, Laitman JT, et al. Postnatal descent of the epiglottis in man. Arch Otolaryngol 1977;103:169.
3. Cote CJ, Todres ID. The pediatric airway. In: Cote CJ, Ryan JF, Todres ID, et al. (eds) A practice of anesthesia for infants and children. 2nd ed. Philadelphia: WB Saunders, 1993.
4. Morgan GAR, Steward DJ. Linear airway dimensions in children: including those with cleft palate. Can Anaesth Soc J 1982;29:1.
5. Eckenhoff J. Some anatomic considerations of the infant's larynx, influencing endotracheal anesthesia. Anesthesiology 1951;12: 401.
6. Boyden EA, Tompsett DH. The changing patterns in the developing lungs of infants. Acta Anat (Basel) 1965;61:164.
7. Dunnill MS. Postnatal growth of the lung. Thorax 1962;17:329.
8. Macklem PT: Airway obstruction and collateral ventilation. Physiol Rev 1971;51:368.
9. Bohn D, Armstrong D, Becker L, Humphreys R. Cervical spine injuries in children. J Trauma 1990;30:463.
10. Lally KP, Senac M, Hardin WE, et al. Utility of the cervical spine radiograph in pediatric trauma. Am J Surg 1989;158:540.
11. Pang D, Wilberger JE. Spinal cord injury without radiographic abnormalities in children. J Neurosurg 1982;57:114.
12. Mansell A, Bryan C, Levinson H. Airway closure in children. J Appl Physiol 1972;33: 711.
13. Anthonisen NR, Danson J, Robertson PC, et al. Airway closure as a function of age. Respir Physiol 1969;8:58.
14. Polgar G. Airway resistance in the newborn infant. J Pediatr 1961;59:915.
15. Wilson TG: Stridor in infancy. J Laryngol Otol 1952;66:437.
16. Wittenborg MH, Gyepes MT, Crocker D. Tracheal dynamics in infants with respiratory distress, stridor, and collapsing trachea. Radiology 1967;88:653.
17. Fearon B, Whalen JS. Tracheal dimensions in the living infant (preliminary report). Ann Otol Rhinol Laryngol 1967;76:965.
18. Maze A, Bloch E. Stridor in pediatric patients. Anesthesiology 1979;50:132.
19. Lazoritz S, Saunders BS, Bason WM. Man-
agement of acute epiglottitis. Crit Care Med 1979;7:285.
20. Schloss MD, Hannallah R, Baxter JD. Acute epiglottitis: 26 years' experience at the Montreal Children's Hospital. J Otolaryngol 1979;8:259.
21. Davis HW, Gartner JC, Galvis AG, et al. Acute upper airway obstruction: croup and epiglottitis. Pediatr Clin North Am 1981;28: 859.
22. Baker SR. Laryngotracheobronchitis—a continuing challenge in child health care. J Otolaryngol 1979;8:494.
23. Cohen SR, Herbert WI, Lewis Jr, GB et al. Foreign bodies in the airway: five-year retrospective study with special reference to management. Ann Otol Rhinol Laryngol 1980;89:437.
24. Stark DCC, Biller HF. Aspiration of foreign bodies: diagnosis and management. Int Anesthesiol Clin 1977;15:117.
25. Mustard WT, Bayliss CE, Fearon B, et al. Tracheal compression by the innominate artery in children. Ann Thorac Surg 1969;8: 312.
26. Bryan AC, Mansell AL, Levison H. Development of the mechanical properties of the respiratory system. In: Hodson WA, ed. Development of the lung. New York: Marcel Dekker 1976;445.
27. Guslits BG, Gaston SE, Bryan MH, England SJ, Bryan AC. Diaphragmatic work of breathing in premature human infants. J Appl Physiol 1987;62:1410.
28. Keens TG, Bryan AC, Levison H, et al. Developmental pattern of muscle fiber types in human ventilatory muscles. J Appl Physiol 1978;44:909.
29. Keens TG, Lanuzzo CD. Development of fatigue-resistant muscle fibers in human ventilatory muscles. Am Rev Respir Dis 1979;(Suppl 119)2:139.
30. Keens TG, Chen V, Patel P, et al. Cellular adaptations of the ventilatory muscles to a chronic increased respiratory load. J Appl Physiol 1978;44:905.
31. Fenner A, Schalk U, Hoenicke H, et al. Periodic breathing in premature and neonatal babies: incidence, breathing pattern, respiratory gas tensions, response to changes in the composition of ambient air. Pediatr Res 1973;7:174.
32. Spitzer AR, Fox WW. Infant apnea. Clin Pediatr 1984;23:374.
33. Rigatto H, Kalapesi Z, Leahy FN, et al. Ventilatory response to 100% and 15% O_2 during wakefulness and sleep in preterm infants. Early Hum Dev 1982;7:1.
34. Frantz III ID, Adler SM, Thach BT, et al. Maturational effects on respiratory responses to carbon dioxide in premature infants. J Appl Physiol 1976;41:634.
35. Brady JP, Ceruit E. Chemoreceptor reflexes in the newborn infant. Effects of varying de-

grees of hypoxia on heart rate and ventilation in a warm environment. J Physiol (London) 1966;184:631.

36. Rigatto H. Apnea and periodic breathing. Semin Perinatol 1977;4:375.

37. Shanon DC, Kelly DH, O'Connor KG. Abnormal regulation of ventilation in infants at risk for sudden infant death syndrome. N Eng J Med 1977;297:747.

38. Hunt CE, McCullough K, Brovillette RT. Diminished hypoxic ventilatory response in near-miss sudden infant death syndrome. J Appl Physiol 1981;50:1313.

39. Unna KR, Glaser K, Lipton EL, Patterson PR. Dosage of drugs in infants and children. I. Atropine. Pediatrics 1950;6:197.

40. Lipton EL, Steinschneider A, Richmond JB. The autonomic nervous system in early life. N Eng J Med 1965;273:147.

41. Codero Jr L, Hon EH. Neonatal bradycardia following nasopharyngeal stimulation. J Pediatr 1971;78:441.

42. Marshall TA, Deeder R, Pai S, et al. Physiologic changes associated with endotracheal intubation in preterm infants. Crit Care Med 1984;12:501.

43. Hawkins J, Van Hare GF, Schmidt KG, Rudolph AM. Effects of increasing afterload on left ventricular output in fetal lambs. Circ Res 1989;65:127.

44. Van Hare GF, Jawkins JA, Schmidt KG, Rudolph AM. The effects of increasing mean arterial pressure on left venticular output in newborn lambs. Circ Res 1990;67:78.

45. Holinger LD. Etiology of stridor in the neonate, infant, and child. Ann Otol 1980;89:397.

46. Backofen JE, Rogers MC. Upper airway disease. In: Rogers MC, ed. Textbook of pediatric intensive care. 2nd ed. Baltimore: Williams & Wilkins, 1992, p. 234.

47. Jones R, Santos JI, Overall JC. Bacterial tracheitis. JAMA 1979;242:721.

48. Kasian GF, Bingham WT, Steinberg J. et al. Bacterial tracheitis in children. Can Med Assoc J 1989;140:46.

49. Bryce DP. Current management of laryngotracheal injury. Adv Otorhinolaryngol 1983; 29:27.

50. Cohn AM, Larson DL. Laryngeal injury. Arch Otolaryngol 1976;102:166.

51. Dalal FY, Schmidt GB, Bennett EJ, Levitsky S. Fractures of the larynx in children. Can Anaesth Soc J 1974;21:376.

52. Mahour GH, Lynn HB, Sanderson DR. Rupture of the bronchus. J Pediatr Surg 1967;2:263.

53. Nakayama DK, Rowe MI. Intrathoracic tracheobronchial injuries in childhood. Int Anesthesiol Clin 1988;26:42.

54. Fein A, Leff A, Hopewell PC: Pathophysiology and management of the complications resulting from fire and the inhaled products of combustion: review of the literature. Crit Care Med 1980;8:94.

55. Vivori E, Cudmore RE. Management of airway complications of burns in children. Br Med J 1977;2:1462.

56. Kosloske AM. Bronchoscopic extraction of aspirated foreign bodies in children. Am J Dis Child 1982;136:924.

57. Rothmann BF, Boeckman CR. Foreign bodies in the larynx and tracheobronchial tree in children—a review of 225 cases. Ann Otol 1980;89:434.

58. Brudno DS, Parker DH, Slaton G. Response of pulmonary mechanics to terbutaline in patients with bronchopulmonary dysplasia. Am J Med Sci 1989;297:166.

59. Wilkie RA, Bryan MH. Effect of bronchodilators on airway resistance in ventilator-dependent neonates with chronic lung disease. J Pediatr 1987;111:278.

60. Helfaer MA, Nichols DG, Chantarojanasiri T, Roger MC. Lower airway disease: bronchiolitis and asthma. In: Rogers MC, ed. Textbook of pediatric intensive care. 2nd ed. Baltimore: Williams & Wilkins, 1992, p. 258.

61. Stempel DA, Mellon M. Management of acute severe asthma. Ped Clin North Am 1984;31:879.

62. Bierman CW, Pierson WE, Shapiro GG. Treatment of status asthmaticus in children. South Med J 1975;68:1556.

63. Wood DW, Downes JJ, Lecks HI. The management of respiratory failure in childhood status asthmaticus. Experience with 30 episodes and evolution of a technique. J Allergy 1968;42:261.

64. Schulaner FA, Mattikoiw MS. Treatment of status asthmaticus: bronchial asthma. Part III. J Med Soc N J 1980;77:501.

65. Petty TL. Oxygen and mechanical ventilation in status asthmaticus. In: Weiss EB, ed. Status asthmaticus. Baltimore: University Park Press, 1978, p. 285.

66. Rice TB, Torres Jr. A. Pneumonitis and interstitial disease. In: Fuhrman BP, Zimmerman JJ, eds. Pediatric critical care. St. Louis: Mosby, 1992, p. 465.

67. Murphy S, Florman AL. Lung defenses against infection: a clinical correlation. Pediatrics 1983;72:1.

68. Moritz AR, Henriques FC, McLean R. The effects of inhaled heat on air passages and lungs: an experimental investigation. Am J Pathol 1945;21:311.

69. Trunkey KK: Inhalational injury. Surg Clin North Am 1978;58:1133.

70. McCarthy PL, Spiesel SZ, Stashwick CA, et al. Radiographic findings and etiology in ambulatory childhood pneumonias. Clin Pediatr 1981;20:686.

71. Riordan JF, Walters G. Pulmonary edema in bacterial shock. 1968;Lancet 1:719.

72. Klein JJ, Haeringen JR, Slinter HJ, et al. Pulmonary function after recovery from adult respiratory distress syndrome. Chest 1976;69:350.

73. Rochester DF, Arora NS. Respiratory muscle failure. Med Clin North Am 1983;67:573.

74. Blesa MI, Lahiri S, Rashkind WJ, et al. Normalization of the blunted ventialtory response to acute hypoxia in congenital cyanotic heart disease, N Eng J Med 1977;296:237.

75. Garg M, Kurzner Si, Bautista D, et al. Hypoxic arousal responses in infants with bronchopulmonary dysplasia, Pediatrics 1988;82:59.

76. Kanter RK. Control of breathing and acute respiratory failure. In: Fuhrman BP, Zimmerman JJ, eds. Pediatric critical care, St. Louis: Mosby, 1992, p. 515.

77. Kewaltramani LS, Tori JA. Spinal cord trauma in children. Neurologic patterns, radiologic features, and pathomechanics of injury. Spine 1980;5:11.

78. Weinstein L. Tetanus. N Engl J Med 1973;289:1293.

79. Alfrey D, Rauscher A: Tetanus. a review. Crit Care Med 1979;7:176..

80. Feigin RD, Guggenheim MA, Johnsen SD. Vaccine-related paralytic poliomyelitis in an immunodeficient child. J Pediatr 1971;79:642.

81. Moore P, James O. Guillain-Barre syndrome: incidence, management and outcome of major complications. Crit Care Med 1981;9:549.

82. Menkes JH. Diseases of the motor unit. In: Menkes JH. Textbook of child neurology. Philadelphia: Lea & Febiger 1975, p. 463.

83. Sellin LC. The action of botulism toxin at the neuromuscular junction. Med Biol 1981;59:11.

84. Johnson RO, Clay SA, Arnon SS. Diagnosis and management of infant botulism. Am J Dis Child 1979;133:586.

85. Long SS, Gajewski JL, Brown LW, Gilligan PH. Clinical, laboratory and environmental features of infant botulism in southeastern Pennsylvania. Pediatrics 1985;75:935.

86. Thompson JA, Glasgow LA, Warpinski JR, Olson C. Infant botulism: clinical spectrum and epidemiology. Pediatrics 1980;66:936.

87. Eisenberg M, Berginer L, Hallstrom A. Epidemiology of cardiac arrest and resuscitation in children. Ann Emerg Med 1983;12:672.

88. Ward Jr JT. Endotracheal drug therapy. Am J Emerg Med 1983;1:71.

89. Ward ME, Roussos C. The respiratory muscles in shock: service or disservice? Int Crit Care Diag 1985;4:3.

90. Rose DK, Byrick RJ, Froese AB. Carbon dioxide elimination during spontaneous ventilation with a modified Mapleson D system: studies in a lung model. Can Anaesth Soc J 1978;25:353.

91. Bishop MJ, Wegmeller EA, Fink BR. Laryngeal effects of prolonged intubation. Anaesth Analg 1984;63:335.

92. Linko K, Paloheimo M, Tammisto T. Capnography for detection of accidental oesophageal intubation. Acta Anaesthesiol Scand 1983;27:199.

93. Kagle DM, Alexander CM, Berko RS, et al. Evaluation of the Ohmeda Biox 3700 pulse oximeter: steady state and transient response characteristics. Anesthesiology 1987;66:376.

94. Rosenberg M, Block CS. A simple, disposable end-tidal carbon dioxide detector. Anesth Prog 1991;38:24.

95. Ko FY, Hsieh KS, Yu CK. Detection of airway CO2 partial pressure to avoid esophageal intubation. Acta Paediatr Sin 1993;34:91.

96. White RD, Asplin BR. Out-of-hospital quantitative monitoring of end-tidal carbon dioxide pressure during CPR. Ann Emerg Med 1994;23:25.

97. Patel R, Lenczyk M, Hannallah RS, McGill WA. Age and the onset of desaturation in apnoeic children. Can J Anaesth 1994;41:771.

98. Videira RL, Neto PP, do Amaral RV, Freeman JA. Preoxygenation in children: for how long? Acta Anaesthesiol Scand 1992;36:109.

99. Khoo ST, Woo M, Kumar A. An assessment of preoxygenation techniques using the pulse oximeter. Ann Acad Med 1992;21:705.

100. Xue FS, Tong SY, Wang XL, Deng XM. Study of the optimal duration of preoxygenation in children. J Clin Anesth 1995;7:93.

101. Hupp JR, Peterson LJ: Aspiration pneumonitis: etiology, therapy, and prevention. J Oral Surg 1981;39(6):430–5.

102. Sladen A, Zanca P, Hadnott WH. Aspiration pneumonitis—the sequelae. Chest 1971;159(4):448–450.

103. Salem MR, Wong AY, Mani M, Sellick BA. Efficacy of cricoid pressure in preventing gastric inflation during bag-mask ventilation in pediatric patients. Anesthesiology 1974;40:96.

104. Admani M, Yeh TF, Jain R, et al. Prevention of gastric inflation during mask ventilation in newborn infants. Crit Care Med 1985;13:592.

105. Moynihan RJ, Brock-Utne JG, Archer JH, et al. The effect of cricoid pressure on preventing gastric insufflation in infants and children. Anesthesiology 1993;78:652.

106. Fanning GL. The efficacy of cricoid pressure in preventing regurgitation of gastric contents. Anesthesiology 1970;32:553.

107. Salem MR, Wong AY, Fizzotti GF. Efficacy of cricoid pressure in preventing aspiration of gastric contents in paediatric patients. Br J Anaesth 1972;44:401.

108. Bloch EC, Ossey K, Ginsberg B. Tracheal intubation in children: a new method for ensuring correct depth of tube placement. Anesth Analg 1988;67:590.

109. Criswell JC, Parr MJ, Nolan JP. Emergency

airway management in patients with cervical spine injuries. Anaesthesia 1994;49:900.

110. Bivins HG, Ford S, Bezmalinovic Z, et al. The effect of axial traction during orotracheal intubation of the trauma victim with an unstable cervical spine. Ann Emerg Med 1988;17(1):25.

111. Majernick T, Bieniek R, Houston J, Hughes H. Cervical spine movement during orotracheal intubation. Ann Emerg Med 1986; 15(4):417.

112. Backofen JE, Rogers MC. Emergency management of the airway. In: Rogers MC, ed. Textbook of pediatric intensive care. 2nd ed., Baltimore: William & Wilkins. 1992.

113. Dauphinee K. Nasotracheal intubation. Emerg Med Clin North Am 1988;6:715.

114. Walker WE, Bender Jr HW. Blind nasotracheal intubation. Surg Gynecol Obstet 1981; 152:87.

115. Iserson KV. Blind nasotracheal intubation. Ann Emerg Med 1981;10:468.

116. Danzl DF, Thomas DM. Nasotracheal intubations in the emergency department. 1980;Crit Care Med 8:677.

117. Jantzen JPAH. Tracheal intubation—blind but not mute [letter]. Anaesth Analg 1985; 64:646.

118. Krishel S, Jackimczyk K, Balazs K. Endotracheal tube whistle: an adjunct to blind nasotracheal intubation. Ann Emerg Med 1992;21:33.

119. Krucylak CP, Schreiner MS. Orotracheal intubation of an infant with hemifacial microsomia using a modified lighted stylet. Anesthesiology 1992;77:826.

120. Weis FR, Hatton MN. Intubation by use of the light wand: experience in 253 patients. J Oral Maxillofac Surg 1989;47:577.

121. Ainsworth QP, Howells TH. Transilluminated tracheal intubation. Br J Anaesth 1989;62:494.

122. Ellis DG, Jakymec A, Kaplan RM, et al. Guided orotracheal intubation in the operating room using a lighted stylet: a comparison with direct laryngoscopic technique. Anesthesiology 1986;64:823.

123. Heller RM, Heller TW. Experience with the illuminated endotracheal tube in the prevention of unsafe intubations in the premature and full-term newborn. Pediatrics 1994; 93:389.

124. Stewart RD: Tactile orotracheal intubation. Ann Emerg Med 1984;13:175.

125. Wijesundera CD. Digital intubation of the trachea [letter]. Ceylon Med J 1990;35:81.

126. Hardwick WC, Bluhm D. Digital intubation. J Emerg Med 1984;1:317.

127. Siddall WJW. Tactile orotracheal intubation. Anaesthesia 1966;21:221.

128. Hancock PJ, Peterson G. Finger intubation of the trachea in newborns. Pediatrics 1992;89:325.

129. McNamara RM. Retrograde intubation of the trachea. Ann Emerg Med 1987;16:680.

130. Cooper CMS, Murray-Wilson A. Retrograde intubation: management of a 4.8 kg, 5-month infant. Anaesthesia 1987;42:1197.

131. Borland LM, Swan DM, Leff S. Difficult pediatric endotracheal intubation: a new approach to the retrograde technique. Anesthesiology 1981;55:577.

132. Audenaert SM, Montgomery CL, Stone B, et al. Retrograde-assisted fiberoptic tracheal intubation in children with difficult airways. Anesth Analg 1991;73:660.

133. Barriot P, Riou B. Retrograde technique for tracheal intubation in trauma patients. Crit Care Med 1988;16:712.

134. Gupta B, McDonald JS, Brooks JHJ, Mendenhall J. Oral fiberoptic intubation over a retrograde guide wire. Anaesth Analg 1989;68:517.

135. Bourke D, Levesque PR. Modification of retrograde guide for endotracheal intubation. Anaesth Analg 1974;53:1013.

136. Graham DR, Hay JG, Clague J, et al. Comparison of three different methods used to achieve local anesthesia for fiberoptic bronchoscopy. Chest 1992;102:704.

137. Spencer CD, Beaty HN. Complications of transtracheal aspiration. N Engl J Med 1972; 286:304.

138. Kalinske RW, Parker RH, Brandt D, et al. Diagnostic usefulness and safety of transtracheal aspiration. N Engl J Med 1967;276: 604.

139. Afilalo M, Guttman A, Stern E, et al. fiberoptic intubation in the emergency department: a case series. J Emerg Med 1993; 11:387.

140. Delaney KA, Hessler R. Emergency flexible fiberoptic nasotracheal intubation: a report of 60 cases. Ann Emerg Med 1988;17:919.

141. Minik, Jr EJ, Clinton JE, Plummer D, Ruiz E. fiberoptic intubation in the emergency department. Ann Emerg Med 1990;19:359.

142. Mulder DS, Wallace DH, Woolhouse FM. The use of the fiberoptic bronchoscope to facilitate endotracheal intubation following head and neck trauma. J Trauma 1975;15: 638.

143. Vauthy PA, Reddy R. Acute upper airway obstruction in infants and children. Evaluation by the fiberoptic bronchoscope. Ann Otol Rhinol Laryngol 1980;89:417.

144. Berthelsen P, Prytz S, Jacobsen E. Two-stage fiberoptic nasotracheal intubation in infants: a new approach to difficult pediatric intubation. Anaesthesiology 1985;63:457.

145. Ovassapian A, Yelich SF, Dykes MHM, Brunner EE. Fiber- optic nasotracheal intubation—incidence and causes of failure. Anaesth Analg 1983;62:692.

146. Nakayama DK, Gardner MJ, Rowe MI. Emergency endotracheal intubation in pediatric trauma. Ann Surg 1990;211:218.

147. Adriani J, Naraghi M, Ward M. Complications of endotracheal intubation. South Med J 1988;81:739.

148. Blanc VF, Tremblay NAG. The complications of tracheal intubation: a new classification with a review of the literature. Anaesth Analg 1974;53:202.

149. Lindgren L, Saarnivaara L. Cardiovascular responses to tracheal intubation in small children. Br J Anaesth 1985;57:1183.

150. Shorten GD, Bissonnette B, Hartley E, et al. It is not necessary to administer more than 10 micrograms.kg-1 of atropine to older children before succinylcholine. Can J Anaesth 1995;42:8.

151. Mirakhur RK, Clarke RS, Elliott J, Dundee JW. Atropine and glycopyrronium premedication. A comparison of the effects on cardiac rate and rhythm during induction of anaesthesia. Anaesthesia 1978;33:906.

152. Barrington KJ, Finer NN, Etches PC. Succinylcholine and atropine for premedication of the newborn infant before nasotracheal intubation: a randomized, controlled trial. Crit Care Med 1989;17:1293.

153. Burney RG, Winn R. Increased cerebrospinal fluid pressure during laryngoscopy and intubation for induction of anesthesia. Anaesth Analg 1975;54:687.

154. Raju TNK, Vidyasagar D, Torres C, et al. Intracranial pressure during intubation and anesthesia in infants. J Pediatr 1980;96:860.

155. Durand M, Bikramjit S, Cabal LA, et al. Cardiopulmonary and intracranial pressure changes related to endotracheal suctioning in preterm infants. Crit Care Med 1989;17:506.

156. Joshi C, Bruce DL. Thiopental and succinylcholine: action on intraocular pressure. Anaesth Analg 1975;54:471.

157. Meyers EF, Krupin T, Johnson M, Zink H. Failure of nondepolarizing neuromuscular blockers to inhibit succinylcholine-induced increased intraocular pressure. A controlled study. Anesthesiology 1978;48:149.

158. Drenger B, Pe'er J, BenEzra D, et al. The effect of intravenous lidocaine on the increase in intraocular pressure induced by tracheal intubation. Anaesth Analg 1985;64:1211.

159. Owen RL, Cheney FW. Endobronchial intubation: a preventable complication. Anesthesiology 1987;67:255.

160. Conrardy PA, Goodman LR, Lainge F, Singer M. Alteration of endotracheal tube position. Flexion and extension of the neck. Crit Care Med 1976;4:8, 1976

161. Todres ID, deBros F, Kramer SS, et al: Endotracheal tube position in the newborn infant. J Pediatr 1976;89:126.

162. Toung TJK, Grayson R, Saklad J, Wang H. Movement of the distal end of the endotracheal tube during flexion and extension of the neck [letter]. Anaesth Analg 1985;64:1029.

163. White SJ. Left mainstem intubation with digital intubation technique: an unrecognized risk. Am J Emerg Med 1994;12:466.

164. Brasch RC, Heldt GP, Hecht ST. Endotracheal tube orifice abutting the tracheal wall: a cause of infant airway obstruction. Radiology 1981;141:387.

165. Redding GJ, Fan L, Cotton EK, Brooks JG. Partial obstruction of endotracheal tubes in children. Incidence, etiology, significance. Crit Care Med 1979;7:227.

166. Miller RD, Hamilton WK. Pneumothorax during infant resuscitation. JAMA 1969;210:1090–1092.

167. Hirschman AM, Kravath RE. Venting vs ventilating. A danger of manual resuscitation bags. Chest 1982;82(3):369–370.

168. Dwyer ME: Pneumothorax. Aust Paediatr J 1975;11(4):195–200.

169. Luck SR, Raffensperger JG, Sullivan HJ, Gibson LE. Management of pneumothorax in children with chronic pulmonary disease. J Thorac Cardiovasc Surg 1977;74(6):834–839.

170. Moylan FMB, Seldin EB, Shannon DC, et al. Defective primary dentition in survivors of neonatal mechanical ventilation. J Pediatr 1980;96:106.

171. Stanievich JF, Marshak G, Stool SE. Airway obstruction in a hemophiliac child. Ann Otol 1980;89:572.

172. Lewis JH. Causes of death in hemophilia. JAMA 1970;214:1707.

173. Othersen Jr HB. Intubation injuries of the trachea in children: management and prevention. Ann Surg 1979;189:601.

174. Fan LL, Flynn JW, Pathak DR. Risk factors predicting laryngeal injury in intubated neonates. Crit Care Med 1983;11:431.

175. Serlin SP, Daily WJR: Tracheal perforation in the neonate: a complication of endotracheal intubation. J Pediatr 1975;86:596.

176. Ducharme JC, Bertrand MR, Debie J. Perforation of the pharynx in the newborn—a condition of mimicking esophageal atresia. Can Med Assoc J 1971;104:785.

177. Szigeti CL, Baeuerle JJ, Mongan PD. Arytenoid dislocation with lighted stylet intubation: case report and retrospective review. Anaesth Analg 1994;78:185.

178. Goitein KJ, Rein AJJT, Gornstein A. Incidence of aspiration in endotracheally intubated infants and children. Crit Care Med 1984;12:19.

179. Galvin AG, Stool SE, Bluestone CK. Pulmonary edema following relief of acute upper airway obstruction. Ann Otol 1980;89:124.

180. Sofer S, Bar-Ziv J, Scharf SM. Pulmonary edema following relief of upper airway obstruction. Chest 1984;86:401.

181. Barin ES, Stevenson IF, Donnelly GL. Pulmonary edema following acute upper airway obstruction. Anaesth Intensive Care 1986;14:54.

182. Warner LO, Beach TP, Martino JD. Negative pressure pulmonary oedema secondary to airway obstruction in an intubated infant. Can J Anaesth 1988;35:507.

183. Kanter RK, Watchko JF. Pulmonary edema

associated with upper airway obstruction. AJDC 1984;138:356.

184. Grande CM, Barton CR. Appropriate techniques for airway management of emergency patients with suspected spinal cord injury [letter]. Anaesth Analg 1988;67: 710–718.

185. Doolan LA, O'Brien JF. Safe intubation in cervical spine injury. Anaesth Intensive Care 1985;13:319.

186. Wright SW, Robinson GG, Wright MB. Cervical spine injuries in blunt trauma patients requiring emergent endotracheal intubation. Am J Emerg Med 1992;10:104.

187. Hastings RH, Marks JD. Airway management for trauma patients with potential cervical spine injuries. Anaesth Analg 1991;73: 471.

188. Wood PR, Lawler PGP. Managing the airway in cervical spine injury: a review of the Advanced Trauma Life Support protocol. Anaesthesia 1992;47:792.

189. Joyce SM. Cervical immobilization during orotracheal intubation in trauma victims [editorial]. Ann Emerg Med 1988;17:88.

190. Knopp RK. The safety of orotracheal intubation in patients with suspected cervical spine injury [editorial]. Ann Emerg Med 1990; 19:603.

191. Rhee KJ, Green W, Holcroft JW, et al. Oral intubation in the multiply injured patient: the risk of exacerbating cervical spine damage. Ann Emerg Med 1990;19(5)45–48.

192. Holley J, Jorden R. Airway management in patients with unstable cervical spine fractures. Ann Emerg Med 1989;18(11): 151–153.

193. Rachesky I, Boyce T, Duncan B, et al. Clinical prediction of cervical spine injuries in children. AJDC 1987;141:199.

PERCUTANEOUS TRANSTRACHEAL VENTILATION

Russell H. Greenfield

INTRODUCTION

The importance of maintaining adequate oxygenation and ventilation for the critically ill child cannot be overstated. In most cases, standard airway interventions, such as bag-valve-mask (BVM) ventilation and endotracheal intubation, can be performed successfully without incident. However, physicians responsible for managing all types of pediatric respiratory distress also must be prepared for those situations in which standard methods are contraindicated or unexpectedly fail. Such circumstances require knowledge of alternative techniques for providing respiratory support. Percutaneous transtracheal ventilation (PTV), also called translaryngeal ventilation or needle cricothyrotomy, is one such technique. Although sometimes a point of confusion, PTV should not be mistaken for high frequency transtracheal jet ventilation, which involves delivering very small volumes of oxygen at extremely high rates. This technique requires special equipment not generally found in the emergency department (ED).

Initial animal studies in the development of PTV dealt with passive transtracheal oxygenation (1). This method, however, was abandoned in favor of intermittent administration of compressed air via a transtracheal catheter, since this provided ventilation as well as oxygenation (2). Successful human studies and various modifications of this technique followed (3, 4), as well as data

showing that transtracheal gas exchange could sustain life for prolonged periods of time (5). Smith (6) and Ravussin (7) subsequently published reports documenting the successful use of PTV in children aged 4 months to 11 years. Although a significant body of literature exists documenting the effectiveness of PTV for adults, a remarkable paucity of data exists concerning the use of this procedure for pediatric patients. Considering the potential complications associated with cricothyrotomy and tracheotomy in young children, PTV represents a useful addition to the options available for managing the difficult pediatric airway.

ANATOMY AND PHYSIOLOGY

The cricothyroid membrane is bound superiorly by the thyroid cartilage and inferiorly by the cricoid cartilage. The cricothyroid arteries typically course through the apical portion of the membrane, although aberrant vessels may rarely complicate procedures in this area (8). For young infants, performing PTV can be difficult due to the small size of the cricothyroid membrane. However, this is also true of other invasive airway techniques, and PTV can often be performed more rapidly with fewer complications. Furthermore, if the cricothyroid membrane of a younger patient cannot be located, the procedure can be performed by introducing the needle through the tracheal cartilage without additional risk to the patient (see below).

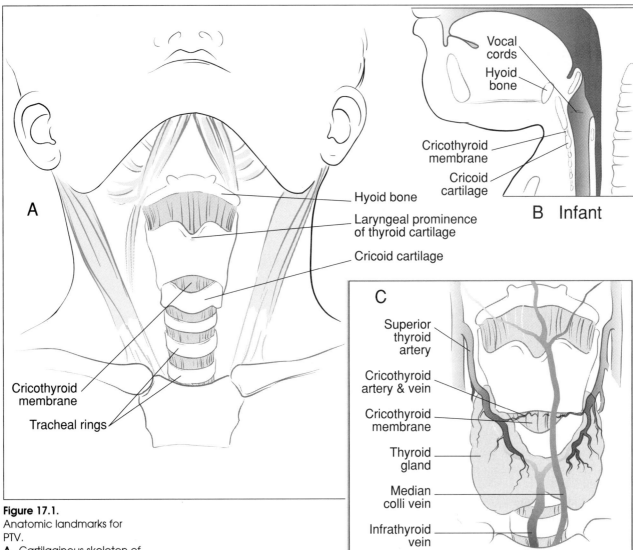

Figure 17.1.
Anatomic landmarks for PTV.
A. Cartilaginous skeleton of the extrathoracic airway. With older children and adolescents, the laryngeal prominence at the superior border of the thyroid cartilage can usually be palpated. The thyroid cartilage is followed inferiorly to locate the cricothyroid membrane.
B. With infants and younger children, the laryngeal prominence is not developed. The rings of the tracheal cartilage are followed superiorly to locate the prominence of the cricoid cartilage. The cricothyroid membrane is just superior to the cricoid cartilage.
C. A midline approach will avoid the normal position of the cricothyroid artery.

The operator must be thoroughly familiar with the anatomy of the anterior neck in order to perform this procedure successfully (Fig. 17.1). Five specific landmarks should be identified: the hyoid bone, the laryngeal prominence of the thyroid cartilage, the cricothyroid membrane, the cricoid cartilage, and the remaining tracheal rings. The laryngeal prominence develops during adolescence and is easily palpable in most adults, whereas the most readily identifiable landmarks in infants and young children are the hyoid bone and cricoid cartilage.

Delivered tidal volume during PTV is affected by a number of factors, including lung compliance, airway resistance, size of catheter, inspiratory pressure, and duration of inspiration (9). Jacobs (10) estimated that a maximum 70% of the volume of oxygen delivered to the catheter tip reaches the lower respiratory tract of adults with normal lung compliance. The remainder passes through the glottic opening and out the nose and mouth, decreasing the efficiency of gas exchange when compared with endotracheal intubation (4, 10–12). Because of the relatively small size of the airways, pediatric patients generally have significantly greater airway resistance than adults. Thus even with a small child, it is important to use a catheter with an adequate luminal diameter and a high pressure oxygen source to effectively perform this procedure. When used with a low pressure oxygen delivery system, PTV provides adequate oxygenation but not ventilation, causing retention of CO_2 over time. An example of such a system would be a bag-valve-mask circuit connected to the catheter via a 3.0 mm ID endotracheal tube adapter (see Equipment). Only when a larger diameter catheter is used with such a setup can hypercarbia be minimized (13).

PTV provides oxygen via intermittent bulk flow of gas under high pressure. Exhalation is achieved passively through the elastic recoil of the chest, with gases being expelled through the mouth and nose. The "ball-valve" effect of most partial laryngeal obstructions permits adequate exhalation during PTV (14), but complete obstruction prevents any egress of gas and results in a dangerously rapid rise in intrapulmonary pressure.

With a 50 psi oxygen source, volumes of 950 mL/sec, 1200 mL/sec, and 1300 mL/sec can be delivered through 16-gauge, 14-gauge, and 13-gauge catheters, respectively (15). These flow rates are more than adequate for maintaining ventilation and oxygenation in adults. Actual peak inspiratory pressures and intratracheal pressures are relatively low even with a driving pressure of 50 psi; however, smaller catheters (16 to 18 gauge) and lower driving pressures (25 to 35 psi) must be used for pediatric patients in order to prevent barotrauma.

The primary drawback to longer term use of PTV is CO_2 retention. For this reason, PTV previously has been viewed only as a temporizing procedure. However, when adequate oxygenation is maintained, even relative high levels of hypercarbia may not be as deleterious as once believed (17, 18). In fact, PTV has been shown to be safe for hours at a time, limited only by the ability of the system used to deliver humidified gases. Only in the setting of increased intracranial pressure or complete airway obstruction should PTV be considered solely as a temporizing measure.

Indications

Indications for the emergent use of PTV are similar to those for cricothyrotomy, i.e., any patient whose airway cannot be maintained with standard interventions should be considered a possible candidate. Potential clinical scenarios include severe maxillofacial trauma, laryngeal foreign bodies, local infections with swelling of upper airway structures such as epiglottitis (16), and congenital anomalies such as Treacher-Collins syndrome or Pierre-Robin sequence. PTV also has been used to provide oxygenation and ventilation before potentially difficult intubations (19), as well as for elective procedures such as head and neck surgery (6–7, 11, 19–20). With younger patients, PTV should be considered before cricothyrotomy, because it is associated with far fewer complications and can be completed in a much shorter period of time. PTV should not be performed when there is known damage to the cricoid cartilage or in the setting of tracheal rupture (21). These situations represent the only absolute contraindications for this procedure. Relative contraindications, such as mild to moderate local swelling or the presence of a hematoma, should be balanced against the potentially devastating complications of failing to provide adequate airway intervention.

Controversy surrounds the use of PTV in the setting of complete upper airway obstruction. A blockage cephalad to the catheter will prevent the passive exhalation of the delivered gases through the mouth and nose during PTV. In a study by Jorden of animals subjected to total airway obstruction, standard PTV caused massive distention of the lungs, severe barotrauma, and subsequent death (22). However, more recent studies have challenged the dogma that PTV is absolutely contraindicated in the presence of complete upper airway obstruction (23–27). The successful use of PTV in animals with complete airway obstruction has been reported using prolonged exhalation times with large internal diameter catheters (25). Frame et al. (27) reported a feline study of total airway obstruction using low flow rates (3 to 5 l/min) in which adequate oxygenation and ventilation were maintained without complication; they hypothesized that these data might be extrapolated to infants. Without the benefit of further studies to settle this issue, it would seem reasonable to use PTV as a temporizing measure for infants and younger children when complete airway obstruction is present only after other methods have been exhausted. In such a situation, prolonged exhalation times, lower oxygen delivery pressures, and the use of larger than normal catheters would all be necessary. For older children and adolescents, cricothyrotomy remains the procedure of choice for emergent alternative airway management in the presence of complete upper airway obstruction.

EQUIPMENT

Because of the lack of controlled data on the use of PTV for children, no definitive standards exist regarding appropriate equipment. However, multiple models have been advocated in the adult literature, and many of these concepts are applicable to pediatric patients. Equipment setups used to perform PTV range from those employing standard materials readily available in any ED to relatively sophisticated, commercially available devices (Fig. 17.2). Universal requirements include (*a*) a high pressure oxygen source (up to 50 psi), (*b*) tubing capable of withstanding high pressures, (*c*) a manual in-line valve to control the intermittent flow of oxygen to the patient, and (*d*) a large bore catheter (Table 17.1).

Oxygen delivered at 50 psi can be obtained directly from a hospital wall outlet (without a regulator), from the flush valve of a mechanical ventilator, or by attaching the tubing directly to an oxygen tank line (without using a flow valve). While high pressures

are necessary to provide adequate ventilation for older adolescents and adults, lower pressures (between 25 and 35 psi) should be used for children in order to prevent barotrauma. Such lower pressures can be obtained by using a standard wall outlet with a regulator set at 10 to 12 L/min. Tubing designed for gas delivery under high pressure must be used throughout the system.

If a permanent valve system is not available for performing PTV, a makeshift inline valve must be fabricated using materials in the ED (Fig. 17.3). This can be easily accomplished by cutting a small hole in the distal end of the tubing to create a side port. The operator can then control the flow of gas by intermittently occluding the port with a finger or thumb. Alternatively, a plastic Y-connector or three-way stopcock (Fig. 17.4) interposed between two pieces of high pressure tubing also permits control of gas flow. Oc-

Figure 17.2.
Permanent inline valve PTV system.

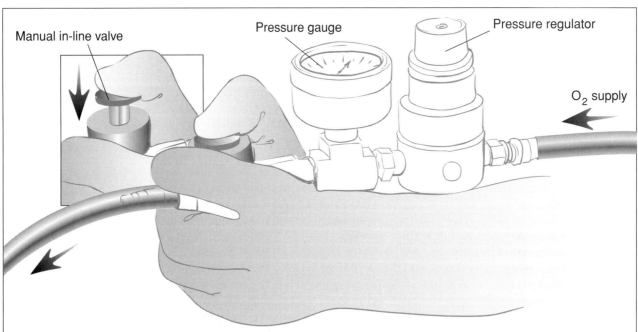

clusion of the open end of the connector or stopcock results in gas delivery to the trachea, while removal of the fingertip allows for exhalation.

Many creative models for performing PTV have been described. Multiple studies have employed mechanical ventilators as the high pressure oxygen source (28–30). Suction tubing (28), an endotracheal tube connector (31, 32), and a syringe with the plunger removed have been interposed between the catheter and oxygen source (Fig. 17.5). Syringes have also been placed in series with endotracheal tube adapters (31), inflated endotracheal tubes (33), and disposable ventilator tubing (34). One commercially produced setup (Instrumentation Industries, Inc., Bethel Park, PA) comes complete with high pressure tubing, permanent inline on/off valve, pressure regulator, and disposable tubing with Luer-Lok for catheter attachment.

The larger the internal diameter of the catheter used, the greater the flow of gas delivered to the trachea. Most studies concerning adult PTV have employed 12-gauge and 16-gauge catheters (internal diameters ranging from 1.5 to 2.8 mm) (35). One commercially available PTV catheter (Acutronic USA Inc., Pittsburgh, PA) is curved for easier placement and has distal side holes which spray the delivered volume of gas over a wider area. Teflon catheters offer the advantage of being kink-resistant. Smaller catheters, in the range of 16 to 18 gauge, should be used for children. A Luer-Lok™ is often used to attach the catheter to the distal end of the high pressure tubing. Prepackaged kits which can be used to obtain tracheal access via a modified Seldinger technique are now widely available. The Pertrach (Pertrach Inc., Bridgeport, WV) is one such kit which in-

cludes three uncuffed tubes ranging in internal diameter from 3.0 to 4.0 mm for use with infants and children up to 10 years of age (Fig. 17.6).

Regardless of the equipment selected, a preassembled system for PTV should be readily available if this procedure will be a potential option for airway management. The moment the equipment is needed is obviously not the time to begin gathering the necessary items. Medical personnel who will be involved with this procedure should also be fully inserviced about the proper use of the equipment.

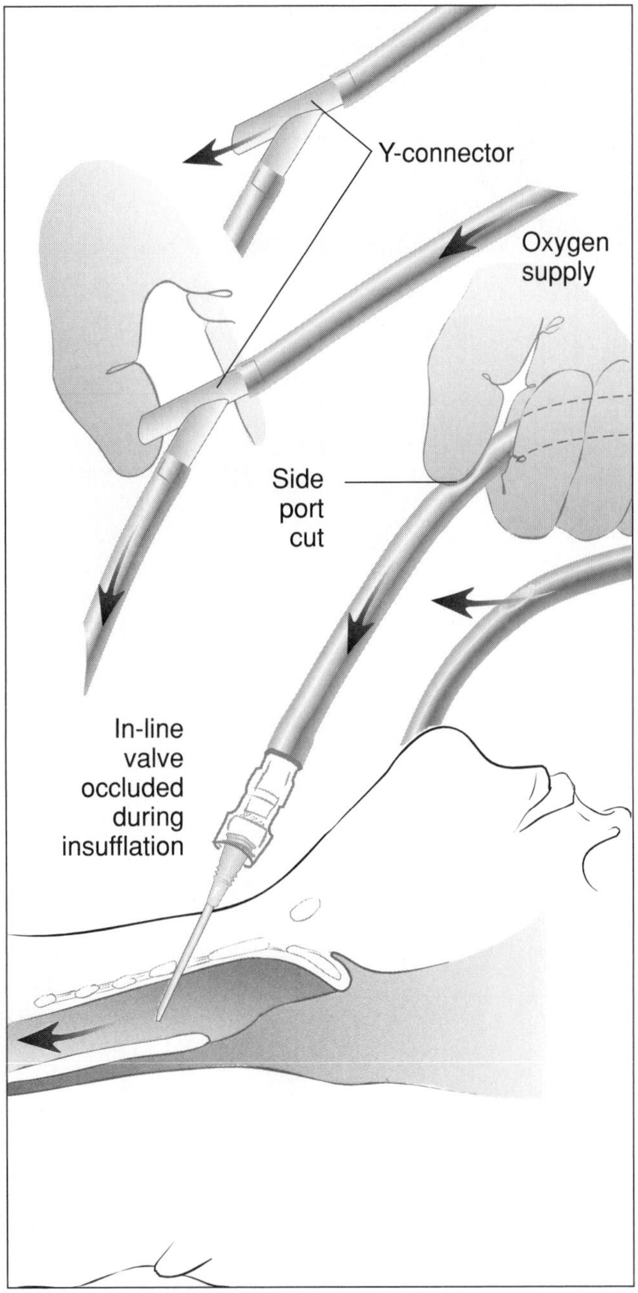

Figure 17.3.
PTV setups utilizing a Y-connector and oxygen tubing with a cut side port.

SUMMARY
1. Attach 3 to 5 mL syringe with a few ml of saline or lidocaine to needle and catheter.
2. Locate cricothyroid membrane, bound by thyroid cartilage superiorly and cricoid cartilage inferiorly.
3. Hold trachea in place and provide skin tension with thumb and middle finger of nondominant hand.
4. Place tip of needle at inferior midline of membrane, directing needle caudally at 30 to 45° angle.
5. Advance needle while pulling back on plunger of syringe. Appearance of air bubbles within syringe confirms intratracheal placement.
6. Slide catheter over needle until hub rests securely on skin surface.
7. Remove needle and syringe as a unit.
8. Connect high pressure tubing and oxygen source to catheter.
9. Confirm correct placement with a few short bursts of oxygen.
10. Ventilate at appropriate rate by opening and closing permanent valve, or occluding side port, stopcock, or Y-connector.
11. Assess patient response.
12. Suture catheter securely in place.

Chapter 17
Percutaneous
Transtracheal
Ventilation

243

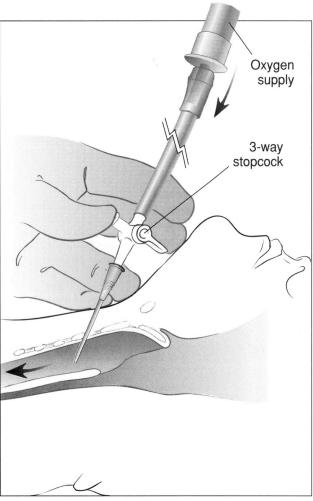

Figure 17.4.
PTV setup utilizing a three-way stopcock.

Figure 17.5.
A syringe with the plunger removed may be used as an adapter between the catheter and a larger endotracheal tube connector. Alternatively, a smaller endotracheal tube connector can be inserted directly into the catheter hub. Both methods can be used to connect the catheter to a standard self-inflating resuscitation bag.

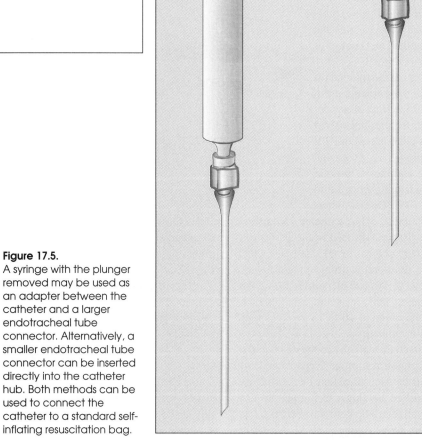

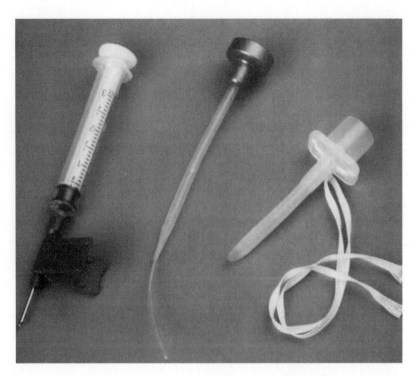

Figure 17.6.
Pertrach kit.

PROCEDURE

The operator can most easily locate the cricothyroid membrane in older adolescents and adults by first running a finger down (caudad) from the laryngeal prominence until he or she feels a small bump (Fig. 17.1), which is the cricoid cartilage. The cricothyroid membrane is appreciated as a subtle depression with slightly more "give" or "bounce" just superior to the cricoid cartilage. However, because the laryngeal prominence does not develop fully until adolescence, this method may not be useful for infants and children. For these patients, the operator's most reliable method for locating the membrane is to run a finger up (cephalad) along the tracheal rings until he or she feels a more prominent bulge representing the cricoid cartilage. Even if the cricothyroid membrane is not palpable, its location can be assumed as just cephalad to the superior margin of the cricoid cartilage. Should the operator be unable to locate the position of the membrane, the catheter can be safely placed in a lower intercartilaginous tracheal space (32). After the cricothyroid membrane has been located, the area should be cleansed with an antiseptic solution. If the patient is alert, the skin overlying the membrane can be anesthetized with lidocaine.

The operator's thumb and middle finger of the nondominant hand hold the trachea in place and provide skin tension as he or she uses the index finger to palpate the cricothyroid membrane (Fig. 17.7.A). A small syringe (generally 3 or 5 ml) containing 2 to 3 cc of saline or lidocaine attached to the needle and catheter is held in the dominant hand. The needle is placed in the midline of the neck at the inferior margin of the cricothyroid membrane (to avoid the normal position of the cricothyroid arteries) and directed caudally at an angle of 30 to 45°. The skin and subcutaneous tissue are then punctured with the needle. The operator may choose to make a small nick in the skin with a scalpel blade to facilitate insertion of the needle (15). While applying continuous negative pressure on the syringe, the operator advances the needle through the membrane until he or she sees air bubbles in the syringe, confirming intratracheal placement. The catheter is then advanced forward off the needle until its hub rests at the skin surface. The needle and syringe are then removed (Fig. 17.7.B). Either the operator or an assistant should hold the catheter securely in place at all times until it can be secured with a suture to reduce the likelihood of causing subcutaneous emphysema. The high pressure tubing and 100% oxygen source are then connected to the catheter (Fig. 17.7.C), and a few short bursts

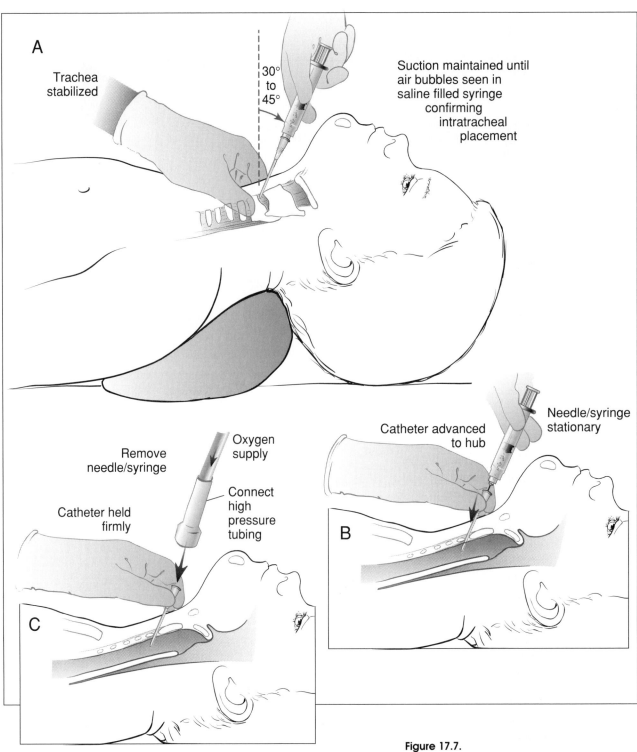

A
Trachea
stabilized

30°
to
45°

Suction maintained until
air bubbles seen in
saline filled syringe
confirming
intratracheal
placement

Remove
needle/syringe

Oxygen
supply

Connect
high
pressure
tubing

Catheter held
firmly

Catheter advanced
to hub

Needle/syringe
stationary

B

C

Figure 17.7.
Performing PTV.
A. The needle is angled caudally at 30 to 45°
and inserted through the cricothyroid
membrane until bubbles are seen in the fluid-
filled syringe, indicating puncture of the
trachea.
B. The catheter is advanced to the hub as
the needle and syringe are removed.
C. The catheter is secured in place and
connected to the oxygen delivery system.

**Chapter 17
Percutaneous
Transtracheal
Ventilation**

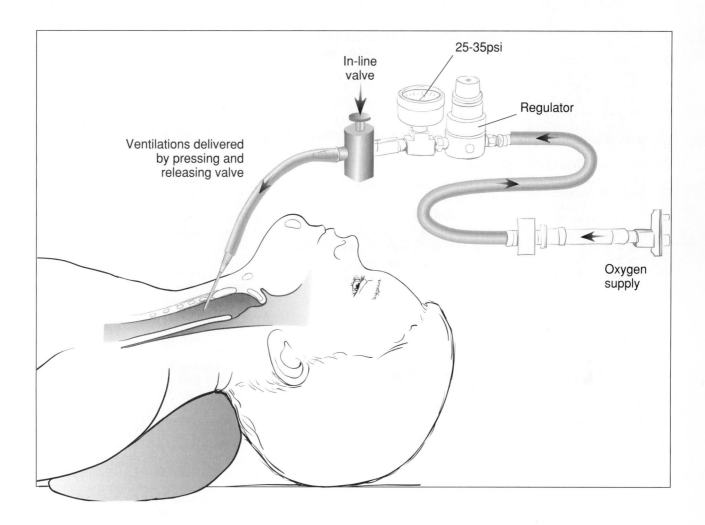

In-line valve

Ventilations delivered by pressing and releasing valve

25-35psi

Regulator

Oxygen supply

of gas are delivered both to reconfirm placement and ensure that the equipment is functioning properly. At this point, the patient can be ventilated by opening and closing the in-line valve apparatus, if such a system is used, or by intermittently occluding the side port, Y-connector, or stopcock (Fig. 17.8).

To date no controlled studies have been performed to determine the optimal I:E ratio for children when performing PTV. Based on published experience in the available literature, the ratios listed in Table 17.2 are recommended. In general, children who have isolated respiratory distress without upper airway obstruction will require a ratio of 1:4 to 1:5 seconds. In the setting of increased in-

tracranial pressure the ventilatory rate should be increased (1:2 to 1:3 seconds). If PTV is performed for a child with partial upper airway obstruction, the rate should be decreased (1:9 seconds) so that the risk of barotrauma to the lungs is reduced. During insufflation, oropharyngeal secretions may be expelled through the patient's mouth and nose with great force. Operators should stand clear and be properly gowned, gloved, and masked.

COMPLICATIONS

The most common complication associated with PTV is subcutaneous emphysema. This can develop both during the procedure as well as after removal of the catheter (15, 36–38), and in some cases can be extensive. This complication is usually associated with difficulty in adequately securing the catheter in place in the anterior neck. The catheter tip is easily kinked or partially dislodged, which

Figure 17.8.
Positive pressure ventilation is administered by pressing and releasing the valve (or opening and occluding the Y- connector, three-way stopcock, etc.). If necessary, a standard self-inflating resuscitation bag can be used as a temporizing measure.

Table 17.2.
Ventilatory Rates (I:E RATIOS)

Standard	1:4 to 1:5 seconds
Elevated ICP	1:2 seconds
Airway obstruction	1:9 seconds

Chapter 17
**Percutaneous
Transtracheal
Ventilation**

247

can result in the rapid accumulation of gases in subcutaneous tissues. Multiple attempts at correct placement of the catheter can also result in localized subcutaneous emphysema, as gas escapes through previous puncture sites and enters the soft tissue (37). The likelihood of subcutaneous emphysema can be reduced by (a) using kink-resistant teflon catheters, (b) assigning one individual to be responsible for holding the catheter hub in place at all times, (c) using one of the commercially available PTV catheters with attached flanges for securing the catheter, and (d) minimizing attempts at catheter placement. On removal of the catheter, a fingertip should be placed firmly over the puncture site and held for a few minutes to prevent air entry into the subcutaneous tissue.

Allowing insufficient time for passive exhalation (i.e., a ventilatory rate that is too rapid) can lead to barotrauma to the lungs with resulting pneumomediastinum and pneumothorax (12, 16, 22, 32, 37, 38). This can also occur if PTV is performed when complete upper airway obstruction is present. Although there have been no reports of perforation of the posterior trachea, this complication would seem more likely with children, as the result of increased compliance of the tracheal cartilages, and should be carefully avoided.

Other reported complications associated with using PTV include minor bleeding from arterial perforation, pneumatocele formation (39), and fire in conjunction with electrocautery (40). It is important to remember that PTV does not provide complete control of the airway, and therefore aspiration is still a possibility. However, at least one animal study has suggested that PTV may provide some protection from aspiration (41).

SUMMARY

Percutaneous transtracheal ventilation is an underutilized technique for the management of the difficult pediatric airway. The indications for PTV are essentially the same as for cricothyrotomy, although cricothyrotomy remains the procedure of choice in older children and adults in the setting of complete airway obstruction. PTV requires no special surgical skills and can be initiated within a matter of moments. Familiarity with alternative methods of

airway management such as PTV can often provide the temporary respiratory support needed for a critically ill child until more definitive measures can be performed.

REFERENCES

1. Jacoby JJ, Hamelberg W, Reed JP, Gillespie B. A simple technique for artificial respiration. Am J Physiol 1951;167:798–799.
2. Reed JP, Kemph JP, Hamelberg W, Hitchcock FA, Jacoby JJ. Studies with transtracheal artificial respiration. Anesthesiology 1954;15:28–41.
3. Spoerel WE, Narayanan PS, Singh NP. Transtracheal ventilation. Br J Anaesth 1971;43:932–939.
4. Jacobs HB. Emergency percutaneous transtracheal catheter and ventilator. J Trauma 1972;12:50–55.
5. Slutsky AS, Watson J, Leith DE, et al. Tracheal insufflation of O_2 (TRIO) at low flow rates sustains life for several hours. Anesthesiology 1985;63:278–286.
6. Smith RB, Myers N, Sherman H. Transtracheal ventilation in paediatric patients: case reports. Br J Anaesth 1974;46:313–314.
7. Ravussin P, Bayer-Berger M, Monnier P, Savary M, Freeman J. Percutaneous transtracheal ventilation for laser endoscopic procedures infants and small children with laryngeal obstruction: report of two cases. Can J Anaesth 1987;34:83–86.
8. Little CM, Parker MG, Tarnopolsky R. The incidence of vasculature at risk during cricothyroidostomy. Ann Emerg Med 1986;15:805–807.
9. Yealy DM, Plewa MC, Stewart RD. An evaluation of cannulae and oxygen sources for pediatric jet ventilation. Am J Emerg Med 1991;9:20–23.
10. Jacobs HB, Smyth NPD, Witorsch P. Transtracheal catheter ventilation: clinical experience in 36 patients. Chest 1974;65:36–40.
11. Wagner DJ, Coombs DW, Doyle SC. Percutaneous transtracheal ventilation for emergency dental appliance removal. Anesthesiology 1985;62:664–666.
12. Ward KR, Menegazzi JJ, Yealy DM, Klain MM, Molner RL, Goode JS. Translaryngeal jet ventilation and end-tidal pCO_2 monitoring during varying degrees of upper airway obstruction. Ann Emerg Med 1991;20:1193–1197.
13. Yealy DM, Stewart RD, Kaplan RM. Clarifications on translaryngeal ventilation (letter). Ann Emerg Med 1988;17:1130.
14. Zornow MH, Thomas TC, Scheller MS. The efficacy of three different methods of transtracheal ventilation. Can J Anaesth 1989;36:624–628.
15. Stewart RD. Manual translaryngeal jet ventilation. Emerg Med Clin North Am 1989;7:155–164.
16. Levinson MM, Scuderi PE, Gibson RL, Comer PB. Emergency percutaneous transtracheal ventilation. JACEP 1979;8:396–400.
17. Cote CJ, Eavey RD, Todres ID, et al. Cricothyroid membrane puncture: oxygenation and ventilation in a dog model using an intravenous catheter. Crit Care Med 1988;16:615–619.
18. Goldstein B, Shannon DC, Todres ID. Supercarbia

in children: clinical course and outcome. Crit Care Med 1990;18:166–168.

19. Benumof JL, Scheller MS. The importance of transtracheal jet ventilation in the management of the difficult airway. Anesthesiology 1989;71: 769–778.

20. Weymuller EA, Paugh D, Pavlin EG, Cummings CW. Management of difficult airway problems with percutaneous transtracheal ventilation. Ann Otol Rhinol Laryngol 1987;96:34–37.

21. Mace SE. Percutaneous translaryngeal ventilation (needle cricothyrotomy). In: Roberts JR, Hedges JR, ed. Clinical procedures in emergency medicine. Philadelphia: WB Saunders 1991:49–56.

22. Jorden RC, Moore EE, Marx JA, Honigman B. A comparison of PTV and endotracheal ventilation in an acute trauma model. J Trauma 1985;25:978–983.

23. Frame SB, Simon JM, Kerstein MD, McSwain NE. Percutaneous transtracheal catheter ventilation (PTCV) in complete airway obstruction—a canine model. J Trauma 1989;29:774–781.

24. Neff CC, Pfister RC, van Sonnenberg E. Percutaneous transtracheal ventilation: experimental and practical aspects. J Trauma 1983;23:84–90.

25. Stothert JC, Stout MJ, Lewis LM, Keltner RM. High pressure percutaneous transtracheal ventilation: the use of large gauge intravenous-type catheters in the totally obstructed airway. Am J Emerg Med 1990;8: 184–189.

26. Campbell CT, Harris RC, Cook MH, Reines HD. A new device for emergency percutaneous transtracheal ventilation in partial and complete airway obstruction. Ann Emerg Med 1988;17:927–931.

27. Frame SB, Timberlake GA, Kerstein MD, et al. Transtracheal needle catheter ventilation in complete airway obstruction: an animal model. Ann Emerg Med 1989;18:127–133.

28. Zucker-Pinchoff B, Ramani T. A simple device for transtracheal ventilation. J Clin Anesth 1992;4:

342–343.

29. Delaney WA, Kaiser RE. Percutaneous transtracheal jet ventilation made easy. Anesthesiology 1991;74:952.

30. Scuderi PE, McLeskey CH, Comer PB. Emergency percutaneous transtracheal ventilation during anesthesia using readily available equipment. Anaesth Analg 1982;61:867–870.

31. Patel R. Systems for transtracheal ventilation. Anesthesiology 1983;59:165.

32. Attia RR, Battit GE, Murphy JD. Transtracheal ventilation. JAMA 1975;234:1152–1153.

33. Gildar JS. A simple system for transtracheal ventilation. Anesthesiology 1983;58:106.

34. Aye LS. Percutaneous transtracheal ventilation. Anaesth Analg 1983;62:619.

35. Yealy DM, Stewart RD, Kaplan RM. Myths and pitfalls in emergency translaryngeal ventilation: correcting misimpressions. Ann Emerg Med 1988;17: 690–692.

36. Koch E, Benumof JL. Percutaneous transtracheal jet ventilation: an important airway adjunct. AANA J 1990;58:337–339.

37. Jorden RC. Percutaneous transtracheal ventilation. Emerg Med Clinics of N.A. 1988;6:745–752.

38. Craig DB. Transtracheal ventilation (letter). JAMA 1976;235:2082.

39. Carden E, Calcaterra TC, Lechtman A. Pneumatocele of the larynx: a complication of percutaneous transtracheal ventilation. Anesth Analg 1976;55: 600–601.

40. Bowdle TA, Glenn M, Colston L, Eisele D. Fire following use of electrocautery during emergency percutaneous transtracheal ventilation. Anesthesiology 1987;66:697–698.

41. Yealy DM, Plewa MC, Reed JJ, Kaplan RM, Ilkhanipour K. Manual translaryngeal jet ventilation and the risk of aspiration in a canine model. Ann Emerg Med 1990;19:1238–1241.

Central Venous Access and Central Venous Pressure Monitoring

Jane Lavelle and Andrew Costarino, Jr.

INTRODUCTION

Central venous cannulation can be defined as the percutaneous placement of a vascular catheter within the lumen of a major high flow vein of the abdomen or thorax. Mastery of central venous cannulation is a crucial skill for any clinician who regularly participates in resuscitation and stabilization of critically ill infants and children.

Development of vascular access tools and techniques came as the result of two motivating forces that continue today: the desire to better understand the circulation and the need to administer intravenous fluids, blood products, and medications. The first recorded central venous catheterization was performed in England by Stephen Hales in 1733. As part of his investigation of the circulation he inserted a glass tube into the jugular vein of a horse to measure the central venous pressure. Later the value of intravenous fluid administration was recognized. In 1833 W.B. O'Shaughnessy described the treatment of cholera victims to replace the lost "neutral saline ingredients" of the water content of serum. Intravenous saline solutions were first used to treat shock associated with surgery by Rudolph Matas in 1891. Progress in intravenous therapy was accelerated in the early 20th century when blood transfusion became an important clinical tool. This came about as a result of the description of the blood types by Landsteiner in 1901 and the development of a method to prevent coagulation in stored blood in 1914. By the mid-1900s intravenous fluids, blood products, and medications were a regular part of clinical practice.

When Seldinger described a practical technique for percutaneous entry to central vessels in 1953, the stage was set for central venous cannulation to became a feasible intervention. By the late 1960s this procedure had gained widespread clinical acceptance. Today the central venous catheter (CVC) is used for a broad range of clinical purposes in adults and children of all ages (1, 2). A technique that is performed exclusively by physicians or supervised physicians-in-training, percutaneous central venous cannulation may be used during initial patient stabilization or as a definitive procedure for long-term patient management. This chapter will review the methods for performing percutaneous central venous cannulation in pediatric patients using the Seldinger technique via the femoral, jugular, and subclavian veins.

ANATOMY AND PHYSIOLOGY

General Anatomic Considerations

Major sites for percutaneous cannulation of the central veins include the internal and ex-

Chapter 18
Central Venous
Access and Central
Venous Pressure
Monitoring

251

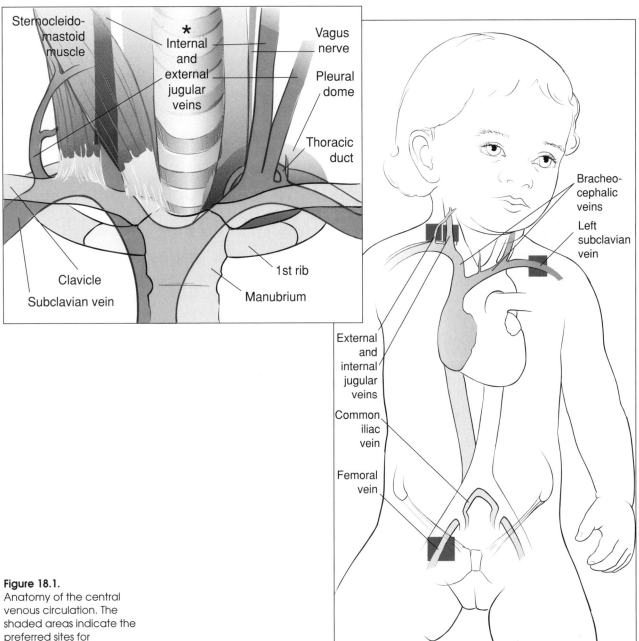

Figure 18.1.
Anatomy of the central venous circulation. The shaded areas indicate the preferred sites for cannulation.

**Chapter 18
Central Venous
Access and Central
Venous Pressure
Monitoring**

ternal jugular veins, the subclavian veins, and the femoral veins. Figure 18.1 illustrates these major vessels and their relation to the abdominal and thoracic vena cava and the heart. Although vascular anatomy is similar in all age groups, some subtle and important differences exist among pediatric patients, particularly young infants. One general difference to consider is that small body size, tissue softness, and compressibility (particularly of the chest) make the body surface landmarks used in locating deep veins less

apparent and more easily distorted in younger patients.

More specific considerations also exist for some of the common central venous cannulation sites. For example, in infants less than 1 year of age anatomic factors make subclavian vein entry significantly more difficult than for older patients. In this age group, the subclavian vein arches more superiorly as it courses to the atrium, causing acute angles that can obstruct catheter placement. The subclavian arch assumes a more typical horizontal position within the chest only after 1 year of age. Additionally, in young infants the notch on the inferior aspect of the first rib, a landmark commonly employed to identify the percutaneous entry site for the subclavian vein, is difficult to identify. Finally, the diameter of the subclavian vein is smaller than that of the internal jugular vein in these patients, and for this reason, many clinicians prefer the jugular site (3–6).

A general anatomic consideration that applies to both children and adults relates to central venous cannulation via the internal jugular veins (IJV) or subclavian veins (SV), namely, these vessels are more easily approached from the right side rather than the left. On the right, the IJV follows a straight course and joins the right SV to form the brachiocephalic (innominate) vein which continues to the superior vena cava (SVC). The left IJV joins the SV at a more acute angle; moreover, the left brachiocephalic forms a sharp angle with the superior vena cava. Adding to these difficulties associated with negotiating vascular turns during left-sided approaches to the SVC are other problems that arise as a result of the lymphatic communications with these veins. The larger left thoracic duct enters the left SV at its junction with the IJV and can hinder venous cannulation. The right lymphatic duct is a much smaller structure which is often congenitally absent. Finally, the left pleural dome is higher than the right, increasing the likelihood of a pneumothorax during the procedure. Although specific clinical situations such as right-sided neck or chest trauma may preclude use of the right-sided vessels, they are preferred whenever possible (3–6).

The femoral vein is relatively easy to identify in children and adults, and no important differences exist when right and left sides are compared. For these reasons, as well as other reasons to be discussed, the femoral vein has become the most popular site for central venous cannulation in pediatric patients.

Anatomy of Specific Sites

Femoral Vein

The femoral vein (FV) travels superficially in the anterior thigh and then passes beneath the inguinal ligament, coursing deep into the pelvis to become the external iliac vein. In the proximal thigh (distal to the inguinal ligament), the FV lies within the femoral sheath where it is medial to the femoral artery which in turn is medial to the femoral nerve. The mnemonic NAVL ("naval") is often used to remember this orientation from lateral to medial: nerve, artery, vein, lymphatic. Thus, the FV can be identified 1–2 centimeters medial to the femoral artery pulse when palpated 1–2 centimeters below the inguinal ligament (4).

The Jugular Veins
Internal Jugular Vein
The right and left internal jugular veins (IJV) exit the skull via the jugular foramina. They follow a straight course through the neck before emptying into the subclavian veins. The right IJV joins the right subclavian vein just lateral to the sternoclavicular joint, forming the brachiocephalic (innominate) vein which continues in a straight path to the SVC. On the left side, the IJV joins the SV at an almost perpendicular angle, as just described. Similarly, the left innominate vein joins the SVC at an acute angle. As the IJV moves caudal in the neck it becomes more superficial to the skin and larger in diameter.

In the cephalad portion of its course on either side of the neck, the IJV is found medial to the sternal (medial) head of the sternocleidomastoid muscle. In the midportion of the neck it is located beneath the line that bisects the angle formed by the sternal and clavicular (lateral) heads of the sternocleidomastoid. In the caudad portion of the neck, it lies just medial to (or sometimes beneath) the clavicular head of the muscle.

Other important structures are adjacent to the IJV. Within the carotid sheath, the carotid artery is medial and posterior to the vein, whereas the vagus nerve is between the carotid artery and IJV. The cervical sympathetic chain and stellate ganglion are deep and medial to the IJV, whereas the brachial plexus is found deep to all these structures. The phrenic nerve is lateral and the laryngeal nerve medial to the carotid/jugular vascular bundle. Lymphatic ducts enter the subclavian veins near the junction of the IJV with the subclavian vein. The right IJV is chosen for cannulation whenever possible (5, 7–9) for the advantages listed previously.

Chapter 18
Central Venous
Access and Central
Venous Pressure
Monitoring

253

External Jugular Vein

The external jugular vein (EJV) drains the structures of the exterior of the cranium and the deep face. It begins within the parotid gland at the angle of the mandible and travels obliquely across the sternocleidomastoid muscle to the middle of the clavicle. Below the clavicle, it empties into the SV at virtually a right angle (5, 7, 8).

Subclavian Vein

The subclavian vein arises from the axillary vein as it passes over the first rib. It continues superiorly, passing anterior to the scalenus anterior muscle, before descending slightly as it joins the IJV to form the brachiocephalic vein, which then empties into the SVC. The SV lies anterior to the subclavian artery and the brachial plexus; it is separated from these structures by the thin scalenus anterior muscle. At this level ventral to the scalenus anterior muscle, the thoracic duct crosses to terminate at the junction of the IJV and the SV. As with the IJV, the right-sided SV is chosen for cannulation whenever possible for reasons described previously (6, 10).

Physiology of Central Venous Pressure Measurement

Central venous catheters are frequently used to measure the vascular pressure—i.e., central venous pressure (CVP) or right atrial pressure (RAP)—in order to assist in judgments regarding intravascular volume and preload of the heart. To use such pressure measurements optimally, the catheter tip should be positioned within the thoracic structures. Any such pressure measurement is an indirect measure of preload and therefore only estimates end diastolic volume in the cardiac chamber. In addition, CVP or RAP reflects function of the right ventricle and is further removed from influence of the left ventricle. Despite these limitations, the CVP provides clinically valuable data to guide fluid resuscitation and other therapies to improve systemic circulation.

With initial incremental administration of intravenous fluid, there may be little change in the CVP readings even though diastolic volume is increasing and cardiac output is improving. Then as the vascular capacitance is filled, the pressure will rise. When the myocardial fibers have reached their optimal length after restoration of intravascular volume, systemic circulation and blood pressure will also be maximized. Further fluid administration—filling the cardiac chambers beyond the optimal state—will result in progressively increasing CVP readings with little improvement in cardiac output. Because this CVP/RAP to end diastolic volume relationship can vary significantly from patient to patient, as well as among various disease states, the change in pressure associated with a therapy (or with time) is more useful clinically than the absolute values. However, a useful guide which is generally applicable for the normovolemic patient is that an infusion of 10 mL/kg of normal saline is expected to increase the CVP by 2 to 4 mm Hg. The pressure returns to baseline over a variable period of time (normally between 10 and 20 minutes) depending on such factors as vascular tone and renal function. A rapid return to baseline or a smaller increase in the CVP readings after a 10 mL/kg fluid bolus suggests a depleted intravascular volume. Greater increases in the CVP reflect an increased intravascular volume or a poorly compliant ventricle. In addition to the CVP, other variables that have a significant effect on cardiac output include the heart rate, myocardial contractility, and afterload.

When interpreting the central venous pressure measurement, it is important to recognize the influence of the pressure measurement reference point. Traditionally, the CVP is "zeroed" to atmospheric pressure at the midaxillary line while the patient is in a supine position (i.e., zeroing to the level of the heart). The pressure measured in the vascular space must therefore be interpreted in relation to atmospheric pressure. For example, a reading of "5" means that the CVP is 5 mm Hg greater than atmospheric pressure at the level of the heart. If the relationship between the patient's thorax and the transducer were to change, the pressure would increase or decrease solely because of this change. Thus, if the transducer were raised above the patient, the zero point is higher than the level of the heart, and the vascular pressure will be decreased as an artifact of the change. Conversely, if the transducer is placed below the

Chapter 18
Central Venous
Access and Central
Venous Pressure
Monitoring

254

patient, the hydrostatic pressure applied to the transducer will be increased and the monitor will falsely indicate that the CVP had increased. It is therefore extremely important to maintain a constant zero point when interpreting serial CVP readings.

Another consideration when using the CVP to estimate filling of the cardiac chambers is the unmeasured effect of intrapleural pressure. A CVP of 5 mm Hg for a patient breathing spontaneously represents a much different right atrial distending pressure (an approximate measure of preload) compared with a patient receiving positive pressure ventilation with the same reading. In the spontaneously breathing child, the mean pleural pressure referenced to atmosphere is -3 mm Hg, and the right atrial distending pressure is 8 mm Hg ($5 - [-3] = 8$ mm Hg). In contrast, the mechanically ventilated patient has mean pleural pressure of $+4$ mm Hg, resulting in a distending pressure of 1 mm Hg ($5 - [+4] = 1$ mm Hg). In estimating pleural pressure in the clinical setting, the clinician must consider the degree of pulmonary pathology. Generally, about two-thirds of the airway pressure is transmitted to the pleural space. For example, a child with severe pneumonia receiving mechanical ventilation with mean airway pressures of 12 mm Hg will have an approximate pleural pressure of 8 mm Hg. This child would need a CVP of 13 mm Hg to maintain a right atrial distending pressure of 5 mm Hg ($13 - [+8] = 5$). Esophageal pressure measurement is occasionally advocated as a way to determine pleural pressure more accurately. However, this is not an essential requirement for using this procedure effectively, because as mentioned previously, relative changes in the CVP are used to guide volume therapy rather than absolute values.

INDICATIONS

General Considerations

Central venous cannulation should be performed by a physician, usually an emergency medicine specialist, intensivist, anesthesiologist, radiologist, or surgeon. The operator should be skilled in the technique and familiar with the indications, anatomy, and potential complications of the procedure, so that the balance of benefit versus risk can be appropriately judged. Indications for percutaneous CVC placement include (a) the need to obtain vascular access for patients with circulatory failure when vasoconstriction or vascular depletion prevent peripheral access (b) facilitating placement of other devices such as a Swan-Ganz catheter or transvenous pacemaker; (c) the administration of vasoactive substances, thrombogenic therapies, or other medications in order to allow more rapid distribution and onset of these therapies, (d) the safe administration of hypertonic fluids or highly concentrated medications into a large volume, high flow body space, (e) assessment of cardiac function and tissue oxygen delivery through CVP measurement and mixed venous blood gas measurement; and (f) providing long-term access to the circulation for repeated administration of medications that may injure a peripheral vein or for repeated blood sampling (Table 18.1). Indications for CVP monitoring include circulatory failure requiring large volume fluid resuscitation or inotropic support in association with respiratory failure.

The only absolute contraindications for CVC placement are vascular disease in the involved extremity and congenital or acquired vascular abnormality. Relative contraindications include acute inflammation or injury to the skin overlying the planned entry site and the presence of a hypercoagulable state or bleeding diathesis. Relative contraindications for specific anatomic sites are described below.

Site Specific Considerations

Femoral Vein
The femoral site has become the first choice for emergent CVC placement in children.

Table 18.1.
Indications for Central Venous Cannulation

Administration of fluids/medications to treat circulatory failure
Administration of vasoactive medications
Administration of hypertonic fluids (TPN, chemotherapy, etc.)
Measurement of venous vascular pressures
Measurement of mixed venous blood gases
Access for Swan-Ganz catheter or pacemaker placement
Long-term vascular access

Chapter 18
Central Venous
Access and Central
Venous Pressure
Monitoring

255

Among the reasons are the easily identifiable anatomic landmarks, ready application of hemostatic pressure in the event of bleeding at the site, and no interference with airway management or chest compressions. Unlike the cervical and thoracic sites for CVC placement, where pneumothorax and other serious acute complications can occur, the femoral site is relatively free of such hazards (4, 10, 12).

The relative contraindications to CVC placement at the femoral site are abnormal vascular status of the lower extremity, congenital malformation of the lower extremity, femoral hernia, abdominal tumor or trauma, abdominal ascites, and anticipated cardiac catheterization.

Jugular Vein

General patient care, movement, and entry site dressing care is made easier when the catheter is away from an extremity. In addition, a site near the chest ensures that the tip of the catheter will lie within the thorax, allowing for accurate CVP measurement. These are the primary advantages that have made the neck and upper chest entry sites popular for CVC placement, especially among adult patients.

Internal Jugular Vein

The anatomic landmarks for internal jugular vein catheterization are similar among infants, small children, and adolescents. In comparison to the EJV, this site has a much higher rate of success for central venous cannulation. Compared to the SV, the IJV approach is associated with a lower risk of causing pneumothorax, but has a higher risk of inadvertent puncture of the carotid artery and stellate ganglion. The proximity of the IJV to the carotid artery makes this site relatively contraindicated for children with any type of coagulopathy (5).

External Jugular Vein

The external jugular vein is occasionally used for access to the central circulation, although it is more commonly used for peripheral access. The primary advantage of this site is that the vessel is located superficially, which reduces the likelihood of pneumothorax, carotid puncture, or injury to the sympathetic chain. In addition, the superficial location of the vein and its distance from the carotid artery may make this a more favorable option for the child with a coagulopathy. The external jugular site has a major disadvantage in that successful central venous cannulation occurs much less frequently than with other approaches. Difficulty in passing catheters into the superior vena cava from an EJV entry site is due to the presence of venous valves, the sharp turns made by the vein as it courses under the clavicle, and its virtually perpendicular angle of entry into the SV (5).

Subclavian Vein

The subclavian vein is the least common site used for percutaneous central venous cannulation in children. Anatomic characteristics of infants and younger children that differ significantly from adults are the major reason for the reluctance of many practitioners to use this approach. The size and softness of the chest and clavicles make the landmarks for the SV more difficult to identify, and the curvature of the anterior chest in the infant reduces the space available for entering the vein without puncturing the lung or artery. Skill and experience are required to perform this procedure without complications.

As with jugular venous cannulation, right-sided subclavian cannulation is favored over the left primarily because of anatomic considerations. The cupola of the lung, which lies inferior to the junction of the IJV and SV and posterior to the subclavian artery, is higher in relation to these vascular structures on the left side as compared to the right. In addition, the left thoracic duct is large and may be injured during cannulation. Finally, the acute angle of entry by the left-sided subclavian/innominate into the SVC place the patient at greater risk for intimal damage and vascular perforation (6).

EQUIPMENT

As shown in Table 18.2, the equipment necessary for CVC placement can be listed in four general categories: (*a*) materials used for establishing an aseptic field and maintaining sterile technique during the procedure (see also Chapter 7); (*b*) the various catheters, needles, wires, and other items needed for placing, securing, and dressing the catheter; (*c*) monitoring equipment necessary to ensure

**Chapter 18
Central Venous
Access and Central
Venous Pressure
Monitoring**

256

Table 18.2.
Equipment Checklist

I. Aseptic technique
   betadine solution
   sterile 4 × 4 gauze
   sterile towels, drapes
   sterile gloves
   sterile gowns, masks
II. Catheter kit, Suturing material
   intravascular catheters (have an extra on hand)
   finder needle (usually 20 to 22 gauge, 1.5 inches)
   flexible guidewire (straight or J-tip, make sure it fits the catheter)
   heparinized saline solution
   syringes, 3 or 5 ml
   silk suture (3.0 or 4.0)
   needle holder
III. Monitoring equipment
   pulse oximeter
   ECG monitor
   impedance pnuemogram
   Dynamapp
   pressure transducer
IV. Medications
   lidocaine 1% (without epinephrine)
   midazolam 0.1 mg/kg
   morphine sulfate 0.1 to 0.15 mg/kg

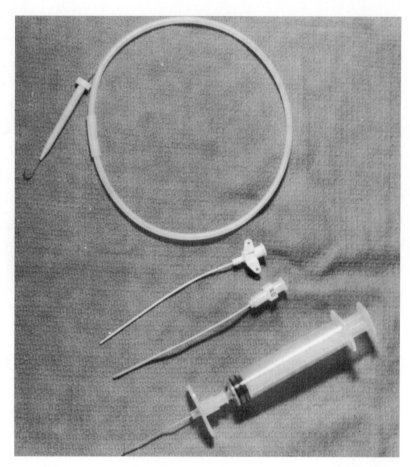

Figure 18.2.
Items in a commercially produced pediatric central venous catheter tray (available from various manufacturers).

patient safety during the procedure and after the catheter is in place (see also Chapter 5); (*d*) medications and other items necessary to ensure patient comfort and cooperation during the procedure (see also Chapter 35).

Ensuring that the proper equipment for CVC placement is available has become a relatively simple task because of the many commercially produced kits for this procedure (e.g., Cooke®, Abbott®, Arrow®, Viggo-Spectramed®) (Fig. 18.2). These kits contain most of the equipment included in the first two categories listed previously. In addition, organizing desired ancillary equipment into prepackaged trays or packets for CVC placement will also improve efficiency and reduce the likelihood of errors.

Types of Catheters

Four types of catheters, corresponding to specific techniques that may be performed have been used most commonly for percutaneous CVC placement. These include (*a*) plain needle, (*b*) catheter passed through a needle, (*c*) catheter passed over a needle, and (*d*) catheter passed over a guide wire (Seldinger technique). More recently plain needle CVC, when a steel needle remains within the ves-

sel, has all but disappeared because of availability of synthetic polymer plastics now used in the manufacture of catheters.

In the catheter-through-the-needle technique, the skin is first punctured with a relatively large, hollow needle (Fig. 18.3). After blood return is observed, a catheter is then passed through the needle lumen and advanced into the vein. Once the catheter is in the proper position, the needle is removed from the skin but remains surrounding the catheter, usually housed in a plastic shield to prevent it from injuring the patient or cutting the catheter wall. With this technique, the catheter commonly contains a wire stylet which confers rigidity as the catheter is advanced into the vein and which is removed before infusion of fluids.

The catheter-over-the-needle technique employs a thin needle housed in a tightly fitting, plastic catheter to puncture the skin and enter the vein (Fig. 18.4). When blood return is apparent, the needle and catheter are advanced an additional 2 to 5 mm, at which

**Chapter 18
Central Venous
Access and Central
Venous Pressure
Monitoring**

257

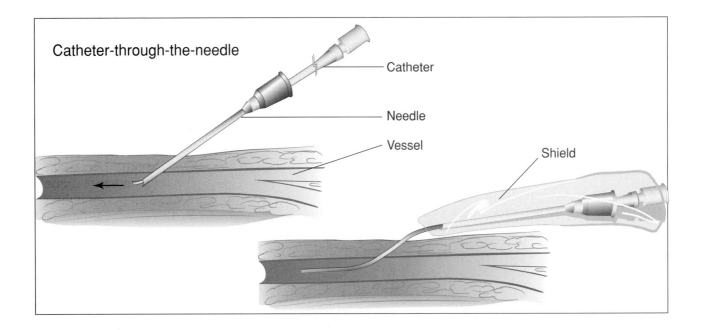

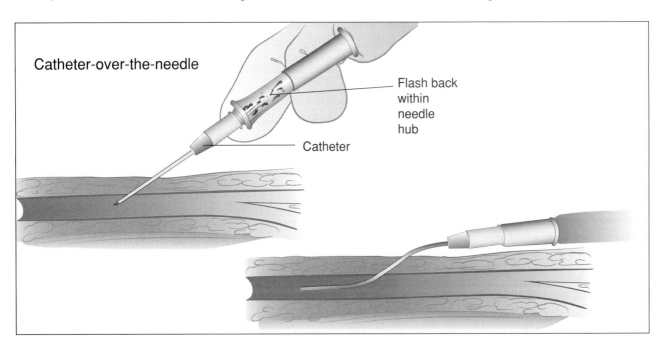

Figure 18.3.
Catheter-through-the-needle technique.

Figure 18.4.
Catheter-over-the-needle technique.

point the catheter is then advanced off the needle and into the vessel.

Seldinger Technique

Although the previously mentioned catheter-through-the-needle and catheter-over-the-needle systems are still favored by some, by far the most widely used technique for children is the catheter-over-the-wire method more commonly known as the Seldinger technique (Fig. 18.5). Described by Sven Ivar Seldinger in 1953 for placement of vascular catheters, this procedure has been so success-ful that systems using its basic principles have now been extended to other procedures such as emergency tracheostomy and nonoperative gastrostomy tube placement. The Seldinger technique utilizes a small gauge entry needle which is used initially to puncture the skin and enter the blood vessel lumen. A guide wire is then threaded through the entry needle into the vessel. The entry needle is removed and a larger caliber vascular catheter is advanced over the wire into the vessel. The entire procedure may be repeated with increasing sizes of wires and catheters to

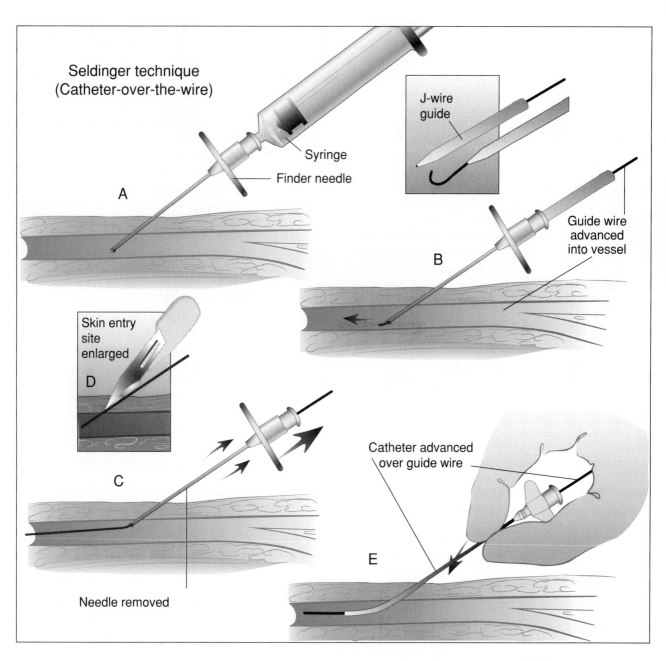

Seldinger technique
(Catheter-over-the-wire)

Syringe
Finder needle

A

J-wire
guide

Guide wire
advanced
into vessel

B

Skin entry
site
enlarged
D

C

Needle removed

Catheter advanced
over guide wire

E

achieve the desired catheter size even when starting with a small entry needle (12).

The guide wires used for the Seldinger technique have both a flexible end and a rigid end. The flexible tip is designed to enter the blood vessel allowing it to negotiate a potentially tortuous blood vessel. Often the tip has a *J* configuration and comes with a plastic sleeve which serves to straighten the tip while the wire is threaded into the entry needle hub. J-wires are particularly useful for situations in which acute angles or sharp turns are encountered within the cannulated blood vessel, as with the EJV approach (see below). The

rigid end of the wire is designed to facilitate threading the stiff catheter over the guide wire.

Catheter Plastics

Catheters used today for central venous cannulation come in a variety of materials, diameters, and lengths, as well as with multiple lumens. The first vascular catheters used for infusions or pressure measurement were made of glass, steel, or natural rubber; therefore it is not difficult to understand why vas-

Figure 18.5.
Catheter-over-the-wire
(Seldinger) technique.
A. The central vein is first
punctured using a needle
and syringe.
B. The syringe is removed
and the guide wire is
inserted through the needle
into the vein.
C. The needle is removed
and the wire is left in place.
D. A small incision is made
at the entry site to facilitate
insertion of the catheter.
E. The catheter is inserted
over the guide wire and
the wire is removed.

cular catheterization was performed infrequently in the past (2). Over the last 30 years, the introduction of various synthetic polymers in the manufacture of biomedical devices has been crucial in the development of vascular catheters which are relatively inexpensive, safe, reliable, and effective.

Synthetic polymers used in biomedical devices are high molecular weight materials composed of a repeating, simple chemical unit (monomer) (13). Monomers may be linked in chains of linear bonds, or they may have branched connections forming a three-dimensional network. The material may contain only one type of repeating chemical structure or may be composed of a combination of two or more chemically different copolymers. The most popular material currently used in vascular catheter manufacture is a family of plastics—the polyurethanes—composed of various copolymers. The chemical and physical properties of the monomers and the nature of the polymeric links determine whether the material is hard or soft, brittle or flexible, how it responds to changes in temperature, and how it is affected by the blood and other tissues. In turn, these features determine how suited the materials are for use in the manufacture of vascular catheters and for what specific purposes the resulting catheters can be employed.

Teflon® was the first material widely used in the manufacture of central venous catheters. Teflon® is strong, which allows for a large internal-to-external diameter ratio and thereby provides the maximal lumen size; this also makes the catheter stiff for easy percutaneous insertion. Radiocontrast material is easily mixed with this polymer, and therefore Teflon® is readily made radiopaque. However, the primary disadvantage of Teflon® catheters is that they kink easily (14). In addition, although the surface of Teflon® is smooth, which reduces the likelihood of thrombus formation, the stiffness of these catheters can lead to endothelial injury and vascular mural thrombi.

Polyvinylchloride is another plastic used in many biomedical devices including vascular catheters. Yet polyvinylchloride has not remained popular for use in long-term vascular catheters for two reasons. The first reason is that the material is associated with high thrombogenicity. Although pulmonary artery (Swan-Ganz) catheters are still often made of polyvinylchloride, they are almost always manufactured with a heparin coating to reduce thrombus formation during the relatively short duration of time that these catheters are designed to be used (15–17). The other major problem limiting the use of polyvinylchloride for vascular catheters is that drugs infused through these catheters adsorb to the plastic (15).

Silicone rubber (Silastic®) is polymerized polydimethylsiloxone, which confers a flexible rubberlike quality, mixed with silica powder, which provides increased hardness. Hickman, and later Broviac, described techniques for providing long-term vascular access using catheters made of silicone rubber which are subcutaneously tunneled proximal to the entry site and into the vein. This remains the primary use of such catheters today (2). Silicone is smooth and soft, giving catheters made of this material a remarkable record of low infection and clotting rates and a low incidence of injury to vascular and cardiac structures. However, the softness of silicone catheters requires surgical incision and dissection for placement and predisposes them to fracture or rupture. Kits designed to overcome the need for surgical placement and allow percutaneous placement have been designed; however, this technique is not practical for emergency catheter placement. The accuracy of vascular pressure measurements obtained using silicone rubber catheters also has been questioned, although some recent observations do not support this contention (18).

In recent years, catheters made of polyurethane have proven to be the most popular. This is because the various polyurethanes currently available provide the best combination of biocompatibility, stiffness (to ease percutaneous placement), softness and smoothness (to reduce vascular injury, thrombosis and infectious complications), a low tendency to kink, the ability to incorporate radiocontrast and low manufacturing costs (14, 19).

Catheter Diameter and Flow Characteristics

The diameter of vascular catheters is designated in one of two measurement systems: gauge or French. In the French measurement

Chapter 18
Central Venous
Access and Central
Venous Pressure
Monitoring

260

Table 18.3.
Catheter Sizes for Pediatric Patients

Age	Average Weight (kg)	Average Height (cm)	Average Catheter Length (cm)		
			IJ	SC	Fem
1 mo	4.2	55	6.0	5.5	15.7
3 mo	5.8	61	6.6	6.0	17.3
6 mo	7.8	68	7.3	6.6	19.1
9 mo	9.2	72	7.6	6.9	20.1
1 yr	10.2	76	8.0	7.3	21.1
1.5 yr	11.5	83	8.7	7.9	22.9
2 yr	12.8	88	9.2	8.3	24.2
4 yr	16.5	103	10.6	9.6	28.1
6 yr	20.5	116	11.8	10.7	31.4
8 yr	26	127	12.9	11.7	34.2
10 yr	31	137	13.8	12.5	36.8
12 yr	39	149	15.0	13.5	39.9
14 yr	50	165	16.5	14.9	44.0
16 yr	62.5	174	17.3	15.7	46.3

scale, each unit is equivalent to 0.33 mm in outer diameter. For example, a 5-French catheter has an outer diameter (OD) of 1.65 mm (5 times 0.33 mm). The gauge system developed in a more empiric fashion, but is now standardized. The OD in millimeters for commonly used pediatric gauge catheters include: 14 gauge = 2.1 mm, 16 gauge = 1.6 mm, 18 gauge = 1.3 mm, 20 gauge = 1.1 mm, 22 gauge = 0.7 mm. Guidelines for selection of catheters based on age, weight, and height are shown in Tables 18.3 and 18.4.

The French or gauge designations always refer to the OD of the catheter. In general, with the plastics used in the manufacture of catheters today, the practitioner can assume that the lumenal diameter is about 40 to 50% of the OD. In multiple lumen catheters, the equivalent OD is often marked on each lumen port. If all ports are of equal size, a reasonable assumption is to divide the overall diameter by the number of lumens to estimate each lumen size.

Catheter diameter and length have a great impact on medical utility. The appeal of central venous cannulas for the treatment of circulatory failure include the ability to (a) bypass local venous constriction present in hypovolemic states, (b) remain relatively unimpeded by patient movement that might otherwise result in altered infusion rates or loss of access, and (c) avoid extravascular infiltration of fluid. The disadvantage of CVCs for these purposes is that the necessary length and diameter of the catheter may reduce the infusate flow rate. Factors that determine flow rate through a catheter are expressed in Poiseuille's law:

$$\text{flow rate} = \pi \cdot (P_1 - P_2) \cdot (R^4 / 8) \cdot v \cdot L$$

where π is the constant pi, P_1 is the hydrostatic pressure driving the fluid into the catheter, P_2 is hydrostatic pressure in the blood vessel outside the catheter tip, R is the radius of the catheter lumen, v is the viscosity of the infused fluid, and L is the length of the catheter. Flow therefore increases in proportion to the 4th power of the lumen radius but decreases in proportion to the length of the catheter. In addition, the rate of flow is inversely proportional to the viscosity of the fluid, so that saline and other crystalloid solutions will flow more rapidly than blood products. Increasing the hydrostatic pressure driving the fluid into the catheter will increase the flow rate. Conversely, high vascular hydrostatic pressure outside the tip of the catheter will reduce flow rate.

Theoretic considerations outlined previously can have important clinical implica-

Table 18.4.
Catheter Diameters for Pediatric Patients

Age	Catheter Diameter (French)		
	IJ	SC*	Fem
0–6 months	3	3	3
6 months–2 years	3	3	3–4
3 years–6 years	4	4	4
7 years–12 years	4–5	4–5	4–5

* For infants and younger children, the subclavian approach should only be performed by highly experienced operators.

Chapter 18
Central Venous
Access and Central
Venous Pressure
Monitoring

261

tions. For example, when a 16 gauge (1.6 mm OD) is used rather than a 14 gauge (2.1 mm OD) during a resuscitation, the operator should be aware that although the catheter diameter is only reduced by 24%, the rate of flow will be decreased by 66%, if all other factors remain constant. Similarly, the number of lumens within a catheter must also be considered. A 14-gauge double lumen catheter, with one lumen 16 gauge and the other 20 gauge (1.1 mm OD), will have a 66% reduction in flow rate if the 16-gauge lumen is used and a 90% reduction in flow rate when the 20-gauge lumen is used when compared to a 14-gauge single lumen catheter.

Although theoretic considerations outlined above are qualitatively true, actual flow measurements in studies of pediatric catheters have demonstrated slightly greater flow rates than are predicted from Poiseuille's law. Changes in length have a linear effect on flow rate; thus if other factors remain constant, a catheter of one-half the length will have twice the maximum flow rate. Although this consideration suggests that large caliber, short peripheral catheters may better serve patients in need of rapid fluid replacement than longer central circulation catheters, experimental data indicates that in children this may not always hold true. Hydrostatic pressure in a tortuous or compressed peripheral vein may explain why comparable flow rates are achieved with longer central venous catheters versus shorter peripheral catheters in these studies.

The driving pressure forcing fluid through the catheter is another important variable determining flow rate through catheters. A 500 mL bag of saline and a standard 200 cm IV tubing exert approximately 85 mm Hg pressure when held 100 cm above the catheter connector. Manually inflated pressure bags generally increase driving pressure to about 300 to 400 mm Hg and in some cases to as high as 700 mm Hg. Pneumatically driven automatic pressure bags achieve pressures above 400 mm Hg whereas a hand-held syringe can achieve pressures as high as 2000 mm Hg (although this is highly variable, because the individual pushing the syringe generally fatigues quickly). Syringe infusion pumps available for clinical use have safety limits to prevent them from generating pressures in excess of 500 to 1200 mm Hg.

In order to put these driving pressure numbers into perspective, the theoretic calculations derived from Poiseuille's equation should be considered in light of experimental data from recent studies on this subject. For example, the total blood volume of a briskly hemorrhaging 40 kg child is approximately 2600 mL. If this patient has a 25-cm, 14-gauge central venous catheter in place, it would take approximately 50 minutes to replace the total blood volume if the bag is simply raised 100 cm above the entry site of the catheter. If a manual pressure bag is applied at 300 mm Hg, replacement time would be reduced to 15 minutes. To replace an ongoing blood loss of 500 mL per minute with the same catheter, 900 mm Hg of pressure would be required continuously to transfuse the patient (20–25).

Monitoring Equipment

Frequent heart rate, blood pressure and pulse oximetry measurements are mandatory during CVC placement. Routine ECG monitoring is desirable in most cases, but it is required if the catheter tip or guide wire is likely to touch the endocardium. For the intubated, mechanically ventilated patient end tidal CO_2 monitoring is also helpful. These monitoring recommendations are based on considerations related to the patient's underlying disease, the sedative or analgesic medicines used to facilitate the procedure, and the likelihood that a good portion of the child's body will be draped obscuring observation during the procedure. Additionally, if the physician primarily responsible for the patient's treatment is also the individual placing the CVC, his or her attention may be focused on performing the procedure. Under these circumstances, the aid of an assistant, in addition to the electronic monitors, is imperative to ensure patient safety.

During catheter placement, a method to determine the vascular pressure at the catheter tip with real-time display of the pressure waveform is optimal for excluding inadvertent arterial puncture and confirming proper venous positioning. Following placement, continuous pressure and waveform monitoring are valuable to detect accidental displacement or occlusion of the line.

The necessary components for central venous pressure measurement are shown in

Chapter 18
Central Venous
Access and Central
Venous Pressure
Monitoring

262

Figure 18.6. The venous catheter is connected via a saline-filled tube to the transducer system. A transducer converts a mechanical force (in this case pressure) into an electronic signal. By coupling the transducer via an electronic amplifier to an monitor, a wave form of pressure versus time can be displayed on the monitor screen and/or the pressure can be digitally displayed. In recent years these systems have been greatly simplified and standardized. Multiple manufacturers now provide setups that include a disposable transducer with necessary tubing and stopcock connections to facilitate connection to the catheter. Such systems are compatible with all clinical monitors. In most cases, these disposable transducers utilize a piezoelectric crystal system that produces a five microvolt voltage change per milliliter of mercury change in hydrostatic pressure. Industry standards for the amplifiers stipulate that this five microvolt change per unit pressure produces a one volt change in output on the monitor screen.

As described previously, it is important to recognize the influence of the pressure measurement reference point. Traditionally, the transducer reference point is set by zeroing the monitor to the midaxillary line on the supine patient (zeroing at the level of the heart). Modern transducer/monitor systems make this a relatively simple process. One of the stopcocks between the catheter and transducer is positioned at the midaxillary line and opened to expose the transducer to atmospheric pressure. Pressing a button on the monitor will then automatically set the electronic scale to zero. Once this is done, the pressure within the vascular space will always be indicated as the value above or below the atmospheric pressure at the level of the heart.

Medications and Equipment for Patient Comfort

Medications and equipment required to ensure patient comfort and cooperation during the procedure include local anesthetic, intravenous sedatives and analgesics, neuromuscular blocking agents, and physical restraints. Obviously, neuromuscular blockade would only be considered for the child who has a definitive airway already in place. Which of

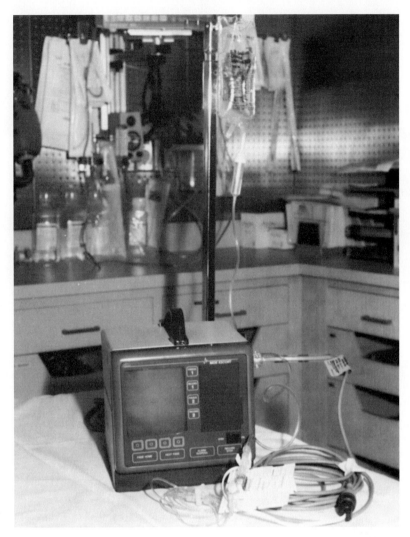

these adjuncts are selected and how they are used will vary from patient to patient, but careful preparation of these items is necessary for successful CVC placement (see also Chapters 35 and 37).

PROCEDURE

Successful central venous cannulation requires careful preparation and attention to the patient and environment before, during, and immediately after the procedure. Some of the more generic issues regarding CVC placement, as well as a description of the steps involved with standard Seldinger technique, are described first. Then important points relating to the specific entry sites that may be used are presented.

Figure 18.6.
Equipment used for central venous pressure monitoring.

Consent

Obtaining consent is always desired before performing any medical procedure. Patients and parents will appreciate a brief discussion of the procedure, including patient positioning, the use of monitoring devices, sterile draping that may cover the child's face, the use of sedation or analgesia, and any potential complications. A note in the chart describing this interaction—or depending on institutional policy, a signed consent form—can be helpful to other professionals involved in the patient's care and may protect the physician and hospital at a later time. The details of these practices vary among different institutions, but the overall principals are generally applicable. Although this may be the desired goal, however, percutaneous CVC placement is often required in urgent or life-threatening situations which preclude obtaining informed consent. In such circumstances, common sense, compassion and clinical judgment must dictate the physician's actions. A brief retrospective discussion of the procedure and its complications is still often helpful to patients and/or their families (see also Chapter 9).

Preparing the Environment

Medications and monitors used to ensure patient comfort and safety during the procedure should all be prepared, convenient to the operator, and functioning properly before medicating or even positioning the patient. Any assistants should be briefed regarding their anticipated roles. As discussed, it is recommended that heart rate, blood pressure, and pulse oximetry be measured and recorded frequently (every 1 to 2 minutes) or displayed continuously during the procedure. A continuous electrocardiogram is required whenever stimulation of the endocardium is possible. Ideally, the pressure transducer and waveform monitor should also be ready before attempting to catheterize the vessel. Finally, it should be emphasized that all the sophisticated electronic monitors available today are no substitute for human observation. Since the physician operator will be concentrating on the procedure, it is important to have one or more experienced assistants who are practiced in the assessment of critically ill children and familiar with the procedure.

Preparing the Patient

Once the equipment, medications, personnel, and monitors are in place, the next step is to properly position the patient. Details of positioning will be addressed below within the discussion of each specific approach, but one general principle is that ensuring patient comfort is a key to success. Medications for analgesia and sedation are helpful in meeting this goal but their use must be individualized to each patient's needs. Patients' underlying medical problems, particularly their circulatory and respiratory function, must be carefully considered in the decision to use these adjuncts.

Most patients will benefit from a local anesthetic used at the point of skin puncture. This is most often provided with 1% lidocaine solution (10 mg/mL) without epinephrine, which will adequately anesthetize the site without exceeding the toxic threshold dose of approximately 7 mg/kg (see also Chapter 37). For the anxious patient with stable circulation, the operator may choose to use intravenous sedatives and/or an analgesic titrated to the desired effect. An effective and commonly used combination is 0.05 to 0.1 mg/kg of midazolam and 0.05 to 0.1 mg/kg of morphine sulfate (see also Chapter 35). Judicious use of restraints—or neuromuscular blockade for mechanically ventilated patients capable of moving suddenly—may also be valuable adjuncts. In addition, the benefit of a soothing voice or gentle touch in helping a child tolerate and cooperate with these procedures should not be underestimated.

Preparing the Site

After the patient is properly positioned, comfortable and cooperative, the cannulation site can be prepared using aseptic technique (see also Chapter 7). The use of sterile gowns, masks, and hats is advocated by some experts, but no data exist to prove these adjuncts decrease infection. These additional precautions, however, may be helpful when placing long catheters or when instructing another physician, as the equipment has a tendency to accidentally touch the operator's chest or arms in such situations.

When cleansing the anatomic site with the antiseptic solution of choice, it is important to clean an area large enough to allow observation and palpation of anatomic landmarks adjacent to the entry site without contaminating the field. Trimming hair with scissors rather than shaving prevents abrading and inflaming the skin, which can lead to an increased incidence of infection. The area should be adequately draped with sterile towels to provide a sterile work space large enough to prevent accidental contamination of the catheter, wire, or other equipment.

Once the area is properly draped and the landmarks reexamined, the skin site is infiltrated with local anesthetic. A generous skin wheal is first made using a short 25-gauge needle, and then the subcutaneous tissues are infiltrated using a slightly longer 21- or 22-gauge needle. With small infants, the cutaneous and subcutaneous injections are easily accomplished in one step using the smaller needle. The syringe should always be aspirated before infiltrating the skin in order to avoid an intravascular delivery of local anesthetic.

Placing the Catheter

Because it is by far the method most commonly used today, the Seldinger technique (catheter-over-the-wire) will be the focus of this discussion (Fig. 18.5). After the anatomic landmarks appropriate for the specific entry site are identified, the skin puncture site is well anesthetized. The entry needle is attached to a small 3 or 5 mL syringe and rinsed with a heparinized saline solution. The small syringe prevents air embolism and the heparin reduces clot formation in the needle. Some experts also recommend ejecting a small volume of fluid (less than 0.5 mL) through the needle just after making the skin puncture to flush out any skin plugs caught in the beveled needle tip. Once through the skin, a small amount of negative pressure is applied to aid blood return as the needle is advanced. When blood return is apparent, the needle should be inserted an additional 1 to 2 mm until a free flow of blood is obtained to ensure that the tip lies well within the vessel lumen.

A few techniques that may be beneficial during this phase of the procedure deserve emphasis. First, using a small syringe with gentle suction while locating the vein will prevent vessel collapse even with a small, hypovolemic child. Second, if blood flow is not obtained after deeply advancing the needle, the needle should be slowly withdrawn to a depth just beneath the surface of the skin while maintaining gentle negative pressure. In this way, if the vessel lumen was inadvertently passed completely through during needle entry, it will be identified as the needle is withdrawn. If blood return into the needle is not noted during this withdrawal procedure, the needle tip is redirected and advanced again. By this slow, careful advance and withdrawal, multiple vein lacerations and hematoma formation are avoided. Third, some clinicians prefer to use a 23- or 25-gauge, 1.5 inch finder needle to locate the vein first before puncturing it with the larger gauge entry needle. They leave the small finder needle in place as a guide until the vein is again accessed with the larger entry needle. This also may prevent unnecessary injury to the vessel. Fourth, inadvertent arterial puncture should be suspected whenever the blood appears redder (oxygenated) than the expected darker venous blood. Occasionally, this may be difficult to determine due to the poor oxygenation status of the patient. If any question remains, a specimen of blood can be sent for blood gas analysis. Finally, use of a non-Luer-Lok syringe prevents accidental dislodgment of the needle out of the vessel as the syringe is removed. Most commercially available kits provide these.

Once the needle successfully enters the vessel, the syringe is carefully detached so that the guide wire can be inserted. After the syringe is removed, and before the wire is inserted, the needle lumen is occluded with the thumb of the operating hand. If the needle hub or catheter is left unoccluded, air embolus or significant blood loss may result. Pulsatile blood flow from the needle indicates arterial puncture. Assuming venous placement, the guide wire is then inserted a short distance beyond the tip of the entry needle. The operator must always ensure that the rigid (proximal) end of the wire is visibly protruding from the hub of the entry needle. Accidental loss of the guide wire in the central circulation is prevented by this method.

If the wire does not pass with minimal resistance, it should be removed. When a guide wires does not pass easily, reconfirmation of the needle position within the vessel

Figure 18.7.
Central venous catheter
with dilator suitable for an
older adolescent or adult.

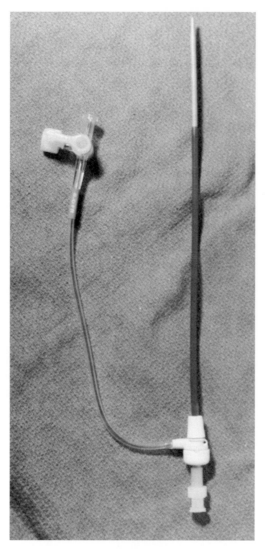

will make it easier to advance the larger caliber catheter into the blood vessel and will protect the catheter tip from fraying. Before advancing the catheter into the vessel, the wire should always be observed to emerge from the proximal end of the catheter, again to prevent accidental loss of the wire into the central circulation. During catheter advancement, the fingertips are positioned close to the catheter tip and steady gentle pressure is applied with a slow, twisting motion. This facilitates controlled insertion of the catheter through the subcutaneous tissues and into the lumen of the vein. If resistance is met at this stage of the procedure, a few additional techniques may be helpful. First, the catheter should be removed so that the tip can be examined. Fraying of the tip will prevent smooth entry into the vessel. If fraying is present, the catheter must be replaced. Before attempting insertion with the new catheter, the operator should repeat the scalpel incision, but this time extending slightly deeper into the subcutaneous tissue. Alternatively, a stiff single lumen dilator may be used to create a tract through which the softer permanent vascular catheter will more easily pass. In fact, some catheters are now packaged with a dilator that is tightly fit within the lumen of the permanent catheter (Fig. 18.7). When using one of these kits, the technique for placement is the same, except that the combined venodilator/catheter is passed over the wire in a single step. The dilator and wire are then removed together leaving the catheter in place. In addition to standard CVC placement, methods just described may also be used to replace an existing catheter with a new one using a guide wire, to place an introducer through which a Swan-Ganz catheter or transvenous pacemaker may be inserted, as well as other maneuvers.

The last step before securing and dressing the catheter is to ensure that the tip is properly positioned. As mentioned previously, determining venous versus arterial placement of the catheter can be made based on the appearance of blood aspirated, blood gas analysis, and/or vascular pressure measurement. These are the only methods required for short catheters placed in the femoral vein. For all other catheters, a portable chest and/or abdominal radiograph are also necessary to confirm proper position. The radiograph should indicate that the

should be attempted by observing for free flow of blood with aspiration of the syringe. Strategies helpful on subsequent attempts include redirection or rotation of the needle bevel, or use of the J-wire. The J-wire should be gently rolled between the operator's thumb and forefinger during advancement to facilitate passage. If the operator ever encounters resistance during wire removal from the entry needle, he or she must withdraw the needle and wire together to prevent shearing of the wire by the beveled tip of the needle.

After the wire is successfully placed in the vessel, the entry needle is removed and a scalpel blade (No. 11) is used to enlarge the skin puncture site. The blade is placed perpendicular to the skin, with the sharp edge pointed away from the wire, and advanced along the path of the guide wire through the skin and subcutaneous tissue. This incision

catheter tip is parallel to the vascular wall. This will prevent inadvertent vessel laceration or endothelial injury with movement of the catheter or the patient. When accessing the central circulation from sites cephalad to the heart, the desired position for the catheter tip is in the vena cava just proximal to the right atrium/vena cava junction. This position ensures that (*a*) the infusions are entering a high volume, high flow space, (*b*) vascular pressure measurements reflect the intrathoracic pressure, and (*c*) myocardial injury will not occur. More proximal catheter tip positions are acceptable as long as the tip/wall orientation remains parallel. Central venous pressure measurements from an infradiaphragmatic tip position (femoral venous entry site) have been shown to correlate with intrathoracic tip measurements as long as a pressure wave form is observed on the monitor. It should be emphasized that the CVC tip should never be allowed to remain within the right atrium. Atrial wall perforation with hemopericardium is a rare but catastrophic complication that is avoided by ensuring that the catheter tip is not located in the heart (26, 27).

Dressing the Catheter

After the catheter is properly positioned it should be sutured in place at the entry site, and the entry wound then dressed. Infection is the most common complication of CVC placement, and the incidence of infection is influenced by the type and care of the catheter wound dressing. Recently, some practitioners have abandoned the conventional dressing technique of sterile gauze held in place with tape for a newer method using a transparent polyurethane sheet (Tegaderm®, Opsite®) placed over the catheter at the skin entry site. Advocates note that these dressing systems allow for continuous inspection of the site while reliably securing the catheter and permitting the patient to more easily bathe. One obvious disadvantage for this newer dressing is its expense, but more importantly, a recent meta analysis of studies comparing this technique with older methods suggest the polyurethane covering is associated with a higher risk of catheter tip infection, bacteremia, and sepsis. Unpublished experience over 2 years in our 33-bed multidisciplinary

pediatric intensive care unit is similar, leading us to prefer the following approach to caring for a CVC wound site. First, a small amount of povidone-iodine ointment is applied to the skin at the entry site. The wound is then covered with a sterile 4 x 4 gauze and secured with silk tape. A label placed on the catheter dressing documents date and time of insertion. Regarding longer-term care, dressing changes should be performed at least 3 times weekly in accordance with CDC guidelines. During the dressing change, the site is inspected for signs of inflammation and then cleansed with povidone-iodine solution following strict sterile technique. Antiseptic ointment is then applied and clean gauze secured. The intravenous tubing is changed every 48 hours unless hyperalimentation solutions are being infused, in which case the tubing is changed every 24 hours. The tubing extending from the hub of each lumen of a multiple lumen catheter is secured to the patient's skin with silk tape or steri-strips. This will prevent accidental dislodgment of the catheter and kinking of the tubing. At our institution, a stopcock/tubing attachment is often interposed between the catheter hub and the intravenous tubing to allow access for multiple medication infusions or the addition of intermittent bolus medications through each lumen (28–35).

Documentation

When the procedure has been completed, the clinician should place a note in the patient's chart including the following information: date and time of catheter insertion, type, gauge and length of catheter placed, any complications encountered, catheter placement confirmation, and the patient's condition.

Selecting the Site

As described previously, the most common sites used for percutaneous central venous cannulation are, in order of preference, the femoral vein, the jugular veins (internal and external), and the subclavian vein. Site selection is influenced by operator experience, preexisting medical conditions of the patient, equipment considerations, indications for placing the catheter, and the urgency of the procedure. Advantages and disadvantages of the potential sites are shown in Table 18.5. Surprisingly, given the widespread use and potential hazards of central catheters, few pediatric studies have been performed to compare the various sites regarding success rates, longevity, and incidence of complications.

The femoral site is so popular for pediatric central venous access that it might well be considered the approach of first choice (see Indications). The primary advantage of this site is that it is farthest away from the head and chest, thereby avoiding interference with evaluation or treatment of the critically ill patient. CVC placement at the femoral site also requires less technical expertise than at the jugular or subclavian sites. For most practitioners, the jugular sites would be considered a secondary choice. At our institution, CVC placement is performed at these sites in 15 to 20% of cases. As discussed previously, the subclavian approach is used infrequently for children, because it requires the highest degree of expertise and is associated with the greatest incidence of

serious complications, such as significant hemorrhage and pneumothorax.

Femoral Vein

Although early reports indicated that femoral venous cannulae had a high rate of complications, experience with pediatric patients over the last two decades has demonstrated the safety and effectiveness of this procedure. As stated previously, among the reasons that account for the popularity of this approach are unimpeded access to the airway and chest, easily identifiable landmarks, ease of hemostasis, and relative absence of serious acute complications. Perhaps the most important advantage of this site, however, is the high rate of successful cannulation. Swanson et al. reported an 89% success rate of percutaneously placed femoral catheters in critically ill ED patients, with the only reported complication being arterial puncture causing a small groin hematoma in one patient (12). Failure was the result of either inability to locate the vein or inability to thread the catheter. Similarly, Kanter et al. found that

Table 18.5.
Advantages and Disadvantages of Specific Sites

Site	Landmark	Advantage	Disadvantage	Complications
FV	Femoral triangle, just medial to femoral artery pulse (if palpable)	Requires least operator experience, fastest, out of the way of resuscitation, anatomy exposed, available for direct compression	Risk of contamination, may be harder to secure, may be more uncomfortable for the pt, difficult in obese patients, need fluoroscopy to place Swan-Ganz catheter	Infection, bleeding, thrombosis
IJV	Angle formed by the two heads of SCM m	Right side offers direct route to SVC, out of resuscitation field, anatomy exposed, available for direct compression	Requires operator experience, generally takes longer, more difficult in children <1 yr with short, fat necks, more difficult in pts with tracheostomy and pts who are not intubated	CA puncture, PTX, on left side risk of thoracic duct injury, cardiac tamponade, multiple neuropathies, thrombosis, infection
EJV	Visible in the neck crossing posteriorly over SCM m	Visible, superficial, available for direct compression, least complications	Difficult to cannulate central circulation from this site, if not visible cannot use this site	Hematoma
SV	Supraclavicular: Lateral to clavicular head of SCM m, above the clavicle Infraclavicular: Just beneath junction of middle and lateral thirds of the clavicle	Right side offers direct route to SVC, vein may be less collapsible	Requires operator experience, may be more difficult in pts <1 yr, no access to control bleeding	PTX, bleeding, tamponade, dysrhythmias, thoracic duct injury, catheter malposition, air embolism, neuropathies

FV (femoral vein), IJV (internal jugular vein), EJV (external jugular vein), SV (subclavian vein), AV (axillary vein), SVC (superior vena cava), CA (carotid artery), PTX (pneumothorax), SCM (sternocleidomastoid)

Chapter 18
Central Venous
Access and Central
Venous Pressure
Monitoring

268

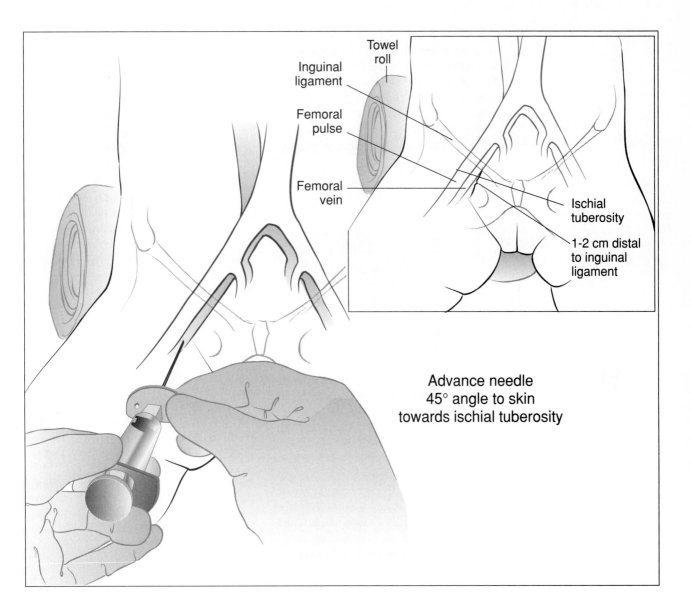

Inguinal ligament

Towel roll

Femoral pulse

Femoral vein

Ischial tuberosity

1-2 cm distal to inguinal ligament

Advance needle
45° angle to skin
towards ischial tuberosity

pediatric residents demonstrated an 86% success rate (11). Remarkably, this physician group, with relatively little previous experience, also achieved a median time to placement of only 5 minutes in a critically ill pediatric population, with 48% of patients demonstrating signs of shock. Furthermore, in this 33-month survey femoral catheters had a complication rate that was no different from central lines placed at other sites.

Although the femoral approach has several advantages, a few relative contraindications do exist to this procedure. These include abnormal vascular anatomy or congenital malformation of the lower extremity, femoral hernia, abdominal tumor or trauma, abdominal ascites, and future plans for cardiac catheterization (see Indications).

Identification of Landmarks
The femoral vein can be identified 1 to 2 cm medial to the femoral artery pulse (when palpated) 1 to 2 cm below the inguinal ligament. When the child has weak or absent pulses, the position of the FV can be located by identifying the point halfway between the pubic tubercle and the anterior iliac spine and 1 to 2 cm below the inguinal ligament (Fig. 18.8).

Procedure
When cannulating the FV, optimal patient position requires abduction and external rotation at the hip. A folded towel placed beneath the patient's ipsilateral gluteal region often improves exposure of the site. The site is located using the landmarks previously de-

Figure 18.8.
Entry site for femoral vein cannulation.

Chapter 18
Central Venous
Access and Central
Venous Pressure
Monitoring

269

scribed. The needle is inserted at a 45° angle 1 to 2 cm below (distal to) the inguinal ligament and advanced in the direction of the ischial tuberosity. At no time should the tip of the needle pass beyond the inguinal ligament, as this can result in bowel perforation or formation of a retroperitoneal hematoma that cannot be adequately controlled with hemostatic pressure (4, 36–39). Catheter insertion is performed using the Seldinger technique as described (see Placing the Catheter).

Jugular Veins

Chest and neck entry sites offer the advantages of being more stable and easily dressed, as well as providing more accurate CVP measurements because the catheter is in the thoracic cavity. They also are generally more comfortable for the patient. For these reasons, many experienced practitioners consider the IJV as the entry site of first choice. Although the EJV is sometimes used to provide access to the central circulation, the success rate for CVC placement at this site is relatively low.

Although the likelihood of complications at the IJV site is somewhat higher than with femoral placement, this approach has a lower incidence of complications than subclavian cannulation. Complications that occur with IJV cannulation include inadvertent carotid artery puncture, pneumothorax, thoracic duct laceration, and stellate ganglion injury. Complications with EJV cannulation are rare and less serious (5–9).

Internal Jugular Vein
Identification of Landmarks. Three possible approaches to cannulating the IJV are commonly referred to as the median, anterior, and lateral approaches. The optimal points of entry used for each of these approaches is determined by the position of the jugular vein as it courses through the neck. In the superior (cephalad) portion of the neck, the vessel lies just medial to the sternal (medial) head of the sternocleidomastoid muscle. In the midportion of the neck, the IJV is located beneath the junction of the sternal and clavicular (lateral) heads of the sternocleidomastoid. In the inferior (caudad) portion of the neck, the IJV lies just medial to (or sometimes beneath) the clavicular head of the sternocleidomastoid (see also Anatomy and Physiology). The most popular site is the median approach (Fig. 18.9). For all methods, the patient's head is turned approximately 30° away from the side of planned entry. To locate the median entry site, an imaginary line is drawn between the sternal notch and the mastoid process. The middle third of this line will cross over the apex of the triangle formed by the two heads of the sternocleidomastoid muscle laterally and the clavicle inferiorly. The IJV is just below the apex of this triangle. It is superficial and lateral to the carotid artery, which can be palpated just medial to this point. The anterior approach is performed less frequently but is also effective. The entry site is located at the medial border of the sternal head of the sternocleidomastoid muscle at the level of the thyroid cartilage. The carotid artery should be palpable just lateral to this point. Although often effective for adult patients, the lateral approach is not recommended for children and is therefore not described.

Procedure. As mentioned, the patient should be placed in the supine position with the head turned 20 to 30° to the contralateral side. Care should be taken not to turn the head too much (greater than 45°), as this will cause the clavicular portion of the sternocleidomastoid muscle to slide over the IJV and block easy entry to the vessel. A small, rolled towel can be positioned between the child's shoulder blades to help accentuate anatomic landmarks. The head of the bed is tilted down 15 to 30° (Trendelenburg) to promote venous distention in those patients who can tolerate this maneuver. Otherwise, the child can be asked to hold his or her breath or perform a Valsalva maneuver during venipuncture, although younger children will obviously be unable to cooperate with this request. If the child is receiving mechanical ventilation, the same effect can be produced by prolonging inspiratory times.

When using the median and anterior approaches, the needle is inserted at a 30° angle to the skin at the appropriate entry site (see above) and directed toward the ipsilateral nipple. The IJV is relatively superficial at the entry sites and consequently the needle must only be inserted 0.5 to 3.0 cm (depending on the child's age and size) in order to enter the vessel. The carotid artery should not be palpated during insertion of the needle, as this will tend to compress the IJV decreasing its diameter. The entry needle is kept at a relatively low angle to the skin during the proce-

Chapter 18
Central Venous
Access and Central
Venous Pressure
Monitoring

270

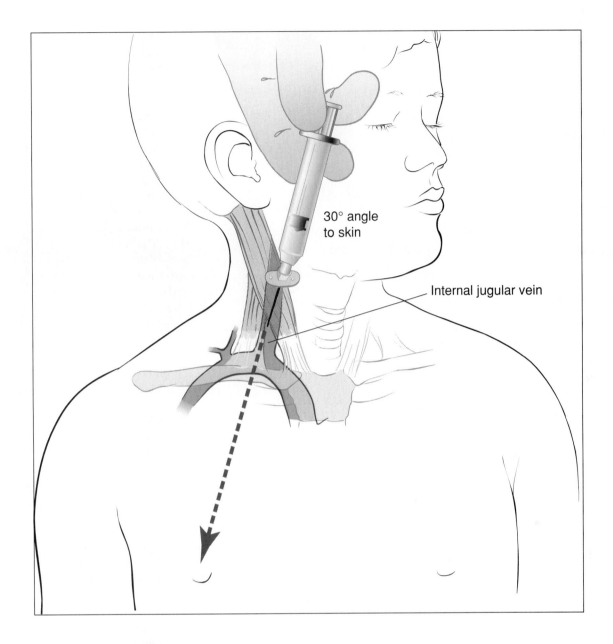

30° angle to skin

Internal jugular vein

dure as this both facilitates threading of the guide wire and reduces the chance of causing a pneumothorax (5, 7).

External Jugular Vein

As described previously, advantages of the EJV site include a low risk of pneumothorax, hematoma, carotid puncture, or injury to the sympathetic chain. However, successful central venous cannulation is much less likely using this approach than with the other sites.

Identification of Landmarks. With the patient in the supine position and the head turned 45° to the contralateral side, the EJV should be identifiable by inspection of the lateral neck (Fig. 18.10). If the vein is not visi-

ble as it crosses the sternocleidomastoid muscle, it is probably best to choose another site of entry.

Procedure. The patient is positioned in 15 to 30° Trendelenburg to promote venous distention. The operator stabilizes the vein by applying gentle traction to the skin cephalad to the point of entry using the nondominant hand. The vein is entered at the point at which it crosses the sternocleidomastoid muscle. The entry needle is inserted bevel up at a shallow (10 to 20°) angle to the skin. Because the EJV is easily compressible, relatively superficial, and highly mobile in the subcutaneous tissue, inserting a needle alone often leads to punc-ture of both walls of the vessel

Figure 18.9.
Median approach for internal jugular vein cannulation.

Chapter 18
Central Venous
Access and Central
Venous Pressure
Monitoring

271

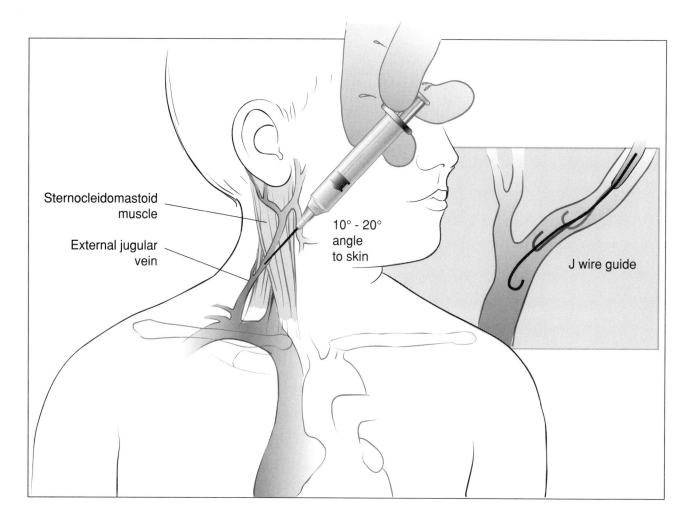

Sternocleidomastoid muscle

External jugular vein

10° - 20° angle to skin

J wire guide

Figure 18.10.
Entry site for external jugular vein cannulation.

leading to a hematoma. Consequently, it is generally advisable to use a short (2 inch) catheter over the needle, which is advanced into the vessel after insertion. Once in place, the short flexible catheter serves as the conduit for the guide wire. The J-wire is used when cannulating the external jugular, because it is more likely to negotiate the tortuous course of the vessel as well as the venous valves. The wire is advanced using a gentle twisting motion. Insertion of the wire may also be facilitated by medial or lateral flexion of the neck and/or abduction with lateral rotation of the ipsilateral arm at the shoulder (5, 7). If central venous cannulation is unsuccessful, the catheter can be left in place to provide peripheral access.

Subclavian Vein
For reasons previously mentioned, the SV is the least common site used for percutaneous central venous cannulation in children. The small size and increased compliance of the

chest and clavicles make identification of the appropriate landmarks more difficult. In addition, a higher incidence of pneumothorax and subclavian artery puncture have been reported.

Identification of Landmarks
Many techniques for cannulating the SV have been described, but they can essentially be divided into two general categories: supraclavicular approaches and infraclavicular approaches. Many clinicians tend to prefer the infraclavicular approaches in the belief that these are associated with a lower risk of pneumothorax and other complications. It is felt that movement of the needle is limited by the rib and clavicle using the infraclavicular approach, whereas the operator must carefully control the needle with the supraclavicular approach. However, studies of SV cannulation have not confirmed this hypothesis. The entry site for the supraclavicular approach is identified by locating the lateral border of the

Chapter 18
Central Venous
Access and Central
Venous Pressure
Monitoring

272

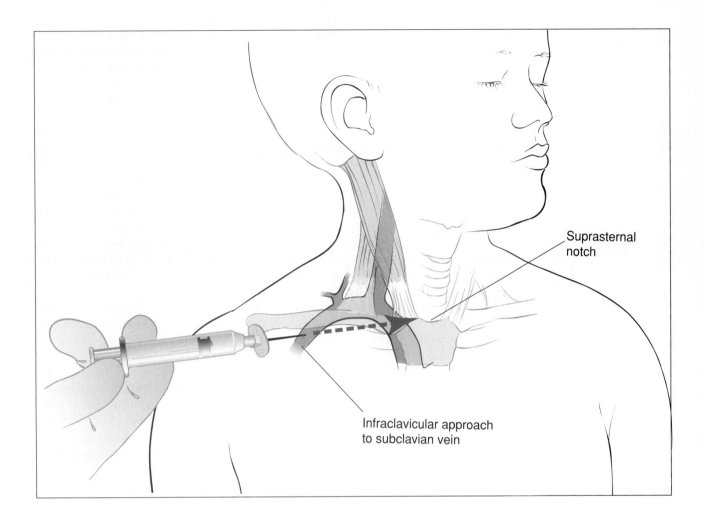

Suprasternal
notch

Infraclavicular approach
to subclavian vein

clavicular head of the sternocleidomastoid muscle and the superior border of the clavicle. The site of skin entry is approximately one finger width lateral to the muscle just above the clavicle. The infraclavicular entry site is found by identifying the clavicle and the suprasternal notch. The skin entry site is located at, or just lateral to, the midclavicular line below the clavicle (Fig. 18.11).

Procedure

The patient is placed in a supine 10 to 25° Trendelenburg position with the head turned slightly away from the planned cannulation site. A rolled towel is positioned longitudinally between the shoulder blades so that the child's shoulders fall posteriorly away from the chest. The ipsilateral arm should be at the child's side; gentle downward traction on this arm may also be helpful. The operator is positioned at the patient's side when using the infraclavicular approach or at the head of the bed when using the supraclavicular approach.

To perform the supraclavicular approach, the entry site is first identified as described previously. The finder needle is then directed so that it bisects the angle formed by the clavicle and the sternocleidomastoid muscle when aimed toward the contralateral nipple. The needle should be angled 10 to 15° above the coronal plane. The bevel of the needle is rotated inferiorly to facilitate catheter insertion into the vein following skin puncture. The catheter is slowly advanced to a distance equal to 2 to 3 times the width of the clavicle. If the operator is unsuccessful with the first pass, the needle is redirected 5 to 10° in the coronal plane and reinserted.

When using the infraclavicular approach, the patient is positioned in the same manner used for the supraclavicular approach and the entry site is located as described above. The needle is advanced slowly just beneath the inferior surface of the clavicle 2 to 4 cm, aiming toward the sternal notch. The needle should be kept as nearly parallel to the

Figure 18.11.
Infraclavicular approach for subclavian vein cannulation.

**Chapter 18
Central Venous
Access and Central
Venous Pressure
Monitoring**

horizontal plane of the chest as possible. If the first pass is unsuccessful, the needle should be withdrawn and only minimally redirected inferiorly before reinsertion. Keeping the initial orientation of the needle near the horizontal plane just under the clavicle and then making small realignments on subsequent passes will minimize the likelihood of subclavian artery puncture and pneumothorax (6, 10, 40, 41).

COMPLICATIONS

Thrombosis, vascular/cardiac perforation, cardiac arrythmia, air embolus, catheter fragment embolus, and infection are complications that can occur with any method of CVC placement (42–50). A rare complication is accidental entry of the guide wire into the central circulation, potentially requiring removal by a vascular or cardiothoracic surgeon. This unusual but significant complication can be avoided by always ensuring that the proximal end of the wire is secured at all times. Site-specific complications involve injury to adjacent structures or unique effects of the more general complications at the individual anatomic locations. The most important factors relating to all complications associated with CVC placement are operator technique during placement and subsequent care (Table 18.4).

Perforation and Erosion

The incidence of perforation and erosion from vascular catheter insertion is low. However, these can be catastrophic complications, resulting in a mortality rate exceeding 60% as a result of hemorrhage or cardiac tamponade. This fact has recently led to stringent FDA guidelines regarding catheter placement. The most critical factor in the occurrence of perforation/erosion is the position of the catheter tip. Other considerations include catheter stiffness, patient movement, and properties of infused solutions. As mentioned previously, the ideal position for a CVC is parallel to the vessel wall of the vena cava outside the reflection of the pericardium (i.e., proximal to the right atria/vena cava junction). A radiograph must always be obtained to confirm appropriate intraluminal placement. If the catheter tip is angulated toward the wall of the vessel or is within the right atrium, the catheter should be repositioned. Perforation is more likely when the left-sided IJV or SV are cannulated, because the catheter tip often lies angled against the vascular wall.

In a recent prospective evaluation of catheter tip placement in adult patients, McGee et al. found that in almost half of the cases using standard methods, the tip was positioned in the right atrium (26). In this study a technique utilizing an electrocardiography lead attached to the catheter to locate the sinoatrial node during insertion, and then withdrawing the catheter 3 cm, resulted in no cases of atrial placement of the catheter tip. It should be emphasized that proper confirmation of the position of a catheter after insertion is an important step that should not be overlooked. With adult patients, it has been shown that neck flexion can result in migration by subclavian/internal jugular catheters of 1 to 3 cm. When cephalic or axillary sites are used, catheter migration can be even greater with arm movement. Confirmation of the catheter position after placement will aid in preventing this problem from going unrecognized (45, 51, 52).

Thrombosis

Catheter-related thrombosis is a common occurrence and ranges in severity from minute fibrin deposition around the catheter tip to formation of vascular wall thrombi of varying sizes, and in more extreme cases, to complete vascular obstruction and collateral vessel formation. The vast majority of thrombi are small and cause no symptoms.

The site of catheter placement has little influence on the incidence of thrombosis. The most important factors are (a) the time elapsed since catheter placement, (b) the use of heparin, and (c) the characteristics of the catheter material. In general, heparin (1.0 IU/mL) should be added to the solutions administered through the catheter if the rate of infusion is less than 3 mL/hr. When there is no continuous infusion, the catheter should be periodically filled with a heparin solution (i.e., "flushed"); this is routinely done once daily and each time blood is aspirated from the catheter. Concentration of the heparin flush should be 100 IU/mL for older patients

Chapter 18
Central Venous
Access and Central
Venous Pressure
Monitoring

274

and 10 IU/mL for children under 1 year of age. Using heparin bonding in the manufacture of catheters reduces catheter-associated thrombosis. Heparin bonding is regularly used in Swan-Ganz pulmonary artery catheters because these catheters are often made of polyvinylchloride, a material that has a high propensity for thrombus formation. The smooth surface of Teflon® catheters allows little thrombus attachment but the stiffness of this material increases the incidence of vascular wall injury and mural thrombosis. Studies over the last decade suggest that when these techniques are used with polyurethane or silicone catheters, the rate of thrombosis is 0.04 ± 0.04 per 100 catheter days (52, 53).

Infection

Vascular catheters, like other prosthetic devices, are prone to bacterial colonization, which in some cases leads to a true infection. Infectious complications include cellulitis at the entry site, thrombophlebitis of the peripheral veins, and even systemic problems such as bacteremia, sepsis, or metastatic infections (endocarditis, abscess, etc.). The most common pathogens are bacteria present on the patient's skin or on the hands of those caring for the patient. Bacteria colonize the thin layer of fibrin that forms over the surface of all vascular catheters shortly after placement. This fibrin layer allows the patient's system to tolerate the foreign body (i.e., the catheter) but may also inhibit immunologic defenses. Some bacteria also have the ability to generate a protective covering of slime that both impedes immunologic recognition and attack by host defenses and provides a barrier to antibiotic penetration. The presence of mural thrombosis can also increase the incidence of infection. Multiple modifications have been attempted to decrease the incidence of bacterial colonization, including antibiotic bonding to the catheter material as well as other coatings such as silver or copper compounds. Although these innovations hold promise, they currently have not found universal application. The importance of good sterile technique and catheter care in preventing infection cannot be overemphasized (42, 52, 54–57).

Site-Specific Complications

Femoral Vein

During FV cannulation, the femoral artery may be inadvertently punctured leading in rare cases to major hematoma formation. However, this complication is generally inconsequential as long as artery puncture is recognized and direct pressure is applied. Infectious and thrombotic complications at this site occur with similar frequency to other sites. However, thrombosis of the iliofemoral vessels may carry more serious implications in terms of potential injury to distal structures than thrombosis of the upper extremities.

It is a commonly held belief that the femoral site for CVC placement is more prone to contamination and potential infection as a result of stool and urine soiling. In fact, multiple studies in both children and adults have indicated that the femoral site carries no overall increased risk of this complication when compared with other sites (4, 36, 38, 39, 58, 59).

Jugular Veins

Arterial puncture and associated sequela are the most common complications of IJV cannulation because of the proximity of the carotid artery. Unlike the femoral artery, applying adequate pressure hemostasis at the carotid artery can sometimes be difficult. In extreme cases, hematoma resulting from arterial puncture in the neck can result in acute airway obstruction. This complication can generally be avoided by using small gauge needles and by observing a venous wave form with respiration. If the artery is inadvertently punctured, fingertip pressure should be applied for at least 20 minutes. Nerve damage is fortunately quite rare, although brachial plexus injury has been reported with IJV cannulation. Cellulitis at the IJV site may result in mediastinitis, and thrombosis can lead to SVC syndrome. Pneumothorax can also occur, but in most cases this is readily treatable without significant complications as long as the needle misplacement is recognized and the appropriate measures are taken (see Chapter 30). Air embolus is prevented by occluding the hub of the catheter after removing the needle and by placing the patient in a head down position, because most pediatric patients cannot perform Valsalva on command.

Chapter 18
Central Venous
Access and Central
Venous Pressure
Monitoring

275

Site-specific complications are not an issue when using the EJV site for central venous cannulation. Hematoma formation here is of little clinical consequence, and nerve injury does not occur. The more generic complications just described are seen at the EJV site with the same frequency as other entry sites (6, 7, 40, 41).

Subclavian Vein

The incidence of complications with SV cannulation is approximately 5% and depends on operator skill and the circumstances under which CVC placement is performed. Pneumothorax and subclavian artery puncture are the most common complications. In cases of arterial puncture, pressure should be applied above and below the clavicle. Rarely, thrombosis can result in SVC syndrome or pulmonary embolus (41, 59).

CLINICAL TIPS

1. Ejecting a small volume of fluid from the entry needle after initial insertion through the skin will clear any skin plugs and facilitate aspiration of blood.
2. The use of a small (3 to 5 mL) syringe to initially locate the vein will prevent collapse of the vessel, even with a small, hypovolemic child.
3. If blood flow is not obtained after deep insertion of the entry needle, the needle should be slowly withdrawn while maintaining negative pressure on the syringe. If the vessel was inadvertently passed through, blood may be aspirated as the needle is withdrawn.
4. In locating the central vessel, the entry needle should be inserted and withdrawn in a slow, methodical pattern in order to prevent multiple vein lacerations.
5. Bright red blood and/or pulsatile flow indicate arterial puncture, although these findings may not be readily apparent when cardiac output is severely compromised. If there is any remaining question about whether the blood aspirated has a venous or arterial source, a specimen can be sent to the laboratory for blood gas analysis.
6. Use of a non-Luer-Lok syringe prevents accidental dislodgment of the needle on removal of the syringe before insertion of the guide wire.
7. After the syringe is removed from the entry needle, but before the guide wire is inserted, the hub of the needle should be occluded by a finger to prevent air embolus and/or blood loss.

CLINICAL TIPS CONTINUED

8. The operator must always ensure that the proximal end of the guide wire is secured at all times to prevent entry of the wire into the central circulation.
9. If resistance is felt with removal of the guide wire through the needle, the wire and needle should be removed together in order to prevent shearing of the wire by the beveled tip of the needle.
10. The catheter tip should not lie within the right atrium, since this may result in erosion and perforation of the atrial wall.
11. To obtain an accurate reading using a central venous pressure monitor, the transducer reference point must first be set by zeroing to the midaxillary line with the patient supine (i.e., zeroing to the level of the heart).

SUMMARY

Central venous access is often a critical component of pediatric resuscitation, providing a means of rapidly delivering necessary fluids and medications. Several potential anatomic locations are available for CVC placement, but the site used most commonly with pediatric patients is the proximal femoral vein. Knowledge of the anatomy, the various approaches, and the potential complications for central venous cannulation, as well as currently available catheter types and materials, is imperative for any physician who must resuscitate critically ill children. Once central venous access is obtained, measurement of the central venous pressure can provide a guide to fluid therapy when a Swan-Ganz catheter setup is not readily available. Clinical experience, coupled with the efforts of manufacturers and researchers, continues to advance the technology underlying the use of these procedures. The ongoing development of new catheter systems and materials will enhance the safety and clinical application of CVC placement for pediatric patients.

REFERENCES

1. Smith RA, Mallory DL, Wilson GL, Veremakis C. Vascular access: past, present, and future. Problems in Crit Care 1988;2:199–216.

Chapter 18
Central Venous
Access and Central
Venous Pressure
Monitoring

276

2. Kalso E. A short history of central venous catheterization. Acta Anaesth Scand 1985; 81(Suppl):7–10.

3. Cobb LM, Vincour CD, Wagner CW, Weintraub WH. The central venous anatomy in infants. Surg Gynecol Obstet 1987;165:230–234.

4. Tribett D, Brenner M. Peripheral and femoral vein cannulation. Problems in Crit Care 1988;2:266–285.

5. McGee WT, Mallory DL. Cannulation of the internal and external jugular veins. Problems in Crit Care 1988;2:217–241

6. Novak RA, Venus B. Clavicular approaches for central vein cannulation. Problems in Crit Care 1988;2:242–265.

7. Nicolson SC, Sweeney MF, Moore RA, Jobes DR. Comparison of internal and external jugular cannulation of the central circulation in the pediatric patient. Crit Care Med 1985;13:747–749.

8. Belani KG, Buckley JJ, Gordon JR, Castaneda W. Percutaneous cervical central venous line placement: a comparison of the internal and external jugular vein routes. Anaesth Analg 1980;59:40–44.

9. Cote CJ, Jobes DR, Schwartz AJ, Ellison NG. Two approaches to cannulation of a child's internal jugular vein. Anesthesia 1979;50:371–373.

10. Venkataraman ST, Orr RA, Thompson AE. Percutaneous infraclavicular subclavian vein catherization in critically ill infants and children. J Pediatr 1988;113:480–485.

11. Kanter RK, Zimmerman JJ, Strauss RH. Central venous catheter insertion by femoral vein: safety and effectiveness for the pediatric patient. Pediatrics 1986;77:842–847.

12. Swanson RS, Uhlig PN, Gross PL, et al. Emergency intravenous access through the femoral vein. Ann Emerg Med 1984;13:243–247.

13. Habal M. The biologic basis for the clinical application of the silicones. Arch Surg 1984;119:843–848.

14. Gingles B, Cooke critical care personal comm. Bloomington, IN, 1994.

15. DiCostanzo J, Sastre B, Choux R, Kasparian M. Mechanism of thrombogenesis during total parenteral nutrition: role of catheter composition. J Parenter Enteral Nutr 1988;12:190–194.

16. Welch GW, McKeel DW Jr, Silverstein P, et al. The role of catheter composition in the development of thrombophlebitis. Surg Gynecol Obstet 1974;138: 421–424.

17. Larm O, Lins LE, Olsson P. An approach to antithrombosis by surface modification. Prog Artifical Organs 1985; 2:313–318.

18. Hutyra J, Bunegin L, Albin MS. Evaluation of pressure recording characteristics of silicone elastomere, polyurethane, and polyethylene catheters. Crit Care Med 1987 April (abstract), pp. 384.

19. Linder LE, Curelaru I, Gustavsson B, Hansson HA, Stenqvist O, Wojciechowski J. Material thrombogenicity in central venous catheterization: a comparison between soft, antebrachial catheters of silicone elastomer and polyurethane. J Parenter Enteral Nutr 1984;8:399–406.

20. Idris AH, Melker RJ. High-flow sheaths for pediatric fluid resuscitation: a comparison of flow rates with standard pediatric catheters. Pediatr Emerg Care 1992;8:119–122.

21. Hodge D, Fleisher G. Pediatric catheter flow rates. Am J Emerg Med 1985;3:403–407.

22. Hodge D, Delgado-Paredes C, Fleisher G. Central and peripheral catheter flow rates in "pediatric" dogs. Ann Emerg Med 1986;15:1151–1154.

23. Mateer JR, Thompson BM, Aprahamian C, Darin JC. Rapid fluid resuscitation with central venous catheters. Ann Emerg Med 1983;12:149–152.

24. Rosen KR, Rosen DA. Comparative flow rates for small bore peripheral intravenous catheters. Pediatr Emerg Care 1986;2:153–156.

25. Spivey WH, Lather CM, Malone DR, Unger HD, Bhatt S, McNamara RN, Schoffstall J, Turner N. Comparison of intraosseous, central, and peripheral routes of sodium bicarbonate administration during CPR in pigs. Ann Emerg Med 1985;14:1135–1140.

26. McGee WT, Ackerman BL, Rouben LR, et al. Accurate placement of central venous catheters: a prospective, randomized, multicenter trial. Crit Care Med 1993;21:1118–1123.

27. Dailey RH. Use of wire-guided (Seldinger-type) catheters in the emergency department. Ann Emerg Med 1983;12:489–492.

28. Hoffman KK, Weber DJ, Samsa GP, et al. Transparent polyurethane film as an intravenous catheter dressing. JAMA 1992;267:2072–2076.

29. Maki DG, Ringer M. Evaluation of dressing regimens for prevention of infection with peripheral intravenous catheters. JAMA 1987;258:2396–2403.

30. Vicari M, Swecker M. Care of venous cannulas. Problems in Crit Care 1988;2:314–323.

31. Maki DG, Ringer M. Evaluation of dressing regimens for prevention of infection with peripheral intravenous catheters—gauze, a transparent polyurethane dressing, and an iodophor-transparent dressing. JAMA 1987;258:2396–2403.

32. Sitges-Serra A, Linares J, Perez JL, et al. Hub colonization as the initial step in an outbreak of catheter-related sepsis due to coagulase-negative staphylococci during parenteral nutrition. J Parenter Enteral Nutr 1984;8:668–672.

33. Maki DG, Ringer M. Evaluation of dressing regimens for prevention of infection with peripheral intravenous catheters. JAMA 1987;258:2396–2403.

34. Viall CD. Your complete guide to central venous catheters. Nursing 1990;2:34–41.

35. Hoffman KK, Weber DJ, Samsa GP, Rutala WA. Transparent polyurethane film as an intravenous catheter dressing. JAMA 1992;267:2072–2076.

36. Williams JF, Seneff MG, Friedman BC, et al. Use of femoral venous catheters in critically ill adults: prospective study. Crit Care Med 1991;19(4): 550–553.

37. Kanter RK, Zimmerman JJ, Strauss RH, Stoeckel KA. Central venous catheter insertion by femoral vein: safety and effectiveness for the pediatric patient. Pediatrics 1986;77:842–847.

38. Swanson RS, Uhlig PN, Gross PL, McCabe CJ. Emergency intravenous access through the femoral vein. Ann Emerg Med 1984;13:244–247.

39. Kanter RK, Zimmerman JJ, Strauss RH, Stoeckel KA. Pediatric emergency intravenous access. AJDC 1986;140:132–134.

40. Groff DB, Ahmed N. Subclavian vein catheterization in the infant. J Pediatr Surg 1974;9:171–174.

41. Irwin G, Fifield G, Clinton J. Emergency catheterization of the superior vena cava in pediatric patients. Am J Emerg Med 1984;2:494–496.

**Chapter 18
Central Venous
Access and Central
Venous Pressure
Monitoring**

277

42. Sitzman JV, Townsend TR, Siler MC, Bartlett JG. Septic and technical complications of central venous catheterization—a prospective study of 200 consecutive patients. Ann Surg 1985;202:766–770.

43. Torramade JR, Cienfuegos JA, Hernandez JL, Pardo F, Benito C, Gonzalez J, Balen E, deVilla V. The complications of central venous access sytems: a study of 218 patients. Eur J Surg 1993;159:323–327.

44. Scott WL. Complications associated with central venous catheters. Chest 1988;94:1221–1224.

45. Langston CS. The aberrant central venous catheter and its complications. Radiology 1971;100:55–59.

46. Walters MB, Stanger HA, Rotem CE. Complications with precutaneous central venous catheters. JAMA 1972;220:1455–1457.

47. Stenzel JP, Green TP, Fuhrman BP, Carlson PE, Marchessault RP. Percutaneous central venous catheterization in a pediatric intensive care unit: a survival analysis of complications. Crit Care Med 1989;17:984–988.

48. Scott Walter L. Central venous catheter complications. Office of Training and Assistance (HFZ-250), Center for Devices and Radiologic Health, Food and Drug Administration, 5600 Fishers Lane, Rockville, MD 20857. Winter 1994.

49. Goutail-Flaud MF, Sfez M, Berg A, Laguenie G, Couturier C, Larrieu B, Saint Maurice C. Central venous catheter-related complications in newborns and infants: A 587 case survey. J Pediatr Surg 1991;26:645–650.

50. Eisenhauer ED, Derveloy RJ, Hastings PR. Prospective evaluation of central venous pressure (CVP) catheters in a large city-county hospital. Ann Surg 1982;196:560–564.

51. Sheep RE, Guiney WB. Fatal cardiac tamponade. JAMA 1982;248:1632–1635.

52. Grisoni ER, Mehta SK, Connors AF. Thrombosis and infection complicating central venous catheterization in neonates. J Pediatr Surg 1986;21:772–776.

53. Ross P, Ehrenkranz R, Kleinman CS, Seashore JH. Thrombus associated with central venous catheters in infants and children. J Pediatr Surg 1989;24:253–256.

54. Centers for Disease Control Working Group. Guidelines for prevention of intravenous therapy-related infections. Infect Control 1982;4:472–473.

55. Collignon P, Soni N, Pearson I, Sorrell T, Woods P. Sepsis associated with central vein catheters in critically ill patients. Intensive Care Med 1988;14(3):227–231.

56. Bozzetti F, Terno G, Bonfanti G, et al. Prevention and treatment of central venous catheter sepsis by exchange via a guidewire. A prospective controlled trial. Ann Surg 1983;198:48–52.

57. McLean RJ, Hussain AA, Sayer M, Vincent PJ, Hughes DJ, Smith T. Antibacterial activity of multilayer silver-copper surface films on catheter material. Can J Microbiol 1993;39:895–899.

58. Stenzel JP, Green TP, Fuhrman BP, Carlson PE, Marchessault RP. Percutaneous femoral venous catheterizations: a prospective study of complications. J Pediatr 1989;114(3):411–415.

59. Stenzel JP, Green TP, Fuhrman BP, Carlson PE, Marchessault RP. Percutaneous femoral venous catheterizations: a prospective study of complications. J Pediatr 1989;114:411–415.

Chapter 18
Central Venous
Access and Central
Venous Pressure
Monitoring

278

CHAPTER 19

VENOUS CUTDOWN CATHETERIZATION

Robert J. Vinci

INTRODUCTION

Obtaining vascular access is an integral component of pediatric resuscitation. It allows for the emergency administration of fluids, blood products, and pharmacologic agents required for treatment and stabilization of the acutely ill patient. In 1945 Kirkham first described the technique for saphenous vein cutdown, and through the years other anatomic locations have been demonstrated as possible sites for performing emergency venous cutdown (1, 2). Although recent advances such as central venous catheterization and intraosseous infusions have diminished the role of venous cutdown, it remains an important option for emergency vascular access in the critical pediatric patient (3).

Venous cutdown catheterization is most often indicated for infants and young children, especially in the face of hypovolemia, because of the difficulty of placing percutaneous intravenous lines in small patients with peripheral vasoconstriction. Clinicians can take advantage of a number of possible anatomic sites, although once the vein is identified, the technique for performing a venous cutdown is similar regardless of which vessel is used. A venous cutdown is best reserved for the hospital setting, because of the time required and the expertise needed to perform the procedure. This procedure is generally performed by emergency physicians, critical care specialists, and surgeons.

ANATOMY AND PHYSIOLOGY

Venous Anatomy and External Landmarks

Distal Saphenous Vein at the Ankle

The distal saphenous vein is the most common site for a venous cutdown. Located just anterior and superior to the medial malleolus, the saphenous vein courses adjacent to the periosteum along the medial aspect of the ankle (Fig. 19.1). After the initial skin incision, blunt dissection is usually all that is necessary to locate the saphenous vein (see below). The saphenous nerve travels adjacent to the vein and can be confused with the vein, especially when the vein is constricted due to hypovolemia. While the position of the saphenous vein remains constant regardless of age, the diameter of the vessel varies greatly and has implications for the size of the catheter chosen for vascular access.

Proximal Saphenous Vein at the Groin

In its proximal location the saphenous vein lies medial to the femoral vein as it courses toward the inguinal region. It passes through the fascia lata of the thigh where it enters the femoral vein, approximately 2 to 3 cm distal to the inguinal ligament. In its proximal location the saphenous vein can be isolated by using the landmark demarcated by the junction of the thigh with the lateral margin of the labial or scrotal folds (Fig. 19.2). The opera-

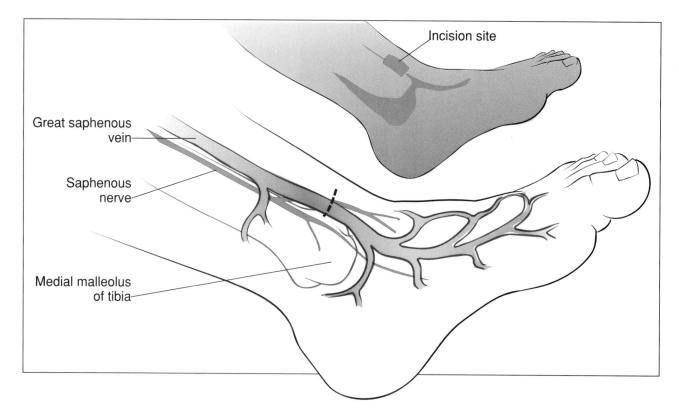

Great saphenous vein

Saphenous nerve

Medial malleolus of tibia

Incision site

Figure 19.1.
Distal saphenous vein cutdown site.

tor must be careful not to enter the femoral sheath during the procedure, so that injury to the adjacent neurovascular structures is avoided. The advantage of the saphenous cutdown at the groin is that the increased diameter of the vessel will allow for a larger bore catheter compared to the saphenous vein at the ankle. This is especially useful when rapid infusion of intravenous fluid is required (4, 5).

Basilic Vein

The basilic vein is a superficial vessel located just proximal to the flexor crease of the elbow (Fig. 19.3). While the distal portion of the basilic vein originates in the medial aspect of the hand, it is too small at this point to be clinically useful. However, above the elbow the basilic vein is joined by the median cubital vein and is accessible to dissection and subsequent venotomy. It can be isolated as it courses between the tendons of the biceps and pronator muscle groups. The median cutaneous nerve of the forearm is often found adjacent to the basilic vein; it should be identified in order to avoid injury to this nerve and resulting damage to the sensory distribution of the medial forearm.

Axillary Vein

Isolation of the axillary vein has recently been described in newborns as another site for venous cutdown (6). The axillary vein of the proximal arm is situated within the axillary sheath as it traverses the inferior surface of the axilla. To localize the axillary vein, a transverse incision can be performed along the midaxillary line in the deepest skin fold of the axilla. Blunt dissection is then performed to extend the incision to the axillary sheath (Fig. 19.4). The axillary sheath encloses the axillary artery and vein as well as the roots of the brachial plexus. Because of these contiguous major neurovascular structures, a cutdown of the axillary vein is associated with a high complication rate and should only be attempted by experienced clinicians.

Circulatory Physiology

A detailed description of the physiologic effects of the shock state on pediatric patients can be found in Chapters 12 and 18. Hypovolemia, tissue hypoxia, and metabolic acidosis are commonly seen in the acutely ill or traumatized pediatric patient. Compensatory

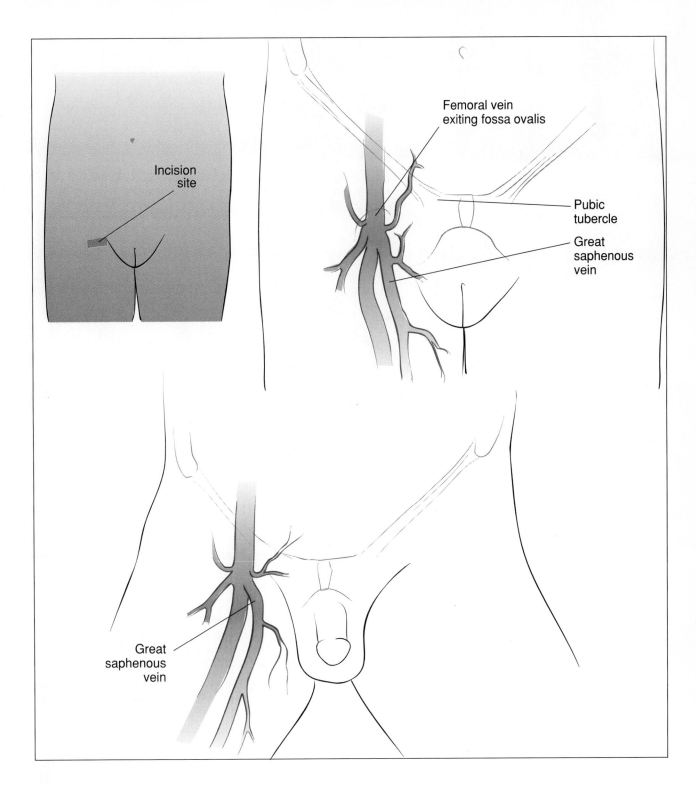

Figure 19.2.
Proximal saphenous vein cutdown site.

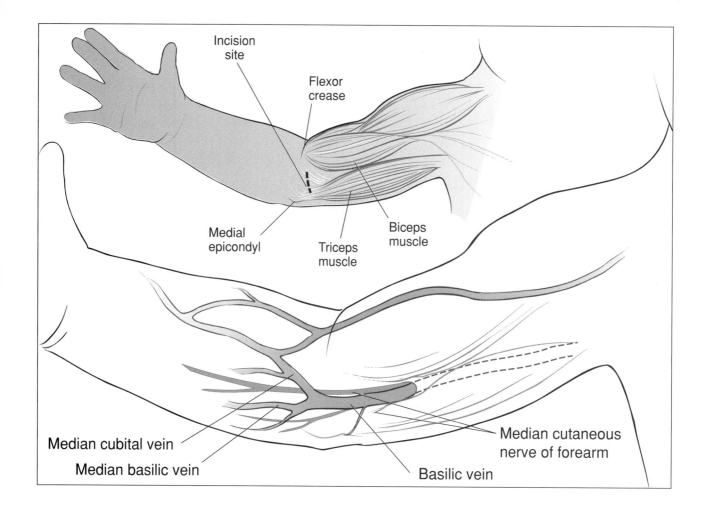

Incision
site

Flexor
crease

Medial
epicondyl

Triceps
muscle

Biceps
muscle

Median cubital vein

Median basilic vein

Median cutaneous
nerve of forearm

Basilic vein

Figure 19.3.
Basilic vein cutdown site.

mechanisms maintain cardiac output by shunting blood away from nonvital organs, producing counterregulatory hormones, and buffering lactic acid resulting from cellular anaerobic metabolism. A properly performed venous cutdown will allow for rapid volume expansion required to restore vascular tone. It also provides entry into the venous circulation for the pharmacologic treatment of the critically ill child.

INDICATIONS

Percutaneous venous cannulation is normally the procedure of choice when establishing venous access in the pediatric patient. However, acute hypovolemia and acidosis can produce extreme peripheral vasoconstriction which may make it impossible to cannulate a peripheral vein during a resuscitation. Although an array of vascular procedures (in-cluding central venous lines and intraosseous infusions) may be initially attempted, a venous cutdown remains a viable therapeutic option. This is especially true when other methods are unsuccessful or contraindicated. Consequently, it is imperative to develop clear written guidelines that delineate the protocol and sequence of vascular procedures during a pediatric resuscitation to ensure that a venous cutdown is properly utilized for the patient requiring vascular access (7).

Peripheral vein cutdown is warranted in any situation that requires rapid volume expansion or treatment of metabolic derangements commonly seen in the acutely ill child. Hypovolemic shock from severe gastroenteritis, thermal burns, or metabolic disorders such as diabetes mellitus require prompt restoration of circulating blood volume. Additionally, acute blood loss from blunt or penetrating trauma and acute hemorrhage secondary to bleeding diathesis, gastric ulcer,

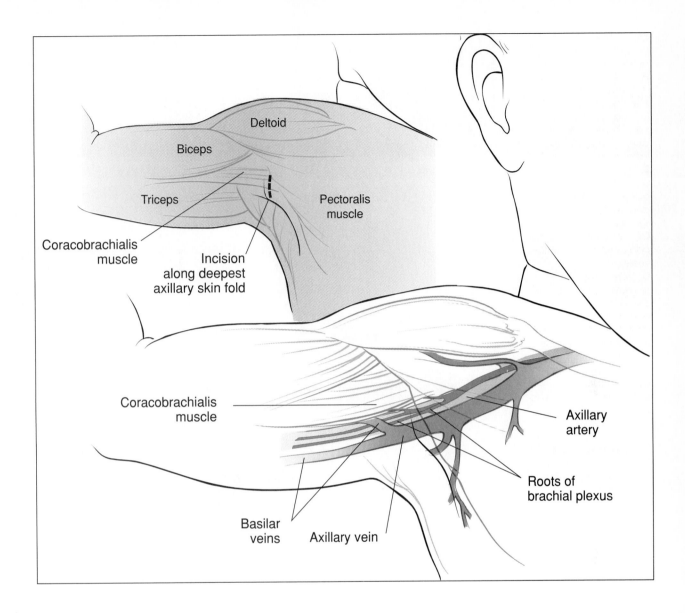

Labels on figure:
Deltoid
Biceps
Triceps
Pectoralis muscle
Coracobrachialis muscle
Incision along deepest axillary skin fold
Coracobrachialis muscle
Axillary artery
Roots of brachial plexus
Basilar veins
Axillary vein

and inflammatory bowel disease may warrant emergency vascular access. Patients with overwhelming infection, sepsis, and cardiopulmonary failure may also require a venous cutdown for emergency treatment. Finally, in selected situations a venous cutdown may be indicated for the ongoing stabilization of a patient or in preparation for interfacility transport.

While there are no absolute contraindications to placement of a venous cutdown, there are a few circumstances when one should consider other options for venous access. Traumatic disruption of the inferior vena cava or vessels proximal to the site of the cutdown may significantly limit the effectiveness of this technique. In addition, local trauma, such as comminuted fracture of the ankle, suspected compartment syndrome, potential damage to the vessel from local trauma and infection at the site of the cutdown require selecting an alternative technique or a different site for venous cutdown. Mast suits are not a contraindication because they have been shown to have only a minimal effect on venous flow rates from a distal saphenous cutdown.

EQUIPMENT

1. Sterile drapes, dressings, gloves, face shields, and 4 x 4 sponges
2. 1% betadine solution or surgical scrub

Figure 19.4.
Axillary vein cutdown site.

Figure 19.5.
Procedure for venous cutdown catheterization.
A. A transverse incision is made at the appropriate site. The incision should extend into the subcutaneous tissue but not deep enough to potentially lacerate the vein.
B. The vein is isolated using blunt dissection. A suture is passed around the vein and cut to give two ligatures.
C. The distal suture is tied and used to stablize the vessel.
D. Venotomy is performed to allow insertion of the catheter. Alternatively the operator may choose to insert the catheter over a needle without performing a venotomy, in a manner similar to percutaneous catheterization.
E. The catheter is inserted into the vein. Placement within the vessel is confirmed by aspirating blood or infusing fluid.
F. The proximal suture is tied and the wound is closed and dressed.

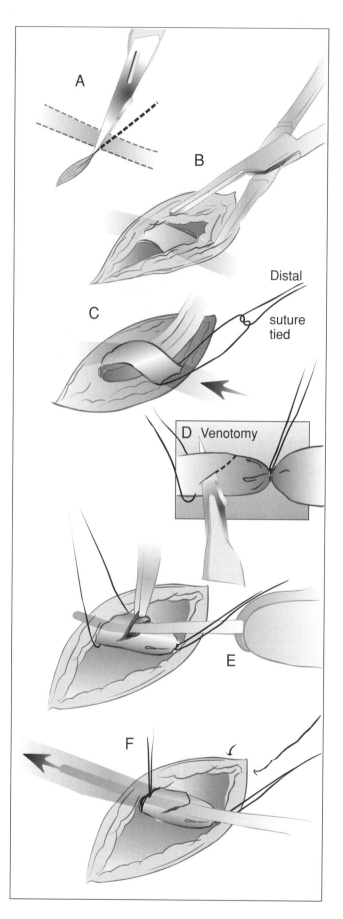

3. Intravenous catheters (14-gauge to 22-gauge) or CVP catheters (3.0–8.0 French)
4. Scalpel handle with a No. 11 blade
5. Hemostats, iris scissors, tissue forceps, and needle holder
6. Lidocaine (1 to 2%) without epinephrine
7. Syringes (3, 5, and 10 mL)
8. Saline solution for flush
9. Intravenous tubing and intravenous fluids
10. Nonabsorbable suture (e.g., silk)

PROCEDURE

Technique for performing venous cutdown catheterization is similar regardless of the site selected (Fig. 19.5). Specific aspects of the procedure relevant to the individual approaches are described in this section.

Saphenous Vein at the Ankle

The ankle should be positioned with lateral deviation of the foot to provide maximum exposure of the medial malleolus. In the awake patient, the foot and lower leg should be restrained to prevent movement. Care must be taken to avoid constricting dressings that may inhibit venous flow. The area is scrubbed with 1% betadine solution or surgical scrub, while surrounding the field with sterile drapes. The site for the skin incision is identified by drawing a line 1 cm superior and anterior to the medial malleolus (Fig. 19.1). A 1 to 2 cm transverse incision should be made beginning 1 cm superior to the medial malleolus just posterior to the anterior margin of the bone. For the child under 1 year of age, a 1 cm incision is often sufficient to locate the vein. The subcutaneous tissue and fat should be separated with a pair of curved forceps. While keeping the forceps parallel to the incision with the curved edge facing upward (toward the skin edge), the operator advances the forceps until contact is made with the tibia. The tissue is elevated and separated from the anterior tibia until the saphenous vein is located. The blunt dissection is continued until the vein is isolated and separated from the surrounding tissue and the saphe-

nous nerve. A nonabsorbable suture (e.g., silk) is placed beneath the vein and the loop of the suture is grasped with a pair of forceps. After pulling the suture beneath the vein, the operator cuts the loop to form two ligatures extending around the vessel. The distal suture is then tied. Using the proximal suture to elevate the vessel, the operator makes a small nick (venotomy) in the vessel through which the catheter is inserted. Alternatively, the operator may choose to insert a catheter over a needle without incising the vessel in a manner similar to placing a standard percutaneous intravenous line. A syringe attached to the catheter is aspirated to determine proper placement within the vessel. With infants or small children, the operator may not see significant blood return with aspiration. If this is the case, he or she can attempt infusion of fluid and check for any leakage or soft tissue swelling. The catheter is secured in place by tying the proximal suture around the vessel and catheter. Skin edges are closed using a nonabsorbable suture. The wound should be covered with an antibiotic ointment such as bacitracin and the foot and ankle immobilized to prevent dislodgment of the catheter.

Saphenous Vein at the Groin

A transverse incision should be made beginning at the point where the scrotal or labial fold meets the thigh (Fig. 19.2). This incision is extended 4 to 6 cm to allow adequate exposure of the area. The lateral margin of this incision should reach an imaginary line drawn perpendicular from the edge of the pubic tubercle. A blunt dissection of the superficial adipose tissue of the thigh is required to locate the proximal saphenous vein. The tissue must be carefully dissected to avoid inadvertent damage or transection of the vein. As the saphenous vein nears the femoral vein it travels through Scarpa's fascia. If the operator reaches the fascia of the adductor musculature, the cutdown is too deep and should be focused at a more superficial level. Isolation of the vein, venotomy, and catheter insertion are performed as previously described (Fig. 19.5). Meticulous wound care is required to avoid bacterial contamination in the inguinal area.

SUMMARY: VENOUS CUTDOWN CATHETERIZATION AT THE DISTAL SAPHENOUS VEIN

1. Scrub medial malleolus and surrounding area with aseptic solution
2. Make 1 to 2 cm skin incision beginning 1 cm superior to medial malleolus and just posterior to anterior margin of bone
3. Bluntly dissect subcutaneous tissue and fat with curved forceps
4. Identify saphenous vein and gently separate it from surrounding tissue
5. Insert loop of nonabsorbable suture around vessel and then cut loop so two ligatures are formed
6. Tie off distal portion of vessel
7. Lift proximal suture to elevate vessel and make small venotomy incision
8. Cannulate vessel
9. Tie proximal suture around catheter and vessel
10. Close skin with nonabsorbable suture
11. Stabilize cutdown site

SUMMARY: VENOUS CUTDOWN CATHETERIZATION AT THE PROXIMAL SAPHENOUS VEIN

1. Begin 4 to 6 cm transverse incision at point where scrotal or labial fold meets thigh
2. Use blunt dissection of adipose tissue to locate proximal saphenous vein just distal to its junction with femoral vein
3. Isolate vein and perform venotomy and catheter insertion as described for distal saphenous vein cutdown

SUMMARY: VENOUS
CUTDOWN CATHETER-
IZATION AT THE BASILIC
VEIN
1. Position arm so elbow
   is extended and fore-
   arm lies supine
2. Make 2 to 3 cm trans-
   verse incision just
   proximal to flexor
   crease and anterior to
   medial epicondyle
3. Using careful blunt
   dissection locate
   basilic vein between
   biceps and triceps muscles
4. Isolate vessel and perform venotomy and
   catheter insertion as
   described for distal
   saphenous vein cut-
   down

SUMMARY: VENOUS
CUTDOWN CATHETER-
IZATION AT THE AXILLARY
VEIN
1. Extend and abduct arm
   using restraint methods
   as necessary
2. Make small transverse
   incision along deepest
   skin fold of axilla and
   identify axillary sheath
   with blunt dissection
3. After isolating axillary
   sheath, use blunt dis-
   section with hemostat
   to enter sheath and isolate axillary vein
4. Separate axillary vein
   by encircling it with a
   suture, and perform
   venotomy and catheter
   insertion as described
   for distal saphenous
   vein cutdown (Note:
   distal end of axillary
   vein is usually not ligated)

Basilic Vein

The arm should be positioned with the elbow extended and the forearm supine. A 2 to 3 cm transverse incision is made at a point 2 cm proximal to the flexor crease and 2 to 3 cm anterior to the medial epicondyle (Fig. 19.3). Using careful blunt dissection, the basilic vein is located as it courses between the biceps and triceps musculature. Once the vessel is identified, venotomy and catheterization are performed as described previously (Fig. 19.5).

Axillary Vein

The arm should be extended and abducted, taking care to provide proper restraint. For the awake patient, local anesthetic should be infiltrated along the midaxillary line in the deepest skin fold of the axilla. A small transverse incision should be made at this site and gentle blunt dissection is utilized to identify the axillary sheath (Fig. 19.4). The axillary sheath is a neurovascular bundle that contains the great nerves and vessels of the arm. The axillary artery is the deepest structure within the axillary sheath and its pulsation can be used to help locate the axillary vein.

The axillary sheath is released from its attachments and entered, using a hemostat to perform blunt dissection, so that the contents can be identified. The axillary vein is the most superficial and inferior structure, and should be separated with blunt dissection to allow placement of sutures around the vessel. A venotomy is performed as described previously, although the distal end of the axillary vein is usually not ligated with a suture. Catheterization is performed as described (Fig. 19.5).

COMPLICATIONS

Complications, although uncommon, can occur after any invasive vascular procedure such as a cutdown. Important safety measures to avoid complications are meticulous sterile technique and wound care, as well as carefully monitoring the cutdown site over time. Common complications include failed cannulation leading to hemorrhage, hematoma, or extravasation of intravenous fluids (3, 8). Phlebitis may be associated with a venous cutdown, but this most commonly occurs after prolonged use of the site (9). Infection can present both as a localized soft tissue infection (cellulitis) or as a suppurative phlebitis (10). Local injury to a contiguous structure such as an artery or a peripheral nerve can also occur, but this can generally be avoided with proper technique. Finally, catheter related sepsis, although less common than with a central venous line, has been reported as a complication of venous cutdown catheterization.

CLINICAL TIPS
1. The most commonly used (and probably easiest) site for performing emergency venous cutdown catheterization is the distal saphenous vein at the ankle.
2. After making the initial skin incision, the remainder of the cutdown should normally be performed using blunt dissection to avoid injury to nerves and vessels.
3. Slipping a loop of non-absorbable suture (e.g., silk) around the vessel and then cutting the loop forms both ligatures needed to perform the procedure in a single step.
4. Once the ligatures are extended around the vessel, they can be used to more easily manipulate the vessel during venotomy and catheterization.
5. A larger diameter catheter (16 gauge or 18 gauge) should be used to maximize intravenous infusion.

Summary

Emergency intravenous access is required for acute management and stabilization during medical or trauma resuscitation of pediatric patients. Venous cutdown catheterization at the saphenous vein in the ankle or groin, as well as the axillary and basilic veins, can be utilized to provide access to administer life-saving intravenous fluids, blood products, and medications. Clinicians responsible for the care of critically ill children should be familiar with at least one method of performing this procedure.

References

1. Kirkham JH. Infusion into the internal saphenous vein at the ankle. Lancet 1945;2:815.
2. Wax PM, Talan DA. Advances in cutdown techniques. Emerg Med Clin North Am 1989;7:65–82.
3. Gauderer MWL. Vascular access techniques and devices in the pediatric patient. Surg Clin of North Am 1992;72:1267–1284.
4. Dronen SC, Yee AS, Tomlanovich M. Proximal saphenous vein cutdown. Ann Emerg Med 1981;10:328–330.
5. Rogers FB. Technical note: A quick and simple method of obtaining venous access in traumatic exsanguination. J Trauma 1993;34:142–143.
6. Stephens BL, Lelli JL, Allen D. Silastic catheterization of the axillary vein in neonates: an alternative to the internal jugular vein. J Pediatr Surg 1993;28:31–35.
7. Kanter RK, Zimmermen JJ, Strauss RH, et al. Pediatric emergency intravenous access. Am J Dis Child 1986;140:132–134.
8. McIntosh BB, Dulchavsky SA. Peripheral vascular cutdown. Crit Care Clin 1992;8(4):807–818.
9. Rhee KJ, Derlet RW, Beal SL. Rapid venous access using saphenous vein cutdown at the ankle. Am J Emerg Med 1989;7(3):263–266.
10. Jupiter JB, Ehrlich MG, Novelline RA, et al. The association of septic thrombophlebitis with subperiosteal abscesses in children. J Pediatr 1982;101:690–695.

INTRAOSSEOUS INFUSION

Dee Hodge III

INTRODUCTION

After ensuring an adequate airway and providing adequate ventilation, assessing circulation and establishing vascular access are the next priorities in pediatric resuscitation. Traditional approaches to vascular access in children (peripheral catheters, central catheters, and cutdowns) may be difficult under any circumstances and may be almost impossible when vascular collapse is present. In one study of pediatric arrests, 24% of the patients required more than 10 minutes before vascular access was achieved (1). Intraosseous infusion is a rapid method of obtaining vascular access during critical situations. Intraosseous lines can be placed quickly and fluids and medications given rapidly via this route.

Intraosseous infusion is an old technique first developed during the 1930s as the preferred route of vascular access in children (2–4). With the advent of butterfly needles and plastic catheters during the 1950s and 1960s, the technique fell out of favor and was rarely if ever performed. The development of advanced pediatric life support interventions brought the need for a rapid, reliable method of vascular access. Intraosseous infusion has filled that need.

The technique is used in the prehospital, emergency department (ED), and hospital settings where critical intravenous IV access is necessary. The procedure is relatively straightforward and can be effectively performed by physicians, physician assistants, nurses, and paramedics (5–7). Intraosseous lines are most commonly placed in children under 3 years of age, because this group usually represents the greatest challenge in obtaining vascular access; however, the technique may be used in any age group (8).

ANATOMY AND PHYSIOLOGY

The marrow space of the long bones functions essentially as a noncollapsible vein (9). Blood flows from the venous sinusoids of the medullary cavity of the long bones to drain into a central venous canal. From the central canal blood drains by nutrient or emissary veins into the central circulation (Fig. 20.1). Absorption from bone marrow into general circulation is quite rapid, although obviously slower than for peripheral or central lines of comparable gauge (3, 10, 15). Intraosseous flow rates are influenced by venous valves, venous tortuosity, venous pressure, and blood flow through the marrow cavity. The tibia and femur are the preferred sites, because the marrow cavity is well developed even in the neonatal period, and the limbs are readily accessible (11). Insertion at the proximal and distal tibia is generally easier than at the distal femur, because of little subcutaneous tissue overlying the bone (Fig. 20.2). To enter the distal femur, the needle must pass through the relatively bulky quadriceps femoris muscle. In addition, the bony cortex is thinner and more easily pierced at the tibial sites.

In case of shock or cardiopulmonary failure, blood flow is shunted away from the periphery to supply vital organs. In early stages of shock due to hypovolemia or pump failure,

Figure 20.1.
Venous drainage from the
medullary cavity.

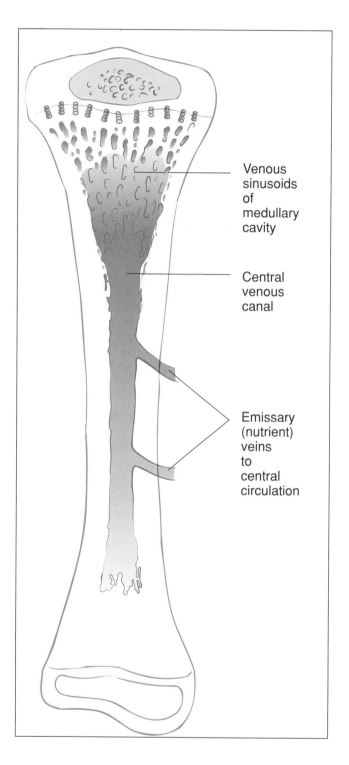

Venous
sinusoids
of
medullary
cavity

Central
venous
canal

Emissary
(nutrient)
veins
to
central
circulation

blood pressure is maintained by increasing the peripheral vascular resistance (see also Chapters 12 and 18). This is largely the result of sympathetic nervous system stimulation and circulating catecholamines. Preload is enhanced by contraction of capacitance veins. This resulting vasoconstriction makes vascular access for the child in shock much more difficult. In addition, obtaining access is generally more problematic for children than adults because of the small size of the vessels and the abundance of subcutaneous fat—both of which make identification of veins by palpation more difficult.

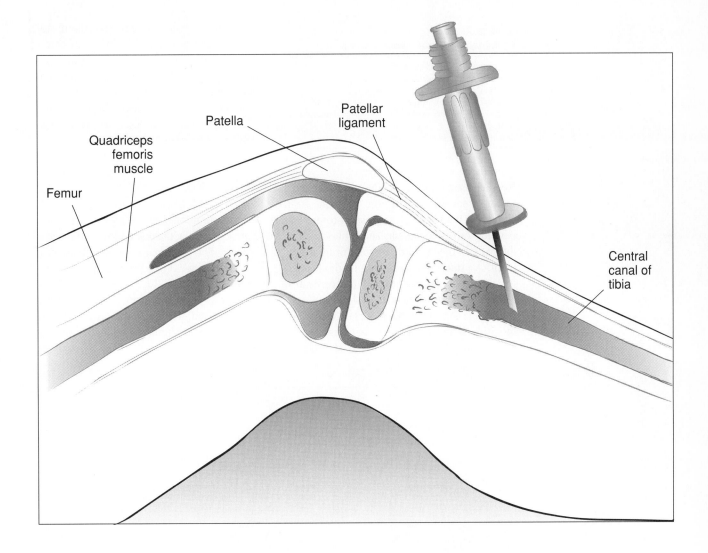

Quadriceps
femoris
muscle

Patella

Patellar
ligament

Femur

Central
canal of
tibia

Figure 20.2.
The proximal tibia is a
preferred site for
intraosseous needle
insertion, because of little
overlying soft tissue.

INDICATIONS

Intraosseous infusion is indicated for those situations when immediate vascular access is required, most often cardiopulmonary arrest and shock (see also Chapter 18). Unlike the administration of medications, many of which can be given through the endotracheal tube or rectally, fluid volume can only be given via vascular access. Because the flow rates achieved are not sufficient to fully treat severe hypovolemic shock, this technique should not be considered "definitive" access. Intraosseous access should be attempted simultaneously with attempts at peripheral and central access. However, often after an initial bolus of fluid via an intraosseous line, the vessels are more prominent and establishing peripheral access then becomes possible. The few absolute contraindications to this procedure include recent fractures in the bone to be used, osteogenesis imperfecta, and osteopetrosis. Cellulitis or an infected burn at the site of insertion are relative contraindications (10–14).

EQUIPMENT

The equipment necessary for performing intraosseous infusion is listed in Table 20.1. Intraosseous needles are manufactured by several companies, with multiple designs incorporating the main desired features. It is useful to have regular in-service training sessions or "mock codes" during which the intraosseous needle is used, so that ED personnel can become familiar with these features.

**Chapter 20
Intraosseous Infusion**

291

Table 20.1.
Equipment for Intraosseous Infusion

Lidocaine 1 to 2% (without epinephrine)
Syringe/needle (25 gauge)
Antiseptic prep solution (e.g., betadine)
Intraosseous or bone marrow aspiration needle (Cook Inc.,®
   Jamshidi,® Medsurg Industries®) or 20-gauge spinal needle
10 cc syringe
Saline/heparinized saline

Figure 20.3.
Entry site at the proximal tibia.

Needles used for the procedure should have a trocar or some method to prevent bone from occluding the needle, a short shaft to prevent bending or displacement, and a hub to fit in the palm of the operator's hand during placement. A protective flange or a method to adjust the depth of penetration of the needle also affords some advantage (Jamshidi®, Cook-Sussmane-Raszynski® model). Many authorities believe threaded needles, which screw into the bone (Cook-Sur-Fast® model)

offer no true advantage and have the disadvantage of not providing the "feel" of entering the marrow cavity. Povidone-iodine (Betadine) is needed for skin preparation and gloves should be worn in observance of universal precautions (see also Chapters 7 and 8). Lidocaine should be used for local anesthesia in awake patients.

PROCEDURE

The most common sites used for insertion are the proximal tibia, the distal tibia, and the distal femur. The proximal tibia may be used in patients up to age 3 to 4 years. After this age, the patient's proximal tibia is more difficult to penetrate, and therefore the distal tibia should be used. To locate the proximal tibia site, the operator should first identify the anterior medial surface of the tibia and palpate

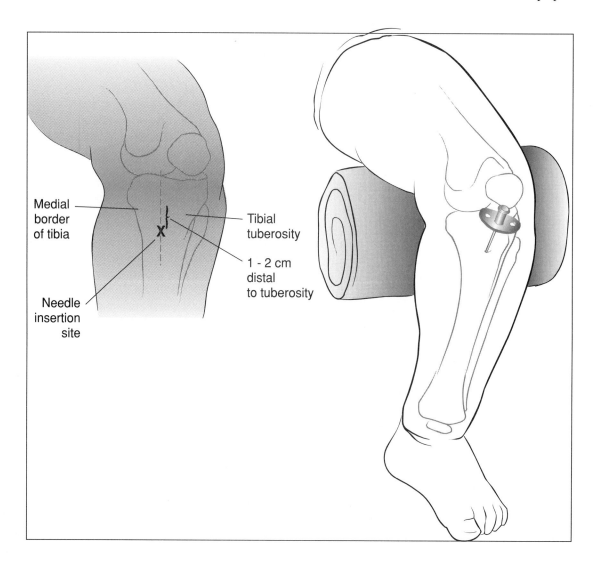

Medial border of tibia

Tibial tuberosity

1 - 2 cm distal to tuberosity

Needle insertion site

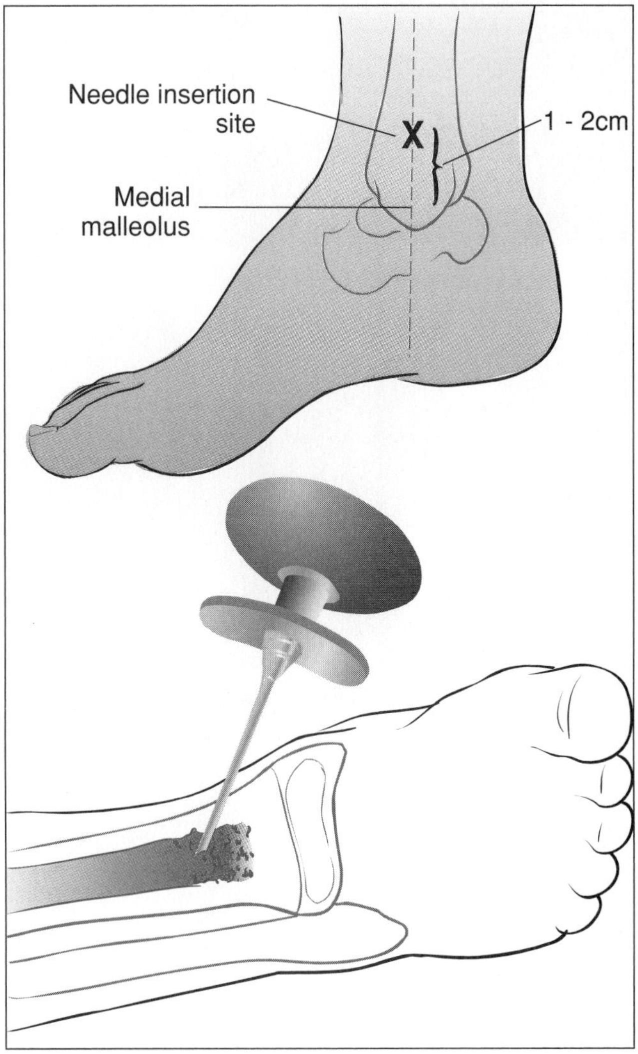

Figure 20.4.
Entry site at the distal tibia.

Needle insertion site

1 - 2cm

Medial malleolus

the tibial tuberosity/plateau. The entry site is halfway between the anterior and posterior border of the tibia and 1 to 2 cm distal to the tibial plateau (Fig. 20.3). For older children, the distal tibial site is used. The site of insertion for this approach is located just proximal to the medial malleolus halfway between the anterior and posterior borders of the bone (Fig. 20.4). The distal femur is used as a secondary site in infants or when the operator fails to enter the tibia. The location of insertion is approximately 1 cm proximal to the femoral plateau (Fig. 20.5).

If the patient is alert, 1 to 2 mL of a local anesthetic should be injected into the skin and periosteum. After prepping the skin with povidone-iodine, the operator stabilizes the leg and/or foot using the nondominant hand. The needle is angled slightly away from the joint space during insertion or, as some more recent sources have recommended, perpen-

dicular to the bone. It is best to hold the intraosseous device so that the hub rests in the palm while the thumb and index finger are 1 to 2 cm from the tip of the needle (Fig. 20.6.A). Gradually increasing pressure is applied with a back and forth rotational motion until the operator feels a sudden decrease in resistance ("trap-door effect") (Fig. 20.6.B). The operator must take care not to insert the needle with the tip angled into the joint space, as this may injure physeal (growth plate) structures. The operator should also avoid rocking the needle from side to side, because this will enlarge the entrance hole and allow for extravasation of administered fluid into the soft tissues. Excessive or sudden force should be avoided at all times, because this will often result in puncture of both cortices. Once the marrow space is entered, the needle need not be advanced further; usually 1 cm beyond the bony cortex is sufficient in infants

**Chapter 20
Intraosseous Infusion**

Figure 20.5.
Entry site at the distal femur.

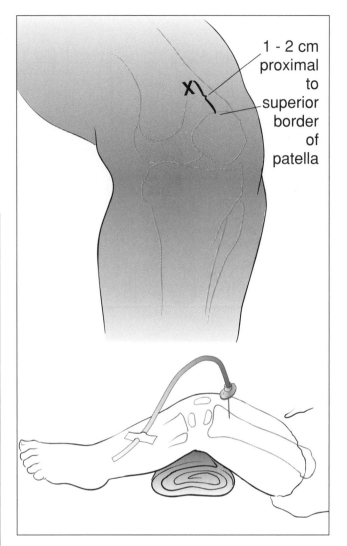

1 - 2 cm
proximal
to
superior
border
of
patella

X

SUMMARY
1. Restrain patient appropriately
2. Prepare field aseptically
3. Provide local anesthesia for awake patient
4. Choose appropriate insertion site: proximal tibia for patients <3 yr, distal tibia for patients >3 yr, or distal femur if failure to insert in tibia
5. Insert needle perpendicular to bony cortex or angled slightly away from joint space
6. Use steady back and forth rotational movement rather than "rocking" needle from side to side
7. Aspirate marrow to confirm needle placement or infuse small amount of saline and aspirate, looking for pink fluid
8. Attach to IV. infusion setup and secure line
9. Monitor for extravasation and swelling of tissues.

and small children. The trocar is then removed leaving the hollow needle in place. To confirm proper needle position a syringe is attached and blood or marrow is aspirated (Fig. 20.6.C). If marrow contents are not aspirated, 2 to 3 mL of sterile plain or heparinized saline is injected. The saline should infuse easily without evidence of extravasation. Alternatively, the operator may choose to reaspirate the injected fluid. If it is pink-tinged, the tip of the needle is probably in the marrow cavity. Once the correct position has been confirmed, the hub is attached to an IV infusion system.

Failure to place the needle in the marrow cavity results in a failure to infuse. If the needle punctures both cortices, fluid will extravasate into the soft tissues. In this situation, continued infusion of fluid under pressure can result in a compartment syndrome. These problems can generally be avoided by ensuring proper needle placement and closely monitoring the insertion site, as well as the calf or lower thigh, for tension or swelling (6, 7, 15). The line may be secured in a manner similar to taping an umbilical line (Fig. 20.7). The line should not be dressed with a bulky dressing or

Figure 20.6.
Procedure for intraosseous infusion.
A. The needle is angled slightly away from the joint space or, as some more recent sources have recommended, perpendicular to the bone.
B. A back and forth "screwing" motion is used to insert the needle. "Rocking" the needle from side to side results in enlargement of the puncture site and extravasation of infused fluid.
C. Intramedullary placement is confirmed by aspirating marrow.

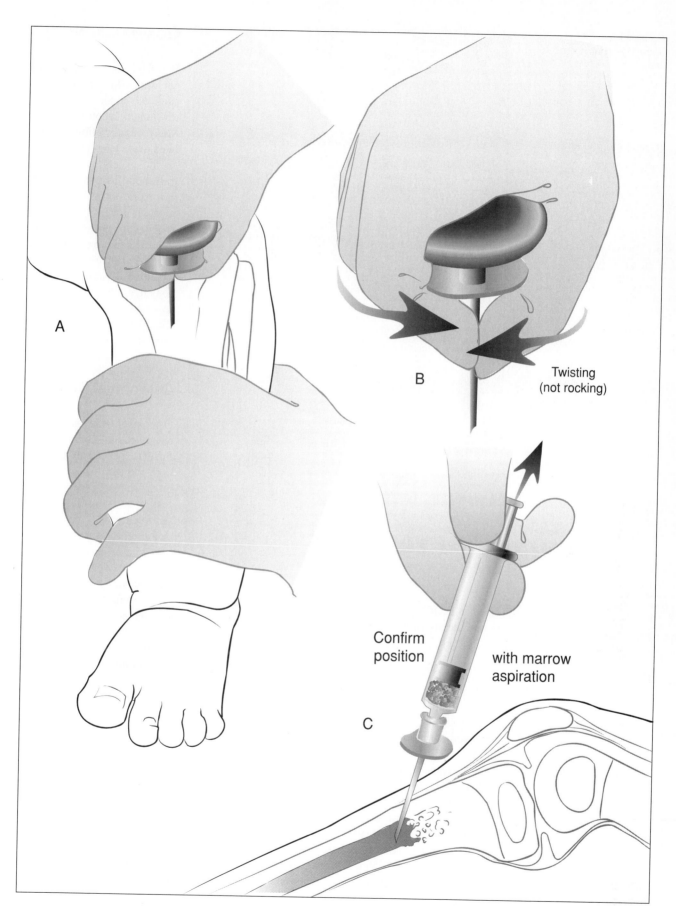

A

B Twisting (not rocking)

C Confirm position with marrow aspiration

Figure 20.7.
Securing an intraosseous line.

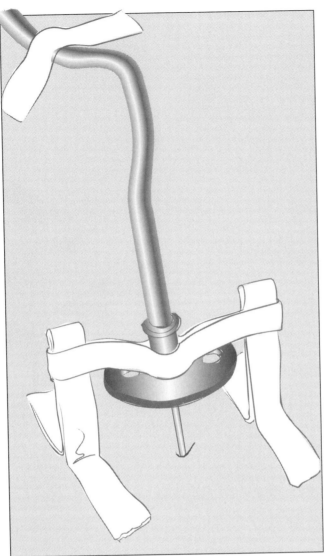

COMPLICATIONS

Based on current and historical data, this technique is safe and associated with a low complication rate (1, 4). Many complications are related to the length of time the needle is left in place. Intraosseous lines should be removed as soon as other stable vascular access is obtained. Whenever possible, lines should be removed within 12 hours. Furunculosis and osteochondritis are complications that are rarely seen but described in the literature (14). Other reported complications are listed below.

Osteomyelitis

Osteomyelitis is the most often discussed complication, but the published rate for both the early literature and more recent experience is less than 1% (1, 4). Osteomyelitis may be avoided with proper skin preparation and with using sterile gloves during needle placement. The rate of osteomyelitis primarily depends on the length of time the intraosseous needle is left in place. Lines left in for over 24 hours have a higher incidence of osteomyelitis. For this reason, many experts advise removing the intraosseous line as soon as other routes of vascular access have been established.

Cellulitis and Subcutaneous Abscess

Both cellulitis and subcutaneous abscess are rare and often associated with extravasation of fluid at the insertion site as well as inadequate skin preparation. Like osteomyelitis, the incidence primarily depends upon the length of time the intraosseous needle is left in place.

taped in such a way that obscures visualization of the insertion site.

Success rate of this procedure is high (5, 6, 15); however, reasons for failure include improper placement, bending of the needle, dense marrow, or an underlying process that results in replacement of marrow by fat or fibrous tissue (6–8, 10, 15). The flow rates achieved with intraosseous infusion vary from 11 to 45 mL/min (16). In addition to volume replacement, all current drugs used in pediatric advanced life support can be given via the intraosseous route at the usual doses (17–23). Blood aspirated from the marrow may be used for laboratory tests such as electrolytes, glucose, BUN, and creatinine but not for a complete blood count. Marrow aspirate may also be used for type and crossmatch (24, 25).

Compartment Syndrome

Compartment syndrome can occur when fluid extravasates or leaks around the insertion site. This may be avoided by proper needle placement and close monitoring of the surrounding tissues. The calf or lower thigh should be serially examined for the development of tension or swelling (26, 27).

Fat Embolus

Although a theoretical complication, no cases of fat embolus have been reported in humans. One study using animals showed no V/Q mismatch (28).

Fracture and Damage to the Growth Plate

Fracture and damage to the growth plate may occur if the patient has osteopetrosis or osteoporosis. Fractures also may occur if too large a needle is used for the relative size of the bone. In addition, if the extremity is not properly stabilized at the time of insertion, fractures may occur (29). Needle insertion through the growth plate should be avoided to prevent damage which may affect normal bone growth. Although a theoretical complication, no cases have been reported in humans and a study using animals showed no growth impairment (30).

Septicemia and Bacteremia

Although a potential complication, septicemia and bacteremia are often seen in patients who were septic as part of their underlying condition. As with other potential complications, this is primarily a risk when intraosseous lines are left in place longer than 12 hours.

SUMMARY

Intraosseous infusion is a rapid method of obtaining vascular access during critical life support situations involving infants and young children. Intraosseous lines can be placed quickly and fluids and medications given rapidly via this route. The most common sites used for insertion are the proximal tibia, the distal tibia, and the distal femur. The procedure is easy to learn and the success rate is high. The technique has been demonstrated as safe with a low complication rate.

REFERENCES

1. Rosetti VA, Thompson BM, Aprahamian C. Difficulty and delay in intravenous access in pediatric arrests. Ann Emerg Med 1984;13:406.
2. Josefson A. A new method of treatment—intraosseous injection. Acta Med Scand 1934;81:550–564.
3. Tocantins LM, O'Neil JF. Infusion of blood and other fluids into circulation via the bone marrow. Proc Soc Exp Bio Med 1940;45:782–3.
4. Heinild S, Soderguard T, Tudvad F. Bone marrow infusion in childhood: experiences from a thousand infusions. J Pediatr 1947;30:400–11.
5. Seigler RS, Tecklenburg FW, Shealy R. Prehospital intraosseous infusion by emergency medical services personnel: a prospective study. Pediatrics 1989;84:173–177.
6. Glaeser PW, Hellmich TR, Szewczuga D. Five-year experience in prehospital intraosseous infusions in children and adults. Ann Emerg Med 1993;22:1119–1124.
7. Smith RJ, Keseg DP, Manley LK, Standeford T. Intraosseous infusions by prehospital personnel in critically ill pediatric patients. Ann Emerg Med 1988;17:491–495.
8. Valdes MM. Intraosseous fluid administration in emergencies. Lancet 1977;1:1235–1236.
9. Drinker CK, Drinker KR, Lund CC. The circulation in the mammalian bone marrow. Am J Physiol 1922;62:1–92.
10. Spivey WH. Intraosseous infusions. J Pediatr 1987;111:639–643.
11. Tocantins LM, O'Neil JF. Complications of intraosseous therapy. Ann Surg 1945;122:266–277.
12. Fiser DH. Intraosseous infusions. N Engl J Med 1990:322:1579–1581.
13. Hodge D III. Intraosseous infusions: a review. Pediatr Emerg Care 1985;1:215–218.
14. Kanter RK, Zimmerman JJ, Straus RH, Stoeckel KA. Pediatric emergency intravenous access. AJDC 1986:132–134.
15. Rosetti VA, Thompson BM, Miller J, Mateer JR, Aprahamian C. Intraosseous infusions. Ann Emerg Med 1985;14:885–887.
16. Hodge D III, Delgado-Paredes C, Fleisher G. Intraosseous infusion flow rates in hypovolemic "pediatric" dogs. Ann Emerg Med 1987;16:305–307.
17. Dubeck MA, Pfeiffer JW, Clifford CB, Runyon DE, Kramer GC. Comparison of intraosseous and intravenous delivery of hypertonic saline/dextran in anesthetized, euvolemic pigs. Ann Emerg Med 1992;21:498–503.
18. Spivey WH, Malone D, Unger HD, et al. Comparison of intraosseous, central and peripheral routes of administration of sodium bicarbonate during CPR in pigs. Ann Emerg Med 1985;14:1135–1140.

19. Orlowski JP, Porembka DT, Gallagher JM, Lockrem JD, Vanlente F. Comparison study of intraosseous, central intravenous, and peripheral intravenous infusions of emergency drugs. AJDC 1990;144:112–117.

20. Sapien R, Stein H, Padbury JF, Thio S, Hodge D III. Intraosseous versus intravenous epinephrine infusions in lambs: pharmacokinetics and pharmacodynamics. Pediatr Emerg Care 1992;8:179–183.

21. Biello JF, O'Hair KC, Kirby WC, Moore JW. Intraosseous infusion of dobutamine and isoproterenol. AJCD 1991;145;165–167.

22. Tobias JD, Nichols DG. Intraosseous succinylcholine for orotracheal intubation. Pediatr Emerg Care 1990;6:108–109.

23. Jaimovich DG, Kumar A, Francom S. Evaluation of intraosseous versus intravenous antibiotic levels in a porcine model. AJDC 1991;145:946–949.

24. Grisham J, Hastings C. Bone marrow aspirate as an accessible and reliable source for critical laboratory studies. Ann Emerg Med 1991;20:1121–1124.

25. Brickman KR, Krupp K, Rega P, Alexander J, Guinness M. Typing and screening of blood from intraosseous access. Ann Emerg Med 1992;21:414–417.

26. Rimar S, Westry JA, Rodriguez RL. Compartment syndrome in an infant following emergency intraosseous infusion. Clin Pediatr 1988;27:259–260.

27. Vidal R, Kissoon N, Gayle M. Compartment syndrome following intraosseous infusion. Pediatrics 1993;91:1201–1202.

28. Orlowski JP, Julius CJ, Petras RE, Porembka DT, Gallagher JM. The safety of intraosseous infusions: risks of fat and bone marrow emboli to the lungs. Ann Emerg Med 1989;18:1062–1067.

29. LaFleche FR, Slepin JM, Vargas J, Milzman DP. Iatrogenic bilateral tibial fractures after intraosseous infusion attempts in a 3-month-old infant. Ann Emerg Med 1989;18:1099–1101.

30. Dedrick DK, Mase C, Ranger W, Burney RD. The effects of intraosseous infusion on the growth plate in a nestling rabbit model. Ann Emerg Med 1992;21:494–497.

CARDIAC PACING

Kathleen P. Kelly and Michael F. Altieri

INTRODUCTION

Emergency cardiac pacing is performed rarely in children but in selected cases can prove life-saving. With increasing prevalence of cardiac surgery among pediatric patients with congenital heart disease, the likelihood of encountering children with arrhythmias in the emergency department (ED) has increased. Emergency cardiac pacing enables the physician to initiate and sustain a cardiac rhythm which will provide perfusion of the vital organs in patients with symptomatic bradyarrhythmias. Clinicians who care for critically ill infants and children should be familiar with the unique aspects of performing cardiac pacing for these patients. Two methods used in the emergency setting are the transvenous and the transcutaneous approaches. Transvenous cardiac pacing involves placement of a pacing wire in direct contact with the myocardium via the central venous circulation. Transcutaneous pacing, which can be performed far more rapidly, utilizes electrodes incorporated into adhesive pads which are applied directly to the external chest wall. Although easier, this method yields less reliable results and is most commonly used as a temporizing measure until transvenous pacing can be performed. Emergency transvenous pacers are inserted by physicians in the ED, intensive care unit (ICU), or operating room. Transcutaneous pacers are technically easier to use and may be applied and operated by physicians, nurses, or paramedics.

The ability to electrically depolarize muscle was first noted over a century ago; however, it was not until 1952 that the clinical utility of cardiac pacing for humans was demonstrated by Zoll. Pacemaker technology advanced from the original devices, which consisted of wires passing through the skin into the myocardium, to a more modern endocardial transvenous pacer introduced in 1959 by Furmkn and Schwedel. The first implantable permanent pacemaker also was developed in 1959. With the creation of the balloon-tip, central venous catheter by Swann in 1970 came the flow-directed transvenous pacers used today. The most recent development in pacing technology is the transcutaneous pacer. Although the initial experiments with transcutaneous pacing actually predated transvenous pacing, this technique was all but abandoned because of the pain caused by severe muscle contractions. This problem now has been overcome primarily with the use of decreased delivered current, an electrode with a larger surface area, and an electrical impulse with a longer duration. Consequently, it is now feasible in many instances to perform cardiac pacing effectively without using an invasive procedure.

ANATOMY AND PHYSIOLOGY

Sites used for transvenous pacer insertion are the femoral, right internal jugular, and left subclavian veins (Fig. 21.1). In adolescents, the right internal jugular vein and, if necessary, the left subclavian vein approaches may be used. Whenever possible, the right internal jugular access site should be used so that the left subclavian vein is preserved for possible long-term pacemaker placement. When in-

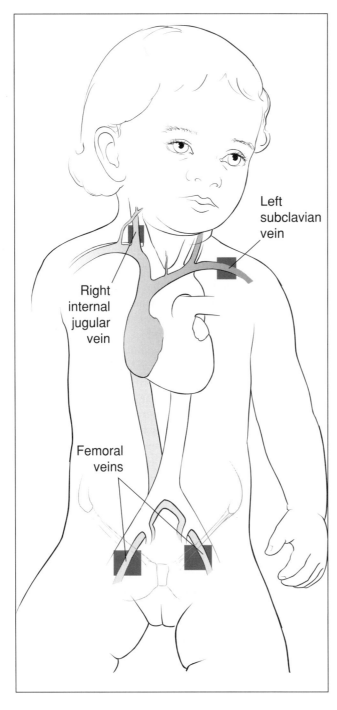

less acute than is encountered with the right subclavian approach. The main disadvantage of subclavian placement is possible pneumothorax.

Because infants and younger children have a relatively short neck and a subclavian vein that is less accessible behind the clavicle, the femoral approach is preferred. Many clinicians use the femoral approach for all pediatric patients. The pacer wire passes along the length of the femoral vein into the inferior vena cava and finally enters the right atrium. The principle disadvantages of this route are an increased risk of thrombophlebitis, a higher incidence of infection, and restricted patient mobility because the catheter is easily dislodged with movement. In addition, the increased distance to the heart from a femoral access site often requires the use of fluoroscopic guidance in a child with poor cardiac output (i.e., when flow-directed catheters are less effective). An alternative approach is via the brachial vein, although this method is seldom used because of the smaller size of the vein and the relative difficulty of this technique. A cutdown is often necessary when using the brachial vein approach. The pacer wire passes along the brachial vein into the subclavian vein and finally through the inferior vena cava into the right atrium. Further discussion of these central venous access approaches is provided in Chapter 18.

Unlike transvenous pacing, transcutaneous pacing is easy to perform with pediatric patients and is often more effective for children than for adults. This is primarily because children have a smaller chest wall mass which results in a lower transthoracic resistance. Transcutaneous pacing can even be used with small children by trimming the adhesive if necessary to keep the pads from touching one another.

Before discussing the applications of cardiac pacing, it is useful to briefly review the conduction system of the heart. Electrical activity is initiated by the sinoatrial node, located at the junction of the superior vena cava and the right atrium (Fig. 21.2). The stimulus is then spread throughout the atria and terminates at the atrioventricular (AV) node in the lower part of the right atrium. From there the electrical impulse is conducted through the bundle of His which divides to form the right and left bundle branches of the ventricles. The bundle branches further divide into the

Figure 21.1.
Preferred approaches for transvenous pacemaker placement. (Note: the left subclavian vein approach is recommended only for adolescents.)

**Chapter 21
Cardiac Pacing**

serted through the right internal jugular vein, the pacer wire has a more or less straight-in approach to the right atrium via the superior vena cava. Disadvantages of this approach include possible carotid artery puncture, dislodgment of the catheter with movement of the head, and an increase risk of thrombophlebitis of the internal jugular vein. When inserted through the left subclavian vein, the angle of entry into the superior vena cava is

Purkinje fibers which penetrate the myocardium, allowing rapid conduction of the impulse throughout the ventricles with resulting contraction.

Most life-threatening arrhythmias in children are bradyarrhythmias. Asystole is also a common terminal rhythm in children although not amenable to pacing. For infants and younger children, cardiac output directly depends on heart rate, and therefore bradyarrhythmias produce a fall in cardiac output and resulting circulatory compromise. Sinus bradycardia (a rate less than 60 bpm) is relatively uncommon in the pediatric age group and generally indicates markedly increased vagal tone. Failure of impulse formation or transmission from the sinus node is referred to as sinoatrial block and may manifest as a nodal rhythm. Complete AV block is usually a congenital condition but can also be seen with digitalis intoxication and rheumatic carditis.

INDICATIONS

Conditions that lead to arrhythmias that require cardiac pacing are relatively uncommon in children. Consequently, this procedure will be indicated only in rare instances. However, in those circumstances where cardiac pacing is necessary, the procedure can be life-saving. In general, the indications for cardiac pacing can be divided into two categories: urgent and emergent. Situations requiring urgent cardiac pacing are those in which a child has a persistent arrhythmia that is refractory to drug therapy. Although minor associated symptoms may exist (e.g., mild dizziness, orthostasis), the cardiovascular status of the patient is otherwise stable. Potential arrhythmias include SVT, which may require overdrive pacing in the ICU, or stable AV dissociation, which may require surgical implantation of a permanent pacemaker. In such cases, transcutaneous pacing should be available in the ED, but transvenous pacing is generally unnecessary as part of the initial management. If transvenous pacing proves to be necessary, this procedure can normally be performed in the radiology suite with the aid of fluoroscopic guidance. Echocardiography is an alternative means of visualizing placement of the pacer wire.

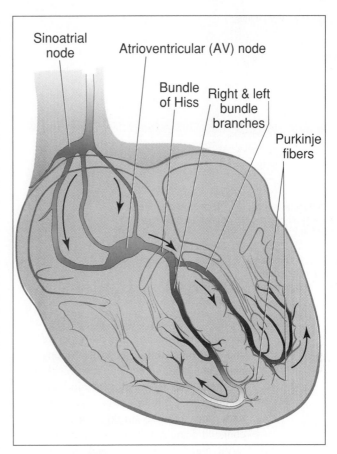

Figure 21.2.
Anatomy of the cardiac conduction system.

Emergent cardiac pacing is the procedure that will be indicated in the ED. In such cases, patients will have significant hypotension associated with a refractory bradyarrhythmia. The most common presenting arrhythmia for these patients is AV dissociation. Transcutaneous pacing can be attempted in such cases, but because these rhythms are generally difficult to manage, this should take place at the time the equipment required for transvenous pacing is assembled and appropriate central venous access is obtained. An algorithm showing the indications for cardiac pacing is presented in Figure 21.3.

The young child with a significant bradyarrhythmia typically shows signs of poor perfusion. The patient may be pale and/or mottled. The extremities are often cool and cyanotic, and capillary refill time may be prolonged. Urine output is decreased or absent. The child will often be lethargic, or in more extreme cases, unconscious.

Congenital heart defects are associated with a variety of clinically significant arrhythmias, including the bradyasystolic rhythms. Such defects include Ebstein's

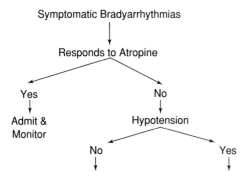

Symptomatic Bradyarrhythmias

Responds to Atropine

Yes → Admit & Monitor

No → Hypotension

No:
- Place transcutaneous pacer leads on chest wall and back
- If necessary, admit and arrange for permanent pacemaker placement

Yes:
- Place transcutaneous pacer and activate
- Obtain central venous access
- Insert transvenous pacemaker

Figure 21.3.
Indications for cardiac pacing.

anomaly, transposition of the great vessels, and congenital mitral stenosis. Among neonates, congenital complete heart block is associated with maternal systemic lupus erythematosus. Pediatric patients who have undergone cardiac surgery for repair of a congenital anomaly (e.g., tetralogy of Fallot, atrial and ventricular septal defects, and endocardial cushion defects) are also at risk for arrhythmias. Acquired processes are also associated with an increased incidence of bradyarrhythmias. These include rheumatic heart disease, myocarditis, cardiac tumors, and certain metabolic and electrolyte disturbances.

In general, infants and younger children requiring emergent transvenous pacing should have the wire inserted via a catheter in the femoral vein, using fluoroscopic guidance as indicated. Older children and adolescents may be managed similar to the adult patient, using the right internal jugular vein or subclavian vein. Although the left subclavian vein provides a more reliable method for insertion of a transvenous pacer, this approach should only be used when absolutely necessary, because the left subclavian is also the preferred site for a permanent pacemaker. A balloon-tipped, flexible catheter should be used to avoid cardiac perforation. A rigid wire is indicated only in an arrest state with no significant blood flow. Because children rarely suffer a full arrest purely on the basis of cardiac dysfunction, using a rigid wire will seldom be appropriate for this patient population.

TRANSVENOUS PACING

Equipment

Pacemakers operate by delivering a small amount of electrical energy to the myocardium, thus stimulating contraction. Some are equipped to sense the patient's cardiac rhythm so that pacing occurs when no rhythm is sensed and is inhibited when a normal rhythm is present. Stimulation of the heart muscle results when the positive pole (anode) and the negative pole (cathode) of the pacemaker battery are briefly connected allowing current to flow. If the energy delivered exceeds the minimum required for cardiac muscle stimulation, a contraction occurs. The completed circuit therefore is composed of two poles of the battery, pacing lead wires, and electrodes as well as the intervening cardiac and body tissues. The pacing systems employ one of two possible electrode configurations: unipolar or bipolar. Unipolar pacing has a single electrode at the cardiac end of the pacing lead and the pulse generator serves as an "indifferent" electrode. During a paced impulse, current flows through the large circuit formed by the components of the pacing system and the body tissue. Bipolar pacing has an additional small ring electrode located on the pacing lead just proximal to the tip of the electrode; current flows between these two electrodes.

Because transvenous pacing can be technically challenging, prior preparation is crucial for this procedure. It is advisable to have available at all times a pediatric central venous access tray, as well as an introducer sheath with a rubber diaphragm which can be easily used for pacer wire placement (see also Chapter 18). The pacemaker and a spare 9-volt battery should be kept on the pediatric code cart, and battery function should be checked initially as well as on a routine basis. Pacing wires also should be stored with the pacemaker and should include both the rigid and the flexible (floating or semifloating) types. Because most children can be paced with a 3- or 4-French pacer wire through a 5- or 6-French sheath, a prepared pediatric pacing tray can be assembled which includes these items as well as necessary equipment for central venous access (Table 21.1).

Medical personnel involved with pacer insertion should be knowledgeable about the specific characteristics of the pacing equipment at their institution. A cardiac emergency obviously does not allow time to become familiar with these items. Pacemakers from a variety of manufacturers are available, but the general design features are similar. The Medtronic 5375 is a typical example (Fig. 21.4). This device has an on/off switch, and when in the on position, releases a spring-loaded button that acts as a safety lock to prevent accidental pacer interruption. It also has an output control that allows for adjustment of the stimulus current amplitude from 0.1 to 20 milliamperes (ma). The rate control dial can be varied from 30 to 180 beats per minute, which is adequate for ventricular pacing in all adults and children. It does not achieve the high rates needed to overdrive pace some children, and therefore is not useful when atrial overdrive pacing, a procedure which would rarely be performed in the ED, is necessary. The device also is equipped with a sensitivity control which controls the magnitude of the R-wave signal required to suppress the pulse generator. In the full counterclockwise position the pacer is not sensing at all and is in an asynchronous mode. The device also has two signal lights, one that indicates sensing and one that indicates pacing. The sensing indicator flashes when a cardiac impulse is sensed. The pacer indicator flashes when a pacing stimulus is generated, although this does not necessarily indicate capture. Finally, the battery test button provides a battery voltage check. When the test button is depressed both the sensing and the pacing indicators flash simultaneously indicating sufficient voltage for use (1).

Pacemaker wires used for emergency transvenous pacing are also available in prepackaged kits from several manufacturers (e.g., Balectrode™ and Medtronic™). These wires come in a variety of sizes, but in general, the 3-

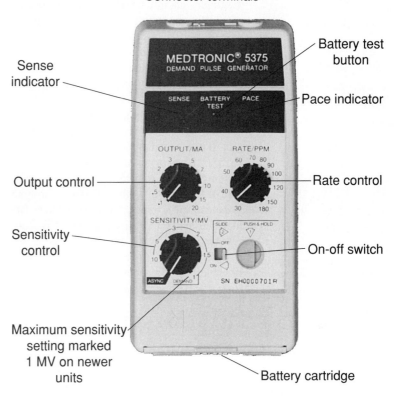

Figure 21.4.
Medtronic cardiac pacer.

or 4-French wire should suffice for most infants and children. The wires are approximately 100 cm in length and are marked at 10 cm intervals to aid with positioning. Many pediatric cardiologists prefer the rigid wire over the floating or semifloating type, due to the controlled setting under which they normally insert pacemakers. It should be pointed out, however, that the rigid wires carry more danger of cardiac perforation (2–4). Without the benefit of visual guidance the semifloating balloon-tip wire may be safer to use in low flow states (5). The balloon is inflated with 1.5 mL of air and "floats" the catheter into the heart if some circulation is present (6, 7). The balloon is checked initially for leaks by inflating it while it is immersed in sterile water. When the patient has no forward blood flow, the balloon is of no use and the rigid catheter should be used.

If the pacemaker is to be inserted using electrocardiographic guidance, then a well-grounded ECG machine (i.e., with a three-pronged plug) must be at the bedside. It should be positioned to allow the operator inserting the pacemaker to watch the changing ECG morphology as the wire passes through the large vessels and cardiac chambers. In addition, a reference depicting the morphology of the QRS

Table 21.1.
Equipment for Transvenous Pacing

9 volt battery

Central venous access tray including introducer sheath with rubber diaphragm suitable for pacer wire placement (see Chapter 18)*

Rigid and flexible (floating or semifloating) pacer wires*

Cardiac monitor

Pulse oximeter

Supplemental oxygen

ECG machine and insulated wire with an alligator clip at each end (optional)

Bedside electrocardiography machine (optional)

* Most children can be paced with a 3- or 4-French pacer wire through a 5- or 6-French sheath.

complex obtained from intracardiac electrocardiography should be kept with the pacing equipment and used as a guide in placing the wire (7, 8–10). An insulated wire with an alligator clip on each end should be available to connect the ECG machine to the pacer wire.

Finally, all patients undergoing pacemaker insertion will require a cardiac monitor, supplemental oxygen, and pulse oximetry monitoring. Pulse oximetry is particularly important if sedation is used (see also Chapter 35). If personnel and equipment for performing bedside echocardiography are available, this can be a highly useful tool for rapid placement of a transvenous pacemaker. The ideal modality to assist placement is fluoroscopy, particularly when the femoral access site is used. However, patients undergoing fluoroscopic pacemaker insertion away from the ED require careful cardiac monitoring and close observation as the incidence of dysrhythmias is high.

Procedure

Pacemakers are placed into the central venous circulation using the internal jugular, femoral, or subclavian approaches. The right internal jugular is a direct approach used primarily with older children and adolescents (Fig. 21.5) For most younger children, the femoral vein is the easiest and safest approach (Fig. 21.6). This is particularly true when chest compressions or airway control must be performed, because the femoral approach does not interfere with these actions. As stated previously, it is best to leave the left subclavian vein available for permanent pacer insertion should that prove necessary (Fig. 21.7).

Figure 21.5.
Transvenous pacemaker placement via the right internal jugular vein.

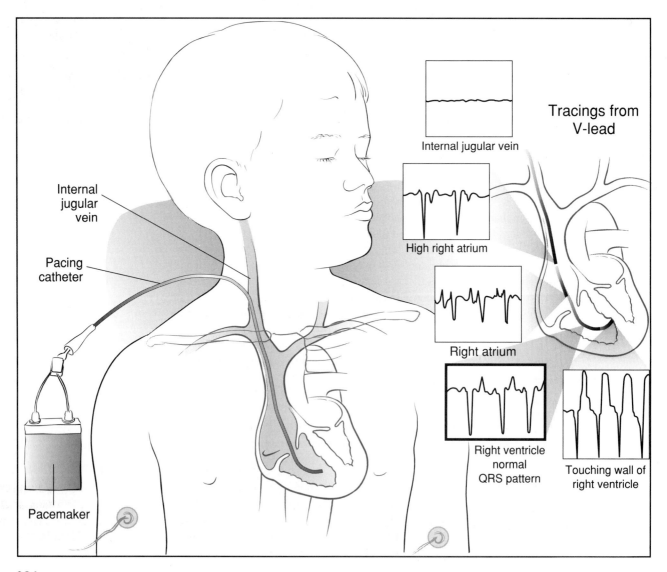

Internal jugular vein

Pacing catheter

Pacemaker

Internal jugular vein

High right atrium

Right atrium

Right ventricle normal QRS pattern

Touching wall of right ventricle

Tracings from V-lead

SUMMARY: TRANSVENOUS PACING USING ECG GUIDANCE

1. Establish central venous access
2. Attach patient to ECG machine using limb leads
3. Insert first 10 cm of pacer wire into catheter sheath
4. Connect negative pole of pacer wire to a V lead of ECG machine by an insulated wire with an alligator clip at each end
5. Turn on ECG machine to read appropriate V lead
6. Advance wire, and if a floating wire is used, inflate balloon when tip has entered vena cava
7. Follow changing patterns of P waves and QRS complexes as wire is advanced through central vessel into right ventricle
8. Once tip of wire is in right ventricle, deflate balloon and further advance until a current of injury (ST segment elevation) is shown on ECG
9. Disconnect from ECG machine and connect to pacemaker
10. Set output to 5 ma, full demand mode, rate appropriate for age, and turn pacer on
11. If capture does not occur, turn off pacemaker and reposition wire
12. Once 100% capture is attained, turn output down until capture is lost. Set output for 2 to 3 times this value (pacing threshold)
13. Check sensor function by turning rate down until below patient's intrinsic rate. If it is sensing appropriately, pacing should stop. Reset at desired minimum heart rate

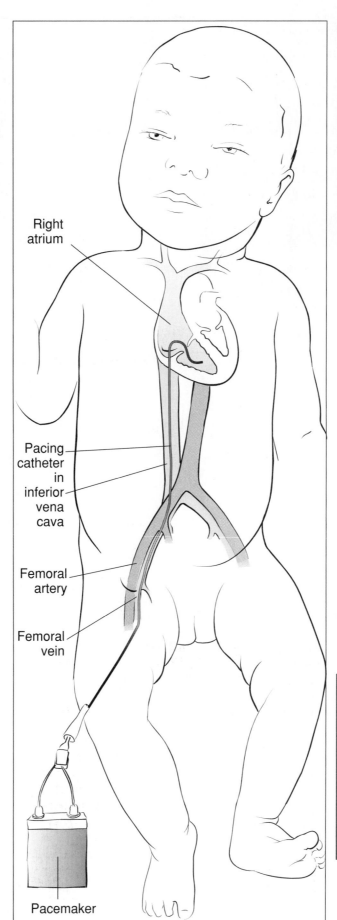

Right atrium

Pacing catheter in inferior vena cava

Femoral artery

Femoral vein

Pacemaker

Figure 21.6.
Transvenous pacemaker placement via the femoral vein. In patients with severe impairment of cardiac output, fluoroscopic guidance may be required to successfully traverse the greater distance from the femoral site to the right ventricle. For blind pacer insertion at the groin, flow-directed catheters are usually necessary, but in a low-flow state such catheters are often ineffective.

SUMMARY: TRANSVENOUS PACING USING ECG GUIDANCE— CONTINUED

14. Suture pacer wire in place
15. Check chest radiograph and ECG for proper placement. The ECG should show LBBB pattern

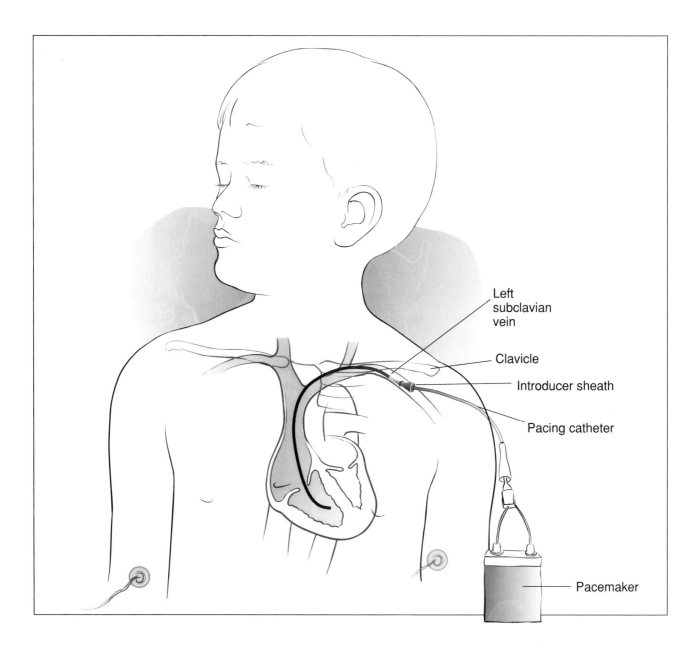

Left
subclavian
vein

Clavicle

Introducer sheath

Pacing catheter

Pacemaker

Figure 21.7.
Transvenous pacemaker placement via the left subclavian vein. (Note: this site should be reserved for later permanent pacemaker placement, if feasible).

Transvenous Pacing Using ECG Guidance

The first step for all pacing methods is to check the equipment. The limb leads of the ECG machine should be attached to the patient. If a balloon is used, it should be deflated as the pacer wire is advanced into the central venous catheter up to the first 10 cm mark. The pacer wire is not connected to the energy source at this time. The distal "negative" terminal (cathode) of the wire should be attached to the ECG machine by an insulated wire with alligator clips at each end. The ECG machine should be turned on and set to the V lead that will be used. It should be emphasized that the ECG machine must be well

grounded (i.e., with a properly functioning three-pronged plug) in order to avoid the risk of inducing ventricular fibrillation. A standard reference should be available showing the expected QRS morphologies that are seen as the pacer wire is advanced from the superior vena cava to the right atrium and finally into the right ventricle (Fig. 21.5).

At this point the pacer wire is inserted into the central vein and gradually advanced. If a balloon is used, it should be inflated after the tip of the pacer wire has entered the vena cava. Once the pacer wire has been advanced into the high right atrium, large negative P waves will be seen. The P waves will become upright and the QRS will become larger as the low right atrium is approached. In the right ventricle, a normal QRS pattern will appear. When the cathode touches the ventricular wall, a current of injury with ST segment elevation will be seen. If the pacer wire is inserted from above, it can (rarely) pass from the superior vena cava directly to the inferior vena cava, rather than into the right atrium. In such cases, the size of the P wave as well as the QRS will suddenly decrease. If the wire enters the pulmonary outflow tract, the P wave becomes negative again and the QRS size diminishes.

Once the pacer wire is in the right ventricle, the balloon should be deflated. The pacer wire is then advanced until it contacts the right ventricle. Again this will appear as a current of injury with ST segment elevation and a left bundle branch block pattern. The position of the pacer wire when contact is made should be noted by checking the 10 cm markings on the wire. The wire is then disconnected from the ECG machine and connected to the pacer source using the receptacles for positive and negative wires. The pacer is set to a rate appropriate for the age of the child and placed in full demand mode with the output at 5 ma. The pacemaker is then turned on. If no evidence of capture is seen or if capture is intermittent, the pacemaker should be turned off and the pacer wire repositioned. Often a clockwise or counterclockwise twist of the catheter will be helpful in this situation. If ventricular ectopy develops, the catheter should be withdrawn until this ceases. If ectopy is frequent, administration of intravenous lidocaine may be necessary before continuing with the procedure.

When the pacemaker appears to be working properly, it can be checked for sensing and pacing thresholds as well as proper positioning. The current should first be decreased until capture is lost. The current is then set to 2 to 3 times the current at which capture was lost. This is called the pacing threshold. The pacing threshold can change in response to certain drugs or as the heart becomes desensitized over time. To check the pacer for appropriate sensing, the rate should be decreased while in the full demand mode until the patient's intrinsic rhythm suppresses the pacer. This ensures that the sensor is working. The rate should be reset to the desired minimal level (7–10, 12).

Failure to capture is the most frequently occurring problem with this procedure, although this can normally be overcome using the methods described previously. Other problems include catheter dislodgment as a result of movement and difficulty in directing the flexible catheters into the right ventricle.

Blind Transvenous Placement

The blind transvenous approach is an alternate method for establishing ED pacing in the emergency department setting. It is best to use a soft floating or semirigid wire to minimize risk. Just as with the electrocardiographic guided technique, this method begins with inserting the pacer wire 10 cm into the central venous catheter. The pacer wire is then connected directly to the pacemaker, rather than an ECG machine. The pacemaker should be turned on and set to twice the patient's heart rate. The output should be set very low. The pacer should be in the full demand mode (pacer senses but does not pace). The wire is then advanced at 10 cm intervals as the operator watches the sensing indicator. When the wire enters the right ventricle, it will sense on every other beat as indicated by the blinking light. If a balloon is used, it should be deflated at this point. The output should then be increased to 4 or 5 ma, and the wire advanced until ventricular capture occurs. The wire should not be advanced more than an additional 10 cm. If capture is not obtained, the wire should be withdrawn slightly, rotated in one direction or the other, and then reinserted until capture occurs. Once capture is achieved, the desired rate should be set and the thresholds checked as previously described (13).

Emergency Blind Transvenous Placement

Emergency blind transvenous placement is indicated in absent cardiac flow states when there is no time to place the pacemaker by other means (i.e., fluoroscopic or ultrasound guided methods). A rigid wire is used without a balloon, because the balloon will be ineffective with no blood flow. The wire is introduced into the central circulation and attached to the pacemaker. The settings for the pacemaker should be asynchronous mode, maximal output, and an appropriate rate for the age of the patient. The wire is advanced until capture occurs. A reasonable estimate of the length of wire needed can be obtained before insertion by measuring the distance that

SUMMARY: BLIND TRANSVENOUS PACING
1. Establish central venous access
2. Advance pacer wire 10 cm into central venous sheath
3. Attach pacer wire to pacer source
4. Set pacemaker to lowest output, full demand mode, and twice patient's rate
5. Turn pacemaker on
6. Advance pacer wire until blinking sensor light corresponds to every other beat, indicating placement in right ventricle
7. Turn output to 5 ma
8. Advance wire until capture takes place (no more than 10 cm)
9. Once 100% capture occurs, set threshold and check sensing
10. Suture pacer wire in place
11. Check chest radiograph and ECG

SUMMARY: EMERGENT BLIND TRANSVENOUS PACING
1. Establish central venous access
2. Measure approximate length of wire needed to reach right ventricle externally before beginning
3. Advance pacer wire into catheter sheath 10 cm
4. Attach wire to pacemaker and set on asynchronous mode, maximum output and average rate for age
5. Advance until capture takes place
6. Withdraw and reposition if unsuccessful
7. If capture takes place set threshold and check sensing
8. Suture pacer wire in place
9. Check chest radiograph and ECG

must be traversed from the point of insertion to the approximate position of the right ventricle. For this approach, the left subclavian provides the most direct route of insertion (9, 14). Using the femoral access site with this technique is usually impossible, since the distance from the groin to the heart is greatly increased and the pathway through the vessels is more tortuous. For this reason, infants and children should normally have pacer insertion via the right internal jugular vein in such situations. The risk of cardiac perforation is high with this method, because it is performed blindly using a rigid catheter.

Postpacemaker Assessment

A chest radiograph must be obtained immediately after placement to assess proper positioning of the pacer wire in the right ventricle. An electrocardiogram should also be performed to identify the characteristic left bundle branch block pattern during paced beats. A right bundle branch block pattern indicates that (*a*) the wire may be in the coronary sinus, (*b*) the wire is positioned too close to the septum in the left ventricle, or (*c*) the wire has perforated the septum and is in the right ventricle. Vital signs should be closely monitored immediately after pacing is initiated as the incidence of complications at this time is increased. Adequate blood pressure and signs of good peripheral perfusion are two of the best indicators that the pacer is functioning properly.

TRANSCUTANEOUS PACING

Equipment

The equipment for transcutaneous pacing is composed of the pacing unit, electrodes, cardiac monitor, and defibrillator. Several transcutaneous pacing models are available that perform only pacing (e.g., Zoll NTP, ZMI Corp., Cambridge, MA). However, many practitioners prefer to use a unit that combines external pacing with cardiac monitoring and defibrillator capabilities (e.g., Lifepak 8, Physio Control, Redmond, WA) (Fig. 21.8). These units are equipped with a dial to control the delivered current and a button to select either the demand or asynchronous modes. The Lifepak 8 has a variable rate control ranging from 40 to 90 bpm (Fig. 21.8). These rates are not high enough for longer term external pacing in infants and most younger children, but may provide temporary support before transvenous pacemaker placement. With older children and adolescents, these rates should be adequate.

The electrodes for transcutaneous pacing are relatively large and at present are available in only one size (Fig. 21.9). They are silver/silver chloride pads measuring 8 cm in diameter with a surrounding adhesive strip which increases the overall size to between 12.5 cm and 16 cm, depending on the manufacturer. The large electrode size was a design modification intended to cause less pain and decrease skeletal muscle stimulation. However, this can sometimes pose a problem when pacing small infants, although in most cases, the two electrodes can be placed on the anterior and posterior chest without contacting one another. The surrounding adhesive area can also be trimmed if necessary. The electrodes have been shown to be safe for both the patient and medical personnel. Minute electrical shocks may be appreciated when accidentally contacting them, but clinicians can normally perform CPR with their hands directly over the electrodes without discomfort.

Procedure

Transcutaneous pacing electrodes are easily applied to the anterior and posterior chest

---

SUMMARY: TRANSCUTANEOUS PACING
1. Sedate patient as indicated
2. Apply adhesive electrodes to anterior and posterior chest walls
3. Connect patient to monitoring system of pacing module
4. Set rate just above patient's rate
5. Set system on demand mode if patient has an intermittently acceptable intrinsic rate; otherwise set system on asynchronous mode
6. Set output to lowest value
7. Turn on pacer
8. Gradually increase output until capture is noted
9. Set output just above pacer threshold
10. Set rate to minimum desired rate
11. Make plans for transvenous pacing

walls using adhesive strips. The normal location of the V3 lead of the ECG is an ideal anterior position while the posterior lead should be placed on the upper back between the scapula (Fig. 21.10). If capture does not occur in these positions, the posterior lead can be moved to a more lateral or even axillary location. If possible, the leads should not be placed over bony structures such as the scapula.

The patient should be monitored using the cardiac monitoring capabilities of the transcutaneous pacer. In general, pediatric patients should be sedated before transcutaneous pacing (see Chapter 35). The rate should be set appropriately based on the age of the child. Assuming there is an intrinsic rate, the pacemaker is set on demand mode, so that pacing will occur only when the patient's own ventricular rate is inadequate. The monitor is turned on with the output at the lowest level, and the output is gradually increased until capture is obtained. The rate is then set to the minimum acceptable heart rate for the patient and the output is set just above the pacing threshold (see Transvenous pacing using ECG guidance). At this point, immediate plans should be made for transvenous pacing.

COMPLICATIONS

Several complications have been associated with emergency transvenous pacing. Ventricular perforation may occur, particularly when a rigid wire is used (2–4). Children are at higher risk for this complication, because they have relatively thin right ventricular walls. Rigid wires only should be passed blindly when there is no discernible cardiac output and when direct visualization with fluoroscopy or echocardiography is impossible. Air embolism secondary to rupture of the balloon in the floating pacer wires has also occurred (15, 16). Checking the balloon for leaks before insertion will limit this problem. Care should also be taken not to overinflate the balloon. Ventricular fibrillation can occur during emergency pacing when the myocardium is exposed to outside electrical current from an ungrounded ECG machine. Most hospitals now use only ECG machines with three-pronged plugs that are inserted

into grounded outlets, thereby eliminating this risk. Only with older equipment is this a significant possibility. Finally, ventricular tachycardia also may result because of irritation of the myocardium by the wire. If persistent ventricular ectopy occurs, the wire should be withdrawn and administration of intravenous lidocaine should be considered before subsequent pacing attempts.

No significant complications are associated with transcutaneous pacing. Muscle damage, burns, and other such injuries associated with cardioversion and defibrillation do not occur, because the energy of the currents delivered is low. Medical personnel also are at no risk from this procedure. The most common difficulty with using the transcutaneous pacemaker is achieving adequate seda-

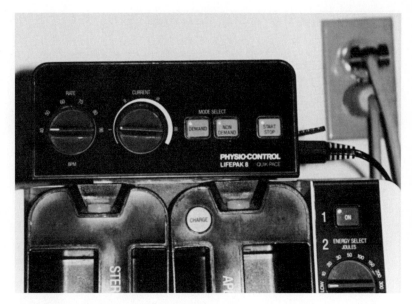

Figure 21.8.
Lifepak 8 transcutaneous pacing unit.

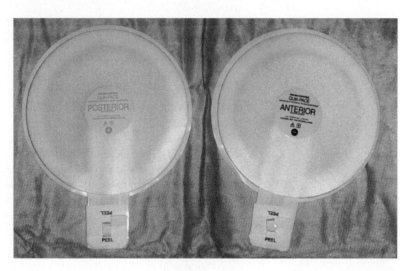

Figure 21.9.
Transcutaneous pacing electrodes.

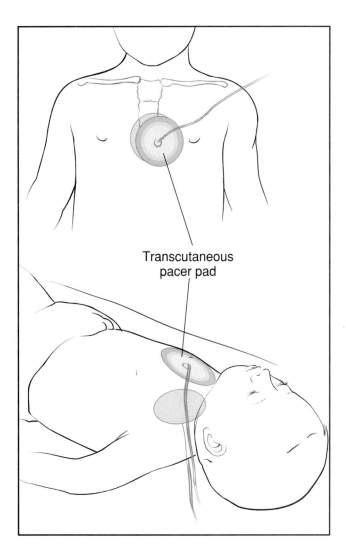

Figure 21.10.
Proper placement of transcutaneous pacing electrodes.

under fluoroscopic guidance is the safest and most effective means of performing emergency pacing. However, when fluoroscopy is not available, blind procedures using a flow-directed (balloon-guided) pacer electrode may be necessary. Emergency transvenous pacing is associated with a variety of potentially serious complications and must therefore be performed only when indicated. Transcutaneous pacing is a relatively simple technique which can be used as a temporizing measure in the treatment of bradyarrhythmias. No significant complications result from the use of transcutaneous pacing.

tion so that the patient can tolerate a current that is effective in pacing the heart.

SUMMARY

Fortunately, emergency cardiac pacing for pediatric patients is rarely indicated, although this may change over time as more children are surviving surgical repair of heart abnormalities. Many such children live in communities far removed from a tertiary pediatric facility. Emergency pacing is indicated for bradycardia resulting in hypotension that is unresponsive to standard medications. It is also indicated for the treatment of hemodynamically significant tachyarrhythmias which do not respond to medications (overdrive pacing), a procedure that will rarely be performed in the ED. Transvenous pacing via the femoral vein using a rigid bipolar catheter

---

CLINICAL TIPS: TRANSVENOUS PACING
1. The natural curve of the pacer wire should be used to aid in positioning the tip in the right ventricle (i.e., curving toward the left side of the chest).
2. The operator should ensure that the catheter sheath is larger than the pacer wire before beginning the procedure.
3. If no evidence of capture exists or if capture is intermittent, the pacemaker should be turned off and the pacer wire repositioned. Often a clockwise or counterclockwise twist of the catheter will be helpful in this situation.
4. If ventricular ectopy develops, the catheter should be withdrawn until this ceases. If ectopy is frequent, administration of intravenous lidocaine may be necessary before continuing with the procedure.
5. The pacer wire should be coiled at the skin surface after suturing to decrease the likelihood of dislodgment.
6. The on/off switch on the pacemaker should be covered at all times to avoid accidental power loss.

CLINICAL TIPS: TRANSCUTANEOUS PACING
1. If possible, the pacer electrodes should not be placed over bony structures such as the scapula.
2. The two pacer electrodes should not touch one another, to prevent a short circuit which could result in a loss of delivered current.
3. It may be necessary to trim the adhesive strips on the pacer electrodes to decrease the size of the pads with infants and small children.

References

1. Medtronic Model 5375 Technical Manual. External demand pulse generator and accessories. Medtronic Inc. 1990:10–12.
2. Goswani M, et al. Perforation of the heart by flexible transvenous pacemaker. JAMA 1971;216:2013.
3. Danielson GK, et al. Failure of endocardial pacemaker due to myocardial perforation. J Thorac Cardiovasc Surg 1967;54:42.
4. Kalloor GJ. Cardiac tamponade. Report of a case after insertion of transvenous endocardial electrode. Am Heart J 1974;88:88.
5. Snag R, et al. The use of the balloon-tipped floating catheter in temporary transvenous cardiac pacing. PACE 1981;4:491.
6. Swan HJ, et al. Catheterization of the heart in man with use of a flow-directed, balloon-tipped catheter. N Engl J Med 1970;283:447.
7. Schnitzler RN, et al. "Floating" catheter for temporary transvenous ventricular pacing. Am J Cardiol 1973;31:331.
8. Kimball JT, Killip T. A simple bedside method for transvenous intracardiac pacing. Am Heart J 1965; 70:35.
9. Harris CW, et al. Percutaneous technique for cardiac pacing with a platinum-tipped electrode catheter. Am J Cardiol 1965;15:48.
10. Escher DJ, Furman S. Emergency treatment of cardiac arrhythmias. Emphasis on use of electrical pacing. JAMA 1970;214:2028.
11. Hazard PB. Transvenous cardiac pacing in cardiopulmonary resuscitation. Crit Care Med 1981;9:666.
12. Goldberger E. Temporary cardiac pacing. In: Goldberger E, ed. Treatment of cardiac emergencies. 4th ed. St. Louis: CV Mosby, 1985:272–274.
13. Benjamin GC. Emergency transvenous cardiac pacing. In: Roberts JR, Hedges JR, eds. Clinical procedures in emergency medicine. 2nd ed. Philadelphia: WB Saunders, 1985:170–191.
14. Rosenberg AS, et al. Bedside transvenous cardiac pacing. Am Heart J 1969;77:697.
15. Campo I, et al. Complications of pacing by pervenous subclavian semifloating electrodes including extraluminal insertions. Am J Cardiol 1970; 26:627.
16. Foote GA, et al. Pulmonary complications of the flow-directed, balloon-tipped catheter. N Engl J Med 1974;290:927.

CHAPTER 22

CARDIOVERSION AND DEFIBRILLATION

Richard J. Scarfone

INTRODUCTION

Synchronized cardioversion is the application of direct current electricity to terminate dysrhythmia. Current is timed (synchronized) so that it is delivered outside the vulnerable phase of the cardiac cycle to minimize risk of precipitating ventricular fibrillation. Types of dysrhythmia seen in children that may require using synchronized cardioversion include supraventricular tachycardia, atrial fibrillation, atrial flutter, and ventricular tachycardia. Defibrillation involves application of a higher initial dosage of direct current electricity which is not timed to the cardiac cycle (asynchronous). A large segment of the myocardium is depolarized, rendering it refractory to further disorganized cardiac conduction. Defibrillation is used in the treatment of ventricular fibrillation or pulseless ventricular tachycardia (1). These procedures are relatively straightforward and are performed by a diversity of health care professionals.

Because the most common cause of cardiopulmonary arrest in children is respiratory failure leading to hypoxemia and asystole rather than primary cardiac dysfunction, cardioversion and defibrillation are not frequently performed for this patient population. However, recent advances in pediatric cardiothoracic surgery have led to significantly higher survival rates among children who undergo repair of congenital abnormalities, and these patients are at increased risk for dys-

rhythmias. In addition, children who accidentally or intentionally ingest excessive amounts of medications such as tricyclic antidepressants or sympathomimetics also develop atrial and ventricular dysrhythmias. These drugs have become more easily available to pediatric patients as increasing numbers of adolescents and adults are treated with antidepressant medications and as albuterol has become a first-line agent in the outpatient management of childhood asthma. For those children who present with cardiac dysrhythmias and hemodynamic compromise, cardioversion and defibrillation often represent life-saving interventions when performed in a timely and appropriate manner.

ANATOMY AND PHYSIOLOGY

Under normal circumstances, the sinoatrial (SA) node, located in the right atrium, serves as the primary source of cardiac impulses (Fig. 22.1). A depolarization wave travels through the atria to the atrioventricular (AV) node at the lower portion of the right atrium. Here conduction of the current is slowed, allowing sufficient time for completion of atrial contraction. The impulse is then conducted along the bundle of His, through the right and left bundle branches to the Purkinje fibers, resulting in an organized ventricular depolarization and contraction.

Tachyarrthyhmia commonly occurs as a result of reentrant conduction (2). As shown

Figure 22.1.
The cardiac cycle and cardiac conduction system.

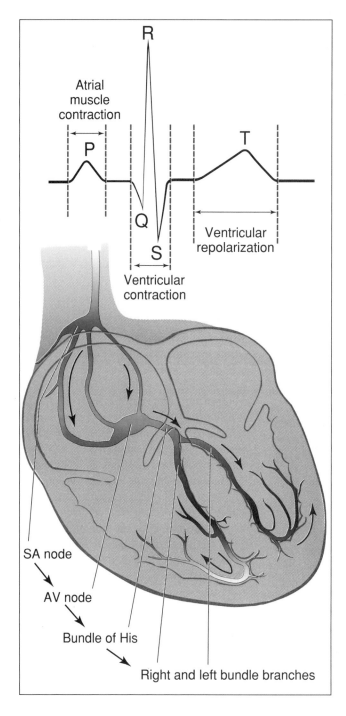

Atrial muscle contraction

P

R

Q

S

Ventricular contraction

T

Ventricular repolarization

SA node

AV node

Bundle of His

Right and left bundle branches

from this reentrant focus produce tachyarrhythmia. Reentry may result in a rapid atrial and/or ventricular rate, depending on the extent of conduction from the atria to the ventricles and the location of the reentrant circuit within the myocardium.

With cardioversion, an externally applied electrical current depolarizes a segment of the myocardium, rendering it refractory to continued depolarization by the reentry impulse. This often allows the SA node to resume its role as pacemaker, because it normally has the greatest intrinsic automaticity. A synchronized cardioversion impulse is timed so that it is not given during the vulnerable period of the cardiac cycle in the phase of early repolarization, represented on the ECG tracing by the beginning of the T wave. An electric shock delivered at this time (the so-called "R on T" phenomenon) can produce ventricular fibrillation (3).

The physiology of fibrillation is not well understood. Factors such as ischemia and acidosis are believed to decrease the refractory period that myocardial cells normally enter following depolarization (4). Numerous depolarization wavefronts which arise outside of the sinus node may then be conducted, begin-

in Figure 22.2, during reentry the usual conduction route for an electrical impulse (path A) is in a state of depressed excitability. While the current travels a more slowly conducted secondary path (path B), path A repolarizes. The current is then conducted along path A, but in a retrograde direction. The resulting pattern of rapidly cycling current (down path B and up path A) is known as circus conduction. Repetitive depolarizations

ning a series of reentry circuits leading to asynchronous activity. Fibrillation may occur in both the atria and the ventricles. In most instances, atrial fibrillation is not a serious dysrhythmia, as long as the resulting ventricular rate maintains a stable blood pressure. Emergent therapy is therefore usually unnecessary. In contrast, ventricular fibrillation is extremely dangerous if untreated. The ventricles contract in an ineffective and

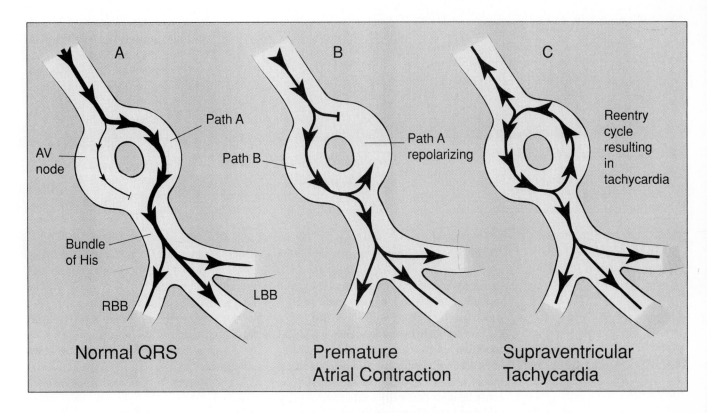

A. Normal QRS

B. Premature Atrial Contraction

C. Supraventricular Tachycardia

(Labels in figure: AV node, Path A, Path B, Bundle of His, RBB, LBB, Path A repolarizing, Reentry cycle resulting in tachycardia)

Figure 22.2.
Schematic anatomy of a reentrant focus (see text for description).

disorganized manner, leading to a rapid progression of diminished stroke volume, inadequate tissue perfusion, hypoxemia, and death. The heart is said to resemble a "bag of worms" during the chaotic depolarizations of ventricular fibrillation. Electrical defibrillation is often the only intervention that will reverse this lethal cascade of events. Defibrillation involves an externally applied asynchronous electrical impulse which results in the depolarization of a large segment of ventricular tissue. After depolarization, these cells are refractory to ectopic impulses. As with direct cardioversion, the SA node can then take over the function of generating cardiac depolarizations, resulting in a resumption of normal sinus rhythm.

INDICATIONS

Many indications for using cardioversion and defibrillation depend on the presence of hemodynamic instability (i.e., hypotension or signs of inadequate cerebral or peripheral perfusion— agitation, lethargy, weak pulses, mottling) or heart failure. With children, proper assessment of blood pressure must be based on the normal range for each age group in question. A listing of normal blood pressure ranges for pediatric patients can be found in Chapter 4.

Supraventricular Tachycardia

Supraventricular tachycardia (SVT) is the most common significant dysrhythmia in children (5). It most often occurs as a result of reentry as described previously, although a nonreentrant ectopic atrial focus also may be the cause. Distinguishing SVT from sinus tachycardia sometimes can be difficult in children, although the degree of tachycardia with SVT is typically more extreme. In infants, the rate of SVT ranges from 220 to 320 bpm, and in older children, from 150 to 250 bpm. Fever, anxiety, pain, and respiratory distress are a few conditions that may contribute to sinus tachycardia, but the heart rate rarely exceeds 200 bpm. In addition to extreme tachycardia, ECG findings consistent with SVT include a regular RR interval that does not vary with respiratory pattern, narrow QRS complexes, and dysmorphic or absent P waves (Fig. 22.3). Causes of SVT in children include congenital heart disease, Wolff-Parkinson-White syndrome, fever, and medi-

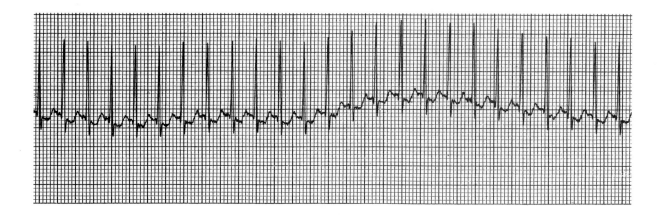

Figure 22.3.
Supraventricular
tachycardia.

cations (most commonly sympathomimetics). Among infants, 50% of cases are classified as idiopathic (5). A recent case report described a child with albuterol-induced SVT, which was terminated with adenosine (6).

Severe tachycardia associated with this condition results in decreased diastolic filling time, leading eventually to congestive heart failure. Adults with SVT will normally become hemodynamically compromised relatively quickly. However, an infant or young child with SVT will usually develop congestive heart failure more gradually, sometimes maintaining adequate tissue perfusion for 24 hours or more. Thus the child with SVT will have a variable clinical presentation, ranging

at the extremes from tachycardia alone to cardiogenic shock, depending on the duration of the dysrhythmia. Signs of congestive heart failure in infants include tachypnea, poor feeding (typically with diaphoresis during feedings), agitation, prolonged capillary refill time, pallor, depressed mental status, and hypotension.

For children with stable hemodynamics, maneuvers designed to increase vagal stimulation to the heart may be both diagnostic and therapeutic in the management of SVT (see Chapter 72). For the child with SVT, vagal maneuvers either will have no effect on the heart rate or will result in an abrupt termination of the dysrhythmia. With sinus tachycar-

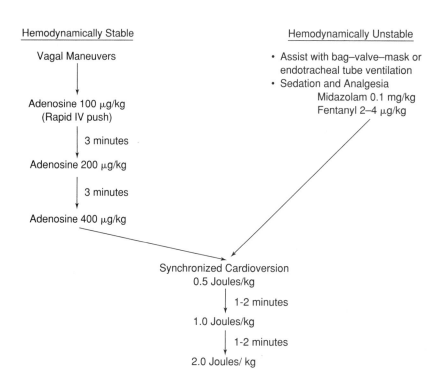

Figure 22.4.
Treatment of SVT.

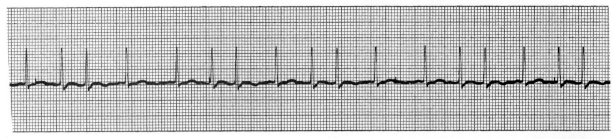

Figure 22.5.
Atrial fibrillation.

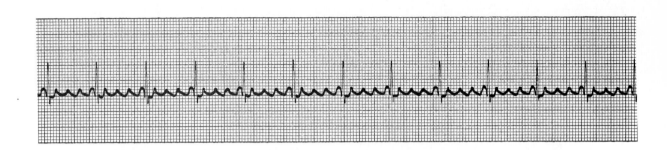

Figure 22.6.
Atrial flutter.

dia, vagal stimulation will result in a gradual decrease in the heart rate, followed by a steady return to the initial rate. If vagal maneuvers are unsuccessful, the next step is to administer intravenous medication. For many years, digoxin and verapamil were used as the primary agents for this presentation. However, digoxin has a relatively slow onset of action, and verapamil can cause an idiosyncratic cardiovascular collapse, particularly among children under 1 year of age. Currently, adenosine is the drug of choice in treating the hemodynamically stable child with SVT (7–16). Synchronized cardioversion is indicated for patients who fail to respond to vagal maneuvers and pharmacologic agents or who manifest signs of hemodynamic instability. One cautionary note regarding the use of synchronized cardioversion is that low energies should be used for the child with SVT who is taking digoxin, because ventricular dysrhythmias may be precipitated in this setting (3). The recommended management approach is shown in Figure 22.4.

Atrial Fibrillation and Atrial Flutter

Although relatively uncommon in children, atrial fibrillation and atrial flutter should be recognized and treated appropriately. Atrial fibrillation appears on the ECG tracing as fine oscillating waves between QRS complexes without definable P waves. The hallmark of atrial fibrillation is an irregular ventricular response (Fig. 22.5). Atrial flutter is characterized by a regular ventricular rhythm with "saw-toothed" waves between each QRS complex (Fig. 22.6). Atrial rates may exceed 400 bpm with either atrial fibrillation or atrial flutter, but since all of the impulses are not usually conducted to the ventricles, the ventricular rate will be considerably less. The clinical state of the patient depends on the rate of the ventricular response, the effects of any underlying heart disease, and the duration of the arrhythmia. With a very rapid ventricular rate, diastolic filling time is diminished resulting in decreased cardiac output.

With atrial fibrillation, ample time is usually available to initiate drug therapy in an attempt to terminate the dysrhythmia. If the patient fails to respond to drug therapy or becomes hemodynamically unstable, however, synchronized cardioversion is indicated. Success rates as high as 90% have been reported for adults with no underlying heart disease who were treated with direct cardioversion for atrial fibrillation (3). On the other hand, synchronized cardioversion is now considered the treatment of choice for atrial flutter,

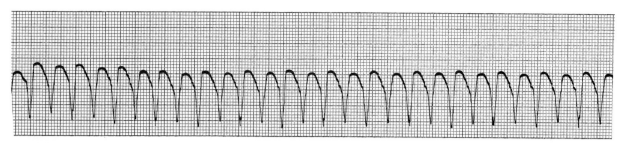

Figure 22.7.
Ventricular tachycardia.

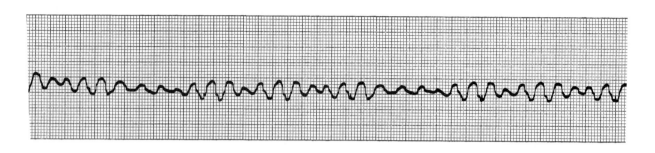

Figure 22.8.
Ventricular fibrillation.

even when the patient is stable (3). This is true because atrial flutter is notoriously difficult to convert with drug therapy, and successful treatment with cardioversion has been reported in 72 to 100% of cases (3).

Ventricular Tachycardia

Ventricular tachycardia (VT) is also an uncommon dysrhythmia in the pediatric population. Conditions that may predispose to VT in children include underlying heart disease, a tricyclic antidepressant overdose, or disease processes leading to hyperkalemia such as renal failure or congenital adrenal hyperplasia.

As with SVT, VT may occur either as the result of reentry or an ectopic focus, although here the abnormality is obviously ventricular in origin. On the cardiogram, the characteristic feature of VT is wide QRS complexes (greater than .12 seconds) with a bundle branch morphology (Fig. 22.7). The rate may vary from 120 to 400 bpm, but is typically 200 to 300 bpm. P waves may be absent, retrograde (i.e., inverted and appearing after the QRS complex), or unrelated to the QRS complex (AV dissociation). SVT with aberrant conduction is virtually impossible to distinguish from VT based on cardiographic appearance. However, because fewer than 10% of children with SVT have aberrant conduc-

tion, the clinician must assume the presence of VT when treating a child with a wide complex tachycardia (17).

Children with VT decompensate far more rapidly than those with SVT. As with SVT, tachycardia can result in a decreased ventricular filling time which in turn leads to diminished stroke volume and cardiac output. Prolonged VT may also degenerate into ventricular fibrillation. For patients who are hemodynamically stable, intravenous lidocaine is the treatment of choice. If the patient fails lidocaine therapy or shows signs of hemodynamic decompensation while still having a palpable pulse, synchronized cardioversion is indicated. For patients with pulseless VT, the most recent American Heart Association (AHA) guidelines recommend immediate asynchronous defibrillation (1). Studies with adults show that cardioversion is successful in converting ventricular tachycardia in over 95% of cases (3).

Ventricular Fibrillation

Myocardial ischemia, a rare condition in children, is the most important factor in lowering the heart's fibrillation threshold (4). For adults, ventricular fibrillation (VF) is the primary cause of sudden cardiac death (18), whereas the most common terminal dysrhythmias in children are asystole and brady-cardia (19). Therefore, those caring for critically ill children are more frequently called on to perform assisted ventilation rather than defibrillation. Reflecting these facts, the most recent basic life support (BLS) guidelines recommend that for the child who suffers an out-of-hospital arrest, cardiopulmonary resuscitation (CPR) should be performed for 1 minute before alerting EMS (19). This is done under the presumption that a primary respiratory insult, which is the most likely cause of the arrest, may be rapidly reversible with adequate CPR. By contrast, it has been convincingly demonstrated that the timeliness of defibrillation is the single most important factor determining prognosis for an adult arrest patient. Therefore, it is recommended that the EMS system should be activated immediately for these patients, before initiating CPR (18).

Ventricular fibrillation is a disorganized depolarization of the entire ventricle caused by multiple reentry circuits. The cardiogram will show a coarse or fine oscillating baseline without QRS complexes and no measurable heart rate (Fig. 22.8). The ventricles contract ineffectively, resulting in no significant cardiac output and pulselessness. If electrical activity consistent with VF is noted on the monitor, the clinician should confirm this finding by examining the patient for palpable pulses, because a disconnected lead or a malfunctioning monitor can sometimes mimic this dysrhythmia. If no pulses are present, defibrillation should be performed immediately. The clinician should not delay defibrillation until an airway or intravenous access is established. Three successive shocks should be administered as needed before any other interventions are performed. In one study of hospitalized children who developed ventricular fibrillation and were promptly treated with defibrillation, 89% were successfully resuscitated (20).

Defibrillation is not effective in the management of children with asystole and is therefore not indicated for this purpose (21). However, fine VF oscillations with an amplitude of 1 mm or less may be mistaken for asystole (22). When using the paddles as "quick look" monitor leads, the operator should rotate the paddles 90° to assess the rhythm in a different plane before assuming the dysrhythmia is asystole (22). If the child

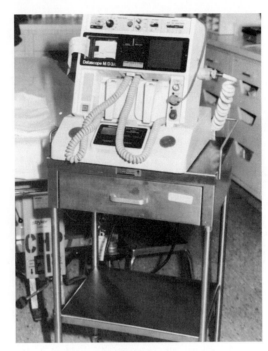

Figure 22.9.
Cardioverter-defibrillator unit.

is connected to a standard cardiac monitor, this can also be accomplished by switching to all the available leads in turn and assessing the rhythm.

EQUIPMENT

The source of the electrical current for all cardioversion devices in clinical use today is a direct current depolarizer. Most modern units can be used for both cardioversion and defibrillation. Cardioversion is performed in synchronous mode, and defibrillation is performed in asynchronous mode. The synchronizer allows discharge of current only after a repetitive series of R waves to ensure that energy is delivered outside of the vulnerable period of the cardiac cycle. Many machines have separate on-off switches for the defibrillator and the oscilloscope screen or monitor. In addition, all cardioverters have a control to select the energy level, a control to initiate charging of the machine, and a light to indicate the machine is fully charged (Fig. 22.9).

The depolarizer delivers energy to the patient via two electrode paddles (Fig. 22.10). Typically, the controls allowing discharge of current are present on the paddle handles, but in some cases, they are on a separate panel located on the machine. The most recent AHA guidelines recommend 4.5 cm

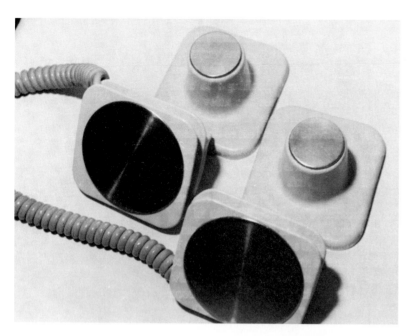

Figure 22.10.
Pediatric and adult electrode paddles.

cumstances (23). Other factors that have been shown to decrease impedance include applying firm pressure when using the paddles and delivering the energy at the end of expiration for the spontaneously breathing patient (24, 25).

PROCEDURE

Preparing the Patient

For all children requiring defibrillation and for many requiring synchronized cardioversion, the unstable clinical condition of the patient necessitates that the procedure be performed immediately. Other interventions such as establishing intravenous access must be delayed until after attempts are made to terminate the dysrhythmia. However, for the stable conscious child who has failed to respond to medications, synchronized cardioversion may be performed as a semielective procedure. In such cases, supplemental oxygen should be provided, and intravenous medications to induce sedation and analgesia should be administered. Short-acting agents such as midazolam (0.1 mg/kg) and fentanyl (2 to 4 µg/kg) are ideally suited for this purpose. Midazolam provides sedative as well as amnestic properties. Fentanyl will potentiate the sedative effects of midazolam while also serving as an analgesic. Both medications should be infused slowly over 30 to 60 seconds to minimize risk of respiratory depression. The reversal agents naloxone and flumazinol should be readily available (see also Chapter 35).

Operating the Machine

Just before turning the machine on, a commercial paste or gel should be liberally applied to the paddles to decrease transthoracic impedance and to minimize the risk of burns. Modern machines used for synchronized cardioversion provide a means of connecting ECG leads to the patient, allowing the operator to select the waveform that will be displayed on the monitor. It is best to choose the lead that produces the tallest R wave when performing synchronized cardioversion to optimize sensing by the machine. This minimizes the likelihood that current will be ad-

diameter paddles for infants and children weighing less than 10 kg and 8 cm (adult) paddles for children over 10 kg (1). The goal is to choose the largest paddle that allows chest wall contact over its entire surface area. The larger the paddle, the lower the impedance and the greater the amount of cardiac muscle depolarized (4). In addition, larger paddles will produce less myocardial injury by allowing the energy to be dissipated over a greater surface area (3). However, if the paddles are too large, they may contact one another when the energy is delivered, creating a short circuit and decreasing the energy delivered to the heart (3).

Energy delivered to the myocardium during cardioversion is directly related to the amount of current applied and the duration of current flow; it is inversely related to the impedance across the chest wall (4). Transthoracic impedance partially depends on the conductive material applied at the paddle-skin interface. Commercial creams, pastes, and gels have been shown to have a lower impedance than bare skin (18). Saline-soaked gauze pads have a higher impedance than commercial products. An additional problem is that the saline from one paddle will often drip and contact the other paddle, causing a short circuit and diminishing the delivered energy. Sonographic gels are unacceptable because they are poor electrical conductors (17). Alcohol pads can cause serious burns and should not be used under any cir-

Table 22.1.
Energy Dosages

Direct cardioversion
0.5 J/kg for initial attempt; then double the dose for subsequent attempts

Defibrillation
2 J/kg for the initial attempt; then 4 J/kg for the second and third attempts

ministered during the vulnerable phase of the cardiac cycle. For defibrillation, the clinician should use the "paddle" electrodes, so that valuable time is not lost placing monitor leads on the patient. The unit is then set on synchronous or asynchronous mode depending on the dysrhythmia being treated.

Selecting the Energy

At this point, the amount of energy to be delivered is set (Table 22.1). The optimum amount of electrical energy for pediatric cardioversion or defibrillation has not been established (23). The most recent AHA guidelines suggest beginning with a dose of 0.5 J/kg for direct cardioversion and doubling the dose on subsequent attempts (1). For defibrillation, the recommended starting dose is 2 J/kg (1). If unsuccessful, the dose is doubled and repeated. A third attempt again should be with 4 J/kg. After three unsuccessful attempts, the operator should focus on treating any processes that may be lowering the fibrillation threshold, such as metabolic acidosis, hypothermia, or electrolyte disturbances. If the rhythm initially terminates, but then reverts to fibrillation, increases in energy are not indicated (1). If multiple shocks are required, the machine must be recharged each time. Once the energy is selected, a separate control is activated to charge the machine; after a few seconds, it will be maximally charged as indicated by a light or audible tone.

SUMMARY: SYNCHRONIZED CARDIOVERSION
1. Assess patient:
   a. For patients who are hemodynamically unstable, perform cardioversion before establishing intravenous access or securing definitive airway
   b. For patients who are stable, administer supplemental oxygen and intravenous sedation and analgesia before performing cardioversion

SUMMARY:SYNCHRONIZED CARDIOVERSION (CONTINUED)
2. Turn cardioverter on
3. Attach ECG leads to patient (if stable)
4. Select lead that displays tallest R wave
5. Set machine on synchronous mode
6. Apply electrode paste or gel to paddles
7. Select energy and charge unit
8. Place paddles firmly on chest in appropriate positions
9. Ensure that operator is not contacting patient and that patient is not contacting any metal parts of stretcher
10. Clear area ("All clear!")
11. Apply current by depressing discharge buttons simultaneously and holding paddles in place for several moments
12. If dysrhythmia persists, double energy level, recharge unit, and apply current after 2-to-3 minute interval (if patient's clinical condition permits)
13. If patient develops postcardioversion dysrhythmia, treat appropriately
14. After patient is stabilized, address other management issues (administration of antiarrythmic agents, correction of metabolic abnormalities, etc.)

SUMMARY: DEFIBRILLATION
1. Perform defibrillation when indicated before establishing intravenous access or securing definitive airway
2. Apply electrode paste or gel to paddles
3. Turn machine on
4. Select "quick look" paddle leads to assess rhythm
5. Apply paddles firmly to appropriate positions on chest
6. If monitor waveform appears to be asystole, rotate paddles 90° to assess rhythm in another plane, since true rhythm may be fine VF
7. Select energy and charge unit
8. Ensure that operator is not contacting patient and that patient is not contacting any metal parts of stretcher
9. Clear area ("All clear!")
10. Apply current by depressing discharge buttons simultaneously
11. If dysrhythmia persists, double energy level, recharge unit, and reapply current
12. After three unsuccessful attempts, focus on correcting underlying process that is lowering fibrillation threshold

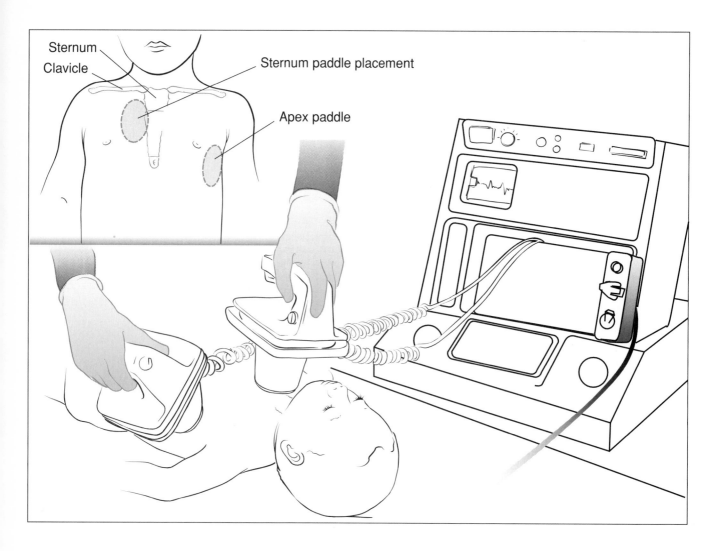

Figure 22.11.
Position of electrode paddles with a supine patient.

Using the Paddles

In most paddle sets, one paddle is labeled "sternum" and the other is labeled "apex." With the patient supine, the "apex" paddle is held in the operator's right hand and placed over the 4th and 5th intercostal spaces, just lateral to the nipple. The opposite paddle is placed just below the right clavicle lateral to the sternum (Fig. 22.11). As mentioned previously, fine ventricular fibrillation may be mistaken as asystole if only one cardiac plane is monitored (22). Before assuming a rhythm as asystole, the paddles should be used as electrodes and rotated 90° to assess the electrical activity in a different plane.

An alternate method of paddle placement is the anteroposterior position. With the patient upright, the "sternum" paddle is pressed directly over the sternum while the "apex" paddle is placed on the back between the scapulae (Fig. 22.12). One study found no difference in the success rate of cardioversion with either method (3). The former position, with the child lying supine, is more practical in most situations. However, anteroposterior placement is preferred when adult paddles must be used for an infant or young child because of the unavailability of appropriate pediatric paddles. This method decreases the likelihood that the large paddles will contact one another on a smaller chest during delivery of the current. With either position, it is important to apply firm pressure with the paddles to decrease transthoracic impedance. In addition, the operator should ensure that the paste from one paddle does not contact that of the other, since the resultant "bridg-

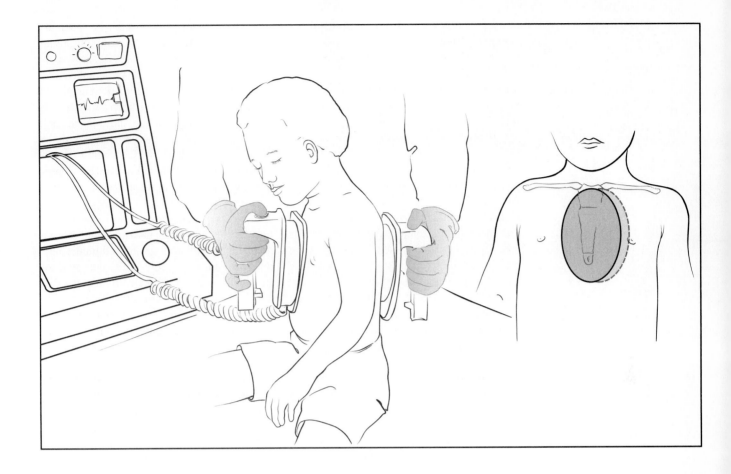

Figure 22.12.
Anteroposterior paddle
placement.

ing" of current will decrease the energy delivered to the heart and increase the risk of skin burns.

Delivering Current

Once synchronous or asynchronous mode has been set, the energy has been selected, the machine has charged, and the paddles are in correct position, the current is then delivered to the patient. Extreme caution must be taken to ensure that all personnel other than the person operating the unit are away from the patient and stretcher and that the child's exposed skin is not in contact with any metal. The standard warning "All clear!" must always be given. The operator must also be careful not to directly contact the patient or the stretcher.

With most units, energy is delivered by simultaneously depressing buttons on the paddle handles. This should be performed as soon as possible after charging to minimize the amount of stored energy that is lost. Delivery of current will be marked by skeletal muscle contraction and a rapid rise and fall of the trunk. One or more factors may explain a failure to deliver current successfully. With synchronized cardioversion, the clinician must ensure that the cardioverter (not just the monitor) is on, that the machine has been charged, that firm contact between the chest wall and the paddles is made, and that the paste or gel from one paddle is not contacting that of the other. In addition, in cases of extreme tachycardia (as often occurs with children), the machine may not be able to properly sense the R waves when set on synchronous mode. The buttons are depressed but no current is delivered, and the assumption is often made that the equipment is defective. In such cases, the operator should depress the discharge buttons with the paddles in firm contact with the chest for a full 10 to 15 seconds before abandoning the attempt. If this fails, it may be necessary to administer an asynchronous discharge when the patient is hemodynamically unstable. The risk of inducing VF by delivering current during the vulnerable phase of the cardiac cycle may be outweighed by the deteriorating clinical condition of the patient.

If after shock delivery the patient remains in the same abnormal rhythm, the dose of energy is doubled, the machine is recharged, and the current is readministered. A delay of 2 to 3 minutes between shocks will generally minimize complications, assuming that the patient's clinical condition permits this. Using repeated shocks is based on the theory that additive amounts of myocardium are depolarized and that multiple shocks decrease transthoracic impedance, increasing the effectiveness of the delivered current (4). After the patient is stabilized, other management issues (administering antiarrhythmic drugs, correcting electrolyte disturbances, etc.) can be addressed. Although rare, the patient undergoing direct cardioversion will sometimes develop VF or asystole. The operator should always be prepared for this potential outcome by having all necessary resuscitation equipment readily available. If the patient develops VF, the machine is recharged and set on asynchronous mode in preparation for immediate defibrillation. Fortunately, the rate of conversion of VF to normal sinus rhythm in such cases is high.

COMPLICATIONS

Complications associated with cardioversion and defibrillation are dysrhythmias, myocardial injury, and skin burns. Risk of complications is increased with higher energy doses, multiple shocks, shorter intervals between shocks, and increased transthoracic impedance (4).

A variety of rhythm disturbances may occur following cardioversion or defibrillation. Sinus bradycardia, VF or VT, and atrioventricular block have all been reported. However, these dysrhythmias are typically transient and do not result in cardiovascular compromise. Asystole may also occur but is rare. The primary factors that increase the likelihood of dysrhythmia are a high dose of delivered energy and the presence of underlying cardiac disease or metabolic derangements. As discussed previously, postcardioversion VF should be treated with immediate asynchronous shock. Because cardioversion is performed in synchronous mode, the operator must make certain to switch the machine to asynchronous mode before administering the current in such cases. Digitalis toxicity is associated with the occurrence of VT and VF following the administration of electrical current (3). Consequently, if a child is suspected of having dysrhythmia secondary to digitalis toxicity, appropriate precautions should be taken. Before cardioversion, the patient should receive lidocaine as well as Digibind, a digitalis antidote. In addition, a low initial energy dose should be used and subsequently increased in small increments. Cardioversion has been shown to be safe for treating supraventricular dysrhythmias in patients receiving maintenance digitalis therapy who have no evidence of digitalis toxicity (3).

Direct injury to cardiac muscle is another potential complication of cardioversion and defibrillation (26–29). Animal studies have shown that injury is usually subepicardial, resulting in ST segment elevation and modest elevations of the CPK-MB fraction (4). These changes are dose-related and associated with using small paddles (30). To minimize cardiac injury, the lowest energy that is therapeutic should be delivered with intervals of 2 to 3 minutes between shocks if the patient's clinical condition allows. Skin burns are another dose-related complication of electrical shock. Burns may result if too little gel or paste is used at the paddle/skin interface. Conversely, if too much gel or paste is used or if liquid (such as sweat or blood) is present on the anterior thorax, the current may pass along the skin surface and produce burns. Alcohol pads must never be used in place of gel or paste, because this can cause serious burns. Burns also may be produced if the paddles are not in firm contact with the skin.

CLINICAL TIPS
1. Hemodynamic instability is indicated by hypotension, signs of inadequate cerebral or peripheral perfusion (lethargy, agitation, weak pulses, mottling, etc.), or heart failure.

SUMMARY

With direct current cardioversion and defibrillation, electricity is administered to a patient to terminate dysrhythmia. These procedures are indicated for patients exhibiting signs or symptoms of cardiovascular compromise resulting from dysrhythmia or for patients who fail to respond to pharmacologic therapy. Although attention should be given to other aspects of patient care such as respiratory or metabolic abnormalities, delay in administering electrical current when indicated for the unstable patient must be avoided. Medical personnel caring for criti-

cally ill children should be knowledgeable about all aspects of cardioversion and defibrillation including sedation methods, selection of correct energy dosage and paddle sizes, and standard operation of the equipment. When properly performed, cardioversion and defibrillation offer a highly effective means of terminating dysrhythmias with a relatively low incidence of complications.

REFERENCES

1. Pediatric Advanced Life Support. JAMA 1992; 268(16):2262–2275.
2. Suddaby EC, Riker SL. Defibrillation and cardioversion in children. Pediatric Nurs 1991;17(5): 477–481.
3. Gazak S. Direct current electrical cardioversion. In: Roberts JR, Hedges JR, eds. Clinical procedures in emergency medicine. 2nd ed. Philadelphia: WB Saunders, 1991, pp. 160–166.
4. Ventriglia WJ, Hamilton GC. Electrical interventions in cardiopulmonary resuscitation: defibrillation. Emerg Med Clin North Am 1983;1(3): 515–534.
5. Gewitz MH, Vetter VL. Cardiac emergencies. In: Fleisher, Ludwig, eds. Textbook of pediatric emergency medicine. 2nd ed. Baltimore: Williams & Wilkins, 1988, pp. 351–390.
6. Cook P, Scarfone RJ, Cook RT. Adenosine in the termination of albuterol-induced supraventricular tachycardia. Annals of Emerg Med. 1994;24: 316–318.
7. DiMarco JP, et al. Adenosine for paroxysmal supraventricular tachycardia: dose ranging and comparison with verapamil. Ann Emerg Med 1990;113: 104–110.
8. Pinski SL, Maloney JD. Adenosine: a new drug for acute termination of supraventricular tachycardia. Cleveland J Med 1990;6383–6388.
9. Owens M, Zellers-Jacobs L. Adenosine: the newest drug for PSVT. RN 1992;38–41.
10. Cairns CB, et al. Intravenous adenosine in the emergency department management of paroxysmal supraventricular tachycardia. Ann Emerg Med 1991;7:717–721.
11. Till J, et al. Efficacy and safety of adenosine in the treatment of supraventricular tachycardia in infants and children. Br Heart J 1989;62:204–211.
12. Ros SP, Fisher EA, et al. Adenosine in the emergency management of supraventricular tachycardia. Ped Emerg Care 1991;222–223.
13. Reyes G, et al. Adenosine in the treatment of paroxysmal supraventricular tachycardia in children. Ann Emerg Med 1992;12:119–121.
14. Litman RS, et al. Termination of supraventricular tachycardia with adenosine in a healthy child undergoing anesthesia. Anaesth Analg 1991;73:665–667.
15. Rossi AF, Burton DA: Adenosine in altering short- and long-term treatment of supraventricular tachycardia in infants. Am J Cardiol 1989;9(64):685–686.
16. Overholt ED, et al. Usefulness of adenosine for ar-

rhythmias in infants and children. Am J Cardiol 1988;2(61):336–340.

17. Cardiac Rhythm Disturbances. American Heart Association. Chameides L, ed. Textbook of pediatric advanced life support, 1988, pp. 61–67.

18. Hedges RJ, Greenberg MI. Defibrillation. In: Roberts, Hedges, eds. Clinical procedures in emergency medicine. 2nd ed. Philadelphia: WB Saunders, 1991, pp. 167–177.

19. Seidel J. Pediatric cardiopulmonary resuscitation: an update based on the new American Heart Association guidelines. Pediatric emergency care, vol 9, no 2. Baltimore: Williams & Wilkins, 1993.

20. Gutgesell HP, Tacker WA, Geddes LA, Davis JS, Lie JT, McNamara DG. Energy dose for ventricular defibrillation of children. Pediatrics 1976;58(6): 898–901.

21. Losek JD, Hennes H, Glaeser PW, Smith DS, Hendley G. Prehospital countershock treatment of pediatric asystole. Am J Emerg Med 1989;7(6):571–575.

22. Ewy GA. Ventricular fibrillation masquerading as asystole. Ann Emerg Med 1984;13(9):811–812. 23. Chameides L, Brown GE, Raye JR, Todres DI, Viles PH. Guidelines for defibrillation in infants and children. News from the American Heart Association, Special Report.

24. Crampton R. Accepted, controversial, and speculative aspects of ventricular fibrillation. Prog Cardiovasc Dis, 1980;23:167–186.

25. Ewy GA. Cardiac arrest and resuscitation: defibrillators and defibrillation. Curr Probl Cardiol 1978; 2:1.

26. Davis JS, Lie JT, Bentinck DC, et al. Cardiac damage due to electric current and energy: light microscopic and ultrastructural observations of acute and delayed myocardial cellular injuries. Proceedings of the Cardiac Defibrillation Converence, Purdue University, West Lafayette, IN, October 1975, p. 27.

27. Dahl CF, Ewy GA, Warner ED, Thomas ED. Myocardial necrosis from direct current countershock: effect of paddle electrode size and time interval between discharges. Circulation 1974;50:956.

28. Sussman RM, Woldenberg DH, Cohen M. Myocardial changes after direct current electroshock. JAMA 1964;189:739.

29. Ehsani AA, Ewy GA, Sobel BE. CPK isoenzyme elevations after electrical countershock. Circulation 1973;48(4):129.

30. Kastendieck JG. Cardiac arrest. In: Rosen P, Baker FJ, Barkin RM, et al. eds. Emergency medicine concepts and clinical practice. St. Louis: CV Mosby, 1988, pp. 103–111.

Trauma Life Support Procedures

Section Editor: Brent R. King

CHAPTER 23

CERVICAL SPINE IMMOBILIZATION AND IMAGING

George A. Woodward and Nanette C. Kunkel

INTRODUCTION

Cervical spine injuries, fortunately, are uncommon in the pediatric population. It has been estimated that cervical spine injuries occur in approximately 1 to 2% of pediatric patients with multiple trauma (1). However, potentially devastating consequences of a cervical spine injury mandate proper immobilization and evaluation of all children with potential cervical spine trauma. The purpose of cervical spine immobilization is to prevent the occurrence or exacerbation of spinal cord injury in the child with a potentially unstable cervical spine. A variety of techniques can be used to attempt cervical spine immobilization, some more effective than others.

Mechanisms of injury most often associated with cervical spine damage in children include motor vehicle accidents, sports (contact, high force activities), falls, diving accidents, and difficult newborn deliveries (breech, forceps)(2) (Table 23.1). All multiple trauma patients and those who have experienced a high risk mechanism of injury should have cervical spine immobilization and evaluation.

To be effective and prevent secondary or ongoing injury, proper immobilization and care of the cervical spine should be started at the scene by bystanders and continued with prehospital and ED personnel. Although cervical spine injuries can be devastating, the clinician should not delay needed airway intervention while awaiting formal cervical spine evaluation. Initiation of airway care, with careful attention to cervical spine stabilization, should take precedence over complete cervical spine evaluation.

Two types of cervical spine immobilization to consider are full immobilization with cervical collars, spine board, and spacing devices, and in-line stabilization for airway control. This chapter will discuss how to immobilize the pediatric cervical spine and assess the adequacy of the immobilization.

ANATOMY AND PHYSIOLOGY

The pediatric cervical spine is similar to the adult's in that it can be anatomically divided into two sections (3). The anterior cervical spine is bordered by the anterior and posterior longitudinal ligaments and contains the bodies of the cervical vertebrae as well as the intervertebral discs. The posterior cervical spine includes the pedicles, lamina, spinous processes, facet joints, and the remainder of the cervical ligaments. Disruption of bony or ligamentous elements can lead to a potentially unstable cervical spine.

The child's cervical spine differs in many ways from that of the adult. (2, 4, 5) (Table 23.2). The infant's large head and relatively weak neck muscles result in the fulcrum of the neck being at C2–3 compared to C5–6 in the adult. Younger children tend to have upper cervical spine fractures whereas older children and adolescents have fractures in lower cervical spine regions, similar to adults. The large amount of cartilage in the

Table 23.1.
High Risk Mechanisms of Injury

Motor vehicle accident
Sports injury
Falls
Dives
Difficult delivery

Table 23.2.
Pediatric Cervical Spine Differences

Higher fulcrum of neck motion
    Large occiput
    Weaker neck muscles
Increased anterior/posterior motion
    Horizontal facet joints
    Increased ligamentous laxity
    Pseudosubluxation
Large cartilage component
    Growth plates
    Tapered anterior vertebrae
    Radiologic artifact
Lack of lordosis until age 6
Soft tissue variability with breathing, vocalization
Congenital abnormalities (clefts, accessory ossicles)

Figure 23.1.
A. Adult's neck in neutral position on spine board.
B. Child's neck in kyphotic position on spine board.

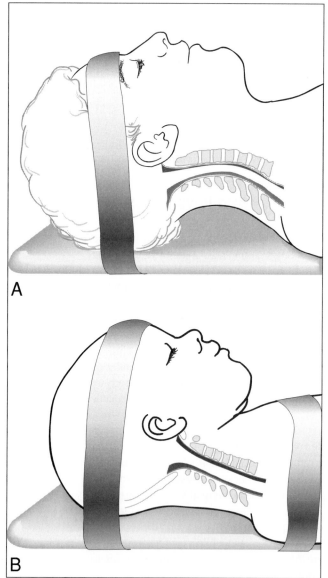

pediatric cervical spine cushions direct vertical forces and limits the occurrence of bursting or compression-type fractures. The radiolucent cartilaginous component of the pediatric cervical spine, however, can make radiographic evaluation challenging. Children have more horizontal facet joints and increased ligamentous laxity allowing for increased anterior and posterior motion of the cervical spine. This flexibility allows for significant spine distortion during the traumatic event which can rebound to appear normal when evaluated radiographically.

Children have relatively large occiputs in comparison to their chest circumference which leads to relative kyphosis of the neck in a supine position (6). An adult who is immobilized on a hard cervical spine board has his or her neck in a neutral (30° lordosis) position. A young child, however, will have his neck forced into relative kyphosis with a similar immobilization technique (Fig. 23.1). At age 8, the disparate growth between the occiput and chest, as well as the other cervical spine differences have diminished and the patient can be immobilized and evaluated as an adult.

INDICATIONS AND RADIOGRAPHIC EVALUATION

As mentioned previously, mechanisms of injury most often associated with cervical spine or cord damage include motor vehicle accidents, sports injuries (contact, high force activities), falls, diving accidents, and difficult newborn deliveries (breech, forceps). Cervical spine immobilization is necessary after all high risk mechanisms of injury and in many other pediatric trauma victims. Often a reliable witness is not available and the full extent of the trauma may initially be difficult to assess. Young children can be difficult to examine, and can be uncooperative, often nonverbal or crying immediately after a traumatic event, and lacking the relatively sophisticated language skills necessary to relay symptoms (weakness, sensory changes) suggestive of a cervical spine injury.

Physical findings suggestive of cervical spine or cord injury include cervical pain (especially midline), traumatic torticollis, limitation of cervical motion, motor weakness, sensory changes, diaphragmatic breathing without retractions, hypotension without tachycardia, bowel or bladder dysfunction, and priapism (5). These patients may or may not have cervical spine immobilization in place on presentation to the ED.

Full cervical spine immobilization (hard cervical collar, spine board, spacers, and straps) should be applied to any patient with an unwitnessed or unclear mechanism of injury, high risk mechanism of injury, head injury involving loss of consciousness or altered mental status, and whenever neurologic deficit or symptoms suggest a cervical cord injury. When the patient requires airway manipulation or intervention, in-line stabilization should be used.

Although cervical spine protection is important, immobilization techniques and cervical spine concerns should not impede airway assessment or intervention. Gentle airway maneuvers such as the chin lift, jaw thrust, suctioning, and cricoid pressure can be performed without worsening an existing cervical injury. Vigorous airway maneuvers can, however, be detrimental to a patient with an unstable cervical spine injury (7).

Once an unstable cervical spine injury has been diagnosed or suspected, neurosurgical consultation may be necessary for evaluation and therapy that will more securely restrict cervical spine mobility. Transport of patients with unstable cervical spines over long distances may require semipermanent immobilization (tongs, traction), and if the equipment and expertise does not exist at the referring hospital, a neurosurgeon may be included with the transport team.

Radiographic options for cervical spine evaluation include routine radiographs, tomograms, computerized tomography (CT), and magnetic resonance imaging (MRI) (5) (Fig. 23.2). The most useful radiograph for cervical spine assessment is a lateral view, often done portably during trauma evaluation. This view should show any persistent dislocation or distraction, but has an injury identification sensitivity of only 80 to 90%. The lateral cervical spine radiograph should be evaluated with regard to alignment, bones, cartilage, and soft tissue. The addition of at least two anterior views, C1–2 (odontoid view) and C3–7 (9), increase the fracture identification sensitivity of the radiographic evaluation to 95 to 99%. Oblique (pillar) views should be considered if the patient has signs or symptoms of cervical spine or cord injury and the initial three-view series does not demonstrate an injury (3). Oblique views will further assess the posterior cervical column (pedicles, lamina, articulating and spinal processes), and complete the five-view trauma series.

The oblique views are potentially dangerous if performed with the standard 15° cranial angulation and neck rotation. Clearly any initial radiographic evaluation should not involve neck motion if a cervical fracture is suspected. Flexion and extension radiographs can be added for the awake patient who has a normal neurologic examination and five-view trauma series, but for whom a persistent concern over possible spinal injury exists.

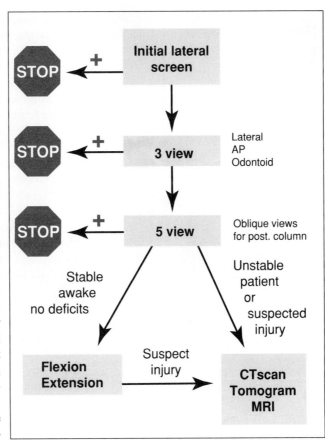

Figure 23.2.
Radiographic scheme for cervical spine evaluation.

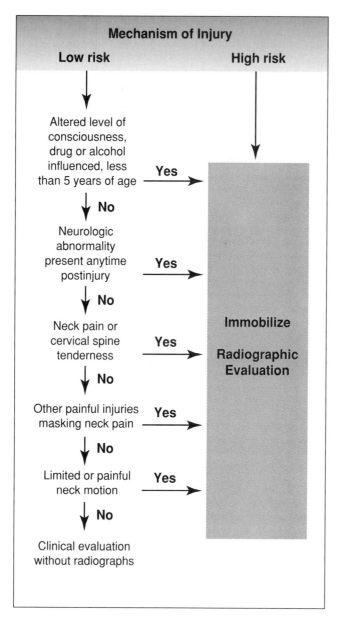

Mechanism of Injury

Low risk   High risk

Altered level of consciousness, drug or alcohol influenced, less than 5 years of age — **Yes** →

No ↓

Neurologic abnormality present anytime postinjury — **Yes** →

No ↓

Neck pain or cervical spine tenderness — **Yes** →

No ↓

Other painful injuries masking neck pain — **Yes** →

No ↓

Limited or painful neck motion — **Yes** →

No ↓

Clinical evaluation without radiographs

Immobilize Radiographic Evaluation

Figure 23.3.
Decision tree for radiographic vs. clinical evaluation of the cervical spine.

alized with routine films, to delineate fractures suspected on radiographs, and to further elucidate an identified injury. A CT scan can be performed quickly and efficiently without neck motion. CT scans done properly can be reconstructed to avoid missing fractures in the horizontal plane.

Tomograms, while providing adequate views of cervical spine fractures, are time consuming and require patient motion, making them less desirable in an acute situation. MRI is helpful if concern exists about blood accumulation (epidural hematoma), ligamentous or cord damage, but is not ideal for evaluation of cortical bone injury. Difficulties of managing acutely ill patients during an MRI scan and need for lack of motion to obtain an effective study limit its usefulness for acute injury evaluation.

The syndrome of spinal cord injury without radiographic abnormality (SCIWORA) is specific to children less than 8 years of age (2, 10). Forces to the child's spine that would result in fracture or dislocation in an adult may not result in an abnormality on radiograph or CT scan, because of the child's ability to realign the flexible cervical spine. The patient may, however, have had significant neurologic compromise. For this reason, all patients should remain immobilized until a normal neurologic examination can be documented.

Medical personnel can consider clinical (without radiographs) "clearing" of the cervical spine if the patient has not been involved in a high risk mode of injury, and is awake, alert, and has normal mental status (not under the influence of head injury, shock, drugs, or alcohol). The child also should be able to have meaningful conversation (at least 4 to 5 years old), no neck pain or tenderness, no other painful injuries that might mask perception or appreciation of neck pain, full range of motion of the neck, a normal neurologic examination (motor, sensory, mental status), and no history of transient neurologic symptoms (11) (Fig. 23.3). The cervical spine should not be cleared, regardless of radiographic findings, in the patient with altered mental status. It is not until the patient is alert and awake and demonstrates normal neurologic status in concert with normal radiographs that the cervical spine should be cleared. If questions arise during the assessment of a child's cervical spine, consultation with a radiologist or neurosurgeon may be helpful.

Flexion and extension are performed by the patient, not by the radiology technician, to the point of mild discomfort. If an abnormality is identified, a search for other injuries which may not be contiguous is still necessary. Further radiographic views of an identified fracture, however, usually are not helpful in the acute evaluation. Importantly cartilage fractures and ligamentous injuries will not be directly visible on the cervical radiograph. These might only be suspected if the patient presents with an abnormal neurologic examination or demonstrates increased soft tissue swelling on the radiograph.

A CT scan of the neck can be helpful to assess areas of the spine not adequately visu-

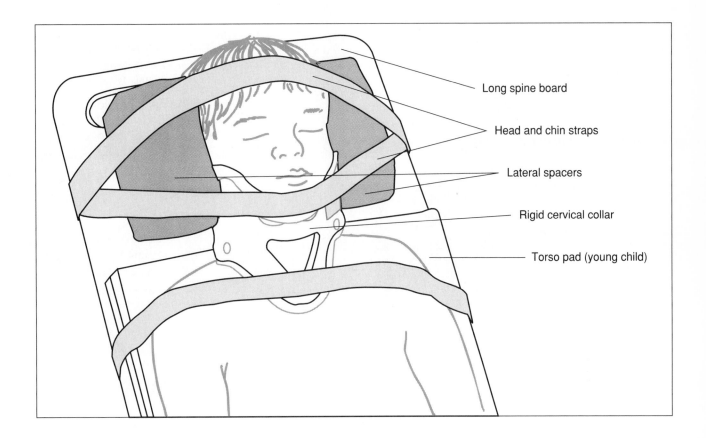

Long spine board

Head and chin straps

Lateral spacers

Rigid cervical collar

Torso pad (young child)

A difficult scenario arises when a child presents hours or days postinjury with neck pain. The type and extent of immobilization that should be placed while awaiting radiographic evaluation is an area open to interpretation. Many authorities recommend at least the placement of a hard cervical collar and a paucity of patient movement during evaluation to help minimize potential risk to the patient and the provider.

EQUIPMENT

Optimal immobilization of the cervical spine requires a spine board, hard cervical collar, soft spacing devices, and straps to help secure the patient to the spine board (12) (Fig. 23.4). A long, rigid spine board is used to immobilize the child's entire body. The head and neck must be kept in a neutral position or one of slight extension. Young children have a prominent occiput which, when lying supine on a rigid surface, may force the neck into flexion. Some spine boards have a cutout space for the occiput of the head, allowing the head to rest at a slightly lower level than the rest of the body, maintaining a neutral posi-

tion for the cervical spine. Other spine boards incorporate padding underneath the torso, elevating the body level to maintain neutral position. Padding underneath the shoulders and upper thorax can be improvised to achieve the same effect, and recent literature advocates a height of approximately 1 inch (13).

The provider should be aware that full cervical immobilization is the best form of initial spinal protection for the patient (14). Heurta demonstrated that a soft cervical collar provided no protection against cervical spine motion, and that the hard cervical collars, when used alone, were not much better (15). A soft cervical collar provides inadequate immobilization, and should not be used in the emergency setting. A hard cervical collar (Stifneck^{TM} or Philadelphia^{TM}) when used in combination with a spine board and spacing devices provides effective immobilization that is easy to implement. These collars are made of a hard foam or flexible plastic with foam lining and velcro attachments (16, 17). They are available in various sizes, and do not interfere with radiographs or resuscitative efforts. With caution, the clinician can proceed with endotracheal intubation while a child is immobilized in a cervical collar, and most col-

Figure 23.4.
Ideal immobilization including long spine board, spacer to elevate torso, hard collar, soft lateral spacers, forehead and chin straps.

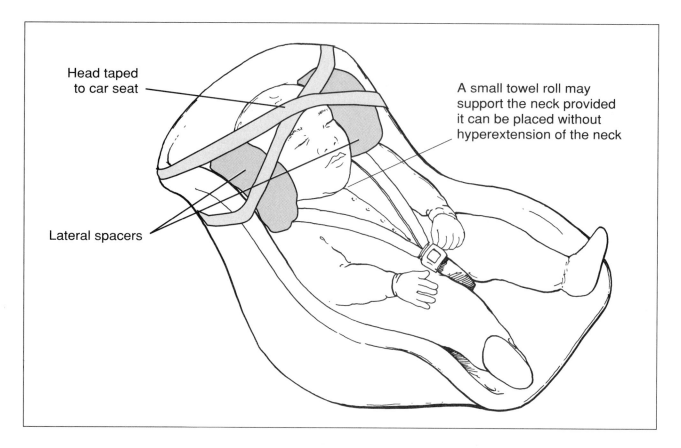

Head taped to car seat

Lateral spacers

A small towel roll may support the neck provided it can be placed without hyperextension of the neck

Figure 23.5.
Infant immobilized in a car seat.

lars have a cutout area in front in the event a surgical airway is necessary.

After a cervical collar is applied, the child must be secured to a long spine board. The spine board serves to immobilize the joints above and below the suspected injury site, an important concept in the splinting of any suspected bony injury. Spine boards may be the traditional adult length or a smaller specialized pediatric board. The length chosen should ensure that the board can accommodate the child's entire body.

Many techniques for securing the patient to the spine board are used. Recently, disposable devices consisting of foam pads placed beside the head, or cardboard barriers to lateral head movement have been developed. If these are not available, towel rolls or i.v. bags placed beside the patient's head can achieve a similar result. Soft spacers are better than heavy sandbags which can cause patient injury if they shift during logrolling of the patient. In all cases, the child's forehead and the chin area of the hard collar are secured to these spacing devices and also to the spine board. Some spine boards come with their own straps. Surgical tape can also be used. Placement of the strap on the chin rather than

on the cervical collar should be avoided because of possible hyperextension of the neck and further injury. The chin strap should be secured to the cervical collar to effectively immobilize both the collar and the patient. In addition to immobilizing the child's head, the rest of the body needs to be secured to the spine board. Straps immobilizing the bony prominences of the shoulders and pelvis are most effective. Straps incorrectly placed or shifted to be around the chest and abdomen can restrict chest wall movement and diaphragmatic excursion, leading to significant respiratory compromise (18).

Young infants pose unique immobilization dilemmas, because they are often too small for a spine board and cervical collar even if spacing devices are used to secure their position. It is possible to partially immobilize the infant's cervical spine while in a car seat using towel rolls and the car seat's own seat belt along with additional tape to secure the infant's head to the car seat (Fig. 23.5). This technique should not be used in an infant who has multiple injuries, has airway compromise, or is unstable in any way.

Immobilized children require constant observation. Suction should always be available. As mentioned previously, chest and abdominal straps can restrict respiration and even properly placed straps can shift causing problems. Children should have cardiorespiratory and oxygen saturation monitors in place during immobilization.

If an unstable cervical spine injury is documented, or highly suspected due to neurologic abnormalities, neurosurgical consultation is recommended. The injury may necessitate using further immobilization and/or fracture reduction in the ED to avoid worsening of the existing injury. Cervical tongs can be applied in the ED, providing weighted skeletal traction which allows for bony reduction and maintenance of neutral alignment of the cervical spine (19, 20). Problems with skeletal traction include difficulties with transport, patient movement, radiographic evaluation, airway intervention (as a result of the traction apparatus), and the need for the patient to remain supine. Other types of immobilization include halos and halo vests which maintain alignment between the head, thorax, and cervical spine (21, 22).

PROCEDURE

Assessing Prior Immobilization

A patient who arrives with cervical spine immobilization in place should have an immediate assessment of that immobilization. The ED personnel should ask the following questions:

Are all the components of full immobilization present?

Is the cervical collar of the correct type and size for the patient?

Is the patient's neck in the neutral position?

Is the patient securely strapped to a long spine board?

Has the patient or the immobilization shifted during transport to diminish the immobilization, cause hyperflexion or hyperextension of the cervical spine, or compromise excursion of the chest with respiration?

Is the immobilization in any way interfering with assessment or management of the ABCs?

If these or any other immobilization difficulties are identified, they should be immediately addressed.

SUMMARY

1. Assess any prior immobilization and correct or modify as necessary.
2. Stabilize head and neck in neutral position using in-line immobilization.
3. Apply cervical collar (best as two-person procedure):
   a. Check collar size
   b. Assemble collar (if necessary)
   c. Slide collar behind neck
   d. Slide chin piece up chest wall
   e. Fasten velcro on collar
   f. Recheck neutral alignment
4. Position patient on spine board.
   If patient is supine:
   a. Logroll child maintaining in-line manual immobilization
   b. Place long spine board under child
   c. Roll child as a unit onto board
   If patient is seated:
   a. Position short spine board behind child
   b. Secure child to short board
   c. Place long spine board alongside child
   d. Pivot and lower child onto long board (knees/hips bent)
   e. Lower child's legs to long board
5. Secure patient to spine board
   a. Place soft spacing devices on both sides of head and neck
   b. Apply forehead strap
   c. Apply chin support strap
   d. Apply shoulder and pelvis straps
6. Evaluate effectiveness of procedure
   a. Maintain head and neck in neutral position
   b. Assess for respiratory/airway compromise
   c. Ensure immobilization prevents any significant movement of head and neck
7. Reassess ABC's
8. Repeat neurologic exam

Application of Full Cervical Immobilization

The initial stage of cervical spine stabilization is in-line immobilization. In-line immobilization (not traction) is applied by placing hands on both sides of the patient's head and holding the head and neck in a neutral position. Cervical collars help to maintain this neutral position. Application of a cervical collar is best accomplished as a two-person procedure, to avoid sudden movements of the neck and potential injury.

Selection of the correct size collar is im-

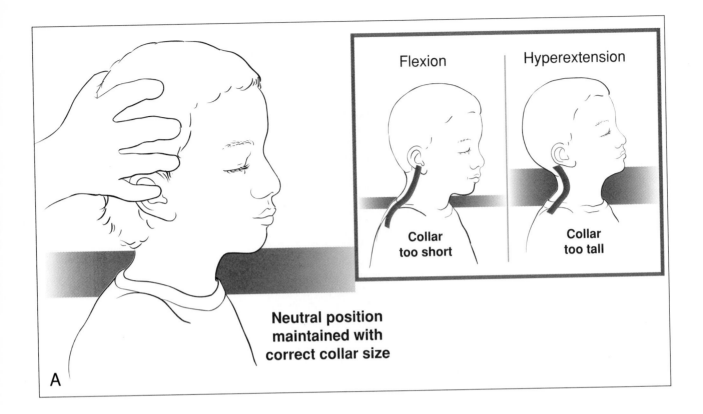

Figure 23.6.
A. Appropriate sizing and
B. Application of
Philadelphia™ collar and
Stifneck™ collar.

portant. A short collar may cause the neck to flex, a tall collar may result in hyperextension. The tallest collar that does not hyperextend the neck is the correct selection. A rapid examination of the neck for injury clues (open wounds, expanding hematomas, subcutaneous air, anatomy distortion, shifted trachea) should precede placement of the collar (Fig. 23.6).

The Stifneck™ collar consists of one piece, with a simple sizing method that uses the distance between the top of the shoulders and the bottom of the chin as a measure for choosing the correct size (23). The collar lies flat for storage and is assembled for use by moving the end of the chin piece and pushing the black fastener through the small hole on the collar, which forms the chin support at the front of the collar. If the child is supine, the back portion of the collar then slides behind the neck. It is helpful to fold the velcro before sliding to avoid it becoming caught on hair or debris. Once the back of the collar is visible on the other side of the neck, the chin piece is fitted by sliding the collar up the chest wall. The chin should be well supported by the collar and should cover the central fastener on the collar. The collar can then be fastened with the velcro, and adjusted if the chin is not

well supported. If tightening the collar will cause hyperextension of the neck, then a smaller size should be selected. If the patient is sitting, the chin support is fitted first, as just described, then the back portion of the collar slides behind the patient's neck.

The Philadelphia™ collar is a two-piece, preformed cervical collar. Again, the proper size is selected to provide adequate chin support avoiding flexion or hyperextension of the neck. The back portion of the collar slides behind the patient's neck. The front portion of the collar moves up the chest wall until the chin support meets the chin. If the chin appears to be well supported, without flexion or hyperextension of the neck, then the velcro attachments are fastened. Neutral alignment must be maintained manually throughout application of any cervical collar. If the patient is wearing a helmet at the time of injury, it should be removed before applying the cervical collar (see Chapter 24).

Once the cervical collar is applied, the supine child is logrolled as a unit maintaining in-line manual immobilization of the head and neck (12). A long spine board is placed behind the patient, with padding as necessary. The child is rolled as a unit onto the long board. If the child is seated, a short spine

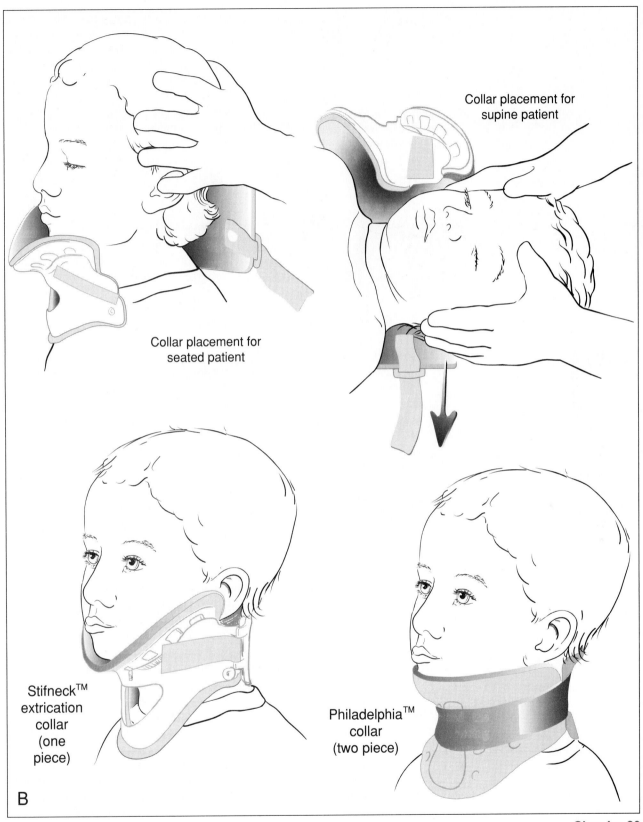

Collar placement for supine patient

Collar placement for seated patient

Stifneck™ extrication collar (one piece)

Philadelphia™ collar (two piece)

B

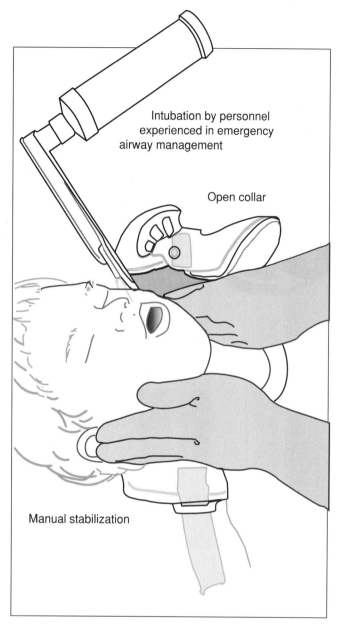

Intubation by personnel
experienced in emergency
airway management

Open collar

Manual stabilization

Figure 23.7.
Manual immobilization from below, with open cervical collar, during intubation attempt.

board is positioned behind the patient who is then secured to that board. Next, a long spine board is placed beside the child. The child is then pivoted and lowered onto the long board, keeping the knees and hips bent at right angles until the child is completely on the board. The child's legs are then lowered and secured to the board.

To secure the child to the spine board and allow the manual immobilization to be released, the soft spacing devices are first placed on both sides of the head and neck. The forehead strap or tape is applied, originating on one side of the board, traveling over the spacers, across the forehead and down the

opposite side. The chin support strap (tape) should originate from the same location on the spine board. It should travel over the spacers, across the chin support of the cervical collar and down the opposite side to meet with the forehead strap on that side. The shoulder and pelvis straps are then applied. If proper equipment is unavailable, any rigid surface can substitute for a spine board, and towel rolls, i.v. bags, or other soft items such as pillows can be used as spacing devices with tape substituting for straps.

Assessment of Cervical Spine Immobilization

Once a child is immobilized, the effectiveness of the procedure must be evaluated. The head and neck must be in a neutral position (slight extension). Respiratory status should not be compromised by the straps or tape. The child may be crying and upset but should not be able to move significantly. Flexion, extension, or lateral movement of the head and neck should be prohibited and prevented. The ABCs should be reassessed after immobilization. Finally, the neurologic examination should be reassessed and hopefully is unchanged or improved after immobilization is in place.

Semipermanent Cervical Spine Immobilization

If the child has evidence of cervical spine injury, with an abnormal radiograph, physical examination, or suggestive symptoms, neurosurgical consultation is required for possible semipermanent cervical spine immobilization. Successful skeletal traction relies more on the principle of application than on using a particular instrument. Contraindications to application of cervical tongs include bony disease leading to brittle or fragile bones and loss of skeletal integrity due to multiple skull fractures or patent sutures.

Cervical tongs are applied to the scalp in the coronal plane with the mastoid processes (19, 20). Hair should be shaved at the tong insertion points, skin prepped with an antiseptic solution, and local anesthesia injected. The tips of the tongs point toward the top of the skull so that increased pressure will direct them inward and avoid slippage of the tongs from the skull. The screws of the tongs (Gardner) are tightened until approximately

30 pounds of squeeze is exerted, indicated by protrusion of the distal spring-loaded points.

Once the tongs are in place, gradual cervical realignment and reduction of the fracture is begun with weights attached to a pulley system and the tongs. Although there is some debate about the rapidity at which reduction should ideally take place, no attempt should be made to immediately reduce the fracture, as the force necessary to do this may cause further spinal cord injury. Frequent neurologic examinations and cervical spine radiographs are necessary to evaluate the effects of the traction. If at any time further symptoms or evidence of neurologic abnormality occur, traction should be reduced and radiographs retaken. Once satisfactory alignment is attained, traction weight is reduced to the minimum required to hold the correct position, which will allow the spinal ligaments to heal. Neurosurgical consultation for the application of skeletal traction should be obtained before its use and continued until final disposition or transport of the patient. Cervical halo/vest combinations are also useful for immobilization of the cervical spine and offer an advantage in that free weights are not needed for reduction (21, 22). This may be important in the patient who needs transport or frequent position changes.

In-line Stabilization for Airway Control

If intubation is required, the oral route is preferred in children. This can be accomplished by having an experienced clinician immobilize the head and neck from above or below (most efficient) to prevent neck flexion or extension during intubation (Fig. 23.7). Excessive force causing neck movement must be carefully avoided. The patient's neck must always remain in a neutral position while airway or other interventions are ongoing (see also Fig. 16.25, p. 201). Although intubation can be performed with the cervical collar in place, it is usually more efficient to open the collar anteriorly to facilitate mandibular motion and visualization of the anterior and cephalad larynx. Nasal intubation can be performed on adults or adolescents but should not be attempted in children. If surgical airway placement is indicated, active neck immobilization must again be performed by an experienced clinician. In addition, the operator performing a surgical airway must be vigilant to avoid applying excessive downward pressure on the neck while making incisions or inserting airway devices.

COMPLICATIONS

A patient with cervical spine immobilization poses risks for several potential complications in management and resultant iatrogenic injury (Table 23.3). Incorrect or inadequate stabilization or a lack of vigilance also could lead to an adverse outcome for the patient.

Airway compromise with vomiting, bleeding, or aspiration can occur while the patient is supine. The child could easily choke, aspirate, or have a respiratory arrest if the airway is not kept free of debris. Children with vomiting need to be logrolled while still immobilized to prevent aspiration (see Fig. 13.10, p. 112). As mentioned previously, cervical spine immobilization may have to be partially removed for airway management and replaced with manual stabilization.

Attempts at placing a cervical collar on a struggling patient may worsen the underlying injury due to patient exertion. In most instances, a patient is better off without formal immobilization if he or she vigorously resists cervical collar application but is otherwise calm.

Incorrect sizing of the cervical collar can lead to hyperextension or flexion of the neck and worsen the underlying injury. Ensuring

Table 23.3.
Potential Complications of Cervical Immobilization

Inadequate immobilization with potential neck mobility
   Use of soft collar for immobilization
   Reliance of hard collar alone for immobilization
Inadequate immobilization with respiratory restriction
   Initial incorrect immobilization
   Shifted patient/immobilization during transport
Incorrect immobilization with hyperflexion/extension
   Incorrect size collar
   Child on hard spine board without torso elevation
   Resistant patient forced into immobilization
Restricted access to immobilized child
   Inability to physically examine/assess neck with collar in place
   Difficult with airway intervention (intubation, surgical airway)
   Difficult venous access (external/internal jugulars)
   Airway compromise with vomiting, bleeding, aspiration, when secured in supine position

the correct size of the cervical collar is imperative to prevent this complication.

The cervical collar, while protecting the cervical spine, may limit visibility of a shifted trachea, expanding neck hematoma, or subcutaneous emphysema. Although not a complication of the immobilization, cervical spine stabilization also limits the accessibility of external or internal jugular catheterization because the clinician cannot manipulate the neck in a lateral or AP direction to facilitate venous access. These procedures are best avoided in a patient suspected of having a possible cervical spine or cord injury.

Inappropriate securing of the patient to the spine board can complicate immobilization. Straps connecting the patient to the spine board that cross the chest, abdomen, neck, or chin may cause problems with ventilation or exacerbation of the spinal injury. This is also true of immobilization that has shifted secondary to motion or vibration during the transport. Frequent reassessments of the patient and the immobilization should help to alleviate these difficulties. Clinicians should also be aware that even a patient in a hard cervical collar, on a long spine board with appropriate spacer devices and properly attached securing straps, still has the potential for neck motion and worsening of an existing injury.

The patient should be firmly secured to the long cervical spine board, so when logrolling is needed in response to emesis, the cervical spine is not subjected to increased lateral motion. As mentioned, soft spacing devices should be used to avoid adding stress to the neck during the logrolling

procedure. Suction should be immediately available to avoid the complication of aspiration.

As mentioned, the immobilization may have to be partially removed for airway management and replaced with manual immobilization. Incorrect manual stabilization or a lack of vigilance could also lead to an undesirable outcome for the patient.

Because of the possibility of SCIWORA in children, radiographs alone are insufficient to "clear" a cervical spine when documentation of a normal neurologic examination is not possible. An unconscious or multiply injured patient with normal cervical spine radiographs should have immobilization maintained until his or her mental status allows for complete neurologic examination. In such cases, cervical spine immobilization should not be removed in the ED setting unless clinical neurologic evaluation is complete and normal. It is vitally important to provide full attention to the patient's cervical spine immobilization and to continue to assess the patient for changes in status, shifting of immobilization, and other clues to ongoing injury.

SUMMARY

All patients with a suspected cervical spine injury, neurologic abnormality, altered level of consciousness, an inability to assess because of young age, mental status changes or other painful injuries, and those with a high risk mechanism of injury or multiple trauma should be immobilized. It is important to realize that immobilization must be complete to be effective. Incomplete or improper immobilization can predispose the patient to secondary injury. Although the incidence of cervical spine injury in children is low, the devastating consequences demand that if an injury is suspected, correct immobilization and evaluation be performed. As in any emergency procedure, a complete evaluation before and after any intervention is important as is proper documentation.

CLINICAL TIPS
1. Cervical injury should always be suspected.
2. The most important initial goals in a trauma resuscitation are to stabilize the primary injury and to prevent secondary injury.
3. Adequate cervical immobilization will only be achieved if the appropriate equipment and proper sizes are used.
4. Effectiveness of cervical immobilization should be reassessed frequently.
5. Neurosurgical consultation should be sought early when indicated.
6. Cervical immobilization should not be removed until clinical and (if necessary) radiographic "clearing," as well as a normal neurologic examination, are completed.

REFERENCES

1. Wilberger J. Spinal cord injuries in children. New York: Futura, 1986.

2. Dickman C, Rekate H, Sonntag V, Zabramski J. Pediatric spine trauma: vertebral column and spinal cord injuries in children. Pediatr Neurosci 1989;15:237–256.

3. Doris P, Wilson R. The next logical step in the emergency radiographic evaluation of cervical spine trauma: the five-view trauma series. J Emerg Med 1985;3:371–385.

4. Jones E, Hensinger R. The x-ray look of young spines. Emerg Med 1982;7:74–87.

5. Woodward GA. Neck trauma. In: Fleisher GR, Ludwig S, eds. Textbook of pediatric emergency medicine. 3rd ed. Philadelphia: Williams & Wilkins, 1993.

6. Herzenberg JE, et al. Emergency transport and positioning of young children who have an injury of the cervical spine. J Bone Joint Surg 1989;71:15–22.

7. Bivins H, Ford S, Bezmalinovic Z, Price H, Williams J. The effects of axial traction during orotracheal intubation of the trauma victim with an unstable cervical spine. Ann Emerg Med 1988;17:53–57.

8. Swischuk L. Emergency radiology of the acutely ill or injured child. 2nd ed. Baltimore: Williams & Wilkins, 1986, pp. 556–599.

9. Harris J. Radiographic evaluation of spinal trauma. Orthop Clin North Am 1986;17:75–8671:15–22.

10. Pang D, Pollack I. Spinal cord injury without radiographic abnormality in children—the SCIWORA syndrome. J Trauma 1989;29:654–664.

11. Jaffe DM, Binns H, Radkowski MA, Barthel MJ, Engelhard III HH. Developing a clinical algorithm for early management of cervical spine injury in child trauma victims. Ann Emerg Med 1987;16:270–276.

12. Spine and spinal cord trauma. In: Manual of advanced trauma life support. American College of Surgeons, 1989, pp. 179–180.

13. Nypaver M, Treloar DJ. Neutral cervical spine positioning in children. Ann Emerg Med 1994;23:208–211.

14. Podolsky S, Baraff LJ, Simon RR, et al. Efficacy of cervical spine immobilization methods. J Trauma 1983;3:461–464.

15. Huerta C, Griffith R, Joyce S. Cervical spine stabilization in pediatric patients: evaluation of current techniques. Ann Emerg Med 1987;16:55–60.

16. McCabe JB, Nolan DJ. Comparison of the effectiveness of different cervical immobilization collars. Ann Emerg Med 1986;15:50–53.

17. Dick T. Prehospital splinting. In: Roberts JR, Hedges JR, eds. Clinical procedures in emergency medicine Philadelphia: WB Saunders, 1985.

18. Schafermeyer RW, Ribbeck BM, Gaskins J, et al. Respiratory effects of spinal immobilization in children. Ann Emerg Med 1991;20:1017–1019.

19. Gardner WJ. The principle of spring-loaded points for cervical traction. J Neurosurg 1973;39:543–544.

20. Crutchfield WG. Skeletal traction in treatment of injuries to the cervical spine. JAMA 1954;155:29–32.

21. Heary RF, Hunt CD, Krieger AJ, Antonio C, Livingston DH. Acute stabilization of the cervical spine by halo/vest application facilitates evaluation and treatment of multiple trauma patients. J Trauma 1992;33:445–451.

22. Chandler DR, Nemejic C, Adkins RH, et al. Emergency cervical spine immobilization. Ann Emerg Med 1992;21:1185–1188.

23. Stifneck™ package insert. California Medical Products, Inc., 1989.

CHAPTER 24

HELMET REMOVAL

Kathleen P. Kelly

INTRODUCTION

Pediatric trauma patients who are injured while involved in sports or recreational activities may present to the ED wearing various types of helmets. In these patients it is important that the helmet be removed by trained personnel in order to prevent injury to the cervical spine. In most cases this will not be necessary before radiographic evaluation. When the airway is compromised, or has the potential to become compromised, the helmet should be removed promptly by using the techniques described in this chapter.

Helmets are being used more frequently by the general population as people are made more aware of injury prevention. This is a positive move toward preventing the devastating effects of traumatic brain injury. As the demand for helmets has increased so has the sophistication of their design, increasingly encompassing more of the head and neck. Medical personnel who deal with trauma victims must be aware of the types of helmets and successful means for removing them without causing spinal cord injury.

Incidence of spinal cord injury is fortunately low in children, occurring in 1 to 2% of multiple trauma victims (1). Injury occurs most commonly in the upper cervical spine in infants and young children. Older children (over age 8) show a pattern of injury similar to the adult with the C5–6 area being most frequently injured. Children engaged in activities that require protective head gear are at increased risk of trauma and spinal cord injury. The helmeted young trauma victim always should be treated as having a possible cervical spine injury.

Helmets and their use in the pediatric population have changed over the years. Previously most helmeted patients were teenage motorcyclists or football players. Now children wear helmets from the toddler age on for bicycles, mopeds, rollerblades, or all-terrain vehicles. Most states now require helmet use for all motorcyclists and their passengers and some jurisdictions have mandatory bicycle helmet laws. This means more helmets on more children and, as mentioned, a necessary awareness of safe helmet removal.

Most injured pediatric patients who are helmeted at the time of injury will arrive immobilized on a spineboard with the helmet still in place. Paramedics as well as athletic trainers often are trained in safe helmet removal to facilitate airway management. The physician assumes responsibility for assessing the patient and directing removal of the helmet once the patient has entered the ED, and must therefore also be aware of safe helmet removal techniques.

ANATOMY AND PHYSIOLOGY

Helmets have been shown to cause cervical flexion in adults when the patient is supine and the helmet is unsupported (2). In-line stabilization of the helmet, however, eliminates this flexion and provides easy control of the cervical spine. Small children have an exaggerated degree of flexion as a result of their prominent occiput. Some elevation beneath the shoulders should help eliminate this problem and aid in maintaining neutral cervical immobilization. It is particularly important not to apply traction while stabilizing the neck of a child, because the spinal cord is vulnerable to further injury by these types of forces.

Cervical spine injury sites vary with age in the pediatric population. Infants and young children injure the upper cervical spine (C2–3) most frequently, because of the larger relative head size, the weaker neck muscles and cartilage, and shorter necks. These anatomic differences cause the forces of extension and flexion to pivot about a higher point in the neck. As children approach 8 years of age the site of cervical spine injury resembles the adult injury site (C5–6) (1) (see also Chapter 23).

The pediatric spine contains more cartilage than the adult. Although this can enable it to be more forgiving to injuries, it may also mean that serious injuries will go undetected by radiographic evaluation. It is for this reason that the appearance of the soft tissues is so important in detecting spinal injury in children.

The pediatric spine has more inherent anterior and posterior movement than the adult spine. It can sustain a significant subluxing injury without any change of alignment on the lateral radiograph. The soft tissue changes and neurologic findings are the only suggestion of injury.

The shorter necks of younger children demand that the clinician be careful not to obstruct the airway with his or her hands while maintaining cervical immobilization. In addition, a larger helmet may compromise central venous access if it covers most of the child's neck and clavicular areas.

As children mature, the nose becomes more prominent and the ear cartilage stiffens. Older children require a technique to remove the helmet that spreads the helmet laterally away from the ears while tilting it backward to clear the nasal prominence.

INDICATIONS

The typical pediatric patient wearing a helmet is brought by EMS on a spineboard with neck and helmet immobilized by sandbags and tape. The patient often comes from the scene of a sporting event or may have sustained a fall while engaged in a low speed recreational activity. Occasionally the pediatric patient is a passenger on a motorcycle involved in a high speed injury, often with devastating consequences.

Children may be wearing the full-faced helmets used by motorcyclists, the open-faced helmets used in football or hockey, or the simple helmets which only enclose part of the skull worn by bicyclists, skateboarders, or rollerbladers. In the case of the latter types of helmets, these frequently have been removed before patients arrive in the ED.

Immediate helmet removal is indicated in the pediatric patient with airway compromise who is wearing a helmet that obstructs airway access. All other patients should be transported with the helmet in place and immobilized with tape, collar, and sandbags. Some support beneath the shoulders such as a small towel roll should be used to maintain a neutral position of the neck.

On arrival at the hospital most patients will require a lateral cervical spine radiograph and a thorough neurologic examination before the clinician attempts to remove the helmet. In some instances the helmet can be removed without radiograph, but it is only advised if the child is alert and over 5 years of age, denies neck pain, has a history of minor trauma without loss of consciousness, and on examination has no neurologic deficits or midline cervical tenderness (1). All children under 5 years of age require spinal radiographs before helmet removal.

Cervical spine radiographs may be obtained through the helmet. Metallic or painted stripes on the helmet may obstruct the view on a lateral radiograph, although these can normally be peeled off without difficulty.

If the pediatric patient has no evidence of neurologic injury and the lateral cervical spine film is normal, then the helmet can be removed while maintaining in-line stabilization as will be discussed in the Procedure section. If evidence of spinal cord injury exists or an abnormal cervical spine film is noted, immediate neurosurgical consultation should be obtained and the helmet removed with a cast saw (3).

Techniques for helmet removal without the cast saw have been shown to cause 10° flexion in adults unless the shoulders were elevated (2). Additionally in studies on cadavers with unstable cervical fractures these techniques caused some degree of subluxation [3]. For this reason all helmets should be removed with a cast saw if neurologic injury or an abnormal radiograph is evident. Only those patients with a normal lateral cervical spine radiograph and normal neurologic examination should have their helmets removed by the two techniques that maintain in-line stabilization. The one-person technique is only illustrated for the rescuer who happened to be the only one available to assist the patient who required urgent removal of his or her helmet. The patient must be alert and cooperative for this technique. In almost all cases in the ED the two-person technique or the technique using the cast saw will be used. The two-person technique is most frequently used and is recommended by the American College of Surgeons [2].

EQUIPMENT

Scissors
3-inch cloth tape
Sandbags
Cast cutters
Size-appropriate cervical collars

PROCEDURE

One-Person Technique

To remove the helmet when alone, the straps should be untied or cut at the D rings. A small towel roll should be used to elevate the shoulders as is described in the two-person technique. The hands should be placed on the helmet at ear level from a cephalad position and the helmet should be spread laterally. Helmets are egg-shaped and fit most snugly at the ears. The helmet should then be slid off while maintaining in-line stabilization. In older children it will be necessary to rock the helmet posteriorly to clear the nose. Once the nose has been cleared the helmet should be returned to a neutral position. As the helmet begins to clear the occiput both hands should be walked to the occiput in slow progressive movements with the heels of both hands still on the rim of the helmet and maintaining stability. As both hands encircle the occiput the helmet should

be pushed off again using the heels of both hands. In-line stabilization must be maintained until immobilization can be secured with collar, tape, and sandbags (Fig. 24.1) [2].

Two-Person Technique

A small towel roll should be slid carefully beneath the shoulders to ensure that the body, neck, and helmet are in the same horizontal plane before beginning the two-person technique. The straps should be loosened by an assistant from a caudal position. One of the hands of this assistant should be placed on the occiput while the second hand is placed on the angle of the jaw with the thumb on one side and the index and middle finger on the other. Care must be taken not to obstruct the airway. The physician should then apply lateral traction to the helmet to spread it over the ears. The physician should begin to slide it over the ears. Notably, the full-faced motorcycle helmets are rigid and do not spread. Most have 1 to 2 inches of foam at ear level, however, which provides for a snug helmet fit but usually gives in to a slow, steady pulling. As the helmet is being removed it should be tilted backward to clear the nose in older children. Tilting of the helmet should begin just before the level of the nose to avoid trauma to the nose. The assistant at the caudal position must be careful to keep the neck from tilting backward with the helmet. Once the nose has cleared the helmet rim the helmet should be returned to a neutral position and then removed. When the physician has removed the helmet, his or her hands should be placed on the occiput and in-line stabilization should be maintained. Cervical collar, sandbags, and tape then should be applied by the assistant (Fig. 24.2) [4].

Bivalve Technique

Bivalve technique, which is the safest method for the known cervical spine injured patient, involves cutting the helmet with a cast saw in the coronal plane. An assistant should be designated to stabilize the neck from the caudal position as indicated in the two-person technique. The helmet should be cut at ear level in the coronal plane. The anterior half should be

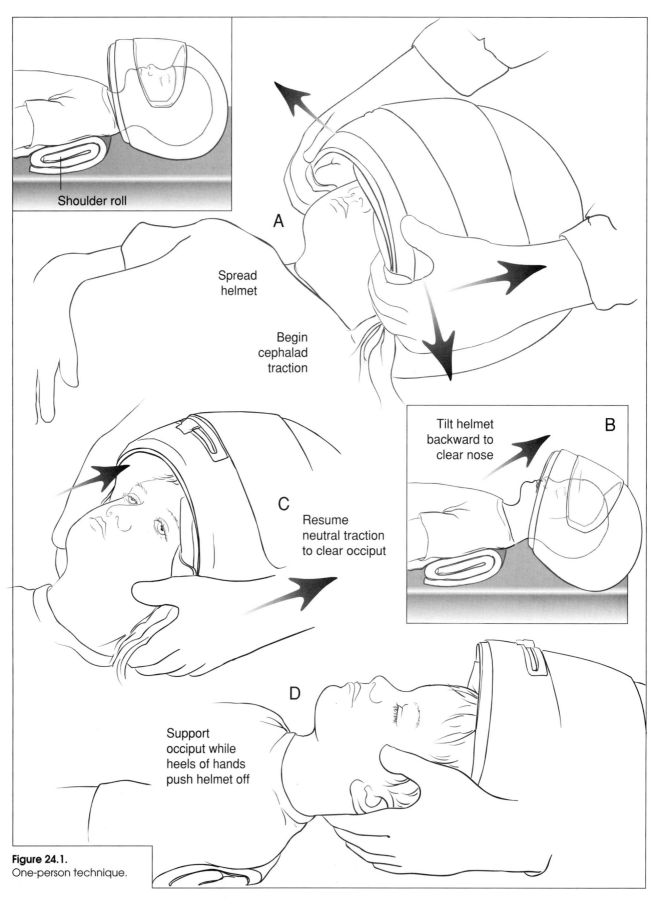

Shoulder roll

A

Spread
helmet

Begin
cephalad
traction

Tilt helmet
backward to
clear nose

B

C

Resume
neutral traction
to clear occiput

D

Support
occiput while
heels of hands
push helmet off

Figure 24.1.
One-person technique.

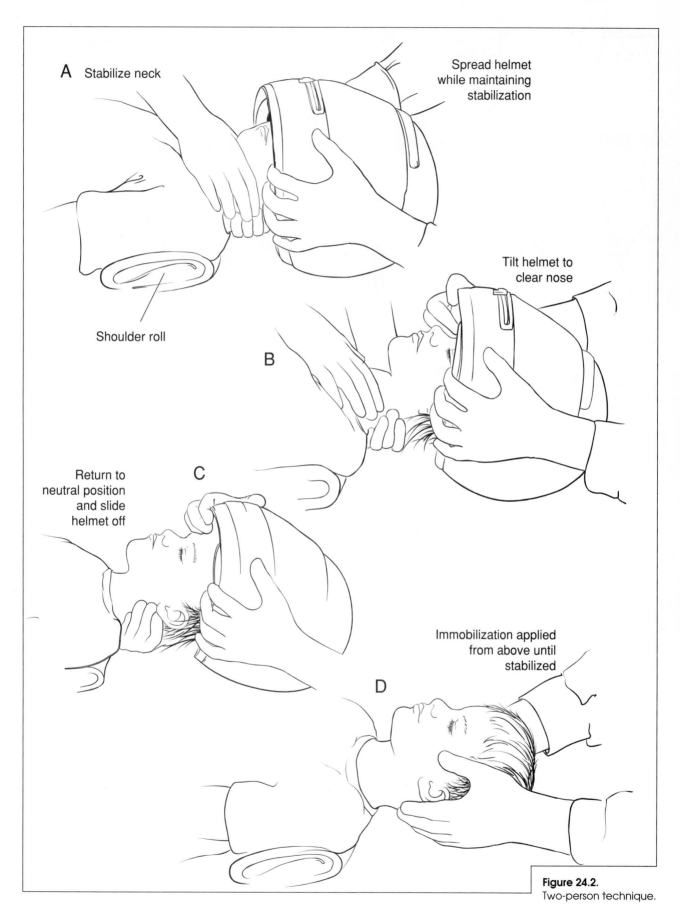

A Stabilize neck

Spread helmet while maintaining stabilization

Shoulder roll

B

Tilt helmet to clear nose

Return to neutral position and slide helmet off

C

Immobilization applied from above until stabilized

D

Figure 24.2.
Two-person technique.

347

Figure 24.3.
Using a cast saw to "bivalve" helmet, facilitating removal.

1. Untie straps
2. Stand at cephalad end of patient
3. Place hands on each side of helmet at ears and spread if possible.
4. Maintain in-line stabilization and begin to slide off
5. Tilt backward to clear nose
6. Return to neutral when nose cleared
7. When occiput cleared, walk hands with slow progressive movements to position where hands are encircling the occiput while heels of hands are on helmet rim.
8. Gradually push off helmet with heels of hands in slow progressive movements
9. Maintain in-line stabilization until able to stabilize

SUMMARY: TWO-PERSON TECHNIQUE
1. Untie straps
2. Person in caudal position places hands on occiput and jaw
3. Second person in cephalad position maintains in-line stabilization while spreading sides of helmet over ears
4. Tilt backward to clear nose and return to neutral position
5. Slide off
6. Second person maintains in-line stabilization
7. First person applies collar, tape, and sandbags

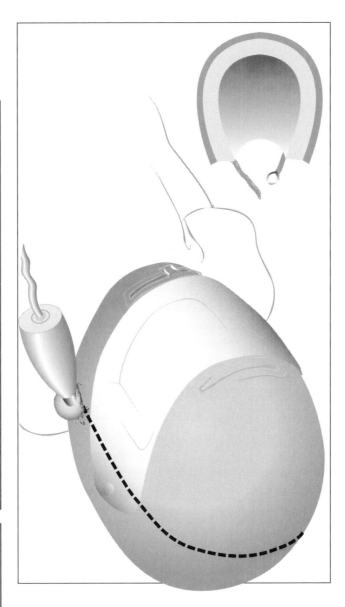

SUMMARY: BIVALVE TECHNIQUE
1. One person maintains stability with hands on jaw and occiput
2. Helmet cut in coronal plane at ear level using cast saw
3. Ties are cut and foam is cut
4. Anterior portion removed
5. Posterior slid off
6. Collar, tape, sandbags

CLINICAL TIPS
1. The clinician should make no attempt to spread a rigid full-faced motorcycle helmet. The foam lining of the interior will yield to gentle pulling.
2. The helmet should be tilted backward before the level of the nose to avoid injury.
3. Shoulders should be elevated because all helmets cause cervical flexion.
4. Metallic strips should be removed before taking the lateral spine radiograph.

removed by cutting the straps and the foam padding. The posterior half should then be slid out. The neck should be stabilized with collar, tape, and sandbags (Fig. 24.3).

Loud noise and vibration may cause significant anxiety and discomfort in the alert child. In this case the benefit of the procedure should be carefully considered. Mild sedation with rigorous monitoring may be an option (see Chapter 35).

COMPLICATIONS

Complications are few but significant if clinicians do not strictly adhere to recommended techniques. Permanent spinal cord injury may be caused or exacerbated by the procedure. If the shoulders are not elevated before attempting the one- or two-person technique some flexion or subluxation may occur. Children's spinal cords are very susceptible to traction injuries. Care should be taken not to add a strong, pulling force to the helmet while maintaining in-line stabilization.

Airway compromise may result from aggressive efforts to maintain cervical immobilization, particularly in the unconscious child. The neck is small and pressure from adult hands can obstruct the airway. The child who is lethargic or unconscious cannot respond appropriately to such inadvertent obstruction and is at increased risk unless carefully monitored.

Careless or aggressive removal of snug-fitting, full-faced helmets can injure tender nasal cartilage or cause fracture. The assistant who is at the caudal position during the two-person removal technique should ensure that the nose and ears are protected.

SUMMARY

Helmet removal will be increasingly necessary in pediatric trauma patients with the increase in patient safety awareness. Most unstable patients will have had their helmets removed in the field to provide airway protection. Those who are stable and arrive with their helmets on should have radiographs of their cervical spines and physical examinations before helmet removal. Helmets can be removed by three different techniques depending on the degree of injury and skill of the people involved. The primary concern of the operator must be to minimize cervical spine movement.

REFERENCES

1. Woodward GA. Neck trauma. In: Fleisher GR, Ludwig S, eds. Textbook of pediatric emergency medicine. 3rd ed. Baltimore: Williams & Wilkins, 1993, p. 1124.
2. Meyer RD, Daniel WW. The biomechanics of helmets and helmet removal. J Trauma 1985;25: 329–332.
3. Aprahamian C, Thompson BM, Darin JC. Recommended helmet removal techniques in a cervical spine injured patient. J Trauma 1984;24:841–842.
4. American College of Surgeons. Helmet removal from injured patients. Bull Am Coll Surg 1980;65:19–21.

CHAPTER 25

SURGICAL CRICOTHYROTOMY

Gary R. Strange and Leo G. Niederman

INTRODUCTION

The majority of children who require airway control or assisted ventilation can be managed with standard means such as bag-valve-mask ventilation or tracheal intubation. However, occasionally these techniques fail or cannot be performed. In these cases, alternative means of airway control must be employed. Three common alternatives to standard airway techniques are surgical cricothyrotomy, percutaneous needle cricothyroidotomy with transtracheal ventilation, and retrograde intubation. This chapter discusses the technique of surgical cricothyrotomy; the other two techniques are discussed in Section 2.

Surgical cricothyrotomy involves dissection of the anterior neck and visualized incision of the cricothyroid membrane. The technique has been well described in the adult population but experience in young children is anecdotal or limited. Furthermore, surgical cricothyrotomy has received little description in standard pediatric emergency medicine texts and ideal training for this procedure in children has not been developed or evaluated.

ANATOMY AND PHYSIOLOGY

Important to understanding any invasive airway procedure is knowledge of the anatomy of the anterior neck, larynx, and trachea (Fig.

25.1). The larynx, which consists of the thyroid cartilage, the cricothyroid membrane, and the cricoid cartilage, lies in the anterior neck, deep to the skin, subcutaneous tissues, and the sternohyoid muscle. The thyroid cartilage is cephalad to the cricothyroid membrane and the cricoid cartilage is caudad to it. The fibroelastic cricothyroid membrane can be palpated as an indentation between the two more prominent cartilage structures.

The cricoid cartilage attaches inferiorly to the tracheal rings. At approximately the same level of the junction of the cricoid membrane and the trachea is the isthmus of the thyroid gland. Care must be taken during dissection to avoid this structure. Additionally, although the cricothyroid membrane is relatively avascular, the superior thyroid artery crosses the superior portion of the membrane and can be damaged during dissection or incision.

In adolescents and adults the cricothyroid membrane is approximately 20 to 30 mm in width and 9 to 10 mm in superior-to-inferior length. In infants and children, the larynx is smaller and positioned more rostrally, making the topical landmarks of the thyroid and cricoid cartilage more difficult to identify. Furthermore, in this population the hyoid bone may be more easily felt than the thyroid cartilage. In infants the cricothyroid membrane is only about 3 mm in rostrocaudal length. For this reason, some medical personnel recommend that alternative techniques be employed in young children (1) (see Indications, this chapter).

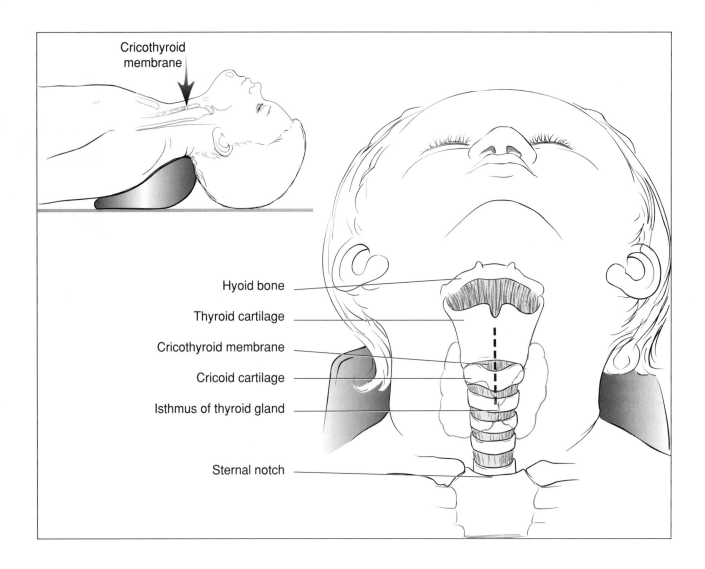

Cricothyroid membrane

Hyoid bone

Thyroid cartilage

Cricothyroid membrane

Cricoid cartilage

Isthmus of thyroid gland

Sternal notch

Figure 25.1.
Anatomical landmarks for surgical cricothyrotomy.

INDICATIONS

Indication for surgical cricothyrotomy is to achieve necessary airway control when less invasive techniques are unsuccessful or contraindicated. In infants and children this will occur most often when an upper airway obstruction occurs either as a result of an unremovable foreign body or of massive edema (such as epiglottitis or Ludwig's angina), or when significant maxillofacial, mandibular, oropharyngeal, or laryngeal trauma has occurred resulting in significant edema or severe anatomic distortion. Usually, masseter spasm or laryngeal spasm in children can be managed by other means such as pharmacologic paralysis and endotracheal intubation. The use of surgical cricothyrotomy in chil-

dren with known or suspected cervical spine injury is controversial. It is an option when BVM ventilation or controlled orotracheal intubation with in-line stabilization of the head and neck cannot be safely accomplished in the apneic or hypoxemic child.

The major contraindication to this technique is the ability to provide adequate oxygenation and ventilation by more standard, less invasive means (see Chapters 13, 14, and 16). Massive trauma to the larynx or the trachea, particularly transecting injury, is also a relative contraindication to surgical or needle cricothyrotomy; these techniques should be attempted under these circumstances only when other means of airway control are impossible and death is imminent. Additionally, because of the small size of the cricothyroid membrane in young children, some medical personnel suggest that this technique not be employed in children less than 5 years of age (1). Needle cricothyrotomy is preferred in younger children.

Other relative contraindications include neck trauma or edema that hinders surgical dissection or landmark identification. Known bleeding diathesis also may increase the risk of failure to obtain airway control rapidly, and increase the risk of other complications.

Surgical cricothyrotomy most often will be performed by physicians; however, in many situations airway control must be accomplished in the field. It is therefore vital that prehospital providers be familiar with this technique or with one of the alternatives discussed in Section 2.

EQUIPMENT

The equipment necessary to perform surgical cricothyrotomy is listed in Table 25.1. As is the problem with other procedures, this technique is rarely employed in children and the equipment available on a surgical airway tray may be inappropriate for use in children. Valuable time may be lost in an attempt to gather the proper equipment when the need for it arises. Therefore, it is important to include pediatric equipment on such trays or to develop a pediatric surgical airway tray. It is particularly important to have the proper size tracheal tubes and/or tracheostomy tubes and a range of tube sizes should be immediately available.

Table 25.1.
Equipment

1. Scalpels with #15 and #11 blades loaded
2. Trachea hook(s)
3. Trousseau dilator (trachea dilator)—Note this device may be too large for young children
4. Curved Mayo scissors
5. Curved hemostats (2)
6. Small vascular clamps (2)
7. Needle holder
8. Suture or circumferential tie for tracheostomy tubes
9. Syringe with 25-gauge needle for lidocaine with epinephrine
10. Sterile gauze pads
11. Sterile drapes
12. Appropriate tracheostomy tubes (Shiley 0 to 6)
13. Appropriate endotracheal tubes (2.5 mm to 7.0 mm ID)

PROCEDURE

Surgical Cricothyrotomy

The cricothyroid membrane should be identified below the tip or notch of the thyroid cartilage and above the cricoid cartilage. As stated previously, these structures can be difficult to palpate in young children but the thyroid cartilage is large enough to be felt in most children. Once this structure is identified its anterior surface should be palpated in a rostrocaudal fashion. The palpating finger should drop into the notch below the thyroid cartilage; this is the location of the cricothyroid membrane. When the thyroid cartilage cannot be identified by palpation, an alternative is to identify the hyoid bone and to then palpate caudally. Either the thyroid cartilage or the cricoid cartilage or both can be identified by this method.

If time permits, adequate surgical preparation and local anesthetic infiltration using lidocaine with epinephrine should be accomplished. A vertical, midline incision is made over the entire cricothyroid membrane (Fig. 25.2.A). The midline incision should protect most of the major neck vessels which are located laterally but some venous bleeding should be anticipated. Limiting the caudad extension of the incision is necessary to avoid the highly vascular thyroid gland. The skin and subcutaneous tissue should be incised and then held open with retractors (Fig. 25.2.B). After this incision, the cricothyroid membrane should be quickly palpated a second time to confirm its position. The sternohyoid muscle then should be carefully incised or separated by blunt dissection exposing the cricothyroid membrane (Fig. 25.2.C). The trachea is stabilized with either a tracheal hook or the fingers of the nonsurgical hand and a short horizontal incision is made with the point of a No. 11 scalpel blade. The incision is made in the lower half of the membrane, near the cricoid cartilage (Fig. 25.2.D). Care must be taken to direct the scalpel blade perpendicular to the frontal plane of the membrane and not to enter too deeply into the trachea, because this could result in injury to the posterior wall of the trachea and the esophagus behind it. Curved Mayo scissors or a curved hemostat is in-

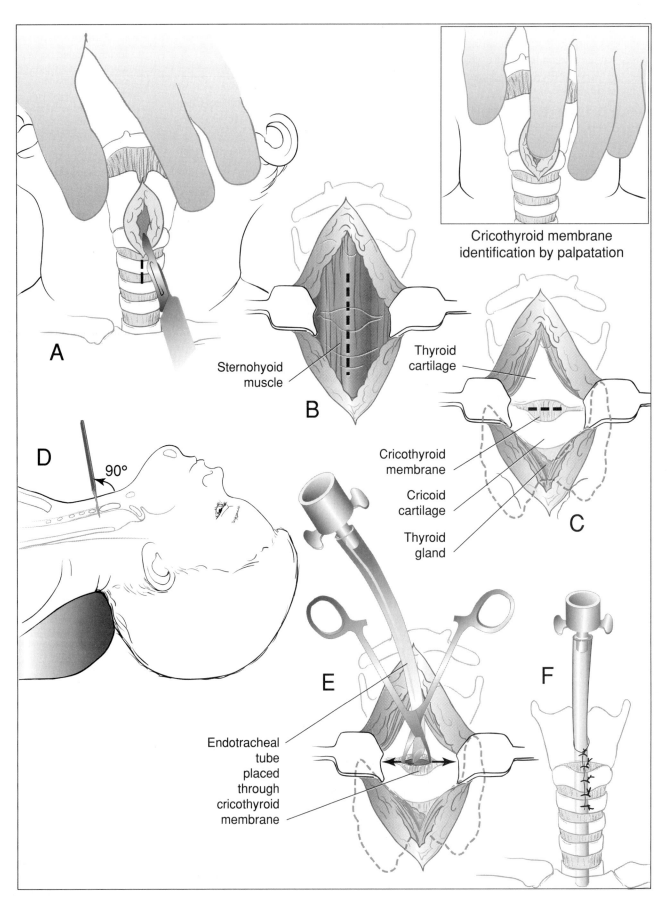

Cricothyroid membrane
identification by palpatation

A

B

Sternohyoid
muscle

Thyroid
cartilage

Cricothyroid
membrane

Cricoid
cartilage

Thyroid
gland

C

D

90°

E

Endotracheal
tube
placed
through
cricothyroid
membrane

F

354

serted into the incision, turned, and spread to widen the opening. While the blades of the scissors or hemostat are used to maintain the opening, the trachea is stabilized and lifted anteriorly and an appropriate size tracheostomy tube or endotracheal tube is inserted between the scissor or hemostat blades and into the trachea (Fig. 25.2.E). Alternatively, a tracheal hook can be inserted into the caudal portion of the incision and used to elevate the cricoid cartilage and trachea. The tube can be passed below the hook and into the trachea. The tube is secured and attached to a bag-valve device and ventilation is assessed (Fig. 25.2.F).

Finally, the above discussion describes the procedure as performed under ideal circumstances. Occasionally, the technique may have to be modified. For example, if bleeding prevents visualization of the cricothyroid membrane, it can be identified using palpation. The membrane has an elastic feel compared to the more rigid cartilage above and below it. Likewise, if, after the membrane is opened it is lost from view, the operator may be able to find it again using escaping air bubbles. In the spontaneously breathing patient these will occur with each exhalation. In the apneic patient pressure should be applied to the chest to force air from the incision (2, 3).

Complications

In adults, complication rates for this procedure have been reported to be as high as 40% (4, 5). Complications include incorrect site of incision or tube placement, prolonged procedure time, hemorrhage, and failure of the procedure to access the airway. Less commonly, esophageal and mediastinal perforation, subcutaneous emphysema, pneumothorax, pneumomediastinum, and laryngeal injury may occur (2–5). Traditional teaching has emphasized the risk of subglottic stenosis after this procedure. However, more recent literature suggests that this complication may occur less frequently than was previously thought (6, 7). Furthermore, some risks that are unacceptable for an elective procedure become quite acceptable in an emergency situation for which the alternative to a relatively high risk procedure may be death. Unfortunately, there are no reports of large series of surgical cricothyrotomy in children but complication rates would be expected to exceed those seen in adult series as a result of the increased technical difficulties involved in working with small structures.

Risk of occurrence of some of the previously mentioned complications can be minimized with careful attention to proper technique. A midline, vertical incision above the level of the thyroid isthmus reduces the chance of inadvertent injury to vascular structures because most of the major vessels lie lateral to the midline. Likewise, when possible puncture of the cricothyroid cartilage should be performed in the inferior portion of the membrane because a portion of the superior thyroid artery sometimes crosses the membrane along its rostral border. The incision should be made under direct vision whenever possible and should be just large enough to permit scissors or vascular clamps to be inserted. The scalpel also should be kept perpendicular to the membrane and not allowed to penetrate too deeply into the larynx. These two precautions help to avoid damage to the vocal cords which lie above the cricothyroid membrane and to the posterior trachea and esophagus which lie posterior to it.

SUMMARY

Surgical cricothyrotomy is a potentially lifesaving technique which can be used to obtain

SUMMARY
1. Alternative means of airway control such as needle cricothyroidotomy or retrograde intubation should always be considered first, particularly if the patient is a young child.
2. The initial incision is made vertical and in the midline. This reduces the risk of damage to vascular structures.
3. In some cases, the cricothyroid membrane may not be easily visualized. In these instances, the membrane should be palpated with a fingertip. "Blind" incision is a technique of last resort because of the risk of damage to vascular structures in the area.
4. A tracheal hook or the blades of the scissors or hemostats should be used to keep the incision open and to maintain location of the incision.
5. If the incision is "lost" bubbles of exhaled air will often identify its location. In the apneic patient these may be produced by pressure on the anterior chest wall.
6. Even a small airway is better than none. If a small endotracheal or tracheostomy tube is all that will pass through the incision, then it should be used until more effective airway control can be established.

Figure 25.2.
A. Initial vertical incision with manual stabilization of the trachea.
B. Skin retraction and exposure of the sternohyoid muscle.
C. Retraction of the sternohyoid muscle and exposure of the cricothyroid membrane (note location of incision is indicated).
D. Horizontal incision through the cricothyroid membrane with the scalpel perpendicular to the membrane.
E. Hemostats or scissors used to maintain the opening in the membrane while a tracheal tube is passed through the incision and into the trachea.
F. Tracheal tube secured in place.

necessary airway control when circumstances prevent the effective use of more traditional and less invasive techniques. This procedure is closely related to both needle cricothyroidotomy with transtracheal ventilation and to retrograde tracheal intubation, both of which are discussed in Section 2. For some patients, particularly for young children, one of these techniques may be preferred.

REFERENCES

1. Tucker JA. Obstruction of the major pediatric airway. Otolaryngol Clin North Am 1979;12:329–341.
2. Mace SE. Cricothyrotomy. J Emerg Med 1988;6: 309–319.
3. Walls RM. Cricothyroidotomy. Emerg Med Clin North Am 1988;6:725–736.
4. McGill J, Clinton JE, Ruiz E. Cricothyrotomy in the emergency department. Ann Emerg Med 1982;11: 361–364.
5. Kress TD, Balsubramaniam S. Cricothyrotomy. Ann Emerg Med 1982;11:197–201.
6. Brautigan CO, Grow JB. Cricothyroidotomy revisited again. Ear Nose Throat J 1980;59:289–295.
7. Brautigan CO, Grow JB. Subglottic stenosis after cricothyroidotomy. Surgery 1982;91:217–221.

DIAGNOSTIC PERITONEAL LAVAGE

Patricia L. VanDevander and David K. Wagner

INTRODUCTION

When assessing children who have sustained blunt abdominal trauma, the emergency physician or surgeon must quickly determine which of these children have sustained a serious injury necessitating emergency surgery and which have not. In some cases this determination can be made on clinical grounds alone but often a diagnostic procedure is required. Diagnostic peritoneal lavage (DPL) is one method by which intraabdominal injuries can be identified (1, 2). Simply stated, this technique involves inserting a catheter into the peritoneal cavity to identify intraperitoneal injury by demonstrating the presence of blood or fecal material. This procedure is accurate and inexpensive. It can be performed at the bedside and is not time consuming. For these reasons, DPL has become one of the gold standard tests in the evaluation of both child and adult trauma victims (3).

However, in this era of new imaging modalities, noninvasive testing, and conservative management of the trauma victim, DPL is rarely performed in children despite its potential advantages. Certain circumstances remain to be discussed, however, in which this procedure can provide valuable information in the evaluation and management of pediatric trauma patients. For this reason, recommended techniques and applications of DPL are presented, with particular emphasis on those aspects that specifically relate to children.

ANATOMY AND PHYSIOLOGY

Because DPL is in many ways a "blind" procedure, it is important to understand the anatomy of the abdomen and especially how the abdominal anatomy of infants and young children differs from that of adults (Fig. 26.1).

The abdominal cavity is continuous with the pelvic cavity. It is bordered superiorly by the muscular thoracoabdominal diaphragm and interiorly by the pelvic diaphragm. The anterior abdominal wall consists of skin and several layers of underlying muscles whose tendinous sheaths fuse together in the midline to form the linea alba. This relatively avascular area is the site for needle insertion into the abdominal cavity. The posterior surface of the anterior abdominal wall has, at the level of the umbilicus, both superior and inferior ligamentous attachments. The superior attachment is the falciform ligament. The falciform ligament extends to and incorporates the ligamentum teres, the remnant of the umbilical vein (4, 5). In young infants this vein may be patent and its inadvertent cannulation should be avoided, if possible.

Inferior to the umbilicus, in the midline, is the attachment of the median umbilical ligament, which extends into the apex of the bladder. This ligament is the remnant of the urachus. In infants and young children the muscles of the anterior abdominal wall are relatively weak when compared to those of adolescents and adults. These muscles, there-

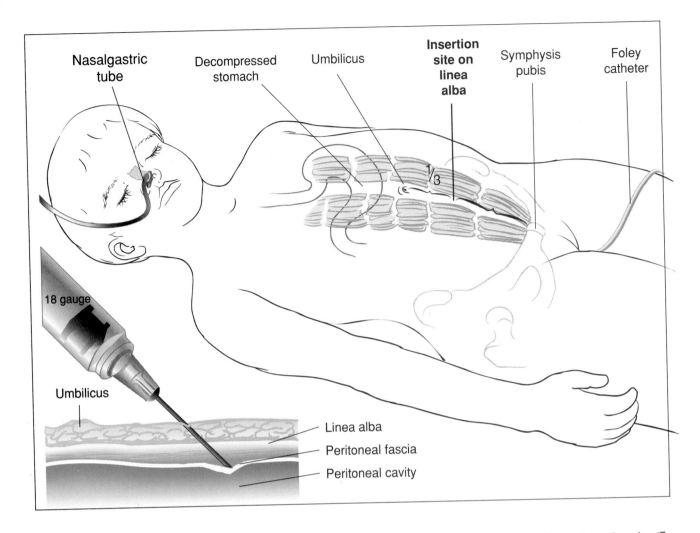

Labels in figure:
Nasalgastric tube
Decompressed stomach
Umbilicus
Insertion site on linea alba
Symphysis pubis
Foley catheter
1/3
18 gauge
Umbilicus
Linea alba
Peritoneal fascia
Peritoneal cavity

Figure 26.1.
Anatomical landmarks for diagnostic peritoneal lavage.

fore, provide less protection for the abdominal organs than the abdominal muscles of older patients.

The intraabdominal organs in children occupy a relatively larger portion of the abdominal cavity than these organs do in adults. The bladder is of particular concern, because in young children the bladder is more an abdominal than a pelvic organ. The stomach, when distended, may extend far into the abdominal cavity. Because young, crying children may ingest large quantities of air, a large, distended stomach should be anticipated. The combination of a relatively large liver and spleen and weak anterior abdominal muscles predisposes the child to splenic and/or hepatic hemorrhage after significant blunt abdominal trauma (6). Additionally, under certain circumstances, such as when a young child is involved in a motor vehicle accident while wearing a standard automobile lap belt, a hollow viscus injury can occur. Such an injury has the potential for leakage of

bowel contents into the peritoneal cavity (7, 8). Other important mechanisms for blunt abdominal injury in children include automobile versus pedestrian accidents and child abuse (9, 10, 11).

INDICATIONS

Clearly, all children who sustain an injury involving the abdomen are not candidates for DPL. Instead, these patients may be considered as part of a spectrum of injury. On one end of the spectrum are the children who are determined to require urgent laparotomy on clinical grounds alone. This group includes those who have sustained gunshot wounds that clearly involve the abdomen and those who have obvious signs of severe injury such as abdominal distension and hypotension (12). On the other end of the spectrum are those children who are awake and alert, have a completely normal physical examination, and no

Chapter 26
Diagnostic Peritoneal
Lavage

358

complaints of abdominal pain. These children likewise do not require DPL. This procedure should instead be reserved for a select group of patients whose presenting signs and symptoms lie between these two extremes.

In the case of blunt trauma, possible pediatric candidates for DPL include: patients who are obtunded; those in whom, as a result of age or developmental factors, an accurate history and physical examination cannot be obtained; those who have persistent abdominal pain and tenderness after significant abdominal trauma; and those patients whose abdominal examination remains equivocal during a period of observation (13).

Penetrating Trauma

Use of DPL in selected cases of penetrating trauma remains somewhat controversial. As previously stated, gunshot wounds to the abdomen usually require laparotomy; the destructive force of firearms places the patient at great risk for significant injury. However, in some cases the bullet pathway is near the abdomen but exhibits little evidence of penetration of the abdominal cavity. In such situations DPL may be helpful in making this determination. Some children who have been stabbed may also be candidates for DPL. These children have no signs of significant organ injury and no cardiovascular instability. DPL should be undertaken in these children only after examination of the stool, urine, and gastric aspirate for blood. In such patients, DPL may serve as an adjunct to local exploration of the wound. However, if evidence of significant injury exists (e.g., blood in the stool), DPL will provide no new information (3, 12, 14, 15).

Additionally, when DPL was introduced, management of suspected intraabdominal injury was by emergency laparotomy. Although DPL certainly reduced the number of exploratory laparotomies for abdominal trauma, patients who had a positive DPL were still managed surgically. Since that time, however, two important changes have occurred that have had a profound effect on the evaluation and management of the potentially injured abdomen. First, advances in imaging technology have provided the latest development in sophisticated and accurate forms of noninvasive imaging devices. Second, the overall trend in management of children with intraabdominal injuries has changed from surgical management to nonsurgical management.

Many children with known liver and spleen injuries are managed by observation and serial examination and most of these children do not ultimately require surgery (16, 17). Under these circumstances, it is important to know not only whether an intraabdominal injury is present but also its location and extent. Computed tomography (CT) of the abdomen enhanced with both intravenous and intragastric contrast material often provides this information as well as images of the retroperitoneal structures (18). Additionally, this technique is relatively noninvasive. For these reasons, in many medical centers CT scanning has all but eclipsed DPL in the evaluation of children who are victims of abdominal trauma (19, 20).

CT scanning, however, is not universally available on an emergent basis. Furthermore, recent studies have questioned the accuracy of abdominal CT scanning (21, 22). CT scanning requires transportation of the patient from the resuscitation area and, in many centers, completely out of the ED. Once on the CT scanner table the management of emergent problems becomes more difficult. For these reasons, some patients are too unstable to undergo this procedure.

Another technique which has been extensively studied in the evaluation of the injured abdomen is abdominal ultrasound (US). This technique has not proved to be as useful as CT scanning in detecting the exact location and extent of injury, but in several studies it has been shown to compare favorably to DPL in detecting the presence of injury (23, 24, 25, 26). Specifically, this technique appears to be extremely sensitive in identifying abnormal intraperitoneal fluid collections. Ultrasound also has the advantage of being noninvasive and, because it is a bedside procedure, no patient transportation is required.

As in CT scanning, US is not universally available on an emergent basis. Furthermore, although both surgeons and emergency physicians have been able to accurately use US and interpret the results, a distinct "learning curve" has appeared. Specific training and supervision is therefore required (25, 26) at least initially. In addition, equipment cost remains beyond the means of many ED budgets.

For these reasons it is important for the

emergency physician to be familiar with the technique of DPL, and its limitations and possible complications. The clinician will often be forced to decide when to employ CT scanning and when to employ DPL or US. Because these methods of evaluating the potentially injured abdomen provide different types of information, they may be considered complimentary (27, 28).

Notably before any imaging technique or DPL is undertaken, ED personnel, if possible, should contact the surgeon who will be responsible for the patient should an injury be identified. The surgeon should be offered every opportunity to participate in the initial evaluation of the patient, particularly if he or she may ultimately have responsibility for the patient's care. Ideally, the surgeon should see and examine the child in the ED. If this is not possible, then the surgeon should at least be contacted (Table 26.1).

When the physician decides to perform DPL, he or she also must determine which of the several described variations is best to use. The original DPL was essentially a "mini laparotomy." This procedure, although still performed in many centers, has some distinct disadvantages. It is somewhat time consuming and it involves an (albeit small) midline incision. This incision creates the potential for bleeding and a false-positive DPL. Making a midline incision also may lead to accidental evisceration or wound dehiscence (29).

The most popular alternative to the classic diagnostic peritoneal lavage is the so-called "closed technique," in which a guide wire passed through a needle is used to direct the lavage catheter (30). Most authorities prefer the closed technique for the pediatric patient. Because this procedure will rarely be performed in children, the clinician is better served to learn and use one approach. Gaining a thorough understanding of a single, reliable method by which to perform this procedure will facilitate success with this and other infrequently performed procedures. Therefore, only the closed technique is described in this chapter. Those wishing to learn either the traditional open approach or other variations are referred elsewhere (14, 31, 32).

Two groups of patients in whom DPL is relatively contraindicated are those who have had previous abdominal surgery and those who are pregnant. If the physician feels that DPL is necessary in a pregnant adolescent, the supraumbilical approach is recommended (33). Ultrasound has obvious advantages for the pregnant patient because it allows evaluation of the fetus and involves no radiation exposure. In the patient who has had previous abdominal surgeries, CT scanning may be a useful alternative. If DPL must be done, the physician should choose the abdominal position (supraumbilical versus infraumbilical) farthest from the previous incision.

EQUIPMENT

Most equipment required for diagnostic peritoneal lavage is readily available in the ED. In fact, many EDs have prepackaged equipment trays designed for this procedure. Although these trays are mainly designed for use in adult patients, they can be adapted for pediatric use with the addition of selected equipment. With increasing popularity of the closed technique for DPL, many commercial kits also have become available. Some of

Table 26.1.
Indications for Diagnostic Peritoneal Lavage

A. General
  1. Other imaging modalities unavailable or yield equivocal results
  2. US unavailable and patient condition prevents transport to CT scanner.
  3. Monitoring difficult or impossible outside of ED as a result of inadequate staffing or available equipment
  4. Surgical backup availability greater than 15 to 30 minutes
B. Significant blunt abdominal trauma with:
  (assumes other imaging modalities unavailable or inappropriate, see above)
  1. Obtundation
  2. Equivocal physical examination
  3. Patient age or developmental level preventing accurate physical examination
  4. Unexplained hypotension
C. Stab wounds: (controversial)
  1. Abdominal stab wound without obvious evidence of intra-abdominal injury, after local exploration of the wound

Table 26.2.
Equipment for Diagnostic Peritoneal Lavage

Povidine solution
1 or 2% lidocaine with epinephrine
Sterile drapes
Introducer needle or angiocatheter—18 or 19 gauge
Guide wire with soft *J* end
No. 11 scalpel blade
Lavage catheter
Normal saline or Ringer's lactate
Syringes

these kits are specifically designed for pediatric use and others can be easily modified. Table 26.2 lists the equipment necessary for the performance of this procedure.

PROCEDURE

In preparation for DPL, sedation may be administered as needed (see Chapter 35). The stomach is decompressed using a nasogastric or orogastric tube (see Chapter 86), and the bladder is emptied using a bladder catheter (see Chapter 98). These procedures decrease the risk of inadvertent puncture of either the stomach or the bladder.

The child is then placed in the supine position with full exposure from the xiphoid to the symphysis pubis. The abdomen is prepared with providine-iodine solution and sterile drapes are applied (see Chapter 7) so that an area approximately 4 cm around the umbilicus is exposed. The usual site for needle insertion is in the midline, below the umbilicus approximately one-third of the distance from the umbilicus to the symphysis pubis. This infraumbilical approach is generally used unless the patient in question is pregnant or has a pelvic fracture, an abdominal wall hematoma, or local skin infection at the infraumbilical site.

The supraumbilical approach is recommended for these patients, but most importantly for infants and young children because it reduces the possibility of accidental puncture of the bladder, which as previously stated, can extend well into the abdomen in these patients. With the supraumbilical approach, the needle is inserted above the umbilicus, approximately the same distance from the umbilicus as for the infraumbilical approach. In adults this distance is usually approximately 3 cm, but will be less in a small child (usually 1 to 2 cm). Using the midline location allows the needle to pass through the relatively avascular linea alba. This helps to prevent bleeding and, therefore, a false-positive result.

Once the patient is prepared and the site of insertion chosen, local anesthetic (Chapter 37) is administered into the skin and down to the fascia. Use of local anesthetic containing epinephrine is recommended to reduce the amount of local bleeding. Using sterile technique, a long 18-gauge angiocath or a thin walled 19- or 20-gauge needle is inserted and gently advanced through the anesthetized tissues in a slightly caudad direction. It is important that the needle not be directed laterally where it might encounter the liver or the spleen. The angiocath is preferred because once the insertion needle is removed, only the relatively blunt plastic catheter remains in the peritoneum.

On insertion, two distinct "pops" should be felt—one as the needle penetrates the linea alba and one as the peritoneal fascia is penetrated. If an angiocath is used, it should be inserted a few millimeters into the peritoneal cavity to ensure that both the needle and the plastic catheter have actually entered the cavity. The insertion needle is then removed and the soft end of a guide wire is advanced through the plastic catheter and into the peritoneal cavity (Fig. 26.2.A). The guide wire should advance smoothly and easily with minimal, if any, resistance. If significant resistance is felt to guide wire insertion then both the guide wire and the insertion catheter (or needle) should be removed and reinserted. Once the guide wire has been successfully advanced into the peritoneal cavity, the plastic catheter (or needle) may be removed. A small puncture is made in the skin with a No. 11 scalpel blade at the site of guide wire insertion (Fig. 26.2.B). The lavage catheter is advanced over the guide wire and into the peritoneal cavity in a slightly caudal direction. Then the guide wire is removed.

When the lavage catheter is in the peritoneal cavity the physician should attempt to aspirate any free peritoneal fluid (Fig. 26.2.D). In the full sized adolescent or adult 5 to 10 mL or more of gross blood aspirated via the lavage catheter is considered a positive result. In children, the amount of blood necessary to consider the procedure positive is unknown. It is safest to assume that any amount of gross blood aspirated from the peritoneum of a child 8 years of age or younger is representative of significant intraabdominal injury (34). Under these circumstances the procedure need not continue. Any gross blood recovered by this initial aspiration should be observed for clotting. In rare instances it is possible to cannulate a vessel in the abdominal wall and to aspirate clotting blood from this vessel; however, blood aspirated from the peritoneal cavity should not clot.

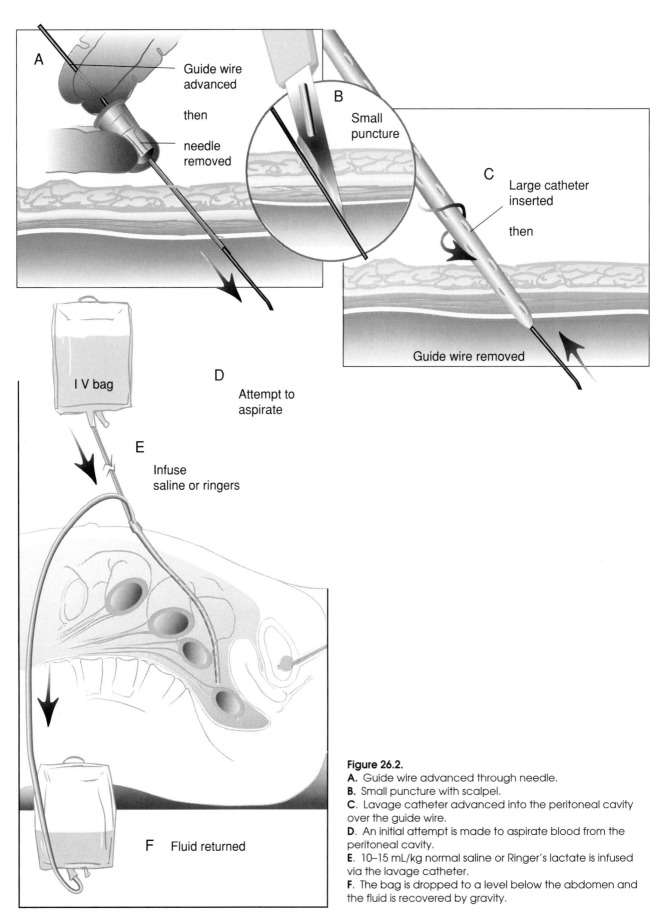

A Guide wire advanced then needle removed

B Small puncture

C Large catheter inserted then

Guide wire removed

D Attempt to aspirate

I V bag

E Infuse saline or ringers

F Fluid returned

Figure 26.2.
A. Guide wire advanced through needle.
B. Small puncture with scalpel.
C. Lavage catheter advanced into the peritoneal cavity over the guide wire.
D. An initial attempt is made to aspirate blood from the peritoneal cavity.
E. 10–15 mL/kg normal saline or Ringer's lactate is infused via the lavage catheter.
F. The bag is dropped to a level below the abdomen and the fluid is recovered by gravity.

If no fluid returns or, in the adolescent, if less than 10 mL of blood is aspirated from the peritoneal cavity, then 10 to 15 mL/kg of normal saline or Ringer's lactate is rapidly infused by gravity into the peritoneal cavity (Fig. 26.2.E). The volume of fluid infused must be limited to 10 to 15 mL per kilogram because infusion of large amounts of fluid into the child's peritoneum may affect diaphragmatic excursion and therefore breathing. Once the fluid is fully infused then, if the patient's condition permits, he or she should be gently rolled onto the right and left sides to allow the fluid to "wash" over the peritoneal cavity. The bag is then dropped to a level below that of the patient's abdomen and the fluid allowed to return to the bag by gravity (Fig. 26.2.F). Although most of the fluid should return to the bag, it is not necessary to recover more than 3 to 5 mL/kg (about 20% of the instilled fluid) (12). If only a small amount of fluid returns, however, then an effort should be made to recover more fluid. This may be accomplished by repositioning the lavage catheter, by rotating the patient from side to side (again, only if his or her condition permits), or, as a last resort, by reinserting the guide wire and replacing the lavage catheter with a new one or a large bore (14- or 16-gauge) angiocatheter.

The fluid recovered should be sent to the laboratory for analysis. Specifically, it should be analyzed for the presence of red blood cells and white blood cells, a Gram stain should be performed to look for bacteria and fecal matter, and the fluid should be tested for the presence of pancreatic amylase/lipase (12, 32, 34, 35). Table 26.3 lists the criteria by which a diagnostic peritoneal lavage is considered to be positive and therefore diagnostic for an intraabdominal injury. To be considered negative, the returned lavage fluid should contain less than 50,000 RBCs per mm^3 and less than 100 WBCs per mm^3. It is

Table 26.3.
Criteria for a Diagnostic Peritoneal Lavage to be Considered Positive

1. Gross blood aspirated from the peritoneal cavity
2. Greater than 100,000 RBCs per mm^3 in returned lavage fluid (blunt trauma)
3. Greater than 5000 RBCs per mm^3 in returned lavage fluid (stab wound)
4. Greater than 500 WBCs per mm^3
5. Fecal material in returned lavage fluid

Table 26.4.
Criteria for a Diagnostic Peritoneal Lavage to be Considered Equivocal

1. 50,000 to 100,000 RBCs per mm^3 in returned lavage fluid
2. 100 to 500 WBCs per mm^3 in returned lavage fluid

possible for the result of the DPL to be equivocal (Table 26.4). In this case, if the patient's condition permits, the operator should consider using a different method of testing which might include computed tomography or ultrasound. Alternative strategies are observation and repeated examinations and, of course, exploratory laparotomy.

Complications

Serious complications associated with diagnostic peritoneal lavage are surprisingly rare (35, 36, 37). The most important complications involve direct injury to an intraabdominal structure. Of all the intraabdominal organs the liver and spleen are the least likely to be injured; however, if the needle is directed laterally, needle puncture of these organs is possible. Even in the unlikely case that one of these organs is hit by the needle no serious injury is likely to occur.

A potentially more serious situation is perforation of bowel by the needle. Although normal intestine should be somewhat resistant to penetration because it is in essence floating and should simply move aside, it is still possible for the needle to enter the bowel lumen. This risk is increased when adhesions have caused the bowel to be relatively fixed in place or to become adherent to the peritoneal lining. Risk can be minimized by using an angiocatheter to introduce the guide wire into the peritoneum. The needle should only be advanced far enough into the peritoneal cavity to allow the blunt plastic catheter to be advanced. If the needle does enter the bowel, the bowel usually reseals itself on removal of the needle but soiling of the peritoneum with resultant peritonitis is possible.

The two organs at greatest risk during DPL are the stomach and the bladder. Nasogastric or orogastric decompression should be used to minimize the size of the stomach. Furthermore, the catheter should not be directed laterally. Although the stomach may reseal itself after penetration with the needle,

SUMMARY
1. Prepare patient by using sedation and restraint as necessary; insert nasogastric or orogastric tube and bladder catheter.
2. Sterilely prep abdomen and apply sterile drapes exposing approximately 4 cm around umbilicus.
3. Select infraumbilical or supraumbilical approach as indicated (see p. 361) then infiltrate selected site with lidocaine with epinephrine.
4. Using 18-gauge angiocatheter, 19-gauge needle, or equipment provided in a commercial kit, enter peritoneal cavity.
5. Pass soft end of guide wire through catheter or needle into peritoneal cavity.
6. Using a No. 11 scalpel blade incise skin where guide wire enters, enlarging hole.
7. Thread lavage catheter onto wire and then, directing it caudally, into peritoneal cavity.
8. Attempt to aspirate fluid from peritoneal cavity—if any frank blood is recovered in a young child, this is deemed to be a positive result and procedure can be terminated.
9. If no frank blood is recovered, then instill 10 to 15 mL/kg of normal saline or Ringer's lacate rapidly by gravity.
10. When all fluid is in peritoneal cavity, patient may be rocked from side to side; bag is then dropped to a level below abdomen.
11. Fluid recovered in bag should be sent to laboratory for analysis.

as does the bowel penetration of the stomach may allow gastric contents into the peritoneal cavity causing potentially serious peritonitis. As previously stated, the bladder in infants and young children can extend quite far into the abdomen placing it at risk for penetration. This is a less serious situation because the relative muscular bladder wall reseals itself readily. In fact, aspiration of urine from the bladder is one means by which sterile urine samples are sometimes obtained in infants (see Chapter 99). Penetration of the bladder, however, can be avoided by decompressing the bladder with a urinary catheter and by using a supraumbilical approach in young infants.

The other potentially serious complication from DPL is injury to vascular structures within the abdominal wall or peritoneal cavity. Such injury rarely leads to significant hemorrhage into the peritoneal cavity, but rather to a false-positive DPL which could result in the child undergoing an unnecessary laparotomy. Using a midline location for needle placement and avoiding lateral direction of the needle are the best ways to avoid this complication. If doubt exists about whether or not blood recovered from the peritoneal cavity represents an actual injury, and the patient's condition permits, then CT or US should be used. If the patient's condition does not permit, the blood must be assumed to represent a significant injury.

Lack of adherence to sterile technique may allow skin flora or other bacteria into the peritoneal cavity with resultant infection (37). DPL is an invasive procedure and therefore strict adherence to sterile technique is mandatory.

CLINICAL TIPS (CONTINUED)

5. Local anesthetic containing epinephrine should be used to decrease bleeding around the site of insertion of the lavage catheter. This helps to reduce the possibility of a false-positive result.
6. The supraumbilical approach should be used for young infants and small children and for those patients who are pregnant, have pelvic fractures, or who have local irritation or skin infection in the infraumbilical area. For patients who have had previous abdominal surgeries, the site farthest from the previous incision is used. The infraumbilical approach is indicated for all others.
7. The needle should be directed slightly caudad. A lateral trajectory of the needle (off the midline) must always be avoided.
8. The guide wire should advance very smoothly. If it does not then both the wire and the insertion needle should be removed.
9. The lavage catheter should be directed caudally during insertion.
10. Infusion of saline or Ringer's lactate into the peritoneal cavity should be limited to 10 to 15 mL/kg to avoid interference with respiratory function.
11. If the clinical condition permits, the patient should be rolled from side to side to allow the lavage fluid to wash over the peritoneal cavity.
12. It is only necessary to recover 3 to 5 mL/kg of fluid. If less fluid is recovered, the patient can be rolled from side to side or the blunt lavage catheter can be repositioned or replaced.

SUMMARY

Diagnostic peritoneal lavage is a time-tested method of determining the presence of significant intraabdominal injury after abdominal trauma. It offers the advantage of being a low cost, bedside procedure that can be performed with readily available equipment. It does not require transportation of the patient from the resuscitation area and the samples of fluid obtained can be easily analyzed by most laboratories. DPL is an invasive procedure, however, and the results offer no information about the location and extent of injury. Furthermore, DPL yields no information about retroperitoneal structures. With the advent of accurate noninvasive imaging techniques and conservative management of children with

---

CLINICAL TIPS

1. Alternative imaging techniques should be considered based on availability and patient condition.
2. Surgical consultation should be obtained early in the management of the patient.
3. Adequate restraint and conscious sedation should be used as needed to minimize risk of injury.
4. A gastric tube and bladder catheter should be inserted to reduce risk of inadvertent puncture of the stomach or bladder.

intraabdominal injuries, indications for DPL in the pediatric population have become fewer. As more EDs obtain ultrasound equipment and more emergency physicians and surgeons become facile in its use, DPL is likely to become a rare procedure. At present, however, emergency physicians should remain familiar with the technique of DPL and its indications.

REFERENCES

1. Root HD, Hauser CW, McKinley CR, LaFave JW, Mendiola RP. Diagnostic peritoneal lavage. Surgery 1965;57:633–637.
2. Civetta JM, Williams MJ, Richie RE. Diagnostic peritoneal irrigation: a simple, reliable technique. Surgery 1970;67:874–877.
3. Powell DC, Bivins BA, Bell RM. Diagnostic peritoneal lavage. Surg Gynecol Obstet 1982;155:257–264.
4. Moore KL. The abdomen in clinically oriented anatomy. 2nd ed. Moore KL, ed. Baltimore: Williams & Wilkins, 1985.
5. Woodburne RT. The abdomen in essentials of human anatomy. 6th ed. Woodburne RT, ed. New York: Oxford University Press, 1978.
6. Richardson JD, Belin RP, Griffen Jr. WO. Blunt abdominal trauma in children. Ann Surg 1972;176:213–216.
7. Newman KD, Bowman LM, Eichelberger MR, Gotschall CS, Taylor GA, Johnson DL, Thomas M. The lap belt complex: intestinal and lumbar spine injury in children. J Trauma 1990;30:1133–1138.
8. Statter MB, Coran AG. Appendiceal transection in a child associated with a lap belt restraint: case report. J Trauma 1992;33:765–766.
9. Hood JM, Smyth BT. Nonpenetrating intraabdominal injuries in children. J Pediatr Surg 1974;9:69–77.
10. Levy JL, Linder LH. Major abdominal trauma in children. Am J Surg 1970;120:55–58.
11. Sivit CJ, Taylor GA, Eichelberger MR. Visceral injury in battered children: a changing perspective. Radiology 1989;173:659–661.
12. Hill AC, Schecter WP, Trunkey DD. Abdominal trauma and indications for laparotomy. In: Mattox KL, Moore EE, Feliciano DV, eds. Trauma. East Norwalk, CT: Appleton & Lange, 1988.
13. Henneman PL, Marx JA, Moore EE, Cantrill SV, Ammons LA. Diagnostic peritoneal lavage: accuracy in predicting necessary laparotomy following blunt and penetrating trauma. J Trauma 1990;30:1345–1355.
14. Coleridge ST, Bell C. Diagnostic peritoneal lavage. In: Roberts JR, Hedges JR, eds. Clinical procedures in emergency medicine. 2nd ed. Philadelphia: WB Saunders, 1991.
15. Lucas CE. The role of peritoneal lavage for penetrating abdominal wounds. J Trauma 1977;17:649–650.
16. Schiffman MA. Nonoperative management of blunt abdominal trauma in pediatrics. Emerg Med Clin North Am 1989;7:519–535.
17. Delius RE, Frankel W, Coran AG. A comparison between operative and nonoperative management of blunt injuries to the liver and spleen in adult and pediatric patients. Surgery 1989;106:788–792.
18. Mohamed G, Reyes HM, Fantus R, Ramilo J, Radhakrishnan J. Computed tomography in the assessment of pediatric abdominal trauma. Arch Surg 1986;121:703–707.
19. Karp MP, Cooney DR, Berger PE, Kuhn JP, Jewett Jr. TC. The role of computed tomography in the evaluation of blunt abdominal trauma in children. J Pediatr Surg 1981;16:316–323.
20. Goldstein AS, Sclafani SJA, Kupferstein NH, Bass I, Lewis T, Panetta T, Phillips T, Shaftan GW. The diagnostic superiority of computerized tomography. J Trauma 1985;25:938–946.
21. Meyer DM, Thal ER, Coln D, Weigelt JA. Computed tomography in the evaluation of children with blunt abdominal trauma. Ann Surg 1993;217:272–276.
22. Frame SB, Browder IW, Lang EK, McSwain Jr. NE. Computed tomography versus diagnostic peritoneal lavage: usefulness in immediate diagnosis of blunt abdominal trauma. Ann Emerg Med 1989;18:513–516.
23. Chambers JA, Pilbrow WJ. Ultrasound in abdominal trauma: an alternative to peritoneal lavage. Arch Emerg Med 1988;5:26–33.
24. Akgur FM, Tanyel FC, Akhan O, Buyukpamukcu N, Hicsonmez A. The place of ultrasonographic examination in the initial evaluation of children sustaining blunt abdominal trauma. J Pediatr Surg 1993;28:78–81.
25. Boulanger BR, McLellan BA, Rizoli SB, Brenneman FD, Hamilton P. A prospective study of emergent abdominal sonography after blunt trauma. Acad Emerg Med 1994;1:A26.
26. Ma OJ, Mateer JR, Ogata M, Kefer M, Wittman D, Aprahamian C. Ultrasonography for trauma patients by emergency physicians. Acad Emerg Physicians 1994;1:A26–A27.
27. Sorkey AJ, Farnell MB, Williams Jr. HJ, Mucha Jr. P, Ilstrup DM. The complementary roles of diagnostic peritoneal lavage and computed tomography in the evaluation of blunt abdominal trauma. Surgery 1989;106:794–800.
28. Thal ER, Meyer DM. The evaluation of blunt abdominal trauma: computed tomography scan, lavage, or sonography? Adv in Surg 1991;24:201–228.
29. Frame SB, Hendrikson MF, Boozer AG, McSwain Jr. NE. Dehiscence with evisceration: a rare complication of diagnostic peritoneal lavage. JEM 1989;7:599–602.
30. Howdieshell TR, Osler TM, Demarest GB. Open versus closed peritoneal lavage with particular attention to time accuracy and cost. Am J Emerg Med 1989;7:367–371.
31. London PS. The surgical management of the severely injured person. In: Kirk RM, Williamson RCN, eds. General surgical operations. 2nd ed. Edinburgh: Churchill Livingstone, 1987.
32. Cocks RA, Yates DW. How to perform a diagnostic peritoneal lavage. Br J Hosp Med 1990;44:122–123.

33. Haycock CE. Blunt trauma in pregnancy. In Haycock CE, ed. Trauma and pregnancy. Littleton, MA: PSG Publishing, 1985.

34. Ziegler MM, Templeton Jr. JM. Major trauma. In: Fleisher GR, Ludwig S, eds. Textbook of pediatric emergency medicine. 3rd ed. Baltimore: Williams & Wilkins, 1993.

35. Fischer RP, Beverlin BC, Engrav LH, Benjamin CI, Perry Jr. JF. Diagnostic peritoneal lavage: fourteen years and 2586 patients later. Am J Surg 1978; 136:701–704.

36. Watson JS, Park PF. Peritoneal lavage in the evaluation of abdominal trauma. Okla State Med Assoc J 1974;67:257–261.

37. Catapano M, Cwinn AA, Marx JA, Moore EE. Toxic shock syndrome following diagnostic peritoneal lavage. Ann Emerg Med 1988; 17:736–738.

CONTROL OF EXSANGUINATING EXTERNAL HEMORRHAGE

John J. Kelly

INTRODUCTION

Recognition and control of significant external hemorrhage becomes an important issue whenever a childhood injury involves the soft tissues or vascular structures. An amount of blood loss that might be considered almost inconsequential in an adult patient may be life-threatening in the child. Furthermore, extensive blood loss can occur in the absence of a single obvious site of major hemorrhage. Therefore, all personnel who care for injured children must be familiar with techniques designed to limit blood loss.

As in the management of all traumatic injury, assessment and management priorities must be established. Control of the airway and ventilation should be undertaken while the temporizing measures to be discussed are initiated to limit external hemorrhage (1). Furthermore, external bleeding, particularly when it appears to involve significant blood loss, may be the parents' primary concern. The clinician must provide reassurance that all injuries, including site of bleeding, will be cared for promptly.

Because control of hemorrhage by definition involves some potential for contact with blood, ED personnel involved in these procedures must pay strict attention to universal precautions (Chapter 8).

ANATOMY AND PHYSIOLOGY

From the standpoint of control of bleeding, children are anatomically similar to adults in most respects. Blood vessels at risk for injury in both children and adults are in two anatomic locations. The peripheral vessels are those that lie beneath the skin and above the fascial layer. Most of these vessels are small and are rarely a source for significant bleeding. However, some larger veins are in this location. Bleeding from these veins is manifested by continuous hemorrhage of dark-colored blood. Most of the major vessels lie deep to the fascia and are at risk from penetrating trauma, significant blunt trauma, and from fractures that may allow fragments of bone to injure these structures. Major arteries are among these deeper vessels. Hemorrhage from these structures is seen as bright red blood that pumps in time to cardiac systole.

Some important differences between adults and children may influence management. First, because young children are simply smaller than adults, energy has less body mass over which to dissipate and therefore significant amounts of force may be directed against a relatively small target area (2). Furthermore, the body habitus of the child is somewhat different (3). The head is relatively large as compared to the rest of the body, which means that the head is at greater risk for injury and also means that more vascular areas such as the face and scalp may be the sites of significant hemorrhage. Injury to scalp veins can result in significant blood loss. Most significant bleeding from head injuries will be the result of bleeding from these structures; however, profuse and uncontrollable venous bleeding after a head injury may rarely be caused by a skull fracture that has torn the dural sinus.

In addition, children's extremities are comparatively small and, compared to those of adults, are thin. Limbs of toddlers lack the potential protection of both subcutaneous fat which is present in babies and well-developed muscles found in adolescents.

Circulating blood volume comprises about 8 to 9% of the child's ideal body weight and is therefore equivalent to 80 to 90 mL/kg ideal body weight (2). The percentage of ideal body weight occupied by blood decreases with age and by adulthood has decreased to 7% or approximately 70 mL/kg. Thus, bleeding that results in 500 mL of blood loss would represent 25% of the blood volume of a 25 kg child and only 10% of the blood volume of an adult.

Children have a unique ability to maintain adequate blood pressure in the face of significant hypovolemia (4). A drop in blood pressure is a late sign of shock in children and may, in fact, signal that the shock state is irreversible (5). It is vital for the ED personnel to recognize early signs of shock such as peripheral pallor, a widened pulse pressure, cool extremities, tachycardia, and decreased urine output and move forward to control hemorrhage at this stage.

INDICATIONS

Lacerations with hemorrhage, bleeding puncture/stab wounds, gunshot wounds, soft tissue injuries, and traumatic amputations are all indications for immediate control of hemorrhage. In fact, any time visual evidence exists of bleeding after an injury, an attempt to control hemorrhage by one of the following methods is required. These methods are presented in order from least to most risky. Obviously, the least potentially dangerous methods should be employed first and

the clinician should only proceed to other methods when these have failed. Also, attempts to control hemorrhage should begin with the child's first encounter with the health care system and as such most of these techniques should be well understood by prehospital personnel, nurses, and physicians.

PROCEDURES

Three important basic maneuvers may be employed to control bleeding. The clinician must recognize that these methods may or may not result in definitive control of bleeding in and of themselves but regardless of the extent of bleeding or the need for further repair, these methods should be attempted first.

Manual Pressure

Direct pressure with gloved fingers controls most bleeding sites as soon as it is initiated (Fig. 27.1). Using a gauze sponge to cover the site while exerting direct pressure helps to absorb the remaining bleeding and may also decrease the risk of infection. However, gauze may also obscure the wound and cause pressure to be directed in the vicinity of, but not directly on, the source of bleeding. Placement of the gauze pad is therefore critical to success. An acceptable alternative is direct pressure with a finger covered by a sterile glove (6, 7). Bleeding from the edge of a large tissue flap may be controlled by pinching the bleeding site between the thumb and the forefinger.

Control of high pressure arterial bleeding may be facilitated by using pressure proximal to the site of bleeding—so-called "pressure points" in addition to direct pressure on the bleeding site. Pressure exerted at these areas obviously serves to reduce blood flow to the site of hemorrhage. The pressure point is identified by locating the arterial pulse proximal to the site of bleeding then compressing the artery with the fingers. The ideal pressure point is an area where the artery passes in close proximity to a bone or other firm anatomic structure against which it may be compressed. It may be necessary for the clinician to palpate along the course of the artery to identify the best site at which to apply pressure (6) (Fig 27.2).

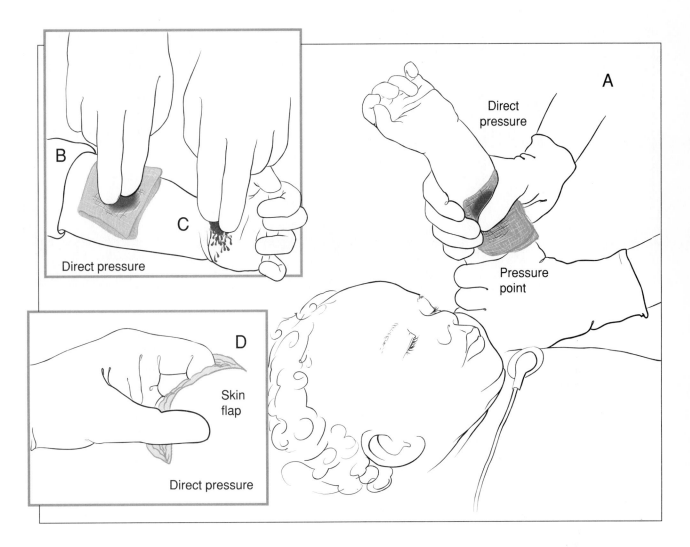

Figure 27.1.
A. Direct pressure applied to the site of bleeding is the initial maneuver in attempts to control external hemorrhage. Direct pressure may be augmented by applying pressure to a proximal "pressure point."
B. Direct pressure at the site of the injury with a sterile gauze pad used to cover the bleeding site.
C. Direct pressure at the site of injury using sterile gloved fingers.
D. Pinching a bleeding skin flap between the thumb and forefingers to control hemorrhage.

Ideally, when either of these methods is used, pressure should be initially applied for a specific period of time, usually 5 to 10 minutes. Time passes slowly when performing a monotonous activity such as holding pressure so it is best to use a timepiece to ensure that pressure is maintained for the desired duration.

Elevation of the Bleeding Area

When possible, elevation of the injured area may reduce hemorrhage by counteracting the forces of gravity. Under optimal circumstances the area should be elevated to a height above the heart. If, however, this is not possible then the bleeding site should be kept level with the rest of the body and not allowed to become dependent (6).

Pressure Bandages

Pressure bandages may be useful in two circumstances. Most commonly they are used to treat significant hemorrhage which is refractory to treatment by elevation and direct pressure alone. However, they may also be used as a temporary alternative to direct pressure when the patient has other, more severe, injuries that require the attention of all available personnel. The procedure is performed by first placing a stack of gauze pads approximately 1 inch thick directly over the site of bleeding. Then an elastic bandage is wrapped over the gauze pads tight enough to provide adequate hemostasis. Some commercial variations of pressure bandages employ a semi-rigid styrene block placed directly over the site of bleeding, which is first covered by a gauze pad. The block is then pressed and molded into the wound by an elastic overwrap (8).

**Chapter 27
Control of
Exsanguinating
External Hemorrhage**

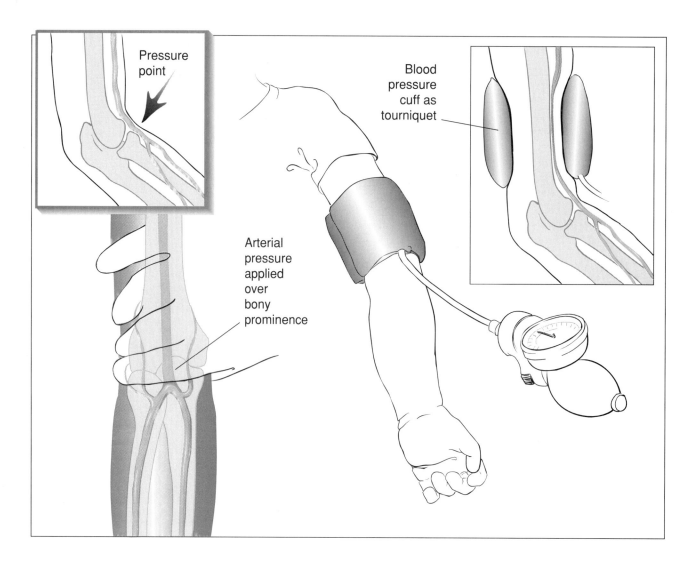

Pressure point

Blood pressure cuff as tourniquet

Arterial pressure applied over bony prominence

Figure 27.2.
Pressure may be applied proximal to a site of bleeding using either manual pressure applied at a pressure point or, in more severe cases, an inflated blood pressure cuff.

Pressure bandages do have potential complications. If wrapped too tightly, they can lead to distal ischemia; therefore, distal perfusion should be monitored frequently while the pressure bandage is in place. When a pressure bandage must be left in place for a protracted period of time (such as during a prolonged transport) then the bandage should be loosened for a few minutes every 30 minutes. Conversely, pressure bandages that are not wrapped tightly enough will not stop the bleeding and will instead allow blood to soak into the gauze pads, giving the clinicians a false sense of security and placing the child in greater jeopardy.

Tourniquets

Procedures just described should control the vast majority of cases of hemorrhage in chil-

dren. However, in extreme cases of uncontrollable hemorrhage a tourniquet may be used. This technique should be reserved for those cases in which it may be acceptable to sacrifice the injured limb in order to save the child's life. When the less extreme methods described previously have failed to control severe hemorrhage, then a tourniquet may be the only alternative and should be employed.

The easiest tourniquet is a blood pressure cuff of the appropriate size for the patient (Fig. 27.2). If two blood pressure cuffs are near the appropriate size then the smaller one should be used for this procedure. The blood pressure cuff is placed on the injured extremity proximal to the site of bleeding and inflated until the bleeding stops. This usually occurs at a pressure just higher than the child's systolic blood pressure (9). Once hemostasis has been achieved, tubing of the blood pressure cuff must be occluded to prevent leakage of air from the cuff. Occlusion is most easily accomplished by cross clamping the tubing with a hemostat.

Some commercially available tourniquets are air inflated and have valves that control air ingress and egress. Because these devices are built for this purpose they leak less frequently than do blood pressure cuffs. Commercial tourniquets are available in many hospital operating rooms where they are used to maintain a bloodless field for extremity surgery. (Tourniquets and elastic wraps may also be used for this purpose in the ED. They can facilitate exploration of wounds. In field situations any device (e.g., belt, necktie, purse strap) that can be placed circumferentially about the injured extremity and tightened to interrupt blood flow may be used as a temporary tourniquet (6).

Application of a tourniquet for control of hemorrhage (other than to facilitate wound exploration as previously described) implies that the medical team has recognized that the injured limb may be sacrificed to prevent death from exsanguination. This decision should be documented in the medical record along with the time at which the tourniquet was placed. This time should also be prominently displayed on the bed sheets or on a sticker placed on the patient. This is particularly important for patients who will be transferred but should be used for every patient on whom a tourniquet is placed. Furthermore, the condition of the extremity distal to the tourniquet should be carefully monitored and the results of this monitoring should be documented. Much like the pressure bandage described previously, when the tourniquet must be left in place for a protracted period of time, it should be loosened after 30 minutes and occasionally thereafter to ensure that it is still required. In an ED setting, it is very unlikely that a tourniquet would ever be required and in no case should a tourniquet be used in the ED for more than 1 hour.

Significant bleeding from a finger injury may be controlled by a Penrose drain or a phlebotomy tourniquet clamped tightly at the base of the finger (10). A wide tourniquet should be used because narrow rubber bands may allow too much pressure to be applied over a small surface area causing pressure necrosis at the site of application. A large clamp should be used so that the presence of a tourniquet is noted by everyone. As stated,

the time of tourniquet application should be prominently displayed on the patient or on the bed and the reasons for tourniquet use should be clearly documented in the patient's medical record. A finger tourniquet should not be left in place for more than 20 minutes in other than exceptional circumstances.

Scalp Lacerations

Scalp lacerations are common in children and most do not pose significant risk to the patient. However, the scalp is a highly vascular structure and large scalp lacerations may cause bleeding to the point of exsanguination. Furthermore, this bleeding may be underestimated because this low pressure, venous bleeding can run beneath the hair and into the child's clothing. Risk from these injuries is increased when the ED is crowded and patients with "routine" lacerations may be forced to wait a significant period of time before treatment.

When direct pressure fails to control hemorrhage from a scalp wound, hemostasis may be attempted with the application of a Penrose drain applied as a snug headband at the level of the forehead and the occiput. This device should compress the scalp vasculature enough to provide hemostasis (11, 12) (Fig. 27.3).

Bleeding from scalp lacerations also may also be controlled by injecting local anesthetic containing epinephrine into the wound edges (13). The local effect of the epinephrine combined with the pressure exerted by the suture should provide adequate hemostasis for the majority of cases. If, however, this technique fails, alternative methods to obtain hemostasis may be attempted. If a specific vessel appears to be the source of the bleeding then this vessel can be clamped with a hemostat and ligated with absorbable suture before wound closure. The vessel should be clamped under direct vision as blind clamping may cause damage to other structures.

An alternative is using a so-called "figure of eight" stitch. Absorbable suture is used and the stitch is placed proximal to the site of bleeding by one of the methods shown in Figure 27.4. This stitch compresses the tissue surrounding the bleeding vessel and tamponades the hemorrhage. Cautery and hemostatic

Figure 27.3.
A Penrose drain used to control hemorrhage from a scalp laceration.

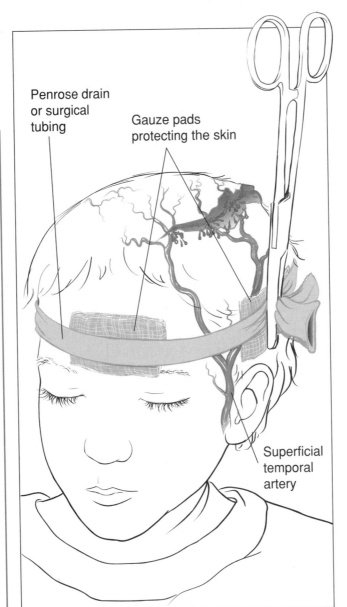

Penrose drain or surgical tubing

Gauze pads protecting the skin

Superficial temporal artery

SUMMARY

1. Perform initial screening examination aimed at identifying sources of bleeding, detecting early evidence of hypovolemia, and documenting neurovascular status of involved area.
2. Use sterile technique and universal precautions to protect both patient and staff.
3. Apply direct pressure to site of bleeding with either gloved fingers or gauze pad. This may be augmented by simultaneous application of pressure at a pressure point. Hold pressure for 5 to 10 minutes by clock.
4. While pressure is being applied, elevate involved area to a higher level than heart, if possible.
5. If direct pressure and elevation fail or if all available personnel are required to address other injuries, then apply a pressure bandage to area. Use commercial pressure dressing or stack of gauze pads approximately 1 inch thick surrounded by an elastic wrap to provide pressure. Check neurovascular status of area distal to dressing frequently after it is applied.
6. In extreme situations when a choice must be made between life and limb, a tourniquet may be used. Apply blood pressure cuff or commercial tourniquet to area proximal to site of bleeding and inflate device until bleeding

SUMMARY CONTINUED

stops. Record time that tourniquet was placed and mark in a prominent location on bed or patient. Carefully monitor neurovascular status of distal extremity subsequent to tourniquet inflation. Carefully document reasons for tourniquet use, time of inflation, and results of ongoing monitoring in medical record.
7. Under certain circumstances and in certain anatomic locations (e.g., the scalp), bleeding vessels may be clamped under direct vision and then ligated or cauterized. These procedures have potential to injure nerves and other tissues and should be used judiciously, if at all.
8. Persistent low pressure bleeding may be controlled using epinephrine soaked pads (1:1000 epinephrine), injection of lidocaine with epinephrine (1:100,000 epinephrine), and by agents such as fibrin or gel-foam applied directly on the site of bleeding.

adjuncts also may be employed for bleeding scalp vessels (see below).

Using scalp clips has been suggested to control excessive bleeding from the scalp (14). The clips are often used by neurosurgeons to obtain hemostasis of scalp vessels during craniotomies. These clips are spring loaded so that they are closed unless pressure is applied on the rear portion of the clip. The clips are placed into a special applicator. When the applicator handles are closed, the clip opens and is then applied to the wound edge. The handles are then released and the clip closes over the wound edge, compressing bleeding vessels between the upper and lower jaws of the clip. Multiple clips may be used, if needed. Exploration and irrigation of the scalp wound may be facilitated by using these devices and they can be easily removed with the applicator when no longer required (Fig. 27.5).

Large scalp lacerations may continue to bleed into the space above the galea aponeurotica even after closure. Although this bleeding is unlikely to be life-threatening, it can result in an uncomfortable and unsightly hematoma. This can be avoided by using interrupted sutures, applying a snug bandage after closure, and by applying ice to the area intermittently in the first 24 hours after wound closure.

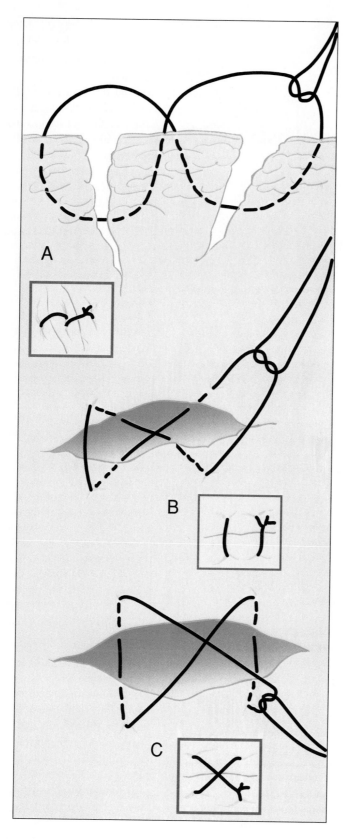

Figure 27.4.
A "figure of eight" stitch may be used to tamponade a bleeding vessel.
A. A vertical "figure of eight" stitch.
B–C. Two types of horizontal "figure of eight" stitches.

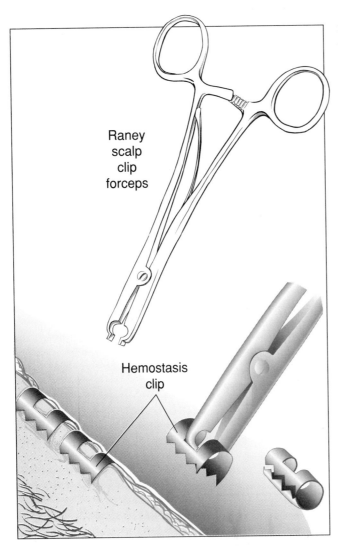

Figure 27.5.
Use of scalp clips to control hemorrhage from scalp lacerations.

Raney scalp clip forceps

Hemostasis clip

Special Situations and Procedures

Clamping Bleeding Vessels
In areas other than the scalp (i.e., the extremities) where significant bleeding has not been controlled by the basic maneuvers previously described, the clinician may be tempted to try clamping the involved vessels. This technique should be avoided if at all possible. Veins, arteries, and nerves are usually found together and blind clamping of a bleeding vessel may result in irreversible damage to the adjacent nerve.

If the clinician feels that clamping is necessary then the following method should be employed. First a tourniquet or some other source of pressure should be used to control blood flow to the area. It also may be necessary to control venous bleeding distal to the injury by wrapping the distal extremity with elastic wrap or by applying several phlebotomy tourniquets. In either case the wrap or the phlebotomy tourniquets should be applied from the distal portions of the extremity proximally and should be placed before the application of the proximal tourniquet or direct pressure aimed at controlling bleeding into the wound.

Once a bloodless field has been established, then pressure can be gradually released proximal to the injury until bleeding appears. By repeating this step as often as necessary it should be possible to identify the bleeding vessel. Once this vessel has been identified, a bloodless field should be reestablished and the vessel should be clamped under direct vision and ligated with absorbable suture. Finally, the clinician should carefully document why clamping was felt to be necessary.

Cautery
Battery-powered, disposable electrocautery units are available in most EDs and may be used to facilitate hemostasis. They are most effective when applied to vessels of less than 2 mm in diameter. As discussed for clamping and ligation, cautery should be used under direct vision. The site of bleeding should be identified and a bloodless field established. The area around the target vessel then should be dried. Finally, the cautery should be applied to the target vessel. Most of these disposable units are activated by pressing and holding a single button. When the button is released the power is turned off and the device cools. Care must be taken to avoid damaging surrounding tissues with this device.

Other Methods
A few uncommonly employed agents may be useful in certain situations and are therefore important for medical personnel to understand. First, epinephrine solution (1:1000) can be applied to gauze pads which are then placed over the wound. This solution works well to control areas of persistent low pressure bleeding particularly when a tissue bed continues to ooze blood. Care must be taken to avoid injection of this solution (lidocaine with epinephrine solution is 1:100,000 epinephrine) and to avoid using large volumes, as epinephrine can be absorbed by the

tissues and can cause clinical effects. This is particularly important in so-called "end organ" areas which are served by the most distal branches of an artery.

A safer alternative to epinephrine solution is using fibrin or gel-foam. These substances are available as a sterile powder or as small sterile strips which may be placed directly on the wound to facilitate clot formation. Like epinephrine solution they are most effective for areas of low pressure bleeding as brisk bleeding tends to dilute them and wash them out of the wound.

COMPLICATIONS

Direct pressure and pressure points, pressure bandages, and tourniquets all carry the risk of ischemia distal to the wound. Areas distal to the injury should be monitored carefully during the application of pressure particularly when tourniquets are applied. Tourniquets should be loosened after 30 minutes to determine whether or not they have been effective and to allow the distal tissues to receive some blood. Pressure, and particularly tourniquets, also carry the risk of compression of nerves. This nerve compression can result in permanent injury that may persist long after the bleeding vessel has been repaired. A carefully documented neurosensory examination and documentation of the need for the tourniquet and ongoing monitoring may be useful later, should a child be found to have sustained nerve damage after an injury.

Direct clamping of vessels and use of electrocautery may both cause injury to other nearby structures. Nerves are particularly vulnerable because of their close proximity to blood vessels. Additionally, clamps can cause crush injury which leads to devitalization of tissues and electrocautery devices may cause burns.

Solutions containing epinephrine can cause vasoconstriction of blood vessels distal to the site of injection and result in distal ischemia on this basis. Care should be taken when epinephrine is employed near areas that are supplied by distal arterial branches and have no collateral blood supply.

Any method involving direct contact with an open wound places the patient at risk for a wound infection and medical personnel at risk for contact with infected blood. Aseptic technique (Chapter 7) and universal precautions (Chapter 8) should be used at all times.

All medical personnel from prehospital providers to emergency nurses and physicians must recognize and address the early signs of hypovolemia in children and must recognize which wounds have the potential to result in significant blood loss.

SUMMARY

Control of significant hemorrhage is of primary importance in the resuscitation of trauma victims. Fortunately, most hemorrhages can be readily controlled by using simple techniques such as application of direct pressure. When bleeding is refractory to minimally invasive measures, however, health care personnel should not hesitate to emply more aggressive means of hemostasis. When these more invasive techniques are used, the reasons for use should be clearly documented. Certain special types of injuries (e.g., flaps) may be best managed using methods specifically designed for their treatment.

REFERENCES

1. American College of Surgeons Committee on Trauma. Initial assessment and management. In: Advanced trauma life support course instructor manual. Chicago: American College of Surgeons, 1989, pp. 9–24.
2. American College of Surgeons Committee on Trauma. Pediatric trauma. In: Advanced trauma life support course instructor manual. Chicago: American College of Surgeons, 1989, pp. 215–234.
3. Ludwig S, Loiselle J. Anatomy, growth, and development: impact on injury. In: Eichelberger MR, ed. Pediatric trauma, prevention, acute care, and rehabilitation. St Louis: CV Mosby, 1993, pp. 39–58.
4. Perkin RM, Levin DL. Shock in the pediatric patient. Part I. J Peds 1982;101(2):163–169.
5. American Heart Association and American Academy of Pediatrics. Recognition of respiratory failure and shock: anticipating cardiopulmonary arrest. In: Chameides L, ed. Textbook of pediatric advanced life support. Dallas: American Heart Association, 1988, pp. 3–19.
6. Boericke PH. Emergency! Part 2: first aid for open wounds, severe bleeding, shock, and closed wounds. Nursing 1975;5(3):40–46.
7. Borja AR, Lansing AM. Immediate control of intermediate vascular bleeding. Surg Gynecol Obstet 1971;132(3):494–496.
8. Safar P, Bircher NG, Yealy D. Basic and advanced

Chapter 27
Control of
Exsanguinating
External Hemorrhage

life support. In: Schwartz GR, Cayten CA, Mangelsen MA, Mayer TA, Hanke BK, eds. Principles and practice of emergency medicine. Philadelphia: Lea and Febiger, 1992, pp. 89–214.

9. Edlich RF, Rodeheaver GT. Scientific basis for wound management. Emerg Med Ann 1983;2:1.

10. Luban JD, Koeneman J, Kosar K. The digital hand tourniquet: how safe is it? J Hand Surg 1985;10(A): 664.

11. Lammers RL. Principles of wound management. In: Roberts JR, Hedges JR, eds. Clinical procedures in emergency medicine. Philadelphia: WB Saunders, 1991, pp. 515–564.

12. Barst HH. Hemostasis for head injuries (letter). Lancet 1968;153;1204.

13. Kirk RM, Williamson RCN. Introduction. In: Kirk RM, Williamson RCN, eds. General surgical operations, 2nd ed. Edinburgh: Churchill Livingstone, 1987, pp. 1–13.

14. Lemos MJ, Clark DE. Scalp lacerations resulting in hemorrhagic shock: case reports and recommended management. J Emerg Med 1988;6:377–379.

CHAPTER 28

USE OF MILITARY ANTISHOCK TROUSERS (MAST)

Sigmund J. Kharasch

INTRODUCTION

The first extensive use of antishock trousers was for field management of trauma during the Vietnam conflict. This device, also known as a pneumatic antishock garment (PASG), was the prototype of the current military antishock trousers (MAST) garment that has been widely used for the last two decades. Until recently, MAST suits were a standard component of prehospital management of hypovolemic shock. Because they are portable and relatively easy to apply, MAST suits have been widely used as a temporizing procedure by emergency medical technicians for prehospital transport of patients with hypovolemic shock.

Emergency department application of MAST suits by physicians and nurses has also been described as an adjunct to blood replacement and definitive surgical management in cases of hemorrhage. The major use of MAST suits has been in the management of hemorrhagic shock secondary to blunt or penetrating trauma. MAST suits have also been reported to be helpful in the treatment of hemorrhage from other causes including pelvic fractures, ruptured ectopic pregnancy, and aortic aneurysms. Recent controlled clinical trials, however, have raised concerns regarding the efficacy of MAST suit use in the prehospital setting. Specifically, for penetrating abdominal injuries with short emergency medical service response times, MAST suits were not associated with improved survival.

For thoracic injury (including cardiac and major thoracic vascular), MAST suit application may actually increase mortality (1, 2).

In view of this information, the 1993 Advanced Trauma Life Support course sponsored by the American College of Surgeons acknowledged that "the efficacy of PASG in-hospital or in the rural setting remains unproven, and in the urban prehospital setting, controversial" (3). Accordingly, the criteria for MAST suit application have been revised by the American College of Surgeons (see Indications in this chapter). Although most studies have been performed on adult trauma victims, MAST suits are available in pediatric sizes and have been used in pediatric trauma victims (4).

ANATOMY AND PHYSIOLOGY

Previous studies suggested that the beneficial effect of MAST suits was mainly the result of an autotransfusion of 750 to 2000 mL of blood from regions covered by the trousers to the upper body. More recent work has demonstrated only a 4 mL/kg autotransfusion effect from antishock trouser inflation (5). It appears most likely that inflation of MAST suits elevates blood pressure by increasing total peripheral resistance rather than by augmenting cardiac output via autotransfusion (6). By decreasing the diameter of blood vessels under the suit, MAST suit inflation temporarily improves coronary and cerebral blood flow.

Another function of MAST suits is that of causing hemostasis in vessels under the garment (7), which is especially important in unstable pelvic fractures. By elevating the pressure surrounding these vessels, both the transmural pressure and the radius of the vessels are decreased. The smaller vessel radius decreases both blood flow through the vessel and the circumferential tension. As circumferential tension decreases, tears in a vessel are minimized and clot formation encouraged. MAST suits have three potential advantages in the treatment of pelvic fractures: (a) they compress the pelvic area and tamponade venous and small arterial bleeding as described previously, (b) they immobilize pelvic fractures, and (c) they may reduce bony displacement and improve pelvic bone alignment (8).

INDICATIONS

There are no absolute indications for use of the pneumatic antishock garment. Certain circumstances exist, however, under which this device may be useful. The MAST suit was originally designed to support failing circulation and it may still be used for this purpose, either as an adjunct to volume infusion or when adequate circulatory access cannot be obtained. Additionally, the pneumatic antishock garment can be used as a splint for lower extremity fractures and to tamponade intraabdominal bleeding. Currently, however, the MAST suit is most useful in the management of unstable pelvic fractures with continuing hemorrhage. When properly applied to a pelvic fracture the suit serves to both stabilize the fracture and to control hemorrhage.

Before the MAST suit is employed, the contraindications to its use must be clearly understood. Only three absolute contraindications to the use of the MAST suit exist. These are (a) the presence of frank pulmonary edema, because the increased peripheral vascular resistance and increased intraabdominal pressure will exacerbate this condition; (b) injury to the diaphragm, because

the increased intraabdominal pressure may force abdominal contents into the thoracic cavity; and (c) uncontrolled hemorrhage in any portion of the body not covered by the garment, because the increased vascular resistance will make this bleeding worse. The pneumatic antishock garment may also be harmful to patients who have significant myocardial dysfunction. The MAST suit is relatively contraindicated in patients who have abdominal evisceration and in those who have objects impaled in the abdomen. Finally, the device is relatively contraindicated in pregnancy. If it is applied to a pregnant woman, only the leg portions should be inflated.

EQUIPMENT

The MAST suit (trade name) consists of a pair of trousers with three inflatable bladders held in place by velcro fasteners or zippers. The suit consists of three components: two legs and an abdominal portion, each of which can be inflated separately. The pants are incomplete in that the perineum is left uncovered. The suit is usually inflated through a foot pump and has pressure gauges or pop-off valves (set at 104 mm Hg) to regulate the pressures generated. MAST suits are also available for pediatric patients (Pedi-MAST, David Clark, Inc.). In the pediatric MAST suit (Fig. 28.1), the level of pressure is determined by positive-end expiratory pressure valves placed in the system.

PROCEDURE

Inflation of MAST Suits

The abdomen, pelvis, and legs should be examined before placement of the MAST suit because further evaluation will be difficult once the suit is applied. If the patient's pants are left on, the pockets should be searched and any contents removed as these might puncture the suit or cause pressure injury

Figure 28.1.
Procedure for inflation of pneumatic antishock garment.

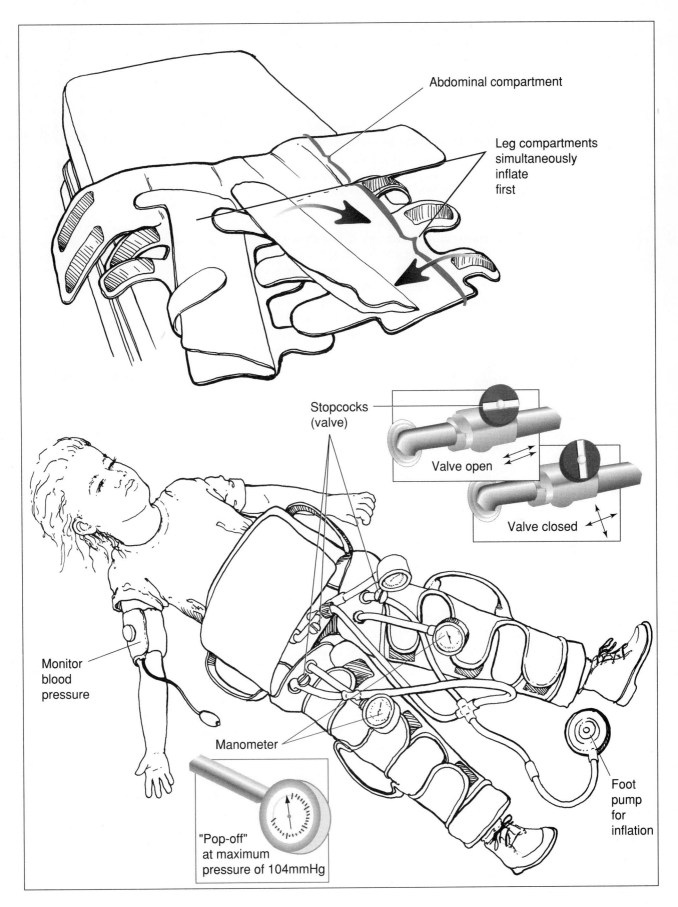

Abdominal compartment

Leg compartments
simultaneously
inflate
first

Stopcocks
(valve)

Valve open

Valve closed

Monitor
blood
pressure

Manometer

"Pop-off"
at maximum
pressure of 104mmHg

Foot
pump
for
inflation

once the suit is inflated. Grossly angulated fractures should be reduced, if possible.

The patient is then placed on the open suit so that it extends from the ankles to the lower border of the lateral rib cage. If suspicion of a cervical spine injury exists, the MAST suit should be slid underneath the patient and standard cervical spine precautions should be taken. The garment should then be snugly fastened with the velcro closures or by zippering closed the separate leg and abdominal compartments.

The hose is connected from the foot pump to the three compartments. Stopcocks to the compartments to be inflated should be opened and those to all other compartments should be closed. The leg portions are inflated first and the abdominal section last.

The compartments are inflated using the foot pump (Fig. 28.1). If a gauge is available, inflation to an initial pressure of 30 to 40 mm Hg is reasonable (10). Higher inflation pressures may be required in severely hypotensive patients. In children, it is usually not necessary to inflate the MAST suit above 50 mm Hg. Blood pressure should be checked frequently. Inflation of the MAST suit can be continued in stepwise increments until systolic blood pressure is adequate for age. When inflation is completed, stopcocks should be closed and pump tubing disconnected. The patient's clinical status must be monitored closely as leakage from the suit can occur.

Deflation of MAST Suits

The abdominal section should be deflated first to avoid a tourniquet effect around the abdomen. Deflation should be a slow, careful procedure accomplished with repeated monitoring of the patient (Fig. 28.2).

Deflation is begun by releasing a small amount of air from the stopcock in the abdominal section. The patient's blood pressure is then checked. If the blood pressure has decreased 5 mm Hg or more, infusion of fluids should be continued until the blood pressure has been restored. If the blood pressure is stable, deflation can be continued in small increments, rechecking the blood pressure after each deflation. After complete deflation of the abdominal portion, the leg compartments can be deflated in a similar stepwise fashion.

SUMMARY

Inflation of MAST Suit:
1. Examine abdomen, pelvis, and legs before placement of MAST suit since further evaluation will be difficult once suit is applied.
2. Place patient on open suit so that it extends from ankles to lower border of lateral rib cage. Fasten snugly with velcro closures or zippers.
3. Attach hose from foot pump to three compartments (Fig. 28.1). Inflate the leg portions first and the abdominal section last. Inflate to initial pressures of 30 to 40 mm Hg (higher pressures may be required in severely hypotensive patients).
4. Check BP frequently. Continue inflation until BP is adequate for age. Close stopcocks and disconnect pump tubing when inflation is complete.

Deflation of MAST Suit:
1. Deflate abdominal section first. Release small amount of air from stopcock in abdominal compartment. Deflation should be a slow, careful procedure accomplished with repeated monitoring.
2. Check patient's BP. If BP has decreased 5 mm Hg or more, continue infusion of fluids until blood pressure has been restored.
3. If BP is stable, continue deflation in small increments, rechecking BP after each deflation. After complete deflation of abdominal portion, leg compartments can be deflated in a similar stepwise fashion.

COMPLICATIONS

Several potential complications of MAST suit inflation exist, the most common of which are:

1. Compartment syndrome (particularly with prolonged inflation of the leg compartments in the patient in shock with extremity trauma).

2. Respiratory distress. If respiratory distress develops after inflation of the abdominal compartment, diaphragmatic rupture should be assumed and the abdominal component deflated. Respiratory distress as a result of decreased diaphragmatic excursion produced by increased intraabdominal pressure within the abdominal compartment is rare with appropriate inflation pressures, but can occur in young children.

3. Hypotension (sudden falls in BP can occur with rapid deflation or deflation before adequate volume replacement).

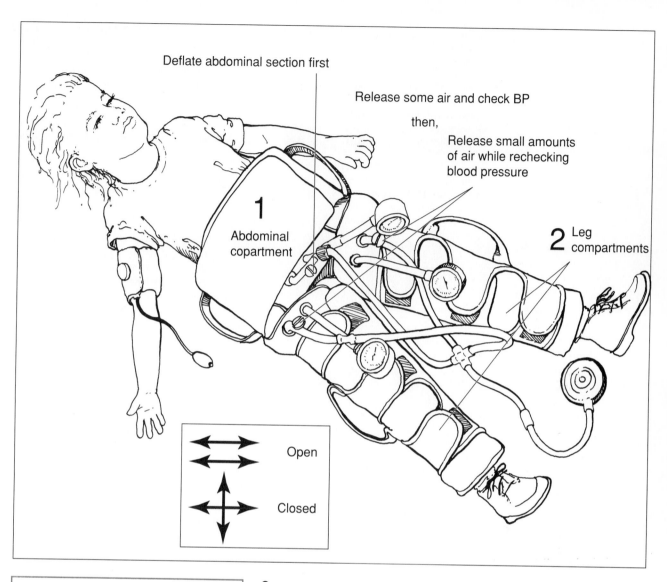

Deflate abdominal section first

Release some air and check BP

then,

Release small amounts
of air while rechecking
blood pressure

1 Abdominal copartment

2 Leg compartments

Open

Closed

CLINICAL TIPS

1. The use of MAST suits must not delay volume replacement or rapid transport.
2. Prolonged inflation of the leg components of the MAST suit can result in compartment syndrome, particularly in the patient in shock with extremity trauma.
3. Inflate the leg compartments first and abdominal segment last.
4. The deflation process is gradual, beginning with the abdominal segment. Air is allowed to escape slowly, while blood pressure is closely monitored. A fall in systolic blood pressure of more than 5 mm Hg is an indication for more fluid resuscitation before continued deflation.
5. If inflation of the abdominal compartment results in respiratory distress, diaphragmatic rupture must be assumed and the abdominal compartment must be deflated (regardless of the patient's blood pressure).
6. In general, if the patient requires transfer to another facility, the garment is left in situ, inflated or deflated as indicated.

SUMMARY

Application of MAST suits can raise systolic pressure by increasing peripheral vascular resistance and myocardial afterload. Primary indications for MAST suit use are currently for hemorrhagic shock associated with intraabdominal trauma and unstable pelvic fractures. Further studies are needed to evaluate the efficacy of MAST suit use in the blunt trauma victim and in the setting of prolonged transports.

REFERENCES

1. Bickell WH, Pepe PE, Bailey ML, et al. Randomized trial of pneumatic antishock garments in the prehospital management of penetrating abdominal injuries. Ann Emerg Med 1987;16:653–658.
2. Mattox KL, Bickell W, Pepe PE, et al. Prospective

Figure 28.2.
Procedure for deflation of pneumatic antishock garment.

mast study in 911 patients. J Trauma 1989;29:
1104–1110.

3. American College of Surgeons. Advanced trauma
life support (ATLS) course. Chicago: American
College of Surgeons Committee on Trauma, 1993,
pp. 89–90.

4. Brunette DD, Fifield F, Ruiz E. Use of pneumatic
antishock trousers in the management of pediatric
pelvic fractures. Pediatr Emerg Care 1987;3:86.

5. Niemann JT, Stapczynski JS, Rosborough P, et al.
Hemodynamic effects of pneumatic external coun-
terpressure in canine hemorrhagic shock. Ann
Emerg Med 1983;12:661–667.

6. Wangensteen SL, Ludewig RM, Eddy DM. The effect of external counterpressure on the intact circulation. Surg Gynecol Obstet 1968;27:253–258.

7. McSwain NE. Pneumatic antishock garment: state
of the art 1988. Ann Emerg Med 1988;17:506–525.

8. Mucha P, Welch TJ. Hemorrhage in major pelvic
fractures. Surg Clin North Am 1988;68:757.

9. Moritz ZM, Templeton JM. Major trauma. In:
Fleisher GR, Ludwig S, eds. Textbook of pediatric
emergency medicine, 3rd ed. Baltimore: Williams &
Wilkins, 1993.

10. Kaback KR, Sanders AB, Meislin HW. MAST suit
update. JAMA 1984;9:2598–2603.

CHAPTER 29

MANAGEMENT OF OPEN CHEST WOUNDS

Richard M. Cantor

INTRODUCTION

Open chest wounds are those that violate the integrity of the chest wall, creating a communication between the pleural cavity and the outlying atmosphere. In common parlance, such wounds are often referred to as "sucking" wounds because air entry during inspiration may be audible as to and fro movement of air through the wound occurs during each phase of respiration. Open chest wounds represent true traumatic emergencies. They may prove fatal if untreated or cared for improperly. The majority of patients who present with open chest wounds will necessitate, after ED stabilization, admission to the hospital for close observation.

Open chest wounds have, throughout the literature, been traditionally reported and investigated during periods of war and combat (1). With the acceleration of urban violence within our country today, however, the emergency physician will often be presented with a child who is the victim of penetrating trauma secondary to assault with firearms or knives. Importantly, although far less common, open chest wounds also may present after blunt pediatric trauma (2). Regardless of the etiology, all open chest wounds should be considered significant trauma because the probability of accompanying cardiothoracic damage is high.

ANATOMY AND PHYSIOLOGY

Any communicating wound of the chest will permit free air to violate the relative vacuum of the pleural space. During inspiration, intrathoracic pressure will rise, causing the ipsilateral lung to collapse. If air is allowed to collect under tension, a shift of all mediastinal structures will occur toward the uninjured pleural segment, preventing the contralateral lung from attaining full expansion. Most importantly, as intrathoracic pressure rises, a diminution of the normal airway pressure gradient is seen which is present within the thoracic cavity. This results in a severe reduction of both ventilatory volume and tidal volume (Fig. 29.1).

In cases when the defect is in the chest wall, which is larger than the glottic aperture, a greater degree of air may enter the thorax through the wound than by the usual mechanisms, causing a "competition" for space between the tidal volume of air and air that enters the defect itself. Concomitant chest wall pain and ineffective cough mechanisms will further impair ventilatory efforts.

As work of breathing increases, expiration is forced, causing the intrathoracic pressure to rise above atmospheric pressure. The lung on the injured side will migrate paradoxically, because its volume is increased during expiration. Gas entry will preferentially be di-

Figure 29.1.
Physiologic effects of an
untreated open chest
wound.

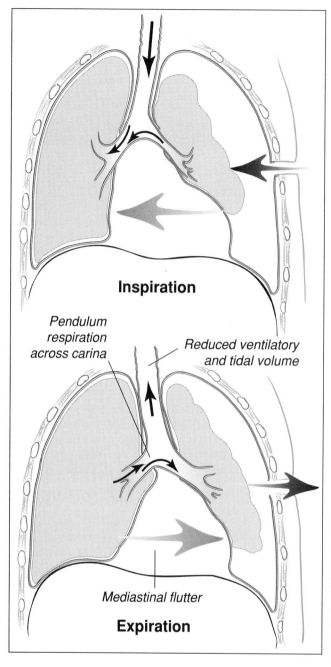

Inspiration

Pendulum
respiration
across carina

Reduced ventilatory
and tidal volume

Mediastinal flutter

Expiration

also greatly affected by the presence of elevated intrathoracic pressure. A reduction in the venous pressure gradient into the thorax compromises venous return. As hypoxemia progresses, pulmonary vascular resistance increases, compromising pulmonary blood flow. As circulatory embarrassment continues, cardiac output and systemic mean arterial pressure will progressively fail. If untreated, metabolic acidosis, shock, and death often result.

Functional anatomy and physiology of the pediatric thorax possesses characteristics that favor the development of intrapulmonary catastrophes in the setting of an open chest wound (3). Children have a more compliant chest wall secondary to a lesser degree of bony ossification when compared to adults. It is intuitive, therefore, that serious intrathoracic injury may be present in the absence of obvious external chest wall injury. The degree of mediastinal flutter is more pronounced in the child because these structures are more mobile, predisposing the pediatric patient to further compromise from tracheal angulation. The absence of anastomotic channels which allow collateral ventilation in the pediatric lung favors the development of atelectasis and interstitial emphysema.

rected from contralateral to ipsilateral lung across the carina, commonly referred to as pendulum respiration. The net effect is the creation of large amounts of intrapulmonary dead space. As the pressure gradient across the mediastinum falls, a shift of all structures occurs back toward the uninjured side. This to and fro motion of the mediastinum is often called mediastinal flutter. Secondary physiologic effects include hypoxia, respiratory acidosis, and eventually shock.

Central and peripheral circulation are

Treatment of open chest wounds is directed at correcting the pathophysiology of thoracic injury (4). Expansion of the lung on the injured side is assisted by the provision of positive intrapulmonary pressure. Containment of the chest wall defect will restore the integrity of the intrathoracic vacuum. Ventilatory volume will increase with pulmonary expansion of both the ipsilateral and contralateral lungs. Respiratory dead space will decrease as well. As pulmonary vascular resistance decreases, pulmonary blood flow will improve, resulting in better air entry in general to the lung and decreasing the vasoconstrictive effects of hypoxemia on the pulmonary vasculature. Restoration of intrathoracic negative pressure will improve both the airway gradient and the tidal volume, resulting in a greater return of blood to the right heart and an increase in cardiac output.

INDICATIONS

Whenever a patient presents either to the ED or in the prehospital phase of care with an open chest wound, treatment is mandatory. In many cases, this treatment will involve placement of a thoracostomy tube (Chapter 30). However, when definitive treatment cannot be instituted immediately, the wound then should be treated as described later in this chapter (see Procedure). Often a patient will have an obvious injury to the chest wall but without direct evidence of penetration of the thoracic cavity. Treatment in this case depends both on treatment environment and on patient condition. In the prehospital environment, the patient should be assumed to have an open chest wound and should be treated accordingly. In the ED, however, stable patients may undergo diagnostic procedures before treatment.

In many EDs initial treatment of an open chest wound will most adequately be performed by an emergency physician or pediatric emergency specialist. As in the prehospital environment, this procedure will be performed by emergency medical technicians, paramedics, or by specialized flight nurses or transport nurses. Depending on institutional protocol, chest tube insertion may be performed by ancillary subspecialist personnel as well. Essentially no contraindications exist pertinent to the treatment of an open chest wound because it most often represents a ventilatory emergency.

EQUIPMENT

Equipment needed for the ED treatment of open chest wounds in children is essentially directed at the two-part approach recommended for definitive therapy. The first phase of treatment involves closure of the chest wall defect itself. The equipment necessary for this initial closure is listed in Table 29.1. The second phase of definitive therapy involves placement of a thoracostomy tube to facilitate resolution of any collection of free air or blood within the thoracic space (5, 6). This technique is discussed in Chapter 30.

The clinician must continually monitor vital signs during the performance of any and all procedures relative to the correction of an open chest wound. Recommended equipment includes cardiac monitoring, a continuous readout with mean arterial blood pressure, and pulse oximetry. Level of consciousness, and respiratory rate and effort should be assessed on an ongoing basis throughout the procedure.

PROCEDURE

In cases of severe respiratory compromise, most patients will benefit by providing positive pressure ventilation. Awake patients may, if capable, be able to provide forcible Valsalva maneuvers during the application of the closure dressing. In patients whose level of consciousness or degree of respiratory sufficiency are inadequate, definitive provision of positive pressure by endotracheal intubation and mechanical ventilation will often be necessary (see Chapter 16).

While positive pressure and pulmonary expansion are maintained, a dressing of multiple layers (three to four) of petroleum gauze should be placed over several layers of dry gauze to cover the chest wall defect. The clinician should cleanse the skin surrounding the dressing with povidone-iodine, after which the site should be allowed to dry. To facilitate adequate adhesion, tincture of benzoin should be applied around the perimeter of the dressing itself. The dressing should be placed with the dry gauze contacting the skin and should be secured on three sides only, leaving the superior margin open (Fig. 29.2). This will allow the escape of intrapleural gas through the wound which facilitates drainage of a tension pneumothorax if it develops. At this point, it is prudent to obtain a chest film to further assess any

Table 29.1.
Equipment Required for Closure of Chest Wall Defect

Betadine solution
Sterile gloves
Vaseline-saturated gauze
Sterile gauze
Tincture of benzoin
Adhesive tape

SUMMARY
1. Monitor and assess patient for oxygenation and ventilation.
2. Provide bag-valve-mask or mechanical ventilation as indicated.
3. Prepare area under sterile precautions.
4. Apply petroleum gauze over dry gauze to chest wall defect.
5. Under adequate adhesion, close all but superior side of dressing sufficiently.
6. Obtain chest radiograph to assess residual intrapulmonary blood or free air.

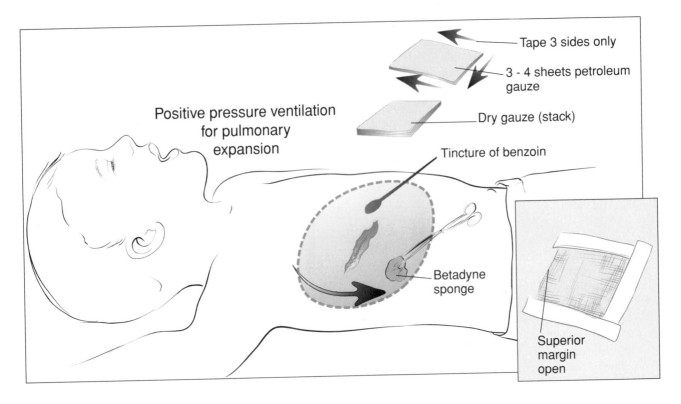

Positive pressure ventilation
for pulmonary
expansion

Tape 3 sides only

3 - 4 sheets petroleum
gauze

Dry gauze (stack)

Tincture of benzoin

Betadyne
sponge

Superior
margin
open

Figure 29.2.
Technique for temporary,
emergency treatment of
an open chest wound.

residual air or blood which may remain within the pleural cavity itself.

COMPLICATIONS

The most significant complication associated with the treatment of open chest wounds occurs when the chest wall defect is closed completely with a dressing and then a significant period of time is allowed to elapse before the placement of a thoracostomy tube. In these circumstances a tension pneumothorax may develop. Therefore, unless the relatively immediate placement of a chest tube is anticipated it is important to close chest wall defects on three sides only. This allows accumulated air within the thoracic cavity to be expelled while minimizing the ingress of air from outside the chest.

Patient monitoring remains the cornerstone of management after the dressing has been placed. It is possible for the open side of the three-sided dressing to become adherent to the chest wall by clotted blood or misplaced benzoin, thus converting the three-sided dressing into a four-sided dressing. As long as the dressing remains in place before the chest tube is placed, the patient should be carefully observed for signs of clinical deterioration.

The clinician must be aware of the secondary development of tension pneumothoraces in patients with open chest wounds. It is inappropriate, therefore, to utilize catheters of insufficient size in treating these patients. Large catheters are often indicated to ensure continued pulmonary expansion.

SUMMARY

Open chest wounds represent true surgical emergencies. Patients who present to the ED with penetrating trauma, or in rare situations, blunt trauma, should be continuously monitored for ventilatory sufficiency. Adequate closure of the chest wall defect will often temporize the further collection of free air within the chest wall cavity. Immediate tube thoracostomy will facilitate correction of any extraneous intrapleural collections of air or blood which may take place in these traumatized patients. Appropriate attention to ongoing monitoring of vital signs, complications of the procedure itself, and assessment for further injuries will help facilitate a favorable outcome in most patients.

REFERENCES

1. Graham BA. Open pneumothorax: its relation to the treatment of empyema; war medicine. Am J Med Sci 1918;156:839.
2. Beaver BL. Pediatric thoracic trauma. Sem Thor Card Surg 1992;4:255–262.
3. Helafer MA. Developmental physiology of the respiratory system. In: Rogers MC, ed. Textbook of pediatric intensive care. 2nd ed. Baltimore: Williams & Wilkins, 1992:104–133.
4. Collins JC. Occult traumatic pneumothorax: immediate tube thoracostomy versus expectant management. Am Surg 1992;58:743–746.
5. Frumkin K. Tube thoracostomy. In: Roberts JR, Hedges JR, eds. Clinical procedures in emergency medicine. 2nd ed. Philadelphia: WB Saunders, 1985, pp. 128–149.
6. Templeton JM. Thoracic trauma. In: Fleischer GR, Ludwig S, eds. Textbook of pediatric emergency medicine. 3rd ed. Baltimore: Williams & Wilkins, 1993, pp. 1336–1360.

Tube Thoracostomy and Needle Decompression of the Chest

Kathleen M. Connors and Thomas E. Terndrup

INTRODUCTION

Tube thoracostomy and needle decompression of the chest are procedures that are used to drain abnormal collections of air or fluid from the thoracic cavity. These are bedside procedures which can be performed rapidly for children in extremis or in a semi-elective fashion for less urgent circumstances while in the emergency department (ED). These procedures are a vital part of the skills required to be performed by practitioners caring for children in the ED. A related procedure, thoracentesis, is discussed in Chapter 83.

Hippocrates was the first to describe entering the pleural space with a metal tube to drain "bad humors" (1). Playfair in 1875 (2) and Hewitt in 1876 (3) described closed chest tube drainage with a tube and an underwater seal. The technique of tube thoracostomy, however, was not widely used until 1917 when it became useful in treating postinfluenza empyema (4). During World War II, tube thoracostomy gained widespread use for the treatment of traumatic hemopneumothorax and empyema. It is now used commonly to treat many types of pleural collections.

A pneumothorax is an abnormal collection of air in the pleural space. When air becomes trapped in the pleural space at pressures greater than atmospheric, a tension pneumothorax has developed. The abnormal collection may contain blood (i.e., hemothorax), blood and air (i.e., hemopneumothorax) or other fluids, generally referred to as pleural effusions (e.g., purulent material or empyema). Pleural air in direct connection with the atmosphere is termed an open pneumothorax. These wounds may be intermittently closed and opened depending on the relative pressures of the atmosphere and the thoracic cavity. An open pneumothorax with ingress of air is sometimes called a "sucking" chest wound.

The importance of these abnormal collections in the pleural space is that they can interfere with respiratory and cardiovascular function. Drainage of the collection by tube thoracostomy can restore cardiorespiratory functions, and may be life-saving. However, not all pleural collections require thoracostomy. Some pleural collections, particularly smaller ones, can be managed by observation alone. In other patients, a needle or catheter aspiration of the collection may alleviate the problem or may temporarily correct the problem.

These procedures are most commonly done in the ED or in the ICU setting by an emergency physician, neonatologist, intensivist, or surgeon. In some areas emergency medical technicians may perform chest decompression during prehospital care. In areas where subspecialty care is not readily available, pediatricians and family practitioners

Chapter 30
Tube Thoracostomy
and Needle
Decompression
of the Chest

389

may be called on to manage a pneumothorax in a child. Needle aspiration of a pneumothorax and tube thoracostomy are relatively simple procedures that can be performed by any of these caregivers.

ANATOMY AND PHYSIOLOGY

The thorax is normally completely filled by lung parenchyma and mediastinal structures. The pleura is a serous membrane consisting of a parietal layer lining the chest wall and a thinner visceral layer covering the lung, diaphragm, mediastinum, and interlobar fissures. The two layers meet at the lung hilum to form the pleural sac. A thin layer of serous fluid in the pleural space serves to lubricate the lungs during the respiratory cycle and maintain contact between the two pleural surfaces. Elastic recoil of the chest wall and lung assists in binding the lung to the chest wall, preventing their separation during subatmospheric pressures generated during spontaneous inspiration. Air or blood may enter the pleural space due to direct trauma to the lung parenchyma, chest wall, thoracic vessels, or other mediastinal structures. In the absence of trauma, a pneumothorax may result from rupture of an alveolus secondary to abrupt increases in intrathoracic or interalveolar pressures against a closed glottis, particularly in cystic lung tissue. Rarely, tears or rupture of the esophagus may produce a pneumothorax or pneumomediastinum.

A variety of abnormal pleural collections can occur in patients (Fig. 30.1). In a simple pneumothorax (Fig. 30.1.A), air in the pleural space allows the lung to lose contact with the chest wall and collapse. As a result, the collapsed lung tissue becomes unavailable to participate in gas exchange and a ventilation-perfusion (VQ) mismatch may develop. A tension pneumothorax is present when the air accumulated in the pleural space is under supraatmospheric pressures (Fig. 30.1.B). This occurs when direct communication exists between the large airways or lung parenchyma and the pleural space. The communication allows air to enter the pleural space without an adequate means of exit, often via a ball-valve mechanism. A tension pneumothorax may shift the mediastinum and interfere with cardiac inflow by "kinking" the vena cava or increased resistance to blood flow, leading to decreased cardiac filling pressures, hypotension, and shock.

Hemothorax results from intrathoracic hemorrhage. This bleeding is usually from the heart, lungs, great vessels or their branches, intercostal arteries or veins, diaphragm, or chest wall vessels. Air and blood present simultaneously in the pleural space create a hemopneumothorax (Fig. 30.1.C). Penetrating trauma that produces a loss of a portion of the chest wall with a direct opening into the thoracic cavity may cause an open pneumothorax with ingress of air (Fig. 30.1.D). An immediate equilibration occurs of intrathoracic and atmospheric pressures. If the opening in the chest wall is of a larger diameter than the airway, air preferentially passes in and out of the chest defect with each respiratory effort, resulting in reduced ventilation of the lung. A to and fro movement of the mediastinum also may occur, and an associated reduction in venous return. Complete sealing of an open pneumothorax may produce a tension pneumothorax (see Chapter 29).

Unique aspects of the physiology and anatomy of the thorax exist in childhood that are relevant to the pathophysiology and management of pneumothoraces. Children have a more compliant, less ossified chest wall which results in a reduced incidence of rib fractures. However, serious intrathoracic injury may be present in the absence of obvious, external signs of chest wall injury. The mediastinum of the child is more mobile, thus cardiovascular and ventilatory compromise from tracheal angulation can occur because of excessive mediastinal shifting (5). During the first 5 years of life the distal airways are relatively narrow creating increased peripheral airway resistance (6). This increase in pulmonary resistance requires greater peak inspiratory pressure during mechanical ventilation, increasing the risk for barotrauma. The infant lung lacks the anatomic channels that allow for collateral ventilation in older children and adults. Without these pathways, infants and young children are at increased risk for atelectasis and emphysematous changes (6). Changes in pulmonary physiology that occur during and immediately after birth cause newborns to have a greater incidence of pneumothorax than any other age group (7). With the first breath, the transpulmonary pressure rises from 40 to as much as

Chapter 30
Tube Thoracostomy
and Needle
Decompression
of the Chest

390

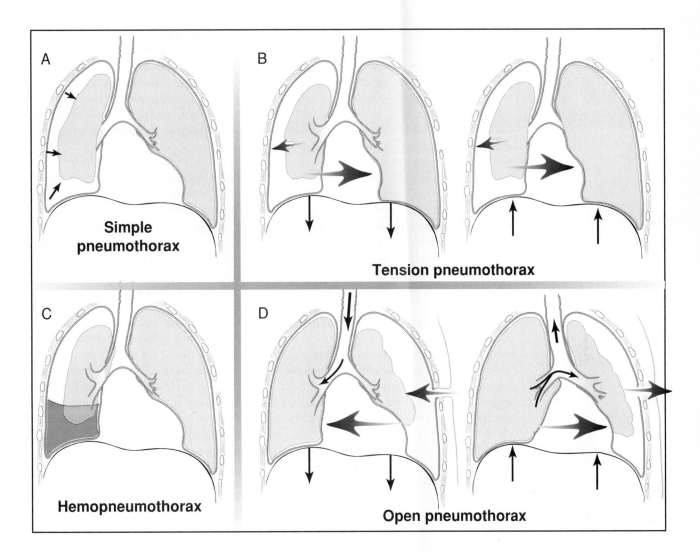

A
Simple
pneumothorax

B
Tension pneumothorax

C
Hemopneumothorax

D
Open pneumothorax

100 cm H_2O. Compression of the chest during vaginal delivery places the diaphragm and the muscles of respiration at a marked mechanical disadvantage because of shortening of the respiratory muscles. In addition, mechanical obstruction of some alveoli can occur following aspiration of amniotic fluid or meconium. Transmission of increased transpulmonary pressures to the alveoli can lead to overdistension, rupture of the alveoli, and development of a pneumothorax (7, 8, 9).

INDICATIONS

Management of an abnormal pleural collection depends on several factors: (*a*) the etiology and size of the lesion, (*b*) the general condition of the patient, (*c*) associated problems, (*d*) the need for patient transport, and (*e*) the need for mechanical ventilation or general

anesthesia. A tension pneumothorax is a life-threatening condition that should be treated immediately with needle decompression. The goal of needle decompression is to rapidly relieve cardiovascular complications of tension pneumothorax by converting it to a simple pneumothorax. Following needle decompression, these patients require tube thoracostomy in order to allow continuous drainage of the pleural space and prevent recurrence of the tension pneumothorax. The most common cause of tension pneumothorax is positive pressure ventilation. Other causes include bronchial injury, major parenchymal trauma, inadvertently sealing a sucking chest wound, or as a complication of a spontaneous pneumothorax.

In contrast to patients with a tension pneumothorax, patients with a simple pneumothorax are often asymptomatic. Spontaneous pneumothoraces, either pri-

Figure 30.1.
A. Simple pneumothorax.
B. Tension pneumothorax in inspiration (left) and expiration (right). Note the shift of the mediastinal structures to the left.
C. Hemopneumothorax.
D. Open pneumothorax ("sucking" chest wound) in inspiration (left) and in expiration (right). Note that the lung is more expanded in expiration.

Chapter 30
Tube Thoracostomy
and Needle
Decompression
of the Chest

mary (without underlying lung disease), or secondary (with underlying lung disease), are often asymptomatic in children. Some iatrogenic pneumothoraces also may be asymptomatic. Patients undergoing central line placement may develop pneumothoraces that are usually immediately evident on a chest radiograph, which are more likely to be asymptomatic than those with a delayed presentation (10). Patients with small traumatic pneumothoraces, particularly those with occult posttraumatic pneumothoraces (i.e., pneumothoraces apparent on CT scans, but not on plain radiographs) may also be asymptomatic (11, 12).

In adult patients, substantial support exists for the conservative management of simple, asymptomatic pneumothoraces. Observation alone is recommended when: (*a*) the patient is otherwise healthy, (*b*) the pneumothorax is unilateral and small, and (*c*) the patient is not likely to require positive pressure ventilation, general anesthesia, or a lengthy transport. Currently no published studies support this observational approach in children.

Opinions about exactly what constitutes a small pneumothorax vary, but is generally believed to be less than 10 to 20% of the thoracic cavity volume (13–17). Several methods exist for measuring the volume of a pneumothorax based on its radiographic appearance. Unfortunately, estimates of the size of a pneumothorax are neither accurate nor reproducible (16). Rhea has determined that a single measurement, the average intrapleural distance, accurately determines pneumothorax size (18). A nomogram derived from this data predicts the percentage of pneumothorax to thoracic cavity better than a best radiologic guess estimate (Fig 30.2). A method for estimating the size of an occult pneumothorax based on a CT scan has also been proposed (19), but has not been substantiated.

The literature also supports management of clinically stable adult patients with a larger, simple pneumothorax by catheter aspiration. Although this literature does not include pediatric patients, this procedure is performed on children. This procedure may sometimes be done in lieu of a tube thoracostomy. When used appropriately, catheter aspiration has several advantages over tube thoracostomy. It is simpler to perform, less traumatic, leaves a smaller scar, and gener-

ally results in less patient discomfort (10, 20, 21). Small catheter aspiration also permits a greater degree of patient mobility (22). In adults, successful outpatient management of a simple pneumothorax using small catheter drainage has been described (23, 24). Many spontaneous or iatrogenic pneumothoraces can be managed in this fashion. Victims of minor chest trauma may also be candidates for this procedure. However, those with tension pneumothorax, hemothorax, persistent air leak, hemodynamic instability, or serious associated injuries requiring surgery are not candidates for this procedure and should receive conventional tube thoracostomy. Underlying lung pathology is also a relative contraindication for this procedure.

Tube thoracostomy is indicated for any abnormal pleural collection that will require continuous drainage for some period of time. Recurrent pleural effusions, empyema, and chylothorax should all be managed with tube thoracostomy. A tube thoracostomy also may be indicated as a prophylactic procedure in patients with evidence of significant chest trauma (e.g., pulmonary contusion or subcutaneous emphysema) without detectable pneumothoraces who will be undergoing prolonged transports, general anesthesia, or mechanical ventilation. Such patients are at high risk for developing a tension pneumothorax when subjected to positive airway pressures.

Hemothoraces or hemopneumothoraces large enough to interfere with respiratory function require drainage with tube thoracostomy. Tube thoracostomy also may be indicated in patients with hemothorax to monitor the rate of hemorrhage or to prevent the formation of a fibrothorax. Early administration of blood components is recommended for patients with massive hemothorax before evacuation is begun. The hemothorax may be functioning to tamponade an otherwise briskly bleeding vessel, and marked hypotension can result if a tube thoracostomy is performed without adequate fluid resuscitation (18, 25). A number of commercial devices are available for the collection, filtration, anticoagulation, and autotransfusion of blood obtained by tube thoracostomy. Autotransfusion is further discussed in Chapter 31.

Chapter 30
Tube Thoracostomy
and Needle
Decompression
of the Chest

392

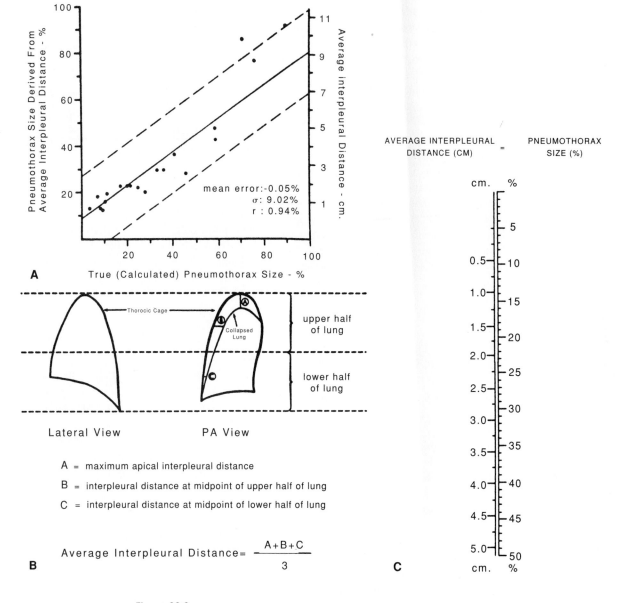

Figure 30.2.
Calculation of percent pneumothorax using the average interpleural distance method.
The number obtained from the calculation on the left (**B**) can be used to obtain a percentage from the nomogram on the right (**C**) (From Rhea JT, Deluca SA, Greene RE. Determining the size of pneumothorax in the upright patient. Radiology 1982;144:733. Reproduced with permission of the Radiological Society of North America, Inc.)

Open pneumothoraces most commonly result from penetrating trauma. In young children, penetrating chest trauma is far less common than blunt trauma in most areas of the country. However, some urban areas report an increasing frequency of penetrating thoracoabdominal injuries in children. Because of the potential for the development of an open pneumothorax with ingress of air, open chest wounds require immediate treatment to allow ventilation of the lung (see Chapter 29).

No absolute contraindications exist to closed tube thoracostomy. The presence of either a hemorrhagic diathesis or a dermatologic disorder is a relative contraindication. However, chest tube drainage is often performed as a life-saving procedure and therefore such relative contraindications are outweighed. If a patient does have a coagulopathy or other complicating factor, at-

Table 30.1.
Other Materials Required for Tube Thoracostomy

Betadine solution
Sterile gloves
Vaseline impregnated gauze
Tape
Lidocaine
Suture apparatus
Drainage apparatus
Adaptors/tubing
Chest tube (appropriate size)*

* See Table 3

Table 30.2.
Tube Thoracostomy Tray

Curved Kelly clamps
Scalpels (#11 and #15 blades)
Sterile basin
Needle holder
Suture scissors
Syringe and needles for infiltration
of local anesthetic
Sterile drapes
Sterile gauze/sponges

tempts should be made to correct or at least improve the disorder, before thoracentesis or tube thoracostomy is performed. The site of insertion can often be moved to avoid problematic skin lesions. Other relative contraindications include multiple adhesions or blebs, recurrent pneumothoraces mandating surgical treatment, massive hemothorax without adequate volume replacement, and the need for an immediate open thoracotomy.

Consultants in cardiopulmonary surgery, trauma surgery, and neonatology may be required when difficulty with tube thoracostomy placement or elective conditions for tube placement exist. Most commonly, cardiopulmonary surgeons are required for significant volumes of tube thoracostomy drainage.

EQUIPMENT

Needle Decompression

Equipment needed for needle decompression depends on the specific technique to be used (see Procedure). At a minimum, a needle and syringe are required, although for evacuation of abnormal pleural collections, a catheter should be inserted once the pleural space is entered with a needle. Commercial kits for both the modified Seldinger and trocar catheter insertion techniques are available. Alternatives for the modified Seldinger technique include a through-the-needle catheter, an intravenous catheter, or a trauma catheter. Alternatives for the trocar insertion method include a through-the-needle catheter, or a needle with a trocar threaded through an intravenous catheter. Additional equipment required for site preparation and anesthesia is similar to that listed for tube thoracostomy (Table 30.1).

Tube Thoracostomy

Most institutions have a prepared tray containing the instruments necessary for tube thoracostomy. The contents of a typical tray are listed (Table 30.2), whereas other supplies often necessary for performing a tube thoracostomy are listed separately (Table 30.1). When time allows, all equipment should be assembled and inspected before be-

Table 30.3.
Chest Tube Size*

Age (50th percentile weight)	Tube Size (French)
Preemie (1–2.5 kg)	10–14
Neonate (2.5–4.0 kg)	12–18
6 mo (6–8 kg)	14–20
1–2 yr (10–12 kg)	14–24
5 yr (16–18 kg)	20–32
8–10 yr (24–30 kg)	28–38

* Adapted from Textbook of Pediatric Advanced Life Support

ginning the procedure. Size of the chest tubes and needles will vary with the patient's age and type of collection to be drained. Larger tubes are required to drain blood or pus than to drain air. Appropriate sizes of chest tubes for different age children are estimated (Table 30.3). The most commonly used tubes (Argyle®, Sherwood Medical, St. Louis, MO) are clear plastic, straight tubes with a series of holes at one end and a radiopaque stripe. Other types of tubes that have been used include Mallinckrodt® (PPI Inc., Irvine, CA) and Foley catheters. Plastic tubes are thought to be superior to rubber because they are less antigenic (15).

In addition to the equipment needed for insertion of the tube, adequate lighting, monitoring equipment, and adequate personnel are required. A continuous readout cardiac monitor and pulse oximetry should be used. Intermittent monitoring of respiratory rate and effort, arterial blood pressure, and level of consciousness also should be performed routinely.

PROCEDURE

Conservative Management

If it has been decided to manage the patient conservatively (without drainage of the collection), an observation period in the hospital is recommended (13). Depending on the amount of air, rate of the air leak, and the condition of the lung parenchyma, the normal pleural blood flow reabsorbs the air at about 1.25% per day and allows the lung to reexpand (26). Supplementary oxygen increases the rate of absorption by as much as sixfold (27). Follow-up radiographs should be done to monitor the progression of the collection.

Needle Decompression of a Tension Pneumothorax

If a tension pneumothorax is suspected, emergency needle decompression is required. This procedure should not be delayed by obtaining a confirmatory chest radiograph. In the emergent situation, using sedation is precluded by time constraints. Restraining the patient may be necessary if he or she is awake and uncooperative. The patient should be placed in the supine position with the head of the bed elevated 30° if possible. The recommended puncture site to relieve a tension pneumothorax in a supine patient is the 2nd intercostal space in the midclavicular line, as free pleural air will normally rise to the anterior upper chest (Fig. 30.3). In a tension pneumothorax, however, the collapsed lung is moved away from the entire ipsilateral chest wall, making a lateral approach possible if the anterior chest is obscured.

The insertion site is swabbed rapidly with antiseptic. If time permits, local anesthesia is appropriate when decompressing a tension pneumothorax. A needle or over-the-needle catheter (usually an angiocatheter) is attached to a 5 to 10 mL syringe also if time permits. Inserting a needle without a syringe or other drainage device in a patient without a pneumothorax may actually create a pneumothorax. The third rib is identified by palpitation. The needle is inserted perpendicularly in the midclavicular line over the upper edge of the rib and "walked" over the superior aspect of the rib into the lower portion of the 2nd intercostal space. If a syringe is attached it should be gently aspirated as the needle is advanced. A loss of resistance and a rush of air will be heard or felt as the pleural space is entered and pressurized air is evacuated. If an over-the-needle catheter is being used, it is advanced over the needle into the pleural space and then removed. If a syringe is attached to the needle, the pressure of the exiting air may drive the plunger down the barrel without manually withdrawing it. If no syringe is attached, a rush of air exiting the chest may be heard in both inspiration and expiration. If a pneumothorax is confirmed, a one-way drainage device should be attached. A marked improvement in the patient's degree of respiratory distress and hemodynamic status will be noted when a tension pneu-

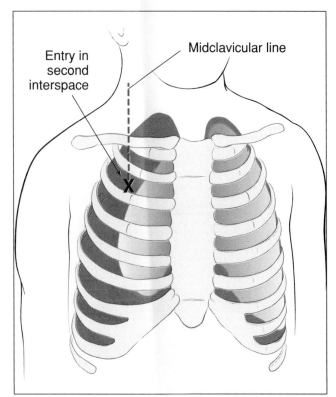

mothorax is decompressed. A tube thoracostomy should then be performed as soon as possible in these patients.

Catheter Aspiration

For smaller catheter aspiration of a pleural collection, the patient is positioned and prepped in the same manner as for tube thoracostomy (see next section). Lidocaine is infiltrated along the planned path of the catheter as is described in the next section. The catheter itself is inserted by using either the trocar or the modified Seldinger technique. For trocar, or through the cannula, making a small incision with a No. 11 blade can ease entry of the catheter assembly. If a small catheter is used, however, it may be possible to insert the assembly without an incision (Fig. 30.4.A, B). Neither method requires the dissecting of soft tissue. A Z-track method (Fig. 30.5) can be used to avoid inadvertent entry of air into the pleural space during removal of the catheter. While the skin is being retracted the catheter assembly is advanced over the superior portion of the anesthetized rib and through the parietal pleura (Fig. 30.4.B). The clinician will feel decreased resistance once

Figure 30.3.
Site for evacuation of a tension pneumothorax: 2nd interspace, midclavicular line.

Chapter 30
Tube Thoracostomy
and Needle
Decompression
of the Chest

395

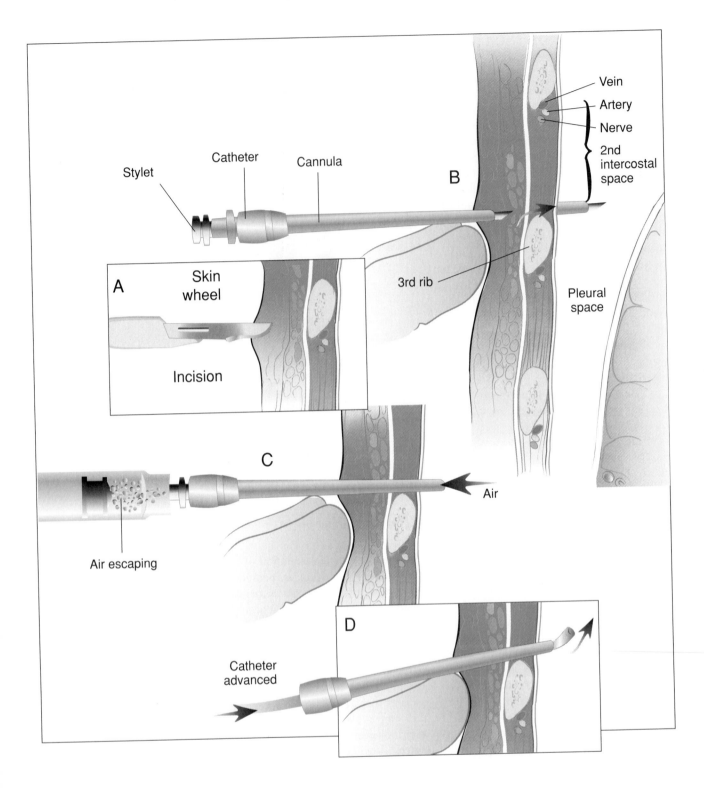

Figure 30.4.
Aspiration of a pneumothorax using the trocar method for catheter aspiration.
A. An incision is made in the skin at the proposed insertion site.
B. The catheter assembly is advanced while the skin is being retracted inferiorly.
C. Aspiration of air confirms pleural drainage.
D. The catheter is slid forward through the cannula into the pleural space.

Chapter 30
Tube Thoracostomy
and Needle
Decompression
of the Chest

396

the assembly enters the pleural space. At this point, the stylet is removed and a syringe attached to the proximal end of the assembly. Aspiration of air confirms placement in the pleural space (Fig. 30.4.C).

Once the assembly is known to be in the pleural space, the catheter should be slid forward slightly while the cannula is held in place (Fig. 30.4.D). If necessary the cannula can be used to guide the catheter apically. The syringe is then detached and the cannula is withdrawn and a two-way stopcock is attached to the proximal end of the catheter. A large, locking syringe is then attached to the stopcock, and the air is manually withdrawn.

In the modified Seldinger technique for small catheter aspiration, a needle attached to a syringe is advanced over the superior margin of the selected rib (Fig. 30.6). Gentle negative pressure on the plunger should be maintained while advancing the needle. When the needle enters the pleural space, air will be aspirated into the syringe (Fig. 30.6.A). It may be helpful to use a partially saline-filled syringe to detect air bubbles. A *J*-tipped guide wire is then inserted through the needle and the needle is withdrawn (Fig. 30.6.B). After a small incision is made with a No. 11 blade (Fig. 30.6.C), a catheter is threaded over the guide wire into the pleural space. The guide wire is then removed. As outlined, a stopcock is added to the catheter and the air is manually removed. (Note: This technique also has been adapted for the placement of larger diameter chest tubes. In order to do this it is usually necessary to pass a series of increasingly larger dilators over the guide wire before passing the chest tube. These steps are shown in Fig. 30.6.D and E)

Once the catheter is in place, air is withdrawn through the syringe until the clinician feels mild resistance. If air cannot be aspirated it may help to have the patient sit upright and cough or take a deep breath. When no additional air can be aspirated a chest radiograph should be obtained to confirm reexpansion of the lung. These patients will need to be followed up to ensure that the collection does not reaccumulate. This usually involves admission to the hospital and serial chest radiographs. Outpatient management after observation in the ED has been described in adults, but not in children. A stepwise process for managing these adult patients has also been described (23).

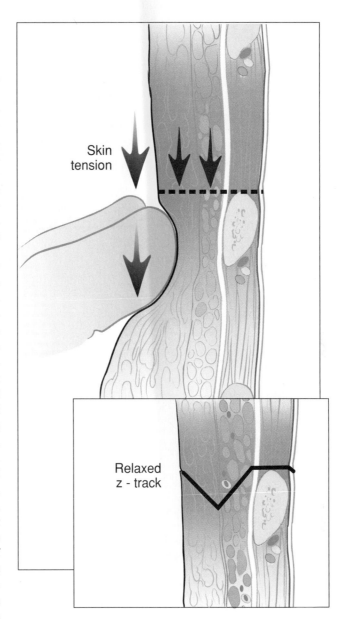

Tube Thoracostomy

Following is a description of standard, ideal technique for placing a chest tube by the blunt dissection method. The patient's clinical condition and the available resources may necessitate modifications of the technique. If the patient is hemodynamically stable and alert, sedation and analgesia should be given. Narcotics and benzodiazepines in appropriate doses are used most commonly. The patient should then be properly positioned. Positioning will depend on the site chosen for insertion of the tube. The site utilized for tube insertion varies with the clinical condition of

Figure 30.5.
Z-track method for insertion of a needle or catheter. Before the catheter is advanced, the patient's skin and subcutaneous tissues are stretched 1 to 2 cm inferior to the proposed point of insertion. This tension is maintained while the needle or catheter is inserted and advanced. Once the tension is released and the needle or catheter is removed, the tract will be discontinuous through the tissue planes.

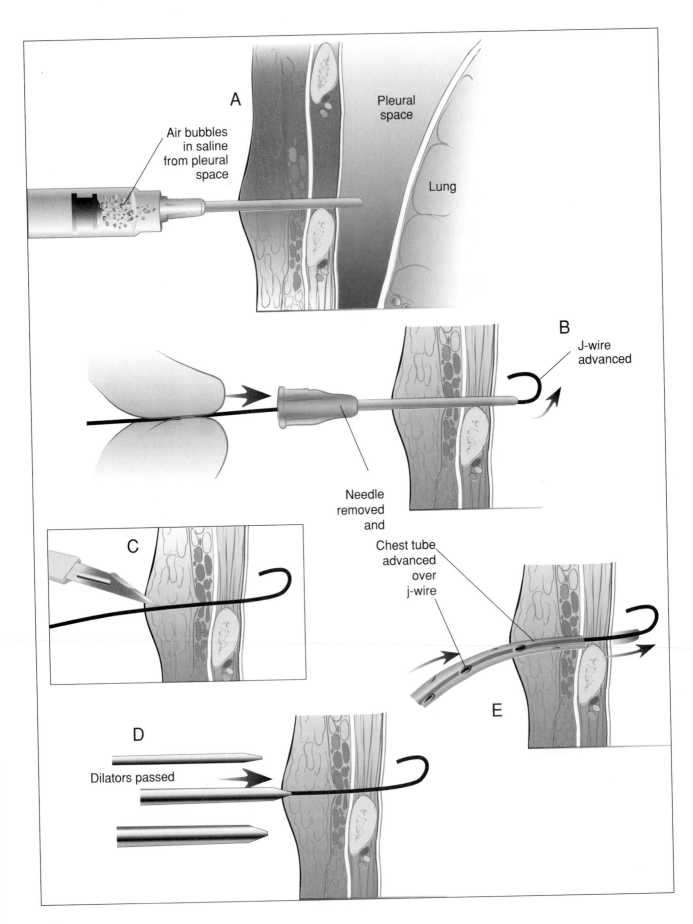

398

the patient and the experience and preferences of the clinician.

Commonly proposed insertion sites are illustrated (Fig. 30.7). The 2nd intercostal space, midclavicular line is the classic site for placing a tube intended to evacuate air alone. However, this site has disadvantages. The penetration of muscle and breast tissue is more difficult to avoid from this position and a cosmetically unappealing scar may result. The evacuation of air or fluid is believed by many to be less effective from this site. Most experts now suggest using a midaxillary approach for draining all collections (13, 14), because it is cosmetically preferable and better tolerated by the patient (13). Most also recommend using the 4th or 5th intercostal space for standard chest tube placement in the ED (13, 14, 17, 28, 29). However, use of the 3rd intercostal space in newborns also has been recommended (8). If an anterior site is to be used then the patient should be supine and restrained with the ipsilateral arm extended over the head. If a midaxillary site is to be used, the patient may be placed on the decubitus position with the involved side elevated, supported by towels or pillows, and with the arm flexed over the head and secured. Stable, older, and more cooperative children may sit straddling a chair. Stable infants may be held by an assistant in the burping position (30).

After the clinician has gowned and gloved, the insertion site should be swabbed with antiseptic and a sterile field prepared with drapes. Local anesthetic (1% lidocaine or equivalent) should then be used to raise a skin wheel. The wheel should be located in the skin one interspace below the planned insertion site. The tunneling over the next rib that this requires is believed to provide a better seal against air leaks, both while the tube is in place and after its removal (i.e. prevention of fistulas). A larger needle should then be used to anesthetize the subcutaneous tis-

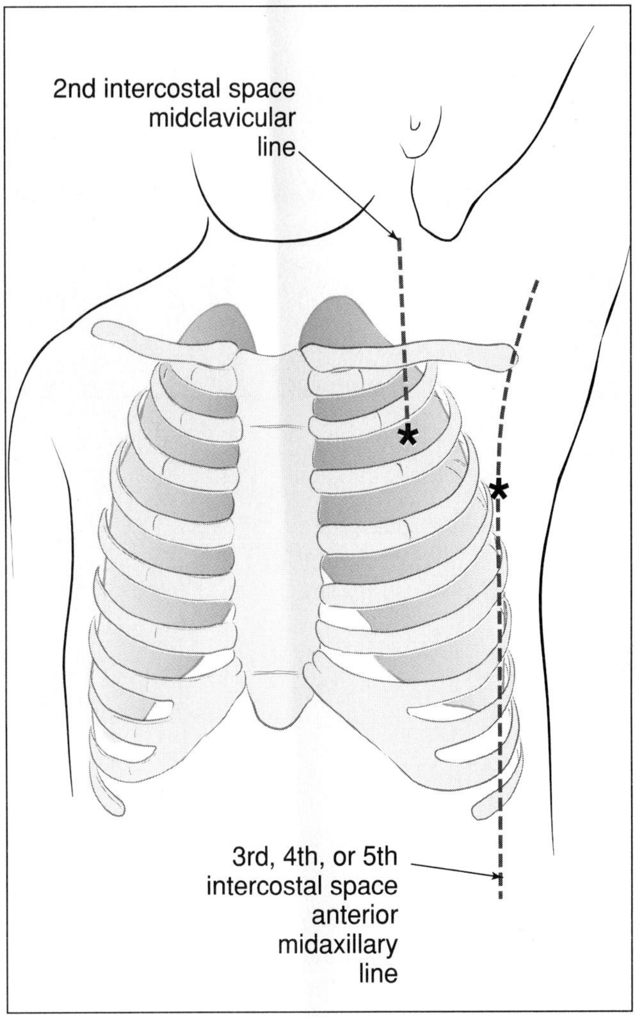

Figure 30.7.
Possible sites for chest tube placement.

sue and the muscle, overlying the rib (Fig. 30.8). The needle is advanced slowly and lidocaine infiltration is alternated with aspiration to confirm that the needle is not in a blood vessel or in the pleural space. When the superior aspect of the rib is reached, the periosteum is infiltrated. The needle is then advanced over the rib into the pleural space. Entry into the pleural space will be indicated by a loss of resistance and easy aspiration of either fluid or air. The needle is then withdrawn

---

Figure 30.6.
Modified Seldinger technique for catheter aspiration of a pneumothorax.
A. A needle attached to a partially saline-filled syringe is advanced over the rib at the proposed site of insertion. Air is aspirated when the needle is in the pleural space.
B. A J-tipped guide wire is advanced through the needle into the pleural space.
C. A catheter is advanced over the guide wire into the pleural space.
D. The operator may also use progressively larger dilators to allow **(E)** insertion of a small chest tube.

Chapter 30
Tube Thoracostomy
and Needle
Decompression
of the Chest

399

Figure 30.8.
Anesthesia for
thoracostomy or catheter
aspiration of a
pneumothorax.

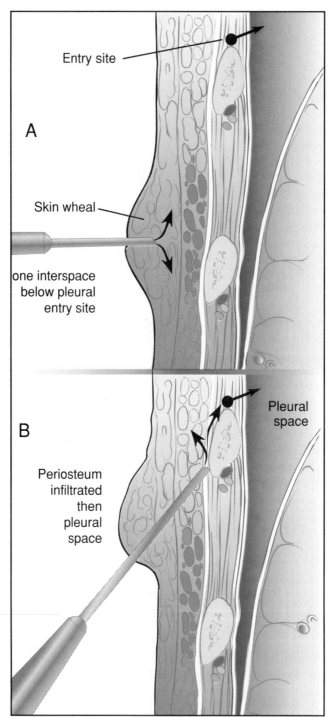

Entry site

A

Skin wheal

one interspace
below pleural
entry site

B

Pleural
space

Periosteum
infiltrated
then
pleural
space

slowly while aspirating the syringe until no fluid or air is returned. At this point lidocaine should be injected to anesthetize the pleural space where the tube will be placed. The clinician should be careful not to exceed 5 mg/kg of total lidocaine in order to avoid systemic toxicity.

Once local anesthesia is sufficient, the clinician makes an incision with a scalpel through the skin and subcutaneous tissue at the site of the skin wheal (Fig. 30.9.A). The incision should be made through the subcutaneous tissue to the level of the skeletal muscle. Length of the incision should vary with the size of the child and the size of the chest tube to be placed. In an infant or a small child a 0.5 to 1 cm incision will be adequate. In a larger child or adolescent, a 2 to 4 cm incision may be needed. Next, a closed curved clamp or hemostat is inserted in the incision and blunt dissection is performed through an opening and closing motion of the clamp. The clinician should dissect through the muscle and fascial layers to the upper surface of the lower rib (Fig. 30.9.B). Care must be taken to avoid the neurovascular structures located on the inferior margin of the upper rib. Proper position is confirmed by palpating the bone with the instrument. The tip of the

Figure 30.9.
Blunt dissection technique for thoracostomy.
A. Incision is made one interspace inferior to proposed point of thoracostomy tube insertion.
B. Blunt dissection through the subcutaneous tissue using a clamp.
C. Clamp spread after entering pleural space.
D. Probing finger inserted to confirm pleural placement and to identify the diaphragm and any adhesions.
E-F. Chest tube grasped with clamp and inserted with the finger as a guide.
G. Tube sutured firmly in place.

Chapter 30
Tube Thoracostomy
and Needle
Decompression
of the Chest

400

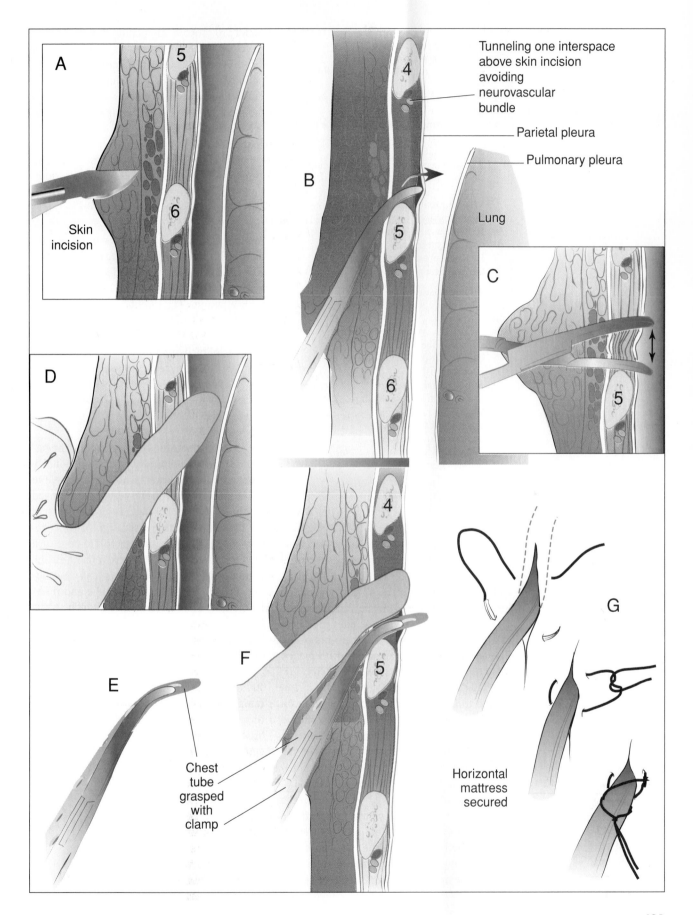

A

Skin
incision

5

6

B

Tunneling one interspace
above skin incision
avoiding
neurovascular
bundle

Parietal pleura

Pulmonary pleura

Lung

4

5

6

C

5

D

E

F

Chest
tube
grasped
with
clamp

4

5

G

Horizontal
mattress
secured

SUMMARY

Needle Decompression

1. Assemble equipment and assign duties to personnel.
2. Explain procedure and obtain consent (as indicated).
3. Position patient, and prepare and anesthetize (as time allows) skin and subcutaneous structures.
4. Advance needle over superior aspect of rib while maintaining negative pressure in syringe.
5. When air return, advance catheter into pleural cavity.
6. Remove needle, attach three-way stopcock and large syringe.
7. Evacuate pneumothorax.
8. Obtain chest radiograph.

Tube Thoracostomy

Steps 1–3 above, but sterile preparation and drape area.

4. Incise skin over rib below interspace of intended tube placement.
5. Bluntly dissect subcutaneously and superiorly.
6. Enter pleural space with clamp tips closed and confirm location by exploration with finger.
7. Insert chest tube directing tube superiorly and posteriorly.
8. Attach to water seal and suction.
9. Secure chest tube with suture, gauze, and tape.
10. Obtain chest radiograph.

clamp is then slid over the superior rib margin, and with firm but controlled pressure, the remaining intercostal muscles and parietal pleura are punctured. A "pop" or sudden loss of resistance should be felt when the pleural is punctured with the clamp. A rush of air or fluid may also occur at this point. The tip of the clamp should not be placed more than 1 cm into the thoracic cavity.

Tips of the clamp should then be spread widely to ensure a large enough opening in the pleura (Fig. 30.9.C). The clamp should then be withdrawn and if the patient is large enough, a finger should be placed into the pleural space to confirm placement and to strip any adhesions between the lung and parietal pleura (Fig. 30.9.D). The chest tube is then inserted into the pleural space. If the patient is too small to allow a finger to pass through the incision site, the tube can be inserted through the tips of the open, curved clamp. The tips of the clamp should be spread

widely to provide an opening through the intercostal muscles and pleura that is at least 1.5 to 2 cm in diameter. Alternatively, if the patient is large enough the chest tube may be grasped with a curved clamp and inserted into the pleural space by guiding it with the probing finger that has been left in the pleural space (Fig. 30.9.E, F).

Direction of insertion of the chest tube depends on the type of collection. For fluid, including blood, a posterior-superior direction is recommended, while an anterior-superior direction is used for air. Regardless of direction, the chest tube should be inserted until all the side holes are within the pleural space. The chest tube is then connected to a drainage system (see below) and the tube is secured with a suture (Fig. 30.9.G). Sterile vaseline gauze is applied over the skin site and the chest tube, and the tube is securely taped. Many clinicians recommend a purse-string-like suture be placed around the chest tube where it enters the chest wall (13, 15). This suture may then serve both to secure the tube and to close the incision when the tube is removed.

After successful tube placement, the patient's cardiorespiratory status usually shows an improvement. This is most notable in the patients who were very compromised by the pleural collection. Improvements in oxygenation and decreased signs of respiratory distress may be noted. In the case of a tension pneumothorax improvement in the patient's hemodynamic status may also occur. Proper placement of the tube and relief of the abnormal collection should be verified by a chest radiograph as soon as possible. Most patients will require serial radiographs to follow the resolution of the pleural collection and to detect a recurrence. Any sudden change in the patient's cardiorespiratory status should be considered to be the recurrence of the collection until proven otherwise. Patients receiving mechanical ventilation are especially at risk for recurrence of the original collection or the development of a new pneumothorax.

Alternative Techniques

Blunt dissection as described previously is the technique commonly recommended by

Chapter 30
Tube Thoracostomy
and Needle
Decompression
of the Chest

402

various authorities on chest tube placement (13, 14, 15, 28, 29). A technique that uses a metal trocar to puncture the pleura is used by some practitioners. Trocar usage has been reported to have a higher incidence of lung and large vessel trauma (13, 4), and a higher incidence of bronchopleural fistula (15).

Small pigtail catheters (6.0 to 8.5 French) have been used successfully in children to drain pneumothoraces (31, 32). This method of pleural drainage is thought to be less traumatic than conventional chest tube placement. It also uses a modified Seldinger technique as described previously for catheter aspiration. After penetrating the pleural space with a 16- to 18-gauge needle attached to a syringe, a wire is passed through the needle into the pleural space and the needle withdrawn. A small scalpel blade is used to pierce the skin adjacent to the guide wire. Dilators may then be passed over the wire to create a larger opening. The pigtail catheter is then threaded over the guide wire until all of the side holes are well within the chest. The wire is then removed. The curve of the pigtail catheter is thought to protect against parenchymal lung injury. The catheter should be secured to the chest wall and connected to a drainage system. Proper placement should be confirmed by chest radiograph. Commercial chest tube kits utilizing the Selding technique are available (Fig. 30.6).

Drainage Systems

All chest tubes will require some type of drainage system. A chest tube left open to atmosphere in a spontaneously breathing patient allows air to enter the pleural space. If the nonpatient end of the tube is placed underwater at a level below the patient's chest, any positive interpleural pressure (e.g., tension pneumothorax) will still be allowed to escape (visualized as bubbles in the water seal), while not allowing air to enter. Any open container with liquid will accomplish this and may be used when no suitable closed system is available.

Because an open container is impractical in anything but an emergency situation, a bottle or closed container with an opening to atmosphere should be used whenever possible (Fig. 30.10.A). Fluid in this bottle should be kept at a depth of 2 to 3 cm H_2O, which is commonly known as a water seal system. A single bottle system will work unless the clinician is draining fluid from the pleural space. In that case, fluid will build up in the bottle, causing the pressure of the water seal system to rise. Any air that subsequently collects in the pleural space will have to overcome a higher pressure (i.e., greater than the height of the fluid in the bottle) to escape. A tension pneumothorax may develop if excess fluid collects in this fashion. The solution to this problem is to add a second bottle to the setup that will allow fluid to collect while still providing an escape for intrapleural air under pressure (Fig. 30.10.B).

In order to improve or increase the rate of drainage of fluid or air it is useful to apply suction to the chest tube. Connecting the tube directly to a wall suction device is dangerous as the pressure generated may injure lung parenchyma and pleura. Adding a third bottle to the above mentioned system can help to avoid this problem. The third bottle is connected to the water seal bottle and filled to a level corresponding to the desired level of suction (usually 15 to 20 cm H_2O). The venting tube (to atmosphere) thus ensures that any suction applied that is greater than the set level will entrain air from outside the bottle (Fig. 30.10.C). Several commercially available plastic chest tube drainage units are equivalent to the three-bottle system (Fig. 30.10.D).

In certain clinical situations a flutter or Heimlich valve may be used in lieu of a water seal drainage system, which is a one-way valve that allows air to exit from the pleural space but prevents reentry during inhalation. It therefore allows the patient's normal respirations to decompress the pneumothorax. A commercially available Heimlich valve is distributed by Bard-Parker (Fig. 30.10.E). Its use in patients with asymptomatic, small, self-limited, simple pneumothoraces has been well described in adults (33, 34, 35). The valve will flutter during exhalation as long as it is in contact with pleural air. Cessation of fluttering indicates either resolution of the pneumothorax or obstruction of the valve. If resolution of the pneumothorax is confirmed by physical examination and a radiograph, the valve may be removed. The ad-

Chapter 30
Tube Thoracostomy
and Needle
Decompression
of the Chest

403

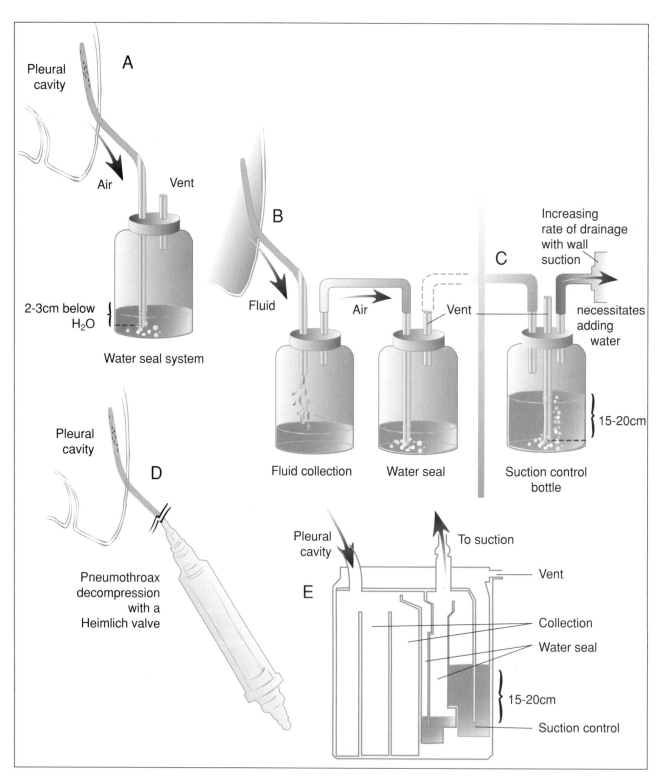

Figure 30.10.
Drainage systems.
A. Single bottle system.
B. Two-bottle system for fluid collection.
C. Three-bottle system allowing fluid collection and regulated suction.
D. The Heimlich valve chest drainage system.
E. Commercially available three-bottle system.

Within the figure:

Pleural cavity

A

Air   Vent

2-3cm below
H₂O

Water seal system

B

Fluid   Air   Vent

Fluid collection   Water seal

C

Increasing
rate of drainage
with wall
suction

necessitates
adding
water

15-20cm

Suction control
bottle

Pleural
cavity

D

Pneumothroax
decompression
with a
Heimlich valve

Pleural
cavity   To suction

E   Vent

Collection

Water seal

15-20cm

Suction control

Chapter 30
Tube Thoracostomy
and Needle
Decompression
of the Chest

404

vantages of this device are that it is small and thus does not limit patient mobility and that it is less expensive than commercially available chest drainage units (34). Disadvantages of this system include the inability to detect a new or progressive pleural air leak, and that it is easily obstructed by serous fluid or blood.

COMPLICATIONS

Complications of tube thoracostomy may occur during penetration of the pleural cavity, during placement of the tube, or after tube placement. Complications that can occur during dissection include damage to the thoracic nerve and intercostal arteries. Damage to the thoracic nerve can result in a winged scapula (36). This can usually be avoided by using only blunt dissection after the skin incision is performed. Injury to the intercostal nerve may also occur and usually results in continued pain or numbness at the thoracostomy site. Excessive bleeding as a result of damage to the intercostal arteries can also occur. Injury to these structures may be prevented by dissecting closely to the superior portion of the rib to avoid the neurovascular bundle on the inferior margin of the ribs.

Complications that can occur during placement of the tube include excessive bleeding secondary to vessel damage and damage to intrathoracic or intraabdominal organs. Penetration of the pulmonary artery, vein, and thoracic aorta can occur. Intercostal artery bleeding can be avoided by placing the tube just superior to the rib and avoiding the inferior margin of the rib above with its underlying neurovascular bundle. Organs that may be perforated by the tube during insertion include the lung, heart, diaphragm, liver, stomach, and spleen (36). The technique of chest tube insertion has been shown to influence the incidence of organ perforation. The trocar insertion method is associated with a much higher incidence (37, 38). When using the blunt dissection technique the tube should pass easily and not be forced through the soft tissue tract or pleural space. Using a finger to explore the dissection tract may help to minimize the risk of diaphragm penetration or other tube misplacement. It is important to remember that on forceful expiration the diaphragm may come up as high as the 4th intercostal space. Abdominal penetration during tube thoracostomy secondary to hemidiaphragm paralysis has been reported (39). A high-lying diaphragm may also be associated with previous thoracotomy, intraabdominal injuries, and the supine position. If a high-lying diaphragm is suspected from the chest radiograph or other clinical information, sitting the patient upright to shift the abdominal contents and diaphragm inferiorly reduces the possibility of injury.

Other complications appear to occur without regard to method of placement, but are directly related to tube location after placement. If the tube is inserted into the subcutaneous tissue or the wrong pleural space the procedure will have to be repeated, causing undue pain and delaying treatment. A tube inserted too far will press against the parietal pleura or thoracic structures, resulting in pain and injury. Cardiogenic shock secondary to right atrial compression can occur (40). Horner syndrome secondary to pressure on the inferior cervical ganglion as a complication of chest tube placement as well as of a tension pneumothorax itself have been described (41, 42). A tube not inserted far enough may cause an air leak and subcutaneous emphysema, if the last hole is outside the pleural space.

Complications may also occur after placement of the tube. A properly placed tube may move or become disconnected. Awareness of this possibility, especially in the event of an abrupt change in the patient's status, and prompt replacement or reconnection of the tube reduces morbidity. Pain at the insertion site and secondary splinting may lead to pneumonia or atelectasis. Intercostal nerve blocks, intrapleural local anesthetics, and use of incentive spirometry may help prevent this complication. Infections around the tube site also may occur. Good sterile technique during insertion and while the tube is in place can aid in avoiding this problem. Reexpansion pulmonary edema and hypotension have been described following drainage of long-standing effusions (43). These complications can be avoided by slower evacuation of larger collections.

CLINICAL TIPS
1. All necessary equipment should be assembled and tube size(s) should be checked before starting.
2. Adequate sedation and analgesia must be provided for the conscious patient.
3. For tube thoracostomy, the incision should be made directly over a rib.
4. Passage of the chest tube should not be attempted through too small an incision.
5. A probing finger should be used whenever possible to verify that the pleural space has been entered and to identify the diaphragm and any adhesions.
6. For needle decompression of a pneumothorax, a saline-filled syringe is used to detect bubbles.

Chapter 30
Tube Thoracostomy
and Needle
Decompression
of the Chest

405

Summary

Abnormal collections in the pleural space can lead to severe compromise of both respiratory and cardiac function. Tube thoracostomy and needle decompression are two bedside procedures that can be used by pediatric emergency care providers to drain these collections and restore compromised cardiorespiratory function. Although common etiologies of pneumothoraces may be different in children than in adults, procedures of thoracostomy or needle drainage of pneumothoraces in children vary little from that performed in adults. Important differences include selecting the properly sized equipment based on the size of the patient and obtaining adequate cooperation through the proper use of sedation and analgesia. Careful use of the blunt dissection technique as described will help to ensure effective performance of the procedure and avoid complications.

References

1. Hippocrates. Genuine works, vol. 2 (translated by Francis Adams). New York: William Wood and Company, 1886, p. 226.
2. Playfair GE. Case of empyema treated by aspiration and subsequently by drainage: recovery. Br Med J 1875;1:45.
3. Hewett FC. Drainage for empyema. Br Med J 1876;1:1317.
4. Graham EA, Bell RD. Open pneumothorax: its relation to the treatment of empyema: war medicine. Am J Med Sci 1918;156:839.
5. Beaver BL, Laschinger JC. Pediatric thoracic trauma. Sem Thor Card Surg 1992;4:255–262.
6. Helafer MA, Nichols DG, Rogers MC. Development physiology of the respiratory system. In: Rogers MC, ed. Textbook of pediatric intensive care. 2nd ed. Baltimore: Williams & Wilkins, 1992: 104–133.
7. Yu VY, Lieu SW, Robertson NR. Pneumothorax in the newborn: changing patterns. Arch Dis Child 1975;50:449.
8. Monin P, Vert P. Pneumothorax. Clin Perinatol 1978;5:535.
9. Wiggllesworth JS. Pathology of the lung in the fetus and neonate, with particular reference to problems of growth and maturation. Histopathology 1987; 11(7):671–689.
10. Plaus WJ. Delayed pneumothorax after subclavian vein catheterization. J Parent Enteral Nutr 1990; 14:414–415.
11. Collins JC, Levine G, Waxman K. Occult traumatic pneumothorax: immediate tube thoracostomy versus expectant management. Am Surg 1992;58:743–746.
12. Wolfman NT, Gilpin JW, Bechtold RE, Meredith JW, Ditesheim JR. Occult pneumothorax in patients with abdominal trauma: CT studies. J Comput Assist Tomagr 1993;17:56–59.
13. Frumkin K, Wright SW. Tube thoracostomy. In: Roberts JR, Hedges JR, eds. Clinical procedures in emergency medicine. 2nd ed. Philadelphia: WB Saunders, 1985, pp. 128–149.
14. Iberti TJ, Stern PM. Chest tube thoracostomy. Crit Care Clin 1992;8:879–894.
15. Silver M, Bone RC. Techniques for chest tube insertion and pleurodesis. J Crit III 1993;8:631–637.
16. Vukick DJ. Diseases of the pleural space. Emerg Med Clin North Am 1989;7(2):309–324.
17. Templeton JM. Thoracic trauma. In: Fleischer GR, Ludwig S, eds. Textbook of pediatric emergency medicine. 3rd ed. Baltimore: Williams & Wilkins, 1993:1336–1360.
18. Rhea JT, Deluca SA, Greene RE. Determining the size of pneumothorax in the upright patient. Radiology 1982;144:733.
19. Garramore JR, Jacobs LM, Sahdev P. An objective method to measure and manage occult pneumothorax. Surg Syn Obstet 1991;173:257–261.
20. Minami H, Saka H, Senda K, et al. Small catheter drainage for spontaneous pneumothorax. Am J Med Sci 1992;304:345–347.
21. Conces DJ, Tarver RD, Gray WC, et al. Treatment of pneumothoraces utilizing small caliber chest tubes. Chest 1988;94:55–57.
22. Bone RC. The technique of small catheter pleural aspiration. J Crit III 1993;8:827–883.
23. Vallee P, Sullivan M, Richardson H, et al. Sequential treatment of a simple pneumothorax. Ann Emerg Med 1988;19:936.
24. Delius RE, Obeid FN, Horst HM, Sorenson VJ, Fath JJ, Bivens BA. Catheter aspiration for simple pneumothorax. Experience with 114 patients. Arch Surg 1989;124(7):833–836.
25. Bayne CG. Pulmonary complications of the McSwain dart. Ann Emerg Med 1982;11:136.
26. Kircher LT, Swartzel RL. Spontaneous pneumothorax and its treatment. JAMA 1954;155:24.
27. Northfield TC. Oxygen therapy for spontaneous pneumothorax. Br Med J 1971;4:86.
28. Symbas PN. Chest drainage tubes. Surg Clin North Am 1989;69:41–46.
29. Miller KS, Sahn SA. Chest tubes: indications, technique, management and complications. Chest 1987;91:258–264.
30. Barkin RM, Rosen P, eds. Emergency pediatrics: a guide to ambulatory care. 3rd ed. St Louis: CV Mosby Co, 1990.
31. Buhrman BP, Landrum BG, Ferrara TB, et al. Pleural drainage using modified pigtail catheters. Crit Care Med 1986;14:575.
32. Lawless S, Orr R, Killian A, et al. New pigtail catheter for pleural drainage in pediatric patients. Crit Care Med 1989;17:173.
33. Bernstein A, et al. Management of a spontaneous pneumothorax using a Heimlich flutter valve. Thorax 1973;28:386–389.
34. Obeid FN, et al. catheter aspiration for simple pneumothorax in the outpatient management of a simple traumatic pneumothorax. J Trauma 1985;25: 882–886.

Chapter 30
Tube Thoracostomy
and Needle
Decompression
of the Chest

406

35. Hamilton AD, Archer GJ. Treatment of pneumothorax by simple aspiration. Thorax 1983;38:934–936.
36. Moore HV. Complications of thoracentesis and thoracostomy. In: Cordell AR, Ellison RG, eds. Complications of intrathoracic surgery. Boston: Little, Brown, 1979, p. 142.
37. Daly RC, Mucha P, Pairolero PC, Farrell M. The risk of percutaneous chest tube thoracostomy for blunt thoracic trauma. Ann Emerg Med 1985;14: 865–870.
38. Fraser RS. Lung perforation complicating tube thoracostomy: pathological description of three cases. Human Pathol 1988;19:518–523.
39. Foresti V, Villa A, Casati O, Parisio E, De Fillippi G. Abdominal placement of tube thoracostomy due to lack of recognition of paralysis of hemidiaphragm. Chest 1992;102:29.
40. Kolleff MH, Dothager DW. Reversible cardiogenic shock due to chest tube compression of the right ventricle. Chest 1991;99(4):976–980.
41. Mahfood S, Hix WR, Aaron BL, et al. Reexpansion pulmonary edema. Ann Thorac Surg 1988;45:340.
42. Cook T, Kietzman L, Leibold R. "Pneumo-ptosis" in the emergency department. Am J Emerg Med 1992;10:431–434.
43. Bertino RE, Wesbey GE, Johnson R. Horner syndrome occurring as a complication of chest tube placement. Radiology 1987;164:745.

Chapter 30
Tube Thoracostomy
and Needle
Decompression
of the Chest

407

AUTOTRANSFUSION

James D'Agostino and Elliott M. Harris

INTRODUCTION

Autotransfusion or autologous blood transfusion is the collection of blood from a hemorrhaging trauma victim, its preparation, and reinfusion. Autotransfusion was first used by Blundell in 1818 and its popularity, once dismal, has now been rejuvenated as a result of the demand for and risks associated with banked blood (1). Collection of blood for autotransfusion can be performed by physicians, nurses, or trained technicians in EDs, operating rooms, or ICUs.

Autotransfusion offers several advantages over transfusion of homologous blood. The patient is not exposed to bloodborne infectious disease, no risk of transfusion reaction exists, and the blood is immediately available. The advantages of recycling fresh, warm, autologous blood outweigh the potential disadvantages of clotting abnormalities, renal and pulmonary complications, and inadvertent infusion of blood contaminated with bacteria.

Equipment needed to perform autotransfusion can be assembled quickly and the process of collection, preparation, and reinfusion of blood can be easily performed even in the traumatized pediatric patient. Finally, autotransfusion may offer the advantage of being lower in cost than transfusion of banked blood. However, this depends on the relative costs of the equipment for autotransfusion compared with those of banked blood. When smaller volumes of blood are transfused, autotransfusion may be slightly more expensive. The physician will have to weigh the higher cost of autotransfusion against the risks associated with the transfusion of banked blood (2).

ANATOMY AND PHYSIOLOGY

In children, as in adults, the trunk is often the target of both intentional and accidental trauma. Traumatic hemorrhage into the thoracic cavity is most often the result of bleeding from the lung parenchyma, intercostal vessels, or the internal mammary arteries (3). However, the source of the bleeding may be the heart or great vessels and, in cases of diaphragmatic injury, from abdominal organs (3). Bleeding into the abdominal cavity can be the result of injury to solid organs such as the spleen and liver or to intraabdominal vessels.

Hemothorax and hemoperitoneum can result in exsanguinating hemorrhage. Additionally, hemothorax may result in raised intrathoracic pressures which, in turn cause impaired venous return to the heart. Finally, hemothorax causes impaired gas exchange secondary to compression of the ipsilateral lung.

The shed blood recovered from the peritoneal and thoracic cavities behaves somewhat differently than blood that is lost to external hemorrhage in that it does not clot as readily (4). This fact favors using intracavitary blood for autotransfusion. Additionally, autotransfused blood has higher levels of 2,3-diphosphoglycerate than banked, homologous blood (5).

INDICATIONS

In addition to patients who are in shock as a result of hemorrhage and have had minimal if any response to crystalloid therapy, blood replacement should be considered for those patients who are deemed to have lost 30% or more of their circulating blood volume as well as those who have lost lesser amounts of blood but have evidence of ongoing hemorrhage (6) (Table 31.1). In adults, 30% of the circulating blood volume is approximately 1500 mL. In children, of course, the amount of blood loss necessary to cause significant hemorrhage varies with both age and size. Circulating blood volume is about 8 to 9% of body weight in young children, as opposed to 7% of body weight found in adults.

In the traumatized adult patient, hemothorax is the most common cause of shock. The major indication for autotransfusion is hypotension associated with hemothorax. Other potential indications include a stable hemothorax, emergency thoracotomy, and intraabdominal injury from hepatic, splenic, or vascular injury without hollow viscous injury.

Autotransfusion is contraindicated when the blood is collected from injuries that are more than 4 hours old or in the presence of large clots. Likewise, contamination of the blood with intestinal contents or a communication between the abdomen and the chest represent contraindications to ED autotransfusion (5, 7, 8). Other conditions that are contraindications to autotransfusion are known coagulopathy, sepsis, and malignant neoplasms. Using blood recovered from traumatic hemoperitoneum is controversial. In most cases, this blood should not be used in the ED setting because it is impossible for the resuscitation team to determine whether or not the blood is contaminated with bowel contents. However, in some circumstances this may be the only blood available for the patient. In such cases, the potential benefits of transfusion clearly outweigh the risks (8). Blood recovered from a hemoperitoneum may be used for intraoperative transfusion.

PROCEDURE

Several autotransfusion devices are commercially available. The following procedure describes the Atrium® 2050 system; however with some minor differences, most systems function similarly. Clinicians should become familiar with the equipment used in their institution. Among the other systems are the Sorensen® device, the Bently® device, the Baylor® Rapid System, and the Haemonics® Cell Saver unit. The Baylor® system has a cell washing step and the Haemonics® unit has both washing and concentrating abilities. The necessity for the cell washing step, at least in the ED setting, has been questioned and many health care centers do not use this step.

Monitoring is important during autotransfusion. Vital signs should be recorded at frequent intervals during the procedure and continuous cardiorespiratory monitoring and pulse oximetry should be performed. Additionally, depending on the volume of blood infused and whether are not anticoagulant is used, CBC, PT/PTT, calcium, and electrolyte may need to be monitored (see Complications).

The first step in the procedure is the insertion of a large bore chest tube such as might be used to treat any hemothorax (see Chapter 30). As the tube is being inserted the Atrium® 2050 or other appropriate blood recovery unit is prepared. This procedure is similar to that employed when a chest tube drainage system is prepared. When the equipment is assembled, the citrate phosphate dextrose (CPD) solution is added to the anticoagulant port of the recovery unit. The manufacturer recommends adding 14 mL CPD solution to each 100 mL recovered autolo-

Table 31.1.
Autotransfusion

Indications
1. Hemothorax with shock unresponsive to crystalloid therapy
2. Hemothorax with loss of at least 30% of the circulating blood volume
3. Loss of less than 30% of the circulating blood volume with ongoing blood loss
4. Open thoracotomy to relieve ongoing intrathoracic bleeding

Contraindications (absolute)
1. Blood greater than 4 hours old
2. Presence of large blood clots
3. Patient with known malignant neoplasm or coagulopathy
4. Blood known or strongly suspected to be contaminated by bacteria (e.g., perforated diaphragm with known intestinal perforation)

Contraindication (relative)
1. Blood recovered from peritoneal cavity (Note: This blood should be used in the ED only when the benefit clearly outweighs the risk of inadvertent infusion of blood contaminated with bacteria.)

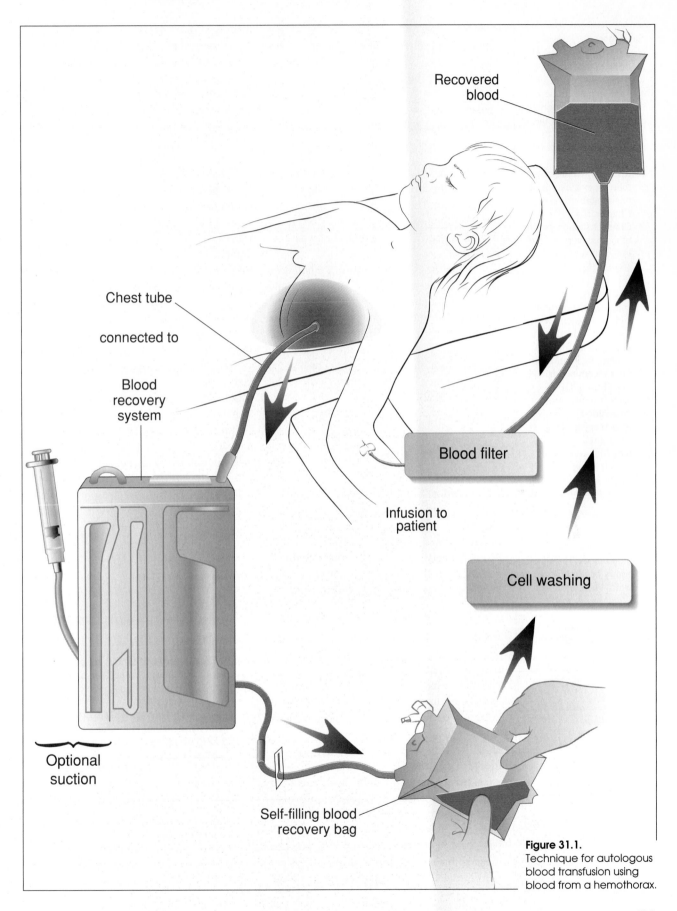

Recovered
blood

Chest tube

connected to

Blood
recovery
system

Blood filter

Infusion to
patient

Cell washing

Optional
suction

Self-filling blood
recovery bag

Figure 31.1.
Technique for autologous
blood transfusion using
blood from a hemothorax.

411

SUMMARY

Note: Clinicians should familiarize themselves with autotransfusion equipment used at their institution. (The procedure described is for the Atrium® system but most systems function in a similar fashion.)

1. Insert large bore chest tube for evacuation of the hemothorax (see Chapter 30).
2. Connect suction port of blood recovery unit to low wall suction (5 to 15 mm Hg).
3. If citrate phosphate dextrose (CDP—anticoagulant) solution is added to system, it should be added at this point; for the Atrium® system, the manufacturer recommends adding 14 mL CDP to each 100 mL autologous blood.
4. Attach chest tube to chest drainage port of blood recovery unit.
5. Attach blood recovery bag to ATS access line located on inferior section of chest drainage unit.
6. Open two clamps and activate self-filling blood recovery bag by gently bending it upward where indicated.
7. When bag is full, remove from recovery system and connect to blood filter and tubing.
8. A cell washing step may be introduced before infusion of recovered blood.

gous blood. Many health care centers do not routinely add anticoagulant to the autologous blood because, as previously stated, blood recovered from body cavities does not clot quickly and forgoing the addition of anticoagulant simplifies the process.

The chest tube is attached to the chest drainage port of the recovery unit. The autotransfusion system (ATS) blood recovery bag is then attached to the ATS access line located on the inferior section of the chest drainage unit. The two clamps are opened and the self-filling ATS blood recovery bag is activated by gently bending it upward where indicated.

When the ATS bag is full, it should be removed and connected to a blood filter and infusion tubing. A cell washing step may be added before infusion into the patient. The ATS recovery bag and filter are then connected to i.v. tubing and air is carefully purged from the tubing. The autologous blood may then be infused through the blood filter (2, 5, 8, 9) (Fig. 31.1).

COMPLICATIONS

Autotransfusion is relatively free of complications. Most complications and potential complications discussed in this chapter are remarkably rare or have never been reported but are theoretically possible. However, this is a potentially dangerous procedure and it is important for the physician to have an understanding of the potential complications involved.

Coagulopathies due to decreased platelets, fibrinogen, or clotting factors may occur and the risk is increased with increasing volumes of transfused blood. To avoid this complication it has been recommended that the amount of autotransfused blood not exceed 2000 mL, however reports have been made of autotransfusion of larger volumes (10). Air embolism has been described during cardiopulmonary bypass and intraoperatively when roller pump type units have been used for autotransfusion (5). This complication has never been described when gravity infusion units such as those described previously have been used. However, prudent practice dictates that air be purged from the system before transfusion. Hyperkalemia from the

hemolysis of red blood cells is another potential complication. Risk of excessive hemolysis may be minimized by using low wall suction to recover the blood and by keeping the suction tip below the surface of pooled blood, if possible. Some authorities recommend using as little as 5 to 15 mm Hg of suction pressure to recover the blood (5).

The citrate buffer CDP used as an anticoagulant in the preparation of the recovered blood places the patient at risk for hypocalcemia when large amounts of blood are transfused. To reduce this risk, the volume of transfused blood should be the minimum amount needed to ensure hemodynamic stability and the amount of CDP added to the recovery unit should be carefully monitored. As previously discussed many authorities believe that the addition of CDP is unnecessary and some newer autotransfusion units do not include this step (5, 8).

Bacteremia is a concern and the physician must avoid collecting blood contaminated with intestinal contents. A cell washing step may decrease the incidence of infection. Fortunately, even when infection occurs, it appears to respond well to antibiotics. Finally, pulmonary and renal complications of autotransfusion have been described, and a cell washing step could potentially remove the unknown factors responsible for this condition (5, 10).

CLINICAL TIPS

1. Autotransfusion is primarily indicated in cases of hemothorax with shock or significant blood loss.
2. Regular in-service sessions for physicians, nurses, and other involved personnel with the appropriate autotransfusion equipment are highly valuable.
3. Hemolysis is avoided when recovering blood by maintaining low suction pressure (5 to 15 mm Hg).
4. If the recovered blood is to be used immediately, adding anticoagulant is probably unnecessary.
5. Cell washing may be used to minimize risk of infection when the transfused blood may be contaminated with bacteria; however, such blood should be used only when the potential benefits outweigh the potential risks.

SUMMARY

Autotransfusion offers a safe alternative to using homologous blood transfusion in the hemorrhaging trauma victim. Because this technique is relatively simple and free from complications, it should be considered for use in pediatric trauma victims.

REFERENCES

1. Blundell J. Experiments in the transfusion of blood. Medico Chir Trans 1818;9:56.
2. Gentilello LM. Autotransfusion in the emergency situation. In: Cameron JL, ed. Current surgical therapy. 5th ed. St. Louis: CV Mosby, 1995.
3. Templeton JM. Thoracic trauma. In: Ludwig S, Fleisher GR, eds. Textbook of pediatric emergency medicine. 3rd ed. Baltimore: Williams & Wilkins, 1993.
4. Broadie TA, Glover JL, Bang N, Bendick PJ, Lowe DK, Yaw PB, Kafoure D. Clotting competence of intracavitary blood in trauma victims. Ann Emerg Med 1981;10:127–130.
5. Kharasch SJ, Millham F, Vinci RJ. The use of autotransfusion in pediatric chest trauma. Pediatr Emerg Care 1994;10:109–112.
6. American College of Surgeons Committee on Trauma. Shock in advanced trauma life support, student manual. Chicago: American College of Surgeons.
7. American Association of Blood Banks. Guidelines for blood salvage and reinfusion in surgery and trauma. Arlington, VA: 1990.
8. Blansfield J. Emergency autotransfusion in hypovolemia. Crit Care Nurs Clin North Am 1990;2:195–199.
9. Atrium(R) 2050 Blood Recovery System. Instructions for use. Hollis, NH: Atrium Medical Corp., 1993.
10. Plaiser BR, McCarthy MC, Canal DF, Solotkin K, Broadie TA. Autotransfusion in trauma: a comparison of two systems. Am Surg 1992;58:562–566.

EMERGENCY THORACOTOMY

Brent R. King and David K. Wagner

INTRODUCTION

Few procedures are as dramatic as open, emergency thoracotomy. When performed for proper indications this technique can save a child from otherwise certain death. This procedure must be used selectively, however, because only a small subset of patients will benefit. This chapter discusses both the indications for and the technique of open thoracotomy as performed in the emergency department (ED).

The purpose of emergency open thoracotomy is to relieve pericardial tamponade, which is usually the result of penetrating injury to the heart, or control of exsanguinating hemorrhage within the thoracic or abdominal cavity. This focus should be kept in mind while performing the procedure. The goal for the ED team is stabilization rather than definitive repair.

The concept of thoracotomy as a method of resuscitation is not new. Original descriptions of the procedure occurred in the late 1800s (1). In the years before the development of closed chest cardio-pulmonary compressions, in-hospital arrests were sometimes managed by direct, open chest, cardiac compressions (2). Since the development of closed chest compressions as a means to perform resuscitation, open thoracotomy has been employed almost exclusively in the resuscitation of trauma victims. It has long been recognized that victims of trauma who succumb during the initial phase of resuscitation have often sustained significant injury to the heart or great vessels (3). In such cases

blood can collect between the heart and the pericardium leading to pericardial tamponade, or the patient can experience exsanguinating hemorrhage into the thoracic cavity. In this situation, immediate thoracotomy to identify and repair injuries may be life-saving. Occasionally, emergency pericardiocentesis (Chapter 73) may provide temporary relief and allow for thoracotomy under more controlled circumstances.

ANATOMY AND PHYSIOLOGY

In terms of anatomy relevant to this procedure a few differences exist between children and adults. For all patients, the wall of the thorax is composed of the muscles of the anterior and posterior chest wall, the ribs, and three sets of intercostal muscles—the external intercostal muscles, the internal intercostal muscles, and the innermost intercostal muscles. The external intercostal muscle exists as a membrane anterior to the midclavicular line and the internal intercostal muscle is a membrane posterior to the midaxillary line. The neurovascular bundles containing the veins, arteries, and nerves lie along the lower margins of the ribs. The ribs themselves are very plastic in infants and young children but in older children and adolescents the ribs are more like those of adults. Deep to the ribs is the parietal pleura, which is adherent to the interior of the thoracic wall, and deep to the parietal pleura is the mediastinum, which contains the heart surrounded by the pericardium and the origins of the great vessels.

Viewed from the standpoint of a thoracotomy, the right ventricle lies anterior, just beneath the sternum with the left ventricle posterior, and slightly lateral, to the right ventricle. The left phrenic nerve lies on the pericardium on the lateral aspect of the left ventricle, placing it at risk during the procedure. Between the superficial tissues and the left ventricle is the left lung which is invaginated by the ventricle. When the standard left lateral thoracotomy is used, the anterior and lateral walls of the left ventricle are visible once the left lung is retracted. Situated in a position cephalad to the heart itself lie the great vessels; lateral and slightly posterior to these are the structures of the pulmonary hili. One distinct, if obvious, difference between adults and children is the size of the structures involved. This procedure can be much more difficult in a small child simply because everything is smaller (4, 5).

The physiologic considerations involved in pediatric thoracotomy are likewise similar to those in the adult procedure. Direct trauma to the heart often allows blood to accumulate between the heart and the pericardial sac, particularly if the hole in the pericardium is small, because the pericardial defect will often partially or fully seal itself. Even a small amount of blood in the space between the heart and the pericardium can restrict cardiac function. In a small child this can be a few milliliters. Fortunately, removal of even a portion of this fluid often results in dramatic improvement in cardiac output. Conversely, if the hole is large or fails to seal, then the blood exits the heart into the mediastinum or the thorax. The child can exsanguinate rapidly in this circumstance.

It is for relief of pericardial tamponade and correction of a direct, penetrating injury to the heart that thoracotomy is most likely to be successful, but it also may be used in cases of direct injury to the great vessels, to highly vascular abdominal structures, or to the pulmonary hilar structures. In the aforementioned situations, thoracotomy is done to halt exsanguinating hemorrhage into the thoracic or abdominal cavities. In cases of intraabdominal hemorrhage, thoracotomy allows the interruption of blood flow to the abdomen (by clamping the aorta) and selective perfusion of the brain and the cardiopulmonary system. Little doubt exists that direct (open) cardiac compressions result in better cardiac output than do indirect (closed) cardiac compressions (6).

INDICATIONS

Emergency thoracotomy became a part of the resuscitation of trauma victims in the 1960s and 1970s, and since then indications for performance of this procedure have been the subject of intense investigation. Initially, virtually any victim of trauma who arrived in full cardiopulmonary arrest, who arrested in the resuscitation area, or who failed to respond to maximal resuscitation efforts was considered a candidate for this procedure. However, with experience, indications for thoracotomy have become more clear (7–19). In virtually all studies of resuscitative thoracotomy, victims of blunt trauma have fared far worse than victims of penetrating trauma. This difference almost certainly reflects both the high incidence of head trauma associated with blunt trauma and the fact that injury in blunt trauma often involves multiple organs. In any case, survivorship with good neurologic outcome is rare for blunt trauma victims who arrest during the prehospital phase of resuscitation.

Victims of penetrating trauma can be further subdivided into victims of shooting and victims of stabbing. While penetrating trauma carries a better prognosis overall, shooting victims are less likely to survive than are victims of stabbing. The most reasonable explanation for this difference in survivorship is that stabbing is a relatively low velocity injury which often results in damage to a single organ, while shooting, primarily because of the higher velocity, often involves multiple organs and far more tissue destruction. In the case of penetrating trauma, survivorship appears to be determined by the time elapsed between the event and the institution of definitive treatment. Most large studies have few survivors who had undetectable vital signs for more than a few minutes.

Unfortunately, little information is found in the medical literature dealing specifically with children (20–23). To date only four studies of resuscitative thoracotomy have been restricted to patients less than 18 years of age. These studies demonstrate a similar outcome pattern to those involving adults, with survivorship being rare in blunt trauma victims. A total of 142 patients in the four studies underwent emergency thoracotomy; 85 sustained blunt trauma and 57 penetrating trauma. Of the 85 victims of blunt trauma 2 survived, whereas 7 children who had a penetrating injury survived to hospital discharge. Of the three studies that specifically list the ages of the involved children, no patient younger than 15 years of age has survived. This reflects both the high incidence of blunt trauma in young children and the little appreciated fact that while children may be better able to resist full cardiopulmonary arrest than adults, once arrested they are unlikely to recover (24, 25). Additionally, these results demonstrate the level of interpersonal violence among teenagers which ultimately leads to penetrating injuries.

Although no doubt an injured child should be given every possible chance to recover and thoracotomy should be used liberally despite the dismal statistics, there are three compelling reasons to limit the application of this technique in children, just as the literature suggests that it be limited in adults. First, this is a highly invasive technique which is often performed under less than ideal circumstances. This combination makes thoracotomy very risky to medical personnel from the standpoint of blood exposure (26). Second, whether successful or not, thoracotomy is costly in financial, emotional, and operational terms. Finally, this procedure may produce a limited period of spontaneous circulation in a patient after a period of protracted arrest. Under such circumstances the outcome will almost certainly be either a protracted death from multiorgan system failure or survival with neurologic devastation.

With this information in mind, some recommendations can be made for patient selection:

1. Victims of blunt trauma who arrest during the prehospital phase of care and who are without detectable vital signs for more than 5 minutes have virtually no chance for intact survival and should not be considered candidates for this procedure.
2. Victims of either penetrating or blunt trauma who have no pulse, no detectable blood pressure, and no organized electrical activity on a cardiac monitor will benefit from thoracotomy only if the procedure is performed promptly. If thoracotomy cannot be undertaken within 5 minutes of the time of arrest, little reason remains in performing it at all.
3. Victims of penetrating trauma, particularly those with penetrating trauma to the chest and upper abdomen, who have short arrest times or arrest en route to the ED, and those who fail to respond to initial resuscitation, should be considered candidates for this procedure.
4. Rarely, a victim of nontraumatic arrest may be considered a candidate for thoracotomy. Medical personnel should consider this technique in cases of severe chest wall abnormality and other situations that make traditional closed chest compressions impossible or ineffective.

EQUIPMENT

The list of necessary equipment for thoracotomy is short. The procedure can be performed with a scalpel and some sort of chest wall retractor. Several other pieces of equipment are useful, however, and these are listed in Table 32.1. Equipment listed in part I of Table 32.1 represents a standard thoracotomy

Table 32.1.
Equipment

I. Equipment for Standard Thoracotomy Tray
  Scalpel—No. 20 blade
  Mayo scissors
  Chest wall retractor ("rib spreaders")—Finichetto's or other type
  Tissue forceps—10 inch
  Vascular (Satinsky) clamps—2 to 4
  Needle holder—10 inch
  Suture—2.0 silk, curved needle
          4.0 silk, vascular needle
  Teflon™ pledgets
  Aortic tamponade instrument
  Vascular tape
  Metzenbaum scissors
  Curved hemostats—4 to 10
  Right angle clamps—2 to 4
  Liebsche knife/sternal osteotome with hammer/sternal saw
  Chest tubes—sizes 20 through 40
  Foley catheters—16 through 24 French
  Sponges
  Drapes/towels
  Sterile suction equipment
  Sterile internal defibrillator paddles—6 inch
II. Additional Equipment for Child/Infant Resuscitation
  Scalpel—No. 15 Blade
  Foley catheters—5 through 12 French
  Chest tubes—10 through 20 French
  Internal defibrillator paddles—2 inch and 4 inch
  Small chest wall retractor

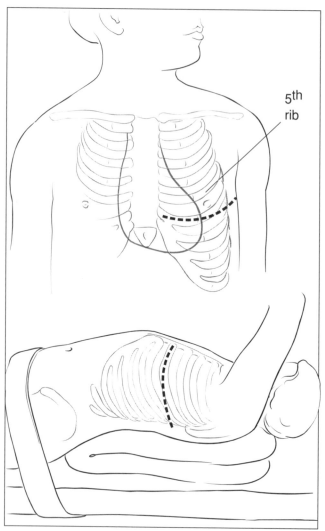

5th
rib

with the equipment before performing the procedure. Adequate assistance also is important for success.

As with all resuscitation efforts, the upper airway should be secured and artificial ventilation begun before the circulatory status of the patient is addressed (Chapters 14 to 17). If enough skilled personnel are available, airway control can be accomplished simultaneously with the initiation of resuscitative thoracotomy. Consideration must always be given to the possibility of lower airway obstruction with concomitant circulatory compromise (i.e., tension pneumothorax), in which case needle decompression of the chest (Chapter 30) should be performed in advance of or concomitantly with upper airway control measures.

Exposure

After rapid preparation with an antiseptic such as povidone-iodine, the skin incision is made at the left 4th or 5th intercostal space from the sternal border to the posterior axillary line. The correct line of incision usually passes just below the left nipple and follows the curve of the rib (Fig. 32.1). In females, breast tissue should be spared by manually retracting the breast superiorly, if necessary. In the young female the clinician should avoid cutting the breast bud. If the correct interspace cannot be identified, then the incision can be started at the posterior axillary line even with the inferior tip of the scapular wing and completed at the sternal border. Once the skin incision has been completed, the intercostal tissue is cut using the Mayo scissors along the upper border of the rib so as not to damage the neurovascular bundle which runs along the lower rib margin.

Once the chest wall is open, the chest wall retractor ("rib spreader") is placed into the incision. Although several types of chest

tray which may be used for large children, adolescents, and adults. Part II lists equipment that is useful for small children and infants. Notably, this procedure is rarely performed in most EDs but the likely candidates for this procedure would be adolescents or adults. It is, therefore, reasonable to maintain a single thoracotomy tray in the ED which contains some equipment for infant and small child resuscitation as well as the more standard equipment for adults and adolescents.

PROCEDURE

Performing an emergency thoracotomy is not as awesome a task as it might seem. The technique is nothing more than a logical sequence of relatively straightforward manual skills. It is important for the emergency physician to be thoroughly familiar with the technique and

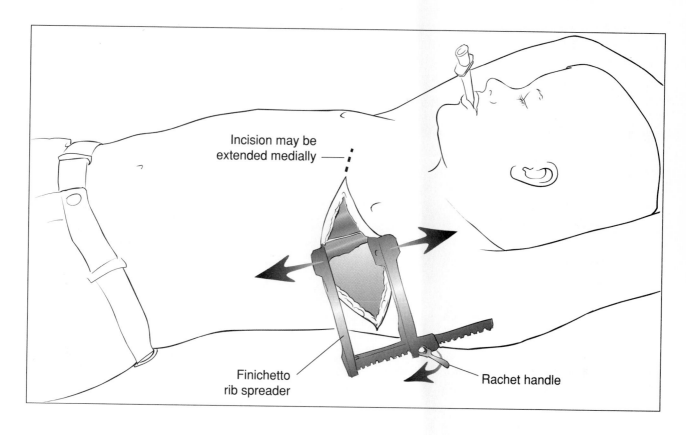

Incision may be
extended medially

Finichetto
rib spreader

Rachet handle

Figure 32.2.
Correct placement of the
Finichetto rib spreader for
emergency thoracotomy.

SUMMARY

1. Rapidly apply sterile povidone-iodine solution to chest wall.
2. Make incision at 4th or 5th costal interspace from sternum, along rib margin to posterior axillary line, cutting through skin and muscles of chest wall.
3. Cut through intercostal muscles with heavy scissors along upper rib margin.
4. Insert Finichetto's chest wall retractor with bar extending into axilla and use ratchet handle to open ribs.
5. Using suction, remove any blood obstructing a clear view of heart—remember that blood can be saved for autotransfusion.
6. Open pericardium anterior to phrenic nerve. Remove any blood or clots and explore myocardium for injuries—remember to keep heart as warm as possible using warm saline and/or heat lamps.
7. Apply direct pressure to any sites of hemorrhage from heart—pressure should be maintained until injury can be definitively repaired.
8. Repair any myocardial injuries, if possible. Be careful to avoid damage to coronary

arteries or phrenic nerve. Atrial lacerations may be repaired with a simple running stitch and ventricular lacerations with interrupted stitches reinforced with Teflon™ pledgets.

9. If no myocardial injury is found, retract left lung out of chest anteriorly and superiorly. Identify aorta, separate it from esophagus and prevertebral fascia and occlude it using fingers, a vascular clamp, vascular tape, or an aortic tamponade device.
10. Extend incision into right chest by making a right-sided thoracotomy incision identical to left-sided one and then cutting sternum with a sternal saw or a Liebsche knife. Ligate internal mammary arteries, if possible.
11. Explore thoracic cavity for other sources of bleeding and apply pressure to any bleeding site identified—vessels that can be exposed may be cross clamped.
12. If heart is beating spontaneously continue resuscitation with fluids and blood. If not, begin open cardiac massage and then defibrillate using internal paddles.

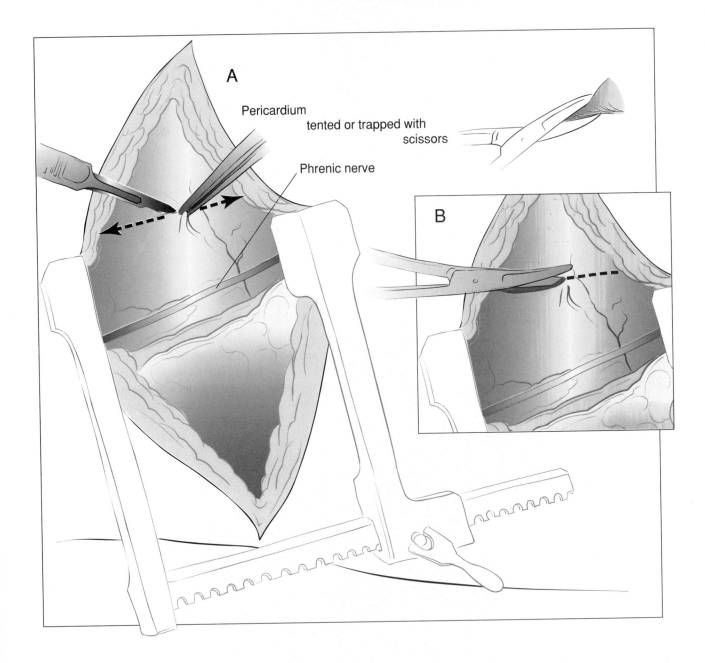

A

Pericardium

tented or trapped with
scissors

Phrenic nerve

B

Figure 32.3.
Techniques for incising the
pericardium.
A. The pericardium may be
grasped with a pair of
forceps and then nicked
with a scalpel.
B. The pericardium may be
trapped between the
blades of a pair of scissors,
then cut.

**Chapter 32
Emergency
Thoracotomy**

wall retractors are available, the Finichetto
device is the most commonly used in adults
and adolescents. The placement of the
Finichetto retractor is critical to the success
of the procedure. The bar and ratchet handle
should be placed so that they are perpendicular to the base of the incision with the bar extending into the axilla as shown in Figure
32.2. Insertion in this fashion allows extension of the incision into the right chest, if necessary. Once the chest wall retractor is in
place the rachet handle is used to open the
ribs.

Exploration

After the ribs are retracted open, the next task
is to control obvious hemorrhage. If an obvious site of bleeding can be readily identified
then direct pressure should be used to stop it
if possible. The source of bleeding may not
be obvious in which case blood should be
evacuated from the chest to allow for better
visualization, a cell saver can be used to collect the blood for use in autotransfusion
(Chapter 31). If, on opening the chest, no
bleeding occurs, then the pericardium should

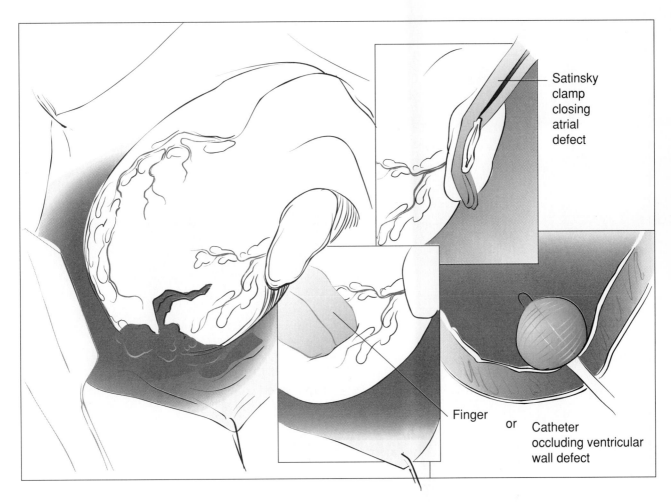

Satinsky
clamp
closing
atrial
defect

Finger   or   Catheter
occluding ventricular
wall defect

be examined and in most cases opened.

Of the several methods described for opening the pericardium, none can be considered absolutely correct; however, the two methods to be described offer advantages over the others. The pericardium should be opened by an initial incision made anterior to the phrenic nerve. This incision can be made by picking up the pericardium with a pair of forceps or a hemostat and then cutting with scissors or a scalpel. When pericardial tamponade is present, the pericardial sac may be so tense that it cannot be grasped. In this case it can be trapped between the blades of a pair of Mayo scissors and incised in this fashion (Fig. 32.3). Once the pericardium is open, the incision should be extended widely, which

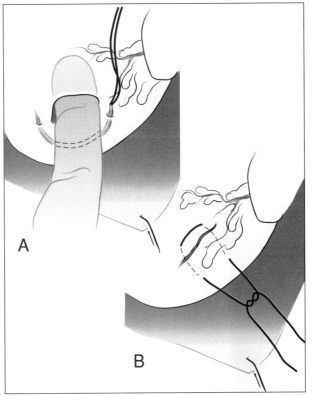

A

B

Figure 32.4.
Techniques for occlusion of a cardiac defect. Initial maneuver should be manual occlusion. Atrial lacerations can be closed with a Satinsky clamp, and ventricular lacerations may be occluded with a Foley catheter.

Figure 32.5.
A. Definitive closure of ventricular defects may be accomplished using a simple nonabsorbable suture.
B. In cases where the laceration is in proximity to one of the coronary arteries or the phrenic nerve, then a mattress stitch should be used.

**Chapter 32
Emergency
Thoracotomy**

421

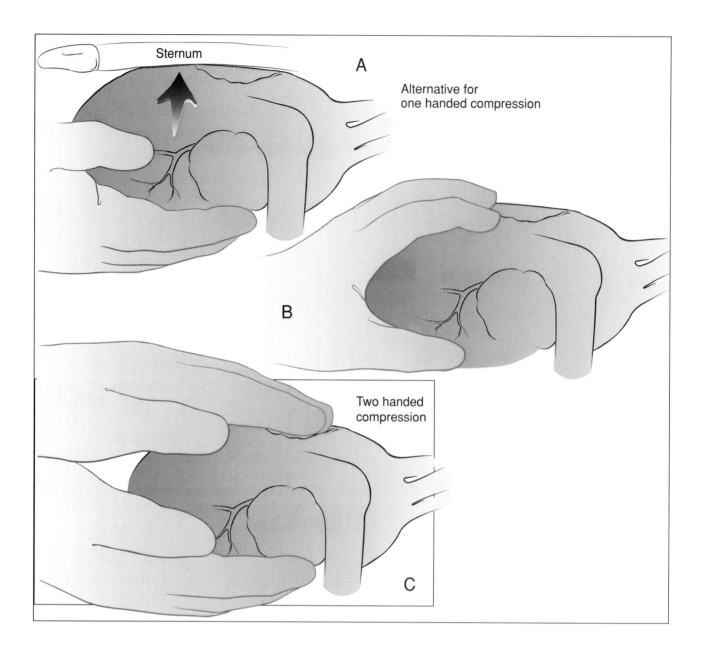

Sternum

A

Alternative for
one handed compression

B

Two handed
compression

C

Figure 32.6.
Techniques for open
cardiac compressions.
A. The heart is compressed
against the sternum.
B. One-handed
compressions.
C. Two-handed
compressions (the
recommended technique).

allows for easy exploration of the myocardium and prevents herniation of the heart through a small opening. Such herniation can inhibit myocardial function by constricting the inflow and outflow tracts of the heart and can be very difficult to relieve.

The next stage of the procedure depends somewhat on the findings after the pericardium is incised. If opening the pericardium relieves a tamponade then all clots should be removed from the pericardial space and the myocardium should be quickly explored to identify the source of bleeding, usually an atrial or ventricular laceration. When such a laceration is found it should be oc-

cluded so as to stop the hemorrhage. For a ventricular injury, the first method to use is to place a fingertip over the bleeding site and apply direct pressure. More protracted occlusion of a ventricular laceration can be accomplished by passing a sterile Foley catheter through the hole, inflating the balloon, and then placing traction on the catheter which, in turn, pulls the balloon against the hole. Additionally, the lumen of the catheter may be used to rapidly infuse large quantities of fluid. In the case of an atrial laceration a vascular (Satinsky) clamp may be used to temporarily close the defect. These techniques are shown in Figure 32.4.

Once the defect has been occluded and resuscitation efforts are well underway, the injury to the heart should be definitively closed with suture material. For atrial lacerations a simple running stitch using 3.0 nonabsorbable suture can be used. Most ventricular lacerations can be closed with simple interrupted sutures (2.0 or 3.0). Nonabsorbable sutures should be used. The suture material is passed beneath the occluding finger or about the Foley catheter and then tied (Fig. 32.5). If a Foley catheter has been used as a temporizing measure, care must be taken to avoid pulling the catheter through the heart wound or puncturing the catheter balloon with the needle. Ventricular wall, like all muscle tissue, separates easily, making suturing somewhat difficult. Some of this difficulty can be overcome by placing Teflon™ pledgets on either side of the laceration to reinforce the tissues. If the laceration is in close proximity to a coronary artery or to the phrenic nerve, then a mattress stitch (Figure 32.5) should be used to prevent ligation of the artery or nerve. Finally, if the heart is beating, the repairs previously described may be difficult or impossible to accomplish. If this proves to be the case, then the temporizing maneuvers should be continued until the patient can be taken to the operating room and placed on cardiopulmonary bypass.

Once pericardial tamponade has been relieved the heart may resume spontaneous activity. If not, then after identifying and closing lacerations as previously described, direct cardiac massage should be started and preparations for internal defibrillation should begin. Internal massage may be correctly performed in three ways. (Fig. 32.6). The heart may be compressed from below against the sternum (unless the incision has been extended through the sternum into the right hemithorax). The heart may be compressed between the two hands of the resuscitator, or a one-handed compression technique may be used. Using the one-handed technique involves a small risk of accidental myocardial damage, usually digital perforation of the thin-walled right atrium. Furthermore, in children, the sternum is often relatively plastic, making compression against it more difficult and less effective. Therefore, two-handed cardiac compressions are preferred.

To correctly perform two-handed compressions, one hand is placed beneath the

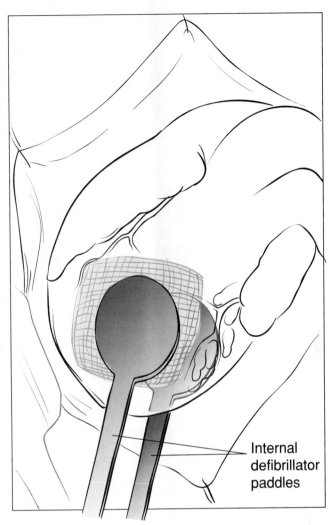

Internal defibrillator paddles

heart and one above it. The apex of the heart lies at the level of the heel of the hands and the base of the heart lies between the fingertips. The heart is compressed between the hands. Starting at the heels of the hands pressure is progressively applied through the palm and to the fingertips. As in closed chest cardiac compression, the rate should be maintained at 100 beats per minute, if possible. During cardiac compressions with the chest open, the heart can become hypothermic relatively quickly. This hypothermia makes the myocardium resistant to defibrillation. Hypothermia can be minimized by intermittently bathing the heart in a direct stream of warm saline and by using some external warming source, such as heat lamps.

If the heart does not resume beating, then the internal defibrillator paddles should be used. The paddle size for an adolescent is 6

Figure 32.7.
Correct placement of paddles for internal defibrillation.

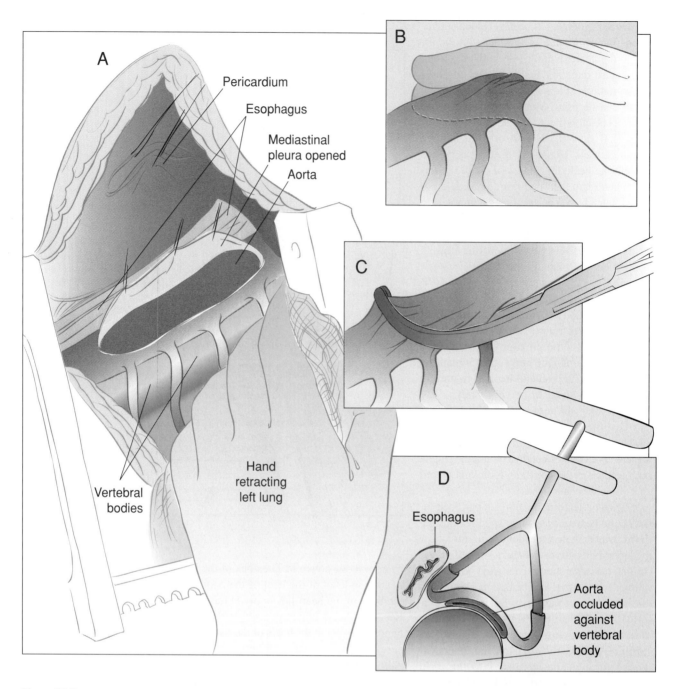

Figure 32.8.
Occlusion of the aorta.
A. Anatomical landmarks visible after the left lung is manually retracted.
B. Manual occlusion of the aorta.
C. Aortic occlusion using a vascular clamp.
D. Aortic occlusion by compression against the vertebral bodies using a compression type aortic occlusion device.

cm, for a child 4 cm, and for an infant 2 cm. The paddles are placed in the chest as shown in Figure 32.7. Using saline-soaked pads as conductive material, one paddle is placed posteriorly, usually behind the left ventricle, and the other is placed anteriorly, over the right ventricle. The ideal defibrillator charge for a child in these circumstances is unknown; however, it has been suggested that starting doses should be in the range of 5 joules (J) and proceed up to 20 J. The starting dose of electricity for an adolescent is 20 J

with subsequent doses of 40 and 60 J, if necessary.

If no pericardial tamponade is present and no cardiac laceration can be identified, then the source of bleeding is either elsewhere in the chest or within the abdominal cavity. Bleeding elsewhere in the chest may be obvious but, if not, then the incision should be extended into the right chest (see below). For suspected bleeding occurring primarily within the abdomen, as well as to improve perfusion to the brain and myocardium,

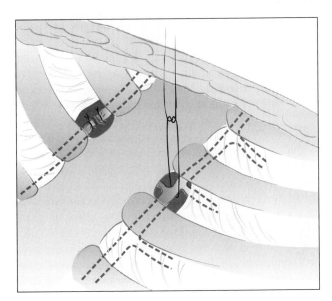

Figure 32.9.
Ligation of the internal
mammary arteries before
extension of the incision
across the sternum.

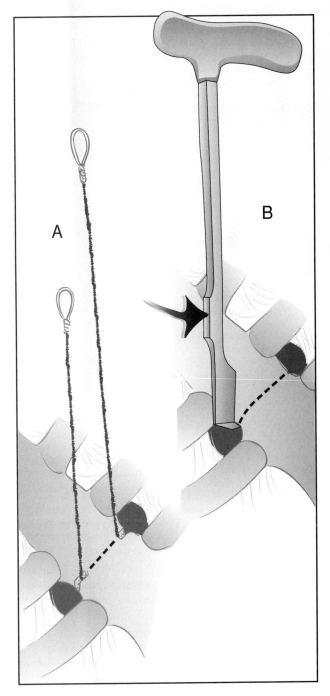

Figure 32.10.
Techniques for dividing the
sternum.
A. Use of a sternal saw.
B. Use of a Liebsche knife.

the aorta should be identified and occluded. This is best accomplished by rotating the left lung anteriorly and superiorly out of the chest so that the aorta can be directly visualized or at least easily identified.

After the aorta is visualized, the mediastinal pleura is incised and, using blunt dissection, the aorta is freed from its anterior attachment to the esophagus and its posterior attachment to the prevertebral fascia. Alternatively, the clinician can palpate along the posterior portions of the ribs until the vertebral bodies are encountered. The aorta lies just anterior to the vertebral bodies. Once this has been accomplished, the aorta can be occluded without risk of damage to the aorta or to the esophagus. The initial technique for aortic occlusion is to trap the aorta between two fingers. If an extended period of aortic occlusion is anticipated, however, the aorta should be either cross clamped using a vascular clamp, tamponaded using a specially designed instrument, or encircled with vascular tape (Fig. 32.8). Aortic occlusion to control suspected intraabdominal hemorrhage should be a prelude to immediate transfer of the patient to the operating room for definitive exploration of the abdomen.

If, on opening the chest, the source of bleeding appears to be from the right chest, then the incision should be extended across the sternum. The right-sided incision is made in exactly the same fashion as the left-sided one. Dividing the sternum in a small child can be accomplished using a pair of heavy scis-

Chapter 32
Emergency
Thoracotomy

426

sors but in the older child or adolescent a sternal saw or the Liebsche knife must be used. Ideally, before the sternum is divided, the internal mammary arteries should be identified and then ligated (Fig. 32.9). However, if this cannot be accomplished quickly, then division of the sternum should proceed. As shown in Figure 32.10, the sternal saw is passed beneath the sternum and the sternum is sawed in half from below using a rapid to and fro motion. Alternatively, when using the Liebsche knife, the sharp, hooked portion of the blade is placed against the sternum and the hammer is used to tap the blade through the sternum by hitting the flat knob extending from the back of the blade. Once the sternum is divided and the incision is extended into the right chest, the right pulmonary hilar area can be explored to rule out hemorrhage from this site. Also the possibility of bleeding from the right subclavian artery should be considered.

If, on exploration of the heart, the injury appears to involve a coronary artery, then the best course available is to apply direct pressure to the artery until the vessel can be closed by a vascular or cardiovascular surgeon. In children the coronary arteries can be quite small, requiring expertise to repair.

COMPLICATIONS

Exigent thoracotomy has many potential complications and careful attention should be given to correct technical performance. However, most of these complications are far less worrisome than the injury which led to the necessity for an open thoracotomy. The most important pitfalls likely to be encountered in the performance of open thoracotomy are: damage to breast tissue with the initial incision; injury to the intercostal vessels or nerves when opening the chest wall; failure to properly insert the Finichetto's chest wall retractor; failure to recognize and relieve pericardial tamponade; and inadvertent ligation of the phrenic nerve or a coronary artery. As previously discussed, care should be taken to avoid injury to the breast tissue in female patients. In young children, the incision should be made so as to avoid cutting the breast bud and in adolescents the breast should be re-

tracted superiorly out of the line of the incision.

The neurovascular bundles of the ribs lie along the lower rib margins. When opening the chest wall, the intercostal tissues should be cut near the upper border of the rib to avoid injury to these structures. Intercostal arteries, if damaged, are a potential source for significant bleeding.

The Finichetto's retractor should be inserted so that the bar and ratchet handle are at the base of the incision with the bar extending into the patient's axilla. This allows the incision to be extended into the right chest if necessary. Placement of this device in the more traditional thoracotomy position with the bar at the top (anterior portion) of the incision prevents extension because the bar blocks any attempt to cut through the sternum.

Pericardial tamponade can be difficult to recognize on inspection alone. Most authorities recommend opening the pericardium in every case so as not to miss this very treatable entity. Once the pericardium is incised, the incision should be extended widely to avoid herniation of the myocardium through the incision with subsequent restriction of myocardial function.

When an injury to the myocardium is near one of the coronary arteries or the phrenic nerve, it must be repaired carefully to avoid accidental ligation of either of these structures. Lacerations should be repaired using a mattress type stitch as shown in Figure 32.5. The suture material is passed beneath the structure and tied parallel to it. Notably, even under the best of circumstances, the child's survival is far from ensured.

SUMMARY

Open resuscitative thoracotomy has the potential to be life saving if employed promptly in properly selected patients. However, success of this technique relies upon rapid exposure of the intrathoracic organs and equally rapid control of hemorrhage. Because correction of cardiac tamponade and direct injury to the heart offers the best chance of survival, exploration of these areas should be undertaken first. If no cardiac injury is present, then the search for another source of intrathoracic bleeding should begin. Cross clamping of the aorta may provide for temporary control of intra-abdominal hemorrhage pending laparotomy. While there are many potential complications of this procedure, even a perfectly performed open thoracotomy offers only a slim chance for long term survival.

REFERENCES

1. Rehn L. Veber penetriren den herzwunden and hertnacht. Arch Clin Chir 1896;55:315.
2. Feliciano DV, Mattox KL. Indications, technique and pitfalls of emergency center thoracotomy. Surg Rounds 1981 Dec;32–37,40.
3. Brewer LA. Wounds of the chest in war and peace. Ann Thorac Surg 1969;7:387–408.
4. Moore KL. The thorax in clinically oriented anatomy 2nd ed. Moore KL, ed. Baltimore: Williams & Wilkins, 1985.
5. Woodburne RT. The chest in essentials of human anatomy. 6th ed. Woodburne RT, ed. New York: Oxford University Press, 1978.
6. Bircher N, Safar P. Manual open-chest cardiopulmonary resuscitation. Ann Emerg Med 1984;13(9 Pt 2):770–773.
7. Mattox KL, Espada R, Beall AC, Jordon GL. Performing thoracotomy in the emergency center. JACEP 1974;3:13–17.
8. Siemens R, Polk HC, Gray LA, Fulton RL. Indications for thoracotomy following penetrating thoracic injury. J Trauma 1977;17:493–500.
9. MacDonald JR, McDowell RM. Emergency department thoracotomies in a community hospital. JACEP 1978;7:423–428.
10. Moore EE, Moore JB, Galloway AC, Eiseman B. Postinjury thoracotomy in the emergency department: a critical evaluation. Surgery 1979;6:590–598.
11. Baker CC, Thomas AN, Trunkey DD. The role of emergency department thoracotomy in trauma. J Trauma 1980;20:848–855.
12. Harnar TJ, Oreskovich MD, Copass MK, Heimbach DM, Herman CM, Carrico CJ. Role of emergency thoracotomy in the resuscitation of moribund trauma victims—100 consecutive cases. Am J Surg 1981;142:96–99.
13. Cogbill TH, Moore EE, Millikan JS, Cleveland HC. Rationale for selective application of emergency department thoracotomy in trauma. J Trauma 1983; 23:453–460.
14. Shimazu S, Shatney CH. Outcomes of trauma patients with no vital signs on hospital admission. J Trauma 1983;23:213–216.
15. Hoyt DB, Shackford SR, Davis JW, Mackersie RC, Hollingsworth-Fridlund P. Thoracotomy during trauma resuscitations—an appraisal by board certified general surgeons. J Trauma 1989;29:1318–1321.
16. Lorenz HP, Steinmetz B, Lieberman J, Schecter WP, Macho JR. Emergency thoracotomy: survival correlates with physiologic status. J Trauma 1992; 32:780–788.
17. Bodai BL, Smith JP, Blaisdell FW. The role of emergency thoracotomy in blunt trauma. J Trauma 1982;22:487–491.
18. Mansour MA, Moore EE, Moore FA, Read RR. Exigent postinjury thoracotomy: analysis of blunt vs. penetrating trauma. SGO 1992;175:97–101.
19. Esposito TJ, Jurkovich GJ, Rice CL, Maier RV, Copass MK, Ashbaugh DG. Reappraisal of emergency room thoracotomy in a changing environment. J Trauma. 1991;31:881–887.
20. Beaver BL, Colombani PM, Buck JR, Dudgeon DL, Bohrer SL, Haller AJ. Efficacy of emergency room thoracotomy in pediatric trauma. J Pediatr Surg 1987;22:19–23.
21. Powell RW, Gill EA, Jurkovich GJ, Ramenofsky ML. Resuscitative thoracotomy in children and adolescents. Am Surg 1988;54:188–191.
22. Rothenberg SS, Moore EE, Moore FA, Baxter BT, Moore JB, Cleveland HC. Emergency department thoracotomy in children: a critical analysis. J Trauma 1989;29:1322–1324.
23. Sheikh AA, Culbertson CB. Emergency department thoracotomy in children: rationale for selective application. J Trauma 1993;34:323–328.
24. Torphy DE, Minter MG, Thompson GM. Cardiorespiratory arrest and resuscitation of children. Am J Dis Child 1984;138:1099–1102.
25. Ludwig S, Fleisher G. Pediatric cardiopulmonary resuscitation: a review and a proposal. Pediatr Emerg Care 1985;1:40–44.
26. McCray E. Occupational risk of acquired immunodeficiency syndrome among health care workers. N Engl J Med 1986;314:1127.

Emergent Radiologic Evaluation of Renal and Genitourinary Trauma

Cynthia C. Hoecker and Richard M. Ruddy

Introduction

Early recognition and treatment of injury to the genitourinary tracts following trauma can prevent significant morbidity. For this reason diagnostic evaluation should be thoughtfully considered in injured patients with hematuria or a high risk mechanism (e.g., crush injury to the pelvis). Excretory urography (IVP) and retrograde urethrocystography are diagnostic procedures which have been used to evaluate the upper and lower urinary tracts following traumatic injury for over three decades (1–6). The history of intravenous urography dates back to the 1920s when scientists in Germany discovered that the kidney and bladder could be visualized following I.V. administration of iodide-containing compounds. The 1930s through the 1950s saw the development of newer and safer iodinated contrast agents and by the 1960s uroradiography was aiding the diagnosis of a multitude of urologic problems.

Today, the development of newer imaging techniques such as computed tomography has led to a decline in the use of the intravenous urogram (7). However, circumstances remain in the emergency setting in which the IVP may yield more rapid diagnosis of an injured kidney or confirm the presence of a functional one. Although contrast-enhanced CT scanning and fluoroscopic-guided studies may yield more complete information, they

may be more time consuming and are generally obtained only with senior radiology presence. In short, the IVP and retrograde cystourethrogram remain "quick and dirty" bedside procedures which can provide important structural and functional information in the emergency department.

Anatomy and Physiology

Characteristics of the kidneys and genitourinary tracts in children may predispose them to traumatic injury in blunt trauma. For example, major renal injury following abdominal trauma is more common in children owing to a proportionately larger kidney size (relative to the abdomen) and less protection from perirenal fat and the lower ribcage. Because the bladder occupies a more abdominal position in young children, it too is more vulnerable to rupture from blunt trauma or lap belt related, motor vehicle injuries. Ureteral injuries are rare following blunt trauma in all ages. However, ureteral avulsion at the level of the ureteropelvic junction occasionally results after extreme extension of the trunk following rapid deceleration mechanisms (e.g., high speed motor vehicle accidents). Urethral injuries are most commonly seen in association with pelvic fractures, straddle injuries, and increasingly from gunshot wounds (1, 5). Another important point is that gross hema-

Chapter 33
Emergent Radiologic
Evaluation of Renal
and Genitourinary
Trauma

429

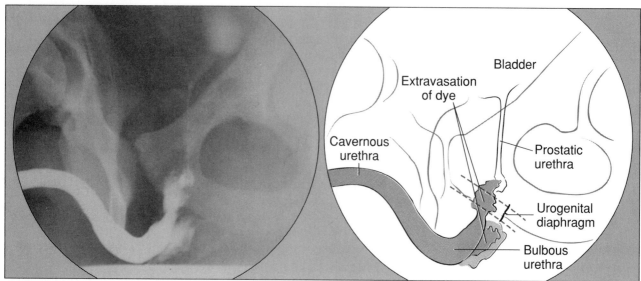

Figure 33.1.
Retrograde urethrogram demonstrating extravasation of contrast material from the proximal urethra.

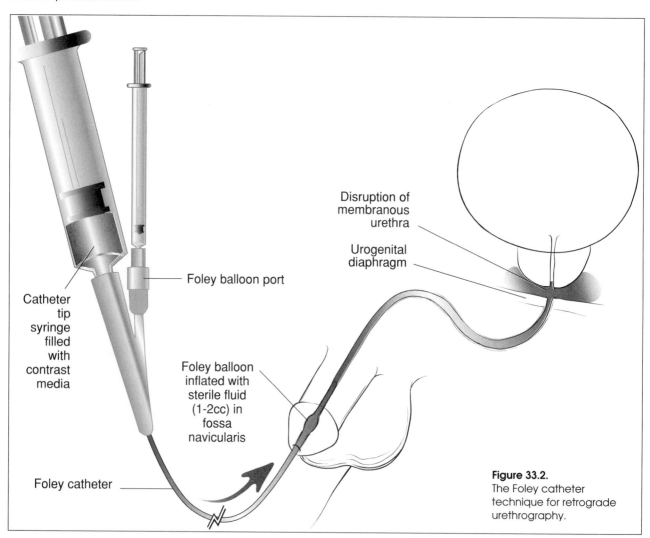

Figure 33.2.
The Foley catheter technique for retrograde urethrography.

turia in a child following relatively minor trauma may be the first sign of an underlying occult renal anomaly or disease of the kidney (e.g., hydronephrosis or Wilm's tumor).

IVP/EXCRETORY UROGRAPHY

Indications

The IVP has been employed in the evaluation of blunt or penetrating abdominal trauma in which injury to the kidney or its collecting system is suspected based on the presence of hematuria (greater than 20 red blood cells per high-powered field), physical examination findings (e.g., ecchymosis over flank), or a high risk mechanism (1, 6). Mechanisms known to be associated with renal and ureteral injury include direct trauma to the back, flank, or abdomen and rapid deceleration injuries resulting in severe flexion of the trunk causing ureteropelvic junction disruption or injury to the renal pedicle.

Information obtained by IVP includes the gross anatomical detail of the renal parenchyma and collecting system as well as a general estimate of renal function. Because a good nephrogram relies on perfusion of the kidneys, reliable information may not be obtained in the hypovolemic, vasoconstricted patient. Furthermore, consultation with a radiologist or urologist, when available, should be sought to aid in the timing and interpretation of this study.

Procedure

With the patient supine, reliable I.V. access should be obtained using a large bore I.V. catheter to facilitate injection of viscous contrast media. The I.V. tubing should be connected with a stopcock or I.V. port close to the hub of the I.V. catheter to minimize the waiting or prolonged flushing of the contrast material in lengthy I.V. tubing (Fig. 33.1). This would be especially important in a smaller child when a smaller volume of contrast media is used. A preliminary AP radiograph of the abdomen (scout film) should be obtained as a baseline comparison study (Fig. 33.2). The go-

nads should be shielded in the male as this should not affect the study. The dose of contrast media in the 30 or 60 mL syringe should be attached to the stopcock or port and the I.V. should be rechecked for the backflow of blood. Once this is confirmed, rapid injection (in less than 1 minute) of the total volume of contrast material through the I.V. should be followed by 5 mL of flush solution. The infusion should be halted if any evidence of local extravasation exists as this may produce pain and tissue necrosis. Serial repeat AP films should then be obtained at 1 minute, 5 minutes, and 10 minutes postinjection looking for a delayed or asymmetric nephrogram, extravasation through the renal capsule, or calyceal defects. Further delayed films also may be required for completion of the study.

RETROGRADE URETHROCYSTOGRAPHY

Indications

This procedure may be emergently indicated in the evaluation of blunt or penetrating trauma to the perineum, penis, or pelvis to evaluate the integrity of the urethra and bladder (9). Urethral tears should be suspected whenever a penetrating injury has occurred to the penis, blood is found at the urethral meatus, or a scrotal hematoma or a history of direct blunt trauma to the perineum (e.g., a straddle injury) is evident. Bladder injuries include bladder contusions and ruptures (intraperitoneal or extraperitoneal). Extraperitoneal rupture is more common and often is seen with pelvic fractures. Intraperitoneal ruptures generally occur at the dome as the result of blunt trauma to the lower abdomen when the bladder is full of urine.

Retrograde urethrography should be performed before cystography in males if the clinician suspects urethral disruption, because urethral injury is a contraindication to transurethral bladder catheterization. In addition, when the clinician encounters difficulty passing a urethral catheter following lower abdominal trauma, no further attempts should be made and prompt consultation with a urologist is indicated.

> **SUMMARY: INTRAVENOUS PYELOGRAM**
> 1. Obtain supine KUB as a scout film (shield gonads in the male).
> 2. Inject I.V. contrast material (2 mL/kg up to 100 mL) rapidly through a working large bore I.V. followed by flush solution.
> 3. Obtain serial AP supine films at 1 minute, 5 minutes, and 10 minutes.

Chapter 33
Emergent Radiologic
Evaluation of Renal
and Genitourinary
Trauma

431

Procedure

Retrograde Urethrography

Check equipment and test Foley catheter balloon with normal saline. The catheter can be wet with normal saline, but generally no lubricant is used. With the patient in a supine position and the penis sterilely draped and cleansed, an appropriate sized feeding tube or Foley catheter already filled with contrast media should be placed (no lubrication) in the distal penile urethra up to the level of the base of the glans penis or just slightly beyond. Patient size and equipment availability may dictate whether a Foley catheter or feeding tube is used. In infants, a small feeding tube may be all that is available (see Table 33.1 for approximate sizes based on patient age). The catheter should fill the urethral lumen so that contrast is less likely to flow distally with injection. In the teenage or adult patient some authorities recommend inflating the Foley balloon in the fossa navicularis with 1 to 2 mL saline to secure the position of the catheter and to prevent leakage of the contrast back out of the meatus. If this practice is elected, extreme caution should be exercised in order to prevent traumatizing the urethra from balloon inflation. If the Foley technique is used the 30 or 60 mL catheter-tipped syringe containing contrast media may be connected to the Foley catheter (Fig. 33.1) If a feeding tube is used as the urethral catheter, it may be connected to I.V. tubing and spiked to a bottle of contrast media or simply attached to a syringe filled with media (Fig. 33.3).

Whichever method is used care should be taken to prime the tubing and catheters so that large amounts of air are not injected into the urethra and bladder. A scout film should be obtained after catheter insertion into the

penis. The urethra should be filled using 15 to 30 mL contrast media (less is necessary in younger patients) while films of the penis and lower pelvis are obtained with the radiograph beam at a 30 or 40° oblique projection. Once the integrity of the urethra has been confirmed radiographically the catheter may be advanced to the level of the bladder for the cystography portion of the study. If the Foley balloon had been inflated it should be deflated before advancement.

Retrograde Cystography

Once the bladder has been catheterized, its contents should be drained and an AP film of the pelvis should be obtained as a scout film. Contrast media is then instilled by gravity from a hanging bottle of contrast media connected to I.V. tubing (Fig. 33.3) or by slow injection (Foley technique) until the patient experiences discomfort or the predicted volume has been instilled (Table 33.2 lists the formula for calculating predicted bladder capacity based on age). If fluoroscopy is used radiation should be brief and intermittent to minimize gonadal irradiation. AP and oblique radiographs of the pelvis should be obtained in an attempt to demonstrate intraperitoneal or extraperitoneal extravasation from bladder rupture. Once adequate films have been obtained with a contrast-filled bladder, the bladder is drained and postdrainage films are obtained to avoid missing extravasation of contrast material which might have been hidden by a contrast-filled bladder.

COMPLICATIONS

The greatest risk associated with IVP is from an anaphylactic reaction to the intravenous

Table 33.1.
Estimated Urethral Catheter Size

Age	Catheter Size
Newborn	5 French (feeding tube)
3 mos	8 French
1 yr	8–10 French
3 yr	10 French
6 yr	10 French
8 yr	10–12 French
10 yr	12 French
12 yr	12–14 French
Teen/adult	16+ French

Table 33.2.
Formula for Predicting Bladder Capacity

Age	Bladder Capacity
<1 yr	wt (kg) $\times$ 10 = mL
>1 yr	(age + 2) $\times$ 30 = mL*

* Maximum volume = 400 mL

Chapter 33
Emergent Radiologic
Evaluation of Renal
and Genitourinary
Trauma

432

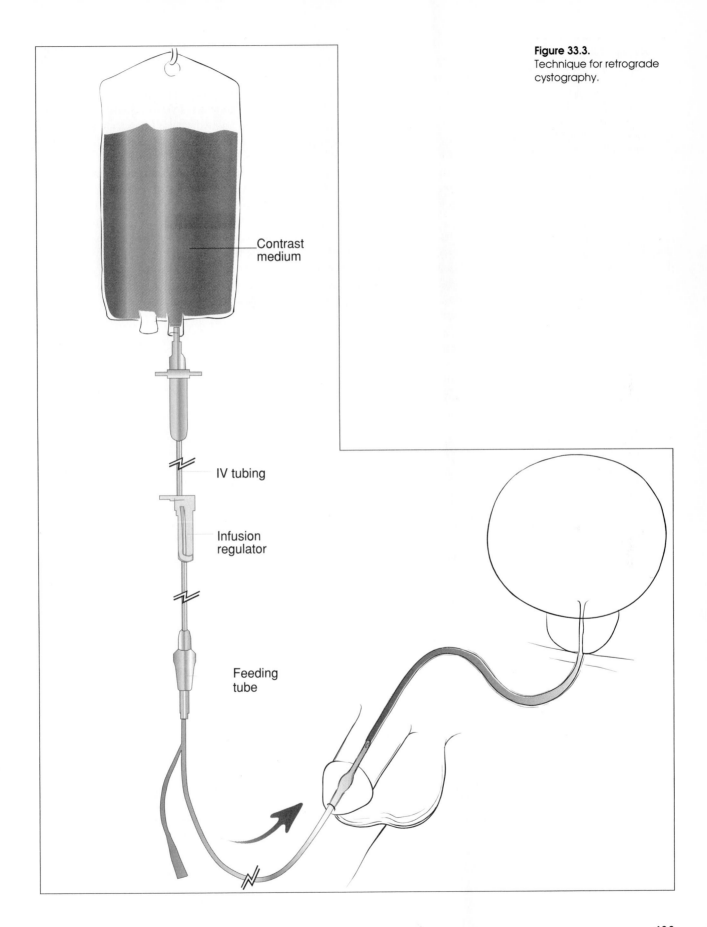

Figure 33.3.
Technique for retrograde cystography.

Contrast medium

IV tubing

Infusion regulator

Feeding tube

contrast material (10). Adverse reactions to I.V. contrast agents occur in approximately 2 to 10% of individuals receiving the higher osmolality agents and is much lower in those receiving nonionic contrast material. Risk factors associated with anaphylaxis include a history of asthma and a prior reaction to iodinated contrast material. High risk patients requiring the study should have only nonionic agents and receive prophylactic parenteral corticosteriods, epinephrine, and antihistamines (e.g., diphenhydramine). Epinephrine should be immediately available. In all cases, these drugs and advanced airway equipment should be available at the bedside during the procedure in the case of an adverse reaction. Nonallergic reactions occasionally occur as a result of direct toxic effects of the contrast media and include nausea, arrhythmias, and contrast nephropathy. Contraindications to intravenous contrast include a history of renal or hepatic insufficiency and shocklike states in which renal perfusion is absent or greatly diminished. In addition to anaphylactic reactions, other known complications associated with intravenous contrast agents include acute renal failure, dehydration as a result of the high osmolality of the agents, and tissue necrosis from local infiltration.

Complications related to retrograde cystourethrography include bleeding and trauma to both the urethra and the bladder, induced during catheter insertion, and a very low but documented risk of allergic reactions to the contrast media. Iatrogenic trauma to the urethra can result later in urethral strictures.

SUMMARY

The techniques described are important adjuncts to the evaluation and stabilization of many trauma victims. Intravenous pyelography is a time-tested means of documenting injury to the urinary system. This technique identifies the presence of an injury and its location, usually within minutes. In many trauma centers, however, the use of computed tomography has replaced intravenous pyelography because CT scanning allows for the evaluation of other retroperitoneal structures and of the abdominal organs.

Retrograde urethrography must be performed prior to instrumentation or catheterization of the urethra in all males suspected of having sustained an injury to the urethra. Failure to identify such injuries may result in significant morbidity.

REFERENCES

1. Allshouse MJ, Betts JM. Genitourinary injury. In: Eichelberger MR, ed. Pediatric trauma: prevention, acute care, rehabilitation, St. Louis: C.V. Mosby, 1993.
2. Amis ES, Newhouse JH. History of uroradiology. In: Essentials of uroradiology. Boston: Little-Brown, 1991, pp. 1–2.
3. Bakht F, Guerriero G. Genitourinary emergencies. Primary Care 1989 Dec; 16(4):905–926.
4. Harwood-Nuss AL, Sandler CM. Genitourinary trauma. In: Rosen P, ed. Diagnostic radiology in emergency medicine. St. Louis: CV Mosby, 1992, pp. 143–158.
5. NormanNoe H, Jenkins GR: Genitourinary trauma in children, from Kelalis PP, King LR, Balman AB ed. Clinical Pediatric Urology, 3rd edition Saunders, Phila. 1992.
6. Murphy JP: Genitourinary trauma. In: Pediatric radiology by Ashcraft, pp. 437–445.
7. Moreau JF, Mazzara L. Intravenous urography. New York: John Wiley & Sons, 1983, pp. 1–17.
8. Neuwirth H, Frasier B, Cochran S. Genitourinary imaging and procedures by the emergency physician. Emerg Med Clin North Am 1989 Feb; 7(1):1–28.
9. Rehm C. Blunt traumatic bladder rupture: the role of retrograde cystogram. Ann Emerg Med 1991 Aug; 20(8):845–847.
10. Weese DL, Greenberg HM, Zimmern PE. Contrast media reactions during voiding cystourethrography or retrograde pyelography. Urology 1993 Jan; 41(1):81–84.

Chapter 33
Emergent Radiologic
Evaluation of Renal
and Genitourinary
Trauma

SECTION FOUR

ANESTHESIA AND SEDATION PROCEDURES

Section Editor: Mark D. Joffe

CHAPTER 34

Pain Management Techniques

Jeffrey R. Avner

"A second of pain lasts as long as a day of pleasure"

—Proverb

Introduction

A large part of emergency care, both diagnostic and therapeutic, centers around the issue of pain. Most injuries are associated with pain and pain is often a marker for serious illness. Acute pain may help the physician localize a fracture, differentiate a cellulitis from an insect bite, or suspect appendicitis. However, although acute pain may serve a function, continued or prolonged pain is rarely warranted in any setting.

Pain can be defined as an unpleasant sensory and emotional experience arising from actual or potential tissue damage (1, 2). In the emergency setting several factors affect the nature of the pain a child experiences. These factors are related to the child, the provider, and the procedure. Child factors include any underlying medical condition, previous painful events, the culture and the environment in which the child is reared, and the developmental, cognitive, and emotional level of the child. Provider factors include the attitude, experience, and the competence of the physician. In addition, the type of procedure, the part of the body involved, the duration of manipulation, and the type of medication used will also affect the child's perception of pain. Clearly pain is multifactorial and sub-

jective (3), but only with the appreciation of the factors involved can the clinician try to relieve or minimize it.

It is important to have a clear understanding of the meaning of the terms used in describing pain control to avoid confusion about their usages. Anesthesia is the loss of all sensation in a part, or in the whole body, induced by the administration of a drug, whereas analgesia is the reduction or elimination of pain sensation (4). Lidocaine is an excellent local anesthetic because infiltration alleviates pain in the area involved. Acetaminophen is a better analgesic because it reduces the general feeling of pain. Sedation is the act of calming usually by quieting nervous excitation (4). Sedation may make it easier for a child to cope with a painful procedure, but does not, by itself, alleviate pain. Conscious sedation is "light sedation" during which the child retains airway reflexes and responds to verbal stimuli (5).

Anatomy and Physiology

The pathway by which pain is transmitted from the skin or other organs to the brain is multifaceted and can be modulated in several ways. A peripheral stimulus for pain is detected by specialized sets of peripheral nerve endings in the skin. One set of these receptors, or nociceptors, is composed of thinly myelinated A-δ fibers that conduct impulses rapidly and are responsible for the initial feeling of sharp or pricking pain. The other set of nociceptors contains unmyelinated C fibers that conduct impulses more slowly and are responsible for longer-lasting burning or dull pain sensations (6). Because the fibers of these nociceptors are unmyelinated, they are more amenable to the effects of local anesthesia (7). A-δ fibers are located in the skin and mucous membranes; C fibers are widely distributed in deep tissues and the skin. In addition to nociceptors, thermoreceptors and mechanoreceptors are composed of A-α or A-β fibers that are responsible for the feeling of touch and light pressure. All these receptors convert a stimulus to electrical activity that is then transmitted through various routes in the spinal cord to the brain. The initial cortical response is probably reflexive but the subsequent response may be altered by cortical activity including inputs from the frontal lobes and the limbic system (8).

Several theories attempt to explain why other cutaneous stimuli and emotional stress can alter the quality and intensity of pain. The gate control theory, hypothesized by Melzack and Wall (9), suggests that collateral input from the A-β touch fibers and collateral input from the A-δ and C fibers have antagonistic effects on so-called "gate cells" in the substantia gelatinosa in the spinal cord (6). This explains, for example, why when a person accidentally bangs an arm, he or she instinctively rubs the affected area (i.e., stimulate the touch fibers that antagonize the pain receptors). This principle can be applied when attempting venipuncture by rubbing or slapping the skin before inserting the needle.

A variety of developmental and psychological factors influence the child's perception of pain and create broad variations in the child's response to pain (10). Appreciation for the child's cognitive developmental level is mandatory for appropriate pain management. For example, it is of limited value to explain to a 3-year-old child that insertion of an intravenous line is important so that he or she can get medication to feel better. At this age, the child does not have the formal logical thinking necessary to understand and accept the pain of a procedure. The explanation

of a procedure must be age appropriate and address the fears of the child. Describing her fear of needles, an 8-year-old girl stated, "The scariest thing about the hospital is needles. They hurt! He said it was gonna be a little pinch, but the little pinch hurt!" (11). A developmental sequence of understanding pain is shown in Table 34.1 (12).

Innate responses combined with responses conditioned by the environment form a child's temperament (13, 14). This temperament is a major factor in determining the child's perception of pain. Because pain is a subjective experience, management must be directed toward the child's perception and not the parents' or the physician's perception. Difficulty in pediatric pain assessment results from inability of the young child to clearly state the degree of pain. Psychological responses do not adequately reflect the child's perception of pain and tend to habituate quite rapidly (15). In infants, indirect measures such as observations of cry, body movement, eye squeeze, heart rate, and especially facial expression have been found to be indicative of pain (16, 17). In the older child, self-report is more useful. For preschool-age children, many self-report scales of pain intensity have been developed including linear analogue scales (18), photographic scale of facial ex-

Table 34.1.
Developmental Sequence of Understanding Pain

Age	Understanding of Pain
0–3 months	No obvious understanding; memory of pain likely but not proven. Pain responses are dominated perceptually.
3–6 months	Infantile pain response persists; initiation of toddler anger response.
6–18 months	Fear response develops. Words for pain appear: "ouchie," "boo-boo," etc. Localization of some pain occurs.
18 months–6 years	Prelogical thinking: concrete, egocentric, transductive logic.
7–10 years	Concrete operational thinking: ability to distinguish self from environment; behavioral coping strategies.
11+ years	Formal logical thinking: abstraction, introspection; cognitive coping strategies.

Adapted from McGrath PJ, Craig KD. Developmental and psychological factors in children's pain. Pediatr Clin North Am 1989;36:826.

pression (Oucher scale) (19), and line drawing of faces (20).

An understanding of some general pharmacologic principles will help determine the type of drug and the route of administration for the drug used for pain control. The speed of onset, peak effect, and duration of action of a drug are determined largely by the rate of absorption and clearance. The rate of absorption is influenced by drug solubility, rate of dissolution, concentration, absorbing surface, circulation to the site of absorption, and route of administration (21). Six common routes of administration of pain medications used in the ED are oral, intramuscular, intravenous, subcutaneous, intranasal, and rectal. Each route has characteristic absorption patterns which may be particularly useful depending on the clinical setting. A general principle in pain management is that the clinician should avoid giving medication to relieve pain by painful injection. The child then may not ask for pain medication, or not admit to being in pain, because of the fear of receiving another painful injection.

The oral route is a convenient and economical route, but absorption may be variable and incomplete. Furthermore, many patients cannot or will not take medication orally. Still, for management of postprocedural pain, especially as an outpatient, the oral route is preferred. Subcutaneous and intramuscular routes provide prompt and sustained absorption of the drug resulting in a smoother induction of analgesia. However, drugs given in this manner cannot be titrated. In addition, under certain conditions, circulation to the site of injection may be poor, thereby leading to erratic absorption. In patients with poor perfusion to an extremity or in patients with large burns, intramuscular and subcutaneous routes may be ineffective for the prompt delivery of pain medications. The intranasal route has been shown to be effective for some medications, including midazolam. The drug is rapidly absorbed from the nasal mucosa; however, it is difficult to deliver large volumes, especially in small children, by this route.

For the management of acute pain in the ED, the intravenous route allows the most rapid delivery of the drug and can provide immediate pain relief. With slow injection the drug can be titrated for the desired effect. However, the physician must be aware of the limitations of using the intravenous route, because it adds an increased risk of adverse effects and, because high concentrations of the drug are achieved rapidly, overdosing may occur. Therefore, intravenous injection should always be given slowly, by an experienced provider, with constant monitoring of the patient (see Fig. 35.1, p. 453).

INDICATIONS

Pain management techniques should be used any time a child complains of pain. Unfortunately, attentiveness to pain control in children is usually inadequate (22–25). Although children, including neonates, exhibit significant stress responses (26, 27), the responses often are not well appreciated by the provider. As opposed to adult patients who clearly verbalize their discomfort, a child's cry is nonspecific and often misinterpreted. This is particularly true in nonverbal children. In a study of analgesic use in the ED, Selbst and Clark (25). found that children were much less likely to receive pain medication than adults, and children under 2 years of age less often than older children.

Many explanations exist for undertreatment of pain in children (28). Physicians often have an exaggerated fear of complications when using pain medication in the pediatric patient, which may lead to using a less potent regimen or an underdosing of medications. With the understanding of how pain medications work, and with proper use of monitoring equipment, side effects such as respiratory depression and hypotension can be avoided. In fact, good pain control and adequate sedation will usually make treatment easier for the provider and less traumatic for the child and the parents.

Another part of the reluctance of ED physicians and pediatricians to use analgesics in children is based on an unfounded fear of addiction to narcotics (29, 30). Children are no more at risk to be addicted to narcotics than adults. In fact, because of their increased ability to clear most medications, children often tolerate large and prolonged doses of pain medications better than adults. Fear of a child becoming addicted to narcotics should not be a concern to the physician in the acute setting.

The method of pain management will depend on the clinical situation encountered. In general, relaxation and behavior therapy should be tried in most situations. The decision to use restraints or pharmacologic therapy is affected by cognitive level and temperament of the child combined with the anticipated or realized pain of the event.

Providing pain medications is rarely contraindicated. Using these medications in situations when the location and severity of pain is used as a clinical indicator of progression of disease is controversial. In the setting of abdominal pain in a child with suspected appendicitis, or headache in a child with head trauma, repeated evaluation often involves assessment of pain. "Masking" symptoms is a concern of some physicians, though others believe a more comfortable patient can better communicate their symptoms and better cooperate during a careful physical examination. Certainly once the diagnosis is established (e.g., deciding to operate on a child with appendicitis) or excluded (a negative head CT scan in a child with head trauma) there is no reason to have the child endure prolonged pain.

EQUIPMENT

Type of personnel and equipment that should be readily available will depend on the drug used for pain management. Nonpharmacologic techniques and common oral analgesics (acetaminophen, ibuprofen) can generally be given without risk of serious side effects. Concentrated sucrose solutions seem to have an analgesic effect on young infants. The more potent analgesics and sedatives, including narcotics and benzodiazepines, should be given by a physician who has had experience using these medications and is familiar with management of complications of these techniques. Both a physician and a nurse must assume responsibility for monitoring the child when these medications are used.

Patient monitoring should be recorded on a sedation or pain-control flow sheet in the medical record. Vital signs, pulse oximeter reading, level of consciousness, response to stimulation, and color should be noted at premedication and at regular intervals (5 to 10 minutes) thereafter. The following should be available at bedside:

Oxygen
Bag-valve-mask
Intravenous line setup
ECG monitoring
Pediatric defibrillator
Reversal agents (naloxone, flumazenil)

Medications

Nonnarcotics

The most common nonnarcotic pain medications used in the ED are aspirin, acetaminophen, and nonsteroidal antiinflammatory drugs (NSAID). These medications are generally weak analgesics and should be reserved for mild to moderate pain such as headache, arthralgias, or for treatment of superficial burns and abrasions. Aspirin is an excellent antiinflammatory drug which is now used less often because of its association with Reye's syndrome. The dose is 10 mg/kg/dose given every 4–6 hours, up to 5 times per day. Aspirin will usually cause some gastrointestinal irritation and may cause bleeding by altering platelet function. Acetaminophen is better tolerated and has less side effects than aspirin. Although acetaminophen is as potent an analgesic as aspirin, it does not have any antiinflammatory properties and therefore may be less useful for management of generalized myalgias and inflammatory arthritides. The dose is 15 mg/kg/dose given every 4–6 hours, up to 5 times per day. NSAIDs are generally used to describe a group of propionic acid derivatives that have aspirinlike properties. The most widely used NSAIDs are ibuprofen and naproxen. NSAIDs have excellent antiinflammatory, analgesic, and antipyretic activities. They are particularly useful in the management of arthritic pain seen with inflammatory diseases. In addition, NSAIDs have become prime drugs in the management of pain associated with viral syndromes, dysmenorrhea, and soft tissue injuries. Although the patient may have some gastrointestinal side effects, NSAIDs are generally better tolerated than aspirin. Furthermore, the longer half-life of NSAIDs allows a longer dosing interval. Ibuprofen in now available in liquid form making it more practical for use in pediatrics; the dose is 10 mg/kg/dose every 6–8 hours, up to 4 times per day.

Because these medications are given orally, the analgesic effects may not be appreciated for 30 to 90 minutes after administration. Therefore, in the management of acute pain, it may be preferable to give these medications at a regular interval, for continuous analgesia, rather than waiting for the child to complain of pain.

Narcotics

Opioids act primarily by binding to μ-receptors in the central nervous system thereby initiating a complex cellular reaction which produces analgesia. Morphine has become the standard drug for comparing the potency and dosing of the other narcotics. All the narcotics are potent analgesics; however, they also share the side effects of respiratory depression, inhibition of gastric motility, and nausea. One advantage to using narcotics is that their potentially adverse effects are reversible with naloxone, a narcotic antagonist. Therefore, naloxone should be readily available whenever narcotics are administered. If a child develops respiratory depression after receiving a narcotic analgesic, naloxone should be given immediately (0.1 mg/kg) either i.v., i.m., or via an endotracheal tube and other measures of respiratory support should be instituted. This dose may be repeated as necessary for all age groups.

The starting dose of morphine is 0.1 mg/kg/dose given i.v., i.m., or subcutaneously every 3 to 4 hours. The route of administration depends on the clinical situation (see Anatomy and Physiology in this chapter). Onset is almost immediate with the peak effect after intravenous administration in 15 to 20 minutes. After peak effect has been reached, supplemental dosing may be needed to achieve the degree of analgesia desired. Morphine may be given as a continuous i.v. infusion at 0.05 to 0.1 mg/kg/hr titrated to the desired effect. Along with respiratory depression, morphine may cause bronchospasm, hypotension in hypovolemic patients, and rarely seizures with large doses.

Meperidine (Demerol) has similar pharmacologic properties to morphine although it is 10 times less potent. It is better absorbed than morphine after intramuscular injection, but also can be given intravenously or even orally. The dose is 1 mg/kg every 3 to 4 hours. One often discussed advantage to meperidine is that it may be less likely to cause spasm of the common bile duct than morphine. However, it is unclear whether this effect is consistent when equianalgesic doses of meperidine and morphine are used (31). In addition to the shared side effects with morphine, meperidine can cause severe reactions—hyperpyrexia, delirium, seizures—when given to a patient using monoamine oxidase (MAO) inhibitors (31, 32).

Fentanyl is 100 times more potent than morphine and its rapid onset of action and quick elimination make it better suited for titration than morphine. Because of its potency, fentanyl is rarely used for isolated pain control but is a superb drug for conscious sedation because it is titratable and does not cause prolonged sedation (see Chapter 35).

On an ambulatory basis, many narcotics can be given orally. Codeine can be as effective an analgesic as morphine. The dosing is 0.5 to 1 mg/kg/dose given orally every 3 to 4 hours. Onset of action is about 20 minutes and the peak effect occurs at 1 to 2 hours. Codeine is often used in combination with aspirin or acetaminophen, since these drugs will potentiate the analgesic effect of codeine. A variety of other oral narcotics—hydrocodone, hydromorphone, oxycodone—also are effective agents.

Other Medications

Other pain medications such as nitrous oxide, ketamine, and the benzodiazepines, have become useful drugs in the management of pain, especially related to procedures. These medications are described in Chapters 35 and 36. In addition, local anesthetics are important adjuncts to pain control in children (see Chapter 37).

PROCEDURES

Preparation and Relaxation

With appreciation of the child's fears and concerns, the clinician should create as relaxed an environment as possible. A quiet examination room should be used—it is difficult to relax when the child hears other children screaming and crying. After the initial examination, overhead lights should be dimmed if possible; a gooseneck or operating room light can be used for illumination. Once the child has been told of an impending painful procedure, long delays should be avoided. All necessary equipment (suture kit, needles, etc.) should be prepared in advance and away from the child's direct sight. Open-

SUMMARY
1. Administer medications under supervision of personnel experienced in sedation and airway management
2. Have following equipment readily available in procedure room:
   Cardiorespiratory monitor
   Pulse oximeter
   Suction
   Oxygen
   Nonrebreather face mask
   Bag-valve-mask
   Airway equipment
3. Ensure monitoring at bedside by experienced physician and/or nurse who is not directly involved in procedure
4. Prepare all equipment and medications in a quiet, darkened room
5. Allow parents at bedside during induction if desired
6. Relax child with guided imagery, behavior therapy, and/or hypnosis
7. Place cardiac monitor leads and pulse oximeter after child is relaxed
8. Begin intravenous line if needed
9. Titrate medications by i.v. route whenever possible
10. Administer local anesthetic if full analgesia is needed
11. Use physical restraint if needed to control random motion
12. Administer oxygen for pulse oximeter reading less than 95%
13. Allow child to remain in quiet room after procedure. Minimize verbal and tactile stimulation during recovery. Continue to monitor vital signs.
14. Discharge criteria:
    Return to pretreatment level of awareness
    Parental recognition
    Purposeful movement
15. Discharge instructions:
    Nothing by mouth for 2 hours
    Careful parental observation
    No independent ambulation for 2 hours

ing needles and unfamiliar equipment in front of the child will no doubt heighten anxiety. All attempts should be made to keep the painful procedure brief.

Many children can be further relaxed through guided imagery. The child's favorite doll or television character in an adventure story can be used, with the hope of focusing the child into the fantasy. These stories should be age appropriate and incorporate the child's interests (Sesame Street or fairy tales for young children; beach scenes or sporting events for the older child).

Parental presence during a painful event may help the child relax, because the parent is often a source of comfort for the child (33). Furthermore, the parents can often accurately predict the child's degree of distress to the painful stimulus (34, 35). Still, the decision to have parents remain in the room for painful procedures will depend on the age and needs of the child as well as the ability of the parent to remain calm. A parent who moans and groans during the procedure will disrupt any chance of relaxation. For very painful procedures it may be best for the parents to wait outside the treatment area (see also Chapter 1).

Behavior Therapy

The provider should never lie, or downplay a child's perception of pain with flippant remarks such as "This won't hurt" or "Oh, come on, that didn't really hurt you." These remarks will only serve to erode the trust between the child and the provider. Children should be encouraged to express their feelings and not be made to feel they must prove how brave or grown up they are by internalizing their emotions (20). Conversely, consistent positive reinforcement is often helpful. Words should be chosen carefully and communicated in an empathetic tone.

Young children think in concrete terms making cognitive-behavioral techniques less applicable. They may not understand that an intravenous line may help them get better, but they may believe that a Band-Aid or a parent's kiss can make the pain go away (21).

Restraint

Despite even the best attempts at relaxation, restraints may be needed for certain procedures. In particular, it is better to restrain a child at the beginning of a procedure than to take a chance that he or she will lay still only to find that three people need to hold the child down in the middle of the procedure. However, using restraints is not a license to abandon other techniques for pain control. Restraints should be used in conjunction with relaxation techniques and an explanation of the restraint to the child. The clinician should avoid wrestling a child into a tight-fitting restraint. Specific types of restraints and their uses are described in Chapter 3.

Hypnosis

Rather than trying to distract the child, hypnosis uses guided imagery to facilitate pain control (36). This approach probably works best with children who have vivid imaginations or are "hypersuggestable." Developmental age of the child will largely determine the most effective hypnotic approach. Various suggestions have been documented (37), including (*a*) direct suggestion—"pretend you are painting numbing medicine on the part of your body that hurts"; (*b*) distancing suggestions—"imagine you are in your favorite place"; and (*c*) suggestions for feeling that are antithetical to pain—"think of the funniest movie you ever saw." Hypnotic techniques are most effective when used in a quiet, comfortable environment, which obviously may be difficult to provide in a hectic ED. Furthermore, although hypnosis can often be a valuable adjunct in pain control, the operator should not refrain from also using pharmacologic agents, when needed.

Medications

As discussed earlier, the type of medication used will depend on the type of painful condition or procedure, the duration of the desired effect, and the experience of the physician. After being placed in a quiet room and relaxed with behavior therapy or hypnosis, the child should be placed on appropriate monitors. Suction, oxygen, bag-valve-mask, and appropriate airway equipment should be available. Medications should be drawn up in a syringe small enough to allow the operator to administer appropriate aliquots. If an antagonist medication is available (such as naloxone), it should be drawn up and ready for immediate use. With continuous clinical one-on-one monitoring at the bedside by a physician and/or nurse, medication should be given by a predetermined route. The preferred route of administration, onset of action, and duration of effect is described elsewhere in this chapter or in the chapter on conscious sedation (Chapter 35). When the child is sedated, additional pain medication can be titrated based on the response of the child to movement or touching of the painful area. Use of local anesthetic may be needed for full analgesia.

After a procedure is completed, the child still must be monitored for continued effects of the analgesic, especially apnea and hypotension. Antagonistic medications should be avoided (unless needed to reverse apnea) so that the child can have a gradual emergence and avoid the agitation that may accompany rapid reversal of a sedative or narcotic agent. The period of sedation may be considered complete when the child returns to pretreatment level of awareness, can recognize his or her parents, and shows purposeful movement.

COMPLICATIONS

Complications during the use of pain medications occur in three major areas—airway compromise with or without respiratory depression, paradoxical drug reactions such as agitation or hallucinations, and abnormal central nervous system activity including seizures. Initial management of any complication is similar for any pediatric emergency; assess airway, breathing, and circulation. Keen awareness of these basic life support measures will avert much of the morbidity that occurs when measures to ensure ventilation, oxygenation, and perfusion are overlooked. Management of airway compromise and basic life support are detailed in Section 2. After stabilization of airway, breathing and circulation, children with paradoxical hyperactivity and/or agitation can be given intravenous benzodiazepines (e.g., diazepam or midazolam 0.1 mg/kg). However, the clinician should be certain that the agitation is secondary to drug reaction and not a sign of hypoxia or inadequate ventilation. Similarly, basic life support measures should precede intravenous benzodiazepines (diazepam 0.1 mg/kg or lorazepam 0.05 mg/kg) in the management of seizures.

SUMMARY

Pain is a frequent and often difficult problem to manage. The clinician must assess a variety of patient and environmental factors, enlist the aid of experienced personnel, be familiar with basic nonpharmacologic techniques, and use effective medications. Sensitivity to the needs of the child and appreciation of the child's fears and apprehensions are of paramount importance. Above all, the clinician should do no harm, and be prepared to act swiftly for any untoward event.

References

1. International Association for the Study of Pain. Pain terms: a list with definitions and notes on usage. Pain 1979;6:249.
2. Merskey H. An investigation of pain in psychological illness. D.M. Thesis, Oxford, 1964.
3. Goodman J, McGrath PJ. The epidemiology of pain in children and adolescents: a review. Pain 1991;46: 247–264.
4. Stedman's medical dictionary. 21st ed. Baltimore: Williams & Wilkins, 1966.
5. Acute Pain Management Guideline Panel. Acute pain management: operative or medical procedures trauma. Clinical practice guideline. AHCPR PUL No. 92-0032. Rockville, MD: Agency for Health Care Policy Research, Pubic Health Service, US Department of Health & Human Service, Feb 1992.
6. Kelly DD. Central representations of pain and analgesia. In: Kandel ER, Schwartz JH, ed. Principles of neural science. New York: Elsevier North Holland 1981, pp. 200–212.
7. Hendler N. The anatomy and psychopharmacology of chronic pain. J Clin Psych 1982;43:15–20.
8. Schechter NL. Pain and pain control in children. Current Prob in Pediatr 1985;15:6–67.
9. Melzack R, Wall PD. Pain mechanism: a new theory. Science 1965;150:971–979.
10. Schechter NC, Berde CB, Yaster M. Pain in infants, children and adolescents: an overview. In: Schechter NC, Bende CB, Yaster M, eds. Pain in infants, children, and adolescents. Baltimore: Williams & Wilkins, 1993, pp. 3–10.
11. Fassler D, Wallace MA. Children's fear of needles. Clin Pediatr 1982;21:59–60.
12. McGrath PJ, Craig KD. Developmental and psychological factors in children's pain. Pediatr Clin North Am 1989;36:823–835.
13. Thomas A, Chess S, Birch HG. Temperament and behavior disorders in children. New York: New York University Press, 1968.
14. Poznanski ED. Children's reaction to pain: a psychiatrist's perspective. Clin Pediatr 1976;15: 1114–1119.
15. McGrath LA. An assessment of children's pain: a review of behavioral, physiological and direct scaling techniques. Pain 1987;31:147–176.
16. Johnston CC, Stranda ME. Acute pain response in infants: a multidimensional description. Pain 1986; 24:373–382.
17. Granau RVE, Craig KD. Pain expression in neonates: facial action and cry. Pain 1984;28: 395–410.
18. Broadman L, Rice L, Hannallah R. Evaluation of an objective pain scale for infants and children. Reg Anesthes 1988;13:45.
19. Beyer J. The Oucher:aA user's manual and technical report. Denver: University of Colorado Health Sciences Center, 1988.
20. LeBaron S, Zeltzer L. Assessment of acute pain and anxiety in children and adolescents by self-reports, observer reports, and behavioral checklist. J Consult Clin Psych 1984;52:729–738.
21. Mayer SE, Melmon KL, Gilman AG. Introduction: the dynamics of drug absorption, distribution, and elimination. In: Gilman AG, Goodman LS, Gilman A, eds. The pharmacologic basis of therapeutics. 6th ed. New York: Macmillian Publishing Co., 1980, pp. 1–27.
22. Swafford LI, Allan D. Pain relief in the pediatric patient. Med Clin North Am 1968;52:131–136.
23. Beyer J, De hood DE, Ashley CC, et al. Patterns of postoperative analgesic use with adults and children following cardiac surgery. Pain 1983;17:71–81.
24. Schechter NC, Allen DA, Hanson K. Status of pediatric pain control: a comparison of hospital analgesic usage in children and adults. Pediatrics 1986;77: 11–15.
25. Selbst SM, Clark M. Analgesic use in the Emergency Department. Ann Emerg Med 1990;19: 1010–1013
26. Arand K. The biology of pain perception in newborn infants. In: Tyler D, Krane E, eds. Advances in pain research and therapy: pediatric pain. New York: Raven Press, 1990, vol.15, pp. 113–122.
27. Arand KJ, Hickey PR. Pain in the fetus and neonate. N Engl J Med 1987;317:1321–1329.
28. Schechter NL. The undertreatment of pain in children. Pediatr Clin North Am 1989;36:781–794.
29. Schechter NL, Allan DA. Physicians' attitudes toward pain in children. J Dev Behav Pediatr 1986;7: 350–354.
30. McCaffery M, Ferrell BR. Opioid analgesics: nurses' knowledge of doses and psycological dependance. J Nurs Staff Dev 1992;8:77–84.
31. Yaster M, Maxwell LG. Opiod agonists and antagonists. In: Schechter NC, Bende CB, Yaster M, eds. Pain in infants, children, and adolescents. Baltimore: Williams & Wilkins, 1993, pp. 145–171.
32. Taylor DC. Alarming reaction to pethidine in patients on phenelzine. Lancet 1962;2:401–402.
33. Bauchner H, Waring C, Vinci R. Parental presence during procedures in an emergency room: results from 50 observations. Pediatrics 1991;87:544–548.
34. Fradet C, McGrath PJ, Kay J, Adams S, Luke B. A prospective survey of reactions to blood tests by children and adolescents. Pain 1990;40:53–60.
35. Schecter NL, Bernstein BA, Beck A, Hart L, Sherzer L. Individual differences in children's response to pain: role of temperament and parental characteristics. Pediatrics 1991;87:171–177.
36. Zeltzer L, LeBaron S. Hypnosis and nonhypnotic techniques for reduction of pain and anxiety during painful procedures in children and adolescents with cancer. J Pediatr 1982;101:1032–1035.
37. Gardner GG, Olness K. Hypnosis and hypnotherapy in children. New York: Grune & Stratton, 1981.

Conscious Sedation

Sandra J. Cunningham and Ellen F. Crain

Introduction

Many painful and anxiety-provoking procedures are performed in children on a routine basis in a pediatric emergency department (ED). In order to provide optimal patient comfort and to ensure the success of the procedure, it is important that the child be as calm and pain free as possible. However, the safety of the patient is of the utmost concern. It is the task of the ED physician to strike a balance that will ensure a safe environment while minimizing the child's pain and anxiety. The ED is not an operating room, and general anesthesia can not be delivered in this setting. The child must always be easily arousable in order to maintain the capacity to protect his or her own airway.

Sedation is a state of calm that can be achieved by a chemical intervention, such as the administration of sedative drugs, or by a psychological intervention, such as hypnosis. A vital difference exists between conscious and unconscious sedation which does not allow for any overlap between the two states. The American Academy of Pediatrics Committee on Drugs defines conscious sedation as "a medically controlled state of depressed consciousness that (*a*) allows protective reflexes to be maintained; (*b*) retains the patient's ability to maintain a patent airway independently and consciously; and (*c*) permits appropriate response by the patient to physical stimulation or verbal command, such as 'open your eyes'" (1).

During unconscious sedation, or general anesthesia, the patient loses control of protective reflexes such as the gag reflex, thereby losing the ability to self-maintain a patent airway (1). Sedation producing this state should only be conducted in an operating room by an anesthesiologist or during rapid sequence intubation in the ED.

Analgesia is accomplished when the perception of pain is blunted; therefore, painful stimuli are not interpreted as pain (see Chapter 34). The physician caring for young children is faced with the difficult task of separating pain and anxiety in the child and discerning which is the predominant contributor to the child's state. In the pediatric ED, the need for pain reduction is often concomitant with the need for anxiety alleviation. Some drug classes, such as benzodiazapines, do not produce analgesia but offer a significant sedative effect. The child in a calm state will allow for a more optimal physical examination and better assessment of the need for analgesia.

No single drug or drug combination in any fixed dose will be successful in every child for a given procedure. It is often necessary to titrate a pharmacologic agent to reach the desired effect of sedation or analgesia. Although this can be accomplished by various routes of administration, the intravenous (i.v.) route lends itself to tighter control of incremental additions to reach the desired endpoint. For example, although a strict protocol is provided for the rate at which fentanyl, a potent narcotic analgesic, should be administered, no fixed total dose is given. The drug can be titrated depending on the degree of pain and anxiety the child is experiencing and the procedure being performed. The physician must appreciate the variations among individual children to achieve optimal results and minimal side effects.

Physicians no longer debate that all children can experience pain, including the neonate (2). Psychological development, pain threshold, and the anxiety level of the individual must be considered on a case by case basis (see Table 34.1, p. 438). A younger child may require sedation for a painless procedure such as a computed tomography (CT) scan whereas an older child may require nothing more than a local anesthetic for wound repair.

ANATOMY AND PHYSIOLOGY

Major anatomic and physiologic differences exist between the child and the adult that affect decision making about the use of sedation in children. Furthermore, major variations exist within the pediatric age group from birth through adolescence. The most obvious age-related difference is size. Although body surface area is the more exact reference measurement for children, for clinical purposes, the child's weight in kilograms (kg) is an appropriate, accessible alternative. Drug dosage is determined on a per kg basis throughout the early pediatric years.

Vital signs differ widely in children of different ages (see also Chapter 4). Average systolic blood pressure in children is 90 + 2(age in years). Minimally acceptable systolic blood pressure is 70 + 2(age in years). Physicians monitoring children receiving conscious sedation must be familiar with normal vital signs for age to recognize abnormalities, should they occur.

Metabolic differences in the renal and hepatic systems exist between infants, children, and adults—all affecting drug dosing, response to drugs, and appropriateness of particular drugs in children of different ages. Pharmacokinetics of a drug include absorption, volume of distribution, metabolism, and excretion. Absorption of a drug depends on factors related to the drug and to the patient. Most drugs administered by the oral route are absorbed by the small intestine. Factors that limit or delay absorption by the oral route include a full stomach, decreased gastric emptying, and reduced small bowel surface area. Many oral medications undergo a first pass effect by the liver where they are metabolized before reaching the systemic circulation. Drugs given by the parental route escape this first pass effect. The clinician must be aware of drug metabolism when choosing a route of administration. For example, meperidine, which is well absorbed from the gastrointestinal tract, has extensive first pass metabolism resulting in significantly lower serum levels when given orally than when the drug is given intramuscularly (i.m.). Basic drugs, such as opiates and benzodiazepines, cross cell membranes easier than acidic drugs because the intracellular pH is more acidic than the extracellular pH. Acidic drugs, such as barbiturates, do not enter cells as readily. The elimination half-life of basic drugs is usually longer because the drugs are more widely distributed (3).

Both the medication chosen and the route of administration will determine the level of sedation. Wide variation in the clinical effects of medications given in similar doses by the same route is the rule, not the exception. Understanding the physiology and pharmacokinetics does not replace careful dosing and close monitoring that can ensure safe, effective conscious sedation for all children.

INDICATIONS

Intravenous sedation should be considered for any child undergoing a very painful procedure, such as closed reduction of a fracture or incision and drainage of an abscess. A deeper and more controlled level of sedation also is useful for procedures requiring meticulous care, such as reimplantation of an avulsed fingertip or complex facial laceration repair. Intravenous sedation will generally provide the deepest, most predictable sedation. Choosing medications with a rapid onset of action given intravenously best enables the physician to titrate the dose as needed. An advantage of the intravenous route is the ability to rapidly administer reversal agents such as naloxone or flumazenil should the need arise.

Intramuscular sedation potentially can provide mild, moderate, or deep sedation. However, it lacks the tight control of the i.v. route and medications given by the i.m. route cannot be titrated. In general, there is less risk of complications at a given dose. The pain of injection to some degree defeats the purpose of the sedation and analgesia.

Oral, intranasal, and rectal agents can be useful for less painful procedures such as routine laceration repair in which local anesthetic will also be given. They are excellent for sedation for diagnostic studies such as MRI or CT scans. The onset, depth, and duration of sedation are less predictable than parenterally administered drugs. Medications given orally to a child with a full stomach may have a delayed onset and reduced efficacy.

An inhalational agent such as nitrous oxide (see Chapter 36) is appropriate for cooperative children who are able to follow directions. It is useful for procedures involving mild to moderate pain of brief duration, or for those procedures that are anxiety provoking.

EQUIPMENT

Monitoring Equipment
    Pulse oximeter
    Cardiorespiratory monitor
Resuscitation Equipment
    Suction (Yankauer)
    Oxygen source
    Bag and mask
    Oral airway
    Endotracheal tubes
    Laryngoscope
    Stylet, tape
    Resuscitation medications
    Reversal agents—naloxone, flumazenil

SPECIFIC AGENTS FOR CONSCIOUS SEDATION

A variety of medications are available to the ED physician to provide conscious sedation. As noted, choice of a particular agent depends on a number of factors including, the age of the child, the degree of pain or anxiety the child is experiencing, the likely duration of the pain produced by the procedure, the routes by which a particular agent can be delivered, as well as physician preference and experience with the drug. Some of the more commonly used drugs are described as follows.

Opioids

Opioids provide strong analgesia for painful procedures, elevating the pain threshold and altering mood. These drugs act at various receptor sites throughout the central nervous system (CNS) designated as μ, δ, κ, and σ. It is at the μ-receptor sites that the classic effects of opioids are seen—analgesia, respiratory depression, and euphoria. Animal studies indicate that the number and sensitivity of receptor sites are age related (2). For example, respiratory depression is more profound in the newborn. An appealing property of opioids is that the effects are reversible with naloxone, a pure opioid antagonist. Naloxone will reverse all effects of opioids including analgesia, respiratory depression, sedation, and gastrointestinal effects. Reversal is almost immediate when naloxone is administered by the i.v. route.

Morphine

Morphine is the principal alkaloid of opium and is the drug by which the potency of other narcotics is compared (2). It is a potent analgesic that works via opioid receptors in the CNS. Morphine is less protein bound in newborns than in adults, resulting in higher "free" morphine levels and greater penetration into the CNS. Clearance of morphine is decreased in infants under 2 months of age. Higher peak levels and decreased clearance justify restriction of morphine use in young infants to carefully monitored settings.

Morphine is an appropriate agent for moderate to severe pain during procedures that require extensive time, making its longer elimination half-life advantageous.

Given intravenously, onset is almost immediate but peak effect is not reached for 15 to 20 minutes. Morphine is less useful for i.v. titration than fentanyl or midazolam, which reach peak effect more quickly. Repeated doses can be given safely after 20 to 30 minutes if the child is still in pain and no adverse reactions have occurred. Elimination half-life is approximately 2 to 3 hours.

Intravenous morphine is given at the T-connector site as a slow i.v. infusion. The dose is 0.1 to 0.2 mg/kg/dose to a maximum of 10 mg. It can also be given intramuscularly or subcutaneously, but these routes of administration are less useful for conscious sedation than for analgesia alone.

With proper dosing and monitoring, clinical complications from morphine are unusual. Administration of morphine does not require the intensive monitoring needed when using more potent opioids such as fentanyl or when combined with benzodiazepines; however, the physician should be prepared to resuscitate as with any sedated patient. Although morphine causes peripheral vasodilation, hemodynamic effects are minimal in the patient who is euvolemic with a normal blood pressure.

Miosis is an expected side effect. Adverse side effects include respiratory depression, vasodilation leading to hypotension in the hypovolemic patient, nausea and vomiting, urticaria, and seizures at toxic doses.

Untoward effects of morphine are reversible with naloxone. The initial i.v. dose of naloxone is 0.01 mg/kg. If desired results are not achieved, the dose can be increased to 0.1 mg/kg and repeated doses given. Subcutaneous or i.m. administration of naloxone are alternate routes but are less desirable. Because serum half-life is approximately 60 minutes, patients must be monitored carefully for return of CNS and respiratory depression.

Fentanyl

Fentanyl is a synthetic opioid which is 25 to 100 times more potent than morphine. Fentanyl alone or in combination with a benzodiazepine provides predictable sedation and analgesia for painful procedures. Similar to morphine, it is reversible with naloxone but does not have as great a hemodynamic effect in hypovolemic patients.

Onset and peak effect is extremely fast as it rapidly enters the CNS (2). Fentanyl is short acting with complete recovery in approximately 30 minutes (4), making it ideal for brief, painful procedures. The dose of fentanyl is 1 to 4 μg/kg, 100 μg maximum. It is infused at a rate of 0.5 μg/kg/min to a maximum of 25 μg/min. Peak effect is in minutes when given intravenously, so titration to the desired depth of sedation can easily be accomplished in a timely fashion. A T-connector must always be used when fentanyl is given. Instilling the drug at a more proximal site in the i.v. line will decrease the physician's control of the infusion rate and potentially cause the administration of boluses of the drug rather than a slow, steady infusion (Fig. 35.1).

Patients receiving fentanyl must be closely monitored. A pulse oximeter and cardiorespiratory monitor are recommended. A physician or nurse responsible for monitoring the patient should remain in close visual contact until the sedative effects are waning.

Fentanyl frequently causes facial pruritus. Children undergoing repair of facial lacerations may contaminate the sterile field as they attempt to rub their face. As with all opioids, respiratory depression is the major complication of fentanyl even in appropriate doses, and can last up to 30 minutes. Most patients who hypoventilate do not need naloxone. They can be awakened with verbal or physical stimulation and will breath deeply on command.

Chest wall rigidity ("wooden chest") is a serious complication that makes ventilation difficult. It occurs with rapid boluses of high doses of fentanyl and is reversible with naloxone, but may require higher doses than normally used. Alternatively, a muscle relaxant or paralytic can be used, but the patient will require mechanical ventilation until the effect of the paralytic has worn off. Hypotension, bradycardia, nausea, and vomiting have been reported.

Fentanyl in combination with midazolam provides excellent sedation/analgesia for painful procedures. When the drugs are used in combination, midazolam should be administered first at a dose of 0.1 mg/kg over 2 to 3 minutes to a maximum of 2.5 mg, followed by fentanyl as previously described. Generally, a lower dose of fentanyl, approximately 50% of the usual dose, is required when used in combination with midazolam. Because both drugs are potential respiratory depressants, the patient must be meticulously monitored until drug effects have worn off.

Meperidine

Meperidine (Demerol) is a synthetic opioid agonist which can be administered by the i.v., i.m., or oral routes (2). It is useful as an analgesic for moderately to severely painful procedures such as foreign body removal, incision and drainage, or burn debridement. Demerol is better absorbed intramuscularly than morphine. The onset of action when given intramuscularly is approximately 10 minutes. The duration of action is 2 to 4 hours. The dose of meperidine is 1 to 2 mg/kg/dose to a maximum of 100 mg every 4 hours.

Major adverse effects of meperidine, as morphine, are respiratory and circulatory de-

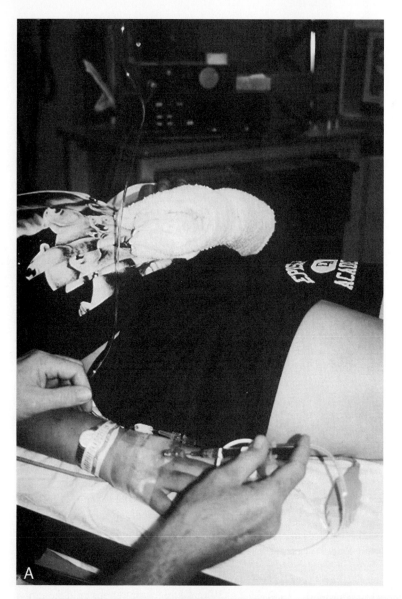

Figure 35.1.
A. Conscious sedation medications being administered to a patient about to undergo fracture reduction, with concurrent monitoring of vital signs and pulse oximetry.
B. Medications being injected via the T-connector in order to enter the venous circulation through as little tubing as possible.

A

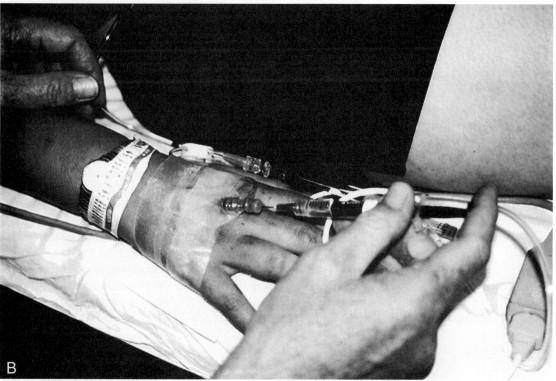

B

pression. Nausea, vomiting, and dizziness are more frequently encountered with meperidine than other narcotics. Large doses can occasionally result in a toxic accumulation of normeperidine, a meperidine metabolite, that can cause CNS excitation and seizures. Meperidine is contraindicated in the presence of head trauma with potential increased intracranial pressure, and in patients receiving monoamine oxidase inhibitors (see Chapter 34, p. 441).

Sedative effects of meperidine are potentiated by hydroxyzine (Vistaril), a piperazine derivative antihistamine which also has antiemetic properties. Hydroxyzine enhances CNS depression of narcotics and, when the two drugs are used simultaneously, the meperidine dose should be decreased by 25 to 50% (0.5 to 1 mg/kg). Hydroxyzine is given as an i.m. injection and can be mixed with the meperidine in the same syringe. It should not be given by the i.v. route. The hydroxyzine dose is 0.5 to 1.0 mg/kg/dose. Adverse side effects are dose dependent and include excessive somnolence and hypotension. The effects of meperidine, but not hydroxyzine, are reversible with naloxone. This combination is rarely recommended in current ED practice.

Benzodiazepines

Benzodiazepines are used for their sedative-hypnotic, anxiolytic, and amnestic effects. Although these drugs have no analgesic effects, amnesia for pain experienced during a procedure is a very desirable property. Using a benzodiazepine in conjunction with a local anesthetic is a good choice in the anxious child undergoing a mildly painful procedure, such as laceration repair. Drugs in this class that are widely used on an outpatient basis include diazepam, lorazepam, and midazolam. To provide sedation for ED procedures, midazolam is an appropriate choice given its potency and short half-life.

Midazolam
Midazolam (Versed) is a short acting benzodiazepine. It provides anxiolysis, sedation and antegrade amnesia. It is often used in combination with a narcotic such as fentanyl or morphine, or as premedication for a procedure when local anesthesia will be used. Several studies have assessed the use of midazolam in the pediatric population and it has been found to be a safe and effective drug for pre-

medication for outpatient procedures (5). The onset of action, when given by the i.v. route, is 3 to 5 minutes. The plasma half-life is approximately 2 hours. Midazolam is an excellent choice for conscious sedation during short procedures in an anxious patient. The dose of midazolam i.v. when used alone is 0.1 to 0.3 mg/kg. Children should be given 0.1 mg/kg as a first dose (maximum of 2.5 mg) given as a slow i.v. infusion over 2 to 3 minutes. The dose may be repeated in 5 minutes to titrate the sedation to the desired level. Midazolam also can be given as an i.m. injection at the same dose.

Midazolam is rapidly absorbed into the systemic circulation from the nasal mucosa, making intranasal administration an effective route of drug delivery (6). It is useful as an anxiolytic for nonpainful procedures such as CT scan or MRI or when additional analgesia will be used. Onset of action is 5 to 10 minutes. The concentrated solution (5 mg/mL) must be used to minimize the volume of fluid instilled into the nostrils. The dose is 0.2 mg to 0.6 mg/kg to a maximum of 6 mg. One-half of the total dose is placed in each nostril. Patients with mucosal secretions may not be able to absorb the drug adequately.

Oral midazolam (0.2 to 0.6 mg/kg) is effective as a premedication when given to children with empty stomachs. In the emergency setting the stomach contents make absorption, onset, and depth of sedation unpredictable.

When using intravenous midazolam in conjunction with fentanyl, the midazolam (0.1 mg/kg) is given first. Often a smaller dose of narcotic is required to reach the desired sedation level when used in this way (see section on fentanyl in this chapter).

The major complication of benzodiazepines given by the i.v. route is respiratory depression. Complications are minimal when the drug is used as a single agent, but are potentiated when it is used in conjunction with other sedative hypnotics or narcotics.

Flumazenil is a benzodiazepine antagonist that blocks the activity of benzodiazepines at CNS receptor sites (7). Its use in the pediatric population has not been widely studied. It is appropriate in iatrogenic overdose or when adverse side effects are experienced, but is not recommended for routine use to reverse the known effects of benzodiazepine administration.

The pediatric dose of flumazenil is 0.02 mg/kg by slow i.v. infusion to a maximum of 1 mg. The onset of action is within 1 to 3 minutes. Patients must be monitored closely for resedation because the effects of flumazenil wear off before the sedative effects of the benzodiazepine.

Barbiturates

Barbiturates are sedative-hypnotics that act as general depressants of the central and peripheral nervous systems, and skeletal, smooth, and cardiac muscle. Depending on the dose, effects vary widely from mild sedation to coma. Barbiturates can be divided into four groups: ultrashort- acting (thiopental and methohexital), short acting (pentobarbital), intermediate (butabarbital), and long acting (phenobarbital). Generally the ultrashort- or short-acting barbitures are utilized in the emergency setting for conscious sedation. When used alone in the proper sedative dose, adverse side effects are rare. Higher doses, for example, a preintubation dose of methohexital, will cause apnea, transient hypotension, and bradycardia.

Barbiturates have no analgesic qualities when used in sedative doses. Analgesia is only provided when high, anesthetic doses are administered. When pain is anticipated, an additional analgesic (parenteral or local) must be used.

Thiopental
Thiopental (pentothal) is an ultrashort-acting barbiturate which for sedation can be administered per rectum (8). It is indicated for use in painless procedures requiring sedation, such as CT scan and MRI, or for procedures in which a local anesthetic will be used, such as in laceration repair.

The onset of action when given rectally is 15 to 30 minutes. The recommended dose is 25 mg/kg PR. Although adverse side effects at this dose are exceedingly rare, some sedation failures do occur. At higher doses, hypotension, bronchospasm, and laryngospasm have been reported.

Pentobarbital
Pentobarbital (Nembutal) is a short-acting barbiturate useful for longer procedures or as a preoperative sedative. It can be used in conjunction with an analgesic for painful procedures. The drug can be given parenterally, orally or rectally. Onset of action is rapid by the i.v. route, with duration about 60 minutes. The onset for oral or rectal administration can be slow, up to 45 minutes. The dose is 3 to 4 mg/kg.

Chloral Hydrate

Chloral hydrate is a sedative, hypnotic CNS depressant widely used in children as a premedication for procedures for CT scan, MRI, or EEG, and in mildly painful procedures such as minor dental work or wound repair when a local anesthetic is used (9). The drug is well absorbed by either the oral or PR routes. The dose is 25 to 75 mg/kg/dose to a maximum of 1.0 gram. Peak therapeutic levels occur in approximately 30 to 60 minutes with rapid absorption from the gastrointestinal tract. Chloral hydrate is metabolized in the liver to its active metabolite trichloroethanol. Elimination half-life of this metabolite is 8 to 12 hours.

Low dose chloral hydrate used for mild sedation (25 mg/kg) does not require monitoring beyond initial and periodic vital signs. Patients given higher doses of the drug (50 to 75 mg/kg) should be monitored with continuous pulse oximetry. Adverse side effects include excessive somnolence and paradoxical excitation. Major disadvantages in using chloral hydrate are sedation is not reversible, onset of action and level of sedation are unpredictable, and half-life is long and requires observation for several hours.

Ketamine

Ketamine is a phencyclidine derivative that acts as a dissociative anesthetic. It produces pronounced sedation and uncouples cortical pain perception. An advantage to ketamine is it causes less cardiorespiratory depression than other sedatives and analgesics (10, 11). Ketamine increases oral and airway secretions, so it is generally given with atropine.

Ketamine is useful as a sedative/analgesic for painful procedures of short duration such as closed fracture reduction, wound repair, and incision and drainage. It is contraindicated in the presence of cardiovascular disease including hypertension, respiratory disease, head injury, or any clinical state with the potential for increased intracranial pressure.

The drug can be given either intravenously, orally, intramuscularly, or by the PR route, and onset and duration of action are route dependent. The intramuscular route appears to be safe and effective and negates the need for intravenous cannulation. The dose of ketamine given intramuscularly is 3 mg/kg. Atropine acts as an antisialagogue and can be delivered in the same syringe at a dose of 0.01 mg/kg to a maximum of 0.5 mg. Midazolam at a dose of 0.05 mg/kg to a maximum of 1.0 mg can also be administered in the same syringe to minimize the emergence reactions associated with ketamine.

Emergence reactions are a major side effect of ketamine and include visual hallucinations, anxiety, and unpleasant dreams. Emergence reactions appear to be more prevalent in older children and adults, and occur more frequently in noisy, chaotic settings such as in an ED. The reaction is minimized by the addition of a benzodiazepine. Laryngospasm has been reported in infants. Restricting the use of ketamine to children between the ages of 6 months and 6 years may help avoid these complications.

Ketamine sedation is not reversible. Major advantages include potent sedation and analgesia, ease of administration, and low complication rate when used properly.

Meperidine, Promethazine, Chlorpromazine

Meperidine (Demerol), promethazine (Phenergan), and chlorpromazine (Thorazine), commonly referred to as DPT, is an i.m. combination that has been used frequently in the outpatient setting for painful procedures. Currently, better alternatives are available for sedation of children. Given its adverse effects, especially prolonged sedation and variability of onset depth of sedative effects, it is not recommended (9).

PROCEDURE

Presedation Assessment

Safety precautions must be adhered to when using any anxiolytic or analgesic agent. Pre-assessment of the child's physical and mental status with attention to significant past medical history, present clinical condition, allergies, medication use, and last oral intake of solids or fluids should be completed in every individual. Vital signs, including heart rate, respiratory rate, and blood pressure, must be measured and recorded before initiating conscious sedation.

According to the American Society of Anesthesiologists, children are appropriate candidates for conscious sedation if they can be classified as a normal healthy patient (Class I) or a patient with mild systemic disease (Class II) (1).

Sedation should be given in a room equipped for resuscitation, should the need arise. Reversal agents (naloxone, flumazenil) should be immediately available.

Medication Types and Routes of Administration

The medication chosen, the dose, and the route of administration will determine the level of sedation. The child's condition and nature of the procedure as well as the age and psychological status of the individual child should be considered when choosing a route for delivery of sedative or analgesic medications (Table 35.1).

Administration of Medications

Sedatives and narcotic analgesics given intravenously should be administered slowly. Medications with a rapid onset, such as fentanyl or midazolam, should be titrated to the desired effect whenever possible. An initial dose at the lower end of the dosage range is given and the child is assessed for degree of sedation after 2 to 5 minutes. If the child is alert, immediately and vigorously responsive to verbal commands, then additional medication is given incrementally, each time waiting 2 to 5 minutes to reassess the degree of sedation. When the eyelids are "half mast" and the child is relaxed but still responsive to verbal commands, an appropriate level of conscious sedation has been achieved. During prolonged procedures reassessment is necessary to determine when additional doses of medication are needed.

Table 35.1.
Commonly Used Sedative/Analgesic Agents

Drug	Dose	Route	Duration	Comments
Morphine	0.1–0.2 mg/kg	i.v., i.m., SC	2–3 hours	Repeat dose in 30 minutes if needed
Fentanyl	1–4 μg/kg	i.v.	15–30 minutes	Titrate, requires close monitoring
Meperidine	1–2 mg/kg	i.v., i.m.	2–4 hours	Better i.m. than morphine
Midazolam	0.1–0.3 mg/kg	i.v.	30 minutes	Titrate
	0.2–0.6 mg/kg	IN, PO	30 mintues	For mild sedation
Thiopental	25 mg/kg	PR	2 hours	Ultrashort onset
Pentobarbital	3–4 mg/kg	PO, PR	2 hours	Rapid onset when i.v.
Chloral hydrate	25–75 mg/kg	PO, PR	3–5 hours	Repeat half dose in 30 minutes if needed
Ketamine	3 mg/kg	i.m.	30 minutes	Give with atropine
				Consider benzodiazepine
Nitrous oxide	50% mixture	inhalation	minutes	

Key: i.v., intravenous; i.m., intramuscular; PO, oral; PR, rectal; IN, intranasal; SC, subcutaneous.

Monitoring During Sedation

Attending to the ABCs of basic life support—airway, breathing, and circulation—throughout a procedure and until the patient has recovered from the effects of the medication will allow the physician to recognize and intervene to prevent potentially life-threatening complications. Respiratory depression and apnea with oxygen desaturation that is detected and treated promptly should not progress to cardiorespiratory arrest. If personnel experienced and comfortable with basic life support and monitoring are not available then conscious sedation should not be undertaken.

Vital signs should be reassessed throughout the procedure at frequencies dependent on the type of medication used and the clinical status of the child. Children receiving conscious sedation intravenously should be on a cardiorespiratory monitor and a pulse oximeter. A designated person should remain at bedside or in close proximity throughout the procedure and during the recovery phase. If the respiratory rate or oxygen saturation drops, the child will often respond to a loud, clear command to take a deep breath. Supplemental oxygen should be administered. If respiratory depression or desaturation continues, bag-valve-mask ventilation with 100% oxygen is begun and an appropriate reversal agent (naloxone and/or flumazenil) is administered.

The period just after completion of the procedure is extremely important for close monitoring. The sedative effects are still quite profound and the child no longer is stimulated by the pain of the procedure. The physician responsible for managing the sedation must avoid the tendency to leave the bedside when the procedure is over. That may be when his or her skills are most needed.

Discharge Criteria

A decision to discharge a child after conscious sedation should be made by someone aware of the details of the individual case. Presedation status, medications and route of administration, time since administration, level of alertness, ability to take oral fluids, and ability to ambulate are all considered before discharge.

COMPLICATIONS

Improper use of drugs given intravenously is more likely to cause oversedation and respiratory depression, which necessitates careful monitoring by experienced personnel, when using the i.v. route. Other anticipated complications, depending on drug type and route, include vomiting and aspiration, allergic reactions, anaphylaxis, and seizures.

SUMMARY

The purpose of conscious sedation is to reduce pain and anxiety in the pediatric patient. Numerous therapeutic options are available and choices should be individualized to the patient, procedure, and circumstances of the case. With meticulous attention to clinical preassessment, dosing, and monitoring, untoward effects of sedation can be minimized and intervention to prevent complication can be prompt and effective.

SUMMARY
1. Explain purpose, type, and anticipated depth of sedation to patient and parent
2. Select medication(s), route of administration, and dose after careful consideration of individual patient and procedure
3. Place child on appropriate monitors; pulse oximeter and CR monitor for i.v. conscious sedation
4. Record vital signs before and during period of sedation
5. Titrate intravenous fentanyl or midazolam to desired level of sedation
6. Administer supplemental oxygen and instruct child to breathe deeply if respiratory rate decreases or oxygen saturation begins to decrease
7. Ventilate with a bag and mask and give naloxone and/or flumazenil if significant respiratory depression occurs.
8. Continue monitoring until sedative effects have diminished
9. Discharge when child is alert, taking oral fluids, and ambulating without difficulty

Chapter 35
Conscious Sedation

453

REFERENCES

1. Committee on Drugs. Guidelines for monitoring and management of pediatric patients during and after sedation for diagnostic and therapeutic procedures. Pediatrics 1992;89:110–115.
2. Yaster M, Deshpande JK. Medical progress. Management of pediatric pain with opioid analgesics. J Pediatr 1988;113:421–429.
3. Ellenhorn MJ, Barceloux DG. Medical toxicology: diagnosis and treatment of human poisoning. New York: Elsevier, 1988.
4. Chudnofsky CR, Wright SW, Dronen SC, Borman SW, Wright MB. The safety of fentanyl use in the emergency department. Ann Emerg Med 1989;18:635–639.
5. Sievers TD, Yee JD, Foley ME, Blanding PJ, Berde CB. Midazolam for conscious sedation during pediatric oncology procedures: safety and recovery parameters. Pediatrics 1991;88:1172–1179.
6. Theroux MC, West DW, Corddry DH, Hyde PM, Bachrach SJ, Cronan KM, Kettrick RG. Efficacy of intranasal midazolam in facilitating suturing of lacerations in preschool children in the emergency department. Pediatrics 1993;91:624–627.
7. Jones RD, Lawson AD, Andrew LJ, Gunawardene WMS, Bacon-Shone J. Antagonism of the hypnotic effect of midazolam in children: a randomized, double-blind study of placebo and flumazenil administered after midazolam-induced anaesthesia. Br J Anaesth 1991;66:660–666.
8. O'Brien JF, Falk JL, Carey BE, Malone LC. Rectal thiopental compared with intramuscular meperidine, promethazine, and chlorpromazine for pediatric sedation. Ann Emerg Med 1991;20:644–647.
9. Committee on Drugs and Committee on Environmental Health. Use of chloral hydrate for sedation in children. Pediatrics 1993;92:471–473.
10. Green SM, Nakamura R, Johnson NE. Ketamine sedation for pediatric procedures: part 1, a prospective series. Ann Emerg Med 1990;19:1024–1032.
11. Green SM, Johnson NE. Ketamine sedation for pediatric procedures: part 2, review and implications. Ann Emerg Med 1990;19:1033–1046.

CHAPTER 36

NITROUS OXIDE ADMINISTRATION

John H. Burton and Christopher King

INTRODUCTION

Nitrous oxide has a long history of utilization and experimentation over the last two centuries. The first documented medical application of a nitrous oxide/oxygen combination was to facilitate a dental extraction in 1840 (1). Nitrous oxide is now widely used for sedation in a variety of clinical settings. The advantages offered by nitrous oxide are a quick onset of action, a low incidence of complications, and the rapid return of the patient's baseline level of consciousness. For the pediatric population, perhaps the greatest advantage is that nitrous oxide can be administered without inflicting pain. The primary disadvantage of nitrous oxide administration is that its clinical effects are sometimes unpredictable; i.e., the degree of anxiolysis and analgesia experienced can be variable. Furthermore, effective delivery of the gas is predicated on the patient's acceptance of the mask and willingness to inhale the gas mixture. Lack of interest and/or cooperation often result in inadequate administration of nitrous oxide and a poor clinical response.

In the pediatric literature, a number of investigations have appeared regarding nitrous oxide utilization (2–6), although the only large study to date that includes pediatric patients was published by Griffin et al. in 1983 (2). In this study, data were reported on over 3000 patients, ranging in age from 16 months to adulthood, for whom nitrous oxide sedation was administered to perform minor outpatient surgery. Nitrous oxide concentrations of 50 to 60% were delivered by nasal mask, and significant relief of pain and anxiety were noted in most patients. Vomiting was cited as the most serious complication (9 of 3000 patients). Smaller studies have reported similar results for a variety of pediatric procedures, including laceration repair (3, 4), venous cannulation (5), and fracture reduction (4, 6–8). Occasional minor side effects of nausea and lightheadedness were observed. In these studies, emesis was a relatively uncommon complication.

Although most published studies have focused on the self-administered delivery of nitrous oxide, physician-assisted delivery of gas to pediatric patients also has proven to be safe and effective (2–5). As described below, this method allows the operator to provide sedation and analgesia to younger children, typically between the ages of 2 and 5 years, who might not otherwise understand or cooperate with self-administration. Using nitrous oxide sedation for children under 2 years of age is uncommon, primarily because of the fact that it is often difficult or impossible to convince a younger child to accept the mask apparatus. Above all, administration of a nitrous oxide/oxygen mixture to pediatric patients requires skill and experience with airway management procedures and a thorough familiarity with the delivery apparatus and the physiologic effects of the gas.

ANATOMY AND PHYSIOLOGY

The obvious unique aspect of nitrous oxide that distinguishes it from other agents used for conscious sedation outside the operating room is that it is a gas. Although a daily activity for the anesthesiologist, the use of gaseous agents by most other practitioners is less common. Consequently, an understanding of the physiologic mechanisms governing the uptake, distribution, and excretion of an administered gas is important when using nitrous oxide.

Inhaled medications must be transferred from a respiratory circuit to the patient's lungs, taken up by the pulmonary vasculature, and distributed to the tissues where it will have an effect, primarily the central nervous system. Several qualities of both gas and patient will govern the uptake and elimination of an inhaled medication. The most important physical property of the gas is its solubility. An insoluble gas is taken up in the lungs much more rapidly than a highly soluble gas. Nitrous oxide is the most insoluble gas used in anesthesia; as a result, a high concentration develops in the alveoli favoring a large concentration gradient to the blood, which in turn causes rapid uptake. A more soluble agent is continually washed out of the lung and therefore produces a lower concentration gradient.

Once the gas is in the lung, the patient's minute ventilation will determine the rate of delivery of gas to the blood. The cardiac output will determine the rate of uptake of gas. A high minute ventilation (which is normal in children) increases uptake of the gas. However, this effect is partially offset by a high cardiac output, which will delay gas uptake. This occurs because the gas is washed out of the lung, producing a lower concentration gradient from the alveoli to the blood. Despite this competing effect, the onset of action of nitrous oxide with a pediatric patient is rapid (2 to 3 minutes) as a result of the low solubility of the gas and a high minute ventilation.

Elimination of a gas (off-loading) occurs in a manner that is essentially the reverse of uptake. In other words, a concentration gradient develops from the blood to the alveoli when gas delivery is discontinued, and the agent is excreted each time the patient exhales. Several factors contribute to the rapid off-loading of nitrous oxide, which normally takes 2 to 5 minutes (9). For one, nitrous oxide is not metabolized before excretion, so that elimination begins immediately. Nitrous oxide also is lipid insoluble and therefore uptake by the muscle, fat, and solid organs is minimal. This lowers the total body stores and makes the gas rapidly available for excretion. Finally, nitrous oxide is not significantly protein bound, which also enhances diffusion of the gas from the blood to the alveoli.

The mechanism of action of nitrous oxide is poorly understood, although it does appear to act directly on the endogenous opioid system (10, 11). This in part accounts for its analgesic properties. Nitrous oxide also acts as an anxiolytic, but the mechanism of this effect is unknown. Despite being a potent CNS depressant, nitrous oxide has been shown to have minimal effects on the normal protective airway reflexes in children (12). As mentioned previously, patients can have a wide range of clinical responses using this agent. Anxiolysis, a sense of detachment, and euphoria are most commonly observed. In addition, the patient is usually amnestic after the procedure. This profile of sedation, analgesia, and amnesia is what makes nitrous oxide an excellent choice in selected cases for pediatric conscious sedation.

INDICATIONS

The typical pediatric candidate for using nitrous oxide is the child who requires a short duration of sedation and/or analgesia during a painful or anxiety-provoking procedure. Nitrous oxide provides a low to moderate depth of sedation in the majority of patients. Specific clinical circumstances in which nitrous oxide might be chosen include foreign body removal, intravenous access with an anxious child, laceration repair, minor joint relocation, incision and drainage of an abscess, or burn debridement. Almost any minor pediatric procedure can be facilitated by nitrous oxide administration. In addition, recent experience has demonstrated that nitrous oxide may be used effectively for fracture reduction in children. The patient should be allowed to inhale the gas for a somewhat longer period of time before performing the reduction, so that adequate analgesia, sedation, and amnesia are achieved (see Procedure). As with any procedure, if the level of sedation proves to be inadequate, another method should be used. One point worth emphasizing is that nitrous oxide should not be used as a replacement for local anesthesia during painful wound management procedures. As with all forms of conscious sedation, a local anesthetic should be administered intradermally or topically whenever possible. The purpose of nitrous oxide sedation is not to remove all sensation of pain, since this depth of sedation is not necessary or desirable. Nitrous oxide should be used as a complement to local anesthesia in such cases.

Contraindications to using a nitrous oxide/oxygen mixture are relatively few. One important concern with this agent is the property of expansion within closed spaces. Nitrous oxide readily diffuses across biologic membranes. This diffusion theoretically continues until equilibrium is reached for the gases contained within any space. Consequently, the volume of gas within a closed space will increase as diffusion of nitrous oxide continues, eventually leading to excessively high pressures. Any known or suspected gaseous pocket in the body has the potential for expansion during the use of nitrous oxide. Nitrous oxide is therefore contraindicated in patients with suspected pneumothorax, bowel obstruction, or with a particularly common pediatric problem, otitis media. Examining the ears and eliciting any history of otalgia is especially important before using this agent with children. Potential adverse consequences include tension pneumothorax, bowel perforation, or tympanic membrane rupture (see also Complications).

Another contraindication to using nitrous oxide is impairment of the patient's level of consciousness. Because safe and effective use of this agent requires significant cooperation, the patient with mental status changes who requires sedation would likely be better managed with an intravenous regimen. For example, the child with a minor head injury who has post-concussive agitation or lethargy would not be an appropriate candidate for nitrous oxide sedation (e.g., to repair a complex facial laceration or to reduce a displaced fracture). In such situations, the patient is unlikely to provide the degree of cooperation necessary to use nitrous oxide appropriately.

EQUIPMENT

Equipment used for nitrous oxide delivery is commercially available from a number of suppliers. Although the specific characteristics of a given delivery system may vary by manufacturer, the units can be divided into two general categories based on the number of tanks required: single tank systems and multiple tank systems. Overall, characteristics of these two types of nitrous oxide delivery systems are similar regardless of the brand.

Single tank systems

These systems normally consist of a tank containing a 50:50 mixture of nitrous oxide and oxygen, a regulator valve apparatus, and a scavenging device (Fig. 36.1). The concentration of nitrous oxide delivered is fixed at 50%. Once the supply of the gas mixture is exhausted, a new premixed tank must be obtained. This type of system is especially pop-

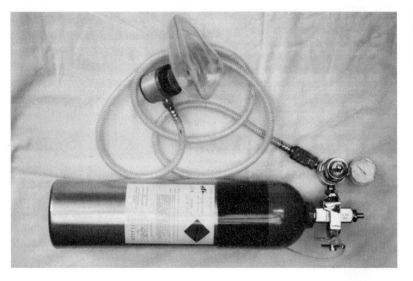

Figure 36.1.
Single tank apparatus for delivering a fixed nitrous oxide/oxygen concentration.

concentration will almost always be adequate to provide sedation.

A potential disadvantage of single tank systems with more serious implications relates to the fact that nitrous oxide is heavier than oxygen, which in a cold environment can cause settling and fractionation of the agents within the tank. It is therefore theoretically possible for the patient to receive a higher concentration of oxygen until the tank is almost empty, and then to receive almost pure nitrous oxide, resulting in profound hypoxemia (see Complications). Although this is only likely with a tank that is both stored and used in cold temperatures (e.g., a prehospital field setting), it is generally a good practice to invert the tank before use to ensure adequate mixing of the agents.

Multiple tank systems

These systems offer the ability to titrate the concentration of nitrous oxide delivered (usually 0 to 70%). Multiple tank setups typically utilize the same D cylinders of nitrous oxide and oxygen commonly found in most hospitals and operating rooms (Fig. 36.2). Although titration of gases may offer the advantage of providing a more gradual induction, evidence suggests that exceeding a 50% concentration of nitrous oxide increases the incidence of complications (e.g., emesis) without significantly enhancing clinical response (2, 5). All systems should have one or more safeguards to prevent delivery of an excessive nitrous oxide concentration. This typically consists of a valve system that will allow a maximum nitrous oxide concentration of 70% and/or a shutoff device that is triggered if the F_iO_2 is ever lower than 30%. Alternative systems also are now available that combine elements of both the single and multiple tank setups. Utilizing a single tank of nitrous oxide, these devices mix an appropriate concentration of oxygen supplied from a standard wall-mounted valve, eliminating the need for tank oxygen.

Most commercially available delivery systems incorporate some type of scavenger system, which provides a means of removing nitrous oxide from the environment (13, 14). Once connected to standard wall suction, the scavenger system will exhaust the gases exhaled by the patient, preventing accumulation of excessive ambient concentrations of nitrous oxide. Prolonged exposure to high lev-

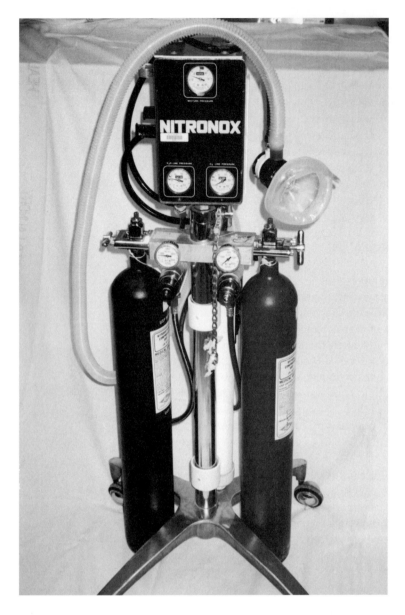

Figure 36.2.
Multiple tank apparatus

ular among prehospital and EMS personnel because of its simplicity, compactness, and light weight. One drawback of a single tank system is that the operator does not have the ability to increase or decrease the nitrous oxide concentration administered, potentially making the level of sedation somewhat more difficult to control. However, in the outpatient setting, titration can usually be carried out effectively by varying the amount of time that the patient is breathing the nitrous oxide/oxygen mixture. When the patient feels more pain, the child is assisted in maintaining a tight mask seal while breathing the gas; when the patient becomes too sleepy, the mask is removed. If a child is likely to have the desired response to nitrous oxide, a 50:50

Table 36.1.
Equipment

1. Commercially available single or multiple tank delivery apparatus.
2. Variety of pediatric face masks and/or nasal masks.
3. Spare cylinders of nitrous oxide and oxygen or premixed single tank.
4. Scavenger device (usually included with delivery apparatus).
5. Flavored scents (Chapstick®) with several options from which the patient can choose.
6. Patient monitoring and resuscitation equipment: pulse oximetry, cardiac and blood pressure monitors, suction, bag-valve-mask, etc.

els of nitrous oxide by medical personnel has been associated with adverse health effects (see Complications).

A variety of standard pediatric nasal or face masks may be used to administer nitrous oxide. The operator should carefully assess the fit and seal of the mask to ensure proper gas delivery. If a nondisposable mask is used, it should be thoroughly cleaned or sterilized between uses. Applying flavored scents (e.g., Chapstick) to the inner lining of the mask will often enhance acceptance by the pediatric patient.

As with all methods of pediatric conscious sedation, the minimum necessary monitoring modalities include cardiac monitoring and pulse oximetry. Any equipment necessary for basic and advanced airway management also must be readily available (Table 36.1). These precautions should be taken even though airway and ventilatory compromise are less likely to occur with nitrous oxide than with other sedation regimens (see also Chapter 35).

PROCEDURE

Administration of nitrous oxide sedation begins with a discussion by the physician with the patient and parents of the procedure, equipment, and likely effects of the agent. A favorable outcome is directly related to the degree of cooperation by the patient. Therefore, time taken to enhance the interest of the child, and to calm any anxieties of the parents, is well invested in increasing the likelihood of success.

Preparation of the delivery apparatus should be routinely performed before each use, which includes checking the function of the tank system and ensuring availability of the proper volume of gas needed for the procedure. A mask should be selected that is appropriate for the size of the patient. Allowing the child to hold and investigate the mask while the procedure is explained often will alleviate any concerns about the equipment. Pointing out the similarity of the mask to a "space mask" or other familiar object also may enhance the child's desire to participate. To give the patient a sense of control with the procedure he or she should select the flavored scent applied to the inside of the mask (orange, cherry, bubblegum, etc.).

Proper positioning should be based on the nature of the procedure and the patient's wishes. A child may initially be fearful of lying supine and should therefore be allowed to remain sitting upright. After the nitrous oxide has been administered for a few moments, the patient will often begin to feel somewhat dizzy or lightheaded and wish to lie down. Acceptance of the gas mixture should be controlled by the patient. Delivery is always optimal with the patient holding the mask and breathing the nitrous oxide as necessary during the procedure (Fig. 36.3). However, younger children often prefer parents to hold the mask, and this should be allowed as long as the parent has a clear understanding that the mask must not be forced on the patient and should be temporarily removed whenever the patient falls asleep.

Individual features of the tank setups vary, but the first step to initiating gas flow is usually to open one or more valves. If the unit has a security system, a key may be required to open the primary regulator valve. The operator should check any gauges on the tanks to ensure that they are reading in the appropriate range for proper gas flow. The dial may be color-coded to indicate the correct range. When available, the scavenger device should be connected to wall suction. Because flow is governed by a demand system, gas is only administered in response to the negative pressure exerted when the patient inspires; otherwise, no gas flow occurs. With a single tank setup, a uniform concentration of nitrous oxide and oxygen is delivered, depending on the fraction of each gas within the tank. As mentioned previously, this is normally a 50:50 mixture. With a multiple tank setup, the relative concentrations of nitrous oxide and oxygen can be adjusted by the operator using the primary regulator valve. For example, if oxy-

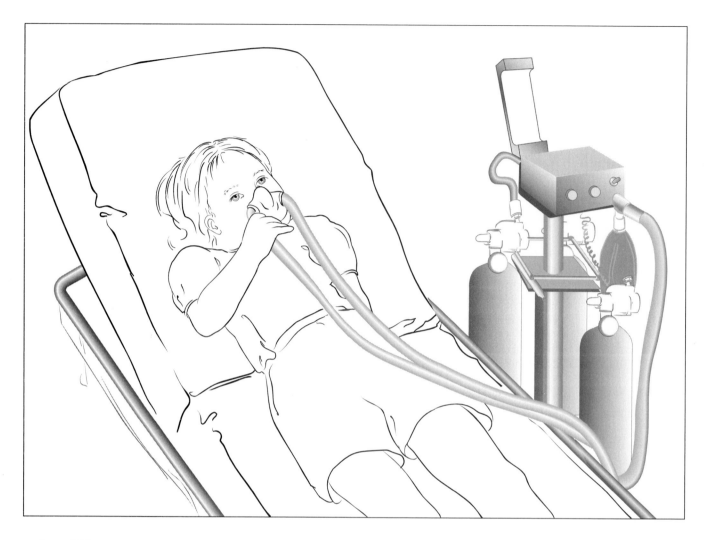

Figure 36.3.
Nitrous oxide delivery is
optimal with the patient
holding the mask. Younger
children may prefer that a
parent or the physician
hold the mask.

gen is flowing at 4 L/min and nitrous oxide is
flowing at 6 L/min, this constitutes a 60% nitrous oxide concentration delivered. With
most systems, the highest allowable concentration of nitrous oxide is 70%, since the minimum flow of oxygen is 3 L/min and the maximum flow of nitrous oxide is 7 L/min.
Because of the risk of hypoxemia with inadequate oxygen flow, nitrous oxide concentrations higher than 70% should not be used for
conscious sedation.

When effects of the gas are apparent, the
concentration of nitrous oxide may then be
titrated (if the system has this option) to the
desired clinical response. Titration is necessary most commonly when the child becomes
overly sedated during the procedure. Should
this occur, the concentration can be decreased
until the desired level of sedation is obtained.
If the tank system does not offer titration as
an option, the seal of the mask can be modified to allow entrainment of air into the mask

and therefore decrease the inhaled nitrous oxide concentration. The mask can also be intermittently removed altogether as needed.
As mentioned previously, nitrous oxide can
have a relatively wide range of clinical effects, from the patient who sleeps quietly
throughout the procedure to a hysterical, un-
controllably giggling patient. However, most
children will lapse into a detached yet alert
state within a few minutes of inhalation.

After the gas has been administered for a
few moments and the child is lightly sedated,
painful procedures such as intradermal administration of lidocaine can be performed. Although the child will feel the pain, anxiety is
normally at a minimum and cooperation greatly
enhanced. More painful procedures (e.g., fracture reduction) should be delayed until 3 to 5
minutes after the initiation of gas administration, so that the patient will be somewhat more
heavily sedated (7). However, the goal should
never be to sedate the child so deeply that all

sensation of pain is eliminated, as this may suppress the normal airway reflexes. Furthermore, because the amnestic effect of the agent usually removes any memory of the painful procedure, deep sedation is unnecessary. As long as the child self-administers the gas mixture, oversedation is highly unlikely.

A calm, reassuring voice is very effective in facilitating the sedation. Guided imagery techniques (telling a story, talking about favorite places, etc.) may be used by a parent or by the operator (see Chapter 34). Questions directed to the child regarding the sensations felt are helpful in assessing the level of anxiolysis and analgesia attained. The patient may experience dizziness, lightheadedness, or a sensation of floating. Reassurance that these are normal effects of the gas is generally the only measure necessary to alleviate any discomfort. Refusal of the nitrous oxide should be allowed at any time during the procedure. However, the patient's interest in the flavored mask scent or the sensation experienced will usually be adequate to maintain cooperation throughout the procedure. If the patient does not respond to the gas in a manner conducive to completion of the procedure, the mask should be removed and an alternate method of sedation used.

Once administration of the nitrous oxide is terminated, the patient should remain in a sitting or supine position for approximately 3 to 5 minutes. Oxygen may be administered during this time, but with healthy children (i.e., no underlying lung disease) this is unnecessary. Patients who rise and attempt to walk will often experience increased vertigo and are at risk for falling. After the effects of the gas subside and the patient's level of consciousness returns essentially to baseline (which generally takes about 20 to 40 minutes), normal activities may be resumed.

COMPLICATIONS

When used appropriately, nitrous oxide has been associated with relatively few complications. A screening physical examination and history will normally identify any patients at risk for gaseous expansion within a closed space (otitis media, pneumothorax, intestinal obstruction, etc.). As mentioned previously, such patients are at risk for exacerbation of

the underlying condition, potentially resulting in tympanic membrane perforation, tension pneumothorax, or bowel perforation (15, 16). Less severe complications such as dizziness or emesis can generally be managed with routine supportive care.

Hypoxemia as a result of improper gas concentrations and/or nitrous oxide delivery is a potential danger that must be avoided. Patient-titrated administration, and when necessary, physician-assisted administration, are the only acceptable methods of delivery. Periodic checks of the delivery apparatus should be made to ensure that safety features designed to prevent this complication are functional. In addition, although clinically significant depression of protective airway reflexes is uncommon with nitrous oxide administration, the response of the patient must be carefully monitored during the procedure. If at any time the patient appears too deeply sedated, administration of the gas mixture should be immediately terminated, which will normally cause the patient to quickly return to a baseline mental status. Appropriate resuscitation equipment should always be readily available whenever conscious sedation is administered to a pediatric patient.

An often repeated concern about the use of nitrous oxide/oxygen mixtures is the phenomenon of "diffusion hypoxia." First described by Fink in 1955 (17), diffusion hypoxia occurs when high concentrations of nitrous oxide in the body rapidly diffuse out of the tissues back into the alveoli on termination of gas administration, potentially displacing oxygen and thereby causing hypoxemia. However, a number of more recent studies have demonstrated that with the concentrations of oxygen and nitrous oxide most commonly used for sedation (i.e., a 50 : 50 mixture), diffusion hypoxia does not occur in healthy patients (18–21). This represents a potential risk only for patients with significant underlying lung diseases or with higher nitrous oxide concentrations. Any risk of this complication can be eliminated if the patient receives 100% oxygen for a few minutes after the procedure.

As mentioned previously, nitrous oxide is heavier than oxygen. If a single tank system is exposed to cold temperatures (less than $-5°C$) for prolonged periods of time, the nitrous oxide will settle to the bottom, resulting in fractionation of the agents. Obviously this

PROCEDURE
1. Discuss with patient and parents typical gas effects and use of delivery apparatus
2. Ensure that nitrous oxide and oxygen supplies are adequate for planned intervention
3. Select proper nasal or face mask for inhalation
4. Position patient for optimum comfort and delivery of gas.
5. Start flow of nitrous oxide/oxygen mixture and check that gauges are reading correctly
6. Allow patient to hold mask and titrate gas inhalation whenever possible. If necessary, physician-assisted administration may be performed with younger patients.
7. Titrate nitrous oxide concentration (if delivery apparatus allows) or occasionally remove/adjust mask seal to provide the appropriate level of sedation.
8. On completing procedure, remove mask and have patient remain in supine or sitting position until effects subside. Administer oxygen for several minutes as patient recovers.

is only likely to be a concern when the tank system is used in a field setting. Furthermore, this problem should be recognized quickly because a high concentration of oxygen will be administered initially, making sedation impossible. However, in the unlikely event that the oxygen is completely vented, the patient could theoretically receive pure nitrous oxide, causing profound hypoxemia. This complication can be easily avoided if the tank is inverted each time before its use to adequately mix the agents.

Recurrent exposure of health care providers to nitrous oxide has been associated with a number of potential health problems, including hepatic dysfunction, neurologic disorders, and reproductive abnormalities (22–24). However, studies on this subject have dealt with exposure to high ambient levels of nitrous oxide over long periods of time. With the intermittent use of nitrous oxide that occurs in most acute care settings, such prolonged and frequent exposures are extremely unlikely. Furthermore, no such risks have been demonstrated for patients who undergo an isolated nitrous oxide sedation. Nevertheless, to reduce any potential risk to medical personnel, nitrous oxide/oxygen mixtures should only be administered in an adequately ventilated room. In addition, it is recommended that all delivery systems used on a regular basis should have a functional scavenging device.

SUMMARY

Nitrous oxide/oxygen mixtures have been shown to be safe and effective when administered to pediatric patients. Subjects generally experience pain relief, anxiolysis, and amnesia. Its relatively rapid onset, short duration of action, and easy use make nitrous oxide sedation an attractive option for the acute care setting. Furthermore, nitrous oxide is especially appropriate for use with children, because unlike other methods of sedation, no pain (i.e., intramuscular or intravenous injection) is associated with administering the medication. Potential side effects with this agent are remarkably few, although the patient may have nausea, vomiting, dizziness, and increased excitability. More serious problems such as oversedation and hypoxemia can be avoided by using proper tech-

nique. Nitrous oxide/oxygen mixtures offer a valuable adjunct in facilitating painful or anxiety-provoking pediatric procedures.

REFERENCES

1. American Dental Association Horace Wells Centenary Committee. Horace Wells, dentist, father of surgical anesthesia. Hartford: Connecticut Printers, 1948.
2. Griffin G, Campbell V, Jones R. Nitrous oxide-oxygen sedation for minor surgery: experience in a pediatric setting. JAMA 1981;245:2411–2413.
3. Gamis AS, Knapp JF, Glenski JA. Nitrous oxide analgesia in a pediatric emergency department. Ann Emerg Med 1989;18:177–181.
4. Etzwiler LS, Fleisher G, McGravey A. Safety and effectiveness of nitrous oxide for sedation and analgesia in the pediatric emergency department (abstract). Ped Emerg Care 1990;6:225.
5. Henderson JM, Spence DG, Komocar LM, et al. Administration of nitrous oxide to pediatric patients provides analgesia for venous cannulation. Anesthesiology 1990;72:269–271.
6. Wattenmaker I, Kasser JR, McGravey A. Self-administered nitrous oxide for fracture reduction in children in an emergency room setting. J Orthop Trauma 1990;4:35–38.
7. Evans JK, Buckley MD, Alexander AH, et al. Analgesia for the reduction of fractures in children: a comparison of nitrous oxide with intramuscular sedation. J Pediatr Orthop 1995;15:73–77.
8. Hennrikus WJ, Simpson RB, Klingelberger CE, et al. Self-administered nitrous oxide analgesia for pediatric fracture reductions. J Pediatr Orthop 1995;14:538–542.
9. Stewart RD. Nitrous oxide sedation/analgesia in emergency medicine. Ann Emerg Med 1985;4:139–148.
10. Gillman MA. Analgesic (subanesthetic) nitrous oxide interacts with the endogenous opioid system: review of the evidence. Life Sci 1986;39:1209–1211.
11. Gilman MA. Opioid action of analgesic nitrous oxide (letter). Ann Emerg Med 1990;19:843.
12. Roberts GJ, Wignall BK. Efficacy of the laryngeal reflex during oxygen-nitrous oxide sedation. Br J Anaesth 1982;54:1277–1281.
13. Dula DJ, Skiendzielewski JJ, Royko M. The scavenger device for nitrous oxide administration. Ann Emerg Med 1981;10:575–578.
14. Dula DJ, Skiendzielewski JJ, Snover SW. The scavenger device for nitrous oxide administration. Ann Emerg Med 1983;12:759–761.
15. Eger EJ, Saidman LT. Hazards of nitrous oxide anesthesia in bowel obstruction and pneumothorax. Anesthesiology 1965;26:61–64.
16. Perreault L, Normandin N, Plamondon L, et al. Tympanic membrane rupture after anesthesia with nitrous oxide. Anesthesiology 1982;57:325–326.
17. Fink BR. Diffusion anoxia. Anesthesiology 1955;16:511–519.
18. Stewart RD, Gorayeb MJ, Pelton GH. Determina-

tion of arterial blood gases before, during and after nitrous oxide: oxygen administration. Ann Emerg Med 1986;15:1177–1180.

19. Murphy IL, Splinter WM. The clinical significance of diffusion hypoxia in children. Can J Anaesth 1990;37:S40.

20. Dunn-Russell T, Adair SM, Sams DR, et al. Oxygen saturation and diffusion hypoxia in children following nitrous oxide sedation. Pediatr Dentistry 1993; 16(2):88–92.

21. Quarnstrom FC, Milgrom P, Bishop MJ, et al. Clin-ical study of diffusion hypoxia after nitrous oxide analgesia. Anaesth Prog 1991;38:21–23.

22. Rowland A, Baird D, Weinberg C, et al. Reduced fertility among women employed as dental assis-tants exposed to high levels of nitrous oxide. N Engl J Med 1992;327:993–997.

23. Yagiela JA. Health Hazards and nitrous oxide: a time for reappraisal. Anaesth Prog 1991;38(1):1–11.

24. Donaldson D, Meechan JG. The hazards of chronic exposure to nitrous oxide: an update. Br Dentistry J 1995;178(3):95–100.

CHAPTER 37

LOCAL AND REGIONAL ANESTHESIA

Lisa Lewis and Maria Stephan

INTRODUCTION

Local anesthesia is useful in treating pediatric patients with a variety of injuries and illnesses. Tissue infiltration, topical application, and regional anesthesia make use of the unique properties of these agents. Physicians and other health care providers with basic knowledge about local anesthesia can administer it safely and effectively. For the sake of clarity, certain types of nerve blocks are discussed elsewhere in this text. The auricular block of the external ear is described in Chapter 58. Nerve blocks of the oral and facial areas are described in Chapter 65.

Cocaine was the first local anesthetic used in medical practice. Halsted showed in the 1880s that nerve conduction could be blocked by cocaine. In the past 50 years local anesthetics and techniques for their use in clinical practice have increased dramatically. Unfortunately, opportunities to minimize pain in pediatric patients are sometimes overlooked. Practitioners in the acute care setting must keep pace with the new and refined techniques for local anesthesia.

GENERAL CONCEPTS

Anesthetic Structure

Local anesthetics are classified on their chemical structure and linkage. This basic chemical structure is:

aromatic segment–intermediate chain–hydrophilic segment (1–4).

The most commonly used anesthetics are aminoesters and aminoamides (1, 2, 4, 5). Procaine, cocaine, chloroprocaine, and tetracaine are examples of aminoesters. Lidocaine, bupivacaine, prilocaine, mepivacaine, and etidocaine are amides. Drugs from the amide group are used more frequently for pediatric patients.

The aromatic moiety of the anesthetic molecule contributes to its lipid solubility: 2-6-dimethylanaline for amides and p-aminobenzoic acid for esters. Changes in the structure of the aromatic portion have effects on lipid solubility and pK_a (4, 6). Local anesthetics are solubilized by combining them with hydrogen chloride to form the salt of a weak acid. The proportion of local anesthetic in the ionized versus nonionized form is determined by its pK_a and the pH of the solution. Neutral or alkaline pH favors the nonionized form, which is more lipid soluble and therefore better penetrates nerve membranes.

Differences in the intermediate chain of the local anesthetic molecule determine its metabolism and clearance (1, 2, 4, 6). Amides are metabolized by the liver through enzymatic degradation, whereas aminoesters are metabolized in the plasma by pseudocholinesterase (2, 6). However, cocaine is an aminoester that undergoes significant metabolism within the liver (1). As expected, patients with pseudocholinesterase deficiency demonstrate decreased metabolism of aminoester drugs, although prolongation of nerve blockade or increased systemic toxicity have not been observed (1).

Molecular Action

The sodium channel plays a central role in the mechanism by which local anesthetics block action potentials along the nerve axons. The nerve axon is surrounded by a membrane consisting of lipid and protein molecules (7), which control passage of small ions such as potassium and sodium. An electrostatic gradient (8, 9) is generated by the sodium-potassium ATPase pump, with high concentrations of intracellular potassium and extracellular sodium and chloride. A resting potential of between −70 to −90 mVs is thereby maintained.

When a nerve impulse is generated, depolarization occurs through a complex process in which membrane proteins ("gates") become permeable to sodium and potassium. As sodium enters the cell, the transmembrane potential reaches a threshold and an action potential is propagated (2, 7, 10, 11). Repolarization occurs as sodium and potassium ions are actively transported by the sodium ATPase pump, reestablishing the resting potential. Local anesthetics interact with the membrane protein gates and prevent sodium entry into the cell, although the precise mechanism of this interaction is not currently known. Without an influx of sodium, the electrochemical gradient does not reach the threshold potential, and no action potential is generated. This effectively blocks transmission of impulses from sensory receptors to the central nervous system.

Nerve Structure

A nerve fiber is composed of the axon and its surrounding Schwann cell sheath. A single Schwann cell may surround several unmyelinated nerve fibers (7). Myelinated nerve fibers often have one Schwann cell wrapped around a single axon. Junctions between the sheaths along the axon are called nodes of Ranvier (1). These myelin-deficient junctions are the sites where sodium channels necessary for depolarization are located. The nodes are more excitable than the rest of the membrane, allowing the impulse to skip from node to node and increasing conduction velocity. As the diameter of the axon increases, the nodes of Ranvier are spaced further apart.

Nerve fibers can be classified into three types: A, B, and C fibers (2, 6, 7, 9, 12). The diameter and degree of myelination of the nerve predict the sensitivity to local anesthetics (12). Thick, type A nerve fibers (motor, proprioception, reflex, pressure, and touch) are less readily blocked than thin, unmyelinated type C fibers (pain and temperature) (2, 3). A variety of factors determine the final concentration of anesthetic presented to the nerve membrane, including dilution of the anesthetic by tissue fluid, fibrous tissue barriers, uptake by fatty surrounding fatty areas, and systemic absorption (1, 2, 9).

Anesthetic Effectiveness

The effectiveness of a local anesthetic is influenced by various properties of the physiologic environment and by the inherent chemical activity of the agent, which largely determines its onset of action, potency, and duration. Diffusion of local anesthetics (and therefore potency) depends on lipid solubility. Local anesthetics with greater inherent lipid solubility are generally more potent. The nonionized form is more lipid soluble. The ratio of ionized to nonionized forms depends on both the pK_a of the parent molecule and the pH of the solution, as described by the Henderson-Hasselbach equation:

$$pH = pK_a + \log (\text{ionized form}/ \text{unionized form}) \qquad (1)$$

Local anesthetics are commercially available as water-soluble salts in an acidic solution, which primarily contain the cationic form of the drug (12, 14, 17). Raising the pH by adding sodium bicarbonate before administration increases the proportion of molecules in the nonionized, more lipid-soluble form, which speeds the onset of action (1, 12, 13). Rate and extent of diffusion also depend on molecular weight and concentration (1, 3, 4). The site of administration also plays an important role. As the amount of tissue or size of the nerve sheath increases, the onset is delayed because of the greater distance the drug must travel to reach its receptor (1, 3, 6).

Protein binding of the anesthetic is an

important factor in determining the duration of action. Binding reduces the amount of free drug available to diffuse onto nerves directly (1, 4, 6, 8, 12). Agents that bind more tightly to the protein receptor remain in the sodium channel longer (10). Vasodilation produced by local anesthetics inversely influences the potency and duration of action (3, 4). Local blood flow competes with nerve tissue and other binding sites for the drug. Vasoconstriction decreases this washout effect, allowing more molecules to remain at the peripheral nerve. In this way, epinephrine added to the local anesthetic solution can increase the potency and duration of anesthesia (3, 6, 12, 18, 19). The duration also varies with mode of administration and dose. Topical application usually produces a shorter period of anesthesia than tissue infiltration. Increasing the concentration of anesthetic, while being cautious to avoid any toxic effects, can prolong the duration.

Significant differences exist in distribution and metabolism of local anesthetics in young children compared with adults. Young infants have a larger volume of distribution, more rapid absorption, and lower plasma levels of albumin and α_1-glycoprotein, which binds lidocaine (1, 20). The activity of plasma pseudocholinesterase and microsomal enzyme systems in the liver are low in this age group (20, 21). Special caution and reduced dosages are warranted when using local anesthetics in young infants. After the first few months of life, children have a greater clearance of local anesthetics than adults (20). Myelination is not complete until age 8 to 12 years. In laboratory studies, young animals are more sensitive to lidocaine due to fewer myelinated type A fibers (9). The difference in myelination of nerve fibers may account for the effectiveness of lower concentrations of local anesthetics in children.

Adverse Reactions

Systemic toxicity may occur by inadvertent intravascular injection or by using excessive extravascular drug. After injection, peak blood levels are reached in 10 to 60 minutes. The more potent agents also are more toxic. Those with high lipid solubility and protein binding tend to become sequestered in tissue and have a slower rate of absorption, which produces a lower blood concentration. Esters are difficult to measure in blood due to their rapid hydrolysis by pseudocholinesterase. The toxic effects seen are usually central nervous system (CNS) or cardiovascular in origin. Local anesthetics are administered to inhibit conduction in the peripheral nerves, but any excitable nerve membrane (e.g., heart, brain, or neuromuscular junction) may be affected if a higher drug concentration is reached (22).

Local anesthetics are lipophilic and cross the blood-brain barrier. As serum concentrations increase, patients initially complain of numbness of the lips and a metallic taste in the mouth. Nystagmus may follow, progressing to muscle twitching, tremors, seizures, and ultimately CNS depression and respiratory arrest at excessive concentrations (1, 2, 12, 22–25). The blood-brain barrier is more permeable in infants than in adults, resulting in greater CNS concentrations of local anesthetic. Infants are therefore more susceptible to systemic complications resulting from use of a local anesthetic (1).

The cardiovascular system seems to be more resistant to toxic effects than the central nervous system (CNS). A decrease in blood pressure, however, may be observed secondary to the negative inotropic action of these agents, which can lead to a diminished cardiac output and stroke volume (1, 2, 12, 15, 22, 23). Cocaine produces its toxic effects on the cardiovascular system by inhibiting reuptake of catecholamines (epinephrine and norepinephrine) at adrenergic nerve endings, leading to increased blood pressure and/or ventricular dysrhythmias.

Allergic reactions to local anesthetics are uncommon. Most reports involve the aminoesters which have a para-aminobenzoic acid nucleus (22, 23). More often, methylparaben, a common preservative found in commercial preparations, is the causative agent for an allergic reaction (22, 26). Local anesthetics are available in preservative-free preparations. Reactions to amide anesthetics are rare. Allergic reactions are manifested by dermatitis, urticaria, anaphylaxis, pruritus, or bronchospasm. Small lacerations in allergic individuals may be repaired without local anesthesia or with normal saline infiltration. Diphenhydramine has also been used as a local anesthetic in a 1% solution (50 mg/mL diluted with 4 mL of normal saline to produce a 1% solution).

Tissue injury can result from injection of anesthetic into a nerve or from passage of the needle. Neuropathy has been reported, especially with direct intraneuronal injection (28). In addition, inflammatory changes in muscle have been observed, but wound healing does not seem to be impaired (27, 29). Tissue ischemia may result when using epinephrine-containing solutions injected in areas perfused by end arteries. Epinephrine administration is therefore contraindicated for use in digits, penis, nasal alae, and pinna. Local anesthetics do not affect the incidence of wound infection (30–31). Lidocaine has some antiseptic properties but this has little effect on wound infection rates. If a wound is to be cultured, however, the swab should be obtained before local infiltration with lidocaine. Vasoconstrictors such as epinephrine have been associated with increased potential for infection in animal studies, but clinical studies in humans show no difference in actual infections. Methemoglobinemia has been described with large doses of prilocaine and benzocaine (1). Toxicity may be controlled by using an appropriate dose and route of administration, and administering vasoconstrictor-containing solutions when not contraindicated.

Selecting a Local Anesthetic

The most common local anesthetics administered to children are lidocaine (Xylocaine(R)) and procaine (Novocaine(R)), accounting for approximately 90% of use. Plain lidocaine may be used up to 5 mg/kg, whereas the addition of epinephrine allows for a maximum dose of 7 mg/kg. Bupivacaine is not recommended for children under 12 years. Table 37.1 summarizes information regarding the most commonly used local anesthetics (2, 12, 23, 26).

For increased safety in using local anesthetics in pediatrics, the following guidelines are recommended (33):
1. Dosage should be reduced to 80% of the maximal allowable dose.
2. Anesthetic should be administered slowly in divided doses when possible.
3. Epinephrine (1 : 100,000 to 1 : 400,000) should be added if not contraindicated.

As mentioned previously, the addition of epinephrine delays absorption but is con-

traindicated in areas where end arteries exist . For most procedures, it is unnecessary to choose a local anesthetic based on onset time. Waiting 5 to 10 minutes will generally obviate the need for additional injections of any local anesthetic.

Minimizing Pain with Injection

Rapid infiltration of an acidic solution of local anesthetic is painful. Decreasing the speed of infiltration can significantly reduce pain during injection (35–37). In addition, buffering the local anesthetic with sodium bicarbonate not only improves potency but also reduces the pain associated with infiltration (37, 38). To buffer a local anesthetic solution, 1 part sodium bicarbonate is mixed with 10 parts anesthetic (by volume) in a syringe. Buffering an entire bottle reduces the shelf life and is not generally recommended (26).

INFILTRATION ANESTHESIA

Wound infiltration is a safe, rapid, and easy method for providing anesthesia and hemostasis to a localized area. It is used for the majority of minor procedures (e.g., laceration repair, wound debridement, foreign body removal, and abscess drainage). Two primary methods of infiltration anesthesia are direct infiltration and parallel margin infiltration.

Direct infiltration involves the injection of an anesthetic agent directly into the tissues and results in the production of localized analgesia at the site of infiltration. Individual nerves are not specifically blocked, but become anesthetized in the tissue planes surrounding the wound. The region is rendered painless by altering the perception of pain, although the sensation of touch may persist. Direct infiltration is the most commonly used technique for administration of local anesthetic for laceration repair.

Parallel margin infiltration (field block) is produced by injecting adjacent tracts of anesthesia parallel to the wounded edge or surgical field. This results in the interruption of nerve impulses from the site to the CNS.

Table 37.1.
Characteristics of Commonly Used Local Anesthetics

Infiltration Anesthetic	Concentration	Physiochemical Properties				Maximum Allowable Dose	
		Lipid Solubility	Relative Potency	Onset of Action (minutes)	Duration (minutes)	mg/kg	mL/kg
Procaine (Novocaine®)	1%	0.6	1	5–10	60–90	7–10	0.7–1
Lidocaine (Xylocaine®)							
—without epinephrine	1%	2.9	2	2–5	50–120	4–5	0.4–0.5
—with epinephrine (1:200,000)	1%	2.9	2	2–5	60–180	5–7	0.5–0.7
Mepivacaine (Carbacaine®)	1%	0.8	2	2–5	90–180	5	0.5
Bupivacaine* (Marcaine®)	0.25%	27.5	8	5–10	240–480	2	0.8

* Some authorities do not recommend bupivacaine for use in children under 12 years of age.

As with direct infiltration individual nerves are not sought specifically; they are anesthetized in the tissue plane in which they lie. This technique is essentially the same as for local infiltration except that the local anesthetic is injected circumferentially at a distance from the wound rather than into the wound margins. Field blocks are preferred for procedures in areas of inflammation or gross contamination. This technique allows for instillation of anesthetic away from acidic, infected areas where local anesthetic has reduced penetration. Parallel margin infiltration also prevents the needle from carrying debris or bacteria from the wound into uncontaminated surrounding tissues. In addition, this technique does not distort tissue planes that must be accurately reapproximated to optimize the cosmetic result of laceration repair. It is therefore preferred over direct wound infiltration when preservation of wound architecture is desired.

Anatomy and Physiology

The skin is composed of the epidermis, dermis, and superficial fascia. Free nerve endings that generate impulses from painful stimuli are plentiful in the dermis and epidermis. The preferred plane of injection is into the superficial fascia, immediately below the dermis, where nerve fibers transmitting painful stimuli are easily blocked by infiltration of local anesthetic. Insertion of the needle through the margin of the wound beneath the majority of free nerve endings is therefore less painful than insertion through intact, densely innervated epidermis. Tissue resistance and pain with instillation of anesthetic

are also less in the subdermal tissue plane than in the epidermis or dermis (39, 40).

As in direct wound infiltration, the plane of injection for a field block is the superficial fascia, just beneath the dermis. Proximal to the laceration, nerves (bundles of nerve fibers) can be blocked producing a field of anesthesia distally. With parallel margin infiltration, the superficial fascial layer is approached through intact skin, parallel to the wound or field edge. As a result, needle insertion with this technique is more painful than direct wound infiltration because it passes through intact skin.

Indications

Direct wound infiltration is indicated for most wounds and lacerations. In highly contaminated wounds, injection through intact skin may be preferred to prevent introducing organisms from the wound margin into the surrounding tissues.

Some tissues, such as the sole of the foot, are difficult to infiltrate because of the fibrous, septated subcutaneous tissue structure. In other areas, swelling and distortion of the anatomy with infiltration make it more difficult to accurately reapproximate tissue planes and optimize the cosmetic result. Nerve blocks described later in this chapter are often superior to infiltration anesthesia in such cases.

Indications for field blocks are local anesthesia for procedures in areas of inflammation or infection (grossly contaminated lacerations, incision and drainage of abscesses, etc.) or for local anesthesia with preservation of the wound architecture.

Equipment

10% povidone-iodine solution

Sterile gauze

Sterile gloves

1% lidocaine (with or without epinephrine, depending on location) 8.4% sodium bicarbonate (1 mEq/mL)

3, 5, or 10 mL syringe

27- or 30-gauge, 1.5 inch hypodermic needle

Procedure

Direct Infiltration

The region is checked for perfusion, sensation, motor function, and associated injuries before anesthetic injection. To minimize patient anxiety, the syringe is filled with buffered lidocaine out of view of the child or before the child enters the treatment room. Whenever possible, the child should not be allowed to see the needle. All materials should be ready to use before the start of the procedure. After an appropriate explanation of the procedure, infiltration should begin without delay. A sensitive, calm, and soothing approach that engages the child in conversation or distraction may avoid the need for sedation. The young child should be immobilized by either an assistant, a papoose restraint, or both (see Chapter 3).

The area surrounding the wound is cleansed with povidone-iodine solution and dried with sterile gauze. A few drops of anesthetic are instilled directly into the wound. A 27- or 30-gauge, 1.5 inch needle is inserted through the subcutaneous tissue exposed by the laceration. Anesthetic solution is slowly injected as the needle is advanced. Alternatively, the needle may be fully inserted and slow injection performed on withdrawal. Aspiration is generally necessary only in the vicinity of major vessels, as only a small amount of anesthetic is injected at any given point while the needle is continually advancing. The needle is removed and then reinserted into adjacent tissue through the subdermis that has already been anesthetized. Reinsertion and slow injection of anesthetic continues sequentially until the entire perimeter of the wound has been infiltrated. Optimal anesthetic effect is reached in less than 5 minutes. The needle can be lightly applied to the skin around the wound site to test for adequate wound anesthesia.

Parallel Margin Infiltration (Field Block)

Preparation for this technique up to the point of needle insertion is the same as for direct infiltration. A 27- or 30-G, 1.5 inch needle is first inserted through the skin to the subcutaneous tissue 1 to 2 proximal to the laceration. Small amounts of anesthetic are injected as the needle is advanced to at least two-thirds its entire length. Slow injection is continued as the needle is withdrawn from the insertion site. The needle is then reinserted at the end of the first wheal where the skin is anesthetized. In similar fashion, the injection is repeated until complete infiltration of the circumference has been achieved. Optimal local anesthesia is achieved in about 5 minutes.

Complications

Direct wound infiltration and parallel margin infiltration are generally safe procedures, as long as correct medication dosages are administered and careful technique is practiced. Complications of both techniques include infection, bleeding, and intravascular injection of anesthetic.

TOPICAL ANESTHESIA

Topical anesthesia is an alternative method to local infiltrative anesthesia. It is used to anesthetize small wounds and intact skin for simple procedures. Topical agents may be advantageous because they are easier and less painful to apply, they do not distort wound margins, and they can decrease the need for sedation and physical restraint of pediatric patients. In clinical use, major limitations to topical anesthesia have been its slow onset, inadequate analgesia, cost, and local or systemic adverse effects.

Tetracaine/Adrenaline/Cocaine

Tetracaine/adrenaline/cocaine (TAC) is a clear solution of 0.5% tetracaine, 1:2000 epinephrine, and 11.8% cocaine. Its anesthetic efficacy was first described by Pryor et al. in 1980 (41). The solution can be prepared easily in the hospital pharmacy and has a shelf life of approximately 3 months. The original solution was arbitrarily composed and recent studies have demonstrated equal efficacy with a 5.9% cocaine concentration or with a half-strength TAC formulation (42, 43). Attempts to remove cocaine entirely from the solution have resulted in reduced anesthesia (44). Although the optimal dose and formulation are still being developed, a dosage of 1 mL per centimeter of wound length (with a total dose not to exceed 0.9 mL per kilogram or a maximum of 4 mL) is generally recommended (42, 45).

TAC topical anesthesia is about as effective as lidocaine infiltration for anesthetizing pediatric facial and scalp lacerations. It is less effective on trunk and extremity lacerations, and in adult patients (45, 46). TAC may be the preferred anesthetic for repair of pediatric facial lacerations less than 4 cm in length that do not involve mucous membranes. Topical application of TAC is advantageous as it is easy, painless, and has been shown to improve patient compliance with the subsequent wound repair procedure (41, 45, 47). The psychological trauma associated with restraint and painful procedures is reduced because of the relative absence of pain. Additionally, topical application avoids the swelling and distortion of wound margins caused by infiltrative anesthesia. This may enhance accurate tissue approximation and cosmetic outcome. TAC does not appear to increase bacterial proliferation or wound infection rates when compared with lidocaine (48).

The major disadvantage of TAC is that its use is limited to highly vascularized, nonmucous membrane regions. Even with selected wounds, inadequate anesthesia may occur. However, subsequent lidocaine infiltration is usually less painful. In addition, when compared with lidocaine, TAC costs significantly more per patient dose and also incurs additional indirect costs associated with using a Schedule II agent (44, 46). Finally, the time for application of TAC is considerably longer than the time for lidocaine infiltration.

Anatomy and Physiology

TAC causes local anesthesia by the diffusion of the topical anesthetic combination through the margins of lacerated tissues. Tetracaine hydrochloride is a long-acting ester group local anesthetic. It acts on the neuronal membrane, interacting with the sodium channel to prevent the generation and conduction of nerve impulses in axons of the peripheral nervous system (46). Cocaine hydrochloride, which is derived from the leaves of the Erythroxylon coca plant, is an ester group local anesthetic with vasoconstrictive properties. Cocaine induces anesthesia by preventing impulse generation and conduction in sensory nerves, and it also blocks the presynaptic reuptake of norepinephrine and other catecholamines. This process results in excess norepinephrine concentrations in the synaptic cleft, and is responsible for the vasoconstrictive properties (46). Epinephrine, an endogenous catecholamine with vasoconstrictive effects, prolongs the duration of action of locally infiltrated anesthetics by retarding drug removal and limiting systemic absorption.

Indications

TAC is used for the repair of wounds less than 4 cm in length that are located in well-vascularized, nonmucous membrane regions. Typically, these are facial and scalp lacerations.

TAC is contraindicated in areas of end-arteriolar supply (pinna of the ear, nasal alae, penis, digits), because vasoconstriction without collateral circulation can result in tissue ischemia. TAC should not be used on mucosal surfaces or on areas of extensively burned or abraded skin, as excessive uptake into the systemic circulation may cause toxicity. In addition, TAC use in or around the eye may result in corneal injury. Other contraindications include an allergy to any of the components of TAC, cholinesterase deficiency, or significant hepatic disease.

TAC should be used with caution in children with underlying seizures or cardiac dysrhythmias, as systemic absorption of the cocaine and lidocaine may exacerbate these conditions.

Equipment

TAC solution (0.5% tetracaine, 1:2000 epinephrine, 11.8% cocaine)
Sterile 3 mL syringe
Sterile cotton ball or gauze
Protective gloves

Procedure

TAC should always be administered with gloved hands as the compound may cause vasoconstriction of normal skin. To maximize TAC penetration, debris, blood clots, and devitalized tissue are removed from the wound surface. TAC is applied directly to the wound surface by dripping it onto the laceration or by "painting" it on with a sterile cotton swab. A portion of the TAC dose can be placed on a sterile cotton ball or gauze and applied to the wound with firm continuous

pressure for at least 10 to 20 minutes. As a safety precaution, a health professional may apply the TAC or carefully supervise parental application. TAC must not inadvertently come in contact with the eyes or mucous membranes where it is more likely to produce complications. Blanching of the skin that surrounds the wound from the vasoconstrictor effect indicates that anesthesia should be adequate. Good anesthesia generally persists for up to 1 hour.

Lidocaine/Adrenaline/Tetracaine

Two recent studies have investigated using lidocaine/adrenaline/tetracaine (LAT) as a topical anesthetic alternative to TAC solution (59, 60). Both studies found LAT to have comparable anesthetic efficacy to TAC in the repair of pediatric facial and scalp lacerations. LAT maintains all the advantages of topical anesthesia, and is considerably cheaper with less abuse potential than TAC. Further studies and greater clinical experience are needed to demonstrate the safety of LAT.

Eutectic Mixture of Local Anesthetics

Eutectic mixture of local anesthetics (EMLA) is a topical anesthetic formulation developed for use on intact skin (61). The term "eutectic" refers to the phenomenon whereby the melting point of the combination of agents is lower after mixing than that of any of the agents alone. The active ingredients of the EMLA mixture are the local anesthetics lidocaine and prilocaine.

EMLA 5% cream produces reliable anesthesia after a 60- to 120-minute application under an occlusive dressing. The onset, depth, and duration of dermal analgesia depends on the duration of application. Rates of percutaneous absorption vary according to the location and condition of the skin. Absorption occurs faster on diseased, facial, or Caucasian skin when compared with normal intact, extremity, or African-American skin (62, 63). After typical application, duration of topical anesthesia is approximately 2 hours

(64). Maximal depth of analgesia to needle insertion is about 5 mm (65).

Using eutectic lidocaine/prilocaine cream to relieve the pain associated with a variety of medical and surgical procedures is well established. EMLA has been demonstrated to have similar analgesic efficacy to lidocaine infiltration and ethyl chloride spray in children undergoing venipuncture and intravenous cannulation (66–71). In children undergoing lumbar puncture, analgesic efficacy of EMLA was significantly better than placebo in double-blind trials (72, 73).

EMLA has been applied to mucosal surfaces without an occlusive dressing. Onset to effective analgesia is approximately 10 to 15 minutes (64). Although EMLA is currently not indicated for application to mucous membranes, its beneficial effect is evident in a variety of ocular, oral, and genitourinary procedures (62).

The major limitation for using EMLA cream in the emergency department (ED) is its slow onset of analgesic action. Although pain was adequately relieved when used before venous cannulation, studies have not demonstrated evidence of improved patient cooperation (67, 71). Some authorities question whether the delay involved with using EMLA cream is justified for an isolated procedure (74). Other shortcomings of topical anesthesia with EMLA include the limited total dose that can be applied, unsatisfactory deep analgesia, and limited current indications. It is possible, however, that EMLA usage will broaden significantly with a wider range of future applications.

Anatomy and Physiology

EMLA results in dermal analgesia through the diffusion of the amide anesthetics (lidocaine and prilocaine) into the epidermal and dermal layers of the skin. The resultant accumulation of anesthetic stabilizes neuronal membranes by inhibiting the ionic fluxes required for impulse conduction.

The amount of lidocaine and prilocaine systemically absorbed from the eutectic mixture is directly related to the area and duration of contact, and the region over which it is applied. Pharmacokinetic studies showed the maximum plasma concentrations of lidocaine and prilocaine to be 10 to 100-fold less than concentrations considered toxic (62).

Indications

Eutectic lidocaine/prilocaine cream is currently approved for topical analgesia only on normal intact skin. The cream has proven useful for venipunctures, intravenous cannulation, superficial surgery, and lumbar punctures in children.

EMLA is contraindicated in patients who have a history of sensitivity to local amide anesthetics or who have congenital or idiopathic methemoglobinemia. The cream is not recommended for use in infants less than 3 months of age and in those under age 12 months who are receiving treatment with methemoglobin-inducing agents.

Equipment

EMLA cream
Occlusive dressing (adhesive bandage, plastic wrap, or duoderm)

Procedure

A thick layer of 5% EMLA cream is applied to intact skin and covered with an occlusive dressing. Dermal anesthesia will increase during the initial 3 hours after application and lasts for 1 to 2 hours after cream removal. Application time should not exceed 4 hours in children under 1 year of age (62).

For minor dermal procedures such as venipuncture or intravenous cannulation, 2.5 g (i.e., one-half of the 5 g tube) of EMLA 5% cream is applied over 20 to 25 cm^2 of skin surface for at least 1 hour before the procedure. For superficial surgeries or procedures that involve a larger surface area of dermis, approximately 1.5 to 2.0 g/10 cm^2 is applied at least 2 hours before the procedure.

Ethyl Chloride (Chloroethane)

Ethyl chloride (chloroethane) is a sterile, colorless, and flammable liquid used as a topical analgesic for superficial procedures. A spray bottle is used to direct pressurized liquid to cool the skin and produce instantaneous anesthesia.

Ethyl chloride has been demonstrated to significantly reduce the pain of venipuncture and lumbar puncture (80, 81). When compared with intradermal lidocaine for venipuncture, ethylchloride produced no difference in the pain of application, although it

1. TAC is primarily useful for lacerations of the face and scalp. Anesthesia achieved for trunk or extremity lacerations is generally inadequate.
2. Lidocaine infiltration may be necessary for trunk and extremity wounds in addition to (or instead of) TAC.
3. Blanching of surrounding skin indicates onset of anesthesia with TAC.
4. Contact with eyes, mucous membranes, and end-arteriolar locations must be avoided when using TAC.
5. When EMLA is used for venipuncture or venous cannulation, additional site(s) are prepared in case the initial attempt is unsuccessful.
6. To be effective, EMLA must be applied at least 1 hour before the painful procedure.
7. When using ethyl chloride, prior application of petrolatum to the skin surrounding the desired area of anesthesia will limit skin exposure.
8. Adequate anesthesia with ethyl chloride is usually indicated by frost formation on the skin.

is less potent in producing skin anesthesia (80). Nevertheless, ethyl chloride does not cause tissue distortion or venoconstriction, and results in less interference with venous cannulation than lidocaine (80).

Ethyl chloride is easy to use, quick, readily accessible, and dependable. The cost is approximately five dollars per multidose bottle (81). However, cooling only results in brief superficial anesthesia, and ethyl chloride should not be used for deeper pain, which is better managed with local infiltration or nerve blockade. Appropriate room ventilation is essential and its use is prohibited near ignition sources.

Anatomy and Physiology
Ethyl chloride is a vapocoolant. The liquid has a boiling point of 12 to 13°C. On contact with skin it vaporizes and cools the surrounding area to −20°C, thereby freezing any water vapor present which crystallizes as white precipitate. The anesthetic action of ethyl chloride rarely lasts for more than a few seconds to a minute.

Indications
The application of ethyl chloride for topical anesthesia is indicated for minor surgical procedures, such as incision and drainage of abscesses, and before needle sticks for phlebotomy, venous cannulation, injections, and arthrocentesis. Ethyl chloride is contraindicated in individuals with a history of ethyl chloride or cold hypersensitivity.

Equipment
Bottle or metal tube of ethyl chloride with metal spray tube.

Procedure
Petrolatum can be applied to areas adjacent to the skin to be anesthetized to limit the area exposed to ethyl chloride. Appropriate restraint and control of the spray can prevent inadvertent eye exposure. All necessary equipment should be readily available before beginning the procedure.

In a well-ventilated room, the bottle of ethyl chloride should be inverted and held 6 to 12 inches from the application site. The spring cap should be depressed completely to allow for a steady stream of ethyl chloride to flow from the bottle directly onto the treatment site. The spray is directed at the site of the procedure for a few seconds. Frost formation as the skin becomes white indicates that the area has been adequately cooled and adequate anesthesia should be achieved. Because anesthesia lasts for a few seconds to 1 minute, the procedure should be performed promptly.

Complications

TAC
Appropriate use of TAC is relatively safe. Patients and their families should be advised that with routine usage blood and urine samples may become positive for cocaine and its metabolites, even without clinical signs of toxicity (49, 50, 51).

Misuse of TAC can lead to serious complications. Most occur through the inappropriate application of TAC on, or in close proximity to, mucosal surfaces resulting in increased absorption. Complications may also occur with excessive amounts (more than 5 mL or repeated dosing) or through use on large areas of burned or abraded skin. Relatively minor reactions include pupillary dilation, agitation, and tachycardia; major complications are seizures, apnea, and death (52–58). These systemic toxicities may be the result of cocaine or tetracaine poisoning, or a combination of all three drugs (46). Corneal abrasions also may result when TAC contacts the eye (54).

Complications of TAC can be minimized by strict adherence to correct application procedures, and by usage only in nonmucous membrane, non-end arteriolar regions. Additionally, using half-strength TAC may decrease the risk of side effects while maintaining adequate analgesia (42).

EMLA
The most frequent adverse effects of topical EMLA cream are mild local cutaneous reactions. Pallor (37%), erythema (30%), altered temperature sensation (7%), edema (6%), itching (2%), and rash (less than 1%) were noted in 56% of over 1300 patients treated (62). Effects are transient and resolve within 1 to 2 hours after cream removal.

Metabolites of prilocaine are capable of inducing methemoglobinemia, and this complication has resulted from using EMLA cream (75). Infants under 3 months of age and children receiving other methemoglobin-producing agents appear to be at particular risk; therefore, using EMLA should be avoided in these individuals. The methemoglobinemia probably develops through the overloading of methemoglobin reductase (76). Recent studies in children 3 months to 6 years of age have demonstrated a twofold increase in methemoglobin levels after treatment with EMLA. Methemoglobin levels remained within the normal range and the elevations were not considered clinically significant (76–78).

Ingestion, and ocular and airway instillation of EMLA cream have occurred through disruption of the occlusive dressing (79). Precautionary measures should be taken to ensure that the young child does not remove the dressing. Although rare, allergic reactions also may occur (64).

Ethyl Chloride
Prolonged spraying with ethyl chloride may result in chemical frostbite, skin ulceration, and muscle damage (82). Rarely, contact dermatitis may occur after topical spray application (83).

Ethyl chloride must always be sprayed in a well-ventilated room, as inhalation may produce narcotic and general anesthetic effects. The solution is highly volatile and should never be used near an open flame or electrical cautery equipment.

NERVE BLOCK ANESTHESIA

Certain instances occur in which local infiltrative anesthesia is impractical or would be excessively painful to administer. Examples include repair of a nailbed laceration, incision and drainage of a paronychia, manipulation of the foreskin when it is tightly entrapped in a zipper, excision of an ingrown toenail, or repair of a large laceration on the palm of the hand or sole of the foot. Adequate local anesthesia of the fingertip, nailbed, or penis may be impossible, and extensive infiltration of the highly innervated palm and sole is usually extremely painful. In such cases, regional anesthesia using an appropriate nerve block can be the best (or only) method for providing effective anesthesia.

Upper Extremity Nerve Blocks

Nerves of the upper extremity most amenable to regional anesthesia in the acute care setting are the median, ulnar, radial, and digital nerves. These nerves innervate the highly pain-sensitive areas of the fingers and hand. Administering one or more nerve blocks to perform painful procedures in these areas often provides excellent anesthesia while minimizing discomfort for the patient.

Median Nerve Block
Anatomy
At the wrist, the median nerve enters the palm through the carpal tunnel and lies deep to the palmaris longus tendon, between the tendons of the flexor digitorum superficialis and flexor carpi radialis. At the proximal end of the tunnel, the location of the nerve is easily identified between the palmaris longus and flexor carpi radialis tendons (Fig. 37.1.A).

Indications
Median nerve block is used to provide anesthesia for procedures to the palmar aspect of the thumb, index and middle fingers, and the radial aspect of the fourth digit. Dorsally, the median nerve supplies the tip of the thumb and the distal portion of the index and middle fingers, as well as the radial side of the fourth finger (Fig. 37.1.B). Median nerve blocks can be combined with radial and ulnar nerve blocks for procedures of the hand. Carpal tunnel syndrome is a relative contraindication to performing median nerve block at the wrist (84).

Equipment
1% lidocaine solution
25- or 27-gauge, 0.5 or 1 inch hypodermic needle
5 mL syringe
10% povidone-iodine or other antiseptic solution
Sterile gauze

Procedure
The area requiring anesthesia is carefully identified. The hand and digits are checked for perfusion, sensation, and motor nerve function before injecting the anesthetic agent. Apposition of the thumb and fifth finger with flexion of the wrist against some resistance

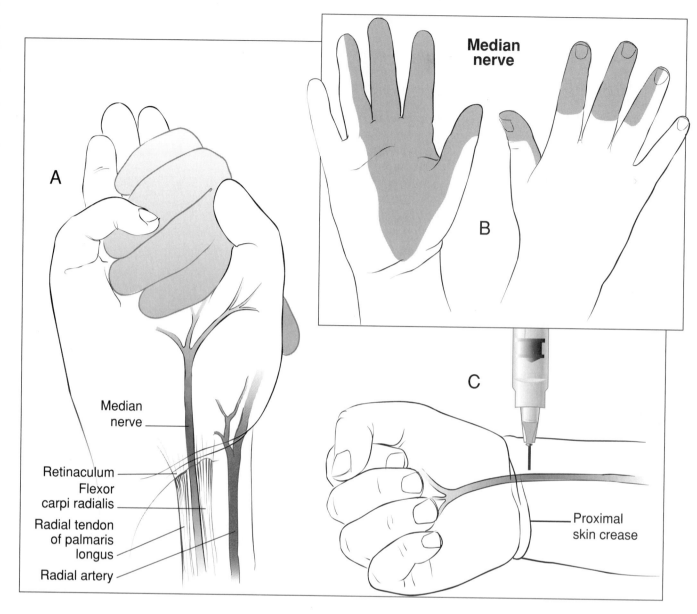

Figure 37.1.
A. The median nerve is located just radial to the palmaris longus tendon at the wrist.
B. Sensory innervation of the median nerve.
C. Median nerve block.

will easily identify the tendon of the palmaris longus, which protrudes from the volar aspect of the wrist. The overlying skin is prepared with povidone-iodine or alcohol.

A 25- or 27-gauge, 0.5 inch needle is inserted perpendicularly, just radial to the palmaris longus tendon at the level of the proximal flexor wrist crease (Fig. 37.1.C). A "pop" may be felt as the retinaculum is pierced (85). Paresthesias (i.e., tingling sensations or jolts in the distribution of the nerve) occur when the needle mechanically stimulates nerve fibers. It may be difficult for a child to cooperate with the physician and distinguish between the pain of needle insertion and the

sensation of paresthesia. If a paresthesia is elicited, the needle tip is certain to be in close proximity to the nerve. The needle is withdrawn slightly to avoid intraneuronal injection, and 2 to 3 mL of anesthetic is injected. If a paresthesia is not elicited, a larger volume of anesthetic (about 3 to 5 mL) is injected to increase the likelihood that the nerve is blocked. Optimal anesthetic effect may take 10 to 20 minutes.

Ulnar Nerve Block
Anatomy
At the level of the elbow, the ulnar nerve lies in the groove between the medial epicondyle

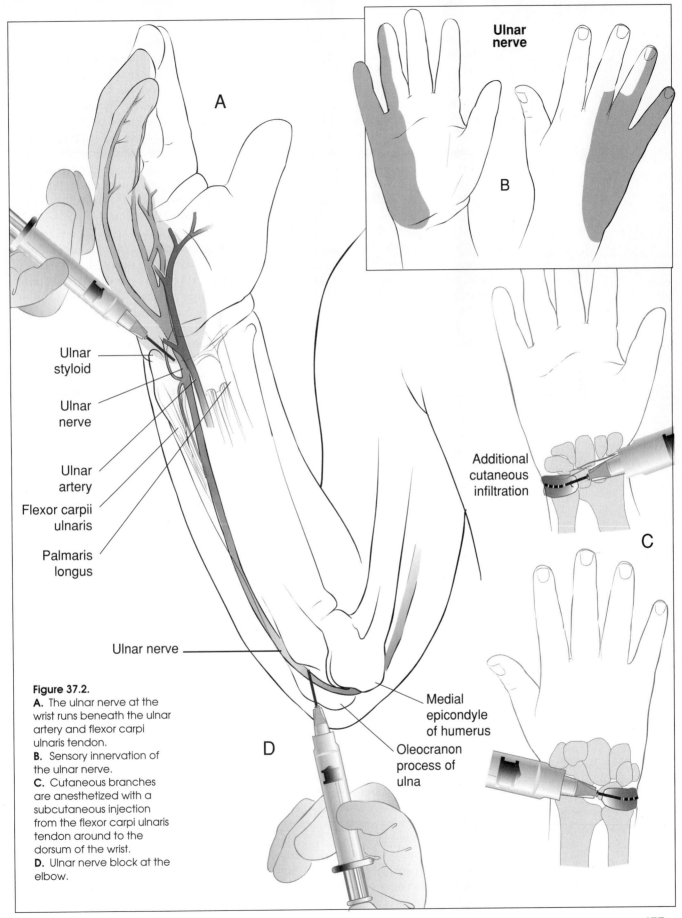

A

Ulnar
nerve

B

Ulnar
styloid

Ulnar
nerve

Ulnar
artery

Flexor carpii
ulnaris

Palmaris
longus

Additional
cutaneous
infiltration

C

Ulnar nerve

D

Medial
epicondyle
of humerus

Oleocranon
process of
ulna

Figure 37.2.
A. The ulnar nerve at the
wrist runs beneath the ulnar
artery and flexor carpi
ulnaris tendon.
B. Sensory innervation of
the ulnar nerve.
C. Cutaneous branches
are anesthetized with a
subcutaneous injection
from the flexor carpi ulnaris
tendon around to the
dorsum of the wrist.
D. Ulnar nerve block at the
elbow.

and the olecranon (Fig. 37.2). As it approaches the middle of the forearm, the ulnar nerve lies between the flexor digitorum profundus and the flexor carpi ulnaris (Fig. 37.2.A). In the lower portion of the forearm, it divides about 0.5 cm proximal to the wrist giving off two cutaneous branches, the palmar cutaneous branch, which provides some sensation to the ulnar side of the wrist and hand, and the dorsal cutaneous branch, supplying the ulnar side of the hand and the dorsum of the fifth and ulnar half of the fourth digits. At the wrist, the ulnar nerve passes between the tendon of the flexor carpi ulnaris and ulnar artery, deep to the artery. Its superficial terminal branch supplies the skin of the anterior fifth digit and ulnar half of the fourth digit in the hand. If local anesthesia is needed throughout the entire ulnar distribution, it is preferable to block at the elbow instead of the wrist (before the nerve subdivides) (87).

Indications

Ulnar nerve block should be used to provide anesthesia of the dorsal and palmar aspects of the ulnar side of the hand, fifth finger, and ulnar side of the fourth finger (Fig. 37.2.B). As with other nerve blocks, this technique is used for painful procedures such as laceration repair, reduction of hand fractures, or removal of a foreign body. It is often used in combination with median and/or radial nerve blocks to achieve a larger field of anesthesia.

Equipment

1% lidocaine solution
25- or 27-gauge, 0.5 or 1 inch hypodermic
    needle
5 mL syringe (for block at wrist)
10 mL syringe (for block at elbow)
10% povidone-iodine or other antiseptic solution
    lution
Sterile gauze

Procedure

Ulnar Nerve Block at the Wrist.   The area requiring anesthetic is carefully identified. The hand and digits are checked for perfusion, sensation, and motor nerve function before injecting the anesthetic agent. A modified Allen test may be used to verify collateral arterial supply to the hand, although this test is not always reliable. The tendon of the flexor carpi ulnaris is located by having the patient flex the wrist against mild resistance. The skin of the lateral wrist is prepared with povidone-iodine or alcohol.

The palmar cutaneous branch of the ulnar nerve is anesthetized by raising a skin wheal at the level of the proximal wrist crease (ulnar styloid), between the tendon of the flexor carpi ulnaris and the ulnar artery. A 25- to 27-gauge needle is advanced through the wheal to a depth of approximately 0.5 cm (just deep to the tendon). Paresthesia indicates proximity of the needle tip to the nerve. After slight withdrawal to avoid intraneuronal injection and aspiration to ensure that the needle is not intravascular, 1 to 3 mL of solution is injected. If a paresthesia is not obtained, a larger volume (3 to 5 mL) of anesthetic solution should be administered. Alternatively, repeated fanned insertions can be done until an ulnar paresthesia is obtained.

If the dorsal cutaneous branch of the ulnar nerve is not adequately anesthetized, additional cutaneous infiltration should be instilled over the dorsal and ulnar aspect of the wrist, at the level of the ulnar styloid (Fig. 37.2.C.). Optimal anesthesia is usually achieved within 10 to 15 minutes.

Ulnar Nerve Block at the Elbow.   Preparations for the ulnar nerve block at the elbow are similar to those used for the wrist. With the elbow flexed, the ulnar nerve is palpable in the groove between the medial epicondyle of the humerus and the olecranon. A 25-gauge needle is inserted approximately 1 to 2 cm proximal and parallel to the course of the ulnar nerve in the groove (Fig. 37.2). Blocking the nerve within the groove is more likely to cause nerve injury, so the needle tip is advanced to the proximal end of the groove. Paresthesias indicate proximity to the nerve, but are not necessary to elicit. If noted, the needle is withdrawn approximately 2 mm to avoid injection into the nerve sheath. An injection of 3 to 5 mL of 1% lidocaine on each side of the groove will block this rather large nerve. Anesthesia is usually achieved in 15 minutes.

Radial Nerve Block

Anatomy

The radial nerve splits into peripheral branches about two-thirds of the way down the forearm. At the wrist, one of the major branches lies lateral to the flexor carpi radialis tendon in close proximity to the radial

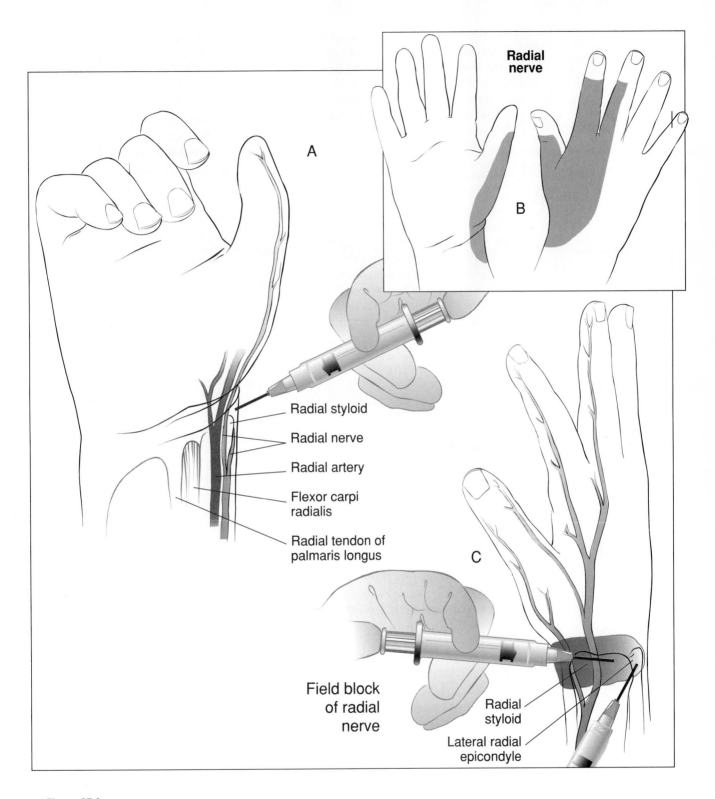

Radial nerve

A

B

C

Radial styloid

Radial nerve

Radial artery

Flexor carpi radialis

Radial tendon of palmaris longus

Field block of radial nerve

Radial styloid

Lateral radial epicondyle

Figure 37.3.
A. The radial nerve at the wrist is blocked just lateral to the radial artery.
B. Sensory innervation of the radial nerve.
C. Cutaneous branches are anesthetized with subcutaneous injection in a cuff-like distribution around to the dorsal midline.

artery (Fig. 37.3). Proximal to the wrist, sensory branches emerge and course subcutaneously around the distal radius to the dorsolateral portion of the wrist and hand. These branches innervate the dorsal aspect of the proximal thumb, and the second, third, and radial portion of the fourth fingers.

Indications

Radial nerve block is used to provide anesthesia for the radial portion of the thenar eminence, dorsal surfaces of the thumb, and proximal two-thirds of the index, middle, and radial aspect of the fourth finger (Fig. 37.3.B). As with other nerve blocks, radial nerve block is useful for procedures such as laceration repair, reduction of hand fractures, and removal of foreign bodies. Combined radial, median, and ulnar nerve blocks provide complete anesthesia of the hand.

Equipment

1% lidocaine solution
25- or 27-gauge, 1 inch hypodermic needle
10 mL syringe
10% povidone-iodine or other antiseptic solution
Sterile gauze

Procedure

The area requiring anesthetic is identified. Perfusion, sensation, and motor nerve function of the hand and digits are checked before injecting the anesthetic agent. The flexor carpi radialis tendon is located by flexing the wrist slightly. The skin over the distal radial portion of the wrist at the level of the skin creases is prepared with alcohol or povidone-iodine.

To anesthetize the major peripheral branch of the radial nerve, the flexor carpi radialis tendon and radial artery are palpated at the level of the proximal palmar crease. A 25- to 27-gauge needle is inserted just lateral to the radial artery to the depth of the artery. Intravascular injection is avoided by aspirating for blood return. Approximately 2 to 4 mL of local anesthetic is injected (Fig. 37.3.A).

To anesthetize the dorsal cutaneous branches of the radial nerve, local anesthetic is infiltrated subcutaneously over the dorsoradial aspect of the wrist in a cuff-like distribution from the initial injection site to the midline of the dorsal aspect of the wrist (Fig. 37.3.C). After the initial injection, the needle

can be repositioned to start the subcutaneous infiltration of the radial aspect of the wrist. A second needle insertion may be necessary to complete the infiltration to the dorsal midline, but pain can be minimized by entering through previously anesthetized skin. Approximately 5 mL are required (3 to 5 mg/kg of lidocaine maximum). Onset of the anesthetic effect generally takes about 10 minutes. The effectiveness of a radial nerve block is assessed by applying a stimulus to the dorsal web space between the thumb and index finger, which is an area of pure radial nerve innervation.

Digital Nerve Blocks of the Hand

Anatomy

Each digit of the hand is supplied by four nerves. In cross-sectional view, the two dorsal digital nerves lie along each phalanx at the 2- and 10-o'clock position, while the palmar digital nerves lie at the 4- and 8-o'clock position (Fig. 37.4).

The palmar or common digital nerves arise from deep branches of the ulnar and median nerves, supplying sensation to the volar skin and interphalangeal joints. These are the principal nerves supplying the digits. The palmar nerves also supply the dorsal distal aspects (fingertip and nailbed) of the second, third, and radial portion of the fourth digits. Therefore, only the palmar digital nerves may require blockade to obtain adequate distal anesthesia in these digits.

The two dorsal digital nerves arise from the radial and ulnar nerves, supplying sensation to the dorsal aspect of all five fingers to the level of the distal interphalangeal joints. The dorsal nerves also supply the dorsal distal aspects (fingertip and nailbed) of the thumb, and fifth digits and ulnar aspect of the fourth finger. In these digits, all four nerves must always be blocked to obtain adequate anesthesia for distal repairs.

Figure 37.4.
A. Anatomy of digital nerves.
B. Web space technique.
C. Dorsal technique for palmar and dorsal digital nerve block.
D. Palmar technique for palmar nerve block.

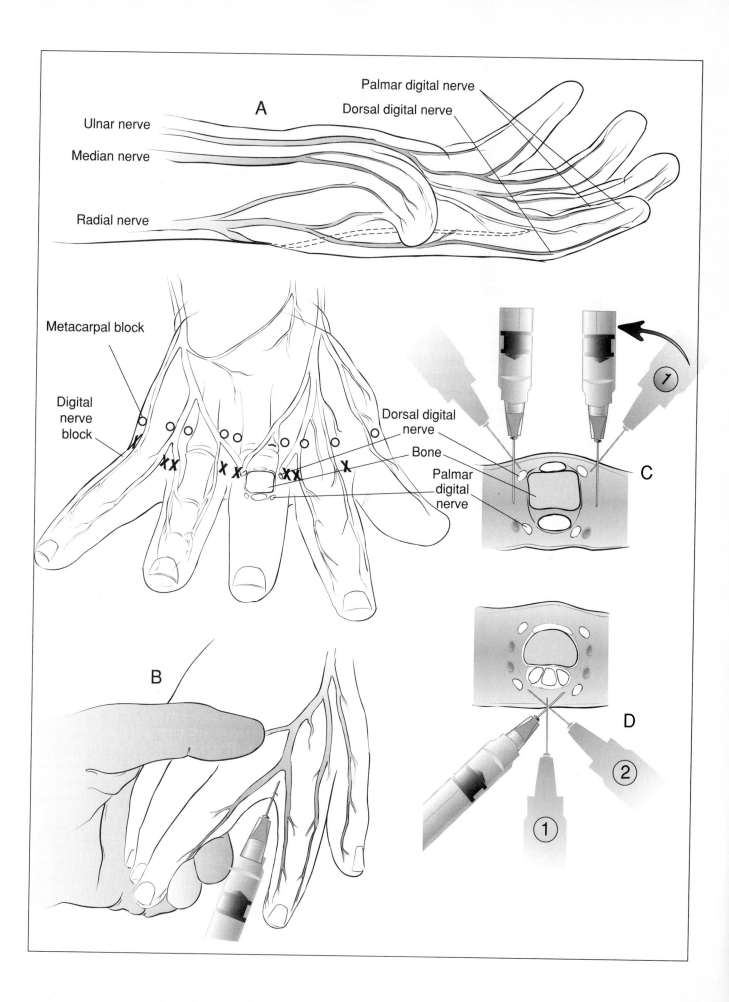

A

Palmar digital nerve
Dorsal digital nerve
Ulnar nerve
Median nerve
Radial nerve

Metacarpal block
Digital nerve block
Dorsal digital nerve
Bone
Palmar digital nerve

B

C

D

Indications

Digital nerve blocks are used to provide anesthesia of the fingers for procedures such as finger laceration and nailbed repair, drainage of a paronychia, and reduction of fractures and dislocations. The digital nerve block is the most common nerve block used by ED physicians for minor wound care (85).

The common digital nerve block can be performed from either the dorsal or the palmar aspects. The dorsal approach is advantageous because injection is considerably more painful through the thicker palmar skin (88). With the palmar approach, however, anesthesia can be achieved with a single needle puncture. The distal digital nerve block at the web space is used to provide anesthesia for procedures to the distal two-thirds of the fingers. Distal digital nerve blockade requires small volumes of local anesthetic infiltration between the skin and the bone. Large volumes are unnecessary and pose an additional risk of vascular compression and patient discomfort. A proximal block at the level of the distal metacarpal may be preferred over the distal digital nerve block, because it reduces the risk of vascular compromise by compression of the arterial supply. It also anesthetizes the entire length of the finger. Only the palmar digital nerves need to be blocked in the middle three fingers to achieve complete anesthesia of the fingertip (85). The first and fifth digits require both palmar and dorsal digital nerve blockade.

Equipment

1% lidocaine solution *without epinephrine*
25- or 27-gauge, 0.5 or 1 inch hypodermic needle
5 mL syringe
10% povidone-iodine or other antiseptic solution
Sterile gauze

Procedure

Preparations for each of the digital nerve blocks are similar. The area requiring anesthetic is first identified. The distal fingers are assessed for perfusion, sensation, and motor nerve function before injection. Because the digital nerve may be injured by the initial finger injury, it is important to determine and document the digital nerve function before

nerve blockade. Sterile injection technique after preparation of the skin with alcohol or povidone-iodine is necessary, but sterile gloves and drapes are not required.

Distal Digital Nerve Block. The interdigital web space skin is prepared with povidone-iodine solution. A 25- or 27-gauge needle is inserted into the dorsal aspect of the web space distal to the metacarpal-phalangeal joint. The needle is advanced toward the bone of the affected finger. If no blood return occurs with aspiration, 0.5 to 1.0 mL of local anesthetic is injected to block the dorsal digital nerves (Fig. 37.4.B). Next the needle is redirected toward the volar surface of the digit and an additional 0.5 to 1.0 mL of solution is deposited to anesthetize the palmar digital nerve. The procedure is repeated on the opposite side of the digit to achieve complete anesthesia of all four digital nerves. Anesthetic effect is usually adequate in 5 to 10 minutes.

Proximal (Common) Digital Nerve Block or Metacarpal Block To perform the dorsal technique of the proximal digital nerve block, the skin over the dorsal surface of the metacarpals is first prepared with alcohol or povidone-iodine. A subcutaneous skin wheal is raised between the metacarpal bones on the dorsum of the hand approximately 1 to 2 cm proximal to the lebspace. With a 1 inch 25-gauge needle, the skin is entered through the wheal and slowly the needle advances to just under the skin on the palmar side. Aspiration to ensure no blood return protects against intravascular injection. Local anesthetic (2 to 3 mL) is deposited. Because the common digital nerve lies just above the flexor retinaculum of the hand, most of the local anesthetic should be delivered close to the palmar surface. The procedure is repeated on the opposite side of the metacarpal to ensure that both sides of the involved digit are anesthetized (Fig. 37.4.C). The block takes effect in 10 to 15 minutes.

To perform the palmar technique of the proximal digital nerve block, the palmar skin over the metacarpal heads is first prepared with alcohol or povidone-iodine. A 25- or 27-gauge, 1 inch needle is inserted at the level of the distal palmar crease, over the center of the metacarpal head (Fig. 37.4.D). Anesthetic solution is injected as the needle is advanced to the bone. The needle is withdrawn slightly, redirected toward the radial aspect of the metacarpal head, and advanced a few millimeters. Aspiration to ensure no blood return protects against intravascular injection. Approximately 1.0 to 1.5 mL of local anesthetic is deposited. The needle is withdrawn a few millimeters, angled toward the ulnar aspect of the metacarpal head, and advanced slightly. An additional 1.0 to 1.5 mL is injected after aspiration (Fig. 37.4.D). The block becomes effective in 10 to 15 minutes.

Lower Extremity Nerve Blocks

Ankle Blocks
Sensory innervation of the foot involves five nerves that course through the ankle. Considerable overlap is evident in the sensory distribution, frequently necessitating more than one nerve block at the ankle for complete anesthesia. Nerve blocks of the deep peroneal, posterior tibial, saphenous, superficial peroneal, and sural can be used alone or in combination for procedures involving the foot. They are often preferable to infiltrative anesthesia because in many areas the skin of the foot is more sensitive than the skin at the ankle, and the dense, septated subcutaneous connective tissue of the foot is not easily infiltrated (89).

The saphenous nerve provides sensation to the medial aspect of the ankle and instep. The superficial peroneal nerve innervates the central dorsum of the foot. Because local infiltrative anesthesia is generally quite successful for lacerations and wound repair in these areas, saphenous and superficial peroneal nerve blocks will not be described.

Anatomy
The posterior tibial and sural nerves supply sensory innervation to the entire sole of the foot (Fig. 37.5). When both nerves are blocked simultaneously, this is often referred to as a posterior ankle block. The posterior tibial is a branch of the sciatic nerve and, at the ankle, runs behind the medial malleolus just posterior to the easily palpated posterior tibial artery. The posterior tibial nerve provides sensation to the medial portion of the sole of the foot anteriorly and the plantar surfaces of the hallux and the second, third, and medial side of the fourth toes. The sural nerve courses with the short saphenous vein behind the fibula and lateral malleolus. It provides sensation to the heel and lateral portion of the sole of the foot anteriorly, and the plantar surface of the lateral aspect of the fourth and entire fifth toes.

The deep peroneal nerve arises from the bifurcation of the common peroneal nerve and is located anteriorly (Fig. 37.6). In the ankle it lies under the extensor hallucis longus tendon continuing to the dorsum of the foot. It innervates the short extensors to the toes, as well as the skin on the lateral side of the hallux and on the medial side of the second toe.

Indications
Ankle blocks are used for performing any painful procedures involving the foot, such as laceration repair, drainage of infections, and foreign body removal. The sural and posterior tibial nerve blocks provide anesthesia of the heel and sole of the foot (Figs. 37.5.A, 37.5.B). The deep peroneal nerve block provides anesthesia of the distal foot at the web space between the great and second toes and is often combined with other ankle blocks (Fig. 37.6.A).

Equipment
1% lidocaine solution
25- or 27-gauge, 1.0 or 1.5 inch hypodermic needle
10 mL syringe
10% povidone-iodine or other antiseptic solution
Sterile gauze

Procedure
Initial preparation for each of the ankle blocks to be described is the same. The area requiring anesthesia is first identified. Perfusion and sensation are assessed before injection of the anesthetic agent. Evaluation for nerve or tendon injury must be performed before nerve blockade.

Posterior Tibial Nerve Block. The patient should be positioned prone, with the foot extending beyond the end of the stretcher and held in slight dorsiflexion (90). The skin over the medial malleolus extending posteriorly to the Achilles tendon is prepared with povidone-iodine. The posterior tibial artery is palpated just posterior to the medial malleolus. A 25- or 27-gauge, 1.0 or 1.5 inch needle is

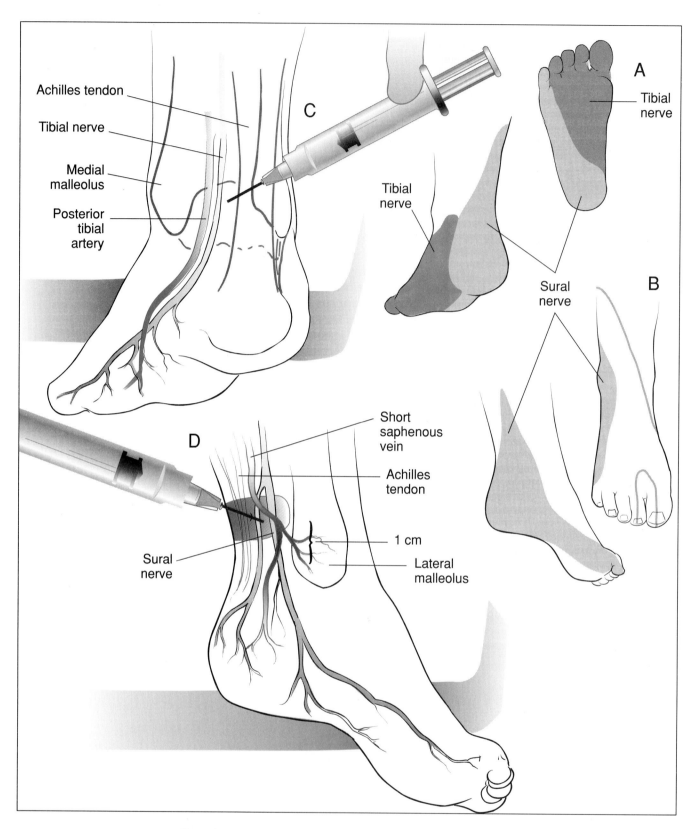

Figure 37.5.
A. Distribution of sensory innervation of posterior tibial and sural nerves (medial and plantar aspects).
B. Distribution of sensory innervation of posterior tibial and sural nerves (lateral and dorsal aspects).
C. Posterior tibial nerve block.
D. Sural nerve block.

inserted perpendicular to the skin, at the level of the top of the medial malleolus just posterior to the pulse of the artery. If the arterial pulse is not palpable, the insertion site is located between the superior border of the medial malleolus and the Achilles tendon (Fig. 37.5.C). The tip of the needle is advanced to a position approximately 1 mm from the underlying tibia. Paresthesias along the sole of the foot may be elicited with movement of the tip of the needle. When this occurs, the needle should be withdrawn 1 to 2 mm to prevent intraneuronal injection. After aspiration to prevent intravascular injection, 3 to 4 mL of anesthetic solution is injected. If no paresthesia is elicited, 5 mL of anesthetic is injected as the needle is slowly withdrawn. Anesthetic effect may be tested in 5 to 10 minutes. A successful block may cause an increase in the skin temperature of the foot due to vasodilation (85, 91).

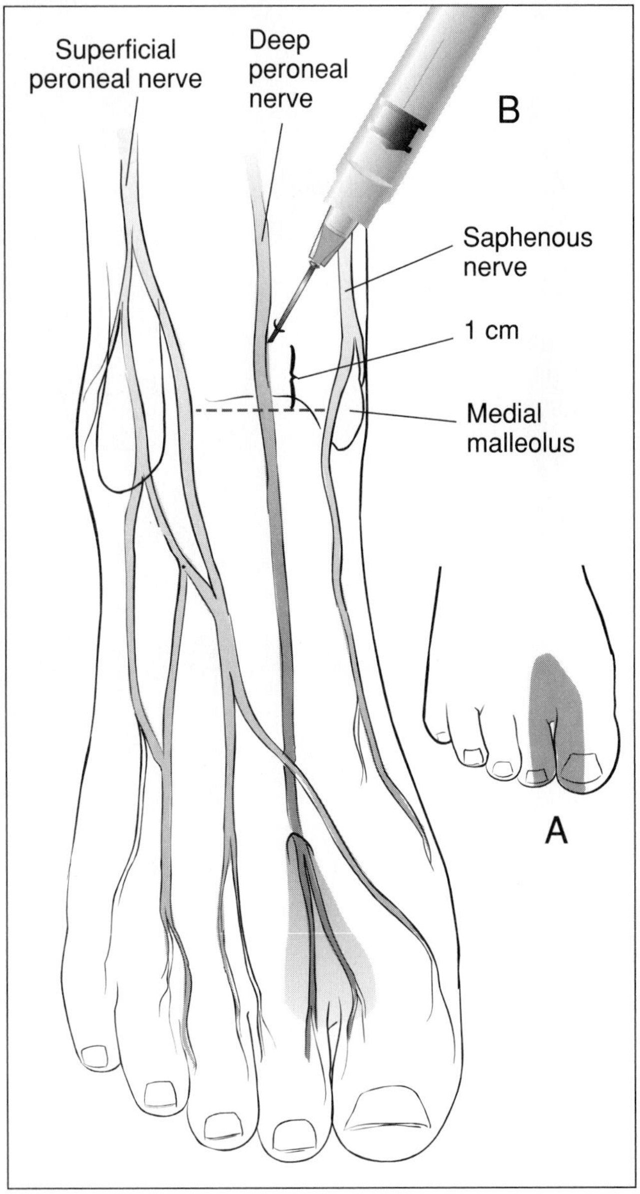

Sural Nerve Block. The patient should be positioned as previously described for the posterior tibial nerve block. The skin over the lateral malleolus extending posteriorly to the Achilles tendon is prepared with povidone-iodine. A 25- or 27-gauge, 1.0 to 1.5 inch needle is inserted just lateral to the Achilles tendon about 1 cm superior to the lateral malleolus. The needle is advanced subcutaneously toward the lateral malleolus (Fig. 37.5.D). After aspiration, the branches of the sural nerve are blocked by creating a subcutaneous band of anesthetic (3 to 5 mL) extending from the posterior aspect of the lateral malleolus to the anterior margin of the Achilles tendon. Anesthetic effect is usually adequate in 5 to 10 minutes. As with the posterior tibial nerve block, the patient may ex-

Figure 37.6.
A. Distribution of sensory innervation of deep peroneal (anterior tibial) nerve.
B. Deep peroneal nerve block.

perience an increase in the skin temperature of the foot due to vasodilation.

Deep Peroneal (Anterior Tibial) Nerve Block. The deep peroneal nerve is blocked anteriorly beneath the extensor hallucis longus and anterior tibial tendons. The patient is placed in the supine position. Dorsiflexion of the great toe can help locate the tendon of the extensor hallucis longus 1 cm above the superior aspect of the medial malleolus (Fig. 37.5.B). The area is prepared with povidone-iodine. With a 1.0 or 1.5 inch 27-gauge needle, a wheal is raised just medial to the tendon of the extensor hallucis longus. The needle is directed 30° laterally, beneath

Figure 37.7.
A. Digital block of toe.
B, C. Digital block of the hallux is achieved with a circumferential ring of anesthetic.

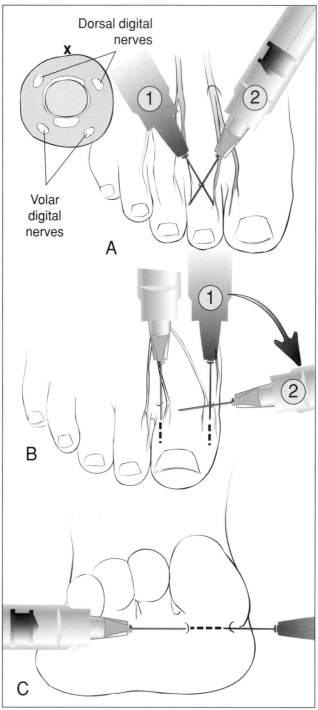

Dorsal digital nerves

X

Volar digital nerves

A

B

C

provide adequate anesthesia. This is particularly true of the volar aspect of the toes and the nailbed. For this reason, a digital nerve block is often superior to local anesthesia for performing painful procedures involving the toes.

Anatomy
Each toe is supplied by four nerves. In cross-sectional view, the two dorsal digital nerves lie along each phalanx at the 2- and 10-o'clock positions, while the volar digital nerves lie at the 4- and 8-o'clock positions (Fig. 37.7). The dorsal digital nerves arise from branches of the deep and superficial peroneal nerves, supplying sensation to the dorsal skin and interphalangeal joints of all five toes. The volar nerves, which are branches of the posterior tibial and sural nerves, supply the volar distal aspects of the toes.

Indications
Digital nerve block is used to provide anesthesia of the toes for painful procedures such as toe laceration and partial amputation repair, drainage of infections, reduction of fractures and dislocations, and repair of nailbed injuries.

Equipment
1% lidocaine solution *without epinephrine*
25- or 27-gauge, 1.0 or 1.5 inch hypodermic needle
10 mL syringe (for hallux)
5 mL syringe (for other toes)
10% povidone-iodine or other antiseptic solution
Sterile gauze

the extensor hallucis tendon, and advanced 0.5 to 1.0 cm until it strikes the tibia. After withdrawing about 1 mm and aspirating, 3 to 5 mL of local anesthetic is deposited. Anesthetic effect at the web space between the hallux and second toe may take 15 minutes.

Digital Nerve Blocks of the Foot
As with the fingers, local infiltration of the toes is generally quite painful and may not

Procedure
The area requiring anesthetic is identified. Perfusion and sensation should be assessed

before injecting the anesthetic agent. As always is important to determine and document the extent of any nerve injury before anesthesia.

The same technique used in digital blocks of the hand may be used to block the metatarsal heads, web spaces, or toes. However, because the proximal portion of the phalanx itself is sufficiently narrow, a single dorsal midline needle insertion site is used to anesthetize both sides (89).

Toe Block. The proximal portion of the toe is prepared with povidone-iodine. A 25- to 27-gauge, 1 inch needle is inserted through the skin on the dorsal aspect of the toe over the middle of the proximal portion of the phalanx (Fig. 37.7.A). The needle is advanced to just under the volar skin surface passing in close approximation to the bone. After aspiration, 1 to 2 mL of anesthetic is injected as the needle is slowly withdrawn. The needle is further withdrawn, without removing it from the skin, and redirected to the opposite side of the phalanx, again advancing it in close approximation to the bone. After aspiration, another 1 to 2 mL is injected as the needle is withdrawn completely. Anesthesia takes effect in 5 to 10 minutes.

Hallux Toe Block. Because of the unique innervation of the hallux, a circumferential ring of anesthetic is necessary for a complete nerve block. The dorsal surface of the great toe is prepared with povidone-iodine. A 1 inch, 25- to 27-gauge needle is inserted in the dorsomedial aspect of the proximal portion of the great toe, extending to the plantar surface (Fig. 37.7.B). After aspiration, 1 to 2 mL of anesthetic is deposited as the needle is withdrawn. Without removing the needle, it is redirected across the dorsal surface of the proximal phalanx laterally, and 1 to 2 mL of solution is injected as the needle is withdrawn completely. The needle is then inserted through the dorsolateral aspect of the proximal portion the great toe that was infiltrated on the first injection. The needle is advanced to the plantar surface, and 1 to 2 mL of anesthetic solution is injected as the needle is removed. To complete a circumferential block of the hallux, the needle is inserted in a medial-to-lateral direction along the plantar surface of the great toe, at the proximal portion of the phalanx. After aspiration, 1 to 2 mL of solution is injected as the needle is removed. Full anesthesia is achieved in 5 to 10 minutes. (Fig. 37.7.C).

Penile Nerve Blocks

Anatomy

The second, third, and fourth sacral nerve roots join to form the sacral plexus. The pudendal nerve arises from this sacral plexus and a deep terminal branch—the dorsal nerve of the penis—furnishes most of the somatosensory innervation of the glans and shaft of the penis. The dorsal nerves of the penis lie just lateral to the midline, adjacent to the dorsal veins and arteries beneath Buck's fascia (Fig. 37.8).

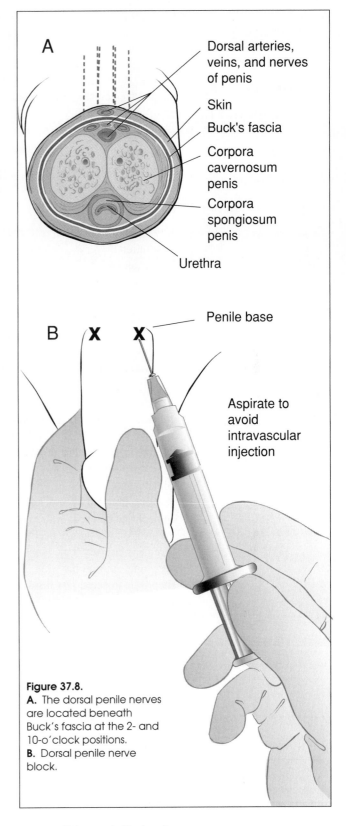

Figure 37.8.
A. The dorsal penile nerves are located beneath Buck's fascia at the 2- and 10-o'clock positions.
B. Dorsal penile nerve block.

1. Cleanse base of penis with povidone-iodine or other antiseptic solution
2. For neonates, use 0.8 mL 1% lidocaine *without epinephrine* in a 1 mL syringe. For older children, use 1 to 5 mL of lidocaine *without epinephrine*. For children over 12 years, use 1 to 5 mL of 0.25% bupivacaine without epinephrine.
3. Insert needle 3 to 5 mm beneath skin, at the junction of the penile base and suprapubic skin at the 10-o'clock position. After a negative aspiration for blood, infiltrate half of the anesthetic dose.
4. Repeat step 3 at the 2-o'clock position and inject remaining anesthetic
5. Wait 5 minutes and test for anesthetic effect before performing procedure

Indications

Penile nerve block is used to provide anesthesia for minor procedures of the penis. In the emergency setting, this block is useful for a dorsal slit, removal of a zipper that has entrapped the foreskin, or paraphimosis reduction.

Equipment

1% lidocaine solution *without epinephrine*
25- to 27-gauge, 1.0 or 1.5 inch hypodermic needle
1 mL or 5 mL syringe
10% povidone-iodine or other antiseptic solution
Sterile gauze

Procedure

Using aseptic technique, the skin at the base of the penis is prepared with povidone-iodine solution. Local anesthetic is drawn into a syringe. In the neonate, 0.8 mL of 1% lidocaine is traditionally used, whereas 1 to 5 mL of lidocaine is used for older children. For the child over 12 years, 1 to 5 mL of 0.25% bupivacaine is preferred to provide longer lasting anesthetic effect. Because the neighboring dorsal penile arteries are end arteries, it is imperative that only local anesthetic without epinephrine be used.

A 25- to 27-gauge needle attached to the syringe is inserted at the junction of the penile base and suprapubic skin. The anesthetic should be injected just inside Buck's fascia, which lies approximately 3 to 5 mm beneath the skin surface. A "pop" is usually felt as the needle pierces Buck's fascia. Aspiration is necessary to avoid intravascular injection in this highly vascular region. Half of the anesthetic is deposited at the 10-o'clock position. The needle is reinserted at the 2-o'clock position (Fig. 37.8.B) and the remaining anesthetic is injected. The injection should occur without resistance.

Alternative methods include injecting a subcutaneous ring of anesthetic around the base of the shaft of the penis. To avoid two needle insertions, a single midline injection technique can be used. The needle is inserted in the midline and advanced perpendicularly through the skin at the lower surface of the symphysis pubis into Buck's fascia. A pop is again felt as the needle traverses Buck's fascia. After negative aspiration for blood, approximately 1 to 4 mL of local anesthetic is deposited. Diffusion of the anesthetic through Buck's fascia to both penile nerves results in local anesthesia. Optimal anesthetic effect is generally achieved in 5 minutes.

Complications

For any nerve block, large doses of local anesthetic injected into the intravascular space can cause systemic toxicity, including seizures and cardiovascular dysfunction (86).

CLINICAL TIPS: NERVE BLOCK ANESTHESIA

1. An anesthetic solution containing epinephrine should never be used for nerve blocks of the fingers, toes, or penis.
2. Nerve blocks are often preferable over local infiltration anesthesia for procedures involving the hands or feet, because insertion of the needle at the appropriate sites for a nerve block is generally much less painful than through the highly innervated skin of the palm of the hand or sole of the foot.
3. For certain procedures (e.g., nailbed repairs, replacing a minor fingertip avulsion, or incision and drainage of a paronychia) a digital block of the finger or toe is always the anesthetic method of choice.
4. When repairing injuries, the sensory and motor function of distal structures should be tested if possible (depending on the child's age), so that no confusion occurs about whether any neurologic damage resulted from the initial injury or the nerve block.
5. To obtain adequate anesthesia of the hand or foot, it is sometimes necessary to combine two or more nerve blocks.
6. Unlike infiltration anesthesia, when performing a nerve block it is generally necessary to wait at least 15 minutes after injection to obtain the full anesthetic effect.
7. If the patient reports numbness and tingling (paresthesias) on insertion of the needle, the needle should be withdrawn 1 to 2 mm before injecting the anesthetic solution, so that intraneuronal injection does not occur. With younger children, the occurrence of paresthesias may be difficult to distinguish from the pain of the injection.
8. Aspiration for blood should always be performed before injecting the anesthetic solution to prevent intravascular injection.

For this reason, it is important to always aspirate the syringe before injecting an anesthetic. In addition, intraneuronal injection can damage the nerve, resulting in either transient or permanent injury. If the patient feels paresthesias, this may indicate that the nerve has been pierced and therefore the needle should be withdrawn somewhat before injecting the anesthetic solution. As with any injection, a small risk of bleeding and infection exists.

Complications from a digital nerve block of the fingers or toes are rare. Intravascular injection may result in blanching of the digit due to ischemia from vasospasm or capillary blood displacement. If this occurs, the injection should be immediately discontinued. The ischemia is usually transient and resolves spontaneously (85). Inadvertent use of an anesthetic containing epinephrine can result in ischemia of the finger or toe, because these are end-arteriolar structures.

Complications from a dorsal penile nerve block also are uncommon and usually clinically insignificant. The most frequent complication is bruising and (rarely) hematoma formation. These are most likely to result from puncture of the penile vasculature (92). As with digital blocks, large volumes of local anesthetic and the use of epinephrine must be avoided in this region to prevent ischemia through compression or vasospasm of end arteries.

INTRAVENOUS REGIONAL ANESTHESIA (BIER AND "MINIDOSE" BIER BLOCKS)

The desire for a rapid, safe, effective, and easy to perform technique to anesthetize extremities for orthopaedic reduction or minor procedures led to the development of intravenous regional anesthesia by Bier in 1908 (93). This procedure involves exsanguination of an affected extremity, through elevation and the application of a tourniquet, followed by distal instillation of intravenous lidocaine. This results in rapid anesthesia and a relatively bloodless field. The technique was later popularized by Holmes in 1963 (94), and its use in the ED was described by Roberts in 1977 (95). A "minidose" Bier block uses half the usual dose of lidocaine compared with the traditional Bier block, and

its safety and efficacy in the ED have been demonstrated (96). This lower dose may decrease the incidence of CNS side effects and is therefore preferred in the emergency setting.

The Bier and minidose Bier blocks provide satisfactory anesthesia and muscle relaxation of the hand and forearm in 95 to 98% of patients (97, 98). This procedure may be used alone or may be supplemented by light sedation. The technique is easily mastered and has a very low failure rate. Although most often performed in the operating room, intravenous regional anesthesia can be used effectively in the ED for fracture reduction, repositioning of dislocations, and repair of multiple or large lacerations. Although most of the literature relates to this technique as it is performed on the upper extremity, it also may be used successfully in the lower extremity for procedures below the knee.

Regional anesthesia such as the minidose Bier block has several advantages over general anesthesia. For one, it is often preferable for an emergency procedure in the patient with a presumed full stomach, because the airway reflexes are obviously not affected. In addition, regional anesthesia is cost effective; the cost of this procedure is less than 20% of the cost for performing general anesthesia (99). Intravenous regional anesthesia also can be accomplished rapidly. For example, the total time from beginning the minidose Bier block to orthopaedic reduction and casting is usually less than 30 minutes (96).

Anatomy and Physiology

The site and mechanisms of action of intravenous regional anesthesia are not completely understood (100–104). The three most probable sites of action are at the sensory nerve endings, the neuromuscular junction, and the nerve trunks. Most likely, a combination of these theories may best explain the clinical findings (105). The anesthetic does not diffuse throughout the extremity distal to the tourniquet, even though anesthesia of the arm or leg is complete. The effects begin distally, suggesting the central portions of the nerve trunks are blocked first. The transient ischemia of the extremity produced by the pneumatic tourniquet also may contribute to the anesthetic effect.

18 gauge needle

Indications

The Bier and minidose Bier blocks may be used to achieve regional anesthesia, muscle relaxation, and/or a bloodless field. This type of anesthesia is effective for procedures of the arm (at or below the elbow) or of the leg (below the midcalf). As mentioned previously, such procedures include reduction of fractures and dislocations, laceration repair, removal of foreign bodies, debridement of burns, and drainage of infection. Intravenous regional anesthesia has been widely used in the outpatient setting for children with upper extremity injuries (98, 99, 106, 107).

Contraindications to these procedures are significant underlying cardiac disease and any allergies to local anesthetics. This method cannot be used in manipulations in which the pulse must be monitored as a guide to reduction (e.g., supracondylar humeral fractures), because the pulse cannot be palpated while the pneumatic tourniquet is inflated. It should also be used with caution for patients with sickle cell disease, as the effects of the ischemic tourniquet on red blood cells have yet to be clarified (95). Because it is generally a safer procedure, using only the minidose Bier block for children in the outpatient setting is recommended.

Equipment

Resuscitation cart (with benzodiazepine anti-convulsants) at bedside
Cardiac and blood pressure monitors
Pulse oximeter
Intravenous catheters
Normal saline solution and intravenous extension tubing
Esmarch™ rubber or Ace™ elastic bandage
Two single pneumatic tourniquets or a double cuff pneumatic tourniquet (Note: standard blood pressure cuffs are not recommended because they often leak, rupture, or may not sustain high pressures for a prolonged period of time.)
Lidocaine 0.5% *without epinephrine* (may dilute 1% lidocaine with sterile saline to form 0.5% solution)
50 mL infusion syringe

Procedure

Informed consent is first obtained. Younger children and those who are overly anxious may benefit from light sedation before performing the procedure. Leads for the cardiac monitor and pulse oximeter are placed on the child. Resuscitation equipment, including anticonvulsant medications, should be readily available. Since the discussion here will be limited to intravenous regional anestesia for pediatric patients, only the minidose Bier block is described.

For a procedure of the arm, intravenous access is obtained in both upper extremities. A large bore intravenous catheter with normal saline solution infusing is established in the unaffected extremity for administration of resuscitation medications should they be needed. The intravenous line in the affected limb is used for lidocaine infusion. This is usually inserted at the dorsum of the hand rather than the antecubital space, because evidence suggests that the procedure is more likely to be successful when the anesthetic is injected distally (108).

A double pneumatic tourniquet or two single pneumatic tourniquets are placed above the elbow (Fig. 37.9). The affected limb is exsanguinated either by elevation for a few minutes or by elevation and wrapping the extremity with an Esmarch rubber or Ace™ elastic bandage in a distal-to-proximal fashion. With the extremity still elevated, the upper or proximal pneumatic cuff is inflated to 50 mm Hg above the systolic blood pressure to occlude the arterial blood supply. The bandage is removed and the extremity is lowered back onto the stretcher.

As described by Farrell (96), a minidose Bier block is performed by first infusing 0.5% lidocaine intravenously into the affected extremity at a dose of 1.5 mg/kg (maximum 100 mg) over 60 to 90 seconds. Using alkalinized lidocaine during intravenous regional anesthesia offers no advantage (109). Tourniquet pressure must be maintained at all times throughout the procedure. In addition, injection of local anesthetic into the limb should be performed slowly to avoid generating supraarterial pressure in the venous system, leading to escape of drug under the tourniquet. Following injection, the skin will

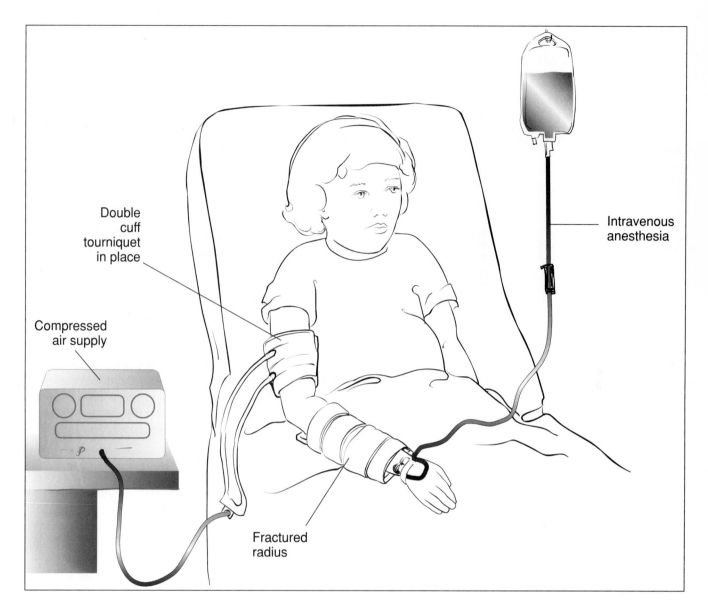

Double
cuff
tourniquet
in place

Compressed
air supply

Intravenous
anesthesia

Fractured
radius

Figure 37.9.
Intravenous regional
anesthesia setup (Bier and
minidose Bier blocks).

often blanch and become erythematous in patches as residual blood is displaced from the vascular compartment. This is not a toxic manifestation and usually signifies success of the procedure.

Over the next several minutes, the patient will experience paresthesias or warmth, beginning distally and spreading proximally. At this point, the lower or distal cuff is inflated to 50 mm Hg above systolic pressure, and the proximal cuff is then deflated. In this way, the tourniquet pressure is now over an area that is already anesthetized, eliminating the pain caused by the proximal tourniquet. Anesthesia, which is usually satisfactory in about 10 minutes, is followed by muscle relaxation. Gentle manipulation of the painful site should be used to test for adequate anes-

thesia. Although pain is eliminated, the patient may still have tactile and proprioceptive sensation and may retain some motor function (96).

An additional 0.5 mg/kg of lidocaine may be used with the minidose Bier block if anesthesia is still inadequate after 15 minutes. However, the overall maximum dose of 100 mg of lidocaine should not be exceeded. Additional lidocaine infusion is required in about 7% of cases (96).

Once adequate analgesia has been reached, the infusion catheter is removed and the site adequately bandaged to prevent extravasation of the anesthetic. The procedure should be performed promptly. For fracture reduction, portable postreduction radiographs should be obtained while the tourniquet is still inflated. This allows for repeat reduction under the same anesthetic if necessary.

With the minidose Bier block, the tourniquet should be left in place a minimum of 15 to 20 minutes, and a maximum of 60 to 90 minutes after the infusion of lidocaine, because peak blood levels are related to the duration of vascular occlusion (110, 111). To

---

SUMMARY: MINIDOSE BIER BLOCK

1. Prepare all necessary items (including resuscitation equipment at bedside) that may be used during procedure
2. Place monitor and pulse oximetry leads appropriately on patient
3. Obtain large bore i.v. access in uninvolved extremity and distal i.v. access in involved extremity
4. Position double tourniquet (just above elbow for upper extremity; no higher than midcalf for lower extremity)
5. Elevate and exsanguinate extremity (optional: wrap extremity with Esmarch™ rubber or Ace™ elastic bandage in a distal-to-proximal fashion to speed exsanguination)
6. Inflate proximal tourniquet to 50 mm Hg above systemic blood pressure and place extremity back on stretcher
7. Gradually infuse 1.5 mg/kg (100 mg max) of 0.5% lidocaine solution (a 1:1 mixture of 1% lidocaine and sterile saline)
8. Inflate distal tourniquet to 50 mm Hg above systemic blood pressure, and when secure, deflate proximal tourniquet
9. Check for adequate anesthesia
10. Perform procedure for which anesthesia has been administered
11. Deflate tourniquet after a minimum of 20 to 30 minutes and a maximum of 60 to 90 minutes via a series of several deflation cycles; each cycle should consist of 5 seconds of deflation time alternating with 1 to 2 minutes of reinflation.
12. Observe patient for 1 hour for possible reaction

---

prevent a bolus of lidocaine from entering the intravascular compartment, the cuff is slowly deflated through a series of cycles. The cuff should be deflated for 5 seconds, then reinflated for 1 to 2 minutes. This cycle is repeated several times until distal perfusion is restored as indicated by capillary refill. After the tourniquet is removed, sensation returns in 5 to 10 minutes. The child should be observed for at least 1 hour after the procedure

before discharge (88).

Complications

Although infrequent, complications can occur without strict adherence to proper technique and meticulous attention to the function of the equipment. The most common complication relating to anesthetic is a rapid systemic vascular infusion. This may occur with rapid intravascular infusion at pressures surpassing tourniquet cuff pressure, tourniquet leakage, blood pressure cuff malfunction, early release of the tourniquet, medication error (i.e., an excessively high dose), or intravenous lines placed in close proximity to the tourniquet. Although the consequences of an inadvertent lidocaine bolus are potentially serious, the minidose technique has been shown to be very safe, because the dosages are similar to therapeutic intravenous boluses given to patients with cardiac dysrhythmias. The extremely low incidence of airway compromise (as compared with conscious sedation) also contributes to the relative safety of this procedure.

A lidocaine bolus into the systemic circulation may result in dizziness, headache, lethargy, and blurred vision. This is reported in 2 to 3% of patients and requires no additional treatment (112). Seizures are quite rare, having been reported in 0.2% of patients (113). Seizures should be managed with standard supportive care and anticonvulsant medications. With massive overdoses of intravenous lidocaine, bradycardia, vasomotor collapse, and cardiac depression or arrest can occur.

Other complications include tissue extravasation of the anesthetic from an infiltrated intravenous catheter and intraarterial injection resulting in distal limb necrosis. If any doubt exists about venous versus arterial placement of the catheter, another line should be inserted. Alternatively, a blood gas analysis can be performed to determine the source of the blood. Allergy to lidocaine is rare. Any history of significant allergic reactions to local anesthetics should cause the operator to consider using another method of anesthesia. Pain at the tourniquet site may also occur. This is more frequent when using a single pneumatic cuff or with prolonged tourniquet times. When regional anesthesia is used in the lower extremity, the patient may develop a phlebitis. In addition, tourniquets must be placed no higher than midcalf to avoid peroneal nerve damage.

sitioned over an area of the extremity that is already anesthetized.

SUMMARY

Infiltration anesthesia is by far the most commonly used method of providing local anesthesia in the ED. The needle is inserted through the subcutaneous tissue exposed by a wound, and the anesthetic solution is slowly injected around the entire margin. It is a straightforward procedure that achieves a high rate of success. Parallel margin anesthesia is similar to infiltration anesthesia, although in this case the needle is inserted in a circumferential fashion through intact skin 1 to 2 cm from the site of the procedure. The primary advantage of this technique is that the wound edges of a laceration are not distorted.

Topical anesthesia is an excellent technique for pediatric patients when it can be used. Currently, the most popular topical anesthetic for wound repair is TAC (tetracaine/adrenaline/cocaine). It can be used alone or in combination with supplemental lidocaine infiltration if necessary. Careful adherence to proper usage will minimize the likelihood of complications. TAC is painless, easily applied, and does not distort the margins of a wound. EMLA (eutectic mixture of local anesthetics) contains lidocaine and prilocaine and is a safe, easy, and effective method for dermal anesthesia of intact skin. The slow onset of action, however, limits its widespread applicability in the emergency setting. Ethyl chloride provides reliable, convenient, and effective dermal analgesia. Its instantaneous onset is useful for minor procedures in the emergency setting, although the short duration and small depth of skin analgesia limit its usefulness.

Regional anesthesia of an entire area of the body can be provided by performing a nerve block or intravenous regional anesthesia. Nerve blocks are useful for anesthesia of especially pain-sensitive structures, primarily the fingers, toes, palm of the hand, and sole of the foot. Injection of anesthetic solution at a more proximal site over the nerve that innervates the desired structures is gen-

---

CLINICAL TIPS: INTRAVENOUS REGIONAL ANESTHESIA

1. Because it is safer as a result of a lower dosage of lidocaine, the minidose Bier block should be used for children in the ED.
2. Rapid administration of lidocaine can cause venous pressures to exceed the pressure of the pneumatic tourniquet resulting in leakage of the lidocaine under the cuff and into the systemic circulation.
3. Intravenous regional anesthesia should not be used for any procedure that requires the pulse to be monitored (e.g., reduction of a supracondylar fracture), because the pulse will be lost when the tourniquet is inflated.
4. Because of the slight possibility of delivering a large bolus of lidocaine to the systemic circulation, resuscitation equipment (including anticonvulsant medications) should always be at bedside during this procedure.
5. Two reliable intravenous lines should be started before performing intravenous regional anesthesia, one distally in the affected limb and one in another limb. In this way, resuscitation medications can be administered if necessary without deflating the pneumatic tourniquet.
6. A double pneumatic tourniquet or two single pneumatic tourniquets are ideal for this procedure. A standard blood pressure cuff is not optimal, because it may leak or rupture.
7. By using two tourniquets, the physician can minimize the pain associated with prolonged pressure on the extremity. The proximal tourniquet is inflated first and the lidocaine is administered. When the anesthesia begins to take effect, the distal tourniquet is inflated and the proximal tourniquet is deflated. In this way, the tourniquet that remains inflated throughout the procedure is positioned over an area of the extremity that is already anesthetized.
8. Children who undergo intravenous regional anesthesia should be observed for 1 hour after the pneumatic tourniquet is deflated so that any adverse reactions can be appropriately managed.

---

erally much less painful. More than one nerve block may be performed to anesthetize a larger area. Intravenous regional anesthesia results in safe and effective analgesia for selected extremity procedures. For pediatric patients, the minidose Bier block is recommended for use in the ED, because it is generally as effective as a standard Bier block and uses a lower dose of lidocaine.

REFERENCES

1. Denson D, Mazoit J. Physiology, pharmacology, and toxicity of local anesthetics: adult and pediatric consideration. In: Prithviraj P, ed. Clinical practice of regional anesthesia. New York: Churchill Livingstone, 1991;73–105.
2. Goth A. Pharmacology of local anesthesia. In: Medical pharmacology: principles and concepts. St. Louis: CV Mosby, 1988, pp. 407–415.
3. Covino B. Pharmacology of local anesthetic agents. Br J Anaesth 1986;58:701–716.
4. Mulroy M. Local anesthetics. In: Regional anesthesia. Boston: Little, Brown & Co., 1989, pp. 1–12.
5. Arthur G, et al. Pharmacology of loocal anesthetics. In: Principles and practice of regional anesthesia. New York: Churchill Livingstone, 1993, pp. 29–46.
6. Tucker G. Pharmacokinetics of local anesthesias. Br J Anaesth 1986;58:717–731.
7. Wildsmith J. Peripheral nerve and local anesthetic drugs. Br J Anaesth 1986;58:692–700.
8. Heavner J. Molecular action of local anesthetics. In: Prithviraj P, ed. Clinical practice of regional anesthesia. New York: Churchill Livingstone, 1991, pp. 67–71.
9. Benzon H, et al. Developmental neurophysiology of mammalian peripheral nerves and age-related differential sensitivity to local anesthetics. Br J Anaesth 1988;61:754–760.
10. Butterworth J, Strichantz G. Molecular mechanisms of local anesthesia: a review. Anesthesiology 1990;72(4):711–734.
11. Hille B. Common mode of action of three agents that decrease the transient change in sodium permeability in nerves. Nature 1966;216:1220–1221.
12. Mather L, Cousins M. Local anesthetics and their clinical use. Drugs 1979;18:185–205.
13. Narahashi T, et al. The site of action and active form of local anesthetics. I. Theory and pH experiments with tertiary compounds. J Pharm Exp Ther 1970;171:32–44.
14. Frazier D, et al. The site of action and active form of local anesthetics. II. Experiment with quaternary compounds. J Pharm Exp Ther 1970;171:45–51.
15. Reiz S, Nath S. Cardiotoxicity of local anesthetic agents. Br J Anaesth 1986;58:736–746.
16. Ritchie J, et al. The active structure of local anesthetics. J Pharm Exp Ther 1965;150:152–159.
17. Moore D. The pH of local anesthetic solutions. Anaesth Analg 1981;60:833–834.
18. Mulroy M. Clinical characteristics of local anesthetics. In: Regional anesthesia. Boston: Little, Brown & Co., 1989, pp. 13–30.
19. Swerdlow M, Jones R. The duration of action of bupivacaine, prilocaine, and lignocaine. Br J Anaesth 1970;42:335–339.
20. Arthur D, McNicol L. Local anesthetic techniques in pediatric surgery. Br J Anaesth 1986;58:760–778.
21. Ecoffey C, et al. Pharmokinetics of lignocaine in children following caudal anesthesia. Br J Anaesth 1984;56:1399–1401.
22. de Jong R. Toxic effects of local anesthesia. JAMA 1978;239:1166–1168.
23. Mulroy M. Complications of regional anesthesia. In: Regional anesthesia. Boston: Little, Brown & Co., 1989, pp. 31–44.
24. Munson E, Embrow P W. Central nervous system toxicity of local anesthetic mixtures in monkeys. Anesthesiology 1977;46:179.
25. Scott D. Toxic effects of local anesthetic agents on the central nervous system. Br J Anaesth 1986;58:732–735.
26. Trott A. Infiltration and nerve block anesthesia. In: Wounds and lacerations: emergency care and closure. St. Louis: CV Mosby, 1991, pp. 30–36.
27. Benoit P, Beit WD. Some effects of local anesthetic agents on skeletal muscle. Exp Neurol 1972;34:264–278.
28. Born G. Neuropathy after bupivacaine wrist and metacarpal nerve blocks. J Hand Surg 1984;9A:109–112.
29. Chvapil M, Haneroff S, et al. Local anesthetics and wound healing. J Surg Res 1979;27:267.
30. Fariss B, Foresman P, Rodeheaver G, et al. Anesthetic properties and toxicity of bupivacaine and lidocaine for infiltration anesthesia. J Emerg Med 1987;5:275–282.
31. Barker W, et al. Damage to tissue defenses by a topical anesthetic agent. Ann Emerg Med 1982;11(6):307–310.
32. de Jong R, Bonin JD: Mixtures of local anesthesiology 1981;54:177–183.
33. Smith RM. Local and regional anesthesia. In: Anesthesia for infants and children. St. Louis: CV Mosby, 1980, pp. 229–233.
34. McLeskey C. pH of local anesthetic solutions. Anaesth Analg 1980;59:892–893.
35. Rund DA. Essentials of emergency medicine. East Norwalk, CT: Appleton-Lange, 1986, p. 274.
36. Wrightman M, Vaughn R. Comparison of compounds used for intradermal anesthesia. Anesthesiology 1976;45:687–689.
37. Christoph R, Buchanan L, Begalla K, et al. Pain reduction in local anesthetic administration through pH buffering. Ann Emerg Med 1988;17(2):117–120.
38. McKay W, Morris R, Mushlin P. Sodium bicarbonate attenuates pain on skin infiltration with lidocaine, with or without epinephrine. Anaesth Analg 1987;66:572–574.
39. Morris R, et al. Comparison of pain associated with intradermal and subcutaneous infiltration with various local anesthetic solutions. Anaesth Analg 1988;66:1180–1182.
40. Arndt KA, Burton C, Noe JM. Minimizing the pain of local anesthesia. Plast Reconstr Surg 1983;72:676–679.
41. Pryor GJ, Kilpatrick WR, Opp AR. Local anesthesia in minor lacerations: topical TAC versus lidocaine infiltration. Ann Emerg Med 1980:568–571.
42. Bonadio WA, Wagner V. Half–strength TAC topical anesthetic. Clin Pediatr 1988;27:495–498.
43. Smith SM, Barry RC. A comparison of three formulations of TAC (tetracaine, adrenaline, cocaine) for anesthesia of minor lacerations in children. Pediatr Emerg Care 1990;6:266–270.
44. Schaffer DJ. Clinical comparison of TAC anesthetic solutions with and without cocaine. Ann Emerg Med 1985;14:1077–1080.

45. Hegenbarth MA, Altieri MF, Hawk WH, et al. Comparison of tetracaine, adrenaline, and cocaine with cocaine alone for topical anesthesia. Ann Emerg Med 1990;19:63–67.

46. Grant SAD, Hoffman RS. Use of tetracaine, epinephrine, and cocaine as a topical anesthetic in the emergency department. Ann Emerg Med 1992;21:987–997.

47. Anderson AB, Colecchi C, Baronoski R, DeWitt TG. Local anesthesia in pediatric patients: topical TAC versus lidocaine. Ann Emerg Med 1990;19:519–522.

48. Martin JR, Doezema D, Tandberg D, Umland E. The effect of local anesthetics on bacterial proliferation: TAC versus lidocaine. Ann Emerg Med 1990;19:987–990.

49. Altieri M, Bogema S, Schwartz RH. TAC topical anesthesia produces positive urine tests for cocaine. Ann Emerg Med 1990;19:577–579.

50. Fitzmaurice LS, Wasserman GS, Knapp JF, Roberts DK, Waeckerle JF, Fox M. TAC use and absorption of cocaine in a pediatric emergency department. Ann Emerg Med 1990;19:515–518.

51. Terndrup TE, Walls HC, Mariani PJ, Gavula DP, Madden CM, Cantor RM. Plasma cocaine and tetracaine levels following application of topical anesthesia in children. Ann Emerg Med 1992;21:162–166.

52. Dailey RH. Fatality secondary to misuse of TAC solution. Ann Emerg Med 1988;17:159–160.

53. Daya MR, Burton BT, Schleiss MR, et al. Recurrent seizures following mucosal application of TAC. Ann Emerg Med 1988;17:646–648.

54. Dronen SC. Complications of TAC (letter). Ann Emerg Med 1983;12:333.

55. Jacobsen S. Errors in emergency practice. Emerg Med 1987;19:109.

56. Tipton GA, DeWitt GW, Eisenstein SJ. Topical TAC (tetracaine, adrenaline, cocaine) solution for local anesthesia in children: prescribing inconsistency and acute toxicity. Southern Med J 1989;82:1344–1346.

57. Tripp M, Dowd DD, Eitel DR. TAC toxicity in the emergency department. Ann Emerg Med 1991;20:106–107.

58. Wehner D, Hamilton GD. Seizures following topical application of local anesthetics to burn patients. Ann Emerg Med 1984;13:456–458.

59. Ernst AA, Marvez E, Nick TG, Chin E, Wood E, Gonzaba WT. Lidocaine, adrenaline, tetracaine gel versus tetracaine, adrenaline, cocaine gel for topical anesthesia in linear scalp and facial lacerations in children aged 5 to 17 years. Pediatrics 1995;95:255–258.

60. Schilling CG, Band DE, Borchert BA, Klatzko MD, Uden DL. Tetracaine, epinephrine (adrenaline), and cocaine (TAC) versus lidocaine, epinephrine, and tetracaine (LET) for anesthesia of lacerations in children. Ann Emerg Med 1995;25:203–208.

61. Evers H, von Dardel O, Juhlin L, et al. Dermal effects of compositions based on the eutectic mixture of lignocaine and prilocaine (EMLA). Br J Anaesth 1985;57:997–1005.

62. Buckley MM, Benfield P. Eutectic lidocaine/prilocaine cream. A review of the topical anaesthetic/analgesic efficacy of a eutectic mixture of local anaesthetics (EMLA). Drugs 1993;46:126–151.

63. Juhlin L, Evers H. EMLA: a new topical anesthetic. Adv Dermatol 1990;5:75–92.

64. Lycka BA. EMLA. A new and effective topical anesthetic. J Dermatol Surg Oncol 1992;18:859–862.

65. Bjerring P, Arendt-Nielsen L. Depth and duration of skin analgesia to needle insertion after topical application of EMLA cream. Brit J Anaesth 1990a;64:173–177.

66. Cooper CM, Gerrish DP, Hardwick M, Kay R. EMLA cream reduces the pain of venipuncture in children. Eur J Anaesth 1987;4:441–448.

67. de Jong PC, Verburg MP, Lillieborg S. EMLA cream versus ethylchloride spray: a comparison of the analgesic efficacy in children. Eur J Anaesth 1990;7:473–481.

68. Hopkins CS, Buckley CJ, Bush GH. Pain-free injection in infants. Use of a lignocaine-prilocaine cream to prevent pain at intravenous induction of general anesthesia in 1- to 5-year-old children. Anaesthesia 1988:43:198–201.

69. Joyce TH, Skjonsby BS, Taylor BD, Morrow DH, Hess KR. Dermal anesthesia using a eutectic mixture of lidocaine and prilocaine (EMLA) for venipuncture in children. Pain Digest 1992;2:137–141.

70. Robieux I, Kumar R, Radhakrishnan S, Koren G. Assessing pain and analgesia with a lidocaine-prilocaine emulsion in infants and toddlers during venipuncture. J Pediatr 1991;971–973.

71. Soliman IE, Broadman LM, Hannallah RS, McGill WA. Comparison of the analgesic effects of EMLA (eutectic mixture of local anesthetics) to intradermal lidocaine infiltration prior to venous cannulation in unpremedicated children. Anesthesiology 1988;68:804–806.

72. Halperin DL, Koren G, Attias D, Pellegrini E, Greenberg ML, et al. Topical skin anesthesia for venous, subcutaneous drug reservoir and lumbar punctures in children. Pediatrics 1989;84:281–284.

73. Kapelushnik J, Koren G, Solh H, Greenberg M, DeVeber L. Evaluating the efficacy of EMLA in alleviating pain associated with lumbar puncture; comparison of open and double-blinded protocols in children. Pain 1990;42:31–34.

74. Yaster M, Maxwell LG, Nicholas EJ. Local anesthetics in the management of acute pain in children: a primer for the nonanesthesiologist. Comp Therapy 1991;17(10):27–35.

75. Jakobson B, Nilsson A. Methemoglobinemia associated with a prilocaine-lidocaine cream and trimethoprim-sulfamethoxazole. A case report. Acta Anaesth Scand 1985;29:253–255.

76. Nilsson A, Engberg G, Henneberg S, et al. Inverse relationship between age-dependent erythrocyte activity of methaemoglobin reductase and prilocaine-induced methaemoglobinaemia during infancy. Br J Anaesth 1990:64:72–76.

77. Engberg G, Danielson K, Henneberg S, Nilsson A. Plasma concentrations of prilocaine and lidocaine and methemoglobin formation in infants after epicutaneous application of 5% lidocaine-prilocaine cream (EMLA). Acta Anaesth Scand 1987;31:624–628.

78. Frayling IM, Addison GM, Chattergee K, Meakin G. Methaemoglobinaemia in children treated with prilocaine-lignocaine cream. Brit Med J 1990;301: 153–154.

79. Norman J, Jones PL. Complications of the use of EMLA (letter). Br J Anaesth 1990;64:403–406.

80. Armstrong P, Young C, and McKeown D. Ethyl chloride and venipuncture pain: a comparison with intradermal lidocaine. Can J Anaesth 1990;37: 656–658.

81. Azppa SC, Nabors SB. Use of ethyl chloride topical anesthetic to reduce procedural pain in pediatric oncology patients. Cancer Nurs 1992;15:130–136.

82. Nielsen AJ. Precautions about ethyl chloride. Phys Ther 1980;60:474–475.

83. Aberer W. Local anaesthesia with chloride freezing: problems despite proper application. Brit J Dermatol 1991;124:113–114.

84. Murphy M. Regional anesthesia in the emergency department Emerg Med Clin North Am 1988; 6(4):783–809.

85. Orlinsky M, Dean E. Local and topical anesthesia and nerve blocks of the thorax and extremities. In: Roberts J, Hedges J, eds. Clinical procedures in emergency medicine. Philadelphia: WB Saunders, 1991.

86. Poulton TJ. Peripheral nerve blocks. Am Fam Phy 1977;16:100.

87. Katz J. Sections on head, upper and lower extremities. In: Atlas of regional anesthesia. East Norwalk, CT: Appleton-Lange, 1994, pp. 1–36, 61–92, 149–174.

88. Stewart S. Local anesthesia. In: Paris P, Stewart S, eds. Pain management in emergency medicine. East Norwalk, CT: Appleton-Lange, 1988, p. 77.

89. Trott A. Infiltration and nerve block anesthesia. In: Wounds and lacerations. Emergency care and closure. St. Louis: CV Mosby, 1991, pp. 30–54.

90. Simon R, Brenner B, eds. Anesthesia and regional blocks. In: Procedures and techniques in emergency medicine. Baltimore: Williams & Wilkins, 1982, pp. 87–122.

91. Locke RK. Nerve blocks of the foot. JACEP 1976;5:698.

92. Snellman LW, Stang HJ. Prospective evaluation of complications of dorsal penile nerve block for neonatal circumcision. Pediatrics 1995;95:705.

93. Bier A. Uber einen neuen Weg Lokalanaesthesia an den Gliedmasses zu erzeugen. Arch Klin Chir 1908;86:1007.

94. Holmes CM. Intravenous regional anesthesia, a useful method of producing analgesia of the limbs. Lancet 1963;1:245.

95. Roberts JR. Intravenous regional anesthesia. JACEP 1977;6:261.

96. Farrell RG, Swanson SL, Walter JK. Safe and effective i.v. regional anesthesia for use in the emergency department. Ann Emerg Med 1985;14:288.

97. Chambers WA, Wildsmith JA. Upper limb. In: Nimmo WS, Smith G, eds. Anesthesia. Oxford: Blackwell Scientific Publications, 1989: 1071–1073.

98. Juliano PJ, Mazur JM, Cummings RJ, McCluskey WP. Low-dose lidocaine intravenous regional anesthesia for forearm fractures in children. J Pediatr Orthop 1992;12(5):633.

99. Barnes CL, Blasier RD, Dodge BM. Intravenous regional anesthesia: a safe and cost-effective outpatient anesthetic for upper extremity fracture treatment in children. J Pediatr Orthop 1991;11(6): 717.

100. Miles DW, James JL, Clark DE, et al. Site of action of intravenous regional anesthesia. J Neurol Neurosurg Psychiatry 1964;27:574.

101. Fleming SA, Veiga-Pires JA, McCutcheon RM, et al. A demonstration of the site of action of intravenous lignocaine. Can Anaesth Soc J 1966;13:21.

102. Raj PP, Garcia CE, Burleson JW, et al. The site of action of intravenous regional anesthesia. Anaesth Analg 1972;51:776.

103. Raj PP. Site of action of intravenous regional anesthesia. Reg Anaesth 1979;4(1):8.

104. Lille PE, Glynn CJ, Femwick DG. Site of action of intravenous regional anesthesia. Anesthesiology 1984;61:507.

105. Rosenberg PH, Heavner JE. Multiple and complementary mechanisms produce analgesia during intravenous regional anesthesia. Anesthesiology 1985;62:840.

106. Olney BW, Lugg PC, TurnerPL, Eyres RL, Cole WG. Outpatient treatment of upper extremity injuries in childhood using intravenous regional anesthesia. J Pediatr Orthop 1988;8:576–579.

107. Colizza WA, Said E. Intravenous regional anesthesia in the treatment of forearm and wrist fractures and dislocations in children. Can J Surg 1993; 36(3):225.

108. Sorbie C, Chacho PB. Regional anesthesia by the intravenous route. Br Med J 1965;1:957.

109. Benlabed M, Jullien P, Guelmi K, Hamza J, Bonhomme L, Benhamou D. Alkalinization of 0.5% lidocaine for intravenous regional anesthesia. Reg Anaesth 1990;15(2):59.

110. Covino BG. Pharmacokinetics of intravenous regional anesthesia. Reg Anaesth 1979;4:5.

111. Tucker GT, Boas RA. Pharmacokinetic aspects of intravenous regional anesthesia. Anesthesiology 1971;34:538.

112. Dunbar RW, Mazze RI. Intravenous regional anesthesia experience with 779 cases. Anaesth Analg 1967;46:806.

113. Van Nierkerk JP, Tonkin PA. Intravenous regional analgesia. S Afr Med J 1966;40:165.

Special Procedures for Neonates

Section Editor: John Loiselle

NEONATAL RESUSCITATION PROCEDURES

Robert J. Vinci and Sigmund J. Kharasch

INTRODUCTION

Neonatal resuscitation is an uncommon event in the emergency department (ED). Although the majority of births do not require advanced life support, those who deliver in the ED are frequently from high-risk groups (i.e., lack of prenatal care, trauma-induced labor, drug abuse) and may be more prone to complications. Asphyxia in the neonatal period continues to be a major problem which in many circumstances can be avoided with prompt, skilled resuscitation. For this reason, current recommendations state that "at least one person skilled in neonatal resuscitation should be in attendance at every delivery and an additional skilled person should be readily available" (1). Recently developed curriculum such as the neonatal advanced life support (NALS) course emphasize the goal of teaching infant resuscitation skills to all appropriate practitioners. Precipitous deliveries can occur anywhere in the prehospital setting including the home, an office practice, or during a prehospital transport. Therefore, it is incumbent for all practitioners, including nurses, physicians, midwives and EMTs to be familiar with the techniques described in this chapter.

ANATOMY AND PHYSIOLOGY

Fetal Transition

Transition from fetal to neonatal life involves a series of rapid anatomic and physiologic adaptations. In fetal circulation, blood flow to the lungs is minimal as a result of high pulmonary vascular resistance, a patent ductus arteriosus, and low resistance of the systemic (placental) circulation. At birth, the fetus must establish the lungs as the site of gas exchange. The circulation, which previously shunted blood away from the lungs, must now fully perfuse the pulmonary vasculature.

Although surfactant production begins at approximately 24 weeks' gestation, adequate amounts of surfactant to open alveoli are generally not present in sufficient amounts until week 34. A combination of events at birth act to initiate respirations. These events include the interruption of umbilical circulation, stimulation of peripheral and central chemoreceptors, and tactile and thermal stimulation. The first few breaths must clear amniotic fluid from the lungs and establish a functional residual capacity. With the onset of respirations and a rise in pH and pO_2, pulmonary vasodilation occurs. A fall in pulmonary vascular resistance decreases the right-to-left shunt through the ductus arteriosus with subsequent closure of the foramen ovale. Fetal circulation now assumes the adult pattern (Fig. 38.1) (2).

Asphyxia

Neonatal asphyxia can result from multiple maternal or neonatal factors (Table 38.1). Asphyxia is the initial event in the cascade that produces pulmonary vasoconstriction and delays closure of the ductus arteriosus. Fetal cir-

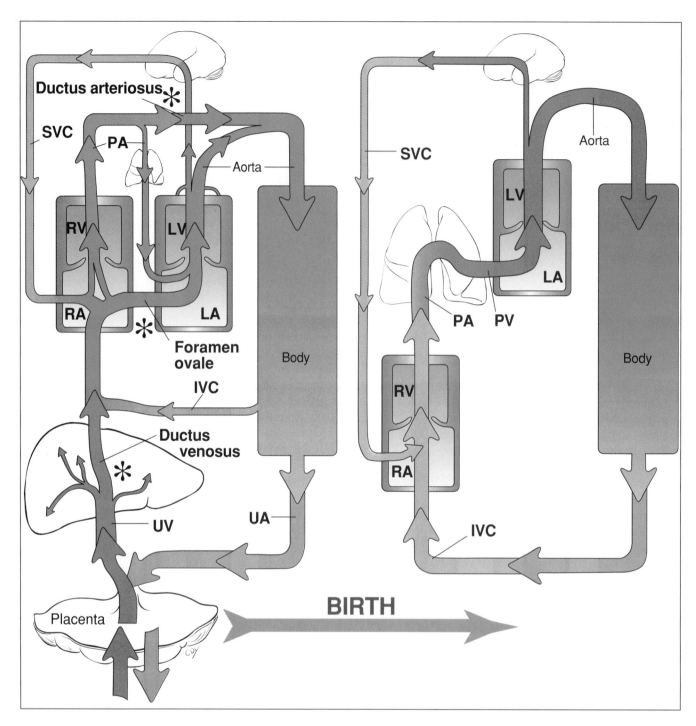

Figure 38.1.
Schematic representation of transition from fetal to neonatal circulation. SVC = superior vena cava; PA = pulmonary arteries; RV = right ventricle; RA = right atrium; LV = left ventricle; LA = left atrium; IVC = inferior vena cava; UV = umbilical vein; UA = umbilical arteries. Shading represents relative oxygen saturation. * Structures marked with an asterisk close soon after birth.

**Chapter 38
Neonatal
Resuscitation
Procedures**

culation is therefore maintained with no increase in pulmonary blood flow. The goal with any asphyxiated infant is to reverse the asphyxia as soon as possible before permanent injury occurs.

When asphyxia occurs (either in utero or following delivery), an initial period of hyperpnea occurs with sinus tachycardia. If hypoxia continues, respiratory effort ceases and bradycardia ensues (primary apnea). Providing oxygen and stimulation during this period in many cases will induce spontaneous respirations. If asphyxia continues, the infant develops gasping respirations, the heart rate continues to decrease, and blood pressure

Table 38.1.
Factors Associated with Neonatal Asphyxia

Techniques involved in neonatal resuscitation are applicable to the delivery of all newborns. More aggressive resuscitation and evaluation of the depressed or asphyxiated newborn can be anticipated in many cases based on information found in the antepartum and the intrapartum histories.

Antepartum Factors
   Maternal diabetes
   Pregnancy-induced hypertension
   Chronic hypertension
   Previous Rh sensitization
   Previous stillbirth
   Bleeding in second or third trimester
   Maternal infection
   Polyhydramnios
   Oligohydramnios
   Postterm gestation
   Multiple gestation
   Size-dates discrepancy
   Drug therapy (reserpine, lithium carbonate, magnesium, adrenergic-blocking agents)
   Maternal drug abuse
Intrapartum Factors
   Elective or emergency cesarean section
   Abnormal presentation
   Premature labor
   Rupture of membranes more than 24 hours before delivery
   Foul-smelling amniotic fluid
   Precipitous labor
   Prolonged labor (greater than 24 hours)
   Prolonged second stage of labor (greater than 2 hours)
   Nonreassuring fetal heart rate patterns
   Use of general anesthesia
   Uterine tetany
   Narcotics administered to mother within 4 hours of delivery
   Meconium-stained amniotic fluid
   Abruptio placenta
   Placenta previa
   Prolapsed cord

(Modified from American Heart Association/American Academy of Pediatrics. Textbook of neonatal resuscitation. Dallas: American Heart Association 1991.)

falls. During this period of secondary apnea, the infant becomes unresponsive to stimulation and positive pressure ventilation (PPV) must be initiated rapidly. The clinician must realize that when he or she evaluates an infant in distress or full arrest, the asphyxiating event may have begun in utero; therefore, apnea at birth should be treated as secondary apnea and resuscitation should begin immediately.

The Environment

Because of a large surface area: mass ratio, the neonate is susceptible to significant heat loss, and because many ED deliveries involve the birth of a premature infant, heat loss may be a significant problem. Newborns and especially premature infants may be unable to effectively modulate their own temperature control. Without appropriate attention to thermal management, hypothermia may occur. Continued careful attention to the thermal environment of the newborn is critical as hypothermic stress in the newborn may contribute to acidosis, hypoglycemia, and respiratory depression.

INDICATIONS

Basic techniques involved in neonatal resuscitation are applicable to the delivery of all newborns. While delivery of a depressed or asphyxiated infant can be anticipated in many cases based on antepartum or intrapartum history (Table 38.1), it may not always be possible to elicit these factors in the ED. Resuscitation is required for about 80% of infants with birth weights less than 1500 g (1). Approximately 5 to 10% of term infants require resuscitation beyond suctioning, drying, and stimulation. Preparation for high-risk situations in the ED requires proper equipment and personnel trained in the techniques of neonatal resuscitation. Because of the difficulty in assessing an accurate gestational age in unanticipated deliveries, initiation of resuscitation is indicated unless it can be reliably determined that the infant is of 23 weeks' gestation or less (3). Neonatology consultation in questionable circumstances should be obtained when possible.

EQUIPMENT

Equipment requirements for more extensive resuscitations can be found in the appropriate chapter as noted.

Suction Equipment

Bulb syringe
Mechanical suction
Suction catheter—10 French
Meconium aspirator (Chapter 39)

Warming Equipment

Radiant warmer
Warm, dry blankets
Stockinette hat

Bag-Mask Equipment

(Chapter 14)

Intubation Equipment

(Chapter 16)

Medications

Epinephrine (1:10,000) 3-mL or 10-mL ampules
Sodium bicarbonate 4.2% (5 mEq/10 mL) 10-mL ampules
Dextrose 10% 250 mL
Naloxone hydrochloride 0.4 mg/mL in 1-mL ampules or 1.0 mg/mL in 2-mL ampules
Normal saline
Volume expander

Additional Equipment

Stethoscope
Cardiac monitor
Umbilical vessel catheterization tray (Chapter 40)
Syringes—1, 3, 5, 10, 20, 50 mL
Needles—25 gauge, 21 gauge, 18 gauge
Intravenous catheters—24 gauge, 22 gauge, 20 gauge, 18 gauge
Adhesive tape
Alcohol pads

PROCEDURE/TECHNIQUE

A summary of the resuscitation process is seen in Figure 38.2. All newborn infants undergo the initial steps of resuscitation, including thermal management, clearing of the airway, and tactile stimulation. These first steps can generally be completed within 20 seconds.

Preventing Heat Loss

Immediate drying of the infant with removal of amniotic fluid will prevent evaporative heat loss. All wet blankets should then be removed from around the infant. An overhead warmer is necessary to minimize radiant and convective heat loss. Initially, the unit should be set to the manual mode at the maximum temperature setting. This will allow for an immediate warm environment for the infant. Eventually the servo mode can be used to allow for the temperature to be modulated by the infant's own body temperature. A tar-geted body temperature (37°C) is selected by adjusting the skin temperature control point setting. With the infant in the supine position, a skin temperature probe is placed on the abdomen between the xiphoid process and the umbilicus so that exposed skin surrounding the probe is in direct line with radiation from the warmer.

Adjunctive measures such as wrapping the infant in warm, dry blankets and covering the infants head with a stockinette hat can be used to prevent evaporative heat loss.

Clearing the Airway

Establishing an open airway is accomplished by positioning the infant correctly and suctioning the nose and mouth. The infant should be placed supine in slight Trendelenburg position with the neck slightly extended (Fig. 38.3). Care should be taken not to hyperextend or underextend the neck because either position may result in decreased air entry. The airway can be cleared with a suction catheter (10 French) or bulb syringe (Fig. 38.4). The mouth should be suctioned first to prevent aspiration should the infant gasp while suctioning the nose. Suctioning of the deep oropharynx or stomach is not routinely recommended because of the likelihood of vagal stimulation.

Tactile Stimulation

Usually drying and suctioning the newborn infant provides enough tactile stimulation to initiate respirations. If not, stimulating the soles of the feet either by slapping or flicking the feet may initiate respirations in the mildly depressed infant (Fig. 38.5). Firmly rubbing the infant's back also is an acceptable method of tactile stimulation in an attempt to initiate respirations. Methods of stimulation used in the past, which include slapping the infant's back, squeezing the rib cage, or forcing the thighs onto the abdomen, can be harmful to the newborn and should not be used. If the infant remains apneic after appropriate techniques are attempted once or twice, tactile stimulation should stop and positive pressure ventilation (PPV) begun immediately.

Further Evaluation

After completing the initial steps in resuscitation, further action will depend on evaluation of respiratory effort, heart rate, and color (Fig. 38.2). If the infant has spontaneous respirations and the heart rate is above 100, the infant's color should be evaluated. If central cyanosis is present, oxygen should be administered via a free flow system. Using a flow of 5 l/min, with either an oxygen tube held one-half inch from the infant's nose or an oxygen mask, will provide an oxygen concentration of approximately 80%.

If the heart rate is below 100, PPV with 100% oxygen is indicated (Chapter 14). Continuous monitoring of the infant's heart rate either with a stethoscope or by palpating the umbilical or brachial artery pulse is critical and will determine the extent of the resuscitation. If the heart rate increases above 100 with PPV and the infant begins spontaneous respirations, PPV can be replaced with free flow oxygen.

If the heart rate is between 60 and 100 and appears to be increasing, PPV should continue until the heart rate is greater than 100 and spontaneous respirations develop. If the infant fails to improve and ventilation is adequate (i.e., sufficient chest movement and good breath sounds), PPV should continue. If at this point the heart rate is less than 80 or at any point below 60 after an initial period of PPV with 100% oxygen, chest compressions should begin immediately (Chapter 12). If the infant's condition continues to deteriorate or fails to

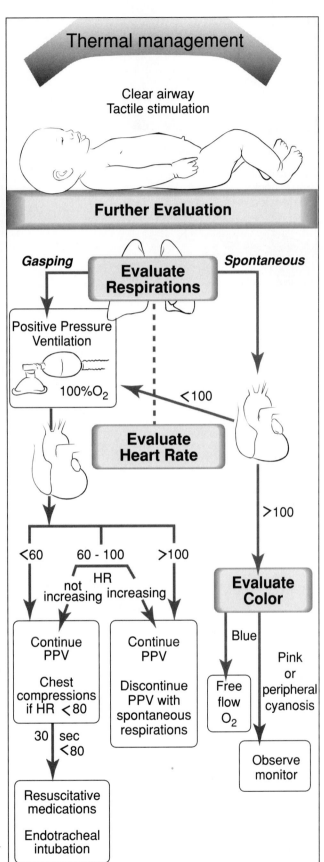

Figure 38.2.
A summary of the resuscitation process.

Figure 38.3.
Positioning the neonatal airway.

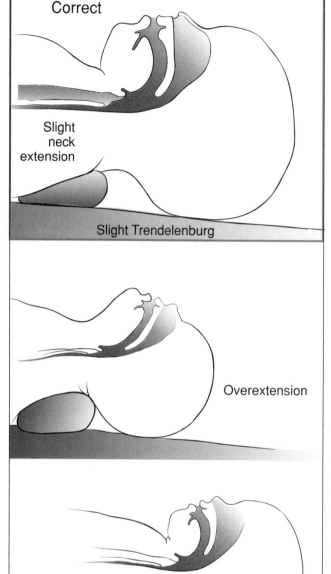

Correct

Slight
neck
extension

Slight Trendelenburg

Overextension

Inadequate
extension

**SUMMARY: INITIAL STEPS
IN RESUSCITATION**
Prevent heat loss:
1. Set radiant warmer in manual mode to maximum temperature
2. Dry infant thoroughly and place stockinette hat to prevent evaporative heat loss
3. Convert warmer to servo mode once ambient temperature has increased and skin temperature monitor has been applied to infant
4. Wrap infant in warm, dry blankets when radiant warmer is unavailable
Clear airway:
1. Place infant in slight Trendelenburg position with neck slightly extended (Fig. 38.3)
2. Gently suction mouth and then nose with bulb syringe or 10 French catheter (Fig. 38.4)
Provide tactile stimulation:
1. Slap or flick soles of infant's feet or firmly rub infant's back to stimulate respiration (Fig. 38.5)

improve despite assisted ventilation and chest compressions, endotracheal intubation (Chapter 16) and administration of resuscitation medications may be required.

COMPLICATIONS

Neonates are more often vulnerable to asphyxia and are far more likely to require resuscitation than any other age group. Efforts to avoid or minimize effects of asphyxia can usually be avoided by (a) having skilled staff readily available who are able to function as a team, (b) having proper equipment available, and (c) recognizing neonatal depression promptly. Complications associated with asphyxia are seen in Table 38.1.

Finally, clinicians who are resuscitating newborns must have a thorough understanding of the techniques described in this chapter. Care should be exercised to suction the airway gently, as vigorous suctioning and stimulation of the posterior pharynx may induce bradycardia and/or apnea. Providing tactile stimulation with methods other than those recommended may result in bruising or fractures. When using an overhead warmer in the servo mode, the skin probe should always remain in contact with the skin and in direct line with radiation from the warmer. Displacement of the probe can result in overheating and possible burning of the infant. Rectal temperature should never be used to control skin temperature. Radiant warming also results in increased insensible water losses, and attention to fluid balance is necessary. During PPV, chest excursions and pressure gauge readings should be closely monitored to avoid pneumothoraces.

SUMMARY

Overall goals of neonatal resuscitation are to assist the newborn in making the transition to neonatal life and to avoid the dire consequences of asphyxia. The uncommon occurrence of ED deliveries mandates an organized and effective approach to the emergent

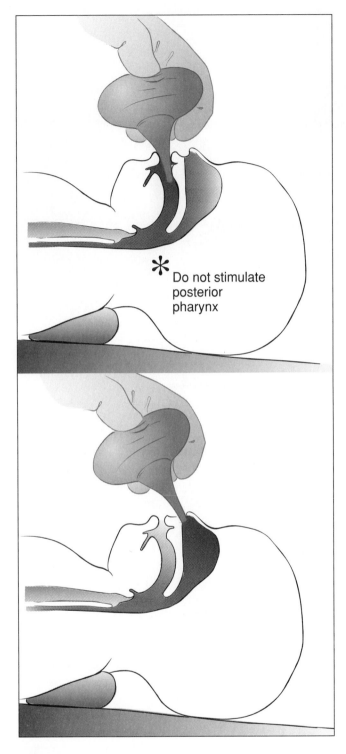

* Do not stimulate posterior pharynx

Figure 38.4.
Suctioning the mouth and nose.

1. Continuously monitor respirations, umbilical or brachial pulse, and color
2. If infant has spontaneous respirations and heart rate above 100, then evaluate color; provide oxygen if central cyanosis is present
3. If infant displays no spontaneous respirations or heart rate below 100, provide PPV with 100% oxygen
4. If infant's heart rate is between 60 and 100 and increasing, continue PPV until it is above 100 and spontaneous respirations develop
5. If the heart rate is below 60 or between 60 and 80 and not increasing despite adequate ventilation, then begin chest compressions
6. If heart rate remains below 80 after 30 seconds then initiate intubation and resuscitation medications

CLINICAL TIPS
1. Activate radiant warmer as soon as delivery is anticipated.
2. Ensure that all resuscitation equipment is available and in working order.
3. Avoid deep suctioning to prevent precipitating vagal-induced apnea and/or bradycardia.
4. Suction the mouth first and then the nose to avoid aspiration.
5. If the infant remains apneic after one or two attempts of tactile stimulation, begin PPV. Continued use of tactile stimulation in an infant who does not respond is not warranted and wastes valuable time.

Chapter 38
Neonatal
Resuscitation
Procedures

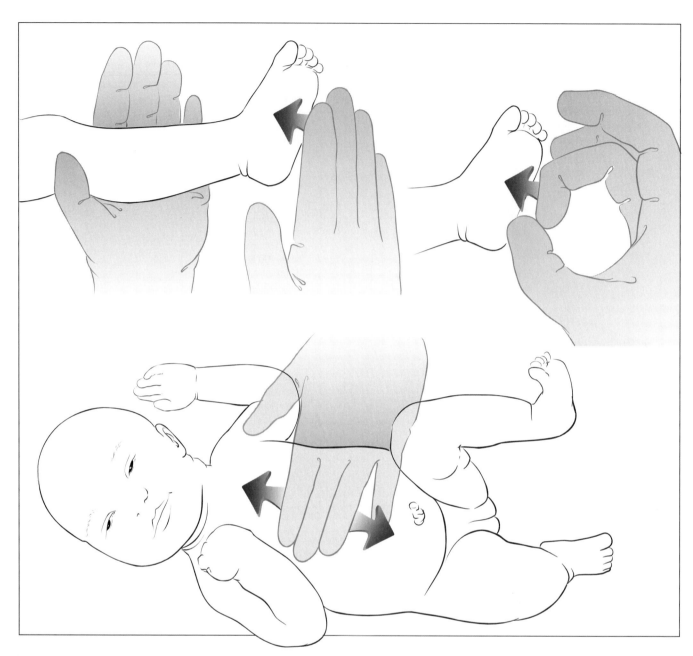

Figure 38.5.
Tactile stimulation of the newborn.

resuscitation of newborns. More specific information and skills that are necessary, including management of meconium aspiration, techniques of intubation, and bag-mask ventilation, are described in great detail in other sections. These should be reviewed to supplement the general approach delineated in this chapter.

REFERENCES

1. Bloom RS, Cropley CS. American Heart Association American Academy of Pediatrics. Textbook of neonatal resuscitation. Dallas: American Heart Association National Center, 1990.
2. Bloom RS. Neonatal-perinatal medicine: diseases of the fetus and infant. 5th ed. Mosby, 1992, pp. 301–323.
3. Allen MC, Donohue PK, Dusman AE. The limit of viability-neonatal outcome of infants born at 22 to 25 weeks' gestation. NEJM 1993, 329:1597–1600.

Prevention and Management of Meconium Aspiration

Jordan D. Lipton and Robert W. Schafermeyer

Introduction

Meconium staining of the amniotic fluid is thought to indicate fetal distress, and is seen predominantly in infants who are postmature or small for their gestational age. It rarely occurs in newborns of less than 38 weeks' gestation. Meconium is present in the amniotic fluid in 11 to 22% of deliveries and (1, 2, 3), is best managed quickly and aggressively when thick meconium is encountered during a delivery room or emergency department (ED) delivery. This is in spite of the fact that meconium aspiration may occur in utero. Meconium aspiration syndrome is defined as the presence of meconium below the vocal cords associated with some degree of respiratory distress and hypoxia. It develops in approximately 0.2 to 1.6% of deliveries, has a mortality rate as high as 40% (2, 3) and a significant incidence of pulmonary complications.

Anatomy and Physiology

Meconium first appears in the fetal ileum between the 10th and 16th week of gestation. It is a viscous liquid composed of gastrointestinal secretions, cellular debris, bile, pancreatic secretions, mucus, blood, hair, and vernix. Passage of meconium before birth may be a normal physiologic event, and the maturation of peristaltic activity may account for the increased incidence of meconium-stained am-niotic fluid seen with increased gestation. An increase in passage of meconium also is associated with fetal asphyxia.

Respiratory movements are normal in utero. General direction of amniotic flow is from the lungs to the amniotic sac. Asphyxia of the fetus stimulates deep breaths and gasping which results in aspiration of amniotic contents into the lungs (Fig. 39.1). As a result, meconium aspiration may occur both in utero and at the time of delivery, and may indicate fetal distress or asphyxia.

Presence of meconium below the vocal cords is associated with a wide range of respiratory symptoms from mild to severe. Meconium has been shown to produce acute airway obstruction, decreased lung compliance, and inflammatory changes. In the most severe cases meconium aspiration results in pulmonary hypertension and persistent fetal circulation with right-to-left shunting. Air leak also has been noted as a common complication of significant meconium aspiration.

Indications

Meconium is a dark brownish-green material. The distinction between thin and thick refers to its density, which varies from liquid to semisolid ("pea soup"). This consistency is dictated by the quantity of meconium that is passed and the amount of amniotic fluid in which it is diluted. With increasing gestational age the relative amount of amniotic

Figure 39.1.
In utero flow of meconium
predisposing to aspiration.

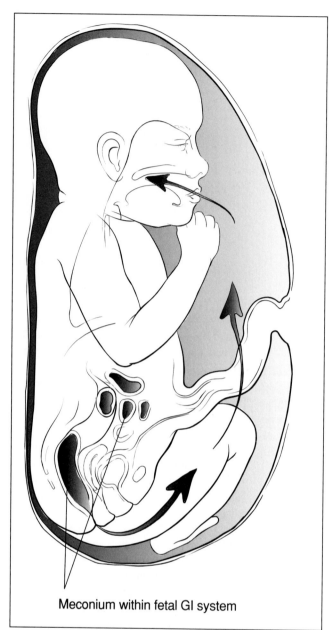

Meconium within fetal GI system

Either of two generally accepted approaches are taken to prevent meconium aspiration (1, 2, 4, 5, 6). The first alternative—selective intubation—involves visualizing the glottis using a laryngoscope followed by intubation and suctioning of the infant. This method applies only if (*a*) meconium is seen at the level of the vocal cords or below, or (*b*) if the infant is severely depressed. This approach is taken by authorities who believe that when signs of distress or presence of meconium at the cords are absent, infants are unlikely to have a significant amount of meconium in the trachea. According to this approach, complications of intubation in this situation may outweigh any benefits. The second option—universal intubation—involves endotracheal intubation and suctioning whenever thick meconium is present in the amniotic fluid. The latter approach has been adopted by various medical centers after one study found that 9% of meconium-stained infants had meconium suctioned from their tracheas when no meconium was visible in the mouth, pharynx, or at the vocal cords (1).

fluid decreases resulting in thicker meconium. Fetal stress also may be responsible for increased passage of meconium and thereby a thicker consistency.

Indications for intubation and active suction of the trachea are controversial. Thin meconium without any particulate matter rarely requires special intervention and, in fact, unnecessary intervention may cause iatrogenic damage. However, thick particulate meconium, especially in association with a depressed neonate, requires removal and clearance from the infant's respiratory tract. It is estimated that 95% of meconium aspiration develops in the presence of thick meconium (3).

Equipment

Suction—capable of generating up to 100 mm Hg negative pressure
¼ inch connective tubing
Suction trap or canister
Suction catheters (10–14 French)
DeLee suction trap apparatus
Bulb syringe
Endotracheal tubes—uncuffed (3.0, 3.5, 4.0 mm)
Endotracheal tube stylettes
Laryngoscope and straight blades (Miller 0 and 1)
Meconium aspirator

PROCEDURE

To prevent aspiration, the oropharynx and nasopharynx of infants born with meconium staining should be suctioned after the head is delivered but before delivery of the thorax (Fig. 39.2). A bulb syringe or wall suction apparatus with suction catheter is used for this process. Suctioning should occur along the buccal mucosa to avoid overstimulation of the posterior pharynx which can result in a severe reflex vagal bradycardia.

Delivery is then completed, the umbilical cord is cut, the infant is placed under a radiant warmer, and residual meconium is suctioned from the hypopharynx under direct vision. Overstimulation, such as vigorous drying, should be avoided during the intubation procedure, as this may promote gasping or deep breathing. Cardiac and oxygen saturation monitoring can be performed by an assistant during the resuscitation, but should not delay resuscitative efforts.

Direct laryngoscopy is performed while maintaining the infant's neck in a slightly extended position. When indicated, the patient is intubated (Chapter 16). Once placed, the tube should be secured with a free hand resting on the infant's head while preparing for suctioning. The entire intubation procedure, excluding suctioning, should be limited to approximately 20 seconds to avoid significant hypoxia. Free flow blow-by oxygen should be provided over the infant's face to minimize hypoxia during suctioning.

Tracheal suctioning should be limited to 10 seconds per pass. Wall suction devices should be set at 60 to 80 mm Hg negative pressure with a maximum of 100 mm Hg. Suction tubing can be connected to a DeLee suction apparatus or directly to the endotracheal tube with a special

adapter called a meconium aspirator. Suction is applied continuously as the endotracheal tube is slowly withdrawn from the trachea (Fig. 39.3). Oral suction through a face mask functioning as a filter with or without a DeLee suction apparatus is no longer a recommended method because of the infectious risks to the physician (chlamydia, *N. gonorrhoeae, T. vaginalis*, group B streptococcus, CMV, HSV, hepatitis, and HIV).

Reintubation and repeat suctioning is necessary until no further meconium is collected in the trap. If the endotracheal tube becomes obstructed with thick meconium, a new one should be used for subsequent intubation. Using a small, disposable plastic catheter to suction through the endotracheal tube is not recommended because the

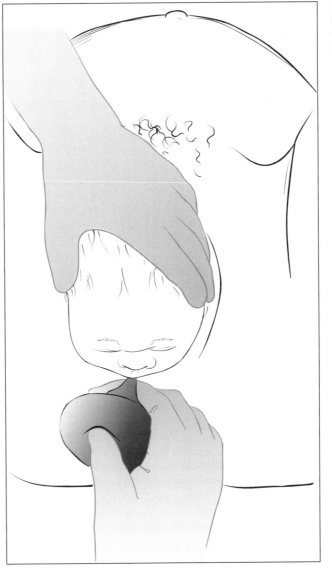

Figure 39.2.
Suctioning of a meconium-stained infant at the perineum.

Chapter 39
Prevention and
Management of
Meconium Aspiration

511

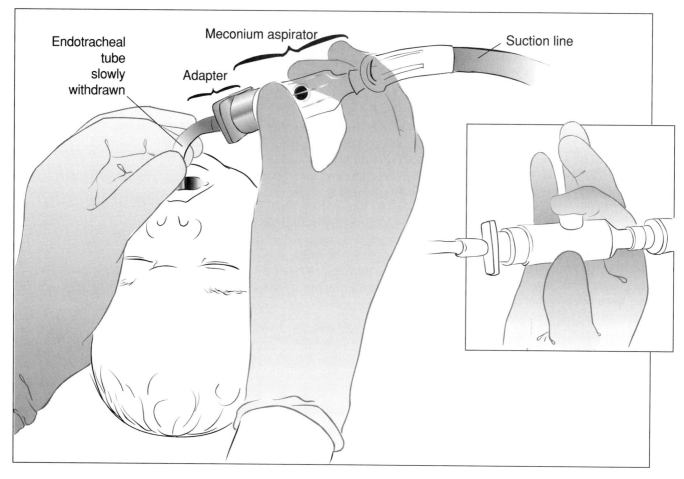

Endotracheal tube slowly withdrawn

Adapter

Meconium aspirator

Suction line

Figure 39.3.
Using the meconium aspirator in suctioning meconium from the trachea of an intubated newborn.

catheter size required to fit through a 3.0 to 4.0 mm endotracheal tube is too small to adequately suction thick meconium. For meconium that is especially tenacious, normal saline lavage and resuctioning through an endotracheal tube can be performed.

After the airway is cleared, standard resuscitation of the newborn is continued, and positive pressure ventilation is begun if needed. The stomach may require suctioning after stabilization of the neonate, because moderate amounts of meconium may remain in the stomach and later be aspirated.

COMPLICATIONS

Complications of tracheal intubation for meconium-stained, amniotic fluid include damage to the alveolar ridge during laryngoscopy and vocal cord or esophageal injury during intubation (Chapter 16). Vagal stimulation with subsequent bradycardia and hypoxia can occur during suctioning or because of esophageal intubation. Injury to the upper

respiratory tract may result in laryngeal stridor or subglottic stenosis. The physician who performs oral suctioning also is at risk of infection. The performance of this procedure results in a delay in the usual resuscitative procedures of the newborn, especially in the provision of adequate oxygenation and ventilation.

SUMMARY

Amniotic fluid stained with thick meconium during delivery generally requires removal and clearance from an infant's respiratory tract. First bulb syringe, or wall suctioning, is performed at the perineum after delivery of the infant's head. Next, the trachea is suctioned using direct laryngoscopy and repetitive endotracheal intubation following delivery of the body. Finally, the stomach is suctioned. Aggressive management is thought to reduce the incidence of meconium aspiration syndrome and its severe complications.

SUMMARY

1. Prepare suctioning and intubation equipment in event of meconium-stained amniotic fluid
2. Deliver head of infant and suction nasopharynx and oropharynx along buccal mucosa with bulb syringe, or wall suction before delivery of thorax
3. Complete delivery, place infant under radiant warmer while avoiding stimulation of infant
4. Perform direct laryngoscopy and endotracheal intubation with 3.0, 3.5, or 4.0 mm endotracheal tube
5. Apply continuous suction at 60 to 80 mm Hg negative pressure to endotracheal tube as it is withdrawn
6. Repeat laryngoscopy, intubation, and tracheal suctioning until no further meconium is suctioned
7. Begin positive pressure ventilation if needed, and resume standard newborn resuscitation
8. Suction stomach for residual meconium
9. For infants who develop meconium aspiration syndrome despite preventive measures, provide warmed nasal or endotracheal oxygen with ventilatory support and transfer to neonatal intensive care unit

CLINICAL TIPS

1. After the head is delivered at the introitus, suction is applied along the buccal mucosa to avoid overstimulation of the posterior pharynx during suctioning.
2. Stimulation before and during intubation should be avoided, as this may promote gasping or deep breathing.
3. The stomach should be suctioned of any residual meconium following stabilization of the neonate.
4. When multiple passes are necessary, the endotracheal tube should be replaced between each attempt.
5. Intubation and suctioning should be repeated until no significant meconium is obtained.

REFERENCES

1. Gregory GA, Gooding CA, Phibbs RH, Tooley WH. Meconium aspiration in infants—a prospective study. J Pediatr 1974; 85:848–852.
2. Holtzman RB, Banzhaf WC, Silver RK, Hageman JR. Perinatal management of meconium staining of the amniotic fluid. Clinics in perinatology 1989;16(4):825–838.
3. Katz VL and Bowes WA. Meconium aspiration syndrome: reflections on a murky subject. Am J Obstet Gynecol 1992;166:171–183.
4. Carson BS, Losey RW, Bowes WA, Simmons MA. Combined obstetric and pediatric approach to prevent meconium aspiration syndrome. Am J Obstet Gynecol 1976;126:712–715.
5. Cunningham AS, Lawson EE, Martin RJ, Pildes RS. Tracheal suction and meconium: a proposed standard of care. J Pediatr 1990;116:153–154.
6. Linder N, Aranda JV, Tsur M et al. Need for Endotracheal intubation and suction in meconium-stained neonates. J Pediatr 1988;112:613–615.

SUGGESTED READINGS

Abramovici H, Brandes JM, Fuchs K, Timor-Tritsch I. Meconium during delivery: a sign of compensated fetal distress. Am J Obstet Gynecol 1974;118: 251–255.

American Heart Association and American Academy of Pediatrics Neonatal Resuscitation Steering Committee. Major revisions to the NRP provider textbook. Dallas: American Heart Association, 1991.

Ballard JL, Musial MJ, Myers MG. Hazards of delivery room resuscitation using oral methods of endotracheal suctioning. Pediatr Infect Dis 1986;5:198–200.

Cordero L, Hon EH. Neonatal bradycardia following nasopharyngeal stimulation. J Pediatr 1971;78: 441–447.

Dillard RG. Neonatal tracheal aspiration of meconium-stained infants. J Pediatr 1977;90:163–164.

Falciglia HS. Failure to Prevent Meconium Aspiration Syndrome. Obstet Gynecol 1988;71:349–353.

Gage JE, Taeusch HW, Treves S, Caldicott W. Suctioning of upper airway meconium in newborn infants. JAMA 1981;246:2590–2592.

Hageman JR, Conley M, Francis K et al. Delivery room management of meconium staining of the amniotic fluid and the development of meconium aspiration syndrome. J Perinatol 1988;8:127–131.

Locus P, Yeomans E, Crosby U. Efficacy of bulb vs De Lee suction at deliveries complicated by meconium-stained amniotic fluid. Am J Perinatol 1990;7:87–91.

Wiswell TE, Tuggle JM, Turner BS. Meconium aspiration syndrome: have we made a difference? Pediatrics 1990;85:715–721.

UMBILICAL VESSEL CATHETERIZATION

Jordan D. Lipton and Robert W. Schafermeyer

INTRODUCTION

Umbilical vessel catheterization has come to be used frequently in the newborn period for transfusion therapy, blood pressure monitoring, emergency delivery of medications and fluids, delivery of parenteral nutrition, and blood sampling. Although most likely to be performed in the neonatal ICU setting or delivery room on preterm infants, arterial or venous catheterization also can be performed in the emergency department (ED) for the resuscitation of infants delivered in the prehospital or ED setting. Peripheral intravenous access should be attempted first; however, this can at times be difficult or impossible to obtain. Umbilical vessel catheterization provides a reliable means of emergency vascular access in the newborn. In addition, the umbilical vein should be considered as an option for emergency access in the neonate up to 2 weeks of age. The procedure is potentially difficult and time consuming, but can be performed rapidly by physicians skilled in the procedure. This method provides the advantage of direct visualization of the vessels to be catheterized while obtaining central venous access.

ANATOMY AND PHYSIOLOGY

The fetal cardiovascular system serves prenatal needs and allows for modifications after birth that lead to a postnatal circulatory pattern (Fig. 40.1) (1). In the fetal circulatory system, well-oxygenated blood (~80% saturated) returns from the placenta through the umbilical vein, which courses through the hepatic sinusoids and ductus venosus to the inferior vena cava. High pressure in the fetal pulmonary vascular system results in the majority of blood being shunted from the right atrium across the foramen ovale into the left atrium. Blood that reaches the right ventricle is distributed one-third to the lungs and two-thirds to the aorta by way of the ductus arteriosus. Umbilical arteries receive approximately 40 to 50% of the mixed blood in the descending aorta (~58% saturated with oxygen) and return it to the placenta where O_2, CO_2, nutrients, and waste products are exchanged. The remainder of the blood from the descending aorta circulates through the gut, kidney, and lower extremities.

Numerous changes occur in the circulatory system following birth. With the first breath and the inflation of alveoli, pulmonary vascular resistance falls. Elevation in PaO_2 and pH further contributes to pulmonary vasodilation. Systemic resistance is immediately increased when the umbilical cord is clamped. These dramatic changes in pressure result in a reversal of the gradient across the atrial septum and closure of the foramen ovale. The ductus arteriosus begins to constrict almost immediately following birth stimulated by increased oxygen tension and prostaglandin release. Complete closure generally occurs 1 to 2 days after birth. The duc-

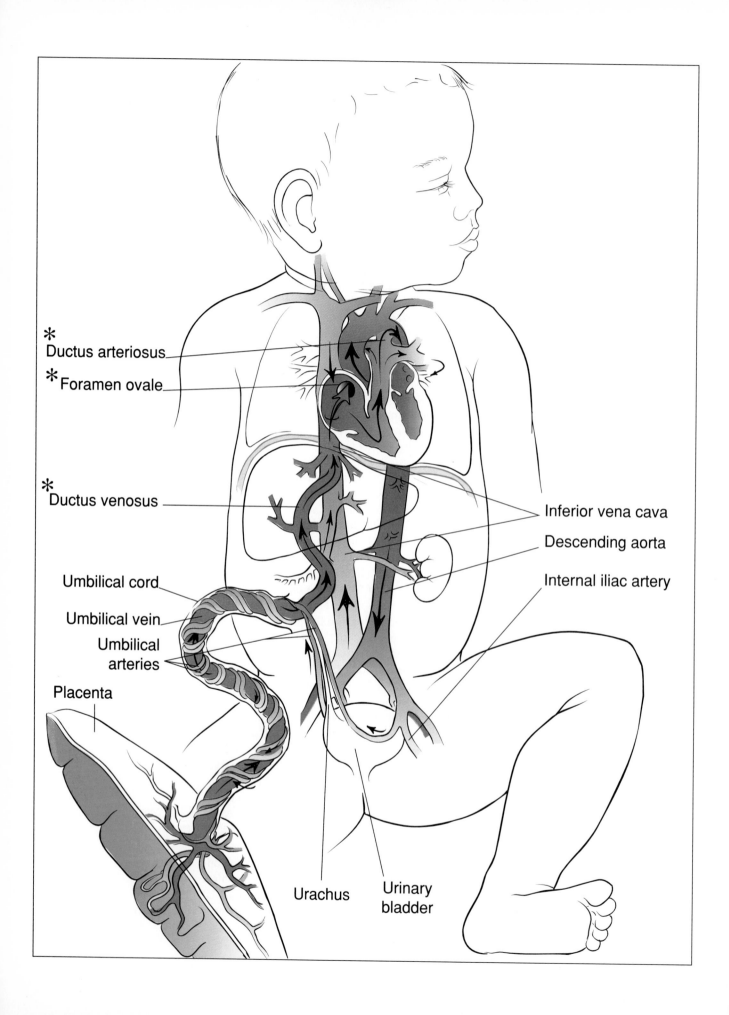

* Ductus arteriosus

* Foramen ovale

* Ductus venosus

Umbilical cord

Umbilical vein

Umbilical arteries

Placenta

Inferior vena cava

Descending aorta

Internal iliac artery

Urachus

Urinary bladder

tus venosus also closes once the umbilical cord is clamped. The umbilical arteries begin to constrict within minutes of birth and close before the umbilical vein. The umbilical vein may retain some degree of patency for up to 2 weeks after the cord is clamped and cut.

The umbilical arteries and vein can be differentiated in a cross section of the umbilical cord based on a number of characteristics. The vein is generally located on the cephalad end of the umbilicus. It is thin walled with a large lumen and only a single vein is present within the cord. The umbilical artery posesses a thicker wall and a smaller lumen. Two arteries generally are present in the umbilical cord; however, approximately 0.5% of newborns will have only one umbilical artery. A patent urachus is a persistent embryologic connection to the bladder which may rarely be present and can appear similar to the umbilical vein, but without bleeding.

INDICATIONS

Umbilical artery catheterization is indicated for newborns with severe cardiopulmonary insufficiency requiring mechanically assisted ventilation. The umbilical artery catheter allows for frequent arterial blood gas determinations, and can be used for administration of fluids, medications, and exchange transfusion. It is usually quite simple to catheterize the umbilical artery in a sick infant during the first hour of life, and most infants can be catheterized within the first 24 hours. Occasionally this route can be used up to 7 days of age.

Umbilical vein catheterization in the ED or delivery room is recommended for emergent situations in which delivery of resuscitative medications, volume expanders, or blood products is the desired goal. Catheterization of the umbilical vein is easiest in newborns, but has been successful in infants up to 2 weeks of age.

An umbilical vessel catheter (arterial or venous) should never be inserted in the presence of omphalitis or impetiginous skin lesions. It is also generally contraindicated

◀
Figure 40.1.
The fetal cardiovascular system illustrating the course of the umbilical vessels. Structures marked with an asterisk (✱) close soon after birth.

when a possibility of intestinal hypoperfusion or necrotizing enterocolitis exists, both of which are often suggested by abdominal distention. Finally, inserting an umbilical catheter for routine administration of parenteral fluids or medications or for routine blood sampling is inappropriate.

EQUIPMENT

Radiant warmer with light source
Prep solution (povidone-iodine), sterile drape, gauze pads
Mask, cap, goggles, sterile gloves, gown
Scalpel—No. 11 or 15
Curved, nontoothed iris forceps (4″) or pointed, solid metal dilator
Small, smooth curved hemostat(s)
Straight Crile forceps
Iris scissors
Needle holder
Nonthrombogenic, molded-tip umbilical catheters (3.5, 4, 5, 8 French with end hole)
3.0 or 4.0 silk suture on curved or straight needle
Linen umbilical tape (~15″)
Adhesive tape
10 cc syringe filled with NS (with or without heparin 1 unit/mL)
D5W, D10W, or NS infusion setup (with heparin 1 unit/mL, unless medications incompatible with heparin)
Fluid chamber, i.v. tubing, infusion pump, 0.22 μ filter
Three-way stopcock
Needle—20 or 22 gauge
Cardiac monitor, pulse oximeter

PROCEDURE

Preparation

Treatment for cardiorespiratory disturbances should begin before commencing the procedure. The child is placed beneath a radiant warmer and the extremities restrained in a supine frog-leg position (Fig. 40.2). The cardiac rate should be monitored and adequate oxygenation should be made available throughout the procedure. The clinician performing the procedure should wear a surgical gown, gloves, cap, mask, and goggles (Chap-

Figure 40.2.
Restraint of the neonate for umbilical vessel catheterization. Note shoulder-to-umbilicus and crown-to-heel or total body length measurements. Shading represents area to be cleansed with bactericidal solution.

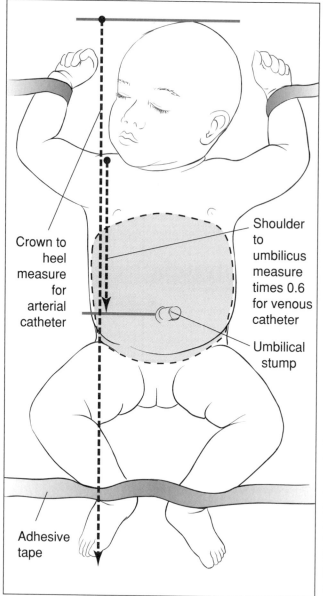

Crown to heel measure for arterial catheter

Shoulder to umbilicus measure times 0.6 for venous catheter

Umbilical stump

Adhesive tape

are used to grasp the umbilical stump, and the vessels are identified.

Arterial Catheterization

A curved hemostat is used to grasp the cut edge of the cord near the artery selected for catheterization, or two hemostats to grasp opposite sides of the umbilicus. The edges are then everted (Fig. 40.3.B). Using curved iris forceps without teeth, approximately 1 cm of arterial lumen is gently dilated by repetitively introducing and opening the tips of the forceps within the lumen. A pointed, solid metal dilator can be used in place of the iris forceps, paying careful attention not to tear the arterial wall.

The catheter, previously flushed with heparinized solution, is grasped approximately 1 cm from its tip with thumb and index finger, or with small forceps, and the tip is inserted into the arterial lumen (Figs. 40.3.C, D, E). A 3.5- to 4-French catheter is used for infants weighing less than 2 kg, and a 5-French catheter for infants weighing more than 2 kg. During insertion, tension is placed cephalad on the cord so that the catheter can be advanced more directly toward the feet. The catheter is passed using gentle, constant pressure to overcome resistance, which is usually felt at two points. Slight resistance is first met at 1 to 2 cm, where the umbilical artery curves toward the feet; placing tension cephalad on the cord helps to reduce this resistance. The clinician will feel greater resistance at the junction of the internal iliac artery at 5 to 6 cm, where the artery turns upward (Fig. 40.1). A slight twisting motion of the catheter will help to overcome resistance. Resistance as a result of vasospasm can sometimes be relieved by removing the catheter, filling its tip with 0.1 to 0.2 mL of 2% lido-

ter 7). The infant's abdomen and remaining umbilical cord is scrubbed with a bactericidal solution such as povidone-iodine, from the xiphoid process to the symphysis pubis. Pooling of solution at the infant's side should be avoided because this may result in skin blistering. The umbilical area is draped in a sterile fashion and the infant's head is left exposed for observation.

A purse-string suture or loosely tied umbilical tape is placed at the base of the umbilical cord to provide hemostasis and an anchor after line placement. The cord is grasped full thickness with forceps between 0.5 to 2 cm from its base and cut transversely at the top edge of the forceps using the scalpel (Fig. 40.3.A). A forceps or thumb and index finger

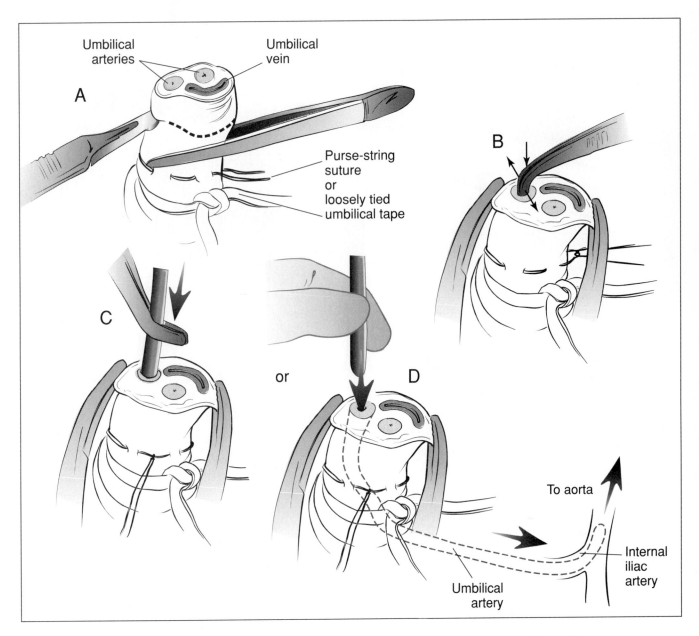

Umbilical arteries
Umbilical vein

A

Purse-string suture or loosely tied umbilical tape

B

C

or

D

To aorta

Internal iliac artery

Umbilical artery

Figure 40.3.
Introduction of the umbilical artery catheter.

caine without epinephrine, and reinserting the catheter. At the point of resistance, the lidocaine is flushed into the vessel, and after 1 to 2 minutes, advancement of the catheter is reattempted.

Resistance at 4 to 5 cm generally indicates that a false tract has been created with subintimal cannulation. If this occurs to both arteries, a vessel may still be cannulated by performing a subumbilical cutdown. This latter procedure does, however, carry the risk of hemorrhage and accidental entry into the peritoneum and should therefore only be performed by personnel experienced with the procedure.

Two insertion depths for the distal end of an umbilical artery catheter are generally accepted. Optimal position above the diaphragm is at the level of the thoracic aorta between the ductus arteriosus and the origin of the celiac axis (spinal level T6-T9). Below the diaphragm, the tip is positioned between the inferior mesenteric artery and the bifurcation of the aorta (spinal level L3-L5) (Fig. 40.4). Data supporting the advantage of one location over the other are equivocal. Nomograms are available that estimate the proper length of umbilical artery catheter insertion based on the vertical distance from the lateral aspect of the clavicle to the level of the um-

Chapter 40
Umbilical Vessel
Catheterization

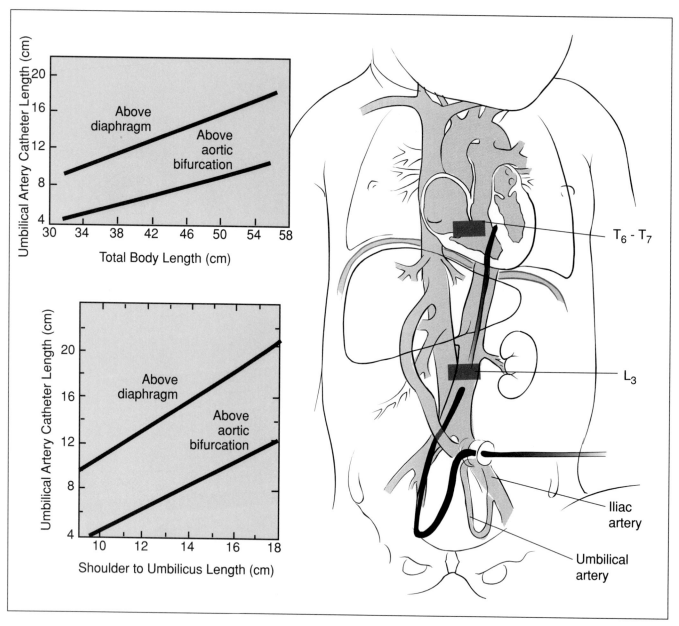

Figure 40.4.

Nomograms for estimating umbilical artery catheter length based on total body or shoulder-to-umbilicus measurements. (Adapted from Dunn PM. Localization of the umbilical catheter by postmortem measurement. Arch Dis Child 1966; 41:69.)

bilicus (shoulder-to-umbilicus length) or the crown-heel length, one or both of which should be measured before commencing with the procedure (Figs. 40.2, 40.4) (2, 3). If the thoracic umbilical artery catheter position is desired and a nomogram is unavailable, an estimate can be obtained using the shoulder to umbilicus length. If the measurement obtained is less than 13 cm, the catheter is inserted that distance plus 1 cm; if greater than 13 cm, it is inserted that distance plus 2 cm. For the subdiaphragmatic position, the arterial catheter is inserted until blood is first obtained, and then advanced an additional 1 cm. These estimated measurements do not in-

clude the additional length of the umbilical stump.

Once the desired position is reached using the aforementioned nomograms or formulas, a radiograph should be obtained to confirm placement. Pending radiographic confirmation, an infusion of D5W or D10W with heparin can be started. In an emergent situation, subdiaphragmatic placement will obviate the need for a radiograph before starting medications and/or fluids. Once sterile technique is broken, the line may not be advanced. Therefore in a nonemergent situation, it is preferable to position the catheter too high and to withdraw it as necessary

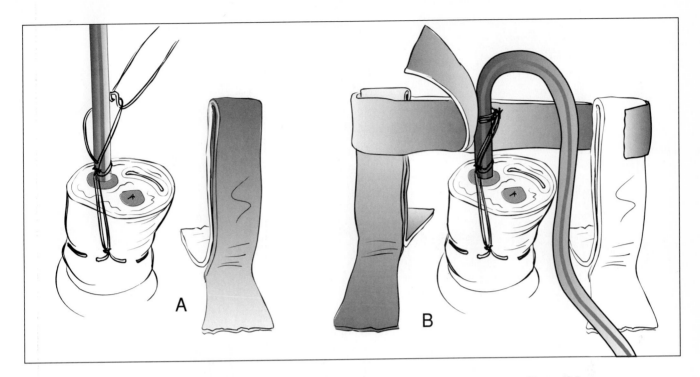

Figure 40.5.
Securing the umbilical
vessel catheter.

based on the radiograph. A radiograph of a properly positioned umbilical artery catheter will reveal the catheter proceeding from the umbilicus caudad toward the pelvis, where it makes an acute turn into the internal iliac artery. From there it continues along the left side of the vertebral column toward the head, past the bifurcation of the aorta, through the abdominal aorta, and into the thoracic aorta.

After the correct position is confirmed, the catheter is secured using the previously placed purse-string suture (Fig. 40.5.A). The original suture or a second one secured to the skin margin of the umbilical stump is tied with a square knot around the catheter in 1 or 2 additional places—at the entrance into the umbilical vessel and/or 2 to 4 cm from the cord. A piece of adhesive tape, incorporating both the catheter and the suture, is placed perpendicular to the umbilical stump. This tape is then secured to the abdominal wall with additional strips of tape (Fig. 40.5.B).

Venous Catheterization

The technique of umbilical vein catheterization is similar to that of arterial catheterization, but because the lumen of the vein is larger, a larger catheter (generally 5 or 8 French) can be used. After positioning and prepping the infant, tying the base of the cord, and identifying the umbilical vessels, the flushed catheter is inserted into the lumen of the umbilical vein. In an emergent situation, the catheter is gently passed 4 to 5 cm or until blood return is noted. This achieves access to the vessel while minimizing the risk of injecting sclerosing solutions directly into the liver. The shoulder-to-umbilicus length multiplied by 0.6 approximates the length of catheter to be inserted to place its tip above the diaphragm at the junction of the inferior vena cava and the right atrium (Fig. 40.6) (4). This distance (10 to 12 cm) will allow for central venous pressure monitoring or infusion of medications or hyperalimentation solutions. However, if obstruction is encountered at 5 to 10 cm, the catheter has likely passed into a branch of the portal vein within the liver, into which the injection of high osmolar solutions can result in hepatic necrosis.

Removal of Catheters

As soon as an umbilical catheter is no longer indicated, it should be removed. In preparation for removal, the stopcock is turned off. Loosely tied umbilical tape is placed around the umbilical stump, and over 3 to 5 minutes, the catheter is gradually withdrawn. If bleeding occurs, the umbilical tape can be tight-

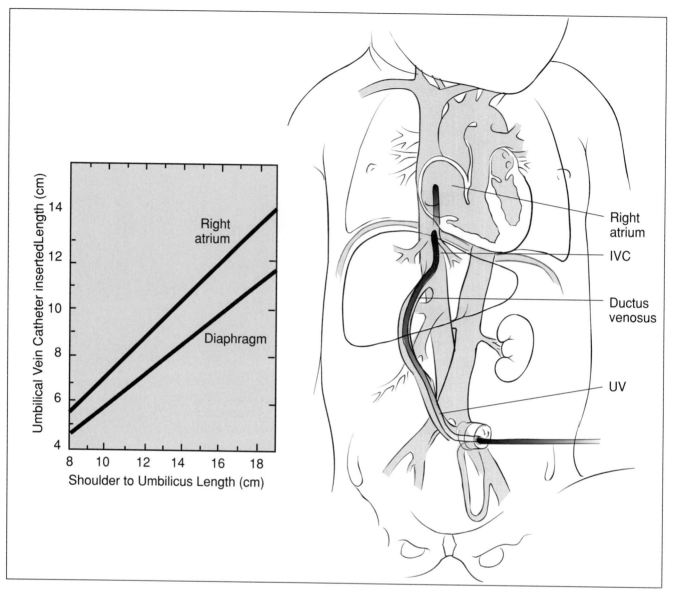

Right atrium

IVC

Ductus venosus

UV

Figure 40.6.
Nomogram for estimating umbilical vein catheter length based on shoulder-to-umbilicus measurement. (Adapted from Dunn PM. Localization of the umbilical catheter by postmortem measurement. Arch Dis Child 1966; 41:69.)

ened. If bleeding persists, the vessel can be grasped with a curved hemostat.

COMPLICATIONS

Lower extremity or buttock ischemia caused by umbilical artery catheters is often the result of vasospasm (5–7). This can often be treated with warm compresses applied to the contralateral extremity triggering a reflex vasodilation in the affected limb. The catheter should be removed if no improvement in limb color or pulse is seen within 15 minutes, which may indicate inadvertent cannulation of the left internal iliac artery. Similarly, ischemia of the bowel or kidneys can occur

with improper positioning of the catheter at the origin of a renal or mesenteric artery (7, 8). This may respond to repositioning of the catheter. Thrombus formation associated with umbilical artery catheters is common (4–9), but risks are minimized by using non-thrombogenic catheters and heparin-containing solutions.

Bacterial colonization of umbilical catheters has been reported with frequencies as high as 57%; however, bacteremia is unusual (4, 7–9). Significant blood loss is most commonly the result of an accidentally dislodged arterial catheter or stopcock, and is much less likely to occur when locking connectors are used and the catheter is sutured and taped securely in place (4–6, 8, 9). Peri-

SUMMARY

1. Place infant under radiant warmer in supine frog-leg position with cardiac monitor
2. Prepare antiseptic field
3. Determine distance to which catheter will be inserted:
   a. Arterial:
   Elective: Use nomogram for umbilicus to lateral clavicle distance, or if <13 cm, insert catheter that distance plus 1 cm; if >13 cm, insert that distance plus 2 cm.
   Emergent: For subdiaphragmatic positioning, insert catheter until blood is obtained, then advance 1 cm.
   b. Venous:
   Elective: Measure vertical distance from umbilicus to lateral clavicle and multiply by 0.6 for inferior vena cava positioning.
   Emergent: Pass the catheter 4 to 5 cm or until blood return is noted.
4. Loosely tie umbilical tape or purse-string suture at base of umbilical cord.
5. Cut cord transversely 0.5 to 2.0 cm from its base, and identify vessels
6. Grasp and evert side(s) of umbilical stump with hemostat(s)
7. Dilate vessel lumen using curved iris forceps to accomodate 3.5- to 5-French catheter (artery) or 5- to 8-French catheter (vein)
8. Insert catheter tip into vessel lumen and pass catheter using gentle, constant pressure
9. Techniques to overcome resistance during arterial catheterization:
   a. Place tension cephalad on the cord
   b. Apply twisting motion to catheter
   c. Flush with 0.1 to 0.2 mL of 2% lidocaine
10. Obtain radiograph of thorax and abdomen to confirm placement
11. Secure catheter in place using purse-string suture and adhesive tape

cardial perforation can occur when an umbilical venous catheter is placed into the right atrium. Systemic hypertension can result from renovascular stenosis or renal artery thrombosis as a result of umbilical vessel catheter placement. Other complications include vessel perforation (6, 7), peritoneal perforation, organ perforation, arrhythmias, aneurysm formation, and portal hypertension.

Air embolism, which is more common with umbilical vein catheters (4, 6, 7–9), can be avoided by flushing the catheter and intravenous tubing with intravenous fluid before insertion, and by using a three-way stopcock.

SUMMARY

Vascular access is frequently difficult to obtain in the newborn. Umbilical vessel catheterization provides a useful alternative to peripheral lines in this age group. Once cannulated, these vessels can be used for transfusion of blood products, blood pressure monitoring, delivery of medications and fluids, and blood sampling.

REFERENCES

1. Moore KL. The developing human: clinically oriented embryology, 5th edition. Philadelphia: WB Saunders, 1993.
2. Dunn PM. Localization of the umbilical catheter by postmortem measurement. Arch Dis Child 1966;41:69–75.
3. Rosenfeld W, Biagtan J, Schaeffer H, et al. A new graph for insertion of umbilical artery catheters. J Pediatr 1980;96:735–737.
4. Prinz SC, Cunningham MD. Umbilical vessel catheterization. J Fam Pract 1980;10(5):885–890.
5. Dorand RD, Cook LN, Andrews BF. Umbilical vessel catheterization—the low incidence of complications in a series of 200 newborn infants. Clin Pediatr 1977;16:569–572.
6. Kitterman JA, Phibbs RH, Tooley WH. Catheterization of umbilical vessels in newborn infants. Pediatr Clin North Am 1970;17:895–912.
7. Tooley WH, Myerberg DZ. Should we put catheters in the umbilical artery? Pediatrics 1978;62:853–854.
8. Cowett RM, Peter G, Hakanson DO, Stern L, Oh W. Prophylactic antibiotics in neonates with umbilical artery catheter placement—a prospective study of 137 patients. Yale J Biol Med 1977;50:457–463.
9. Thomas DB. Umbilical vessel catheterization. Med J Aust 1974;1:404–407.

SUGGESTED READINGS

Chameides L, ed. Textbook of pediatric advanced life support. Dallas: American Heart Association, 1990.
Harris MS, Little GA. Umbilical artery catheters: high, low, or no. J Perinatal Med 1978;6:15–21.
Klaus MH, Fanaroff AA. Care of the high-risk neonate. Philadelphia: WB Saunders, 1986.
Paster S, Middleton P. Roentgenographic evaluation of umbilical artery and vein catheters. JAMA 1975;231:742–746.

CLINICAL TIPS

1. In an emergent situation, subdiaphragmatic placement of an umbilical artery catheter is recommended and will obviate the need for a radiograph before starting medications and/or fluids.
2. During emergent umbilical vein catheterization, the catheter is passed cephalad for 4 to 5 cm or until blood return is noted.
3. The umbilical artery can occasionally be accessed in neonates up to 7 days of age, the umbilical vein in neonates up to 14 days of age.
4. A twisting motion of the catheter will often help to overcome resistance when inserting an umbilical artery catheter.
5. Resistance as a result of vasospasm can sometimes be relieved by removing the catheter, filling its tip with 0.1 to 0.2 mL of 2% lidocaine, reinserting the catheter to the point of resistance, flushing the lidocaine into the vessel, and waiting 1 to 2 minutes before reattempting to advance the catheter.
6. Resistance at 5 to 10 cm in umbilical vein catheterization suggests the incorrect cannulation of a branch of the portal vein.
7. Vasospasm as a result of umbilical artery catheters often can be relieved with warm compresses applied to the contralateral extremity.

CHAPTER 41

EMERGENCY MANAGEMENT OF SELECTED CONGENITAL ANOMALIES

Gail S. Rudnitsky and Sonia O. Imaizumi

INTRODUCTION

Congenital anomalies requiring surgical intervention in the immediate postnatal period are not uncommon, occurring in 2 to 3% of all malformations (1). With improvements in monitoring capabilities and increased use of high resolution ultrasonography, most babies with congenital anomalies are diagnosed in utero and delivered in a tertiary care center with the appropriate specialists standing by to care for these high-risk infants. However, unforeseen circumstances, such as lack of prenatal care or unexpected premature deliveries, may result in an infant being born in an emergency center or delivery room of a hospital not equipped to care for an infant with such an anomaly. Therefore, it is necessary for the treating physician to be able to stabilize an infant before transport to a hospital that is capable of caring for an infant born with a congenital malformation. Stabilization should include standard neonatal resuscitative measures (Chapter 38), including stabilizing the airway and cardiovascular system when necessary, keeping the infant warm, and preventing any exposed organs from injury or drying out. The accepting hospital should be a tertiary care center with the appropriate surgeons and subspecialists available to provide definitive care for these children. Discussion in this chapter will be limited to several of the more common and severe malformations which require immediate attention.

Abdominal Wall Defects

Anatomy and Physiology

The more common abdominal wall defects include gastroschisis, omphalocele, bladder exstrophy, and cloacal exstrophy. All these defects require immediate intervention to prevent loss of heat and fluids and to minimize the chance of fatal infections.

Gastroschisis

Gastroschisis is a full-thickness defect of the abdominal wall, varying from a few centimeters in length to a large defect that extends from the xiphoid process to the pubic symphysis with herniation of uncovered intestinal contents through the defect (3) (Fig. 41.1.A). The origin of this disorder is still unknown. The most commonly accepted theory is that the defect arises from a rupture of a hernia of the umbilical cord at the site of the involution of the vestigial right umbilical vein. This anomaly can be differentiated from an omphalocele by the generally smaller size of the defect which is located lateral to the umbilicus. In gastroschisis the umbilical cord is normally attached to the abdominal wall to the left of the defect (1). Because no amniotic or peritoneal sac covers the bowel, it is exposed

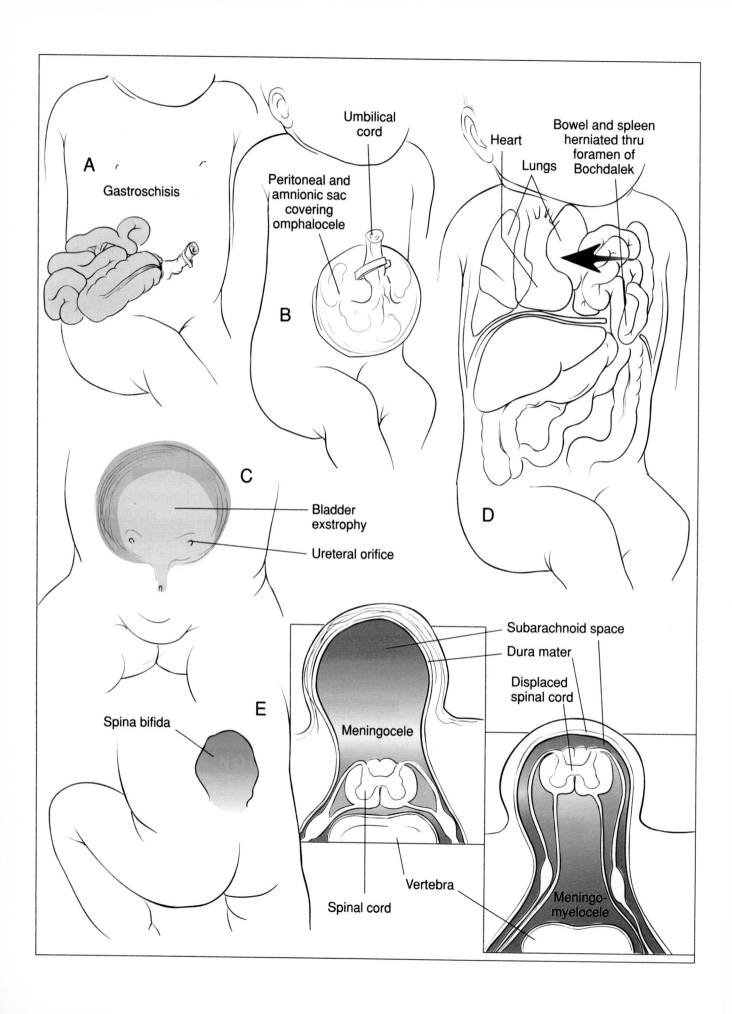

A Gastroschisis

B Umbilical cord

Peritoneal and amnionic sac covering omphalocele

C Bladder exstrophy

Ureteral orifice

D Heart

Lungs

Bowel and spleen herniated thru foramen of Bochdalek

E Spina bifida

Meningocele

Spinal cord

Subarachnoid space

Dura mater

Displaced spinal cord

Vertebra

Meningo-myelocele

to the chemical irritation of amniotic fluid in utero and is often edematous, matted together, and covered with a gelatinous exudate (2). All infants have nonrotation and abnormal fixation of the intestines. Of infants with gastroschisis, 16% will have gastrointestinal malformations consisting of atresias and stenoses. Other associated congenital anomalies are rare (6). The incidence of gastroschisis is approximately 1/10,000 live births (5).

Omphalocele

Omphalocele, by contrast, is a 2 to 15 cm defect of the umbilical ring resulting from failure of fusion of the four somatic folds that define the abdominal wall early in gestation, (1), with herniation of varying amounts of abdominal viscera into a sac composed of amnion and peritoneum (Fig. 41.1.B). This sac may be ruptured before or at the time of delivery exposing the viscera to amniotic fluid or the ambient environment. The size of the defect and covering sac determines the amount of viscera that is herniated. Omphalocele may be associated with other abnormalities (cardiac, neurologic, genitourinary, skeletal, and chromosomal) as well as the following syndromes: Beckwith Wiedemann syndrome, Prune Belly syndrome, trisomies 13, 18, and 21, and Pentalogy of Cantrell (3).

Indications

These defects in the abdominal wall should be readily apparent on observation. Management of gastroschisis and omphalocele from delivery to transport is nearly identical and should be initiated once either diagnosis is suspected.

Equipment

Radiant warmer
Routine neonatal resuscitation equipment (Chapter 38)
Sterile gauze
Sterile saline
Sterile intestinal bag
Plastic film wrap (such as Saran® or Glad®)
Nasogastric tube (8–10 French)

Figure 41.1.
Selected congenital anomalies.
A. Gastroschisis.
B. Omphalocele.
C. Exstrophy of the bladder.
D. Diaphragmatic hernia.
E. Spina bifida.

Procedure

In addition to routine neonatal resuscitative measures outlined in Chapter 38, the goals of stabilizing these infants are to minimize heat and fluid loss and to prevent desiccation, injury, or infection of the exposed viscera. Care must be taken in placing the umbilical cord clamp so as to avoid injury to the herniated intestine.

The infant is placed under a radiant warmer and the exposed viscera is protected with a warm, sterile saline-soaked dressing. The exposed viscera should be inspected to ensure that it is not twisted or kinked to prevent vascular or caval obstruction. A change in color of the exposed bowel from pink to grey may indicate the presence of such an obstruction. Tension on the mesentery may be reduced by supporting the bowel on packs of warm, sterile wet gauze (3). As soon as possible, the infant should be placed in a sterile intestinal bag with the drawstring tied around the chest (Fig. 41.2.A). If the infant is small, the arms also can be enclosed (1). This clear plastic bag has the following advantages: heat and fluid loss are minimized, and it allows the physician to observe the color of the bowel, looking for signs of ischemia. An 8- to 10-French nasogastric tube should be placed to free drainage and should be aspirated every 10 to 15 minutes to prevent vomiting and to keep the bowel decompressed. Fluid resuscitation should be initiated with 10 to 20 mL/kg of colloid, Ringer's lactate, or normal saline solution. Maintenance fluids of D10 1/4 normal saline should be started at twice the calculated normal maintenance volume and continued until the urine output is 2 to 3 mL/kg/hr (2). Broad spectrum antibiotics (ampicillin and gentamicin) should be started after a baseline blood culture is obtained. Transport should be promptly arranged to a tertiary care center with an available neonatologist and pediatric surgeon.

Gastroschisis is considered a surgical emergency and should be corrected as soon as possible. In the surgical management of these defects the infant is stabilized either by fascial or skin closure or with construction of a prosthetic sac, which is called a silo, enclosing the herniated viscera (6). Small omphaloceles (≤ 5 cm) usually can be closed primarily. Larger defects are repaired either by closing skin leaving a vertical hernia that can be repaired later, or a silo is constructed

Chapter 41
Emergency
Management of
Selected Congenital
Anomalies

527

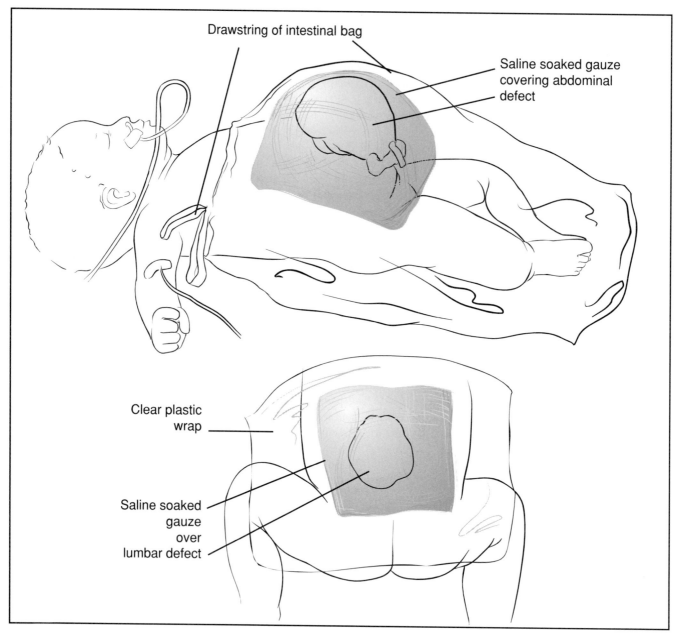

Drawstring of intestinal bag

Saline soaked gauze covering abdominal defect

Clear plastic wrap

Saline soaked gauze over lumbar defect

Figure 41.2.
Initial management of selected congenital anomalies.
A. Gastroschisis and omphalocele.
B. Neural tube defects.

Chapter 41 Emergency Management of Selected Congenital Anomalies

that is compressed on a daily basis. When the contents of the site are completely reduced into the abdomen (usually in 7 to 10 days), fascial closure is possible (6).

Complications
Despite the measures already described, the infant may arrive at the accepting hospital with problems related to hypothermia, volume depletion, acidosis, or all three (3). Insensible fluid loss is minimized by the overlying plastic wrap, but must be watched closely to avoid drying of the viscera or hypovolemia in the patient. Excessive handling of the bowel may predispose to infection or injury.

Bladder Exstrophy
Exstrophy of the bladder occurs in 1/10,000 to 1/50,000 live births and results from incomplete fusion of the caudal fold, abnormal development of the cloacal membrane, and failure of anterior closure of the pelvis at the symphysis pubis (2) (Fig. 41.1.C). Classic exstrophy of the bladder, with the bladder open on the lower abdominal wall, is usually associated with some degree of epispadias of the male or female genitalia. The ureteral orifices are usually plainly visible with a continuous dribble of urine covering the exposed bladder (8). At birth, the bladder mucosa is thin and smooth, but with exposure, becomes

hyperemic, thickened, and friable (3). The kidneys and ureters are usually normal at birth but may become secondarily dilated by reflux and infection or by fibrosis of the ureteral openings.

Procedure

The bladder should be covered by plastic film wrap such as Saran® or Glad®, or vaseline gauze (2). Antibiotics are not necessary. The infant should be transferred to a neonatal unit for further evaluation. Repair is done electively in stages beginning in the neonatal period with the ultimate goal of closing the bladder, reconstructing the abdominal wall, genital reconstruction, and eventual urinary continence.

Cloacal Exstrophy

Cloacal exstrophy or vesicointestinal fissure is a complex abnormality consisting of a large omphalocele beneath which lies the open bladder. The bladder is divided in half by a zone of intestine with an upper orifice leading to the terminal ileum and a lower orifice leading to a short colon (5 cm) which ends blindly (3, 8). Almost all infants with this defect have either a meningomyelocele or a tethered cord (3, 8). Other associated anomalies include undescended or absent testes, bicornate uterus, absent or duplicated vagina and epispadias. In addition, 50% of infants have abnormalities of the kidneys or ureters (3). Cardiovascular, musculoskeletal, diaphragmatic, and other small intestinal abnormalities may occur (3).

Management

Complete functional repair is difficult or impossible (8). However, without surgical intervention, infants with cloacal exstrophy usually die shortly after birth (3). Because of the ethical and moral issues involved, these children should be treated as previously described in the section on omphalocele and should be transferred to a tertiary care center where the staff is available to give the parents complete information concerning the infant's condition and long-term prognosis.

Neural Tube Defects

Defects in enclosure of the neural tube are the most common of the major malformations of the central and peripheral nervous systems. They include meningocele, meningomyelocele, myeloschisis, and spina bifida occulta. The latter is not functionally or cosmetically obvious and, as a result, is not diagnosed until later in life (30% are diagnosed in adults) (1).

The incidence of open neural tube defects vary from 1/3000 live births in the United States to 1/1000 in Great Britain (2). with 85% located in the lumbosacral region (5).

Anatomy and Physiology

The neural tube is formed during the 3rd and 4th week of gestation by differentiation of the neural plate with subsequent invagination and closure. The neural tube closes initially in the region of the medulla and proceeds rostrally and caudally. Interruption of this process results in a variety of midline defects of the neural elements and their coverings including the meninges and the overlying bones (1).

Spina bifida refers to a deficit in the closure of the spinal canal and can be classified into four types of abnormalities. Meningocele consists of a cystic dilation of the meninges and a deficit in the overlying skin (Fig. 41.1.E). No neurologic deficit is present because the spinal cord and nerve roots are normal. Meningomyelocele is identical to a meningocele but is associated with abnormalities of the spinal cord and nerve roots (Fig. 41.1.E). Neurologic deficits occur below the level of the lesion. Myeloschisis is a spina bifida with exposure of the spinal cord and nerve roots but without a cystic covering of meninges. Neurologic deficit is present below the lesion. Spina bifida occulta is nonfusion of one or more of the posterior arches of the spine usually in the lumbosacral region. This lesion may be associated with an underlying diastematomyelia, spinal lipoma, or dermoid (1). Some other anomalies associated with meningomyelocele include club feet, hip dislocation, rib anomalies, kyphoscoliosis, horseshoe kidney, and neurogenic bladder (2). The quality of survival depends on prompt management by an experienced and skilled team. The level of the lesion determines the degree of neurologic deficit. Preservation of existing function of the lower extremities is enhanced by surgical correction within the first 48 hours although with higher lesions, earlier surgery does little to improve quality of survival (1). The deci-

Chapter 41
Emergency
Management of
Selected Congenital
Anomalies

529

sion to repair a high meningomyelocele or myeloschisis involves moral and ethical considerations beyond the scope of this chapter. With immediate closure, infants born with spina bifida have a 90% chance of survival (1). Without repair, many die from untreated hydrocephalus, infection, or renal failure secondary to their neurogenic bladder.

Indications

Initial management of neural tube lesions is conservative, noninvasive, and not associated with adverse effects and is therefore indicated in those instances in which the diagnosis is known or suspected. Early temporizing measures are important in avoiding infection, desiccation and injury to the involved structures and in improving the eventual outcome. The physical finding of a midline defect along the back is the most obvious suggestion of such a lesion. In cases of meningomyelocele or myeloschisis, neurologic abnormalities in the lower extremities such as decreased tone and lack of spontaneous movement may be noted at birth.

Equipment

Radiant warmer
Sterile saline
Sterile gauze
Clear plastic film wrap (such as Saran® or Glad®)
Support (intravenous fluid bags)
Intravenous access equipment (Chapters 40, 75)
Intravenous antibiotics (ampicillin, gentamicin)

Procedure

Immediately following delivery, if no other resuscitation measures are needed, the infant should be placed in a prone position, and the meningomyelocele or meningocele protected from drying, trauma, or infection. This is generally accomplished with saline-soaked sterile gauze covered by a clear plastic wrap (5) (Fig. 41.2.B).

If active airway management or umbilical vessel catheterization is required, the infant can be maintained in the supine position by raising the shoulders with bilateral support using, for example, bags of intravenous fluids (Fig. 41.3). Once the necessary procedures have been completed, the child can be placed

in the prone position. Parenteral use of antibiotics usually varies from unit to unit and with the existing flora. Ampicillin and gentamicin are generally adequate before transport. Intravenous hydration should be initiated at normal maintenance for transport.

Complications

Excessive handling or force may result in perforation of the cystic lesion, introduction of infection, or further injury to involved neurologic structures.

Diaphragmatic Hernia

Anatomy and Physiology

When the fusion of the diaphragmatic leaflets fails to happen by 8 weeks' gestation, a defect occurs in the diaphragm which can vary from several centimeters to complete absence of the involved hemidiaphragm (1). Of these, 85% are left sided at the foramen of Bochdalek, and 1% are bilateral and uniformly fatal. They occur as an isolated defect in 1 to 2/1000 live births (1, 5).

Major morbidity and high fatality rates of infants with diaphragmatic hernia occur because of the effects of the herniated abdominal viscera into the thoracic cavity and interference with the normal development of the lungs (Fig. 41.1.D). The severity of the defect is related to the timing and degree of the prenatal visceral herniation (1). The subsequent lung hypoplasia is more severe on the side of the hernia, but the contralateral side also is affected. An infant with congenital diaphragmatic hernia suffers both hypoperfusion and hypoventilation of the lungs by the herniated bowel (2). The latter occurs as a result of the arrested development (hypoplasia) and compression of the lung (2). Hypoventilation leads primarily to hypoxia, hypercarbia, and acidosis, decreasing further the already compromised pulmonary blood flow by increasing the pulmonary vascular resistance.

Pulmonary hypoperfusion is a result of a decrease in the cross sectional arterial surface area and from vascular smooth muscle cell hyperplasia. Both contribute to the exaggerated vasoconstriction caused by the hypoxia and acidosis. Cardiac dysfunction with a subsequent increase in pulmonary venous pressure and decrease in systemic pressure may

Chapter 41
Emergency
Management of
Selected Congenital
Anomalies

530

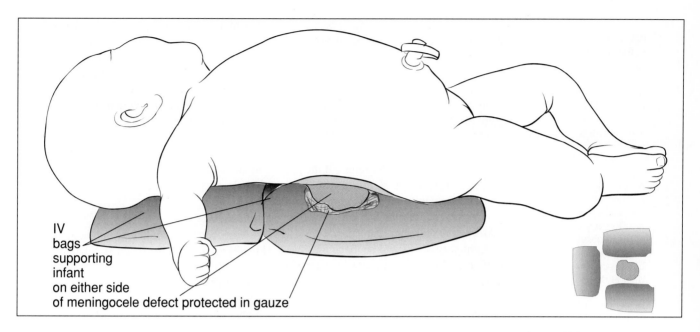

IV
bags
supporting
infant
on either side
of meningocele defect protected in gauze

Figure 41.3.
Support for infant with a
neural tube defect
requiring supine positioning.

occur as a consequence of the hypoxia or the associated left-sided cardiac hypoplasia (2).

Indications

A diaphragmatic hernia should be considered in infants who develop respiratory distress within the first day of life. These infants clinically may have a scaphoid abdomen and an asymmetric or distended chest (6). As the infant feeds or swallows air, the herniated bowel becomes distended and the infant's clinical condition deteriorates. Tachypnea and cyanosis may occur (cyanosis without dyspnea is more commonly associated with a congenital heart lesion) (3). On physical examination, the apex of the heart is frequently displaced to the right. Breath sounds may not be heard on the affected side, although this may be difficult to appreciate as transmitted breath sounds from the opposite side are frequently heard. Retractions and grunting may be present. Bowel sounds in the chest are not a reliable finding (3).

Diagnosis of a diaphragmatic hernia is usually made by a plain radiograph of the chest and abdomen showing intestinal loops in the chest cavity on the affected side and the lung compressed into a small area at the apex. Placement of a nasogastric tube before the radiograph may aid in the diagnosis if the stomach is in the chest. If in doubt, a small amount of contrast material can be given through the nasogastric tube.

Equipment

Standard neonatal resuscitation equipment (Chapter 38)

Endotracheal intubation equipment (Chapter 16)
8- and 10-French nasogastric tubes
Umbilical vessel catheterization equipment (Chapter 40)
Sedative agent
Paralytic agent
Tolazoline
Dopamine and dobutamine

Procedure

All infants should be intubated and ventilated with 100% O_2. If diagnosis is suspected, bag-valve-mask (BVM) ventilation should be avoided to prevent filling the intestines with air. Some authorities recommend paralysis with pancuronium to prevent swallowing and noncompliance with ventilation (3). Sedation with fentanyl as necessary may be an alternative to paralysis. High inspiratory pressures are often necessary for lung inflation; however, pneumothoraces are a frequent complication, and physicians should be prepared to insert thoracostomy tubes when necessary (Chapter 30). An 8- or 10-French nasogastric tube should be placed and the stomach deflated by intermittent or continuous suctioning. Positioning of the infant in reverse Trendelenburg also may decrease pressure of the abdominal contents on the lungs. Umbilical arterial (UA) and venous lines should be placed immediately. The venous line provides access for resuscitation. The arterial line minimizes repeated punctures for blood sampling as these can cause the infant to desaturate. Oxygenation can be determined with arterial blood gases drawn either from the right radial artery (preductal) or a pulse oximeter probe placed on the right hand. This should be compared with postductal measurements from the UA line. Blood pH should be kept greater than or equal to 7.40, and the $PaCO_2$ should be kept at 25 to 30 torr and PaO_2 at 100 +/–20 torr range. If the preductal PaO_2 is less than 80 torr, a vasodilator such as prescoline (tolazoline) may be used. Dopamine and dobutamine are generally used for blood pressure maintenance.

Arrangements should be made for transfer of the infant to a neonatal center with extracorporeal membrane oxygenation (ECMO) capabilities, because adequate oxygenation and ventilation of these infants is difficult, if not impossible. ECMO has improved the survival rates of infants diagnosed with a diaphragmatic hernia to 67% (7).

Complications

Infants with congenital diaphragmatic hernias require accurate diagnosis and aggressive management to survive. Diagnosis can be confused with eventration of the diaphragm, Pentalogy of Cantrell, an esophageal hiatus, Morgagni hernia, and congenital cystic disease of the lung (6). The stomach bubble in the chest may be misdiagnosed as a pneumothorax followed by inappropriate chest tube insertion. High inspiratory pressures necessary to adequately oxygenate and ventilate infants with diaphragmatic hernias place them at high risk for pneumothoraces. Using tolazoline may precipitate hypotension, which can be treated with volume infusion, administration of pressors, or interrupting the infusion of tolazoline. Additional complications are the same as those associated with individual procedures.

Choanal Atresia

Anatomy and Physiology

Choanal atresia is theorized to be the result of a failure of the invaginating nasal pits to rupture through the oronasal membrane separating the nasal pits from the oral cavity. This process normally occurs during the 7th week of gestation. Choanal atresia occurs in approximately 1 per 8000 live births and can be unilateral or bilateral although the unilateral form is more common. Obstruction generally occurs at a distance of approximately 3 cm from the opening of the nares (1). Ninety percent of the time the obstruction is bony and is membranous in the remainder (2). Associated anomalies are common. If diagnosis is missed, infants with choanal atresia are at risk for developing respiratory insufficiency if they do not establish oral breathing (1).

Indications

Because newborn infants are obligate nasal breathers, if the obstruction is bilateral, infants with choanal atresia will present immediately after birth with a cyclic respiratory obstruction pattern that improves when the infant cries or when an oral airway is in place (2). Diagnosis is suspected by failure to pass a 6-French suction catheter down the infant's nostril. A wisp of cotton also can be placed in front of the infant's nostril while occluding the opposite nostril and mouth. If the nostril is patent, the cotton should move toward the nose with inspiration and away with expiration (2). Confirmation is by computerized tomography.

Procedure

If the emergency physician suspects the diagnosis, an oral airway can be placed or endotracheal intubation may be performed as temporizing measures in the distressed infant until surgery. Unilateral choanal atresia may remain undetected for years.

SUMMARY

Initial management of infants with congenital anomalies follows standard resuscitation procedures. In addition, certain exposed structures will require protection from desiccation, infection, and injury. Early temporizing measures are crucial in determining the eventual outcome of patients with congenital anomalies, independent of the definitive surgical procedures. Management can be performed with equipment available in the standard ED or delivery room. Infants diagnosed with congenital anomalies require timely transport to tertiary care centers equipped with experienced surgeons and subspecialists capable of providing definitive care.

SUMMARY

Abdominal Wall Defects

1. Place infant under radiant warmer
2. Keep viscera moist with sterile, saline-soaked gauze dressings
3. Ensure that bowel or sac is not kinked
4. Place infant in sterile intestinal bag
5. Insert 8- or 10-French nasogastric tube
6. Initiate fluid resuscitation with 10 to 20 mL/kg normal saline followed by D10 ¼ normal saline at twice maintenance rate
7. Start antibiotics (ampicillin and gentamicin) after baseline blood culture is obtained
8. Arrange transport to tertiary care center

Neural Tube Defects

1. Place infant in prone position for initial resuscitation
2. If intubation or umbilical vessel catheterization is required, place infant in supine position with bilateral support to prevent pressure against lesion
3. Apply saline-soaked sterile gauze to lesion
4. Cover area with clear plastic wrap
5. Begin broad spectrum antibiotics (ampicillin and gentamicin)
6. Initiate D10 ¼ normal saline maintenance intravenous hydration

Diaphragmatic Hernia

1. Intubate and ventilate with 100% oxygen; avoid BVM ventilation.
2. Paralyze or sedate infant
3. Place 8- or 10-French nasogastric tube to continuous or intermittent suction
4. Place infant in reverse Trendelenburg position
5. Place umbilical artery and umbilical vein lines
6. Obtain preductal arterial blood gas or pulse oximeter reading from right arm
7. Maintain pH at 7.40 and $PaCO_2$ at 25 to 30 torr, PaO_2 at 100 $\pm$ 20 torr
8. Consider tolazine if the $PaO_2 < 80$
9. Maintain blood pressure with dopamine or dobutamine

Choanal Atresia

1. Assess nasal airway with 6-French catheter or respiratory motion of cotton wisp
2. Relieve respiratory distress with oral airway or endotrocheal intubation as necessary

REFERENCES

1. Fanaroff AA, Martin RJ. Neonatal-perinatal medicine, diseases of the fetus and infant. St. Louis: Mosby, 1991.
2. Donn SM, Faix, RG. Neonatal emergencies. Mount Kisco, NY: Futura Publishing Co. Inc., 1991.
3. Lister J, Irving IM. Neonatal surgery. London: Butterworth Co. Ltd., 1990.
4. Stringer MD, Brereton RJ, Wright VM. Controversies in the management of gastroschisis: a study of 40 patients. Arch Dis Child 1991;66:34–36.
5. Seeds JW, Azizkhan RG. Congenital malformations, antenatal diagnosis, perinatal management and counseling, Rockville, MD: Aspen Publishers, 1990.
6. Altman PR, Stylianos S. Pediatric surgery. Pediatr Clin of North Am 1993 Dec; 4016.
7. Mems KP, Van MD, Newman KD, Anderson KD, Short BL. Effect of ECMO on survival of infants with congenital diaphragmatic hernia. J Pediatr 1990;117:954–960.
8. Raffensperger JG. Swenson's pediatric surgery. 5th ed. Norwalk, CT: Appleton & Lange, 1990.

Chapter 41
Emergency
Management of
Selected Congenital
Anomalies

533

CHAPTER 42

HEEL STICKS

Susan Duffy and Dale Steele

INTRODUCTION

Capillary blood sampling by means of a heel stick is used to obtain blood for hematologic, biochemical, and blood gas analysis in elective and emergent situations. It is most useful in young infants in whom venous access is difficult or limited. It is a relatively simple procedure that can be performed by physicians, nurses, EMTs, or other trained personnel.

ANATOMY AND PHYSIOLOGY

The primary arterial and venous blood supply for the heel skin is located at the junction of the dermis and subcutaneous tissues. In infants the distance from the surface of the heel to this junction is quite constant at 0.35 to 1.6 mm (1). The distance to the calcaneus from the heel surface increases with infant weight. The mean depth from the skin to the calcaneus is deeper in the medial and lateral portions of the heel than in the posterior aspect (4). Calcaneal depth also increases with growth; however, after 1 year of age callus formation in the heel precludes using this site.

Boundaries of the calcaneus can be located by extending a line posteriorly from between the fourth and fifth toes running parallel to the lateral aspect of the heel, and a line extending posteriorly from the middle of the great toe running parallel to the medial portion of the heel. To avoid calcaneal puncture, heel sticks should be performed only in the areas delineated in Figure 42.1.

INDICATIONS

Heel puncture samples are useful for most common laboratory studies that require frequent measurement, including hemoglobin/hematocrit and electrolyte determination. It is most practical in the newborn and especially the premature infant, but can be performed in children up to 1 year of age. If hemolysis, venous stasis, or bacterial contamination will interfere with interpretation, samples are better obtained by vascular puncture.

Heel puncture is not recommended when poor peripheral perfusion (e.g., shock) is present, or compromised blood flow to an extremity, local infection or edema, significant polycythemia, or there is a need for an accurate measurement of PaO_2.

EQUIPMENT

Gloves
Warm, wet towel or hot pack
Alcohol swab
Sterile petroleum jelly
Sterile gauze
Detachable capillary blood collector
Collection tubes
    capillary blood gases: heparinized glass capillary tubes
    chemistries: microtainer tube with serum separator available
    complete blood count: microtainer tube with heparin or EDTA
    hemoglobin/hematocrit (spun): heparinized glass capillary tube

Figure 42.1.
Acceptable sites for heel
stick puncture illustrated by
shaded area.

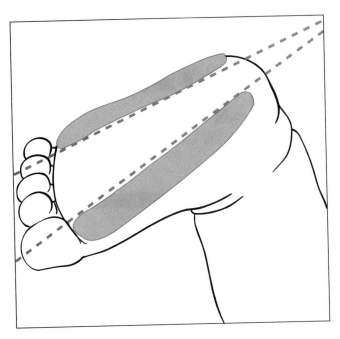

Capillary cap adapters
Clay pad
Incision device
    #11 surgical blade
    lancet
    automated disposable incision device
    (e.g., Tenderfoot®, Surgicutt®)

The blade and the lancet are subject to variability in operator technique and lack features to control puncture depth. The lancet compresses the dermis and does not allow for free flow of blood. Automated heel stick devices allow collection of increased volumes of blood more quickly with reduced hemolysis (2).

PROCEDURE

A warm, wet towel is applied to the heel for approximately 5 minutes before the procedure to increase blood flow to the skin surface. The heel is cleansed with alcohol and allowed to dry (alcohol on the skin may lead to erroneously high glucose values). The leg is held in a dependent position while the patient is supine. The heel is held at an 80 to 90° angle to the leg. The incision device is then used to puncture the heel perpendicular to the skin on the most medial or lateral portion of the heel as demonstrated in Figure 42.2.A. The posterior curve of the heel should not be punctured and any previous puncture sites that may be infected should be avoided. The

puncture should not exceed 2.5 mm in depth. Milking the heel may activate clotting and cause hemolysis.

The first drop of blood is wiped away with gauze (Fig. 42.2.B) and subsequent drops are collected using the plastic lip on the capillary blood collector (Fig 42.2.C). A thin layer of sterile petroleum jelly promotes droplet formation on the skin surface and facilitates collection. Once collection is completed, the clinician applies pressure to the puncture site with a sterile gauze for 2 to 3 minutes. The detachable capillary blood collector is removed with a twisting motion and the specimen is capped (Fig. 42.2.C).

For collection in a glass capillary tube, one end of the heparinized capillary tube is touched to the drop of blood. The tube is held at about a 20° angle from horizontal, and fills by capillary action (Fig. 42.2.C). Both ends of the tube should remain unoccluded during the collection. For blood gas sampling the tube should be filled as completely as possible to minimize exposure to the external air. Once the tube is full, the free end is occluded with a gloved fingertip to prevent air entry when removing it from the site. The collection end of the tubes for chemistry or hematocrit samples is inserted into clay to form a

Figure 42.2.
A. Heel puncture in safe area.
B. Collection of specimen.
C. Capping of specimen.

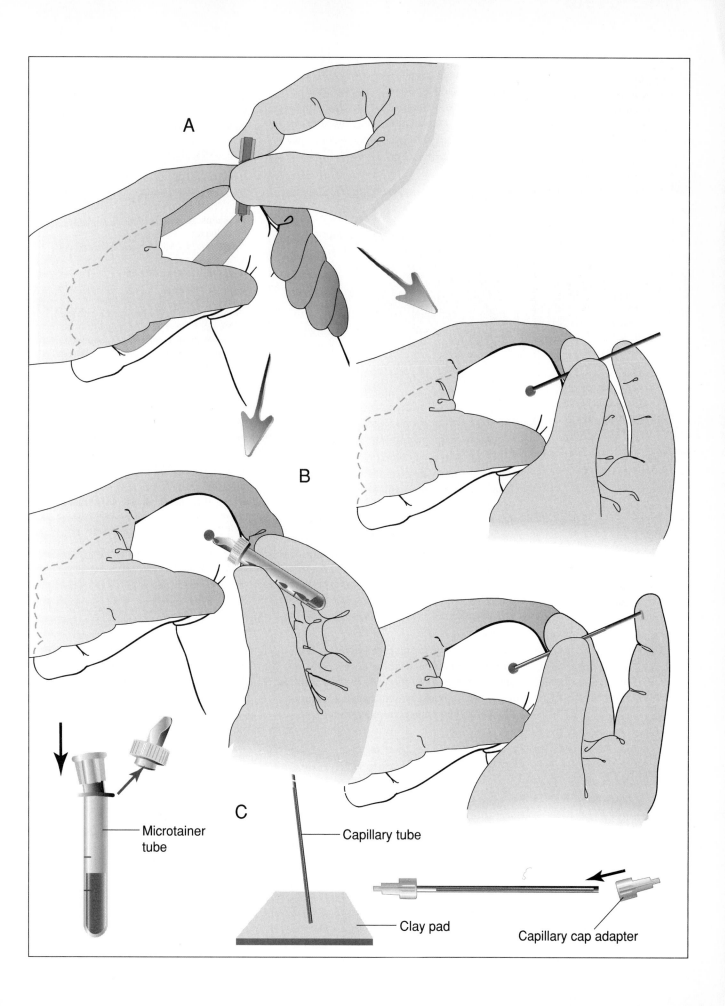

A

B

C

Microtainer
tube

Capillary tube

Clay pad

Capillary cap adapter

plug. Both ends are plugged for blood gases. Plugging should be done gently to avoid inadvertant tube breakage. Alternatively, plastic capillary cap adapters may be used in place of clay but must be applied to both sides of the capillary tube (Fig. 42.2.C).

COMPLICATIONS

The most significant potential complication from heel puncture is infection subsequent to puncture of the calcaneus. This can result in necrotizing chondritis or osteomyelitis. Additional complications include (*a*) calcified nodules of the heel, (*b*) hemolysis of the blood sample resulting in falsely elevated bilirubin and potassium levels, (*c*) erroneously high glucose values secondary to alcohol from the swab, (*d*) inaccurate pCO_2 and pO_2 values from poor blood flow, (*e*) elevated hematocrit from hemoconcentration, and (*f*) pain from the procedure (3, 5–7).

An inadequate volume of blood collected for a complete blood count in relation to the amount of anticoagulant may result in an inaccurately low hematocrit and hemoglobin. An excessive volume will frequently result in clotting of the specimen. Capillary tube breakage during plugging may result in injury and percutaneous blood exposure to the physician

SUMMARY

Heel puncture is a quick and simple procedure that is particularly useful in young infants. When performed correctly it is a safe method for obtaining interpretable laboratory samples when venipuncture is difficult.

REFERENCES

1. Blumenfeld TA, Turi GK, Blanc WA. Recommended site and depth of newborn heelstick punctures based on anatomical measurements and histopathology. Lancet 1979 1:230–233..
2. Paes B, Janes M, Vegh P, LaDuca F, Andrew M. A comparative study of heel stick devices for infant blood collection. AJDC 1993 March;147:346–348.

3. Boris LC, Helleland H. Growth disturbance of the hind part of the foot following osteomyelitis of the calcaneus in the newborn. J Bone Joint Surg 1986;68A(2):302–305.
4. Reiner CB, Meites S, Hayes JR. Optimal sites and depths for skin puncture of infants and children as assessed from anatomical measurements. Clin Chem Aeta 1990;36(3):547–549.
5. McLain BI, Evans J, Dear PR. Comparison of capillary and arterial blood gas measurements in neonates. AJDC 1988;63:743–747.
6. Lauer BA, Altenberger KM. Outbreak of staphylococcal infections following heel puncture for blood sampling. AJDC 1981;135(3):277–278.
7. Sell EJ, Hansen RC, Struck-Pierce S. Calcified nodules on the heel: a complication of neonatal intensive care. J Pediatr 1980;96:473–475.

SUGGESTED READINGS

Burns EJ. Development and evaluation of a new instrument for safe heel stick sampling of neonates. Lab Med 1981 July;20(7):481–483.
Short BL, Avery GB. Capillary blood sampling. In: Fletcher MA, MacDonald MG, Avery G, eds. Atlas of procedures in neonatology. Philadelphia: JB Lippincott, 1983, pp. 68–74.

NEUROLOGIC AND NEUROSURGICAL PROCEDURES

Section Editor: James F. Wiley II

CHAPTER 43

LUMBAR PUNCTURE

Kathleen M. Cronan and James F. Wiley II

INTRODUCTION

Lumbar puncture (LP) is used to obtain cerebrospinal fluid (CSF) for diagnostic and therapeutic purposes. A relatively simple procedure, it is most commonly performed in neonates and infants who, due to anatomic characteristics and the nature of their illness, are prone to respiratory compromise during the procedure (1, 2). The potential for complications during and following lumbar puncture therefore dictates that it be performed in an area equipped for resuscitation and by a health professional well trained in the procedure and well versed in the appropriate indications and contraindications for lumbar puncture. In some patients, lumbar puncture can only be safely performed after brain imaging indicates that increased intracranial pressure or a space-occupying brain mass is not present. In other patients with shock or respiratory compromise, in whom meningitis or encephalitis is suspected, stabilization of the patient and presumptive antibiotic therapy must precede lumbar puncture. These considerations require careful patient evaluation before performing LP.

ANATOMY AND PHYSIOLOGY

The CSF resides in the space between the pia mater and the arachnoid mater that surrounds the brain, spinal cord, ventricles, aqueduct, and the central canal of the spinal cord. The majority of CSF is formed in the choroid plexuses of the lateral ventricles. After formation, CSF travels out the foramina of Luschka and Magendie into the subarachnoid space, around the spinal column, and over the cerebrum. The CSF is primarily absorbed by the arachnoid villi located adjacent to the sagittal sinus and returned to the venous circulation (3).

Average total volume of CSF in children is 90 mL; in full-term infants it is 40 mL. One quarter of the CSF is located in the ventricles and the remainder in the subarachnoid space. It provides physical cushioning between bony structures and the brain and spinal cord (4). CSF expands and contracts to buffer intracranial changes in the size of brain, as well as arterial and venous volumes in pathologic conditions such as cortical atrophy or parenchymal injury (5). CSF also has an important role in transferring chemical by-products from the brain to the venous circulation (6).

At birth, the inferior end of the spinal cord is opposite the body of the third lumbar vertebra (L3). As the child's spinal cord grows, the vertebral column grows more rapidly. In the adult, the caudal aspect of the cord lies opposite the inferior border of the first lumbar vertebra. Notably the spinal cord rises slightly when the trunk of the body is bent forward (3).

Structures pierced during median lumbar puncture are (in order): skin, subcutaneous fat, supraspinal ligament, interspinal ligament, ligamentum flavum, dura mater, and arachnoid mater (Fig. 43.1). In older patients, supraspinal and interspinal ligaments may be calcified, which requires a lateral approach (Fig. 43.2). This situation, however, is rare in

Figure 43.1.
Anatomy of the lumbar
spine.

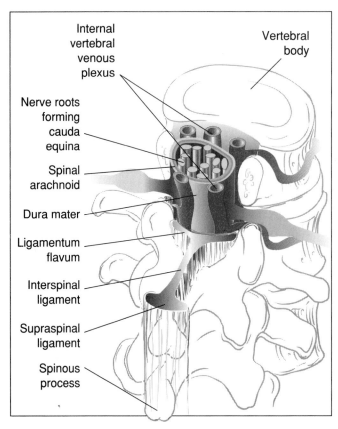

Internal
vertebral
venous
plexus

Vertebral
body

Nerve roots
forming
cauda
equina

Spinal
arachnoid

Dura mater

Ligamentum
flavum

Interspinal
ligament

Supraspinal
ligament

Spinous
process

children and the median approach is most commonly used (7).

INDICATIONS

In the pediatric patient, the primary emergent reason for LP is suspicion of CNS infection. Fever, paradoxic irritability (increased crying when held), or bulging anterior fontanel are classic findings associated with bacterial meningitis in the infant. Fever, headache, neck pain, confusion, or meningismus manifested by Brudzinski sign (pain on flexion of the neck) or Kernig sign (pain on extension of the knee when the hips are flexed to 90°) are commonly present in older children with bacterial meningitis. Signs of meningeal irritation may be subtle in neonates, young infants, and in patients on oral antibiotics with partially treated meningitis (8). Furthermore, patients with viral meningitis often have fewer clinical signs. Patients with a facial cellulitis caused by *Haemophilus influenzae* type B or with a complex febrile seizure are also at increased risk for concurrent meningitis (9). It is important to remember that meningismus

may not be present in a comatose patient or when neurologic impairment exists. Furthermore, meningismus may be present in the absence of meningitis in children with posterior fossa brain tumor, retropharyngeal abscess, upper lobe pneumonia, cervical diskitis, and pyelonephritis (8).

Suspected spontaneous subarachnoid hemorrhage constitutes another urgent indication for lumbar puncture. Patients with suspected intracranial bleeding should have a brain imaging study before LP in most instances. A small percentage of subarachnoid hemorrhages are not detectable on CT scans of the head and LP would be the sole method of diagnosing this problem (10). Lumbar puncture also is performed in a variety of nonacute situations such as instillation of chemotherapeutic agents, administration of radiopaque dye for spinal cord imaging, diagnosis of CNS metastases, treatment of pseudotumor cerebri, and measuring of opening pressure to rule out specific disease entities (9).

Contraindications to lumbar puncture include the presence of infection in the tissues near the proposed puncture site, cardiorespiratory instability of the patient, an uncorrected severe coagulopathy, evidence of spinal cord trauma or spinal cord compression, and signs of progressive cerebral herniation. In these situations the LP should be withheld. If infection is suspected, then appropriate antibiotic therapy should be given presumptively.

When an elevation in intracranial pressure exists as a result of space-occupying lesion, the clinician must use extreme caution and in most instances should not perform LP. Presence of a brain tumor, cerebral hemorrhage, cavernous sinus thrombosis, brain abscess, and epidural or subdural collection comprise the most common diagnoses in this group. Focal neurologic findings in conjunction with these conditions should be interpreted as a sign of impending herniation and contraindicate LP. Dexamethasone or mannitol infusion may be helpful if increased intracranial pressure from an unsuspected mass lesion is encountered or signs of cerebral herniation occur during or after LP (11, 12).

Patients with a known spinal column deformity should have the procedure performed under fluoroscopy. Lumbar puncture cannot access the subarachnoid space in patients who have undergone posterior spinal fusion in the lumbar region. These patients require a cisternal tap for CSF collection which should be performed by a neurosurgeon. In all situations presented here, risks and potential benefits of LP must be evaluated thoroughly before performing the procedure.

Equipment

Sterile gloves
Betadine solution
Lumbar puncture tray:
    Sterile drapes
    Betadine swabs or tray to pour betadine
    Sterile sponges for preparing the puncture site
    Lidocaine 1% without epinephrine and/or EMLA cream (eutectic mixture of lidocaine 2.5% and prilocaine 2.5%)
    Sterile 3 mL syringe with needle for lidocaine injection
    Sterile collecting tubes
    Sterile spinal needle (Table 43.1)
    Manometer (may be a separate sterile item to be added to tray)

Procedure

Indication for lumbar puncture and potential complications should be explained fully to the patient (if appropriate) and the parents. Many institutions require written informed consent before the procedure. Monitoring of heart rate, respirations, and oxygen saturation should be strongly considered during the procedure, particularly in neonates, young infants, and children with any degree of cardiorespiratory compromise. Airway and resuscitation equipment should be immediately available. If the lumbar puncture is being performed for elective reasons, EMLA cream may be applied over the puncture site (see Figure 43.3) approximately 60 minutes before the procedure (see also Chapter 37).

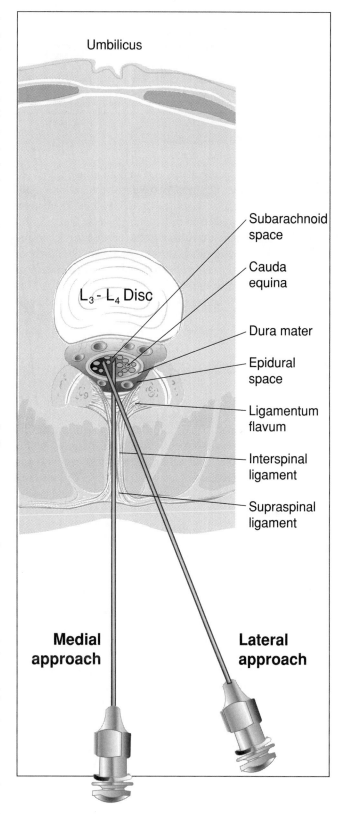

Figure 43.2.
Spinal needle access into the subarachnoid space by the median or lateral approach.

Table 43.1
Spinal Needle Size by Age

Premature infant	22 gauge or smaller, 1.5 inch, plastic hub preferred
Neonate–2 yr	22 gauge, 1.5 inch, plastic hub preferred
2–12 yr*	22 gauge, 2.5 inch
Over 12 yr	20 or 22 gauge, 3.5 inch

* May need larger needle depending on patient habitus.

Achieving and maintaining proper patient position is the most crucial and challenging aspect of LP in children. The patient is placed on the examining table and the clinician performing the procedure is seated comfortably next to the table. The goals of positioning are to stretch the ligamenta flava and to increase the interlaminar spaces. The two positions most widely used in the pediatric population are the lateral recumbent and the sitting position (Fig. 43.3). For the lateral recumbent position, the patient lays on his or her side near the edge of the examining table next to the clinician performing the procedure. The neck is flexed and the knees are drawn upward by placing one arm under the child's knees and the other arm around the posterior aspect of the neck. By grasping his or her own wrists, the assistant can maintain a greater degree of control over the restraint of the child. The assistant also should ensure that the shoulders and hips are perpendicular to the bed, thus keeping the spinal column in line without rotation. To increase the size of the interlaminar spaces, the cooperative patient can be asked to fully bend his or her back toward the physician.

Lumbar puncture can be done in the sitting position in older children who are cooperative and in very young infants who are unlikely to struggle and may have increased respiratory distress in the lateral recumbent position (2). An older child may sit with feet over the side of the bed and with neck and upper body flexed over a pillow or a pile of blankets held in the lap. With an infant, the assistant holds the patient in a sitting position with an arm and a leg in each hand while supporting the head to prevent excess flexion of the neck (Fig. 43.3).

Once the patient is positioned, the upper aspect of the posterior superior iliac crests are palpated and an imaginary line between them is pictured. This line intersects the midline just above the fourth lumbar spine. The inter-spaces between L3-L4 and L4-L5 can then be located, and one site is chosen for puncture (Fig. 43.3). In children outside infancy, the interspace between L2-L3 also may be used for LP.

After the puncture site has been selected, it should be cleansed with iodine-soaked, sterile gauze using an enlarging circle that begins with the precise puncture site. The betadine solution may then be removed with alcohol in the same manner. Sterile towels are draped around the operative site allowing for

SUMMARY
1. Determine patient ability to safely undergo lumbar puncture
2. Explain procedure to parents and patient (if applicable)
3. Correctly position patient in lateral recumbent or sitting position
4. With patient positioned, choose puncture site by lining up upper aspects of superior posterior iliac crests and finding L3-L4 or L4-L5 spinal interspace
5. Cleanse area with iodine solution, drape, and relocate puncture site
6. Anesthetize skin and subcutaneous tissue with 1% lidocaine infiltration (Chapter 37)
7. For median approach (preferred if no ligamenous calcification), identify interspace with thumb of one hand and direct needle:
   Lateral recumbent position—parallel to bed and cephalad (toward umbilicus)
   Sitting—perpendicular to skin (slightly caudad)
8. For lateral approach, puncture skin just above transverse process of L3 or L4 and direct it medially and upward (cephalad)
9. Keeping stylet in place, advance spinal needle until a loss of resistance or a "pop" is felt; in infants, a pop may not be felt and the spinal needle should be advanced approximately 1 to 2 cm
10. If performing manometry, attach manometer and stopcock to spinal needle; extend patient's neck and legs as much as possible and read the CSF pressure
11. Remove stylet or manometer and collect fluid in sterile tubes
12. Once fluid is obtained, remeasure CSF pressure (if indicated), replace stylet, and remove spinal needle
13. Dress lumbar puncture site with adhesive bandage.

Figure 43.3.
Lateral recumbent and sitting positions for lumbar puncture.

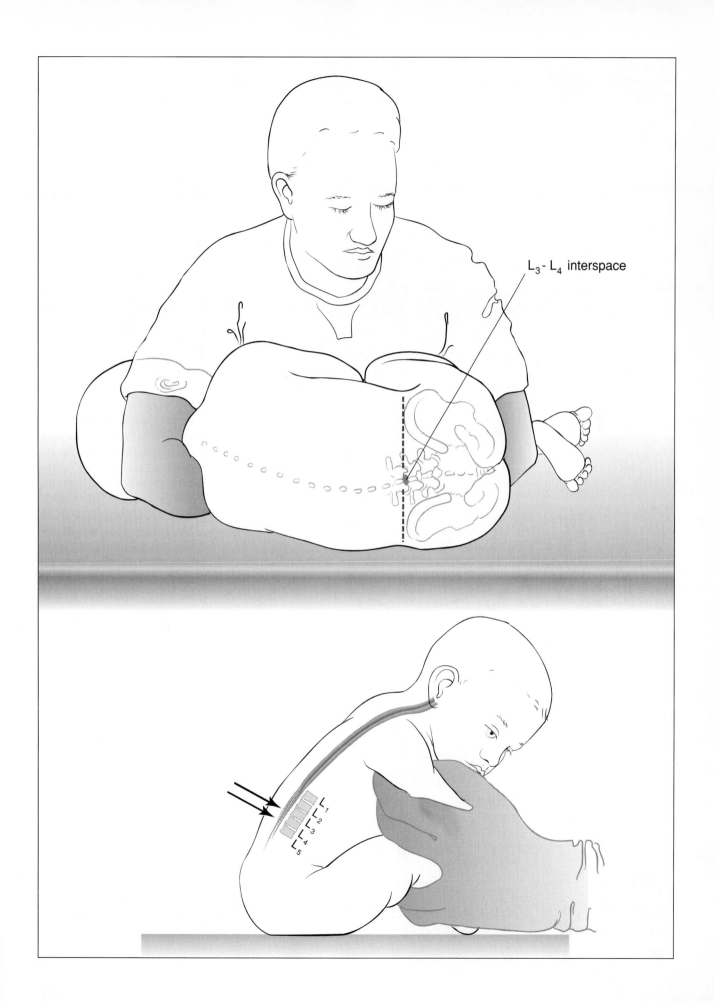

L_3 - L_4 interspace

L_1
L_2
L_3
L_4
L_5

Figure 43.4.
Spinal needle placement
using one or two hands.

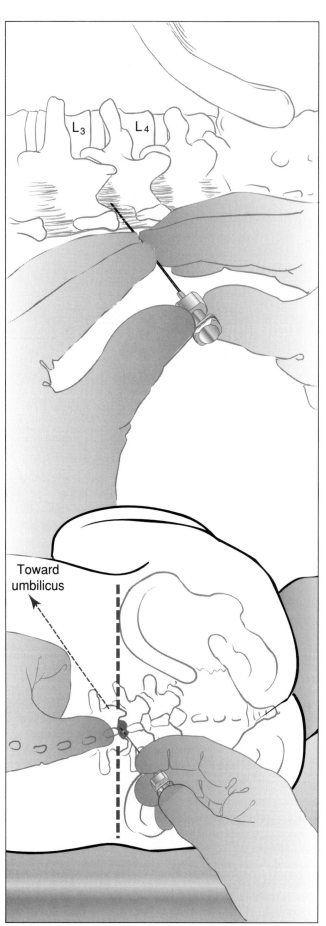

Toward
umbilicus

good exposure. The puncture site should be relocated as previously described, and the site can be marked with a fingernail depression in the skin.

The skin and subcutaneous tissues are then anesthetized using 1% lidocaine (Chapter 37) or the EMLA patch is removed. The practice of withholding local anesthesia for this procedure is strongly discouraged. Local anesthesia has been shown to decrease the pain response to LP without hampering its successful completion in neonates (13). Benefits of local anesthesia for LP become even clearer for older children. In rare instances, sedation is required to adequately perform the LP (Chapter 35).

When placing the spinal needle, two possible approaches can be used. The median approach positions the needle through the supraspinal ligament and the lateral approach places the needle just lateral to the ligament (Fig. 43.2). In both cases the needle may be held in one hand or with both hands. When the needle is held in one hand, the clinician can ensure good alignment of the needle by placing the tip of the thumb of the noninserting hand on the spinous process above the space being entered. When holding the needle with both hands, the thumbs are placed on either side of the needle hub and the index fingers are used to support the needle (Fig. 43.4).

In the median approach, the needle with the stylet in place is positioned exactly in the midline. The bevel of the spinal needle should be positioned horizontally if the lateral recumbent position is used or vertically if the sitting position is used so that the dura mater is pierced parallel to its fibers which run longitudinally down the spinal cord. This precaution decreases the amount of CSF leak and postspinal headache (4). The needle is then inserted cephalad toward the umbilicus if the patient is in the lateral recumbent position or slightly caudad if the patient is in the sitting position. In the lateral approach, the needle should be inserted lateral to the upper border of the spinous process of L3 or L4. It should then be directed slightly medial and slightly upward (cephalad) to avoid contact with the supraspinal ligament.

With either the median or the lateral approach, a degree of resistance during insertion of the needle is appreciated. When the ligamentum flavum is penetrated a loss of resistance may be felt, especially in older children. This change in resistance is again experienced when the dura is penetrated. This second loss of resistance is often referred to as a "pop." If a pop is felt, the stylet is removed from the needle and fluid is obtained. In neonates and infants, the pop may not be evident and the stylet should be removed after advancing the needle an appropriate distance (approximately 1 to 2 cm in infants under 6 months) to check for fluid return. Depth of needle insertion also may be calculated using the body surface area: depth (in cm) = 0.77 + [2.56 × BSA], where BSA is body surface area in m^2 (14). The spinal needle should be supported with one hand during fluid collection (particularly in infants) to prevent dural tugging, a potential source of local pain and post-spinal CSF leak.

Measurement of CSF opening pressure is recommended during any LP in which it can be accurately performed. The struggling infant or child precludes the accurate measurement of opening pressure. The measurement is most reliable in a relaxed patient who is in the lateral recumbent position. When a free flow of CSF is obtained, the pressure manometer should be immediately attached to the needle hub via a three-way stopcock. CSF then fills the manometer column and is measured as the highest level achieved in the column. This measurement should not end until respiratory variation (rise and fall of the fluid meniscus with breathing) is attained (Fig. 43.5). Normal pressure is 5 to 20 cm H_2O in a relaxed patient who has neck and legs extended and 10 to 28 cm H_2O in a re-

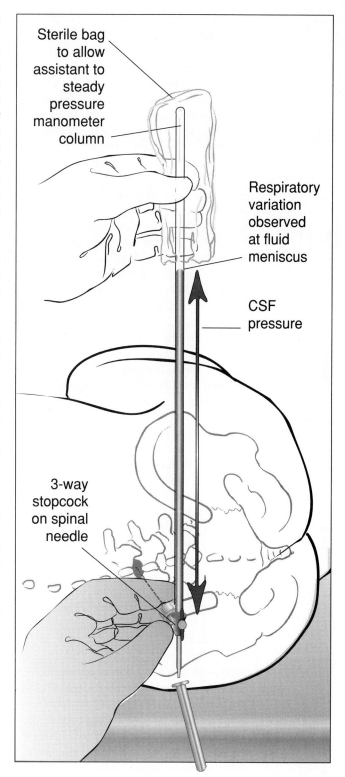

Figure 43.5.
Manometer measurement of CSF pressure.

laxed patient who has neck and legs flexed (15). The manometer should be supported at the connection to the spinal needle and at the top of the measuring column. It is helpful to have an assistant hold the top of the manometer column so that the clinician performing the procedure can make the measurement and manipulate the stopcock for fluid collection. CSF pressure also may be estimated based on drops of CSF counted over time (16).

The CSF should be collected in a series of sterile tubes. Approximately 1 mL/tube is required for standard studies. The first tube specimen should be sent for Gram stain and bacterial culture, the second for CSF glucose and protein, and the third for CSF cell count and differential. Additional tubes may be obtained for viral culture, fungal culture, bacterial antigens, cell pathology, or special chemistries as needed. After fluid collection, closing pressure may be measured as previously described. The spinal needle is removed with stylet in place. The puncture area should be cleansed and a sterile dressing applied.

If fluid does not flow, the stylet should be rotated 90°. If the rotation of the needle does not result in CSF flow, the stylet should be replaced and the needle advanced a little farther. If spinal fluid is not obtained at this point, the procedure should be attempted again by removing the spinal needle with the stylet in place to just under the skin and redirecting it or by removing the needle entirely and starting with an unused spinal needle at a different site. Occasionally in dehydrated infants, CSF may flow slowly in the lateral recumbent position. Moving the patient to a sitting position may increase flow in this situation.

Occasionally, bony resistance is felt upon spinal needle placement. This situation may occur when the skin is punctured over the spine of the vertebral body instead of the vertebral interspace or when the patient's position does not achieve adequate spinal flexion to open the interlaminar space. If bony resistance is felt superficially, then puncture over the spinous process is likely and the needle should be withdrawn to just below the skin and redirected through the interspace. If bony resistance is felt more deeply, then inadequate spinal flexion is likely. Directing the needle more cephalad in conjunction with improved positioning usually overcomes this problem.

A traumatic tap occurs when the needle penetrates the dura too far to one side into an epidural venous plexus or when the needle is advanced through the subarachnoid space into or adjacent to the vertebral body. If blood is seen during fluid collection but the spinal needle is in proper position, the CSF will usually clear and the specimen does not clot. If the bloody fluid does not clear and clots in the collection tube, then the spinal needle is in the wrong place indicating that the spinal needle should be removed. The puncture should be repeated at a different interspace with an unused needle. A traumatic puncture can usually be avoided by proper patient and needle positioning.

Complications

Lumbar puncture is frequently associated with minor complications of localized back pain without neurologic abnormalities, transient paresthesia during the procedure, and postspinal headache. Localized back pain typically resolves with symptomatic treatment such as acetaminophen and applied heat. Severe back pain associated with neurologic signs such as decreased sensation or incontinence may be indicative of a subdural or epidural spinal hematoma and requires emergent investigation and treatment. Paresthesias may occur as the spinal needle contacts nerves in the cauda equina and are ameliorated by repositioning of the spinal needle. Permanent peripheral nerve damage is unusual in this setting because the spinal needle does not pierce the nerve but may move or stretch the nerve (4). Postspinal headaches occur most commonly in children over 10 years of age with an incidence from 10 to 70%, depending on technique (17, 18, 19, 20). Postspinal headaches are caused by continued leakage of spinal fluid through the dural hole, which decreases the cushioning of intracranial contents. Associated symptoms include vertigo and tinnitus induced by decreased endolymph volume in the semicircular canals as well as diplopia and blurry vision induced by stretching of cranial nerve VI as it passes over the petrous portion of the temporal bone (21). Headache is best prevented by using the smallest spinal needle possible and limiting the amount of cerebrospinal fluid removed. Headache occurs as frequently as 80% of the time after LP with a 16-gauge needle whereas only 1% of the time after puncture with a 25-gauge needle (21, 22). Placing the patient supine immediately following LP does not prevent postspinal headache (23). Treatment of postspinal headache depends on its severity. Bed rest and symptomatic treatment of pain and nausea suffice in most cases. Severe or prolonged (longer than 4 to 5 days) symptoms have been successfully treated with intravenous caffeine in adults and epidural blood patching in adults and children (21). Epidural blood patching requires the injection of 5 to 15 mL of autologous fresh blood into the epidural space at the same level as the previous LP. The epidural patch approaches an efficacy of 90% in relieving postspinal headache in adults (21).

Major complications after LP include LP-induced meningitis, epidural/subdural hematoma, acquired epidermoid tumor, damage to adjacent structures (disk herniation, retroperitoneal abscess, spinal cord hematoma), and cerebral herniation. As previously discussed, the lateral recumbent position for LP can cause respiratory obstruction, hypoxemia, and cardiovascular instability, particularly in the young infant (2).

Lumbar puncture through an area of cellulitis predictably causes meningitis. For this reason, cellulitis overlying the LP site is an absolute contraindication to performing the procedure. Lumbar puncture in children with bacteremia has been associated with meningitis (23). However, analysis of risk factors found that the development of bacterial meningitis in children with occult bacteremia was very strongly related to the infecting organism but not with performance of a lumbar puncture (24). Eng et al. reported the incidence of LP-induced meningitis to be no greater than 2.1% which does not exceed the incidence of spontaneous meningitis in patients with bacteremia. They also found possible LP-induced meningitis to be most common in critically ill patients who underwent multiple LPs (25). Although LP may lead to meningitis in a small portion of children with bacteremia, LP-induced meningitis is a rare event and should not deter the physician from performing the procedure if clinically indicated.

Subdural or epidural hematoma following LP has been reported with all forms of bleeding dyscrasias. Subdural spinal hematoma has been reported in thrombocytopenic children with leukemia, cancer, or ITP who had platelet counts from 1000 to 73,000/mm^3. Signs and symptoms of spinal cord compression including pain, sensory deficits, paralysis, and incontinence developed 1 hour to 6 days after the procedure. In most cases, the LP was difficult and yielded bloody fluid. In these patients, platelet counts were low or falling, and platelet transfusion was not provided before LP (26). Epidural spinal hematomas have occurred spontaneously after anticoagulation in patients who did not receive lumbar puncture, after epidural anesthesia, and after lumbar puncture in an infant with undiagnosed hemophilia A (26, 27). Lumbar puncture can be performed safely in patients with thrombocytopenia if they receive transfusion to a peripheral platelet count greater than 100,000/mm^3 and in patients with coagulopathy after appropriate correction of factor deficiency (28).

Acquired epidermal spinal cord tumors can arise from implantation of epidermal material into the spinal canal during LP. The tumor manifests as gait disturbance, pain, and neurologic dysfunction occurring 1.5 to 23 years after lumbar puncture. Experimental and clinical evidence strongly suggest that these tumors can be avoided if a spinal needle with a tight fitting stylet is used during LP (29, 30). Osteomyelitis, diskitis, herniated vertebral disk, and spinal cord hematoma all have been described as complications of LP and can be avoided by strict adherence to sterile technique and by careful attention to proper puncture site selection and to needle placement depth (31).

Cerebral herniation leading to sudden death is the most feared complication from LP. Patients with an intracranial space-occupying lesion (abscess, hematoma, tumor) are at greatest risk. Patients with focal neurologic signs before LP may have as high as a 40% risk of death (32). Conversely, in 1053 patients with papilledema or documented increased intracranial pressure (manometry greater than 20 cm H_2O) and no focal neurologic findings, only 5 or 1.2%, respectively, had possible complications from their LP, regardless of the etiology of their intracranial hypertension (33). Risk of herniation in an infant with an open fontanel *and* no focal neurologic findings is probably much lower. In most patients, the safety of lumbar puncture can be made on clinical grounds. Patients who have a history of focal neurologic symptoms (seizures, visual change), focal neurologic findings on physical examination, or papilledema should have brain imaging before LP. If meningitis or other CNS infection is strongly considered, the patient should receive appropriate antibiotic therapy before an imaging study. Infants in whom the fundus cannot be visualized can undergo LP if no neurologic focality is suggested by history or physical examination. Patients with altered mental status alone should have an LP performed early in their evaluation and before brain imaging as long as no focal neurologic signs or evidence of increased intracranial pressure exist.

SUMMARY

Lumbar puncture is commonly performed in the care of sick infants and children. The potential for cardiorespiratory decompensation during the procedure, especially in neonates and young infants, requires that it be performed in an area equipped for resuscitation. Its successful completion depends on proper positioning, judicious analgesia, and a thorough knowledge of the anatomy of the lumbar spine. Complications may be avoided by careful clinical assessment of the patient before LP and strict adherence to proper technique.

REFERENCES

1. Weisman LE, Merenstein GB, Steenbarger JR. The effect of lumbar puncture position in sick neonates. Am J Dis Child 1983; 137:1077–1079.
2. Gleason CA, Martin RJ, Anderson JV, Carlo WA, Sanniti KF, Fanaroff AA. Optimal position for a spinal tap in preterm infants. Pediatrics 1983;71:31–35.
3. Barr ML. The human nervous system. 3rd ed. Hagerstown: Harper & Row Publishers, 1979.
4. Swaiman KF. Spinal fluid examination. In: Swaiman KF, ed. Pediatric neurology: principles and practice. 2nd ed. St. Louis: Mosby, 1994.
5. Truex RC, Carpenter MB. Cerebrospinal fluid. In: Truex RC, Carpenter MB, eds. Human neuroanatomy. Baltimore: Williams & Wilkins, 1971.
6. Hochwald GM. Cerebrospinal fluid. In: Baker AB, Baker LH, eds. Clinical neurology. New York: Harper & Row, 1984.
7. Lachman E. Case studies in anatomy. 2nd ed. New York: Oxford University Press, Inc., 1978.
8. Fleisher GR. Infectious disease emergencies. In: Fleisher GR, Ludwig S, eds. Textbook of pediatric emergency medicine. 3rd ed. Baltimore: Williams & Wilkins, 1993.
9. Ward E, Gushurst CA. Uses and technique of pediatric lumbar puncture. Am J Dis Child 1992;146:1160–1165.
10. Earnest MP. Safe and effective use of lumbar puncture. In: Earnest MP, ed. Neurologic emergencies. New York: Churchill Livingstone, 1983.
11. Clarke MA. Timing of lumbar puncture in severe childhood meningitis. BMJ 1985;291:899.
12. Horwitz SJ, Boxerbaum B, O'Bell J. Cerebral herniation in bacterial meningitis in childhood. Ann Neurol 1980;7:524–528.
13. Pinheiro JMB, Furdon S, Ochoa LF. Role of local anesthesia during lumbar puncture in neonates. Pediatrics 1993;91:379–382.
14. Bonadio WA, Smith DS, Metrou M, DeWitz B. Estimating lumbar puncture [sic] depth in children. [Letter] N Eng J Med 1988;319:952–953.
15. Ellis III RW. Lumbar cerebrospinal fluid opening pressure measured in a flexed lateral decubitus position in children. Pediatrics 1994;93:622–623.
16. Ellis III RW, Strauss LC, Wiley JM, Killmond TM, Ellis Jr. RW. A simple method of estimating cerebrospinal fluid pressure during lumbar puncture. Pediatrics 1992;89:895–897.
17. Vandam LD, Dripps RD. Long-term follow-up of patients who received 10,098 spinal anesthetics. JAMA 1956;161:586–591.
18. Bolder PM. Postlumbar puncture headache in pediatric oncology patients. Anesthesiology 1986;65:696–698.
19. Scher C, Amar D, Ginsburg I, et al. Postdural puncture headache in children with cancer. [Abstract] Anesthesiology 1992;77:A1183.
20. Tobias JD. Postdural puncture headache in children: etiology and treatment. Clin Pediatr 1994;33:110–113.
21. Crawford JS. The prevention of headache consequent upon dural puncture. Br J Anaesth 1972;44:598–600.
22. Carbaat PAT, Van Crevel H. Lumbar puncture headache: controlled study on the preventive effect of 24 hours' bed rest. Lancet 1981;2:1133–1135.
23. Teele DW, Dashefsdy B, Rakusan T, Klein JO. Meningitis after lumbar puncture in children with bacteremia. N Eng J Med 1981;305:1079–1081.
24. Shapiro ED, Aaron NH, Wald ER, Chiponis D. Risk factors for development of bacterial meningitis among children with occult bacteremia. J Pediatr 1986;109:15–19.
25. Eng RHK, Seligman SJ. Lumbar puncture-induced meningitis. JAMA 1981;245:1456–1459.
26. Edelson RN, Chernik NL, Posner JB. Spinal subdural hematomas complicating lumbar puncture: occurrence in thrombocytopenic patients. Arch Neurol 1974;31:134–137.
27. Faillace WJ, Warrier I, Canady AI. Paraplegia after lumbar puncture in an infant with previously undiagnosed hemophilia A: treatment and perioperative considerations. Clin Pediatr 1989;28:136–138.

28. Silverman R, Kwiatkowski T, Bernstein S, Hilgartner M, Cahill-Bordas M, Jackson K, Lipton R. Safety of lumbar puncture in patients with hemophilia. Ann Emerg Med 1993;22:1739–1742.

29. Batnitzky S, Keucher TR, Mealey J, Campbell RL. Iatrogenic intraspinal epidermoid tumors. JAMA 1977;237:148–150.

30. Gibson T, Norris W. Skin fragments removed by injection needles. Lancet 1958;2:983–985.

31. Dripps RD, Vandam LD. Hazards of lumbar puncture. JAMA 1952;247:1113–1122.

32. Duffy GP. Lumbar puncture in the presence of raised intracranial pressure. BMJ 1969;1: 407–409.

33. Korein J, Cravioto H, Leicach M. Reevaluation of lumbar puncture: a study of 129 patients with papilledema or intracranial hypertension. Neurology 1959;9:290–297.

CHAPTER 44

EVALUATION OF VENTRICULAR SHUNT FUNCTION

George A. Woodward and Carolyn M. Carey

INTRODUCTION

Ventricular, subdural, and cystic shunts are used to drain fluid from their respective areas to the peritoneum, atrium, or pleural cavity. Unfortunately, these shunts may malfunction with potential life-threatening consequences. Mechanical malfunction will account for the majority of shunt problems, with infection also being a concern (1, 2). In one study of 1719 pediatric patients with hydrocephalus, the probability of shunt malfunction by 10 years of age was 70% (80% by 12 years), with the highest risk occurring in the immediate postoperative period (3). By comparison, the probability of infection in the same group of patients was only 9% in 10 years (3). Morbidity of shunt malfunction can be high and mortality has been reported as greater than 1%. Improvements have been made in shunt design and surgical technique over the past several years in an attempt to prevent these complications. This chapter will discuss assessment of function of central nervous system (CNS) shunts. Diagnostic and therapeutic sampling of fluid from the shunts will be discussed in Chapter 45.

ANATOMY AND PHYSIOLOGY

Shunts are used to transport fluid from one anatomic cavity to another when the body is unable to do so on its own. Accumulation of fluid in the ventricles or other areas within the rigid cranial vault can lead to signs, symptoms, and consequences seen with hydrocephalus and increased intracranial pressure.

Shunts are inserted in a sterile operative environment, and may be located in several different cranial areas. Portions of the shunt are usually available for palpation as part of the evaluation process. The palpable external shunt hardware includes the tubing exiting from the burr hole, the reservoir (often placed directly above the burr hole or directly beneath the skin incision), the valve, and that portion of the tubing that travels across the cranium and down the neck to the point of entry into the chest or abdomen. A palpable antisiphoning device also may be distal to the shunt valve (Fig. 44.1).

Many different ventricular shunts are available, and evaluation of a particular shunt becomes easier if the clinician knows the type of shunt the patient has in place (4). Variations include multiple or single component systems, single or double reservoirs, and shunts with programmable flow capability. Knowledge of the location and function of the shunt (ventriculoperitoneal, ventriculoatrial, ventriculopleural, or drainage of other fluid collection) is of lesser importance during initial evaluation.

Malfunctions can occur proximally or distally in a ventricular shunt. Proximal malfunctions can be categorized as (*a*) disconnection, (*b*) kinking of the catheter, (*c*) blockage by blood, infection, or CNS tissue, and (*d*) ventricular contraction with catheter pen-

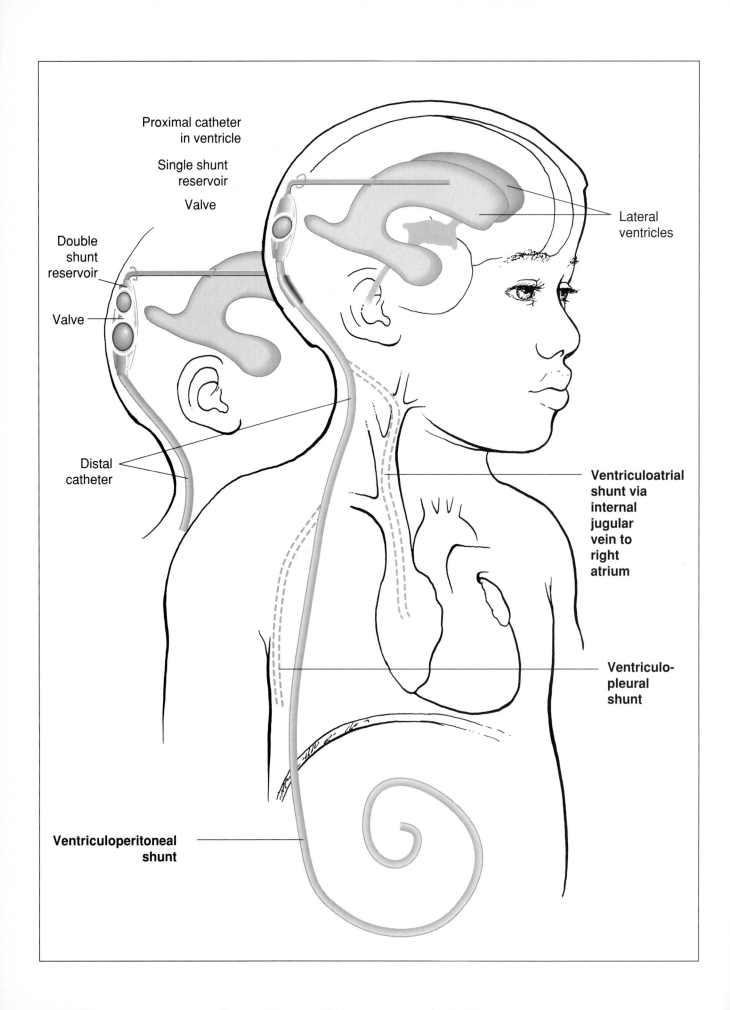

Proximal catheter
in ventricle

Single shunt
reservoir

Valve

Double
shunt
reservoir

Valve

Distal
catheter

Lateral
ventricles

**Ventriculoatrial
shunt via
internal
jugular
vein to
right
atrium**

**Ventriculo-
pleural
shunt**

**Ventriculoperitoneal
shunt**

Table 44.1.
Possible Locations of Shunt Malfunction

Proximal shunt tubing:
  Disconnection
  Kinking of catheter
  Catheter blockage (CSF, blood, proteinaceous material, infection)
  Overdrainage (slit ventricles, subdural hematoma, craniosynostosis)
Valve:
  Disconnection
  Failure
Distal shunt tubing:
  Disconnection
  Migration
  Catheter blockage (tissue, infection)

etration or perforation into or through the ventricular wall. Distal malfunctions may occur at the level of the valve (disconnection, valve failure) or the distal catheter (disconnection, migration, blockage). Overdrainage can occur and lead to sequela of slit ventricle syndrome (symptoms of shunt malfunction associated with small, often noncompliant, slit-like ventricles), subdural and epidural accumulations of blood or fluid, and craniosynostosis (Table 44.1) (1, 5, 6). Infections can be classified as external (erythema, warmth over the shunt tubing with involvement of the subcutaneous tissues) or internal (often with Staphylococcus epidermidis) (5, 7).

INDICATIONS

Signs and symptoms that may suggest shunt malfunction or infection include:
1. swelling, fluid collection or erythema around the shunt tubing,
2. full or bulging anterior fontanel,
3. increasing head circumference with suture separation,
4. fever, headache, or pallor,
5. personality change or change in school performance,
6. irritability, nausea, papilledema, or vomiting, and
7. lethargy, gait disturbance, neck pain, visual difficulties, and sepsis (8).

Signs suggestive of more serious complications include cranial nerve palsies, loss of consciousness, respiratory abnormalities, seizures, coma, posturing, and hemiparesis with potential progression to herniation and death. These symptoms can be nonspecific and mimic or coexist with viral and other types of illness. Other complications of ventricular shunts depend on the shunt location. Peritoneal shunts have been associated with inguinal hernias, hydroceles, ascites, intraabdominal cyst formation, viscus perforation, neoplasm, and peritonitis (5). Vascular shunts have been associated with vascular thrombi, endocarditis, dysrhythmias, cardiac tamponade, and embolization of detached distal shunt tubing (5). Shunt malfunction may be intermittent rather than an all-or-none phenomenon, which can confuse the diagnosis. Prompt evaluation, recognition, and management of a malfunctioning shunt is imperative to optimal outcome for the patient.

If a child with a shunt presents with any of the previously mentioned signs or symptoms, an evaluation of shunt function should be initiated. Shunt malfunction can occur as a result of incorrect placement, hardware failure, kinks in the tubing, disconnection, migration of the proximal or distal segment from the intended drainage cavity because of growth or other reasons, blockage with blood or proteinaceous material, pseudocysts around the ends of the shunt, incorrect programmable flow (if a programmable shunt), or infection. Unfortunately, in a patient with signs and symptoms of shunt malfunction, no definitive, inexpensive technique exists for evaluation in the majority of cases. Radiographic and fluid evaluation often need to be considered in the process of assessing shunt function. In a febrile patient with a shunt, the clinician must consider shunt infection as a possible source of the fever, although other causes should first be considered. Diagnosis of a shunt infection requires obtaining and evaluating shunt fluid (see Chapter 45).

EQUIPMENT

No special equipment is needed for the external evaluation of the shunt. Radiographic equipment (plain radiographs, CT scan) availability is necessary for shunt visualization, assessment of shunt continuity, and ventricular size assessment.

Figure 44.1.
Selected ventricular shunt components.

SUMMARY

1. Determine type of ventricular shunt by history, physical examination, radiographs and neurosurgical consultation
2. Assess integrity of shunt system by palpating around burr hole, reservoir, valve, and distal tubing looking for fluid collections or erythema

Single reservoir shunt

1. Compress reservoir and observe time for refilling
2. Resistance on reservoir compression suggests distal malfunction
3. Diminished or absent reservoir refilling suggests proximal malfunction

Double reservoir shunt

1. Compress proximal reservoir (closest to burr hole)
2. While continuing to compress proximal reservoir, compress distal reservoir
3. Release proximal bubble and observe time for refilling
4. Release distal bubble
5. Increased resistance when compressing distal reservoir suggests distal obstruction
6. Delay in proximal reservoir filling (>1 second) suggests proximal obstruction unless shunt has been pumped recently

Procedure

Shunt evaluation involves a working knowledge of the variety of shunts available and, if possible, the specific type of shunt the patient has in place. It is helpful to know if the shunt consists of a multiple or single component system. As mentioned, knowledge of the location and function of the shunt (ventriculoperitoneal, ventriculoatrial, ventriculopleural, or drainage of other fluid collection) is not of critical importance, although ventriculoatrial shunts may be associated with a higher incidence of life-threatening infection (9). The first step in diagnosing a shunt malfunction is recognizing that the patient has a shunt and that it may be responsible for the patient's condition (see Indications).

Many different types and configurations of shunts are available. Each physician should be aware of the most common shunts used in or evaluated at his or her hospital. When available, neurosurgical consultation will be useful in assessing the specifics of a shunt with which the practitioner is unfamiliar. A plain radiograph may be beneficial to identify specifics of an individual shunt and also will be useful for the neurosurgical consultant.

The type of shunt the patient has and whether a reservoir is in place will determine the specifics of the evaluation. Before evaluating the function of the shunt, the clinician should assess the external tubing, reservoir, and valves for any obvious disconnection. Swelling around the shunt tubing or reservoir(s) suggests a fluid leak from a shunt that has lost its continuity. This usually occurs if the shunt is broken or if a connecting site is not intact. Erythema and warmth tracking along the catheter suggest a shunt infection.

In the single reservoir type shunt, simply pressing on the reservoir and observing its return to baseline position can help identify a shunt blockage and determine if the malfunction is proximal (before the reservoir) or distal (post-reservoir). Resistance to compressing the reservoir suggests a distal malfunction as fluid is impeded from leaving the reservoir, whereas diminished or absent refilling of the reservoir suggests a proximal malfunction (Fig. 44.2).

In a double reservoir (double bubble) type system, the same principles apply, although the clinician uses both bubbles to evaluate shunt function. The clinician must first compress the proximal bubble (closest to the shunt skull entrance), which in effect empties the proximal bubble and fills the distal bubble for the next step. While continuing to compress the proximal bubble, the distal bubble is compressed. A normally functioning distal valve should offer no resistance to compression and emptying of fluid through the distal tubing. Increased resistance suggests a distal shunt malfunction (blockage, disconnection, insufficient length). The clinician then releases the proximal bubble, which should fill with fluid from the shunted cavity. Any delay in filling (more than 1 second) suggests a malfunction of the proximal shunt tubing (Fig. 44.2). If the shunt has been pumped recently, however, the amount of fluid may not be enough to fill the reservoir immediately or the fluid flow may be temporarily impeded by the choroid plexus abutting the intracranial tip of the shunt. A one-way valve is located in the distal tubing that prevents retrograde fluid flow. The proximal tubing is without a similar type of valve, which allows for repeated testing of the proximal tubing and reservoir without draining excessive fluid from the ventricle. Unfortunately, the sensitivity of shunt pumping has recently been shown to be less than 40% in identifying a malfunctioning shunt. The predictive value of a negative test was between 65 and 81% (10).

Programmable shunts can be identified by history and radiographic evaluation, but this is difficult without prior experience. As these shunts become more prevalent, or if they are used in a given medical facility, the clinician should become familiar with the specifics of their evaluation.

Shunt integrity also can be assessed radiographically or by manometric fluid measurement. Radiographic options include plain films which demonstrate the full length and integrity of the shunt, and should include skull, neck, chest, and abdominal views. Obvious disconnections should be visible, although the clinician must be careful not to mistake the radiolucent areas that signify the connection between the proximal, distal, and valve segments as disconnections.

A CT scan can be useful in the evaluation of shunt function, especially if previous CT scans are available for comparison. Evi-

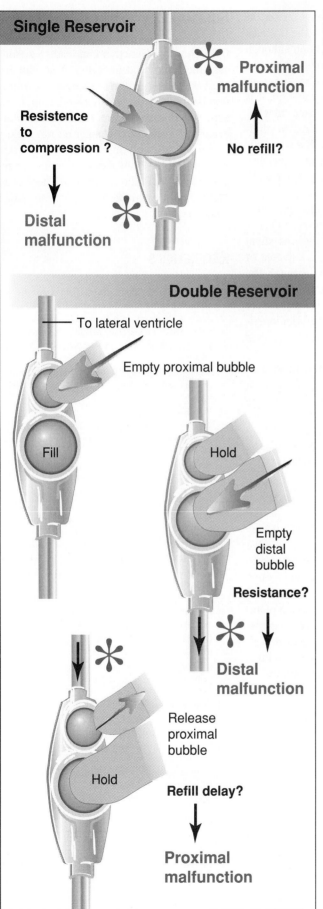

Figure 44.2.
Pumping technique for single
reservoir and double reservoir
ventricular shunts.

Single Reservoir

Resistence
to
compression ?

↓

**Distal
malfunction**

*

**Proximal
malfunction**

↑

No refill?

*

Double Reservoir

— To lateral ventricle

Empty proximal bubble

Fill

Hold

Empty
distal
bubble

Resistance?

↓   *   ↓

**Distal
malfunction**

Release
proximal
bubble

Hold

Refill delay?

↓

**Proximal
malfunction**

dence of enlargement or a change in size of the fluid spaces or ventricles on the CT scan suggests a malfunction of the shunt, although location of the malfunction usually cannot be determined. Although this may be an expensive method to evaluate shunt function, it is the gold standard to document ventricular enlargement suggesting malfunction. The clinician must be aware, however, that some patients have slit or noncompliant ventricles, and that shunt malfunction may occur without evidence of enlarged ventricles.

Radionuclide imaging techniques also are available for shunt evaluation (11). Radioactive material is injected into the shunt reservoir and its flow noted. Assessment of the cerebral spinal fluid flow through the shunt tubing is available with this modality. Evaluation of cerebrospinal fluid pressure can be performed simply by a ventriculoperitoneal shunt tap. This technique is described in detail in Chapter 45.

As in the evaluation of all illness, the history is important, and if it suggests a shunt malfunction, definitive diagnosis should be aggressively pursued. If the ED evaluation is inconclusive, in-hospital observation and shunt externalization or replacement should be considered.

COMPLICATIONS

Complications of shunt evaluation involve failing to recognize the possibility that presenting signs or symptoms are secondary to a shunt malfunction, or misinterpreting those signs and symptoms as being the result of another process. One potential area of diagnostic misinterpretation involves the patient with slit ventricle syndrome, in whom the shunt is assumed to be functionally intact because no radiographic evidence of increased fluid collection exists (2).

SUMMARY

CNS shunt malfunction can lead to significant morbidity and mortality. The clinician must make every effort to identify a malfunction before serious symptoms develop. If the approach discussed here and fluid sampling discussed in the next chapter do not yield a definitive answer, in-hospital observation with possible shunt externalization or replacement should be considered. These decisions should be made in conjunction with a neurosurgeon.

REFERENCES

1. Sainte-Rose C. Shunt obstruction: a preventable complication? Pediatr Neurosurg 1993;19:156–164.
2. Aldrich EF, Harmann P. Disconnection as a cause of ventriculoperitoneal shunt malfunction in multicomponent shunt systems. Pediatr Neurosurg 1990;16: 309–312.
3. Sainte-Rose C, Piatt JH, Renier D, et al. Mechanical complications in shunts. Pediatr Neurosurg 1991–92;17:2–9.
4. Post EM. Currently available shunt systems: a review. Neurosurg 1985;16:257–260.
5. McLaurin RL. Ventricular shunts: complications and results. In: McLaurin RL, Schut L, Venes JL, Epstein F, eds. Pediatric neurosurgery: surgery of the developing nervous system. 2nd ed. Philadelphia: WB Saunders Co., 1989.
6. Kalia KK, Swift DM, Pang D. Multiple epidural hematomas following ventriculoperitoneal shunt. Pediatr Neurosurg 1993;19:78–80.
7. Renier D, Lacombe J, Pierre-Kahn A, Sainte-Rose C, Hirsch JF. Factors causing acute shunt infections: computer analysis of 1174 operations. J Neurosurg 1984;61:1072–1078.
8. Sekhar LN, Moossy J, Guthkelch AN. Malfunctioning ventriculoperitoneal shunts. J Neurosurg 1982;56:411–416.
9. Olson L, Frykberg T. Complications in the treatment of hydrocephalus in children: a comparison of ventriculoatrial and ventriculoperitoneal shunts in a 20-year material. Acta Paediatr Scand 1983;72: 385–390.
10. Piatt JH. Physical examination of patients with cerebrospinal fluid shunts: is there useful information in pumping the shunt? Pediatrics 1992;89:470–473.
11. Blair K, AuCoin R, Kloiber R, Molnar CP. The complementary role of plain radiographs and radionuclide shuntography in evaluating CSF-VP shunts. Clin Nuclear Med 1989;4:121–123.

VENTRICULAR SHUNT AND BURR HOLE PUNCTURE

Ann-Christine Duhaime and James F. Wiley II

INTRODUCTION

Children with ventricular shunts can present to the emergency department (ED), office, or clinic with signs or symptoms of two major shunt complications—obstruction or infection. Shunt puncture or "tapping" the shunt refers to withdrawing cerebrospinal fluid (CSF) from the shunt apparatus percutaneously to aid in diagnosing a shunt malfunction or infection. In some cases, high intracranial pressure may be acutely relieved by removing some ventricular fluid. However, because shunt puncture carries a risk of approximately 1% of introducing an infection, and because improperly performed taps can damage certain types of shunt components, the physician should try to identify shunt problems without tapping the shunt, if possible (1). Ideally, shunt punctures should be performed by a neurosurgeon who is familiar with the particular type of shunt in question, and who has assessed the patient and can weigh the relative risks and benefits to be derived from a shunt tap. Because some shunt problems require immediate attention, however, the goal of this chapter is to review the basics of shunt anatomy and evaluation and to describe the indications and techniques for shunt puncture and burr hole puncture when the neurosurgeon is unavailable. Because of the potential for cardiorespiratory instability in the child with a shunt obstruction or infection, a physician should only perform this procedure in an area where monitoring, resuscitation equipment, and personnel are sufficient to handle sudden decompensation such as in the EDs, intensive care unit, or operating room.

ANATOMY AND PHYSIOLOGY

The majority of shunts placed for hydrocephalus consist of the following four main components (Fig. 44.1):
1. a proximal catheter, usually in the lateral ventricle;
2. a distal catheter, usually in the peritoneal cavity or, less commonly, in the right atrium, pleural cavity, or other site;
3. a reservoir, which is usually a single or double bubble or button, often located on the head near the burr hole entry site of the proximal catheter;
4. a valve to control flow, which may be a device located within or adjacent to the reservoir or may be part of the distal catheter (slit valve).

Shunts are named according to their proximal and distal drainage sites; therefore, a VP shunt drains from the ventricle to the peritoneal cavity, a VJ or VA shunt drains the ventricle through the jugular vein into the right atrium, and an LP shunt drains the lumbar subarachnoid space into the peritoneum.

Pumping the shunt to assess its function (see Chapter 44) involves pressing on the reservoir or valve, depending on the particular shunt type. Tapping the shunt requires

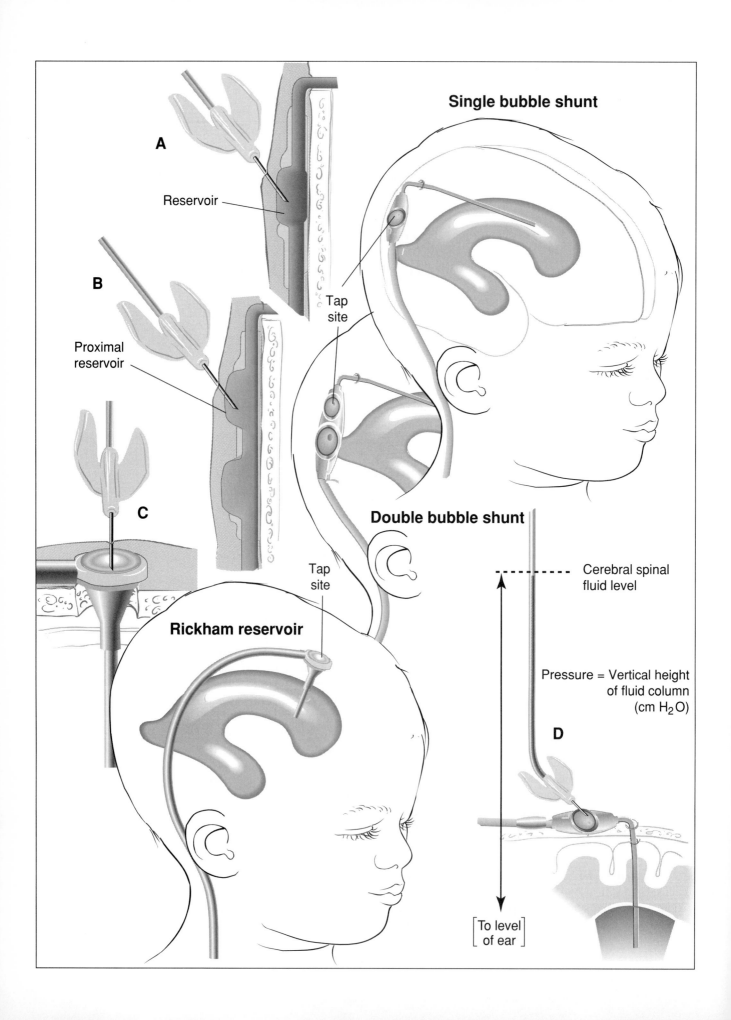

Single bubble shunt

Reservoir

Tap site

A

Double bubble shunt

Proximal reservoir

B

Tap site

C

Rickham reservoir

Cerebral spinal fluid level

Pressure = Vertical height of fluid column (cm H$_2$O)

D

[To level of ear]

identifying the reservoir, which is specifically designed for this purpose. A shunt survey (radiograph of the shunt along its course) will usually show its location. The part of the shunt that is pumped usually but not always is the part that is tapped. For example, with a Holter type valve, a separate (Rickham) reservoir is usually placed in the burr hole itself (Fig. 45.1); tapping the pumping chamber of the cylindrical Holter valve may cause it damage.

As always, there are exceptions and variations in shunt components. Proximal catheters are sometimes multiple and may drain other cavities such as cysts, a trapped fourth ventricle, or the subdural space. Some shunts do not have reservoirs or valves, and some components may be radiolucent on radiograph. The neurosurgeon can usually help sort out these less common situations.

INDICATIONS

Shunt Malfunction

Children with a ventricular shunt malfunction often present with signs and symptoms of increased intracranial pressure such as headache, vomiting, irritability, or lethargy. Sunsetting (inability to look up) or crossed eyes may be seen, and in infants the fontanel may be full. Occasionally, less common symptoms will herald malfunction, such as seizures or other neurologic symptoms. In severe cases, coma, herniation, arrest, and death can occur (2). Families often recognize and diagnose shunt problems with a high degree of accuracy, especially because each shunt malfunction tends to present with the same signs in a given child. Their opinion is a valuable resource not to be overlooked.

Shunt malfunction may result from obstruction of the proximal catheter (usually with choroid plexus) or the distal catheter, from malfunction of a valve, or from discon-

Table 45.1.
Indications for Ventriculoperitoneal Shunt Puncture*

Malfunction
1. Problem not clear by the physical examination and radiographs (see Chapter 44)
2. Severe symptoms of elevated intracranial pressure which cannot be managed medically until definitive repair

Infection
Ventriculoperitoneal shunt
1. Persistent fever without known source
2. Fever with recent (< 6 mo) shunt surgery or recent shunt tap
3. Suspected intraabdominal soilage/contamination
4. Incisional CSF leakage or exposed shunt
Ventriculojugular/atrial shunt
1. Fever without known source
2. Sepsis
3. Suspected shunt nephritis

* Individual exceptions may occur and should be discussed with the patient's neurosurgeon.

nection. Proximal obstructions are diagnosed by a slowly refilling shunt in the presence of ventricular enlargement on CT scan. Shunt disconnections or insufficient distal length are diagnosed by shunt survey. The remaining problems are usually distal obstructions (2). In general, proximal obstructions cause the most acute neurologic symptoms, and may require urgent surgical correction, because a high-grade proximal obstruction precludes relief of pressure by a shunt puncture. If the problem is elsewhere in the shunt, or if the proximal obstruction is partial, tapping the shunt will usually allow withdrawal of sufficient CSF to relieve the more severe symptoms temporarily until definitive surgical repair can be performed. The CSF pressure and the ease with which fluid can be withdrawn also help evaluate shunt function. If symptoms are mild, and if the diagnosis is clear by noninvasive means (see Chapter 44), temporary medical management with diuretics such as acetazolamide is preferred until surgical correction is accomplished, as the risks associated with shunt puncture can thus be avoided (Table 45.1).

Shunt Infection

Shunt infections nearly always present with fever, which may be low grade, intermittent, or high. Abdominal pain or, uncommonly, frank peritonitis may be seen with infected

Figure 45.1.
Ventricular shunt tap and measurement of intraventricular pressure.
A. Single reservoir shunt
B. Double reservoir shunt
C. Rickham reservoir
D. Measurement of CSF pressure during ventricular shunt tap.

SUMMARY: VENTRICULAR SHUNT PUNCTURE

1. Position child:
   Supine for frontal shunt
   Lateral for posterior parietal shunts
2. Clean shunt site and adjacent scalp with isopropyl alcohol
3. Clip or shave a dime-sized area over reservoir
4. Carefully clean site for several minutes with betadine and allow to dry
5. For dome-shaped pumping reservoirs, insert needle tangentially approximately 2 to 5 mm; Rickham reservoirs should be punctured perpendicular to scalp
6. Measure opening pressure by holding butterfly tubing perpendicular to floor and measuring from ear to top of CSF column in tubing
7. Remove CSF until ventricular pressure is approximately 10 cm H_2O (10 to 20 mL) (Remember that slow flow may indicate a proximal obstruction and pressure measurement may be inaccurate in this setting.)
8. Transfer CSF into sterile test tubes for further studies
9. Remove butterfly needle and apply sterile dressing

VP shunts. Redness or tenderness over the shunt may appear. In VA shunts, nephritis is a rare but serious complication of shunt infection. Although a severe shunt infection may lead to obstruction and shunt failure, the majority of infected shunts continue to function so that increased intracranial pressure is not a part of the usual picture of shunt infection (2).

Bacteria causing VP shunt infections almost always seed the shunt at the time of surgery. Therefore, infections present as fever within the first few months after an operation. If it has been more than 6 months since any invasive VP shunt procedures, fever is highly unlikely to be the result of a shunt infection (3). Exceptions include obvious contamination of the shunt by an intraperitoneal process such as a ruptured appendix or erosion of a shunt component through the skin. Shunts in the bloodstream may become contaminated by any bacteremia, and thus are suspect as a source of fever regardless of time of last revision (4).

Children with shunts who present with fever and who demonstrate an obvious source, such as otitis media, or who present with concomitant upper respiratory or gastrointestinal viral symptoms, can be treated for the presumed medical problem. Tapping the shunt in this setting is usually unnecessary (Table 44.1).

As mentioned, infection can be introduced by shunt puncture. Shunts should never be tapped through compromised or inflamed skin. Partial shunt obstructions can be worsened by forceful suction on the choroid plexus. Withdrawal of a large volume of fluid before CT scan may compromise interpretation of ventricular size, so therefore tap should be withheld until after imaging unless symptoms are severe.

Cerebral Herniation

Burr hole puncture can be a lifesaving procedure in the setting of a complete proximal shunt obstruction with high intracranial pressure. The goal is to relieve intracranial pressure acutely by inserting a spinal needle directly into the ventricle using the burr hole through which the shunt enters the skull.

A ventricular tap through the burr hole almost always damages the ventricular shunt and carries a significant risk of parenchymal brain injury, intracranial hemorrhage, and infection. It should *only* be performed if cerebral herniation is occurring despite medical management of increased intracranial pressure and no alternative, such as immediate surgery, is available.

VENTRICULAR SHUNT PUNCTURE

Equipment

Isopropyl alcohol
Betadine
23-gauge butterfly needle
Sterile test tubes or syringe with cap
Razor

Procedure

Although a shunt puncture is not painful, reassurance is in order. The child is placed in the lateral position for posterior shunts and supine for frontal shunts. In small children this can be accomplished in the parent's lap, which aids in controlling crying and facilitates a more useful pressure measurement. Contamination is prevented by keeping the child calm and stationary; the use of surgical drapes and towels is usually unnecessary. Although most neurosurgeons prefer that the tap site be shaved, some believe that shaving increases the risk of infection and prefer to cleanse the hair. In either case, the first step is to clean and degrease the scalp with alcohol, in an area including the part of the shunt to be tapped and a surrounding margin of several centimeters. The hair is then clipped or shaved, if desired; a dime-sized area is all that is required. A thorough, repetitive, center-to-circumference betadine cleansing is then performed for several minutes. Importantly, a shunt tap breaches a foreign body—three brief wipes with the LP tray sponges is not adequate preparation for this procedure. Ideally, the betadine should then be allowed to dry on the skin while equipment is readied.

As mentioned, the reservoir is the component to puncture. For most dome-shaped pumping reservoirs, the needle should be inserted tangentially to a depth of a few millimeters (Fig. 45.1). The clinician should feel the needle pop through the reservoir dome. If the needle is advanced too far, it may embed in the back wall of the reservoir and become occluded. Firm, button type reservoirs (usually Rickham reservoirs) are situated in the burr hole. These are most easily punctured straight down, perpendicular to the scalp.

Once CSF flow is established and the child is reclining and quiet, the butterfly tubing is held perpendicular to the floor. If fluid does not immediately flow, gentle syringe suction is then applied. An assistant can measure the distance between the ear and the top of the CSF column in the butterfly tubing with a metric rule or tape measure after the syringe is removed from the tubing. This is easier than using a manometer and provides an accurate opening pressure.

Rapid flow of CSF under pressure suggests a shunt obstruction distal to the reservoir with a patent proximal shunt catheter. Slow or absent flow in the presence of large ventricles (relative to the patient's baseline) indicates a proximal shunt obstruction, and pressure measurements are not accurate in this setting. Slow flow, with good respiratory variation and a normal pressure, is usually normal in the setting of small ventricles seen on brain imaging.

If the ventricles are large, the proximal catheter is unobstructed, and the pressure is high, at least 10 mL of fluid can be withdrawn through a syringe to acutely lower the pressure. Small ventricles or a partially occluded proximal catheter will result in slow flow, and fluid is best removed by gentle suction through a small (5 mL or less) syringe. Only a small amount of fluid can be obtained in this case. After fluid is withdrawn, specimens are transferred to sterile tubes or the syringe is tightly capped. Helpful laboratory tests include CSF cell count, Gram stain, and culture.

If the shunt tap is not successful, and if severe symptoms of increased intracranial pressure exist and are not amenable to medical management (hyperventilation and diuretic therapy), then a ventricular tap through the burr hole should be performed.

Burr Hole Puncture

Equipment

Isopropyl alcohol
Betadine
3.5-inch, 21-gauge spinal needle
Razor
Sterile towels

Procedure

After shaving and cleansing the scalp thoroughly with isopropyl alcohol and betadine, the burr hole is palpated, and a 3.5, 22-gauge needle is slowly inserted straight in, perpendicular to the skull through either a frontal or occipital burr hole (Fig. 45.2). In some shunts, the burr hole will contain a reservoir, and this also is punctured by the spinal needle. The ventricle usually will be reached by a depth of 5 cm. The stylet is withdrawn after advancing the needle and fluid is allowed to drain spontaneously until it begins to slow down, indicating relief of pressure. The stylet is replaced and the needle is slowly withdrawn along its entry tract. Most patients will then proceed directly to the operating room for definitive shunt repair (5).

COMPLICATIONS

Ventricular shunt puncture and burr hole puncture carry a significant risk for complications. The abrupt change in relative pressure among brain compartments as a result of rapid relief of ventricular pressure can cause significant upward, lateral, and subdural fluid shifts. Upward and lateral pressure gradients can cause rapid intraparenchymal brain expansion with bleeding and edema. Rapid removal of ventricular fluid can cause shrinkage in brain size, which leads to tearing of subdural bridging veins and results in subdural hematoma formation. These complications may be difficult to avoid in the patient who requires ventricular fluid removal to avoid cerebral herniation. With a diagnostic ventricular shunt puncture, limiting the amount of cerebrospinal fluid removed and collecting the fluid without using excessive suction should avoid most of the dangers related to fluid shifts. A ventricular puncture through the burr hole carries a much greater risk for intraparenchymal damage than a shunt puncture. For this reason, close monitoring of clinical findings and reassessment by computed tomography or magnetic reso-

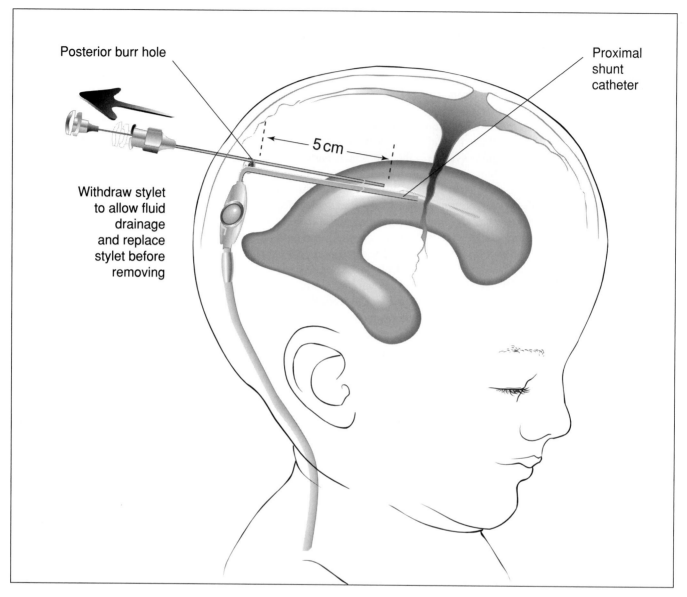

Posterior burr hole

Withdraw stylet
to allow fluid
drainage
and replace
stylet before
removing

5 cm

Proximal
shunt
catheter

Figure 45.2.
Ventricular puncture
through the burr hole.

**Chapter 45
Ventricular Shunt and
Burr Hole Puncture**

nance imaging must ensue following a burr hole puncture.

Risk of ventriculitis after a shunt tap approaches 1%. Staphylococcus epidermidis is the most common pathogen isolated when a shunt is infected (2, 4, 6, 7). A ventricular tap through the burr hole adds the potential for intracerebral abscess with extension into the ventricle. Infectious complications of these procedures underscore the need for strict adherence to sterile technique.

A ventricular shunt puncture can break a functioning shunt if the wrong component is entered. For this reason, it is essential that the shunt mechanism is understood before the procedure. In some instances, the choroid plexus adheres to the proximal shunt catheter after fluid removal despite correct technique.

Shunt revision may be required to reposition or replace the blocked catheter. As previously noted, a ventricular puncture through the burr hole almost always shears the proximal catheter and necessitates immediate proximal shunt revision.

CLINICAL TIPS: BURR HOLE PUNCTURE
1. The direction of the spinal needle should not be changed during the puncture to avoid shearing of brain parenchyma.
2. Burr hole puncture inevitably damages the shunt, necessitating operative intervention soon after alleviation of ventricular pressure.
3. Risk of intracranial injury after a ventricular puncture through the burr hole necessitates close observation and brain imaging after the procedure.

Summary

Correct performance of a ventricular shunt tap requires a knowledge of proper indications and an understanding of the shunt mechanism. In most cases, careful clinical and radiographic examination precede the procedure. A shunt tap may diagnose a malfunction or infection and alleviate signs of increased intracranial pressure until definitive neurosurgical treatment can be arranged. Occasionally, a shunted patient seeks medical attention and has severe signs of increased intracranial pressure. In this setting, a ventricular shunt tap may be life saving.

Ventricular tap through the burr hole is indicated in a shunted patient with cerebral herniation who has a proximal shunt obstruction. When successful, this procedure is also life saving but must be immediately followed by revision of the ventricular shunt. Both procedures have significant complications including intracranial bleeding, subdural hematoma, shunt infection, ventriculitis, and parenchymal brain injury.

References

1. Noetzel MJ, Baker RP. Shunt fluid examination: risks and benefits in the evaluation of shunt malfunction and infection. J Neurosurg 1984;61:328–332.
2. Kanev PM, Park TS. The treatment of hydrocephalus. Neurosurg Clin North Am 1993;4:611–619.
3. Michell JJ, Ward JD. Evaluation and treatment of increased intracranial pressure. In: Practice of pediatrics. Philadelphia: Harper & Row, 1987;9:28–29.
4. McLaurin RL. Ventricular shunts: complications and results. In: Schut L, Venes JL, Epstein F, eds. Pediatric neurosurgery. 2nd ed. Philadelphia: WB Saunders Co., 1989, pp. 219–229.
5. Duncan CC. Management of proximal shunt obstruction. J Neurosurg 1988;68:817–819.
6. Odio C, McCracken GH, Nelson JD. CSF shunt infections in pediatrics: a 7-year experience. Am J Dis Child 1984;138:1103–1108.
7. Yogev R. Cerebrospinal fluid shunt infections: a personal view. Pediatr Infect Dis 1985;4:113–118.

CHAPTER 46

SUBDURAL PUNCTURE

George A. Woodward and Carolyn M. Carey

INTRODUCTION

A subdural tap is used to evacuate subdural blood or fluid. This procedure can be performed on infants when a subdural fluid collection is causing the child to experience symptoms of increased intracranial pressure. The procedure also can be used for diagnostic purposes in a child with infected cerebrospinal fluid (subdural empyema and meningitis with effusions). Neurosurgical consultation should always be obtained before this procedure whenever possible. The recommended age group for subdural taps is infants, preferably those with an open fontanel. The procedure can also be performed in patients with fibrous or split sutures (to approximately 18 months).

ANATOMY AND PHYSIOLOGY

The subdural space lies beneath the skin, subcutaneous tissue, skull, and dura (Fig. 46.1). The major landmark for a subdural tap is the lateral margin of the anterior fontanel which is formed by the coronal suture. Subdural fluid collections can be acute, subacute, or chronic (1). They result from trauma or infection. Disruption of the cerebral veins that traverse the dura is a major factor leading to subdural hematomas (2). Dural or sinus tears, and repeated needle punctures of the fontanel also are known causes. Transudates and exudates can occur and may be loculated. Identification of a subdural fluid collection as the etiology of increased intracranial pressure

can allow rapid reversal of symptoms with the successful removal of fluid.

INDICATIONS

Physiologic parameters that suggest the therapeutic need for a subdural tap include those signs and symptoms associated with increased intracranial pressure. These are mental status changes, irritability, somnolence, pallor, lethargy, vomiting, full or bulging fontanel, third or sixth nerve palsies, respiratory irregularity, unconsciousness, coma, posturing, seizures, hypotonia, hemiparesis, or spasticity (see also Chapters 44 and 45). The fluid can be an acute or subacute blood collection from trauma or a transudate/exudate that accompanies a central nervous system infection. The subdural tap can be used as a therapeutic and/or diagnostic tool to verify and identify the type of fluid, and to decrease the intracranial pressure (3, 4). This invasive procedure should be reviewed with a neurosurgical consultant before proceeding if time allows. Ultrasound, computed tomography, or magnetic resonance imaging should be used before undertaking this procedure whenever possible. A magnetic resonance image of the head before the tap can be especially useful in cases of suspected intentional trauma to document the presence and age of the blood collection before evacuation. Repeated subdural taps to remove residual fluid are rarely indicated. Generally a drain will be placed if the fluid reaccumulates. Contraindications to initiating the subdural tap include

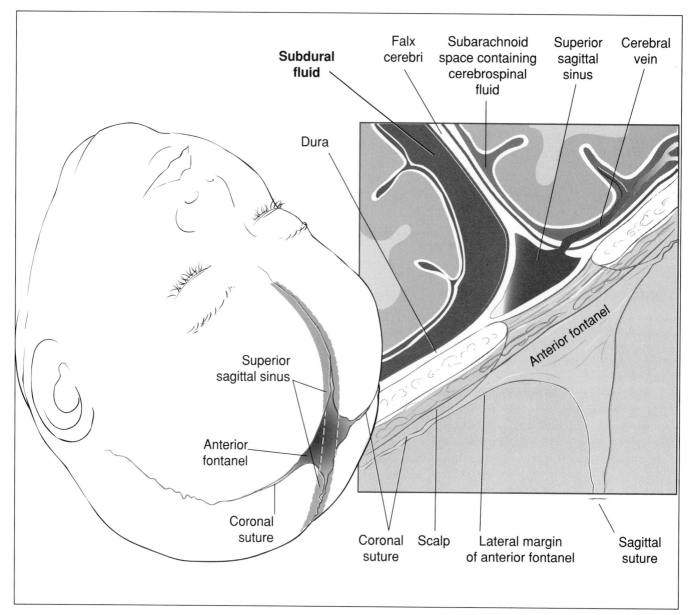

Figure 46.1.
Anatomy of the subdural space adjacent to the anterior fontanel.

bleeding abnormalities, overlying infected skin, and age outside the infant/toddler group.

EQUIPMENT

Sterile gloves, drapes
Mask
Immobilizer (papoose board) (see Chapter 3)
Povidone-iodine solution
Alcohol
Subdural or spinal needle (22 gauge, 1.5 inch)
Local anesthetic (lidocaine)
Sterile gauze, cotton

Dressing material
Cardiac monitor, pulse oximeter
Resuscitative equipment, personnel as needed

PROCEDURE

The child should be in the supine position and secured in an immobilizer with additional head stabilization by an experienced assistant. Resuscitative equipment should be identified and readily available for immediate use as needed. All appropriate resuscitative maneuvers should have been attended to before this point. The patient should be physically and mechanically monitored at all times during the procedure. A small area of hair should be clipped or shaved around the intended puncture site. The skin is then cleansed with povidone-iodine or other appropriate sterilizing solution. Local anesthetic can be infiltrated in the skin at the area of intended puncture. Strict aseptic technique should be observed, including sterile gloves, masks, instruments, and field.

Once the area has been prepared, a subdural needle (22 gauge, 1.5 spinal needle) should be inserted at a 90° angle through stretched skin at the lateral margin of the anterior fontanel. This can be identified where the coronal suture forms the lateral margin of the anterior fontanel (Fig. 46.2). If the anterior fontanel is small, the physician can make the puncture 5 to 10 mm laterally in the coronal suture (at least 2 cm from the midline) to avoid entering the sagittal sinus. By stretching the skin before inserting the needle through the fontanel, the physician will effectively establish a Z-track and help minimize the possibility of post-procedure fluid leak. The needle should be secured in the physician's hand with the heel of the hand against the infant's scalp to prevent a deep puncture with inadvertent head or table motion. The needle should be advanced slowly through the skin and suture line until the subdural space is entered. The physician may feel de-

Figure 46.2.
Subdural puncture.

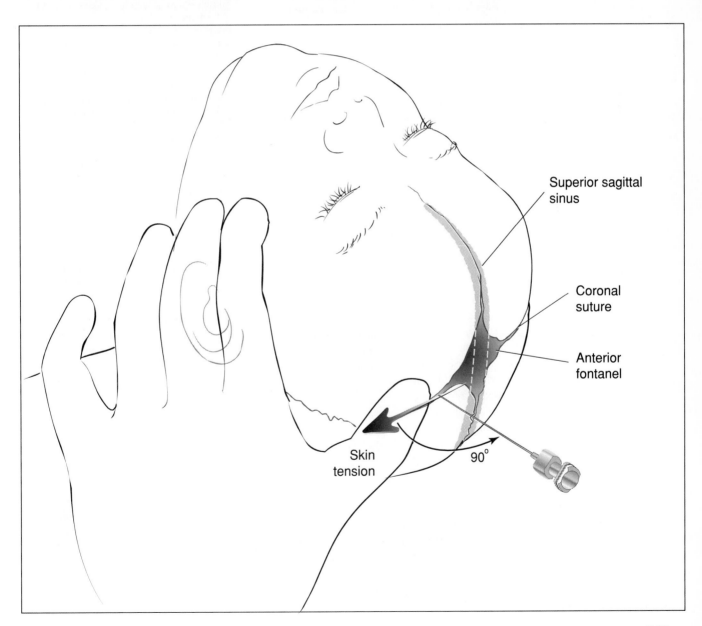

Superior sagittal sinus

Coronal suture

Anterior fontanel

Skin tension

90°

creased resistance as the needle enters the subdural space. This should be at a distance of approximately 5 to 10 mm. Once obtained, correct positioning of the needle can be maintained by clamping the needle at the skin with a hemostat. This will avoid inadvertent and potentially dangerous advancement of the needle. The fluid should drain spontaneously. Extension tubing placed on a T-connector may assist drainage by the siphoning effect. Suction should not be applied to the needle. The cessation of fluid flow does not necessarily indicate complete emptying of the subdural space, but rather that pressures are now equal between the intracranial and extracranial areas. A gentle pressure dressing should be applied to the needle site once the procedure is completed (3, 5).

The fluid should be collected for laboratory tests (hematocrit, bacterial or fungal culture, Gram stain, glucose, protein, cell count, differential) as indicated. The procedure can be performed on the opposite side, although most subdural cavities will communicate and bilateral taps are rarely needed. Repeated subdural taps, if indicated, should be accomplished under the direct guidance of a pediatric neurosurgeon. External drain placement should be considered if repeated subdural taps are necessary and a shunt may be required if external drainage fails (4, 6).

COMPLICATIONS

Suction applied to the indwelling subdural needle or inadvertent vessel puncture can cause vascular tears or lacerations and increase the blood component of the already compromised subdural space. In addition, overly rapid decompression of the cerebral cortex may cause cerebral edema (3). However, a pial vessel, if lacerated, will usually stop bleeding without intervention. A persistent leak can occur from the site of the subdural puncture. If this occurs, a gentle pressure dressing with cotton or collodion will usually suffice to seal such a leak.

Other complications include contusion or laceration of the underlying cerebral cortex and the introduction of infection. Notably, a subdural tap in the recommended location may not identify localized or loculated occipital or basal subdural fluid collections.

SUMMARY
1. Ensure that subdural puncture is appropriate; consider neurosurgical consultation, if time allows
2. Immobilize patient in supine position and ensure appropriate monitoring, ancillary personnel, and resuscitation equipment
3. Don a surgical mask and sterile gloves
4. Prepare puncture site (lateral margin of the anterior fontanel) by shaving a small area of hair
5. Vigorously clean the site with povidone-iodine solution applied in a circular fashion from puncture site outward
6. Drape area with sterile surgical towels
7. Inject local anesthetic intradermally; be sure to aspirate to ensure that inadvertent subdural injection does not occur
8. Stretch skin overlying puncture site to aid in formation of Z-track
9. Insert spinal needle and release skin
10. Advance needle slowly to a maximum depth of 1 cm at lateral margin of anterior fontanel at a 90° angle to the skull. If the fontanel is closed but the suture is fibrous (up to 18 months), insert needle in similar fashion 2 cm from the midline through the coronal suture.
11. Secure needle in place with hemostat applied at base of spinal needle
12. Allow fluid to drain without using suction
13. Apply gentle, sterile pressure dressing when procedure is completed

---

CLINICAL TIPS
1. If possible, a cerebral imaging study should be performed before subdural puncture, especially when intentional head trauma (child abuse) is suspected.
2. Bilateral or repeated subdural punctures are rarely needed.
3. Consultation with a pediatric neurosurgeon is indicated before a diagnostic or emergent subdural puncture, if time allows and if subdural fluid reaccumulates.

SUMMARY

A subdural tap can be a lifesaving procedure to remove fluid from the subdural space in infants. The procedure should be accomplished in a sterile fashion, with an awareness for the complications that may be encountered. As in all invasive pediatric procedures, resuscitative personnel and equipment should be immediately available if needed.

REFERENCES

1. McLaurin RL, Towbin R. Posttraumatic hematomas. In: McLaurin RL, Schut L, Venes JL, Epstein F, eds. Pediatric neurosurgery. 2nd ed. Philadelphia: WB Saunders Co., 1989.
2. Choux M, Lena G, Genitori L. Intracranial hematomas. In: Raimondi AJ, Choux M, Di Rocco C, eds. Head injuries in the newborn and infant. New York: Springer-Verlag, 1986.
3. Ingraham FD, Matson DD. Subdural hematoma in infancy. J Pediatr 1944;24:1–37.
4. Till K. Subdural hematoma and effusion in infancy. Br Med J 1968;3:400–402.
5. McLaurin RL. Posttraumatic hematomas. In: Section of pediatric neurosurgery of the American Association of Neurologic Surgeons, ed. Pediatric neurosurgery: surgery of the developing nervous system. New York: Grune & Stratton, 1982.
6. Collins WF, Pucci GL. Peritoneal drainage of subdural hematomas in infants. J Pediatr 1961;58:482–485.

CHAPTER 47

VENTRICULAR PUNCTURE

James F. Wiley II and Ann-Christine Duhaime

INTRODUCTION

Ventricular puncture refers to the removal of cerebrospinal fluid directly from the intracranial ventricular system by way of an open fontanel or suture. The procedure is appropriate for young patients with signs of impending brain herniation from acute untreated hydrocephalus. Once excess fluid is removed, definitive treatment with a ventriculoperitoneal (VP) shunt follows. A ventricular puncture requires a thorough knowledge of anatomy and an understanding of the risks and benefits of the procedure. Ideally, a neurosurgeon should perform a ventricular puncture. When the neurosurgeon is unavailable, only the most experienced physician should attempt this procedure. The need for a ventricular puncture implies that the patient is unstable from untreated intracranial hypertension. For this reason, the physician should perform the procedure in an area where acute decompensation can be quickly managed such as the emergency department (ED), intensive care unit, or operating room.

ANATOMY AND PHYSIOLOGY

The anterior horn of the lateral ventricle lies directly beneath the lateral border of the anterior fontanel before its closure around 12 to 18 months (Fig. 47.1). This area corresponds to the coronal suture, approximately 2 cm from the midline in an older child. In a patient with hydrocephalus, dilation of the ventricles creates a large potential site for puncture.

Most importantly, the physician must not puncture too close to the sagittal midline where the venous sagittal sinus is located (Fig. 47.1).

Hydrocephalus occurs under two conditions—obstructive hydrocephalus in which a physical blockage of the ventricular system is present, and communicating hydrocephalus in which the capacity to absorb cerebrospinal fluid is exceeded by the production of cerebrospinal fluid. Common causes of chronic obstructive hydrocephalus include congenital aqueductal stenosis, posterior fossa tumors, and other congenital anomalies such as the Dandy-Walker malformation. Meningitis is the most common cause of communicating hydrocephalus. Acute decompensation with cerebral herniation is more likely to occur in a patient with acute obstructive hydrocephalus, which may complicate head trauma, intracranial hemorrhage, and space-occupying lesions that impinge on the ventricular system such as a brain abscess or brain tumor (1).

INDICATIONS

Cerebral herniation, unresponsive to hyperventilation and diuretics, in a child with an open fontanel or coronal suture is the primary indication for a ventricular puncture. Physical findings in such a child would include unilateral or bilateral pupillary dilation, ocular cranial nerve abnormalities, focal neurologic findings and decorticate or decerebrate posturing (see also Chapters 44 and 45). Before performing the procedure,

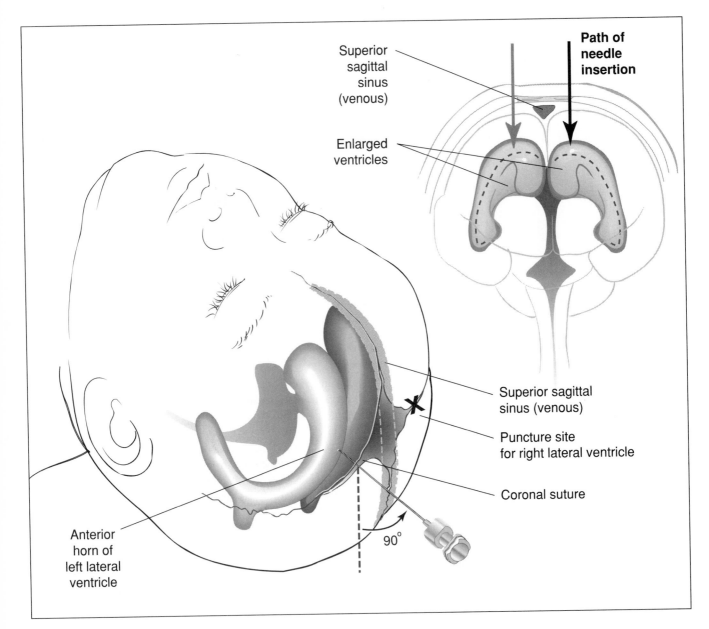

Figure 47.1.
Ventricular puncture.

Superior sagittal sinus (venous)

Enlarged ventricles

Path of needle insertion

Superior sagittal sinus (venous)

Puncture site for right lateral ventricle

Coronal suture

Anterior horn of left lateral ventricle

90°

the physician must consider other potential etiologies for which this procedure would not be indicated such as brain tumor, head trauma with cerebral edema, subdural hematoma, and epidural hematoma. Consultation and concurrent management with a neurosurgeon, as well as imaging studies (computed tomography of the head or cerebral ultrasound) should precede the procedure if at all possible.

This procedure is not indicated for the patient with hydrocephalus who is asymptomatic. A patient with a closed fontanel and sutures requires a surgical approach to the ventricular system.

EQUIPMENT

Isopropyl alcohol
Betadine
18-gauge, 2.5 spinal needle
Sterile 10 mL syringe
Sterile test tubes
Sterile towels

PROCEDURE

Because performance of this procedure assumes ongoing herniation, the patient should be positioned head up at 30°. The child must

**Chapter 47
Ventricular Puncture**

be restrained to prevent inadvertent movement (see Chapter 3). The site should first be cleansed with alcohol. The hair may be clipped or shaved to provide a 2 cm area at the lateral border of the anterior fontanel or over the coronal suture approximately 2 cm from the midline. Next the site should be thoroughly cleansed with betadine using repetitive center-to-circumference motions.

The needle enters the skin perpendicular to the skull at the lateral border of the anterior fontanel or through the coronal suture at least 2 cm from the sagittal midline (Fig. 47.1). The needle is advanced slowly checking for fluid return every centimeter. The direction of the spinal needle should not be changed while it is advanced. Alternatively, the stylet may be removed from the spinal needle after the skin is punctured and a syringe is attached which is then advanced with gentle suction until cerebrospinal fluid is obtained. Enough fluid is removed to reverse the signs and symptoms of hydrocephalus (2).

COMPLICATIONS

A ventricular puncture carries a high risk of potentially life-threatening complications such as cerebral abscess, intracranial hemorrhage, parenchymal damage, and subdural hematoma. Cerebral abscess and ventriculitis may occur following a ventricular puncture if a lapse in sterile technique occurs. Inadvertent puncture of the sagittal venous sinus results from a ventricular puncture that is too close to the midline. Subsequent bleeding

may be difficult to control, potentially leading to severe brain injury or death. By necessity, a ventricular puncture causes damage to brain parenchyma. This damage can be increased if the spinal needle is passed in multiple directions with shearing of the brain matter. Finally, rapid removal of fluid may lead to a shrinkage in brain size which can cause transection of subdural bridging veins with subdural hematoma formation. The serious nature of potential complications after a ventricular puncture dictates close assessment of the patient after the procedure, ideally with immediate imaging by computed tomography, once the patient is stabilized.

SUMMARY

A ventricular puncture is indicated for a patient with hydrocephalus and an open anterior fontanel or coronal suture who shows advanced signs of cerebral herniation unresponsive to hyperventilation and diuretic therapy. This procedure may be life-saving in this setting but carries significant risks of infection, parenchymal brain damage, and intracranial bleeding. After a ventricular puncture, the patient requires close observation and immediate brain imaging.

REFERENCES

1. Milhorat TH. Acute hydrocephalus. N Engl J Med 1970;283:857–859.
2. Perret G, Meyers R. Neurosurgery in infants and children. Pediatr Clin North Am 1960;7:543–582.

SUMMARY
1. Restrain patient to prevent inadvertent motion
2. Position patient with head up at 30°
3. Prepare site (lateral border of anterior fontanel or coronal suture 2 cm from midline) using alcohol
4. Shave or clip hair to provide 2 cm diameter site
5. Cleanse puncture site vigorously with betadine
6. Stretch skin over puncture site
7. Puncture skin at lateral border of anterior fontanel or through coronal suture 2 cm from midline with 18-gauge, 2.5 or 3.5-inch spinal needle
8. Release skin, direct and advance needle perpendicular to skull (straight in)
9. Advance needle slowly checking for fluid return every centimeter OR remove stylet and attach syringe and advance slowly with gentle suction
10. Remove fluid until signs and symptoms of herniation subside
11. Withdraw spinal needle slowly

CLINICAL TIPS
1. Once symptoms are relieved, the needle should be removed slowly until CSF flow ceases. The needle length is marked from skin edge to tip, thus estimating cortical width.
2. The direction of the spinal needle should not be changed nor should the needle be rotated in the skull. To change direction of puncture, the spinal needle must be removed to skin level.

OPHTHALMOLOGIC PROCEDURES

Section Editor: Mark D. Joffe

GENERAL PEDIATRIC OPTHALMOLOGIC PROCEDURES

Alex V. Levin

INTRODUCTION

Physicians caring for children will be confronted with a number of ocular problems including trauma, infection, inflammation and ocular manifestations of systemic disease. Although management of some ocular conditions will require consultation by an ophthalmologist (1), initial diagnosis and management can be greatly facilitated by a familiarity with basic ocular procedures that lie within the skills of the nonophthalmologist.

OPENING THE LIDS

One of the most challenging procedures is to adequately visualize the external ocular structures when obscured by lid swelling or when a noncompliant, fearful child refuses to voluntarily allow the eyeball to be viewed. Selection of the appropriate technique depends on circumstance and equipment availability. Once the eyeball is visualized, the examiner then can make the appropriate triage: ophthalmology consultation (hyphema, full thickness or lid margin laceration, corneal ulcer), treatment (bacterial conjunctivitis, corneal abrasion), or observation (viral conjunctivitis). The eye can be evaluated in a logical, progressive anatomical fashion considering each structure separately and in order—eye movements, visual acuity, conjunctiva, cornea, anterior chamber, pupil, lens, optic nerve, and retina.

Anatomy and Physiology

Skin of the eyelids is quite loose and redundant, which allows for the marked accumulation of fluid. As the tissues become increasingly distended, the lids become tense and more difficult to open. The eyelashes are inserted in the lid margin—a firm, densely packed area at the edge of each lid. The lid margin acts as a focal point for the application of mechanical devices designed to separate the lids for visualization of the underlying eyeball (Fig. 48.1). Forced lid closure is largely accomplished by voluntary (and at times involuntary) contraction of the orbicularis oculi muscle. If the examiner places pressure on the bony origins and insertions of this muscle, its contractile force is greatly disadvantaged.

Manual Lid Opening

Indications
This technique is best used for the noncompliant child who is firmly squeezing the eyelids closed. It also can be used to facilitate the instillation of eye drops or ointments.

Equipment
None

Procedure
With the child's head gently restrained in the supine position (or when available in an ex-

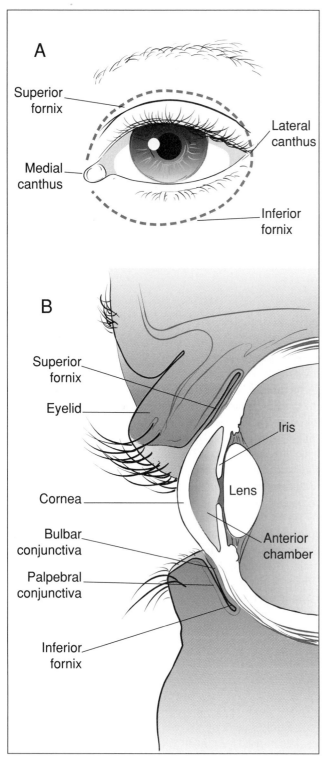

Figure 48.1.
Anatomy of the eye.

**Chapter 48
General Pediatric
Ophthalmologic
Procedures**

thumb on the infraorbital rim. Pressure is applied at these two locations compressing the underlying muscle firmly against the bone (Fig. 48.2). This is not a painful procedure. While pressure is being applied, the thumbs and underlying tissue are moved superiorly and inferiorly thus dragging the lids open. The thumbs should not be placed on the eyelids as this may cause lid eversion or pressure on the eyeball. This procedure also can be used in any type of lid swelling as it allows for the lids to be opened without putting undue pressure on the globe.

Complications
The major complication of this technique is extrusion of intraocular contents if an underlying unrecognized laceration of the globe is present.

Summary
Manual lid opening is an excellent technique requiring no equipment which allows for the opening of virtually any lids. Care must be taken in a trauma setting to avoid putting manual pressure on a ruptured globe.

Lid Opening with Cotton-Tipped Swabs

Indications
Although this procedure can be very useful in opening swollen or forcibly closed lids, particularly in infants, it should *not* be used in the traumatized eye until the presence of a ruptured globe has been ruled out, as this procedure will put pressure on the globe.

Equipment
The examiner should use a cotton-tipped applicator of the usual bulk, but with a short wooden or plastic stick. If only applicators with long sticks are available, then the examiner should either break the stick to within a few inches of the tip or be sure to grasp the stick close to the tip. This helps to avoid potentially harmful breakage of the stick during the procedure.

Procedure
While standing beside the supine patient's head, ipsilateral to the eye to be examined, and with the child's head gently restrained,

amining chair with the head tilted back), the palm of one hand is placed on the forehead and the fingers of the other hand are used to grasp the lower face, taking care not to obstruct the airways but allowing for the head to be stabilized. The upper thumb is placed on the supraorbital rim (eyebrow) and the lower

one applicator tip is placed on the mid body of the upper lid, and the other in a similar position on the lower lid (Fig. 48.3.A). With just enough pressure to engage the skin, the swabs are rotated approximately one-quarter turn in the direction of the lashes (Fig. 48.3.B). This will begin to draw the lid margins apart. The tips are then depressed with some firmness posteriorly (in the direction of the underlying globe), thus engaging the entire thickness of the lid, and then simultaneously the swabs are separated from each other in the direction of the orbital rims—the upper lid swab moving superiorly and the lower swab inferiorly (Fig. 48.3.C).

Complications

If the swabs are not applied firmly to the lids or if the rotation is in the wrong direction, the lids will evert thus making visualization even more difficult. If the swab sticks are too long, they may break during the procedure possibly causing injury to the globe. Rolling the swabs too far toward the eyelid margin might allow the swabs to roll onto the corneal surface and can result in a corneal abrasion.

Summary

Using cotton-tipped swabs allows for wide, controlled separation of the lids. Swabs should not be used in the traumatized eye until rupture of the globe has been excluded.

Lid Specula

Indications

Virtually no contraindications exist to speculum insertion. Specula do not put pressure on the globe and can therefore be used to open lids swollen by trauma.

Equipment

A variety of pediatric lid specula are commercially available. When purchasing a

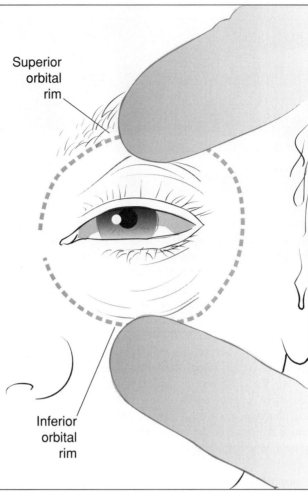

Superior orbital rim

Inferior orbital rim

speculum, considerations should include tensile strength (to resist spontaneous extrusion with the child's voluntary forced lid closure), size (to allow easy insertion particularly in infants), cost, and ease of handling. The Alfonso eye speculum is useful in the greatest number of situations because it has good tensile strength, a small open blade which can be inserted into palpebral openings of virtually any size, reasonable cost, and a thumb rest to facilitate ease of handling. Specula that are bulky or that require screw mechanisms to keep them in place are usually not desirable in the emergency setting and require more skill to insert. Specula and retractors should be sterilized between patients.

Procedure

Before inserting the speculum, the child should be supine and gently restrained to prevent spontaneous movement of the head. A drop of topical anesthetic (proparacaine or

**Chapter 48
General Pediatric
Ophthalmologic
Procedures**

581

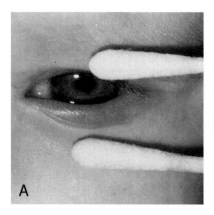
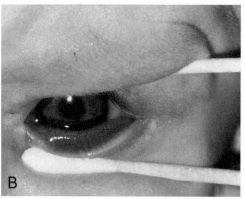
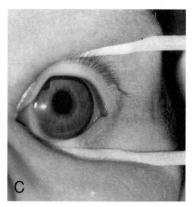

Figure 48.3.
Opening eye with cotton-tipped swabs.
A. Swabs are placed against upper and lower lids.
B. Gentle pressure and a one-quarter rotation toward the lid margin engages the upper lid without eversion. A similar procedure will engage the lower lid.
C. Swabs are separated to visualize the eyeball.

tetracaine) must be instilled. Onset of action of these drugs is within 30 seconds. Arms of the speculum are grasped between the thumb and forefinger. The first blade can be inserted into either the upper or lower lid. The examiner should gently retract the lid away from its fellow lid to expose the lid margin, so that the corresponding speculum blade can be placed on the lid margin (Fig. 48.4). The speculum is then compressed while pushing the engaged lid away so that the fellow lid can then be engaged with the remaining speculum blade on the lid margin. The speculum is then slowly and gently released to allow the lids to separate with it.

Complications
Although specula are fashioned in such a way that, with the assistance of the normally present corneal tear film, they glide easily over the ocular surface, they may on rare occasion induce corneal abrasion. Despite using topical anesthetic, some patients object to the periocular "stretching" sensation which might in turn increase agitation and combative behavior. Specula also may cause the extension of a preexisting lid laceration.

Summary
Specula are more expensive but provide an easy and effective way to achieve lid separation. They can be used in any situation to facilitate examination of the eyeball.

Lid Retractors

Indications
Retractors can be used in virtually any situation when the lids need to be separated in an assisted fashion. They tend to be less disturb-

ing to the agitated patient as they cause less stretching discomfort than a speculum.

Equipment
Lid retractors operate on only one lid at a time although two can be used simultaneously to retract both lids. The most commonly used commercial type is the Desmarres retractor, which is available in a number of sizes. A small (size 1) Desmarres is perhaps most practical in the pediatric emergency setting because it can be used on any size patient. If this commercial retractor is too costly or not available, the examiner can easily construct a disposable retractor out of paper clips (Fig. 48.5.A). The paperclip type chosen for this usage should be smooth metal, and not coated. The coating on some clips may fragment when the clip is bent, creating particles which can disperse onto the conjunctiva or cornea. After bending, it would be prudent to double-check the bent clip to be certain no such particles have formed. Such paperclip retractors are intended for single usage, and should be prepared by cleansing with an alcohol swab prior to use. Like specula, retractors do not put pressure on the globe.

Procedure
The patient is positioned and the eye anesthetized topically in the same fashion as just described for using specula. The retractor can be held either like a pencil or with the thumb and forefinger, approaching one lid (usually the upper) at a 90° angle to the lid margin. The margin is then engaged by the retractor blade and pulled back away from the fellow lid while being careful not to lift the lid too far off the surface of the eyeball (Fig. 48.5.B). If needed, it can be helpful to have an assis-

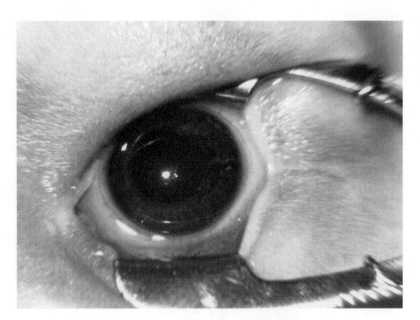

tant hold the retractor in place while the eyeball is then examined. If paper clips are used as retractors, they can be taped to the forehead (upper lid) and cheek.

Complications

Like specula, retractors can result in corneal abrasion or extension of a preexisting lid laceration. Paper clip retractors may allow for the deposition of tiny particulate matter loosened from the clip surface when it is bent into position.

Summary

Retractors offer the examiner a handy, painless way to move the lids away from the eyeball. When used properly, retractors are safe even in the setting of eye trauma.

Everting the Upper Eyelid

Introduction

This is a basic technique that should be mastered by all primary care physicians and emergency personnel. It allows for rapid inspection of the undersurface of the upper lid with minimal discomfort.

Anatomy and Physiology

The upper lid contains a band of dense collagenous tissue (tarsal plate) which spans the majority of the horizontal width of the lid and rises to occupy approximately 60% of the lid height from the lid margin upward. By applying pressure to the lid just above the superior border of this plate, a fulcrum point is created whereby the lower section of the lid can be rotated upward, thus folding the lid back on itself so that its undersurface (the palpebral conjunctiva) comes into view.

Indications

Eversion of the eyelid is useful when the examiner wishes to view the palpebral conjunctiva of the upper lid. The lid is everted to search for foreign bodies, to facilitate complete lavage following chemical exposure, and to visualize changes diagnostic of various types of conjunctivitis.

Procedure

The key to success when performing upper lid eversion is to have the child keep the eyes in down gaze (Fig. 48.6.A). Repetitively reminding the child to keep looking down is very helpful. The procedure is extremely difficult in the noncompliant child who is crying or refusing to open the eyes. Examination with sedation or ophthalmology consultation may be required. In the compliant patient, the lid can be everted with the patient supine, cradled in the arms of the parent, or sitting.

A cotton-tipped applicator (vide supra) is placed on the mid body of the upper lid with just enough pressure to engage the skin (Fig. 48.6.B). The applicator is rotated in position toward the lid margin which will draw the skin up under the applicator causing the lid margin and lashes to rotate away from the

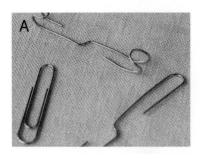

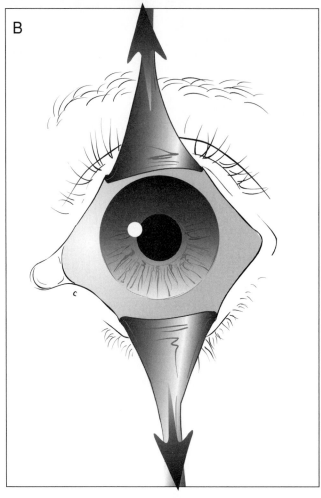

If a foreign body is seen, it can be removed gently with a cotton swab or, if embedded, plucked away with a nontoothed forceps (Chapter 50). This type of manipulation usually requires topical anesthetic.

Complications

Lid eversion is a painless procedure when done properly, although it may be associated with an unfamiliar and uncomfortable sensation. Instillation of topical anesthetic may be helpful in such patients. Extension of a lid laceration can occur.

Summary

Lid eversion is a technique used for inspection of the undersurface of the upper lid, particularly when searching for a foreign body or during ocular lavage. It is simple and very useful in the emergency care of children.

Visual Acuity Testing

Introduction

Visual acuity testing is the foundation of the eye examination. However, a basic understanding of the pediatric visual system and age-related behavioral patterns is important for optimizing the usefulness and accuracy of this procedure.

eyeball (Fig. 48.6.C). The lashes are grasped between the thumb and forefinger, and then simultaneously pulled upward (towards the forehead) while pushing the applicator tip into the body of the lid in a downward direction (Fig. 48.6.D, E). The lower half of the lid should abruptly "flip" over the swab. The examiner can then use the thumb of the hand holding the lashes to pin the lashes against the superior orbital rim or eyebrow while the examination is conducted (Fig. 48.6.F). At this point, the swab is removed by pulling it straight laterally away from the face, which may require a firm tug.

Anatomy and Physiology

Visual acuity testing is based on a construct that specifies "normal" as the ability to read a certain size letter from a certain distance, which in turn is based on the assumption that there is a normal or average shaped eye which is capable of performing this visual task without any assistance. Such an eye is said to see 20/20 (metric equivalent 6/6). However, if an otherwise perfectly healthy eyeball is a bit longer (nearsightedness, myopia), shorter

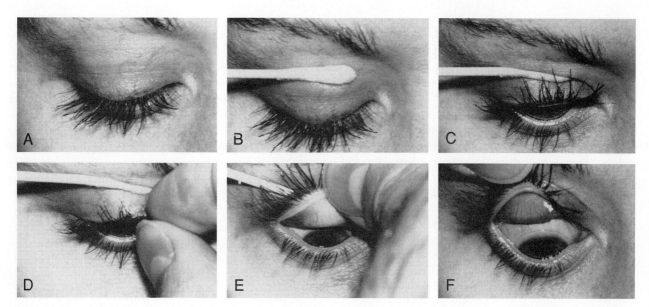

Figure 48.6.
Upper eyelid eversion.
A. The child is asked to look downward.
B. A cotton-tipped applicator is placed on the mid body of the upper lid.
C. The applicator is rotated toward the lid margin causing the lid margin and lashes to rotate away from the eyeball.
D., E. The lashes are grasped between the thumb and forefinger, pulled upward while pushing the applicator tip into the body of the lid.
F. The thumb pins the lashes against the superior orbital rim while the examination is conducted.

(farsightedness, hyperopia), or the surface of the eye is not perfectly round (astigmatism), then the abnormal eye shape will result in images that are not focused on the desired spot on the retina. This results in a blurry image. For example, a person who sees 20/80 has to stand at 20 feet to see what the normal 20/20 individual can see standing from 80 feet. Glasses can correct this problem by altering the pathway of light so that the image that is being viewed is redirected to fall crisply on the retina. It is this corrected visual acuity that is the true measure of ocular health. Only if an organic abnormality exists (retinal trauma, optic nerve problem, cataract, hyphema) will a reduction occur in the best corrected visual acuity.

Although the visual acuity of each eye is essentially independent from its fellow eye, another important consideration is the unconscious desire for the immature pediatric visual system to use the better eye. Not only will children demonstrate behavioral alterations when their better eye is covered, but they also may engage in somewhat unconscious behaviors in an attempt to use their better eye for testing, despite the efforts of the examiner to prevent this from occurring. As a result, the child will capitalize on any breech in technique to allow the better eye to become the seeing eye. The child will look around a handheld occluding device, look through the tiny gaps between the fingers in the hand that is covering an eye, or turn the face to look around an occluding device or hand while reading a chart straight ahead. The examiner must constantly be alert for these behaviors to avoid inaccuracy. It is this demanding preference for the better eye that results in amblyopia, a condition unique to the developing visual system.

Indications

Virtually all patients who present with an ocular complaint (and many who present with neurologic complaints) should have their visual acuity measured. Even the preverbal patient or the supine patient, both of whom are unable to read the standard wall chart, should have some estimation made of their visual acuity.

Equipment

Occlusion of the eye that is not being tested is perhaps best achieved by covering this eye with a broad (2 inch), lightly adhesive, hypoallergenic tape. In the absence of tape, or when the child objects to the application of tape, the palm of an examiner or caretaker's hand can be used.

Selection of a testing chart is based on the child's developmental age and reading capabilities. The illiterate child can be tested with an Allen picture chart in black and white which uses standardized figures representing a cake, car, hand, telephone, and man on a horse. Color picture charts are available for use but it is recommended that the yellow figures be ignored, as low contrast differential between the yellow and background white, particularly in a brightly lit emergency department, can lead to errors not reflective of the true visual acuity. Other charts are available for the illiterate child, in particular the tumbling E chart, in which the child is asked to indicate the direction in which a capital letter E is pointing. However, this can often be quite confusing to younger children, who are not yet able to describe and point appropriately. Matching systems, such as the HOTV card of the Sheridan Gardiner testing cards, allow the child who is entering the age of literacy to use a rudimentary knowledge of letters to match the chart letter with a card held in his or her own hand which contains identical letters. This is also particularly helpful in children between the ages of 3 and 6 who are capable of performing visual recognition and identification but too frightened or developmentally immature to venture a spoken guess. For children who are fluently familiar with the letters of the alphabet, the standard Snellen letter chart is recommended. Although the charts are available in different sizes, a standard chart designed to be read at 20 feet (6 meters) can be used at virtually any distance. If the chart location only permits the patient to stand at 10 feet, then the value of each line is doubled (the 20/20 line would have a 20/40 value).

Procedure

With visual acuity testing, the unaffected eye is tested first. This is particularly helpful in young children who may be fearful or shy. They can become familiar with the testing procedure and gain confidence in their performance using their better eye. The appropriate chart is selected and the desired eye occluded. When using occluding tape the examiner must ensure that the child is not able to peek out medially or laterally around the edge of the tape, which should be pressed firmly against the bridge of the nose and the lateral orbital rim. The patient should be placed at the proper distance while the examiner stands next to the wall chart. This allows the examiner to observe the child during testing to ensure that no cheating by the better eye occurs.

The examiner should have no need to go through every letter on the chart. In fact, when testing the better eye, the examiner can start with the 20/20 line and ask the child to identify the first one or two letters. If the child fails this line, then the examiner can back down to a line with larger print to avoid losing the child's attention as the examination proceeds. Likewise, the examiner should indicate that all guesses the child makes, particularly in younger children, are correct even when they are not. Using cheerful, positive reinforcement encourages the child's best performance. Telling the child that he or she is wrong repeatedly may inhibit the child from volunteering responses on lines that he or she is able to see.

Testing of both eyes allows for comparison. If, for example, both the injured eye and the uninjured eye have poor vision, then the examiner might suspect that the poor vision is unrelated to the trauma (the child may simply need glasses). Likewise, children should always have their vision tested when wearing their glasses. This allows for measurement of the best corrected visual acuity. If the child does not have the glasses along, the examiner can try testing the vision while the child views the chart through pinholes. Any vision that gets better while viewing through a pinhole is indicative of a refractive error (need for glasses) rather than an organic problem. Although commercially available pinhole occluders can be purchased, the examiner can take any piece of paper, create a cluster of holes using an 18-gauge needle, and then hold this up to the tested eye. For example, if the traumatized eye initially reads 20/400 and the vision then improves to 20/25 or 20/30 (often the best testable using this crude pinhole method), then the examiner knows that the child has no serious visually compromising injury. Although a numerical visual acuity cannot be generated for a preverbal child, the examiner can alternately cover each eye looking for an adverse change in behavior (irritability, pushing the examiner's hand away) when the better eye is covered, thus forcing the child to view with the weaker eye.

If the injured or ill child is unable to stand while using a chart, a commercially available near card can be used to test the vision. If the child is able to see the 20/20 line at near, it is highly unlikely that any serious visually disturbing abnormality is present. If a near card is not available, the child can then be asked to identify letters on any form of common use print which is usually roughly equivalent to the 20/60 line. If a child is unable to read print, the examiner should at least indicate the presence or absence of vision (light perception versus no light perception), a test which can be done even through a closed lid with the use of a bright light. The child who is able to see light can then be asked to identify a hand moving in front of the affected eye and perhaps to count the fingers on that hand, noting the distance at which the child is still able to count fingers (counting fingers at 2 feet).

A critical part of visual acuity testing is the recording of the results. The examiner should indicate the numerical value of the visual acuity and the type of method used for testing. When quantitative acuity is not possible, gross acuity is recorded as a preference for either eye (preverbal), counting fingers distance, hand motions, light perception, or no light perception.

Complications

Perhaps the greatest risk of visual acuity testing lies in obtaining an inaccurate measurement. The examiner also must be careful that the occlusion of the injured eye does not lead to further discomfort or harm. In children with infectious conjunctivitis, tape used to cover the eye should be discarded to prevent fomite transmission.

Summary

Visual acuity testing is an essential part of any emergency examination of the eyes. Both eyes should be tested with the patient wearing his or her glasses. Proper attention to testing procedures will lead to optimal accuracy.

Direct Ophthalmoscopy

Introduction

Direct ophthalmoscopy is the procedure used to view the optic nerve and the posterior retina (Fig. 48.7).

Anatomy and Physiology

The optic nerve enters the sclera nasal to the center of vision—the fovea. The optic nerve carries with it the retinal blood vessels which fan out onto the surface of the retina. The region temporal to the optic nerve between the major superior and inferior vessels (superior and inferior arcades) is the macula. The fovea appears as a small, dark area in the center of the macula, and is used for straight ahead fixation. The optic nerve usually appears pinkish and contains a central white area called the cup, which contains the emerging retinal vessels. The size of the cup in children is quite variable. In papilledema, swelling of the optic nerve fibers causes the cup to be obliterated. The optic nerve margin should be sharply demarcated. Otherwise the examiner might suspect the presence of papilledema. Sometimes a normal variant collection of hyper- or hypopigmentation occurs around the nerve.

The basic principle of direct ophthalmoscopy relies on the illumination of the interior of the eye posterior to the iris which would otherwise appear black.

Indications

Direct ophthalmoscopy is used to look for abnormalities of the optic nerve (papilledema), retinal hemorrhages (as in shaken baby syndrome), or other abnormalities of the posterior retina.

Equipment

Several direct ophthalmoscopes are commercially available. It is beyond the scope of this chapter to discuss their relative merits. How-

Figure 48.7.
Normal posterior retina.
Large arrow—Sharp optic disk margin.
Small arrow—Optic cup.
Triangles—Branching vessel can be followed proximally to locate optic nerve.

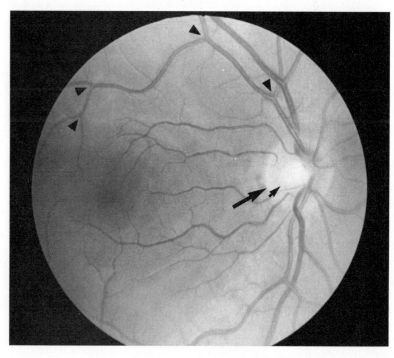

ever, it is recommended that the chosen brand be full size, easily rechargeable, and equipped at least with a blue light (for the detection of fluorescein staining of a corneal abrasion) and at least two sizes of illuminated circular spot beams.

Occasionally, the child's pupil will be too small to allow for an acceptable view of the optic nerve with the direct ophthalmoscope. Under these circumstances, phenylephrine 2.5% and cyclopentolate 1% eye drops can be used to dilate the pupil.

Procedure

The examiner may use the direct ophthalmoscope with or without glasses or contact lenses. The instrument is held in the hand that corresponds to the eye being examined (right hand for right eye, left hand for left eye). The examiner stands on the side of the patient ipsilateral to the eye being examined. The cooperative patient should be asked to sit on an examining table and to fixate on a distant target. This method allows the child to keep the eyes still while the examiner looks in through the pupil. However, if the examiner's head blocks the view of the eye not being examined, then the child's eyes may wander. To avoid this complication, the examiner's face should approach the child's face with the direct ophthalmoscope in front of the same eye of the examiner as the eye being examined (the examiner's right eye is used to examine the patient's right eye) and the examiner's head should be parallel to the child's head. This method prevents obstruction of the other eye by the examiner's head. If the child is seated below the standing examiner, then the examiner can either sit in a chair facing the child or lean over from a standing position while tilting the child's head away, so that when the examiner bends over, his or her head is still parallel to that of the child.

In infants, the examiner cannot hope for continued fixation with the unexamined eye. It is usually easiest to have the infant in the supine position. The examiner should simply be in a position as close to the examined eye as possible and patiently wait for the optic nerve to move briefly, albeit intermittently, into view. The examiner should not "chase" the optic nerve with the movements of the eye as this is usually futile and frustrating. Phar-

macologic dilation of the pupil is helpful in examination of the optic nerves of infants and toddlers.

The examination is facilitated by darkening the room as much as possible to induce natural pupillary dilation. It is best to use the smallest circle of light provided by the direct ophthalmoscope to maximize the amount of light entering the pupil and to minimize the amount of light not entering the pupil, which reflects off the iris causing glare to the examiner.

The direct ophthalmoscope focusing wheel is set on zero. Standing approximately 1 foot away from the patient, the examiner should look through the direct ophthalmoscope while shining the light in the eye to be examined to obtain a red reflex. As the examiner moves closer to the patient, a retinal blood vessel will be sighted within this red reflex and followed toward the optic nerve. The apex of branches in the vessel always points in the direction of the optic nerve and therefore guides the examiner in the proper direction, like arrows pointing the way. The examiner moves closer to the patient, ultimately arriving at a distance of less than 3 inches from the eye. The focusing wheel may be turned in either direction to keep the retinal blood vessel that is being tracked in focus.

Once the optic nerve is localized, its circumferential border is identified and assessed for clarity and sharpness. To view the macula and fovea, compliant children can be asked to look directly into the direct ophthalmoscope.

Complications

Occasionally, particularly in younger children, the direct ophthalmoscope may increase anxiety and induce photophobia (particularly in the presence of ocular surface disease). Although dilating drops may sting when administered, they have virtually no contraindications in children with the exception of ectopia lentis, previously diagnosed narrow angle glaucoma (dilation may occur in other forms of childhood glaucoma), or known allergy to the drops—all of which are rare. If the child has a neurologic disorder or injury, it may be wise to consult with a neurologist, neurosurgeon, and/or ophthalmologist before dilating the pupils so the dilation is not misinterpreted.

Summary

Direct ophthalmoscopy is a critical tool in the evaluation of many ocular disorders, brain injury, and neurologic conditions. Proper preparation will help to ensure an optimal view.

Direct Ophthalmoscope as a Handheld Magnifier

Introduction

The direct ophthalmoscope also can be used in the emergency setting as a high-power magnifier to view the front surface of the eye.

Anatomy and Physiology

The cornea is a clear dome covering the anterior segment of the eye with dimensions that appear to match that of the iris. The space between the iris and the inner corneal surface (endothelium) is filled with optically clear fluid (aqueous humor). The aqueous can become contaminated with red (hyphema) or white (iritis) blood cells. The pupil is a central hole in the iris which should appear round and reactive. Of normal individuals, 20% may have a slight difference in pupil size between the two eyes (anisocoria). It is also common to find that the pupil margin is lined with chocolate brown tissues regardless of the color of the rest of its surface. When the cornea is lacerated, fluid from the anterior chamber will leak out through the hole. The rapid change in hydrostatic pressure will cause the iris to come forward to plug the leak. Therefore, any change in iris anatomy or pupillary roundness may be a sign of a ruptured globe, an indication to stop further examination and seek urgent ophthalmologic consultation.

The lens is also optically clear. It is positioned behind the pupil. When a cataract is present, the pupil may appear white rather than the usual black.

Indications

As a magnifier, the direct ophthalmoscope is helpful in assessing the conjunctiva, cornea, and anterior chamber structures for the presence of abrasions, foreign bodies, lacerations, blood in the anterior chamber (hyphema), or cataract.

Equipment

Direct ophthalmoscope
Lid speculum or lid retractors (see specific sections in this chapter)

Procedure

The examination should be conducted with the patient's glasses off, but contact lenses can be left in place (provided the clinician finds no other reason to remove them). Once the lids are opened to allow a view of the eyeball, the examiner may approach the ocular surface from any close distance (within inches) by dialing in the green or black numbers on the focusing wheel (color of numbers depends on the brand of ophthalmoscope) while viewing through the direct ophthalmoscope. These "plus" lenses will convert the instrument into a handheld magnifier. When looking for a conjunctival or corneal abrasion that has been stained with fluorescein, the largest spot beam is used with a blue light. In the absence of a blue light, a white light is used rather than the green (red free), which may obscure the characteristic yellow-green fluorescence. When looking for a small hyphema clot in the anterior chamber, the examiner concentrates on the peripheral iris moving from the superior (12 o'clock) position in a clockwise pattern for 360°. Following trauma, subtle irregularities in pupil shape may be a sign of more serious injury such as a subluxed lens or a ruptured globe.

The conjunctiva and corneal surface also can be scanned for foreign bodies with the direct ophthalmoscope. Lateral, inferior, and superior conjunctival recesses (fornices) must be carefully inspected, lashes also can be inspected (for trichiasis).

Complications

Provided that the ocular surface is not touched, no complications other than photophobia should occur.

Summary

The direct ophthalmoscope can be used as a high-power, handheld magnifier to assess the anterior structures of the eye.

Red Reflex Test

Introduction

The red reflex test allows for rapid screening of the visual axis to ensure that light is passing clearly without obstruction by ocular abnormalities.

Anatomy and Physiology

The visual axis consists of the central cornea, anterior chamber, pupil, central lens, vitreous, and fovea. An opacity can occur anywhere along this path. For example, a corneal scar, hyphema, pupil pulled out of position by ruptured globe, cataract, vitreous hemorrhage, or retinal detachment can obstruct the visual axis.

Indication

The red reflex is a rapid screening test that should be part of virtually every examination for an ocular emergency. It is particularly helpful in the noncompliant child, and following trauma.

Equipment

Direct ophthalmoscopy
Lid speculum or lid retractors (see specific
    sections in this chapter)

Procedure

The examiner should stand approximately 3 feet (1 meter) away from the patient. While sighting through the direct ophthalmoscope, the entire face is illuminated with the largest spot beam. The examination should be conducted with the patient's glasses off, but contact lenses can be left in place. The red reflex of both eyes should be assessed simultaneously to allow for comparison, while the patient is looking directly at the ophthalmoscope light. The red reflex is actually red, pink, orange, yellow, or some combination of these colors. The color is less important than the symmetry between the eyes. Any black area within the reflex is abnormal and should prompt closer inspection of the anterior segment, optic nerve, and posterior retina as discussed previously. The most common cause of a black reflex is small pupils or a patient who is not looking at the examiner. In the former case, the reflex can be rechecked after instillation of di-

lating drops. The reflex also is enhanced by turning off the room lights.

Any frank white area also is abnormal, usually indicating the presence of an abnormality that would require ophthalmologic consultation (cataract, retinal detachment, retinoblastoma).

Complications

Photophobia is the only complication that may occur.

Summary

The red reflex test is an essential tool to rule out abnormalities in the visual axis.

Instillation of Ophthalmic Drops and Ointments

Introduction

Many children seem to fear the installation of ophthalmic medications as much as needles. With refinement of technique, the examiner can accomplish this task quickly and efficiently, thus minimizing the child's discomfort and anxiety. It also may teach parents how to properly instill these medications for home use.

Indications

Topical medications are used to treat a wide variety of ophthalmic conditions. However, neither drops nor ointments should be instilled when the clinician suspects that the globe has been ruptured. This recommendation is made not because the medications are particularly injurious, but rather because the clinician should try to avoid *all* manipulations of the eye until an ophthalmologist arrives.

Equipment

Ophthalmic drops or ointment

Anatomy and Physiology

The ocular surface, including the inner aspect of each eyelid, is lined with nonkeratinized epithelium which helps to make it remarkably absorbent. Only approximately 20% of each drop, however, can be utilized by the eye. For these reasons, an instilled drop need not touch the eyeball and only one drop, if administered correctly, is necessary. The drop can be instilled onto the inner surface (palpebral conjunctiva) of the lower lid, where it will act just as effectively as if it was dropped directly on the cornea. Absorption is rapid and the drops cannot be rubbed out of the eye immediately after instillation. Because the conjunctival recesses can only use a portion of each drop that is instilled, it is expected that some of the dose will drip down onto the patient's cheek. This should be of no concern.

Many drops sting the eye when instilled. Many children react with a reflex resistance to administration of eye medications with forceful, voluntary contraction of the orbicularis oculi muscle making instillation difficult. Although technically it is preferable to have a 5-minute waiting period between ocular instillation of different medications, the minimal benefit is probably outweighed by the increased anxiety and discomfort for the child. Rapid instillation of two different medications, one right after the other, will still create acceptably effective dosing in most clinical situations.

Procedure

The technique of manual opening of the eyelids (see specific section in this chapter) is particularly useful when strong contraction of the orbicularis oculi muscle is evident. Once *any* conjunctival surface is viewed, a drop can be instilled. The procedure is made easier by using an assistant to instill the medication once the lids are separated.

Alternatively, the clinician can hold the bottle between the forefinger and thumb in one hand while using the ulnar side of that hand to place pressure on the orbicularis either above or below the palpebral fissure (replacing the use of the thumb by that hand as explained in the manual lid opening section in this chapter). The examiner then can accomplish both eye opening and drop instillation without an assistant. If the child is resisting, it may be helpful to have both the child and his or her head restrained by an assistant or caretaker. Many children are comforted after the procedure by being allowed to use a tissue or their hand to rub the eyes.

In the extremely noncompliant patient, when the examiner feels that achieving any eye opening using the manual technique is impossible and/or when specula or retractors are either not available or not desired, he or

she can try an alternative method to get the drops onto the ocular surface. The child is placed in the supine position with eyes closed. A single drop can then be placed into the sulcus between the medial corner of the palpebral fissure (medial canthus) and the ipsilateral side of the nose. Eventually, the child will open the eye and the drop will run onto the ocular surface, provided that the child is kept in the supine position.

Topical ophthalmic ointments are instilled by pulling down the lower lid and expressing an approximately 1 to 2 cm strip onto the lower lid palpebral conjunctiva. This procedure is made easier by having the compliant patient look upward. After the ointment has been instilled, many patients find it more comforting to close their eyes for a few

SUMMARY
Opening the Eye
1. Manually compress orbicularis muscle against bones and separate lids
2. Use cotton swabs with short sticks and roll skin toward lid margin to avoid eversion
3. Instill topical anesthetic before using lid specula or lid retractors
Upper Lid Eversion
1. Recommended for lavage and identification of foreign body under lid
2. Have child look downward
3. Gently press cotton-tipped swab into body of upper lid and pull lashes to fold back upper lid
Visual Acuity Testing
1. Assess in all patients with ocular complaints
2. Test each eye with glasses on; use pinhole if glasses are not available
3. Occlude eye not being tested with tape to prevent cheating
4. Choose appropriate chart for child's developmental stage and degree of literacy
5. Record results clearly
Direct Ophthalmoscopy
1. Assess visual axis by checking red reflex with largest circle of light from 1 meter
2. Examine optic nerve and retina in darkened room with smallest circle of light
3. Use "plus" lenses (green or black numbers) as a magnifier to examine anterior structures
Drop and Ointment Instillation
1. Do not instill any medications until rupture of globe is excluded
2. Open eye and apply one drop to any conjunctival surface
3. Apply 1 cm of ointment to the lower lid palpebral conjunctiva

CLINICAL TIPS
Opening the Eye
1. Manual—no equipment, no pressure on globe
2. Cotton-tipped swabs—inexpensive, exerts pressure on globe
3. Lid specula—specialized equipment, no pressure on globe
4. Lid retractors—moderate expense, less discomfort than speculum—may fashion from paperclips
Upper Lid Eversion
1. Keep reminding patient to look down during procedure.
Visual Acuity Testing
1. Positive reinforcement improves cooperation.
2. Assess light perception or finger counting if standard test cannot be administered.
Direct Ophthalmoscopy
1. Minimize ambient light to dilate pupils.
2. Smallest circle of light decreases glare on retinal examination.
3. For infants, do not chase the moving eye. Hold position and wait for optic nerve to move into view.
Drop Instillation
1. One drop is enough.
2. Conjunctival application is sufficient.

minutes as the ointment begins to melt on the ocular surface. The child should be warned that when the eyelids open, he or she may feel a sticky sensation with some temporary blurring of vision. Excess ointment on the lashes can be wiped away with a tissue.

One special situation deserves mention. Fluorescein is sometimes delivered in the form of an impregnated paper strip. This strip should be wetted (with saline or topical anesthetic) before instillation. Dry, stiff paper in contact with the cornea can cause an abrasion.

Complications

Although each drop and ointment have their own associated side effects, instillation of drops should be atraumatic. Anxiety and fear are usually short lived. The clinician must be careful not to scratch the ocular surface with the tip of the bottle or tube. Likewise, the medication bottle or tube should not be contaminated by the lid, tears, or conjunctiva.

Summary

Instillation of topical ophthalmic medication is an essential process which can be done effectively while minimizing discomfort and anxiety for the child.

REFERENCES

1. Levin AV. Eye emergencies: acute management in the pediatric ambulatory care setting. Pediatr Emerg Care 1991;7:367–377.
2. Levin AV. Ophthalmic emergencies. In: Fleisher GR, Ludwig S, eds. Textbook of pediatric emergency medicine. 3rd ed. Philadelphia: Williams & Wilkins, 1993, pp. 1363–1370.

CHAPTER 49

SLIT LAMP EXAMINATION

Alex V. Levin

INTRODUCTION

Slit lamp biomicroscopy is a diagnostic procedure that requires familiarity and experience. It is unlikely that the majority of physicians will have the opportunity to repetitively use the slit lamp enough to acquire and refine the skills to fully use the slit lamp in many situations. Therefore, this chapter will address the basic theory and practice of slit lamp illumination along with a few common applications that may fall into the scope of practice of nonophthalmologists treating children in the emergency setting. It would of course be appropriate to seek ophthalmology consultation whenever the physician does not feel comfortable in using the slit lamp, when the diagnosis remains in question, or when the evaluation and treatment of the patient requires slit lamp techniques beyond the basics discussed herein.

Purchasing a slit lamp is an individual decision that should take into account cost, need, and the frequency of use. If it is unlikely to be used often, then it is unlikely that the physicians will have the opportunity to acquire the skills necessary for proper use. In this setting, it may be more harmful than beneficial. The slit lamp is best placed in a dedicated area, with the correct adjustable chair, and with ocular medications, forceps, and swabs readily available. Purchasing a slit lamp on wheels is an alternative. Another consideration is the utility of having the slit lamp available on site for the consulting ophthalmologist. In some situations, this may obviate the need for the patient to make a trip to the ophthalmologist's office and may allow the ophthalmologist to optimize the examination on site.

ANATOMY AND PHYSIOLOGY

Light can only be seen when it is reflected off an object. If a person were to hold a flashlight and shine it into an endless vacuum, the beam of light emanating from the bulb would be invisible. Only if a person were to place a substance or object within the path of the light, would the light become visible. For example, if smoke or dust were allowed to enter our theoretical vacuum, the beam of light would readily become apparent as it is reflected by the particles. This is called the Tyndall phenomenon. Likewise, if a person were to erect a several centimeter thick piece of Plexiglas™ in the vacuum and several meters thereafter erect a cement wall, the beam of light would now become visible as it strikes the Plexiglas™, as it moves through the Plexiglas™ (being reflected by the continuous substance of the Plexiglas™), and again as it hits the cement wall (Fig. 49.1.A). Because the vacuum itself contains no reflective materials, however, the beam would remain invisible at all other places.

These principles are directly applicable to the eyeball. If a person shines a beam of light (in this case, the slit lamp beam) into the eyeball, it will only be visible where it is reflected. Between the bulb and the eyeball it is invisible as, for the most part, air is relatively nonreflective from an optical standpoint. As

Figure 49.1.

A. A person shines a flashlight through Plexiglas™ onto a wall. The beam is only visible as it passes through the Plexiglas™ and on the wall—it is not visible between the flashlight and the Plexiglas™ or between the Plexiglas™ and the wall because air is optically clear.

B. Slit lamp beam from 45° angle is visible as an arc of light on the curved surface of the cornea and on two sides of the iris. The beam passes invisibly through the optically clear aqueous humor. The lens located just behind the pupil is also visible.

C. Schematic drawing of B.

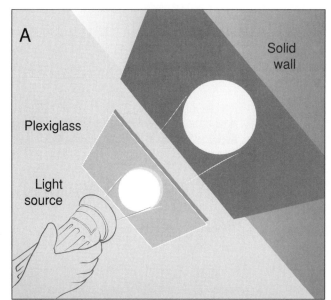

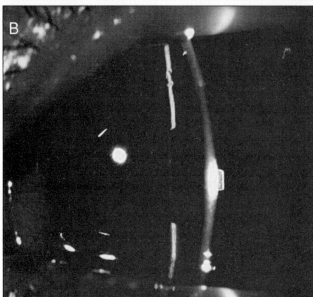

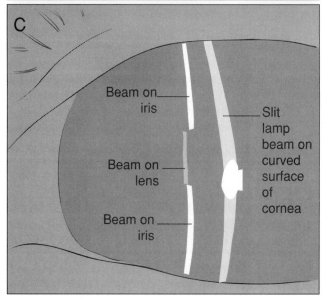

the beam hits the surface of the cornea, however, it can be seen (Fig. 49.1.B, C). As it passes through the corneal substance it is continuously visible, just as the light that passed through the Plexiglas™ in the previous example. The beam then becomes invisible as it leaves the back of the cornea and travels to the surface of the iris where it is once again reflected and therefore visible to the observer. The space between the back of the cornea and the iris (anterior chamber) is filled with optically clear fluid (aqueous humor) which prevents the beam from being visualized. The pupil is simply a hole in the iris through which the beam continues to pass, invisible to the observer until it strikes the front surface of the lens which is just beyond the pupil. Again, the beam becomes visible as it passes through the substance of the lens. Visualization of the interior of the lens is difficult without pharmacologic dilation of the pupil, but the anterior surface is easily seen with the pupil in its usual state. After pupillary dilation, the skilled observer can also visualize strands of vitreous behind the lens. Using special handheld or slit lamp mounted lenses, the ophthalmologist also can direct the slit lamp beam to allow visualization of the posterior vitreous, optic nerve, and retina.

The slit lamp is given its name because of its ability to create a slit beam of light. Using a slit allows for a topographic appreciation of a surface because the light appears to wrap around the curvature of that surface being reflected to the observer's view only where that surface exists. The observer can appreciate the corneal curvature, the iris architecture, and the curved surface of the lens (Fig 49.1). In disease states, the observer can assess the elevation and contour of ocular structures. The slit beam also allows for the delineation of the internal anatomy of translucent structures such as the cornea and lens. The skilled observer can visually distinguish the corneal layers and therefore recognize the depth of a lesion, such as foreign body or corneal laceration.

When the aqueous humor loses its optical clarity, the beam of light becomes visible as it passes from the cornea to the iris and lens. This occurs with iritis and hyphema. The white blood cells of iritis and the red blood cells of hyphema reflect the beam to the observer so that the particles can actually be seen floating in the aqueous. Likewise, protein, which has leaked from iris vessels as part of the inflammatory process of iritis, makes the aqueous turbid, allowing the entire beam to become visible such as the beam of an automobile headlight in the fog. This phenomenon is referred to as flare.

INDICATIONS

It is likely that the slit lamp will be most useful to the physician as a unique diagnostic magnification system to examine the ocular surface, in particular for the identification of corneal injury or foreign bodies. For the physician who is well-versed in slit lamp techniques, it also may be helpful for minor procedures such as foreign body removal (Chapter 50) and for the diagnosis of iritis and microscopic (no clot) hyphema.

EQUIPMENT

Slit lamps are available in many models from several manufacturers (TOPCON, Haag-Streit, Reichert, Zeiss). The Zeiss slit lamp has a different configuration from the other three, but the discussion here should be applicable to all slit lamps. If emergency personnel elect to purchase a slit lamp for their emergency department, clinic, or office, it is advisable to examine a least two models and to request the sales representative to loan a sample for trial use. All potential examiners should become familiar with the purchased

model before using it on patients, and perhaps with the repeated assistance of volunteer adult subjects. Exercises that may be helpful include identification of the corneal layers, grasping eyelashes with a forceps, identifying a contact lens on the cornea, and especially, manipulation of the slit lamp beam up, down, from side to side, and from cornea to iris while maintaining a well-focused view. Only after these skills are mastered should the examiner begin using the slit lamp on pediatric patients.

PROCEDURE

For the most part, successful use of the slit lamp requires a compliant patient. This large machine is often quite imposing for the young child. Examination of infants and those toddlers who are unable to follow directions well and easily get their chin to the head rest should be deferred to the ophthalmologist. Very compliant toddlers, sometimes as young as 2 or 3 years old, will cooperate, particularly if they are allowed to sit on their parent's lap. This is often facilitated by telling the child that the slit lamp is a type of television in which the child can see his or her favorite character. Fortunately, the child's imagination will allow him or her to see the imaginary figure promised! Another approach is to tell the child that slit lamp examination is like riding a bicycle or motorcycle. Most slit lamps have handles for the patient which stick out from either side. These can be likened to handlebars and, with the appropriate noises and encouragement from the examiner, can lead to some fun role playing for the child when being examined.

All of these techniques are made easier by using an electric examination chair which can be raised or lowered by foot pedal or hand control to place the child at a comfortable height. Most slit lamps have an adjustable headrest which is moved up or down so that the eyes of the patient are level with an indicator line or next to the face to ensure optimal ease of focus and adjustment. Slit lamps have a plastic chin rest for the patient, usually with a vertical stop to prevent the child's face from moving too far forward toward the beam. Likewise, they have a forehead bar or band which accomplishes the same purpose. The patient's forehead must be against this

SUMMARY

1. Child may sit on caretaker's lap for comfort; position chin on rest with forehead fully forward
2. Use lowest magnification and illumination that is adequate for examination
3. Examine structures systematically—conjunctiva, cornea, aqueous humor, iris, lens
4. Use fluorescein plus blue light to identify abrasions, foreign bodies, herpetic lesions on corneal surface.
5. For epilation grasp lash at its base and pull sharply along axis of hair shaft
6. Use red-free light to differentiate red and white blood cells in anterior chamber
7. Consult ophthalmology with diagnostic uncertainty, a foreign body not easily removed, a noncompliant patient, hyphema, iritis, herpetic keratitis, corneal laceration, abnormal pupil or other anatomic structures or when the examiner is unfamiliar with slit lamp use.

bar even if it requires gentle pressure on the occiput by the parent.

Once in position, the slit lamp is turned on; usually it has a power switch for which several levels of voltage may be available. Using the lowest setting is both adequate and adds to bulb longevity. Filter switches change the intensity of the illumination and also allow for other options (red-free light). A knob will be available to change the height of the beam (usually using a fully extended vertical height is easiest for the nonophthalmologist) and another knob for adjustment of beam width. A beam of 2 to 3 mm width is usually the best for the nonophthalmologist. For simple magnification of the eyeball without the need for assessing corneal layers or aqueous clarity, the beam can be opened fully in its horizontal direction until it becomes a large circle. Slit lamps also have variable magnification controlled by a knob or lever. The lowest power is usually adequate and easiest to use.

The part of the machine from which the beam emanates may be moved through a 180° arc between the patient and the examiner. In general, the patient's eye is examined with the beam swung to the side ipsilateral to that eye and projected onto the eye at approximately 45° from the visual axis. This allows maximal illumination of the ocular structures while optimizing the observer's ability to sense depth in the cornea, anterior chamber, and lens. The slit beam becomes "a slice of light" imaging a section of each structure as it passes through. The observer's view is then somewhat oblique to the beam allowing its full anterior-to-posterior course to be appreciated as it passes through a structure such as the cornea.

Focusing the beam onto a structure of interest is usually the most difficult task for the beginner. The slit lamp is equipped with a joy stick or adjusting knob(s) that allow the projecting mechanism to be elevated, lowered, moved from side to side, or toward and away from the patient. As the machine is moved, the relationship between the beam and the surface of the eye is changed, causing alterations in focus. Also, because the beam is projected onto the eye from an angle, as the machine is moved forward the beam will move to the side such that the object of regard is no longer illuminated in the same location. Coordination of focus and beam movement is

not one which can be taught in the text of a chapter. Rather, this is a skill that can be acquired only through practice.

Although the slit lamp offers the ophthalmologist the opportunity to perform a multitude of procedures under high magnification, only physicians with considerable experience should attempt the following procedures.

Special Uses

Iritis and Hyphema

Photophobia is often the first obstacle to recognizing iritis or hyphema. Using a lower power of illumination, narrower beam, and/or beam of reduced height may be helpful. Sometimes the cells and flare are best appreciated using a vertically short, moderately wide, bright beam. The examiner should try to focus on the midaqueous with the beam coming from an angle in such a way that the observer's line of sight would be extrapolated into the pupil. The black of the pupil then serves as a backdrop which makes appreciation of the aqueous abnormalities easier.

When looking for hyphema, the physician should be sure to examine the entire iris surface, in particular its far peripheral edges, for tiny adherent clots. It is helpful to do this in a systematic fashion starting superiorly (12 o'clock) and working around the iris clockwise. The slit lamp provides a green colored light, which is a red-free beam. Red blood cells are only visible by virtue of their reflecting red wavelength light. By using a red-free beam, the red blood cells become invisible. Any remaining visible cells are either liberated pigment cells (as in trauma) or white blood cells (as in iritis). This technique, although reserved for the experienced and skilled observer, can be helpful in distinguishing iritis from a microhyphema (no clot). In both situations, management requires ophthalmology consultation.

Corneal Abrasion

The slit lamp provides the observer with a blue beam (cobalt blue) that can be used to examine the cornea after instillation of fluorescein. The blue light causes the fluorescein to fluoresce such that it will appear yellow-green. This technique is useful for viewing surface abnormalities such as corneal and conjunctival abrasion, foreign bodies, and lesions associated with corneal herpetic infection (dendritic keratitis).

Intraocular Pressure Measurement

All slit lamps are capable of measuring intraocular pressure by Goldmann applanation tonometry, which is presented elsewhere (1). This advanced technique is particularly difficult in children, noncompliant patients, and photophobic patients—the very patients that are most likely to be encountered in an emergency setting.

Epilation

An eyelash may be turned toward the cornea such that its tip rubs the corneal epithelium causing microscopic abrasions that can be quite irritating and even painful. This is called trichiasis. The lash can be grabbed at its base with a fine, nontoothed forceps (epilation forceps are available), and quickly tugged along the line of origin away from the lid margin. The lash will come out with its root. Care must be taken not to twist the forceps or pull in a direction that is not parallel to the lash's origin as this will fracture the lash leaving a stub that is more difficult to grasp and may be even more injurious to the corneal surface. The procedure may be facilitated by the instillation of a topical anesthetic. The physician also must be sure to establish the cause of the trichiasis to prevent recurrence. The lash will grow back.

Removal of Foreign Body (See Chapter 50)

COMPLICATIONS

Slit lamp biomicroscopy is usually free from complication with the exception of induced photophobia and anxiety. The procedure should be otherwise painless, although some children may need to be held in place. Care must be taken not to back the machine away while the child is still on the chin rest. This could result in the child falling forward. When not in use, the tonometer should be moved laterally to its resting position to avoid trauma to the cornea when moving the machine from one eye to the other.

Epilation can cause mild pain. Corneal or conjunctival abrasion or perforation can occur during attempted removal of a foreign body, particularly if the examiner is using a needle or pointed forceps, is not well versed in the procedure, or if the child moves unexpectedly forward should the forehead be allowed to drift away from the rest. Deeply embedded foreign bodies should not be removed because of the possibility of an unrecognized perforation of the globe.

SUMMARY

The slit lamp can be a valuable tool in the emergency setting for diagnosis of ocular disorders affecting the conjunctiva, cornea, or anterior segment. An understanding of the theory behind slit lamp use helps the physician utilize the considerable capacity of the machine. Proper use requires experience that this chapter cannot provide. Children are not usually compliant patients, making their ocular evaluation with a slit lamp more difficult. Ophthalmologic consultation will frequently be necessary for full evaluation of children with ocular complaints.

REFERENCES

1. Brubaker RF. Tonometry. In: Tasman W, Jaeger EA, eds. Duane's clinical ophthalmology. Philadelphia: JB Lippincott, 1994; 3(47):1–7.

CLINICAL TIPS

1. Slit lamp use requires practice, understanding of the theory of operation, and a steady hand.
2. Consult ophthalmology for noncompliant patients.
3. A smaller, less intense beam is better tolerated by photophobic patients.
4. Look for small clots of hyphema carefully around 360° of the iris. Red cells opacifying the aqueous humor represent hyphema without clot.
5. Red-free light can help distinguish red blood cells from white blood cells and liberated pigment cells.

CHAPTER 50

Ocular Foreign Body Removal

Jennifer Pratt Cheney

Introduction

Foreign bodies commonly become lodged on the eye surface, whether blown in by wind or propelled at high velocity. Foreign bodies may be located superficially in the cornea or conjunctiva, or may be embedded. It is important to distinguish a superficial foreign body from a penetrating eye injury. Superficial foreign bodies may be removed by nurses, EMTs, or physicians trained in the procedure, and this may be performed in the outpatient setting. Embedded foreign bodies are generally removed by a physician.

Removal of ocular foreign bodies may be challenging in children. Irrigation does not require full cooperation, however, if an instrument is used for removal, the child must be completely still. For children in whom irrigation is not successful, sedation or even general anesthesia is occasionally required.

Anatomy and Physiology

The conjunctiva covers the sclera and lines the inner surfaces of the upper and lower eyelids (Fig. 48.1). It secretes a mucous film that helps to capture particulate matter on the eye surface. The cornea is a tough covering over the iris a few millimeters thick, and consists of three layers. The outer surface is composed of five layers of epithelial cells, which unlike the skin epithelium, is not keratinized. Below this, the stroma gives the cornea structural integrity. It is this layer that glows yellow-green when a corneal abrasion is stained with fluorescein. A single-cell layer of endothelium below the stroma regulates fluid and nutrient supply.

The eye will respond to the presence of a foreign body with injection of the conjunctiva, tearing, and blinking. The patient usually has associated pain; however, not all foreign body injuries, even with globe perforation, are associated with pain. Visual acuity may be affected if the foreign body is in the visual axis or if associated corneal edema is present (1).

Intraocular foreign bodies of inert materials, such as some plastics or glass, may be well tolerated and may not necessitate immediate removal. Metallic foreign bodies precipitate inflammatory reactions that can further damage the eye, whereas organic materials increase the risk of infection (2).

Indications

All foreign bodies in the eye must be removed; however, not all are removed immediately. In some circumstances, such as with the uncooperative child or when equipment is needed that is not available, removal may best be performed in an ophthalmologist's office or in an operating room. A corneal foreign body is best removed as soon as possible, because the cornea may epithelialize over the foreign body in several hours (1) and make removal more difficult.

Foreign bodies may be located on the inner surface of the eyelids, in the fornices, on bulbar conjunctiva and sclera, on the cornea, or may have penetrated the globe. Corneal foreign bodies are most commonly found on the lower two-thirds of the cornea.

Examination to rule out foreign body is indicated when a child complains of foreign body sensation. Foreign body sensations are not uncommon, however, and may represent other conditions such as conjunctivitis. A patient may complain of foreign body sensation when the foreign body is no longer in the eye but has resulted in a residual corneal abrasion.

Vertical, linear corneal abrasions often result when foreign bodies adherent to the inside of the upper lid injure the cornea during blinking. If noted on eye examination with fluoroscein, a thorough search for ocular foreign body is indicated.

The presence of a metallic foreign body in the eye, even for a few hours, may result in a brownish rust ring at the site of the injury. Removal of the foreign body and the rust ring is required, but the rust ring can be removed at follow-up by an ophthalmologist (see Complications in this chapter).

Attempts at foreign body removal by the emergency physician is contraindicated if a ruptured globe is suspected, if patient cooperation precludes safe removal, or if the foreign body appears to be embedded. In these circumstances, and when attempts at foreign body removal are either unsuccessful or the foreign body is incompletely removed, immediate referral to an ophthalmologist is indicated. When the possibility of ruptured globe exists, the eye should be protected with an eye shield. This keeps the patient from rubbing the eye and prevents any contact of the eye that can cause extrusion of orbital contents.

Indications for immediate ophthalmologic consultation include the presence of an embedded foreign body, unsuccessful foreign body removal attempts, a patient who is unable to cooperate with the procedure, any indication of possible ruptured globe such as hyphema or an irregular or sluggish pupil, or a decrease in visual acuity.

EQUIPMENT

Visual acuity chart
Topical anesthetic drops (proparacaine HCl 0.5%)
Sterile water, syringe, and plastic catheter
Sterile cotton-tipped applicators
Fluorescein drops or strips
Wood's lamp or slit lamp
Eye spud or 25-gauge needle on 3 mL syringe
Topical dilating drops (homatropine 5%)
Antibiotic ointment or drops
2 eye patches
Tape

PROCEDURE

Evaluation for Ocular Foreign Body

Emergency personnel should ask the child or parent how the foreign body entered the eye. An object blowing or falling into the eye is unlikely to penetrate the globe, whereas an object entering the eye at high velocity, such as when hammering on metal or working with industrial tools, should alert the clinician to possible rupture of the globe.

Before the eye is anesthetized, the physician may ask the older child where the foreign body sensation is located. Kaye-Wilson demonstrated that adult patients indicating a foreign body sensation in either the temporal, nasal, or central regions were generally correct in identifying the area of the cornea where a foreign body was located. Localization to the lower lid indicated a foreign body in the lower half of the cornea. Localization of the foreign body sensation to the upper lid was less reliable, and foreign bodies were located in any region of the cornea. This information may be particularly useful to the physician who does not have access to a slit lamp (3).

It is often difficult for children to cooperate with techniques involving direct removal of ocular foreign bodies. Minimal cooperation may be required for the irrigation technique. Conscious sedation can be helpful in children who may be able to remain still during foreign body removal (Chapter 35).

Using conscious sedation requires a physician trained in its use and careful monitoring of the patient. If the patient is sedated and the attempt at foreign body removal is unsuccessful, immediate ophthalmologic referral is indicated.

A thorough examination of the eye is necessary for all children in whom a foreign body of the eye is suspected (Chapter 48). Any associated injuries, especially ruptured globe, must be identified before attempts to remove an ocular foreign body are made. Intraocular foreign bodies (within the globe rather than superficial) may be subtle in up to 20% of patients (6) and should be suspected if the patient has a history of high-velocity injury. Diffuse, chemotic subconjunctival hemorrhage raises the suspicion of corneal laceration and therefore ruptured globe (6, 7).

Careful observation of pupil size, shape, and reactivity are critical. Prolapse of the iris with distortion of pupillary shape indicating a ruptured globe may look deceptively like a foreign body. If a ruptured globe is clinically suspected, a metal shield is placed over the eye with no pressure applied to the eye; an eye patch is contraindicated. No drops or ointments are instilled in the eye. The patient is instructed to have nothing by mouth. Broad-spectrum intravenous antibiotics and tetanus immunization, if needed, are given and urgent ophthalmologic consultation obtained. Plain radiographs and computerized tomography may be helpful in ruling out intraocular foreign body, but magnetic resonance imaging should be avoided if any possibility of intraocular metal foreign body exists (8).

A small but reactive pupil may indicate traumatic iritis. A pupil with abnormal reactivity may indicate intracranial injury or optic nerve injury from blunt or penetrating trauma (2).

Once the possibility of a ruptured globe is excluded, two drops of topical anesthetic (proparacaine 0.5%) are instilled in the eye. Prompt relief of pain after topical anesthetic drops should be noted. In adults, Sklar et al. (4) found that pain relief in response to topical anesthetic was more likely when pain was the result of corneal injury (foreign body or abrasion) rather than conditions such as iritis or conjunctivitis.

The patient should not be sent home with topical anesthetics. Not only do they delay corneal reepithelialization, but the anesthetized eye is prone to further injury (4). Systemic analgesics may be necessary when a significant corneal abrasion has resulted.

When possible, visual acuity should be assessed in each eye, before the injured eye is manipulated. If the child is unable to cooperate, the ability to follow objects or response to light perception is noted. Routine use of glasses or contact lenses should be documented.

The eye should then be examined after instillation of fluorescein. A corneal foreign body will often be surrounded by a circular area of fluorescein staining. Vertical abrasions on the cornea are typical of foreign bodies located on the undersurface of the upper lid, which scrape the corneal surface during blinking. A positive Seidel test, with a stream of aqueous humor stained with fluorescein draining from the site of corneal injury, indicates globe perforation. In this situation a shield is placed immediately over the eye with care not to place pressure on the globe, and immediate ophthalmologic consultation is obtained.

The eye is examined carefully for location of one or more foreign bodies. Both eyelids are everted (Chapter 48) and the undersurface examined. Tiny foreign bodies may not be visible in the upper fornix, but the object may be discovered and removed during gentle wiping across the fornix with a moistened cotton swab (5).

Localization of the foreign body is assisted with the use of a slit lamp, loupes (magnifying lenses worn by the physician), or other magnification when available. Indirect lighting, by shining a light at an angle, may cast a shadow from the foreign body. The conjunctival cul-de-sacs and the undersurface of the lids (Fig. 48.1) must be carefully inspected. The anterior chamber is examined for evidence of hyphema or foreign body; if either is found, the eye is protected with an eye shield and immediate ophthalmologic consultation is obtained.

Plain films of the orbit may be indicated if the patient has a history of a high-velocity type injury (BB pellet, metallic splinter propelled during hammering, etc.). The history of a high-velocity type injury, especially combined with an inability to locate the foreign body on physical examination, is an indication for radiography. Plain radiographs may reveal radiopaque foreign bodies such as metallic fragments. Computerized tomography is very useful for foreign body localization, and sonograms may be used in some institutions. The patient with a suspected metallic intraocular foreign body should not undergo magnetic resonance imaging. The history of a blast injury should alert the physician to the possibility of multiple foreign bodies.

Foreign Body Removal

Several techniques are used for foreign body removal. Choice of technique depends on the location and nature of the foreign body. Superficial foreign bodies are often most easily removed with irrigation, whereas embedded foreign bodies may require using a spud or needle for removal.

Superficial Foreign Bodies
Small foreign bodies on the surface of the eye can often be removed most easily by simple irrigation with sterile water or a commercially prepared eye solution (Chapter 51). Irrigation may be performed with an irrigation solution bag attached to intravenous tubing.

A cotton swab premoistened with sterile saline is best reserved for foreign bodies on the bulbar or palpebral conjunctiva. The cotton swab, especially if dry, may cause damage if used on the cornea.

Embedded Foreign Bodies
Removal of an embedded foreign body in a child may be challenging, and often is best left to an ophthalmologist. Embedded corneal foreign bodies generally require using either a 25- or 27-gauge needle on a small syringe or an eye spud device (Fig. 50.1). In a cooperative older child, the head should be secured against a slit lamp frame and the child instructed to focus on an object in the distance. The spud is held tangentially to the eye while the foreign object is gently scooped off the cornea (Fig. 50.2). The physician's hand may be braced against the child's face during foreign body removal.

If difficulty is encountered in removing the foreign body, penetrating ocular trauma should be suspected and immediate referral to an ophthalmologist is indicated. Incomplete foreign body removal also necessitates referral to an ophthalmologist. An eye shield may be placed over the eye to prevent the child from rubbing, thereby forcing a foreign body deeper into the eye or causing extrusion of ocular contents when the globe is ruptured.

After Foreign Body Removal

When the foreign body has been successfully removed, an examination with fluorescein is useful to determine if a corneal abrasion has resulted. The presence of a corneal abrasion requires that the eye be examined again within 24 to 36 hours to ascertain the degree of healing. Patients with larger or deeper corneal abrasions should receive follow-up evaluation by an ophthalmologist.

Figure 50.1.
Spud devices used for removing embedded foreign bodies. A hypodermic needle on a syringe also can be used.

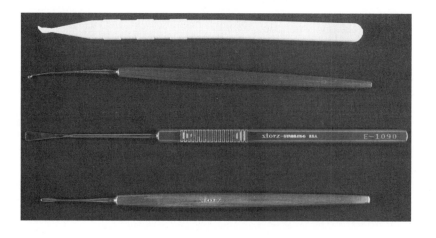

Ciliary spasm or iritis may cause pain after foreign body removal. A drop of topical cycloplegic (e.g., homatropine 5%) can reduce this discomfort. For reasons stated previously, patients should not be discharged with a topical anesthetic agents such as proparacaine. Pain should instead be managed with oral narcotics, if cycloplegics and nonnarcotic analgesics prove ineffective. Instillation of antibiotic solution or ointment may help prevent infection. Risk of infection is increased when the foreign body is of organic material or the patient is a contact lens wearer.

Patching of the eye if corneal abrasion is evident (Chapter 52) may be considered. Although this has frequently been recommended (5, 8, 9), some authorities question its usefulness and caution that infection may go undetected when covered by an eye patch (9). Conjunctival abrasions do not require patching (5).

Patching of the eye after foreign body removal without corneal abrasion is controversial. Patching prevents movement of the lid from denuding the new epithelial layer over the wound. It may, however, increase the risk of infection, particularly in a patient who is a contact lens wearer or when the foreign body is of plant or animal matter (1) (see Chapter 52 for a detailed discussion of eye patching).

COMPLICATIONS

Complications may occur as a consequence of either the foreign body or the removal procedure. Infection may occur as simple conjunctivitis; however, infection resulting after a corneal abrasion may be more severe and should be referred to an ophthalmologist.

Metallic foreign bodies may leave rust rings staining the cornea (See Indications in this chapter). Application of antibiotic ointment may loosen the rust ring and cause it to spontaneously fall out. If after 3 days the ring has not disappeared, the rust ring should be removed. Children may be uncooperative for rust ring removal and most should be referred to an ophthalmologist. Physicians with experience in rust ring removal and with a highly cooperative child may attempt removal in the emergency setting.

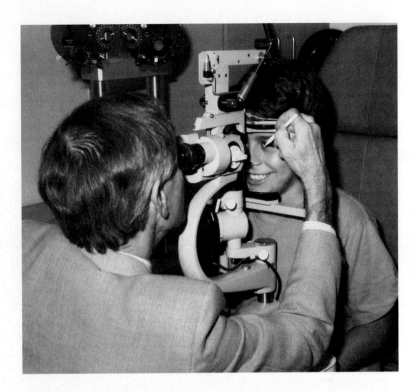

Figure 50.2.
A physician with experience uses a spud device held tangential to the eye with the slit lamp to remove an embedded foreign body in a cooperative child.

Retained foreign bodies may be surprisingly well tolerated (7). Foreign bodies may have penetrated into but not through the corneal stroma. In this case, some inert substances such as glass or sand are relatively inert, whereas organic materials such as plant or insect matter and ionizing metals precipitate an inflammatory reaction. Foreign bodies composed of organic material have an increased risk of infection. Retained intraocular foreign bodies may be suspected when either a history of high-velocity injury or an irregularly shaped pupil is found.

Although not common, vigorous attempts at foreign body removal with a needle or spud in uncooperative, poorly restrained children may cause corneal abrasion or penetrating trauma. This emphasizes the need for good judgment in deciding which children to refer and which to sedate for ocular foreign body removal. Consultation with an ophthalmologist should be readily employed. Recurrent abrasions may occur later in an area of corneal injury, particularly at night when lubrication from tears is decreased (7, 10).

Allergic reactions to anesthetics and antibiotics may occur. Topical antibiotics containing neomycin may be particularly sensitizing. A history of medication allergies, if present, can prevent these reactions.

SUMMARY

1. Obtain a history. High-velocity injuries often result in penetration of the globe.
2. Assess for a ruptured globe. If at any point a penetrating injury is suspected, stop, shield the eye and immediately call an ophthalmologist.
3. Anesthetize the eye.
4. Perform a thorough physical examination of the eye including visual acuity testing and fluorescein examination.
5. Locate the foreign body. Evert the eyelids and inspect with magnification. Tiny foreign bodies adherent to the conjunctiva may be found by wiping a moist, cotton-tipped applicator across the superior fornix.
6. Remove superficial foreign bodies with irrigation.
7. Conjunctival foreign bodies may be removed with a moistened cotton-tipped applicator.
8. Embedded corneal foreign bodies in cooperative children may be removed with a 25 gauge needle on a syringe, or with a spud device.
9. Perform a fluorescein examination after foreign body removal to detect a corneal abrasion.
10. Relieve pain of ciliary spasm or iritis with a drop of topical cycloplegic (homatropine 5%)
11. Prevent infection with instillation of antibiotic ointment or drops.
12. Consider patching of the eye for corneal abrasions not caused by organic matter.
13. Arrange for reevaluation of the patient in 24 hours.

SUMMARY

Ocular foreign bodies must be removed, although not all are appropriate for removal in the emergency setting. Before foreign body removal, a careful eye examination must be performed to rule out associated injuries, in particular ruptured globe and intraocular foreign body. Children with foreign body sensation in the eye need a thorough examination to locate material that may be in the recesses of the upper or lower fornices or embedded in the cornea. Some children with foreign body sensation may have corneal abrasions, conjunctivitis, or other eye injuries without foreign bodies being present.

Removal of ocular foreign bodies may be accomplished by irrigation, or by using a cotton swab for conjunctival foreign bodies or a needle or spud for corneal foreign bodies. Care must be exercised to avoid damage to the eye. Many children will require ophthalmologic consultation for foreign body removal.

REFERENCES

1. Santen SA, Scott JL. Ophthalmologic procedures. Emerg Med Clin North Am 1995;13(3):681–701.
2. Linden JA, Renner GS. Trauma to the globe. Emerg Med Clin North Am 1995;13(3):581–605.
3. Kaye-Wilson LG. Localization of corneal foreign bodies. Br J Ophthalmol 1992;76:741–742.
4. Sklar DP, Lauth JE, Johnson DR. Topical anesthesia of the eye as a diagnostic test. Ann Emerg Med 1989;18(11):1209–1211.
5. Barr DH, Samples JR, Hedges JR. Ocular foreign body removal. In: Roberts JR, Hedges JR, eds. Clinical procedures in emergency medicine. 2nd ed. Philadelphia: WB Saunders, 1991, pp. 1002–1005.
6. Shingleton BJ. Eye injuries. N Engl J Med 1991;325(6):408–413.
7. McMahon TT, Robin JB. Corneal trauma: I-classification and management. J Amer Optom Assoc 1991;62(3):170–178.
8. Janda AM. Ocular trauma. Triage and treatment. Postgrad Med 1991;90(7):51–60.
9. Hulbert MFG. Efficacy of eyepad in corneal healing after corneal foreign body removal. Lancet 1991;337:643.
10. Elkington AR, Khaw PT. ABC of eyes. Injuries to the eye. Br Med J 1988;297(6641):122–125.

IRRIGATION OF CONJUNCTIVA

Mananda S. Bhende

INTRODUCTION

Eye irrigation is the crucial first step in the treatment of chemical injuries to the eye. Chemical burns are among the most urgent of ocular emergencies. The procedure dilutes the chemical (acid or base) and, if accomplished within seconds or minutes after the event, can decrease the damage caused by the chemical and improve the long-term prognosis.

Chemical burns are more common in adult patients and may occur as industrial accidents, or in agricultural work or in the household. In children, household accidents are the most common source of ocular chemical exposure. Ideally, irrigation of the eye begins at the location where the incident occurred, and is continued by EMTs and then completed in the hospital emergency department. The procedure can be performed by the parent, the patient, a bystander, EMTs, nurses and doctors (1–3).

Chemical injuries to the eye can occur accidentally in all age groups and also may occur intentionally in adolescents. Because household agents are a major cause of chemical burns of the eye, active toddlers and preschoolers are at particular risk (Table 51.1).

ANATOMY AND PHYSIOLOGY

The conjunctiva is a thin, transparent mucous membrane that covers the posterior surface of the lids (the palpebral conjunctiva) and the anterior surface of the sclera (the bulbar con-junctiva) (Fig. 48.1). It is continuous with the skin at the lid margin and with the corneal epithelium at the limbus (sclero-corneal junction). The palpebral conjunctiva is firmly adherent to the tarsus. At the superior and inferior margins of the tarsus, the conjunctiva is reflected posteriorly at the superior and the inferior fornices, and attaches to the sclera to become the bulbar conjunctiva, which is loosely attached to the orbital septum in the fornices and the sclera. The fornices and the medial and lateral canthus are locations where chemicals can pool or become trapped, especially if in the solid state. The eye, therefore, must be irrigated well in these difficult to reach areas (4).

The cornea is a transparent, avascular membrane that functions as a refracting and protective window through which light rays pass en route to the retina. The epithelium comprises the outer layer of the cornea and the endothelium lines the anterior chamber of the eye. Chemical or physical damage to the endothelium of the cornea is far more serious than epithelial damage, and can cause marked swelling, scarring and loss of transparency which can lead to loss of vision. Therefore it is vital to limit damage to the cornea during chemical exposure by prompt and thorough irrigation.

The irrigation process is more difficult in a child who is uncooperative. Such a child may need to be immobilized for the procedure; however, sedation is rarely indicated.

The severity of a chemical burn varies depending on the nature of the chemical, its volume, concentration, duration of contact,

Table 51.1.
Common Household Agents Capable of Causing Chemical Burns to the Eye

Household ammonia (ammonium hydroxide 9%—pH 12.5)
Other ammonia-containing agents—window cleaner, jewelry cleaner
Dishwasher detergent (sodium tripolyphosphate—pH 12)
Drain cleaner (sodium or potassium hydroxide—pH 14)
Oven cleaner (sodium hydroxide—pH 14)
Toilet bowl cleaner (sulfuric acid 80%—pH 1.0)
Battery fluid (sulfuric acid 30%—pH 1.0)
Pool cleaner (sodium or Ca hypochlorite 70%)
Bleaches (sodium hypochlorite)
Disinfectants
Deodorizing cleaners
Automotive cleaners and degreasers
Whitewall tire cleaners
Lime (calcium hydroxide) and plaster

and reaction with tissue components. Gases are less injurious than liquids or solid particles.

Alkaline substances are usually more damaging to the ocular structures than acids. Acids with pH of 2.5 or less precipitate tissue proteins, which create a physical barrier against further penetration. Buffering by surrounding tissue proteins also helps localize damage to the initial area of contact. Exceptions include burns from hydrochloric acid and from acids containing heavy metals which rapidly penetrate the cornea.

Alkali burns are usually more severe because they react with fats to form soaps, which damage cell membranes and allow further penetration of the alkali into the eye (1, 3).

INDICATIONS AND CONTRAINDICATIONS

Any suspected contact with the eyes by a caustic or irritant warrants irrigation. Children with acute onset of burning, pain, itch, or redness should have the affected eyes irrigated for possible chemical exposure.

Small foreign bodies of the conjunctiva that are not embedded often can be removed with irrigation. Children with foreign body sensation in the eye without a visible foreign body also may benefit.

For moderate or severe burns, irrigation should begin immediately on arrival to the ED. Consultation with ophthalmology should occur promptly. Irrigation is indicated in children with suspected chemical exposure of the

eye even if the parent or prehospital care providers have already irrigated.

Irrigation of the eye is not contraindicated when penetrating injury occurs to the eye, but extra care must be taken to avoid exerting any pressure on the globe (5).

EQUIPMENT

Normal saline solution (1L bags at room temperature)
Intravenous tubing or cystotubing
Towels or linen saver pads
Emesis basin, pail, or bucket
Topical anesthetic (proparacaine 0.5%)
pH paper
Papoose board, if needed
4×4 gauze
Eyelid retractor—rarely needed
Moist cotton-tip swabs
Gloves
Fluorescein strips
Morgan® Therapeutic lenses (optional)

PROCEDURE

Irrigation with water or saline is the first step in diluting the chemical in the eye so as to decrease the duration of exposure. At home or in the workplace eye irrigation can be accomplished by placing the patient's face in a bowl of water with eyes open and by frequently changing the water. Alternatively, tap water can be run over the patient's open eyes. The water need not be sterile. In the ED setting, using isotonic saline is ideal.

Before the procedure, both the parents and the child should be given a brief explanation about what is going to be done. Although it is important to explain the details, prolonged description should not delay the procedure. Time is of the essence. Parents usually know that the chemical substance has to be washed off the eye. While preparing the child and the equipment for irrigation, parents can be informed about the procedure. Signed informed consent is usually not necessary. Parents should be offered the option of remaining with their child during the irrigation (see Chapter 1).

A quick history and brief physical examination is performed while the equipment is prepared. Gloves should be worn because of the potential contact with a caustic substance. Immobilization is appropriate if the child is uncooperative.

Older children can lie on the examining table with their head just beyond the end. This enables the irrigant fluid to be collected in a pail placed directly underneath the eye.

The pH should be measured if a strip is easily available. Measurement is accomplished by simply placing the strip into the pocket that is formed when the lower eyelid is retracted. This baseline value, though not crucial, will help to determine the effectiveness of therapy. Instillation of a topical anesthetic (proparacaine 0.5%) also is advisable but the search for pH paper and topical anesthetic must not delay the irrigation. For this reason it is advisable to keep these materials together in a single location.

Irrigation is begun by holding the end of the intravenous tubing just above the eyeball and allowing free flow of saline (Fig. 51.1). During irrigation the eyelids must be held open. This is best accomplished by an assistant rather than the physician performing the irrigation. Gauze pads enable the holder to better grip the wet, slippery eyelids. If retractors are necessary (Chapter 48) the physician must ensure that the eye is well anesthetized.

Alternatively, a Morgan® lens can be inserted into the anesthetized eye. This device is a large, soft contact lens with an irrigation nipple extending from its anterior aspect. The nipple is connected to a bag of saline and the saline drains into the eye. The

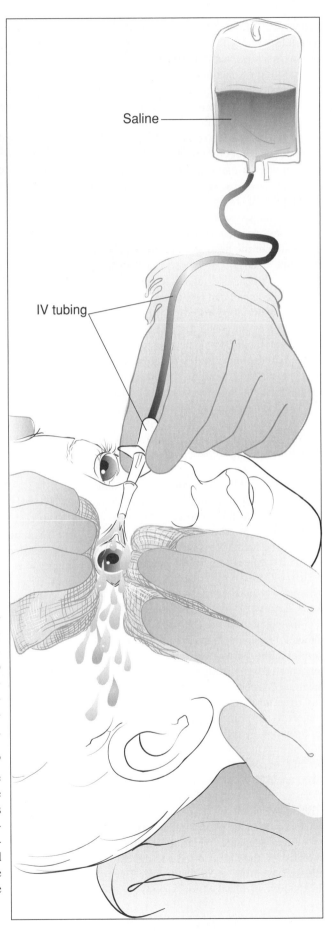

Saline

IV tubing

**Chapter 51
Irrigation of
Conjunctiva**

SUMMARY

1. Obtain brief history and examination as equipment is prepared
2. If necessary, secure child and separate eyelids manually with gauze pads
3. Check pH of conjunctivae
4. Instill topical anesthetic
5. Sweep away any particulate matter with moistened cotton-tipped swabs
6. Irrigate with 1 to 2 L isotonic saline for about 20 minutes; direct saline over globe, into upper and lower fornices, and over canthi
7. Measure pH of tears; if still alkaline or acidic, continue until pH normalizes to 7.4
8. Recheck pH in 20 minutes
9. Check for corneal abrasions with fluorescein
10. Assess visual acuity
11. Consult ophthalmology as needed and arrange for follow-up

CLINICAL TIPS

1. If in doubt—IRRIGATE.
2. Hold lids open with gauze pads.
3. Remove particulate matter from fornices.
4. Measure pH on completion and 20 minutes after irrigation.
5. Remember to assess for visual acuity and corneal abrasion.

Chapter 51
Irrigation of
Conjunctiva

patient can close the lids around the lens without affecting the irrigation. Some concern exists, however, that this device may allow pooling of chemicals beneath the lens. Some authorities therefore recommend using the lens when prolonged irrigation is required after the more traditional technique (Fig. 51.1) has been performed. Additionally, maximum patient comfort during lens irrigation requires a well-anesthetized eye. The lens causes topical anesthetic to be rapidly washed out of the eye and recurrent dosing (which is not without risk) may be necessary.

Towels or linen pads should be placed on either side of the head to catch the irrigating fluid, and an emesis basin also can be used. If the patient's head is extended beyond the end of the table, a pail can be placed on the floor to catch the drops of irrigating fluid.

Saline exiting from the intravenous tubing or cystotubing should be directed over the globe, into the upper and lower fornices, and over the canthi. The saline should flow from medial to lateral so it can be easily collected. The child is instructed to look straight up and then to move his or her eyes in all directions—medial, lateral, up, and down—allowing all areas of the conjunctival sac to be well irrigated.

Care should be taken not to cause trauma to the cornea by touching it with the tubing, retracting the eyelids, or forcing the saline directly against the cornea.

Particulate matter is swept from the conjunctival fornices, medial or lateral canthus with moistened cotton-tipped applicators. This may require eversion of the upper lid (see Chapter 48).

Irrigation with 1 to 2 L of saline over 20 minutes is usually more than adequate. Severe alkaline burns may benefit from prolonged irrigation with larger volumes. As mentioned, a scleral contact lens for continuous irrigation may be used. The pH in the conjunctival fornices should be measured after irrigation. If still alkaline or acidic, irrigation should continue until pH normalizes (normal ocular pH is 7.4). The pH is measured again in 20 minutes to make sure it remains normal. Delayed pH changes are usually the result of incomplete irrigation or residual particulate matter in the fornices.

When adequate irrigation has been accomplished, the face is dried and the child is released from the securing device. The patient's eyes are checked for corneal abrasion with noncontaminated fluorescein liquid or fluorescein strips. It is extremely important to test for visual acuity and document the findings in the record. This is usually done after irrigation to avoid a delay and prolonged chemical contact with the eye.

Ophthalmologic consultation should be sought immediately for all serious injuries. Follow-up for ophthalmologic evaluation should be recommended for all but the most minor injuries (1–3, 5).

COMPLICATIONS

Complications from irrigation of the eye are rare. Most injuries noted after irrigation are the result of the injury for which irrigation was performed. Irrigation may cause abrasion of the cornea or conjunctiva. A linear abrasion may occur from attempts to keep the eyelids open, or a fine punctate keratitis from the force of the irrigation fluid on the cornea. Superficial corneal abrasions are treated in the usual manner. Deep or penetrating injuries are likely to be the result of the chemical and require immediate ophthalmologic evaluation (1, 3, 5).

SUMMARY

Eye irrigation is a useful, easy procedure with minimal complications. If any doubt exists as to whether a patient may benefit from irrigation it should be performed. Omission of this vital procedure permits progression of eye injury and can affect long-term prognosis.

REFERENCES

1. Ervin-Mulvey LD, Nelson LB, Freeley DA. Pediatric eye trauma. Ped Clin North Am 1983;30:1177–1178.
2. Simon JW. Trauma to the globe and adenexa. In: Harley RD, ed. Pediatric ophthalmology. 2nd ed. Philadelphia: WB Saunders, 1983;(2):1202–1204.
3. Nelson LB. Management of ocular trauma. In: Nelson LB, ed. Pediatric ophthalmology. Philadelphia: WB Saunders, 1984, pp. 227–228.
4. Nelson LB. Functional anatomy of the eye. In: Nelson LB, ed. Pediatric ophthalmology. Philadelphia: WB Saunders, 1984, pp. 1–18.
5. Barr DH, Samples JR, Hedges JR. Ophthalmologic procedures. In: Roberts JR, Hedges JR, eds. Clinical procedures in emergency medicine. 2nd ed. Philadelphia: WB Saunders, 1991, pp. 998–1002.

Eye Patching and Eye Guards

Michael Shannon

INTRODUCTION

The eye is frequently injured because of its prominence and delicacy. These injuries occur despite protective mechanisms and structures including the eyelids and eyelashes, the tarsal plates, the orbicularis oculi muscles, the lacrimal apparatus, the corneal reflex, and the lid reflexes. Visual injury can lead to significant disability, especially if the injury is bilateral. Evaluating eye injuries in children is often challenging. The goal is to identify the type and severity of injury without causing further damage. Eye guards play an important role in preventing further injury, whereas eye patching may reduce discomfort and promote healing. Proper use of these techniques and appropriate consultation with an ophthalmologist are important in optimizing outcomes in patients with eye injuries.

ANATOMY AND PHYSIOLOGY

The most important ocular structures to identify are the conjunctivae (bulbar and palpebral), the cornea, the iris, the ciliary apparatus, and the anterior chamber (Fig. 48.1). The epithelium of the cornea is directly continuous with the conjunctiva. The cornea is extensively innervated by the ciliary nerves. It is unique in being avascular, having no direct blood supply. Oxygen and nutrients are supplied by tears and diffusion from the ciliary circulation. Nonetheless, after corneal in-

juries, healing and reepithelialization occur rapidly. Proper patching prevents opening and closing of the eye, which may decrease trauma to the cornea and facilitate healing.

Full-thickness laceration of the cornea or sclera allows extrusion of aqueous or vitreous humor. The underlying iris or choroid often plugs the wound, preventing ongoing leakage. Further trauma or pressure on the globe, or physical agitation can disrupt this delicate protective mechanism and cause further extrusion of intraocular contents. Keeping the child as calm as possible and placing an eye guard protects the ruptured globe from additional injury. Eye patches are to be distinguished from eye guards or shields, which are fenestrated metal guards used to protect the eye from further injury, rather than to maintain the eye in a closed position. Eye patches put pressure on the globe, which can worsen the eye injury.

INDICATIONS AND CONTRAINDICATIONS

Two indications for eye patching are to provide comfort and to facilitate healing. Eye patching can reduce photophobia (light-induced ciliary spasm) and pain with blinking by keeping the eyelid closed. Patching may facilitate healing of corneal injuries by preventing the surface abrasion that may occur during eye blinking. Eye patches are contraindicated in (*a*) patients with possible pen-

Figure 52.1.
The purpose of an eye patch is to hold the eyelid tightly closed.
A. Two pads are placed over the eye with the lid closed.
B. Tape is applied from the center of the forehead to the zygomatic arch on the affected side and continued until the patch is securely taped. In contrast to patching, the purpose of the eye shield is to prevent the application of undue pressure to an injured eye.
C. The shield is placed over the eye and tape is placed along the edges of the shield securing it against the underlying bone. Pressure directly over the eye must be avoided. If an eye shield is unavailable a plastic, paper, or styrofoam cup may be used as a substitute.

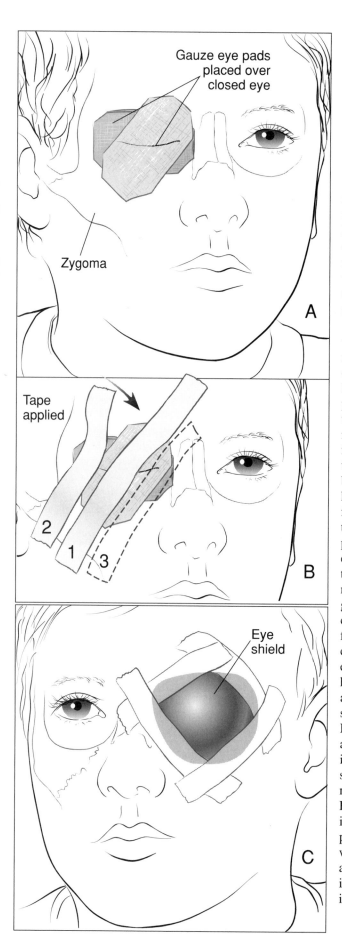

Gauze eye pads placed over closed eye

Zygoma

A

Tape applied

2
1
3

B

Eye shield

C

etrating eye injury or open globe, (b) patients with glaucoma, (c) the patient after instillation of corticosteroid ophthalmic solutions, (d) wearers of extended contact wear lenses, and (e) patients with chemical eye injuries during transport when eyes should remain open to allow residual chemical to drain before thorough irrigation. Patches also are relatively contraindicated in the treatment of abrasions secondary to contact lens wear (see Complications in this chapter).

Although eye patching is virtually always recommended in the treatment of corneal abrasion, almost no literature demonstrates that patching has advantages over treatment without patching in minor corneal abrasions. In fact, some studies indicate that patients who have not been patched have faster healing and are more comfortable (2, 3). Furthermore, the possibility exists that patching may predispose the eye to infection by creating the type of warm, moist environment that favors bacterial growth. Placing antibiotic cream into the eye provides a false sense of security because effective antibiotic levels in the eye fall within 6 hours after cream instillation and within 2 hours after instilling antibiotic eye drops. In adolescents, patching has another disadvantage because it causes the loss of stereoscopic vision increasing the risk of automobile accidents. Reading is also difficult or impossible with a patch in place. If a child or adolescent who has a simple corneal abrasion will not keep a patch in place or finds a patch too inconvenient or uncomfortable, then he or she should be treated without one.

In emergency care, eye guards are used for patients awaiting or being transported for ophthalmologic evaluation with a known or suspected rupture of the globe (1–3, 6).

EQUIPMENT

Eye pads
Gauze, cut into ovals if pads are not available
Eye guard or shield
Tape

PROCEDURE

Eye Patching

The only equipment necessary for eye patching are eye pads and tape. Gauze cut into an oval shape is an acceptable alternative to an eye pad. Before the eye is patched, a thorough ophthalmologic examination should be performed which includes assessment of visual acuity, pupil shape and light response, extraocular movements, inspection for a retained foreign body, and examination of adjacent bony structures (Chapter 48). An ophthalmologist should be consulted before eye patching in patients with chemical eye injuries, suspicion of penetrating globe injuries, or with identified abnormalities of extraocular movement or pupillary action. If warranted, ophthalmic medications (cycloplegics, antibiotics) are applied before patching.

At least two eye pads should be placed against the closed eyelid. The pad is applied on a slant, with the narrow end toward the nose (Fig. 52.1.A). Tape is applied from the center forehead to the cheek overlying the zygoma of the affected side (Fig. 52.1.B); benzoin may be necessary to improve tape adhesion. In young children, instructions for patch reapplication and extra pads and tape should be provided to the parents when possible, in the event the patch falls off or is removed. An improperly placed patch may be worse than no patch at all. If the patch will not maintain the eyelid in the closed position then treatment without a patch should be considered (1, 4, 5).

Eye Shielding

The eye guard is positioned over the injured eye avoiding direct contact with the eyelid or globe. The edges are placed against the underlying bone of the nose, supraorbital ridge, and zygoma. Tape is applied from the forehead to the cheek of the affected side and the guard is checked to ensure that it is firmly positioned without contact with the orbital structures (Fig. 52.1.C).

Occasionally eye shielding is required in the absence of a plastic or metal eye shield. In these cases a plastic, paper, or styrofoam cup may be used as a temporary alternative, provided that the cup is large enough to protect the eye without putting pressure on the globe itself (1, 4).

COMPLICATIONS

Eye patches are always removed 24 to 48 hours after initial application for reexamination of the eye. Complications from eye patching are rare but include corneal drying or abrasion secondary to forced partial opening, infection (particularly in extended wear contact lens wearers), and intraocular hypertension. Eye patches also are relatively contraindicated in the treatment of corneal abrasion secondary to contact lens use. These injuries are predisposed to *Pseudomonas* infections and patching appears to increase the risk of this devastating condition (6).

Improper placement of an eye guard can further injure the affected eye, especially if the globe is ruptured.

REFERENCES

1. Catalano RA. Eye injuries and prevention. Ped Clin North Am 1993;40:827–840.
2. Kirkpatrick JN, Hoh JB, Cook SD. No eye pad for corneal abrasions. Eye 1993;7(Pt 3):468–471.
3. Hulbert MFG. Efficacy of eye pad in corneal healing after corneal foreign body removal. Lancet 1991;337:643.
4. Barr DH, Samples JR, Hedges JR. Ophthalmologic procedures. In: Roberts JR, Hedges JR, eds. Clinical procedures in emergency medicine. 2nd ed. Philadelphia: WB Saunders, 1991, pp. 1005–1007.
5. Buttaravoli PM, Stair TO. Corneal abrasion. In: Buttaravoli PM, Stair TO. Common simple emergencies. Englewood Cliffs: Brady Communications Company Inc., 1985, pp. 40–42.
6. Schein O. Contact lens abrasion and the nonophthalmologist. Am J Emerg Med 1993;11:606.

SUMMARY

Eye Patching
1. Thoroughly examine eye before patching
2. Use at least two eye pads
3. Place over closed eyelid on angle with narrow end toward nose
4. Apply tape from forehead to zygoma using benzoin if better adhesion is needed

Eye Shielding
1. Place eye guard as soon as ruptured globe is suspected
2. Ensure that eye guard does not contact eyelid or globe
3. Apply tape from forehead to zygoma

CLINICAL TIPS
1. Do not place an eye patch on a child who may have a ruptured globe.
2. If the eye patch will not keep the eyelid completely closed, consider treatment without a patch.
3. Secure tape on eye patches and eye guards firmly. Supply parent with tape and patches in case the patch needs to be replaced.
4. If a patient with a simple corneal abrasion cannot or will not wear a patch then he or she should be managed without a patch.

**Chapter 52
Eye Patching and
Eye Guards**

CHAPTER 53

CONTACT LENS REMOVAL

Timothy G. Givens

INTRODUCTION

As the number of persons wearing contact lenses steadily increases, so does the chance that a physician in the emergency department (ED) will encounter problems related to contact lens use. Familiarity with indications and techniques of contact lens removal is therefore essential. These skills also may prove valuable for the office-based practitioner.

Contact lens use requires a certain level of maturity, so children do not usually become contact lens wearers until approximately 10 years of age. At that age children are less likely to be meticulous in regard to the proper wear, removal, and cleaning of their lenses. They are therefore at increased risk of complications such as eye trauma or infection. Children also are less likely to be cooperative with contact lens removal, which can make this procedure much more challenging.

ANATOMY AND PHYSIOLOGY

The cornea is a transparent window at the most anterior portion of the eye (Fig. 48.1). It is a dense layer of tissue that is uniformly about 1 mm thick. Because it has a greater curvature than the sclera, the cornea resembles a watch crystal. The cornea is avascular and receives nutrients from the capillaries associated with the anterior ciliary arteries at its margin. It is well supplied with sensory nerves from the ciliary nerves. Aside from the cornea, the remainder of the visible portion of

the anterior eyeball is covered by the conjunctiva. The conjunctiva joins the corneal epithelium at the limbus, or corneal margin. The conjunctiva and cornea are lubricated by mucous-containing secretions from the lacrimal gland and from the conjunctiva itself (1, 2).

A contact lens is designed to float on the tear film overlying the surface of the centrally located cornea and modify its refractive power. When the lens slides out of position and is lost in the eye, it may commonly hide on the undersurface of either eyelid, especially in the fornices, which are the upper and lower recesses where the conjunctiva reflects onto the eyeball. Tinted lenses are usually easy to locate and remove, but localization and recovery of a clear lens may require topical anesthesia and slit lamp examination (1, 3, 4).

Lack of vascularity of the cornea makes it dependent on the movement of tears beneath the contact lens for oxygen delivery. Both hard and soft contact lenses may, with prolonged wear, cause mechanical irritation, hypotonic tear production, and resultant corneal edema. The subsequent reduction in oxygen-rich tear flow can produce ischemia of segments of the cornea. The symptoms of this overwear syndrome are similar to a foreign body sensation and include eye pain, redness, itching, and tearing. Symptoms may not appear until several hours after removal of the contact lens from the eye, as a result of transient anesthesia of the eye caused by buildup of anoxic metabolites over the course of wear. Chemical irritants such as cigarette smoke, and anything that decreases blinking and normal tear flow such as the ingestion of sedatives (e.g., alcohol), also may produce a similar syndrome of corneal edema and ischemic injury.

The cornea is easily abraded by trauma to the eye, whether it be from a fingernail during contact lens insertion or removal, or from foreign material trapped beneath the improperly cleaned lens. Many abrasions and foreign bodies are visible to the naked eye with fluorescein staining and a Wood's (UV) lamp, although a complete examination should involve using a slit lamp. Mechanical trauma to the cornea may predispose to infection and ulceration if untreated. Few organisms are capable of penetrating an intact corneal epithelium without antecedent injury (1–5).

Soft contact lenses, made of a hydrophilic gel that may contain in excess of 60% water, carry added risk in terms of predisposition to infection. Soft lenses readily absorb water and along with it, pathogenic organisms. Even minor trauma caused by simple lens insertion and wear may provide a portal of entry for organisms which then invade the cornea and lead to the development of a bacterial or fungal corneal ulcer. In the contact lens wearer who presents with eye pain, tearing, photophobia, and/or decreased vision in the affected eye, a suspicion of a corneal ulcer should be raised. The lens should be removed and a fluorescein slit lamp examination performed. Corneal opacity with shaggy debris and a flocculent stromal infiltrate indicate an ulceration. Such a lesion represents an emergency and requires immediate ophthalmologic consultation for appropriate cultures and antimicrobial therapy (5).

Soft contact lenses also may be associated with other forms of nonemergent ocular injury, including corneal neovascularization, giant papillary conjunctivitis, or sensitivity reactions to contact lens solutions (2).

INDICATIONS

The emergency physician may need to remove a contact lens from a patient's eye for several reasons. The first is to allow for a more detailed evaluation of the eye. This is especially true for the contact lens wearer who sustains trauma to the eye with a lens in place. The lens should be removed before a more thorough inspection of the patient's cornea, including instillation of fluorescein. Contact lenses, particularly the soft variety, absorb stains and chemicals and will become permanently stained if fluorescein is instilled before their removal from the eye (1, 6).

Complaint of eye pain in a contact lens wearer is a second common indication for lens removal. Because of the cornea's rich nerve supply, pain is the classic presenting symptom of corneal injury. Photophobia also may be a significant component if the abrasion is large or is present for an extended period of time. As discussed previously, pain may represent traumatic injury to the eye, presence of a foreign body, infection, or the overwear syndrome (1, 6).

Inability of the patient to remove a contact lens is a third indication for removal by a physician. The patient with an altered sensorium who may not be able to express the need to have his or her lenses removed, the patient who needs assistance in locating a lost contact lens in the eye, and the patient who cannot physically remove a lens as a result of corneal edema from prolonged wear all fall into this category. All patients who are unconscious on presentation to the ED should undergo an examination of the eyes aimed at identifying eye injuries and locating and removing contact lenses (1, 6).

The only relative contraindication to contact lens removal is the presence of a corneal perforation. Pressure on the globe must be avoided in this setting. Removal by an ophthalmologist using the suction cup technique is preferred.

EQUIPMENT

Sterile gloves
Sterile saline or lubricating eye drops
Topical anesthetic solution
Several cotton-tipped applicators
A rubber-tipped suction cup device (DMV Corporation)
Pincer type device for removal of soft contact lenses
Penlight
Slit lamp

PROCEDURE

If possible, visual acuity should be assessed in each eye before contact lens removal. If perforation of the globe is suspected, an eye shield should immediately be placed and ophthalmologic consultation sought. Hands should be clean and/or sterile gloves worn when removing a lens. Because most pediatric patients wearing contact lenses will be 10 years of age or older, restraint is seldom necessary if the patient is approached calmly and all procedures are explained beforehand. However, patients with altered mental status or in severe pain as a result of eye trauma may require appropriate restraint devices. Slit lamp examination is impossible for the patient who must remain supine because of immobilization for trauma or other reasons. Unless contraindicated, topical ophthalmic anesthetic should be used before attempts to remove the lens (1, 6).

Hard Contact Lens

If the patient is alert and cooperative, his or her face should be held over a table surface or a clean cloth. The thumbs are placed on the upper and lower eyelids from the lateral palpebral margin and pulled to secure the lids tightly against the edges of the contact lens (Fig. 53.1). The patient is instructed to look toward the nose and then downward. This maneuver allows the lower eyelid to work itself under the lower lens edge and lift the lens off the eye (1).

If the patient is uncooperative or must remain supine, the physician can actively remove the contact lens with a modification of

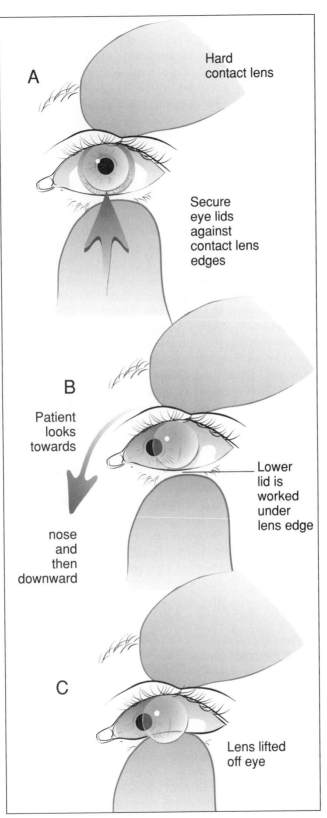

A Hard contact lens

Secure eye lids against contact lens edges

B Patient looks towards

nose and then downward

Lower lid is worked under lens edge

C Lens lifted off eye

Figure 53.1.
Removal of a hard contact lens.
A. Using the thumbs of both hands, pull the eyelids apart and then bring the lids down, trapping the lens between the lids.
B. If possible, have the patient look downward and medially as the lower lid is worked under the lower edge of the lens.
C. The lower edge of the lens will lift off the eye as the lid passes beneath it.

SUMMARY

All Lenses/All Patients
Check patient's visual acuity and do complete eye examination
Appropriately restrain patient, if necessary

Hard Contact Lens:
Cooperative patient
Pull eyelids from lateral palpebral margin to secure lids tightly against edges of contact lens
Instruct patient to look toward nose, then downward
Grasp lens as it flips off eye
Alternatively, use suction device to remove lens

Hard Contact Lens:
Uncooperative patient
Place thumbs on upper and lower eyelids at lid margins
Open eyelids beyond margins of contact lens
Press both eyelids firmly on globe so lid margins touch contact lens edges
Press slightly more firmly on lower lid to work lower lid margin under lens edge
Move lids together so contact lens slides out and is able to be grasped
Alternatively, use suction device to remove lens

Soft Contact Lens
Pull down lower eyelid with middle finger
Place tip of index finger on lower edge of contact lens
Slide lens downward onto sclera and pinch between thumb and index finger or use pincer type removal device

this technique. The location of the lens may be identified by shining a pen light across the surface of the eye from the lateral side. (This should be done in all unconscious adolescents once they are stable.) If the lens is in proper position, the thumbs are placed on the upper and lower eyelid near the margins. The eyelids are opened so that the lid margins pull away beyond the lens edges. Both eyelids are then pressed gently but firmly on the globe so that the lid margins just touch the contact lens edges. Firmer pressure on the lower lid will manually work the lid margin under the bottom lens edge. As the lower lens edge tips away from the surface of the eye, the lids are moved together and the contact lens slid out to where it may be grasped (1, 6).

Alternatively, the lens can be removed from the cornea with a cotton-tipped applicator. After a drop of topical anesthetic solution is placed into the eye, the lens is moved laterally onto the sclera and the tip of the applicator worked beneath a lens edge, lifting the lens off the eye. Applicator contact with the cornea may cause an abrasion.

If available, a moistened suction cup device applied directly to the contact lens allows for easy removal from the cornea. Suction cup devices appropriate for this purpose should be stocked in all EDs (1, 6). A reasonable substitute that may be effective is a drop of honey on a gloved fingertip or cotton-tipped applicator. The honey can be later removed from the lens by simple washing (1).

If the lens is present but not in proper position, a drop of sterile saline or lubricating eye drops may be used to "float" it into a better location (6).

Soft Contact Lens

The lower eyelid is pulled down with the examiner's middle finger (Fig. 53.2). Placing the tip of the index finger on the lower edge of the contact lens, the examiner then slides the lens downward onto the sclera and is able to pinch the lens between the thumb and the index finger. The soft lens will fold, allowing easy removal from the eye. An alternative is to use a specially designed rubber tweezer made for this purpose. The tweezer serves the same purpose as the thumb and index finger, pinching the lens and causing it to fold. If the lens is dry and therefore relatively adherent to

the eye, a drop of saline or an eye drop may be used to moisten and loosen it (1, 6).

The Lost Contact Lens

Occasionally a patient presents with a complaint that he or she is unable to locate the contact lens and is uncertain whether it remains in the eye. As in all other eye examinations, evaluation must begin with an assessment of visual acuity in both eyes. The eye is then directly inspected for the contact lens. Though transparent, when appropriately located over the cornea, a lens is readily visible as a fine line on the sclera a few millimeters peripheral to the limbus. Shining a light from the lateral margin of the eye (sidelighting) may help to identify the location of a lens. If the lens is not apparent on initial inspection, topical anesthetic should be instilled and the eyelids should be everted (Chapter 48) as in a search for a foreign body and an attempt to locate the lens beneath the lids is made. If the lens is not found, then, with the patient looking toward his or her chin, the examiner should sweep over the fornix with a moistened cotton-tipped applicator. If the lens remains elusive yet the patient insists that it is present in the eye, a fluorescein examination may be performed. The fluorescein will pool around the outside of the lens and its location will become apparent. It is important to inform the patient that the dye will permanently stain the soft contact lens if it is present.

If after an exhaustive search the contact lens is not found, the patient should be reassured that a thorough examination has not located the missing lens. It is useful to check that the patient has not inadvertently placed one contact lens over the top of the other in the same eye (1, 6).

COMPLICATIONS

Complications of contact lens removal include the production of a corneal abrasion and contamination of the eye with bacterial or viral organisms. Risk can be minimized by using sterile technique and exercising care in gently removing lenses. A fluorescein examination of the eye is indicated in the evaluation of all suspected abrasions, foreign bodies, or eye infections. Thus any patient who is symptomatic either before or following contact lens removal should undergo a fluorescein examination. Typically, injury to the cornea from overwear results in a centrally located, brightly stippled staining pattern, referred to as superficial punctate keratitis. This is in contrast to the usual sharp, linear staining pattern typical of mechanical trauma, such as might be caused by lens removal itself. Nevertheless, management of both types of corneal abrasions is the same.

Pressure on the globe can extrude intraocular contents and worsen the outcome in patients with perforation of the eye. Contact lens removal should be deferred until an ophthalmologist is present if perforation is suspected.

SUMMARY

Contact lenses are worn by a considerable number of children. With proper technique, removal of a contact lens is rarely difficult. Contact lens removal is necessary to fully evaluate patients with ocular trauma or ocular symptoms. Techniques for removal of hard and soft lenses, and lost lenses require a minimum of equipment and are important skills for those who care for pediatric patients. Thorough evaluation for associated eye pathology can be undertaken after contact lenses are successfully removed.

REFERENCES

1. Barr DH, Samples JR, Hedges JR. Ophthalmologic procedures in Roberts JR, Hedges JR, eds. Clinical procedures in emergency medicine. 2nd ed. Philadelphia: WB Saunders, 1991, pp. 1007–1011.

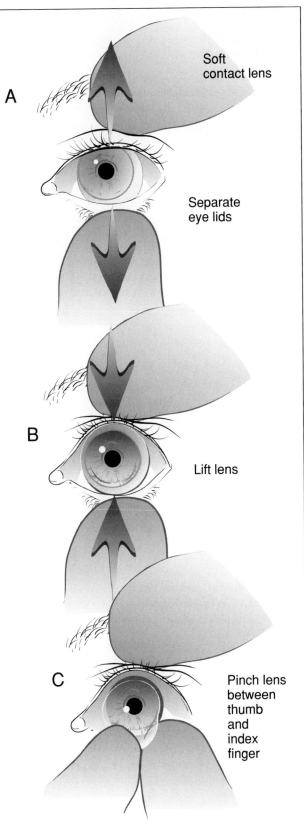

A

Soft contact lens

Separate eye lids

B

Lift lens

C

Pinch lens between thumb and index finger

Figure 53.2.
Removal of a soft contact lens.
A. Have the patient look downward and medially and separate lids.
B. Use the index finger to work the lens onto the sclera. If the lens proves difficult to move, it may be moistened with a drop of saline.
C. Pinch the lens between the thumb and forefinger and remove it.

CLINICAL TIPS

1. Assume that all unconscious adolescents are wearing contact lenses until an appropriate examination proves otherwise.
2. If the patient feels a foreign body in his or her eye, always determine the approximate location of the sensation before instilling of topical anesthetic.
3. Do not hesitate to use fluorescein if a lens cannot be located. This will stain a soft contact lens but finding the displaced lens is more important.
4. Ensure that a proper eye examination is performed after the lens is removed. If the lens has been overworn an underlying corneal infection is possible and should be diagnosed.

2. Paton D, Goldberg MF. Management of ocular injuries. Philadelphia: WB Saunders, 1976, p. 194.
3. Mandell RB. Contact lens practice. Springfield, IL: Charles C Thomas, 1981, pp. 142–168, 496–513.
4. Krezanoski JZ. Physiology and biochemistry of contact lens wearing. In: Encyclopedia of contact lens practice. Vol. 4. South Bend, IN: International Optic, 1959, pp. 18–26.
5. Bohigian GM. Management of infections associated with soft contact lenses. Ophthalmology 1979;86: 1138.
6. Buttaravoli PM, Stair TO. Contact lens overwear, removal of dislocated contact lens, and removal of contact lens in unconscious patient. In: Buttaravoli PM, Stair TO. Common, simple, emergencies. Englewood Cliffs: Brady Communications Company, Inc., pp. 47–52.

Otolaryngologic Procedures

Section Editor: Mark D. Joffe

ACUTE UPPER AIRWAY FOREIGN BODY REMOVAL—THE CHOKING CHILD

Michael P. Poirier and Richard M. Ruddy

INTRODUCTION

Annually in the United States more than 300 deaths of children are due to choking secondary to upper airway obstruction (1). These incidents are usually due to foods, toys, or other small objects. More than 90% occur in infants and children younger than 5 years of age and 65% in infants younger than 2 years of age. Foods continue to be the most common object involved in reported choking episodes in the infant and the child, with round or cylindrical foods most often cited (2) (Table 54.1).

In 1979, the U.S. Consumer Product Safety Commission passed regulations to control the marketing of nonfood choking hazards (3). Small toys, rubber balloons, nails, tacks, and bolts are the main objects responsible for nonfood-related choking episodes in children (4–9). Rubber balloons are the leading cause of choking deaths from toys. Of these deaths 25% are in children over 6 years of age (10).

Treating the child with an acutely obstructed airway is an emergent procedure. Although usually performed in the prehospital setting, it may be necessary to perform the procedure in the emergency department. The first aid approach is routinely taught to the lay public by emergency medicine and other health care providers. The laryngoscopic pro-

cedure may be performed by any qualified physician.

ANATOMY AND PHYSIOLOGY

The nose, mouth, and pharynx comprise the upper airway. The upper airway has numerous functions which include acting as a filter to prevent foreign material from entering the lower airway, humidifying and heating inspired gases, and acting as a conducting system for inspired gases to the lungs.

Ciliated and nonciliated mucous cells line the nose. The function of these cells is to help humidify inspired gases and to filter foreign material. Hair follicles and thick, sticky mucous secretions of the nose also help filter foreign material from the upper airway.

The laryngopharynx extends from the base of the tongue to the esophagus which lies posterior to the trachea. The closure of the glottis protects the tracheobronchial tree from foreign material. This mechanism is crucial in protecting the airway during the process of swallowing. Patients with neuromuscular illness, anatomically abnormal airways, or poorly protected airways are at the highest risk for foreign body aspirations and choking episodes.

The trachea begins at the level of the cricoid cartilage; it descends in the middle of

Table 54.1.
Specific Foods Causing
Choking Episodes
in Children

Hot dog	17%
Candy	10%
Peanut/nut	9%
Grape	8%
Cookie/biscuit	7%
Meat	7%
Carrot	6%
Apple	5%
Popcorn	5%
Peanut butter	5%
Bean	4%
Bread	4%
Macaroni/noodle	3%
Chewing gum	3%
Others	7%

Tinsworth DK. Analysis of choking-related hazards associated with children's products. Washington, DC: U.S. Consumer Product Safety Commission, 1989

the neck to the level of the fifth to sixth thoracic vertebra and then bifurcates into the right and left bronchi. Unlike adults, the angle of takeoff at the carina is almost equal on both sides in young children. In the older child and young adult the trachea at the bifurcation is slightly angled to the right making the opening to the right bronchi a less acute angle.

The airway has protective mechanisms in place that continuously remove foreign debris. Tiny foreign bodies are continually swept up by cilia and mucus to the supraglottic region where they can be swallowed down the esophagus. Coughing is an important means to expel secretions and foreign material from the airway. Through stimulation of receptors in the mucosa of the large respiratory passages, the cough reflex protects the airway from foreign material. Coughing begins with a deep inspiration followed by a forced expiration against a closed glottis. The glottis is then suddenly opened producing a forceful outflow of air.

INDICATIONS

Four assumptions form the rationale for the current recommended treatment of acute airway obstruction in infants and children (11). First, airway obstruction with secondary cardiac arrest is far more common in pediatric patients than sudden cardiac arrest with secondary airway obstruction as seen in adults. Second, a foreign body completely obstruct-

ing the upper airway is an immediate threat to life and must be removed. Third, if the child can speak, breathe, or cough, the foreign body is only partially obstructing the airway, yet it may be dislodged or moved to a position that totally obstructs the airway. This can make first aid airway maneuvers potentially dangerous. Finally, partial airway obstruction with poor air exchange, or complete airway obstruction with cyanosis, requires immediate relief.

Importantly, any child who has choked on a foreign body and who is coughing, crying, or speaking is best left initially to his or her own reflexes to relieve the obstruction. If the child or infant is unable to make sounds, if complete obstruction develops, or if no evidence of respiratory air movement is evident, immediate first aid to establish a patent airway and deliver basic life support is required to avoid permanent disability or death (12).

The abdominal thrust (Heimlich) maneuver is thought to be the most effective method of relieving complete airway obstruction in children greater than 1 year of age (13). This method is based on several physiologic factors: 80% of respiratory effort is from diaphragmatic contraction; abdominal inward pressure compresses the diaphragm upward, thereby raising intrathoracic pressure; a sudden, rapid increase in intrathoracic pressure may expel the obstructing object; and unconscious patients becoming hypoxic from obstruction lose their muscle tone which improves the result of the maneuver (13). The abdominal thrust maneuver may therefore be ineffective initially in a conscious child, but may be completely successful minutes later as the patient loses consciousness (12). The combination of these factors enhances the success of this maneuver in expelling the foreign body from the obstructed airway.

The American Academy of Pediatrics (AAP), the American Heart Association (AHA), and the Red Cross recommend that the abdominal thrust maneuver be used in children greater than 1 year of age for complete airway obstruction. Controversy exists, however, about which maneuver—the abdominal thrust or the back-blow and chest thrust—is the best in the choking infant under 1 year of age. In infants, the stomach, liver, and spleen are relatively large compared with older children. Damage and even rupture of abdominal organs with the abdominal thrust

Chapter 54
Acute Upper Airway
Foreign Body
Removal—The
Choking Child

622

technique has been reported (14, 15). Another point to be considered is greater chest wall compliance in the infant as compared with an older child. A compliant chest wall absorbs some of the energy from the abdominal thrust maneuver leading partially to chest wall expansion rather than lung and airway compression. This can make the abdominal thrust maneuver less effective in producing pressure changes adequate to expel a foreign object from the obstructed airway.

In infants less than 1 year of age, the technique currently recommended by the AAP and AHA involves two steps: first, the head-down back-blow maneuver, followed by second, the chest thrust maneuver (12). The head-down back-blow maneuver is designed to compress the chest from the posterior force while the anterior chest is held. Ideally this will generate a rapid increase in intrathoracic pressure which will move the foreign body along the airway and out (16). Similarly, the chest thrust maneuver uses sternal compression to increase intrathoracic pressure in an effort to expel the foreign object from the infant's airway. This maneuver is much like performing chest compressions in cardiopulmonary arrest. A concern raised by some authorities is that the sudden acceleration that occurs with the back-blow maneuver in an awake patient may actually cause an object to travel further distally in the airway. Back blows in an awake patient could stimulate inhalation at the same time as the pressure is increased, possibly opening distal airways through which the foreign body may further lodge. Researchers have reported that the back-blow maneuver may cause caudal movement of the object in concordance of Newton's third law of motion, i.e., "to every action there is always an opposed equal reaction" (17). Nevertheless, it appears that in infancy, when the maneuver is performed with the infant held head-down and prone over the rescuer's leg (Fig. 54.1), further intrusion of the foreign body is unlikely (12).

Equipment

No specific equipment is needed to manage a pediatric patient with an obstructed airway in the field. Prehospital interventions consist of abdominal thrusts, back blows, and chest compressions, as well as other basic life support maneuvers (see Chapter 12). For this reason, any qualified medical professional or trained lay person can perform the necessary procedures without specialized devices. In the ED or other hospital setting, supplementary oxygen, laryngoscope with appropriate size blades, forceps for removing the foreign body if visualized, bag-valve-mask, suctioning equipment, and capabilities for ensuring an emergent airway must be readily available (see also Chapters 13 through 17 for details of equipment needs associated with these interventions).

PROCEDURE

The following recommendations of the AAP and AHA for the acute treatment of the choking child are made based on current consensus within the pediatric and emergency medicine community (12).

The Infant Younger Than 1 Year of Age

The following steps should be performed immediately in the field to relieve the airway obstruction. The infant is initially held prone, resting on the rescuer's forearm. The infant's head is supported by firmly holding the jaw. The rescuer's forearm should lie on his or her thigh to support the infant, with the patient's head lower than the trunk. Second, the five back blows are delivered forcefully between the infant's shoulder blades, using the heel of the hand (Fig. 54.1.A). After delivering the back blows, the rescuer's free hand is placed on the infant's back, holding the infant's head. The patient is thus held between the two hands of the rescuer—one hand supporting the neck, jaw, and chest, while the other supports the back. The infant is turned while the head and neck are carefully supported, and the infant is held in the supine position across the rescuer's thigh. The infant's head is turned to one side and held lower than the trunk. Five quick, downward chest thrusts are performed in the same location as external chest compressions (lower half of the sternum, approximately one fingerbreadth below the nipple line), but at a slower rate. The rescuer should use two or three fingers to compress the sternum approximately one-third to one-half the depth of the

Chapter 54
Acute Upper Airway
Foreign Body
Removal—The
Choking Child

623

Figure 54.1.

Figure 54.1.
A. Back blows and **B.** chest thrusts are attempted to relieve foreign body airway obstruction in the infant.

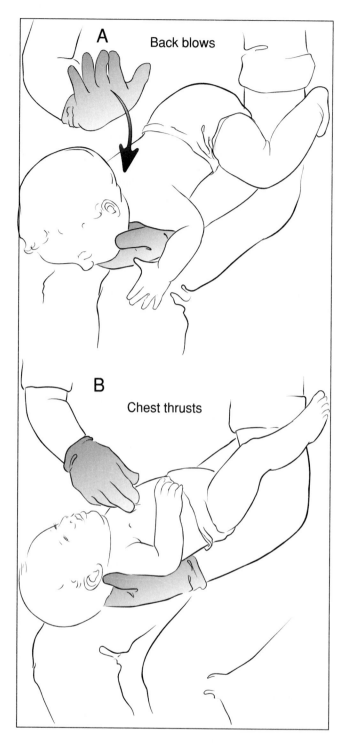

A Back blows

B Chest thrusts

chest, or 0.5 to 1.0 inch (Fig. 54.1.B). Attempts should then be made to provide rescue breathing. If the infant becomes unconscious, the rescuer may attempt a tongue-jaw lift, and if a foreign body is visible in the posterior pharynx, an effort can then be made to remove it with a finger sweep. If the airway remains obstructed, the maneuvers as described are repeated in sequence.

The Child Older Than 1 Year of Age

Abdominal Thrust
With a Conscious Victim

These thrusts are performed with the rescuer standing behind the victim, who may be sitting or standing. The rescuer positions his or her arms directly under the victim's axilla, and

Chapter 54
Acute Upper Airway
Foreign Body
Removal—The
Choking Child

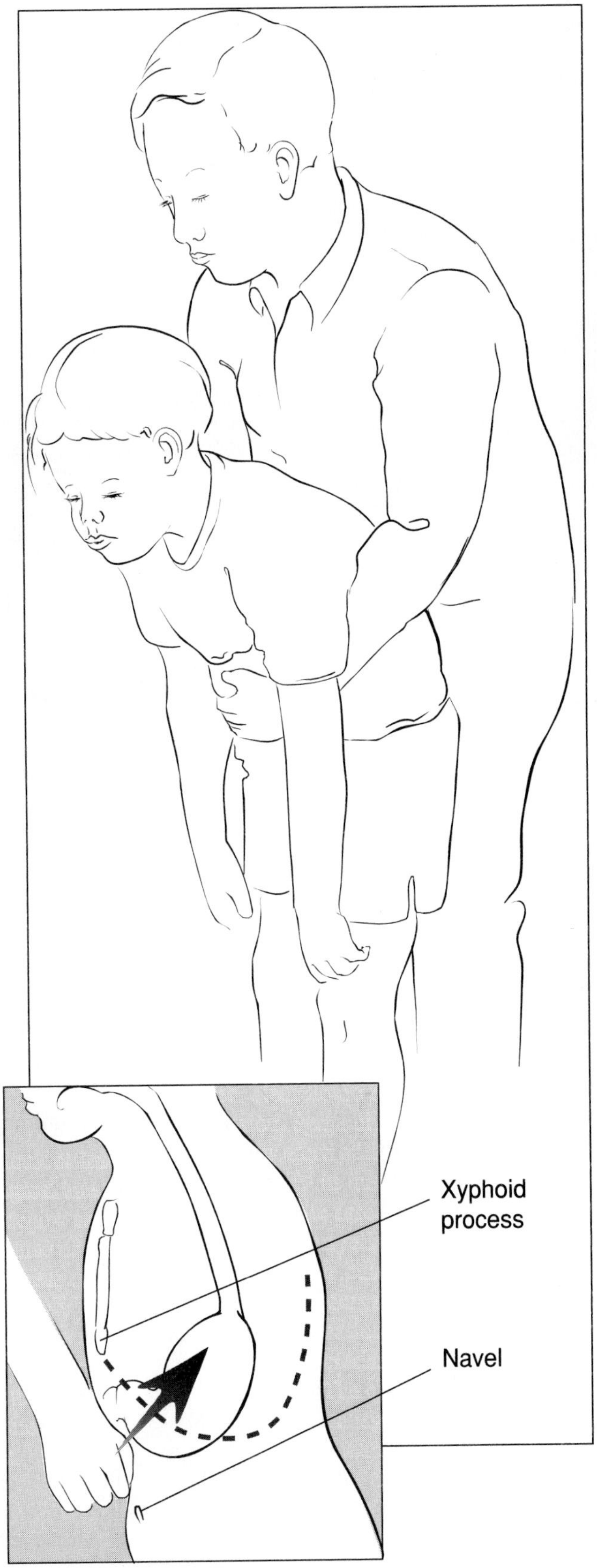

Figure 54.2.
Abdominal thrusts with older conscious child standing or sitting.

Xyphoid process

Navel

1. Hold infant head downward prone, resting on EMT's forearm, with head supported
2. Deliver five back blows between infant's shoulder blades, using heel of hand (Fig. 54.1.A)
3. Place free hand on infant's back, and infant is turned supine, with head dependent, across EMT's thigh
4. Perform five quick downward chest thrusts in same location as external chest compression (lower half of sternum, approximately one finger breadth below nipple line) but at a slower rate (Fig. 54.1.B.)
5. Attempt to provide rescue breathing. If airway remains obstructed and infant becomes unconscious, the EMT should attempt to visualize foreign body and remove manually, then repeat sequence as necessary.

* Adapted from AAP, 1993 (12).

**Chapter 54
Acute Upper Airway
Foreign Body
Removal—The
Choking Child**

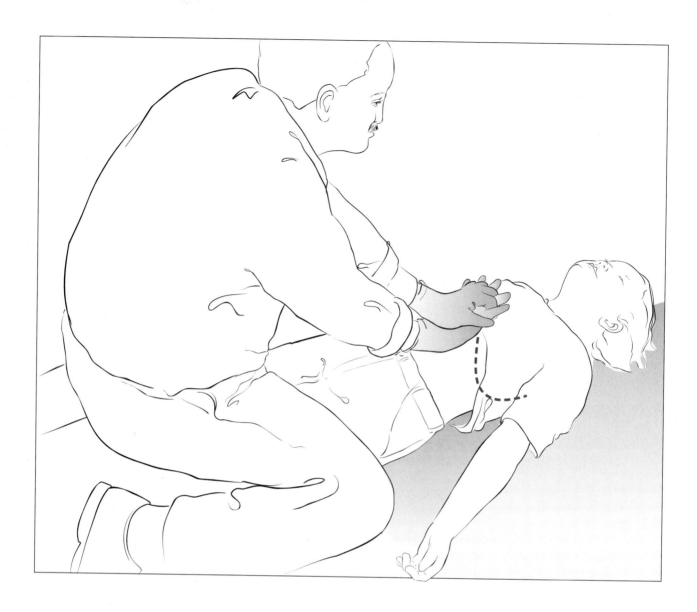

Figure 54.3.
Abdominal thrusts with
older child lying (conscious
or unconscious).

**Chapter 54
Acute Upper Airway
Foreign Body
Removal—The
Choking Child**

encircles the victim's chest (Fig. 54.2). The thumb side of one fist is placed against the victim's abdomen in the midline, slightly above the navel and well below the tip of the xyphoid process. The rescuer grasps this fist with the other hand and administers five quick, upward thrusts. The fist should not impact on the xyphoid process or the lower costal margins, because force applied to these structures may damage internal organs. Each thrust should be a separate, distinct movement. The thrusts are continued until the foreign body is expelled, or five thrusts are completed. Again, the rescuer should attempt to provide rescue breathing. If the airway remains obstructed, this sequence is repeated. If the victim becomes unconscious, the rescuer proceeds with the protocol for the unconscious victim.

**Abdominal Thrust With Unconscious
Victim or Conscious Victim Lying Down**

The victim is placed in the supine position for abdominal thrusts to be performed. The rescuer should kneel close to the victim's side or straddle the victim's hips (Fig. 54.3). The rescuer opens the victim's airway using a chin lift or jaw thrust. The heel of one hand is placed on the child's abdomen in the midline slightly above the navel but well below the costal margins and xyphoid process. The other hand is placed on top of the first. Both hands are pressed into the abdomen with a quick upward thrust. A series of five thrusts is performed as necessary, with each thrust a separate and distinct movement. Thrusts are directed upward in the midline, and not to either side of the abdomen. After five abdominal thrusts, the rescuer attempts rescue breathing. In the unconscious victim, the rescuer makes an effort to visualize an obstructing foreign body and remove it manually if possible. If the airway remains obstructed, these maneuvers are repeated.

Manual or Forceps Removal

If back blows, abdominal thrusts, or chest thrusts are unsuccessful, the rescuer should attempt manual removal of the foreign body in the nonbreathing, unconscious victim. If proper equipment is readily available, as in the ED, this would be optimally achieved with a clamp or forceps under direct visualization by laryngoscopy.

In the absence of appropriate equipment, manual removal should be attempted by grasping the tongue and lower jaw between the gloved thumb and fingers and lifting the mandible (tongue-jaw lift, see Fig. 12.4). Such action may itself partly relieve the obstruction. A towel roll placed under the shoulders in young children may further open the airway and afford visualization. If the foreign body becomes visible, the rescuer should attempt to remove it by sweeping the index finger of the other gloved hand across the posterior pharynx (only in an unconscious victim). Blind finger sweeps of the oropharynx to remove a nonvisible foreign body should not be performed.

With the availability of appropriate equipment, removal under direct visualization should be attempted (18). The laryngoscopy (Chapter 16) should be performed while carefully visualizing the oropharynx, so the laryngoscope blade does not push a foreign body partly obstructing the airway further down and cause complete obstruction. Most such foreign objects are located at the base of the tongue or around the tonsillar pillars. If the foreign body is visualized, the Magill forceps (or a Kelly clamp, if the Magill is not readily available) is used in an attempt to grasp the foreign body and extract it (Fig. 54.4.A). Occasionally, it is useful if the foreign body is not visualized at the time of initial laryngoscopy, it is sometimes helpful to have an assistant perform abdominal or chest thrusts in an effort to move the foreign body further proximally, where it can be visualized and grasped.

Short of creating a surgical airway, endotracheal intubation (Chapter 16) may force the subglottic foreign body distally enough to partially ventilate a child through one mainstem bronchus until rigid bronchoscopy can be emergently performed (Fig. 54.4.B). In this context, the pop-off valve of the bag-valve system should be occluded to deliver sufficient volume for effective oxygenation and ventilation. If these attempts fail to oxygenate the patient, the physician should proceed to create a surgical airway immediately (Chapters 17 and 25).

SUMMARY: FIRST AID FOR THE CHOKING CHILD OVER 1 YEAR OF AGE*

Abdominal Thrust With a Conscious Patient Sitting or Standing
1. Stand behind child with arms directly under child's axilla and encircling chest (Fig. 54.2)
2. Place thumb side of one fist against patient's abdomen in midline, just above navel but below tip of xyphoid process
3. Grasp fist with other hand and exert five quick, upward thrusts
4. Continue thrusts until foreign body is expelled or five thrusts are completed. Attempts are made to provide rescue breathing. If airway remains obstructed, repeat sequence. If patient becomes unconscious, make an attempt to visualize foreign body and remove manually. If unsuccessful, modify approach as described in next section.

Abdominal Thrust With Unconscious or Conscious Patient, Lying Down
1. Place patient supine, with EMT at patient's side or straddling patient's hips (Fig. 54.3)
2. Open patient's airway using chin lift or jaw thrust
3. Place heel of one hand on child's abdomen in midline just above navel and below costal margins and xyphoid. Place other hand on top of first hand
4. Press both hands into abdomen with quick upward thrust in midline. If necessary, perform a series of five thrusts, with each thrust a separate and distinct movement
5. After delivery of five abdominal thrusts, attempt rescue breathing. If airway remains obstructed, the EMT should attempt to visualize and remove foreign body manually. If unsuccessful, repeat sequence

* Adapted from AAP, 1993 (12).

Chapter 54
Acute Upper Airway
Foreign Body
Removal—The
Choking Child

627

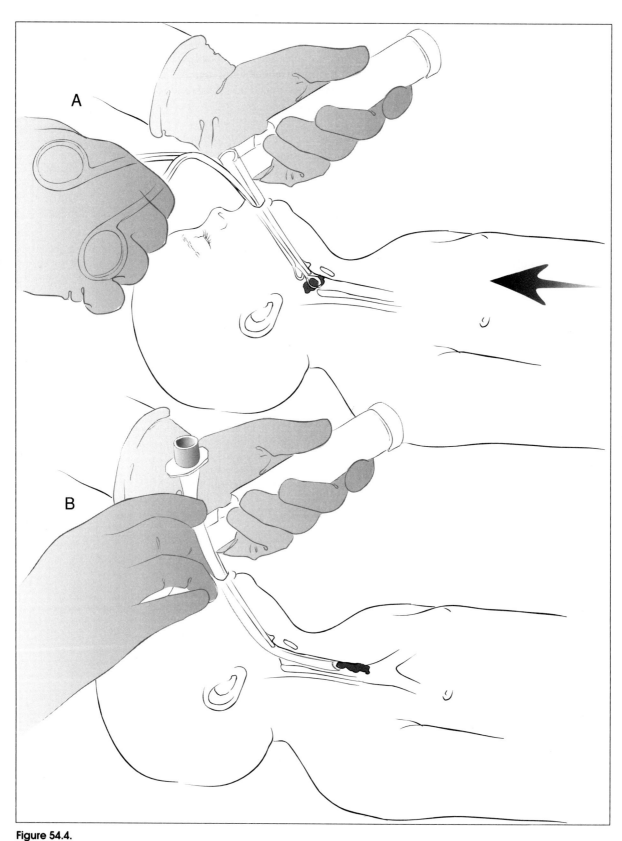

Figure 54.4.
A. The Magill forceps is used to extract a foreign body visualized by direct laryngoscopy.
B. Endotracheal intubation may force the foreign body distally into one mainstream bronchus.

COMPLICATIONS

Although rib and cardiac damage is a theoretical risk of the chest compression maneuver in infants and small children, a large review of infants that underwent chest compressions found no significant rib injuries or fractures (19). Severe complications have been reported when the Heimlich maneuver was performed incorrectly in the emergent treatment of airway obstruction (20). Reported complications include pneumomediastinum, ruptured stomach, and a thrombosed aorta. A possible explanation for these complications is that as many as 70% of maneuvers are done by untrained individuals and 50% of the individuals learned the technique in lay magazines or newspapers. For example, one male infant is reported to have suffered a nonfatal pneumomediastinum as a result of a "bear hug" attempt at the Heimlich maneuver by his father (20). When performed properly, the complication rate of the abdominal thrusts appears to be quite low, particularly given the life-threatening potential of airway obstruction. Complications related to forceps removal of a foreign body under direct visualization should be largely related to those of instrumenting the airway, and are detailed in Chapter 16.

SUMMARY

Despite advances over the past decade through changes in product regulation and increased awareness in first aid, choking deaths still remain a significant problem. Primary prevention and anticipatory guidance play a key role in addressing this problem. Secondary prevention by understanding and using the recommended emergent maneuvers for the obstructed airway can be life saving. In the prehospital setting, when airway equipment is unavailable, the rescuer must rely on the first aid measures for choking as delineated by the AHA and AAP. Techniques for abdominal thrust, chest thrust, back blow, and finger sweep maneuvers should be acquired through appropriate training courses. In the emergency department, or in any setting with access to proper equipment, laryngoscopy and forceps extraction under direct visualization must be rapidly undertaken when indicated.

REFERENCES

1. National Safety Council. Accident facts. Itasca, IL: National Safety Council, 1992: p. 5.
2. Harris CS, Baker SP, Smith GA, Harris RM. Childhood asphyxiation by food; a national analysis and overview. JAMA 1984;251:2231–2235.
3. U.S. Consumer Product Safety Commission. Method for identifying toys and other articles intended for use by children under 3 years of age which present choking, aspiration, or ingestion hazards because of small parts (16 CFR 1501). Washington, DC: General Services Administration, 1979.
4. Tinsworth DK. Analysis of choking-related hazards associated with children's products. Washington, DC: U.S. Consumer Product Safety Commission, September 1989.
5. Becker PG, Turow J. Earring aspiration and other jewelry hazards. Pediatrics 1986;78:494–496.
6. Press S, Liberman JG. Aspiration through a "sip-up" straw. Am J Dis Child 1986;140:1090–1091.
7. Ross MN, Janik JS. "Foil tab" aspiration and retropharyngeal abscess in a toddler. JAMA 1988;260:3130.
8. Arnold RW, Hoffman AD, Brutinel WM, et al. Barbie doll curler aspiration into the upper trachea. Am J Dis Child 1987;141:1325–1326.
9. Myer CM. Foreign body aspiration. Am J Dis Child 1988;142:485–486.
10. Ryan CA, Yacoub W, Paton T, Avard D. Childhood deaths from toy balloons. Am J Dis Child 1990;144:1221–1224.
11. Committee on Accident and Poison Prevention. Revised first aid for the choking child. Pediatrics 1986;78:177–178.
12. Committee on Pediatric Emergency Medicine. First aid for the choking child. Pediatrics 1993;92:477–479.
13. Heimlich HF. A life-saving maneuver to prevent food choking. JAMA 1975;234:398–401.
14. Visintine RE, Baick CH. Ruptured stomach after Heimlich maneuver. JAMA 1975;234:415.
15. Croom DW. Ruptured stomach after attempted Heimlich maneuver. JAMA 1975;234:415.
16. Gordon AS, Belton MK, Ridolpho PF. Emergency management of foreign body airway obstruction. In: Safar PJ, Elam JO, eds. Advances in cardiopulmonary resuscitation. New York: Springer-Verlag, 1977, pp. 39–50.
17. Day RL, Crelin ES, Dubois AB. Choking: the Heimlich abdominal thrust vs. back blows: an approach to measurement of inertial aerodynamic forces. Pediatrics 1982;70:113–119.
18. Young GP, Pace SA. Esophageal foreign bodies. In: Roberts JR, Hedges JR, eds. Clinical procedures in emergency medicine. Philadelphia: WB Saunders, 1985, p. 638.
19. Spevak MR, Kleinman PK, Belanger PL, Primack C, Richmond JM. Cardiopulmonary resuscitation and rib fractures in infants. JAMA 1994;272:617–618.
20. Fink JA, Klein RL. Complications of the Heimlich maneuver. J Pediatr Surg 1989;24:486–487.

Otoscopic Examination

Hnin Khine and Holly W. Davis

Introduction

Symptoms referable to the ears account for over one-third of all pediatric visits, and ear, nose, and throat disorders combined prompt over 50% of visits (1, 2). Patients can present with localized symptoms such as otalgia or otorrhea, or with nonspecific complaints such as fever or irritability. For this reason, the pediatric physical examination is not complete without an otoscopic examination. Pediatricians, emergency physicians, and family practitioners must therefore be skillful with the techniques of assessment. Otoscopic examination is used not only as a diagnostic procedure for external auditory canal problems and middle ear disease, but it also can serve as an indirect evaluation of intracranial injury. Other indications for otoscopic examination include hearing impairment, nystagmus, and vertigo.

Anatomy and Physiology

The external ear includes the pinna, auricle and outer cartilaginous canal, the inner bony canal, and the outer surface of the tympanic membrane (Fig. 55.1). The middle ear includes the inner portion of the tympanic membrane, the three ossicles, and the mastoid air cells (Fig. 55.2). The inner ear is composed of semicircular canals, cochlea, and the seventh and eighth cranial nerves. The eustachian tube connects the middle ear with the nasopharynx. When functioning nor-

mally, the eustachian tube vents the middle ear, serves as a conduit for drainage of middle ear secretions, and protects the middle ear from nasopharyngeal sound pressure and secretions (1, 3). In infancy, the tympanic membrane is tilted at a 130° angle, making visualization of landmarks more difficult (1, 2).

The external auditory canal is often slightly angulated in infancy and early childhood, which necessitates applying gentle lateral traction on the auricle to help visualize the tympanic membrane (1, 2, 4). During the first 4 to 6 months of life, the canal mucosa is somewhat loosely attached to supporting structures and moves readily on insufflation. If care is not taken to inspect the canal as the speculum is inserted to ensure that the transition between the canal wall and tympanic membrane is visualized, movement of the canal wall during insufflation may be mistaken for a normally mobile drum (1, 2).

The wall of the external auditory canal is protected by a waxy layer of cerumen, formed by a combination of viscous secretions from sebaceous glands, watery secretions of apocrine glands, and exfoliated epithelial cells. While the canal is colonized by normal skin flora, the acidic pH of the secretions acts as a chemical barrier against infection (1, 3, 5). Repeated wetting of the canal wall from swimming, bathing, or high humidity alters the protective coating of wax and renders the surface susceptible to infection. Conditions causing excessive dryness, underlying skin disorders (e.g., eczema or psoriasis), and trauma to the external canal (e.g., from fingernails, cotton swabs, or the

Figure 55.1.
Anatomy of the external ear.

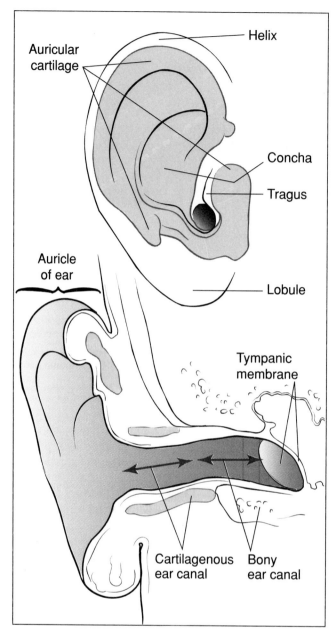

Figure with labels: Helix, Auricular cartilage, Concha, Tragus, Auricle of ear, Lobule, Tympanic membrane, Cartilagenous ear canal, Bony ear canal

genic when the normal equilibrium is disturbed (2, 5).

Acute otitis media or middle ear infection consists of inflammation of the mucoperiosteal lining of the middle ear. Its high incidence in young children who are otherwise healthy partly reflects the fact that the eustachian tube of the young child is shorter, wider, straighter, and more horizontal than that of the older child, thus allowing organisms from the nasopharynx to reach the middle ear region more easily (1–3, 6). Furthermore, infants and young children are prone to functional obstruction of the eustachian tube, as lack of stiffness in the cartilaginous supporting structures predisposes to collapse of the tube, reducing venting of the middle ear (4). As oxygen is absorbed by mucosal cells, negative pressure develops. When venting of air eventually does occur, the vacuum created then facilitates aspiration of nasopharyngeal secretions into the middle ear (4). The anatomic and physiologic abnormalities associated with cleft palate and other craniofacial anomalies result in similar functional obstruction (1–3, 6). The tonsils and adenoids enlarge over the first 8 to 10 years of life and then gradually decrease in size. When markedly enlarged, they can cause mechanical obstruction of the eustachian tube, further predisposing to infection. Less commonly, nasopharyngeal tumors may be the source of mechanical obstruction (1–3, 6). Occasionally, organisms enter the middle ear space from the external canal through a tympanic membrane perforation or via hematogenous spread (1, 6).

Bacteria can be isolated from middle ear fluid in about two-thirds of patients with acute otitis media. The organisms found consist primarily of respiratory pathogens—*Streptococcus pneumoniae, Haemophilus*

presence of a foreign body) also predispose to infection. Perforation of the tympanic membrane in a patient with otitis media may produce infection by releasing purulent material into the external auditory canal (1, 2, 3, 5).

Common pathogens responsible for infection of the external canal (otitis externa) include *Staphylococcus aureus* and *Pseudomonas aeruginosa*, but cultures often grow mixed flora with Gram-negative enteric and Gram-positive organisms. Thirty percent of children are colonized with fungi—mainly *Candida albicans* and *Aspergillus niger*—which have the potential to become patho-

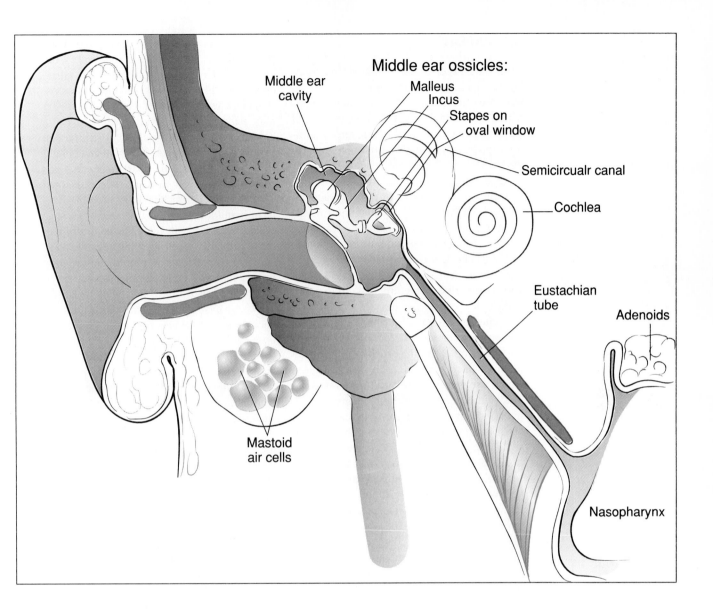

Middle ear ossicles:

Middle ear cavity

Malleus
Incus

Stapes on oval window

Semicircualr canal

Cochlea

Eustachian tube

Adenoids

Mastoid air cells

Nasopharynx

influenzae (nontypeable), *Moraxella catar-rhalis*, and *Streptococcus pyogenes*. Respiratory viruses are also believed to be responsible for a significant proportion of acute otitis media (1, 2, 6–8).

Colonization of the nasopharynx by pathogenic bacteria is thought to be the initial event in the pathogenesis of acute otitis media. Concomitant viral infection then induces respiratory epithelial injury, leading to eustachian tube inflammation and varying degrees of obstruction, impairing middle ear drainage. The mucosal lining becomes inflamed and weeps, resulting in accumulation of mucopurulent material in the middle ear space (1, 2, 6). As pressure in the middle ear increases, the membrane tends to bulge, and

rupture may occur when increased pressure is great enough to cause ischemic necrosis. When the middle ear is filled with fluid, tympanic membrane mobility is markedly reduced on both positive and negative pressure. If, however, some venting of the eustachian tube occurs, air and fluid may be present with only a mild decrease in mobility (2, 9).

Serous effusion of the middle ear occurs in children with eustachian tube dysfunction or following resolution of an acute infection. It may persist for weeks to months. The high negative middle ear pressure typically associated with this condition is reflected by greater movement of the tympanic membrane when applying negative pressure during pneumatic otoscopy (1, 2, 6).

Figure 55.2.
Cross-sectional anatomy of the ear.

**Chapter 55
Otoscopic
Examination**

INDICATIONS

Otitis media is common in infancy and childhood. Given the fact that presenting symptoms are often nonspecific, otoscopic examination is indicated as part of the evaluation of any infant or young child with fever, irritability, upper respiratory symptoms, or sore throat (1, 2, 6). Symptoms specific to the ear such as otalgia, otorrhea, auricular swelling, hearing loss, tinnitus, vertigo, nystagmus, and ear injury are also obvious indications. Furthermore, any patient being evaluated for head and/or facial trauma must undergo otoscopy to check for canal laceration, hemotympanum, or CSF leak which may be seen with a basilar skull fracture. Patients exposed to the severe concussive force of an explosion also must be assessed for traumatic perforation and hearing loss (1, 2, 5, 6).

Acute otitis externa usually starts with an itching sensation and feeling of fullness which progresses to severe throbbing pain. The pain is exacerbated by movement of the pinna, which is a distinguishing feature. The canal is filled with exudate and the mucosal surface is inflamed and friable. In severe cases, attendant edema may produce marked narrowing. The discharge is usually white or yellow, but may become bloody with severe inflammation and tympanic membrane perforation. Prolonged presence of a foreign body may produce a foul-smelling discharge (2, 5). To adequately assess the source, the canal must be cleared of discharge with gentle suction or by careful wiping with cotton wicks. When drainage is persistent or fails to clear with therapy, culture is indicated (2, 5).

Acute otitis media can present in a variety of ways (1, 2, 6). It can occur de novo in a previously healthy child or can follow the onset of an upper respiratory infection by a few to several days, often heralded by a secondary temperature spike. Patients may complain of specific symptoms of otalgia and/or otorrhea, but as mentioned previously, in many cases only nonspecific symptoms of fever and/or irritability are present. Other patients may complain of pain referred to the throat, and some may simply complain of a sensation of fullness, popping, or decreased hearing. Classic findings on physical examination are an erythematous, thickened, opaque tympanic membrane bulging outward with a decreased light reflex, obscured landmarks, and markedly decreased mobility (1, 2, 6, 9, 10). This picture, however, is only one possibility (1, 2, 6, 9, 10). In some cases, the drum appears markedly injected and hyperemic with dilated vessels or frankly hemorrhagic, whereas in other patients erythema may be minimal or even absent. In some cases, the fluid may be clear; in still others, yellow or white pus can be visualized behind the membrane (1, 2, 6, 9, 10). When bubbles or an air-fluid level are seen, reflecting some venting of the eustachian tube, mobility may be only mildly decreased. In cases when negative pressure has developed, the drum may move primarily when applying negative pressure (2). Occasionally, painful bullae may form within the tympanic membrane due to acute infection resulting in a bullous myringitis (1, 2, 6). Notably erythema alone does not necessarily confirm the presence of infection, because high body temperature or excessive crying also can produce this finding. Asymmetry in the degree of erythema and mobility of the tympanic membrane from one ear to the other are useful indicators of infection in such cases.

With serous otitis media, the membrane may appear full, retracted, or normal depending on the chronicity of the disease. The color of the fluid may be yellow, amber, or gray. Mobility is reduced and often greater when applying negative pressure on pneumatic otoscopy (1, 2, 6).

Injury to the external auditory canal or tympanic membrane from foreign objects (such as cotton swabs) can produce abrasions, superficial lacerations, or even tympanic membrane perforation. Concussive forces from severe blows to the side of the head or explosions also can cause perforation. Direct trauma to the middle ear or a basilar skull fracture can result in hemotympanum. The appearance may vary depending on elapsed time since injury, with the color of the membrane ranging from blue to purple (2).

Oral antimicrobial therapy is indicated for all patients with acute otitis media (1, 6). This includes children with fever, upper respiratory symptoms, and/or otalgia who are found to have an inflamed tympanic membrane and fluid or pus behind the tympanic membrane. These patients should be seen in follow-up 3 weeks after treatment is initiated. Topical antimicrobial therapy is indicated for patients with external otitis and canal wall trauma, and in conjunction with an oral agent in children with otitis media and a tympanic membrane perforation. In severe cases of external otitis with marked canal wall swelling, it is often necessary to insert a wick (a short segment of plain gauze packing) to serve as a conduit for the otic drops until the edema subsides (5). Parenteral antimicrobial therapy is indicated for extension of infection resulting in mastoiditis or auricular and periauricular cellulitis.

Indications for consultation and/or referral to an otolaryngologist include (*a*) frequent recurrences of acute otitis media (more than three in a 6-month period), (*b*) persistent effusion for over 3 months despite adequate antimicrobial therapy, (*c*) persistent tympanic membrane perforation following otitis, (*d*) otologic trauma other than canal wall abrasions, and (*e*) presence of any suppurative complications of otitis media (e.g., mastoiditis, intracranial abscess) or of otitis externa (auricular or periauricular cellulitis).

EQUIPMENT

The pneumatic otoscope with 3.5-V halogen illumination and an airtight head and bulb insufflator is the best diagnostic tool available for otoscopic examination (Fig. 55.3). An equipment checklist for this procedure is presented in Table 55.1. Before otoscopic examination, the equipment should be tested for adequate air seal. The speculum is attached to the head of the otoscope, the tip is occluded with the thumb or finger, and positive pressure is applied by pressing on the bulb. No air leak should occur. The clinician also should test the light source on the otoscope. With a wall mounted unit, no light when the device is turned on usually means that the bulb is out and should be replaced. With a battery operated unit, a dim yellow light indicates that the batteries must be replaced or recharged. An adequate light source is essential to obtaining a good otoscopic examination.

The largest speculum that can be inserted to about one-third the distance into the ear canal should be used. Neonates and young infants may require a 2 mm aural speculum. The ear canal of an older infant or toddler usually will accommodate a 3 mm speculum. For children 2 to 7 years of age, a 4 mm speculum is usually appropriate whereas older children and adolescents may require a 5 mm speculum. Putting a piece of rubber tourniquet tubing around the end of the speculum may give a better seal if the clinician encounters a significant air leak in attempting to examine older children with a 4 or 5 mm speculum (2, 11). Extra caution should be taken to avoid inserting the speculum deep into the bony part of the canal because this can be painful.

PROCEDURE

Otoscopic examination of infants and young children can prove challenging, as patients often vigorously resist the procedure, especially if they have had a prior painful experience. In such cases, effective restraint is necessary to prevent injury and another bad experience. Nevertheless, with the toddler or preschool age child it is best to start by attempting the examination with the patient sitting in the parent's lap, using a puppet, stuffed animal, or tongue blade with a face drawn on it as distractors. Gradual introduction of the equipment also is helpful. The clinician can ask preschoolers to try to catch the light as it is moved around or to blow it out as the clinician turns off the light source. The parent or physician also can serve briefly as "patient" while the child is offered a look. Then the clinician takes a turn (see also Chapter 2). If these efforts fail, or when cleaning of

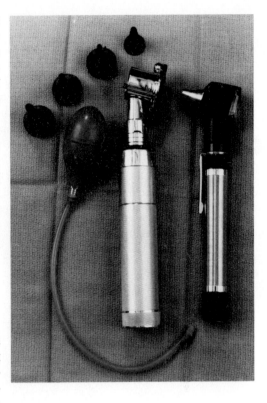

Figure 55.3.
Equipment used for pneumatic otoscopy.

Table 55.1.
Equipment

Pneumatic otoscope
Insufflator bulb
Specula (sizes 2, 3, 4, 5)
Surgical otoscope head (optional)
Rubber tubing
Blunt cerumen curette
3% hydrogen peroxide solution
20 mL syringe, 23-gauge butterfly
    without the needle
Suction

the external canal is necessary, restraint should be used.

When restraint is needed, different positions should be considered for children of different developmental ages (2, 4). When examining a neonate, infant, or young toddler, it is best to position the patient either supine or prone on the examining table. In the supine position, the child can be restrained by an assistant at the head end of the table, holding both upper arms to the side of the head (Fig. 55.4.A). The body and lower extremities can be restrained by a parent who leans over the legs while pressing down on the hips. In the prone position, the parent can hold the arms and body from the caudal end while leaning over the child. The clinician then stabilizes the head using the hand that holds the pinna of the ear.

Toddlers and preschoolers sometimes can be restrained in a sitting position on the mother's lap. The child's legs are secured between the parent's legs. The arms and body are held tightly against the parent's chest using one arm while the other arm stabilizes the child's head against the parent's chest (Fig. 55.4.B). Although this may work for examination, the degree of restraint afforded often is not adequate for cleaning the external auditory canal.

Examination begins with inspection of the auricle and periauricular tissues. The external auditory canal is then viewed as the speculum is gradually inserted. Adequate vi-

Figure 55.4.
A. Restraint in the supine position for otoscopic examination. This method is often most effective for an infant or younger child. A similar approach with the child in the prone position also can be used.
B. Restraint by a parent for otoscopic examination.

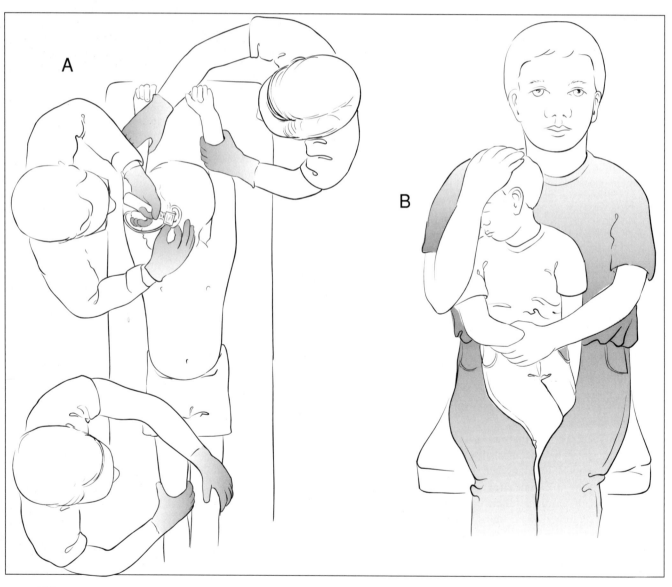

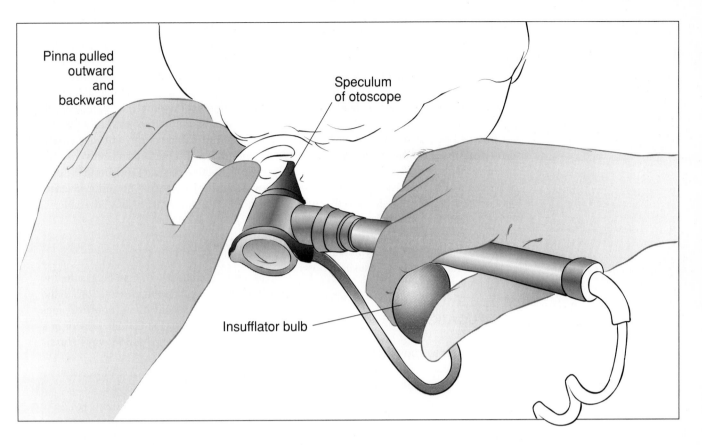

Pinna pulled outward and backward

Speculum of otoscope

Insufflator bulb

Figure 55.5.
Proper hand position for pneumatic otoscopy. Holding the otoscope like a pencil allows the clinician to squeeze the insufflator bulb with the thumb and index finger. The free hand can then be used to gently pull back the auricle to straighten the external canal.

sualization often necessitates removal of cerumen. When the cerumen is soft or flaky, it usually can be removed easily using a blunt cerumen curette. This can be done through a pneumatic otoscope head by partially removing the lens, or more conveniently, through a surgical otoscope head. The curette is carefully inserted beyond the wax and then gently pulled back bringing out the wax. Care should be taken to watch the curette during this procedure to avoid touching the sensitive canal wall. Wet wax or discharge may require suction or wicking for removal. When cerumen is hard and impacted, an effective technique is to instill 3% hydrogen peroxide into the ear and leave it in place for 15 to 20 minutes. The ear is then irrigated with lukewarm water to remove the wax (see also Chapter 56).

To examine the right ear, the otoscope is held in the right hand like a pencil, with thumb and forefinger around the handle near the junction of the barrel and otoscope head (Fig. 55.5). The ulnar aspect of the clinician's right hand rests on the child's cheek to prevent deep insertion of the speculum with sudden movement of the child's head. With the left hand, the pinna is pulled outward and backward to straighten the canal for better visualization. To examine the left side, the clinician changes hands to hold the otoscope with the left hand and the pinna with the right. The clinician should look through the otoscope lens as the speculum is inserted, taking care to ensure that the transition between the canal wall and the tympanic membrane is seen clearly. Once the membrane is visualized, three characteristics should be assessed—color, position, and condition of the membrane (translucency, thickness, scarring, fluid, and air-fluid or air-pus levels). The clarity of the light reflex and the bony landmarks also should be noted (1, 2, 4, 6, 9, 10).

The next task is to check the mobility of the tympanic membrane (2, 4, 6, 9–11). Using the insufflator bulb while at the same time holding the otoscope and the ear is the most difficult step to master in this procedure. The bulb of the insufflator can be held between the fingers or in the palm of the same hand that holds the otoscope. While maintaining the view of the tympanic membrane, the bulb should be pressed gently to create positive pressure in the canal. In a normal ear, this causes the tympanic membrane to move briskly backward. When the bulb is released, negative pressure is applied and the drum moves forward toward the clinician. A normal membrane moves about 1 to 2 mm in each direction. Movement is decreased or absent when middle ear effusion is indicated. A retracted or scarred membrane may have decreased mobility on insufflation whereas a thinned or dimeric area (often formed when a perforation reseals) may have exaggerated movement (1, 2, 4, 6, 9–11). It should be remembered that a true assessment of the mobility of the tympanic membrane will only be obtained when a good seal is maintained between the speculum and the external canal. If the seal is inadequate, the tympanic membrane will not move with insufflation even though it may be healthy.

COMPLICATIONS

The only common complication of otoscopy is nicking the canal wall as a result of forceful insertion of a speculum or overly vigorous curettage of cerumen causing pain and bleeding. This incidence is minimized with proper preparation, positioning, and restraint, as well as careful visualization and avoidance of abrupt movement. If bleeding should occur, instillation of hydrogen peroxide (which is then wicked out with cotton) followed by instillation of Cortisporin™ otic suspension can minimize discomfort and prevent secondary infection. Using Cortisporin™ for a few days after extensive cleaning, even if bleeding does not occur, also is advisable.

SUMMARY

The child complaining of an "ear ache" is one of the most common presentations in the emergency department, clinic, or office practice. However, otitis media may present in a number of other, more subtle ways (fussi-

SUMMARY
1. Select speculum of proper size for patient.
   2 mm for neonate or young infant,
   3 mm for older infant or toddler,
   4 mm for children ages 2 to 7 years, and
   5 mm for older children and adolescents
2. Test equipment—occlude tip of speculum with one finger and apply positive pressure with insufflator bulb to ensure that no air leak occurs. Ensure that otoscope provides high intensity light source.
3. Restrain patient appropriately if necessary
4. Inspect auricle and periauricular tissues
5. Examine right ear by holding otoscope in right hand and examine left ear by holding otoscope in left hand
6. Pull pinna outward and posteriorly to straighten canal if necessary
7. Examine external auditory canal while inserting speculum
8. Remove cerumen if necessary to visualize tympanic membrane
   A. With soft or flaky cerumen, use cerumen curette
   B. With liquid cerumen or debris, use wicking or suction
   C. With cerumen impaction, instill 3% hydrogen peroxide, leave in place for 15 to 20 minutes, and then irrigate ear with warm water
9. Assess color, position, and condition of tympanic membrane, and light reflex and bony landmarks
10. Assess movement of tympanic membrane by pressing and releasing insufflator bulb

CLINICAL TIPS
1. The external auditory canal should be carefully examined as the otoscope is inserted to ensure that the transition between the canal wall and tympanic membrane is visualized. Movement of the canal wall during insufflation may be mistaken for a normally mobile drum.
2. Any patient being evaluated for head and/or facial trauma must undergo otoscopy to check for canal laceration, hemotympanum, or CSF leak.
3. With serous otitis, mobility of the tympanic membrane is reduced and often greater when applying negative pressure on pneumatic otoscopy.
4. Putting a piece of rubber tourniquet tubing around the end of the speculum may give a better seal if a significant air leak is encountered in attempting to examine an older child or adolescent with a 4 or 5 mm speculum.
5. The largest speculum that can be inserted to about one-third the distance into the ear canal should be used. Extra caution should be taken to avoid inserting the speculum deep into the bony part of the canal because this causes pain.
6. A normal tympanic membrane moves approximately 1 to 2 mm in each direction. Movement is decreased or absent when a middle ear effusion is indicated. When a child cries, both tympanic membranes may appear erythematous. Asymmetry of movement between the two sides often indicates the presence of an effusion in this situation.

ness, fever, crying) particularly in younger children. For this reason, the pediatric physical examination is not complete without an otoscopic evaluation. In addition, findings such as hemotympanum and tympanic membrane perforation (e.g., due to a blow to the side of the head) also must be recognized. For older children, making the examination a game will often convince the child to cooperate. With toddlers, it may be necessary to enlist the aid of a parent or other assistant to restrain the child appropriately to perform an adequate otoscopic examination. Taking extra care to avoid causing any real pain (as opposed to the psychological pain of being restrained and having one's ears "invaded") may help reduce the child's fear of subsequent examinations.

REFERENCES

1. Bluestone CD, Klein JO, eds. Otitis media in infants and children. 2nd ed. Philadelphia: WB Saunders, 1995.
2. McBride TP, Davis HW, Reilly JS. Pediatric otolaryngology. In: Zitelli BJ, Davis HW, eds. Atlas of pediatric physical diagnosis. 2nd ed. Philadelphia: JB Lippincott, 1992.
3. Durrant JD. Physiology of the ear. In: Bluestone CD, Stool SE, Scheetz MD, eds. Pediatric otolaryngology. 2nd ed. Philadelphia: WB Saunders, 1990.
4. Bluestone CD, Klein JO. Methods of examination. In: Bluestone CD, Stool SE, Scheetz MD, eds. Pediatric otolaryngology. 2nd ed. Philadelphia: WB Saunders, 1990.
5. Bergstrom L. Diseases of the external ear. In: Bluestone CD, Stool SE, Scheetz MD, eds. Pediatric otolaryngology. 2nd ed. Philadelphia: WB Saunders, 1990.
6. Bluestone CD, Klein JO. Otitis media, atelectasis and eustacean tube dysfunction. In: Bluestone CD, Stool SE, Scheetz MD, eds. Pediatric otolaryngology. 2nd ed. Philadelphia: WB Saunders, 1990.
7. DelBeccaro MA, Mendelman PM, et al. Bacteriology of acute otitis media: a new perspective. In: Lim DJ, Bluestone CD, Klein JO, Nelson JD, Ogra PL, eds. Recent advances in otitis media with effusion. Toronto: BC Decker, 1993.
8. Casselbrant ML, Mandel EM, et al. Incidence of otitis media and bacteriology of acute otitis media during the first 2 years of life. In: Lim DJ, Bluestone CD, Klein JO, Nelson JD, Ogra PL, eds. Recent advances in otitis media with effusion. Toronto: BC Decker, 1993.
9. Karma PH, Sipila MM, et al. Pneumatic otoscopy and otitis media. II. Value of different tympanic findings and their combinations. In: Lim DJ, Bluestone CD, Klein JO, Nelson JD, Ogra PL, eds. Recent advances in otitis media with effusion. Toronto: BC Decker, 1993.
10. Otoendoscopic examination: test videotape 3. Pittsburgh: Kaleida PH, Hoberman A, 1995.
11. Cavanaugh Jr. RM. Obtaining a seal with otic specula: must we rely on an air of uncertainty? In: Lim DJ, Bluestone CD, Klein JO, Nelson JD, Ogra PL, eds. Recent advances in otitis media with effusion. Toronto: BC Decker, 1993.

REMOVAL OF CERUMEN IMPACTION

Ron S. Fuerst

INTRODUCTION

Removing cerumen from the external auditory canal of pediatric patients is a procedure that is performed daily in the emergency department (ED) and a variety of other medical settings. Authorities estimate that cerumen removal by syringing occurs 150,000 times per week. Visualization of the tympanic membrane is critical for completing a physical examination in pediatric patients presenting with symptoms where the underlying cause may involve the middle ear or tympanic membrane.

The two basic methods for cerumen removal are syringing and debridement. Syringing uses an emulsifying agent to soften and break up cerumen, followed by irrigation. Debridement is performed using either a blind technique or by direct visualization with a light source.

ANATOMY AND PHYSIOLOGY

The ear is divided into internal, middle, and external portions (Figs. 55.1 and 55.2). The internal ear is composed of a system of tubes and spaces called the membranous labyrinth that are contained within the bony labyrinth. The middle ear is composed of three ossicles. From lateral to medial they are the malleus, incus, and stapes. All three are contained within the tympanic space, but only the malleus contacts the tympanic membrane. The border separating the middle ear and the external ear is the tympanic membrane. The external auditory canal and the auricle comprise the external ear.

Cerumen is a mixture of desquamated keratin, hair, dust and debris, and secretions from ceruminous and sebaceous glands in the ear canal (1, 2, 3). Long-chain fatty acids, alcohols, squalene, and cholesterol form the major organic components of cerumen (2). Cerumen type is an inherited trait. Wet cerumen is autosomal dominant and is found in most African-Americans and Caucasians. It is soft, sticky, and yellow-gold colored. Dry cerumen is most common in Asians. It crumbles easily and is light gray. The lysosomes, immunoglobulins, and proteins contained in cerumen are believed to have bacteriostatic or bacteriocidal activity (1).

Indications

Clear visualization of the tympanic membrane is indicated for any complaint that may stem from middle ear pathology. In children, this would most commonly be otitis media or tympanic membrane perforation. Symptoms may include ear pain or fullness, hearing difficulty, drainage from the ear canal, and headache. Fever, vomiting, diarrhea, poor appetite, ear pulling, cough, and irritability are nonspecific symptoms that may be seen in infants and toddlers with middle ear infections. Symptoms of cerumen impaction alone include vertigo, hearing loss, cough, tinnitus, ear pain, and fullness (1, 4, 5).

Syringing and debridement with direct visualization work best in older, cooperative pediatric patients. Blind debridement, although sometimes necessary in the older patient, is normally best used for infants and toddlers. Syringing is a less painful procedure than blind debridement and has fewer iatrogenic risks, but is often unsuccessful. Debridement by direct visualization can many times be accomplished without pain. Advantages of debridement are that it is less time consuming and has a higher success rate.

A suspected perforated tympanic membrane, tympanostomy tubes, and an uncooperative patient are contraindications to cerumenolytics and syringing. History of otitis externa, single hearing ear, and previous ear surgery are relative contraindications to syringing (6). Bleeding disorders are a relative contraindication to blind debridement. Introducing fluid into the middle ear through an open tympanic membrane during syringing may cause a new infection or worsen a preexisting one. Disruption of the ossicles also may occur. Debridement may cause an abrasion or laceration of the skin of the external auditory canal. This skin is extremely thin and bleeds readily. Syringing is the preferred method for patients with a bleeding disorder because trauma to the ear canal is avoided.

EQUIPMENT

Several compounds emulsify and lubricate cerumen to enable easier dislodgment from the ear canal (Table 56.1). Sodium bicarbonate 10% and vegetable oils are popular noncommercial products. Paradichlorobenzene 2%, chlorbutal 5%, oil of terebinth 5% (Cerumol™), triethanolamine polypeptide oleate-condensate 10%, and chlorbutanol 0.5% in propylene glycol (Cerumenex™) are the most popular commercial products.

Irrigation is usually performed with a catheter and syringe. Dental type, jet irrigation devices also have been recommended for ease of use in the patient with a normal, healthy tympanic membrane (7, 8, 9).

The choice of curette material and shape is largely a personal one (Fig. 56.1). The metal curette is best for the novice due to its heavier weight which allows the clinician to gently guide the instrument into the auditory canal as opposed to the lightweight plastic curette which frequently must be pushed into the canal with the subsequent risk of perforation. With its plastic tip, the plastic curette has less potential to cause bleeding from abrading the lining of the auditory canal during cerumen removal. Other necessary equipment is listed in Tables 56.2 and 56.3.

Table 56.1. Cerumenolytics (12–14)

Glycerine
Vegetable oils
Spirit of turpentine
Formaldehyde 10%
Alcohol 95%
Mineral oil
Propylene glycol
Water
Sodium bicarbonate 5%, 10%, 15%
Hydrogen peroxide 3%
Sialic acid 2.5%
Buro-sol™ (0.5% aluminum acetate, 0.03% benzothonium chloride)
Cerumenex™ (triethanolamine polypeptide oleate-condesate 10%, chlorbutanol 0.5% in propylene glycol)
Cerumol™ (paradichlorobenzene 2%, chlorbutal 5%, terebinth 5%)
Auralgan™ (benzocaine 14 mg and antipyrine 54 mg in glycerine made up to 1 mL)
Waxsol™ (docusate sodium 0.5% in a water miscible base)
Exterol™ (urea hydrogen peroxide 5% in glycerin)

Table 56.2. Syringing Equipment

Warm water or saline
Emulsifying agent
Syringe
Intravenous catheter
Otoscope
Cotton
Emesis basin or bowel
Towel
Gauze

Table 56.3. Debridement Equipment

Direct Visualization	Blind Technique
Light source	Otoscope
Alligator forceps	Cerumen curette
Cerumen curette	Gauze or towel
Gauze or towel	Auralgan™

PROCEDURE

Syringing

Patients should wear a hospital gown and be placed in the lateral decubitus position with the affected side up. The emulsifying agent of choice is gently placed in the ear canal until the ear canal is full. A compacted piece of cotton is placed in the canal to prevent the solution from dripping out. The other ear canal also may be treated in a similar fashion and the emulsifying solution given a minimum of 20 minutes to work. Ideally, patients should have an emulsifying agent placed for 2 to 7 days before syringing, but this is unrealistic for most ED patients.

The ear canal is now ready to be irrigated. Commonly used agents include saline, water, or a 50 : 50 mixture of saline or water with hydrogen peroxide. All solutions should be warmed to body temperature to minimize discomfort. Some clinicians prefer to use a Frazier suction catheter to remove the emulsifying agent at this point; however, noise from the suction catheter frequently frightens children and may make them less cooperative with the procedure. The patient should now be placed in the supine position so that the irrigating solution will easily spill out of the ear. It is important that the irrigating fluid easily exit the ear canal and not be blocked by the irrigating equipment because perforation may result. An emesis basin or several towels may be held next to the patient's mastoid region to catch excess irrigating solution. A syringe with an attached 16- or 18-gauge intravenous catheter (or a short section of tubing and attached hub cut from a butterfly needle) is used with mild to moderate force to irrigate the canal. The volume of the syringe should be a minimum of 20 mL to generate adequate pressure. The catheter tip should be inserted approximately 1.0 to 1.5 cm into the ear canal and directed toward the posterior, superior wall of the canal (Fig. 56.2). The stream of fluid should never strike the tympanic membrane directly. Often the clinician will observe that pieces of cerumen may fall

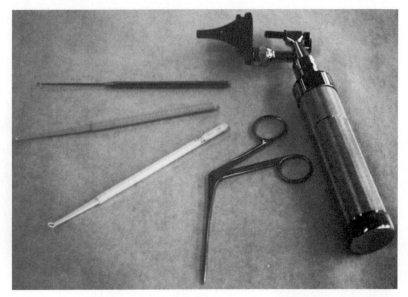

Figure 56.1.
An operating otoscope with (clockwise) an alligator forceps, two flexible plastic cerumen spoons, and a metal cerumen spoon.

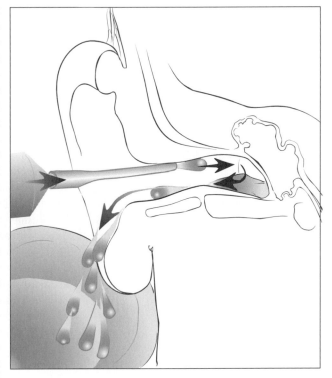

Figure 56.2.
Syringing cerumen or a foreign body from the auditory canal with an intravenous catheter attached to a 20 mL syringe. The irrigating stream is directed at the posterior, superior wall of the canal.

**Chapter 56
Removal of Cerumen Impaction**

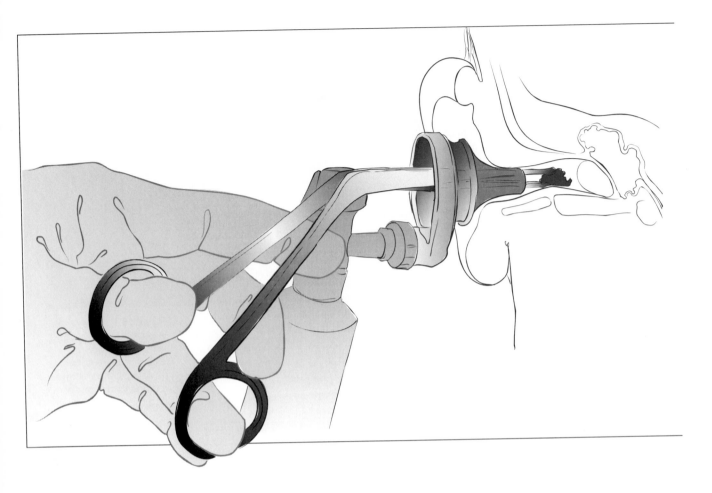

Figure 56.3.
Cerumen or a foreign body
is removed from the
auditory canal under direct
visualization with an
alligator forceps and an
operating head otoscope.

out of the ear. However, even if this is not the case, the ear should still be frequently examined with the otoscope during the procedure because the cerumen may partially dislodge, allowing the clinician to visualize a section of the tympanic membrane. In many cases, this will allow an adequate examination. It is important to always visualize the tympanic membrane when syringing is completed to check for iatrogenic tympanic membrane rupture.

Debridement

Debridement may be accomplished by either direct visualization or the blind method. Direct visualization (Chapter 55) requires a light source, preferably a head mirror, or an operating otoscope (Fig. 56.1). The patient is positioned in either the lateral decubitus position or sitting upright against a headrest. Parents (and patients) should be forewarned that

a minimal amount of unavoidable discomfort may occur, and that some bleeding postdebridement is not uncommon but is rarely serious. The clinician applies traction to the auricle by grasping the helix to straighten the external auditory canal and allow visualization. Cerumen that is visible may now be removed with alligator forceps or a curette (Fig. 56.3). This technique requires a high degree of patient cooperation, and thus is not the method of choice in the very young child.

The blind method is the quickest and most commonly used method of cerumen removal in infants and small children. It is imperative that the child be well restrained with the head rotated so that the opposite ear is held against the stretcher. Some clinicians recommend a drop of an emulsifying agent and then a drop of antipyrine/benzocaine solution (e.g., Auralgan™) a few minutes before the procedure. When ready to proceed,

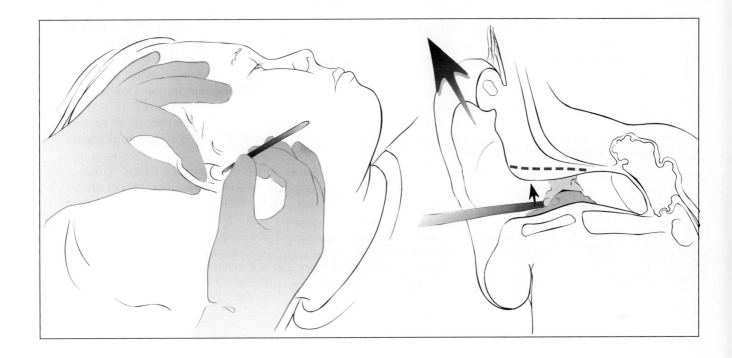

the helix of the auricle is gently retracted to straighten the auditory canal and to briefly visualize the location of the impacted cerumen. This may help identify where the curette can most easily pass beyond the impaction. The cerumen spoon is then grasped with the tips of the thumb, index and middle fingers, and the ulnar side of the hand is braced against the child's head. This position will prevent the curette from plunging deeper into the ear if an unexpected movement occurs. The curette is then gently introduced into the external auditory canal (Fig. 56.4). A plastic cerumen spoon will require some gentle downward pressure before scooping out the cerumen, and therefore this technique requires patience and practice to be done safely. A metal cerumen spoon will pass through the canal by gravity alone due to its heavier weight.

If the clinician is successful in retrieving a piece of cerumen, the spoon is wiped off on a towel or piece of gauze. The clinician should frequently attempt to visualize the tympanic membrane due to the pain associated with this procedure. Visualization should be attempted even when no cerumen is found on the end of the spoon because many times a partial dislodgment of cerumen will enable the clinician to see enough of the tympanic membrane to make a diagnosis.

SUMMARY
Syringing
1. Syringing solution may be saline or tap water at body temperature
2. Necessary equipment includes 20 cc syringe attached to 16- to 18-gauge intravenous catheter or short section of butterfly needle tubing with attached hub
3. Insert catheter 1.0 to 1.5 cm into auditory canal
4. Direct stream posteriorly and superiorly

Debridement
1. Initial attention to proper patient preparation and restraint will ultimately result in a quicker, less traumatic, and much more likely successful procedure. Parents (and patients) should be warned that a certain minimal amount of unavoidable discomfort will occur, and bleeding postprocedure is common but generally not serious.
2. In blind debridement, brace hand holding curette against child's head, with child securely restrained and head held firmly against stretcher
3. Gently lower curette into canal to estimated level of cerumen impaction, and then withdraw with scooping motion
4. Frequently examine canal to ascertain if tympanic membrane is visible, even in absence of overt cerumen removal
5. Debridement under direct visualization requires full patient cooperation, and thus is rarely chosen for infants or toddlers. With visualization, cerumen may be removed by curette or alligator forceps.

Figure 56.4.
A. Blind debridement of cerumen is accomplished with the child well restrained and the clinician's hand braced against the child's head.
B. The cerumen spoon passes the impaction and then is withdrawn while scooping out the cerumen.

Chapter 56
Removal of Cerumen
Impaction

Complications

Complications of cerumen removal include contact dermatitis, infection, tympanic membrane perforation, ossicle disruption, bleeding, vertigo, vomiting, pain, and even cardiac arrest (7, 10, 11). It is estimated that the complication rate of ear syringing is 1 in 1000 (6). Iatrogenic perforation of the tympanic membrane during syringing, or syringing an ear with preexisting tympanic membrane perforation may cause a middle ear infection, disruption of the ossicles, or both. Overzealous use of the cerumen spoon may cause tympanic membrane perforation, significant pain, and bleeding. A case of cerumenolytics causing contact dermatitis has also been reported (15).

Bleeding and pain are not uncommon complications, and are usually caused by abrasion of the external auditory canal. Bleeding can become serious in the patient with a bleeding disorder. Extra care or syringing should be considered for these patients. Blind debridement almost always causes some discomfort. Pain and bleeding episodes will diminish as the clinician gains experience. If the ear canal is abraded, some clinicians advocate the prophylactic use of otic antibiotic drops.

Summary

Cerumen removal is a common procedure in the ED and other outpatient settings. Removal may be performed by direct or indirect debridement or by syringing. Blind debridement is the method most commonly used in infants and small children in the ED because it is the quickest and most reliable method.

Care should be taken to prevent iatrogenic injury and to minimize discomfort.

References

1. Hanger HC, Mulley GP. Cerumen: its fascination and clinical importance: a review. J R Soc Med 1992;85(6):346–349.

2. Okuda I, Bingham B, Stoney P, Hawke M. The organic composition of earwax. J Otolaryngol 1991 Jun;20(3):212–215.

3. Naiberg JB, Robinson A, Kwok P, Hawke M. Swirls, wrinkles and the whole ball of wax (the source of keratin in cerumen). J Otolaryngol 1992;21(2):142–148.

4. Harkess CK. Clearing the occluded auditory canal. Pediatr Nurs 1982;8(1):23–25.

5. Raman R. Impacted ear wax—a cause for unexplained cough? [letter] Arch Otolaryngol Head Neck Surg 1986;112:679.

6. Sharp JF, Wilson JA, Ross L, Barr-Hamilton RM. Ear wax removal: a survey of current practice. Br Med J 1990;301(6763):1251–1253.

7. Dinsdale RC, Roland PS, Manning SC, Meyerhoff WL. Catastrophic otologic injury from oral jet irrigation of the external auditory canal. Laryngoscope 1991;101(1 Pt 1):75–78.

8. Marcuse EK. Removal of cerumen (letter). JAMA 1984;251(13):1681.

9. Watkins S, Moore TH, Phillips J. Clearing impacted ears. Am J Nurs 1984;84(9):1107.

10. Lindsey D. It's time to stop washing out ears! (letter). Am J Emerg Med 1991;9(3):297.

11. Drysdale AJ. Ear wax removal (letter). Br Med J 1991;302(6769):182.

12. Robinson AC, Hawke M. The efficacy of cereminolytics: everything old is new again. J Otolaryngol 1989;18(6):263–267.

13. Andaz C, Whittet HB. An in vitro study to determine efficacy of different wax-dispersing agents. J Otorhinolarygol Relat Spec 1993;55(2):97–99.

14. Mehta AK. An in vitro comparison of the disintegration of human ear wax by five cerumenolytics commonly used in general practice. Br J Clin Pract 1985;39(5):200–203.

15. Shreeve C. Ear wax solvents. Nurs Mirror 1984; 159(5):33.

CHAPTER 57

Foreign Body Removal from the External Auditory Canal

Dale Steele

Introduction

Foreign bodies in the external ear canal (EAC) are a frequent problem in children. The most common foreign objects requiring removal are roaches, paper, toy parts, earring parts, hair beads, and eraser tips (1). Pain from preexisting otitis media may occasionally be the cause for placing foreign bodies in the ear. Older children sometimes present after cockroaches have crawled into the EAC during sleep. Up to 80% of foreign bodies of the ear can be removed successfully without otorhinolaryngologic consultation.

Anatomy and Physiology

The external auditory canal has bony and cartilaginous portions (see also Chapter 55). Objects frequently lodge at the narrow junction of the cartilaginous and bony portions of the EAC. Pulling the pinna superiorly and laterally will straighten the external auditory canal for adequate visualization (see Fig. 55.5). Skin over the bony canal lacks subcutaneous tissue and is tightly adherent to the periosteum. The canal is exquisitely sensitive to touch with sensory innervation supplied by branches of the vagus and trigeminal nerves (2). Nerve blocks of the external ear canal require painful, four-quadrant injections which are impossible to perform without significant emotional distress in an awake child and should not be attempted. Topical anesthesia is not effective due to the impermeable keratinized epithelial surface of the EAC.

Indications

The most common presenting complaints are pain and decreased hearing. Live insects in the EAC cause extreme discomfort. Objects may be found on routine examination, and asymptomatic patients may have been observed putting something in the ear. Foreign bodies that are symptomatic should be removed as soon as feasible to alleviate symptoms. Button batteries may cause erosive injury to the canal or perforation of the tympanic membrane and require prompt removal.

Equipment

Most equipment for foreign body removal is readily available (Table 57.1). The diagnostic type otoscope head commonly available is not ideal for direct visualization during instrument removal. The operating type head (see Fig. 56.1) facilitates introduction of the instrument under continuous direct visualization.

Papoose board
Largest possible ear speculum
20-mL syringe
Butterfly tubing with needle cut off
Water, body temperature for
    irrigation
Suction catheters
Alligator forceps
Blunt right angle hooks
Wire loops or plastic ear curette
Cyanoacrylate glue (Super Glue)
Wooden stick cotton swabs

PROCEDURE

Preparation

For frantic children with live insects in the ear it is reasonable to instruct parents and triage nurses to instill mineral oil (e.g., baby oil) to kill the insect. Mineral oil is superior to lidocaine in its ability to kill insects rapidly (3).

Patient cooperation is the critical factor for success. The first attempt should be the best attempt. Stimulation of the exquisitely sensitive ear canal will quickly reduce the level of cooperation in even the most tractable patient. Younger children should be restrained by first wrapping in a sheet and then applying the papoose board with an assistant to immobilize the head. Parents should be warned that a small amount of bleeding may occur. Sedation should be considered before any subsequent attempts at removal using instruments if the object is not easily grasped on the first attempt (see Chapter 35). For foreign body removal by irrigation or by instrumentation under direct visualization, the approaches follow closely the analogous procedures for cerumen removal, which are discussed and illustrated in Chapter 56.

Irrigation

Irrigation is the technique of choice for the smooth, nonvegetable foreign body not easily grasped with forceps. Irrigation is better tolerated than instrumentation and does not require direct visualization. Pneumatic otoscopy should be done in an attempt to document an intact tympanic membrane before irrigation, particularly when patient his-

tory suggests self-instrumentation or prior blind removal attempts. Water at body temperature will minimize vestibular stimulation. Irrigation is done through a 1 to 2 inch section of butterfly needle tubing, or a 16- to 18-gauge intravenous catheter, attached to a 20-mL syringe. This apparatus is used to produce a pulsatile stream directed against the posterior, superior canal wall (see Fig. 56.2). Irrigation for vegetable foreign bodies is relatively contraindicated due to the risk of the object swelling, making subsequent attempts more difficult. One authority suggests irrigating vegetable foreign bodies with a solution of isopropyl alcohol and water to minimize swelling of the object (2).

Instrument Removal

An alligator forceps can be introduced under direct vision via an operating otoscope head to remove irregular objects such as insects or paper (see Fig. 56.3). Bayonet forceps are useful for superficial irregular objects. For smooth, round objects such as beads, a right-angle hook or plastic ear curette often can be passed beyond the object which, if superficial, may not require otoscopic visualization (see Fig. 56.4). Hair beads can be rotated until the central hole is lined up with the ear canal allowing removal with a straightened paper clip.

Blind attempts using instruments may push objects deeper into the canal, are less likely to be successful, and increase the pain and risk of injury to the tympanic membrane and middle ear structures.

Miscellaneous Techniques

Suction can be used for removal of foreign bodies for which irrigation is inappropriate or has failed. Continuous wall suction is attached to a handheld suction catheter with a soft tip. Frazier suction catheters can be modified by attaching a segment of intravenous tubing or a tympanostomy tube to the end (2). A commercial soft-tipped catheter is available (Foreign Body Remover, Smith & Nephew Richards, Memphis, TN (800)238-7538).

Cyanoacrylate glue (super glue) was reported to have been successful removing an impacted soy bean (4). The glue is applied to the blunt end of a wooden cotton swab stick which is then introduced into the EAC and held to the foreign body surface for about 1 minute. A firm bond will form which allows subsequent withdrawal of the stick with the foreign body attached. This technique has been recommended especially for removing impacted smooth objects in the EAC and for removing intranasal foreign bodies (see Chapter 62) (4). Inadvertent contact of the stick with the EAC surface may result in transient adherence, but this can usually be easily overcome with application of acetone, alcohol, or mineral oil (5).

Postprocedure Care and Referral

Regardless of the technique used it is essential to set reasonable limits for time and number of attempts and to recognize defeat. After failed removal children should be referred to an otolaryngologist, who may choose to perform the procedure with the aid of general anesthesia. Button batteries in the EAC have potentially corrosive effects and should be removed as soon as possible.

Follow-up evaluation should include postprocedure pneumatic otoscopy to document successful removal and an intact tympanic membrane (see Chapter 55). A topical antibiotic/corticosteroid such as Cortisporin® otic suspension should usually be prescribed.

SUMMARY
Syringing (Fig. 56.2)
1. Irrigation is best used for nonvegetable foreign bodies
2. Syringing solution may be saline or tap water at body temperature
3. Necessary equipment includes 20-mL syringe attached to 16- to 18-gauge intravenous catheter or short section of butterfly needle tubing with attached hub
4. Insert catheter 1.0 to 1.5 cm into auditory canal
5. Direct stream posteriorly and superiorly
Instrument removal (Fig. 56.3)
1. Perform under direct visualization for foreign body removal
2. Using curette, gently insert instrument into canal and attempt to pass hooked end beyond foreign body; after rotation, use hooked end to pull out object
3. Alligator forceps are used optimally for irregular, graspable objects
4. Suction and cyanoacrylate techniques are described for resistant cases

---

COMPLICATIONS

A small amount of excoriation and minimal bleeding from the EAC are common after foreign body removal. Hematoma formation and iatrogenic perforation can occur. Failure frequently occurs with firmly impacted and smooth objects deep in the EAC. Prior attempts at removal by the patient, parents, or referring physician decrease the chances of success and increase risk of complications. Poor cooperation in toddlers may necessitate deep sedation. Depending on the clinical setting and the time of the patient's last meal, removal may be best accomplished with such patients under anesthesia in the controlled setting of the operating room. Patients who present with or develop middle ear symptoms (severe bleeding, marked hearing loss, vertigo, or facial paralysis) require immediate consultation as do patients with button batteries that cannot be removed or have already had corrosive effect.

SUMMARY

Foreign bodies in the EAC are a common problem. Most can be removed in the ambulatory setting without consultation. The smooth, deeply embedded foreign bodies in the toddler represents a challenge. To avoid complications, the first attempt should be the best one, reasonable limits on time and number of attempts are set, and using good restraint with direct visualization is recommended.

REFERENCES

1. Baker MD. Foreign bodies of the ears and nose in childhood. Pediatr Emerg Care 1987;3:67–70.
2. Fritz S, Kelen GD, Sivertson KT. Foreign bodies of the external auditory canal. Emerg Med Clin North Am 1987;5(2):183–193.
3. Leffler S, Cheney P, Tandberg D. Chemical immobilization and killing and intraaural roaches: an in vitro comparative study. Ann Emerg Med 1993;22(12):1795–1798.
4. Pride H, Schwab R. A new technique for removing foreign bodies of the external auditory canal. Pediatr Emerg Care 1989;5(2):135–136.
5. Bock GW. Skin exposure to cyanoacrylate adhesive. Ann Emerg Med 1984;13:486.

CLINICAL TIPS
1. Initial attention to proper patient preparation and restraint will ultimately result in a quicker, less traumatic and much more likely successful procedure.
2. Parents (and patients) should be warned that a certain minimal amount of unavoidable discomfort will occur, and bleeding postprocedure is common but generally not serious.
3. Reasonable limits must be set on time and number of attempts to retrieve foreign body. Sedation or even general anesthesia should be considered after a failed attempt at instrument removal.
4. Live insects are optimally first killed with mineral oil which will quickly reduce patient discomfort and anxiety.
5. Button battery impaction is an emergency and requires immediate otolaryngologic consultation if ED removal is unsuccessful, as does any evidence of middle ear pathology.

Chapter 57
Foreign Body Removal
from the External
Auditory Canal

EXTERNAL EAR PROCEDURES

Mary Clyde Pierce

INTRODUCTION

Injuries to the structures of the external ear are common among children, due both to the relatively high incidence of head injury in pediatric patients and the exposed and essentially unprotected position of the ear. The anatomy of the ear makes it vulnerable to complications from even seemingly insignificant trauma. Potential injuries to the external ear include auricular hematomas, simple lacerations, and lacerations that involve cartilage (1). Auricular hematomas result from blunt trauma and require prompt drainage, the proper dressing, and careful follow-up to minimize complications. Lacerations of the external ear vary greatly in their complexity. When extensive cartilage injury is present, a specialist in plastic surgery or ENT surgery should be consulted. Simple lacerations, however, without significant cartilage involvement should be within the emergency physician's skills to perform. Proper mastoid or pressure dressing must then be placed following all procedures to the external ear to help optimize outcome.

ANATOMY AND PHYSIOLOGY

The external ear is divided into the auricle and the external auditory canal (see Fig. 55.1). The auricle is composed of elastic cartilage bound by perichondrium and skin. The avascular cartilage derives its blood supply from the adjacent perichondrium. The lobule is without cartilage and is made of soft tissue and skin only. Anteriorly, the skin of the helix and antihelix region is firmly adherent to the cartilage. Posteriorly the auricle has a subcutaneous layer that separates the skin from the cartilage (2). The lateral (or most external) one-third of the ear canal near the meatus is cartilaginous and the medial two-thirds toward the eardrum is bony. The abundant vascular supply to the external ear comes from the posterior auricular, superficial temporal, and deep auricular branches of the external carotid artery (3, 4). Sensory innervation to the auricle and external auditory canal is provided primarily by branches of the fifth, seventh, and tenth cranial nerves (5).

The perichondrium of the ear supplies nutrients and oxygen to the underlying cartilage. Blunt trauma to the ear may result in partial or complete separation of the cartilage from the perichondrium, which can disrupt the normal relationship between these two structures and lead to significant local injury. Blunt force can tear vessels in the perichondrium and result in further separation that may then result in cartilage infection or necrosis (2). If the resulting hematoma becomes infected, frank perichondritis may occur. Replacement of an auricular hematoma by fibrous tissue can cause thickening as new cartilage is laid down, resulting in a deformity known as "cauliflower ear" (1, 2).

Hemostasis within the auricle can be a problem, and blood or serous fluid accumulation may result in a seroma or other ear deformity. This tends to occur with either lacerations or auricular hematomas but can generally be prevented with proper dressing and early follow-up (1, 2).

INDICATIONS

Children requiring anesthesia and/or repairs of the external ear may present after a wide variety of injury mechanisms. Falls, motor vehicle related crashes, fighting or wrestling, and direct penetrating trauma account for most of the injuries. The patient will generally have an injury to the pinna that is immediately obvious on inspection. Less obvious will be unexplained bleeding from the external canal which may indicate a skull fracture. Malaligned cartilage can result in ear notching (7), inappropriate cartilage debridement can result in a significant gap in the ear (6), exposed cartilage can lead to infection and significant ear deformities (2), and missed or mismanaged auricular hematomas can lead to loss of the external ear (8). Any trauma to the ear can result in perichondritis which in turn can result in necrosis of ear cartilage and a severely deformed ear (8). When chondritis does occur, *Pseudomonas aeruginosa* is present in 95% of cases and is mixed with *Staphylococcus aureus* in greater than 50% of cases (2). This can be rapidly progressive and may result in total loss of the ear cartilage and a small, deformed pinna. Treatment must be prompt and aggressive to avoid serious deformity (2). All patients with ear trauma should be instructed regarding the signs and symptoms of perichondritis, which include increasing ear pain over several hours, progressive swelling, redness, tenderness, and warmth (2, 8).

Fighting or wrestling is the most common cause of an auricular hematoma. Blunt trauma to the ear causes sheared vessels between the perichondrium and cartilage to bleed into the tightly adherent skin, resulting in a hematoma. The patient presents with moderately painful swelling that obliterates the normal contours of the anterior or lateral surface of the ear. The formation of the hematoma may occur immediately or several hours after the trauma. To prevent cartilage damage, any hematoma of the ear must be promptly drained and a pressure dressing must then be applied. Follow-up in 24 hours is important as reaccumulations of fluid are common. When bruising without hematoma formation is present no treatment other than observation for infection is necessary. Abrasions require frequent cleaning and antibiotic ointment application to prevent infection. All abrasions must be carefully followed until complete healing has occurred (2).

Lacerations to the ear are common and are usually obvious unless located behind the ear on the posterior aspect of the auricle. In any trauma, the auricle should be carefully examined for cuts or for exposure of the perichondrium because concomitant scalp lacerations may bleed extensively, resulting in obscuring of the auricular injury. Lacerations to the ear should be closed primarily and care must be taken to not leave any exposed cartilage as this increases the risk for chondritis. Because of the excellent blood supply to the ear, complex lacerations often can be repaired with good tissue survival (1). Lacerations involving or exposing the cartilage may not do as well since cartilage is avascular, therefore increasing the risk for infection (2). Simple skin closure is usually adequate for small lacerations of the auricle even if the cartilage is involved (6). The placement of sutures through the cartilage is not recommended due to a higher complication rate from tearing or infection in the avascular layer. Sutures within cartilage do not reabsorb well and may result in malformation or infection (2, 6, 7). A few sutures may be placed into the cartilage if support is needed (1, 2). If cartilage sutures are required, consultation with a surgeon is generally advisable. Complex cartilage injuries always require consultation as do lacerations that traverse the external ear canal, because stenosis of the canal is likely without prolonged stinting and careful follow-up (2, 6). Consultation also is recommended when cartilage debridement may be necessary or when a skin avulsion results in significant cartilage exposure where skin grafting may be required (1).

Anesthetizing the ear for repair can be

challenging but is important in obtaining a good result. A regional auricular block is indicated when the laceration is extensive and local infiltration would be too cumbersome, or when wound edge distortion from local infiltration would make closure too difficult. Otherwise, local infiltration into the skin, if used in small amounts, should be adequate and not too distorting. It should be noted, however, that meatal lacerations may require local infiltration in addition to the regional block due to vagal nerve sensory innervation (6).

The proper dressing or bandage must be placed after any external ear procedures are performed. A mastoid or pressure dressing is indicated for all external ear laceration repairs and hematoma evacuations to prevent bleeding or fluid accumulation between the cartilage and perichondrium. Initial follow-up should be within 24 hours to check for accumulation of fluid that could potentially compromise the cartilage. The wound should then be rechecked within a few days to evaluate for perichondritis and proper healing.

EQUIPMENT

Auricular Block
Antiseptic solution
10-mL syringe
Needle, 25 to 27 gauge
Lidocaine 1% without epinephrine, 10 to 15 mL

External Ear Laceration Repair
Antiseptic solution
Syringe
Needle, 25 to 27 gauge
Lidocaine 1% without epinephrine
Sterile water for irrigation
Skin sutures, 6.0 nonabsorbable monofilament
Cartilage sutures, 5.0 absorbable vicryl

Auricular Hematoma Aspiration
Antiseptic solution
Lidocaine 1% as local if needed
10-mL syringe
Needle, 18 gauge
No. 15 blade (if needle aspiration inadequate)
Curved hemostat

Mastoid or Pressure Dressing
Cotton balls soaked in saline or petroleum gauze
Gauze sponges, 4- 4×4 with partial cut in center
Gauze sponges, 4- 4×4 without center cut
Gauze wraparound bandage, 4 inch

PROCEDURE

Regional Auricular Block

To anesthetize the ear for laceration repair or hematoma drainage, either local infiltration or a regional block is used. For simple laceration repair or needle drainage of an auricular hematoma, skin infiltration can be done using 1% lidocaine without epinephrine, taking care not to overly distort the wound edges. To obtain an auricular block, the ear and the surrounding skin are first prepared with an antiseptic solution. A 10 mL syringe with a 1.5 inch 27-gauge needle is filled with 1% lidocaine without epinephrine and is used to inject a track of lidocaine around the entire ear (Fig. 58.1). This can be accomplished by first entering a point just above the ear and fully inserting the needle along the back of the ear. Lidocaine (3 to 5 mL) is injected as the needle is withdrawn. Without withdrawing the needle from the skin a second track is made in front of the ear by inserting the needle completely along the skin edge and again injecting the lidocaine as the needle is withdrawn. Similar tracks are made at the bottom of the ear by entering the skin just below the lobe in the sulcus. Injections are made both anteriorly and posteriorly to the ear, leaving a V-shaped track of anesthetic. Maximum anesthetic effect occurs in approximately 10 to 15 minutes (6).

Auricular Laceration Repair

When repairing ear lacerations, the skin is first cleansed using an antiseptic solution and the ear is anesthetized using one of the described techniques. The wound should be thoroughly irrigated using an ample amount of saline solution. Removing debris and contamination and reducing bacterial counts on wound surfaces are best accomplished with wound irrigation (6). If cartilage is not involved or only minimally involved, simple skin edge closure with 6.0 nonabsorbable monofilament sutures should suffice (2, 6). If necessary, a few absorbable 6.0 vicryl sutures can be placed in the cartilage to add support (1). Cartilage should not be debrided because

Auricular Hematoma Drainage

To evacuate an auricular hematoma (Fig. 58.2), the area to be drained is first prepared using aseptic technique. An anesthetic may not be necessary if only a single needle aspiration is to be performed. An 18-gauge needle attached to a 10-mL syringe is inserted into the area of the hematoma that is most fluctuant. The hematoma is then evacuated by applying negative pressure with the syringe and by milking the hematoma using the thumb or index finger. Pressure is then applied to the area for 3 to 5 minutes. If clot formation has occurred and complete evacuation is not possible by needle aspiration alone, a small incision is made using a No. 15 blade. A curved hemostat can then be used to break up the clot. Complete evacuation is necessary to prevent potential cartilage necrosis. After the auricle hematoma has been drained, a pressure dressing is applied to prevent reaccumulation of fluid and to add support to the ear. A repeat examination is required within 24 hours to check for reaccumulation of fluid. If this does occur, the ear must again be drained (2, 7, 9).

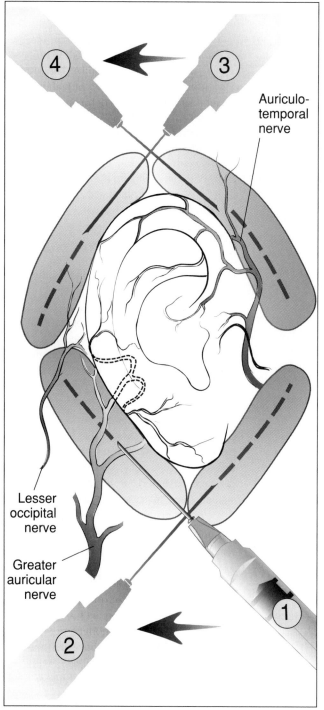

Figure 58.1.
Regional auricular block.

Pressure Dressing Application

A pressure dressing is placed to prevent fluid accumulation and to add structural support. Application can be accomplished using two to four 4×4 gauze pads with the centers cut out so they can be placed around the entire ear (Fig. 58.3). This helps provide support behind the ear and prevents contortion of the ear or excessive pressure. Several saline-

its absence leaves defects or causes notching. Care must be taken to not leave any cartilage exposed, as this increases the likelihood of chondritis and ear deformities. Sutures should be removed in 5 days. Complex cartilage lacerations require consultation (2, 6).

soaked cotton balls or petroleum gauze are placed and molded to fit all contours of the external ear. Two to four intact sponges are placed over the entire ear and a 4-inch gauze bandage is brought around the head and over the ear several times. The desired effect is to apply even pressure without compromising blood flow (6). This dressing should be used for any complicated ear injury. Discharge instructions must include an explanation of the signs and symptoms of perichondritis or chondritis.

SUMMARY

Regional Auricular Block

1. Restrain child appropriately and aseptically prepare the involved area
2. For local anesthesia, infiltrate wound edges using 1% lidocaine so as to not distort wound edges
3. For regional anesthesia of the ear, inject skin surrounding ear as discussed
4. Wait several minutes for local anesthetic and 10 to 15 minutes for regional anesthetic to have maximum effect

Auricular Laceration Repair

1. Restrain child adequately
2. Anesthetize wound as indicated
3. Prepare area using aseptic technique and obtain sterile field
4. Clean and thoroughly irrigate wound
5. For simple lacerations involving skin only, or with only minimal cartilage involvement, approximate wound edges using 6.0 nonabsorbable sutures
6. Cartilage lacerations that require suturing should have a minimum number of 5.0 vicryl sutures placed using large bites to prevent cartilage tearing
7. In general, do not debride cartilage or leave any exposed
8. Complicated auricular lacerations with extensive cartilage involvement or skin avulsions where cartilage is exposed require consultation with ENT surgery
9. Apply pressure dressing and follow-up within 24 hours to check for accumulation of fluid and early signs of infection

Auricular Hematoma Drainage

1. Properly restrain child
2. Prepare area to be drained using aseptic technique and obtain sterile field
3. If necessary, anesthetize area to be drained (frequently not required)
4. Drain hematoma completely using 18-gauge needle or No. 15 blade
5. Apply manual pressure for 3 to 5 minutes and then place pressure dressing
6. Follow-up within 24 hours to check for reaccumulation of fluid and/or blood

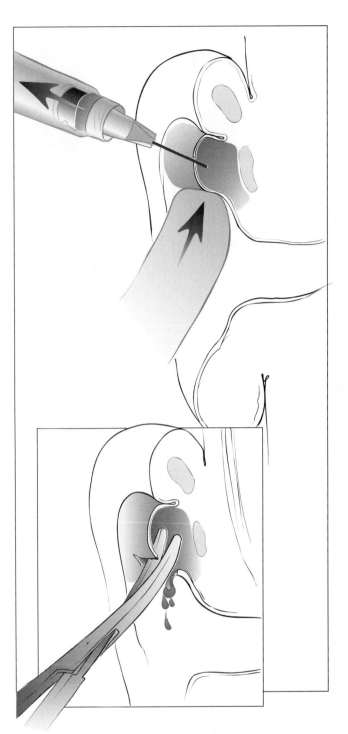

Figure 58.2.
Evacuation of auricular hematoma.

COMPLICATIONS

Complications of an auricular hematoma are related to incomplete drainage or reaccumulation that can result in an infected hema-

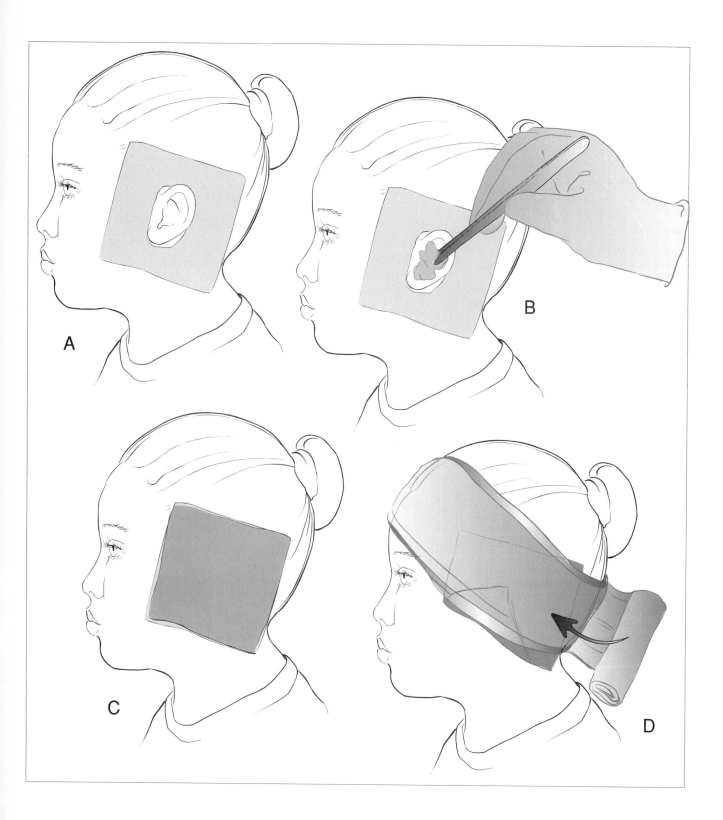

Figure 58.3.
Application of mastoid
(pressure) dressing.

**Chapter 58
External Ear
Procedures**

toma leading potentially to perichondritis, cartilage distruction, and deformity or loss of parts of the external ear (2).

Complications of laceration repair include malalignment resulting in ear notching (7), loss of cartilage from improper cartilage

debridement or suture placement, or infection. Complications from repair of lacerations can be avoided by meticulous cleansing and irrigation before skin closure, careful wound edge alignment, avoidance of cartilage suture placement, careful examination for areas of exposed cartilage (i.e., abrasions or skin avulsions) and early consultation if the laceration is extensive.

Any patient with external ear trauma also should be examined for a hemotympanium, a perforated tympanic membrane with possible CSF leakage, and a Battle's sign to evaluate the possibility of a basilar skull fracture (7). The physician should also make a clinical assessment of the hearing status of each ear.

SUMMARY

The ears are in an exposed position and are subject to trauma that produces both hematomas and lacerations (1). Simple external ear lacerations that do not require extensive cartilage suturing or debridement can normally be repaired by the primary caregiver or emergency physician or other physicians who are skilled at wound management. Complex lacerations of the external ear—particularly those with cartilage involvement—require consultation with a surgeon. An auricular hematoma must be adequately drained and then rechecked for reaccumulation of fluid within 24 hours. Failure to do so may result in perichondritis and significant ear deformities. Extensive laceration repairs warrant an auricular regional block for adequate and nondistorting anesthesia of the wound. A mastoid or pressure dressing should be applied to any ear that has had a hematoma drained or laceration repaired. Any external ear trauma that results in an abrasion, a hematoma, or laceration requires early follow-up and careful instruction of the patient regarding the signs and symptoms of perichondritis.

REFERENCES

1. Serafin D, Georgiade NG. Pediatric plastic surgery. Vol 2. St. Louis: CV Mosby, 1984, pp. 648–651.
2. Templer J, Renner GJ. Injuries of the external ear. Otolaryngol Clin North Am 1990;23:1003–1018.
3. Kenna MA. Embryology and developmental anatomy of the ear. In: Bluestone CD, Stool SE, eds. Pediatric otolaryngology. 2nd. ed. Philadelphia: WB Saunders, 1990, pp. 77–79.
4. Hollinshead WH, Tosse C. Textbook of anatomy. 4th ed. Philadelphia: Harper & Row, 1985, pp. 944–946.
5. Paugh RP, Telian SA. Emergencies of the eyes, ears, nose, and throat: ear infections. In: Schwartz GR, et al., eds. Principles and practice of emergency medicine, 3rd ed. Philadelphia: Lea & Febiger, 1992, pp. 2177–2178.
6. Trott A. Wounds and lacerations: emergency care and closure. St Louis: CV Mosby, 1991, pp. 41–42, 55–63, 163–168.
7. Rahman WM, O'Connor TJ. Facial trauma. In: Barkin RM, et al., eds. Pediatric emergency medicine concepts and clinical practice. St Louis: CV Mosby, 1992, pp. 222.
8. Bergstrom LV. Diseases of the external ear. In: Bluestone CD, Stool SE, eds. Pediatric otolaryngology, 2nd ed. Philadelphia: WB Saunders, 1990, pp. 331–339.
9. Ruddy RM. Procedures. In: Textbook of pediatric emergency medicine, 3rd ed. Baltimore: Williams & Wilkins, 1993, pp. 1602–1603.

CLINICAL TIPS

1. Complete drainage of hematoma is mandatory for good outcome.
2. Follow-up should occur within 24 hours to check for reaccumulation fluid.
3. Placement of sutures into cartilage should be avoided if possible. Consultation should be obtained if cartilage sutures are necessary.
4. Extensive cartilage lacerations, those that traverse the external canal, or extensive skin avulsions exposing cartilage require consultation with a specialist in plastic surgery or ENT surgery.
5. Cartilage debridement should be minimal and is best left to the consultant.
6. All patients should be educated about the signs and symptoms of perichondritis and/or chondritis—increasing pain over several hours, progressive swelling, redness, tenderness, and warmth.

CHAPTER 59

TYMPANOCENTESIS

Mary Clyde Pierce

INTRODUCTION

Tympanocentesis involves needle aspiration of the middle ear contents to obtain middle ear fluid for culture to provide symptomatic relief in cases of painful otitis media. It can be performed by the emergency physician or by other qualified physicians in the outpatient setting (1).

Otitis media is one of the most common childhood infections with approximately 80% of children having at least one episode by 3 years of age. Otitis media denotes inflammation of the middle ear, while acute otitis refers to a suppurative middle ear infection of recent onset. Otitis media with effusion and secretory otitis are more chronic conditions and usually follow an acute episode (2). Middle ear fluid can persist 3 months beyond the initial presentation in as many as 10% of children.

Middle ear infection must be effectively treated to prevent conductive hearing loss with possible speech development problems, to prevent tympanic membrane damage from perforation and scarring, and to prevent extension of inflammation beyond the middle ear into the mastoids or intracranial structures. Systemic antibiotics are generally effective in empiric therapy. In specific situations, when the exact etiology of the otitis needs to be determined, tympanocentesis can be of benefit. If more chronic drainage is desired, then myringotomy or ventilatory tubes may be indicated (1, 3).

ANATOMY AND PHYSIOLOGY

The structure of the middle ear is illustrated in Figure 55.2. The tympanic membrane is composed of three layers: the outer epithelial layer, the middle fibrous layer, and the inner mucosal layer. The membrane inserts into the tympanic ring which is formed from an ossification center in membranous bone. The middle ear consists of the tympanic membrane and cavity, three ossicles, two muscles, tendons, nerves, and the eustachian tube (4, 5). The ossicles and nerves, including a branch from the facial nerve, lie within the superior quadrant of the tympanic membrane and are a major reason why this area should be avoided during tympanocentesis. Landmarks and quadrants of the tympanic membrane which should be clearly identified before performing tympanocentesis include: (*a*) the lateral process of the malleus, which can be seen as a protrusion at the top of the malleus pointing toward the anterior quadrant; (*b*) the manubrium of the malleus, which is the long translucent structure that bisects the membrane into anterior and posterior portions; and (*c*) the umbo, which is the tip of the manubrium delineating the superior from inferior quadrants. The four quadrants of the tympanic membrane are created by drawing one line through the manubrium of the malleus and a second perpendicular line through the umbo of the malleus. An important bony landmark of the tympanic membrane is the long process of the malleus with the umbo at the inferior tip (6, 7). The inferior-posterior quadrant is below this landmark and it is here that the quadrant tympanocentesis should be performed. At birth the tympanic membrane lies nearly horizontal as is the eustachian tube. The eustachian tube connects the nasopharynx with the middle ear cleft and functions to aerate the middle ear on yawning and swallowing. As the eustachian tube further develops, the tympanic membrane becomes more vertical, resulting in fewer middle ear problems.

Eustachian tube dysfunction may result in negative middle ear pressure, tympanic membrane retraction, and collection of fluid into the middle ear (6). Most cases of otitis media occur as a result of an abnormally functioning eustachian tube. The eustachian tube normally permits equilibrium of middle ear pressure with atmospheric pressure, protects the middle ear from reflux of nasopharynx secretions, and drains secretions from the middle ear into the nasopharynx. If external obstruction of the eustachian tube occurs from either a tumor or adenoid tissue, or if abnormal patency of the tube is seen (as in the Native American population), middle ear effusion or otitis media may result. Furthermore, if abnormal compliance of the tube or an abnormal opening mechanism is present, a functional obstruction may result as is commonly seen in young children and in children with cleft palates (2).

INDICATIONS

The uncomplicated case of otitis media does not require aspiration because cultures demonstrate common pathogens. Diagnosis of the etiologic organism becomes necessary in complicated cases of otitis media such as in the immunocompromised child or the septic-appearing child with an obvious ear infection. Because a poor correlation exists between bacterial cultures of the nasopharynx and those of middle ear fluid, tympanocentesis must be performed to diagnose the organism causing the middle ear infection (1, 2). Antibiotics should be withheld until a middle ear culture is obtained unless the patient is toxic appearing or at high risk for sepsis, in which case antibiotics should rapidly be empirically administered.

Possible indications for needle tympa-

nocentesis or myringotomy include serious illness or toxicity in a patient with otitis; suppurative complications such as mastoiditis, meningitis, or brain abscess (1); and otitis media in the ill-appearing neonate (8), the immunocompromised patient, and the patient on a mechanical ventilator (2). Tympanocentesis also may be required in the patient who develops otitis media while already receiving systemic antibiotics (1), or in the patient who fails to respond to multiple trials of antibiotics. Occasionally a patient will present with an extremely painful case of otitis when tympanocentesis may be warranted to provide immediate pain relief (9, 10).

Tympanocentesis is contraindicated in the patient with a bleeding diathesis. It is not recommended in the patient with severe bone marrow suppression, when manipulation from the procedure could lead to septicemia. The clinician should consult with an ENT specialist if mastoiditis, meningitis, or brain abscess occurs in conjunction with otitis.

EQUIPMENT

Restraint system and/or setup for conscious sedation
70% alcohol
22 gauge, 3.5 inch spinal needle bent 3 to 4 cm from tip
1 mL tuberculin syringe
Otoscope with operator head or oto-microscope
Nonbacteriostatic saline

PROCEDURE

The child should be restrained well and conscious sedation should be performed as necessary. Cerumen in the canal should be removed and the external canal should be cleansed with 70% alcohol. An otoscope with an operating head will assist in obtaining a clear view of the entire tympanic membrane and will help ensure that the alcohol has been removed. A 3.5 inch 22-gauge spinal needle with the stylet removed is bent approximately 30° 3 to 4 cm from the tip (Fig. 59.1). Bending the needle in this way allows a better view of the tympanic membrane during the procedure and thereby facilitates puncturing the

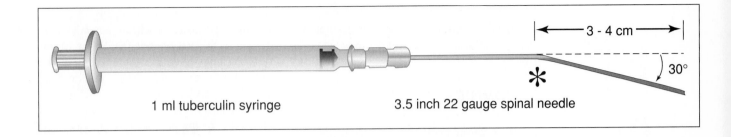

3 - 4 cm

30°

✱

1 ml tuberculin syringe

3.5 inch 22 gauge spinal needle

tympanic membrane in the posterior-inferior quadrant. A 1-mL tuberculin syringe is then attached to the end of the spinal needle and the syringe plunger is used to apply negative pressure during the procedure (11, 12).

The entire tympanic membrane needs to be visualized (Fig. 59.2.A). While the clinician directly visualizes down the ear canal, the spinal needle should be advanced down the inferior aspect of the canal to the inferior-posterior quadrant of the tympanic membrane, as described previously (see Anatomy and Physiology). The membrane is then punctured in the inferior-posterior quadrant and negative pressure is applied on the syringe to obtain a middle ear aspirate (Fig. 59.2.B). If continued drainage is desired, the procedure of choice is a myringotomy, and an otolaryngologist should be consulted (1, 11). After the procedure is completed the ear

Figure 59.1.
Spinal needle on 1 mL syringe.

Figure 59.2.
A. Tympanic membrane at point of puncture through operating otoscope.
B. Tympanic membrane puncture through posteroinferior quadrant.

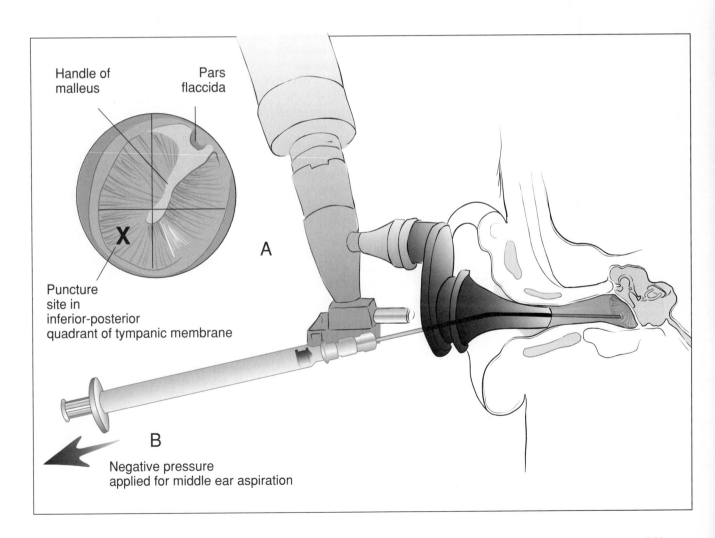

Handle of malleus

Pars flaccida

X

A

Puncture site in inferior-posterior quadrant of tympanic membrane

B

Negative pressure applied for middle ear aspiration

SUMMARY

1. Obtain 22-gauge 3.5-inch spinal needle bent 30° 3 to 4 cm from distal end attached to 1-mL syringe
2. Restrain patient well and use sedation if needed
3. Prepare external canal by removing cerumen and then cleanse canal with 70% alcohol
4. Visualize tympanic membrane using otoscope with operator head
5. Insert needle with direct visualization of landmarks along inferior aspect of ear canal
6. Pierce membrane in inferior-posterior quadrant and apply negative pressure
7. Send aspirate for Gram stain and culture using nonbacteriostatic saline as needed to obtain small amount from spinal needle.

CLINICAL TIPS

1. Control of the child to avoid an unexpected movement is critical during tympanocentesis. Appropriate restraint is essential, and conscious sedation should be considered if necessary.
2. The superior quadrants of the tympanic membrane must be carefully avoided to prevent injury to important middle ear structures.
3. If continued drainage of the ear is desirable, consultation with an otolaryngologist should be sought for possible myringotomy.

should be rechecked for bleeding or signs of significant tympanic membrane trauma, and a procedure note should be completed.

COMPLICATIONS

The superior quadrants of the tympanic membrane must always be avoided because behind these areas lie bones, nerves, and vessels, which can easily be injured. If the needle is incorrectly placed into the superior quadrant and an ossicle is dislocated, a significant hearing loss can result. Also located in the superior quadrant is a branch of the seventh cranial nerve. Piercing this nerve can result in a transient or permanent peripheral seventh nerve palsy. Bleeding into the middle ear can also be a major concern if tympanocentesis is done in the superior quadrant, because several blood vessels traverse that area. It is difficult for the clinician to provide hemostasis in the middle ear. By performing the procedure in the correct quadrant the morbidity of excessive bleeding, hearing loss, facial nerve palsy, or ossicle dislocation can be greatly reduced. Proper restraint of the child is key to avoiding complications from tympanocentesis. Movement at an inopportune moment can result in a tear in the tympanic membrane or penetration into another location. Other complications include a persistent perforation and continued contamination of the middle ear with bacteria from the external canal (1, 2). By using a small needle for aspiration, perforations that persist after 10 to 14 days are unusual but should be rechecked in follow-up visits. Sterile technique should help prevent contamination of the middle ear with bacteria. When tympanocentesis is performed correctly complications are rare.

SUMMARY

Otitis media is one of the most common childhood infections. In cases with complications, when the child is critically ill or immunocompromised or when a potentially resistant organism is present, middle ear aspiration can help determine the etiology of the otitis. Furthermore, tympanocentesis can be useful for providing immediate relief of pain in the unusually severe earache. It is a valuable skill for the primary care provider and the emergency physician.

REFERENCES

1. Bluestone CD, Klein JO. Otitis media, atelectasis and eustachian tube dysfunction. In: Bluestone CD, Stool SE, eds. Pediatric otolaryngology. 2nd ed. Philadelphia: WB Saunders, 1990, pp. 390–453.
2. Kline, MW. Otitis Media. In: Oski FA, et al., eds. Principles and practice of pediatrics. 2nd ed. Philadelphia: JB Lippincott Co., 1994, pp. 974–976.
3. Le CT, Freeman DW, Fireman BH. Evaluation of ventilating tubes and myringotomy in the treatment of recurrent or persistent otitis media. Pediatr Infect Dis 1991;10:2–11.
4. Hollinshead, WH, Rosse C. Textbook of anatomy. 4th ed. Philadelphia: Harper & Row, 1985, p. 945.
5. Kenna, MA. Embryology and developmental anatomy of the ear. In: Bluestone CD, Stool SE, eds. Pediatric otolaryngology. 2nd ed. Philadelphia: WB Saunders, 1990, pp. 77–79.
6. Paugh DR, Telian SA. Emergencies of the eyes, ears, nose, and throat: ear infections. In: Schwartz GR, et al., eds. Principles and practice of emergency medicine. 3rd ed. Philadelphia: Lea & Febiger, 1992, pp. 2177–2180.
7. Clemente CD. Anatomy: A regional atlas of the human body. 3rd ed. Baltimore: Urban & Schwarzenberg, 1987, fig 786.
8. Burton DM, et al. Neonatal otitis media. Arch Otolaryngol Head Neck Surg 1993;119:672–675.
9. Cahill L., Jehle D. Eyes, ears, nose, and throat: otitis. In: Reisdorff E.J., et al. Pediatric emergency medicine. Philadelphia: WB Saunders, 1993, pp. 617–619.
10. Kaplan SL, Feigin RD. Simplified technique for tympanocentesis. Pediatrics 1978;62:418–419.
11. Rowe PC. Pediatric Procedures. In: Oski FA, et al., eds. Principles and practice of pediatrics. 2nd ed. Philadelphia: JB Lippincott, 1994, pp. 2207–2208.
12. Ruddy RM. Procedures. In: Fleisher GR, Ludwig S, eds. Textbook of pediatric emergency medicine. 3rd ed. Baltimore: Williams & Wilkins, 1993, pp. 1600–1601.

CHAPTER 60

Management of Epistaxis

Susanne I. Kost and J. Christopher Post

Introduction

Epistaxis is a common complaint in the pediatric population, especially among toddlers and school-aged children. Most episodes of bleeding from the nose will resolve before the child arrives at a medical care facility, but persistent or recurrent bleeding requires intervention (1, 2). Because specialized equipment is needed for visualization and treatment of epistaxis, a definitive procedure should not be attempted in the prehospital setting. Prehospital management of a nosebleed should consist of applying pressure to the external nares and providing supportive care as necessary. The child who is still bleeding upon arrival at a medical care facility can usually be managed by cautery or anterior packing. An emergency physician or an experienced pediatrician or family practitioner should be capable of performing both of these procedures. Certain properly trained physician extenders also may be qualified to assess and provide minor treatment for anterior epistaxis in children (3). In the unusual situation when posterior packing is required for a pediatric patient, otorhinolaryngologic (ORL) consultation should be obtained whenever possible (4).

Anatomy and Physiology

The relatively high incidence of epistaxis in otherwise healthy children can be explained by a combination of physiologic and behavioral factors. The nasal mucosa is lined with a rich vascular network, which facilitates warming of inspired air. In children, this mucosa is thinner and more likely to bleed than in adults. Children also are prone to manipulate the septal mucosa (nose picking) and are therefore predisposed to anterior bleeding. The most common source of epistaxis is Kiesselbach's plexus in Little's area of the anterior septum (Fig. 60.1). Attempts to localize and treat the typical nosebleed in a child should focus on this area (1, 2, 5).

In addition to minor trauma from nose picking, both local and systemic factors may influence the incidence of epistaxis. Inflammation from viral or bacterial infection, foreign body reaction, or allergic rhinitis increases the friability of the anterior mucosa (6, 7). Dry heat in the winter also irritates the mucosa, a condition known as rhinitis sicca. Although much less common, lesions such as polyps, vascular malformations, and tumors may act as focal points for anterior or posterior bleeding in children (1, 2, 5).

Conditions that may produce or exacerbate epistaxis include hypertension, hematologic disease, menstruation, or the use of anticoagulant medication. Extensive testing for systemic illness should not be undertaken unless current or past medical history, family history, or physical examination leads to suspicion of a systemic disorder. Although hypertension is unusual in children, blood pressure should be measured routinely in a child presenting with epistaxis. Anxiety over the nosebleed and the hospital environment may cause transient hypertension; consequently, a finding of elevated systemic pressure should

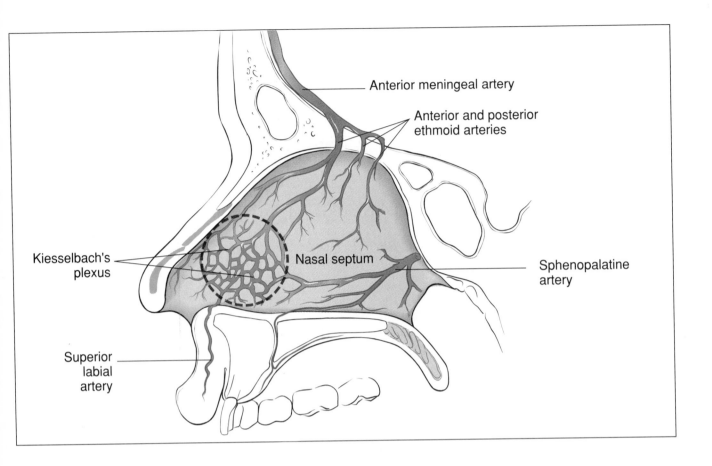

Figure 60.1.
Anatomy of nasal septum.

be confirmed with a repeat reading and then evaluated appropriately on an acute and/or outpatient basis. Hematologic disease may include congenital coagulation defects or acquired conditions such as idiopathic thrombocytopenic purpura or malignancy (6, 8). Assessing the child for bruising, petechiae, and lymphadenopathy therefore should be included as part of the physical examination. Vicarious menstruation should be suspected in an adolescent female with episodes of epistaxis that coincide with menses. Ingestion of drugs that affect coagulation (e.g., coumadin or aspirin) should be suspected in a setting where these drugs are available, especially in the toddler age group (1, 2, 9).

INDICATIONS

Any child who continues to bleed after properly applied nasal pressure, or a child with recurrent episodes of bleeding over a period of hours or days, deserves a more definitive procedure. An adequate trial of nasal pressure consists of 10 to 15 minutes of squeezing the

cartilaginous segment of the nares together between a thumb and finger. Using a rolled gauze pad to compress the upper lip (and thus the labial artery) also may be performed if the child is cooperative. Nasal cautery is performed to prevent further bleeding or if minor bleeding persists. Continued epistaxis from an anterior site despite nasal cautery requires placement of an anterior nasal pack. The persistent appearance of blood in the hypopharynx with no identifiable anterior source indicates a posterior site of epistaxis and necessitates placement of a posterior nasal pack.

When the patient has a known history of an intranasal lesion (e.g., a polyp or hemangioma) or a known bleeding disorder, ORL consultation should be sought before attempting to cauterize or pack the affected area (6). Attempts at cauterization in a patient with a bleeding diathesis may exacerbate the bleeding. These patients require treatment with packing and replacement of the appropriate blood product (factor or platelets). Consultation also is recommended if a posterior site of bleeding or a facial fracture is suspected. In addition, immediate consultation should be obtained in the rare instance of a severe nasal bleed resulting in unstable vital signs or signs of hemorrhagic shock (4, 5, 9).

EQUIPMENT

General
  Adequate light source
  Suction with Frazier tip
  Nasal speculum (small, medium, large)
  cotton pledgets
  bayonet forceps
  alligator forceps
Cautery
  Topical vasoconstrictors and anesthetics
    phenylephrine 0.25% (Neosynephrine™)
    oxymetazoline 0.05% (Afrin™)
    cocaine 1 to 5% (maximum dose 3 mg/kg)
    lidocaine 2 to 4% (maximum dose 7 mg/kg)
    epinephrine 1:1000
  Silver nitrate sticks
  Trichloroacetic acid
  Petroleum or KY jelly
Anterior packing
  Vaseline gauze—$^1/_4''$ and $^1/_2''$ strips
  Topical antibiotic ointment
  Nasal tampon (Merocel™)
  Oxycellulose (Surgicel™)
Posterior packing
  Small red rubber catheters
  Hemostat
  Silk ties or umbilical tapes
  Foley catheters (10 to 16 gauge)
  Syringe 30 mL
  Gauze—2×2, 4×4
  Plastic cuff (2″ length of suction tubing)
  Hoffman clamp

PROCEDURE

Examination and Preparation

The most important task in the treatment of epistaxis is locating the site of bleeding. In an ideal situation, the patient sits upright, leaning slightly forward looking directly at the clinician, although with many pediatric patients, this will not be possible. An adequate light source is essential for good visualization of the nasal mucosa. A headlight provides di-

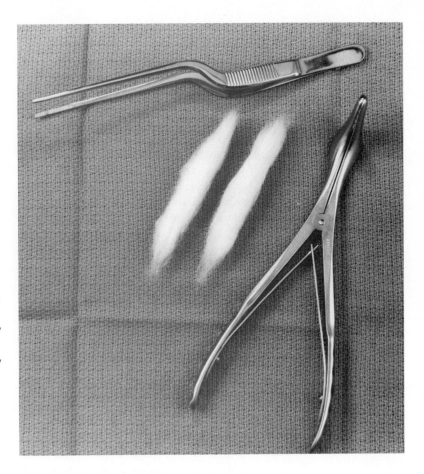

Figure 60.2.
Bayonet forceps, nasal speculum, and cotton pledgets.

rect illumination of the nose and frees both hands for treatment. Young or uncooperative patients may require conscious sedation before the procedures described in this section can be performed successfully (see Chapter 35). Uncooperative or sedated patients must be positioned supine on a stretcher using appropriate restraint (e.g., a papoose) with an assistant stabilizing the head. Once the patient is calm and positioned properly, the clinician can use a nasal speculum to visualize the anterior septum. The speculum blades should be opened vertically rather than horizontally so that the septum is better visualized without being directly instrumented. Keeping the speculum blades slightly open on insertion and removal will prevent plucking nasal hairs. Clots are carefully suctioned from the nose until the source of bleeding can be identified. If active bleeding obscures the septal mucosa, cotton pledgets soaked in a topical vasoconstrictor may be inserted with bayonet forceps (Fig. 60.2). If cautery or packing is anticipated, an anesthetic may be mixed with the vasoconstrictor and applied simultaneously. Phenylephrine or oxymetazoline will provide vasoconstriction but not anesthesia. Oxymetazoline is preferred when available because it has no effect on systemic blood pressure. Cocaine provides excellent vasoconstriction and anesthesia; however, a total dose over 3 mg/kg (e.g., 3 mL of a 4% solution in a 15 kg child) can cause seizures and circulatory compromise. A mixture of lidocaine and epinephrine (0.25 mL of epinephrine 1:1000 in 20 mL of 4% lidocaine) also has been recommended. The maximum allowable dose of lidocaine is 7 mg/kg. Although total systemic absorption of cocaine or lidocaine does not occur after topical administration, the maximum doses should not be exceeded. After 5 to 10 minutes of proper application of the vasoconstrictor, a persistent anterior source of bleeding should be visible (4, 10).

Cauterization

Cautery is recommended as the first-line treatment of persistent or recurrent epistaxis. After adequate anesthesia and hemostasis are obtained and the source of bleeding is visualized, the excoriated area may be chemically cauterized with silver nitrate or trichloroacetic acid. Chemical cautery is preferred over electrocautery in a pediatric outpatient setting, because the latter is more painful and requires proper grounding of equipment. The silver nitrate stick should be applied to the affected area in concentric circles, starting at the outer limits of the area and working inward. If the affected area is small, the end of the stick may simply be rolled over the excoriation or vessel. Petroleum jelly or a water-based jelly (e.g., KY) smeared on the unaffected areas of mucosa will prevent unwanted exposure to the chemical (5). Areas in contact with the silver nitrate will turn gray or black. If the nostril is too small to allow adequate passage of the silver nitrate stick, a small cotton-tipped applicator or a wisp of cotton wrapped around a metal applicator may be soaked in trichloroacetic acid and applied in the same concentric manner. Cauterization alone will not always stop active bleeding; adequate hemostasis with a topical vasoconstrictor before cautery is usually an essential step. Notably, bilateral cauterization of the septum may cause ischemia and septal necrosis. In addition, circumferential cautery of a naris may lead to scarring and stenosis (5, 10).

Anterior Packing

If epistaxis recurs after cautery or if the site of bleeding cannot be located, then anterior nasal packing is indicated. Whenever possible, the site of bleeding should be located and cauterized before the pack is placed. A pack placed blindly is less likely to control bleeding; in fact, it may actually exacerbate bleeding by creating friction against the septal mucosa. If the site of bleeding cannot be visualized, topical thrombin provides a useful alternative to cautery. Thrombin is applied directly on the bleeding septal mucosa in powdered form or as a spray to achieve hemostasis.

The traditional method of anterior packing consists of layering Vaseline gauze ($1/4''$ or $1/2''$) in accordion fashion (Fig. 60.3). The patient is positioned and the mucosa is prepared as described previously. A length of Vaseline gauze is first coated with antibiotic ointment. It is then grasped with bayonet forceps 5 to 7 cm from the end and placed straight back on the floor of the nose. Approximately 2 to 3 cm of gauze should protrude from the nostril to keep the pack from sliding posteriorly into the pharynx. After the first layer is placed, the nasal speculum should be withdrawn and replaced on top of the gauze to gently pack it down while the next layer is placed in accordion fashion. Alligator forceps may be used instead of bayonet forceps in patients with a small nasal opening. Layering the gauze in this manner should continue until the nasal cavity is filled. A piece of tape applied to the protruding gauze end will help stabilize the pack (4, 5, 10).

Alternatives to the layered Vaseline gauze pack include the Merocel™ nasal tampon and oxycellulose (Surgicel™). The nasal tampon, which is available in several sizes, consists of dehydrated material that expands when exposed to moisture, filling the surrounding cavity. It is inserted with bayonet forceps along the floor of the nose. Insertion must be rapid as the material expands almost immediately on contact with fluid. Coating the tampon with antibiotic ointment will fa-

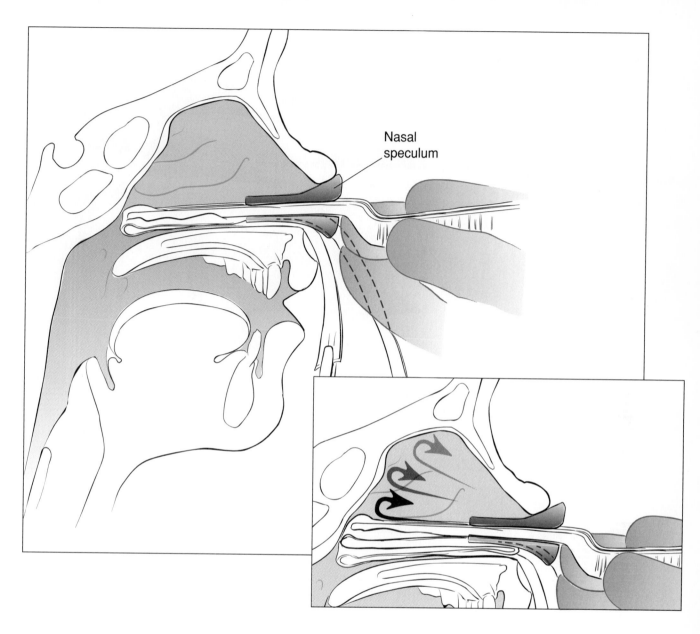

Nasal
speculum

cilitate both insertion and later removal (4, 9, 10). Oxycellulose is supplied as knitted fabric strips in a variety of sizes which can be cut for a custom fit. This material differs from mechanical packs in that it requires contact with blood to form a clot, it provides intrinsic bacteriostatic action, and it is spontaneously absorbed. Notably, previous mucosal cautery or applying antibiotic ointment to oxycellulose will interfere with the action and absorption of this product. A small amount of the material is applied directly to the site of bleeding until hemostasis is obtained. Oxycellulose should not be confused with the absorbable gelatin sponge (Gelfoam™), which although

having similar properties, potentiates bacterial growth and has been associated with toxic shock syndrome (11).

Because anterior nasal packs are foreign bodies which lead to stasis of nasal secretions, patients with a pack in place for more than a few hours should be placed on oral antibiotics to prevent sinus infection and toxic shock syndrome. Nonabsorbable packing material should be removed within 3 to 5 days. Ideally, the child should be reevaluated on an outpatient basis within 24 hours. Absorbable packing material residue should be left in place, as attempts to remove it may cause rebleeding (4, 9, 10).

Figure 60.3.
Traditional method of placing an anterior nasal pack using Vaseline gauze. A bayonet forceps is used to insert the gauze straight back along the floor of the nasal cavity. The speculum is removed after each layer is applied and then reinserted to gently pack the gauze down. The gauze is layered in accordion fashion until the nasal cavity is filled.

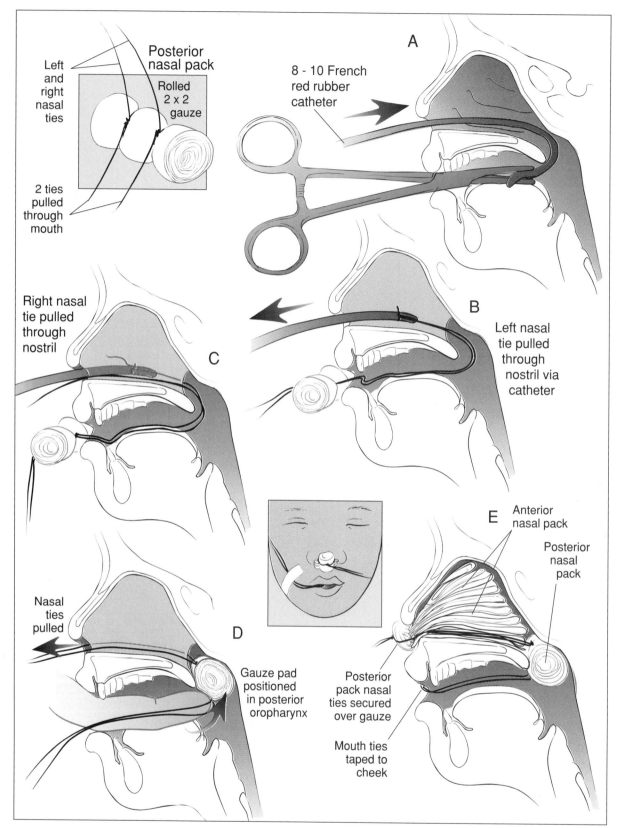

Figure 60.4.
Traditional method of placing a posterior nasal pack using gauze pads.
A. A small catheter is inserted into one nostril, advanced to the posterior pharynx, and withdrawn through the mouth.
B. One end of a tie is then fastened to the end of the catheter and the catheter is removed to pull the tie out through the nose.
C. This is repeated on the opposite side using one end of the other tie.
D. The pack is drawn into the posterior pharynx by pulling both ties and positioned manually against the vomer. An anterior nasal pack is then applied.
E. The ends of the ties protruding from the mouth are taped to the cheek. The ends protruding through the nostrils are tied around a gauze pad under the septum of the nose.

Posterior Packing

If packing of both anterior chambers fails to stop an episode of epistaxis, a posterior pack may be required. ORL consultation is always advisable in this situation. Either the rolled gauze or the inflatable balloon method may be used. The balloon method has become more popular because it is technically easier and is somewhat more comfortable for the patient. Because both methods are painful, adequate analgesia and sedation are always recommended before placing a posterior pack.

The traditional posterior pack is made from cylindrically rolled 2×2 gauze pads or an open gauze pad wrapped around cotton filling (Fig. 60.4). Two silk ties (#0) or umbilical tapes are tied around the gauze roll, leaving a long (8 to 12″) length of tie on each end. A small (8 or 10 French) red rubber catheter is inserted into one nostril, advanced to the posterior pharynx, and withdrawn through the mouth with a hemostat. One end of a tie is fastened to the end of the catheter that protrudes from the mouth. The nasal end of the catheter is then withdrawn from the nose, pulling out the tie with it. This is repeated on the other side, so that one end of each tie protrudes through the nose. The pack is drawn into the posterior pharynx by pulling both ties and quickly positioned manually against the vomer. The opposite ends of the ties (protruding from the mouth) are taped to the cheek, so that they can be used later in removing the pack. The anterior nose is then packed as previously described, and the nasal ties from the posterior pack are tied over a second rolled gauze pad under the nostrils to hold the pack in place. This second pad should be snug against the nose but not tight enough to cause ischemia and potential necrosis of the nasal cartilage. An alternative method of placing the pack is to insert a red rubber catheter in each nostril, fasten each tie separately to a catheter, and withdraw both catheters simultaneously (4).

A Foley catheter also may serve as a posterior pack (Fig. 60.5). The catheter size should approximate the diameter of the external nares (10 to 16 gauge). Before using the catheter, the balloon should be inflated to ensure that no air leak is present, and the end of the catheter distal to the balloon should be cut

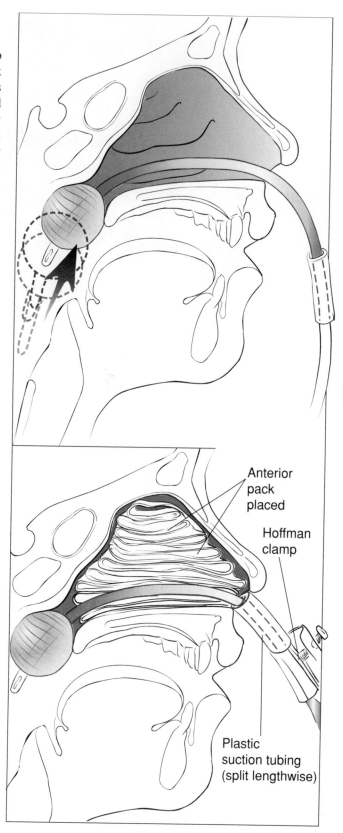

Figure 60.5.
Posterior nasal pack using a Foley catheter.

Anterior pack placed

Hoffman clamp

Plastic suction tubing (split lengthwise)

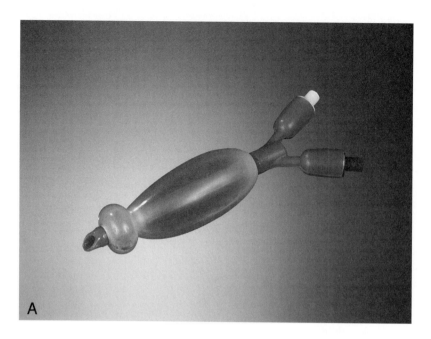

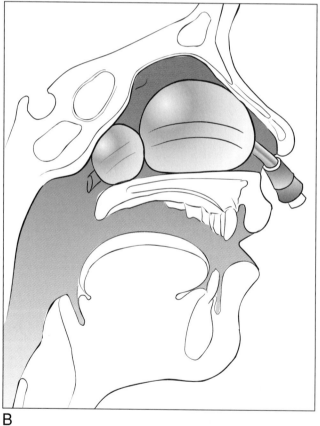

Figure 60.6.
Xomed Epistat anterior and posterior nasal tamponade device (balloons inflated).

A

B

off to prevent irritation of the posterior pharynx. The catheter is lubricated with antibiotic ointment and inserted into the anesthetized bleeding nostril until the balloon is visible in the posterior pharynx. The balloon is then inflated with 10 to 15 mL water or saline, and the proximal end of the catheter is withdrawn until the balloon is snug against the vomer. If the pressure exerted by the balloon causes any significant pain, the balloon should be deflated slightly. The catheter may be secured by placing a length of plastic suction tubing, split lengthwise, around the catheter just under the nostril. A Hoffman clamp, umbilical clamp, or hemostat fastened under the plastic cuff will hold the catheter in place. An anterior pack should then be placed around the Foley catheter (5, 9, 10).

An alternative to placing both anterior and posterior packs separately is to place a double balloon tamponade device, such as the Gottschalk Nasostat™ or the Xomed Epistat™ (Fig. 60.6). Such systems, which consist of both an anterior and a posterior balloon, are inserted in a manner similar to using a Foley catheter as a posterior pack. The posterior balloon is inflated first, the device is withdrawn to secure the posterior balloon against the vomer, and then the anterior balloon is gradually inflated. As with a Foley balloon, pain associated with inflation of either segment of the tamponade device requires that the balloon be deflated slightly (5, 9).

Patients with posterior packs should be monitored in the hospital. Posterior packs are known to cause hypoxia and hypoventilation, and may cause significant pain, dysphagia, and infection. In addition, accidental dislodgment of the pack into the hypopharynx can cause airway compromise. Because of the potential for respiratory complications, patients with posterior packs should be sedated with caution.

COMPLICATIONS

Complications of the procedures described in this chapter are chiefly related to ischemia, scarring, infection, and airway control. Overzealous cauterization or packing under pressure can lead to septal ischemia with possible necrosis. Circumferential cautery of a nostril can lead to scarring and stenosis. Both anterior and posterior packs lead to stasis of nasal secretions and potentiate bacterial growth. Using topical and systemic antibiotics is recommended in patients with nasal packs to reduce the likelihood of this complication. The risk of developing toxic shock syndrome may be minimized with anti-staphylococcal antibiotics and timely removal of the packing material (generally

SUMMARY

Anterior Nasal Packing

1. Position patient sitting upright facing clinician whenever possible. Younger patients who are unable to cooperate may be positioned supine with appropriate restraint. A sedative may be administered as needed.
2. Apply topical vasoconstrictor and topical anesthetic to nasal mucosa
3. Locate site of bleeding and cauterize as well as possible
4. Coat Vaseline gauze ($^1/_4''$ or $^1/_2''$) with antibiotic ointment
5. Insert nasal speculum into nostril and open vertically to expose septum
6. Grasp gauze with bayonet forceps 5 to 7 cm from end and insert it straight back on floor of nose. Approximately 2 to 3 cm of gauze should protrude from nose
7. After first layer is placed, remove speculum and replace it on top of gauze to gently pack it down as next layer is placed in accordion fashion
8. Continue applying layers of gauze until nasal cavity is filled
9. Place a piece of tape on gauze protruding from nose to stabilize pack.

Posterior Nasal Packing*

1. Position patient sitting upright facing clinician whenever possible. Younger patients who are unable to cooperate may be positioned supine with appropriate restraint. A sedative may be administered as needed.
2. Apply topical anesthetic to nasal mucosa
3. Tie two silk sutures or umbilical tapes around cylindrically rolled 2×2 gauze pads or an open gauze pad wrapped around cotton filling, leaving a long (8 to 12'') length of tie on each end
4. Insert small (8 or 10 French) red rubber catheter through anesthetized bleeding nostril until it can be retrieved from posterior pharynx through mouth
5. Fasten one end of a tie to catheter and withdraw catheter so tie protrudes from nostril
6. Repeat same procedure on opposite side using one end of other tie
7. When one end of each tie protrudes through each nostril, draw pack into posterior pharynx and quickly position it manually against vomer
8. Tape opposite ends of ties (protruding from mouth) to cheek, so that they can be used later in removing pack
9. Pack anterior nose
10. Secure nasal ties of posterior pack over a rolled gauze pad placed under nostrils

*A more simplified method of placing a posterior nasal pack using a Foley catheter is described in the text (see also Fig. 60.6).

1. When the patient has a known history of an intranasal lesion (e.g., a polyp or hemangioma) or a known bleeding disorder, ORL consultation should be sought before attempting to cauterize or pack the affected area.

2. When using a speculum to examine the nose, the blades should be opened vertically rather than horizontally so that the septum is better visualized without being directly instrumented.

3. When using silver nitrate to perform chemical cautery, it should be applied to the affected area in concentric circles, starting at the outer limits of the area and working inward. Cautery of both sides of the septum can lead to necrosis. Circumferential cautery around the entire margin of one nostril can lead to scarring and stenosis.

4. Patients with packs in place for more than a few hours should be placed on oral antibiotics to prevent sinus infection and toxic shock syndrome.

5. Posterior nasal packs are known to cause hypoxia and hypoventilation, and may cause significant pain, dysphagia, and infection. In addition, accidental dislodgment of the pack into the hypopharynx can cause airway compromise. Patients with a posterior pack should therefore be monitored in the hospital.

6. The risk of rebleeding after treatment may be minimized by having the parents humidify the child's home environment, by lubricating the anterior septum with petroleum or water-based jelly, and by preventing the child from picking the nose.

7. With younger patients who are unable to cooperate, it may be necessary to administer conscious sedation to successfully perform the procedures used for managing epistaxis.

8. Although complete systemic absorption of cocaine and lidocaine does not occur after topical administration, the maximum allowable doses of these agents (3 mg/kg for cocaine and 7 mg/kg for lidocaine) should not be exceeded.

within 3 days). Improperly secured nasal packs, especially posterior packs, create a risk for aspiration of packing material. Personnel caring for patients with a traditional gauze posterior pack should be instructed to remove the pack immediately with the mouth tie if the patient develops any signs of airway obstruction. All patients with bilateral anterior packs or posterior packs in place should be constantly observed for respiratory complications. Nasal packing also may interfere with the obligatory nasal breathing pattern in young infants.

Although sedation often is necessary to place a nasal pack, it should be used with caution in the setting of potential airway and breathing disturbances. In addition, patients with epistaxis are prone to nausea and vomiting as a result of swallowed blood, thus increasing the risk of aspiration (2, 4, 5, 9, 10).

SUMMARY

The vast majority of epistaxis in the pediatric population stems from an anterior source of bleeding, and most episodes can be managed with nasal pressure and reassurance. In children with persistent or recurrent bleeding, application of a topical vasoconstrictor helps locate the site of bleeding and permits treatment with cauterization. If cautery fails to control the bleeding, placement of an anterior nasal pack is indicated. Posterior packing may be required as a last resort if the source of bleeding is not visible and/or bleeding persists after appropriate placement of an anterior pack. Consultation is recommended if posterior packing is performed.

The risk of rebleeding after treatment may be minimized by having the parents humidify the child's home environment, by lubricating the anterior septum with petroleum or water-based jelly, and by preventing the child from picking the nose. ORL referral and laboratory evaluation for a bleeding disorder are not necessary unless the bleeding is severe or the history and/or physical examination are abnormal.

REFERENCES

1. Henretig FM. Epistaxis. In: Fleisher GR, Ludwig S, eds. Textbook of pediatric emergency medicine. 3rd

ed. Philadelphia: Williams & Wilkins, 1993, pp. 175–177.

2. Mulberry PE. Recurrent epistaxis. Pediatr Rev 1991; 12:213–216.

3. Wolff R. Protocol: pediatric epistaxis. Nurse Pract 1982;7:12–16.

4. Potsic WP, Handler SD. Otolaryngology emergencies. In: Fleisher GR, Ludwig S, eds. Textbook of pediatric emergency medicine. 3rd ed. Philadelphia: Williams & Wilkins, 1993, pp. 1377–1379.

5. Culbertson MC, Manning SC. Epistaxis. In: Bluestone CD, Stool SE, Scheetz MD, eds. Pediatric otolaryngology. 2nd ed. Philadelphia: WB Saunders, 1990, pp. 672–679.

6. Guarisco JL, Graham III HD. Epistaxis in children: causes, diagnosis, and treatment. Ear Nose Throat J 1989;68:522, 528–30, 532.

7. Randall DA, Freeman SB. Management of anterior and posterior epistaxis. Am Fam Physician 1991;43: 2007–2014.

8. Bennett JD, Giangrande PL. Nosebleeds: the importance of taking a history. J R Army Med Corps 1990; 136:167–169.

9. Josephson GD, Godley FA, Stierna P. Practical management of epistaxis. Med Clin North Am 1991; 75:1311–1320.

10. Abelson TI, Witt WJ. Otolaryngologic procedures. In: Roberts JR, Hedges JR, eds. Clinical procedures in emergency medicine. 2nd ed. Philadelphia: WB Saunders, 1991, pp. 1029–1037.

11. Physicians' desk reference. 1993 ed.

Drainage and Packing of a Nasal Septal Hematoma

Daniel J. Isaacman and J. Christopher Post

Introduction

A nasal septal hematoma forms when blood collects in the potential space between the nasal cartilage and the overlying mucoperichondrium of the septum. The presence of a hematoma impairs blood flow into the septal cartilage and can thereby lead to necrosis. Blunt trauma is by far the most common cause of a septal hematoma (1). In children, the most common causes of nasal trauma are domestic (household) injuries and sports injuries (2). Provided no reaccumulation of blood occurs, drainage and packing of a septal hematoma is a curative procedure.

Drainage and packing of a septal hematoma is moderately complex and requires good technical skill. It fulfills the criteria for minor surgery and therefore should be performed by physicians only. Septal hematomas occur in all age groups. The difficulty of treating a septal hematoma in a pediatric patient is usually inversely proportional to the age of the child. For a very young or extremely fearful child, this procedure is often most easily done in the operating room. However, if timely treatment by an otolaryngologist is unavailable, drainage and packing of a septal hematoma can be performed with such patients using conscious sedation techniques (Chapter 35). For a cooperative adolescent, the procedure normally can be successfully accomplished using local anesthesia alone and no sedation.

Anatomy and Physiology

The nasal septum consists of a thin cartilaginous plate with a closely adherent perichondrium and mucosa (Fig. 61.1). Because of the lack of ossified structures in and around the nose, the nasal septum is often damaged by bending or buckling. Forces generated by nasal trauma cause a separation of the perichondrium from the cartilage and the resulting potential space may fill with blood. A septal hematoma is commonly associated with other injuries to the nose, including nasal fractures, septal deviation, and intranasal lacerations (3). Children may develop significant cosmetic and functional abnormalities if such additional injuries are not properly diagnosed and treated (3–8).

Without incision and drainage, a septal hematoma exerts increasing pressure which impedes blood flow to the nasal cartilage, potentially resulting in necrosis of the septal cartilage and a permanent deformity (saddle nose). Drainage of the hematoma improves blood flow to the area but may not reverse antecedent cartilage destruction. An untreated septal hematoma also may result in abscess formation (9).

Indications

Any child who sustains trauma to the nose or midface should be carefully examined to ex-

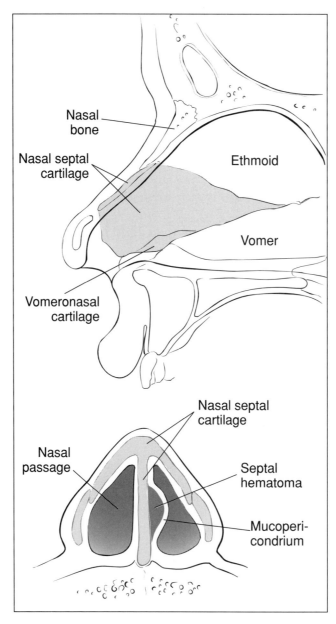

Figure 61.1.
Anatomy of the nose with location of nasal septal hematoma.

clude the presence of a septal hematoma or other injuries to the nose. Because of the potential for adverse long-term sequelae with such injuries, this aspect of the overall physical examination must not be overlooked. A septal hematoma will appear as a discolored (usually dark blue or purple) fluctuant bulge on one or both sides of the nasal septum. Whenever a septal hematoma is identified on examination it should be drained.

Because septal hematomas occurring in young or extremely fearful children are most easily treated under general anesthesia, these cases are usually managed in the operating room. If drainage is attempted using conscious sedation, great care must be taken to prevent any movement of the patient during the procedure so that inadvertent perforation of the septum does not occur.

Although deviation of the nasal bone and/or nasal septum are not necessarily contraindications for drainage, they do increase the complexity of the procedure and are more likely to require a surgical intervention. A septal hematoma associated with these findings merits appropriate consultation (10-12).

EQUIPMENT

Topical anesthesia—4% cocaine (maximum dose 3 mg/kg) or 4% lidocaine (maximum dose 7 mg/kg)
Topical vasoconstrictor—0.25% phenylephrine (Neo-synephrine®)
Scalpel—No. 15 blade
Wall suction, tubing, and Frazier tip suction catheter
Sterile rubber band
Sterile gauze
Anterior nasal pack (Chapter 60)
Light source (a head lamp is ideal)
Nasal speculum
Monitoring and resuscitation equipment for conscious sedation, as needed (Chapter 35)

PROCEDURE

Draining a septal hematoma in an awake patient should be done with the patient in a seated position, which minimizes the discomfort and any potential for swallowing or aspirating blood during the procedure. A young or fearful child who requires conscious sedation should have the procedure performed in the supine position using appropriate restraint techniques (Chapter 3). For these patients, standard monitoring equipment for conscious sedation should be used and necessary resuscitation equipment must be readily available. Reversal agents also should be drawn up in labeled syringes (Chapter 35). An older, cooperative child will not generally require sedation or any extensive monitoring.

Even for the patient undergoing conscious sedation, adequate anesthesia of the nasal mucosa is crucial. Sudden movement by the patient can result in iatrogenic perforation of the nasal septum, and it is therefore essential to minimize painful or noxious stimuli. Local anesthesia is achieved with topical application of 4% cocaine or 4% lidocaine using a cotton pledget inserted in the nose (see also Fig. 60.2). Although unlikely with topical application, the clinician should ensure that the toxic doses for these agents (3 mg/kg for cocaine and 7 mg/kg for lidocaine) are not exceeded. A topical vasoconstrictor such as 0.25% phenylephrine (Neosynephrine®) can then be instilled. The local anesthetic and vasoconstrictor should be applied approximately 10 minutes before performing any instrumentation of the nasal mucosa so that peak effects of these agents are achieved. For all patients, oxygen and suction should be readily available.

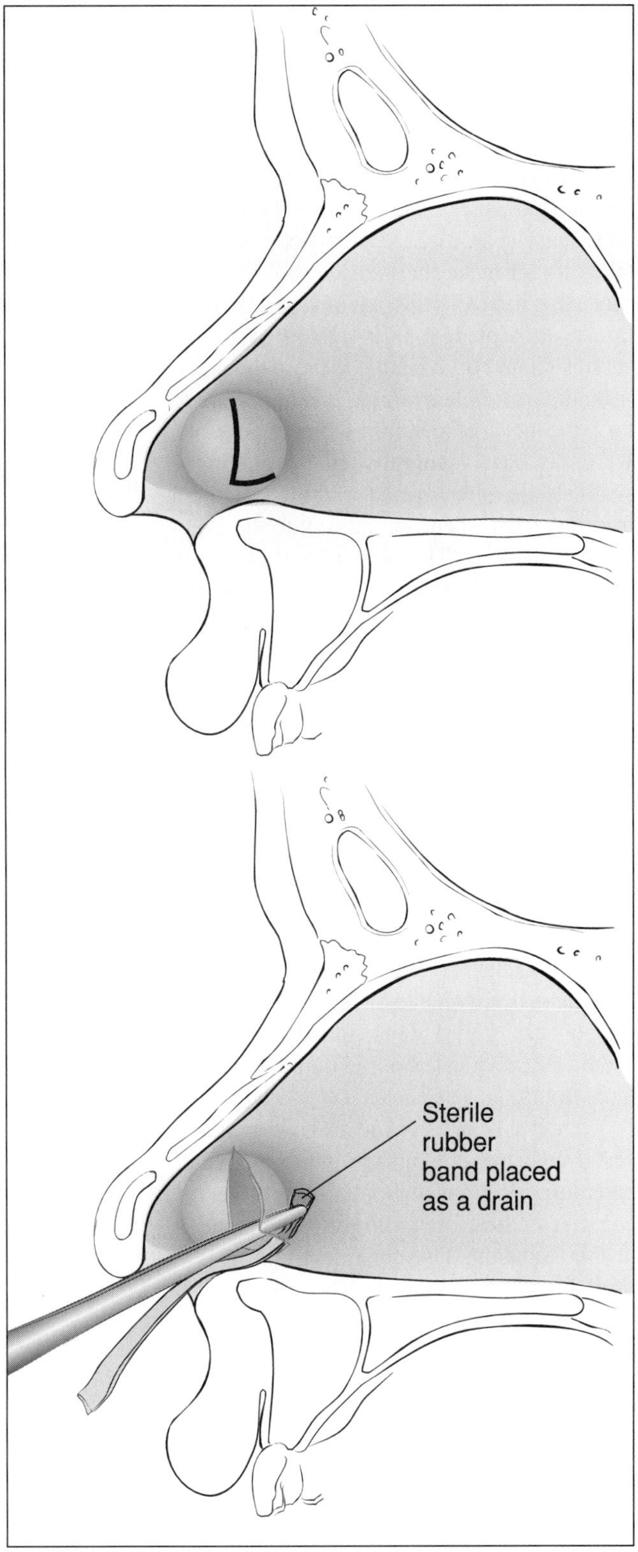

To ensure good visualization of the hematoma, a high intensity, easily directed light is essential. A head lamp with an attached light source is ideal. A nasal speculum should be used to open the nare and provide exposure to the area of interest. The speculum blades should be opened vertically rather than horizontally so that the septum is better visualized without being directly instrumented. Leaving the speculum blades slightly open on insertion and removal will avoid plucking nasal hairs.

Figure 61.2.
Incision and drainage of a septal hematoma.
A. An L-shaped incision is made through the hematoma and the blood is suctioned from the nasal cavity.
B. A sterile rubber band (or a small segment trimmed from a penrose drain) is inserted through the incision to prevent closure of the wound. The anterior nose is then packed as described in Chapter 60.

Sterile rubber band placed as a drain

When available, an assistant should be enlisted to hold the speculum in place, so that both hands of the clinician are free to perform incision and drainage.

At this point, a vertical incision is made into the hematoma with a No. 15 scalpel. The incision is then extended posteriorly to make an L shape (Fig. 61.2). Extreme care must be taken to not make the incision too deep, because this increases the risk of septal perforation. Cotton pledgets, 4×4 gauze pads, and suction should be available to drain the blood from the incised hematoma. It is important to keep the incision open for as long as possible, which is best accomplished by placing a small sterile rubber band (or a small segment trimmed from a penrose drain) into the evacuated hematoma. The rubber band is simply held with a forceps and inserted deep into the incision. It can then be secured in place with an anterior nasal pack or Merocel sponge (Chapter 60). To ensure that the drain stays in place, the clinician must apply the nasal pack securely against the overlying nasal mucosa. It is preferable to insert a nasal pack into both nostrils to avoid creating a deviation of the septum. Because placement of an anterior nasal pack may be associated with sinusitis and toxic shock syndrome, all patients should be started on an oral antibiotic with anti-staphylococcal coverage. Nonabsorbable packing material should be left in place for no longer than 3 to 5 days. Ideally the child should be reevaluated on an outpatient basis in 24 hours.

If the patient is found to have bilateral septal hematomas, drainage involves greater potential risk. Consultation with an otolaryngologist is therefore strongly recommended in this situation. Two treatment options are available for these patients. The primary goal with both methods is to achieve bilateral drainage without causing a permanent septal perforation. The first option involves making an incision through both the hematoma and the septal cartilage from one side. This permits drainage of the contralateral hematoma through the septum from one incision site. When this method is used, it is extremely important not to penetrate the overlying mucosa of the opposite side. The second option is to create L-shaped incisions on both mucosal surfaces, leaving the septal cartilage intact. The incisions must be staggered (offset) somewhat, because placing them directly opposite one another increases the chances of developing a permanent septal perforation.

COMPLICATIONS

As described previously, an untreated septal hematoma can progress to abscess formation and/or necrosis of the septal cartilage with resultant nasal deformity. One primary error of management when dealing with this problem is a delay in diagnosis and treatment due to an inadequate examination of the nose or misidentification of the physical findings (11, 13, 14). The importance of making the diagnosis on the first patient encounter to avoid an adverse outcome cannot be overemphasized. Unfortunately, a nasal deformity may occur despite early and complete drainage of the hematoma. This can result from reaccumulation of blood or preexisting necrosis of the cartilage at the time of treatment (1, 3). Consequently, close follow-up of these patients is essential.

A serious but avoidable complication is the development of a permanent septal perforation, potentially leading to cosmetic deformity and chronic nasal whistling (1, 9). This can generally be prevented by using great caution to incise only the overlying perichondrium without extending the incision into the septal cartilage. Even if a small incision is inadvertently made in the septal cartilage, a permanent septal perforation is unlikely as long as the mucosa on the opposite side re-

---

SUMMARY
1. Perform conscious sedation as necessary (Chapter 35)
2. Apply topical anesthetic (4% cocaine or 4% lidocaine) and topical vasoconstrictor (Neosynephrine®) and allow 10 minutes for peak effect
3. Position patient upright if procedure is performed without sedation; position patient supine with appropriate restraint if procedure is performed using conscious sedation
4. Expose septum using nasal speculum
5. Make vertical incision through hematoma with No. 15 scalpel
6. Extend incision in anterior to posterior direction to make an L shape
7. Place sterile rubber band through incision to serve as drain
8. Apply anterior nasal pack to one or both nares (Chapter 60)

mains intact. However, the septum should be avoided to the extent possible. Clearly, the technical precision required to prevent this complication underscores the importance of having a motionless patient during the procedure. It is in part for this reason that treatment of very young patients in the operating room is recommended whenever possible. Otherwise, restraint techniques and conscious sedation should be used effectively as indicated.

Infection introduced during the procedure can remain localized (septal abscess) or can extend to adjacent cartilage (perichondritis) (9). If left unchecked, infection can progress, leading to such complications as cavernous sinus thrombosis or meningitis. Reevaluation of the incision and drainage site within 24 to 48 hours will generally allow the clinician to identify these problems and initiate early treatment as needed.

As with any invasive procedure involving the airway, the potential exists for aspiration of blood into the lungs during drainage and packing of a septal hematoma. Bleeding associated with this procedure is normally minimal, with only the small amount of blood in the hematoma being evacuated. Careful suctioning will generally be adequate to avoid any complications. With more extensive bleeding, pinching the nose as with any other anterior epistaxis will usually provide adequate hemostasis. In those rare cases when bleeding persists despite an adequate trial of nasal pressure (e.g., an unrecognized coagulopathy), consultation and evaluation of the patient by an otolaryngologist will be necessary.

CLINICAL TIPS

1. The most important aspect of managing a nasal septal hematoma is making the initial diagnosis. Delayed treatment can lead to cosmetic and functional abnormalities of the nose. Any child with nasal or midfacial trauma must have a thorough examination of the septum and nasal cavity.
2. Minimizing any patient movement is essential to avoid perforating the nasal septum. With younger children, this is accomplished by performing conscious sedation and restraining the patient appropriately (e.g., a papoose board). If the patient continues to move despite these measures, the procedure should be performed in the operating room.
3. Enlisting the aid of an assistant to hold the nasal speculum frees both hands of the clinician to perform the procedure and apply necessary hemostasis. With younger children, a second assistant should hold the patient's head completely still.
4. Adequate lighting is essential. A head lamp with a high intensity light source is ideal.
5. Any continued bleeding after drainage of the hematoma can normally be controlled by simply pinching the nose for 5 to 10 minutes. Persistent bleeding after an adequate trial of nasal pressure necessitates evaluation by an otolaryngologist.
6. Although total systemic absorption of cocaine and lidocaine does not occur after topical administration, the maximum allowable doses of these agents (3 mg/kg for cocaine and 7 mg/kg for lidocaine) should not be exceeded.

---

dation methods or under general anesthesia. Careful technique and close follow-up are the most effective means of avoiding potential complications.

SUMMARY

Drainage of a septal hematoma involves making an L-shaped incision into the involved area, inserting a small drain to keep the incision open, and placing an anterior nasal pack to tamponade the bleeding and secure the drain. Caution must be used to avoid incising the cartilaginous nasal septum, as this can lead to a permanent septal perforation. This procedure requires good technical skill and optimal patient cooperation. On younger or uncooperative patients, this procedure is often best done using conscious se-

REFERENCES

1. Kryger H, Dommerby H. Hematoma and abscess of the nasal septum. Clin Otolaryngol 1987; 12: 125–129.
2. East CA, O'Donaghue G. Acute nasal trauma in children. J Pediatr Surg 1987; 22:308–310.
3. Olsen KD, Carpenter III RJ, Kern EB. Nasal septal injury in children. Diagnosis and management. Arch Otolaryngol 1980; 106:317–320.
4. Colton JL, Beekhuis GJ. Management of nasal fractures. Otolaryngol Clin North Am 1986;19:73–85.
5. Renner GJ. Management of nasal fractures. Otolaryngol Clin North Am 1991; 24:195–213.
6. Martinez SA. Nasal fractures. What to do for a successful outcome. Postgrad Med 1987; 82:71–74, 77.

7. Dommerby H, Tos M. Nasal fractures in children—long-term results. ORL J Otorhinolaryngol Relat Spec 1985; 47:272–277.

8. Grymer LF, Gutierrez C, Stoksted P. Nasal fractures in children: influence on the development of the nose. J Laryngol Otol 1985; 99:735–739.

9. Olsen KD, Carpenter III RJ, Kern EB. Nasal septal trauma in children. Pediatrics 1979;64:32–35.

10. Votey S, Dudly JP. Emergency ear, nose and throat procedures. Emerg Med Clin North Am 1989; 7:130–154.

11. Altreuter RW. Nasal trauma. Emerg Med Clin North Am 1987; 5:293–300.

12. White MJ, Johnson PC, Heckler FR. Management of maxillofacial and neck soft-tissue injuries. Clin Sports Med 1989; 8:11–23.

13. Wilson SW, Milward TM. Delayed diagnosis of septal hematoma and consequent nasal deformity. Injury 1994; 25:685–686.

14. Facer GW. Symposium. ENT for nonspecialists. Management of nasal injury. Postgrad Med 1975; 57:123–126.

Chapter 61
Drainage and
Packing of a Nasal
Septal Hematoma

680

CHAPTER 62

Nasal Foreign Body Removal

Daniel J. Isaacman and J. Christopher Post

Introduction

Nasal foreign bodies are a common problem among pediatric patients. Children have a sincere curiosity about placing objects in body orifices, and the nose seems to be a favorite choice for this behavior. At times the diagnosis will be obvious, as the parent's presenting complaint will be "He stuck something in his nose." The task at that point is to find and remove the offending object. Diagnosis of an intranasal foreign body in a child, however, can be more subtle when the parent has not witnessed the object being inserted. The classic presentation in this situation is an unexplained, foul-smelling nasal discharge which is unilateral and persistent. Other less specific complaints include chronic sinusitis, recurrent epistaxis, and halitosis (1-4). Body odor in a child also has been reported as a presentation for intranasal foreign body (5, 6). In addition, objects may be found incidentally, often during routine radiographic procedures (7, 8). It is not unusual for the patient to be seen on multiple occasions with the same symptoms before the correct diagnosis is made. The physician must therefore maintain a high index of suspicion to detect this problem.

A veritable encyclopedia of small objects has been removed from the noses of children (9, 10). Common items include toy parts, beads, tissue paper, and foam rubber (2). More recently, button batteries (i.e., those used in watches, electronic toys and games, and calculators) have been increasingly found as intranasal foreign bodies (11, 12). These small alkaline batteries are a special concern, as they can cause liquefaction necrosis leading subsequently to severe local tissue destruction (11). Objects that are hygroscopic, such as seeds or beans, may enlarge substantially as they absorb moisture from the nasal cavity, making extrication more difficult. Less commonly, animate objects (insects) also may be retrieved from the nose (13).

Goals for the physician suspecting this diagnosis are threefold: to conduct a thorough inspection of the nasal cavity, to maximally visualize the object (assuming one is found), and to remove the object while causing as little trauma (both physical and emotional) as possible. The difficulty of achieving these goals depends on several factors, including size, shape, and location of the object; level of cooperation from the child; and skill of the physician. In cases of pediatric nasal foreign bodies, 90% occur in children under 4 years of age (2). Achieving adequate cooperation with these younger patients often is the primary factor determining the success or failure of the procedure.

Several techniques have been advocated for removing nasal foreign bodies. Most are at least similar to those methods used for retrieving foreign bodies from the external auditory canal (Chapter 57). In general, removal should be performed only by a physician, because a failed attempt can result in advancing the object further into the nasal cavity, making subsequent attempts far more difficult. In addition, younger children become much more fearful and uncooperative after an initial attempt is unsuccessful. The procedure should be performed in a setting that has proper lighting, suction, and a variety of specialty instruments including a right angle, an alligator forceps, and a curette. Airway equipment also should be readily available in the unlikely event that an object is aspirated into the proximal airway.

ANATOMY AND PHYSIOLOGY

A good view of the nasal cavity should always be obtained before any instrumentation. Blind passage of removal devices is rarely successful and increases the risk of injury. One of the most important points about the anatomy of the nasal cavity from a clinical standpoint is that the turbinates are essentially perpendicular to the face rather than parallel to the nasal bone (Fig. 62.1). Instruments inserted into the nose should therefore be oriented in an anterior-posterior (i.e., straight in) direction, per-pendicular to the plane of the face. Notably, objects lodged superiorly and medially to the middle turbinate are precariously close to the cribriform plate. The clinician should not attempt removal from this area without involving an otolaryngologist.

The length of time an object has been in the nose largely determines the difficulty in extraction. The mucosa is prone to bleeding when the foreign body has been present over a longer period. In such cases, it is generally a good idea to warn parents of this possibility before attempting removal. Frequently the child may develop sinusitis due to obstruction of the sinus ostia by the foreign body (3). Persistent nasal discharge after the clinician is sure that the foreign body has been completely removed may be due to this cause. The patient should be started on an appropriate oral antibiotic regimen after the possibility of a retained foreign body has been excluded.

INDICATIONS

A thorough inspection of the nasal cavity is obviously indicated whenever a child has re-

Figure 62.1.
Anatomy of the nasal cavity.

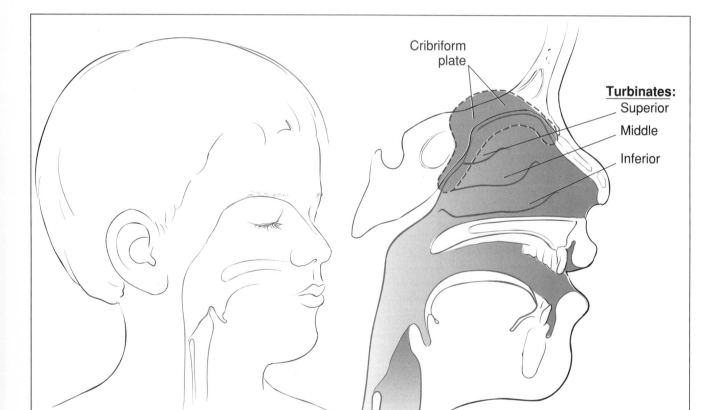

portedly placed a foreign body in the nose. This information may come from a parent or other caretaker, a sibling, or the child. As described previously, other complaints that should prompt suspicion of an intranasal foreign body include a persistent nasal discharge (particularly when unilateral), recurrent epistaxis, or halitosis (1-4). Diagnosis of clinical sinusitis, a common finding in the outpatient setting, is often based on a history of purulent nasal discharge for longer than 7 to 10 days. These children also should be routinely evaluated for a nasal foreign body (3). A more exotic presentation such as body odor, which is unusual before the development of apocrine glands during adolescence, should cause the physician to at least consider the diagnosis of a nasal foreign body as one possibility (5, 6).

In a review of 212 cases of ear and nose foreign bodies in children presenting to an urban ED, Baker (2) found that approximately 90% of the objects could be removed by ED personnel with readily available equipment. If necessary, conscious sedation may be performed in the ED to facilitate the procedure with a young or fearful child (see Chapter 35). Referral to an otolaryngologist, however, is indicated for any case in which the clinician is not confident of successful removal. In the combative young child who may be difficult to sedate adequately, a few minutes of general anesthesia often is preferable to a prolonged and potentially unsuccessful struggle. In addition, cases that are appropriate for immediate referral include embedded foreign bodies, penetrating injuries, patients with a bleeding diathesis, and any evidence of respiratory distress. As mentioned, foreign bodies located superiorly and medially to the middle turbinate should be avoided, because the potential exists for inadvertent puncture of the cribiform plate. Removal of objects in this location should be performed by an otolaryngologist.

EQUIPMENT

Lighting (head light, operating microscope, or surgical lamp)
Nasal speculum
4% cocaine (maximum dose 3 mg/kg) or 4% lidocaine (maximum dose 7 mg/kg)
0.25% Neosynephrine®

Suction (Yankauer and/or silastic catheter)
Right angle
Alligator forceps
Papoose board
Fogarty catheter (optional)
Histacryl blue ("super glue")

PROCEDURE

The clinician should first explain to the parents the planned approach and outline the risks of the procedure. As with any procedure, parental concerns should be completely discussed before proceeding. For this procedure to be successful, it is particularly important that the child remain still, and therefore every attempt should be made to calm the patient. Atraumatic removal is rarely accomplished with a struggling child. If the child is verbal, honestly explaining what should be expected and assuring the child that no needles will be used to remove the object can be helpful. With older children, applying a topical anesthetic is often the only measure needed to minimize pain sufficiently to allow removal. The clinician must ensure that the toxic dose of the anesthetic based on body weight is not exceeded. For younger or fearful children, administration of rectal midazolam also may be required to facilitate the procedure, and in some cases, standard intravenous conscious sedation techniques will be necessary (Chapter 35). Patients should be positioned supine with appropriate restraint. Restraining an older child may only require gently holding the arms down to avoid having the patient grab the clinician's hands as the foreign body is manipulated. Younger children should generally be placed in a papoose or other comparable restraint device (Chapter 3). Above all, the clinician must ensure that the head will be completely immobilized during the procedure. Assigning one assistant to concentrate solely on stabilizing the head will greatly enhance the likelihood of successful removal on the first attempt.

As mentioned, several techniques have been described for removing an intranasal foreign body (14-17). In many cases, the nature of the foreign body will determine the optimal method of removal. For example, firm or rounded foreign bodies can generally

SUMMARY
1. Ascertain nature of foreign body (if possible)
2. Explain procedure to parent and child
3. Assemble necessary equipment
4. Restrain child appropriately; assign one assistant to stabilize child's head
5. Perform conscious sedation as necessary (Chapter 35)
6. Insert nasal speculum and visualize object to determine size, location, and orientation
7. Apply topical anesthesia (4% cocaine or 4% lidocaine) as needed
8. Apply topical vasoconstrictor (0.25% Neosynephrine®) as needed
9. Remove foreign body
   A. For hard, smooth foreign bodies, insert removal instrument parallel to nasal turbinates (straight in) until tip is behind object and pull outward
   B. Grasp soft objects with forceps and remove
10. Reinspect nasal cavity after removal to ensure that object(s) are completely removed and mucosa has not been injured

Figure 62.2.
Removal of an intranasal foreign body.
A. A right angle curette can be used to remove firm or rounded objects.
B., C. A forceps (bayonet or alligator) can be used to remove softer materials (e.g., rubber or paper).

be extracted by placing a right angle or curette behind the object and gently pulling it out (Fig. 62.2.A). Alternatively, histacryl blue ("super glue") can be used with this type of foreign body. The glue is first applied to the tip of a wooden stick which is then pressed directly to a surface of the foreign body. Great care must be taken to avoid touching the interior of the nasal cavity, as the glue also will bond to the mucosal surfaces. The stick should be kept in place against the foreign body for 15 to 30 seconds to allow a strong bond to form. The object can then be retrieved by slowly withdrawing the stick. Another option with firm or rounded foreign bodies is to insert a Fogarty biliary

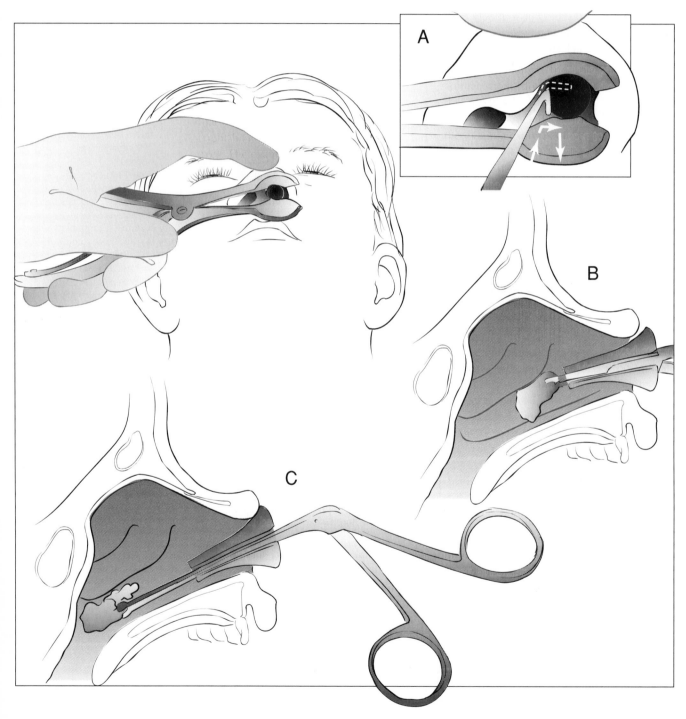

catheter beyond the object, inflate the balloon, and then gently remove the catheter. Foreign bodies made of softer materials (e.g., rubber or paper) can generally be grasped with a forceps and removed (Fig. 62.2.B,C). For some shallow foreign bodies, instructing the patient to cover the unaffected nostril and blow out of the nose may be enough to dislodge the object. Once the approach and instrument have been chosen, the clinician should proceed with removal as quickly and efficiently as possible. It is important to give the patient positive feedback for cooperating and to let the patient know when the procedure is drawing to a close. As described, removing the object on the first pass is highly desirable, as cooperation will quickly diminish after an initial failed attempt, particularly with younger patients.

Using a fiberoptic headlight allows two-hand manipulation, which is a distinct advantage. A nasal speculum should be placed in the nose to open the nostril and maximize visualization. The speculum is held between the palm of the hand and the third, fourth, and fifth fingers. The thumb and index fingers are used to stabilize the instrument against the nose (Fig. 62.2). It is important that the blade of the speculum open in a cephalad-caudad (superior-inferior) orientation, so as to not put pressure on the nasal septum. If significant edema or blood is present, the clinician should administer a vasoconstrictor such as Neosynephrine® and allow 10 minutes for maximal clinical effect. Once the object is adequately visualized, the clinician should assess its size and orientation. Occasionally, an irregularly shaped foreign body will have to be manipulated to ensure that the long axis is parallel to the direction of removal. It is important to emphasize that objects should never be pushed deeper into the nose to move them into the oropharynx, as the risk for aspiration is significant. The procedure should be terminated if the object is being inadvertently pushed deeper into the nose, if adequate visualization of the object is lost, or if significant bleeding occurs. After removing the object, the nares should be reinspected to confirm complete patency, because the object may have broken into pieces or more than one foreign body may have been inserted. Generally, no specific follow-up is required for the asymptomatic patient. Parents should be instructed to return for any signs or symptoms of a retained foreign body, primarily a persistent purulent nasal discharge or recurrent epistaxis.

COMPLICATIONS

A few important complications are associated with this procedure. One is local trauma to the nasal mucosa. It is quite common to induce minor epistaxis during removal of an intranasal foreign body, particularly one that has been present for a long time. The formation of granulation tissue in the area can result in transient bleeding when the object is extricated. Abrasion or laceration of the mucosa also can occur if the child moves suddenly during instrumentation. If histacryl blue is used, inadvertent application of glue to the interior of the nasal cavity can cause mucosal injury. Although bleeding is usually self-limited, the clinician should carefully avoid traumatizing the richly vascularized nasal septum, as this can lead to more extensive epistaxis. Applying a topical vasoconstrictor before the procedure will often limit any bleeding. If cocaine is used for this purpose, the clinician must ensure that the maximum allowable dose based on the child's body weight is not exceeded. This also should be done when lidocaine is used as a topical anesthetic. Toxicity due to either cocaine or lidocaine can produce seizures and circulatory compromise. Unless the child has a congenital or acquired coagulopathy, bleeding can normally be stopped without difficulty by pinching the cartilaginous portion of the nose for 5 to 10 minutes. If necessary, an anterior nasal pack can be applied (Chapter 60).

As mentioned previously, the clinician should be cognizant of the proximity of the superior aspect of the nasal cavity to the intracranial cavity. Overzealous instrumentation with a metal probe can result in fracture of the thin cribiform plate, producing a cerebrospinal fluid leak and allowing entry of bacteria into the cranium. The area superior and medial to the middle turbinate is immediately adjacent to the cribiform plate and as such represents a danger zone. A foreign body lodged in this position should only be removed by an otolaryngologist.

One significant but avoidable complication is aspiration of the foreign body into the proximal airway. This normally results when the object is pushed backward into the nasal cavity during attempts at removal or realignment. Sudden deep inspiration by the patient (e.g., crying) also may contribute to this complication. If the clinician finds that the foreign body is progressively moving posteriorly as it is manipulated, the procedure should be terminated and appropriate consultation sought. In the unlikely event that aspiration of the foreign body does occur, standard methods of addressing this problem must be performed (see Chapter 54).

CLINICAL TIPS

1. A nasal foreign body should never be intentionally pushed back into the hypopharynx in an attempt to remove it, as this may result in aspiration of the object into the proximal airway.
2. If it is apparent that a foreign body is only being pushed further into the nasal cavity during attempted removal, the procedure should not be continued. In such cases, removal by an otolaryngologist in the operating room will likely be necessary.
3. Visualization of the object can generally be improved by (a) applying a topical vasoconstrictor to the nasal mucosa, (b) using a high intensity light source (a head lamp is ideal), and (c) using suction to remove any blood or secretions.
4. The child must be very still during this procedure to prevent injury to the nasal cavity, and the clinician should take appropriate measures to accomplish the goal (restraint, administration of rectal midazolam, conscious sedation). If the clinician is not confident that the child will remain motionless, the procedure should likely be performed in the operating room.
5. With a verbal child, explaining each step of the procedure in a friendly, calming voice is often the most effective means of avoiding any sudden movements by the patient.
6. A firm, smooth foreign body that cannot be readily removed using a curette or right angle can often be retrieved by applying histacryl blue ("super glue") to the tip of a wooden stick, pressing the tip against the object for 15 to 30 seconds to form a secure bond, and then slowly withdrawing the stick.
7. Although total systemic absorption of cocaine and lidocaine does not occur after topical administration, the maximum allowable doses of these agents (3 mg/kg for cocaine and 7 mg/kg for lidocaine) should not be exceeded.

A final complication concerns the emotional trauma caused by an injudicious use of force to remove the foreign body. Unlike many procedures performed in the acute care setting, time is not a factor when removing an intranasal foreign body. Therefore the clinician should try to minimize the discomfort experienced by the child as much as possible. Attempts at simply overpowering a struggling child often are met with failure and subject the patient to needless anxiety and fear. In addition, should the procedure prove unsuccessful, subsequent efforts to remove the foreign body will be complicated by the distrust and apprehension of the patient. For this reason, some authorities recommend conscious sedation to facilitate this procedure for young or extremely fearful children, unless the object is in a shallow position and easily retrievable with one quick pass. If conscious sedation is not feasible in this situation, then removal should be performed in the operating room by an otolaryngologist. In all cases, time spent preparing the child by explaining what can be expected in a calm and nonthreatening manner often will be rewarded with a successful procedure which causes a minimum of emotional distress to both patient and family.

SUMMARY

Removing a foreign body from a child's nose is a skill frequently performed in the outpatient setting. Success primarily depends on the size and location of the object, the duration of time it has been in the nose, and the ability to adequately immobilize the child during the procedure. As with most procedures, proper lighting and the appropriate instruments are essential. Above all, the physician should make a judgment about the difficulty of the procedure before undertaking removal and proceed only when confident of success on the first attempt.

REFERENCES

1. Brownstein DR, Hodge D. Foreign bodies of the eye, ear, and nose. Pediatr Emerg Care 1988; 4:215–218.
2. Baker MD. Foreign bodies of the ears and nose in childhood. Pediatr Emerg Care 1987;3:67–70.
3. Fireman P. Diagnosis of sinusitis in children: emphasis on the history and physical examination. J Allergy Clin Immunol 1992; 90:433–436.

4. Bennett JD. An unexpected cause of halitosis. J R Army Med Corps 1988; 134:151–152.

5. Eun HC, Kim KH, Lee YS. Unusual body odor due to a nasal foreign body in a child. J Dermatol 1984; 11:501–503.

6. Wesley RE, Arterberry JF. Soft tissue intranasal foreign bodies. Ann Emerg Med 1980;9:215–217.

7. Kittle PE, Aaron GR, Jones HL, Duncan NO: Incidental finding of an intranasal foreign body discovered on routine dental examination: case report. Pediatr Dent 1991; 13:49–51.

8. Jones DC, O'Bree WD, Macintyre DR. Intranasal foreign body: an incidental radiographic finding. Dent Update 1987; 14:408.

9. Harun S, Montgomery P, Ajulo SO. An unusual oronasal foreign body. J Laryngol Otol 1991; 105: 1118–1119.

10. Fosarelli P, Feigelman S, Pearson E, Calimano-Diaz A. An unusual intranasal foreign body. Pediatr Emerg Care 1988; 4:117–118.

11. Gomes CC, Sakano E, Lucchezi MC, Porto PR. Button battery as a foreign body in the nasal cavities. Special aspects. Rhinology 1994; 32:98–100.

12. Palmer O, Natarajan B, Johnstone A, Sheikh S. Button battery in the nose—an unusual foreign body. J Laryngol Otol 1994; 108:871–872.

13. Werman HA. Removal of foreign bodies of the nose. Emerg Med Clin North Am 1987;5:253–263.

14. Backlin SA. Positive-pressure technique for nasal foreign body removal in children. Ann Emerg Med 1995; 25:554–555.

15. Nandapalan V, McIlwain JC. Removal of nasal foreign bodies with a Fogarty biliary balloon catheter. J Laryngol Otol 1994; 108:758–760.

16. Cohen HA, Goldberg E, Horev Z. Removal of nasal foreign bodies in children (letter). Clin Pediatr 1993; 32:192.

17. Wavde V. Removal of foreign body from nose or ear. Aust Fam Physician 1988; 17:904.

PHARYNGEAL PROCEDURES

Richard A. Saladino

INTRODUCTION

Two pharyngeal problems in children that may be treated in the emergency department (ED), tonsillar foreign body and peritonsillar abscess, require careful and complete historic investigation and physical examination before any ameliorative procedure.

Foreign body ingestion is a not an uncommon problem in both the pediatric and adult age groups. However, tonsillar foreign body is an infrequent finding, although in older children and adolescents it is no less common than in the adult population. Jones et al. described 388 patients aged 0 to 90 years, in whom 60 of 121 foreign bodies retained in the throat were located in the tonsil and 67 of 71 fishbones were found in the tonsil or posterior third of the tongue (1).

Peritonsillar abscess (quinsy), one of the most common abscesses of the head and neck, is thought to be rare in children younger than 8 years, but has been reported in children 4 (2) and 15 months (3) of age. In fact, in one study of children with peritonsillar abscess, 31% of patients were younger than 10 years of age (4), whereas in another, the mean age was 10 years (range 3 to 16 years) (5).

Management of a tonsillar foreign body depends on the particular foreign body and its location, but often is a straightforward procedure performed by the emergency physician. In contrast, management of peritonsillar abscess has undergone considerable and controversial change over the last century. Management options include medical (antibiotic) treatment, transmucosal needle aspiration, in-cision and drainage, acute tonsillectomy, or delayed tonsillectomy (6–9). The emergency physician will be involved in medical treatment and, in selected cases, may perform needle aspiration or incision and drainage prior to or instead of admission to the hospital. When available, consultation with an otolaryngologist should be sought in such cases.

ANATOMY AND PHYSIOLOGY

The palatine tonsils—the lateral component of Waldeyer's ring of lymphatic tissue (composed of the palatine, lingual, and pharyngeal tonsils)— lie in the tonsillar fossa (Fig. 63.1) (10). The deep or lateral surface of the palatine tonsil is a fibrous connective tissue capsule which opposes the superior constrictor muscle; the palatopharyngeal muscle lies posteriorly and the palatoglossal muscle lies rostral (11, 12). Importantly, the tonsillar and ascending palatine branches of the facial artery are just lateral to the constrictor muscle, whereas the internal carotid artery is no more than 2 cm dorsal and lateral.

Tonsillar Foreign Body

Up to 12% of foreign bodies found in the aerodigestive tract of children are fish or chicken bones (11). Although the majority of objects that children swallow are not retained in the throat, foreign bodies with a spicular shape may be retained in the tonsil: fishbones,

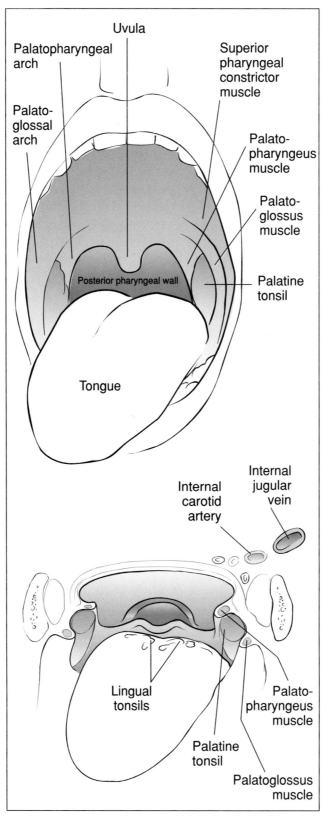

Figure 63.1.
Anatomy of the palatine tonsils and associated structures.

Uvula

Palatopharyngeal arch

Palato-glossal arch

Superior pharyngeal constrictor muscle

Palato-pharyngeus muscle

Palato-glossus muscle

Palatine tonsil

Posterior pharyngeal wall

Tongue

Internal jugular vein

Internal carotid artery

Lingual tonsils

Palato-pharyngeus muscle

Palatine tonsil

Palatoglossus muscle

meat bones, hard seed husks, and man-made objects such as glass, plastic toothbrush bristles, straight and safety pins, ballpoint pen caps, and countless other spicate household items that arouse the curiosity of children (12–15).

Tonsilloliths, most commonly seen in young adults with chronic or recurrent tonsillitis, are composed of retained caseous secretions in exaggerated tonsillar crypts that may contain vegetable matter and calcium salts. Tonsilloliths are therefore often rocklike and radiopaque (16–18).

Peritonsillar Abscess

Peritonsillar abscess is the most common complication of tonsillitis (4, 20) and is a result of suppurative infection of the tonsil. This infection penetrates the tonsillar capsule and extends into the connective tissue space between the fibrous wall of the capsule and the posterior wall of the tonsillar fossa overlying the superior constrictor muscle. Localized pus extends superiorly into the soft palate. Although 85 to 90% of abscesses occur in the superior pole of the tonsillar space (7, 20, 21), pus can accumulate in the mid-aspect or lower pole. Peritonsillar abscess is almost always unilateral (21, 22). Further dissection of the infected space may result in extension of organisms through the constrictor muscle and deep neck infection if a peritonsillar abscess remains untreated.

Streptococcus pyogenes is one important pathogen associated with tonsillitis with the microbiology of peritonsillar abscess cultures being polymicrobial in 30 to 75% of aspirates (5,

23). In several recent series of pediatric patients, *Streptococcus pyogenes* was isolated in 25 to 30% of aspirate cultures, other *Streptococcus* species in 20 to 40% of cases, and anaerobic pathogens in 12 to 33% (4, 5, 7). In two of these studies, 30% of aspirate cultures yielded both aerobic and anaerobic bacteria such as *Streptococcus* and *Bacteroides* species (4, 7). Notably, 20 to 35% of abscess cultures will not grow bacterial pathogens (4, 5, 7, 24).

INDICATIONS

Tonsillar Foreign Body

Older patients with tonsillar foreign bodies will report swallowing a foreign body or choking on food with spicular bones or fragments. Most will have sudden onset of discomfort, and as many as 68% of patients who localize their pain to the tonsil have been found to have foreign bodies (1). Otalgia is not uncommon, and odynophagia can progressively worsen. Foreign body sensation is not reliably reported (11). Younger (especially preverbal) children may have subtle presentations, such as an unwitnessed or unexplained choking episode during a meal or while playing with small objects. Children with mental or developmental retardation are at higher risk for foreign body ingestion (1, 11) with late presentation not uncommon.

Careful inspection of the tonsillar fossae and palate will detect most tonsillar foreign bodies. Using an indirect mirror or fiberoptic nasopharyngoscopy will provide a more optimal examination when the foreign body cannot be adequately or fully visualized (see Chapter 64). Radiographs will corroborate clinical findings of radiopaque foreign bodies such as meat and poultry bones, pins, and most glass. Of note, not all fish species bones are radiographically visible. Ell and Sprigg assessed the radiopacity of the bones of 14 species of fish in a swine head and neck preparation. On plain radiograph, bones of the cod, gunard, haddock, cole fish, lemon sole, monk fish, and red snapper were moderately or clearly visible in the tonsil, larynx, vallecula, and esophagus (Fig. 63.2). In con-

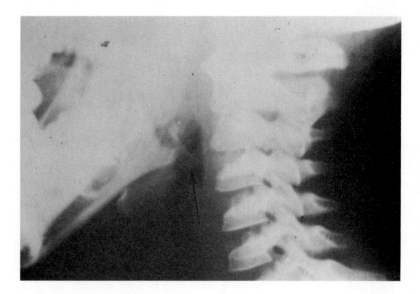

Figure 63.2.
Radiograph of a fish bone lodged in the palatine tonsil and hanging into the hypopharynx of a 3-year-old boy.

trast, bones of the salmon, trout, pike, mackerel, herring, and plaice were not radiopaque (19).

The uncooperative patient or young child with a tonsillar foreign body should be examined carefully by both the emergency physician and a consulting otolaryngologist. Removing a foreign body in such a patient may require general anesthesia in an operating suite. In the older and cooperative patient, removal is straightforward, if the site and depth of the foreign body is established. A lateral radiograph of the soft tissues of the neck can be helpful before removal.

Contraindications for removal of a tonsillar foreign body in the ED include an uncooperative or young child, difficulty visualizing the appropriate anatomy or the foreign body, and anticipation of a difficult removal or difficult management of the airway.

Peritonsillar Abscess

The child with peritonsillar abscess will report sore throat, and a mild fever of a few or several days' duration will be noted. Dysphagia and odynophagia can worsen acutely and changes in phonation can progress to a "hot potato" voice (8, 22). Pyrexia increases and trismus can develop due to spasm of the internal pterygoid muscle (22). Tender cervical adenopathy accompanies the tonsillopharyngitis and inflammatory torticollis is occasionally seen (25).

Figure 63.3.
A. Normal tonsil.
B. Peritonsillar abscess. The tonsil is displaced forward and inferomedially, the uvula is deviated toward the unaffected tonsil, and the soft palate is edematous and ruborous.
C. Acute tonsilitis.

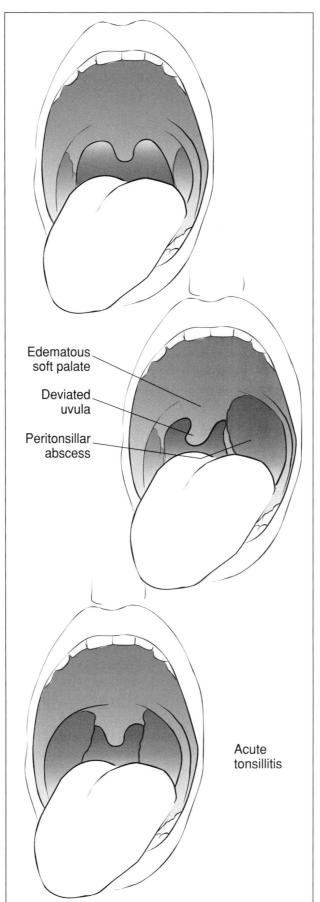

Edematous
soft palate

Deviated
uvula

Peritonsillar
abscess

Acute
tonsillitis

Physical examination of a patient with a peritonsillar abscess reveals a mildly to moderately ill-appearing febrile child. Swallowing may be difficult or painful and the patient may drool as a result (8, 22). Trismus often limits examination, but an exudative tonsillopharyngitis is usually present on inspection of the pharynx. The abscess usually displaces the affected tonsil forward and inferomedially, and the uvula is consequently deviated toward the unaffected tonsil (22) (Fig. 63.3). The soft palate is red and swollen. Halitosis often is present with tender ipsilateral cervical adenopathy.

These findings do not always differentiate peritonsillar cellulitis from abscess (26), although the pharyngotonsillar bulge is usually of greater magnitude with abscess (8). Gentle palpation with the examiner's gloved finger inserted into the patient's mouth will normally reveal fluctuance when a true abscess is present. Consultation with an otolaryngologist is mandatory if the clinician is unsure of the diagnosis. Other diagnostic considerations also should be made, including severe tonsillopharyngitis, retropharyngeal abscess, lymphoma, deep neck tumor, or carotid artery aneurysm. In the pediatric patient, some authorities favor hospitalizing patients with potential peritonsillar abscess for intravenous antibiotic therapy. Those patients who do not respond within 24 to 48 hours undergo acute tonsillectomy (6, 8). The management strategy used should be individualized, and postprocedure care plans should be made in consultation with an otolaryngologist.

Transmucosal needle aspiration or incision and drainage

in the ED is a safe alternative for acute management of the nontoxic, cooperative patient with peritonsillar abscess. Ill-appearing or uncooperative patients, and very young children should be admitted to the hospital with consideration of operative or closely supervised sedation for the procedure.

The cure rates for incision and drainage versus needle aspiration of peritonsillar abscess have been compared in several studies. Stringer et al. found similar cure rates for needle aspiration and incision and drainage of peritonsillar abscess (22 of 24 versus 26 of 28 patients) (27), as did Spires et al. (39 of 41 versus 21 of 21) (22). Likewise, Ophir et al. studied 104 patients with abscesses who had needle aspiration attempted (24). Of 104 patients, 75 had positive aspirations; of these 64 (85%) resolved with oral antibiotic treatment and only 9 required hospitalization.

Transmucosal needle aspiration of a peritonsillar abscess in children was recently studied by Weinberg et al. (7). Of 41 patients with suspected abscess, 31 had pus obtained on aspiration. Of the 31 patients, 27 (87%) had resolution of the abscesses after aspiration and parenteral antibiotics. Of the 10 children with negative aspirates, 7 resolved with parenteral antibiotics.

Current management strategies differ between institutions, although these and other data indicate the safety and efficacy of needle aspiration and antimicrobial treatment of peritonsillar abscess in children. In general, management strategies include parenteral antibiotic therapy and either transmucosal needle aspiration or incision and drainage of the abscess. Some otolaryngologists will, however, recommend incision and drainage if purulent fluid is obtained by needle aspiration.

Contraindications for performing needle aspiration or incision and drainage of a peritonsillar abscess in the ED include uncertainty of the diagnosis, an uncooperative or very young child, and anticipation of a difficult-to-manage airway. Any patient with a potential coagulopathy should have correction before the drainage procedure. Such cases are often best managed in the operating room using general anesthesia.

EQUIPMENT

Tonsillar Foreign Body

Specific equipment for removing a tonsillar foreign body depends on the type of foreign body. Most can be managed with a fine-tipped biopsy (alligator) forceps or straight or curved hemostat. Mishandling a tonsillar foreign body or tonsillolith can result in airway compromise. Equipment required for management of the airway always should be at bedside and is summarized in Table 63.1. Using topical or local anesthesia also is sometimes a helpful adjunct for removing a foreign body, and is similar to that used in treatment of peritonsillar abscess.

Peritonsillar Abscess

Equipment used for transmucosal needle aspiration or incision and drainage of a peritonsillar abscess also is listed in Table 63.1. As with removal of a tonsillar foreign body, air-

Table 63.1.
Equipment for Pharyngeal Foreign Body Removal and I & D of Peritonsillar Abscess

	Equipment	Comments
Airway management	Oxygen	Place at bedside
	Bag-valve-mask apparatus	
	Oral, nasal airways	
	Endotracheal tubes	
	Suction apparatus	Large tonsil (Yankauer) suction tube
Anesthesia	Topical: anesthetic spray, viscous lidocaine 4%, cocaine 4%	
	Injectable: lidocaine 1%, 2%	Luer-Lok syringe
		3-inch dental needle
Removal of tonsillar foreign body	Fine-tipped biopsy (alligator) forceps	
	Straight hemostat; curved hemostat	
Transmucosal needle aspiration of a peritonsillar abscess	3.5-inch, 20-gauge or 22-gauge needle	Use a needle guard
Incision and drainage of a peritonsillar abscess	No. 11 or 12 surgical blade	Use a blade guard
	Curved hemostat	

1. Place required equipment at bedside
2. Have patient seated with head firmly against headrest
3. Firmly grasp spicular foreign bodies with fine-tipped biopsy (alligator) forceps or straight or curved hemostat
4. Carefully loosen non-regular foreign bodies and tonsilloliths with probe and grasp with hemostat or forceps and gently remove
5. Be prepared to manage a compromised airway, and have all equipment at hand—have suction readily accessible

way equipment should be ready at the bedside. Needle and surgical blade guards should be prepared before beginning the procedure.

PROCEDURE

A thorough inspection of the neck, cervical lymph chain, ears, nose, paranasal sinuses, dentition, and the nasopharynx, oropharynx, and hypopharynx is mandatory when a pharyngeal procedure is being considered. Chronic or acute examination findings, and associated disease may impact on management strategy.

Examination of the oropharynx is especially threatening to the young child. Time spent establishing rapport and trust with the patient is imperative for cooperation during examination and subsequent procedures. External examination (neck, ears, nose, paranasal sinuses) should precede oropharyngeal manipulation. Explanation of different phases of the examination and instruments used will allay some children's fears and will also enhance parental acceptance of the examination and procedure. Inspection of the oral cavity and pharynx is aided by using a wooden tongue blade and should include assessment of the floor of the mouth, the gingiva, palate, dentition, and retropharynx. Because both procedures involve the oral airway, it is important to have suction and airway equipment (bag-valve-mask and high flow oxygen) prepared and available at the bedside.

Tonsillar Foreign Body

The patient should be sitting upright with the head firmly back against a headrest. Younger or less cooperative children may require gentle, firm restraint. Using anesthesia such as a spray or viscous lidocaine will aid removal of a tonsillar foreign body. A tongue blade should be used to fully depress the tongue and expose the foreign body.

Fishbones, meat bones, pins, and plastic spicular matter should be grasped firmly with a straight or curved hemostat or fine biopsy forceps and gently removed. Nonregular, man-made, and vegetable matter foreign bodies and tonsilloliths can be loosened with a probe and then grasped with a hemostat or forceps. Care should be taken to protect the

airway during the entire procedure. Removal of a tonsillolith by a surgeon is sometimes necessary to establish a diagnosis. The differential diagnosis of tonsillolith by a surgeon includes granulomatous disease (tuberculosis, syphilis, actinomycosis) and infection.

Peritonsillar Abscess

Evaluation and management of a peritonsillar abscess requires careful examination of the oropharynx and should take place in an examining chair with a headrest or in the lap of the parent who can stabilize the child's head. Optimal visualization requires good light; direct lighting is provided by a handheld source or headlight, and indirect lighting by a head mirror. Careful inspection of tonsils and peritonsillar region should note size, symmetry, and displacement, surface appearance, and the presence of rubor, pus, a site of an abscess point, or foreign body. The uvula also should be inspected and deviation from the midline noted.

Before transmucosal needle drainage or surgical incision and drainage, application of topical or local anesthesia will reduce the risk of the child moving during the procedure. Topical anesthesia is preferred over injection to avoid contamination of uninvolved tissues; application of viscous lidocaine or cocaine solution with a cotton pledget or a cotton-tipped swab or spraying anesthetic liquid will reduce both the pain of incision and the gag reflex. The glossopharyngeal nerve can be anesthetized by an injection of lidocaine through the mucosa and into the tonsillar fossa (28). A Luer-Lok syringe and 3-inch dental needle (22 gauge) can be used to inject 1% lidocaine, although anesthesia can be incomplete due to the low pH in the abscess. Adequate local anesthesia often is not attainable in young children or uncooperative patients, and conscious sedation may be necessary. The child must be continuously monitored with heart rate, pulse oximetry, and frequent vital signs. In such cases, it may be advisable to consult an otolaryngologist for possible incision and drainage in the operating room.

Transmucosal needle aspiration is a straightforward procedure, but requires a cooperative patient. The patient should be sit-

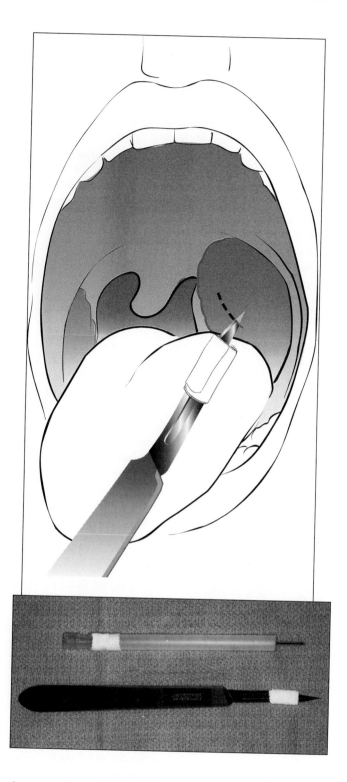

Figure 63.4.
The depth of the needle and blade is controlled using a needle guard or an adhesive tape blade guard.

SUMMARY: PERITONSILLAR ABSCESS

1. Place required equipment at bedside
2. Have patient seated with head firmly against headrest
3. Use needle guard or tape No. 11 or 12 blade to control depth of needle or incision
4. Usual approach for transmucosal needle aspiration is three point. Insert the needle 0.5 to 1 cm and aspirate first at superior pole; aspirate as much pus as possible. If unsuccessful, insert needle 0.5 to 1.0 cm inferior to initial site. If again unsuccessful, aspirate at inferior pole (yield is lower at this relatively inaccessible location)
5. Incision and drainage of a peritonsillar abscess: Make a 1 to 2 cm vertical incision through mucosa overlying area of greatest pharyngotonsillar bulge. Insert curved hemostat through incision and gently spread to break loculations of pus. Suction with rigid suction as necessary.
6. Send both aerobic and anaerobic cultures of aspirated pus or of incision cavity contents

ting up, with the head firmly against a headrest. A 3.5-inch 20-gauge or 22-gauge needle (a spinal needle will suffice) with a needle guard taped in place is attached to a Luer-Lok 3 or 5 mL syringe. A needle guard is used to limit the depth of needle insertion during aspiration—the terminal portion of the plastic needle cover is trimmed beyond which 0.5 to 1.0 cm of the needle will protrude (Fig. 63.4). Up to 90% of abscess collections are located in the superior pole of the peritonsillar space (7, 21). The first attempt in the typical three-point needle aspiration (22) is therefore made at the supratonsillar area of the greatest pharyngotonsillar bulge. This is superior and medial to the tonsil, at the junction of the an-

1. Maintain a high degree
   of suspicion during the
   investigation of a re-
   tained foreign body,
   especially in young,
   preverbal children or
   those with motor retardation.
2. Acute onset and pro-
   gressive discomfort
   and odynophagia are
   often present.
3. Most foreign bodies in
   the tonsil are spicular;
   most, but not all, are
   radiopaque. Obtain a
   lateral radiograph of
   the soft tissues of the
   neck to identify the
   shape, size, and loca-
   tion of a foreign body;
   not all fish species
   bones are radiographi-
   cally visible.
4. The differential diag-
   nosis of tonsillolith includes infection and
   granulomatous disease.

terior tonsillar pillar and the soft palate (Fig. 63.5). A second aspiration is made 0.5 to 1.0 cm below the first if pus is not obtained; a third may be attempted 0.5 to 1.0 cm lower, near the inferior pole. As much purulent fluid as possible should be drained, and the aspirated fluid should be sent for aerobic and anaerobic culture.

The site for incision and drainage is similar to that used for aspiration; the point of maximal fluctuance is normally the best site for incision. A No. 11 or 12 surgical scalpel blade is used for incision and drainage of an abscess. Adhesive tape is wrapped 0.5 cm from the point of the blade to control the depth of incision as shown in Figure 63.4. The tip of the scalpel blade is used to incise 1 to 2 cm of mucosa overlying the area of greatest pharyngotonsillar bulge. A curved hemostat is then placed through the incision and gently spread to extend the incision and break

loculated abscess pockets. The abscess cavity should be swabbed for cultures. Large amounts of drainage should be suctioned using a rigid Yankauer suction device.

During either needle aspiration or incision and drainage, great care should be taken to avoid the arterial vessels just lateral to the constrictor muscles. This is accomplished by accurately controlling the direction and depth of the needle or incision with both hands and maintaining complete control of the patient's head at all times.

COMPLICATIONS

Tonsillar Foreign Body

Although unlikely, aspiration of the foreign body by the patient is the most significant risk. The clinician must carefully grasp the object with whatever instrument is used and ensure that the child remains motionless. A rare complication is the puncture of or erosion into peritonsillar vessels by the foreign body resulting in significant hemorrhage. This is a much greater risk for chronic foreign bodies. Prompt direct pressure should be applied to any bleeding that occurs. If bleeding cannot be controlled in this fashion, exploration of the bleeding site is performed by the otolaryngologist in an operating suite.

Peritonsillar Abscess

Local bleeding usually occurs at the site of aspiration or incision and drainage of a peritonsillar foreign body, but this should be brief in duration. Hemorrhage from the carotid or jugular vessels may result from direct surgical injury or from erosion of the vessel wall due to the abscess itself, although this is rare (29). Direct pressure should

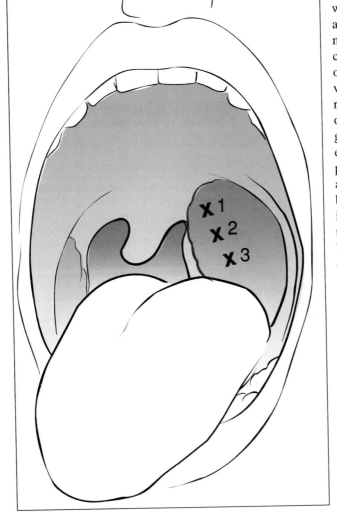

Figure 63.5.
Recommended sites for three-point needle aspiration of a peritonsillar abscess.

Chapter 63
Pharyngeal
Procedures

be applied to any bleeding site. Surgical exploration is indicated if bleeding cannot be controlled easily in 5 to 10 minutes or if it is severe. The patient may aspirate blood or purulent material and this should be anticipated with ready access to suction equipment.

SUMMARY

Procedures involving the pharynx that are most commonly performed on an outpatient basis by physicians who care for children and adolescents include removal of a tonsillar foreign body and needle aspiration or incision and drainage of a peritonsillar abscess. These procedures often provide definitive treatment of the presenting conditions. In most cases, the techniques involved are straightforward, particularly when the patient is cooperative. The physician can usually enhance patient cooperation by liberally anesthetizing the oropharyngeal mucosa with a topical agent and by carefully explaining the procedure in a calm, reassuring manner. Conscious sedation can also be used for a more anxious child. Because the patient must remain motionless during these procedures, younger children who clearly cannot cooperate are usually best managed by an otolaryngologist in the operating room. In the outpatient setting, airway equipment and suction should be readily available when any procedure involving the oropharynx is performed.

REFERENCES

1. Jones NS, Lannigan FJ, Salama NY. Foreign bodies in the throat: a prospective study of 388 cases. J Laryngol Otol 1991; 105:104–108.
2. Lapetus VF. Peritonsillar abscess in a 4-month-old child. J Laryngol Otol 1987; 101:617–618.
3. Shenoy P, David VC. A case of quinsy in a 15-month-old child. J Laryngol Otol 1993; 107: 354–355.
4. Dodds B, Maniglia AJ. Peritonsillar and neck abscesses in the pediatric age group. Laryngoscope 1988; 98:956–959.
5. Holt GR, Tinslet PP. Peritonsillar abscesses in children. Laryngoscope 1981; 91:1226–1230.
6. Parker GS, Tami TA. The management of peritonsillar abscess in the 90s: an update. Am J Otolaryngol 1992; 13:284–288.
7. Weinberg E, Brodsky L, Stanievich J, Volk M. Needle aspiration of peritonsillar abscess in children. Arch Otolaryngol Head Neck Surg 1993; 119: 169–172.
8. Brodsky L, Sobie SR, Korwin D, Stanievich JF. A clinical prospective study of peritonsillar abscess in children. Laryngoscope 1988; 98:780–783.
9. Sexton DG, Babin RW. Peritonsillar abscess: a comparison of a conservative and a more aggressive management protocol. Int J Pediatr Otolaryngol 1987; 14:129–132.
10. Clemente CD, ed. Gray's anatomy. 30th ed., Philadelphia: Lea & Febiger, 1985.
11. Binder L, Anderson WA. Pediatric gastrointestinal foreign body ingestions. Ann Emerg Med 1984; 13: 112–117.
12. Gracia C, Frey CF, Bodai BI. Diagnosis and management of ingested foreign bodies: A 10-year experience. Ann Emerg Med 1984; 13:30–34.
13. Norris CM. Foreign bodies in the air and food passages; a series of 250 cases. Ann Otol Rhinol Laryngol 1948; 57:1049–1071.
14. Osborne EA. Unusual foreign body in tonsil. Case report. J Laryngol Otol 1966; 80:962–963.
15. Pruett CW, Duplan DA. Tonsil concretions and tonsilloliths. Otolaryngol Clin North Am 1987; 20: 305–309.
16. Dale JW, Wing G. Clinical and technical examination of a tonsillolith: a case report. Austral Dental J 1974; :84–87.
17. Shrimali R, Bhatia PL. A giant radiopaque tonsillolith. J Indian Med Assoc 1972; 58:174–175.
18. Marshall WG, Irwin ND. Tonsilloliths. Oral Surg Oral Med Oral Pathol 1981; 51:113.
19. Ell SR, Sprigg A. The radiopacity of fishbones-species variation. Clin Radiol 1991; 44:104–107.
20. Maisel RH. Peritonsillar abscess: tonsil antibiotic levels in patients treated by acute abscess surgery. Laryngoscope 1982; 92:80–87.
21. Zalzal GH, Cotton RT. Pharyngitis and adenotonsillar disease. In: Cummings CW, Fredrickson JM, Hanker CA, Krause CJ, Schiller DE, eds. Otorhinolaryngology-Head and Neck Surgery, 2nd ed. St. Louis: CV Mosby, 1993, pp. 1180–1198.
22. Spires JR, Owens JJ, Woodson GE, Miller RH. Treatment of peritonsillar abscess. A prospective study of aspiration versus incision and drainage. Arch Otolaryngol Head Neck Surg 1987; 113: 984–986.
23. Brook I, Frazier EH, Thompson DHL. Aerobic and anaerobic microbiology of peritonsillar abscess. Laryngoscope 1991; 101:289–292.
24. Ophir D, Bawnik J, Poria Y, Porat M, Marshak G. Peritonsillar abscess: a prospective evaluation of outpatient management by needle aspiration. Arch Otolaryngol Head Neck Surg 1988; 114:661–663.
25. Bredenkamp JK, Maceri DR. Inflammatory torticollis in children. Arch Otolaryngol Head Neck Surg 1990; 116:310–313.
26. Shoemaker M, Lampe RM, Weir MR. Peritonsillitis: abscess or cellulitis? Pediatr Infect Dis J 1986; 5: 435–439.
27. Stringer SP, Schaefer SD, Close LG. A randomized trial for outpatient management of peritonsillar abscess. Arch Otolaryngol 1988; 114:278–298.
28. Scott BA, Stiernberg CM. Deep neck space infections. In: Bailey BJ, ed. Head and neck surgery-otolaryngology. Philadelphia: JB Lippincott, 1993.
29. Blum DJ, McCaffrey TV. Septic necrosis of the internal carotid artery: a complication of peritonsillar abscess. Otolaryngol Head Neck Surg 1983; 91: 114–118.

CLINICAL TIPS: PERITONSILLAR ABSCESS

1. Signs and symptoms characteristic of a peritonsillar abscess include trismus, dysphagia, odynophagia, drooling, fever, "hot potato" voice, deviation of the uvula away from the abscess, bulging of the posterolateral soft palate.

2. It is sometimes difficult to differentiate peritonsillar abscess from cellulitis and often requires aggressive management: parenteral antibiotic therapy and hospitalization. The decision to perform needle aspiration or incision and drainage should be made in consultation with an otolaryngologist.

3. Up to 90% of peritonsillar abscesses are localized in the superior pole; this is the optimum site for aspiration or incision.

4. Take care during these procedures to avoid laterally directed aspiration or incision. Branches of the facial artery are just lateral to the constrictor muscles and the carotid vessels are located no more than 2 cm lateral to the tonsillar fossae.

5. Be prepared to manage a compromised airway and have all equipment at hand. Have suction readily accessible.

DIAGNOSTIC LARYNGOSCOPIC PROCEDURES

J. Christopher Post and Clark A. Rosen

INTRODUCTION

The larynx, hypopharynx, and posterior nasopharynx cannot be adequately visualized by simple examination, and results obtained on plain radiographs may be incomplete or misleading. Special equipment and techniques are therefore necessary to gain accurate information regarding the anatomy and function of these structures. Children who present with complaints such as recurrent or persistent stridor, chronic hoarseness, or a suspected airway foreign body (without respiratory distress) are candidates for these procedures. A preliminary evaluation in the emergency department (ED), office, or other outpatient setting can aid the physician in determining the appropriate management and follow-up for the patient. Thus diagnostic laryngoscopy is a valuable skill for emergency physicians, pediatricians, and family physicians.

Indirect laryngoscopy involves visualization of the glottis, vocal cords, and supraglottic structures using an angled mirror placed above the patient's larynx. An external light source is provided by the reflection from a mirror worn over the physician's eye or by an electric head lamp. By contrast, direct laryngoscopy is performed with either an angled telescope or a flexible fiberoptic laryngoscope. Using these methods, the larynx is directly visualized through an eyepiece and the light necessary for examination is

emitted through the distal end of the instrument. Advances in fiberoptic technology have led to the development of progressively smaller devices which provide excellent image resolution. The availability of these instruments has broadened the options available to the physician for examining pediatric patients. Both direct and indirect techniques allow the clinician to visualize the anatomy of the extrathoracic airway and to assess the function of the vocal cords. Only direct laryngoscopy with the flexible fiberoptic laryngoscope can be used to examine the nasal cavity.

Any pediatric age group can be examined satisfactorily. Although neonates, infants, and toddlers cannot provide the level of cooperation needed to perform the indirect approach, these patients may be successfully examined using a fiberoptic laryngoscope. Older children and adolescents usually can tolerate an indirect laryngoscopic examination if the procedure is thoroughly explained and carefully performed. In addition, direct laryngoscopy can almost always be performed for these patients without difficulty as long as the mucosal surfaces are adequately anesthetized.

Although generally straightforward, the procedures described in this chapter are intended only to enhance the outpatient diagnostic evaluation of children who appear well. If the patient shows signs of respiratory distress, diagnostic laryngoscopy should be performed by an otolaryngologist, preferably in the operating room. Furthermore, even with a healthy child the clinician using a flexible fiberoptic laryngoscope should be fully prepared to secure the airway if necessary, because inadvertent contact with the larynx can in rare instances precipitate laryngospasm. All necessary airway equipment must always be readily available when this procedure is performed. Selected interventional laryngoscopic procedures, which share certain common elements with diagnostic laryngoscopy, are discussed elsewhere in this text. Chapter 54 describes direct laryngoscopy using a standard laryngoscope blade and handle for removing a foreign body in the extrathoracic airway. Emergent endotracheal intubation using a flexible fiberoptic laryngoscope is described in Chapter 16.

ANATOMY AND PHYSIOLOGY

A detailed discussion of distinguishing features of pediatric airway anatomy can be found in Chapter 16. Structures of greatest interest during diagnostic laryngoscopy are the posterior nasopharynx and adenoids, the hypopharynx, and the vocal cords and supraglottic region (Figs. 64.1 and 64.2). The ade-

noids (pharyngeal tonsils) are located primarily along the posterior wall and roof of the nasopharynx. Similar to other lymphoid tissues, the adenoids serve to protect against infection although they also commonly become a site of acute or chronic infection. Adenoidal hypertrophy can occur with or without infection of these tissues. Extensive hypertrophy of the adenoids can result in complete blockage of the nasal cavity. Obstruction of the eustachian tube orifice by enlarged adenoids prevents normal venting of the middle ear, often resulting in recurrent cases of otitis media. In addition, obstructive sleep apnea due to prolonged adenoidal hypertrophy can lead to pulmonary artery hypertension and ultimately cor pulmonale. Although performed less frequently than in the past, adenoidectomy is generally indicated when children develop such symptomatology.

The hypopharynx and supraglottic region are common sites for embedded foreign bodies (see also Chapter 63). Sharp objects that partially penetrate the mucosa of these areas (e.g., a wooden splinter, a fish bone, or a piece of chicken bone) may be missed on simple examination of the oropharynx. Furthermore, such objects may not have suffi-

Figure 64.1.
Anatomy of the nasal cavity.

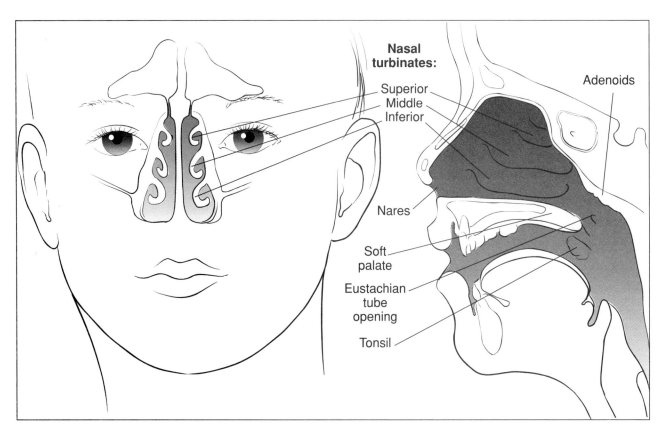

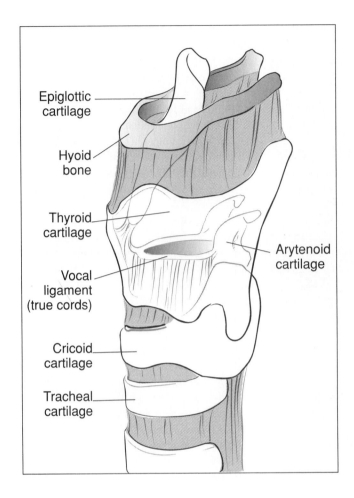

Figure 64.2.
Anatomy of the larynx.

Labels in figure:
Epiglottic cartilage
Hyoid bone
Thyroid cartilage
Vocal ligament (true cords)
Cricoid cartilage
Tracheal cartilage
Arytenoid cartilage

cient density to be visible on a plain radiograph of the neck. Indirect or direct laryngoscopy often are the only reliable means of detecting this type of foreign body.

The vocal cords are paired, V-shaped structures with the point facing anteriorly (Fig. 64.2). Phonation results from a series of minute changes in muscular tension exerted on the vocal cords as air is forced out through the glottic opening. The vocal cords vibrate to produce the sound of the voice. Abnormalities in vocal cord function result in chronic hoarseness and/or stridor. In children, common causes of these symptoms include laryngomalacia, vocal cord paresis or paralysis, subglottic hemangioma, vocal cord nodules, and juvenile laryngeal papilloma (1-3). Infants with a low pitched or breathy cry who have findings suggestive of a neuromuscular disorder, a congenital anomaly of the mediastinum (e.g., tracheoesophageal fistula, vascular ring), or Arnold-Chiari malformation should be suspected of having unilateral or bilateral cord paralysis. The large, floppy

epiglottis of an infant often will fall back and forth over the glottis during respiration, giving the clinician an intermittent view of the vocal cords on laryngoscopy.

INDICATIONS

A variety of presenting complaints may serve as indications to perform indirect or direct laryngoscopic procedures (Table 64.1). The safety of these techniques when performed

Table 64.1.
Indications for Diagnostic Laryngoscopy

Acute change in voice
Unusual cry (low pitched or breathy)
Chronic hoarseness
Persistent stridor
Chronic mouth breathing
Snoring respirations while sleeping
Chronic nasal discharge
Persistent odynophagia
Chronic cough
Suspected exposure to hot fumes or gases (e.g., a house fire)

properly has been demonstrated in both the inpatient and outpatient settings (4-8, 13-18). In general, any child with persistent symptoms referable to the nasopharynx, supraglottic region, or vocal cords that are not adequately explained by a more limited head and neck examination are candidates for these procedures.

Complaints such as voice changes, chronic stridor or hoarseness, an unusual cry, or persistent odynophagia should generally prompt the physician to examine the vocal cords and supraglottic region using indirect or direct laryngoscopy. Any abnormalities of vocal cord function or the presence of a penetrating foreign body lodged in the airway mucosa warrant evaluation by an otolaryngologist. One relatively common cause of stridor in infancy is laryngomalacia. Infants with laryngomalacia will typically present with positional inspiratory stridor and little or no stridor during expiration. The infant will usually have increased symptoms when placed in the supine position and decreased symptoms when prone. Feeding difficulties are rare. Laryngoscopy will reveal the epiglottis and arytenoids collapsing into the glottis with inspiration. Notably children exposed to hot fumes or gases (e.g., during a house fire) may have no stridor or voice changes initially despite the presence of vocal cord or supraglottic edema due to thermal injury. In such cases, a laryngoscopic examination that reveals edema or carbonaceous deposits in the extrathoracic airway requires close observation of the patient and possibly early endotracheal intubation.

Children with chronic mouth breathing, snoring respirations, or a persistent nasal discharge often require an examination of the nasopharynx with a fiberoptic laryngoscope (9-12). Obstruction of the nasal cavity in children is commonly caused by adenoidal hypertrophy. The finding of significantly enlarged adenoid tissue, particularly when the orifice of the eustachian tube is occluded, is an indication for referral to an otolaryngologist. Chronic nasal obstruction also may be due to nasal polyposis, a problem that may be associated with cystic fibrosis. Polyps appear as gray, grapelike masses filling the nasal cavities. In general, children with nasal polyposis should routinely be evaluated for cystic fibrosis, even if they do not have a history of pulmonary or gastrointestinal symptoms. During examination of the posterior nasal cavity with a fiberoptic laryngoscope, the clinician may find an intranasal foreign body not visible on a more limited examination. It is not unusual for children with this problem to have multiple evaluations before the correct diagnosis is made (see also Chapter 62). In such cases, the clinician must take care to not push the object posteriorly into the oropharynx, as this could potentially result in aspiration.

As mentioned previously, indirect laryngoscopy can be performed in most older children and adolescents. A relatively high degree of cooperation is required, but this technique usually will be successful if the clinician thoroughly explains what should be expected and is careful to not stimulate the patient's gag reflex. With infants and younger children, laryngoscopy should be performed with the patient supine and appropriately restrained using a flexible fiberoptic laryngoscope. Although the child often will cry during the procedure, a good examination usually can be obtained. Whenever visualization of the nasopharynx is necessary, using the fiberoptic laryngoscope is obviously required regardless of the patient's age. If the equipment necessary to safely perform these techniques is not available, the patient should be referred to an otolaryngologist for further evaluation. In addition, a significant percentage of patients will have a lesion below the level of the cords which will not be visible on indirect or direct laryngoscopy. For this reason, children with no abnormal findings who have persistent symptoms also should be seen by an otolaryngologist.

Diagnostic evaluation in the ED or office using laryngoscopic techniques is contraindicated for the patient with respiratory distress. For example, the child with a high grade obstruction of the extrathoracic airway due to a foreign body is not a candidate for diagnostic laryngoscopy outside the operating room. The patient's marginal respiratory status may be further compromised as he or she struggles during the procedure. Furthermore, total obstruction may result if the object is inadvertently advanced into the proximal airway. In such situations, the stable patient should be immediately transferred to the operating room where rigid bronchoscopy and emergent tracheostomy can be performed as indicated. An unstable patient should undergo direct laryngoscopy using a standard laryngoscope blade and handle for removing the foreign body (see Chapter 54). Direct diagnostic laryngoscopy also is contraindicated in situations when advanced airway management techniques would not be possible. Although a rare complication, laryngospasm can result when a fiberoptic laryngoscope is inadvertently introduced below the level of the vocal cords. For this reason, the clinician must be fully prepared to secure the airway by emergent intubation or surgical techniques if necessary.

EQUIPMENT

Indirect Laryngoscopy

Examination chair
Light source (two options):
    Head mirror with high intensity lighting
        behind patient
    Electric head lamp
Angled mirror
Laryngeal mirror warmer or other defogging
    device
Gauze to hold patient's tongue
Cetacaine™ spray

Direct Laryngoscopy

Topical vasoconstrictor:
    For infants, 0.25% phenylephrine
    For children, one of the following:
        0.5% phenylephrine (Neosynephrine™)
        or
        1% ephedrine
        or
        0.05% oxymetazoline (Afrin™)
Topical anesthetic (one of the following):
    2% pontocaine hydrochloride
    4% lidocaine (maximum dose 7 mg/kg)
Cotton pledgets or spray device
Forceps—bayonet or alligator
Nasal speculum
Pulse oximeter
Angled telescope
Flexible fiberoptic laryngoscope

The equipment necessary to perform indirect laryngoscopy can be found in most hospital EDs. If a laryngeal mirror warmer is not available, the angled mirror can be placed under warm running water and then dried before use to prevent fogging. Cotton pledgets containing topical anesthetic and topical vasoconstrictor can be placed in the nose before flexible fiberoptic laryngoscopy using a nasal speculum and forceps (see Fig. 60.2). If necessary, diagnostic laryngoscopy can be performed using almost any type of chair (or stretcher); however, the procedure is greatly facilitated by an examination chair that can swivel, has a headrest for the patient, and has a foot pedal allowing the clinician to automatically adjust the height.

Advances in fiberoptic technology have led to the development of smaller laryngoscopic devices suitable for use with any pediatric age group (19). Manufacturers of pediatric units include Machida, Olympus, and Welch-Allen. The basic elements of a fiberoptic laryngoscope are the eyepiece, through which the image is visualized, and the insertion tube containing the fiberoptic bundles (Fig. 64.3). The insertion tube must hold at least two fiberoptic bundles—one that transmits light to illuminate the structures being viewed and another that transmits the desired image back to the eyepiece. The number of glass strands in each bundle largely determines the image quality (and price) of the laryngoscope. If available, a portable light source permits the clinician to use a fiberoptic laryngoscope in any room of the ED. Some units also have the capability for video monitoring and recording, which can be useful for teaching purposes and documenting the examination.

The tip of a flexible fiberoptic laryngoscope is directed by the clinician using a combination of two motions. Rotating the eyepiece along its axis translates to rotation of the entire insertion tube. The flexible tip of the insertion tube also can be directed back and forth along a single plane using a control lever on the eyepiece. By systematically deflecting the tip and rotating the insertion tube, the clinician can obtain a complete view of the airway. Currently, fiberoptic laryngoscopes with an outer diameter of 2.2 mm are available, a size that can easily be passed through the nasal cavity of an infant. The primary drawback of these smaller devices is the lack of a suction port to allow removal of se-

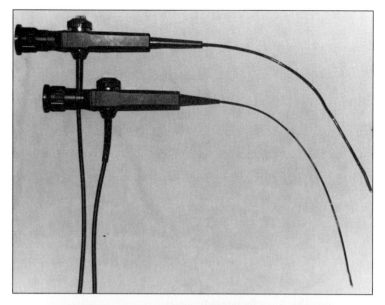

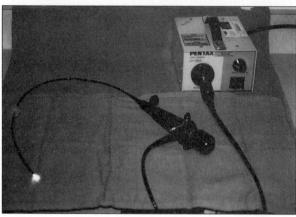

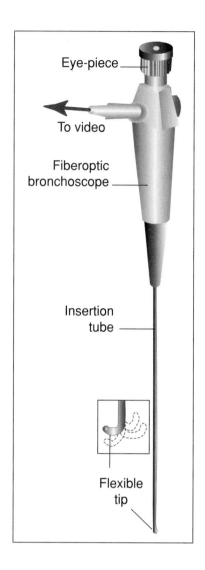

Eye-piece

To video

Fiberoptic
bronchoscope

Insertion
tube

Flexible
tip

Figure 64.3.
Flexible fiberoptic
laryngoscopes for pediatric
use.

cretions, which can make visualization of the airway anatomy more difficult.

After each use, the fiberoptic laryngoscope should be immediately cleansed with a detergent solution to prevent drying of secretions on the insertion tube. The laryngoscope is then sterilized according to the manufacturer's instructions. Not surprisingly, inadequate cleaning and sterilization have been demonstrated to cause transmission of a variety of infectious agents among patients (20, 21).

Special care must be taken when wiping the insertion tube. Grasping the laryngoscope with a gauze and pulling vigorously causes the material covering the fiberoptic bundles to bunch at the tip, making subsequent passage difficult. In addition, bending the insertion tube excessively can cause breakage of the glass bundles. Disposable sheaths for sin-

gle use are available from commercial suppliers for fiberoptic laryngoscopes.

PROCEDURE

Indirect laryngoscopy offers the advantage of providing a wide panoramic view which is not achievable with direct techniques. This procedure, however, requires significant cooperation from the patient and ongoing practice by the clinician to be successful. As mentioned, indirect laryngoscopy is unsuitable for neonates, infants, and young children. Examination using the flexible fiberoptic laryngoscope is often better tolerated by children of all age groups. With proper training and experience, any physician can become adept at performing a preliminary examination of

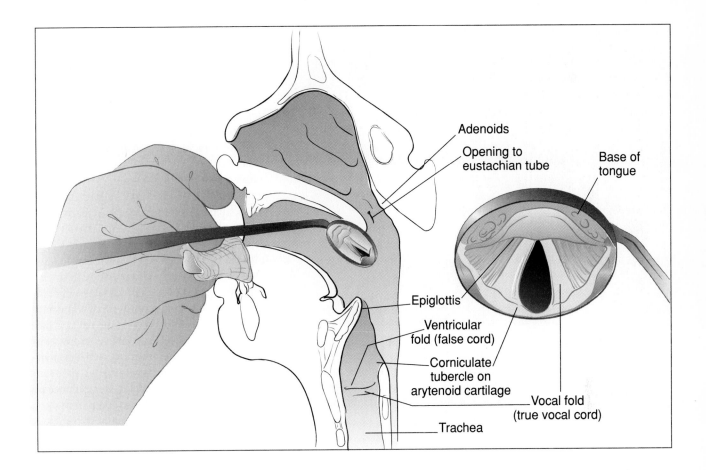

Adenoids

Opening to
eustachian tube

Base of
tongue

Epiglottis

Ventricular
fold (false cord)

Corniculate
tubercle on
arytenoid cartilage

Vocal fold
(true vocal cord)

Trachea

the nasopharynx, supraglottic region, and vocal cords using fiberoptic laryngoscopy. The most important point is that patients must be referred for follow-up evaluation by an otolaryngologist when necessary. With either technique, the physician should wear gloves and eye protection, as the patient may cough or vomit during the procedure.

Indirect Laryngoscopy

The patient should be seated, leaning forward, in the sniffing position, i.e., the head slightly extended (rotated) and the neck flexed. Spraying cetacaine or another topical anesthetic may be helpful in controlling the patient's gag reflex. If a head mirror is used to illuminate the airway, a strong light source should be positioned over the patient's shoulder, so that the light can be reflected from the mirror into the patient's mouth. For the physician who performs this technique less frequently, an electric headlight provides ex-

cellent illumination and is usually much easier to use. The laryngeal mirror should be warmed to prevent fogging. The temperature of the mirror is tested against the back of the clinician's hand before use to avoid burning the patient.

The patient is first instructed to breath in and out through the mouth during the entire procedure. This may be better understood if the child is periodically reminded to pant "just like a dog." Next the tongue is grasped with gauze and gently pulled forward. The clinician inserts the mirror into the patient's mouth and positions it over the back of the tongue (Fig. 64.4). Care must be taken to avoid contacting the tongue or posterior pharyngeal wall with the mirror, as this usually will induce gagging. The light source is directed onto the mirror and down the airway. The larynx and surrounding structures then can be visualized by tilting the mirror back and forth as necessary. Vocal cord function is initially assessed by observing as the patient says "EEEEE," which should cause the cords

Figure 64.4.
Indirect laryngoscopy.

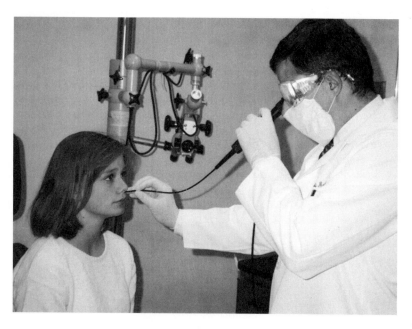

Figure 64.5.
Positioning for flexible fiberoptic laryngoscopy.

to adduct. The clinician then can ask the patient to hum a tune, which results in adduction and abduction of the cords throughout their full range of motion.

Direct Laryngoscopy with an Angled Telescope

The patient is positioned in the same manner as with the indirect technique. The angled telescope is passed into the patient's mouth until the tip is over the base of the tongue. As with using an angled mirror, the best way to prevent gagging and emesis is by avoiding inadvertent contact with the tongue and posterior pharynx. For this reason, the clinician should not look through the eyepiece until the instrument is in the proper examination position. The angled telescope should rest on the back of the clinician's hand to maintain a steady position. The larynx and hypopharynx can then be viewed. Vocal cord function is assessed as with indirect laryngoscopy.

Direct Laryngoscopy with a Flexible Fiberoptic Laryngoscope

The clinician first should examine the patient's nose to determine the more patent side,

which is done by simply occluding each nostril in turn to identify any obstruction to air flow. The laryngoscope is passed on the more patent side. If the nasal cavity is a primary area of interest, the clinician will insert the laryngoscope into both nares during the examination.

The topical vasoconstrictor and anesthetic are applied to one or both nares using cotton pledgets or by spraying. As mentioned previously, 1% ephedrine sulfate and 2% pontocaine hydrochloride are effective for this purpose. The clinician should wait 5 to 10 minutes after application to achieve the full effects of these agents. Most local anesthetics are bitter, and the patient often will complain of the taste. The clinician should explain that it is not harmful to swallow any medicine that accumulates in the back of the patient's throat. It also is advisable to warn the patient that the resulting sensation of numbness may make swallowing or even breathing seem more difficult. Reassurance is all that is necessary for these complaints.

A cooperative patient can be positioned sitting upright with the neck flexed and the head slightly extended (rotated), similar to indirect laryngoscopy (Fig. 64.5). As mentioned previously, infants and younger children should be supine and appropriately restrained. Before inserting the fiberoptic laryngoscope, the clinician should view an object through the eyepiece to ensure that the tip is clean and the focal length is correct. The tip also should be manipulated to determine how much force is needed to move it a given amount. As mentioned, great care must be taken to not bend the laryngoscope excessively, as this can cause the fiberoptic bundles to break. While viewing through the eyepiece, the clinician inserts the fiberoptic laryngoscope along the floor of the nasal cavity parallel to the septum and medial to the inferior turbinate (Fig. 64.6). Importantly, the laryngoscope should never be advanced blindly, because this increases the likelihood of causing injury to the nasal or pharyngeal mucosa. If the landmarks are lost during insertion, the clinician should withdraw the laryngoscope until recognizable structures are again seen. Likewise, if the tip of the laryngoscope fogs, the patient should be instructed to breathe in and out through the mouth until the image reappears. The laryn-

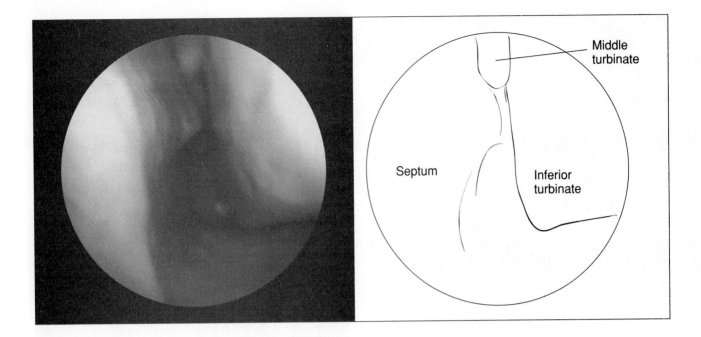

goscope then can be advanced once again under direct visualization. As appropriate, the clinician should carefully examine the posterior nasal cavity to identify adenoid hypertrophy (Fig. 64.7), the orifice of the eustachian tube, nasal polyps, and/or the presence of an intranasal foreign body.

As the posterior nasal cavity is approached, the tip of the laryngoscope should be deflected inferiorly so that it can be passed atraumatically over the posterior aspect of the soft palate. Injury to the posterior pharyngeal wall can be avoided by maintaining direct visualization at all times and never using excessive force to advance the laryngoscope. Once this turn is negotiated, the base of the tongue will come into view. By rotating the laryngoscope from side to side, the clinician also can identify the medial aspect of each tonsil. The laryngoscope is then further advanced until the larynx can be fully visualized (Fig. 64.8). As mentioned previously, the clinician must be careful to avoid contacting the vocal cords with the tip of the laryn-

Figure 64.6.
View of the nasal cavity with fiberoptic laryngoscopy.

Figure 64.7.
Adenoid hypertrophy.

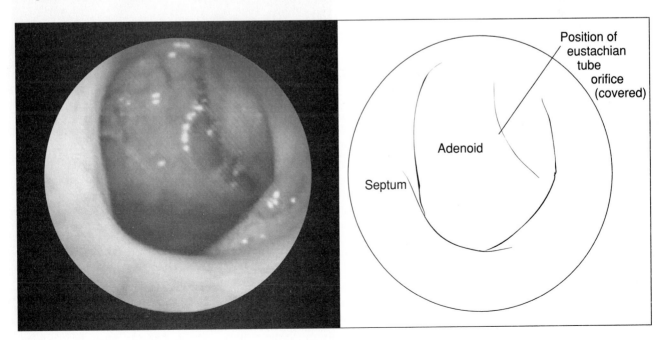

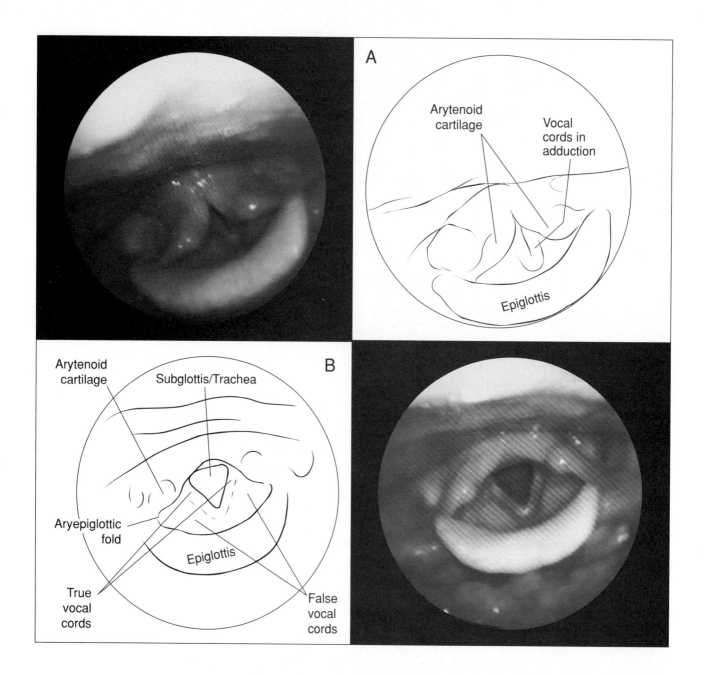

Figure 64.8.
View of the larynx with
fiberoptic laryngoscopy.
A. Adduction of vocal
cords
B. Abduction of vocal
cords.

**Chapter 64
Diagnostic
Laryngoscopic
Procedures**

goscope, as this can precipitate laryngospasm. Vocal cord function is assessed by having the patient say "EEEEE" and whistle (or hum) a tune as with indirect laryngoscopy. With younger children who are unable to cooperate, the cords are observed for any abnormal movement as the patient phonates or cries. Polyps or other lesions of the vocal cords should be noted. In addition, the clinician should carefully examine the epiglottis and arytenoid cartilages. Because a complete view of the entire supraglottic region is not obtainable in one field of vision, the clinician must systematically rotate the laryngoscope while deflecting the tip to visualize all the important structures. Any edema, erythema, bleeding, or disruption of the mucosa should be noted. All areas also must be examined to exclude the presence of a foreign body.

COMPLICATIONS

Although indirect and direct laryngoscopy have proven to be safe when used appropriately, certain hazards must be avoided.

Proper patient selection is one of the most important factors in reducing the risk of complications. Any child with severe respiratory distress is not a suitable candidate for diagnostic laryngoscopy outside the operating room. Conditions such as epiglottitis, high grade airway obstruction due to a foreign body, or an expanding hematoma in the supraglottic region can cause a tenuous respiratory status. Agitating a child in this situation may lead to full respiratory arrest. Generally, diagnostic laryngoscopy in the outpatient setting should only be performed on patients who are well-appearing with no airway compromise.

Complications that are less severe but are more frequently encountered relate to problems with technique. Mucosal injuries of the airway can result when a fiberoptic laryngoscope is passed blindly, (i.e., without maintaining direct visualization through the eyepiece). As with blind nasal passage of an endotracheal tube, abrasions and lacerations of the soft tissues can occur at multiple sites, typically the nasal turbinates, adenoids, and posterior pharynx. Bleeding induced by this type of injury often makes further examination impossible. If airway anesthesia is inadequate or the clinician inadvertently contacts the posterior hypopharynx with an instrument, the patient may cough, gag, or vomit. Although this does not generally lead to any serious consequences as the patient's normal airway reflexes are preserved, subsequent examinations of a previously cooperative child who has been badly gagged are likely to be more difficult.

As mentioned previously, one significant complication related to poor technique is laryngospasm due to accidental passage of a fiberoptic laryngoscope below the level of the vocal cords. Care must therefore be taken to advance the laryngoscope only as far as necessary to fully visualize the larynx and supraglottic region. Although a rare occurrence, the risk of laryngospasm requires that all equipment necessary for advanced airway interventions must be available whenever this procedure is performed.

Assuming that patients are selected appropriately, the risk of complications associated with indirect and direct laryngoscopy can be minimized if the clinician is properly trained and routinely practices these procedures on an ongoing basis. Periodically examining colleagues or other normal subjects is an excellent way to maintain and enhance necessary skills. Clearly, familiarity with the normal anatomy is key to making any meaningful clinical decisions. In addition, honestly explaining what should be expected to older children and adolescents in a calm and unhurried manner often will reduce the likelihood of complications. Because diagnostic laryngoscopy requires significant cooperation, gaining the trust and compliance of a pediatric patient is usually the most important factor in obtaining a successful and atraumatic examination.

SUMMARY: DIAGNOSTIC LARYNGOSCOPY USING A FLEXIBLE FIBEROPTIC LARYNGOSCOPE

1. Apply topical vasoconstrictor and anesthetic to one or both nares using cotton pledgets or a spray device—1% ephedrine sulfate and 2% pontocaine hydrochloride is a good combination. Allow 5 to 10 minutes to achieve full effects of these agents.
2. Before inserting fiberoptic laryngoscope, view an object through eyepiece to ensure that tip is clean and focal length is correct
3. Deflect tip back and forth using control lever on head of laryngoscope to determine force necessary to move tip a given amount
4. While viewing through eyepiece, insert fiberoptic laryngoscope along floor of nasal cavity parallel to septum and medial to inferior turbinate. Examine entire nasal cavity, noting adenoid size, patency of eustachian tube orifice, nasal polyps, etc.
5. At posterior nasal cavity, deflect tip of fiberoptic laryngoscope inferiorly and advance tip around posterior aspect of soft palate. Landmarks at this point are base of tongue and medial aspect of each tonsil.
6. Advance laryngoscope into supraglottic region and carefully examine all important structures. Deflect tip and rotate laryngoscope in a systematic fashion to obtain a complete view of area. Note any abnormal lesions, injuries, presence of a foreign body, etc.
7. Assess vocal cord function. With infants and younger children, observe movement of cords with phonation or crying. With older children and adolescents, have patient say "EEEEE" and whistle (or hum) a tune.

CLINICAL TIPS

1. Because indirect laryngoscopy with an angled mirror requires significant cooperation from the patient, this procedure is not appropriate for infants and younger children. These patients generally can be examined successfully using a flexible fiberoptic laryngoscope.
2. Diagnostic laryngoscopy should not be performed in the outpatient setting when the patient is in significant respiratory distress due to airway obstruction. In such cases, the patient should be transferred to the operating room where rigid bronchoscopy and emergent tracheostomy can be performed if necessary.
3. Significant adenoid hypertrophy, particularly when the orifice of the eustachian tube is occluded, warrants referral to an otolaryngologist.
4. Foreign bodies of the supraglottic region not identifiable on plain radiographs (e.g., a wooden splinter, fish bone) are commonly found using diagnostic laryngoscopy.
5. Inadvertently introducing a fiberoptic laryngoscope at or below the level of the vocal cords can in rare cases precipitate laryngospasm. Consequently, this procedure is contraindicated in situations when advanced airway management techniques would not be possible.

SUMMARY

Diagnostic laryngoscopy for pediatric patients of all ages may be performed in the outpatient setting by emergency physicians, pediatricians, and family physicians with proper training and experience. These techniques are performed to obtain a preliminary evaluation of patients with hoarseness, chronic nasal discharge, a suspected foreign body, and other common complaints. Referral to an otolaryngologist for a more definitive examination should be arranged when necessary. Indirect laryngoscopy gives a panoramic view of the larynx but requires practice and is not suitable for infants and younger children. Direct laryngoscopy with a flexible fiberoptic laryngoscope can be used to examine the nasal cavity, supraglottic region, and vocal cords in any patient age group. Although complications with these procedures are unlikely, good technique and proper patient selection are essential. Children with respiratory distress are not appropriate candidates for outpatient diagnostic laryngoscopy. A thorough knowledge of the anatomy, a gentle technique, and practice will allow the physician to successfully complete this examination.

REFERENCES

1. Swift AC, Rogers J. Vocal cord paralysis in children. J Laryngol Otol 1987; 101:169–171.
2. Grundfast KM, Harley E. Vocal cord paralysis. Otolaryngol Clin North Am 1989; 22:569–597.
3. McBride JT. Stridor in childhood. J Fam Pract 1984; 19:782–790.
4. Riley RH, Dally FG, Fisher PH. Fiberoptic techniques in the emergency department [letter]. N Z Med J 1991; 104:296.
5. Schafermeyer RW. Fiberoptic laryngoscopy in the emergency department. Am J Emerg Med 1984; 2: 160–163.
6. Handler SD. Direct laryngoscopy in children: rigid and flexible fiberoptic. Ear Nose Throat J 1995; 74: 100–104,106.
7. Hocutt Jr JE, Corey GA, Rodney WM. Nasolaryngoscopy for family physicians. Am Fam Physician 1990; 42:1257–1268.
8. Lancer JM, Jones AS. Flexible fiberoptic rhinolaryngoscopy. Results of 338 consecutive examinations. J Laryngol Otol 1985; 99:771–773.
9. Ransom JH, Kavel KK. Diagnostic fiberoptic rhinolaryngoscopy. Kans Med 1989; 90:105–108, 115.
10. Chait DH, Lotz WK. Successful pediatric examinations using nasoendoscopy. Laryngoscope 1990; 101:1016–1018.
11. Wang DY, Clement P, Kaufman L, Derde MP. Fiberoptic examination of the nasal cavity and nasopharynx in children. Acta Otorhinolaryngol Belg 1991; 45:323–329.
12. Weir N, Bassett I. Outpatient fiberoptic nasolaryngoscopy and videostroboscopy. J R Soc Med 1987; 80:299–300.
13. Selkin SG. Clinical use of the pediatric flexible fiberscope. Int J Pediatr Otorhinolaryngol 1985; 10: 75–80.
14. Hawkins DB, Clark RW. Flexible laryngoscopy in neonates, infants, and young children. Ann Otol Rhinol Laryngol 1987; 96:81–85.
15. Wood RE, Postma D. Endoscopy of the airway in infants and children. J Pediatr 1988; 112:1–6.
16. Selner JC. Concepts and clinical application of fiberoptic examination of the upper airway. Clin Rev Allergy 1988; 6:303–320.
17. Holinger LD. Diagnostic endoscopy of the pediatric airway. Laryngoscope 1989; 99:346–348.
18. McDonald RJ. Flexible fiberoptic bronchoscopy in children. West J Med 1990; 153:646–647.
19. Bailey BJ, Strunk CL, Jones JK. Methods of examination. In: Bluestone CD, Stool SEW, eds. Pediatric otolaryngology. 2nd ed. Philadelphia: WB Saunders, 1990.
20. Wheeler PW, Lancaster D, Kaiser AB. Bronchopulmonary cross colonization and infection related to mycobacterial contamination of suction valves of bronchoscopes. J Infect Dis 1989; 159:954–958.
21. Hanson PJV, Jeffries DF, Batten JC, Collins JV. Infection control revisited: dilemma facing today's bronchoscopists. Br Med J 1988; 297:185–187.

DENTAL PROCEDURES

Section Editor: John Loiselle

OROFACIAL ANESTHESIA TECHNIQUES

Zach Kassutto and Mark L. Helpin

INTRODUCTION

Orofacial nerve blocks and infiltrations can be used for regional anesthesia in the event of orofacial pathologies such as dental caries, tooth and alveolar fractures, or soft tissue trauma to the lower half of the face. These procedures are most commonly performed by dentists and oral surgeons in the outpatient setting. Patients requiring these types of procedures also are seen regularly in the emergency department (ED). Given the numerous approaches and types of procedures available, this chapter will review only those procedures that have the greatest utility, success rate, and the lowest rate of complications.

When used for the relief of preexisting pain, these procedures are temporizing only. Using a longer-acting anesthetic agent can extend their effect. These procedures can be performed successfully in children of any age. In younger and uncooperative children, the procedures are more difficult to carry out. Adjuncts to the procedure include emotional preparation and support (Chapter 34), conscious sedation (Chapter 35), appropriate restraint (Chapter 3), and mucosal topical anesthetics. Honesty and sincerity also must be used, as they are perhaps the most important preparation for any procedure with pediatric patients.

ANATOMY AND PHYSIOLOGY

Orofacial anesthesia blocks transmission of painful stimuli via one or several afferent branches of the 5th cranial (trigeminal) nerve. Three primary divisions of the 5th cranial on each side of the face are designated as V_1, V_2 and V_3 (Fig. 65.1).

V_1, the ophthalmic division, supplies structures above the mouth. V_2, or the maxillary division, as its name suggests, supplies sensory fibers to the various structures in and around the maxilla. These include all the maxillary teeth and their associated gingivae, the entire palate and tissues posterior to this including the tonsilar region, the lower eyelid, the side of the nose, the upper lip, and the mucous membranes of most of the nasal cavity. The palatine branches (greater, lesser, and nasopalatine nerves) branch off before the nerve enters the infraorbital canal. These nerves innervate the soft tissue structures of the posterior mouth and the throat.

The posterior superior, middle superior, and anterior superior alveolar nerves are the next branches of V_2. The posterior superior alveolar nerve branches off before entering the infraorbital canal, and innervates the maxillary sinus and the maxillary molars and their gingivae. The middle superior and anterior superior alveolar nerves separate from

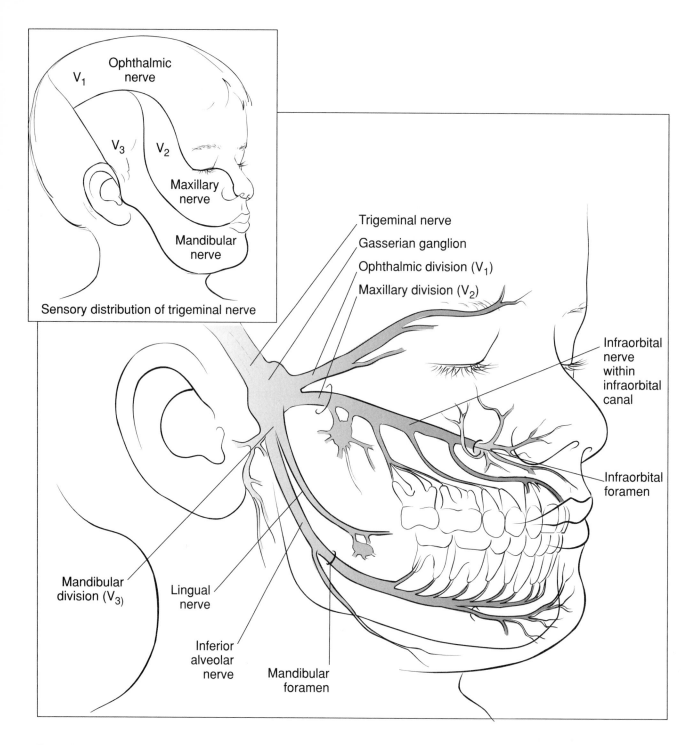

Labels in the inset box:
Ophthalmic nerve — V_1
V_3 — V_2
Maxillary nerve
Mandibular nerve
Sensory distribution of trigeminal nerve

Labels in the main figure:
Trigeminal nerve
Gasserian ganglion
Ophthalmic division (V_1)
Maxillary division (V_2)
Infraorbital nerve within infraorbital canal
Infraorbital foramen
Mandibular division (V_3)
Lingual nerve
Inferior alveolar nerve
Mandibular foramen

Figure 65.1.
Anatomic and sensory distributions of the trigeminal nerve.

**Chapter 65
Orofacial Anesthesia
Techniques**

the maxillary nerve trunk as it traverses the infraorbital canal (where it is called the infraorbital nerve). Together, these nerves supply the anterior maxillary teeth and their associated structures as far posterior as the maxillary premolars or primary molars. The infraorbital nerve exits the skull via the infraorbital foramen and its terminal branches innervate the lower eyelid, the ala of the nose, and the upper lip. Anesthetic applied at the infraorbital foramen allows repair of the alae or upper lip without the swelling associated with direct infiltration.

The mandibular division, or V_3, supplies motor innervation to the muscles of mastication and sensory fibers to the mandible. The inferior alveolar nerve is the largest branch of the mandibular nerve. It enters the mandible via the mandibular foramen which is located on the internal surface of the ramus. It then traverses the mandible through the mandibular canal where the nerve and its branches innervate all the teeth of the mandible on each respective side. The lingual nerve is an early branch of the mandibular division. This branch travels with the inferior alveolar nerve until it enters the mandibular canal. Then the lingual nerve enters the base of the tongue. There it supplies sensory fibers to the anterior two-thirds of the tongue, the floor of the mouth, and the lingual aspect of the mandibular gingivae. Anesthetic applied near the mandibular foramen will usually anesthetize both the lingual and inferior alveolar nerves.

The alveolar bone of the pediatric patient is usually less dense than that of the adult. This advantage allows for more rapid and complete dissemination of the anesthetic solution when infiltration anesthesia is used (1, 2).

INDICATIONS

Orofacial anesthesia can be used for pain relief (e.g., dental abscess or caries) or for the prevention of pain (e.g., tooth extraction, facial and/or oral laceration repair, facial and/or dental abscess drainage). Procedures can further be classified as nerve blocks or direct infiltration.

Nerve blocks allow the use of small amounts of anesthetic applied to a small area for anesthesia of larger areas. In this way manipulation of infected tissues can be avoided and anatomical landmarks are not distorted. An example is using an infraorbital nerve block for repair of the vermilion border in upper lip lacerations. Nerve blocks also decrease the risks of using larger amounts of anesthetic, and avoid the need for injection of anesthetic in areas that are more susceptible to pain. Infiltration anesthesia is used when smaller areas of anesthesia are needed. Examples include tooth pain from caries or isolated tooth injury from trauma. Nerve blocks and infiltrate anesthesia for other parts of the body are described in Chapters 37 and 58.

Need for consultation depends on the patient's exact injury and the practice at a given institution. Possible consultants include dentists, oral surgeons, otorhinolaryngologists, or plastic surgeons. Consultation should be considered for cases involving mandibular fractures, nerve injury from trauma, difficulty achieving anesthesia, or any contraindications to the procedure.

Absolute contraindications to the procedures in this chapter include known allergy to the anesthetic agent and grossly distorted anatomical landmarks. Injecting through infected tissue (e.g., tooth abscess) is a relative contraindication (2). Local anesthetics are less effective when applied in regions of inflammation (3). Manipulating a needle through infected tissues also increases the risk of spreading the infection to other adjacent areas or into the blood stream. Whenever possible, a nerve block (as opposed to direct infiltration) should be used in this type of situation.

EQUIPMENT

Equipment needed for orofacial anesthesia is shown in Table 65.1. A large-bore suction device such as a Yankauer device is preferred to remove any secretions, blood, or emesis (see Chapter 13). Orofacial anesthesia can be performed using medical syringes and needles commonly available in the ED, but is more easily accomplished using dental equipment specifically designed for this task. i.e., an aspirating dental syringe that uses cartridges (carpules) of anesthetic solution and disposable needles (4). This type of syringe affords the physician a better grasp of the instrument and the ability to aspirate with the same hand that is holding the syringe. This frees the other hand to hold, stabilize, and retract the involved tissues.

Various suggestions have been made as to the best sized needle to use for the procedure. Large bore needles make the procedure unduly painful and could compromise exact

Table 65.1.
Equipment for Orafacial Anesthesia

1 × 1 sterile gauze pads
Cotton-tipped applicators
Suction
Supplies for universal precautions (latex gloves, protective eye wear, surgical mask, and moisture-repellent gown)
Anesthetic agents
Sterile syringe and needle
Resuscitation equipment

placement of the needle tip. Narrower needles make aspiration more difficult and increase the risk of needle breakage. Some authorities believe that a needle smaller than 25 gauge may increase the risk of inadvertent intravascular injection (i.e., no blood on aspiration despite the needle being inside a vessel). Others believe that this risk is small, and that slow injection after aspirating further minimizes this risk. Most sources recommend a 27 gauge "short needle" (1 inch) for most infiltrations and blocks, and a 27 gauge "long needle" (1.25 inch) for older adolescents.

Orofacial anesthesia techniques in children differ from adults because of the smaller size of the skull and characteristics of the bone. In general, depth of needle insertion needs to be adjusted for the size of the child's anatomy. Relevant variations in size will be discussed under each procedure.

Commercial topical dental anesthetics are available in liquids, gels, ointments, and sprays. The most commonly used preparations contain benzocaine (e.g., Hurricane, a flavored preparation of 20% benzocaine). If a specific dental preparation is unavailable, 5 to 10% lidocaine or 20% benzocaine can be used. Less concentrated anesthetics usually prove to be ineffective (4).

The oral mucosa is supplied by a rich vascular network. Anesthetics applied topically may be absorbed into the systemic circulation. The dose of topical anesthetic, although often difficult to quantify, must be considered when calculating the overall dose of anesthetic that a patient receives. Benzocaine is the preferred agent because it has virtually no systemic absorption when applied topically (5). Anesthetic sprays are discouraged because they tend to cover larger areas than required for the procedure.

Many dental anesthetics are commercially available for injection in dental anesthetic carpules. These carpules each contain 1.8 mL of anesthetic and insert into standard dental aspirating syringes. They cannot be directly adapted for use with other injecting devices commonly available in EDs. The contents, however, can be drawn into a standard disposable syringe through the carpule's rubber stopper. Care must be taken to use sterile technique when doing this. The standard solution used by dentists is 2% lidocaine with epinephrine 1 : 100,000. In cases when a prolonged effect is desired, longer-acting agents such as bupivacaine also are available. These agents are usually avoided for intraoral anesthesia when the oral mucosa or tongue may be involved (e.g., inferior alveolar block). This is especially important in preadolescent or developmentally delayed children who may self-inflict injury by biting their numbed oral tissues. Less commonly used agents include novocain, prilocaine, and etidocaine.

Anesthetics are available with or without vasoconstrictors. Most practitioners prefer using a vasoconstrictor (such as epinephrine 1:100,000 or 1:50,000) as it slows anesthetic absorption into the surrounding tissues. This allows injection of smaller doses of anesthetic, prolongs the anesthetic effect, and provides for hemostasis. For patients in whom vasoconstrictors are contraindicated (as with certain cardiac anomalies or conduction abnormalities), 3% mepivacaine without epinephrine is the agent of choice. Some dentists advocate warming anesthetic solutions to body temperature before injection to make the injection less painful and anesthesia onset more rapid.

Standard cardiopulmonary resuscitation equipment should be readily available in the unlikely event of an adverse reaction to the medications or procedure.

PROCEDURE

Topical anesthesia of mucous membranes can reduce the pain associated with orofacial anesthesia, and should be considered before any intraoral injection. In the apprehensive patient, the physician must weigh the extra time involved in undertaking this procedure versus the transient pain of passing a thin needle through the oral mucosa. Most topical anesthetics are pleasant tasting, but if unpleasant, can increase the patient's apprehension (5).

First, the area to be injected must be dried with gauze. The anesthetic is applied to a cotton-tipped swab or a small piece of cotton or gauze. The dose of topical anesthetic should be included in calculating the total anesthetic dose that the patient receives. Application of the anesthetic to the mucosa is limited to the site where the needle is expected to pass. According to the manufacturer topical anesthesia should occur within 15 to 30 seconds of using 20% benzocaine. Others have suggested that it takes at least 2 minutes for this drug to exert its effect (2). Application of the anesthetic to the tongue should be avoided, as this may result in excessive salivation. Before injection, any residual topical anesthetic should be removed with gauze.

Infraorbital Nerve Block

An effective infraorbital nerve block places local anesthetic at the infraorbital foramen. This nerve block should effectively anesthetize the anterior and middle superior alveolar nerves which innervate the anterior maxillary teeth. Also anesthetized are the terminal branches of the infraorbital nerve which innervate the upper lip, the nasal alae, and the lower eyelid (Fig. 65.1.B). This block is especially useful for repair of facial lacerations. It avoids the distortion of anatomy usually associated with direct infiltration of the soft facial tissues. This block can be performed by either an extraoral or an intraoral approach. For the sake of clarity, only the latter technique will be described here.

The physician and the patient must be seated comfortably with bright overhead lighting that can be directed into the oral cavity. Ideally the patient sits semi-reclined in a dental chair that supports the head and can tilt the maxillary occlusal plane to about 45° relative to the floor. This position allows for control of the head to reduce movement and is advantageous should the patient have a vasovagal reaction (2). The physician is seated so as to be above the patient's mouth and to have easy access to the equipment. Whenever possible, the help of an assistant who is familiar with the equipment and the procedure should be obtained. If a dental chair is unavailable, the above positioning can be attained with a cooperative patient using an adjustable reclining stretcher. In younger or uncooperative children, the patient should be restrained with a papoose board or bed sheet. The procedure can then be carried out with the patient supine on a stretcher. Ideally, the clinician should be positioned on the side of the patient that will be anesthetized.

The patient's supraorbital and infraorbital notches are palpated. An imaginary line between these two landmarks should cross the patient's pupil (6) (Fig. 65.2.A). Further inferiorly, this line will cross the bicuspid teeth and the mental foramen. About 0.5 cm inferior to the infraorbital notch, a shallow depression can be palpated. The infraorbital foramen lies within this depression. One finger is used to mark the site of the foramen while the other fingers of the same hand retract the lip. The exact position of the physician's hand will depend on his or her handedness and the side of the patient on which the physician is standing. The foramen can be marked with either the thumb or middle finger. In either case the lip is retracted with the index finger. Topical mucosal anesthesia can be applied as previously described. The syringe is best held in the dominant hand. The needle is inserted in the mucolabial fold (where the mucosal aspect of the upper lip meets the maxillary bone) just anterior to the apex of the first premolar tooth. The needle tip should be advanced along the axis of the tooth toward the infraorbital foramen. The digit over the foramen helps direct the needle tip into contact with the bone at the opening of the foramen (Fig. 65.2.B). Advancing the needle into the foramen should be avoided, as this may damage the nerve (3). If the patient complains of paresthesias before the injection of anesthetic, the needle has entered the nerve and must be withdrawn slightly. After aspirating to exclude intravascular needle placement, about 1 to 2 mL of anesthetic is slowly deposited. The needle should be advanced no more than 0.5 to 0.75 inch (1 to 2 cm) from the insertion point. It is important to limit the depth of needle insertion and to mark the infraorbital foramen with a digit, as these precautions prevent accidental entrance of the needle into the orbital cavity. If the location of the needle tip is uncertain, the needle should be withdrawn and insertion reattempted.

If the needle is angled excessively toward the skull, the malar eminence will prevent the advancement of the needle to the foramen. If this occurs, a less acute angle of needle insertion should be used.

The anesthetic requires about 5 minutes to take effect. Effective anesthesia is confirmed by a subjective feeling of numbness or

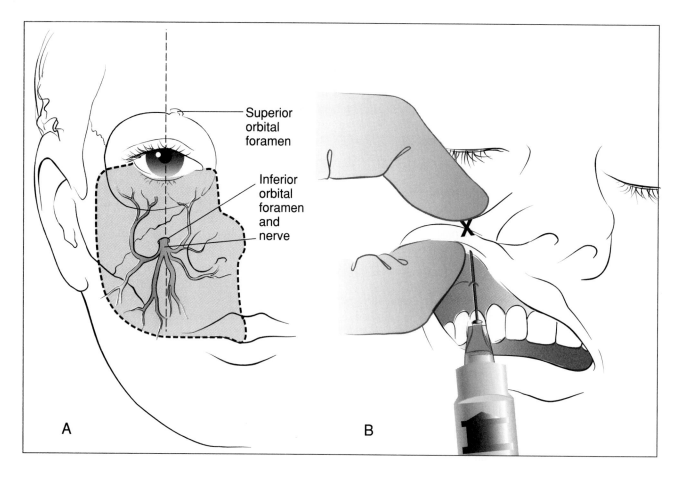

Figure 65.2.
A. Anatomic landmarks
and needle position for
infraorbital nerve block.
B. Localization of
infraorbital nerve.

tingling, and absence of pain with manipulation of the targeted tissues.

Inferior Alveolar Nerve Block

The inferior alveolar nerve block is difficult to perform successfully without practice. Even in the most experienced hands, failure rate is approximately 15%. Failures are mostly the result of improper technique. Anatomical variation and accessory innervation play less of a role. It is recommended that this technique be practiced initially under experienced supervision.

A well-placed inferior alveolar nerve block eliminates pain sensation from all the mandibular teeth, as well as the skin of the chin and lower lip on the side of the block. Because of its proximity, the lingual nerve is almost always anesthetized when attempting a block of the inferior alveolar nerve. This results in anesthesia to the tongue on the side of the block. The buccal mucosa also may be

anesthetized by blocking the long buccal nerve which lies just lateral to the lingual nerve.

The goal of this block is to place the anesthetic in the mandibular sulcus, the notch that funnels into the mandibular foramen. This is where the inferior alveolar nerve enters the mandible. The location of these structures is best approximated by conceptualizing the inner surface of the mandibular ramus roughly as a rectangle (Fig. 65.3.A). The target site for injection is the intersection of two imaginary lines. The horizontal line is identified relative to the occlusal plane of the teeth or relative to the deepest portion of the anterior aspect of the ramus of the mandible. This depression is sometimes called the coronoid notch. The vertical line is at the midpoint of the rectangle and is approximated by the midpoint between two fingers grasping the ramus from either side. To identify the coronoid notch, the ramus of the mandible is clasped between the thumb and index fingers. One finger grasps the extraoral posterior ramus while the other palpates the intraoral anterior

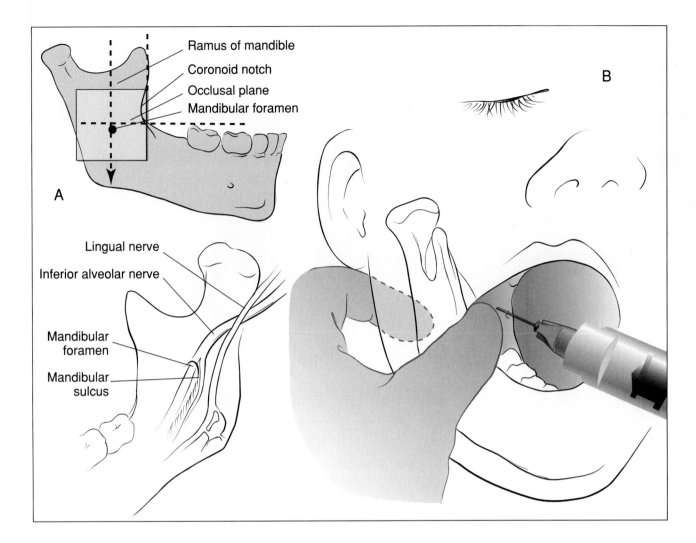

Figure 65.3.
A. Localization of inferior alveolar nerve.
B. Hand and needle positions for inferior alveolar nerve block.

ramus. The intraoral digit slides up and down the anterior border of the ramus of the mandible. The deepest area is the coronoid notch. A horizontal line through the middle of the coronoid notch should transect the mandibular sulcus. The same digit that marks the coronoid notch is used to retract the soft tissues of the cheek outwardly, thus exposing the injection site. The tip of the intraoral digit should remain in contact with the coronoid notch. To confirm the horizontal position of the mandibular foramen, the clinician should note its location relative to the occlusal plane. In children, the mandibular foramen is located below the occlusal plane of the primary teeth. Toward adulthood its location rises to several millimeters above the occlusal plane (1, 3, 5). No age-related difference is found in the anterior-to-posterior location of the foramen.

The patient is positioned and restrained as previously described. Topical anesthesia is applied and maximal exposure is gained by having the patient open his or her mouth as wide as possible. The syringe is held with the dominant hand and the injection site is approached from the opposite side of the patient's mouth (Fig. 65.3.B). The barrel of the syringe should lie over the primary molars of the opposite side of the mouth. The needle should be directed slightly below the occlusal plane of the mandibular teeth in children and at the occlusal plane in older adolescents and adults. The needle is inserted at a point that bisects the coronoid notch and is midway between the intraoral and extraoral digits that are grasping the mandible. The needle is advanced gently until it contacts the bony surface of the inner aspect of the mandible. Penetration depth should be about 15 mm, although this may vary from patient to patient. This site should closely approximate the mandibular sulcus, where the inferior alveolar nerve enters the mandible (Fig.

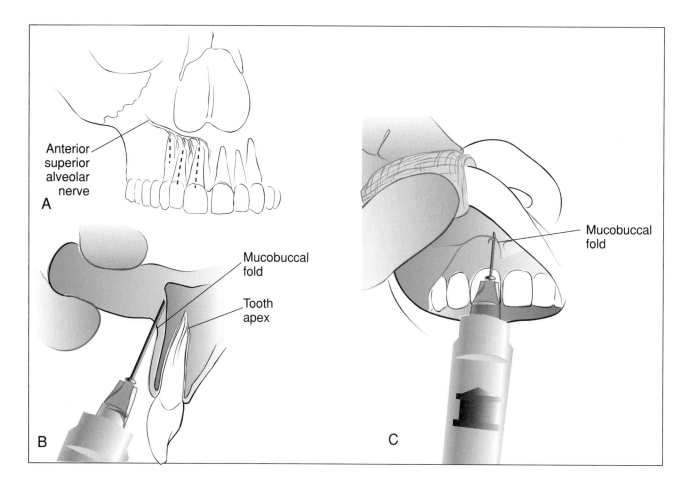

Figure 65.4.
Supraperiosteal infiltration.
A. Nerve supply of maxillary teeth.
B. Needle insertion at the mucobuccal fold allows deposition of anesthesia close to the tooth apex.
C. Minimal depth of needle insertion (about 2 mm) is required for the anterior primary maxillary teeth.

65.3.C). The needle is withdrawn slightly (about 1 mm). Intravascular needle placement is excluded by aspirating, and then up to 1.8 mL of anesthetic (or maximum dose based on patient's weight) is injected over 30 to 60 seconds. Injecting more rapidly may cause unnecessary pain. If the patient complains of paresthesias before the injection of anesthetic, the needle has entered the nerve and must be withdrawn slightly.

Approximately 5 minutes is necessary for complete anesthetic effect. Effective anesthesia is confirmed by a subjective feeling of numbness or tingling, and absence of pain with manipulation of the lower lip on the side of the injection.

Infiltration Anesthesia (Supraperiosteal Infiltration)

Using infiltration technique, anesthetic is deposited near the periosteum of the bone that supports a given tooth. Solution then diffuses through the periosteum and underlying bone and contacts the nerve supplying that tooth (Fig. 65.4.A). The maxillary bone remains relatively porous throughout life thus allowing easy permeability of anesthetic. The mandibular bone is more dense and less permeable to anesthetic. As a result of these characteristics, this procedure is limited in adults to anesthesia of maxillary teeth. In children, the mandible is less dense and therefore allows for the additional use of this technique for anesthesia of the anterior primary teeth or their surrounding gingivae.

The patient is positioned and topical anesthesia is applied as described previously. The lip in front of the involved tooth is grasped with a dry gauze to prevent slippage. The lip is retracted from the mouth to best expose the mucobuccal fold (Fig. 65.4.B). The bevel of the needle is oriented toward the bone to avoid scraping the periosteum with the needle point (2). The needle is introduced through the mucobuccal fold and advanced slowly along the anterior or buccal surface of the tooth toward its apex. The needle is inserted about 1 cm in a preschool child, and about 1.5

cm in a school-aged child (about half the length of a short dental needle). When anesthetizing the anterior primary maxillary teeth, the needle must be inserted only a short distance past the mucobuccal fold (2 mm at most), because the apices of primary teeth are at this level (Fig. 65.4.C). Resistance is felt on contact with the periosteum, and the needle should then be withdrawn slightly. Aspiration excludes intravascular needle placement; 1 to 2 mL of anesthetic is injected over about 1 minute. The anesthetic should be deposited close to the bone. Approximately 5 to 10 minutes is necessary for the full anesthetic effect. It should be remembered that time is required for the anesthetic to diffuse across the bone to the nerve. Anesthesia is confirmed by the absence of pain in the soft tissues surrounding the tooth.

Permanent central and lateral incisors pose a potential problem, in that they occasionally receive additional innervation from the opposite side. Anesthetic placed at the apex of the adjoining central incisor should anesthetize these accessory fibers. Alternatively, additional anesthetic can be placed just lateral or medial to the apex of the targeted tooth.

COMPLICATIONS

Anesthetic Reactions

A larger percentage of dental anesthesia morbidity and mortality occurs in children as compared with adults. This is probably related to overdosing of local anesthetic. Since the introduction of the amide local anesthetics (e.g., lidocaine, mepivicaine) (Table 65.2), allergic reactions have been less frequent. Ester anesthetics (e.g., Novocain) are more likely to cause allergic reactions and are therefore used infrequently.

As with other uses of local anesthetics, the total dose of drug administered must be monitored to avoid systemic toxicity. Care must be taken to avoid intravascular injection. Even with careful aspiration technique, inadvertent intravascular injection may occur and result in a systemic reaction. It is therefore essential that the total dose of anesthetic be measured for every pediatric patient. A maximum lidocaine dose of 2 mg/lb (about 4 mg/kg) is recommended (1). This dose applies to lidocaine with or without epinephrine. Percentage concentrations of anesthetics refer to gram percentage. A 2% concentration of anesthetic contains 2 g/100 mL or 20 mg/mL.

Dose-related toxicity involves the nervous and/or the cardiovascular systems. This can include hypotension, asystole, respiratory arrest, and seizure. Allergic reactions unrelated to dose are rare and include rash, urticaria, edema, or anaphylactoid reactions (3). Most local anesthetics have toxicities qualitatively comparable to those seen with lidocaine.

Anesthesia of Nontargeted Tissues

Soft Tissues

Orofacial anesthesia may result in lip, tongue, facial, or buccal mucosal numbness. This can result in inadvertent tissue damage by the patient's own teeth. This type of injury is more likely to occur in the young, or men-

Table 65.2.
Characteristics of Common Dental Anesthetics

Anesthetic Agent	Relative Toxicity*	Maximum Dose (mg/kg)	Maximum Total Dose (mg)	Class
Lidocaine 2%	2	4.0	300	Amide
Lidocaine 2% with epinephrine	2	4.0	500	Amide
Mepivacaine 3%	1.5	6.6	400	Amide
Mepivacaine 2% with epinephrine	1.5	6.6	400	Amide
Bupivacaine 0.5%	3 +	2	175	Amide
Bupivacaine 0.5% with epinephrine	3 +	2	225	Amide
Novocain 4%	1	20	1000	Ester**

* Refers to cardiac and neurologic toxicities.
** The esters have a much greater allergic potential than the amides.
Adapted from: Bennett CR. Monheim's local anesthesia and pain control in dental practice. 7th ed. St. Louis: CV Mosby, 1984.

**Chapter 65
Orofacial Anesthesia
Techniques**

tally or physically disabled. These injuries can be minimized by selecting shorter-acting anesthetic agents or anesthetics without vaso-constrictors. The patient and the family should be carefully instructed to avoid solid foods and hot substances by mouth for as long as anesthesia persists (5).

Other Nerves

Nontargeted nerves may inadvertently be anesthetized. Examples of this include inadvertent anesthesia of the facial nerve with attempted infraorbital nerve block (3) or anesthesia of the lingual nerve with inferior alveolar nerve block.

Bleeding/Hematoma

Puncture or laceration of blood vessels by the needle tip is uncommon with proper technique. Clinically significant bleeding from application of dental anesthesia is rare (2). In the rare event that a blood vessel is entered, direct pressure should be applied to the site for 2 to 5 minutes. The patient and family should be instructed to watch for signs of soft tissue swelling as a result of extravasation of blood.

Infection

Like bleeding, infection is a theoretical concern that rarely occurs. Injecting through infected tissues, however, should be avoided. This may serve to spread the infection, and anesthesia may be less effective because of the low pH in infected areas.

Neuronal Damage

If the patient experiences paresthesia over the distribution of the targeted nerve before the injection of anesthetic, the needle tip is in the nerve. Anesthetic should not be injected at this point, as permanent nerve damage may result. The needle should be withdrawn 0.5 to 1.0 mm, and then the anesthetic is injected.

Needle Breakage

As with any procedure involving hypodermic needles, the needle has the potential to break

while still in the patient. Although this is a rare occurrence, care must be taken to properly restrain the patient to avoid sudden unexpected movements.

SUMMARY

Orofacial nerve blocks and anesthetic infiltrations are not commonly used in the pediatric emergency setting. When indicated, however, these nerve blocks allow for the temporary relief of pain, greater patient comfort, and improved outcomes with several orofacial procedures.

REFERENCES

1. Malamed SF. Handbook of local anesthesia. 3rd ed. St. Louis: CV Mosby, 1990.
2. Evers H, Haegerstam G. Introduction to dental local anaesthesia. 1st ed. Switzerland: Mediglobe SA, 1990.
3. Haglund J, Evers H. Local anaesthesia in dentistry. 9th ed. Sweden: Astra Lakemedel AB, 1988.
4. Roberts JR, Hedges JR. Clinical procedures in emergency medicine. 2nd ed. Philadelphia: WB Saunders, 1991.
5. McDonald RE, Avery DR. Dentistry for the child and adolescent. 5th ed. St. Louis: CV Mosby, 1988.
6. Brammer-Graham K. Local anesthesia and pain control: A modular approach (video handbook). Kansas City: Kansas City School of Dentistry, 1979.
7. Bennett CR. Monheim's local anesthesia and pain control in dental practice. 7th ed. St Louis: CV Mosby, 1984.

INCISION AND DRAINAGE OF A DENTAL ABSCESS

Elliott M. Harris[a]

INTRODUCTION

A dental abscess is an area of localized infection involving the structures surrounding the teeth. Often this becomes a fluctuant swelling that requires drainage to promote healing. Usually dental abscesses are seen in older children and are more likely to involve the permanent dentition. However, abscesses may be seen in younger patients with poor oral hygiene and carious teeth. Although the vast majority of cases are managed by a dentist or an oral surgeon, the emergency physician is occasionally called on to perform incision and drainage for patients with simple abscesses when referral is delayed. Emergency care will help speed the recovery process and provide some relief from pain. Further dental care will normally be needed once the infectious process subsides.

The most common types of dental abscesses include periapical and periodontal abscesses. The periapical abscess is by far the most common dental abscess in children and results from spread of infection or inflammation from the pulp to the periapical tissues via the apical foramen of the tooth. Periodontal abscesses, which involve the periodontal structures (such as the gingivae or periodontal ligament), are more common in adults and

are usually a complication of periodontal disease. When seen in children, periodontal abscesses are most often the result of a foreign body introduced into previously healthy periodontal tissue.

ANATOMY AND PHYSIOLOGY

The most common predisposing factor to formation of a dental abscess in children is the presence of caries. Once the carious process has extended through the hard structures of the tooth (the enamel and the dentin) and into the pulp cavity (Fig. 66.1), pulpal infection and/or inflammation occur. This process usually results in pulp necrosis. The inflammatory process then extends to the periapical tissues via the apical foramen, leading to the formation of a periapical abscess. Although caries is the most common predisposing factor, any other process that causes pulp necrosis (e.g., trauma) may lead to abscess formation.

Primary teeth have thinner enamel than permanent teeth, and therefore the pulp of the primary dentition has relatively less protection. In addition, because of a more abundant blood supply, the pulp of primary teeth tends to have a greater inflammatory response to injury. One advantage primary teeth have is that they are better at forming dentin beneath carious lesions. This provides some extra protection for the pulp in the face of the poor oral hygiene practiced by many children.

[a] Special thanks to Theodore C. Eckermann, Jr., DDS for his assistance in preparing this manuscript.

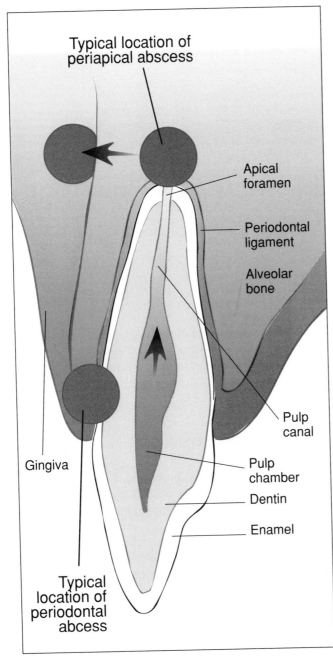

Figure 66.1.
Location of periodontal and periapical abscess.

plicated by spread of infection through the soft tissue planes of the head and neck via paths of least resistance. Infection of the orbit, maxillary sinuses, infratemporal fossa, sublingual and submandibular regions may result from untreated dental abscesses. Chronically draining fistulas also may occur. The buccinator muscle often serves as a barrier to the spread of infection to other areas of the head and neck. In children (who have a shorter facial height), the apices of the teeth—especially the permanent first molars, incisors, and canines—lie outside the muscle attachments. This leads to an increased risk of extraoral spread in younger patients.

Bacteria in dental abscesses tend to correspond to normal oral flora. Gram-positive cocci and anaerobes are the usual pathologic bacteria with *Streptococcus viridans* being the most frequently cultured organism. Penicillin is considered by most to be the drug of choice when antibiotics are required, with erythromycin as a second-line agent for patients allergic to penicillin.

INDICATIONS

All dental abscesses will require drainage at some point. The question is: when does this need to occur? The vast majority should be handled by expedient referral to a dentist or an oral surgeon. However, abscesses that have become fluctuant but are not yet draining in a stable patient, in whom referral might be delayed, may be treated in the emergency department (ED). Reasons the procedure would be desirable include relief of pain and prevention of spontaneous drainage with resulting formation of a chronic sinus tract. Even if incision and drainage are performed by an emergency physician, referral will still be required for definitive treatment and/or follow-up in virtually all patients.

With periapical abscesses, the pulp is almost always nonvital. This necessitates either tooth extraction or endodontic treatment. If the initial procedure permits sufficient drainage, definitive therapy may wait until the infection is under control. For periodontal abscesses, initial treatment may be definitive, but a retained foreign body may still need to be removed to prevent recurrence.

The only absolute contraindication to

As mentioned previously, periodontal abscesses in children, unlike in adults, are not associated with periodontal disease. Often a cause cannot be elucidated, but frequently they are due to impaction of a foreign body in the periodontal tissues. In contrast to periapical abscesses, periodontal abscesses are associated with vital teeth.

Dental abscesses may be found on either side of the gingiva, but lesions are found more frequently on the buccal aspect than on the lingual side. Such infections can be com-

performance of incision and drainage in the ED is a patient who cannot be adequately sedated and/or restrained so that the procedure can be performed safely. Such patients may require general anesthesia to perform the operation and thus are not amenable to treatment in the emergency setting. Relative contraindications to the procedure are patient toxicity and nonfluctuant lesions. The emergency physician needs to determine the risks versus the benefits of proceeding in these situations.

EQUIPMENT

1% lidocaine

3 or 5 mL syringe for anesthetic administration

25-gauge needle

20-gauge angiocath and 10-mL syringe (wound irrigation)

Saline for irrigation

Scalpel with No. 11 blade (may substitute No. 15 blade if preferred)

Small, curved hemostat

10 2 × 2 gauze sponges

Forceps (without teeth)

Suction tip connected to suction

Culture swab

Bite block or mouth prop for uncooperative patients

Monitoring equipment (if sedation is to be used)

Plain gauze or petroleum gauze

Optional equipment (if drain is to be placed):
    T-drain (T-shaped latex drain), small Penrose drain
    Suture kit
    3.0 nonabsorbable (silk) suture

PROCEDURE

Anesthesia is difficult to achieve in an area of infection due to the acidic nature of pus. Liberal application of a topical anesthetic such as benzocaine may help. In many cases a regional block (Chapter 65) may be more effective, but usually the procedure can be accomplished with local infiltration. A topical disinfectant such as chlorhexidine may be used, but this practice is rare. Infiltration into the buccogingival fold or circumferential to the lesion should be accomplished with lidocaine (Fig. 66.2.A). This should be done slowly to minimize patient discomfort. The anesthetic requires several minutes to work. The level of anesthesia should be tested before proceeding.

For uncooperative patients it may be necessary to use either a bite block (a rubber block that is placed between the molars) or a mouth prop (an adjustable metal prop). As this is usually a relatively short procedure, these items are needed infrequently once anesthesia is established. The physician needs only to visualize the lesion. Lip retraction is usually of little added benefit.

With the scalpel blade perpendicular to the bone, a horizontal incision made through the area of fluctuance. The incision should extend down to the level of the alveolar bone if dealing with a periapical abscess (Fig. 66.2.B and C), and should be long enough to allow proper drainage without premature closure. Entry into the abscess cavity is sufficient for periodontal lesions. Gauze sponges or suction should be readily available to remove the pus to avoid the possibility of aspiration. The incision should be widely opened by dissection using the hemostat along the abscess tract. For periapical infections, the dissection should proceed through the bone to the periapical area to allow drainage of the source of infection (Fig. 66.2.D). A culture should be obtained and the wound thoroughly irrigated with saline through a 20-gauge angiocath. Lidocaine may be added to the irrigation solution to decrease sensitivity if desired.

Although most dental texts recommend using a drain, many dentists feel this may not be necessary in all cases. Using a drain tends to be reserved for very extensive abscesses or those with extraoral spread (e.g., those with periorbital or malar swelling). The wound can be packed with either iodoform or petroleum gauze which should be changed within 24 to 48 hours postprocedure. If a latex drain is to be used, it will need to be sutured in place to prevent dislodgment. A single stitch to the gingival surface is generally sufficient. The drain should remain in place for 24 to 48 hours.

The patient should be started on a 5-day course of systemic antibiotics (penicillin, erythromycin) after the procedure. A longer course may be needed if the patient has systemic signs of illness. Local care consists of warm water rinses every 4 hours for 1 day.

Figure 66.2.
Incision and drainage of a
periapical abscess.
A. External appearance of
a periapical abscess.
B., C. Incision of a
periapical abscess.
D. Dissection along abscess
tract.

SUMMARY
1. Provide sedation when
   necessary
2. Apply topical anesthe-
   sia followed by local
   infiltrative anesthesia
   or regional nerve block
3. Make horizontal inci-
   sion through area of
   fluctuance; have suc-
   tion or gauze sponge
   ready to catch any pus
   and extend incision to
   bone for periapical abscess
4. Widen incision with
   hemostat; dissect
   through bone for peri-
   apical abscess when
   possible
5. Irrigate wound with
   saline through a 20-
   gauge angiocath
6. Place drain or packing
   (if desired); suture
   drain into place
7. Begin 5-day course of
   oral antibiotics
8. Encourage warm water
   rinses for first 24 hours
9. Refer for dental fol-
   low-up at 24 to 48
   hours

Chapter 66
Incision and Drainage
of a Dental Abscess

728

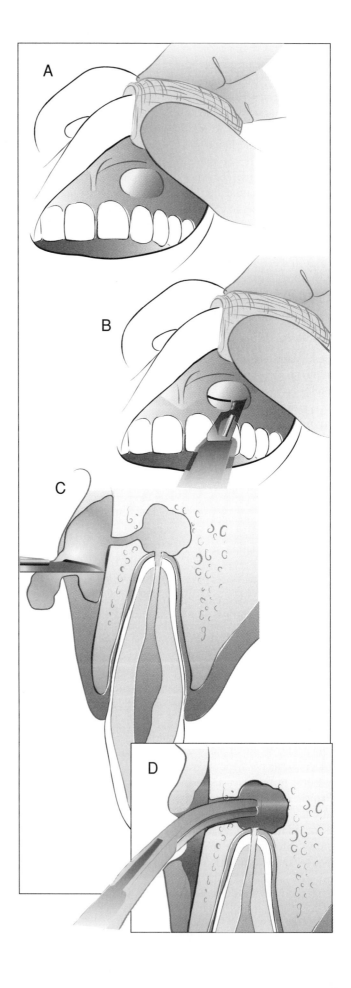

Dental follow-up will be needed in 24 to 48 hours for drain removal (if placed) and more definitive care.

COMPLICATIONS

As with any intraoral procedure, the risk of bacteremia is present. Although for most patients this is rarely a problem, the American Heart Association guidelines should be followed for patients with heart disease that puts them at risk for endocarditis.

The incision must be large enough to promote proper drainage. If drainage is inadequate the infection may worsen and may spread to other areas of the face, leading to more serious soft tissue infections.

Despite optimal care, most teeth with periapical abscesses will die due to necrosis of the pulp. Follow-up care with a dentist is required to more fully evaluate the tooth and determine if it can be salvaged.

Good patient cooperation is essential; therefore, it is important to attain good anesthesia. Younger patients may require sedation (Chapter 35). If the patient remains uncooperative, dental referral would be appropriate.

SUMMARY

Dental abscesses are not uncommon in the pediatric population. In children, periapical abscesses are more common and are usually the result of pulpal inflammation secondary to caries. Although this procedure is usually left to the dentist or oral surgeon, incision and drainage can be performed by the emergency physician on stable patients for whom referral might be delayed. The procedure is done to relieve pain and to prevent the spread of infection to other areas of the head and neck. Close follow-up and dental referral for definitive treatment are imperative.

REFERENCES

1. Braham RL, Morris ME, eds. Textbook of pediatric dentistry. 2nd ed. Baltimore: Williams & Wilkins, 1985.
2. Comer RW, Caughman WF, Fitchie JG, Gilbert BO. Dental emergencies: management by the primary care physician. Postgrad Med. 1989;85(3):63–77.
3. Fleming P, Strawbridge J. Lateral periodontal abscess in a child. J Pedodontics 1989;13(3):280–283.
4. Ingle JI, Taintor JF, eds. Endodontics. 3rd ed. Philadelphia: Lea & Febiger, 1985.
5. McDonald RE, Avery DR, eds. Dentistry for the child and adolescent. 5th ed. St. Louis: CV Mosby, 1987.
6. Thoma KH. Oral surgery. 5th ed. St. Louis: CV Mosby, 1969.

CLINICAL TIPS
1. Acute drainage in the ED is indicated only in stable patients for whom dental referral will be delayed or when pain relief is necessary and a dentist is unavailable.
2. Carious teeth are suggestive of a periapical rather than a periodontal abscess.
3. Good anesthesia is crucial. Treatment is rarely successful if a child feeels any significant pain.
4. All patients will require dental follow-up for more definitive treatment.

CHAPTER 67

MANAGEMENT OF DENTAL FRACTURES

John Loiselle and Mark L. Helpin

INTRODUCTION

Certain tooth fractures are considered dental emergencies. Fractures can occur as the result of isolated mouth trauma or as part of multisystem injury. The severity of fractures ranges from minor cracks to complex transections of the tooth. The primary goal in the acute management of tooth fractures is to maintain the vitality of the pulp, which is the neurovascular tissue within the tooth. Viability of the tooth in many cases is time dependent and prognosis is best when treatment is initiated shortly after the injury (1, 2).

Three peak ages predict when pediatric dental trauma is most likely to occur. The first peak is between 1 and 3 years of age when the child is learning to walk. Bicycle and playground injuries predominate in the 7- to 10-year-old age group. The onset of athletic endeavors and aggressive or violent activities bring the third peak at ages 16 to 18 (3).

Patients commonly seek treatment for dental injuries in the emergency department (ED) although it is not unusual to see these injuries in the office or outpatient clinic setting. Optimal management of a tooth fracture is immediate evaluation by a dentist capable of performing a definitive restoration of the tooth. This approach should be taken when it is available. However, in considering time constraints involved with tooth viability and potential inability to obtain timely dental consultation during off hours, emergency physicians should be familiar with early management options for these injuries. Applica-

tion of a protective covering as described in this chapter is a temporizing procedure performed before eventual aesthetic restoration of the tooth as an outpatient.

ANATOMY AND PHYSIOLOGY

The primary (deciduous) teeth and the secondary (permanent) teeth share a common anatomy, as illustrated in Figure 67.1. The external anatomy of the tooth is divided into two segments, with the gingival margin serving as the dividing line. The clinical crown is the part of the tooth exposed above the margin, whereas the remainder of the tooth below the margin comprises the root. Each tooth is composed of several layers. The external coating of the crown is the enamel, which is the hardest substance in the body. The underlying calcified layer is the dentin. The neurovascular supply, or pulp, is located in the center of the tooth and runs the length of the root. The cementum is an outer layer of calcified material on the root of the tooth. Each tooth is supported in the alveolar bone by fibrous connective tissue known as the periodontal ligament.

Several characteristics including size, shape, and color help to distinguish primary from secondary teeth (Table 67.1). This differentiation can frequently be an issue with anterior teeth in the presence of a mixed dentition. The age of the child also is a helpful indicator of tooth type. Eruption of the permanent central incisors and first molars generally does not occur until the child has

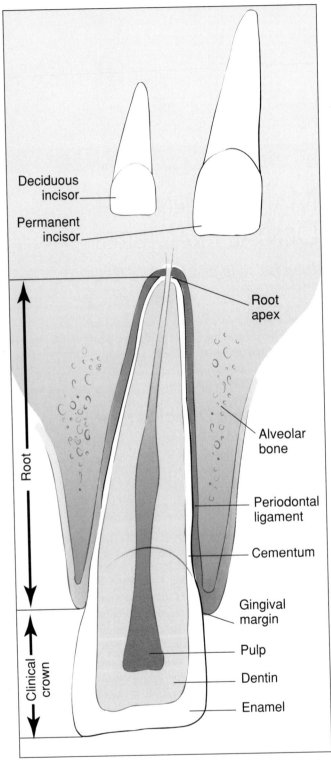

Figure 67.1.
Basic tooth anatomy.

Labels on figure:
Deciduous incisor
Permanent incisor
Root apex
Alveolar bone
Periodontal ligament
Cementum
Gingival margin
Pulp
Dentin
Enamel
Root
Clinical crown

Table 67.1.
Differentiating Characteristics of Primary and Secondary Teeth

Characteristics	Primary Teeth	Secondary Teeth
Age	<6 yr	>6 yr
Color	milky white, opalescent	white to yellowish grey
Size	smaller	larger
Clinical crown length	shorter	wider
Shape	smooth	ridged
Radiographic appearance	developing permanent tooth visible	no apical structures visible

the name "milk teeth." Primary incisors tend to have a smooth incisal edge in contrast to the permanent incisors which are often ridged, especially on the incisal surface. In questionable cases a radiograph may be useful in demonstrating the presence or absence of a developing permanent tooth.

The maxillary central incisors are the most prominent teeth and consequently the most commonly fractured (4–8). Children with excessive protrusion of the maxillary incisors are especially susceptible to injury. Teeth can fracture in a number of ways (Fig. 67.2). Fractures are classified as complicated or uncomplicated depending on whether the pulp is exposed or not (9). The simplest fractures are those involving only the enamel. Fractures that involve the dentin can be identified by the presence of a yellow area within the fracture site and an associated sensitivity of the tooth. Fractures resulting in pulp exposure are identified by the presence of a pink area or an actual bleeding spot located in the center of the tooth. Because dentin consists of microtubules that communicate with the pulp, exposure of dentin allows insult to the

Table 67.2.
Eruption Schedule for Secondary Dentition

	Age (yr)	
	Lower	Upper
Central incisors	6–7	7–8
Lateral incisors	7–8	8–9
Cuspids	9–10	11–12
First bicuspids	10–12	10–11
Second bicuspids	11–12	10–12
First molars	6–7	6–7
Second molars	11–13	12–13
Third molars	17–21	17–21

Adapted from Law, Lunt. JADA 1974;89:872.

reached 6 to 8 years of age (Table 67.2). Permanent teeth are larger than primary teeth and their color ranges from white to a yellowish gray. Primary teeth are a milky, opalescent white and have therefore acquired

pulp which can result in inflammation, infection, and eventual necrosis. Early treatment is therefore crucial in preserving the viability of these teeth (10). Crown-root fractures are visible above the gingiva but extend into the root of the tooth. They involve the enamel, dentin, cementum, and frequently the pulp. Management of these complicated fractures is best handled through dental referral. Root fractures are classified according to their location along the length of the root. They may be classified as cervical, middle, or apical based on their location in relation to the crown of the tooth (Fig. 67.2). The cervical third is adjacent to the clinical crown and the apical third is located at the root apex.

Despite timely management of tooth injuries, death of the pulp may be unavoidable. The initial traumatic event can result in a disruption of blood flow to the pulp which is not detectable at the time of presentation. Fractures that expose the dentin or pulp are associated with a risk of inflammation and infection, which can progress to pulp necrosis and eventual loss of the tooth. Infection and death of the pulp when left untreated can lead to a local abscess or cellulitis.

Tooth discoloration can occur following fractures as breakdown products of hemoglobin become deposited in the microtubules of the dentin. In some cases this staining resolves over time. Pulp damage can result in permanent discoloration of the tooth due to tissue necrosis.

INDICATIONS

Treatment of tooth fractures with the goal of improving tooth survival is generally limited to the secondary dentition (Table 67.3). Survival of a primary tooth, once a significant fracture has occurred, is not significantly improved by immediate active interventions. Normal exfoliation of these teeth means that cosmetic appearance is only a temporary condition.

Fractures that are limited to the enamel require minimal intervention in the acute care setting, and patients can generally be referred to dental follow-up for aesthetic repair.

Fractures through dentin (identified by

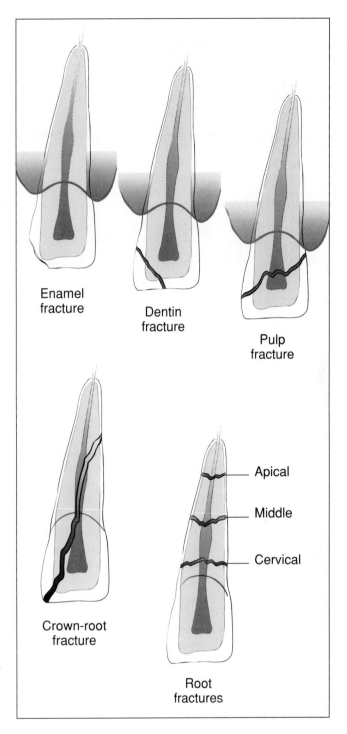

Figure 67.2.
Fractures through various layers of the tooth and location of root fractures.

its yellowish tint) but which do not involve the pulp, also can be referred to a dentist for definitive treatment. Damage with deep or large areas of exposed dentin is not irreversible if care is obtained within 24 to 48 hours of the injury.

Tooth fractures that result in frank pulpal exposure or occur adjacent to the pulp, as suggested by the presence of a pink area or

SUMMARY
1. Account for any missing tooth fragments
2. Use restraint, conscious sedation, and a bite block as needed
3. Inject regional or local anesthesia
4. Irrigate fractured tooth and surrounding area with normal saline
5. Dry fractured tooth and surrounding area with suction and gauze pads
6. Apply calcium hydroxide or glass ionomer product to fracture with applicator stick or wooden end of a cotton-tipped swab.

Table 67.3.
Emergency Department Management of Dental Fractures

Injury Type	Clinical Findings	Treatment Options
Primary teeth	see Table 67.1	• Extraction • Dental referral
Secondary teeth		
Enamel	• Chip of top layer	• Dental referral
Dentin	• Exposed yellow area below enamel • Tooth sensitivity	• Dental referral • Temporary Ca(OH)$_2$ or glass ionomer coating
Pulp	• Exposed pink area • Frank bleeding dot • Tooth sensitivity	• Temporary Ca(OH)$_2$ or glass ionomer coating
Crown-root fracture	• Fracture line visible above gingiva and extends into root	• Dental referral
Root fracture	• Tooth mobility • Bleeding at gingiva • Fracture on radiograph	• Splinting for cervical and middle third root fractures

frank bleeding dot, require emergent dental treatment. Pulp exposure to the oral environment and surrounding bacteria should be minimized by applying a temporary protective coating. Management of crown-root fractures are best handled through dental referral. Root fractures are not visible on the exposed portion of the tooth. The diagnosis is suggested by mobility of the tooth and is confirmed with radiographs. Acute management of cervical and middle third root fractures of the permanent dentition consists of stabilization through splinting, a process which is generally not practical in the primary dentition (4, 7). Fractures in the apical third of the root often do not require splinting, as mobility is minimal and approximation and healing of segments do occur (5, 11).

Teeth with fractures exposing large areas of pulp and in which treatment is delayed for several hours, or in which the pulp appears grossly contaminated, have a low rate of survival and do not benefit from applying a protective coating in the ED (1, 2). Treatment of dental injuries may be deferred to the inpatient setting when associated with more urgent medical priorities (11).

EQUIPMENT

Mouth mirror
Gloves
Protective eyewear
Dental explorer
Cotton rolls
Calcium hydroxide or glass ionomer product
Calcium hydroxide applicator
Mixing pad
Gauze rolls
Cotton pliers
Cotton pellets
Suction catheter
Aspirating syringe
25-gauge 1.5″ needles
Local anesthetic (2% lidocaine with epinephrine 1:100,000)
McKesson or Molt mouth prop
Monitoring as needed for conscious sedation

PROCEDURE

All tooth fragments must be accounted for, because they may become lodged in lacerations, aspirated, or swallowed. A chest radiograph is indicated in the event of a missing tooth fragment. Radiographs which include the lip or tongue are necessary to rule out the presence of tooth fragments within lacerations of these structures.

Young children and the occasional older child may require some combination of restraint and/or conscious sedation for this procedure. For those patients in whom cooperation is hard to obtain, a mouth prop should be inserted to allow adequate visualization and working space. In the most common scenario of a maxillary central incisor injury, the patient is placed in a supine position with the physician seated at the head or side of the bed where control and access are greatest. Both

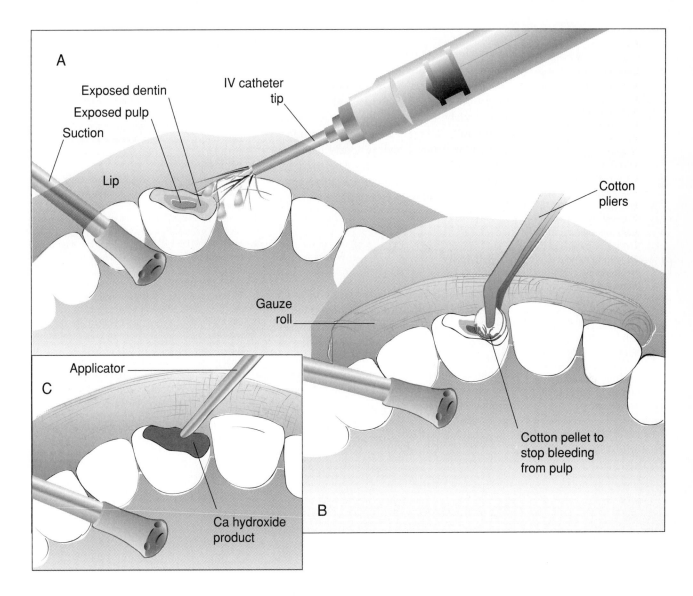

the dentin and the pulp can be extremely sensitive and regional anesthesia may be required before initiating the procedure (Chapter 65). The area around the fractured tooth is irrigated with normal saline through a syringe and intravenous catheter or Splashshield® while simultaneously using oral suction to remove any loose material or blood (Fig. 67.3.A). Once the area has been cleaned, it is dried but not dessicated, using a combination of a suction catheter and gauze pads. Gauze rolls are placed between the lip and tooth and generous oral suction is used to prevent obstruction or contamination of the field by oral secretions. Any bleeding from the pulp can usually be controlled with pressure from cotton pellets on the end of the cotton pliers (Fig. 67.3.B). Calcium hydroxide base and catalyst

or glass ionomer product is mixed on a mixing pad and a thin layer applied directly to the pulp and the surrounding 2 mm of dentin using the applicator instrument or the wooden end of a cotton-tipped swab (Fig. 67.3.C). This is *only* a temporizing measure and follow-up with a dentist should occur within 24 hours. A soft diet is recommended until that time. Prophylactic antibiotics are of unproven benefit in acutely traumatized teeth and should not be given unless other indications are present for antibiotics (9, 10).

COMPLICATIONS

A poor outcome is more likely to result from failure to provide timely treatment or irre-

Figure 67.3.
Application of a temporary protective coating for a tooth fracture.
A. Saline irrigation of fractured tooth.
B. Drying and hemostasis.
C. Application of protective coating.

versible damage occurring at the time of the injury, than from poor technique in applying the protective coating.

Excessive stimulation or drying of the pulp during the procedure may adversely affect its viability. Inadequate coverage of the pulp results in continued exposure to infection and irritation which seriously harm the tooth's chance for survival. The need for early dental referral to minimize these complications cannot be overemphasized.

SUMMARY

Children experience a wide variety of tooth fractures. A fracture of a permanent tooth in which the pulp is exposed is considered a true dental emergency and survival is time dependent. When a dentist is not immediately available, application of a protectivve covering of a calcium hydroxide or glass ionomer product may temporarily preserve the viability of the tooth. Follow-up by the dentist is necessary for definitive repair.

REFERENCES

1. Basrani E. Fractures of the teeth. Philadelphia: Lea & Febiger, 1985.
2. Klokkevold P. Common dental emergencies, evaluation and management for emergency physicians. Emerg Med Clin North Am, 1989 Feb.; 7(1):29–63.
3. Berkowitz R, Ludwig S, Johnson R. Dental trauma in children and adolescents. Clin Pediatr 1980; 19(3):166–171.
4. Andreasen JD, Andreasen FM. Essentials of traumatic injuries to the teeth. Copenhagen: Munksgaard, 1990.
5. Comer RW, Fitchie JG, Caughman WF, Zwemer JD. Oral trauma. Postgrad Med, 1989;85(2):34–41.
6. Josell SD, Abrams RG. Managing common dental problems and emergencies. Pediatr Clin North Am 1991;38(5):1325–1342.
7. Josell SD, Abrams RG. Traumatic injuries to the dentition and its supporting structures. Pediatr Clin North Am 1982;29(3):717–741.
8. McDonald RE, Avery DR. Dentistry for the child and adolescent. 6th ed., 1993 St. Louis, CV Mosby Co.
9. Andreasen JD. Traumatic injuries of the teeth. 2nd ed. Copenhagen: Munksgaard, 1981.
10. McTigue DJ. Management of orofacial trauma in children. Pediatr Ann 1985;14(2):125–129.
11. Dierks EJ. Management of associated dental injuries in maxillofacial trauma. Otolaryngol Clin North Am 1991 Feb.; 24(1):165–179.

REIMPLANTING AN AVULSED PERMANENT TOOTH

Bruce L. Klein and Bernard J. Larson[a]

INTRODUCTION

An avulsed tooth is a tooth that has been totally displaced from its socket. Children and adolescents sustaining this type of injury commonly present to the emergency department (ED). If the tooth is part of the permanent (secondary) dentition, the physician may be able to salvage it. It is emphasized that avulsion of a permanent tooth is a true dental emergency. When avulsed teeth are reimplanted within 30 minutes, 90% survive; when they remain out for several hours, less than 5% exhibit long-term viability (1).

ANATOMY AND PHYSIOLOGY

Maxillary central incisors are avulsed most frequently, followed by maxillary lateral incisors (2). Children with prognathism (buck teeth) are particularly prone to incur such injuries (3). Canines and mandibular incisors are avulsed less often, and posterior teeth only rarely (2).

The emergency physician must distinguish an avulsed deciduous (primary) tooth from a permanent one, because management differs greatly (Table 67.1). Deciduous incisors are smaller and have less pronounced serrations along the edges. In addition, a de-

ciduous maxillary central incisor is approximately the same size as its lateral counterpart, whereas a permanent maxillary central incisor is noticeably larger than the corresponding lateral incisor. Another clue is that deciduous incisors are most often exfoliated between 6 and 9 years of age. Mandibular central incisors are shed first (6 to 7 years of age), followed by maxillary central and mandibular lateral incisors (7 to 8 years of age), and maxillary lateral incisors (8 to 9 years of age) (Table 67.2) (4).

Avulsions of permanent teeth occur most often in 7- to 10-year-old boys (3, 5, 6, 9). Bicycle accidents, playground and sports injuries, and fights are the typical causes. Several factors predispose to exarticulations at this age. Between 7 and 10 years of age, the roots of the permanent teeth are immaturely formed, the periodontal ligaments are loosely structured and weakly connect the roots to the alveolar bone, and the alveolar bone is relatively soft (see also Fig. 67.1) (6, 8). In contrast, older individuals with mature roots, strong periodontal ligaments, and hard alveolar bone are more likely to sustain a dental fracture rather than an avulsion. Fortunately, teeth with immature roots are more likely to be reimplanted successfully.

The key to successful reimplantation is maintaining the viability of the periodontal ligament fibers. These surround the root and secure it to the adjacent alveolar bone. Following a traumatic avulsion, some fibers remain attached to the root whereas others re-

[a]Special thanks to George Acs, D.M.D., M.P.H. for reviewing this manuscript.

SUMMARY
1. Always handle tooth by its crown
2. Inspect it for fractures
3. Cleanse tooth by gently swirling it in normal saline solution or a commercial medium
4. Locate empty socket; for better visualization, lightly suction or swab surrounding area
5. Position tooth at socket opening
6. Reinsert it smoothly, applying firm but gentle pressure
7. Hold tooth in place manually or have child bite on gauze pad until dentist arrives

main on the surrounding alveolus. To avoid traumatizing the periodontal ligament fibers, the physician should only handle the tooth by its crown. In addition, the fibers are quite sensitive and do not tolerate drying or prolonged lack of nutrition. Therefore, if for some reason the tooth cannot be reimplanted immediately, it must be stored in a suitable liquid medium. Although a commercially prepared medium such as Hank's balanced salt solution is best, this type of solution is rarely available, even in the ED (11). Milk, which is readily available in the home, is a good second choice, followed by normal saline solution and intraoral saliva (3, 5-7). Studies show that storing the tooth in water is especially damaging and therefore should be avoided (12).

INDICATIONS

The sole indication for reimplantation is avulsion of a permanent tooth that is not severely fractured. In general, a tooth with a root fracture or a vertical fracture more than half its length should not be reimplanted. Because the long-term success rate of reimplantation is inversely related to the time the tooth remains out of its socket, the tooth must be reimplanted as rapidly as possible, although it is still worthwhile even if 12 or more hours have elapsed. An immature permanent tooth—that is, one with an incompletely formed root—is most able to withstand a prolonged extraoral period.

An avulsed deciduous tooth should not be reimplanted, because its root may damage the developing permanent tooth bud during reimplantation (3, 5-9). Potential sequelae to the immature permanent tooth include enamel dysplasia, root deformation, and discontinuance of tooth development (10). It is suggested that the child place it under a pillow for the tooth fairy instead.

EQUIPMENT

Hank's balanced salt solution, milk, or normal saline solution
Light source
Mouth prop (commercial version or taped stack of tongue depressors)
Sterile gauze

Sterile gloves
Suction (wall or portable)
Suction catheter (Yankauer)
Tongue depressor

PROCEDURE

The avulsed tooth must be located first. This seems obvious, but sometimes a frantic parent forgets to search for the tooth, rushing the child to the ED without it. If the tooth cannot be found at the scene, it may be embedded in the child's lip or the child may have aspirated or swallowed it.

Whenever possible, the parent should be instructed to reimplant the tooth before leaving for the ED. However, this is not always feasible. Often the parent does not call the ED before leaving, or the parent is simply too upset to reinsert the tooth at home. Similarly, if the physician thinks the child may aspirate the tooth en route, it is safest to defer this procedure. In such cases, the tooth should be transported to the ED in milk. An alternative is for the child or parent to hold it under the tongue or in the buccal pouch. Although acceptable, this is less optimal, both because saliva is contaminated by bacteria and because the carrier might aspirate or swallow the tooth.

To minimize damage to the periodontal ligament, the tooth must always be handled by its crown, never by its root. After identifying it as a permanent tooth, it should be inspected for fractures. Reimplantation is contraindicated if a root fracture or a vertical fracture more than half its length is discovered. The best way to cleanse debris off the tooth is to hold it by the crown and gently swirl it in Hank's balanced salt solution, normal saline solution, or milk (Fig. 68.1.A). If necessary, the tooth can be rinsed under slowly running water, although this should obviously never be done over an open drain. Importantly, the tooth must never be scrubbed, because this will injure the periodontal ligament fibers.

Before reimplanting the tooth, the empty socket from which it was avulsed must be located. When multiple teeth have been avulsed, this may not be a trivial task. A hematoma or ecchymosis of the mucosa apical to the socket suggests the possibility of an alveolar bone fracture. To help visualize the socket better, the surrounding area can be

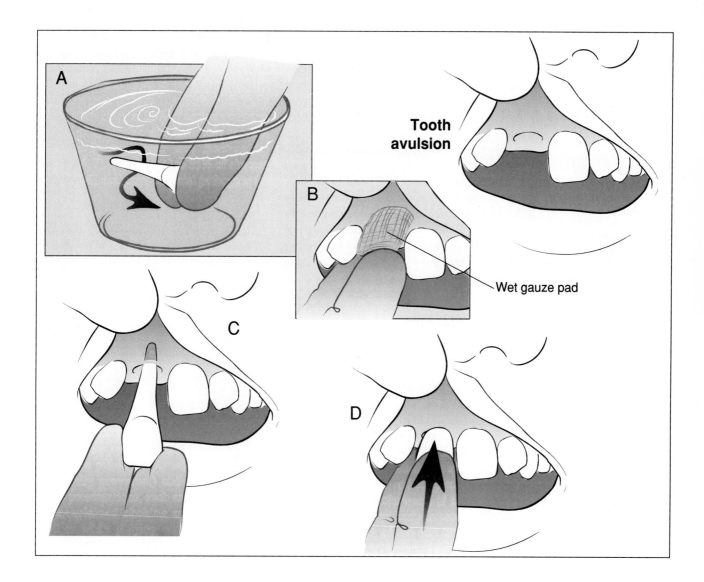

Tooth avulsion

Wet gauze pad

gently swabbed with a wet gauze or cleared with low suction (Fig. 68.1.B). Usually the socket itself does not require suctioning, even when a clot has formed, because young clots tend to be soft and displace easily during reimplantation. When the patient has delayed seeking care, however, suction may be necessary to disrupt and dislodge the clot.

Reimplanting the avulsed tooth is actually a relatively simple procedure. First, the tooth is positioned and aligned correctly at the socket opening. Then, with firm but gentle pressure, it is reinserted into the depth of the socket (Fig. 68.1.C). Administering a sedative or local anesthetic usually is not indicated. If the child resists reinsertion, the alveolus should be inspected for fractures. When present, the displaced alveolar bone can be repositioned using a flat instrument

placed inside the socket. Often the reimplanted tooth protrudes a little more than its nonavulsed equal. The tooth must be stabilized manually until the dentist arrives; the child can bite on a gauze pad, or a responsible adult can hold the tooth in place with finger pressure (Fig. 68.1.D).

Emergency dental consultation is mandatory. Even when the tooth has been reinserted, it remains unstable. To secure it better, the dentist must splint it to the adjacent teeth; an acid etch splint is ideal for this purpose. A dental radiograph is generally taken to confirm proper tooth positioning and to diagnose any associated alveolar bone fractures.

Inflammatory root resorption is greatly reduced when systemic antibiotics are administered following reimplantation (13). Therefore the recommended prescription is a 10-

Figure 68.1.
Reinserting an avulsed tooth.
A. Cleansing the avulsed tooth;
B. Clearing blood and secretions from the socket;
C. Reimplanting the tooth;
D. Stabilizing the reimplanted tooth.

Chapter 68
Reimplanting an
Avulsed Permanent
Tooth

day regimen of prophylactic penicillin which is started before discharge. The patient should also be started on a soft diet and given an analgesic prescription. A tetanus booster should be given if required. A follow-up appointment with the dentist should be scheduled for 7 days. At this visit, the splint is removed and endodontic therapy is usually begun. In an older child or adolescent, root canal treatment is essential because the neurovascular structures of the pulp are virtually always destroyed and will not regenerate. In contrast, a 6- to 8-year-old child may not need endodontic therapy; the root of an immature permanent tooth still retains an open apex, so revascularization is possible.

COMPLICATIONS

Local infection, especially abscess formation, is the principal short-term concern. The most important long-term complications are ankylosis of the reimplanted tooth to the surrounding bone and inflammatory root resorption (13, 14). Ankylosis, which may occur within months, is a particular problem in adolescents because it can result in alveolar growth discrepancies. Severe root resorption can develop within weeks and result ultimately in loss of the tooth. Finally, inadequate endodontic therapy is a cause of tooth discoloration.

SUMMARY

The prognosis for an avulsed tooth need not be grim; in fact, most such teeth can be reimplanted successfully. A favorable outcome is particularly likely when the patient seeks care immediately after the accident occurs and the clinician adheres strictly to the protocol described in this chapter. Most importantly, saving an avulsed tooth spares the child lifelong functional and cosmetic consequences.

REFERENCES

1. Andreasen JD, Hjorting Hansen E. Replantation of teeth. Radiographic and clinical study of 110 human teeth replanted after accidental loss. Acta Odontol Scand 1966;24:287.
2. Coccia CT. A clinical investigation of root resorption rates in reimplanted young permanent incisors: a 5-year study. J Endod 1980;6:413.
3. Henry RJ. Pediatric dental emergencies. Pediatr Nurs 1991;17:162.
4. Johnson KB, ed. The Harriet Lane handbook. St. Louis: CV Mosby, 1993, p. 216.
5. Mueller WA. Emergency dental care. Pediatrician 1989;16:147.
6. McIlveen LP. Orofacial trauma in children. Pediatr Basics 1990;54:7.
7. Nelson LP. Pediatric emergencies in the office setting: oral trauma. Pediatr Emerg Care 1990;6:62.
8. Dierks EJ. Management of associated dental injuries in maxillofacial trauma. Otolaryngol Clin North Am 1991;24:165.
9. Josell SD, Abrams RG. Managing common dental problems and emergencies. Pediatr Clin North Am 1991;38:1325.
10. Holan G, Topf J, Fuks AB. Effect of root canal infection and treatment of traumatized primary incisors on their permanent successors. Endod Dent Traumatol 1992;8:12.
11. Krasner P, Person P. Preserving avulsed teeth for replantation. JADA 1992;123:80.
12. Lindskog S, Blomlof L. Influence of osmolarity and composition of some storage media on human periodontal ligament cells. Acta Odontol Scand 1982;40:435.
13. Hammarstrom L, Blomlof L, Feiglin B, Andersson L, Lindskog S. Replantation of teeth and antibiotic treatment. Endod Dent Traumatol 1986;2:51.
14. Andreasen JD. Traumatic injuries of the teeth. Philadelphia: WB Saunders, 1981, p. 203.

MANAGEMENT OF SOFT TISSUE INJURIES OF THE MOUTH

Peter D. Quinn and John Loiselle

INTRODUCTION

The physician who deals with the pediatric age group is frequently called on to evaluate oral trauma (1, 2). Children often present to the emergency department (ED) after apparently minor trauma with fractured teeth or lacerations to the oral soft tissues.

Blunt trauma is the most common source of orofacial injuries in children, and is usually the result of falls. In the younger age groups the possibility of child abuse should always be considered (3). Animal bites are another frequent cause. Children are at greater risk than adults for being the victim of an animal bite. Three-fourths of all bites involve the extremities; however, because of their small size, children are more likely to suffer bites to the face. Bites to the lips are particularly common, sustained while "kissing" an animal (4).

Electrical burns of the lips and tongue are not an uncommon injury among young children, who seem predisposed to licking electrical outlets or gnawing on electrical cords. It is important to elicit an adequate history relative to the nature of the trauma, because these scenarios will differ in pattern and extent of injury (5).

Closure of oral mucosal lacerations will result in decreased healing time, decreased propensity for infection, and adequate hemostasis and cosmesis (5–7). The issue of cosmesis is one of utmost importance for the parent and patient. Injuries to the orofacial area result in greater anxiety than any other location.

The complexity of injuries varies greatly. The majority heal well without intervention. Those that require repair can, in most cases, be handled by any experienced physician. A small number require surgical expertise. Most facial lacerations are not complicated by associated injuries and are easily managed by ED personnel, although other medical priorities may necessitate deferring treatment to the inpatient setting. Extensive facial lacerations are preferably closed by a specialist in the operating room. Consultants may include a general, plastic or oral surgeon, a dentist, or an otorhinolaryngologist.

ANATOMY AND PHYSIOLOGY

The generous blood flow to the face and mouth contributes to its excellent healing potential (Fig. 69.1). The upper lip is supplied by the superior labial arteries, which branch from the facial arteries. The lower lip also is supplied by branches of the facial artery known as the inferior labial arteries. The labial arteries join and form a ring about the mouth. The inferior labial arteries have anastamoses with the mental and submental arteries, which are branches of the maxillary and facial arteries respectively.

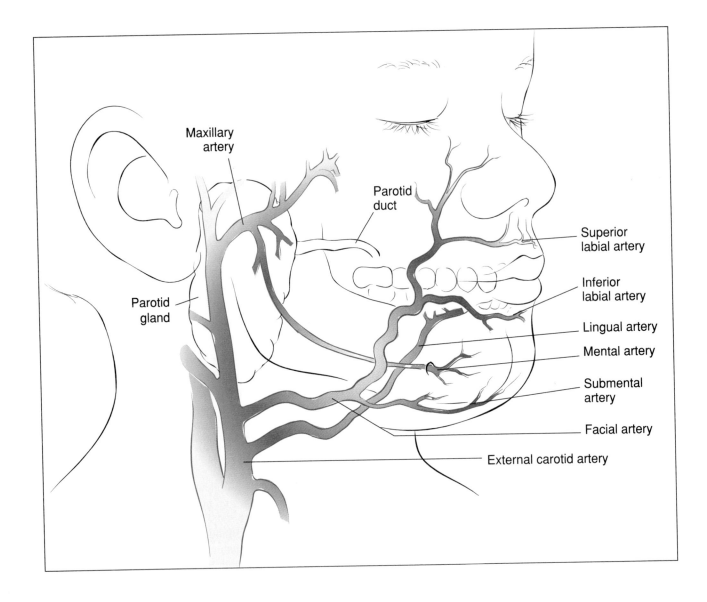

Figure 69.1.
Blood supply to the face
and mouth.

The tongue receives its main blood supply from the lingual arteries. Branches of the lingual artery and the inferior alveolar artery provide blood supply to the mucosa of the floor of the mouth. The maxillary and palatal mucosa are supplied by branches of the maxillary arteries. The buccal mucosa is supplied by branches of both the facial and maxillary arteries (8).

Nerve supply to the area is equally complex. The maxilla and upper lip are innervated by branches of the maxillary division of the trigeminal nerve (Fig. 65.1). The anterior palate derives sensation from the nasopalatine nerve which passes through the incisive canal. The posterior palate is innervated by the greater palatine nerves which exit the greater palatine foramina. The maxillary dentition

and buccal gingiva are innervated by the posterior, middle, and anterior alveolar nerves.

The mandible and lower lip are innervated by branches of the mandibular division of the trigeminal nerve. The mandibular dentition derives sensation from the inferior alveolar nerve. The latter gives rise to the mental nerve which innervates the lower lip and buccal gingiva anterior to the second primary molar. Sensation to the buccal mucosa and buccal gingiva posterior to the primary molars is derived from the long buccal nerve.

The lingual gingiva is innervated by the lingual nerve which also gives sensation to the mucosa of the floor of the mouth and the anterior two-thirds of the tongue. The chorda tympani nerve courses within the sheath of the lingual nerve and is the nerve of taste for

Chapter 69
Management of Soft
Tissue Injuries of the
Mouth

742

the anterior two-thirds of the tongue. The posterior two-thirds of the tongue derives sensory innervation from the glossopharyngeal nerve and the superior laryngeal nerve. The latter provide some small branches to the base of the tongue near the epiglottis (8).

The structure of a lip is multilayered as shown in Fig. 69.2. The skin comprises the external layer and the mucosa the internal layer. The middle layer is composed of muscle (the orbicularis oris), which encircles the mouth. A fibrofatty junction borders both the inside and the outside surfaces of the muscle. Between the inner fibrofatty junction and the mucosa, a layer of submucosal or minor salivary glands is present.

The vermilion border is the mucocutaneous junction of the lips where the mucosa meets the skin. The most common lip injury treated in ED is a through-and-through laceration. These lacerations often involve the vermilion border which is a fixed and obvious landmark.

The tongue is composed almost entirely of eight separate muscle groups which confer a wide variation of movement. It is covered on the dorsal and inferior surfaces by mucous membrane. The anterior two-thirds of the dorsal surface contains the numerous papillae or taste buds.

When a child licks an electrical outlet or two bared wires, saliva will complete the arc. A spark burn will result. Fortunately, the immediate reaction of the victim is to jerk away. When a child bites into a cord, current courses through the soft tissue and produces a muscle contraction. The victim is unable to release the cord because of the ongoing perioral muscle contraction, and the burn progresses (5).

Spark burns produce a limited white blister and will not result in much deep tissue necrosis. Current burns appear more diffuse. Necrosis of deep tissues will occur and the eschar will break down approximately 5 to 10 days post-injury. Without vital connective tissue support, damaged circumoral vessels also will necrose, tear, and bleed (5, 9). Parents should be alerted to the possibility of delayed bleeding and the need to seek medical attention at the first indication of bleeding (10). Alternatively, admission of current burn victims should be considered approximately 4 to 5 days following the injury to observe for

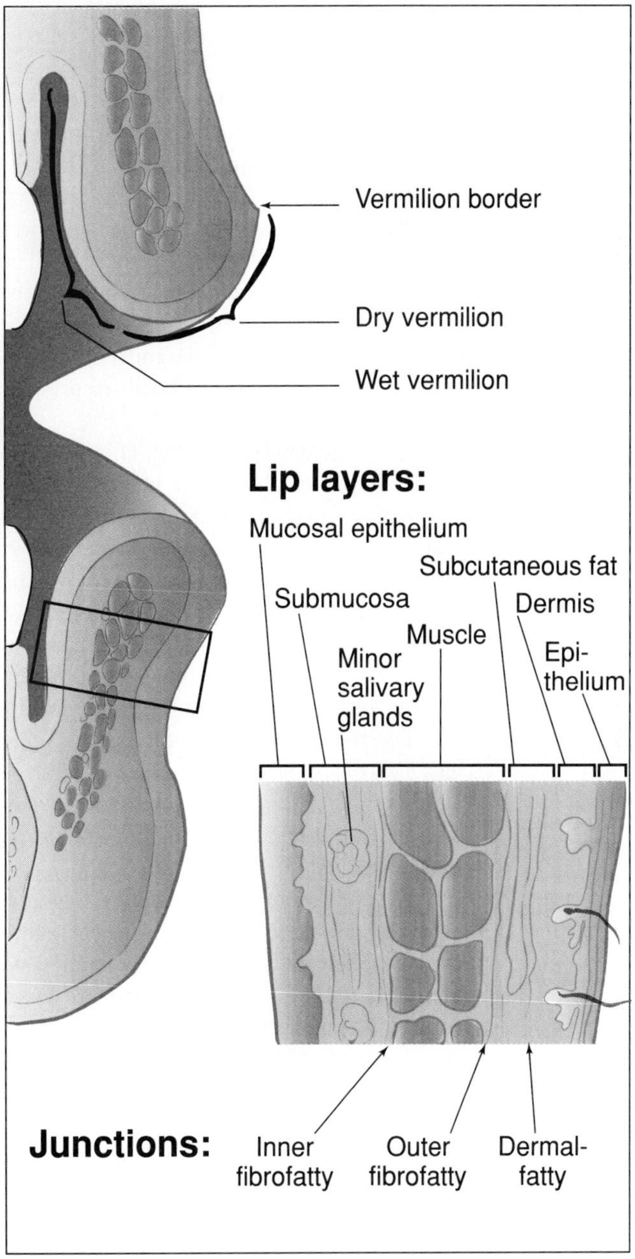

Figure 69.2.
Anatomy of the lip.

bleeding. Pain and edema may prevent adequate oral hydration or, in more severe cases, result in airway compromise.

The parotid duct is an additional structure within the mouth that may be injured. It originates at the anterior parotid gland and courses anteriorly. The duct turns medially at the anterior border of the masseter muscle and penetrates the buccinator muscle. It then courses obliquely forward to exit the mucosa at Stensen's papillae opposite the maxillary second molar (8).

INDICATIONS

The generous blood supply of the face and mouth allows the vast majority of intraoral lacerations to heal well on their own. This benefit is counterbalanced by the fact that even the smallest lacerations in the facial area can leave cosmetically disfiguring scars. The elapsed time from wound occurrence and the degree of contamination of wound are additional concerns. These issues must be considered when deciding on the need for primary closure.

A few general recommendations can be made regarding closure of lip lacerations. Lacerations that are greater than approximately 2 cm, especially when they occur on the dry mucosa, will heal more rapidly and with less distress to the patient if sutured. All lacerations involving the vermilion border should be closed. Through-and-through lacerations of the lip will require suture repair.

The tongue also is composed of highly vascularized tissue, and hemostasis may be an issue in the decision to close a tongue laceration. Full thickness lacerations should, in most cases, be repaired. Lacerations that result in a division of a free edge of the tongue have the potential to heal with a persistent cleft and therefore require approximation. In addition, tongue lacerations that are large enough to entrap food particles heal more slowly and should be sutured.

Through-and-through lacerations of the oral mucosa should be closed. Lacerations that result in a flap may require suture repair if they are at risk of further trauma from biting. Hemostasis also may be an issue in these injuries. Lacerations producing communication between the oral cavity and nasal passages or sinuses require closure and should be referred to an otolaryngologist or oral surgeon.

Injury to Stensen's duct should be suspected with any laceration crossing the middle third of a line drawn from the tragus to the central portion of the upper lip, or if paralysis of the buccal branch of the facial nerve is present. Flow of irrigant into a wound from a 22-gauge intravenous catheter that is cannulating Stensen's papillae confirms parotid duct injury. Such lacerations should be referred for definitive treatment to avoid adverse post-injury sequelae (11). Burn injuries of the mouth

should not be excised nor should primary repair be attempted. Involvement of the labial commissure necessitates referral to a specialist who can fabricate a dental appliance to stent the commissure and prevent contracture.

Tear wounds from animal bites about the face and mouth can be closed as any other laceration, although debridement of devitalized tissue is more likely to be necessary. True puncture wounds should not be closed, but allowed to granulate. Because of the rich vascular supply to the face and mouth, human bite wounds to this region, treated within 24 hours of injury, may be closed primarily. This is unlike human bites to other regions of the body, which are not closed and allowed to granulate. If more than 24 hours has elapsed since the injury, delayed primary closure of facial bite wounds is performed after resolution of infection.

EQUIPMENT

Dental anesthetic syringe or 5 mL Luer-Lok syringe
25 gauge or smaller, 1.5" needle
Yankauer and Frazier suction catheters
1 or 2% lidocaine with or without 1/100,000 epinephrine
Gauze sponges
Bite block
Suture tray (fine scissors, needle holder, nontraumatic forceps)
Saline for irrigation
20-mL irrigation syringe
Splashshield or 18-gauge intravenous catheter tip
Resorbable sutures 3.0 and 4.0 chromic gut, vicryl, dexon
Nonresorbable sutures 5.0 nylon, ethilon, prolene

PROCEDURE

The approach to these injuries, as with all trauma, is to initially assess for concurrent life-threatening injuries to the airway, cervical spine, or brain. Once these injuries have been stabilized, a regional head and neck examination should evaluate for signs and symptoms of facial bone or skull fracture such as hemotympanum, paresthesia of the divisions of the trigeminal nerve, diplopia, cerebrospinal fluid rhinorrhea, cerebrospinal fluid otorrhea, trismus, malocclusion, temporomandibular joint pain, or deviation of the mandible on opening (11). Injuries to the temporomandibular joints or mandibular condyles should be suspected in patients who have sustained blows to the mental symphysis region.

Intraoral examination should evaluate for the integrity of the oral and/or pharyngeal mucosa, the stability of the occlusion, and the presence of luxated, mobile, fractured, or avulsed teeth. Ecchymosis of the floor of the mouth or near the ramus of the mandible may indicate an underlying mandibular fracture. Similarly, palatal ecchymosis or ecchymosis near the zygomatic buttress suggests a maxillary fracture. When the presence of occult facial bone fractures has been excluded, treatment can turn to facial and mucosal lacerations (11).

Oral mucosal lacerations frequently contain tooth fragments and other foreign bodies such as glass and gravel. These must be identified either through direct or radiographic examination and removed before proceeding with the repair. Oral mucosal lacerations can also be quite painful, and administration of regional anesthetic blocks before examination may be helpful. Sensory and motor examinations of the cranial nerves should be documented before the administration of anesthetics. Placement of a bite block or a taped stack of tongue depressors may improve exposure for intraoral procedures.

Anesthesia

Clinical evaluation of the child's interaction with the physician may be helpful in determining the need for restraint. Thorough evaluation and treatment of oral injuries is difficult with an uncooperative child. If necessary, restraint should be used, physically by a papoose board and/or pharmacologically through conscious sedation (Chapters 3 and 35).

Upper Lip
The infraorbital nerve block is the preferred method for obtaining anesthesia in this region (see also Chapter 65). A regional block will cause minimal distortion of the vermilion border and will result in anesthesia of the lower eyelid, the skin overlying the malar prominence, and the skin and mucosa of the upper lip from commissure to midline on the injected side.

Supraperiosteal infiltration in the mucobuccal fold over the laceration also will provide anesthesia of the skin and mucosa of the lip directly distal to the injection site (Chapter 65). This method results in greater distortion of the vermilion border and soft tissue landmarks than an infraorbital block. Several injections will be needed. Injections should be made above the apex of each tooth to which the laceration is adjacent.

Direct infiltration of the laceration margins (Chapter 37) will provide adequate anesthesia and hemostasis, but also will result in the greatest distortion of the vermilion border. If epinephrine is contained in an anesthetic solution used for direct infiltration, blanching of the mucosa will occur, which may result in obliteration of the vermilion border (12).

Lower Lip
A regional nerve block is again the preferred method for anesthesia of the lower lip region. As with the upper lip, a regional nerve block will produce less distortion of soft tissue landmarks, and requires less total anesthetic injection than the techniques of supraperiosteal injection and direct infiltration.

A mental nerve block will result in anesthesia of the buccal gingiva anterior to the mental foramen, as well as the mucosa and skin of the lower lip from the midline to the labial commissure on the side of the injection. The mental nerve can be palpated near the apex of the second primary molar of a young child or near the apex of the second premolar of an adolescent (Fig. 69.3). The lip and buccal tissues are tautly retracted with fingers of the clinician's nondominant hand. A 25-gauge or smaller needle penetrates the mucosa directly over or slightly anterior to the mental foramen. The needle is advanced approximately 5 mm. If no blood is aspirated, 0.5 to 1.0 mL of 1% lidocaine is injected.

An inferior alveolar or mandibular block will result in a distribution of anesthesia which encompasses the region anesthetized by a mental block. In addition, the remainder of the buccal mucosa, the lingual gingiva, the

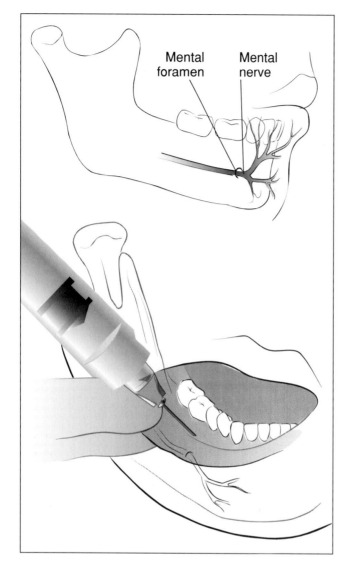

tained in the anesthetic solution will have minimal hemostatic effect on the mucosa and muscles of the tongue.

A 25-gauge or smaller needle is inserted through the mandibular mucosa immediately posterior and medial to the most posterior tooth in the arch (Chapter 65). The needle should penetrate to a depth of approximately 5 mm. If aspiration is negative for blood, 0.5 to 1.0 mL of anesthetic is injected. A mandibular block as previously described also will result in block of the lingual nerve.

Direct infiltration of laceration margins with an anesthetic solution containing a vasoconstrictor will provide both anesthesia and hemostasis. Tongue lacerations can bleed quite briskly. The added hemostatic effect of a vasoconstrictor, although temporary, can aid visualization when suturing (12).

Direct infiltration of the buccal and palatal mucosal soft tissues will provide anesthesia, hemostasis (if vasoconstrictors are used), and will not distort any vital landmarks. Although techniques of regional anesthetic blocks exist, their use in the ED will be rare and therefore these methods are not described.

Repair

The basic principles of suturing are described in Chapter 111. The following discussion is limited to specific techniques for closure of oral soft tissue wounds.

Lip

Repair of a lip laceration should be performed layer by layer from the inside out, and from the wound apex to the free margin (5, 6). It is of paramount importance to identify the vermilion border before initiating infiltration anesthesia or wound debridement. Regional block anesthesia can be administered without distortion of the vermilion border. Some clinicians advocate approximation of the vermilion border with a tacking stitch (5.0 or 6.0 nonabsorbable suture) at the outset. Others recommend simply marking the junction with a pen or scratch from a needle tip or back of a scalpel blade (5, 6).

Once the vermilion border is marked, the wound is debrided and any obviously tramatized minor salivary glands are removed. If these remain in a wound, delayed formation

Figure 69.3.
Administration of a mental nerve block.

anterior two-thirds of the tongue, and the dentition on the side of the injection will be anesthetic. The target area for this block is the mandibular foramen, where the inferior alveolar nerve enters the mandibular canal (Chapter 65).

Supraperiosteal injections and direct infiltration techniques also may be used in anesthesia of the lower lip, although they have the same caveats as those described for the upper lip (12).

Tongue

A lingual nerve block will provide anesthesia to the anterior two-thirds of the tongue, lingual gingiva, and mucosa of the floor of the mouth on the side injected. Although this technique will provide excellent anesthesia in the region described, vasoconstrictors conof a mucocele is likely to occur. Any obviously necrotic tissue should be excised. The face has a rich vascular supply with a tremendous healing potential. Tissue with a minimal blood supply can survive and become revascularized. Care should be taken not to excise tissue that contains the vermilion cutaneous junction. The wound should be thoroughly inspected for foreign bodies, particularly tooth fragments, and all foreign material should be removed. Once debridement is complete, the wound is irrigated with a copious amount of saline and the surrounding skin is prepped with betadine.

Closure of a through-and-through lip laceration occurs in three layers (Fig. 69.4). As described previously, a stitch that aligns the vermilion border may be placed at the beginning of the closure. The inner fibrofatty junction at the wound apex is then reapproximated, using a resorbable 3.0 or 4.0 suture. Interrupted sutures with inverted knots will provide adequate reapproximation without protrusion of the knots through the wound. The outer fibrofatty junction is approximated next, and the two fibrofatty junctions are united at the free edge. If the muscle is not approximated both anteriorly and posteriorly, it will contract away from the wound edge. This will produce an unobtrusive scar with the lip at rest, but when the lip is in function, a contraction will produce an obvious ridging or depression of the scar. If suturing of the inner and outer fibrofatty junctions is not joined at the free edge, a notch in the scar over this region will develop (5).

The dermal-fat junction is then closed with an inverted interrupted stitch using resorbable 4.0 suture. Alignment of the vermilion border must remain perfect before and after this layer is sutured. The presence of any malalignment neccesitates removal of the sutures and reapproximation of the tissue until alignment is achieved.

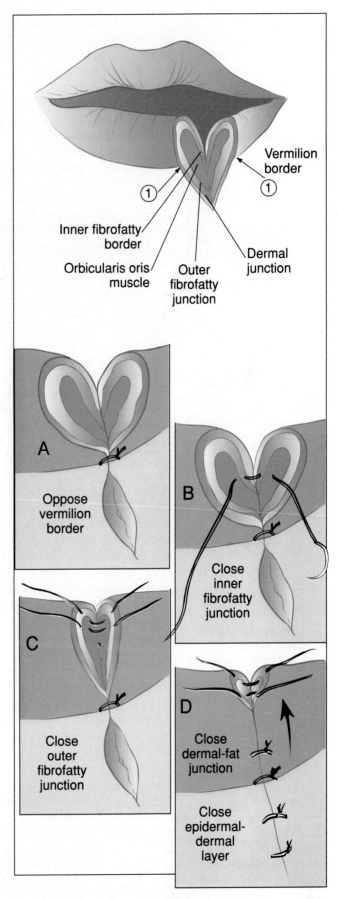

Figure 69.4.
Three-layer repair of a through-and-through lip laceration.
A. Opposition of vermilion border.
B. Closure of the inner dermal-fat junction.
C. Closure of the outer dermal-fat junction.
D. Closure of the epidermal layer, with joining of the dermal-fat junction at the free wound edge.

SUMMARY
1. Assess and stabilize life-threatening injuries
2. Examine injuries for presence of underlying fractures or foreign bodies
3. Document sensory and motor examinations of cranial nerves
4. Administer conscious sedation as needed
5. Physically restrain patient with papoose board if necessary
6. Place bite block or stent mouth open with taped tongue depressors
7. Administer regional nerve block or local infiltrative anesthetic as indicated
8. Carry out any necessary debridement or excision
9. Irrigate wound with saline

Lip Lacerations
1. Identify and mark vermilion border before initiating anesthesia or debridement
2. Prepare wound borders with betadine
3. Reapproximate vermilion border
4. Reapproximate inner fibrofatty junction with resorbable 3.0 or 4.0 suture using interrupted stitches with inverted knots
5. Close outer fibrofatty junction in same manner
6. Unite fibrofatty junction at free edge
7. Close dermal-fat junction with inverted interrupted resorbable 4.0 sutures
8. Ensure vermilion border is reapproximated exactly
9. Close epidermal-dermal layer sewing "away from" vermilion border using 5.0 nonresorbable sutures

**Chapter 69
Management of Soft Tissue Injuries of the Mouth**

The final epidermal-dermal layer is approximated by sewing "away from" the vermilion-cutaneous junction toward the wound apex in the skin using a 5.0 nonresorbable material such as nylon.

If the laceration is limited to the dry vermilion (Fig. 69.2), nonresorbable suture material may be used. If the laceration extends onto the wet vermilion 4.0 chromic gut is used in an interrupted or continuous stitch.

Some clinicians prefer an alternative or simple three-layered closure (13). Using this technique, the outer fibrofatty junction is approximated as previously described. Next, the mucosa and the inner fibrofatty layer are closed as a unit. A 3.0 chromic gut suture is used to penetrate the mucosa, engage the fibrofatty layer on both sides of the laceration, and then exit the mucosa on the other side of the wound. The skin is approximated as previously described.

A two-layer closure, in which the skin and outer fibrofatty layer are closed as a unit and the mucosa and posterior fibrofatty layer are closed as a unit, is not recommended as it can result in great variability in the approximation of tissue layers.

Tongue

With small lacerations, all layers can be closed with interrupted sutures penetrating through mucosa and muscle. Sutures should be inverted to avoid untying of knots. A 4.0 or 3.0 resorbable suture material such as vicryl or chromic gut should be used. Because the tongue is slippery and difficult to grasp, it may be helpful to place one 3.0 silk suture through the tip of the tongue and pull it gently through the open mouth to obtain better exposure of the wound.

Gingiva

Gingival lacerations should be closed using interrupted simple sutures with multiple knots to avoid untying. A 3.0 or 4.0 chromic gut is an ideal choice.

Buccal Mucosa

Through-and-through lacerations should be closed in layers as described for lip lacerations. When possible only the external surface is closed. When both surfaces must be sutured, the inner surface is closed first. The wound is irrigated thoroughly through the external open wound. The muscle layer and then the skin should be closed sequentially. Lacerations involving only the oral mucosa should be closed with 3.0 or 4.0 chromic gut in a continuous or interrupted fashion. Again, multiple knots will prevent untying.

Considerable controversy exists over proper use of antibiotics in patients with facial lacerations. Because of the high bacterial count within the mouth, most intraoral lacerations are considered to be contaminated. Prophylactic use of oral penicillin may reduce the incidence of infection following intraoral wound repair. The incidence of infection is relatively low in lacerations involving only the mucosa. The infection rate is higher in through-and-through laceractions and patients with these wounds may benefit more from prophylaxis (14). Antibiotics are considered more effective before or during ED procedures, but are often not administered until the procedure has been completed. No evidence indicates the superiority of a cephalosporin over penicillin or clindamycin, as long as the antibiotic used is given in high enough concentration to be effective (5).

Patients should be advised to adhere to a soft diet for 24 to 48 hours following repair. In addition only liquids should be taken until the anesthetic has completely worn off. All patients should have a tetanus booster administered if needed.

COMPLICATIONS

Obliteration of landmarks secondary to infiltration anesthetics resulting in volume distortion and blanching of the vermilion mucosa can result in suboptimal repair of this sensitive area. Knots are more likely to become untied when they are placed in the mouth. The occurrence of untying can be lessened with the inversion of knots and tying of multiple knots.

Repeat injury to anesthetized tissues postrepair can occur secondary to cheek and lip biting. This is especially problematic in the young child who may not comprehend the consequences of this action. Extensive manipulation of tissues or anesthetic infiltration may result in airway compromise secondary to edema or excessive hemorrhage. Mucocele formation may result from damage to minor salivary glands and ducts in the lips.

SUMMARY

Orofacial injuries are common in the pediatric age group. While these injuries are of great cosmetic importance to both the patient and the parent, most heal well because the area is highly vascularized. The majority of injuries requiring surgical repair can be closed by an experienced physician. Success is largely dependent on the ability to accurately visualize and assess the injury. Administration of local or regional anesthesia,

with the use of concious sedation when necessary, will greatly facilitate this task in young children. A layered closure of deep wounds with accurate approximation of key landmarks like the vermilion bordetr is essential for a good functional and cosmetic outcome. Although antibiotic prophylaxis is controversial, penicillin is commonly prescribed following intraoral repairs.

REFERENCES

1. Nelson LP. Pediatric emergencies in the office setting: oral trauma. Pediatr Emerg Care 1990;16(3–4): 147–152.
2. Berkowitz R, Ludwig S, Johnson R. Dental trauma in children and adolescents. Clin Pediatr 1980;3: 166–171.
3. Maniglia AJ, Kine SN. Maxillofacial trauma in the pediatric age group. Otolaryngol Clin North Am 1983 August;16(3)717.
4. Newton E. Mammalian bites. In: Schwartz CR, Cayten CG, Mangelsen MA, Mayer TA, Hanke BK, eds. Principles and practice of emergency medicine. 3rd ed. Philadelphia: Lea & Febeiger, 1992, pp. 2750–2761.
5. Dushoff IM. About face. Emerg Med. 1974 Nov.;25–77.
6. Dushoff IM. A stitch in time. Emerg Med 1973 Jan.; 21–43.
7. Potsic WP, Handler SD. Primary care pediatric otolaryngology. New York: Macmillan, 1986, pp. 116–119.
8. Goss CM, ed. Gray's anatomy. 29th ed. Philadelphia: Lea & Febeiger, 1973.
9. Hammond JS, Ward GG. Burns of the head and neck. Otolaryngol Clin North Am 1983 August;16(3):679.
10. McDonald RE, Avery DR, Hennon DK. Management of trauma to the teeth and supporting tissues. In: McDonald RE, Avery DR, eds. Dentistry for the child and adolescent. 6th ed. St. Louis, CV Mosby Co 1993.
11. AAOMS. Oral and maxillofacial surgery services in the emergency department. Rosemont, Illinois: American Association of Oral and Maxillofacial Surgery, 1992, pp. 4–5.
12. Malamed SF. Handbook of local anesthesia. St. Louis: CV Mosby, 1980.
13. Peterson LJ. Contemporary oral and maxillofacial surgery. St. Louis: CV Mosby, 1988, pp. 554–555.
14. Steele MT, Riedel C, Robinson WA, Salomone JA, Elenbaas RM. Prophylactic penicillin for intraoral wounds. Ann Emerg Med 1989;18(8)847–852.

REDUCTION OF TEMPOROMANDIBULAR JOINT DISLOCATION

William Ahrens and John Loiselle

INTRODUCTION

Temporomandibular joint dislocation is the displacement of the mandibular condyle from the mandibular fossa rendering the patient unable to achieve reduction without assistance. It is an uncommon condition in children but may occur in adolescents. Due to the associated pain and anxiety, patients typically present in the acute period to the emergency department (ED) or to a dental or primary care office.

The procedure for reducing a temporomandibular joint dislocation has changed little since Hippocrates, who is generally credited with the earliest description of the technique.

The goal in treatment is to reduce the dislocation, restore function, and alleviate pain. The earlier the reduction is attempted, the better the likelihood of success (1, 2). Reduction is most frequently performed in the office or ED setting by a physician, dentist, or oral surgeon and is relatively uncomplicated assuming that proper technique is followed.

ANATOMY AND PHYSIOLOGY

The temporomandibular joint consists of the head of the mandibular condyle sitting within the mandibular fossa of the temporal bone (Fig. 70.1.A). The articular surfaces are lined by a synovial membrane and separated by a disc or meniscus composed of fibrous connective tissue. The structure of the joint allows for hinge, gliding, and side-to-side motions. The capsular ligament attaches to both the mandibular fossa and the neck of the condyle. Its laxity allows for the flexible movement of the joint. The joint is also supported by two ligaments on the medial surface, the sphenomandibular and stylomandibular ligaments, and one on the lateral surface, the temporomandibular ligament. Recurrent dislocation may be associated with excessive laxity in these ligaments as occurs in Ehlers-Danlos or Marfan's syndrome.

The lateral pterygoid muscle and several neck muscles are responsible for opening the jaw. Closure is controlled by the masseter, medial pterygoid, and temporalis muscles.

Acute dislocation of the temporomandibular joint occurs most frequently in an anterior direction causing the mandibular condyle to become locked in front of the articular eminence (Fig. 70.1.B). Dislocation can occur bilaterally or unilaterally. Spasms of the lateral pterygoid and temporalis muscles maintain the dislocation and often make reduction difficult. Conditions that predispose to dislocation include prior stretching of

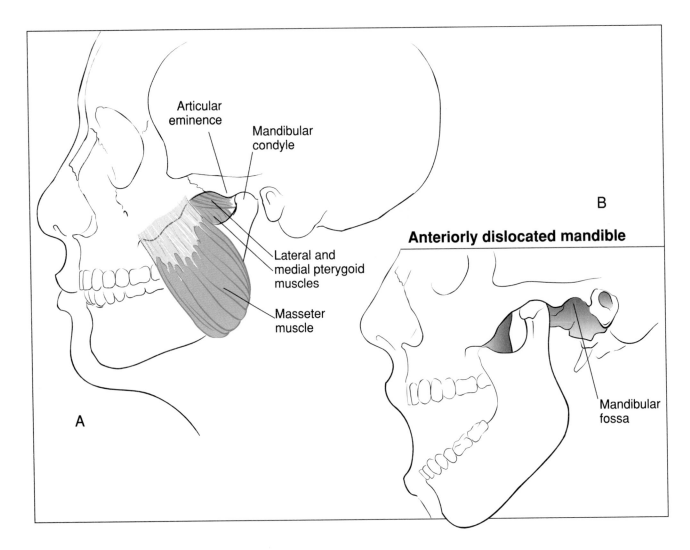

Figure 70.1.
A. Anatomy of the temporomandibular joint.
B. Anterior dislocation of the temporomandibular joint.

Labels in figure: Articular eminence, Mandibular condyle, Lateral and medial pterygoid muscles, Masseter muscle, A

B Anteriorly dislocated mandible, Mandibular fossa

Chapter 70
Reduction of
Temporomandibular
Joint Dislocation

the joint capsule, a low articular eminence, increased tonicity of the muscles of mastication, or excessive ligamentous laxity.

A number of mechanisms are associated with anterior dislocation including extreme mouth opening as occurs during episodes of laughing, yawning, or vomiting, and prolonged mouth opening with tonsillectomy or dental therapy (1, 3). Dislocation also can occur as a result of convulsions, dystonic reactions, or trauma.

Although unusual, posterior and superior dislocations may be seen. Posterior dislocation is generally the result of trauma and often is associated with damage to the nearby auditory system. Disruption of the external auditory canal or fracture of the temporal plate is common (4). Superior dislocation occurs with severe trauma and is associated with fractures of the mandibular fossa. Lateral dislocations occur only with concomitant fractures of the mandibular body (5).

INDICATIONS

Patients with an acute anterior dislocation of the temporomandibular joint complain of severe pain in the preauricular area. They present with an open mouth, protruding mandible, and an inability to occlude the anterior teeth. A visible depression is evident in the preauricular area. In the case of a unilateral dislocation, the jaw will be displaced toward the unaffected side.

Before attempting reduction, radiographs should be obtained to confirm the dislocation and exclude any associated fractures. A panoramic view is considered best for this purpose, although transcranial, transpharyngeal, or transorbital temporomandibular joint views are generally adequate. A dislocation associated with a fracture of the mandibular condyle often requires open reduction and internal fixation. Referral to an oral surgeon is recommended in this situation.

Damage to the cartilage within the temporomandibular joint can produce a hemarthrosis and a subsequent subluxation, but not a true dislocation of the mandible. Attempts at manual reduction will fail for obvious reasons and are contraindicated if this condition is recognized.

EQUIPMENT

Gauze—preferably with an attached string or trailing appendage to avoid aspiration
Gloves
Local anesthetic equipment
2% lidocaine with 1:100,000 epinephrine
3-mL syringe
21- or 25-gauge 1.5" needle
Suction equipment
McGill forceps

PROCEDURE

The patient is positioned in a chair facing the physician performing the reduction (1). The head is held firmly by an assistant or stabilized posteriorly against a wall or head rest. Alternatively, the patient may be placed in a supine position with the physician located at the head of the bed. In the seated patient, further control is gained by straddling the patient's lap (Fig. 70.2.A). Both thumbs are swathed in gauze to avoid injury when the mandible snaps back into place. The thumbs are placed against the surface of the lower molars as far posteriorly as possible. The fingers of each hand are wrapped under the angle and body of the mandible with the elbows flexed at a 90° angle. Pressure is applied first in a downward motion to release the condyle from the articular eminence, and then posteriorly to move the condyle back into the fossa (Fig. 70.2.B). A less common but also effective method is performed by seating the patient upright in a chair and standing behind the patient. The physician presses downward with his or her thumbs over the posterior lower molars. The physician's fingers are used to provide counteraction by pulling upward along the inferior aspect of the patient's anterior mandible. In this way, the patient's

head can be braced against the physician's abdomen, thereby minimizing any movement. Care must be taken to avoid a crushing injury to the fingers or teeth once reduction is achieved. Placing the thumbs in the buccal aspect of the mandibular ridge rather than on the surface of the molars may avoid this risk but provides less leverage for the reduction. When severe muscle spasm is present, reduction may be facilitated by gently rocking the mandible back and forth until the muscles fatigue. With a bilateral dislocation, reducing one side at a time may prove easier and more successful (3, 6).

Because significant pain and anxiety inevitably accompany this condition, using conscious sedation is recommended in reducing both the level of anxiety and the degree of muscle spasm (Chapter 35). Frequently, reduction may not be possible without the concomitant use of anesthetic agents to facilitate patient cooperation and muscle relaxation. In some cases intraarticular or intramuscular administration of lidocaine may aid reduction by relaxing the lateral pterygoid and temporalis muscles, which tend to force the mandible forward (6, 7).

Displacement of the meniscus may simulate temporomandibular joint dislocation and is an additional cause for reduction failure. Patients with temporomandibular joint dislocation that fails to reduce should be referred to an oral surgeon for closed or open reduction under general anesthesia.

Patients who have undergone a successful reduction should be warned against opening the mouth widely for approximately 3 weeks to allow the involved ligaments and muscles to resume their normal tone and strength. The mandible should be supported when yawning. The patient should be started on a mild analgesic and advised to eat a soft diet (8).

COMPLICATIONS

Complications associated with the reduction of a temporomandibular joint dislocation are mainly related to the muscular spasm that accompanies the dislocation. Muscles controlling the mandible are capable of generating forces in excess of 300 lb/in^2 (9). If reduction does not occur in a controlled fashion, these

SUMMARY
1. Administer conscious sedation as needed
2. Position patient upright in chair and straddle patient's lap
3. Protect thumbs by generously wrapping them in gauze
4. Place thumbs against lower posterior molars and wrap fingers around angle and body of mandible
5. Apply slow steady pressure first downward and then posteriorly

CLINICAL TIPS
1. Using sedation is highly recommended to alleviate anxiety and decrease the degree of muscle spasm.
2. Stimulation of the gag reflex has been described in adults as a successful alternative to manual reduction.
3. Gentle rocking of the mandible or digital massage may fatigue muscles that are in spasm and ease reduction.
4. With a bilateral dislocation, reduction of one condyle at a time may be useful when spasm is severe.
5. Dislocations associated with fractures should be referred to an oral surgeon for reduction.

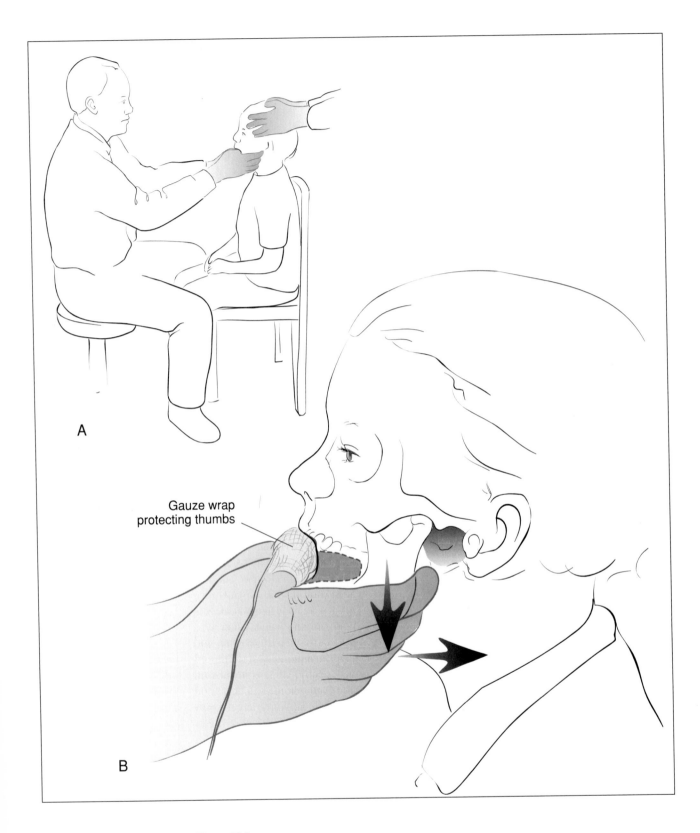

Gauze wrap
protecting thumbs

A

B

Figure 70.2.
A. Position of the patient, assistant, and physician in preparation for reduction.
B. Application and direction of forces in the reduction of an anteriorly dislocated temporomandibular joint.

forces are capable of producing crush injuries of the physician's thumbs and fractures of the patient's teeth.

Aspiration of gauze used as protection for the physician's thumbs has been described (10). The reflex withdrawal of the thumbs on reduction may result in gauze that is not tightly bound to the thumbs remaining in the posterior pharynx. The sedated patient is at additional risk for this problem. Suction and airway equipment, including McGill forceps, should therefore always be available. Using gauze with trailing appendages may decrease the risk of this complication (11).

SUMMARY

Temporomandibular joint dislocation is a painful and anxiety-provoking condition that occurs only rarely in children. Those afflicted generally seek immediate care in the office or ED. Unilateral and bilateral anterior dislocations of the mandible are the most common presentations, and most can be manually reduced. Other dislocations have a higher incidence of associated fractures and complications and require the expertise of an oral surgeon.

REFERENCES

1. Kruger GO. The temporomandibular joint. In: Kruger GO. ed. Textbook of oral and maxillofacial surgery. St. Louis: CV Mosby, 1979.
2. Upton LG. Management of injuries to the temporomandibular joint. In: Fonseca RF, Walker RV, eds, Oral and maxillofacial trauma. Philadelphia: WB Saunders, 1991.
3. Wessberg GA. Mandibular condylar dislocation. Hawaii Dent J 1987:9–11.
4. Bradley PF. Injuries of the condylar and coronoid process. In: Rowe NL, Williams JL, eds. Maxillofacial injuries. Edinburgh: Churchill Livingstone, 1985.
5. Lentrodt G. Treatment of dislocation of the TMJ. In: Kruger E, Schili W, Worthington P, eds. Oral and maxillofacial traumatology. Chicago: Quintessence Publishing Co., 1986.
6. Luyk NH, Larsen PE. The diagnosis and treatment of the dislocated mandible. Am J Emerg Med 1989; 7:329–335.
7. Littler BO. The role of local anesthesia in the reduction of long-standing dislocation of the temporomandibular joint. Br J Oral Surg 1980;18:81–85.
8. Dolwick MF. Management of temporomandibular joint disorders. In: Peterson LJ, Ellis E, Hupp JR, Tucker MR, eds. Contemporary oral and maxillofacial surgery. St. Louis: CV Mosby, 1993.
9. Awang MN. A new approach to the reduction of acute dislocation of the temporomandibular joint: a report of three cases. Br J Oral Maxillofac Surg 1987;25:244–249.
10. Wagner DK, ed. 1985 year book of emergency medicine. Chicago: Year Book, 1985.
11. Mariani PJ. Avoiding "death in the dental chair" (letter). Am J Emerg Med 1989;8:85.

CARDIOVASCULAR PROCEDURES

Section Editor: Richard M. Ruddy

THE ELECTROCARDIOGRAM IN INFANTS AND CHILDREN

Michele R. Wadsworth and Benjamin K. Silverman

INTRODUCTION

The surface electrocardiogram (ECG) remains an efficient and inexpensive aid in the initial and emergent evaluation of dysrhythmias, conduction disturbances, myocardial damage, and chamber hypertrophy and dilatation. Important differences exist between children of various ages and adults in both the procedure for obtaining an ECG and in its interpretation. This chapter provides guidance for efficient use of the electrocardiograph, indications for obtaining a pediatric ECG, and interpretation of some of the more commonly seen tracings in the pediatric acute care setting.

ANATOMY AND PHYSIOLOGY

The anatomy of both the chest wall and heart of the pediatric patient differs from that of an adult in a number of ways which directly affect the recording of the ECG. The heart of an infant or child is larger relative to the size of the thoracic cavity. The normal adult heart occupies about half of the transverse diameter of the thorax, whereas the normal pediatric heart occupies up to two-thirds of this space, depending on the age of the child. Generally, the younger the patient, the larger the area that the heart occupies. This proportionately wider anterior chest surface area is compensated for when recording an electro-cardiogram by adding one or two extra right-sided chest leads and, if necessary, an extra left-sided lead in infants and younger children (see Procedure later in this chapter).

The right ventricle is the dominant ventricle until the child is at least 3 years of age and occasionally even older. As a result, a right axis deviation is generally normal in the child under 3 years, and the unipolar aVR lead usually has a dominant R wave. The QRS progression across the chest leads most often begins with a dominant R wave in V_4R, has equivoltage R and S waves in the transitional area, and has either a dominant R wave or dominant S wave at V_6 or V_7.

Many of the primary differences between adult and pediatric tracings occur because of age-related variations in relative thickness of the ventricular walls and the position and orientation of the heart within the thorax. For example, T waves are normally inverted in the right-sided chest leads in infants and younger children, because the position of the heart and the right ventricular dominance results in the T vector lying leftward and posteriorly. The right-sided T waves also may be inverted in adolescents but eventually become upright in adults, as the T vector gradually shifts from posterior to anterior. T waves also may be inverted in lead III in infants and young children.

An exhaustive explanation of the physiologic and electromechanical principles of electrocardiography and vectorcardiography are beyond the scope of this chapter. Several excellent references provide a more detailed explanation of these principles (1).

To briefly review normal conduction, the cardiac beat begins with spontaneous depolarization of a single "slow response" (calcium channel) cell of the sinus node and spreads by contiguous activation through the sinus node to the "fast response" (sodium channel) cells of the atria (resulting in the P wave). The sequence continues with deactivation of the atrioventricular (AV) node and the bundle of His and Purkinje fibers (during the P-R interval). Depolarization of the ventricles then occurs through the right and left bundle branches, with sequential progression through the septum, the apices, and the ventricular walls (the QRS complex). Ventricular repolarization subsequently follows (T wave) (see also Chapters 21 and 72).

INDICATIONS

The most common indications for obtaining an ECG in the pediatric patient are listed in Table 71.1. History of palpitations, heart racing, and fluttering of the heart should lead the clinician to consider an underlying electrocardiac abnormality or a structural lesion. Tachycardias, bradycardias, or irregular rates and/or rhythms should be detectable on examination of the patient, and the ECG can be used as a confirmatory and diagnostic tool.

Signs of cardiac failure may be subtle in infants and young children, and the differentiation from primary pulmonary disease may be difficult. Patients in failure may manifest nonspecific electrocardiographic changes, and specific cardiac changes associated with an underlying cardiac lesion. An electrocardiogram can be helpful in determining previ-

ously undiagnosed congenital heart disease or onset of acquired heart disease, and can aid in the diagnosis of pericarditis or myocarditis.

In general, significant murmurs, such as heard with underlying cardiac disease, are determined by the intensity, radiation, and point of maximum loudness. Children in a high output state, such as hyperpyrexia, may present with a loud murmur that does not prove to be significant. If the patient has no known prior history of murmur and the clinical picture cannot be defined, an ECG may be helpful.

Cyanosis related to pulmonary disease usually improves significantly with oxygen. Cyanosis not ameliorated by oxygen may be related to methemobloginemia but also may be related to previously undiagnosed cyanotic congenital heart disease. An electrocardiogram can be helpful in excluding the cardiac causes of cyanosis.

The differential diagnosis of chest pain in children is a long list, but is uncommonly related to cardiac disease. The most common causes are functional, musculoskeletal, costochondritis, and respiratory problems. If cardiac disease is suspected, however, an ECG should be obtained which may show signs of cardiac strain, ischemia, or angina. Syncope in children is most commonly related to vasovagal episodes, orthostatic syncope, and breath-holding spells. An electrocardiogram should be performed if the history is not consistent with one of the above mentioned diagnoses, or an abnormality is found on physical examination. On occasion, chest pain without overt palpitations will be found in children with an aberrant atrial pathway, such as Wolff-Parkinson-White syndrome. Syncope is occasionally the only manifestation of prolonged QT syndrome.

Table 71.1.
Indications for ECG Tracing in Pediatric Acute Care

- Extreme tachycardia
- Extreme bradycardia
- Irregularity of rhythm, palpitations, sensation of fluttering of heart
- Clinical suggestion of cardiac failure
- Clinical suggestion of myocarditis or pericarditis
- Significant murmur not readily explainable
- Cyanosis not ameliorated by oxygen
- Chest pain and/or syncope
- Suspected calcium or potassium abnormalities
- Ingestion of cardiac toxic drug and any symptomatic overdose

EQUIPMENT

The essential piece of equipment for recording the ECG is the electrocardiograph and its associated equipment (Table 71.2). These machines have evolved over the years from Einthoven's galvanometer to today's electronically complex computers that do all the recording work when programmed properly. Many of the remaining older, more labor in-

Table 71.2.
Equipment for Recording an Electrocardiogram

Electrocardiograph
  Fully automated and computerized (Fig. 71.1)
  Manually directed
  Semiautomated
Electrode wires, appropriately labeled
Electrodes
  Prepackaged, imbued with adherent conducting substance, possibly with conducting button or clip holder; or
  Metal, requiring electrode gel or paste
Recording paper

tensive, manually operated machines have been relegated to use in the ED, although they are becoming increasingly rare. For this reason, the design and operation of these older electrocardiographs will be reviewed along with the features of the more modern machines. The keyboard, monitor, and simultaneous three-channel paper recording of an automated modern electrocardiograph are shown in Figure 71.1. These machines must be preprogrammed but thereafter are relatively simple to operate.

Electrodes are now conveniently prepackaged. They are coated on one side with an adherent conducting material that holds the electrode in place on the patient's chest. They also have a conducting button or clip holder on the other side that attaches to the electrode wires. The older metal electrodes still require electrode paste or jelly for conduction. The appropriate electrode wires, recording paper, and plugs are supplied with the machine.

PROCEDURE

The patient should be lying on an examining table or crib that is free of vibration, or electrical or human contact. The usual array of distractors and tricks may calm the crying infant or frightened child. If not, sedation may be required (Chapter 35) depending on the urgency with which the tracing is indicated and the general clinical status of the patient.

The proper sites for placement of the electrodes are listed in Table 71.3, and they are demonstrated in the diagram shown in Figure 71.2. Proper placement is essential, particularly when sequential ECG tracings will be required over time for a given patient.

Figure 71.1.
Keyboard and monitor of fully automated electrocardiograph.

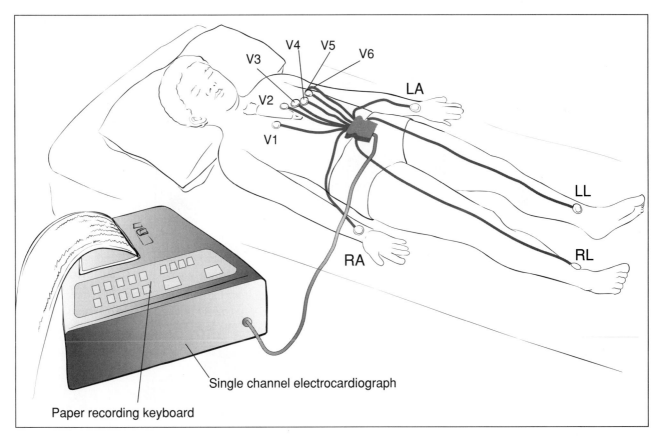

Single channel electrocardiograph

Paper recording keyboard

Table 71.3.
Electrode Location

Extremity Leads
  RA and LA*—anywhere on the right and left arms. In infants less than 1 year of age, place midway between elbow and shoulder
  RL and LL*—anywhere on the right and left legs. In infants place above knee and close to hip
Chest Leads
  V_4R—Midclavicular line (MCL) in right 5th intercostal space (ICS)
  V_3R—Halfway between V_4R and V_1
  V_1—4th ICS at right border of sternum
  V_2—4th ICS at left border of sternum
  V_3—Halfway between V_2 and V_4
  V_4—MCL in 5th left ICS
  V_5—Left anterior axillary line (AAL) on same horizontal level as V_4
  V_6—Left midaxillary line (MAL) on same horizontal level as V_4
  V_7—Left posterior axillary line (PAL) on same horizontal level as V_4

* RA, LA, RL, LL—right and left arms and legs

Figure 71.2.
Correct sites for electrode placement (see Table 71.1 for description).

It may be necessary to clean the skin to remove oils with isopropyl alcohol before placement of the electrodes so that the leads will stay attached during the procedure. Some adolescents will have enough body hair that the electrode sites may be abraded slightly by rubbing with dry gauze or, rarely, shaved. This is not a concern for infants and younger children. As mentioned, most electrodes are now coated with adherent conducting material, but some require application of electrode paste or jelly at each electrode site for adequate electrical contact. Ultrasound gel is nonconducting and is not a substitute for electrode paste.

The number and sites of electrode placement for the chest leads depend on the age of the patient. For infants and children up to approximately 1 year of age, the electrodes

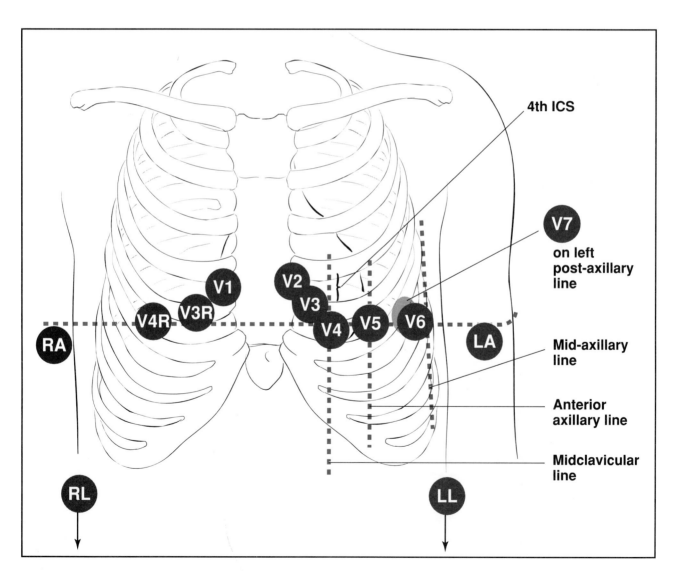

shown in Figure 71.2 will normally be required. Children between 1 and 12 years of age should have leads V_4R through V_6 recorded. For patients older than 12 years of age, only leads V_1 through V_6 are necessary.

Depending on the design of the machine, the electrode lead wires must be attached to the electrode by the appropriate clip, button, or probe. The wires are marked near their distal ends with symbols corresponding to those in Figure 71.2 and Table 71.3. In the more current electrocardiographs, a lead wire is dedicated for each of the chest leads. Modern machines that are designed primarily for adult usage have chest lead wires that are only dedicated for leads V_1 through V_6, and an additional "nondedicated" wire is available for V_4R, V_3, and V_7. Other machines have only a single chest lead wire, which is usually marked with a *C* or a *V*, and which must be disconnected and reattached to the appropriate electrode after each chest lead is recorded. To obtain an interpretable tracing, insertion of the proper lead wire at its correct electrode is essential.

The connector located at the proximal end of the lead wires should be inserted into the designated socket on the electrocardiograph. The power switch should then be turned on and the operator should check the machine for sufficient recording paper. Paper speed is normally set to the standard rate of 25 mm/sec. For older machines, sensitivity should be checked and adjusted by manipulating the sensitivity switch and the 1 mV switch, so that a vertical stylus deflection of 10 mm is equivalent to 1 mV. The patient's name and other pertinent data is then entered.

On modern machines (Fig. 71.1), pressing a single button labeled "Record" will print the entire ECG. Such machines are usually preprogrammed for automatic recording. They are usually set to record one to three leads simultaneously for *X* number of seconds (usually 2.5 to 3 seconds), and they will automatically identify the leads on the recording paper. These machines often store readings that can be sent by modem to the ECG laboratory as a permanent electronic record.

Older semiautomated machines require closer monitoring and greater manual operation. These machines often have to be started and stopped after each lead is recorded. The six limb leads must be selected in sequence by pressing the appropriate button on the keyboard. For each of the chest leads to be recorded, the lead selection switch must be set on *V,* and the chest lead wire must be moved to the appropriate electrode position. Most such machines have a mechanism for marking the leads as they are recorded using a dot-dash system. In others, this can be done manually after the tracing is completed. With the less automated machines, it may be necessary during the recording to adjust the sensitivity from the standard of 10 mm = 1 mV to 5 mm = 1 mV (½ sensitivity) if the stylus deflections exceed the vertical limits of the paper. The leads in which this is done should be identified as "½ sens."

SAMPLE PEDIATRIC ELECTROCARDIOGRAMS

Figures 71.3 through 71.11 show examples of some of the more common findings which may be discovered when obtaining a pediatric ECG. For most examples, only a single lead (Lead II) is reproduced to demonstrate the finding. It should be cautioned that the patient's entire tracing should be examined, and measurements made of P-R interval (Table 71.4), QRS complex, QT interval (Table 71.5), and ST segment depression or elevation. Tracings should be evaluated in the context of the patient's clinical condition and age with reference to a good cardiology text (1) and tables (2, 3, 4). (Table 71.6). In addition, several methods for determining the heart rate are shown in Table 71.7. These methods are discussed more fully with reference to the following specific tracings.

Extreme Tachycardia

Sinus Tachycardia
Figure 71.3 shows the tracing of a child with an extremely rapid heart rate. To measure the actual heart rate using Method 1 in Table 71.7, approximately 3.75 R-R intervals are in six large divisions, so the patient's rate is 188 ($3.75 \times 50 = 188$). Notably, a P wave occurs before every QRS complex, and the P-QRS-T complexes are normal and regular. In general, rates above 160 in a resting neonate, 150 in an infant, and 110 in a child are considered tachycardic. Sinus tachycardia rarely exceeds 220 at any age.

SUMMARY
1. Attempt to calm patient before proceeding, or other appropriate techniques to have child lie still
2. Place electrodes in proper positions
3. Attach distal ends of electrode wires properly onto electrodes and insert proximal plug into machine socket
4. Turn power on
5. Check and adjust sensitivity and paper speed
6. Enter appropriate patient data
7. Record cardiogram, stopping and starting as indicated for semi-automated and manual machines
8. Move and reattach chest electrode wire for each chest lead, if necessary
9. If tracing is not satisfactory, recheck and repeat steps 2–9
10. Identify recorded leads on tracing (using the dot-dash or other method) if not done automatically

Chapter 71
The
Electrocardiogram in
Infants and Children

Figure 71.3.
Sinus tachycardia in a
2-month-old child.

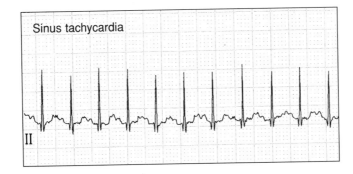

Figure 71.4.
Supraventricular tachy-
cardia in a 7-month-old
child.

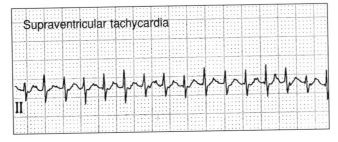

Figure 71.5
Wolff-Parkinson-White
syndrome after conversion
from SVT in 14-year-old
child.

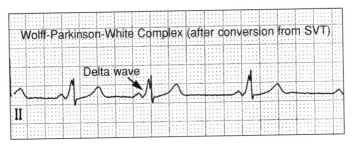

Figure 71.6.
Ventricular tachycardia in
a 2-year-old child.

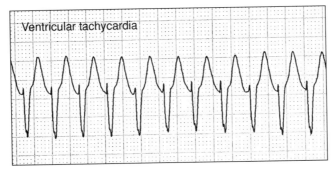

Figure 71.7.
Sinus bradycardia in a 14-
year-old child.

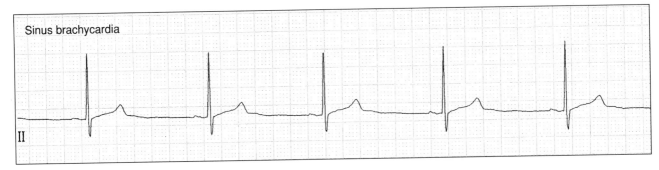

Chapter 71
The
Electrocardiogram in
Infants and Children

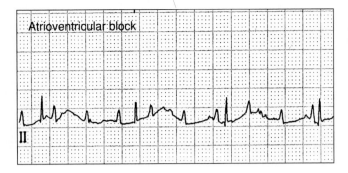

Figure 71.8.
Complete atrioventricular block seen in a 3-month-old child.

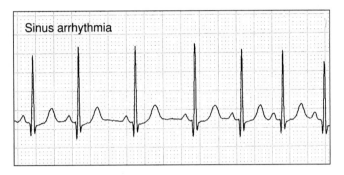

Figure 71.9
Tracing from a 5-year-old child.

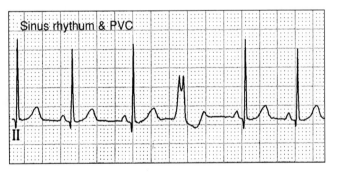

Figure 71.10.
Sinus rhythm with a premature ventricular contraction seen in a 2-year-old child.

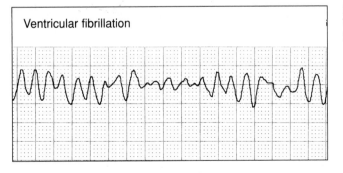

Figure 71.11.
Ventricular fibrillation seen in a 10-month-old child.

Table 71.4.
Normal P-R Intervals with Rate and Age

Rhythm P-R Interval with Rate, Age, and (Upper Limits of Normal)

Rate	0–1 mo	1–6 mo	6 mo–1 yr	1–3 yr	3–8 yr	8–12 yr	12–16 yr	Adult
<60						0.16 (0.18)	0.16 (0.19)	0.17 (0.21)
60–80					0.15 (0.17)	0.15 (0.17)	0.15 (0.18)	0.16 (0.21)
80–100	0.10 (0.12)				0.14 (0.16)	0.15 (0.16)	0.15 (0.17)	0.17 (0.20)
100–120	0.10 (0.12)			(0.15)	0.13 (0.16)	0.14 (0.15)	0.15 (0.16)	0.15 (0.19)
120–140	0.10 (0.11)	0.11 (0.14)	0.11 (0.14)	0.12 (0.14)	0.13 (0.15)	0.14 (0.15)		0.15 (0.18)
140–160	0.09 (0.11)	0.10 (0.13)	0.11 (0.13)	0.11 (0.14)	0.12 (0.14)			(0.17)
160–180	0.10 (0.11)	0.10 (0.12)	0.10 (0.12)	0.10 (0.12)				
>180	0.09	0.09 (0.11)	0.10 (0.11)					

Modified from Guntheroth WG: Pediatric Electrocardiography. Philadelphia: WB Saunders Co, 1965.

Supraventricular Tachycardia

The tracing in Figure 71.4 also shows a tachycardia. Again using Method 1 from Table 71.7, approximately 5.3 R-R intervals are in six large divisions. Therefore the patient's heart rate is 265 (50×5.3 = 265). This rate is higher than what is generally expected for a normally conducting heart, and a form of tachyarrhythmia should be suspected. The QRS complexes are slightly narrowed but otherwise normal, and the P waves are not seen because they are buried in the QRS complexes. When P waves are seen with supraventricular tachycardia (SVT), they are usually inverted and may actually follow after the QRS complex. Adenosine is the drug of choice to treat SVT if the patient is stable. For the unstable patient who is hypotensive or manifests signs of congestive failure (tachypnea, pulmonary crackles, cyanosis, hepatomegaly), immediate cardioversion is necessary. After conversion to sinus rhythm, an underlying Wolff-Parkinson-White complex may be seen as in Figure 71.5. In this tracing, the P-R interval is noted to be shortened, the initial deflection of the QRS complex is sloped (delta wave), and the QRS is widened.

Ventricular Tachycardia

Although demonstrating a tachycardia, the tracing in Figure 71.6 appears markedly different from those shown previously. Once

again using Method 1 from Table 71.7, approximately 3.8 R-R intervals are in six large divisions, giving an underlying rate of 190 (3.8×50 = 190). The rhythm is regular and rapid, with a wide QRS. No correlation exists between the QRS complexes and the P waves, which are difficult to discern. Although the possibility of an SVT with aberrant conduction (right or left bundle branch block) exists, this is a rare occurrence in infants and children. In such cases, the clinician should always assume that the underlying rhythm is ventricular tachycardia unless compelling evidence suggests the contrary (e.g., evaluation in the ED by the patient's cardiologist).

Extreme Bradycardia

Sinus Bradycardia

Figure 71.7 shows the tracing of a child with a slow heart rate. Using Method 2 from Table 71.7, 6.7 large divisions are in 1.0 R-R interval. Thus the heart rate is 44 (300/6.7 = 44). As with sinus tachycardia, the P-QRS-T complexes are normal and regular. Each P wave is followed at a fixed interval by a QRS complex. In general, rates less than 100 in the

Table 71.5.
Corrected QT interval (QT$_c$)

$$QT_c = \frac{\text{measured QT (sec)}}{\text{square root of R-R interval (sec)}}$$

QT$_c$ should not exceed: 0.45 in infants under 6 mo
0.44 in children
0.425 in adolescents and adults

Table 71.6.
Normal Heart Rates for Infants and Children

Age	Heart Rate (beats/min)		
	Resting (awake)	Resting (sleeping)	Exercise (fever)
Newborn	100–180	80–160	Up to 220
1 wk to 3 mo	100–220	80–200	Up to 220
3 mo to 2 yr	80–150	70–120	Up to 200
2 yr to 10 yr	70–110	60–90	Up to 200
10 yr to adult	55–90	50–90	Up to 200

Table 71.7.
Methods for Determining Heart Rate

1. Count R-R intervals in six large divisions (equivalent to 1.2 seconds) and multiply by 50 (best method for fast rates).

OR

2. Count number of large divisions in one R-R interval and divide into 300 (best method for slow rates).

OR

3. Count R-R intervals in 15 large divisions (3 seconds) and multiply by 20 (best for irregular rhythms).

OR

4. Heart rates of 300, 150, 100, 75, 60, 50 have approximate R-R intervals of 5, 10, 15, 20, 25, and 30 small spaces respectively.

OR

5. Use calibrated ECG ''ruler'' for direct reading.

neonate, 80 in the young child, 60 in the older child, and 50 in the adolescent are considered bradycardic. A relatively frequent cause of significant sinus bradycardia in children occurs with unintentional ingestion of cardiac medications such as beta-blockers. Occasionally, an athletic adolescent may have a normal resting heart rate of less than 50. In such cases, the clinician should be guided by symptomatology.

Complete Atrioventricular Block

Figure 71.8 also shows a bradycardia. Using Method 2 from Table 71.7, five large divisions are in 1.0 R-R interval, giving a ventricular rate of 60 (300/5 = 60). Two large divisions are in 1.0 P-P interval, giving an atrial rate of 150 (300/2 = 150). The QRS complexes are regular and narrow, but have no fixed relation to the P waves. This is a complete block at the nodal level. If the block were below the node at the bundle of His, the QRS complexes would be wide and the QRS rate would likely be even slower.

Irregular Rhythm

Sinus Arrhythmia

As shown in Figure 71.9, the R-R intervals are of inconstant duration but each QRS is preceded by a P wave of the same morphology. The P wave is upright in the lead II tracing, indicating a sinus origin of the rhythm.

Premature Ventricular Contractions

The underlying rhythm in Figure 71.10 is sinus. Interspersed are wide QRS complexes occurring before the next anticipated P wave

and followed by an inverted T wave. A series of three or more PVCs in succession is considered ventricular tachycardia.

Ventricular Fibrillation

The QRS complexes in Figure 71.11 occur irregularly and in rapid sequence. They are of varying deflection amplitude and morphology. P waves are not discernible. Immediate defibrillation and drug therapy are essential.

ECGs Demonstrating Other Cardiac Findings

The sample tracings shown in Figures 71.12 through 71.14 demonstrate the pediatric electrocardiographic pictures of ventricular and atrial hypertrophy and of myocardial strain.

RV Hypertrophy

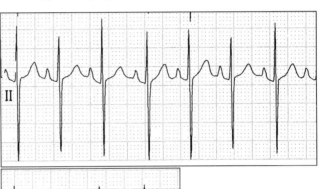

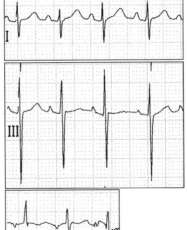

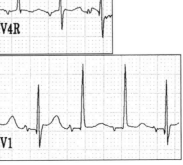

Figure 71.12.
Right atrial and right ventricular hypertrophy in a 5-month-old child.

Chapter 71
The
Electrocardiogram in
Infants and Children

Biventricular hypertrophy

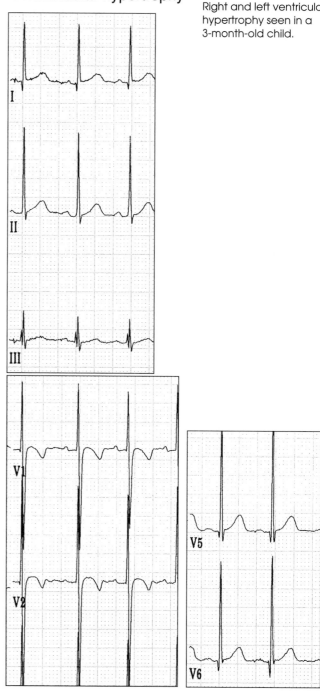

Figure 71.14.
Right and left ventricular hypertrophy seen in a 3-month-old child.

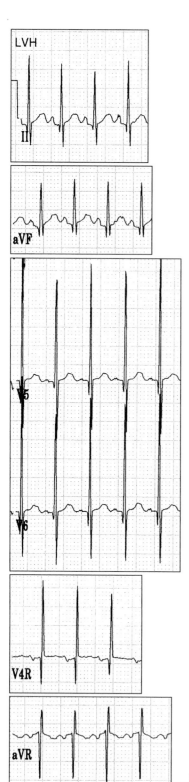

Figure 71.13.
Left ventricular hypertrophy seen in a 4-year-old child.

Importantly, many of these findings vary markedly with the age of the patient and may need pediatric cardiology consultation for definitive interpretation.

Right Ventricular and Right Atrial Hypertrophy

As shown in Figure 71.12, the P-wave deflection in lead II is greater than 3 mm and its shape is pointed, which is diagnostic of right atrial hypertrophy (RAH). Right axis deviation is present, with dominant S in lead I and dominant R in lead III, and positive R deflection in V_4R indicates right ventricular dominance. Although this is not necessarily a pathologic finding in this infant, the S waves in V_6 and V_7 are abnormally deep, suggestive of true right ventricular hypertrophy (RVH). The T waves in V_4R and V_1 are upright and therefore compatible with RVH at this age. A tracing of this sort in an infant is related to increased right ventricular and right auricular pressure due to obstruction to right-sided outflow. Early echocardiography and cardiology consultation are indicated.

Left Ventricular Hypertrophy (LVH)

The cardiogram shown in Figure 71.13 demonstrates tall R waves in lead II, aVF, and the left-sided chest leads of this infant. The S wave is deep in V_4R and dominant in aVR, indicating absence of the normal RV dominance expected at this age. This tracing might be associated with aortic stenosis or primary myocardial disease.

Combined Ventricular Hypertrophy

As shown in Figure 71.14, abnormally tall R waves occur in leads I, II, and III, and in the left-sided and right-sided chest leads in this infant. Deep S waves may also occur in lead I and in the right-sided chest leads. These findings suggest combined ventricular hypertrophy and may be associated with left-to-right shunting or truncus arteriosus, among other lesions.

SUMMARY

In summary, the electrocardiogram remains an efficient and inexpensive aid in evaluating children with arrhythmias, cardiac failure, chest pain, syncope, drug ingestions, and cyanosis. Many differences are found between a child's ECG and an adult's ECG, as outlined in Clinical Tips at the end of this chapter. The electrocardiograph used for a child's and an adult's ECG is basically the same; however, depending on the age of the child, different leads are obtained as explained previously in the Procedure section. The procedure used in obtaining an ECG is described in the Procedure Summary at the end of this chapter. The interpretation of the pediatric ECG can be challenging; however, an orderly approach and remembrance of the difference in a child's anatomy and physiology will enable the clinician to correctly identify abnormalities.

REFERENCES

1. Walsh EP. Electrocardiography and introduction to electrophysiologic techniques. In: Fyler DC, ed. Nadas' pediatric cardiology. Philadelphia: Henley & Belfus, 1992.
2. Park MK, Guntheroth WG. How to read pediatric ECGs. 3rd ed. St. Louis: CV Mosby, 1992.
3. Silverman BK. Patients with heart murmurs. In: Fleisher G, Ludwig, S, eds. Textbook of pediatric emergency medicine. 3rd ed. Baltimore: Williams & Wilkins, 1993, p. 233.
4. Garson A. The electrocardiogram in infants and children: a systematic approach. Philadelphia: Lea & Febiger, 1983, pp. 19–35.

CLINICAL TIPS

1. The pediatric heart fills a greater portion of the chest.
2. Right ventricular dominance is common until approximately 3 years of age.
3. T-wave vector of the right chest may be inverted through much of childhood.
4. In children less than 1 year of age, obtain ECG with additional chest leads—V_3R, V_4R, and V_7.
5. In children 1 to 12 years of age, obtain V_4R through V_6.
6. Heart rate above 220 rarely indicates sinus tachycardia.
7. Bradycardia generally is below 100 in the neonate, 80 in the young child, 60 in the older child, and 50 in an adolescent or adult.

Converting Stable Supraventricular Tachycardia Using Vagal Maneuvers

Kathy N. Shaw

Introduction

Many different vagal maneuvers have been available to convert stable supraventricular tachycardia (SVT). The procedures are relatively simple and can be performed by a variety of medical personnel including physicians, physicians-in-training, nurses, and paramedics. However, because these techniques may in rare instances result in profound bradycardia or asystole, supervision by individuals experienced in pediatric resuscitation would be best. Vagal maneuvers are usually temporary measures to establish sinus rhythm because medication is usually required to maintain the child in normal sinus rhythm.

SVT is an abnormal tachycardia (narrow complex in 90%) usually due to a reentrant mechanism. In older children and adolescents, SVT may be present at rates above 150 beats per minute (bpm). In infants, the heart rate is usually at or above 240 bpm, but may be as high as 300 bpm. SVT must be distinguished from sinus tachycardia (ST) which is usually less than 200 bpm, but can occasionally produce heart rates of up to 265 bpm in infancy. However, signs of fever, hypovolemia, or sepsis usually are present (1, 2). It is important to distinguish SVT from ventric-ular tachycardia (VT). In general, the patient with wide complex tachycardia in the range of 150 to 240 must have an assessment to determine there is a risk factor for VT such as cardiac disease, electrolyte abnormality or overdose. If a past history of SVT is indicated, it is usually easier to assume the patient is in SVT.

SVT is the most common significant dysrhythmia in children. Its incidence ranges from 1:1000 to as high as 1:250. The majority of children presenting with SVT will be under 1 year of age, and close to half of the cases will occur in infants less than 4 months of age. These young babies usually have a normal underlying heart with occasional predisposing factors such as myocarditis, drugs, congenital heart disease, thyrotoxicosis, or sepsis (2). Of interest is that a number of infants present after using an over-the-counter cold preparation or other medication with sympathomimetic properties.

Anatomy and Physiology

The majority of infants and children with SVT have an accessory atrioventricular (AV) pathway. This developmental abnormality may change the heart's electrophysiologic

Chapter 72
Converting Stable
Supraventricular
Tachycardia Using
Vagal Maneuvers

771

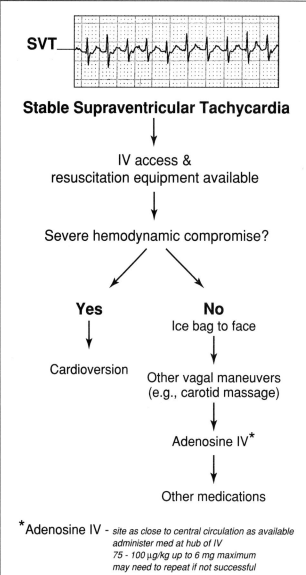

SVT —

Stable Supraventricular Tachycardia

↓

IV access &
resuscitation equipment available

↓

Severe hemodynamic compromise?

Yes   **No**
Ice bag to face

↓   ↓

Cardioversion   Other vagal maneuvers
(e.g., carotid massage)

↓

Adenosine IV*

↓

Other medications

*Adenosine IV - *site as close to central circulation as available*
administer med at hub of IV
75 - 100 μg/kg up to 6 mg maximum
may need to repeat if not successful

Figure 72.1.
Approach to stable
supraventricular
tachycardia (SVT).

**Chapter 72
Converting Stable
Supraventricular
Tachycardia Using
Vagal Maneuvers**

usually successful in converting SVT in young children (3). The diving reflex, which occurs in many aquatic mammals and also in young children, is a very potent stimulus to the afferent limb of this vagally mediated reflex (4).

INDICATIONS

Vagal maneuvers should be used only in children with stable SVT who do not exhibit signs of severe hemodynamic compromise. Patients with congestive heart failure or shock should have immediate cardioversion (Chapter 22) (5). In stable SVT, vagal maneuvers often are tried first. If unsuccessful, adenosine is then used (Fig. 72.1) (5).

All children with SVT deserve a pediatric cardiologist consult even after an uncomplicated return to sinus rhythm. Vagal maneuvers may only be effective temporarily. Further diagnostic work-up may be indicated including electrophysiologic studies. Long-term medical treatment is often indicated.

EQUIPMENT

Table 72.1 lists the equipment used for conversion of stable supraventricular tachycardia. All children should have an intravenous

**Table 72.1.
Equipment**

Monitor:
   Electrocardiographic machine
   Cardiac monitor
   Oximetry
   Bag-valve-mask for age, suction
     equipment
Intravenous access:
   Intravenous catheter
   Alcohol swab
   Normal saline
Resuscitation medications:
   Epinephrine 1:10,000
   Atropine
   Lidocaine
Defibrillator/cardioversion machine:
   Pediatric paddles
   Electrode gel
Ice bag:
   Plastic bag
   Water
   Ice
Gagging or rectal stimulation:
   Sterile tongue depressor
   Gloves
   Lubricating jelly

characteristics during the child's growth (1). At birth, autonomic cardiovascular control is not fully developed and may be under hormonal control. This concept of autonomic imbalance or immaturity is one hypothesis of why SVT is more common in young infants (3). SVT from AV node reentry or primary atrial tachycardia is more common after infancy or postcardiac surgery (1).

Parasympathetic stimulus via the vagus nerve to the sinus and AV nodes slows heart rate. At birth, the infant has a predominance of vagal tone due to an immature sympathetic system. However, despite this parasympathetic predominance, with the exception of the diving reflex, few vagal maneuvers are

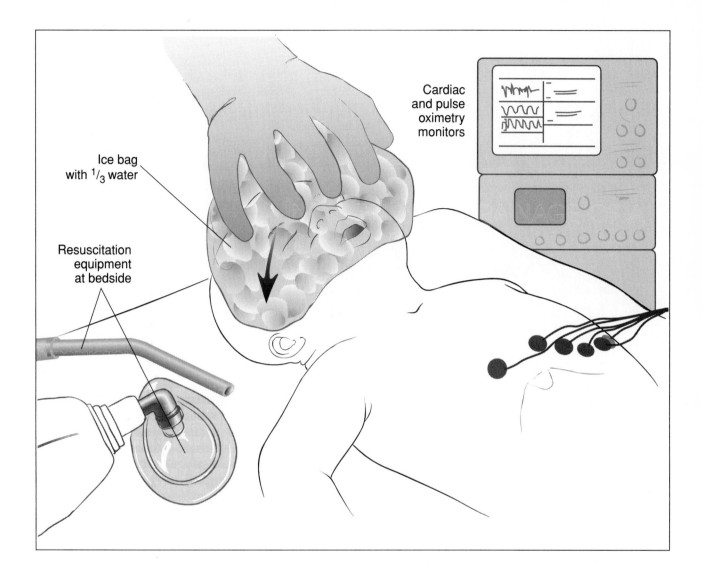

Ice bag
with ¹/₃ water

Resuscitation
equipment
at bedside

Cardiac
and pulse
oximetry
monitors

Figure 72.2.
Ice bag application to the
face to stimulate the diving
reflex.

line placed, and resuscitation drugs and emergency airway equipment available.

PROCEDURE

Vagal maneuvers include facial immersion in cold water or saline, applying an ice bag on the face, carotid sinus massage, valsalva maneuvers, rectal stimulation, eliciting a gag reflex with a tongue depressor, induction of vomiting with ipecac, breath holding, coughing, and using antishock trousers (Table 72.1) (2–9). Ocular pressure also has been used but is not recommended due to risk of eye injury including retinal detachment.

Unfortunately, vagal maneuvers, with the exception of applying the ice bag to the face, are not usually successful in children under 4 years of age (2). Additionally, breath holding, facial immersion in iced saline, coughing, valsalva maneuvers, carotid massage to children with a short neck, and using antishock trousers are impractical in the infant or uncooperative young child. Thus applying the ice bag to the face is the preferred technique. An attempt at gentle rectal stimulation with a gloved, lubricated finger, induction of the gag reflex with a tongue blade, or brief carotid massage also may be attempted before using adenosine. Parenteral use of adenosine is now recommended in children for conversion of stable SVT and is usually successful (10, 11).

Ice Bag Technique

The infant or child should have intravenous access, continuous ECG monitoring, and

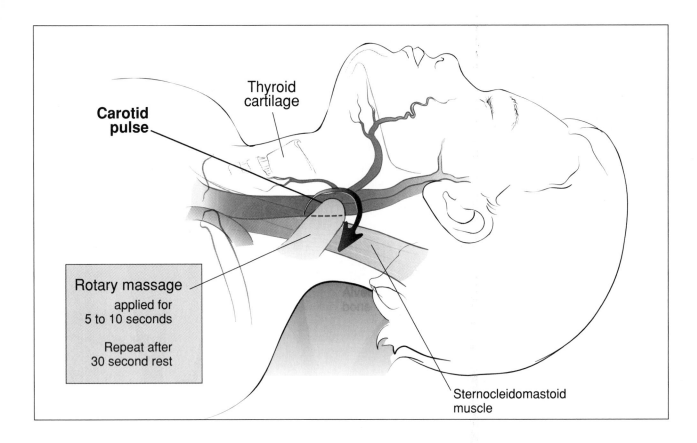

Carotid pulse

Thyroid cartilage

Rotary massage
applied for
5 to 10 seconds

Repeat after
30 second rest

Sternocleidomastoid
muscle

Figure 72.3.
Carotid massage
technique.

pulse oximetry. Resuscitation equipment and medications should be available at bedside. A plastic bag is filled with one-third water and then an equal volume of ice. The bag should be large enough to completely cover the child's face and overlap to the preauricular area. As the procedure is explained to older children they are asked to hold their breath in end inspiration. Young children are immobilized. The bag is applied so that it covers the areas of the nose and mouth and prevents breathing for a maximum of 15 seconds (Fig. 72.2). If conversion to sinus rhythm is noted earlier, the bag is immediately removed (2, 4).

Carotid Massage

Carotid massage is most effective in older children with long, narrow necks who will be cooperative and remain relaxed. Intravenous access should be obtained and normal saline available to treat hypotension. Monitoring and resuscitation equipment and medications are at bedside. To apply carotid massage, the child's head is turned to the left and tilted backward slightly. The carotid pulse is lo-

cated just below the angle of the mandible at the upper level of the thyroid cartilage and anterior to the sternocleidomastoid muscle. Firm but gentle rotary motion or massage is applied with the fingertip for 5 to 10 seconds without complete occlusion of the pulse (Fig. 72.3). If unsuccessful, the procedure may be repeated after 30 seconds of rest. Simultaneous, bilateral carotid pressure or massage should never be used. The procedure also should not be performed if digitalis toxicity is suspected (5, 7).

COMPLICATIONS

No child should have vagal maneuvers tried without first obtaining intravenous access, with ongoing continuous cardiac and pulse oximetry monitoring, and all necessary resuscitation medications and equipment available. Asystole and other dysrhythmias are potentially unavoidable side effects from vagal maneuvers. Usually asystole is brief with spontaneous conversion to sinus rhythm (6). Complications and adverse effects of each of the vagal maneuvers are listed in Table 72.2.

**Chapter 72
Converting Stable
Supraventricular
Tachycardia Using
Vagal Maneuvers**

774

Table 72.2.
Vagal Maneuvers: Complications

Vagal Maneuver	Advantage	Possible Disadvantage
All (5, 6)	**Noninvasive**	• **Transient effect** • **Asystole** • **Dysrhythmias**
Ice bag to face (4)	Most successful	• Apnea • Unpleasant
Immersion of face in iced saline with breathing holding (2)	Older children can perform themselves	• Unpleasant • Aspiration
Carotid massage (5–7)	Easy to perform on older children	• Transient ischemic attack/CVA • Not with digoxin toxicity
Rectal stimulation (8)	Can be used in noncooperative or young child	• Tissue trauma • Unpleasant
Valsalva (6)	Older, cooperative child	• Subconjunctival hemorrhages • Rupture of tympanic membrane • Syncope
Antishock trousers (9)	Easy to use	• Limited from toddler size and older
Coughing	Older, cooperative child	• Aspiration • Subconjunctival hemorrhage • Ruptured tympanic membrane • Syncope
Gag reflex	Easy to perform on all ages	• Tissue trauma • Emesis/aspiration • Unpleasant

SUMMARY

Vagal maneuvers often are not effective in young infants with supraventricular tachycardia. In older children, especially with recurrent SVT, the maneuvers often are successful. However, an attempt at using the diving reflex or other vagal maneuvers can be tried before using adenosine. Proper monitoring, intravenous access, and resuscitation equipment and medications should be available for the uncommon, but serious, complication of prolonged asystole.

REFERENCES

1. Kon Ko J, Deal BJ, Strasburger JF, Benson DW. Supraventricular tachycardia mechanisms and their age distribution in pediatric patients. Am J Cardiol 1992;69:1028–1032.
2. Ludomirsky A, Garson A. Supraventricular tachycardia. In: Gillette PC, Garson A, eds. Pediatric cardiac dysrhythmias. New York: Grune and Stratton Publishers, 1990, pp. 380–514.
3. Perry JC, Garson A. Diagnosis and treatment of arrhythmias. Adv Pediatr 1989;36:177–200.
4. Bisset GS, Gaum W, Kaplan S. The ice bag: a new technique for interruption of supraventricular tachycardia. J Pediatr 1980;97:593–595.
5. Emergency Cardiac Care Committee and Subcommittees, American Heart Association. Pediatric advanced life support. JAMA 1992;268(16):2262–2274.
6. Waxman MB, Wald RW, Sharma AD, Huerta F, Cameron DA. Vagal techniques for termination of paroxysmal supraventricular tachycardia. Am J Cardiol 1980;46:655–664.
7. Gazak S. Carotid sinus massage. In: Roberts JR, Hedges JR, eds. Clinical procedures in emergency medicine. Philadelphia: WB Saunders, 1985, pp. 150–159.
8. Roberge R, Anderson E, MacMath T, Rudoff J, Luten R. Termination of paroxysmal supraventricular tachycardia by digital rectal massage. Ann Emerg Med 1987:16;1291–1293.
9. Walder LA, MacMath TL, Chipman H, Bvayne E. MAST application in the treatment of paroxysmal supraventricular tachycardia in a child. Ann Emerg Med 1988;17;529–531.
10. Till J, Shinebourne EA, Rigby ML, Clarke B, Ward DE, Rowland E. Efficacy and safety of adenosine in the treatment of supraventricular tachycardia in infants and children. Br Heart J 1989;62:204–211.
11. Overholt ED, Rheuban KS, Gutgesell HP, Lerman BB, Dimarco JP. Usefulness of adenosine for arrhythmias in infants and children. Am J Cardiol 1988;61:336–340.

Chapter 72
Converting Stable
Supraventricular
Tachycardia Using
Vagal Maneuvers

775

PERICARDIOCENTESIS

Scott D. Reeves

INTRODUCTION

Pericardiocentesis is the use of a needle-syringe system to aspirate fluid from the pericardial space. Although not often required in the emergency department (ED), the prompt and efficient removal of pericardial fluid can be life saving in cases of cardiac tamponade. Pericardiocentesis also may be performed electively as a diagnostic procedure in cases of pericardial effusion and as a means for improving cardiac output in chronic pericardial accumulations. The technique for pericardiocentesis is relatively straightforward, but studies in both children and adults report variable success rates in the emergency setting. In addition, a number of severe complications have been reported and the overall complication rate is fairly high. For these reasons, emergent pericardiocentesis should be performed only by physicians who are comfortable managing critically ill children and when its performance is necessary to improve cardiac output in the face of life-threatening cardiac tamponade.

ANATOMY AND PHYSIOLOGY

The pericardial sac is a thin, transparent fibrous membrane that surrounds the heart and the trunk of the great vessels. The sac comprises two layers, the visceral and the parietal pericardium. The interface of these two layers is a potential space which when filled with fluid becomes the pericardial space. The nor-

mal pericardium may contain 20 to 30 mL of free fluid if it is accessed by a surgical procedure.

Animal studies have shown that large volumes of fluid may occupy the pericardial space with relatively little impairment of cardiac function. This is especially true in subacute accumulations, when the pericardial space can be greatly expanded in the face of increasing fluid volume. At some point, however, relatively small increases in pericardial fluid volume lead to marked increases in pressure, with a resultant decrease in cardiac filling and cardiac output. The end result of this chain of events is sudden hemodynamic compromise, cardiac tamponade, and shock. The point at which this decompensation occurs depends primarily on three factors: the absolute volume of pericardial fluid, the rate of accumulation of pericardial fluid, and the compliance of the pericardium. In trauma, rapid accumulation of pericardial blood in a space where compliance may play a less important effect leads to rapid deterioration. In collagen vascular disease or chronic infection, the slower accumulation may allow the compliant pericardium to expand to much larger volumes of fluid with less clinical symptoms.

In addition, the pressure-volume relationship of the pericardium demonstrates hysteresis; that is, removal of a given amount of fluid diminishes intrapericardial pressure more than its addition raised the pressure. Prompt drainage of intrapericardial fluid capitalizes on these characteristics. Removal of even small amounts of fluid may dramatically lessen intrapericardial pressure and restore cardiac output to an acceptable range.

Accumulation of pericardial fluid will alter the clinician's findings on physical examination and detailed cardiac evaluation. On auscultation, changes may be as subtle as minimal reduction of the amplitude and tone of the heart sounds (such as muffling). In the subacute effusion, a pericardial friction rub may occur from the movement of the heart within the inflamed fluid and sac, which may translate to reduced voltages on the cardiac monitor and ECG leads. As the fluid further increases, findings begin to further reflect the impact of reduced cardiac filling with reduced stroke volume and compensatory tachycardia, narrowing of the pulse pressure, pulsus paradoxus, and eventually reduced cardiac output and poor perfusion. In trauma, these physiologic changes may occur in minutes to hours whereas in less acute problems this may occur over hours to days. Beck's triad (distant heart sounds, distended neck veins, and hypotension) is the classic sign of cardiac tamponade; however, these findings are both late and inconsistent indicators of tamponade. Although 90% of patients with tamponade will display at least one characteristic of the triad, fewer than one-third of patients exhibit the full triad on diagnosis.

EQUIPMENT

The necessary equipment is listed in Table 73.1. The needle system can be a standard over-the-needle catheter, or in more chronic effusions, it can be beneficial to insert an over-the-wire catheter. This allows the catheter to remain in place to continue drainage in an ongoing process. In trauma, a needle alone is sufficient because it is usually necessary to have an immediate operative thoracotomy or pericardial window.

INDICATIONS

The only emergent indication for pericardiocentesis is the development of cardiac tamponade that is endangering the patient's life. A slightly less urgent indication is to obtain pericardial fluid for diagnostic testing, especially culture in patients with effusion but not in tamponade.

Pericardial effusions leading to cardiac tamponade are commonly divided into two categories—traumatic and atraumatic. This classification scheme emphasizes the importance of traumatic tamponade as a rapidly developing form of tamponade which often poses an immediate threat to the patient's life. Traumatic tamponade commonly is the result of direct penetration of the pericardium, such as by a knife blade. This results in the rapid accumulation of blood in the pericardial space and the sudden onset of cardiac decompensation. Less commonly, traumatic tamponade may develop as the result of blunt trauma, such as that produced by a vehicular crash. These are a result of rapid acceleration-deceleration injuries when the chest impacts against a hard surface (e.g., steering wheel, handle bars, or solid ground). In any case, prompt attention to the historical features—signs and symptoms of traumatic tamponade—is imperative for successful management.

Atraumatic tamponade occurs less frequently than traumatic tamponade and tends to be less acute. This is primarily the result of the slower rate of accumulation of atraumatic effusions, which allows the pericardium to compensate for the increased volume with a proportionately lesser increase in pressure. This slower rate of accumulation has clinical implications for the emergency physician. Many patients with atraumatic effusions can

Table 73.1.
Equipment

All Children	Infants/ Young Children	Older Children
Sterile drapes	20-gauge spinal needle	1.5″ 16- to 18-gauge over-the-needle catheter
Betadine solution	1.5″ 18- to 20-gauge over-the-needle catheter	50 mL syringe
Local anesthetic 3 syringes (10, 20, 50 mL) 3-way stopcock Alligator clip Flexible guide wire Scalpel blade 22-gauge needle ECG monitor	1.5″ 16- to 18-gauge over-the-needle catheter	

be managed without emergent ED drainage or at least undergo pericardiocentesis in a more controlled fashion than those with traumatic tamponade.

Causes of atraumatic pericardial effusions are numerous and varied. A complete discussion is beyond the scope of this chapter. Neoplasm, infection, connective tissue disease, drugs, and metabolic disorders are the most common causes. Of particular interest in the pediatric population is purulent pericarditis, an inflammation of the pericardium secondary to pyogenic bacteria (most commonly *Staphylococcus aureus*). Purulent pericarditis affects younger children predominately, with one-third of all patients less than 6 years of age.

It must be emphasized, however, that any patient with evidence of hemodynamic instability secondary to tamponade, whatever the etiology, should undergo prompt drainage of the pericardial space. Contraindications to pericardiocentesis in the unstable patient are few. Perhaps the most reasonable contraindication is the availability of a better form of therapy (e.g., immediate pericardial window or thoracotomy for the unstable trauma patient). If immediate therapeutic alternatives are lacking, however, no absolute contraindications to pericardiocentesis exist. An important consideration in patients with pericardial effusion or tamponade is whether they have problems with coagulation which could make hemorrhage more likely with pericardiocentesis if the hemostatic disorder is not corrected.

PROCEDURE

Before initiating pericardiocentesis, the physician should ensure that the patient's airway is patent and secure. Parenteral sedation with a short-acting reversible agent may be required in all but the most critically ill patients. Use in injured patients needs to be weighed against possible central nervous system injury or impending shock. The patient should be placed supine, either parallel to the floor or slightly in reverse Trendelenburg. ECG, vital signs and oxygen saturation should be monitored continuously throughout the procedure.

After any necessary management and patient positioning, the operator should gown, glove, and mask for the procedure. The needle entry site (just inferior and to the left of the xiphoid process) is prepped with povidone-iodine (Fig. 73.1.A). If time permits, infiltrative local anesthesia may be used, taking care to anesthetize the muscular layer as well as the skin. After the area is anesthetized, the appropriate sized needle (Table 73.1) is attached to a large syringe (20, 35, or 50 mL). An alligator clip should then be attached to the hub of the needle and connected to a grounded precordial lead on an ECG monitor. The skin is entered approximately 1 cm to the left and immediately inferior to the xiphoid process, with the needle aiming cephalad at a 45° angle to the skin surface. The needle is slowly advanced and directed toward the tip of the patient's left scapula. The plunger of the syringe should be withdrawn slightly and continuously as the needle is inserted. The needle should be advanced until pericardial fluid is obtained or ECG changes are observed. If fluid is obtained, the clinician should drain as much as possible. Pericardial fluid is typically clear and nonclotting. It has a lower hematocrit than venous (ventricular) blood. In patients to be managed nonoperatively, a catheter may then be inserted into the pericardial space using a guide wire by the Seldinger technique. The catheter is then attached to a stopcock, which may be opened and aspirated if symptoms of tamponade recur.

Acute ECG changes during attempted aspiration indicate contact with the ventricular wall (Fig. 73.1.B). These usually appear as either ST-T wave changes, QRS widening, or premature ventricular beats with wide complexes. If ECG changes are encountered, the needle should be withdrawn a small distance until the original electrical pattern returns, then slightly redirected. If ECG changes do not disappear, the needle should be completely withdrawn.

In some cases, the patient's clinical condition may preclude ECG monitoring on the needle during the procedure. In these instances the procedure needs to be performed blindly, using the landmarks outlined previously. An assistant should continuously observe the cardiac monitor to immediately visualize any rhythm disturbance. The best indicator of successful pericardiocentesis is rapid improvement in the patient's hemody-

SUMMARY
1. Assess patient—airway, breathing, circulation
2. Recognize presence of cardiac tamponade
   a. Beck's triad—distant heart sounds, increased jugular venous distention, hypotension
   b. Suspect in appropriate clinical setting in absence of Beck's triad
3. Position patient in reverse Trendelenberg to maximize success rate
4. Select appropriate sizes of equipment for age; consider using catheter-over-wire system if chronic effusion to allow continued drainage
5. Attach needle to grounded ECG lead (if time allows) using chest lead
6. Insert needle at 45 8 angle 1 cm to left of xiphoid process; consider parasternal approach in adolescents
7. Advance needle (with constant traction on plunger) until fluid is obtained and withdraw needle a short distance if ECG changes occur; redirect when ECG changes are sure
8. Assess patient response
   a. Pulses, blood pressure
   b. Heart sounds
   c. Jugular venous distention
9. After procedure, follow up with appropriate monitoring in critical care setting or operative intervention

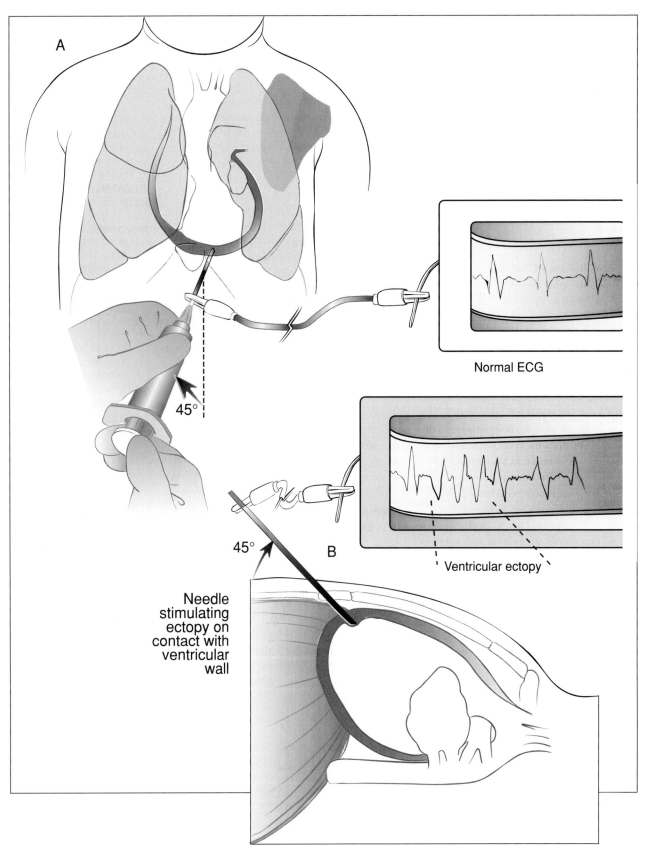

A

Normal ECG

45°

45°

B

Needle
stimulating
ectopy on
contact with
ventricular
wall

Ventricular ectopy

Figure 73.1.
Pericardiocentesis in child
from substernal approach.

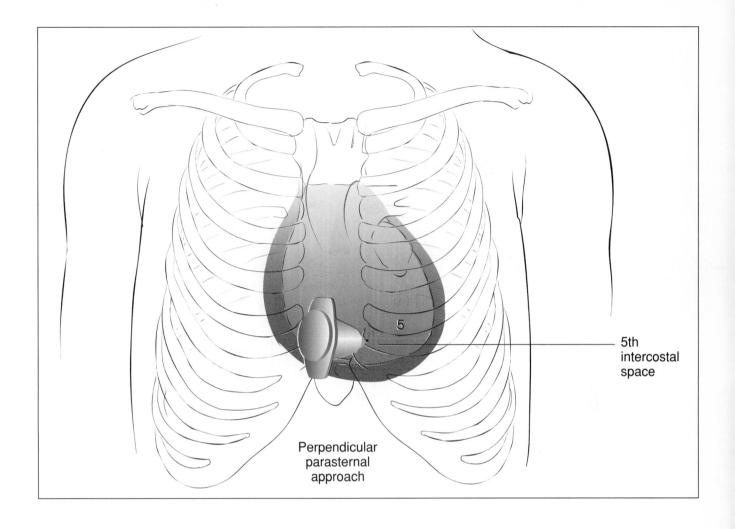

5th
intercostal
space

Perpendicular
parasternal
approach

namic condition after withdrawal of fluid or blood.

Recent adult studies (using echocardiographic guidance) have advocated the parasternal approach as having a higher success rate and a lower complication rate. Using this approach, the needle is inserted perpendicular to the skin surface into the left 5th intercostal space (Fig. 73.2). Insertion should occur at a point just lateral to the sternum. This approach has not been validated in children, but its use can be considered in the older adolescent.

Following the procedure, the patient should be carefully monitored. An upright chest radiograph should be obtained to rule out a pneumothorax and to assess heart size. Finally, arrangements should be made for transfer to a unit or facility that is appropriately equipped to provide ongoing intensive care.

COMPLICATIONS

Pericardiocentesis can be a risky procedure. Complication rates as high as 15% have been reported. Known complications include dysrhythmias, puncture of the ventricle, hemopericardium, and pneumothorax. Almost any vascular structure in the thorax (including coronary arteries and the inferior vena cava) may be punctured or lacerated. In addition, the esophagus, diaphragm, and peritoneal cavity may be penetrated. Delayed complications include pericardial leak, cutaneous fistula formation or local infection.

Many of these complications can be avoided by the routine use of two-dimensional echocardiography while the procedure is being performed. Although not routinely available in the ED or for acute trauma, its use is strongly encouraged when appropriate equipment and personnel are at hand (see also Chapter 135).

Figure 73.2.
Pericardiocentesis in adolescent from parasternal approach.

SUMMARY
1. Assess patient—airway, breathing, circulation
2. Recognize presence of cardiac tamponade
   a. Beck's triad—distant heart sounds, increased jugular venous distention, hypotension
   b. Suspect in appropriate clinical setting in absence of Beck's triad

**Chapter 73
Pericardiocentesis**

SUMMARY

Pericardiocentesis is an infrequently performed but potentially lifesaving procedure. Although not technically difficult, its high complication rate dictates that it be performed only when absolutely indicated. Two-dimensional echocardiography can be a helpful adjunct to minimize complications.

REFERENCES

1. Wong B, Murphy J, Chang CJ, Hassenein K, Dunn M. The risk of pericardiocentesis. Am J Cardiol 1979;44:1110–1114.
2. Krikorian JG, Hancock EW. Pericardiocentesis. Am J Med 1978;65:808–814.
3. Morgan CD, Marshall SA, Ross JR. Catheter drainage of the pericardium: its safety and efficacy. Can J Surg 1989;32:331–334.
4. Ruddy R, ed. Pericardiocentesis. In: Fleisher GR, Ludwig S, eds. Textbook of pediatric emergency medicine. 3rd ed. Baltimore: Williams & Wilkins, 1993, pp. 1630–1631.
5. Callaham ML. Pericardiocentesis. In: Roberts JR, Hedges JR, eds. Clinical procedures in emergency medicine. 2nd ed. Philadelphia: WB Saunders, 1991, pp. 210–228.
6. American College of Surgeons. Advanced trauma life support course for physicians—student manual. Chicago: ACS, 1993, pp. 139–140.
7. Noren GR, Staley NA, Kaplan EL. Nonrheumatic inflammatory diseases. In: Adams FH, Emmanoulides GC, Riemenschneider TA, eds. Heart disease in infants, children and adolescents. 4th ed. Baltimore: Williams & Wilkins, 1989, pp. 740–746.
8. Pories W, Goudiani A. Cardiac tamponade. Surg Clin North Am. 1975;55:573.
9. Shoemaker W, Carey S, Yao S. Hemodynamic monitoring for physiologic evaluation, diagnosis and therapy of acute hemopericardial tamponade from penetrating wounds. J Trauma 1973;13:36.

ARTERIAL PUNCTURE AND CATHETERIZATION

Susan B. Torrey and Richard Saladino

INTRODUCTION

Arterial blood sampling is necessary in the evaluation and management of many seriously ill or injured children (1, 2). Precise measurement of pH, pO_2, and pCO_2 are important adjuncts in assessing respiratory and acid-base status. Venous measurements of pH and pCO_2 can be inaccurate and an arterial sample may be required to clarify an abnormal pulse oximetry reading or to obtain blood samples in patients with difficult venous access. Arterial puncture is used for limited sampling and is a routine procedure as a part of the management of critically ill and injured children.

Repeated access to arterial blood is best accomplished by catheterization of an artery. Indwelling catheters have long been used to monitor critically ill patients in intensive care units (2–4), and logically, monitoring the unstable ill or injured child in the emergency department (ED) is made easier when arterial catheterization has been accomplished (1). The most common indications for arterial catheterization are continuous blood pressure monitoring and repeated sampling of blood. Data from both pediatric ICUs and EDs show that arterial catheterization in children is appropriate and that complications are few (1–4).

Arterial puncture is of moderate technical complexity. Nurses and respiratory therapists have been trained to perform this procedure in many institutions; however, it is more difficult to perform in infants and smaller children. Arterial catheterization in children is technically complex and should be performed by health care providers specifically trained in the technique, usually physicians. Both arterial puncture and catheterization can be performed in children of all ages as indicated by their clinical condition.

ANATOMY AND PHYSIOLOGY

Radial Artery

The radial artery is the most frequently used for both puncture and cannulation. Collateral circulation in the wrist and hand is provided by the superficial and deep palmar arches (5). The superficial palmar arch is formed by the superficial branch of the radial artery which communicates with the terminal aspect of the ulnar artery. The deep palmar arch is likewise a communication of the deep branches of the radial and ulnar arteries.

The strongest radial artery impulse is felt at its most superficial course on the volar aspect of the wrist (Fig. 74.1), lateral to the flexor carpi radialis tendon and median nerve, and medial to the superficial radial nerve and lateral radius, just before the artery descends under the extensor pollicis brevis and abductor pollicis longus tendons to the anatomical snuffbox area. This usually corresponds to a site just lateral to the flexor carpi

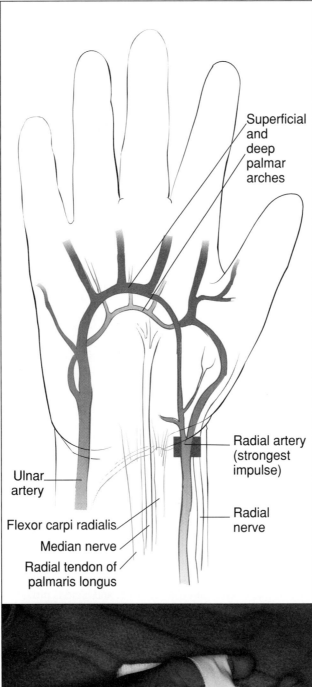

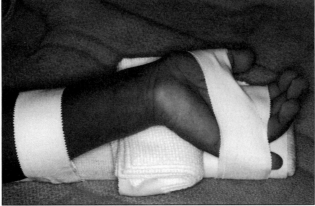

radialis tendon at the second skin crease proximal to the hand. In children, it is often helpful to stabilize the hand and wrist on an armboard, placing the wrist in approximately 30 to 45° extension over several gauze pads.

Femoral Artery

The femoral artery is a common site for arterial and venous access in children, although the over-a-wire catheter technique is primarily used owing to the relatively deeper location of the femoral vascular bundle. The femoral artery courses though the anterior thigh as a continuation of the iliac artery, into the inguinal region after passing under the inguinal ligament (5). In particular, its most superficial and easily palpated course lies in the femoral triangle, bounded above by the inguinal ligament, laterally by the sartorius muscle, and medially by the adductor longus muscle. This site is most easily located as the midpoint between the anterior superior iliac spine and the symphysis pubis (Fig. 74.2). Finally, the operator should keep in mind the close proximity of the laterally related femoral nerve and the medially related femoral vein. In addition, the femoral head lies posterior to the femoral triangle and can be potentially traumatized during femoral artery puncture.

In children, optimal positioning is achieved by externally rotating the leg at the hip and comfortably flexing the leg at the knee before femoral site preparation (Fig. 74.3). With proper sterile preparation, placement technique, and proper nursing care, the potential duration in situ and complication rates

Figure 74.1.
Radial artery anatomy.

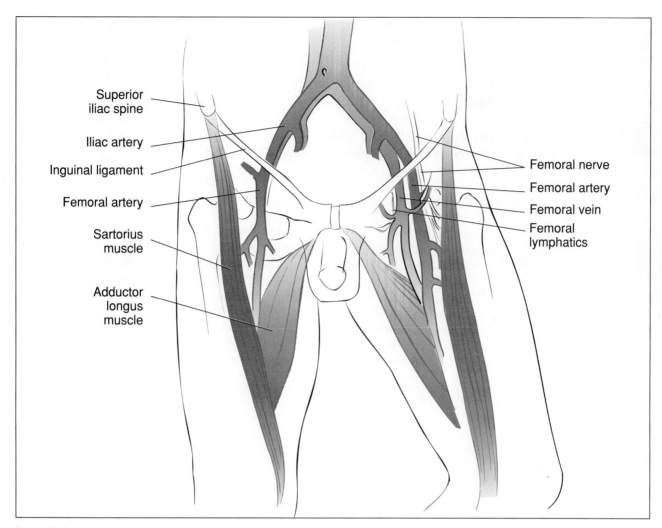

Figure 74.2.
Femoral artery anatomy.

Labels:
- Superior iliac spine
- Iliac artery
- Inguinal ligament
- Femoral artery
- Sartorius muscle
- Adductor longus muscle
- Femoral nerve
- Femoral artery
- Femoral vein
- Femoral lymphatics

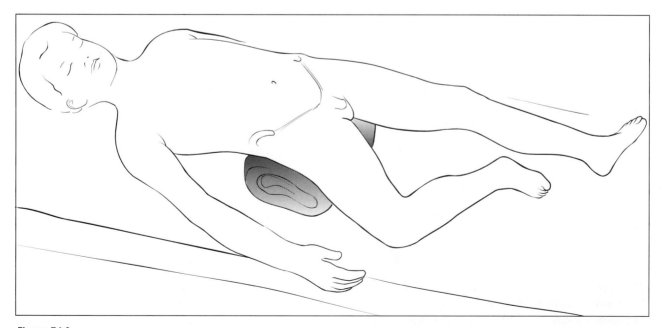

Figure 74.3.
Positioning of the patient for femoral arterial placement.

of femoral vessel cannulations are no different than at any other site.

Posterior Tibial and Dorsalis Pedis Arteries

The posterior tibial artery courses the posterior aspect of the leg as the posterior branch of the popliteal artery, terminating in the plantar arteries and arch (5). Its most superficial and accessible site is a point between the medial malleolus and the calcanean (Achilles) tendon (Fig. 74.4). Cannulation of the posterior tibial artery is usually straightforward and facilitated by holding the foot in comfortable dorsiflexion.

The dorsalis pedis artery is a direct continuation of the anterior tibial artery and passes down the dorsum of the foot to the proximal end of the first intermetatarsal space (5). Cannulation of the dorsalis pedis

artery should be done at the dorsal midfoot where the artery is most easily palpated; this is medial to the extensor hallicus longus and the extensor digitorum longus of the second toe (Fig. 74.5). Cannulation of the dorsalis pedis artery is not complicated if the pulse is easily palpated, and best approached with the foot in mild plantar flexion.

Axillary Artery

The subclavian artery becomes the axillary artery at the lateral border of the first rib which becomes the brachial artery at the tendon of the teres major tendon muscle (5). It is important to locate the most superficial course of the axillary artery so as to avoid trauma to the terminal branch nerves of the brachial plexus. With the patient supine, the arm is positioned in 90° abduction with the dorsum of the hand on the examination table, preferably near the ipsilateral ear or under the occiput. The axillary arterial pulse is palpated high in the axilla medial to the pectoralis major muscle insertion.

In medical literature, more data are available regarding cannulation of the axillary vein (6–8) than the artery. Reports by Cantwell (9) ($n=11$) and Lawless (10) ($n=16$) document the safety of axillary arterial catheterization in children. In the pediatric patient, though, axillary artery catheterization is infrequently indicated. The over-a-wire catheter technique is the preferred method for cannulation of the axillary vessels. This site is technically difficult to access by that technique, and hence, in the ED should be used only when all other sites have been tried.

Brachial Artery

The brachial artery can be easily palpated in the antecubital fossa where it lies atop the brachialis muscle (5). The me-

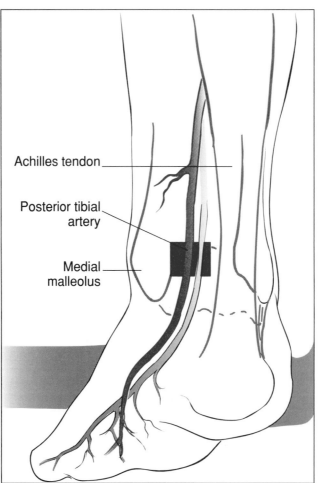

Figure 74.4.
Posterior tibial artery anatomy.

Achilles tendon

Posterior tibial artery

Medial malleolus

dian nerve is located along the medial side of the artery. Although puncture of the brachial artery appears to be relatively safe, little collateral circulation occurs in this area and it should therefore be avoided.

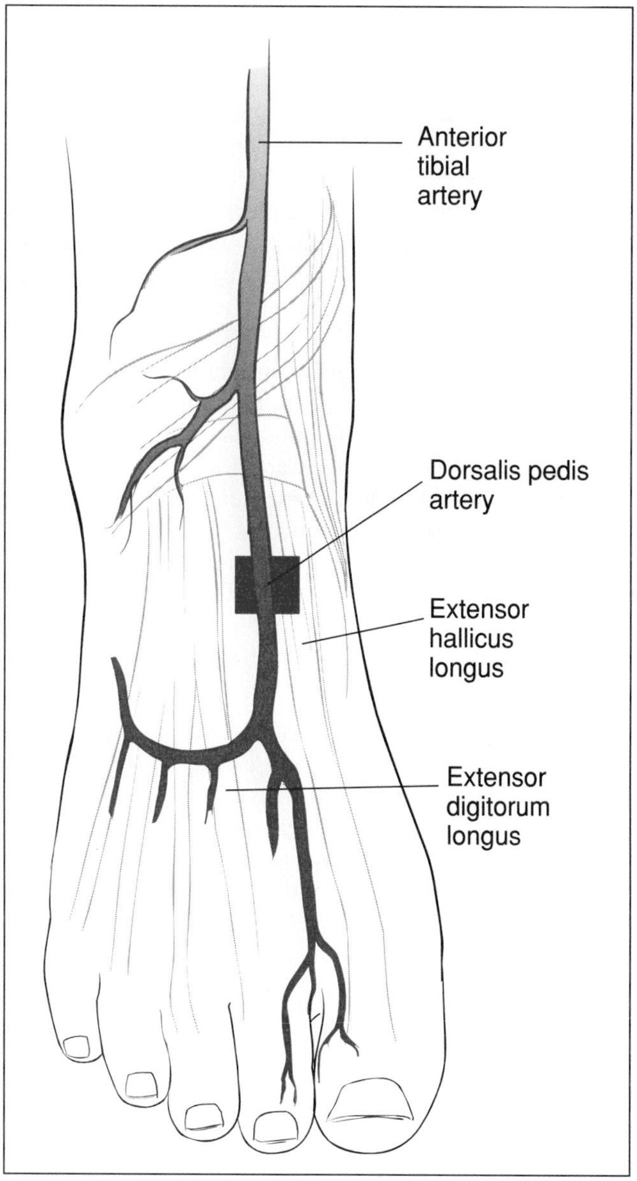

Umbilical Artery

Catheterization of the umbilical vessels in the neonate is useful and possible for hours to days after delivery. A full discussion is provided in Chapter 40.

Temporal Artery

In neonates requiring arterial cannulation, the umbilical artery is the preferred vessel, although this may not be possible in 5 to 10% of neonates who require catheterization (11). In addition, after 4 to 7 days, a catheter in the umbilical artery should be discontinued (12) and a peripheral site selected. Although the radial or posterior tibial arteries are commonly used (if needed) after discontinuation of an umbilical catheter, some data support the usefulness and safety of temporal artery cannulation (3, 12). The superficial temporal artery, a terminal branch of the external carotid artery, ascends through the parotid gland, crosses the zygomatic arch, and terminates in the frontal and parietal branches (5). The course of either branch is palpated and percutaneous catheterization is performed (13). Proper immobilization and care of the catheter is necessary for optimal usefulness and duration in situ.

INDICATIONS

An arterial blood sample for analysis of pH, pO_2, and pCO_2 is mandatory in any patient who may have respiratory compromise. Although pulse oximetry (SaO_2) has become an important tool in the assessment of oxygenation, it provides limited information. Patients with a low SaO_2 require additional oxygen and further clarification of their respiratory status with an arterial specimen. Hypoventilation may be difficult to assess clinically and be present in the absence of hypoxia. This frequently occurs in a postictal child who is receiving supplemental oxygen but has an inadequate tidal volume. Finally, many conditions require an accurate assessment of acid-base status for optimal management, including diabetic ketoacidosis, shock, dehydration, metabolic diseases, and certain drug overdose and poison ingestions.

The most common indications for arterial catheterization are continuous blood

Figure 74.5.
Dorsalis pedis artery anatomy.

Anterior tibial artery

Dorsalis pedis artery

Extensor hallicus longus

Extensor digitorum longus

pressure monitoring and serial blood sampling (1–3, 13). In particular, repeated arterial puncture may injure a vessel, resulting in thrombosis, infection, or arterio-venous fistulae. Serial blood pH and gas tension analysis are easily performed after arterial cannulation; likewise, repeated blood samples can be obtained for other indications via an indwelling arterial catheter.

Puncture or cannulation of an artery is contraindicated if compromise of arterial circulation will result. These situations are unusual but must be considered. Examples include anatomic variants and patients with artificial arteriovenous shunts. Care must be taken when performing these procedures on anticoagulated patients or those with a bleeding diathesis.

EQUIPMENT

Arterial puncture can be performed with a minimum of equipment, although prepackaged kits are available that include a needle and a heparinized syringe. A 25-gauge needle should be used in the newborn whereas a 23-gauge needle is appropriate for older infants and small children. The procedure is most easily performed with a 1 inch butterfly needle. A heparinized syringe must then be prepared by aspirating 1 mL heparinized saline (1000 units/mL) into a syringe, coating the barrel with the solution and then expelling it. If too much heparin remains, the measured pCO_2 may be falsely low (14).

The equipment required for percutaneous arterial cannulation includes supplies to ensure aseptic technique and catheters of appropriate size and length for the age and size of the patient (Table 74.1). Equipment also is required for maintenance of the indwelling catheter or measurement of pressure or both. Prepackaged kits include some or all of the necessary equipment to perform arterial catheterization by the over-a-wire catheter technique (e.g., Cook® Critical Care, Bloomington, IN, or Arrow® International, Reading, PA) (Fig. 74.6).

PROCEDURE

Site Selection

The radial artery is the most frequently used artery for both arterial puncture and cannulation (1–3). It is convenient both for performing the procedure and for maintaining an indwelling line. Catheterization of the femoral artery is technically straightforward and is the site frequently chosen in unstable patients (1, 2). In general, using this artery is discouraged because of the possibility of traumatizing the head of the femur. Axillary artery cannulation is rarely indicated in the pediatric patient. This site is technically difficult to access and should only be attempted in the ED when all other options have been applied. Although the dorsalis pedis and posterior tibial arteries are quite suitable for cannulation, they are easier to use for puncture. The brachial artery should only be used for puncture when other sites are unavailable and should not be used for cannulation. Temporal artery cannulation is indicated in the young

Table 74.1.
Arterial Catheter Sizes by Site and Body Weight

| Site* | Infants <10 kg | | 10–40 kg | | >40 kg | |
	Catheter Size	French Size**	Catheter Size	French Size	Catheter Size	French Size
RA, PTA, DPA, TA	Angiocath 24/22g		Angiocath 22g		Angiocath 22/20g	
Femoral artery, axillary artery	Angiocath 20/18g	3.0/4.0	18/16g	4.0/5.0	18/16/14g	5.0/5.5 6.0
Umbilical artery		Umbilical catheter 3.5/5.0				

* RA = radial artery; PTA = posterior tibial artery; DPA = dorsalis pedis artery; TA = temporal artery.
** Single lumen central catheters are manufactured in standard French size and lengths: 3.0 French (5 or 8 cm); 4.0 French (12 cm); 5.0 French (15, 20, or 25 cm); 5.5 French (5 cm with introducer); 6.0 French (15, 20, or 25 cm). The diameter of wires used for over-a-wire catheter technique correspond to the inner diameter of the catheter used: 3.0 French: 0.018 inch; 4.0 French: 0.021 inch; 5.0 French: 0.035 inch; 6.0 French: 0.035 inch.

infant only when other attempts at sites that are technically less difficult and easier to secure have failed.

In particular, if the radial artery is selected for puncture or catheterization, adequacy of the palmar arterial arch should be assessed. Collateral flow has been shown to be adequate in approximately 93 to 98% of patients tested (15, 16). In 1929, Allen described a method for diagnosis of occlusion of the radial or ulnar artery distal to the wrist (17) which can, with slight modification, be performed even in young or uncooperative patients. The Allen test can be used to assess collateral flow in the hand; in particular, the Allen test will indicate adequacy of ulnar collateral flow such that the radial artery can safely be punctured or cannulated. The patient clenches the fist to exsanguinate the hand. Firm digital pressure (16) is used to occlude the radial and ulnar arteries at the pulse over the wrist. Failure to accurately and completely occlude arterial flow at each artery will result in unreliable results of the Allen test (18). The hand is opened without hyperextending the fingers (19) and the occlusion of the ulnar artery is released. The open hand is observed for return of perfusion (rubor) (Fig. 74.7.B). The Allen test is normal if pallor resolves and rubor returns within 5 seconds, indicating adequate collateral flow. The Allen test is considered abnormal if pallor persists beyond 5 seconds, indicating inadequate palmar arch collateral circulation, and radial arterial puncture should not be performed at that site. The test should be repeated releasing digital pressure over the radial artery so as to assess the radial arterial flow and to ensure that the radial artery pulsation is not due solely to ulnar flow (20). In the young, uncooperative or unconscious patient, occlusion of the arteries is preceded by manual exsanguination, either by "milking" a manually clenched hand by a second individual or by using an elastic bandage wrapped around the hand. Distal arterial flow also may be assessed using a pulse oximeter on the thumb or finger, although this modification may not be reliable (21–25). The Allen test, or a modification thereof, should be performed and documented in the medical record before attempting radial arterial puncture or catheterization.

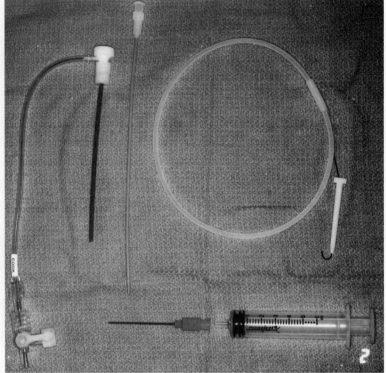

Figure 74.6.
Catheterization tray equipment for arterial line placement by Seldinger technique.

Technique for Arterial Puncture

Once a site is chosen, the most superficial course of the artery is identified by palpation using the nondominant hand. The skin is cleansed with alcohol or iodophor solution. A small amount of 1% lidocaine without epinephrine is used as a local anesthetic with a 27- or 30-gauge needle. A small intradermal wheal can be created at the puncture site, taking care not to obscure the pulse proximally. The artery is palpated continuously just proximal to the puncture site. Using an uncapped butterfly needle or a prepackaged syringe, the skin is approached at a 30 to 45° angle to the horizontal aiming the needle toward the pulse identified by the proximal finger (Fig. 74.8).

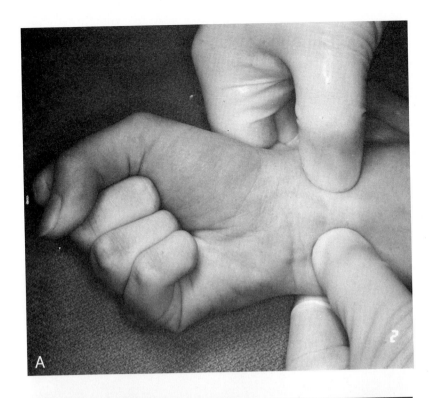

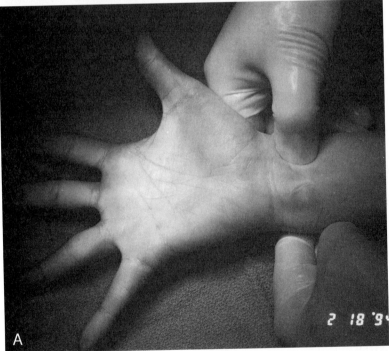

Figure 74.7.
Demonstration of the Allen test for ulnar arterial collateral flow.

The needle is advanced slowly toward the pulse until arterial blood flows into the butterfly tubing. At this point, the heparinized syringe is attached to the butterfly needle tubing and the appropriate volume of blood is aspirated. If using a prepackaged syringe, blood will passively flow into the syringe once the needle has punctured the artery. The needle is withdrawn once the desired amount of blood is obtained. After the needle is withdrawn, manual pressure must be applied to the puncture site for a full 5 minutes to prevent leakage from the puncture site and subsequent hematoma formation.

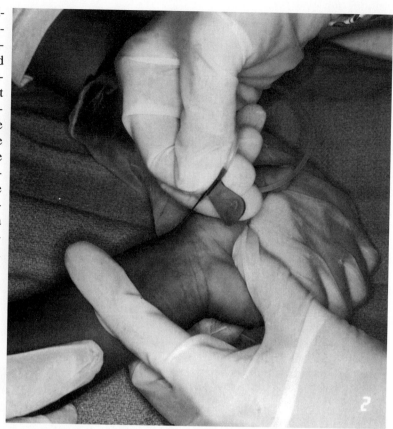

Peripheral Arterial Catheterization

Once the site for arterial catheterization has been selected, the skin should be made sterile with an iodophor solution and meticulous aseptic technique should be maintained throughout the procedure. The approach is at a 30 to 45° angle to the skin (Fig. 74.9.A), entering the artery with the over-a-needle catheter as described for puncture. Bright red blood should appear in the transparent flash chamber of the catheter. It is helpful to slightly lower the angle of the catheter and advance slightly to ensure that the catheter itself enters the lumen of the vessel. The catheter is advanced over the stabilized needle. Pulsatile blood will appear through the hub of the catheter as the needle is withdrawn. If blood does not appear, it may be that puncture of the back wall of the vessel

has occurred. In this case, the catheter should be withdrawn slowly until pulsatile flow is noted, and the catheter is then advanced into the lumen. In fact, this is an alternate method of catheterization: the operator may puncture both walls of the artery, withdraw the needle, slowly withdraw the catheter, and advance into the lumen when pulsatile flow is detected in the hub of the catheter.

The catheter is secured using nylon or silk (4.0 or 5.0) suture material. Sutures are placed in the skin, tied, then looped around the suture ring of the hub of the catheter or through the fenestrations in the wing clips of the catheter (Fig. 74.9.B). Antibiotic ointment may be applied to the catheter entry site, over which a transparent sterile dressing (e.g., OpSite™, Smith and Nephew; Tegaderm™, 3M Health Care) is placed. The catheter hub and extension tubing are further secured with tape.

The catheter is attached to tubing appropriate for pressure transduction if arterial access is to be used for continuous blood pressure monitoring. A three-way stopcock is attached to the tubing proximal to the patient whereas the pressure transducer is located

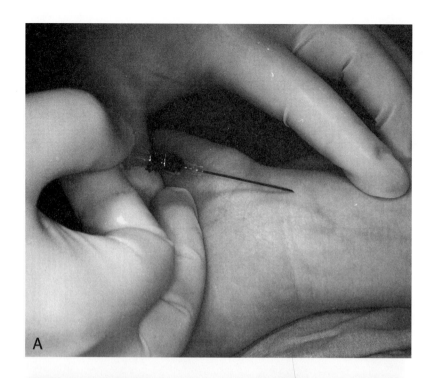

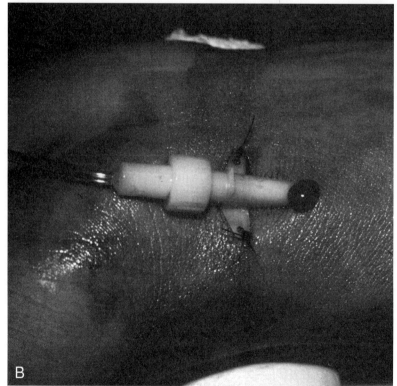

Figure 74.9.
A. Catheter over needle arterial line placement.
B. The catheter is secured by silk sutures and a transparent sterile dressing.

Chapter 74
Arterial Puncture and
Catheterization

distally. Blood sampling is possible from this stopcock system. Care must be taken to draw adequate waste blood before the sample and to avoid air embolism (26). Continuous flushing (2 to 4 mL/hr) of the arterial catheter with heparinized saline (2 units/mL) to prevent clotting is accomplished

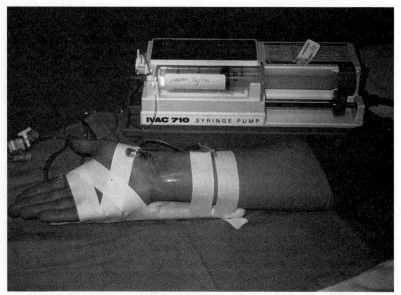

via a pump system distal to the transducer (Fig. 74.10).

Over-A-Wire Catheter Technique

An alternative method of arterial catheterization uses the Seldinger technique of introducing a catheter over a guide wire (Fig. 74.11) (27). This procedure is also discussed in detail in Chapter 18. Briefly, an introducer needle attached to a non-Luer Lok syringe is placed into the lumen of the selected artery, stabilized on aspiration of arterial blood into the syringe, and the syringe disconnected. A guide wire is directed through the introducer needle into the lumen of the artery. The needle is then withdrawn over the guide wire, taking care to control both the proximal and distal ends of the wire. A catheter is then threaded over the guide wire into the artery, keeping the distal end of the guide wire beyond the hub of the catheter. The guide wire is removed and the catheter is connected to the appropriate tubing.

COMPLICATIONS

The most serious complication of arterial puncture is permanent damage to the artery interrupting the arterial supply to the distal extremity. With selection of an appropriate puncture site and proper technique, this is an

CLINICAL TIPS
Arterial Puncture
1. Site selection is important; know the anatomy. The most commonly used sites in the child include the radial, femoral, and posterior tibial arteries.
2. Failure to detect a pulse may be due to low blood pressure, occlusion of an artery by firm pressure by the assistant, or ill-timed inflation of a blood pressure cuff.
3. Perform and document an Allen test for ulnar collateral flow if the radial artery is to be used for puncture or catheterization.
4. Local infiltration of lidocaine may optimize success of arterial puncture or catheterization.
5. After puncture, apply direct pressure over any arterial site after catheter withdrawal for a full 5 minutes.

Arterial Catheterization
1. Once a flash of blood appears in the transparent chamber, lower the angle of the catheter to the skin and advance 1 to 2 mm to ensure that the catheter is in the lumen of the artery.
2. Do not withdraw the needle; stabilize the needle while advancing the catheter over the needle into the artery.
3. Failure to observe pulsatile blood flow from the catheter may indicate that the back wall of the artery has been punctured. Slowly withdraw the catheter and advance again when pulsatile blood appears in the hub.
4. Secure the catheter with a transparent dressing such that a "window" is available to observe blanching of the skin around the site of the catheter.

SUMMARY
1. Assess indications and contraindications for arterial puncture or catheterization
2. Identify optimal site for arterial access
3. Maintain sterile preparation and technique throughout procedure
4. Use finger of nondominant hand to locate most superficial (easily palpable) course of artery
5. Approach skin at 30 to 45° angle from horizontal; when attempting catheterization, lower angle slightly once flashback is observed and advance catheter into lumen of artery
6. Advance catheter over needle; do not withdraw needle until hub of catheter is at skin
7. Secure catheter to skin with nylon or silk suture material (4.0 or 5.0) and sterile transparent dressing
8. Connect catheter to appropriate extension or pressure tubing
9. Use heparinized (2 units/mL) saline to prevent clotting of catheter

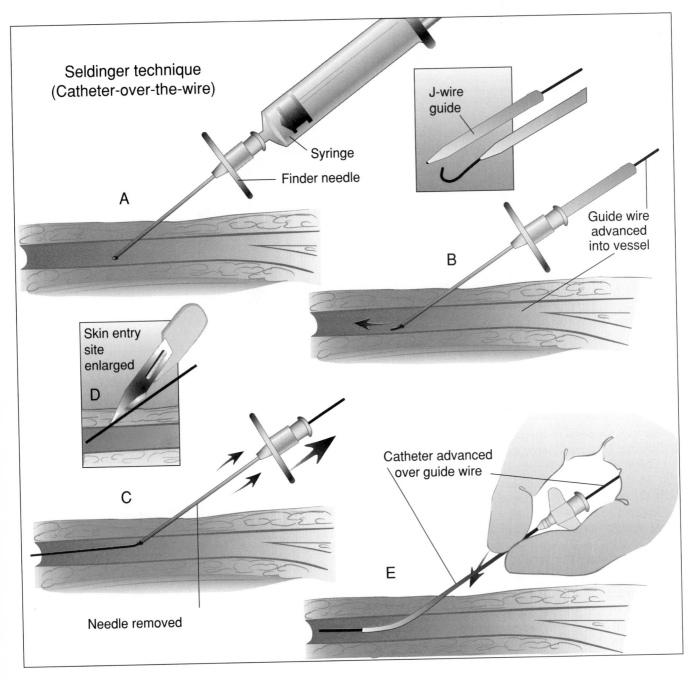

**Seldinger technique
(Catheter-over-the-wire)**

Syringe

Finder needle

A

J-wire
guide

B

Guide wire
advanced
into vessel

Skin entry
site
enlarged

D

C

Needle removed

Catheter advanced
over guide wire

E

Figure 74.11.
Arterial line placement
using the Seldinger
technique.

**Chapter 74
Arterial Puncture and
Catheterization**

exceedingly rare occurrence. Arterial spasm may temporarily impede distal circulation. Injury to the adjacent nerve or underlying bony structures may cause pain temporarily. Hematoma formation at the site also may be uncomfortable.

Complications during or after arterial catheterization include entry into a false lumen in the intima surrounding the vessel, puncture of the artery by the guide wire during its use, kinking or shearing of the catheter, air embolism, and arterial spasm, hematoma, or thrombus formation (1–4, 27,

28, 29). Bedford (30) demonstrated that thrombosis is inversely related to catheter diameter, so care must be taken in appropriately selecting catheter size. Local skin necrosis or infection also may occur secondary to poor technique or arterial spasm or occlusion (3, 4, 30–32).

SUMMARY

Arterial puncture and catheterization are important procedures in the care of critically ill or injured children. When performed properly, these procedures are safe, and the blood sampling and monitoring provided may be valuable adjuncts to the management of patients with impending respiratory and/or cardiovascular failure.

REFERENCES

1. Saladino R, Bachman D, Fleisher G. Arterial access in the pediatric emergency department. Ann Emerg Med 1990;19:382–385.
2. Sellden H, Nilsson K, Larsson L, Ekstrom-Jodal B. Radial arterial catheters in children and neonates: a prospective study. Crit Care Med 1987;15:1106–1109.
3. Randel SN, Tsang BHL, Wung JT, Driscoll JM, James LS. Experience with percutaneous indwelling arterial catheterization in neonates. AJDC 1987;141:848–851.
4. Smith-Wright DL, Green TP, Lock JE, Egar MI, Puhrman BP. Complications of vascular catheterization in critically ill children. Crit Care Med 1984;12:1015–1017.
5. Clemente CD, ed. Gray's anatomy, 30th ed. Lee & Febiger, Philadelphia: 1985.
6. Metz RI, Lucking SE, Chaten FC, Williams TM, Mickell JJ. Percutaneous catheterization of the axillary vein in infants and children. Pediatrics 1990;84:531–533.
7. Oriot D, Defawe G. Percutaneous catheterization of the axillary vein in neonates. Crit Care Med 1988;16:285–286.
8. Martin C, Eon B, Auffray JP, Saux P, Gouin F. Axillary or internal jugular central venous catheterization. Crit Care Med 1990;18:400–402.
9. Cantwell GP, Holzman BH, Caceres MJ. Percutaneous catheterization of the axillary artery in the pediatric patient. Crit Care Med 1991;18:880–881.
10. Lawless S, Orr R. Axillary arterial monitoring of pediatric patients. Pediatrics 1989;84:273–275.
11. Barr PA, Sumners J, Wirtschafter D, Porter RC, Cassady G. Percutaneous peripheral arterial cannulation in the neonate. Pediatrics 1977;59(S):1058–1062.
12. Gauderer M, Holgerson LO. Peripheral arterial line insertion in neonates and infants: a simplified method of temporal artery cannulation. J Pediatr Surg 1974;9:875–877.
13. Filston HC, Johnson DG. Percutaneous venous cannulation in neonates and infants: a method for catheter insertion without "cutdown." Pediatrics 1971;48:896–901.
14. Roberts JR, Hedges JR, eds. Clinical procedures in emergency medicine. 2nd ed. 1991, pp. 255–287. Philadelphia: WB Saunders.
15. Hosokawa K, Hata Y, Yano K, Matsuka K, Ito O, Ogli K. Results of the Allen test on 2940 arms. Ann Plast Surg 1990;24:149–151.
16. Gelberman RH, Blasingame JP. The timed Allen test. J Trauma 1981;21:477–479.
17. Allen EV. Thromboangiitis obliterans: methods of diagnosis of chronic occlusive arterial lesions distal to the wrist with illustrative cases. Am J Med Sci 1929;178:237–244.
18. Hirai M, Kawai S. False positive and negative results in Allen test. J Cardiovasc Surg 1980;21:353–60.
19. Greenhow DE. Incorrect performance of Allen's test: ulnar artery flow erroneously presumed inadequate. Anesthesiology 1972;37:356–357.
20. Meyer RM, Katele GV. The case for a complete Allen's test. Anaesth Analg 1983;62:947–948.
21. Rozenberg B, Rosenberg M, Birkhan J. Allen's test performed by pulse oximeter [letter]. Anaesthesia 1988;43:515–516.
22. Duncan PW. An alternative to Allen's test [letter]. Anaesthesia 1986; 41:88.
23. Spittell Jr JA, Juergens JL, Fairbairn II JF. Radial artery puncture and the Allen test [letter]. Ann Intern Med 1987;106:771–772.
24. Levinsohn DG, Gordon L, Sessler DI. The Allen test: analysis of four methods. J Hand Surg 1991;16:279–292.
25. Fuhrman TM, Reilley TE, Pippin WD. Comparison of digital blood pressure, plethysmography, and the modified Allen's test as means of evaluating the collateral circulation to the hand. Anaesthesia 1992;47:959–961.
26. Chang C, Dughi J, Shitabata P, Johnson G, Coel M, McNamara JJ. Air embolism and the radial arterial line. Crit Care Med 1988;16:141–143.
27. Seldinger SI. Catheter replacement of the needle in percutaneous angiography: a new technique. Acta Radiol 1953;39:368.
28. Brown MM. Another complication of arterial cannulation. Anaesthesia 1991;46:326.
29. Pettenazzo A, Gamba P, Salmistraro G, Feltrin GP, Saia SO. Peripheral arterial occlusion in infants—a report of two cases treated conservatively. J Vasc Surg 1991;14:220–224.
30. Bedford RF. Radial artery function following percutaneous cannulation with 18- and 20-gauge catheters. Anesthesiology 1977;47:37–39.
31. Furfaro S, Gauthier M, Lacroix J, Nadeau D, Lafleur L, Mathews S. Arterial catheter-related infections in children. A 1-year cohort analysis. Am J Dis Child 1991;145:1037–1043.
32. Ducharme FM, Gauthier M, Lacroix J, Lafleur L. Incidence of infection related to arterial catheterization in children: a prospective study. Crit Care Med 1988;16:272–276.

CHAPTER 75

VENIPUNCTURE AND PERIPHERAL VENOUS ACCESS

Mananda S. Bhende

INTRODUCTION

Peripheral venous access and blood sampling by venipuncture remains one of the most common but most challenging procedures in pediatrics. Many professionals who do not deal with infants and children on a regular basis do not feel comfortable performing the procedure. Children, parents, and health care professionals alike may be anxious about the procedure.

Venipuncture continues to be a preferred method of obtaining blood samples in children, often preferred to finger stick, heel stick, or arterial punctures. When more than 1 mL is required for the test, when venous blood is required for blood cultures, or when venous samples better represent the test required, venipuncture is performed. In difficult venous access or when the patient has very few veins, arterial puncture is used for obtaining blood. Venous access is performed to obtain entrance into the circulatory system to provide an avenue for maintaining or replacing body stores of fluids, restoring acid-base balance, replacing blood volume, or administering medications. Historically, blood letting has been described since times immemorial and can be traced back to Hippocrates' time. Some form of intravenous access and treatment has been described since the 17th century. Plastic catheters were introduced in the 1950s for continuous infusion and in most part have replaced those made of metal.

These procedures are commonly performed by many health care professionals, including physicians and nurses, phlebotomists, nurse practitioners, and paramedics. They are performed in prehospital and in-hospital settings, outpatient offices and facilities, emergency departments, inpatient units, operating rooms, or intensive care units and lifesquads. Currently, home care has brought this into the homes of many children who require testing or intravenous medication. Venous access can be an elective procedure such as before surgery or could be an emergent procedure in the field or the ED. If peripheral venous access is not easily obtained in emergent settings, alternative routes include central venous, intraosseous, or venous cutdown (see Chapters 18 to 20).

Currently, peripheral venous access is a short-term, definitive procedure good for 48 to 72 hours. After that time, access needs to be changed because of increased incidence of thrombophlebitis and infection. Long-term intravenous lines and ones for hyperosmolar solutions are best as central lines. These procedures are performed in all age groups.

ANATOMY AND PHYSIOLOGY

Many sites are available for peripheral venous cannulation and venipuncture in the upper extremity, lower extremity, scalp, and the external jugular vein. In adults the veins are usually larger and more easily defined. The

Figure 75.1.
Veins of the upper
extremity.

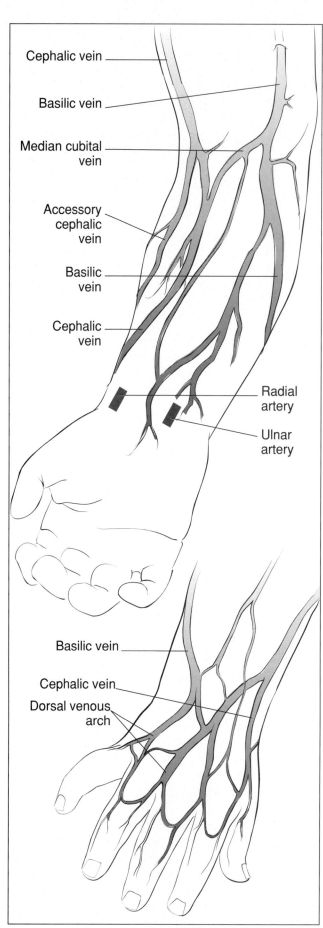

Cephalic vein

Basilic vein

Median cubital
vein

Accessory
cephalic
vein

Basilic
vein

Cephalic
vein

Radial
artery

Ulnar
artery

Basilic vein

Cephalic vein

Dorsal venous
arch

well-nourished toddler with
chubby hands and feet masking
the veins can make intravenous
access difficult for even the
most experienced personnel.

Upper Extremity

On the dorsum of the hand, the
most commonly used veins are
the tributaries of the cephalic
and basilic veins and the dorsal
venous arch (Fig. 75.1). The
cephalic vein which is located
on the radial border of the forearm just proximal to the thumb
is predictable in its location. It
is a large vein that is well secured to the fascia, making it
unlikely to move during venous cannulation and is a good
choice for intravenous placement. The cephalic, basilic, and
median cubital veins in the
forearm may be difficult to locate and cannulate in the well-
nourished child or chubby toddler. In addition, veins on the
inner side of the wrist, if visible, can be cannulated. It is important to avoid puncturing the
radial or ulnar arteries or
nerves which lie in close proximity to these vessels. The axillary vein is a continuation of
the basilic vein and should be
used with caution in peripheral
venous cannulation.

Lower Extremity

The saphenous vein which is
situated about 1 cm above and
in front of the medial malleolus
is a good choice for peripheral
intravenous cannulation (Fig.
75.2). It is large and well secured by fascia, which prevents
it from rolling when cannulation is attempted. Because of
its predictable location, it is
one of the few veins to attempt
access by location—the "blind

stick." The median marginal veins and the veins of the dorsal arch of the foot also may be accessed for cannulation. The anterior and posterior tibial veins form the popliteal which continues as the femoral vein. The long saphenous drains into the femoral vein. When the patient is critically ill and peripheral venipunctures are unsuccessful, the femoral vein which is a site for central catheterization may be used for venipuncture. In the femoral triangle, the anatomic relationship from lateral to medial is nerve, artery, vein, and lymphatics (NAVL). Therefore, if the clinician can palpate the arterial pulsations, the vein lies immediately medial to the pulsations. The femoral artery lies midway between the anterior superior iliac spine and the pubic symphysis 1 cm below the inguinal ligament. Using this anatomic landmark, the femoral vein can be punctured if the artery is not palpable. Cannulation of the femoral vein, a venous cannulation, is described in Chapter 18.

Scalp Veins

Scalp veins are prominent in infants especially under 3 months of age and may be used in infants to approximately 9 months especially when the scalp is not covered by much hair. The scalp veins are closer to the surface and are supported underneath by the bony cranium (Fig. 75.3). They are easily accessed for both venipuncture and venous access. They are not generally accessed when airway management is in progress such as during CPR. Scalp arteries and veins should be differentiated by palpation. Arteries are generally more tortuous than veins. Blood flow through the

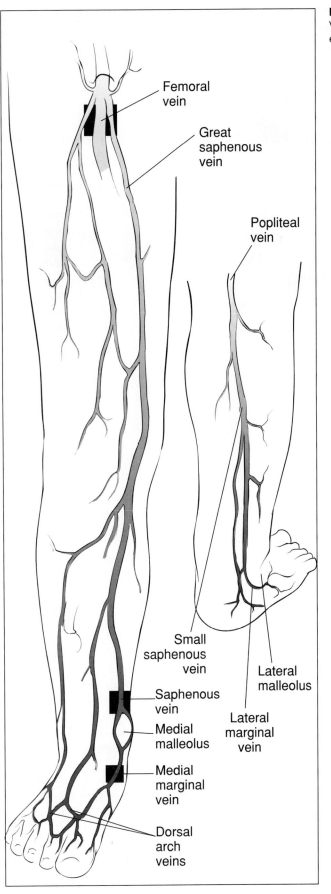

Figure 75.2.
Veins of the lower extremity.

Femoral vein

Great saphenous vein

Popliteal vein

Small saphenous vein

Lateral malleolus

Saphenous vein

Lateral marginal vein

Medial malleolus

Medial marginal vein

Dorsal arch veins

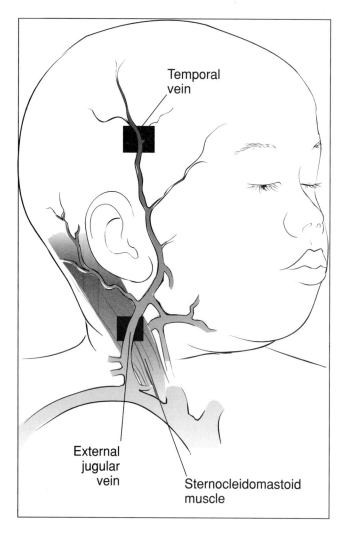

Temporal vein

External jugular vein

Sternocleidomastoid muscle

Figure 75.3.
Scalp vein anatomy and external jugular anatomy.

sors, being careful to hold both ends so it does not snap the infant with one or both ends.

External Jugular Vein

The external jugular vein is usually cannulated by physicians and not by nurses because of its location (Fig. 75.3). Although it is an excellent port close to the central venous circulation because it drains into the subclavian vein, it is a peripheral vein. It is used only when cannulation of other peripheral sites is unsuccessful or when access to it may save considerable time in a critically ill infant or child. It is a difficult site during resuscitative efforts because it comes in the way of airway management. It extends from the lower lobe of the ear to the medial clavicular head across the child's sternomastoid and can be visualized easily with the patient in the Trendelenburg position with the head turned away from the site to be punctured.

INDICATIONS

Venipuncture is indicated whenever blood sampling is needed for laboratory analysis and more than 1 mL is required, or when venous blood is necessary.

Venous access is performed when medications, fluids, transfusions, etc. are required by venous route in the patient. This usually occurs when medication and hydration requirements are not satisfied by the enteral route. For example, excessive vomiting in gastroenteritis, shock, or respiratory distress may preclude the oral route for treatment. A septic child will need parenteral antibiotics and the intravenous route is more effective than intramuscularly. Sometimes peripheral intravenous access is required for intravenous sedations or pain relief. Before rapid-sequence endotracheal intubation, intravenous access is needed to administer the paralytic and sedative agents. Any potentially life-threatening condition requires placement of a peripheral intravenous line as a means of ensuring adequate venous access should a complication develop.

In pediatric resuscitation, peripheral venous access is the accepted mode to treat the patient. In adults during resuscitation, central

arteries also is away from the heart but toward the heart in veins. The clinician can lightly press the vessel with fingers and block the blood flow at two points. Releasing one vessel and then the other will reveal the direction of the blood flow as the clinician watches the vessel refill. If an artery is cannulated by mistake, fluid instillation will cause immediate blanching in the surrounding area, which will indicate that the catheter should be removed. The temporal veins anterior to the earlobe are the largest and the easiest to locate. The frontal vein down the middle of the forehead is another good choice.

A rubber band is convenient to use as a tourniquet on the scalp around the head to distend the veins. Make sure that it is removed immediately after cannulation. Slip tape over the rubber band to assist in removal. It should be carefully slipped over the catheter or butterfly needle or cut with scis-

venous drug administration may provide more rapid onset of action and higher peak concentrations than peripheral venous administration (8). This has not been demonstrated in pediatric arrest models. In pediatric animal and human resuscitation, peripheral, central, and intraosseous administration result in comparable onset of drug action and peak drug levels, particularly if the drug is followed by a bolus of several milliliters of normal saline (1).

CONTRAINDICATIONS

Using peripheral intravenous lines in an extremity that is poorly perfused, edematous, has significant burns, or has a traumatic injury because of the problem of fluid extravasation or inadequate flow should be avoided. They should not be started in areas of cutaneous infection, or if phlebitis or thrombosis is present in the veins. In a patient with neck or upper chest trauma, the ipsilateral arm should not be used to place an intravenous line because the integrity of the proximal veins cannot be ensured. With a gunshot wound or massive trauma to the abdomen, intravenous lines should preferably be started in the upper extremities and not in the lower extremities for the same reason.

Care must be taken in starting intravenous lines in patients with coagulation defects or abnormal blood vessels.

EQUIPMENT

It is important to have all the equipment ready so that the clinician does not have to look for necessary things when doing the procedure. Mobile intravenous carts that have all the equipment stored in one place are a good solution (Table 75.1). These carts should be stocked at least daily. The top of the cart is the designated area where equipment needed for the patient can be placed. The cart comes with its own sharps disposal unit. Having all necessary equipment in one place makes it easier for the nurses and doctors to perform the procedure.

Tourniquets can be rubber tubing, round or flat. They are used proximal to the desired vein so that it causes temporary venostasis by occlusion. Tourniquets should not be tied too

Table 75.1.
Intravenous Cart Equipment List

Tourniquet or rubber bands (for scalp veins)
Povidone-iodine (Betadine) wipes or sticks
Alcohol wipes (70% alcohol)
Butterfly needles—different sizes 21, 23, 25 (large to small)
Over-the-needle catheters (intracaths, angiocaths)—various sizes 14, 16, 18, 20, 22, 24, 26 (large to small)
Normal saline (nonbacteriostatic)
3 and 5 mL syringes
T-connectors
Tape—½-inch, 1-inch, 2-inch (tapes cut and kept ready on the side)
2″ × 2″ sterile gauze packets
4″ × 4″ unsterile gauze
Transparent dressing (Tegaderm®)
Padded arm boards (infant, pediatric, and adult size)
Razors
Betadine ointment
Gloves—sterile and nonsterile
Intravenous infusion microtubing setup
Vacutainers for blood samples for different studies
Plastic medicine cups cut lengthwise in half and sharp edges protected by tape to act as transparent covering for i.v. sites in infants and children in order to protect i.v.
Intravenous infusion pumps on stands

tightly to cause arterial occlusion. When scalp veins are to be punctured or catheterized, rubber bands are used. A small piece of tape is placed around one end with its two sticky ends holding it together, so that the clinician can pull the rubber band off using this tape as a handle, while preventing the rubber band from snapping against the infant's head. Ten percent povidone-iodine prep pads or sticks (Betadine) which are antiseptic and microbicidal are used to first prepare the area. The 70% alcohol pads are used to clean off the Betadine, which allows for visualizing veins. Using alcohol pads alone has been shown to be no different than not using any cleaning agent in terms of infectious complications. Povidone-iodine has been shown to be superior to alcohol alone as an antiseptic agent (9).

Butterfly needles are fine metal cannulas also known as scalp needles. They were once synonymous with pediatric vascular access, and range in size from 19 gauge (largest) to 25 gauge (smallest). Butterflies are useful for venipunctures and short-term vascular access. In children they are preferred over a needle attached to a syringe for venipuncture. It is easier to manipulate a butterfly into tiny veins, and it offers better control while drawing the blood. It is not the preferred method for vascular access because any movement can lead to vessel perforation by the sharp needle tip even after securing it in place.

Intravenous over-the-needle catheters are the most commonly used for venous access. They are composed of thin-walled, semiflexible plastic tubing over hollow needles. Once inside the vein, the plastic coverings are threaded in the veins and the needles withdrawn and discarded. They come in different sizes, from 14 to 26 gauge (large to small). Both 22- and 24-gauge intracaths are the most commonly used in infants and 20, 22, 24 gauge in young children. Both 18 and 16 gauge are used in adolescents. In shock and trauma in adolescents, larger catheters—14 to 16 gauge—are preferred. Over-the-needle infusion catheters cause minimal endothelial irritation and therefore are the most popular choice for peripheral venous access. They are not indicated for long-term use. Many different brands are available, such as Quick-Cath® (Baxter) and Insyte-W® (Becton-Dickinson). Some nurses and doctors prefer one type over the other, but it is usually a matter of personal preference. In patients with tough skin, the soft plastic may cut and fray at the catheter tips. Stiffer catheters have a little more strength but are not as gentle to the veins. Attention to blood and body fluid precautions have led to the development of closed systems where blood stays within the capped tubing (10) (see also Chapter 8).

Padded armboards of different sizes permit the right size to be chosen for immobilizing an extremity from an infant to an older child or adolescent. Sterile gauzes (2×2) are placed near the intravenous site, but around the taping area 4×4 unsterile gauzes are used. In the past 5 years adhesive, sterile, see-through occlusive dressings have greatly improved immobilizing the catheter while allowing visualization of the puncture site and of the area where the intravenous line would infiltrate. Monitoring equipment is only necessary if the child requires it for the severity of the underlying condition.

PROCEDURE

Choosing the Vein

During cardiopulmonary resuscitation, the largest bore vein that does not interfere with resuscitation should be accessed (1). For intravenous access in stable patients, more distal veins such as on the dorsum of the hand and feet should be attempted before using proximal ones—so that proximal veins can be saved for later use, especially in chronically ill children. The clinician should try not to use the child's dominant hand because this may be an unnecessary hardship for activities or thumbsucking. For obvious reasons, it may be wise to avoid the feet of active toddlers. However, the clinician may not have this luxury because only a few veins may be accessible. Except in critical emergencies, it is important to look at intravenous sites before the first attempt to maximize the chances of success. Avoid initiating intravenous lines over joints because movement may dislodge the line and make stabilization more difficult. When veins cannot be visualized, it is advisable to attempt ones with a fixed anatomic location such as saphenous, median cubital, and cephalic vein just proximal to the thumb.

Preparing the Patient— Psychosocial Issues

Verbal consent is usually all that is necessary before venipuncture or placement of a peripheral intravenous catheter. It is essential to prepare the patient and the parent for the procedure which they may view as an ordeal. In the emergent situation (i.e., arrest, seizing child), the clinician cannot take time to explain all details of the procedure. A quick explanation that an intravenous line needs to be started to give medications is sufficient. This can be explained by an assistant helping with the care of the patient (11).

For the patient in whom the intravenous access is not emergent, it is important to discuss with the parents and patient in terms they understand the reason for these procedures. Taking time, when possible, to allay parental concern and to prepare the child will not eliminate the pain of venipuncture, but it can make the procedure less traumatic.

Parents and child should be told that the intravenous stick is a "pinch" when the needle and plastic catheter go into the vein. Explain that the needle is removed, leaving only the catheter in the vein to give fluids and medications. The child may understand better if told that it is like a straw through which "drinks and medicines that will make the child better" can be given directly to the child. Because the pinch hurts, the child should be told that it is okay to cry, but that it is important to hold still. If time allows, explaining with dolls or stuffed animals may help. This is usually possible in elective procedures done outside the ED and occasionally in the urgent setting.

Parents should be encouraged to remain in the room for the procedure if they so desire. They should be told that it is helpful for them to remain calm and supportive. Anxiety and agitation can be conveyed to the child, who would become even more apprehensive and fearful. The child should remain in a parent's arms for as long as possible while the clinician prepares for the procedure (see Chapter 1).

It is important to get a good look at potential intravenous sites. While looking around, it is important for the clinician to explain to the child what he or she is doing and that the tourniquet will be used to choose the best site. The clinician should explain when possible each aspect of the procedure as he or she goes along.

The clinician should not offer a choice to the child as to where the intravenous line can be placed unless the clinician is ready to comply with the choice. Parents may be told that hopefully only one stick is necessary, but that success may require more than one attempt. This will prepare them in case the intravenous line or blood is not obtained on the first attempt.

Speaking in a calm and soothing manner throughout the procedure also assists in relaxing the child. It is important to avoid giving the child food or a bottle to drink during the procedure to reduce the risk of choking. Lastly, praise the child after the procedure regardless of difficulty.

Of course, an extremely critical situation allows no time for such psychological preparation. Showing concern for the parents and child can make the start of an intravenous line a bit easier on everyone.

Methods for Making Veins Prominent

Applying a tourniquet around the extremity just proximal to the vein makes it more prominent by blocking the venous return. This should not be kept on longer than 3 to 5 minutes because prolonged pressure can make the vein tortuous and fragile. The tourniquet should not be so tight as to impede arterial flow. After choosing the vein, it is important to remove the tourniquet and reapply just before venipuncture or catheter placement.

Besides tourniquets, other techniques may assist in enhancing visualization of the vein. Tapping the vein gently often makes it more prominent by increasing vasodilation. Keeping the extremity in a dependent position also helps to fill the vein. Using warm compresses for a few minutes helps dilate the vein. In patients with darker pigmented skin, wiping with betadine swabs reportedly helps the clinician see veins more easily.

In children with chubby hands, it is useful to press the skin with alcohol swabs and release it to allow brief visualization of the vein as it fills. To keep the location of the vein in mind, make a superficial thumbnail impression or keep the alcohol gauze at the specific point. In the antecubital fossa, it is easy to palpate a cordlike structure. By rotating the arm back and forth it can help distinguish the tendon from a vein because the tendon rolls as the arm is rotated.

Another method is to turn the lights off and place a flashlight under the hand or wrist to help illuminate small veins. It is also helpful in finding a vein in a hand darkened by a hematoma from prior sticks, because the linear vein still looks darker than the hematoma. The Landry light for visualization of veins has been found to be useful in identifying veins (12, 13, 14).

In infants, 4% nitroglycerin ointment applied on the area for 2 minutes has been shown to cause local venodilation and help in venous catheterization (15) In adults, a venous distension device with a vacuum system has been studied. This may not be feasible for children because of the infant's fragile veins.

Methods of Pain Relief During Venous Cannulation

The pain and fear of intravenous cannulation or venipuncture can be significant and provokes anxiety and crying even before the procedure. A few methods help to decrease pain perception (see also Chapter 37).

Eutectic mixture of local anesthetics (EMLA cream), such as prilocaine and lidocaine, is able to be absorbed into the intact dermis and induce local anesthesia (16). The disadvantage in the ED setting is that it takes approximately 1 hour for the skin to become anesthetized. It is definitely useful in elective procedures. In children with chronic conditions requiring venipuncture or intravenous access (i.e., hemophiliacs, sickle-cell patients), parents can administer it at home before coming to the office or ED. Unfortunately, if the clinician is unsuccessful in the anesthetized area, another area that is not anesthestized would have to be used. Local injection of bacteriostatic saline 0.5 mL can cause a temporary local anesthetic effect. Sometimes before large bore catheter placement lidocaine injected intradermally with a small bore needle (27 to 30 gauge) can decrease the pain. Lidocaine, alkalinized with sodium bicarbonate (9:1), may reduce the sting of lidocaine infiltration. Local anesthetic patches applied by iontophoresis are being studied to see how effective and within what time period they can anesthetize the skin. Biofeedback, music therapy, and hypnotherapy have been studied in other settings to decrease pain of intravenous lines in patients with chronic illness.

Nitrous oxide inhaled with oxygen also has been shown to be useful in alleviating anxiety and pain of venipuncture and venous cannulation (17) (see also Chapter 36).

Setting up the Equipment

All equipment should be assembled next to the child's bedside (Table 75.1), including cut tape and intravenous fluids. A specific size intravenous line is selected.

Immobilization

Usually two health care staff members are necessary for starting an intravenous line in a child. If the child is uncooperative and strong, more assistants may be needed. It is best but not always possible to have an adult other than the parent assist in restraint of the child. Parents should provide support for calming their child.

If the dorsum of the hand is used, it should be flexed at the wrist, and the fingers should also be flexed at the metacarpophalangeal joints (Fig. 75.4.A). Small infant hands can be held between the thumb and the fingers of the nondominant hand of the person performing the procedure. In slightly older children, the restraining person can hold the forearm and the fingers. The clinician putting in the line should be able to manipulate well for the procedure. Hand position is a matter of personal preference. To make the antecubital veins more prominent a towel can be placed beneath the elbow.

For the foot (Fig. 75.4.B), the ankle should be extended so as to be able to visualize the veins and, if the long saphenous vein is to be cannulated, then the foot also should be turned laterally.

For scalp veins, the head should be immobilized—the veins distended by using a rubber band and the head turned to the opposite side so it lies flat against the bed.

The external jugular vein is sometimes cannulated when other peripheral veins are not accessible. The child should lie in a Trendelenburg position with the head lower than the rest of the body and the neck rotated to the opposite side. Placing a towel under the shoulders or moving the child to the head of the bed and having an assistant hold the head beyond the bed accomplishes this. The clinician is able to visualize the vein crossing the sternocleidomastoid muscle from the angle of the jaw to the lower one-third of the muscle.

For femoral venipuncture, which is done only when the patient is critical, the thigh is abducted and held by the restrainer, and the vein lies medial to the palpable pulsating artery.

The clinician should remember that adequate immobilization is critical to establishing an intravenous line or performing a venipuncture in an efficient, minimally uncomfortable manner.

PROCEDURE

Both the restrainer and the technician starting the intravenous line should don clean gloves. Universal precautions should always be followed.

A tourniquet should be applied proximal to the selected vein. It should not be applied

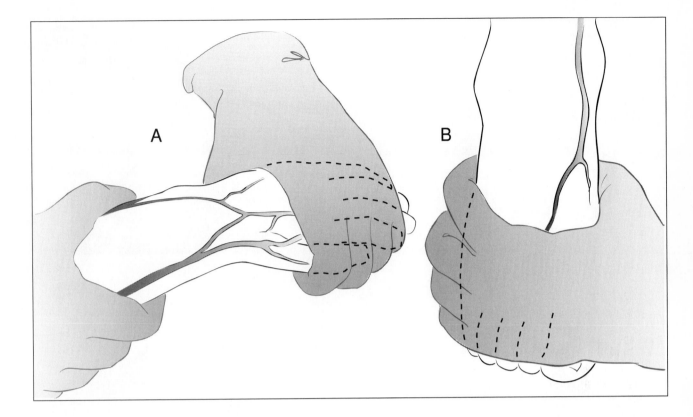

Figure 75.4.
A. Immobilization of the hand for intravenous line placement.
B. Immobilization of the foot for intravenous line placement.

so tightly that it obstructs the arterial supply. To prevent the tourniquet from pinching the skin or pulling hair, it is useful to place a 4×4 gauze under the area where the tourniquet is applied with a slip knot.

The area should be cleansed with providone-iodine swabs starting from the central area where the skin is going to be pierced and in a circular fashion on a radius of 3 to 4 cm. This should dry for a minute to allow it to be bactericidal before cleansing with alcohol swabs. The site should be cleansed in a similar manner for obtaining blood cultures. For venipuncture, the area is usually cleansed with only alcohol swabs unless obtaining a culture of the blood.

Butterfly Needles

The butterfly needle is often the preferred method of venipuncture for obtaining blood samples (Fig. 75.5). The butterfly tubing is attached to a syringe. Usually size 23 or 25 is used, but the clinician may also use the larger size 21 for bigger veins in school-aged children.

Tension is applied to the skin and vein distal to the puncture site so that the vein is straightened. This affords easier penetration,

decreases the chance of puncturing the posterior vessel wall, and also increases visualization of the vein. At this time, the patient should be reminded of the upcoming "little pinch."

The tip of the needle is placed about 0.5 to 1 cm distal to the site selected for entering the vein. With the the needle held at a 30 to 45° angle above the skin surface, the skin and underlying tissue are firmly pierced (Fig. 75.5.A). The angle of the needle is then made closer to parallel to the skin surface, so that the needle is parallel to the vein, and the vein is entered slowly. Entry into the vein is verified by the flashback of blood into the clear plastic tubing of the butterfly set. For intravenous placement, the needle is advanced carefully, lifting the butterfly upward by the wings to avoid piercing the posterior vessel wall. For venipuncture, the needle is advanced only if required to improve blood flow, and then the syringe is attached. If this is awkward for the clinician performing the procedure, an assistant can attach the syringe and withdraw the blood by slowly applying suction. Aspirating the syringe with much negative pressure should be avoided, as the vein may collapse. The clinician may place a piece of clear tape over the butterfly wings

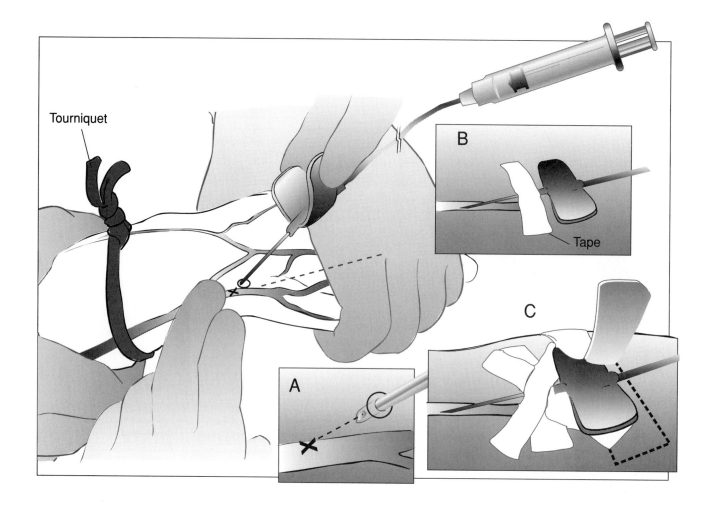

Tourniquet

B

Tape

C

A

Figure 75.5.
Using butterfly needle for
intravenous access or
blood sampling.

when drawing the sample to help stabilize the needle (Fig. 75.5.B).

Sometimes blood will drip from the tubing, but cannot be aspirated. In those cases, the blood may be allowed to drip directly into the specimen tubes. This should not be done for a blood culture however, when the blood must be aspirated into a sterile syringe.

When blood drawing is complete, the tourniquet is removed. The butterfly needle is withdrawn from the skin and pressure is applied to the venipuncture site with a 4×4 gauze. If blood is aspirated from the antecubital veins, holding pressure on the site with the elbow extended is believed to cause a smaller hematoma and less bruising than holding gauze or cotton with the elbow flexed.

If the butterfly is to be converted to an intravenous site, a syringe of normal saline is attached to the butterfly tubing. If the saline flushes easily and no bubble is formed at the

needle tip, the clinician knows that the cannulation is intact.

Unfortunately, it is difficult to maintain butterfly needles as indwelling intravenous lines for prolonged periods. Generally, the site that is most successful in this context is in the scalp veins. Taping and immobilization are illustrated in Figure 75.5.C and described below on page 807 in the section "Securing the Intravenous Line."

Over-the-Needle Catheters

An over-the-needle catheter insertion is the preferred type of intravenous placement in most instances, but not for blood sampling alone. The sizes most commonly used in infants and children are 22 and 24 gauge, and occasionally 20 gauge. In older children during trauma, resuscitation, or shock when large volumes need to be given, large bores such as 14, 16, or 18 gauge are used.

The limb is positioned optimally and the

skin stretched taut (Fig. 75.6.A). The needle cover is removed and the needle enters the skin about 0.5 to 1 cm below the intended site of entry into the vein, holding the catheter needle at about a 30 to 45° angle. The bevel should be kept up to ensure smooth entry through the skin. In small veins, some experts advise entering the vein with the needle bevel down, so that once the vein is entered, the chance of tearing the opposite wall is reduced (18). This works best when the catheter appears larger than the vein.

Next, the operator should lower the angle of the needle so the catheter is almost parallel to the skin surface and advance slowly to puncture the vein (Fig. 75.6.B). The operator should verify entry of the catheter into the vein by visualizing a flashback of the blood inside the clear hub. The device is advanced 1 to 2 mm to ensure that the catheter also has entered the vein and not the needle tip only.

The operator should feed the catheter over the needle while holding the needle steady, so that only the catheter advances into the vein. The thumbnail of the nondominant hand may fit between the needle and the catheter to advance the catheter (Fig. 75.6.C). Sometimes when the catheter tip is against a valve or wall of the vein, feeding it in the vein may be difficult. In that case, either rotating the catheter or the needle while flushing with normal saline as the catheter is advanced may help. When flushing, the needle is removed before the flushing. Then a T-connector is attached and the line is flushed with saline to ensure the catheter is in the vein.

Blood can be aspirated into the syringe for specimens with slow, negative pressure. In small hand veins, some authorities prefer to have the specimen drip directly from the intravenous hub to the sample microtainers or to a syringe for blood culture. Care must be taken to avoid having blood in the intravenous line or system clot, with resulting loss of the line. If not enough blood returns, the tourniquet is removed, and the extremity is "milked" by applying and releasing pressure alternately to obtain blood, followed by reapplication of the tourniquet. If too much suction is used, the vein may collapse which will preclude specimen collection. Before flushing with intravenous fluids, the tourniquet or rubber band is removed. Otherwise distending the fragile vein against pressure will infiltrate the tissue.

After the catheter is inserted into the vein and the needle is removed, it is unwise to place the needle back into the catheter to help thread it. This may cause shearing of the plastic catheter tip and may lead to catheter embolism or intravenous infiltration.

The thumb of the nondominant hand of the clinician placing the intravenous line can be used to physically secure the line until it is taped well in place (Fig. 75.6.D). Sharps should be discarded immediately in the sharps container to avoid accidental needle puncture. It is also useful to limit intravenous attempts to 2 or 3 sticks per clinician, if a more experienced person is available to make additional attempts. In children with difficult veins, such as those with chronic illness, the more experienced clinician technically should consider trying first.

Securing the Intravenous Line

Two general methods are applied to securing the intravenous catheter. A preferred method now is to use clear plastic skin (i.e., Tegederm, Opsite) which will stick to the skin and allow ready visualization of the site. When using one of these products place 2 to 3 small pieces of tape in standard fashion to secure the line as described in the following section. Choose either a piece cut to size or a ready-made one close to the size necessary to completely cover the catheter including the skin puncture site.

The second method is the standard and acceptable taping of the site. Start with a horizontal piece of tape placed above the intravenous line entrance site. A second piece of small tape is placed under the hub with the adhesive side away from the skin and then crossed over above the catheter or butterfly needle (Figs. 75.5.C, 75.6.D). This may be repeated, but ensure that the area of skin over the tip of the needle or catheter in the vein can be visualized to detect early infiltration or phlebitis.

Either approach to securing the intravenous line may be preceded by placement of antibiotic ointment at the puncture site. The T-connector or tubing of the butterfly is taped at least 2 cm away from the intravenous site (Fig. 75.5). If the line is accidentally pulled on, the catheter may remain securely in place.

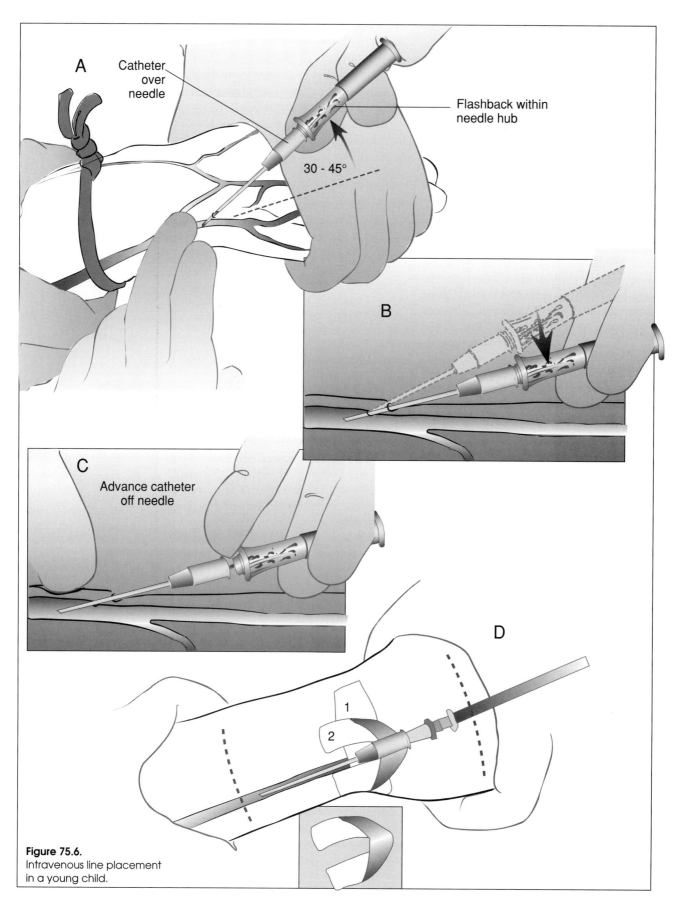

A Catheter over needle

Flashback within needle hub

30 - 45°

B

C Advance catheter off needle

D

1

2

Figure 75.6.
Intravenous line placement in a young child.

The extremity is then placed on a soft board, usually covered with gauze for comfort and taped above and below the intravenous site. To prevent the tape from irritating the skin, gauze can be placed below the tape that circles the extremity to the arm board. When securing the hand, the fingers are allowed to curl up under the board and are taped over the distal metacarpals. It is best to allow the thumb to remain unrestrained. It is important to tape the extremity in as much a functional position as possible to minimize discomfort.

Instead of the clear plastic "skin," a plastic "house" fashioned from medicine cups (see Table 75.1) can be placed on top of the intravenous line which allows visualization of the site. This is used mostly on the scalp, or when the line is placed in a site where the child may hit it routinely.

Parents should be instructed how to assist in caring for the intravenous line. This also can be explained to the child, if possible. This may help the intravenous site stay protected and avoid undue pulling at the site.

COMPLICATIONS

Complications of venipuncture include hematoma formation, injury to the structures adjacent to the vessels such as nerves and tendons, local infection, phlebitis, cellulitis, and thrombosis. All except small hematoma formation are fairly uncommon. Puncture of vessels of the neck, such as the external jugular, may be close to internal structures where injury could lead to serious problems. Related problems include those enhanced by inadvertent injection of intravenous fluids or of therapeutic agents which are sclerosing into the subcutaneous tissue with resultant necrosis or sloughing of the skin. Rarely, air embolism may complicate the injection of air in a peripheral line. Catheter embolism is rare from peripheral intravenous lines with the increased use of over-the-needle catheters.

SUMMARY

Venipuncture and peripheral intravenous access are commonly performed procedures in all pediatric age groups. They are vital procedures in critically ill children to obtain blood for laboratory analysis and ensure direct access for administering parenteral fluids and medications. They are performed by multiple health professionals not only as emergent but also as elective procedures in the ED, hospital wards, operating room, and outpatient settings. The practice of a calm, methodical ap-

SUMMARY

1. Prepare patient and equipment at bedside. Ensure good lighting and appropriate assistance to maximize immobilization
2. Look for best vein before starting
3. Always follow universal precautions—don gloves
4. Immobilize and then apply tourniquet/rubber band to best visualize vein
5. Clean area with betadine and allow to dry, then cleanse with alcohol; make skin taut
6. Insert needle 0.5 to 1 cm distal to actual point of entry "bevel up." When vein is collapsed or small, a "bevel down" entry is recommended
7. Puncture vein and after flashback, insert device into vein 1–2 mm more to ensure that both needle tip and catheter end are in vein
8. Thread catheter in vein by feeding catheter over needle by thumbnail of non-dominant hand while stabilizing needle
9. Attach hub to T-connector and syringe, after flushing with saline. Flush catheter to make sure catheter is still in vein
10. If blood needs to be drawn, then T-connector is not purged beforehand and it is attached to a syringe and blood is drawn into syringe by slow negative suction. Alternatively, blood samples can be collected from blood dripping from catheter hub
11. Secure intravenous site—either with adhesive tape alone or tape and a clear dressing. Tape T-connector tubing away from intravenous site
12. Tape extremity to i.v. board when necessary
13. Consider protecting site with plastic cover, especially on scalp
14. Attach to intravenous fluids or convert i.v. to heparin lock

CLINICAL TIPS

1. Prepare the parents and patient to help things go smoother.
2. Prepare all necessary equipment beforehand. Ensure good lighting.
3. Immobilize the patient well.
4. Clinician should be comfortable.
5. Choose the best vein available, using peripheral veins first. Try not to use the hand of thumbsuckers, a toddler's feet, or a vein that crosses joints.
6. To increase visualization of the vein:
   a) Use tourniquet on extremities or a rubber band on the scalp.
   b) Tap vein gently to enhance filling.
   c) Keep extremity in dependent position.
   d) Apply warm compresses to possibly enhance vasodilation.
   e) In a darkened room, place flashlight under extremity to light blood in vein.
   f) Dab of 4% nitroglycerin cream to possibly cause vasodilation.
7. If veins are not visualized at all, veins with relatively fixed locations can be used for attempts (i.e., long saphenous, median cubital, or cephalic vein proximal to the thumb).

8. After flashback of blood is seen, enter 1–2 mm more into the vein to ensure that the intracath also has entered the vein and not only the needle tip.

9. When the clinician has difficulty feeding the catheter over the needle, rotating the catheter or flushing with saline helps make feeding the catheter into the vein easier.

10. Secure with tape and a transparent dressing (i.e., Tegaderm®).

proach by preparing the patient and being prepared with all the necessary equipment will go a long way in successful and efficient completion of the procedure.

REFERENCES

GENERAL

1. Chameides L, Hazinski MF. Textbook of pediatric advanced life support. AHA, 1994.
2. Engle WA, Frederick JR. Vascular access and blood sampling techniques in infants and children. In: Roberts JR, Hedges JR, eds. Clinical procedures in emergency medicine. Philadelphia: WB Saunders, 1991, pp. 268–287.
3. Hambrick ED, Benjamin GC. Peripheral intravenous access. In: Roberts JR, Hedges JR, eds. Clinical procedures in emergency medicine. Philadelphia: WB Saunders, 1991, pp. 288–300.
4. Hutchinson DB. Pediatric I.V. therapy: starting the line. RN 1991 Dec; 43–47.
5. O'Brien R. Starting intravenous lines in children. J Emerg Nurs 1991;17:225–231.
6. Campbell LS, Jackson K. Pediatric update—starting intravenous lines in children: tips for success. J Emerg Nurs 1991;17:177–178.
7. Millam DA. How to insert an i.v. Am J Nurs 1979 Jul;1268–1271.

SPECIFIC

8. Hedges JR, Barsan WB, Doan LA, Joyce SM, Lukes SJ, Dalsey WC, et al. Central versus peripheral intravenous routes in cardiopulmonary resuscitation. Am J Emerg Med 1984;2:385–390.
9. Jacobsen C-JB, Grabe N, Damm MD. A trial of povidone-iodine for prevention of contamination of intravenous cannulae. Acta Anaesthesiol Scand 1986;30:447–449.
10. Friedland LR, Brown R. Introduction of a "safety" intravenous catheter for use in an emergency department: a pediatric hospital's experience. Infect Control Hosp Epidemiol 1992;13:114–115.
11. Frederick V. Pediatric i.v. therapy: soothing the patient. RN 1991 Dec;40–42.
12. Zimerman E. The Landry vein light: increasing venipuncture success rates. J Ped Nurs 1991; 6:64–66.
13. Nager AL, Karasic RB. Use of transillumination to assist placement of intravenous catheters in the pediatric emergency department [abstract]. Pediatr Emerg Care 1992;8:307.
14. Sieh A, Brentin L. A little light makes venipuncture easier. RN 1993 Mar;40–43.
15. Vaksmann G, Rey C, Breviere G-M, Smadja D, Dupuis C. Nitroglycerine ointment as aid to venous cannulation in children. J Peds 1987;111:89–91.
16. Cooper CM, Gerrish SP, Hardwick M, Kay R. EMLA cream reduces the pain of venipuncture in children. Eur J Anaesth 1987;4:441–448.
17. Henderson JM, Spence DG, Komocar LM, Bonn GE, Stenstrom RJ. Administration of nitrous oxide to pediatric patients provides analgesia for venous cannulation. Anesthesiology 1990;72(2):269–71.
18. Filston HC, Johnson DG. Percutaneous venous cannulation in neonates and infants: a method for catheter insertion without "cutdown." Pediatrics 1971;48:896–901.

CHAPTER 76

ACCESSING INDWELLING CENTRAL LINES

Susan M. Fuchs

INTRODUCTION

In children, numerous illnesses exist that require long-term parenteral pharmacologic or nutritional therapy and repetitive blood drawing. Several central venous access devices (indwelling lines) have been developed that allow the administration of antibiotics, chemotherapy, blood, or hyperalimentation and fluids often on an outpatient basis. Whenever children with such devices are examined in the emergency department (ED), it is important to be able to access them for blood drawing and the administration of fluids, antibiotics, blood, or other parenteral medication.

Because these devices directly access the central circulation, it is important to realize that sterile procedures should be followed to reduce the risk of infection. Air embolism and central vein thrombosis are additional risks.

TYPES OF EQUIPMENT

Several catheter devices are currently on the market, and it is important to become familiar with the ones currently being used in a particular medical center. Some variations between them include access, flushing, and aftercare.

The first partially implanted catheter was developed in 1973 by Broviac and consisted of a Silastic® catheter that was used to admin-

ister total parenteral nutrition (TPN). The Broviac® catheter was 18 gauge (1.0 mm) and was inserted into the external jugular, subclavian, or cephalic vein, with the distal tip positioned in the right atrium. The proximal end was tunneled under the skin to exit on the chest (1). The same procedure for placement exists today. A Dacron® cuff is located on the catheter and is positioned in the subcutaneous tunnel. It serves two purposes: a fibrin sheath develops around it in approximately 2 weeks and serves to anchor the line in the tunnel, and it acts as a mechanical barrier to infection (1). In 1979, Hickman enlarged this catheter (16 gauge, 1.6 mm) to administer chemotherapy and to facilitate blood drawing (1, 2). More recent advances have included single, double, and triple lumen catheters, with a wider range of sizes (0.5 to 2.6 mm inner diameter). Names of some of the commonly used catheters include Broviac® (Evermed), Hickman®, Leonard®, Raaf®, Hermed®, and Corcath® (Fig. 76.1) (2, 3). Another recent advance has been the Groshong® catheter, which has a three-position slit valve near the distal (implanted) tip. The slit opens outward for administrating fluid, inward for aspirating blood, and otherwise remains closed (Fig. 76.2). The benefit of this type of catheter is that blood does not remain in the lumen of the catheter after it is flushed, so only saline flushes (no heparin) are used (3). Another type of central venous access device was introduced in 1982 that is a totally implantable device. It consists of a

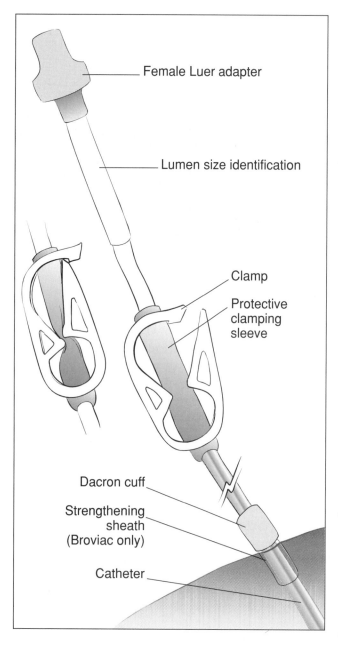

Figure 76.1.
Schematic of Hickman® and Broviac® single lumen catheters.

Female Luer adapter

Lumen size identification

Clamp

Protective clamping sleeve

Dacron cuff

Strengthening sheath (Broviac only)

Catheter

tip and a side hole opening. Most have a 90° bend although some are straight (1, 4). (Fig. 76.4). The reservoirs are made of plastic, stainless steel, and titanium. The plastic and titanium are light and do not interfere with magnetic resonance imaging studies (3). The Port-A-Cath (Pharmacia) comes in two sizes, for infants (outer diameter 2 mm, inner 0.5 mm) and children (outer 2.8 mm, inner 1 mm) (1, 4), but other manufacturers and names include Infuse-A-Port® and Mediport®.

ANATOMY AND PHYSIOLOGY

The basic principle in using these catheter systems is to have an intravenous line distally in a central vein but proximally tunneled under the skin where it can be easily punctured for use. The decision about which type of catheter to use is based on several factors, including age and developmental level of patient, frequency of access necessary, patient and parent desires, and the comfort issues regarding the necessary flushes and dressing changes. For the external catheters, the most common sites include the external jugular, subclavian, or cephalic vein. For the implantable device, the catheter is usually placed in the subclavian vein, but the internal jugular vein also can be used. The distal tips of both catheters are advanced until they are either at the junction of the superior vena cava and right atrium or in the right atrium (2, 3).

Benefits of accessing the central circulation over a peripheral vein include the infusion of some antibiotics and chemotherapeutic agents, which may cause sclerosis of veins, or the administration of solutions which can safely contain a higher dextrose or potassium concentration when infused into a central vein.

INDICATIONS

Central venous access lines are frequently placed in children undergoing chemotherapy, those with a chronic illness that often require long-term intravenous antibiotic therapy (i.e., cystic fibrosis with pulmonary infection or children with osteomyelitis), those who re-

silastic catheter attached to a subcutaneous injection port or reservoir (Fig. 76.3). The catheter is placed in a central vein until the distal tip is at the junction of the superior vena cava and right atrium. The proximal portion is tunneled under the skin, but rather than exiting the skin, it is attached to the reservoir, which is placed in and sutured to a subcutaneous pocket on the chest (1). The reservoir is covered with a thick silicone septum that is self-sealing, where a special needle (Huber® needle) is used for access (Fig. 76.3). This needle is noncoring with a solid

quire parenteral nutrition due to short-bowel syndrome, malnutrition, or other gastrointestinal or hepatic disorders, and selected patients with difficult venous access.

In the ED, access of these lines can be accessed for phlebotomy, fluids, antibiotic therapy, medication, and blood product administration. Other catheter-related problems that may result in ED visits include catheter occlusion or breakage, unintentional displacement, or skin irritation and/or infection at the site of insertion.

Contraindications to access for therapy would include if a catheter is dislodged, if proper placement of an implantable device cannot be confirmed, or if a high risk of significant clot or infection is indicated within the catheter which may be dislodged with use.

EQUIPMENT

Partially Implantable (Broviac®, Hickman®) Catheters

1. Sterile gloves (two pair), mask, gown, and eyewear
2. 10% povidone-iodine solution (betadine) or alcohol
3. Sterile drapes
4. 10 mL syringe filled with normal saline
5. One 10 mL syringe containing 5 mL heparin flush (100 U/mL)
   (**Note:** for the Groshong® catheter, 5 mL saline is used to flush the catheter, not heparin flush)
6. Catheter clamp or hemostat *without teeth*
7. Fluids and medications to be administered
8. Dressing and tape for procedure completion (gauze or transparent dressing—Opsite®, Tegaderm®), providone-iodine ointment
9. 10 mL syringes (2 to 3 empty) (if blood drawing is desired)
10. Heparin lock flush and cap

Totally Implanted Devices (Port-A-Cath®)

1. Sterile gloves (two pair), mask, gown, and eyewear

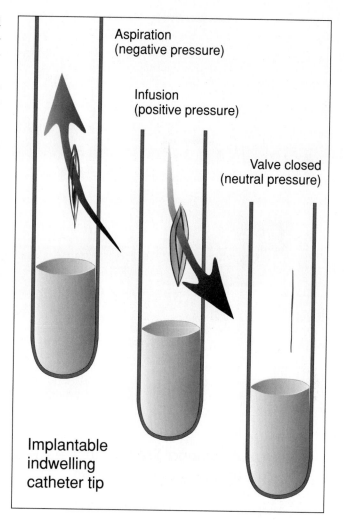

Figure 76.2.
The Groshong® three-position valve.

2. 10% povidone-iodine solution and alcohol
3. Sterile drapes
4. 10-mL syringe filled with normal saline
5. 10 mL syringe containing 5 mL heparin (100 U/mL)
6. Two noncoring needles: Huber® needles with a 90° bend. Preferred sizes are 20 gauge for drawing blood, 22 gauge for administration of intravenous fluids or medications, 19 gauge for administration of blood. (In an emergency, a standard 19 gauge needle can be used.)
7. T-extension tubing with side clamp
8. Several sterile gauze squares (2×2 inch) to stabilize needle
9. Tape
10. Gauze dressing for procedure completion
11. 10 mL syringes (2 to 3 empty) (if blood drawing is desired)

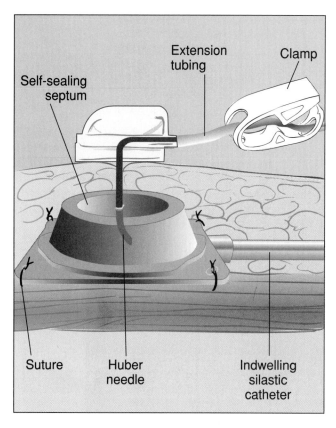

Self-sealing septum

Extension tubing

Clamp

Suture

Huber needle

Indwelling silastic catheter

Figure 76.3.
Implanted indwelling catheter.

Additional Equipment Needed for Special Procedures

Dissolving a Clot in the Catheter:
Urokinase (5000 U/mL)—0.5 mL

Broken Catheter Repair:
Catheter repair kit (Evermed®)
(contains plastic clamps, silicone adhesive, injection caps, and 12-French catheter replacement segment). Three sizes of catheter repair kits are available, based on the internal diameter of the patient catheter—0.8, 1.0, or 1.3 mm.

PROCEDURE

Because any access of these catheters involves risk of infection, air embolism, embolization of catheter thrombus, perforation of external catheter, or displacement, having the appropriate equipment available and ready is important. Maintaining a sterile procedure is important to reduce the risk of line infection.

Several key points should be made before access: (*a*) maintain sterile procedures

and field during the entire procedure; (*b*) do not use acetone or tincture of iodine on the external catheter; (*c*) povidone-iodine is acceptable; (*d*) acetone or tincture of iodine can lead to drying and cracking of the catheter (10); (*e*) do not use forceps with teeth on the external catheter, as these can injure the catheter and cause breakage or make holes; (*f*) always have this clamp nearby when accessing partially implantable devices; (*g*) only 10 mL syringes should be used to draw fluid or flush the catheter; (*h*) smaller syringes generate higher pressure when withdrawn which can rupture the catheter; (*i*) have parenteral fluids to be administered and heparin flush ready; (*j*) do not administer fluids through a catheter if no blood return is obtained after flushed; and k) the clinician should infuse 10 mL of saline flush between any medications to flush the catheter (2, 3, 8, 9).

Accessing Partially Implantable (Broviac®, Hickman®) Catheters

The nurse or physician (i.e., the clinician) should prepare all the necessary equipment, then wash his or her hands, and don sterile gloves. The clinician should clamp the catheter at least 3 inches from cap. Most patients will have their own clamp, but hemostats without teeth also can be used. (If only hemostats with teeth are available, wrap the teeth in gauze to reduce the risk of damaging the catheter.) The clinician should then position a sterile towel under the catheter and remove the cap at the end of the catheter. Then it is time to attach a 10 mL syringe filled with normal saline. The catheter is unclamped and 3 to 5 mL saline is slowly injected into the catheter. Aspiration of fluid back into the syringe is done to check for blood return. If resistance to the instillation of saline is met, or no blood is aspirated, the clinician should reclamp the catheter and attempt maneuvers described in the next section (procedure for establishing patency). Fluids or medications should not be injected if resistance is met or no blood is aspirated. If a blood return has been achieved, the clinician should inject the remaining 5 to 7 mL of fluid into the catheter, reclamp the catheter, and remove the syringe. The intravenous fluid tubing is attached to the catheter. Always be sure to purge the tubing of any air bubbles. The catheter is unclamped and fluids administered. After completion of the procedure, the clinician should inject 3 to 5 mL heparin saline into the catheter, replace the cap, and apply the preferred dressing (gauze must be changed daily, whereas a transparent dressing can be changed weekly). Flush the catheter with heparin flushes on a daily basis, except the Groshong® catheter requires 5 mL of saline weekly.

Accessing Totally Implanted Devices (Port-A-Cath®)

If access of a totally implantable device is not needed emergently, because this procedure involves a skin puncture, a topical anesthetic should be applied over the site. Palpate the reservoir before this to assist in landmark identification. Using eutectic mixture of local anesthetics (EMLA) cream to the skin overlying the reservoir, then covering with an occlusive dressing for 30 to 60 minutes, reduces the discomfort of skin puncture for children when accessing the catheter.

Necessary equipment should be prepared beforehand by the nurse or physician. If EMLA cream and dressing was applied to the patient's access site, the dressing should be removed and the cream wiped away with gauze pad. The clinician should wash his or her hands and don sterile gloves. The clinician should prepare the overlying skin by washing in a circular motion from the center of the device outward with povidone-iodine. After the site dries, he or she should do the same with an alcohol swab. A 10 mL syringe filled with saline should be attached to T-connector tubing and flushed through the tubing. The extension tubing is attached to the Huber® needle, and the needle is flushed with saline to remove air. The extension tubing should then be clamped and set on a sterile field. The clinician should then don a new pair of gloves and other sterile apparel and locate the center of the septum (or reservoir membrane). The clinician should next stabilize the reservoir with the thumb and index finger (Fig. 76.5). With slow but firm pressure, the needle is inserted through the septum to the posterior wall of the reservoir without penetrating the posterior wall. The

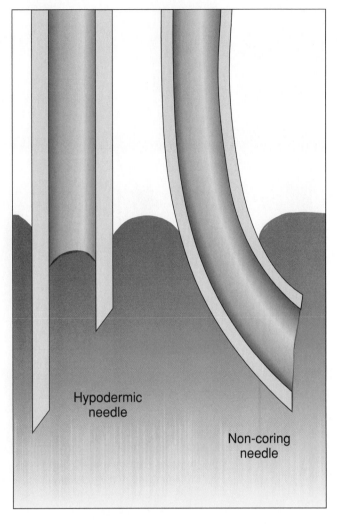

extension tubing is unclamped and 2 mL saline slowly instilled. Do not force fluid into the reservoir if resistance is met; reclamp the extension tubing and use the procedure for establishing patency. If no resistance is met when injecting saline, another 3 mL should be infused into the port. Aspirate the syringe back to check for a blood return. If blood appears, the remaining 5 mL of saline should be injected into the reservoir. The needle is then taped in place, maintaining it at a right angle to the septum. This is best done with gauze pads placed around the needle and then tape reinforced. A sterile dressing should be placed over the needle when in use. The extension tubing should be reclamped and the syringe removed. The intravenous fluid tubing is attached to the catheter, after being sure to purge the tubing of any air bubbles. The catheter is unclamped and fluids adminis-

Figure 76.4.
Hypodermic needle (*left*).
Noncoring needle (*right*).

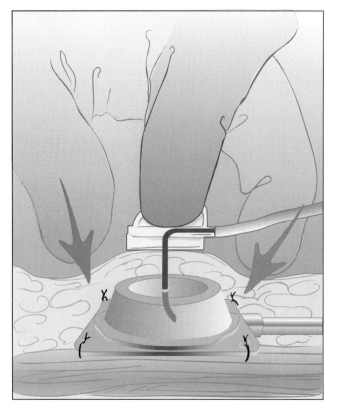

Figure 76.5.
Stabilizing a reservoir with thumb and index finger while accessing an implanted device.

tered. After completion of the procedure, 3 to 5 mL heparin solution should be injected into the catheter through the extension tubing and Huber® needle, the extension tube clamped, and then the needle removed. The preferred dressing should be applied and left in place for 24 hours (for gauze or adhesive strip: heparin flushes are required every 3 to 4 weeks).

If no blood return is seen, the clinician should reclamp and refer to the following procedure for establishing patency. The clinician should not administer fluids or medications through the reservoir or catheter if no blood return is seen.

Establishing Patency

Resistance to saline instillation or a failure to see a blood return can be due to catheter malposition (against a vein wall), catheter malfunction, or a fibrous clot at the distal tip. Noninvasive methods to evaluate for this include altering the patient's position, raising the patient's hands above his or her head, having the patient cough or performing a Val-

salva maneuver, or placing the bed in reverse Trendelenburg. All these may affect changing the venous pressure gradient along the catheter and improve patency (8, 11).

Importantly, the clinician should not try to flush the catheter by forcefully pushing saline into it or by overzealous withdrawal, but rather instill saline or aspirate for blood after trying one or more of the previously mentioned maneuvers.

If fluid cannot be instilled or no blood returns, either a clot in the catheter or a fibrin clot at the tip may be present. In such cases, attempts to declot the catheter should be attempted, unless the patient is actively bleeding or has cerebrovascular disease. (It is the practice in some hospitals to require a physician to directly perform this procedure.) One method is to use a fibrinolytic such as urokinase (5000 U/mL), reconstituted according to package instructions (8, 12). The dose of urokinase used is based on the size of the catheter, using 0.5 mL for a 3 to 4 French catheter and 1 mL for catheters over 4 French size. The clinician should draw the required dose into a 3 mL or larger syringe (do not use a TB syringe) and slowly inject into the catheter. Allow urokinase to remain in catheter for 30 minutes, then attempt to aspirate blood and clot, using a 5 mL syringe or larger. If not successful, this procedure (and the urokinase dose) can be repeated. Urokinase has less antigenic activity than streptokinase and is preferred (3, 9).

If the clot is thought to be secondary to mineral precipitates on the catheter (i.e., calcium, phosphorus), 0.1 normal hydrochloric acid (0.5 mL) can be used. The clinician can slowly inject this into the catheter and allow it to remain in the catheter for 20 minutes, then attempt aspiration. This method may be repeated up to three times within 2 hours (9).

Some centers have used ethanol to dissolve waxy clots secondary to hyperalimentation and intralipids. A 70% ethanol in water mixture is instilled into the catheter and allowed to remain for 1 hour, then aspirated (9). This solution is used once, and if not successful, 0.1 normal hydrochloric acid can then be attempted.

Generally, using hydrochloric acid or ethanol to improve patency needs to involve the primary physician who is involved with the catheter placement and ongoing care.

Drawing Blood from a Partially Implantable (Broviac®, Hickman®) Catheter

The clinician should prepare any necessary supplies and arrange them on a sterile field. The catheter is then clamped and the cap of the catheter is removed and discarded. An empty 10 mL syringe is attached and the catheter unclamped. Approximately 8 to 9 mL of blood is withdrawn, the catheter is reclamped, and the syringe discarded. An empty syringe is attached, the catheter unclamped, the desired amount of blood is withdrawn, and then the catheter is clamped. It is best to reclamp the catheter each time before a syringe is removed. A 10 mL syringe filled with saline is attached, the catheter unclamped, and saline is injected slowly into the catheter. The catheter is clamped once again, the syringe removed, and a new heparin cap attached. Then the cap is swabbed and injected with 1 to 2 mL of 100 U/mL heparin (2, 8, 9).

Drawing Blood from a Totally Implanted Device (Port-A-Cath®)

The clinician should prepare all the supplies and follow steps previously outlined in accessing a line. An empty 10 mL syringe is attached to the extension tubing and the tubing unclamped. Approximately 8 to 9 mL of blood is withdrawn, the tubing is reclamped, the syringe removed, and the blood discarded. The clinician should attach another empty syringe and withdraw the desired amount of blood, and remember to reclamp the extension tubing every time before a syringe is removed. A 10 mL syringe filled with normal saline is attached, the tubing unclamped, the saline is slowly injected into the reservoir, and the extension tubing should then be reclamped. The clinician should mix 1 mL 100 U/mL heparin with 4 mL saline in a 10 mL syringe and attach the syringe to the extension tube, unclamp the tubing, and instill the flush into the reservoir. The tubing is then clamped and the Huber® needle is pulled straight out. If no bleeding occurs, a gauze dressing or adhesive strip can be applied and left in place for 24 hours (2, 8, 9).

Catheter Breakage

This can result inadvertently from cutting the catheter with a scissors while trying to remove the dressing, from a needle piercing the catheter, from a child pulling away during access, from children who play with the implantable port site (Twiddler's syndrome) (3), or from injury to it from contact sports. The catheter can separate from the port of the implanted device. For partially implantable devices, it is important to clamp the catheter proximal to the break and cover the torn region with a sterile gauze if available. If no external catheter is present, pressure should be applied at the catheter entrance site into the vein (not at the exit site) (2, 9, 11). Repair kits are available for partially implantable catheters. For totally implanted devices, a radiograph should be obtained to determine the integrity of the system. Both the primary physician and the surgeon need to be contacted.

Aftercare Instructions for Partially Implantable (Broviac®, Hickman®) Catheters

Always keep the site covered and dry. Change the dressing every other day (gauze), weekly (transparent), and as necessary to reduce risk of contamination. Flush the line daily with heparin solution (100 U/mL). If this cannot be done, notify the physician most responsible for the catheter. Look for bruising, bleeding, or signs of infection (redness, pain, purulent drainage, fever) each day. If present, call a physician immediately (2, 3, 8, 9, 11).

Aftercare Instructions for Totally Implanted Devices (Port-A-Cath®)

Avoid direct pressure over device (includes seat belts with shoulder harness). Flush line at least weekly. If this cannot be accomplished, then notify a physician. Look for bruising, bleeding, or signs of infection (redness, pain, purulent drainage, fever) every day. If present, call the child's physician immediately. Patients do not have to wear a dressing over the device, and swimming and bathing is allowed (2, 3, 8, 9, 11).

Medication Incompatibility

Two medications that possibly should not be administered by central access lines are diazepam and phenytoin. It is thought that these medications interact with the silicone lining of the catheter and could crystallize with it. This cannot be reversed by fibrinolytic agents. Because debate exists around this issue, it is probably beneficial to find another method of administration if these medications are required. It is also important to avoid administering agents that are not compatible with each other (i.e., calcium and bicarbonate) without an adequate saline flush between them.

SUMMARY
Accessing Partially Implantable (Broviac®, Hickman®) Catheters
1. Prepare equipment
2. Wash hands and don sterile gloves
3. Clamp catheter at least 3 inches from cap. Most patients will have their own clamp, but hemostats without teeth also can be used. (If only hemostats with teeth are available, wrap the teeth in gauze.)
4. Position sterile towel under catheter
5. Remove cap at end of catheter and attach 10 mL syringe filled with normal saline
6. Unclamp catheter and slowly inject 3 to 5 mL of saline into catheter
7. Aspirate fluid back into syringe to check for blood return
8. If resistance is met to instillation of saline, or no blood is aspirated, reclamp catheter and attempt maneuvers described below (procedure for establishing patency). Do not inject fluids or medications if resistance is met or no blood is aspirated.
9. If blood return has been achieved, inject remaining 5 to 7 mL of fluid into catheter, reclamp catheter, and remove syringe
10. Attach intravenous fluid tubing to catheter, (be sure to purge tubing of any air bubbles), unclamp catheter, and administer fluids

SUMMARY
(CONTINUED)
11. After completion of procedure, inject 3 to 5 mL of heparin into catheter, replace cap, and apply preferred dressing (gauze dressing should be changed daily, whereas a transparent dressing can be changed weekly—although heparin flushes are required daily, except the Groshong® catheter requires 5 mL of saline weekly)

Accessing Totally Implanted Devices (Port-A-Cath®) (2, 3, 8, 9)
When access of a totally implantable device is not needed emergently, a topical anesthetic should be applied over the site before skin puncture. Using EMLA cream to the skin overlying the reservoir, under an occlusive dressing for 30 to 60 minutes, reduces discomfort for children.
1. Prepare equipment
2. If EMLA cream and dressing was applied, remove dressing and swab cream away with gauze
3. Wash hands and don sterile gloves
4. Palpate reservoir and prepare overlying skin by washing in circular motion from center of device outward with povidine-iodine, then alcohol
5. Attach 10 mL syringe filled with saline to T-connector tubing and flush saline through tubing; set on a sterile field.
6. Attach extension tubing to Huber® needle and flush needle with saline to remove air. Clamp the extension tubing closed; set on sterile field.
7. Don a new pair of gloves and other sterile apparel
8. Locate center of septum and stabilize reservoir with thumb and index finger
9. Slowly but firmly insert needle through septum to back of reservoir
10. Unclamp extension tubing and slowly instill 2 mL saline
11. If resistance is met, do not force fluid into reservoir. Reclamp extension tubing and see procedure for establishing patency (below)
12. If no resistance is met injecting saline, infuse another 3 mL into port
13. Aspirate fluid back into syringe and check for blood return
14. If blood is seen, inject remaining saline into reservoir, tape needle in place, maintaining it at a right angle to septum. This can be done by applying gauze pads around needle with tape reinforcement. A sterile dressing should be applied over needle while in use. If no blood return is obtained, reclamp extension tubing and refer to procedure for establishing patency

15. Reclamp extension tubing and remove syringe
16. Attach intravenous fluid tubing to catheter (be sure to purge the tubing of any air bubbles), unclamp catheter, and administer fluids
17. After completion of procedure, inject 3 to 5 mL heparin into catheter through extension tubing, and Hubert needle, clamp extension tube, then remove needle. Apply preferred dressing for 24 hours (gauze or adhesive strip: heparin flushes are required every 3 to 4 weeks)

Drawing Blood from a Partially Implantable (Broviac®, Hickman®) Catheter (2, 8, 9).

1. Prepare supplies and arrange on sterile field
2. Clamp catheter
3. Remove cap and discard
4. Attach an empty 10 mL syringe and unclamp catheter
5. Withdraw 8 to 9 mL of blood, reclamp catheter, and discard syringe
6. Attach empty syringe, unclamp catheter, and withdraw desired amount of blood, then clamp catheter. Remember to reclamp catheter each time before syringe is removed
7. Attach 10 mL syringe filled with saline and unclamp catheter. Slowly inject saline into catheter
8. Reclamp catheter, remove syringe, and attach new heparin cap (swab cap and inject with 1 to 2 mL 100 U/mL heparin)

Drawing Blood from a Totally Implanted Device (Port-A-Cath®) (2, 8, 9)

1. Prepare supplies
2. Follow steps 2–9 from Accessing Totally Implanted Devices
3. Attach empty 10 mL syringe to extension tubing and unclamp tubing
4. Withdraw 8 to 9 mL blood, reclamp tubing, and remove syringe and discard blood
5. Attach another empty syringe and withdraw desired amount of blood. Remember to reclamp the extension tubing every time before a syringe is removed
6. Attach 10 mL syringe filled with normal saline, unclamp tubing, slowly inject into reservoir, and reclamp extension tubing
7. Mix 1 mL of 100 U/mL heparin with 4 mL saline in a 10 mL syringe
8. Attach syringe to extension tube, unclamp tubing, and instill flush into reservoir
9. Clamp tubing, pull Huber® needle straight out
10. If no bleeding is noted, a gauze dressing or adhesive strip can be applied and left in place for 24 hours

COMPLICATIONS

Infection

One of the main risks of a central line is that of line infection. This occurs at increased risk if sterile technique is not maintained during procedures. Though accessing a line or withdrawing blood can introduce organisms into the line, infection from the line also may be the presenting problem. Precipitating organisms cultured from infected lines include *S. aureus, S. epidermidis, S. viridans, P. aeruginosa, Klebsiella pneumoniae, Escherichia coli, Enterobacter cloacae* as well as fungi (2, 5–7). The risk of introducing line infection is still present in patients even with sterile technique done well.

Catheter infections include line sepsis (at least bacteremia) and skin infections at the skin exit site, subcutaneous tunnel, or the skin overlying the implanted devices. Common organisms implicated in skin infections include *S. aureus* and *S. epidermidis* (5–7). Skin infections involving Gram-negative bacilli such as *Pseudomonas aeruginosa* appear to be more likely in neutropenic patients (5, 6). Management should involve obtaining a blood culture from both the line and a peripheral site. Appropriate intravenous antibiotic therapy is initiated and a decision about exploring for distal sites of infection required.

Air Embolism

Because these catheter systems end in blood vessels near the heart, the risk of air embolism is present. It is vital to keep the system clamped whenever instillation of fluid or withdrawal of blood is not taking place to minimize this risk. Signs and symptoms of air embolism include the sudden onset of tachypnea, hypotension, and loss of consciousness (2). Treatment includes clamping the system immediately, placement of the patient on the left side in a Trendelenburg position, oxygen, and intravenous access (2, 11).

Catheter Occlusion and Embolization of a Catheter Thrombus

A risk of thrombus formation exists at the tip of the catheter. Studies have shown fibrin sheaths around occluded catheters, and one study measured thrombi that were aspirated from occluded catheters after the instillation of urokinase. These thrombi can occlude the catheter or increase the risk of embolization. Although these thrombi are small fragments, a large one can result in pulmonary embolism if dislodged during flushing. Signs and symptoms include tachycardia, tachypnea, hypoxemia, and chest pain. Diagnosis can be confirmed by a ventilation perfusion scan, and therapy initiated (2, 3, 9).

Other catheter-related complications result from catheter migration. These include arrhythmias, cardiac tamponade, pneumothorax, and superior vena cava syndrome (2).

SUMMARY

Many central venous access devices are currently used by children on an outpatient basis. When problems develop due to the device or to their underlying illness, these children will present for emergency evaluation. It is essential to be familiar with the specific devices currently being used in the region, so the necessary equipment and access techniques are available. Aseptic technique, and knowledge and recognition of potential complications, are required.

REFERENCES

1. Bothe A, Piccione W, Ambrosino JJ, Benotti PN, Lokich JJ. Implantable central venous access system. Amer J Surg 1984;147:565–569.
2. Howell JM. Accessing indwelling lines. In: Roberts JR, Hedges JR, eds. Clinical procedures in emergency medicine. 2nd ed. Philadelphia: WB Saunders, 1991, pp. 357–363.
3. Marcoux C, Fisher S, Wong D. Central venous access devices in children. Pediatr Nurs 1990; 16(2):123–133.
4. McGovern B, Solenberger R, Reed K. A totally implantable venous access system for long-term chemotherapy in children. J Pediatr Surg 1985;20: 725–727.
5. Johnson PR, Decker MD, Edwards KM, Schaffner W, Wright PF. Frequency of Broviac catheter infections in pediatric oncology patients. J Infect Dis 1986;154:570–578.
6. Olson TA, Fischer GW, Lupo MC, Garcia VF, Maybee DA, Keiser J, et al. Antimicrobial therapy of Broviac catheter infections in pediatric hematology oncology patients. J Pediatr Surg 1987;22:839–842.
7. Wurzel CL, Halom K, Feldman JG, Rubin LG. Infection rates of Broviac-Hickman catheters and implantable venous devices. AJDC 1988;142: 536–540.
8. Taylor JP, Taylor JE. Vascular access devices: uses and aftercare. J Emerg Nurs 1987;13:160–167.
9. Dyer BJ, Gardner Weiman M, Ludwig S. Central venous catheters in the emergency department: access, utilization, and problem solving. Pediatr Emerg Care 1995;11:112–117.
10. Howser DM, Meade CD. Hickman catheter care: developing organized teaching strategies. Cancer Nurs 1987;10(2):70–76.
11. Karrei I. Hickman catheters: your guide to trouble-free use. Can Nurs 1982 December; 25–27.
12. Zureikat GY, Martin GR, Silverman NH, Newth CJL. Urokinase therapy for a catheter-related right atrial thrombus and pulmonary embolism in a 2-month-old infant. Pediatr Pulmon 1986;2:303–306.

Pulmonary Procedures

Section Editor: Richard M. Ruddy

CHAPTER 77

USE OF PULSE OXIMETRY

Ronnie S. Fuerst

INTRODUCTION

The pulse oximeter is an electronic monitor used to noninvasively measure arterial oxygen saturation and is standard equipment in emergency departments and other monitoring units such as the operating room, intensive care unit, and outpatient settings where the information would be valuable for patient care. An understanding of its applicability, interpretation, and limitations is essential in the modern practice of emergency medicine.

The origin of this technology began in the 1930s when the first in vivo device to measure oxygen saturation by transillumination was developed. The 1970s heralded two important developments. First was the discovery of arterial pulsations in the microvasculature and second was the use of light-emitting diodes (LEDs) as a light source and photodiodes as light detectors. These latter findings assisted greatly in overcoming the size and weight problems associated with previous devices. In the early 1980s microprocessors had been added for self-calibration and improved accuracy (1).

The pulse oximeter now has distinct advantages over other measures of oxygenation. First, it is at most an uncomfortable attachment to an extremity, but can measure both absolute SaO_2 and trends on patients requiring monitoring for acute medical and traumatic illness in an emergency setting. It can be a stand-alone monitor or integrated into more complex monitoring of patients vital functions. Standard pulse oximeters self-calibrate, which is a distinct advantage over

many traditional monitoring systems. Probably its only disadvantages are that it is unable to distinguish other molecules attached to the hemoglobin moiety, such as carboxyhemoglobin or methemoglobin, so it can read a normal value in their presence. Also, in low perfusion states or when monitoring sites are vasoconstricted for other reasons, the tracing may be unreliable.

ANATOMY AND PHYSIOLOGY

Pulse oximetry is a measure of the percent saturation of hemoglobin by the oxygen molecule. This is only one part of the oxygen transport system (Fig. 77.1) and other methods of observation and monitoring are required to evaluate other aspects of oxygen delivery (2). The remainder of this section presents a review of the physiology of hemoglobin saturation and the oxyhemoglobin dissociation curve followed by a review of the mechanism of the equipment function.

The hemoglobin molecule is almost entirely responsible for oxygen transport when oxygen is within the cardiovascular system. Less than 2% of oxygen present is dissolved in plasma. Hemoglobin saturation (SaO_2) is the amount of oxygenated hemoglobin (O_2Hb) compared with the total amount of hemoglobin available for oxygenation, expressed as a percentage (3):

$$SaO_2 = \frac{\text{Oxygenated hemoglobin}}{\text{(Oxygenated hemoglobin} + \text{Reduced hemoglobin)}} \times 100$$

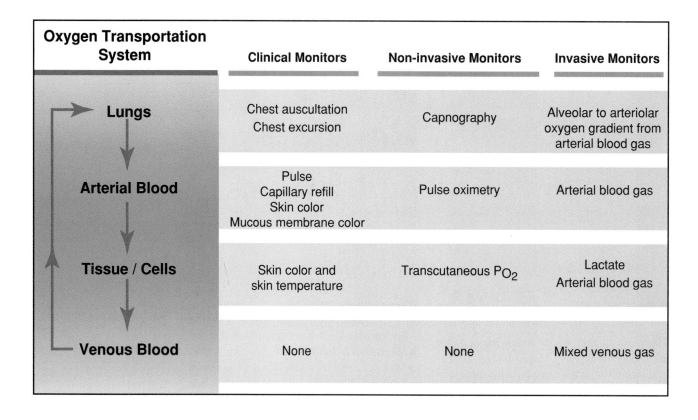

Oxygen Transportation System	Clinical Monitors	Non-invasive Monitors	Invasive Monitors
Lungs	Chest auscultation Chest excursion	Capnography	Alveolar to arteriolar oxygen gradient from arterial blood gas
Arterial Blood	Pulse Capillary refill Skin color Mucous membrane color	Pulse oximetry	Arterial blood gas
Tissue / Cells	Skin color and skin temperature	Transcutaneous P_{O_2}	Lactate Arterial blood gas
Venous Blood	None	None	Mixed venous gas

Figure 77.1.
Oxygen transport system.

The oxyhemoglobin dissociation curve (Fig. 77.2) demonstrates the nonlinear relationship between hemoglobin saturation and the partial pressure of oxygen in plasma (pO_2). Normal SaO_2 is between 95 to 100% and hypoxemia is defined as pO_2 less than 70 mm Hg (SaO_2 below 90%). Small changes in the SaO_2 in the upper, flat part of the oxyhemoglobin dissociation curve result in larger changes in pO_2. In the steep part (lower and middle of the curve), large changes in the SaO_2 result in small changes in pO_2. Under normal physiologic conditions the body operates at the upper portion of the curve as depicted in Figure 77.2. Changes in the oxyhemoglobin dissociation curve either to the left or to the right change the relationship of SaO_2 to pO_2. The factors that shift the oxyhemoglobin curve to the left and increase the affinity of oxygen to hemoglobin at lower pO_2 are increased pH, decreased temperature, decreased pCO_2 and decreased 2,3-DPG. The 2,3-DPG levels are altered by a number of physiologic effects and increases of 2,3-DPG are seen when anemia, chronic hypoxemia, high altitude adaptation, chronic alkalosis, and hyperthyroidism are present.

Pulse oximetry uses the principles of spectrophotometry and the Beer-Lambert law together with complex signal processing algorithms and calibrations to calculate percentage of oxyhemoglobin concentration. Four types of hemoglobin are clinically significant to pulse oximetry. These are oxygenated hemoglobin (O_2Hb), reduced hemoglobin (Hb), carboxyhemoglobin (COHb), and methemoglobin (MetHb). For the purposes of pulse oximetry, both fetal hemoglobin and sickle hemoglobin are assumed to have the characteristics of adult hemoglobin. The oximeter emits two wavelengths of light—one in the red region (660 nm) and one in the infrared region (920 nm)—to differentiate the absorption of light by the oxygenated and deoxygenated hemoglobin species in the microcirculation. Figure 77.3 demonstrates the wavelength absorption of different hemoglobin moieties as they relate to this phenomenon.

Carboxyhemoglobin (COHb) behaves as O_2Hb in regard to its absorption spectra and so the oximeter misinterprets the CoHb and reads a falsely high SpO_2. Methemoglobin (MetHb) absorbs light at both wavelengths emitted by the LED. Therefore, MetHb will always cause a falsely high SpO_2, but as MetHb levels rise the SpO_2 level measured will be less because of the effects on both wavelengths where it causes interference. When the MetHb reaches 30%, the SpO$_2$ will not be above 85% and will remain at that level regardless of increasing MetHb concentrations. Other dyshemoglobinemias may not reliably quantitate the actual oxyhemoglobin percentage. In patients suspected of MetHb or COHb, an ABG should be sent with cooximetry to assess concentrations of those in the blood. The pulse oximeter also must measure absorption differences between the maximal and minimal arterial pulsations to enable it to separate the signals from arterial blood and exclude the background (i.e., venous blood and tissues). After obtaining the separate signals for bound and unbound hemoglobin, the formula previously listed can calculate the percentage saturation of hemoglobin in the circulation measured. Pulse oximeters commonly used in the ED have been found to correlate with arterial blood gas oxygen saturation (SaO$_2$) in patients with systolic blood pressures between 80 and 206 mm Hg, heart rates between 40 and 180 beats per minute, and hematocrits between 20 and 56% (4). The reported accuracy of pulse oximeters by manufacturers with a 95% confidence interval is $\pm$ 4% when the SpO$_2$ is above 70%, $\pm$8% when the SpO$_2$ is 50 to 70%, and unspecified accuracy rate when below 50% (2). This suggests that the trend of readings is more accurate than the individual SpO$_2$ readout. Other technical issues important in this technology include several worth discussing (5–10) Mo-

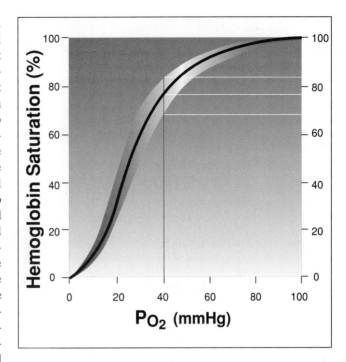

Figure 77.2.
Oxyhemoglobin dissociation curve.

tion near the sensor site may mimic the pulsations of small arteries and affect the reading. In this instance the pulse on the oximeter will not produce a normal curve and will not trace the patient's actual heart rate. In low flow states, the lack of blood flow in the vessels may not transmit sufficient change in light emittance for the monitor to sufficiently read the saturation. This may be demonstrated by the monitor indicating "pulse search." During high venous pressure the ve-

Figure 77.3.
Absorbance spectrum curves for O$_2$Hb and COHb.

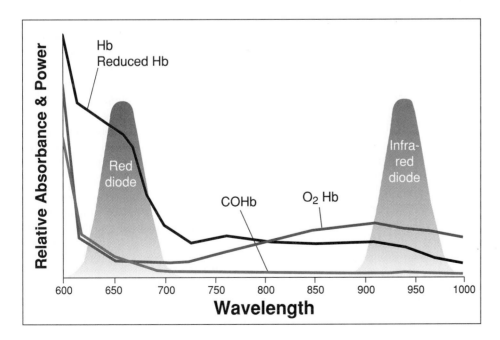

Table 77.1.
Indications for Use
of Pulse Oximetry

nous pulsation may transmit falsely low SpO_2 to the monitor. In children this rarely occurs in heart failure, but may be present in traumatic venous obstruction or when a manometer cuff is inflated or a tourniquet is applied. Lastly, other ambient light sources such as sunlight, warming lights, phototherapy, or bright fluorescent bulbs may interfere with the reading by increasing the light to the photodetector. The patient ought to have the sensor shielded with a more light-resistant covering.

INDICATIONS

Three common indications for using pulse oximetry in the emergency setting are use for monitoring during a clinical procedure, as an indicator or baseline for a patient's clinical respiratory state, and to ascertain to therapy which affects oxygen delivery. Table 77.1 lists the most common indications for pulse oximetry. In monitoring of procedures, it is part of the American Academy of Pediatrics guidelines for the sedation of pediatric patients (11). It is particularly useful to monitor closely with SaO_2 during the use of sedative agents with pain relief in reduction fractures and in the use of anxiolysis in complex laceration repair. Young infants, potentially septic, ought to have continuous SaO_2 during all procedures and observation, but particularly during lumbar puncture when observation for apnea may be difficult. All patients with the need of airway intervention, endotracheal intubation, use of nasopharyngeal and oropharyngeal airways ought to have continuous SaO_2. As listed in Table 77.1, several categories of emergency patients ought to have continuous SaO_2 for monitoring of the child's clinical status. Lastly, a number of illnesses are better managed when the SaO_2 is monitored either continuously or intermittently. Illnesses at risk of leading to hypoxemia in childhood include clinically significant upper airway obstruction, pneumonia, bronchiolitis, and asthma. The list also includes the baby with apnea, and congenital heart disease, including both congestive heart failure and cyanotic heart disease. These illnesses for which acute therapy may reverse the process, such as asthma, are best continuously monitored to evaluate improvement and exacerbation or worsening obstruction. It is key

to remember that SaO_2 measures the oxygen saturation and not the ventilation. Therefore children with upper airway obstruction and large airway-lower airway disease may have normal SaO_2 until late in a deterioration. In acute asthma, patients with moderate obstruction of their airways may demonstrate reduction of the SaO_2 after bronchodilators which will be missed if pulse oximetry is not monitored continuously. Pulse oximeters should be used for transfer of high-risk pediatric patients between medical units, such as the ED to operating room or intensive care unit and for interhospital transfer. In many cities, prehospital care services carry pulse oximeters that enable the paramedics to assess for hypoxia, which may have been difficult to recognize clinically (12).

EQUIPMENT

Pulse oximeters found in EDs are usually freestanding portable devices or integrated into remote patient monitors. The typical unit will display heart rate and arterial oxygen saturation (Fig. 77.4.A). Some units display the wave form or plethysmograph. Typical controls include a power on/off switch, an alarm on/off switch, and a high/low alarm limit control for both pulse rate and saturation level. Many freestanding units have internal battery power for transport. The externally attached component is the probe which is placed on the patient and connected to the oximeter with a standard adapter. Most manufacturers make only probes that are compatible with their own instrument. The probe is made of an LED (light-emitting diode) and a sensor (photodiode). Probes can be reusable in that they are usually clipped on to a toe or finger. The disposable probes are typically held to the extremity with a mild adhesive and are malleable. The latter has distinct advantages because the disposable probes often conform to different children's fingers or toes better and lead to less false alarms from loss of the signal transduction.

PROCEDURE

Orientation to the operation of the pulse oximeter can be accomplished in just a few

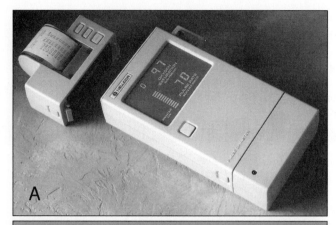

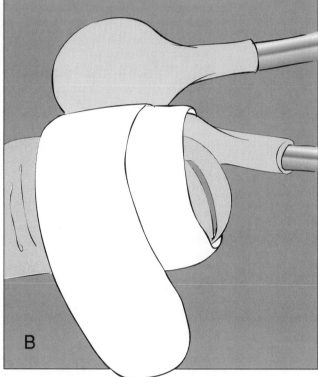

Figure 77.4.
A. Pulse oximeter.
B. Pulse oximetry probe attached to finger of child.

minutes. The operator must first decide on a location for the sensor placement. The sensor must be placed on a part of the body that will allow light to pass through from one side to the other. Fingers, toes, and the earlobe are the most common sites for children and adults. Due to the small size, the hand, foot, nose, lip, or penis also may be used. Most operators initially attempt placement on a finger or toe. Once the site has been chosen, the appropriate size sensor must be selected. The available sizes include infant, child and adult depending on the model available. Nondisposable clip-on sensors are self-aligning, but at times more difficult to use in young children. Disposable sensors are placed in a circular or longitudinal fashion, with care to ensure that the LED is aligned directly across the digit from the light detector (Fig. 77.4.B).

After the sensor has been placed, the unit is turned on and observed for capture of the signal. If the oximeter is able to detect pulsations it will display the rate of pulsations (equivalent to the heart rate) and an SpO_2 value. If no signal is captured, the oximeter may print a message such as "pulse search" or display a heart rate that will not correlate with the true heart rate or not display the SpO_2. If a disposable sensor has been re-used, it is often of value to re-attempt monitoring with a new sensor.

After the signal is picked up, alarm limits for the rate and the SpO$_2$ may need to be set. Alarm limits are a subject for varied opinion, but should be set to the patient's age and clinical condition to warn health care providers of possible adverse values. Most clinicians would set the lower limit SpO$_2$ to at least 90% and as high as 94%. As a general guideline, an SpO$_2$ of 95% is close to a pO$_2$ of 75, an SpO$_2$ of less than 90% correlates with a pO$_2$ of approximately 60 indicating moderate hypoxemia. At 90%, in most circumstances, the level is at the top of the steep portion of desaturation where hypoxemia is defined. It is important to verify that the alarm switch is in the desired position should the clinician walk away from the bedside of the child.

If any doubt exists about the accuracy of the pulse oximeter, or if no correlation is found between the clinical situation and the oximeter reading, an arterial blood gas should be obtained. It must be remembered that the pulse oximeter yields information regarding oxygenation without reflection of ventilation. Therefore when the patient is receiving supplemental oxygen, the reduction in oxygen saturation reflecting hypoxemia may be late with upper and lower airway obstruction.

COMPLICATIONS

Modern pulse oximeters are extremely safe devices with few reported complications. Thermal burns have been reported from connecting the sensor of one manufacturer to an instrument from a different manufacturer (13). Theoretically, ischemia could be induced by applying disposable sensors too tightly. The most common complications observed can be over reliance on the device in place of clinical judgment or the misinterpre-

tation of the data obtained from it. This is especially true in clinical states when hypoxemia may be masked by falsely elevated SpO$_2$, in CO poisoning, or in states of methemoglobinemia.

REFERENCES

1. Tremper KK, Barker SJ. Pulse oximetry. Anesthesiology 1989;70:98–108.
2. Ehrenwerth J, Eisenkraft JB. Anesthesia equipment: principals and applications. St. Louis: CV Mosby, 1993, pp. 249.
3. Scanlan CL, Spearman CB, Sheldon RL. Egan's fundamentals of respiratory care. St. Louis: CV Mosby, 1990, pp. 212–222.
4. Jones J, et al. Continuous emergency department monitoring of arterial saturation in adult patients with respiratory distress. Ann Emerg Med 1988;17: 463–468.
5. Barker SJ, Tremper KK, Hyatt J. Effects of methemoglobin on pulse oximetry and mixed venous oximetry. Anesthesiology 1989:70:112–117.
6. Barker SJ, Tremper KK, Hyatt J. The effect of carbon monoxide inhalation on pulse oximetry and transcutaneous pO$_2$. Anesthesiology 1987;66: 677–679.
7. Tremper KK, Hustedler SM, Barker SJ, Adams AL, Wong DH, Zaccari J, Benik K, Lemons V. Accuracy of a pulse oximeter in the critically ill adult: effect of temperature and hemodynamics. Anesthesiology 1985;63:3A.
8. Scheller MS, Unger RJ, Kelner MJ. Effects of intravenously administered dyes on pulse oximetry readings. Anesthesiology 1986;65:550–552.
9. Veychemans F, Baele P, Guillaume JE, Williams E, Clerbaux T. Hyperbilirubinemia does not interfere with hemoglobin saturation measured by pulse oximetry. Anesthesiology 1989;70:118–122.
10. Lawson D, Norley I, Korbon G, Loeb R, Ellis J. Blood flow limits and pulse oximetry signal detection. Anesthesiology 1987;67:599–603.
11. Committee on Drugs, American Academy of Pediatrics. Guidelines for monitoring and management of pediatric patients during and after sedation for diagnostic and therapeutic procedures, 1992;89: 1110–1113.
12. McGuire TJ, Pointer JE. Evaluation of a pulse oximeter in the prehospital setting. Ann of Emerg Med 1988;17:1058–1062.
13. Murphy K, Secunda JA, Rockoff MA. Severe burns from a pulse oximeter. Anesthesiology 1990;73: 350–352.

END TIDAL CO$_2$ Monitoring

Javier A. Gonzalez del Rey

INTRODUCTION

Measurement of variations in the respiratory cycle of the expired CO$_2$ either by displayed waveform or by absolute numerical values is defined as capnography and capnometry. Measurement of exhaled CO$_2$ at the level of upper airway at the end of the expiration (when CO$_2$ is at its maximum level) is referred to as end tidal CO$_2$ (EtCO$_2$) (1, 2, 3). This noninvasive measurement of blood gases has been used since the 1950s. Initially described by Luft in 1943 (4), it was not until this past decade when its clinical applications made this technique popular in the intensive care unit and operating room setting. Primitive attempts at crude CO$_2$ measurement were made in the anesthesia suite by the barium hydroxide agglutination reaction and the Einstein CO$_2$ detector which was capable of sensing 4 to 6 volume percentage (volume %) CO$_2$ (5). Modern technology designed monitors that use infrared absorption spectroscopy to measure the amount of CO$_2$ in an exhaled breath. These sensors may be located in the patient's artificial breathing circuit (mainstream) or remote from the patient as part of the CO$_2$ monitoring circuit system (sidestream).

In the late 1980s, another practical method that documents concentrations of CO$_2$ usually present in the trachea was introduced. It is based on the device demonstrating colorimetric changes for levels of carbon dioxide above 2%. This technique has been particularly useful for documentation of endotracheal tube (ETT) placement in emergency situations.

Transcutaneous CO$_2$ monitoring, a technique developed in the 1970s primarily for the neonatal intensive care patient, has not been proven useful in the ED setting. This is because transcutaneous CO$_2$ measurements take time to calibrate and skin thickness in older children or adults makes the test inaccurate.

With the development of emergency and transport medicine, EtCO$_2$ measurement has become a very popular and useful tool for both monitoring ventilated patients and as a means for confirming ETT placement. Portable and disposable units have been designed making the technology user friendly and less costly.

All critically ill or injured children requiring ventilatory support, in particular those cases in which outcome may be affected by adequacy of ventilation or special techniques (i.e., acute head trauma, status epilepticus, and in the transport of ventilated patients), should ideally be monitored by pulse oximetry and capnography. Physicians, nurses, and respiratory therapists managing these patients in the ED should be familiar with this technique.

ANATOMY AND PHYSIOLOGY

Carbon dioxide (CO$_2$), one of the waste products of cellular metabolism, is transported in blood predominantly in the form of bicarbonate ion (60%). One-third of CO$_2$ is bound to blood proteins and the rest is carried as dissolved gas in plasma (pCO$_2$). The dissolved

Figure 78.1.
Physiology of lung
ventilation and perfusion.

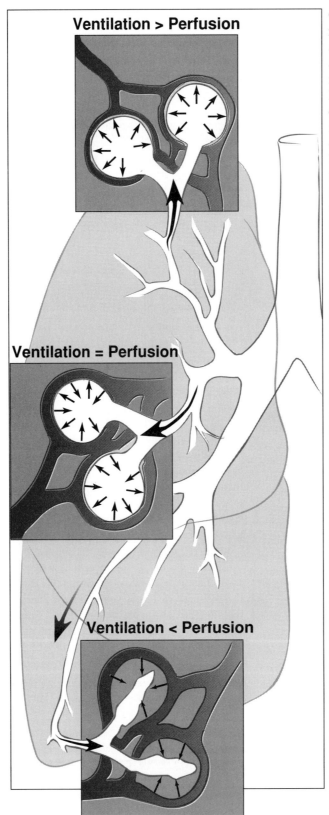

Ventilation > Perfusion

Ventilation = Perfusion

Ventilation < Perfusion

CO_2 concentration in the arterial end of the skin capillaries approximates the pCO_2 of an arterial sample. Carbon dioxide then diffuses in lung capillaries to the alveolar unit and enters the gaseous phase. During exhalation the pCO_2 concentration at the end of each breath will be nearly equal to the $PaCO_2$, if the ventilation and perfusion (V/Q) are well matched. $EtCO_2$ represents the approximation of pCO_2 from all ventilated alveoli regardless if they are perfused. $PaCO_2$ represents the pCO_2 of perfused alveoli. In normal conditions end tidal CO_2 is 2 to 6 mm Hg less than arterial pCO_2 (6).

To further understand the $EtCO_2$ concept, it is important to understand the physiology of lung ventilation and perfusion. Normal lungs (Fig. 78.1), have a tendency for the apical segments to be more aerated relative to perfusion. At the base, secondary to the opposite phenomenon, the lung is more perfused and not as well aerated. The V/Q constant in most individuals is 0.8 (4 parts ventilation to 5 parts perfusion). The normal respiratory cycle has nonused or wasted ventilation. Some of this is alveolar gas which does not get exchanged (alveolar dead space). Other gas travels only within the large or conducting airways and also is not part of the CO_2 exchange (main airway dead space). The sum of these is the physiologic dead space. The $EtCO_2$ concentration is related to the arterial carbon dioxide tension ($PaCO_2$), the segmental perfusion of lung units, and the percent of dead space ventilation.

For example, in cases when pulmonary capillary bed perfusion is less than normal but ventilation is normal, the $EtCO_2$ may significantly underestimate $PaCO_2$. In airways with no perfusion, CO_2 will approach zero if ventilation is adequate, whereas perfused airways will diffuse CO_2. The net effect is that the end tidal CO_2 will represent the combination of normal and close to zero CO_2 and thereby underestimate $PaCO_2$. Conditions that affect a V/Q mismatch include shock, heart failure, pulmonary emboli or thrombi, cardiac arrest, pneumothorax or hydrothorax, or patients persistently in lateral decubitus position. This V/Q mismatch develops because inadequate perfusion to well-ventilated areas results in a widened difference between the arterial pCO_2 ($PaCO_2$) and alveolar CO_2. In these cases $EtCO_2$ underestimates $PaCO_2$ because of the effect of abnormal perfusion.

A different scenario occurs when the lung has adequate perfusion but inadequate ventilation (shunt perfusion). Conditions that reduce alveolar ventilation or increase the production of carbon dioxide will elevate the arterial CO_2, decreasing the V/Q ratio. Although the $EtCO_2$ rises as $PaCO_2$ does from this state, $EtCO_2$ may underestimate $PaCO_2$ because the contribution of dead space ventilation makes it difficult to have a time steady state $EtCO_2$. This is frequently observed in patients with asthma, atelectasis, mucous plugging, right main stem bronchial intubation, emphysema, pneumonia, pleural effusion, and pneumothorax.

During normal respiration, some dead space ventilation travels through the esophagus instead of down the airway. In the proximal esophagus, the measured CO_2 closely correlates with the concentration in inhaled air. It correlates poorly in tracheal trauma or tracheoesophageal fistulas which may raise the concentration of CC_2 to levels closer to that in the airway.

Endotracheal intubation is associated with a complication rate reported as high as 26% (7). Unrecognized esophageal intubation is probably the most serious of these. Utting et al. in 1979 reported that 15% of anesthesia-related accidents resulting in brain injury or death were the result of unrecognized esophageal intubation (8). In the pre-hospital setting, Stewart et al. and Shea et al. noted a 1.8% and 2% incidence of recognized esophageal intubation, respectively (9, 10). In recent years the colorimetric $EtCO_2$ detector has become available, which indicates the presence of CO_2 by a color change. The premise is that with intact pulmonary circulation, CO_2 is present in the trachea but not in the esophageal gas reflux. Studies have revealed that the gastric CO_2 expired is lower and usually less than 0.7 volume % (mL/100 mL) (11, 12). Initially the waveform during esophageal intubations may appear normal, but with successive ventilations (3 to 6) it dissipates. This occurs even under the influence of carbonated beverage consumption or the presence of antacids in the stomach (13–16).

INDICATIONS

Indications and uses of capnography are multiple and based on the determination of $EtCO_2$. Its use in the operating room is primarily to monitor intubated patients during anesthesia, alerting physicians to inadequate ventilation, circuit disconnection or airway leaks. Most importantly it can detect inadvertent placement of the endotracheal tube in the esophagus. In the ED it can be used to assess effectiveness of cardiopulmonary resuscitation, monitoring of ventilated patients due to trauma or respiratory failure, or status epilepticus. It is important during the delivery of special ventilatory therapy, such as controlled hyperventilation in head trauma. Most recently esophageal $EtCO_2$ monitoring has been used in the monitoring of patients under conscious sedation for a procedure or diagnostic study and in the evaluation of patients in impending respiratory failure from pneumonia, asthma, and neurologic illness.

EQUIPMENT

End tidal CO_2 partial pressure can be measured either by mass or by infrared spectroscopy. Mass spectroscopy separates and counts ionized molecules of the gas to determine its concentration. Most commonly used is the infrared spectroscopy which compares the amount of infrared light (IR) absorbed by the sample with that absorbed by a noncarbon-dioxide-containing chamber. Carbon dioxide strongly absorbs infrared light at a wave length of 4.28 nm. In the sample chamber, CO_2 absorbs the light energy emitted by the IR source corresponding to its wave length. At the end of the chamber, a detector

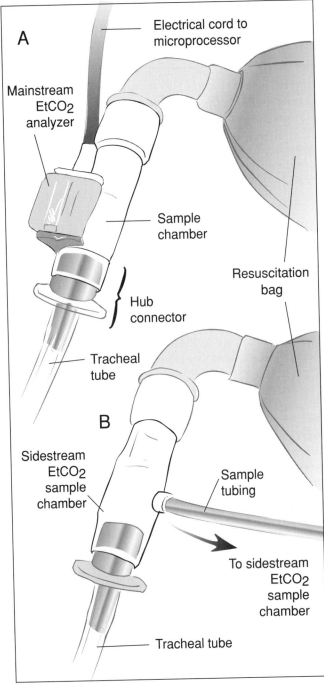

volume % at an atmospheric pressure of 760 mm Hg.

The gas sample may be obtained from the patient's airway using either a mainstream or a sidestream method (Fig. 78.2). Mainstream sampling places a chamber in the airway (between the patient and the ventilatory unit). The sidestream aspirates gas from the ventilatory system and draws the gas sample to the analyzer via the side sample tubing. The advantages in using the mainstream system are mostly related to the location of the infrared source. Because it is placed in the airway in series, no mixing of gases occurs, nor is there aspiration of secretions into the side circuit. Continuous reading of the CO_2 concentration also occurs avoiding lag time to measurement.

The sidestream method collects a sample of gas from the patient's airway and withdraws it down the side tubing to the analyzer. Its advantages are that it does not add weight to the airway, it provides minimal dead space addition in the ventilation system, and it has less risk of contamination with secretions and moisture because the optical sensor is not directly in line with the airway. Some of its disadvantages may include a slight delay in measurement due to the distance between the patient's airway and analyzer. A small risk of sidestream tubing obstruction and falsely low CO_2 values are present due to mixture of exhaled and inhaled gases when the tidal volume is small and flow rates are high.

Several disposable end tidal CO_2 detectors have been recently developed. As discussed previously, they use a chemically treated foam indicator that changes color in the presence of CO_2. This pH-sensitive indicator is contained under a transparent dome mounted in a housing that functions as an endotracheal tube elbow adapter. The minimum concentration of CO_2 required to detect a color change is 0.54% with a range of 0.25 to 0.6% (17). This unit cannot detect hypercarbia or hypocarbia, right main stem bronchus intubation or oropharyngeal intubations in a spontaneously breathing patient. It can verify position of the ETT within the trachea by color change after being in contact with several breaths of CO_2 directly from the airway (3, 18). A new product recently introduced in the market has a crush capsule solution attached to the device that changes in color after contact with CO_2 (Fig. 78.3).

Figure 78.2.
Gas sampling methods.
A. Mainstream.
B. Sidestream.

converts the light energy into an electrical signal proportional to the intensity of the incidental radiation reflecting in this way the EtCO$_2$ of the sample. Most capnometers will usually report concentrations of end tidal expired CO_2 in mm Hg or percentage volume CO_2 by dividing the CO_2 partial pressure by the atmospheric pressure. The normal concentration is approximately 38 mm Hg, or 5

The increase in dead space once the indicator is attached to the airway can be of concern in small infants. Bhende et al. demonstrated in animal studies and in infants and children that disposable CO_2 detectors can be safely used in patients weighing as little as 2 kg (19). Most of the available products have a limited time of use per patient. Overall, these disposable CO_2 detectors are sensitive and can provide vital information for confirming endotracheal tube position after intubation and transport.

PROCEDURE

Capnography should always be used in conjunction with good clinical judgment and management. If not familiar with the equipment or when concerned about proper function of the equipment, the clinician may often be better off to not use them at all.

Appropriate and repeated clinical evaluation of the ABCs is indicated even when $EtCO_2$ monitoring is indicated or available. In the prehospital care setting, the colorimetric capnometers are very practical. Once a patient is intubated, the clinician should ensure that the ETT is in the correct place clinically, which is accomplished by assessing the patient's responsiveness, chest movements, breath sounds, and condensation of air in the ETT. If a disposable detector is available, the clinician should attach it to the ETT and then connect the ambu bag to it. If CO_2 is present in concentrations indicating exhaled air from the trachea, the color will change after several breaths confirming the position of the ETT within the trachea. These disposable units have some limitations. Because they may be affected adversely by humidity, they should not be used continuously for more than 2 hours. If used in conjunction with humidified oxygen, the disposable units may not remain reliable after 15 minutes of continuous use (20).

If a portable unit with mainstream or sidestream sampling is available, turn the unit on and insert the analyzer (mainstream) or sampler (sidestream) in series with the ETT. After several breaths the analyzer should be equilibrating $EtCO_2$. In this case the reading is presented to the operators on liquid display bar graphs in either mm Hg or volume %

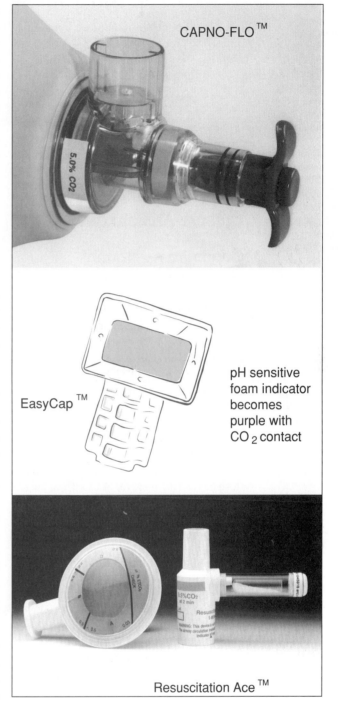

pH sensitive foam indicator becomes purple with CO_2 contact

CO_2. Waveforms will be discussed in the following section on clinical applications.

In the hospital setting, $EtCO_2$ modes have been incorporated to the ICU, OR, and ED monitors. Different $EtCO_2$ manufactures have different ways of initiating or activating the $EtCO_2$ probe. The operator should be familiar with the monitors used in his or her institution. These monitors usually have the

Figure 78.3.
Capnometers using color change from CO_2 detection to verify endotracheal intubation.

**Chapter 78
End Tidal CO_2
Monitoring**

SUMMARY

1. Once patient's airway has been secured and position of ETT has been clinically confirmed, clinician may use $EtCO_2$ monitor to reconfirm position and monitor ventilation

2. If disposable colorimetric $EtCO_2$ monitor is used, it must be attached to ETT and it would take approximately six breaths to change color of membrane in presence of CO_2. If no changes in color are noted, patient's airway should be evaluated immediately and if in doubt, removal of ETT and bag mask ventilation initiated

3. If infrared capnometer is used, operator should evaluate quality of curve and numeric values in relation to clinical presentation before making any changes in patient's management

capability to provide numerical and trend information about the monitored ventilatory status. The process is the same. Once the airway has been established and clinically checked for position, the adaptor is attached to the end of the ETT and then connected to the ambu bag or ventilator. In nonintubated patients, sidestream technology is more convenient. A nasal probe is placed in the patient's nostrils to collect gases for monitoring.

CLINICAL APPLICATIONS

Capnogram—Normal Waveform

A normal capnogram is shown in Figure 78.4. It includes a zero baseline (or phase I) which represents most of the early exhalation. This is followed by a sharp ascent (phase II) which indicates presence of CO_2 as the result of combined alveolar and dead space gas during midexhalation. Phase III represents the plateau; during this period alveolar gas is measured. The end of this steady state represents the maximum CO_2 concentration exhaled. After this point, inspiration will bring fresh gas and the removal of CO_2 from the analyzer making a sharp downstroke and return to baseline (phase IV). The continuous recording of these changes generates a CO_2

trend. In monitoring ventilated patients, the trend may be more critical to assess patient's ventilation than the actual absolute value of expired CO_2 at a given time. This trend is a useful tool to evaluate the significance of sudden changes in the graph with specific events sometimes not clinically apparent.

Abnormal Capnograms

Abnormal $EtCO_2$ wave patterns have been associated with specific clinical situations. Elevations in the baseline from zero are unusual and generally not a risk for the patient, and indicates that CO_2 is being reinspired. This could represent a malfunction in the artificial ventilating system, slow flow rate in the circuit, or extremely shallow respiration causing the rebreathing of exhaled CO_2.

Decrease in the $EtCO_2$ waveform (phases II, III, and IV) may be sudden or exponential (Fig. 78.5). Both cases indicate an immediate danger or potential high-risk event. An $EtCO_2$ wave that maintains near zero values could be the result of ventilator malfunction, patient extubation (esophageal intubation), or an obstructed ETT (Fig. 78.5.A). In cases when pulmonary perfusion is compromised (i.e., shock, pulmonary embolism, cardiac arrest), an exponential decrease occurs (Fig. 78.5.B) in the $EtCO_2$ waveform as the result of a functional in-

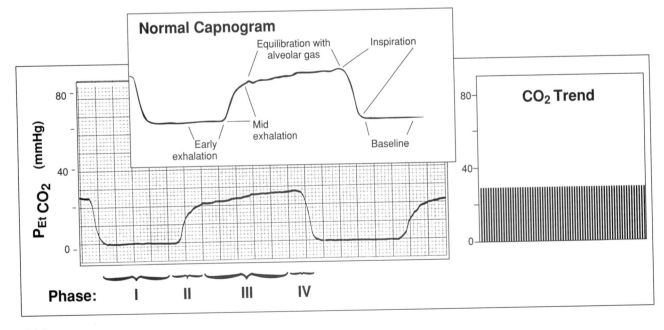

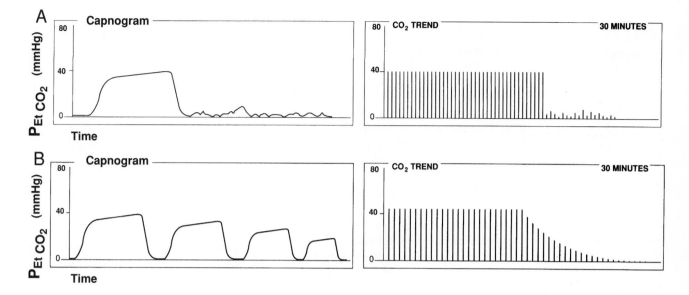

Figure 78.5.
A. Capnogram showing sudden decrease in the waveform.
B. Capnogram with exponential decrease in the waveform.

crease in dead space ventilation from lung units not being perfused.

Steady rises in the CO_2 trend may be associated with hypoventilation, partial airway obstruction, or an increase in CO_2 production as associated with a rising body temperature or increased metabolism. If the trend shows a rapid rise in $EtCO_2$, malignant hyperthermia should be considered as a possibility (Fig. 78.6.A). Conversely, a low $EtCO_2$ trend may indicate hyperventilation or a situation in which an increase in dead space ventilation

occurs, such as asthma, pneumonia, or pulmonary embolism (Fig. 78.6.B).

COMPLICATIONS

As with other monitoring equipment, most of the problems or complications associated with $EtCO_2$ monitoring are directly related to a mechanical malfunction or misinterpretation of data by the operator. Most of these situations such as esophageal intubation, ven-

Figure 78.6.
A. Capnogram with rise in CO_2 trend.
B. Capnoagram with low CO_2 trend.

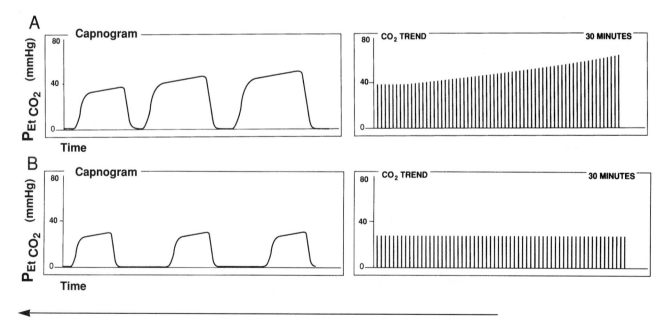

Figure 78.4.
Normal capnogram: phase I, baseline during inspiration; phase II, CO_2 ascent during exhalation; phase III, plateau of CO_2 measurement; phase IV, CO_2 descent during early inspiration.

tilator malfunction, complete or partial obstruction of the ETT, and rebreathing of CO_2 have been discussed previously. The other problem occurs when the operator does not understand changes in baseline or waveforms based on physiology of gas exchange and reacts inappropriately to the data.

Initial capnometers were impractical for pediatric patients. Ones using mainstream sampling had a bulky airway adaptor positioned on the endotracheal tube that added significant weight to the endotracheal tube, which may increase the risk of unplanned extubation or changes in ETT location. The adaptor required to accommodate the sensor housing also may create a problem by increasing the dead space in the ventilator circuit when it is attached in series on the circuit. This is of concern especially in small children. New designs have made available disposable and portable equipment that have minimized or solved these problems. All capnography readings should be correlated with the clinical presentation and the clinical evaluation be used to intervene when in doubt. Capnometers using sidestream sampling have a main disadvantage if water and mucus obstructing the flow of gas to the analyzer occasionally give falsely low $EtCO_2$ readings. It is also important to note that if ventilator flow rates are high and the tidal volume small, some of the inhaled gases will be aspirated with the exhaled gas and may give a falsely low CO_2 reading. In general, patients with severely diminished pulmonary flow (during CPR) may present with false low $EtCO_2$ results (21–24).

Problems associated with the disposable colorimetric units are related to duration of use. Although they are not affected by temperature, they are affected by humidity. For this reason if used for too long, they will not give accurate results. In cases when humidified O_2 is used, they may not be accurate after 15 minutes. Contamination of the indicator with secretions, gastric contents, or endotracheal drugs used during resuscitation can produce permanent yellow decoloration of the detector. In this case, a new detector should be used (22, 25–27).

SUMMARY

The combination of capnography with pulse oximetry provides a complete and continuous (noninvasive) gas monitoring for the critically ill or injured ventilated patient in the pediatric emergency department. It can be used to great advantage in the intubated patient to follow continuously the patient's ventilatory function, to assess immediately the response to a therapeutic intervention on ventilation, or to follow the effectiveness of therapies during cardiopulmonary resuscitation. In the prehospital or ED setting during emergent endotracheal intubations, the monitoring or detection by colorimetric changes of $EtCO_2$ is valuable in assessing the patency or adequate placement of the endotracheal tube.

REFERENCES

1. Sanders AB. Capnometry in emergency medicine. Ann Emerg Med 1989;18:1287–1290.
2. Nobel JJ. Carbon dioxide monitors: exhaled gas (capnographs, capnometry, end tidal CO_2 monitors). Pediatr Emerg Care 1993;9:244–246.
3. Gravenstein JS, Paulus DA, Hayes TJ. Clinical indications. In: Gravenstein JS, Paulus DA, Hayes TJ, eds. Capnography in clinical practice. Stoneham, MA: Butterworth Publishers, 1989, pp. 43–49.
4. Kalenda Z. Capnography during anesthesia and intensive care. Acta Anaesth Belgium 1978;29:3.
5. Berman ILA, Fuirgiure II, Marx GF. The Einstein CO_2 detector. Anesthesiology 1984;60:613–614.
6. Burton GW. The value of CO_2 monitoring during anesthesia. Anaesthesia 1966;21:173–183.
7. Craig I, Wilson ME. A survey of anesthetic misadventures. Anaesthesia 1981;36:933–936.
8. Utting IE, Gray TC, Shelley FC. Human misadventure in anesthesia. Can Anaesth Soc I 1979;26:472–478.
9. Stewart RD, Paris PM, Winter PM, et al. Field endotracheal intubation by paramedical personnel. Success rates and complications. Chest 1984;85:341–343.
10. Shea SR, MacDonald IR, Gruzinski G. Prehospital endotracheal tube airway or esophageal gastric tube airway: a critical comparison. Ann Emerg Med 1985;14:102–112.
11. Linko K, Paloheim M, Tammisto T. Capnography for detection of accidental esophageal intubation. Acta Anaesthiol Scand 1983;27:199–202.
12. Triner L. A simple maneuver to verify proper position of an endotracheal tube. Anesthesiology 1982;57:548–549.

13. Sum Ping ST, Mehta MP, Symreng T. Reliability of capnography in identifying esophageal intubation with carbonated beverage or antacid in the stomach. Anaesth Analg 1991;73:333–337.

14. Garnett AR, Gervin CA, Gervin AS. Capnograph waveforms in esophageal intubation—effect of carbonated beverages. Ann Emerg Med 1989;18: 387–390.

15. Ping STS. Esophageal intubation (letter). Anaesth Analg 1987;66:483.

16. Zbinden S, Schupfer G. Detection of esophageal intubation: the cola complication. Anaesth Analg 1987;66:483.

17. Jones BR, Dorsey MJ. Disposable end tidal CO_2 detector: minimal CO_2 requirements. Anesthesiology 1989;71:A358.

18. Bhende MS, Thompson AE, Orr RA. Utility of an end tidal CO_2 detector during stabilization and transport of critically ill children. Pediatrics 1992;89: 1042–1044.

19. Bhende MS, Thompson AE, Howland DF. Validity of a disposable end tidal CO_2 detector in verifying endotracheal tube position in piglets. Crit Care Med 1991;19:566–568.

20. Ponitz AL, Gravenstein N, Banner MJ. Humidity affecting a chemically based monitor of exhaled carbon dioxide (abstract). Anesthesiology 1990; 73:A515.

21. MacLeod BA, Heller MB, Gerard J, et al. Verification of endotracheal tube placement with colorimetric end tidal CO_2 detection. Ann Emerg Med 1991; 20:267–270.

22. Ornato J, Shipley J, Racth EM, et al. Multicentre study of a portable, hand-size, colorimetric end tidal carbon dioxide detection device. Ann Emerg Med 1992;21:518–523.

23. Varon AJ, Morrina J, Civetta JM. Clinical utility of a colorimetric end tidal CO_2 detector in cardiopulmonary resuscitation and emergency intubation. J Clin Monit 1991;7:289–293.

24. Bhende MS, Gavula DP, Menegazzi JJ. Comparison of an end tidal CO_2 detector with a capnometer during CPR in a pediatric asphyxial arrest model (abstract). Pediatr Emerg Care 1991;7:383.

25. Bhende MS, Thompson AD. Gastric juice, drugs and end tidal carbon dioxide detectors (letter). Pediatrics 1992;90:1005.

26. Muir JD, Randalls PB, Smith GB. End tidal carbon dioxide detector for monitoring cardiopulmonary resuscitation (letter). BMJ 1990;301:41–42.

27. Hayes M, Higgins D, Yau EHS, et al. End tidal carbon dioxide detector for monitoring cardiopulmonary resuscitation (letter). BMJ 1990;301:42.

PEAK FLOW RATE MEASUREMENT

Niranjan Kissoon

INTRODUCTION

Peak expiratory flow is the greatest flow that can be obtained during a forced expiration starting from full inflation of the lung (i.e., total lung capacity). It is the most convenient of all indirect tests of ventilatory capacity. Peak expiratory flow rate (PEFR) assessment is an excellent tool for monitoring the severity of respiratory insufficiency from airway obstruction and for following the progress of children with lower airway obstruction. The procedure is relatively simple to perform using a handheld spirometer. PEFR assessment can be performed by the physician, nurse, or respiratory therapist in the emergency department (ED) or office setting, or by a properly trained parent at home or at school. To obtain reliable results, full cooperation of the patient is required and hence the test is generally useful only for children older than about 5 years of age. The ability to successfully complete the procedure varies widely in the 5 to 7 year age group. Results may not reflect the severity of airway obstruction in patients who are not fully cooperative and delivering a full effort. PEFR should not be attempted in severely symptomatic patients before emergency bronchodilator therapy.

PEFR measurement has been endorsed by the National Asthma Education Program (1) for assessing the degree of airflow obstruction and severity, for monitoring response therapy, and for diagnosing exercise-induced asthma for detecting asymptomatic deterioration. To help asthma patients use home PEFR monitoring, a system of PEFR zones can be established, based on their personal best PEFR or the predicted value for the child's height (2, 3). When the zone system is adapted to a traffic light pattern for the zones, it may be easier to use and remember. The following are the common guidelines used: green (80 to 100% of personal best) signals all is clear (i.e., no asthma symptoms are present); yellow (50 to 80% of personal best) signals caution (i.e., an acute exacerbation may be present), and red (below 50% of personal best) signals a medical alert. A medical alert indicates that a bronchodilator should be administered immediately and a clinician should be notified (1).

In the ED, PEFR assessment on a cooperative, trained patient is obtained with the help of a respiratory therapist, emergency physician, or nurse. The PEFR is an effort dependent maneuver which means that the best result at a given degree of large airway obstruction requires a fully cooperative patient. A supervisor needs to closely monitor and give cues that coach the optimal performance.

ANATOMY AND PHYSIOLOGY

The airway and lung anatomy of children differs somewhat from that of adults. An important fact is that the chest wall in young children is more compliant than adults. This tends to enhance ventilation by requiring small efforts for tidal breathing in the healthy child. As children grow, the chest wall becomes more stiff (less compliant) and recoil of the lung on expiration is more effortless. The pressure necessary to expand the lungs is increased in pathophysiologic states that reduce the lung compliance or increase the "stiffness" of the lungs. Airflow resistance also is an important part of respiration. This is greatest in inspiration in the upper and nasal airway and greatest on expiration in the intrathoracic airways. In addition, the airways of young children are relatively narrow compared with adults. The growth of the distal airways lags behind that of the proximal airway in the first 5 years of life. This narrow peripheral airway accounts for high peripheral airway pressures necessary to optimal air flow. Because flow is related to the radius of the airway to the 4th power, small reductions in the airway caliber secondary to inflammatory processes greatly reduces the flow of air per given amount of generated work. In the healthy state, these differences lead to minimal effort in chest expansion and airway ventilation. In infancy, this is particularly important because the infant is prone to exhaustion sooner than older children and adults.

In processes that cause lower airways disease such as asthma or acute bronchiolitis, airway narrowing is indicated which is caused by bronchial smooth muscle constriction, airway inflammation, and increased mucous production in airway and cells. Partial blockage occurs distal to the airways which leads to larger residual volume at the end of expiration. This inflammation affects more distal small airways not measurable by the PEFR. Small airways measurements, such as the midexpiratory flow rate (FEF_{25-75}), more accurately relate to the small airways where inflammation is greater and airway diameter affected. Air trapping associated with airway obstruction of the small airways places the initiation of inspiration and the end of inspiration with lung volumes higher on the flow/volume curve where more effort is used for a given tidal volume change. The exhalation of a breath from maximal inspiration (from total lung capacity) through the narrowed airways cannot produce the same maximal flow with a patient's best effort that occurs without this obstruction. The point of maximal flow in expiration (PEFR) is almost at the onset of expiration. It is effort dependent and really is a measure of large airway flow rates.

INDICATIONS

Although it does not provide sophisticated pulmonary function information testing, PEFR provides objective evidence of severity of lower airway obstruction and assists in judging the response to therapy to reverse the obstruction. Several indications for ED use are listed in Table 79.1. It can also provide warning signs of increasing severity of asthma or resistance to bronchodilator therapy. PEFR should be undertaken in all asthmatics in the ED who are able to perform this maneuver. In the ED, the PEFR will be useful as an adjunct in determining the need for ongoing therapy or admission. Outside the ED, many patients and physicians find it useful to have children with asthma monitor PEFR at home and at school.

Peak flow monitoring in the ED is useful in addition to clinical findings such as dyspnea, accessory muscle use, and decreased S_aO_2. It is also useful to guide therapy and when referring these patients to specialists and in discussion of these patients via telephone. The importance to PEFR to document and quantitate airway obstruction cannot be overemphasized because patients' reports of their symptoms and physicians' physical findings may not correlate with the variability and severity of airflow obstruction (4, 5). However, peak flow assessment should not be attempted in the severely compromised patient who can be very dyspneic or in impending respiratory failure. Under these circumstances, therapy should be initiated by clinical findings and other ancillary data such as transcutaneous oxygen saturation monitor-

Table 79.1.

Indications for Peak Flow Testing in the ED (Age >5–7 years)

1. Acute asthma in the cooperative patient to grade severity.
2. Monitor the response to therapy of the patients with acute asthma.
3. Confirm the findings of home asthma program in acute asthma patients in the ED.
4. Acute respiratory symptoms or signs suggestive of lower airway obstruction on a pre- and postbronchodilator response.

ing. Measurement of PEFR can follow the improvement to demonstrate response.

Children will present to the ED because of increasing severity of symptoms or more commonly in status asthmaticus not responding to home therapy. Cough, dyspnea, and wheezing are the major clinical features but presentation may vary with age. In some cases children may present with persistent cough at night or during exercise. In others, shortness of breath may be the predominant symptom. The degree of wheezing does not correlate well with the severity of the attacks but the relative absence of wheezing in the presence of respiratory distress, poor air entry, or hypoxia signifies severe obstruction. The use of accessory muscles of respiration and the presence of pulsus paradoxus are other indicators of marked severity.

EQUIPMENT

A standard office peak flow meter is the simplest and easiest to use (6). Several peak flow meters are commercially available (Table 79.2). Specific instructions including a step-by-step chart to assist in performing the maneuver are contained in the literature accompanying each meter. Because different brands and models of peak flow meters often yield different values when used by the same person, children should be encouraged to use the same model in the home, in the clinician's office, and possibly in the ED. Although meters may have different configurations, they all usually have a disposable mouthpiece and gauge (upright, horizontal, balls, arrows, etc.) and function on the same principle (see Procedures in this chapter).

PROCEDURE

PEFR measurement is one of a series of measurements that can be obtained from a full and maximal expiratory maneuver from full inspiration. The moment of most rapid expiratory flow, the peak flow, is brief and occurs early in the maximal expiratory effort (Fig. 79.1). As shown in the graph, peak flow occurs early and at high lung volume. Variability and dependency on both patient effort and muscular strength are evident. In addition, chest wall restriction from pain or tight clothing also may result in a suboptimal effort. The importance of these factors is underlined by the fact that a 10 to 15% variance of PEFR may be indicated on a given subject on repeated best efforts. Therefore, a minimum increase of 15% after β-agonist is necessary to substantiate clinically relevant improvement. Because it occurs in the effort dependent portion of the maneuver, it is as reproducible as other measures. PEFR may be underestimated if the patient does not generate an adequate effort, if air leaks occur from the corners of the mouth (inadequate seal), or if the mouthpiece is blocked by the tongue. Conversely, a tremendous effort by a patient with lower airways obstruction may produce a close to normal peak flow by expulsion of air

Table 79.2.
Commercially Available Spirometers for PEFR Assessment

Name	Types	Manufacturer
Assess Peak Flow Meter	Low range (50–390 L/min)	Health Scan Products Inc.
	Standard range (100–890 L/min)	Cedar Grove, NJ
Personal Best Peak Flow Meter	Full range (90–810 L/min)	Health Scan Products Inc.
	Low range (50–390 L/min)	Cedar Grove, NJ
Pulmo-Graph™ Peak Flow Meter	Standard range (50–750 L/min)	DeVilliss Health Care
	Low range (50–250 L/min)	Somerset, PA
Pocket Peak	Low range (90–400 L/min)	Hudson RCI
	Universal (90–720 L/min)	Temecula, CA
Wright	Standard range (2 scales)	Clement Clark Inc.
	(a) Wright-McKerrow scale (60–800 L/min)	Columbus, OH
	(b) American Thoracic Society scale (60–880 L/min)	
Wright	Low range (2 scales)	
	(a) Wright-McKerrow scale (30–370 L/min)	
	(b) American Thoracic Society scale (30–400 L/min)	

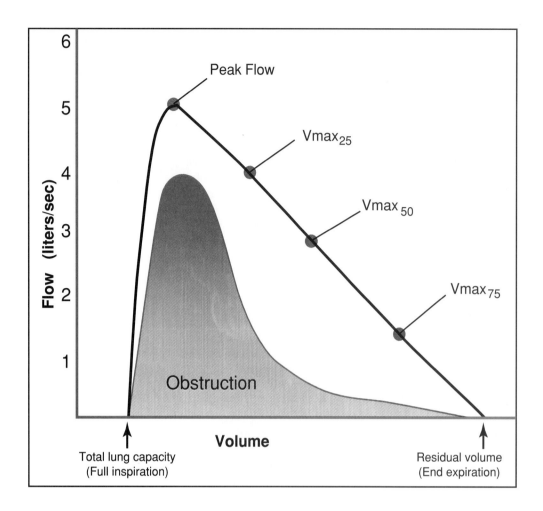

Figure 79.1.
Flow volume loop, showing normal effort and one with reduced flow from lower airway obstruction.

from compressible airways and may give the impression of better ventilation than is the case. Despite these limitations, PEFR can correlate well with other measures of lower airway obstruction such as forced expiration volume (FEV) in 1 second (7, 8).

The patient's demographic data (age, sex, height, weight) needs to be obtained. PEFRs measured are compared with the standard values for the same height and sex or with baseline values established by the patient during a healthy period between attacks (9, 10) (Table 79.3). The patient should be educated and prepared before PEFR testing. It is important to explain that the test is painless and to position the patient in a comfortable position. In addition, articles of clothing that may restrict respiration such as tight vests, belts, or restrictive outer garments should be removed. PEFR testing requires full patient cooperation and relies on the deepest breath possible and maximal forced expiration. Children who are obese or under 12 years old obtain better results if standing

while performing the test. It is also beneficial to perform the test in a quiet, calm environment.

The maneuver should be demonstrated to the child. It is helpful to explain the impor-

Table 79.3.
Predicted Average Peak Expiratory Flow for Normal Children and Adolescents L/min

Height (inches)	Males & Females	Height (inches)	Males & Females
43	147	56	320
44	160	57	334
45	173	58	347
46	187	59	360
47	200	60	373
48	214	61	387
49	227	62	400
50	240	63	413
51	254	64	427
52	267	65	440
53	280	66	454
54	293	67	467
55	307		

Adapted from: Polger G, Promedhat V. Pulmonary function testing in children: techniques and standards. Philadelphia: WB Saunders, 1971.

Chapter 79
Peak Flow Rate
Measurement

tance of a maximal, prolonged effort to squeeze as much air out of the lungs as possible. It is a good idea to demonstrate by blowing into a similar mouthpiece reserved for that purpose. The child should then be instructed to take a few slow breaths and then breathe in as far as possible. The child should then hold his or her breath and concentrate on proper placement of the mouthpiece (Fig. 79.2A, B). The mouthpiece should be placed in the mouth and the lips closed around it to prevent air from escaping between the tight closed lips and the meter. It also should be placed on the top of the tongue so that the tongue will not obstruct the meter. The hole at the back of the meter from which the breath exits should not be obstructed by the patient's hands when the meter is held properly. The child then should blow out as hard as possible.

During the procedure verbal prompting and cheerleading such as "start now, blast off, hard and fast" usually results in a greater effort during exhalation. The operator should maintain close attention to the patient to discourage distractions such as looking at the graph during the procedure. A useful trick to maximize effort may be to ask the child to take a deep breath in and "blow out the candles on a birthday cake" a few feet away.

The goal of testing is to obtain at least two test results that appear acceptable and reproducible. Because it is common for variation in testing to be up to 10% of the obtained value, results that are closer to each other for several attempts are of the greatest value. From a practical standpoint, the highest PEFR obtained is considered to be the most representative. Problems that may produce unacceptable results include a slow start of exhalation, coughing during the procedure, and premature termination of the effort. Recognition of

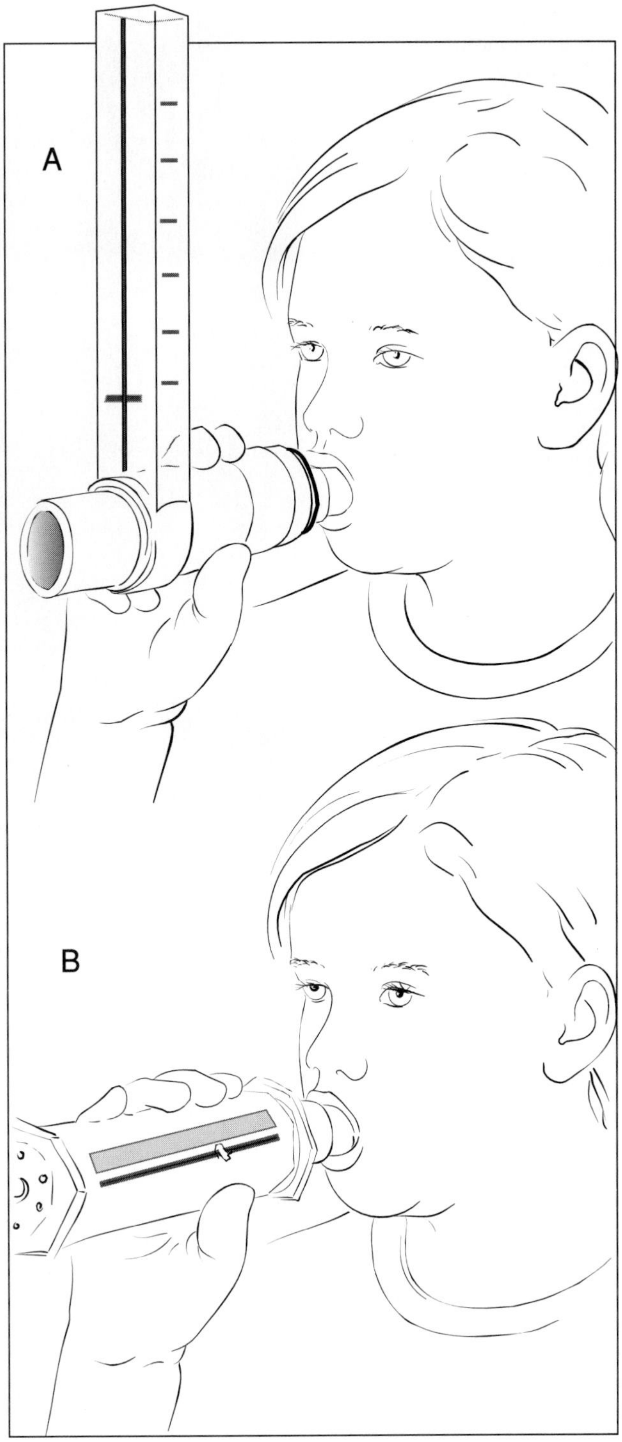

Figure 79.2.
A. Use of peak flow meter by 8-year-old boy.
B. Peak flow meter with targeted green and red zone for a normal and reduced PEFR.

these are important for successful testing. These faults should be identified and explained to the patient in an effort to eliminate them on the next try. PEFR testing is sometimes useful in determining efficacy of bronchodilator therapy (Fig. 79.3). In these instances, the best of three measurements as previously outlined should be accepted as the

Chapter 79
Peak Flow Rate
Measurement

SUMMARY

1. Perform clinical evaluation including degree of airway obstruction. If moderately severe obstruction is present, administer β-agonist aerosol or subcutaneously with supplemental oxygen to patient

2. Determine if patient is capable of performing maneuver. Has the patient done the procedure before? Exclude all children <5 years of age except in elective procedure

3. Obtain demographics—age, sex, height, weight—to enable review of standard for the particular patient

4. Review procedure with patient including demonstration on how to hold meter, purse lips about the meter, and how to perform maximal inspiratory effort and expiratory maneuver

5. Have patient take a few normal breaths

6. Have patient take a maximal inspiratory effort and hold it at full inspiration

7. Have patient place meter in mouth and over tongue

8. Have patient *maximally exhale* to full end expiration; coach patient to best effort

9. Breathe normally for a minimum of 30 to 60 seconds

10. Repeat PEFR 2 to 3 times to obtain best result

11. Assume largest PEFR obtained is patient's current PEFR

12. Establish percentage predicted from chart

Chapter 79
Peak Flow Rate
Measurement

Figure 79.3.
Peak flow meter with side measure of zone clips to assist in setting levels of management.

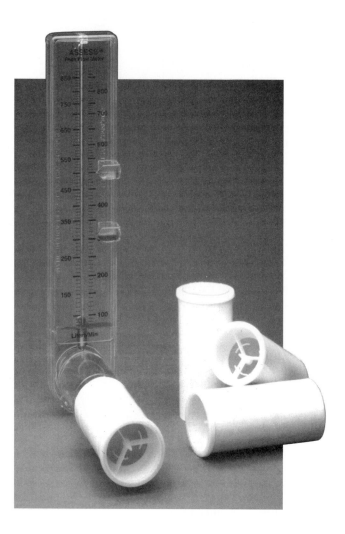

PEFR. This should be done a minimum of 10 minutes after inhaled bronchodilators or at the end of the time of observation before another intervention or before discharge.

COMPLICATIONS

Spirometry may provoke an increase in airways obstruction in asthmatics. Although a small risk, it should be immediately brought to the attention of a physician. An inhaled bronchodilator may be necessary to relieve this obstruction. If obtained before acute bronchodilator therapy in an emergency setting, spirometry can delay administration of bronchodilators or supplemental oxygen which can be harmful in very ill asthmatics.

Close attention should be given to proper technique as incorrect results may lead to over- or undertreatment with bronchodilators.

SUMMARY

Peak flow measurement is a relatively simple and useful objective measurement of large airway obstruction in the lower airways. It can be done by an older patient (5 years of age) independently and is useful in titration of therapy and early identification of worsening of symptoms. Proper performance of this test relies on the cooperation of the patient and is generally not possible in children less than 5 years of age.

REFERENCES

1. Guidelines for the diagnosis and management of asthma. National Asthma Education Program, National Institutes of Health, Bethesda, Maryland 20892. Publication 91-3042A, 1991.

2. Plaut TF. Children with asthma: a manual for parents. Amherst, MA: Pedipress, 1988, pp. 94–108.

3. Hargeave FE, Dolovich J, Newhouse MT. The assessment and treatment of asthma: a conference report. J Allergy Clin Immunol 1990;85(b): 1098–1111.

4. McFadden ER, Kiser R, DeGroot WJ. Acute bronchial asthma: relationships between clinical and physiologic manifestations. N Engl J Med 1973; 288:221.

5. Shim CS, Williams H. Relationship of wheezing to the severity of obstruction in asthma. Arch Intern Med 1983;143:890–892.

6. Enright PL, Hyatt RE. Office spirometer: a practical guide to the selection and use of spirometers. Philadelphia: Lea & Febiger, 1987.

7. Nowak RM, Pensler MI, Parker DD. Comparison of peak expiratory flow and FEV: Admission criteria for cute bronchial asthma. Ann Emerg Med 1982; 11:64–69.

8. Eichenhorn MS, Beauchamp RK, Harper PA, et al. An assessment of three portable peak flow meters. Chest 1982;82:306–309.

9. Weng T, Levison H. Standards of pulmonary function in children. Am Rev Respir Dis 1969;99:879.

10. Rarey KP, Youtsey JW, eds. Pulmonary function testing in respiratory patient care. Englewood Cliffs, NJ: Prentice Hall, 1981, pp. 328–330.

CLINICAL TIPS

1. Avoid the maneuver in patients with severe airway obstruction as it may worsen bronchospasm acutely.

2. Do not attempt in children less than 5 to 7 years of age unless a child has previous experience before present ED visit.

3. Review the procedure before the patient performs it.

4. Be sure the patient has a tight seal on the mouthpiece, the exhalation hole on the meter is not blocked, and the meter measuring gauge is unimpeded by the patient.

5. Coach the patient with encouraging words during the maneuver.

6. Take the best of three measures for the peak flow.

7. If done after a bronchodilator, wait 10 to 15 minutes to obtain an adequate clinical response. Adequate difference from bronchodilator is at or above 15% change.

8. Check the result to standards for this child or to the standard nomograms for the patient's size.

9. Observe the technique for:
   a) Poor maximal inspiration of initiating a breath
   b) Less than maximal effort
   c) Occlusion of exhalation hole or gauge
   d) Premature cessation of the exhalation

CHAPTER 80

Use of Metered Dose Inhalers, Spacers, and Nebulizers

Morton E. Salomon

INTRODUCTION

Respiratory diseases such as asthma, croup, and bronchopulmonary dysplasia (BPD) are among the most common childhood diseases and account for 10 to 15% of visits to the emergency department (ED) each year. Medications delivered by inhalation are being used with increasing frequency to treat respiratory disease both acutely and on maintenance basis. Aerosol therapy permits the delivery of small quantities of medication directly to the site of action (1–3).

Studies comparing the effectiveness of medications delivered via inhalation with that of oral or parenteral delivery have demonstrated that the inhalation route provides more rapid onset, equal duration of activity, and comparable improvement in pulmonary function testing, with fewer side effects (2–5). Because inhalation therapy can be administered without painful or invasive procedures, it also has the added benefit of less enhancement of the fear a child experiences when visiting the ED. Inhalation treatment should be viewed as a significant therapeutic advance and is now the mainstay of our treatment for many respiratory illnesses, particularly asthma.

ANATOMY AND PHYSIOLOGY

Lung Receptor Pathophysiology

The human respiratory system is under the control of the nervous system through autonomic nerve fibers from cranial nerve X. It is also controlled by multiple receptor sites with or without accompanying nerve fibers.

Autonomic influences on the lung are contributed by parasympathetic (cholinergic) forces and by sympathetic (adrenergic) receptors. The adrenergic system contains both α- and β-receptors.

Parasympathetic innervation is provided by fibers of the vagus nerve. Stimulation of the parasympathetic efferent fibers causes bronchoconstriction of the large and midsize airways, increased mucous gland secretion, and vascular dilatation. Postganglionic parasympathetic fibers terminate in bronchial smooth muscle, mucus secreting goblet cells, and mast cells. These parasympathetic nerve fibers are present from the trachea to the bronchioles but are found in greatest density in midsize airways 3 to 8 mm in diameter. These same parasympathetic effects also can be induced by direct administration of cholinergic agents such as acetylcholine and metha-choline (6).

The parasympathetic nervous system plays a role in airway response to irritants through what is referred to as the vagally mediated "cholinergic reflex." When specific irritants activate receptors in the airways, these receptors initiate impulses via afferent fibers of the vagal system. The afferent vagal stimuli trigger reflexive responses via efferent fibers releasing acetylcholine at multiple neuroeffector sites, leading to bronchoconstriction, mucus secretion, and mediator release from mast cells and cell membranes. This cholinergic reflex can be triggered by immunologic or nonimmunologic stimuli. The role of this parasympathetic reflex in chronic hyperreactive airway diseases, such as bronchitis and asthma, is not well defined and likely to vary from one patient to another. The cholinergic reflex is not the only mechanism by which irritants exert influence on the airways (6).

Sympathetic nerve fibers have not been found in the tracheobronchial tree of the human lung. Adrenergic influences on the lung are exerted at α- and β-receptor sites that receive no neuronal innervation. These adrenergic receptors are found in bronchial smooth muscle, blood vessels, and goblet cells, and can be stimulated by either endogenous sympathomimetic agents (e.g., epinephrine) or similar exogenous agonists (e.g., terbutaline).

In contrast to parasympathetic receptors, adrenergic receptors are mostly concentrated in the smaller peripheral airways. Stimulation of β-receptors produces smooth muscle relaxation and subsequent bronchodilatation β-agonists also are potent inhibitors of mast cell release which exerts a strong antiinflammatory effect. This antiinflammatory control is most effective in the earliest phases of inflammation. Prolonged inflammation, with late phase reaction, is not as responsive to β-agonist stimulation. Glucocorticoids, in fact, exert some of their antiinflammatory effect by restoring the availability and binding affinity of β-receptors (6).

At the intracellular level, cholinergic and adrenergic receptor stimulation is mediated by alterations in cyclic AMP and cyclic GMP. Increases in cyclic AMP (c-AMP) relax bronchial smooth muscle and inhibit mast cell degranulation. Increases in cyclic GMP (c-GMP) exert the opposite effect, contracting smooth muscle and stimulating mast cell release. Stimulation of parasympathetic effectors produces increases in intracellular c-GMP. Conversely, β-adrenergic stimulation increases c-AMP, whereas α-receptor stimulation decreases c-AMP (6). Thus, β-sympathomimetic activity produces bronchial relaxation, whereas both parasympathetic and α-sympathetic activity produce bronchoconstriction. Predominant mechanisms in different respiratory patients with hyperreactive airways may contribute much of the problem to excessive parasympathetic tone, excessive α-sympathetic stimulation, or β-sympathetic blockade.

Two common categories of medication available by aerosol and used to treat common pulmonary illnesses are β-adrenergic agonists and parasympathetic antagonists. β$_2$-Agonists relax bronchial smooth muscle producing bronchodilatation, inhibit inflammatory mediator release from mast cells, and stimulate mucociliary clearance. These effects are produced by activating adenyl cyclase with subsequent increase in c-AMP release.

Parasympatholytic agents include atropine and its derivatives. They are competitive inhibitors of acetylcholine at the neuroeffector junction, and block the cholinergic reflex and parasympathetic receptor stimulation, thereby preventing a rise in intracellular c-GMP. The net effect, therefore, is to inhibit bronchoconstriction. Anticholinergic agents currently available for aerosolized treatment include atropine sulfate which may lead to significant side effects when used in therapeutic respiratory doses, and ipratropium, a quaternary derivative of atropine which has a much wider therapeutic margin. Theoretically, α-adrenergic blocking agents should have a beneficial effect in the treatment of bronchoconstrictive respiratory diseases. By blocking α-stimulation and thereby inhibiting decreases in c-AMP, α-blockers should enhance bronchodilation. To date, however, α-receptor blockers have not been shown to have a convincing role in treating asthma or bronchitis. Their application is usually reserved for the patient with severe disease who is already being treated maximally with other agents (6).

It is key to understand that inflammation, not bronchospasm, is the basic pathologic condition encountered in chronic asthma. Airway inflammation results from injury to the lung which might be caused by trauma, inhalation of noxious or toxic or allergic substances, respiratory infection, or even systemic infection. The most common chronic inflammatory disease of the lung is asthma.

Once triggered by injurious stimuli, the inflammatory process starts with the release of several chemical mediators from mast cells, leukocytes, and endothelial cell phospholipids. Chemical mediators in turn activate specific receptor sites on the cell wall surface of the lung. These receptors then decrease c-AMP concentration or increase calcium ion concentration inside the cell. The net result includes smooth muscle contraction, chemotaxis of inflammatory cells, microvascular leaks, increased mucus secretion, and parasympathetic neuronal reflex stimulation. The immediate response to fast-acting inflammatory mediators, such as histamine, is primarily bronchoconstriction. This reaction often responds to bronchodilators. If the inflammatory response continues and the slower-acting metabolites of arachidonic acid accumulate, mucosal swelling, mucus secretion, and desquamation of cells occur. This produces a late phase inflammatory response that is less sensitive to bronchodilator therapy (6).

Corticosteroids exert an antiinflammatory response principally by stabilizing mast cells. They also restore the availability and sensitivity of β-agonist receptors. The glucocorticoids currently used for aerosol therapy are synthetic analogs of hydrocortisone. When compared with cortisol or dexamethasone, they have the distinct advantage of having less systemic absorption, rapid inactivation when reaching the central circulation, high local potency in the lung, and less systemic potency. The aerosolized glucocorticoids currently in use in the United States via metered dose inhalers include beclomethasone, triamcinolone, and flunisolide.

Aerosols

An aerosol is a suspension of either solid particles or liquid droplets in a stream of air. By incorporating medication in these droplets, aerosols can deliver therapy directly to the lung. Large droplets are often trapped and filtered by the upper airway. To be effective in treating respiratory illnesses, the droplets must reach their receptor sites in the smaller airways. Drug delivery to the peripheral lung depends on three factors: aerosol droplet size, inspiratory flow, and disease state in the lung (1, 2).

Droplets created by jet nebulizers and metered dose inhalers vary in size. Droplets greater than 8 μ (microns) are always deposited in the mouth and nasopharynx by inertial impaction. β-Agonists are not well absorbed by this mucosa and therefore will not exert any demonstrable effects (1).

To reach the distal airways, droplets must be less than 5 μ in size. Once they reach the bronchiole they settle out by gravitational sedimentation. However, smaller droplets (less than 1 μ) generally remain suspended in the airstream and are exhaled without deposition on the tissue surface (1).

Regardless of droplet size, particles are unlikely to get beyond the oropharynx if significant turbulence occurs in the airstream. Turbulence can be created by rapid inspiratory flow rates, partial mechanical obstructions, or sudden changes in airstream direction. Inspiratory flow rates through the patient's airways greater than 1.0 L/sec will create turbulent airflow. Under these conditions, inertial forces keep droplets from remaining suspended in the mainstream and droplets of any size will deposit on the nasal and oropharyngeal airways. At slower inspiratory rates—generally less than 0.5 L/sec—laminar airflow is evident and the droplets may reach the peripheral lung units. The airstream slows even further on reaching the smaller airways allowing the droplets to deposit by gravitational sedimentation. Sedimentation can be further enhanced by breath holding at the end of inspiration, which postpones the reversal of airflow. Slow flow rates of less than 0.5 L/sec are best achieved by inhalations of 6-second duration (1, 2).

Airflow through diseased airways, narrowed by spasm, edema, or mucus, is much more turbulent than through healthy airways. More drug is deposited before reaching the targeted airways. Therefore, treatment of the patient with acute respiratory illness may require larger doses of aerosolized medication to create the same therapeutic effect.

INDICATIONS

Aerosol therapy is most commonly applied in pediatric emergency settings to the treatment of asthma, bronchiolitis, bronchopulmonary dysplasia (BPD), and laryngotracheobronchitis (LTB).

Asthma is the most common chronic disease of childhood affecting up to 10 to 15% of the pediatric population in the United States. It is characterized by hyperresponsive airways that are prone to develop edema, mucus hypersecretion, and muscular constriction in response to offending stimuli. Triggers most commonly associated with airways inflammation in asthmatics include inhaled irritants such as cigarette smoke, changes in weather, exposure to cold air, exercise, environmental allergens, and minor respiratory illnesses such as sinusitis and otitis. Patients with asthma generally manifest their airway hyperactivity with symptoms such as cough and wheezing. In more severe cases, patients also will have shortness of breath, tachypnea, retractions, diminished peak expiratory flow rates, and hypoxia. Aerosolized medications are currently the mainstay of bronchodilator therapy for asthma. Metered dose inhalers of corticosteroids and sodium cromolyn are antiinflammatory agents that are commonly used in children to reduce the inflammatory aspects of exacerbations. Inhaled β-agonists, such as albuterol, are used as both prophylactic and acute therapy. Using β-agonists during maintenance therapy is becoming more controversial. The role of inhaled anticholinergic agents in the treatment of acute childhood asthma is not as well substantiated, although these agents are known to have measurable bronchodilator effect. Atropine sulfate is available only as a nebulizer solution. Ipratropium bromide, an anticholinergic agent with much fewer side effects than atropine, is now available in the United States as a metered dose inhaler and nebulizer solution (7). A recent study with ipratropium demonstrated added benefit in children with acute severe asthma (8). Less admissions were noted in the severe patients receiving ipratropium with each dose of albuterol than albuterol alone.

Bronchiolitis is a pulmonary infection generally occurring in late fall and winter that mostly affects young children. Its peak incidence occurs between the age of 2 and 8 months. Bronchiolitis is characterized by coryza and cough progressing to wheezing, prolonged expiration, and respiratory distress. Most cases of bronchiolitis are caused by respiratory syncytial virus (RSV), but other viruses such as parainfluenza can be isolated from patients with this illness. Mild bronchiolitis has been treated with nebulized bronchodilators, such as albuterol, and improved symptoms and signs in subgroups of patients. Corticosteroids have not proven to be a benefit. In some children, however, it is difficult to differentiate acute asthma from bronchiolitis, because the symptoms are so similar. Children are often treated with some form of systemic steroid. Aerosolized ribavirin, 1-β-D-ribofuranosyl-1,2,4-triazole-3-carboxamide, can be effective in ameliorating the course of severe bronchiolitis caused by RSV when administered continuously over a 3- to 5-day period (9, 10). Using this antiviral agent is generally reserved for patients with severe respiratory compromise or an underlying illness such as congenital heart disease or BPD (7, 10).

Bronchopulmonary dysplasia is a chronic pulmonary disorder of infancy that follows treatment by mechanical ventilation of hyaline membrane disease or other congenital lung disorders. It generally occurs only in newborns undergoing prolonged ventilation during the first several weeks of life. Approximately 15% of premature infants develop BPD. Its etiology has been ascribed to many factors including high concentrations of oxygen and barotrauma from positive pressure ventilation. Infants with BPD often have chronic tachypnea, wheezing, and asymmetric breath sounds. In more severe cases, arterial blood gases show chronic hypercarbia and hypoxia. Chest radiographs done on BPD patients will show characteristic overaeration and interstitial nodularity or multiple cystic areas. Home management of patients with BPD and treatment of acute exacerbations of respiratory difficulties can be similar to the treatment of asthma. These patients are frequently helped with daily nebulized β-agonists and occasionally by aerosolized corticosteroids. Acute exacerbations are treated by intensified β-agonist treatment, systemic steroids, and other therapies as necessary (7).

Laryngotracheobronchitis (LTB), also known as croup, is a viral infection of the large airways affecting the larynx, trachea, and bronchi. Sixty percent of cases appear to be caused by parainfluenza virus, mostly in early fall. Influenza virus, adenovirus, and RSV also have been recovered from croup patients. LTB is characterized by mild to moderate fever, barking cough, and inspiratory stridor. Croup is the most common cause of stridor in childhood. Milder cases can be treated simply with humidified normal saline mist. Moderate to severe bouts of LTB receive treatment with either racemic or L-epinephrine in a nebulized format. Nebulized corticosteroids may have a role in this disease as studies are now demonstrating (11).

N-acetylcysteine (Mucomyst®) is used as a mucolytic agent in the maintenance and treatment of patients with cystic fibrosis. Similarly, aminoglycosides can be aerosolized to suppress *Pseudomonas aeruginosa* and other organisms. Aerosolized pentamidine is indicated for prophylaxis against PCP in patients over the age of 5 years, with AIDS, who are unable to tolerate trimethoprim-sulfa (7).

Table 80.1 summarizes the medications available in metered dose inhaler (MDI) format, in nebulized solution, or in both. A large variety of adrenergic medications are available by metered dose inhaler, including nonselective β_1- and β_2-agonists such as epinephrine, isoproterenol, and metaproterenol and β_2-selective agents such as terbutaline, pirbuterol, and albuterol. Corticosteroids are currently only available in metered dose inhaler form for inhalation therapy. These preparations have been difficult to aerosolize when incorporated into nebulizer solutions.

All adrenergic drugs available in metered dose inhaler are also available for nebulization. Ipratropium, sodium cromolyn and N-acetylcysteine (NAC) are similarly available in both MDI and nebulizer formats. However, at this time some drugs come only in nebulizer format. These include atropine, ribavirin (which requires a special particle generator), pentamidine, racemic, or L-epinephrine, and nystatin suspension (for laryngeal candidiasis) (1–3). Cromolyn powder also can be delivered using a spinhaler.

Spacers are small canisters that attach to MDIs to allow for younger or less cooperative patients who cannot easily hold their breath while inspiring the medication. Spacers are indicated for use with metered dose inhalers in patients who are likely to have difficulty correctly coordinating the MDI inhalation, such as younger patients (generally less than 10 years of age), neurologically impaired patients, patients with arthritis of the hands, and adults who are unable to master the MDI technique. Spacers also are helpful for patients of all ages with significant acute distress, who are more likely to have difficulty taking slow deep breaths and breath holding at the end of inspiration. This may include anyone with acute bronchospasm (see Equipment section for a more detailed discussion of spacers).

Indications for nebulizer use are similar to those for spacer need. Nebulizers are indicated for younger patients, patients with coordination problems, and those with moderate to severe acute asthma (see Equipment section for a more detailed discussion of nebulizers).

Patients who are maintained chronically on β-agonist therapy by MDI or by nebulizer at home often require higher doses with more frequency during acute exacerbations of bronchospasm. Home use should not exceed a frequency of every 3 hours without physician contact. Failure to seek hospital care in a timely manner in patients on bronchodilators without antiinflammatory therapy is an important contributor to asthma mortality. In the

Table 80.1.
Medications Currently Available for Inhalation

Available in Both MDIs and Nebulizer Solutions
   β_1 and β_2 agonists
   β_2 selective agonists
   Sodium cromolyn
   N-acetylcysteine
   Ipratropium
Available Only in MDIs
   Corticosteroids
Available Only in Nebulizer Format
   Atropine
   Nystatin suspension
   Pentamidine
   Racemic and L-epinephrine

monitored setting, such as the hospital, metered dose inhalers can be used with significantly more intensity. One hospital regimen that has been suggested is four puffs over 2 minutes followed by one puff every minute until dyspnea is relieved or the patient develops a significant tremor (1). It is key to augment the therapy of β-agonists with antiinflammatory therapy early in episodes (see Equipment section for a detailed discussion of MDIs).

Continuous nebulization therapy (CNT) should be applied only to patients with severe asthma and its use restricted to the ED or the intensive care unit. Indications for CNT might include patients whose chests are too tight to perform peak flow testing, patients with $PaCO_2$ greater than 40, or patients with Wood-Downe's scores greater than or equal to 5. CNT is also indicated for hospitalized patients who repeatedly deteriorate clinically between their every 1- to 2-hour β-agonist treatments (14). (see Equipment section for a detailed description of CNT).

EQUIPMENT—TECHNICAL CONSIDERATIONS

Metered Dose Inhalers

A metered dose inhaler is an inhalation device that contains medication dissolved or suspended in a pressurized solution of chlorofluorocarbons (CFCs). The MDI has two components—the drug canister and the inhalation device (Fig. 80.1). Within the canister, the therapeutic medication is mixed with the CFC propellant at high pressure to maintain a liquid phase. The inhalation device consists of a hollow canister holder, an actuator, a valve, and a mouthpiece with cover. The actuator, when depressed, opens the valve. The valve is designed to release a precise, premeasured amount of aerosol with each actuation.

Sudden decompression of the liquid in the canister produces an aerosol of propellant plus medication. As the liquid exits the mouthpiece, hetero-disperse (varying size) particles average 35 μ in diameter. These large droplets travel away from the mouthpiece at a high velocity and the propellant

evaporates within a few centimeters, leaving smaller droplets consisting primarily of medication.

When the drug is released from the MDI approximately 5 to 10% is deposited on the inhaler device or escapes into the atmosphere, another 80% is deposited in the oropharynx and eventually swallowed. This means that only 10 to 15% of the drug released actually reaches the lung, even under ideal conditions. It is likely that only 3% of the total dose reaches the bronchioles and alveoli. The proportion of drug reaching the lung is greatly influenced by the patient's technique. Factors such as the position of the inhaler at the mouth, slow inspiratory flow rate, adequacy of breath holding, adequate interval between puffs of at least 1 minute, and volume of air inhaled can all influence the delivery of medication to the peripheral lung visits (2).

Most package inserts instruct the patient to close the lips around the mouthpiece of the inhaler. However, the open mouth technique can deliver up to twice as much medication to the lower lung. By holding the inhaler 1 to 2 inches (two adult fingerbreadths) away from the mouth, less medication is deposited on the oropharynx. Studies have demonstrated that the open mouth technique produces less oropharyngeal deposition, more peripheral lung delivery, and better pulmonary function response (2). A variation on the open mouth technique has the patient hold the MDI between opened lips, which reduces the problems of improper aiming and provides the same pharmacologic benefits (2).

As mentioned, slow inspiratory flow rates create more laminar flow and deliver more drug to the distal airways. Ideally the patient should inhale the released medication for a minimum of 6 seconds (2). Breath holding at the end of inhalation allows more time for the inhaled medication to sediment on the lung surface. Breath holding has been shown to incrementally increase drug absorption for up to 10 seconds. Beyond 10 seconds breath holding does not add benefit (2). If the patient is unable to breath hold for 10 seconds, the patient should hold his or her breath for as long as is comfortably possible. Larger, deeper breaths bring a larger tidal volume into the lung and more medication with it. Optimal dosing can be achieved beginning by

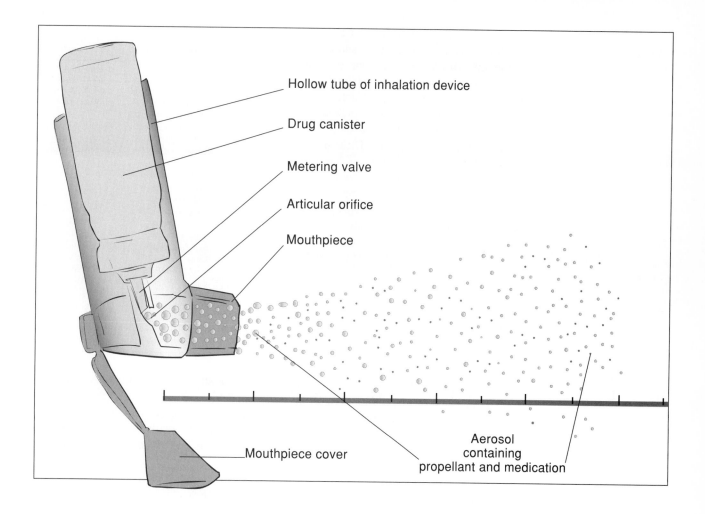

Mouthpiece cover

Aerosol containing propellant and medication

a full exhalation to functional residual capacity, then inhaling. Maneuvers to reach total lung volume, however, are unnecessary and are likely to cause additional turbulence or coughing (1).

Theoretically, waiting several minutes between puffs of bronchodilator aerosol should enhance delivery of drug. The minimum time recommended is 1 minute. Allowing time for the first puff to exert some therapeutic effect should open the airway to deeper penetration by subsequent bursts. Moreover, if the patient is to receive both bronchodilator therapy and antiinflammatory therapy, it would be logical to suppose that bronchodilator therapy should precede antiinflammatory therapy. This would allow the antiinflammatory to penetrate deeper after the bronchodilator exerts its benefit.

Although the mechanisms for optimizing drug delivery in metered dose inhalers are understood in some detail, studies have estimated that only 11 to 40% of adult patients use MDIs correctly (2, 3).

Spacer Devices

Spacer devices are holding systems or reservoirs that collect the aerosol from an MDI, momentarily, before inhalation. The spacer-holding chamber varies in volume, but can be as large as 750 mL. An inlet at one end allows for the insertion of the metered dose and a mouthpiece at the other end allows for the patient to use the inhalation. Possibly within the mouthpiece is a one-way valve that allows aerosol out of the chamber but blocks return of exhaled breath. A whistle or alarm sounds when the patient inhales too rapidly (usually greater than 0.3 L/sec). Each brand of spacer has some combination of these features, but not all. Moreover, spacers are not interchangeable on all commercially available inhalers.

Figure 80.1.
Metered dose inhaler with aerosol cloud

Once the medication is discharged from the MDI into the chamber it is held in place while the patient takes one or two slow breaths, or several normal tidal breaths. A spacer device offers several advantages over the MDI without a spacer attached. The chamber slows down the propellant giving the droplets time to evaporate. These smaller, slower droplets are less likely to deposit on the oropharyngeal mucosa (2). The spacer removes the need to coordinate inhaler activation with inspiration. Thus they are especially useful to children, patients with neurologic impairment or arthritis, or patients having difficulty with correct MDI technique (1–3, 12).

Spacer devices have allowed children as young as 2 or 3 years of age, with stable asthma, to use metered dose inhalers effectively (12). When fitted with a face mask attached to the mouthpiece, spacers can even be used with infants as young as 4 months (13, 14). However, the mask deposits aerosol on the face and increases nasal filtration, thereby reducing lung delivery to some extent.

Because they slow the propellant down, evaporate the particles, and reduce oropharyngeal deposition of the medication, it is expected that spacers increase the dose of medication reaching the lung. However, it has not been proven that the amount of medication reaching the alveoli is increased. In terms of clinical benefits, studies have mixed results when comparing the bronchodilating effects of MDIs with spacers against MDIs used alone. Currently, it appears that spacer devices do not add any measurable clinical benefit, when the MDI without spacer is used properly (1). Even results in children are inconclusive. However it is safe to say that in both children and adults there is no drawback to spacer use and they are likely to produce equivalent or better lung function with generally greater convenience (12).

By decreasing the oropharyngeal deposition of the medication, the spacer provides two particularly significant advantages when used with inhaled corticosteroid. It reduces the incidence of oropharyngeal candidiasis. In one study the incidence decreased from 22% without spacer to 0% with spacer use (2). Moreover, spacers also seem to decrease the systemic absorption of the steroid, as measured by reduced hypothalamic-pituitary-adrenal suppression (15, 16).

Table 80.2.
Available Spacer Devices

Brand Name	Special Features	Disadvantages
Aerochamber	Adapts to most MDIs Inhalation valve Flow indicator whistle	Rigid: Not collapsible
Aerochamber w/mask	Can be used for infants	Not collapsible
Breathancer	Retractable for portability	No inhalation valve
Ellipse	Inhalation valve Stores MDI inside chamber	
Inhal-aid	Large volume (700 mL) chamber Inhalation valve Built-in spirometer	Bulky and rigid: Not collapsible Valve requires replacement
Inspir-ease	Large volume (700 mL) chamber Collapsible for easy carrying Flow indicator whistle	Bag must be replaced every few weeks
Nebuhaler	Large volume (750 mL) Inhalation valve	Rigid and bulky: Not collapsible

Table 80.2 lists the commonly available spacer devices, at this time, and the particular advantages and disadvantages of each device. Of the currently available spacers, the Aerochamber® is one of the best devices available for use with children. It adapts to the widest variety of metered dose inhalers and it contains a flow indicator whistle that warns the child if he or she is inhaling too rapidly. The Aerochamber® is also available with a face mask for use in children under 3 years of age.

Nebulizers

Technically, a nebulizer is any device that produces aerosols. When commonly used, the term nebulizers usually refers to jet nebulizers. These devices create aerosols by passing a gas stream (either air or oxygen) through a fluid. When the fluid is released into the jet of gas the liquid is shattered into small particles and an aerosol of various size particles is created (1, 17). To produce droplets small enough to reach the distal lung, nebulizers commonly use a high gas flow rate and baffling devices. Slow gas jets will produce only large particles. To obtain particle size in the 1 to 5 μ range a gas jet must generally exceed 12 L/min. A baffle—any object placed within a container that obstructs the path of the aerosol particles—will generate smaller particles at lower flow rates. Large particles "rain out" and the smaller particles continue on in the gas stream (1, 17).

Jet nebulizers are considerably easier to use than metered dose inhalers. They deliver significant amounts of medication to the lung without any special respiratory maneuvers. Moreover, they can be used with normal tidal breaths and no coordination between activation and inhalation. They are probably even more effective if the patient takes slow inhalations and breath holds at the end of inspiration. With a face mask attached, nebulizers also can deliver medication to less cooperative patients such as infants.

Even nebulizers are relatively inefficient with more than 90% of the drug not reaching the desired site of delivery. About one-third of the nebulized medication is deposited on the apparatus and another third is lost to the atmosphere. Attaching a face mask reduces this environmental loss, but deposits more drug on the face and the nasopharynx. Less than 10% of the drug reaches the lower airways and a much smaller proportion reaches the distal airways (1). To minimize this dissipation, medication being aerosolized in a jet nebulizer is usually diluted to a total of 3 to 5 mL with normal saline. Ready-made diluted unit dose medication is available for most bronchodilators.

Continuous Nebulization

Continuous nebulization therapy (CNT) uses large volume aerosol generators (up to 240 mL) to deliver β-agonists continuously for as long as 24 hours to asthmatic patients in severe distress. Because they do not require repeated filling, CNT nebulizers are more convenient and can be more cost effective than intermittent nebulizer therapy (INT). They require significantly less respiratory therapist time with the equipment but patients generally need closer observation because they are sicker.

CNT provides a mechanism for maximizing the dose response curve, without exceeding tolerable side effects. When used with patients in impending respiratory failure, CNT may avoid more toxic treatments such as intravenous β-agonist therapy or mechanical ventilation (18).

When CNT is compared with INT for the treatment of acute asthma, clinical outcomes are generally similar. Intermittent therapy is more likely to cause more acute elevations in heart rate (18). Moreover, when used in the ED, CNT appears to reduce ICU admission (18) and, in adults, may increase the likelihood of discharge home (19).

Devices most widely used for continuous nebulization are the high-output extended aerosol respiratory therapy (HEART) nebulizers by Vortran. These nebulizers, which come in large and mini sizes, produce a high density aerosol of small particles using a sonic spray and baffle. The MiniNEB® (also called the MiniHEART®) is especially suitable for use in children (Fig. 80.2). These nebulizers contain a 30 mL reservoir, operate

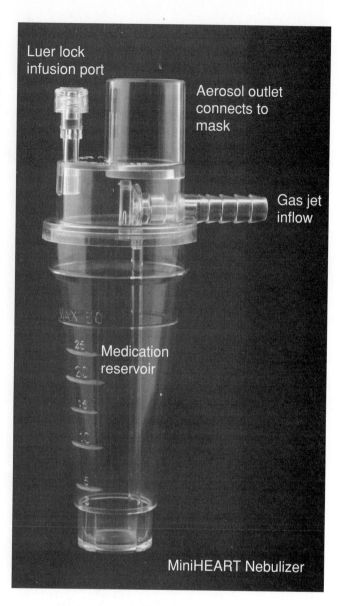

Luer lock infusion port

Aerosol outlet connects to mask

Gas jet inflow

Medication reservoir

MiniHEART Nebulizer

Figure 80.2.
Continuous nebulizer canister–MiniHEART® or MiniNEB® by Vortran®.

at flow rates as low as 1.0 to 2.5 L/min, generate particularly small particles (1.0 to 2.5 μ), can operate from 3 to 10 hours depending on chosen flow rate, have a Luer-Lok intravenous adapter port that permits medication refill without interruption of therapy, and can be connected via an adapter to a mechanical ventilator.

Intermittent Positive Pressure Breathing

Intermittent positive pressure breathing (IPPB) devices automatically coordinate a jet nebulizer aerosol burst with the patient's inspiration. As a result, the patient does not have to learn special techniques to use the device and the medication is not wasted by continuous gas flow.

However, both short- and long-term studies have failed to demonstrate any clinical advantage of IPPB therapy over ordinary jet nebulization in the treatment of asthma or chronic obstructive pulmonary disease (COPD). Moreover, IPPB therapy is more expensive than nebulization and has a greater risk of barotrauma and infection than nebulization (1). Consequently, IPPB devices are no longer routinely used for the treatment of common respiratory illnesses.

Aerosol Therapy for Intubated Patients

Children with respiratory diseases frequently require intubation with mechanical ventilation. Aerosol medication can be delivered to the intubated patient, but only with some technical difficulty. Sidestream actuators have been designed that use jet nebulization to produce aerosol near the origin of the endotracheal tube. However, studies of these actuators demonstrate that only 11 to 66% of the particles produced are in the 1 to 5 μ range. The larger particles created impact on the adaptor and endotracheal tube, without entering the patient's lower airways (20). Moreover, high inspiratory flow rates of the mainstream air flow delivered by the ventilators themselves also lead to significant upper airway deposition of medication due to turbulence and inertial forces. Therefore, less than

3% of the dose arrives in the lung even if the nebulizer adaptor is placed immediately adjacent to the endotracheal tube. Larger doses of medication are needed to achieve the same efficacy (1).

In-line metered dose inhalers appear to be more efficient than jet nebulizers in treating the intubated patient. If the MDI is activated during the inspiratory flow stream of the ventilator, drug delivery is enhanced. To maximize therapy the ventilator should be set at a slower than normal flow rate, with large inspiratory volume, and an inspiratory pause (3, 21). Even though aerosol treatment from metered dose inhalers in the intubated patient is probably more effective than jet nebulizer treatment, the efficiency of drug delivery is still less than that obtained from normal MDI use in the nonintubated patient (21).

Nebulizers Versus MDIs for Acute Attacks

Metered dose inhalers have many obvious advantages over nebulizers. They are less expensive, require less time to deliver a therapeutic dose, are more portable and more convenient to use, and they are less likely to become contaminated. Moreover, at the present time, MDIs are available with a wider variety of respiratory medications than the nebulizer (3, 12).

Conventional wisdom holds that MDIs are better for the provision of maintenance therapy in the stable patient, but the nebulizer may be required for the treatment of acute exacerbations. This belief, however, is not supported by the literature. Whether studied in adults or in children, in the ED or the inpatient wards, there seems to be no difference in mild to moderate asthma in clinical outcome or adverse effects between nebulizer therapy and MDI with spacer therapy (12, 22).

The argument has been made that tachypneic and dyspneic patients might do better with nebulizers because they are unable to use the metered dose inhaler during the attack with the correct technique. However, a spacer can overcome the impediments to proper technique. If jet nebulizers are perceived by some patients to be more effective, this is probably because a much larger dose of medication is used in nebulizers, especially for acute attacks. The standard nebulizer dose is 10 times the dose of β-agonist in the nebulizer than in the metered dose inhaler.

It should also be pointed out that studies comparing the financial cost of MDIs plus spacers to nebulizers in the treatment of hospitalized patients have estimated that patients treated with MDIs required 80% less respiratory therapist time and have their respiratory supply charges reduced by 75% (1, 3). Nebulizers may have the additional disadvantage of carrying a greater risk of infection to the patient, especially if they are not adequately cleaned between usage when colonization rises. Also, in-hospital use of MDIs with spacers—either in the ED or inpatient ward—provide an excellent opportunity to train patients in proper technique for outpatient use. In conclusion, it seems likely that MDIs with spacer devices provide comparable efficacy in the treatment of acute bronchospasm and have several secondary advantages over nebulizers (1, 23).

day, they are washed with dishwashing soap and water along with the medication dropper or syringe. Once a week these components should be soaked in white vinegar and water (1:2 solution) for 30 minutes. Air compressors should be covered after each use to prevent dust accumulation.

MDIs, spacers, and nebulizer masks are designed for single patient use and should not be shared.

Determining How Much Medication Is Left in MDI

The number of aerosol puffs in an MDI canister varies with the type of medication. Most β-agonist canisters contain 200 puffs. Figure 80.3 illustrates how to approximate the amount of medication left in a canister by floating it in water. This method does not apply to all canisters, so the patient should consult the package insert.

Cleaning the Equipment

Metered dose inhalers should be cleaned once a day by removing the canister and rinsing the inhaler, mouthpiece, and cap in warm water and then air dry before using again. Twice a week the mouthpiece should be cleaned with a dishwashing soap and then rinsed.

The spacer mouthpiece should be rinsed in warm running water once a day, taking care not to damage the one-way inhalation valve. The reservoir should be rinsed with warm water at least once a week to remove medication buildup. Both components should be shaken and air dried after cleaning. Never clean a spacer device in a dishwasher.

The facemask or T-piece used with a nebulizer is rinsed under running warm water then air dried after each use. Once a

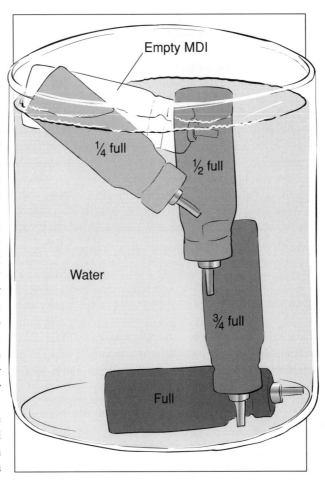

Empty MDI

¼ full

½ full

Water

¾ full

Full

Figure 80.3.
MDI canisters floating in tap water to demonstrate amount of medication remaining in the canister.

PROCEDURE

Metered Dose Inhalers

Before starting, the patient should ensure that the canister is inserted properly into the inhaler mechanism. The patient should remove the cap from the mouthpiece of the inhaler and inspect for foreign materials. The canister-inhaler assembly is shaken immediately before each puff.

Holding the inhaler upright (mouthpiece is below canister), the patient breathes out fully without forcing exhalation. The head is tilted back slightly and the mouthpiece of the inhaler is placed 1 to 2 inches away from the mouth or, alternatively, between open lips (Fig. 80.4.A, B).

The patient or assistant presses down on the canister fully with his or her index finger while the patient starts to breathe in slowly at the same time. The patient should inhale the medication as slowly as possible, taking up to 6 seconds for inspiration. Once the medication is inhaled, the patient holds his or her breath as long as is comfortable and up to 10 seconds. Having completed the breath holding, the patient then exhales.

If additional puffs are required, the patient should wait at least 1 minute between the puffs and then repeat the procedure starting with shaking the canister and ending with exhaling. Once the medication is completely administered, the patient replaces the cap over the mouthpiece and stores the inhaler in a clean, dry place. If corticosteroid inhalers are used, the patient should rinse the mouth with water after treatment to avoid oral candida infection.

Spacer Use

The patient using a spacer device with the MDI should prepare for medication administration by first removing the dust cap from the spacer mouthpiece and inspecting the spacer for foreign material. The patient should then remove the cap from the mouthpiece of the MDI and look for foreign material here as well. Some MDIs adapt to spacers by attaching the canister directly to the spacer device without using the MDI mouthpiece. If this is the case, the canister should be removed from the MDI and inspected for foreign materials. The entire MDI (or just the canister) is then inserted into the spacer in an upright position.

The patient starts the treatment by breathing out fully without forcing exhalation, then places the spacer mouthpiece in the mouth and closes the lips snuggly around it (Fig. 80.4.C). One puff of medication is released into the spacer reservoir by pressing down fully on the inhaler canister with the index finger. The patient then breathes the medication in slowly from the reservoir up to 6 seconds. A whistle sound indicates that the patient is breathing too rapidly and should slow down the rate of inhalation. At the end of inhalation, the patient holds his or her breath as long as is comfortable or up to 10 seconds. The patient then breathes out with the lips closed around the mouthpiece into the reservoir. To complete the inhalation of the first puff of medication, the patient must breathe in slowly, breath hold, and exhale a second or perhaps a third time. If additional puffs of medication are required, the patient then repeats all of the previous steps waiting at least 1 minute between puffs.

Once the medication is fully administered, the patient removes the inhaler from the spacer and replaces the mouthpieces of both the spacer and the inhaler with the dustcaps.

Notably, some authorities advocate discharging all puffs of the medication into the spacer device in rapid succession and then inhaling these puffs together (12). Breathing each puff individually probably delivers more drug to the lung, though the differences between the two approaches may not be significant (2).

Figure 80.4.
A. MDI usage with open mouth technique (1 to 2 inches from mouth).
B. MDI usage with canister mouthpiece surrounded by lips.
C. MDI usage with a spacer attached.

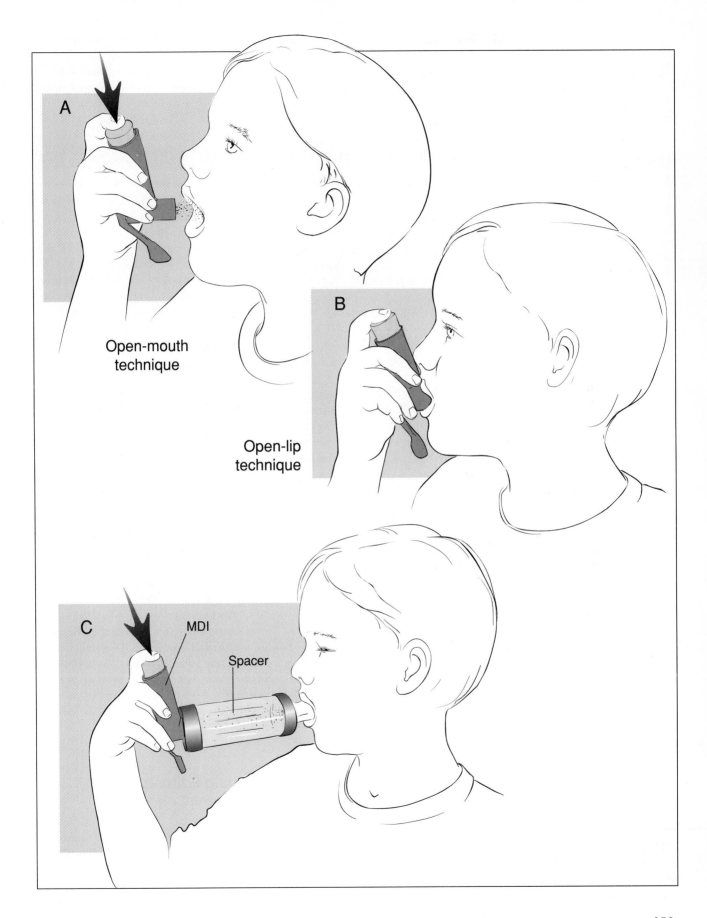

A

Open-mouth
technique

B

Open-lip
technique

C   MDI

Spacer

Nebulizer Use

Starting with a clean medication reservoir, the clinician measures the correct amount of normal saline (usually 3 mL) and places it in the reservoir, and then adds the measured amount of medication to the saline. Once the medication is in the reservoir, the reservoir can be attached to its jet source (air compressor or oxygen line) using gas tubing. The T-connector mouthpiece for the face mask is attached to the other end of the medication cup. It is better to use a T-connector and mouthpiece than a face mask if the patient is able to cooperate with the breathing in of the medication. Face masks deposit a large portion of the aerosol on the face and in the nasopharynx. T-connectors with a mouthpiece waste less medication than face masks and are the device of choice in cooperative patients.

Once the mask is placed around the face or the T-connector mouthpiece set is placed in the mouth, the clinician turns on the jet source. Taking deep breaths the patient inhales slowly (over 6 seconds if possible), and then holds each breath as long as is comfortable (up to 10 seconds). The patient continues inhaling in this manner until all fluid is gone from the reservoir. After the treatment is completed the compressed air or oxygen is turned off.

Continuous Nebulization Therapy—Operating the Vortran MiniHEART® Nebulizer

To prepare for continuous nebulization treatment with a mininebulizer, the clinician connects a low flow oxygen meter (0 to 3 L/min) to the oxygen source. Because continuous nebulization therapy is reserved for severely ill patients, oxygen should always be used as the jet source. The oxygen is connected to the medication reservoir using gas tubing. The reservoir is filled with a mixture of β-agonist and normal saline through the aerosol outlet at the top (up to a maximum 30 mL of solution). The aerosol outlet port is then connected to a face mask and the face mask is placed on the patient. It should be noted that T-connectors are usually not used in continuous nebulization therapy because it would be impractical to expect the patient to hold the T-connector in the mouth for prolonged periods of time.

The oxygen jet should be run at 1.0 to 2.0 L/per min to produce an aerosol output on the MiniHEART® as follows:

    1.0 L/min = 4.5 mL/hr
    1.5 L/min = 6.0 mL/hr
    2.0 L/min = 8.0 mL/hr

This aerosol output will provide continuous nebulization for several hours depending on the oxygen flow rate and the amount of medication initially placed in the reservoir. If the clinician wishes to provide continuous nebulization beyond the capacity of the MiniNEB® reservoir, he or she can mix β-agonist with respiratory NS in the medication bag and place this mixture on an infusion pump. The infusion pump is then connected with intravenous tubing to a LuerLok inlet on the MiniNEB®. The fluid infusion rate is adjusted to match the aerosol output rate, thus keeping the reservoir fluid level at a steady 10 to 20 mL. For infection control precautions, the MiniNEB® reservoir, tubing, and mask should be changed every 24 hours.

Notably, the absolute dose of continuous nebulization medication for children and adults has not been determined. The dosage delivered should be titrated to the individual patient's tolerance of the β-agonist. As a rule of thumb, however, the clinician can start the patient on an hourly dose of β-agonist that is 3 times the usual single intermittent dose. For example, if using 0.15 mg/kg (.03 mL/kg) of 5% albuterol and 3 mL of NS as a single dose, start the patient on 0.45 mg/kg (.09 mL/kg) in 9 mL of NS per hour.

For the adult size patient the clinician can use the full size HEART® nebulizer instead of the MiniHEART®. The HEART® nebulizer does not require a low flow oxygen meter and can be run at an oxygen flow rate of 9 to 10 L/min to produce 20 mL of aerosol per hour.

Teaching Patients to Use Equipment Correctly

A survey from a general medical practice in 1989 indicated that only 25% of adult MDI users had perfect technique whereas more than a third had poor technique (24). Therefore, every medical visit including visits to the ED should be viewed as an opportunity to demonstrate correct technique. It is preferable to use a placebo inhaler and observe the patient's use of it (2). The teaching should emphasize using the open mouth technique, the coordination of inhalation with activation, slow inspiration, and breath holding.

For the patient using a spacer device, teaching should emphasize placing the lips tightly around the mouthpiece, inhaling slowly, and breath holding at the end of inhalation. These same points also should be emphasized for the patient using a home nebulizer, as well as correct measurement of medication.

COMPLICATIONS

Complications of inhalation therapy are limited and are mostly the complications seen with the actual medications. For example, the principal complications of β-agonist inhalation are tremor, hypokalemia, tachycardia, and dysrhythmias. Abuse of β-agonist MDIs has been associated with a higher incidence of asthma deaths but this is probably caused, in part, by delays in seeking care and lack of early treatment with antiinflammatory therapy (25). Similarly, principal complications of corticosteroid inhalation are oral thrush and hypothalamic-pituitary-adrenal suppression. A few complications have been associated with the actual inhalation devices but not the medication they are delivering.

One of the principal concerns raised about metered dose inhalers is their use of chlorofluorocarbons (CFCs) and the environmental effects. Although CFCs from MDIs contribute only a small percentage of the total CFC burden in the environment, this environmental impact is undesirable. Additionally, CFCs, like other halogenated hydrocarbons, can sensitize the myocardium to the effects to catecholamines. It has been estimated that a patient must use an inhaler 20 times over 2 minutes before the CFC concentration in the blood becomes great enough to make the myocardium irritable (3). It also should be noted that inhalation of the dustcap of a metered dose inhaler with subsequent airway obstruction has been reported. Using the MDI with the open mouth technique provides a chance that the patient will misdirect the burst of aerosol. Spraying into the eyes can be a particular problem, especially with ipratropium. This has been reported to cause blurry vision when squirted in the eye (2). To avoid this complication, it is recommended that the closed mouth technique be used for ipratropium MDIs.

A theoretical complication of all aerosol therapies is infection. The small aerosol particles can carry microorganisms far into the airways. In practice, this seems to be principally described as a complication of nebulizers and to a lesser extent spacers. The problem here is probably related to poor cleaning of the reservoirs and mouthpieces. With regard to spacers, those devices made with one-way inhalation valves can cause difficulty for patients with severe airway obstruction. These patients cannot mount enough expiratory pressure to close the valve (1).

Continuous nebulizer therapy carries the most risk of medication toxicity because of the high doses of β-agonist that are used. In addition to tremor, muscle cramps with elevation in CPK (MM fraction) and LDH have been reported. Moreover, one patient was reported to develop unifocal PVCs on high dose therapy. Mild hyperglycemia with blood glucose in the 200 to 250 mg/dL range and hypokalemia have also been reported. These latter two complications can be easily corrected with adjustments in intravenous fluids (18). Other complications are likely to be reported as CNT becomes more widely used in adult patients. Conversely, CNT has not been found more toxic than frequent intermittent treatments.

SUMMARY

The advent of inhalation therapy has made it possible to treat a variety of respiratory illnesses with fewer side effects by delivering small doses of medication directly to their site of action. Metered dose inhalers are capable of delivering a wide variety of medications to the lungs, in a convenient and cost-effective manner. However, their effectiveness is dependent on their being used with correct technique. For those patients unable to use MDIs with ideal technique, spacer devices offer an effective adjunct. MDIs with spacers seem to be at least as effective as nebulizers, even in the treatment of acute asthma and these devices have even been successfully

SUMMARY
MDI Use
1. Shake canister immediately before each aerosol release
2. Breathe out fully without forcing exhalation
3. Hold MDI with mouthpiece down and canister above
4. Place mouthpiece of inhaler 1 to 2 inches away from open mouth or between open lips
5. Pressing canister down with index finger to release measured medication burst, start inhaling slowly over 6 seconds
6. Hold breath to 10 seconds
7. Wait at least 1 minute between each puff
8. If using a corticosteroid inhaler, rinse mouth after each treatment

Spacer Use with MDI
1. Close lips snuggly around spacer mouthpiece
2. Place one puff of medication in reservoir at a time
3. Breathe in medication slowly over 6 seconds
4. If whistle sounds, slow down rate of inhalation
5. Hold breath as long as possible up to 10 seconds
6. Repeat steps 3–5 one or two times more for each aerosol puff taken
7. Wait at least 1 minute before inhaling an additional burst of medication

used in very young children. Conversely, for the treatment of severe bronchospasm, continuous nebulization therapy might prevent the need for intubation with mechanical ventilation and even intensive care admission.

REFERENCES

1. Lee DKP, Ingbar DH. Aerosol delivery: what's best for your patient? J Respir Dis 1989;10:97–116.
2. Whelan AM, Hahn NW. Optimizing drug delivery from metered dose inhalers. DICP, Ann Phamacother 1991;25:638–645.
3. Hofford JM. Metered dose inhaler therapy for asthma, bronchitis and emphysema. J Fam Pract 1992;34:485–492.
4. Kemp JP, Meltzer EO. β_2 adrenergic agonists—oral or aerosol for the treatment of asthma. J Asthma 1990;27:149–157.
5. Kelly HW, Murphy S. β-adrenergic agonists for acute, severe asthma. DICP, Ann Pharmacother 1992;26:81–91.
6. Rau JL. Respiratory care pharmacology. 4th ed. St. Louis: CV Mosby, 1994.
7. Kulick RM, Ruddy RM. Allergic emergencies. In: Fleisher GR, Ludwig S, eds. Textbook of pediatric emergency medicine. 3rd ed. Baltimore: Williams & Wilkins, 1993, pp. 858–873, and Baker MD, Ruddy RM. Scanlin TF. Part A—Pulmonary emergencies. Part B—Cystic fibrosis. In: Fleisher GR, Ludwig S, eds. Textbook of pediatric emergency medicine. 3rd ed. Baltimore: Williams & Wilkins, 1993, pp. 874–895.
8. Schuh S, Johnson DW, Callahan S, Canny G, Levinson H. Efficacy of frequent nebulized ipratropium bromide added to frequent high-dose albuterol therapy in severe childhood asthma. J Pediatr 1995;126:639–645.
9. Hall CB, McBride JT, Walsh EE, Bell DM, et al. Aerosolized ribivirin treatment of infants with respiratory syncytial viral infection. New Eng J Med 1983;308:1443–1447.
10. Feldstein TJ, Swegarden JL, Atwood GF, Peterson CD. Ribivirin therapy: implementation of hospital guidelines and effect on usage and cost of therapy. Pediatrics 1995;96:14–17.
11. Klassen TP, Feldman ME, Watters LK, et al. Nebulized budesonide with mild to moderate croup. New Eng J Med 1994;331:285–289.
12. Karem D, Levinson H, Schuh S, et al. Efficacy of albuterol administered by nebulizer versus spacer device in children with acute asthma. J Pediatr 1993;123:313–317.
13. Noble V, Ruggins NR, Everard ML, Milner AD. Inhaled budesonide for chronic wheezing under 18 months of age. Arch Dis Child 1992;67:285–288.
14. Conner WT, Dolovich MB, Frame RA, Newhouse MT. Reliable salbutamol administration in 6- to 36-month-old children by means of a metered dose inhaler and Aerochamber with mask. Pediatr Pulmonol 1989;6:263–267.
15. Selroos O, Halme M. Effect of volumatic spacer and mouth rinsing on systemic absorption of inhaled corticosteroids from a metered dose inhaler and dry powder inhaler. Thorax 1991;46:891–894.
16. Farrer M, Francis AJ, Pearce SJ. Morning serum cortisol concentrations after 2 mg inhaled beclomethasone diproprionate in normal subjects: effect of a 750 mL spacing device. Thorax 1990;45:740–742.
17. Mc Pherson SP. Respiratory therapy equipment. 4th ed. St. Louis: CV Mosby, 1990, pp. 93–107.
18. Portnoy J, Nadel G, Amado M, Willsie-Ediger S. Continuous nebulization for status asthmaticus. Ann Allergy 1992;69:71–79.
19. Rudnitsky G, Eberlein RS, Schoffstall JM, Mazur JE, Spivey WH. Comparison of intermittent and continuously nebulized albuterol for treatment of asthma in an urban emergency department. Ann Emerg Med 1993;22:1842–1846.
20. Bishop MJ, Larson RP, Buschman DL. Metered dose inhaler aerosol characteristics are affected by the endotracheal tube actuator-adapter used. Anesthesiol 1990;73:1263–1265.
21. Crogan SJ, Bishop MJ. Delivery efficiency of metered dose aerosols given via endotracheal tubes. Anesthesiology 1989;70:1008–1010.
22. Kisch GL, Paloucek FP. Metered dose inhalers and nebulizers in the acute setting. DICP, Ann Pharmacother 1992;26:92–95.
23. Zainudin BM, Biddiscombe M, Tolfree SE, Short M, Spiro SG. Comparison of bronchodilator responses and deposition patterns of salbutamol inhaled from a metered dose inhaler as a dry powder and as a nebulizer solution. Thorax 1990;45:469–473.
24. Buckley D. Assessment of inhale technique in general practice. Irish J Med Sci 1989;158:297–299.
25. Spitzer WO, Suissa S, Ernest P, et al. The use of β-agonists and the risk of death and near death from asthma. New Eng J Med 1992;326:501–506.

SUCTIONING THE TRACHEA

Mary E. Lacher

INTRODUCTION

Suctioning is a technique used to maintain airway patency by removing pulmonary secretions, blood, vomitus, saliva, or other foreign material (1–5). Removal of these materials allows for the maintenance of gas exchange to provide adequate oxygenation and ventilation. In addition, suctioning removes potentially infective material from the upper airway and trachea. Suctioning may be nasal, oral, nasopharyngeal, or tracheal depending on the patient's particular problem. Tracheal suctioning has been performed since the 1950s concurrent with the development of positive pressure ventilation.

Even though suctioning is a common, basic procedure it is associated with complications and risks if not performed appropriately. It is frequently performed in pediatric patients of all age groups and may be done by health care providers with different training backgrounds (EMTs, RNs, MDs, and respiratory therapists). Suctioning the upper airway is detailed in Chapter 13, pp. 110–112.

ANATOMY AND PHYSIOLOGY

The upper airway includes the nose, mouth, and pharynx (Fig. 81.1). The upper airway has several functions including (*a*) acting as a conduction system for inspired gases to the lungs, (*b*) acting as a filter to prevent foreign material from entering the lower airway, and (*c*) humidifying and heating inspired gases.

The nose is lined with ciliated and nonciliated mucous cells. These cells help humidify inspired gases and filter foreign material. The filtering of foreign material is aided by the hair follicles and the thick, sticky mucous secretions of the nose. When an artificial airway (i.e., endotracheal tube or tracheotomy) is in place, the protective mucociliary clearance system is bypassed leading to a reduction in airway humidity with drying and thickening of the secretions. The generous blood supply to the nares helps to warm and humidify inspired gases. As much as 1000 mL of water per day humidifies the inspired air by mucous and serous secretions (1). These glands also are stimulated to produce more secretions from inflammatory processes such as respiratory infections, allergies, or inhalation of toxic substances (i.e., smoke, chemicals).

From the base of the tongue, the laryngopharynx extends to the esophagus which lies posterior to the trachea (Fig. 81.1). The proximity and function of these structures around the larynx serve to protect the airway from microbial organisms. Closure of the glottis during swallowing prevents food or other substances from contaminating the tracheobronchial tree. Patients with neuromuscular illness, anatomically abnormal airways or poorly protected airways, are at greatest risk of the aspiration of gastrointestinal contents.

Within the neck the trachea begins at the

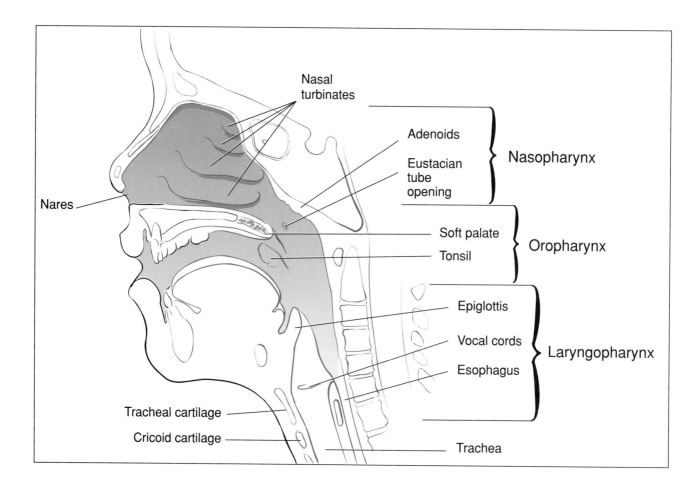

Figure 81.1.
Anatomy of the upper
(pharyngeal) airway.

Nasal
turbinates

Adenoids

Eustacian
tube
opening

Nasopharynx

Nares

Soft palate

Tonsil

Oropharynx

Epiglottis

Vocal cords

Esophagus

Laryngopharynx

Tracheal cartilage

Cricoid cartilage

Trachea

level of the cricoid cartilage. The trachea descends in the middle of the neck to the vertebral level of T5–T6 and bifurcates into the right and left bronchi. This bifurcation is positioned slightly angled to the right making the opening to the right bronchi a less acute angle. This allows an endotracheal tube or suction catheter to enter the right mainstem bronchus if passed beyond the carina.

Gas flow during respiration in normal healthy airways occurs by laminar flow with the molecules traveling parallel to the walls of the airway. Laminar flow is governed by the law of Poiseuille which states that at a constant driving pressure, the resistance to flow of a gas will vary with the 4th power of the radius of the tube it transverses. For example, if the internal diameter of the tube is halved, resistance to flow will be increased 16-fold. Small changes in airway caliber, even in local parts of the tracheobronchial tree (such as secretions or debris causing obstruction, or the insertion of a suction catheter) can greatly increase resistance to gas exchange.

Airway secretions can affect respiratory function in several ways (Fig. 81.2) (1). Initially these secretions may provoke a local inflammatory response leading to increased resistance to airflow by the narrowing secondary to hyperemia and edema. This increases the work of breathing necessary to move gases past the secretions and inflamed airways. Ventilation-perfusion mismatch occurs because plugging, inflammation, and retained secretions lead to uneven distribution of oxygen reaching the distal pulmonary bed. Perfused lung segments may not receive fresh air, which leads to hypoxemia and triggers increased ventilatory effort to attempt compensation. If retained secretions cause total plugging of bronchioles, atelectasis, further reduction in lung compliance, and worsening of ventilation-perfusion mismatch will occur. Atelectatic or inflamed lung segments also continue to produce secretions that further act as a culture media for bacteria.

Defense mechanisms exist to remove foreign debris and excess secretions from the airway that are caused by artificial airways or

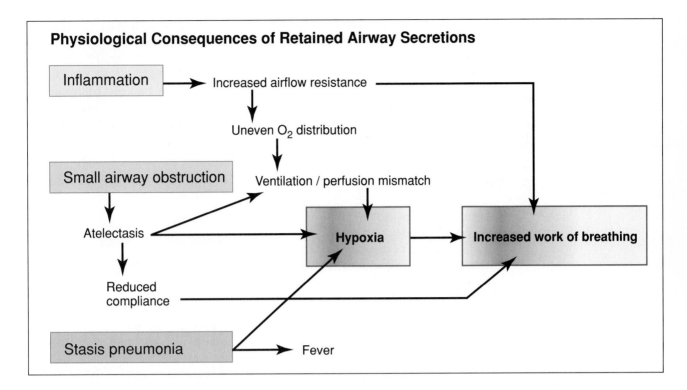

Physiological Consequences of Retained Airway Secretions

Inflammation → Increased airflow resistance

Uneven O$_2$ distribution

Small airway obstruction

Ventilation / perfusion mismatch

Atelectasis

Hypoxia

Increased work of breathing

Reduced compliance

Stasis pneumonia → Fever

primary disease. Small amounts of foreign material are continually swept up by cilia and mucus to the supraglottic region where they can be swallowed down the esophagus. Coughing also is a means through which the secretions and foreign material can be expelled from the airway. Receptors in the mucosa of the large respiratory passages are stimulated by irritation from secretions or foreign material producing cough. Coughing begins with a deep inspiration followed by a forced expiration against a closed glottis. The glottis is then suddenly opened producing a forceful outflow of air.

Endotracheal or tracheotomy tubes tend to reduce effective cough and ciliary clearance potentially leading to further inspissation of secretions. This is in part due to the need for a closed glottis for truly effective cough to be maintained. This is not possible with an endotracheal tube (ETT) in place. Because the normal upper airway humidification systems are bypassed, secretions may be drier and thicker with artificial airways. The ETT impedes ciliary function. A foreign body can stimulate increased secretions.

INDICATIONS

Tracheal suctioning may be necessary any time foreign material is interfering with ade-

quate ventilation or oxygenation of a patient with natural or artificial airways. A number of medical conditions affect production and clearance of secretions to the degree that tracheal suctioning is indicated. Children with pneumonia or cystic fibrosis often have increased, thick secretions that are difficult to clear. Victims of smoke inhalation or other inhalational injury may have edema and increased secretion production. Head injury or intoxicated patients may have reduced or absent protective reflex mechanisms to assist maintaining a clear airway. Patients with poor pulmonary mechanics (due to thoracic-abdominal surgery, rib fracture or chest trauma, neuromuscular disorders such as muscular dystrophy) may not be able to clear their secretions. In addition to suctioning to clear the airway, sputum may be obtained by suctioning to be used diagnostically for culture.

Patients with artificial airways (tracheostomy cannula or endotracheal tube) have a routine need for suctioning. It is common for children with small artificial airways (ETT size 2.5 to 4.0) to require more frequent suctioning than older children or adults with larger airways just to ensure continued patency of the smaller tube.

Suctioning is performed frequently in the ED setting in patients with increased se-

Figure 81.2.
Physiologic consequences of retained secretions. (Adapted from Shapiro B et al. Clinical applications of respiratory care. St. Louis: CV Mosby, 1991.)

cretions or foreign material in the airway. The most common form is oral and nasopharyngeal suctioning (Chapter 13, pp. 110–112). Suctioning is routinely performed when intubating a patient to better visualize landmarks and after the artificial airway is in place to maintain its patency and provide adequate oxygenation and ventilation.

EQUIPMENT

The necessary equipment needed for suctioning is outlined in Table 81.1. Various types of catheters are available depending on the type of suctioning to be performed (Fig. 81.3). Two major types include a disposable, vented, polyvinyl chloride plastic catheter (Fig. 81.3.A) or a Yankauer type tube (Fig. 81.3.B). When suctioning the upper airway, the catheter should be soft and pliable but not collapsible when suction is applied. The distal end should be open with at least two holes and smooth edges. The catheter should allow for intermittent suction with a thumb control valve (Fig. 81.3.C). With this valve, no suction occurs when the valve port is open. To create suction, the clinician places the thumb over the valve opening. The Yankauer catheter is frequently used to suction the pharynx before endotracheal intubation or when initially clearing the oropharynx in children who are at risk of aspiration. In these instances after intubation of the airway, the soft, vented polyvinyl catheter is used.

Catheter size is important for this procedure to be most successful. Too small a catheter may not successfully clear sections. Too large a catheter can induce mucosal trauma and contribute to hypoxia. For endotracheal or tracheotomy tube suctioning, the catheter should be one-half the size of the inner diameter of the tube into which the clinician is suctioning. (For intraoral suctioning, the larger the catheter the better, especially if clearing vomitus. A Yankauer type catheter is recommended for vomitus or large amounts of blood or other material in the oropharynx (Table 81.2).

PROCEDURE

Tracheal Suctioning (via Endotracheal Tube or Tracheotomy Site)

Ideally, two people should be available to assist in the tracheal suctioning. One assistant monitors oxygenation and ventilation and assists in positioning the child while the other assistant performs the procedure. Because the area below the pharynx is sterile, it is important to use aseptic technique to reduce the risk of airway colonization or nosocomial infection.

In an awake patient, the clinician should explain the procedure to the patient and family beforehand. After washing the hands, it is important for the clinician to don protective equipment (gloves, eyewear, mask). The clinician should then set up the necessary equipment using aseptic technique and assess the patient's cardiorespiratory status noting color, auscultatory findings, oxygen saturation, respiratory rate, and heart rate (blood pressure is optional). At the start, the clinician should hyperoxygenate the patient with 100% oxygen by bag-valve ventilation for several minutes. The amount of hyperoxygenation should be lengthened in the extremely ill patient. After removing the bag, the clinician should gently insert the catheter without suction, advancing it a short distance past the distal end of the artificial airway (Fig. 81.4). When the clinician meets resistance (typically at the carina) he or she should pull back the catheter slightly (0.5 cm). While occluding the suction, the clinician should gently and slowly withdraw the catheter. Most authorities suggest using a rotating motion between the thumb and forefinger as the catheter is withdrawn. No more than 5 consecutive seconds of suction should be applied

Table 81.1.
Equipment

1. Pair of sterile gloves, protective eyewear, and mask
2. Appropriately sized suction catheter (Table 81.2) (2, 3).
3. Resuscitation (ambu) bag with high flow oxygen supply
4. Wall suction or portable suction device with age-appropriate pressure setting (infants 60 to 80 mm Hg, children 80 to 100 mm Hg, adolescent–adult 100 to 150 mm Hg) (4)
5. Sterile saline or water to flush catheter (minimum 100 mL)
6. Small vial (3 to 5 mL) or syringe of sterile saline or water for instillation into airway
7. Pulse oximeter and cardiac monitors

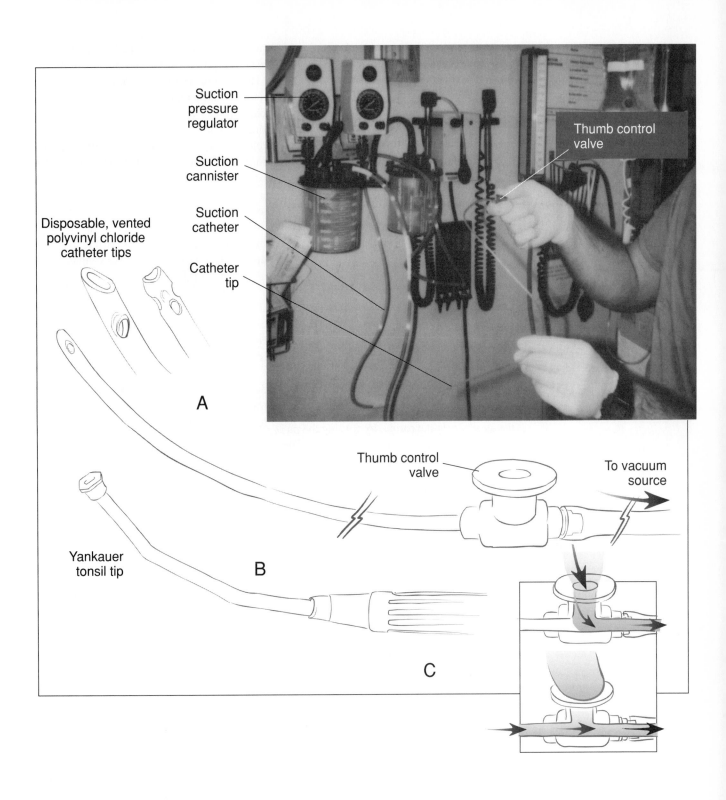

Suction pressure regulator

Suction cannister

Suction catheter

Catheter tip

Thumb control valve

Disposable, vented polyvinyl chloride catheter tips

A

Thumb control valve

To vacuum source

Yankauer tonsil tip

B

C

and a total of 10 seconds with the catheter within the airway is allowed. After the catheter is removed, hyperoxygenation should be repeated with 100% oxygen and manual bag inflation. The procedure should be repeated until the secretions or foreign material are sufficiently cleared. If secretions are particularly thick, sterile saline may be placed down the endotracheal tube followed by a few spontaneous or assisted breaths (saline vol-

Figure 81.3.
Equipment used for suctioning.

**Chapter 81
Suctioning the
Trachea**

SUMMARY

1. Explain procedure
2. Wash hands and wear protective equipment
3. Set up equipment
4. Assess patient's cardiorespiratory status
5. Hyperoxygenate with 100% oxygen (minimum of six breaths)
6. Insert catheter without suction applied to just past distal end of artificial airway or just above carina
7. Withdraw catheter with intermittent suction (total time less than 10 seconds to have catheter in airway)
8. Repeat hyperoxygenate with 100% oxygen
9. Repeat steps 4–8 as necessary and reassess patient

CLINICAL TIPS

1. Have assistant if possible
2. If bradycardia occurs, try oxygen first, then atropine
3. Limit time (less than 10 seconds) and pressure (less than 100 torr)

Table 81.2.
Suggested Age/Weight Appropriate Sizes of Suction Catheter and Endotracheal Tubes

Age/Weight	Endotracheal Tube Internal Diameter (mm)	Suction Catheter
< 1000 g	2.5	5 F
1000–2000 g	3.0	6 F
2000–3000 g	3.0–3.5	6–8 F
Term newborn	3.0–3.5	6–8 F
6 mo	3.5	8 F
12–18 mo	4.0	8 F
3 yr	4.5	8 F
5 yr	5.0	10 F
6 yr	5.5	10 F
8 yr	6.0	10 F
12 yr	6.5	10 F
16 yr	7.0	12 F
Adult (F)	7.5–8.0	12 F
Adult (M)	8.0–8.5	14 F

ume: neonates 0.25 to 0.5 mL, 0.5 to 1.0 mL for infants; 1 to 3 mL for older children; 5 to 10 mL for adolescents and/or adults). If necessary, the clinician can selectively suction the airway past the carina, by varying the patient's head position from side to side. The clinician also can facilitate entry into the left mainstem bronchus by turning the patient's head to the right and the right mainstem bronchus with the patient's head to the left (1).

COMPLICATIONS

Some potential complications can be minimized or prevented with monitoring and technique. The most common potential complication is hypoxemia. Risk is increased with failure to adequately hyperoxygenate and/or by prolonged duration of the suctioning (6–9. Hypoxia may manifest itself as a significant reduction in oxygen saturation (less than 85%), cyanotic color, altered mental status, and/or cardiac dysrhythmia. Initially, tachycardia may be present, but many young infants develop bradycardia (especially in the neonate).

Bradycardia secondary to vagal stimulation may be the result of overstimulation of the gag reflex or secondary to hypoxemia. Hemodynamic changes (hypertension or hy-

potension) and dysrhythmia have been noted secondary to hypoxia or vagal stimulation (10). If bradycardia occurs, the clinician should immediately hyperoxygenate the child. If the patient does not respond and continues to have symptomatic bradycardia, the clinician needs to consider atropine at 0.02 mg/kg i.v. (maximum of 2 mg) because the bradycardia may be secondary to vagal stimulation. It is important to consider hypoxemia as the cause before giving atropine, because atropine will increase the heart rate even in hypoxic patients. Cardiac output may decrease secondary to decrease in venous return if the patient is hyperventilated.

Improper technique by overzealous suctioning can more infrequently lead to airway collapse or atelectasis. This can be avoided by choosing the correct catheter size and limiting the amount of time suction is applied.

Tissue injury or hemoptysis may on occasion be caused by excessive pressure, local trauma, too large a caliber catheter, or prolonged duration of suctioning. Using pressure greater than 100 torr can damage mucosal tissue and denude airways of cilia. Bronchoconstriction may be seen from the irritative stimulation of bronchial smooth muscle but may be present as the primary problem and not specifically from suctioning. A risk of introducing infectious material leading to nosocomial infections is also present. Transient increases in intracranial pressure during or from tracheal suctioning also have been noted (11) which can be minimized in patients requiring suctioning with intracranial problems by careful techniques, sedation, or using prophylactic therapy.

SUMMARY

Suctioning is an important procedure to maintain a patent airway, and oxygenate and ventilate patients with impaired pulmonary function, excessive secretions, and/or artificial airways. It carries the potential serious risk of hypoxemia or local airway injury. The procedure should be performed only by a trained individual with strict adherence to proper technique.

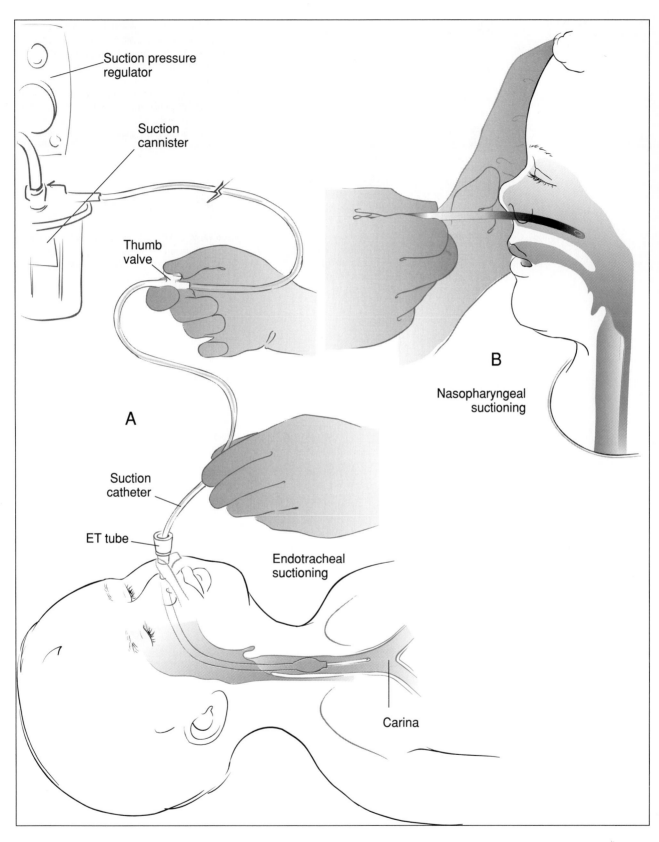

Suction pressure regulator

Suction cannister

Thumb valve

A

Suction catheter

ET tube

Endotracheal suctioning

Carina

B

Nasopharyngeal suctioning

Figure 81.4.
Proper techniques for endotracheal and nasopharyngeal suctioning.

References

1. Shapiro B, et al. Clinical applications of respiratory care. St. Louis: CV Mosby, 1991.
2. Standards for CPR and ECC. JAMA 1986; 255(21):2962.
3. American Heart Association. Textbook of pediatric advanced life support, 1988, p. 26.
4. Koff P. et al. Neonatal and pediatric respiratory care. St. Louis: CV Mosby, 1988, pp. 252–254.
5. Burton G, et al. Respiratory care: a guide to clinical practice. Philadelphia: Lippincott-Raven, 1991, pp. 498–502.
6. Langrehe EA, et al. Oxygen insufflation during endotracheal suctioning. Heart Lung 1981;10:1029.
7. Skelley BF, et al. The effectiveness of preoxygenation methods to prevent endotracheal suction induced hypoxemia. Heart Lung 1980;9:316.
8. Naigow D, et al. The effects of different endotracheal procedures on arterial blood gases in an controlled experiment model. Heart Lung 1977;6:808.
9. Barnes CA, et al. Minimizing hypoxemia due to endotracheal suctioning: a review of the literature. Heart Lung 1986; 15:164.
10. Shim C, et al. Cardiac arrhythmias resulting from tracheal suctioning. Ann Intern Med 1969;71:1140.
11. Rudy EB, et. al. The relationship between endotracheal suctioning and changes in intracranial pressure: a review of the literature. Heart Lung 1986;15: 488.

Suggested Readings

Pierson D, et al. Foundations of respiratory care. New York: Churchill Livingstone, 1922.
Eubansk D, et al. Comprehensive respiratory care. St. Louis: CV Mosby, 1985.

REPLACEMENT OF A TRACHEOSTOMY CANNULA

Jean Marie Kallis

INTRODUCTION

Replacing a tracheostomy cannula is typically a routine and simple procedure. Parents of children with tracheostomies perform this task on a regular basis without the assistance of a health care professional (1).

Although the actual skills involved are generally no more complicated than those used by parents at home, the degree of anxiety present in an emergent situation can make this task more challenging. A calm, methodical approach is usually the key to success. In addition, with those children who present acutely in the ED for cannula replacement, other factors may be present that increase the complexity of the procedure. These include such things as recannulation in the very young infant, a tracheostomy performed in the previous week or two, the absence of an alternative upper airway, and certain underlying airway conditions.

ANATOMY AND PHYSIOLOGY

A tracheostomy is designed to bypass the upper airway and to provide a direct opening to the trachea. Tracheostomies are performed after endotracheal intubation or for an immediate airway because of three broad and often overlapping clinical problems: acute or chronic airway obstruction, prolonged assisted ventilation, and problems requiring improved pulmonary toilet (2–5). Following a tracheostomy, a tract of healing tissue forms between the cervical epithelium and the tracheal endothelium (6). Until this is well granulated recannulation may be difficult (3, 5). Patients are usually hospitalized for a number of days, often in an intensive care setting, to reduce the risk of accidental decannulation and to allow sufficient healing and for the primary process to be better controlled (1, 3, 5, 6). Except in unusual circumstances, ED physicians tend to deal with the more mature tracheostomies which makes reinsertion easier.

The younger the patient the more likely the occurrence of accidental decannulation or obstruction. Infants have short, thick necks that make them prone to dislodgment of the tracheostomy tube (7, 8). Tracheostomy ties may not be snug enough to prevent decannulation. The smaller tracheostomy tubes of young infants also have a narrower internal lumen, making the tubes more susceptible to acute obstruction. Mucous plugging occurs when viscous upper airway secretions occlude the lumen of the cannula, which may already be narrowed by secretions that have previously accumulated and dried. Because infants have less fully developed intercostal and diaphragmatic musculature, they are more likely to be unable to adequately clear a mucous plug from the cannula when it occurs.

INDICATIONS

The need for replacing a tracheostomy cannula in the ED typically occurs after accidental decannulation or obstruction of the tracheostomy tube (secretions, mucous plug, foreign body) (9). The pediatric patient who decannulates or obstructs a tracheostomy tube while being managed in the ED for another problem can normally be managed routinely. However, the child who is brought to the ED for the specific purpose of replacing a tracheostomy cannula may be in significant respiratory distress. The patient may arrive via ambulance, or a worried parent may run into the ED carrying the child. As mentioned previously, the physician who is calm and unhurried, armed with an awareness that the skills required to manage this situation are relatively straightforward, will generally be most effective.

EQUIPMENT

The equipment required for tracheostomy replacement is listed in Table 82.1, with sizes for different ages in Table 82.2. As in airway procedures, the setup of suction, oxygen, and bag-valve-mask for ventilation is key. Appropriate size airway equipment should be immediately available. In critical emergencies, the physician should have endotracheal tubes the same size and one size smaller available (Table 82.2 for exchange sizes). Lastly, set up the equipment necessary to secure the new airway.

PROCEDURE

Initial assessment of the patency or placement of the tracheostomy tube requires

Table 82.1.
Equipment for Tracheostomy Change

Suction—source, catheters
Oxygen—high flow source of 100% O$_2$ (preferably humidified)
Bag-valve-mask—appropriate sizes to cover mouth and nose
Tracheostomy cannulas—appropriate sizes
Endotracheal tubes—appropriate sizes
Laryngoscope—blade, handle, bulb, battery
Tape—tracheostomy twill tape, ''cloth tape''
Bandage scissors
Sterile saline

proper positioning. The patient should be positioned with the head and neck hyperextended to expose the tracheostomy site and improve accessibility of the tracheocutaneous fistula (3–5, 9, 10). In the nondistressed, alert, cooperative patient it is wise to have the parent assist in finding the best position for the child. This may reduce the child's anxiety when the physician accesses the airway. Oxygen should be delivered by face mask over the nares and mouth or tracheostomy stoma. The physician needs to evaluate the patient for signs of tracheostomy cannula dislodgment or obstruction (discussed in Indications in this chapter). If the child is unstable, assistance should be obtained to provide immediate advanced life support.

Replacing Cannula after Accidental Dislodgment

Accidental decannulation is obvious—the cannula is no longer in the stoma (a partial dislodgment should not be overlooked). Ideally a new tracheostomy cannula of the same size and model should be reinserted, but if not immediately available the former tube can be used if it is patent. The obturator should be placed within the outer cannula before insertion, removing the inner cannula first, if present (Fig. 82.1). If time allows, lubricating or wetting the tip of the cannula with a lubricating gel or sterile saline may help ease passage (10, 11). The cannula is most easily manipulated by holding it with the dominant hand either by the flange or like a pencil. It is then gently inserted in a posterior then caudal direction in a single sweeping motion (Fig. 82.2) (10, 12). Once the tracheostomy tube is in place the obturator is removed and the inner cannula (if needed) is reinserted. A bag should then be attached with high flow oxygen and manual breaths provided to check patency and hyperoxygenate.

If resistance is met when reinserting, care must be taken not to force the tube in place creating a false passage in the subcutaneous tissues of the neck. This may have potentially devastating consequences (subcutaneous air, pneumomediastinum, pneumothorax) (11). Notably, the stoma may close after decannulation, even if the tube has been out for only a few hours (9, 11). A smaller

Table 82.2.
Approximate Size of Tracheostomy Cannulas, Endotracheal Tubes, Suction Catheters

	Shiley	Holinger	Portex*	Bivona*	Berdeen*	ETT*	Suction Cath
Premature	00**	00	3.0	2.5–3.0**	—	2.5–3.0	6 Fr
Newborn	0	0	3.0	3.0–3.5	3.5	3.0–3.5	6 Fr
NB–6 mo	0–1	1–2	3.5	3.5–4.0	3.5–4.0	3.5–4.0	6–8 Fr
6–12 mo	1–2	2–3	4.0	4.0–4.5	4.0–4.5	4.0–4.5	8 Fr
12 mo–2 yr	3	3	4.5	4.5–5.0	5.0	4.5–5.0	8 Fr
3–6 yr	4	4	5.0	5.0	5.0	5.0	8–10 Fr
7–10 yr	4	5	5.0	5.0–6.0	6.0	6.0	10 Fr
10–12 yr	6	6	6.0	6.0–7.0	6.0	7.0	10 Fr
12–14 yr	6	6	7.0	7.0	7.0	7.5	10 Fr

* Based on internal diameter in millimeters
** Have neonatal series with shorter lengths
*** **NOTE:** Tracheostomy tubes in infants and young children are usually uncuffed because the airway lumen is small with the cricoid ring as the narrowest portion.

size tracheostomy cannula or an endotracheal tube may be used if the physician is unable to pass the original size cannula (7, 9, 12). When using an endotracheal tube, it is advisable to compare it with the tracheostomy tube length and note the markings to assist in determining the depth of insertion. A more appropriate cannula can be placed at a later time after dilation of the tract.

Another aid for reinsertion for a difficult recannulation involves the passage of a small suction catheter attached to an oxygen source (approximately 0.5 to 1.0 L/min) a short distance into the trachea (4, 6, 9–11). After oxygenation via the catheter, it is necessary to cut the catheter proximally leaving a length of it outside the stoma to thread through a tracheostomy or endotracheal tube. Care should be taken not to let go of the catheter. This is then used as a stylet for the advancement of the new tracheostomy or endotracheal tube over it to avoid creating a false passage (Fig. 82.3). Once the tube is in place the patient must be reevaluated to

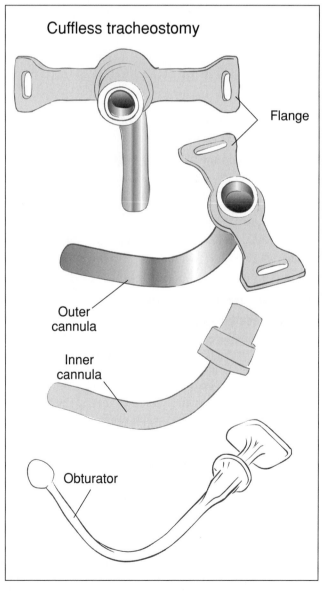

Cuffless tracheostomy

Flange

Outer cannula

Inner cannula

Obturator

Figure 82.1
Tracheostomy tubes with tube, inner cannula, and obturator. (If tracheostomy tube is rigid at the distal end, an obturator is necessary to pass the cannula with risk of minimal tissue damage. Softer cannulas may not require using an internal obturator.)

Chapter 82
Replacement of a
Tracheostomy
Cannula

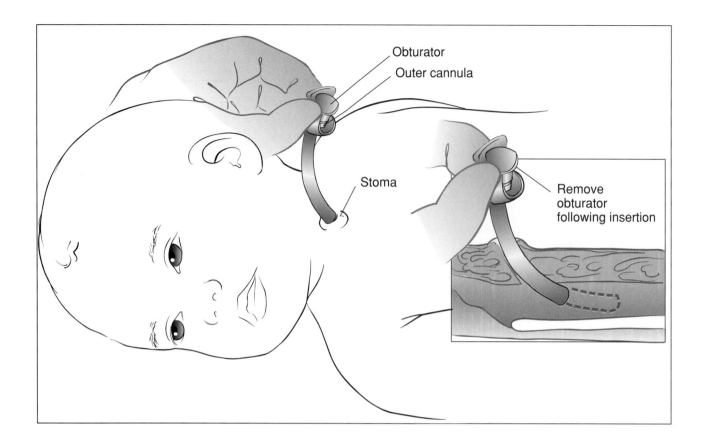

Obturator
Outer cannula
Stoma
Remove obturator following insertion

ensure the adequacy of the airway. If all attempts at recannulation fail, the patient usually can be ventilated via the nose and mouth with a bag and mask with the stoma occluded with a gloved finger and further airway management is undertaken with assistance as needed.

Replacing an Obstructed Tracheostomy Cannula

A child presenting to the ED with a tracheostomy tube in place experiencing respiratory distress, inadequate oxygenation, or ventilation should be assumed to have a mechanical obstruction of the cannula until proven otherwise (9, 11, 12). The patient should be properly positioned and oxygen delivered as previously described. An immediate effort to carefully pass a suction catheter and clear the offending obstruction is made. If this is unsuccessful, 1 to 4 mL sterile saline can be instilled into the tube in an attempt to thin secretions and allow effective clearing of the obstruction with further suctioning. Suctioning should not be ex-

tended for more than 10 seconds after insertion of the catheter into the distal trachea, as longer periods of suction may precipitate hypoxia and cardiac arrest (8, 10). The patient should be ventilated with 100% oxygen between suctioning attempts. The inner cannula can be removed, if present, to aid in relieving the obstruction. The clinician should not hesitate to remove the entire tracheostomy tube if the above-mentioned measures are unsuccessful or immediately if the patient is decompensating. Most patients will breathe easier through just the stoma than a significantly obstructed cannula.

A new tracheostomy cannula is inserted as described earlier. Often the parents have a spare tube, if another of the same size and type is not readily available in the ED. Once the cannula is in place, the patient should be reassessed to check for correct positioning (breath sounds, oxygenation, ventilation).

Securing the Airway

An appropriate method for securing the tube is essential to prevent extubation. Trache-

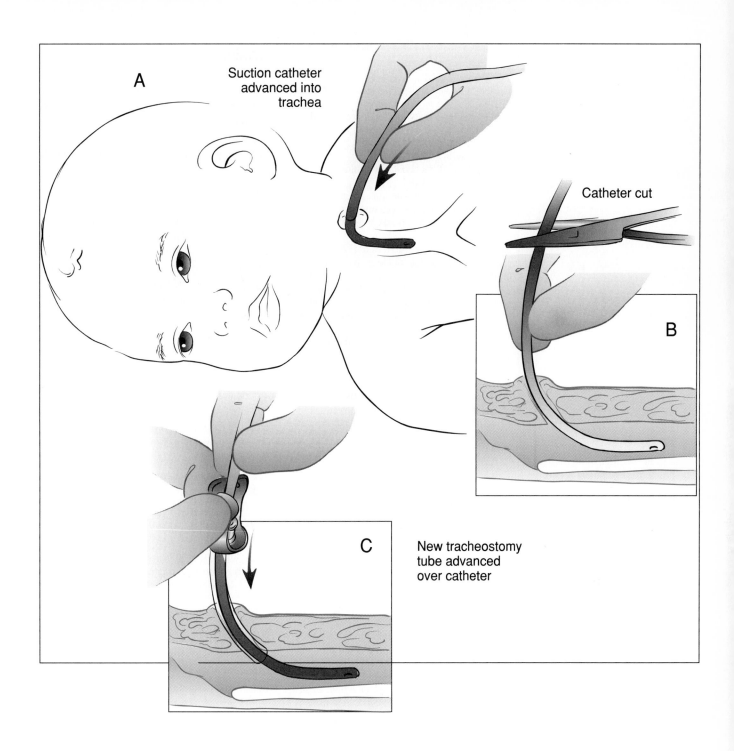

A

Suction catheter
advanced into
trachea

Catheter cut

B

C

New tracheostomy
tube advanced
over catheter

ostomy twill tape is used and should be cut at a length long enough to wrap around the patient's neck twice and an additional 6 to 8 inches for tying. Cutting the ends diagonally will aid insertion through the eyelets of the flange. One end of the tie is threaded through the eyelet and then the ends are pulled even. Both ends of the tape are then slid behind the head and around the neck and one tie is

threaded through the second eyelet. With the neck in a flexed position, the ends are pulled snugly and secured to the flange with a square knot, allowing space for only one finger under the tape once it is tied (9, 10). After the tube is secured and the patient stabilized, a chest radiograph can be obtained to check placement of the distal tip and assess for any pulmonary parenchymal changes.

Figure 82.3
Inserting tracheostomy over red rubber catheter into the airway through the stoma.

**Chapter 82
Replacement of a
Tracheostomy
Cannula**

COMPLICATIONS

Complications are rare if decannulation or obstruction are promptly identified and properly managed. Certainly if adequate oxygenation and ventilation are not provided in a timely fashion, hypoxia and hypercarbia can ensue. It is imperative that both nurses and physicians recognize a patient with a compromised airway and intervene immediately. In a patient with a tracheostomy this should include attempting to clear the obstruction, replacing the cannula, and/or providing bag and mask ventilation until further airway management is undertaken.

Life-threatening pneumomediastinum and pneumothorax can potentially result from false tracking in the subcutaneous tissues of the neck (2, 4, 5, 8). This is more likely to occur in the operative or immediate postoperative period, with interruption of a tissue plane outside the tracheal lumen. In the ED, disruption can be avoided by never attempting to force the cannula into place.

Occasionally granuloma or stricture formation at the stoma or where the tip of the tube meets the tracheal wall can lead to localized bleeding with manipulation of the cannula (2–5, 8). This small amount of bleeding is typically not a problem. Erosion into the innominate artery is a rare occurrence (2, 3, 6, 11), usually related to a inferiorly located tracheostomy stoma and not a consequence of replacement of a tracheostomy cannula.

SUMMARY

In the emergency department, replacing a tracheostomy cannula is frequently performed under anxiety-provoking circumstances. When the physician remains calm, this task is often no more difficult than a routine tracheostomy tube change. Certain factors may contribute to making recannulation more challenging. The goal in any case is to allow for adequate oxygenation and ventilation, whether by clearing the obstruction, replacing the cannula, or providing bag and mask ventilation until further airway management is undertaken.

If the clinician elects to replace the cannula he or she needs to remember to properly position the patient and use correct technique

---

SUMMARY

1. Assess patient—airway, breathing, circulation
2. Position—head and neck hyperextended (roll under shoulder)
3. Oxygenate—100% O_2 via nose, mouth, and/or stoma
4. Determine if tracheostomy cannula is dislodged or obstructed
    a. Attempt to pass suction catheter
    b. Try to ventilate via cannula
    c. Remove inner cannula and repeat steps a. and b.
5. Remove complete tracheostomy tube if dislodged or unable to clear obstruction
6. Recannulate
    a. Select tracheostomy tube, preferably same size and model as original tube (parents often carry a spare one) (Table 82.2)
    b. Remove inner cannula of new tube, if present, and place obturator within outer cannula before insertion
    c. Lubricate tip of cannula
    d. Insert gently in a posterior then caudal direction in one sweeping motion
    e. Remove obturator and replace inner cannula (if needed)
    Note: DO NOT FORCE cannula into place
7. If difficult insertion
    a. Use smaller size tracheostomy tube or endotracheal tube
    b. Consider passing catheter (ideally connected to oxygen source) and use as a stylet. Insert it and oxygenate; cut it longer than cannula length outside of stoma entry and pass tube or cannula over it into airway.
    c. If unsuccessful, bag and mask from above while stoma is covered, until further airway management is undertaken
8. Secure tracheostomy cannula
    a. Cut cloth tape at a length long enough to wrap around neck two times allowing an additional 6 to 8 inches to tie (cut ends on diagonal)
    b. Thread one end through an eyelet and pull ends even (hemostats can assist threading)
    c. Slide both ends under head and around neck, then thread one end of tie through second eyelet
    d. Pull ends snugly with neck in FLEXED position (leaving space for only an index finger snugly under tie)
    e. Secure with a square knot
9. Check for proper placement of new tracheostomy cannula
    a. Auscultate breath sounds
    b. Assess oxygenation and ventilation
    c. Chest radiograph to check distal tip placement

CLINICAL TIPS

1. Have equipment set up before elective procedure.
2. In critical airway obstruction, most children can be oxygenated by bag-valve-mask from the natural airway.
3. To maximally open the tracheostomy stoma, hyperextend the child's neck by placing towel rolls under it.
4. Choose appropriate size equipment. When it is unavailable, remember parents may have a spare tracheostomy tube.
5. If tracheostomy is unavailable, use endotracheal tube through the stoma of same or smaller diameter (Table 82.2).

Chapter 82
Replacement of a Tracheostomy Cannula

to increase the ease and success of insertion. Care must be taken not to force the cannula into place, potentially leading to further complications. Once the cannula is successfully replaced, it must be adequately secured. The patient should be repeatedly assessed to ensure proper positioning of the cannula allowing for optimal oxygenation and ventilation.

REFERENCES

1. Duncan BW, Howell LJ, DeLorimier AA, et al. Tracheostomy in children with emphasis on home care. J Pediatr Surg 1992;27:432–435.
2. Caldwell SL, Sullivan KN. Artificial airways. In: Burton GG, Hodgkin JE, eds. Respiratory care: a guide to clinical practice. 2nd ed. Philadelphia: JB Lippincott, 1984, pp. 493–521.
3. Jardine DS, Crone RK. Specific diseases of the respiratory system: upper airway. In: Fuhrman BP, Zimmerman JJ, eds. Pediatric critical care. St. Louis: CV Mosby, 1992, pp. 425–434.
4. Stool SE, Roland DE. Tracheotomy. In: Bluestone CD, Stool SE, Scheetz MP, eds. Pediatric otolaryngology. Philadelphia: WB Saunders, 1990, pp. 1226–1243.
5. Waring WW. Diagnostic and therapeutic procedures. In: Chernick V, Kendig EL, eds. Disorders of the respiratory tract in children. 5th ed. Philadelphia: WB Saunders, 1990, pp. 77–96.
6. Backofen JE, Rogers MC. Emergency management of the airway. In: Rogers MC, ed. Textbook of pediatric intensive care. 2nd ed. Baltimore: Williams & Wilkins, 1992, pp. 52–74.
7. Perry AG, Potter PA. Clinical nursing skills and techniques. 3rd ed. St. Louis: CV Mosby, 1994, pp. 435–447.
8. Seid AB, Gluckman JL. Tracheostomy. In: Paparella MM, Shumrick DA, Gluckman JL, Mayehoff WL, eds. Otolaryngology. Philadelphia: WB Saunders, 1991.
9. Handler SD. Replacement of a tracheostomy cannula. In: Fleisher GR, Ludwig S, eds. Textbook of pediatric emergency medicine. 3rd ed. Baltimore: Williams & Wilkins, 1993, pp. 1621–1623.
10. Lichtenstein MS. Pediatric home tracheostomy care: a parent's guide. Pediatr Nurs 1986;12:41–48, 69.
11. Katz RL. Tracheotomy care. In: Roberts JR, Hedges JR, eds. Clinical procedures in emergency medicine. 2nd ed. Philadelphia: WB Saunders, 1991, pp. 60–64.
12. Thompson AE. Pediatric airway management. In: Fuhrman BP, Zimmerman JJ, eds. Pediatric critical care. St. Louis: CV Mosby, 1992, pp. 111–128.

SUGGESTED READINGS

Bernahard WN, Yost L, Joynes D, et al. Intracuff pressures in endotracheal and tracheostomy tubes. Chest 1985;87:720–725.
Irving RM., Jones NS, Bailey CM, Melville J. A guide to the selection of paediatric tracheostomy tubes. J Laryngol Otol 1991;105:1046–1051.
Prescott CA. Peristomal complications of pediatric tracheostomy. Int J Pediatr Otorhinolaryngol 1992;23: 141–149.

CHAPTER 83

Thoracentesis

Gregg A. DiGiulio

Introduction

A pleural effusion is a collection of fluid in the potential space that exists between the visceral and parietal pleuras of the lung. The causes of an effusion are varied. In the pediatric patient, acute pulmonary infection is the most common etiology of a pleural effusion, whereas some of the other less common etiologies include collagen-vascular disease, congestive heart failure, hypoalbuminemic states, trauma, or neoplasm (1, 2). Table 83.1 lists some of the various etiologies of pleural effusions. Children with an effusion are usually older than 2 years of age but may be younger especially if it is a parapneumonic effusion (1, 3).

A thoracentesis is a method to remove fluid or air from the pleural space (4). In this chapter, the discussion will be limited to removal of fluid from the pleural space. A discussion relevant to the appropriate management and approach to the treatment of a pneumothorax is described in Chapter 30.

Indications for a thoracentesis include to remove fluid that has caused respiratory embarrassment and to determine the etiology of the effusion (5). Depending on the volume and the characteristics of the pleural fluid, the procedure itself may be either definitive or temporizing. A tube thoracostomy is considered the definitive therapy when an empyema is present or when continued bleeding into the thoracic cavity occurs, as in a traumatic hemothorax (4, 5). The thoracentesis is most frequently performed on a semi-elective basis in a monitored setting. If the effusion is causing significant respiratory distress, however, a more urgent procedure is required.

Anatomy and Physiology

The pleural space is a potential space that exists between the visceral and parietal pleura. Normally this space contains less than 15 cc of pleural fluid (6). The formation of pleural fluid is controlled in part by the effect of Starling forces. The forces affecting net fluid movement across the pleura depend on the capillary and intrapleural hydrostatic pressures, the plasma and intrapleural oncotic pressures, and the capillary filtration coefficient. These forces are summarized in Figure 83.1. In a healthy person, the forces are such that protein-free extracellular fluid enters the pleural space from the parietal pleura and is absorbed at the visceral pleura (6, 7, 8). A small amount of protein in the pleural space leaks into the space from the pleural capillaries. Approximately 10% of the pleural fluid and the protein leave the space through the rich lymphatic supply (7).

In the healthy state, no net accumulation of fluid is evident because of a balance between the Starling forces. A pleural effusion develops when various disease processes alter these forces and lead to net fluid accumulation (7, 8). For example, in the hypoproteinemic state, a decrease in the serum oncotic pressure leads to a gradient favoring fluid transport to the pleural space. Pleural fluid collects in inflammatory diseases, such as pneumonia or serositis due to a collagen vascular disease, through an alteration in the capillary filtration coefficient. A pleural effusion also may develop if obstruction of the lymphatic drainage would occur as with traumatic rupture of the thoracic duct.

Fluid collecting in the pleural cavity affects normal respiratory physiology and may interfere with normal respiratory function. If the effusion is large or has expanded rapidly, it may clinically cause respiratory embarrassment (9). The pleural fluid initially reduces the lung volume and consequently diminishes the vital capacity. If sufficient fluid accumulates, the vital capacity and the functional residual capacity can decrease to the point where distal lung units collapse (i.e., atelectasis). The enlarging effusion also impedes diaphragmatic function and reduces chest wall compliance increasing the work of breathing and making deep sigh breaths more difficult. The final outcome is an impairment of alveolar gas exchange.

INDICATIONS

When the etiology of the pleural effusion is unknown or when respiratory embarrassment occurs because of the effusion, a thoracentesis should be performed. In certain circumstances it may be reasonable to defer thoracentesis and institute therapy when the cause of the effusion is readily apparent. This would be the case in nephrotic syndrome with effusion or from left ventricular heart failure (10). Before attempting the procedure, it may be helpful to consult a specialist in pediatric pulmonary medicine or infectious disease to review issues and determine which laboratory studies should be obtained on the fluid.

Clinical suspicion of a pleural effusion arises when a child presents with pain on inspiration, shortness of breath, dyspnea, decreased breath sounds, and dullness to percussion over the affected area. Occasionally, a pleural friction rub is heard.

An upright PA and lateral chest radiograph will confirm the clinical impression. When the effusion is small, the only radiographic abnormality may be a meniscus or "blunting" at the costophrenic angle on up-

right chest radiograph (11). This occurs with small or large amounts of fluid (i.e., 175 cc to 525 cc) (12). As the effusion enlarges, there is extension of the fluid up the lateral chest wall on the upright view (11). Large effusions may appear to be consolidation or "white out" of the entire lung and may include mediastinal shift away form the affected side (11). In the latter case, ultrasound can be helpful in differentiating an effusion draping the lungs from a complete consolidation of the lung (11).

The appearance of a pleural effusion is somewhat different in recumbent films. If the fluid collection is less than 125 cc, a recumbent film may appear normal despite the presence of an effusion (13). Moderate size effusions appear as a homogeneous density in the lower lung fields, and as the collection enlarges, the entire lung field takes on a ground glass appearance (13). For all suspected pleural effusions, a lateral decubitus radiograph is extremely useful. This radiograph helps identify questionable effusions and also aids in determining whether an effusion is free flowing or loculated (10). Loculated pleural fluid does not shift with position changes. When the fluid appears loculated, consideration should be given to a radiologically guided procedure to ensure proper drainage and decrease the incidence of complications.

The most frequent indication for performing a thoracentesis is as a diagnostic aid. In adults, results of a thoracentesis give diagnostic or clinically useful information in over 90% of examinations when taken in context of the clinical presentation (14).

Once fluid is obtained the most useful information to be determined is whether the fluid is a transudate or an exudate. An exudate implies a breakdown of vascular integrity as seen in infection, neoplasms, or other inflammatory processes as opposed to a transudate which is an ultrafiltrate of plasma. Table 83.1 categorizes the etiologies of pleural effusions as to whether they are associated with an exudative or a transudative process.

Although the laboratory diagnosis of an exudate is not absolute, the criteria established by Light and his colleagues are generally accepted to define an exudative process (10). Light et al. defined an exudate as having any one of the three following characteristics:

1. a pleural/serum protein ratio of >0.5;
2. a pleural/serum LDH ratio of >0.6; or
3. a pleural fluid LDH of more than two-

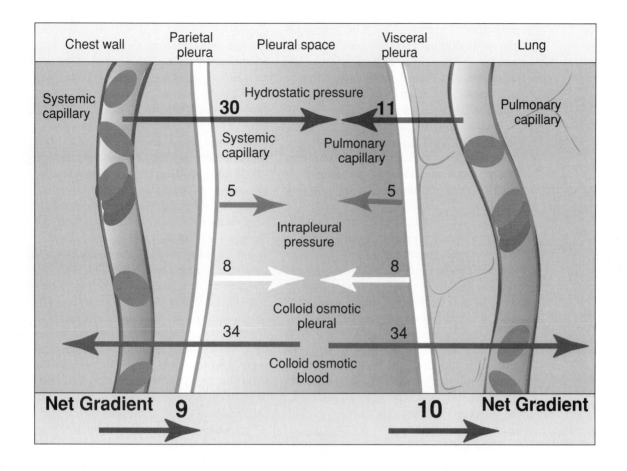

Figure 83.1

Below the figure (labels within the schematic):

Chest wall | Parietal pleura | Pleural space | Visceral pleura | Lung

Systemic capillary

Hydrostatic pressure

30   **11**

Systemic capillary   Pulmonary capillary

Pulmonary capillary

5   5

Intrapleural pressure

8   8

Colloid osmotic pleural

34   34

Colloid osmotic blood

Net Gradient   **9**   **10**   **Net Gradient**

thirds the upper limits of normal for the serum LDH (15).

A transudate will have none of these characteristics. In the initial study by Light et al., sensitivity and specificity of the criteria approached 100%. Later studies on unselected populations have confirmed the high sensitivity of these criteria (16, 17).

If initial studies indicate that the effusion is a transudate, some authorities have suggested that further laboratory evaluation of the fluid is costly and does not increase the diagnostic yield (17, 18). These authorities suggest a two-step approach where the initial laboratory studies are sent to determine whether an exudate or a transudate exists. During the initial collection of fluid, samples should be "held" so that they can be used at a later time. If the laboratory evaluation suggests an exudative process, the history and physical examination should guide further laboratory and diagnostic evaluation. For a transudate, the physician should treat the underlying disease process (5).

Pleural Fluid Laboratory Studies

This section reviews the potential laboratory studies that can be performed in the evaluation of pleural fluid. This is not meant to imply that all studies need to be sent on every patient. Clinical circumstances should guide the subsequent laboratory evaluation.

The gross appearance of the pleural fluid can be helpful. Transudates are often pale yellow. Milky white fluid suggests a chylothorax. Bloody fluid has been associated with neoplasms, pulmonary infarction, or trauma. This finding is tempered by the fact that 2 mL of blood into 1000 mL of fluid can give a bloody appearance (19). A thick, purulent fluid is diagnostic of an empyema.

Pleural fluid is frequently sent for cytologic examination. Some authorities question the utility of cytologic examination for red and white blood cells (10, 19, 20). Light et al. in a prospective study of 182 patients concluded that a red cell count of above 100,000/mm^3 suggested neoplasm, pulmo-

Figure 83.1
Schematic of Starling forces on formation of pleural fluid.

nary infarct, or trauma, but RBC counts between 10,000 and 100,000/mm^3 were not specific for any disease process (19). They also concluded that the absolute white blood cell count is of limited utility due to a lack in both sensitivity and specificity. The differential count, however, may be helpful. A predominance of polymorphonuclear cells usually results from an acute inflammatory process such as pneumonia, pulmonary infarction, or a sympathetic effusion from pancreatitis. The presence of more than 50% lymphocytes strongly correlates with the presence of a malignancy or tuberculosis in patients with exudative effusions. The study did confirm the utility of cytologic examination for malignant cells with a sensitivity of 77% when performed on one sample and of 90% when performed on three samples (19).

Although serosanguineous fluid has no predictive value (10, 19), truly bloody fluid may indicate a traumatic hemothorax. If the hematocrit of the bloody fluid approaches that of serum, a traumatic hemothorax should be suspected and tube thoracostomy considered (5).

The pH, glucose, and Gram stain of the pleural fluid aid in discriminating between complicated parapneumonic effusions (effusions behaving like empyemas and requiring chest tube drainage for resolution), and uncomplicated parapneumonic effusions (that can be managed expectantly with antibiotic therapy). Unfortunately, clinical and radiologic indicators are not sufficiently distinct to separate those children with uncomplicated effusions from those with empyema (2). A pleural fluid pH of less than 7.0 to 7.2, a glucose less than 40 mg/dL, or a positive Gram stain suggests a complicated parapneumonic effusion requiring tube thoracostomy (21, 22). Pleural fluid glucose levels also are decreased in tuberculosis, malignancy, and rheumatoid diseases (5, 23).

When differential diagnosis of the pleural effusion includes parapneumonic effusion or an empyema, a Gram stain and aerobic culture, with consideration of anaerobic culture, should be obtained (10). *Staphylococcus aureus* and *Streptococcus pneumoniae* cause the majority of empyemas in children and adolescents (1, 2, 3, 24, 25). *Streptococcus pyogenes*, Gram-negative bacteria, and now *Haemophilus influenzae* are found less frequently (1, 25). In adult patients, anaerobic bacteria frequently are found alone or in a mixed infection (26). Their role in childhood empyemas is less clear although some authorities suggest that anaerobes may play a significant role when aspiration pneumonia, lung abscess, subdiaphragmatic abscess, or abscesses of dental origin are the underlying cause of the empyema (25).

If tuberculosis is suspected, mycobacterial culture and acid-fast staining of the fluid should be performed. A culture of the pleural fluid for mycobacteria is of low yield, and the diagnosis is best confirmed by acid-fast staining of a needle biopsy of the pleura, sputum culture, or skin test conversion (10, 27).

Several other tests may be helpful in certain clinical circumstances. The amylase will be elevated in effusions caused by acute pancreatitis or esophageal rupture (7, 8). In patients with a malignant effusion the amylase is elevated 10% of the time (7). A creatinine level of the fluid may be elevated in urinothorax from genitourinary injury to the ureter or bladder (5). In patients with a pleural effusion due to lupus erythematosis, an antinuclear antibody titer is frequently greater than 1:160 and the LE cell prep may be positive. Complement levels may be decreased in lupus or other rheumatoid diseases. An elevated rheumatoid factor suggests an effusion due to rheumatoid arthritis (28). A true chylothorax will have triglyceride levels above 110% of the serum triglyceride level and a Sudan III stain of fluid positive for chylomicrons (15).

Relative contraindications to performing a thoracentesis include an uncooperative patient, skin infection at the insertion site, bleeding diathesis, or an insufficient volume of pleural fluid (5, 10). Pleural adhesions increase the risk of pneumothorax, and therefore a thoracentesis should be performed cautiously in these patients (4).

EQUIPMENT

Assemble the necessary equipment listed in Table 83.2. Use the thoracentesis needle on the tray or the largest over-the-needle-catheter possible for the thoracentesis, which is usually an 18- to 22-gauge catheter depending on the size of the child. Commercial kits are available that contain a similar list of supplies.

PROCEDURE

The following method is recommended when an effusion is felt to be free flowing. If the effusion is loculated, one should strongly consider performing the procedure with ultrasound or fluoroscopic guidance to more successfully obtain fluid and decrease the risk of complication (11, 29, 30).

The physician and nurse should explain the procedure to the child in an age-appropriate manner. The time spent preparing the child is well worth the cooperation that the physician will gain. A peripheral intravenous catheter is started in the event that a complication arises. A venous blood sample is drawn to determine the serum LDH and protein levels and other studies as indicated. Monitoring includes continuous pulse oximetry and heart rate with frequent vital signs. Supplemental oxygen is supplied for hypoxemia and the hypoxemia that can arise after the procedure (see Complications in this chapter). For the younger or anxious child, mild, short-acting sedation may be considered. If conscious sedation is used, follow the appropriate monitoring guidelines as established by the American Academy of Pediatrics (31) (see Chapter 35 for sedation guidelines).

A thoracentesis is usually performed with the child in a sitting position (Fig. 83.2). This is best accomplished by having the child lean forward over a pillow that is placed over the back of a chair or table. If the child is unable to sit, the procedure is performed in the lateral decubitus position. The level of dullness is percussed and a chest radiograph is used to identify the best location to perform the thoracentesis. The midscapular line is frequently used although the posterior axillary line also is acceptable (4). When choosing which intercostal space to use, it is important to recall the level of the diaphragm throughout the respiratory cycle. Specifically, the height of the diaphragm is most superior during expiration. The right arch is higher than the left because of the size of the liver. During maximal expiration, the level of the right dome is at the 4th costal cartilage anteriorly,

at the 6th rib laterally, and at the 8th rib posteriorly. The dome of the left arch is one to two ribs below that of the right (32). Overall, the 7th intercostal space posteriorly is a reasonable place to attempt a thoracentesis most of the time and will help prevent accidental puncture of the liver or spleen. When a child raises his or her arm, the tip of the scapula lies at the level of the 7th intercostal space in the posterior axillary line (6).

The area is widely prepared in a sterile manner with an antiseptic. Sterile towels are used to drape the area. With a 27-gauge needle attached to 5-mL syringe filled with local anesthetic, such as 1 or 2% lidocaine with epinephrine, a wheal is raised over the insertion site as identified by the rib below the desired intercostal space. The needle is removed and changed to a 22-gauge needle. Entering directly over and perpendicular to the rib and through the previously raised wheal and by slowly advancing and injecting, one should anesthetize to the periosteum. Then, one should "walk" the needle over the superior margin of the rib, infiltrate, and proceed to aspirate while advancing the needle. The clinician needs to remember to keep the needle perpendicular to the skin surface to minimize the risk of accidental laceration of one of the intercostal arteries that lie along the inferior border of the rib superior to the entry site. Once fluid is aspirated, the physician should stop infiltrating and mark the depth of the needle at the skin surface by cross clamping the needle with a hemostat or a metal spring. The needle, hemostat, and syringe together are then removed from the entry site.

If no fluid is aspirated on entering the pleural space, it is sometimes necessary to enter one intercostal space inferior to the previously selected one. Again the clinician needs to recall the levels of the diaphragm during the respiratory cycle to minimize the risk of injury to the abdominal contents.

A 15- or 30-mL syringe and an over-the-needle catheter are now attached to a three-way stopcock. The previously identified depth of insertion is transferred to this needle by marking the level by grasping the needle between the index finger and thumb. The skin is entered through the anesthetized area and gentle negative pressure applied (Fig. 83.2). Follow the same procedure as was outlined in

Table 83.2. Equipment and Supplies

For procedure:
- Pillow
- Sterile gloves
- Povidone-iodine solution
- Sterile gauze sponges
- Sterile basin for skin preparation
- Sterile towels or drape
- 5-mL syringe
- 27- and 22-gauge needles
- 1% lidocaine
- Hemostat or metal spring
- 15-mL or 30-mL syringe
- One 14-gauge to 22-gauge angiocath or a thoracentesis needle
- Three-way stopcock
- Intravenous tubing—optional
- Vacuum bottle—optional
- Sterile dressing
- Tape to secure bandage

For specimen collection:
- Aerobic and anaerobic culture bottles
- Sterile tubes for mycobacterial or fungal cultures
- Sterile tube for cytology
- Blood gas syringe
- Specimen tube for hematology
- Specimen tube for chemistry
- Other specimen tubes as needed

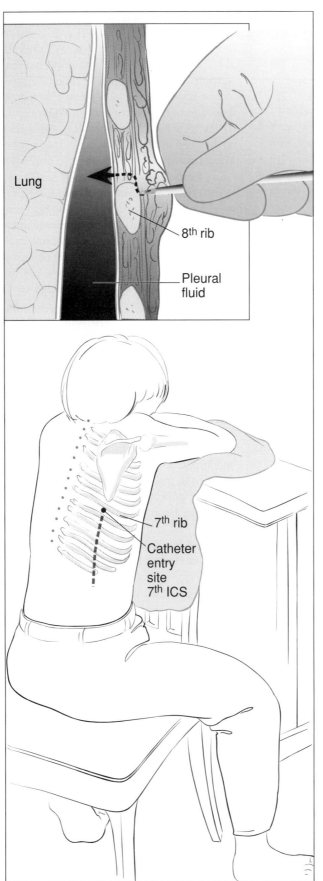

the previous paragraph to advance the needle. Once fluid is obtained, the needle is advanced slightly to ensure that the tip of the catheter is in the pleural space. The catheter is advanced over the needle. One should withdraw the needle and place a finger over the open end of the catheter to prevent the aspiration of air. The syringe and stopcock apparatus are reattached and fluid withdrawn. Although 15 to 30 mL is usually adequate to establish a diagnosis, it may be useful clinically to withdraw more fluid when it appears the fluid is causing respiratory embarrassment. If malignancy is suspected, fluid for cytology requires a volume of 20 to 30 mL. Tubing attached to a vacuum bottle and the open end of the stopcock may help to evacuate a large amount of fluid. Withdraw the fluid into the syringe and expel it into the vacuum bottle.

If the fluid is not free flowing, the child may lean back or to one side. Some commercial, over-the-needle thoracentesis catheters have sideports which may make fluid retrieval easier (Fig. 83.3.A). The catheter is removed and a sterile dressing applied. An urgent upright chest radiograph is obtained looking for an iatrogenic pneumothorax.

Needle Thoracentesis

The above-mentioned procedure also may be done with a needle rather than an over-the-needle catheter. The procedure is performed as previously described except that

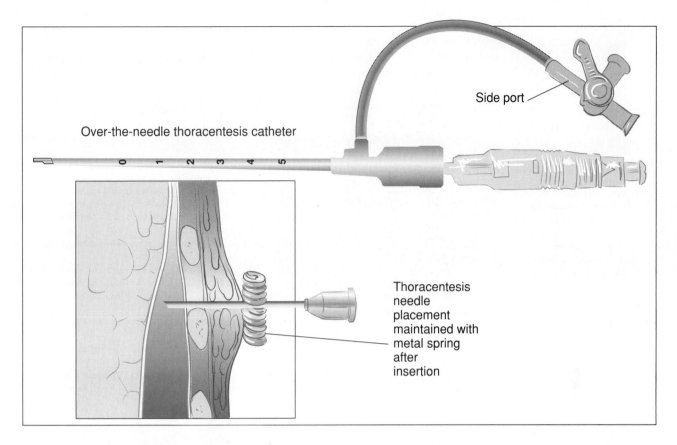

Over-the-needle thoracentesis catheter

Side port

Thoracentesis
needle
placement
maintained with
metal spring
after
insertion

Figure 83.3
Needle thoracentesis with
spring and thoracentesis
catheter.

after the depth of the needle is identified during anesthetic infiltration, this depth should be transferred to the thoracentesis needle by placing a hemostat or metal spring across the thoracentesis needle (Fig. 83.3.B). This will help prevent accidental advancement of the needle into the lung and subsequent pneumothorax. The level of the hemostat sometimes needs to be adjusted slightly.

Other Techniques

Other techniques include using pigtail catheters (29, 33) or semiflexible catheters (34, 35) for the thoracentesis. These can be performed under ultrasound or fluoroscopic guidance (29) or directly if the fluid is free flowing (33). The catheters are introduced into the thoracic cavity via the Seldinger technique. An advantage of this technique is that the catheters, once in place, can be attached to water seal suction drainage and provide continuous drainage (29, 33, 36). The patient can be moved with minimal risk of puncture or injury to the underlying lung.

Otherwise, patient preparation and follow-up is as described previously.

COMPLICATIONS

A diagnostic thoracentesis does carry the risk of significant complications. The most frequent major complication is a pneumothorax, which occurs in up to 11 to 30% of procedures (14, 30, 37). Risk is reduced when the procedure is performed by a clinician well trained in the technique and in a monitored setting with cooperative patients (38). Ultrasound guidance of the procedure appears to significantly decrease the rate of pneumothorax (30). Using mild sedation and measures to suppress the child's cough may lessen the risk of pneumothorax. Other less common complications include laceration of the intercostal vessels and subsequent hemothorax, laceration of the liver or spleen, cough, vasovagal reactions, or persistent local pain (5, 14, 38).

In an adult, no more than 1000 to 1500 mL of fluid should be removed at a time. Re-

Summary

1. Identify effusion and whether it is free flowing with PA and lateral decubitus chest radiograph
2. Monitor with pulse oximetry and frequent vital signs
3. Consider pharmacologic sedation as necessary
4. Position child in sitting position leaning forward over chair
5. Identify insertion site—frequently 7th intercostal space in posterior or posterior axillary line
6. Prepare sterile field and anesthetize skin and tissue to pleura
7. Attach needle or angiocath to three-way stopcock and syringe and walk needle over top of rib while applying negative pressure to syringe
8. Once fluid is obtained, thread angiocath into pleural space
9. Reattach syringe and stopcock to catheter and remove pleural fluid
10. Remove catheter and cover with dressing
11. Obtain chest radiograph looking for iatrogenic pneumothorax
12. Send pleural fluid for protein and LDH. Send patient's serum for protein and LDH. "Hold" other samples in appropriate containers
13. If a transudate is identified, treat underlying cause
14. If an exudate is identified, consider further laboratory analysis relative to presenting history and physical examination

expansion pulmonary edema or severe hypotension has been described if larger volumes are removed (5, 10, 39). Larger volumes can be safely removed if intrapleural pressure is monitored during the procedure and kept above –20 cm H_2O (39). No comparable data are available for children.

Hypoxemia predictably occurs after thoracentesis and correlates directly with the volume of fluid removed (40). Hypoxemia resolves after 24 hours and supplying oxygen during and after the procedure prevents this complication.

Summary

When used to remove pleural fluid causing respiratory embarrassment, a thoracentesis is considered therapeutic. When used to assist in identifying the underlying cause of the effusion, it is considered diagnostic. Important information to obtain is whether the effusion is an exudate or a transudate. The causes of a pleural effusion are diverse, and the evaluation of pleural fluid is particularly useful when taken in context of the clinical presentation. The procedure itself is straightforward and either a needle or a flexible catheter can be used. No matter which method is used, care must be taken so that the risk of pneumothorax is minimized.

Clinical Tips

1. A lateral decubitus chest radiograph identifies free-flowing pleural fluid.
2. A loculated effusion is best approached with an ultrasound-guided thoracentesis.
3. The neurovascular bundle lies along the inferior border of the rib.
4. The 7th intercostal space posteriorly is a safe landmark to attempt a thoracentesis and is located at the tip of the scapula when the arm is completely abducted.
5. If the pleural fluid does not flow freely, try having the child lean back or to the side. If using the needle approach, care must be taken to prevent accidental puncture of the underlying lung. Commercial thoracentesis needles with sideports may ease fluid retrieval.
6. Empyemas and hemothorax require tube thoracostomy.

References

1. Wolfe WG, Spock A, Bradford WD. Pleural fluid in infants and children. Am Rev Respir Dis 1968;98:1027–1032.
2. Chonmaitree T, Powell KR. Parapneumonia pleural effusion and empyema in children. Clin Pediatr 1983;22:414–419.
3. Freij BJ, Kusmiesz H, Nelson JD, McCracken GH. Parapneumonia effusions and empyema in hospitalized children: a retrospective review of 227 cases. Pediatr Inf Dis 1984;3:578–591.
4. Ross DS. Thoracentesis. In: Roberts JR, Hedges JR, eds. Clinical procedures in emergency medicine. 2nd ed. Philadelphia: WB Saunders, 1991, pp. 112–128.
5. Jay SJ. Diagnostic procedures for pleural disease. Clin Chest Med 1985;6:33–48.
6. Zeitlin PL. Pleural effusions and empyema. In: Laughlin GM, Eigen H, eds. Respiratory disease in children. Baltimore: Williams & Wilkens, 1994, pp. 453–463.
7. Light RW. Pleural effusions. Med Clin North Am 1977;61:1339–1352.
8. Sahn SA. The pathophysiology of pleural effusions. Ann Rev Med 1990;41:7–13.
9. Pagtakhan RD, Chernick V. Liquid and air in the pleural space. In: Chernick V, ed. Kendig's disorders of the respiratory tract in children. 5th ed. Philadelphia: WB Saunders, 1990, pp. 545–557.
10. Health and Public Policy Committee, American College of Physicians. Diagnostic thoracentesis and pleural biopsy in pleural effusions. Ann Intern Med 1985:103:799–802.
11. Swischuk LE. Emergency radiology of the acutely ill or injured child. 3rd ed. Baltimore: Williams & Wilkins, 1994.
12. Collins JD, Burwell D, Furmanski S, Lorber P, Steckel RJ. Minimum detectable pleural effusions: a roentgen pathology model. Radiology 1972:105:51–53.
13. Woodring JH. Recognition of pleural effusion on supine radiographs: how much fluid is required. AJR 1984;142:59–64.
14. Collins TR, Sahn SA. Thoracentesis: clinical value, complications and experience. Chest 1987;91:817–822.
15. Light RW, MacGregor I, Ruchsinger PC, et al. The diagnostic separation of transudates from exudates. Ann Intern Med 1973:132:854.
16. Romero S, Candela A, Martin C, et al. Evaluation of different criteria for the separation of pleural transudates from exudates. Chest 1993;104:339–404.
17. Peterman TA, Speicher CE. Evaluating pleural effusions: a two-stage laboratory approach. JAMA 1984;252:1051–1053.
18. Sahn SA. The differential diagnosis of pleural effusions. West J Med 1982;137:99–108.
19. Light RW, Erozan YS, Ball WC. Cells in pleural fluid: their value in differential diagnosis. Arch Intern Med 1973; 132:854–860.
20. Dine DZ, Pierce AV, Franzen SS. The value of cells in the pleural fluid in the differential diagnosis. Mayo Clin Proc 1975;50:571–572.
21. Houston MC. Pleural fluid pH: therapeutic, and prognostic value. Am J Surg 1987;154:333–337.

22. Light RW, Giraud WM, Jenkinson SG, et al. Parapneumonia effusions. Am J Med 1980;69:507–512.

23. Lillington GA, Carr DT, Mayne JG. Rheumatoid pleurisy with effusion. Arch Intern Med 1971;128:764–768.

24. Fajardo JE, Chang MJ. Pleural empyema in children: a nationwide retrospective study. South Med J 1987;80:593–596.

25. Brook I. Microbiology of empyema in children and adolescents. Pediatrics 1990;85:722–726.

26. Bartlett JG, Gorbach SL, Thadepalli H, Finegold SM. Bacteriology of empyema. Lancet 1974;1:338–339.

27. Van Hoff DD, LiVolsi V. Diagnostic reliability of needle biopsy of the parietal pleura. Am J Clin Pathol 1975;64:200–203.

28. Halla JT, Schrohenloher RE, Volanakis JE. Immune complexes and other laboratory features of pleural effusions. Ann Intern Med 1980;92:748–752.

29. Westcott JL. Percutaneous catheter drainage of pleural effusion and empyema. AJR 1985;144:1189–1193.

30. Grogan DR, Irwin RS, Channick R, et al. Complications associated with thoracentesis: a prospective randomized study comparing three different methods. Arch Intern Med 1990;150:873–877.

31. Committee on Drugs. Guidelines for monitoring and management of pediatric patients during and after sedation for diagnostic and therapeutic procedures. Pediatrics 1992;89:1110–1115.

32. Pick TP, Howden R, eds. Gray's anatomy. Philadelphia: Running Press, 1974.

33. Fuhrman BP, Landrum BG, Ferrara TB, et al. Pleural drainage using modified pigtail catheters. Crit Care Med 1986;14:575–576.

34. Cooper CMS. Pleural aspiration with a central venous catheter. Anesthesia 1987;42:217.

35. Clarke JM. A new instrument for thoracentesis. Surg Gyne Obst 1984;159:587–588.

36. Crouch JD, Keagy BA, Delany DJ. "Pigtail" catheter drainage in thoracic surgery. Am Rev Respir Dis 1987;136:174–175.

37. Seneff MG, Corwin W, Gold LH, Irwin RS. Complications associated with thoracentesis. Chest 1986;89:97–100.

38. Bartter T, Mayo PD, Pratter MR, et al. Lower risk and higher yield for thoracentesis when performed by experienced operators. Chest 1993;103:1873–1876.

39. Light RW, Jenkinson SG, Minh V, George R. Observations on pleural fluid pressures as fluid is withdrawn during thoracentesis. Am Rev Resp Dis 1980;121:799–804.

40. Brandstetter RD, Cohen RP. Hypoxemia after thoracentesis. JAMA 1979;242:1060–1061.

INTRODUCTION TO MECHANICAL VENTILATION

Joseph W. Luria

INTRODUCTION

The appropriate use of mechanical ventilation is a requisite skill for all physicians caring for children who are critically ill. The first widespread use of ventilators in a nonoperative setting occurred during the polio epidemic of the 1950s. Since that time, ventilators and ventilation strategies have become more sophisticated and, for some, more challenging. Although ventilators may seem to be complex machines, a few basic principles govern their function. Once these principles are understood and applied correctly, ventilator management can proceed in an effective manner.

ANATOMY AND PHYSIOLOGY

The respiratory cycle consists of inspiration and exhalation. Inspiration is an active process initiated by contraction of the intercostal musculature and diaphragm. The actions of these muscles cause an expansion of the chest cavity, which generates a negative transpleural pressure. Air flows along the resultant pressure gradient (between the atmosphere and pleural space) through the airways and into the lungs. Exhalation, which eliminates air after alveolar gas exchange, is largely a passive process due to the elastic recoil of the lung.

The two forces that affect airflow through the respiratory tree are compliance and resistance. Compliance represents the elasticity of the respiratory system and is defined as the unit change in lung volume per unit change in pressure. When respiratory compliance decreases, the lung is often described as being "stiff." The lung and chest wall have their own respective compliances and each contributes to the total compliance of the respiratory system. Adult respiratory distress syndrome (ARDS), neonatal RDS, and the presence of pulmonary edema are examples of clinical scenarios in which respiratory compliance is decreased.

Resistance describes the impedance of airflow due to friction. It is defined as the unit change in pressure per unit change in gas flow. Respiratory resistance is greatest in the airways. Processes that cause a narrowing of the airways, such as asthma or viral croup, will increase respiratory resistance.

Work of breathing is the amount of effort required to overcome both the respiratory compliance and resistance. Processes that decrease compliance or increase resistance will increase the total work of breathing. In these settings, patients will compensate by adopting a respiratory pattern that minimizes their work of breathing. Generally, acute lung processes that decrease compliance are associated with rapid, shallow breathing. In contrast, processes that increase respiratory resistance are associated with slow, deep breathing. These breathing patterns can be useful clinical clues when determining a patient's underlying pathophysiology.

The volume of air that is moved into the lungs during a normal inspiration is termed the tidal volume. Normal tidal volume at all ages is 6 to 8 mL/kg. Functional residual capacity (FRC) or resting volume is the amount of air remaining in the lungs at the end of a normal, quiet exhalation. FRC is determined by two opposing forces that are equal at the end of exhalation. These are the elastic properties of the lung and chest wall. At FRC, the elasticity of the lung exerts a force that favors a reduction in lung volume. The elastic force of the chest wall favors expansion. Processes that alter the relationship between these two forces will alter the FRC. Closing capacity is the volume of air in the lung below which small airways begin to collapse. Any disease state that increases the closing capacity or decreases the FRC can result in airway collapse and atelectasis. One objective of mechanical ventilation is to optimize the relationship between closing capacity and FRC. For example, closing capacity occurs at greater lung volumes in premature infants with surfactant deficiency (RDS). The goal of positive pressure ventilation in this setting is to increase the FRC above closing capacity by using positive end-expiratory pressure (PEEP). This will prevent further atelectasis and assist in the reexpansion of collapsed segments of the lung. These lung volumes are illustrated in the spirogram in Figure 84.1.

The central nervous system (CNS) coordinates the actions of the respiratory muscles. The respiratory muscles are responsible for the bellowslike action that brings oxygen into the lungs and expels carbon dioxide. The lungs provide the interface for the transfer of oxygen into the blood and the removal of carbon dioxide. The circulatory system is responsible for delivering oxygen to the tissues and bringing carbon dioxide back to the lung for removal. In a simplistic manner, this describes the big picture of normal respiration. Processes that depress the CNS (i.e., traumatic brain injury, narcotic intoxication), weaken the respiratory musculature (i.e., Guillain-Barré syndrome, poliomyelitis, myopathies), or affect the lung or heart can lead to respiratory failure.

A large number of pulmonary and cardiac processes can result in respiratory failure. The end result of these processes is impaired pulmonary gas exchange with or without increased work of breathing. Impaired gas exchange results in the inability of the circulation to deliver adequate amounts of oxygen to peripheral tissues. To meet the oxygen demands of the body, minute ventilation and/or cardiac output must be increased. To accomplish this, the respiratory and cardiac musculature are forced to work harder. This additional work of breathing increases the oxygen consumption of the cardiopulmonary system. To meet the higher oxygen demand, minute ventilation and/or cardiac output must be further increased. If the underlying insult is severe or is not corrected, this cycle will continue until demand cannot be met. Then it will not be possible to meet the oxygen requirements of the body, the respiratory musculature will fatigue, and respiratory failure will ensue. This concept as it pertains to specific pathophysiologic processes is discussed in the Procedure section later in this chapter.

INDICATIONS

Respiratory failure is the primary indication for initiating mechanical ventilation. Respiratory failure is characterized as the inability to maintain adequate oxygenation and/or ventilation despite using more conservative respiratory therapies. Traditionally, hypoxemic respiratory failure is defined as a P_AO_2 of less than 55 to 60 torr in the face of inspired oxygen con-

Figure 84.1
Spirogram illustrating lung volumes. ERV, expiratory reserve volume; FRC, functional residual capacity; IRV, inspiratory reserve volume; TV, tidal volume. (Adapted from Rogers MC, ed. Textbook of Pediatric Intensive Care. Baltimore: Williams & Wilkins, 1987:115.)

**Chapter 84
Introduction to
Mechanical
Ventilation**

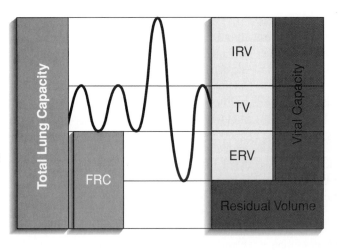

centrations of greater than 60%. Inadequate ventilation is defined as the presence of respiratory acidosis, elevated P_ACO_2, with an arterial pH of less than 7.2 to 7.25. These numbers are guidelines and should not be used as absolute values. The clinician in his or her decision to begin mechanical ventilation should consider the disease process present and its anticipated progression, the patient's clinical assessment and response to other therapies, and the risks associated with mechanical ventilation.

Impending respiratory failure with or without increased work of breathing constitutes a relative indication for mechanical ventilation. It is always preferable to initiate mechanical ventilation under controlled conditions rather than to wait for worsening acidosis, exhaustion, or cardiorespiratory collapse.

In some medical and surgical conditions, it may be best for a patient to assume a specific respiratory pattern. When this occurs, mechanical ventilation can be used to achieve this goal. The most common example of this is the need for hyperventilation in a patient with intracranial hypertension. Table 84.1 reviews these indications for initiating mechanical ventilation.

Mechanical ventilation may be an indicated treatment in a number of clinical diseases. Specific details of ventilator management are highly dependent on the disease state present and its severity; therefore, specific pathophysiologic processes and how they relate to ventilator management will be discussed in the Procedure section later in this chapter.

Table 84.1.
Indications for Initiating Mechanical Ventilation

Absolute Indications:
  Apnea
  Inadequate oxygenation (despite F_1O_2 >60%)
  1. PaO_2 <55–60 torr
  2. O_2 saturation <90%
  Inadequate ventilation—Respiratory acidosis (hypercapnia; pCO_2 >50) with pH <7.2–7.25
Relative Indications:
  Increased work of breathing
  1. Circulatory insufficiency
  2. Prolonged respiratory distress
  Need to control respiratory pattern—Intracranial hypertension

Adapted from Rogers MC, ed. Textbook of Pediatric Intensive Care. Baltimore: Williams & Wilkins, 1987.

EQUIPMENT

To use a ventilator effectively, it is important to have a basic understanding of how it works and a common vocabulary for describing its function. Similar to spontaneous respiration, mechanical breaths may be divided into four phases: transition from exhalation to inspiration, inspiration, transition from inspiration to exhalation, and exhalation. The goal of the operator is to select ventilator settings to perform these phases of respiration in a manner that is optimal for the patient.

Transition from exhalation to inhalation refers to the way in which a ventilator initiates a mechanical breath. For practical purposes, initiation of a mechanical breath can be controlled by either time or pressure. When a breath is initiated because a preset time has elapsed, the ventilation is said to be time triggered. A pressure-triggered breath is initiated in response to a spontaneous respiratory effort. Contraction of the respiratory musculature from a spontaneous breath results in a negative transpleural pressure. This negative pressure is transmitted through the respiratory tree to the endotracheal tube, and into the ventilator circuit. The ventilator will sense this decrease in the circuit pressure and a positive pressure breath will be delivered.

Once a mechanical breath has been initiated, the ventilator must deliver an effective tidal volume, which is accomplished by preselecting limits for the inspiration. For instance, if the inspiratory pressure reaches a constant value before inspiration ends, it is a pressure limited breath. If a constant volume or flow rate is reached before the end of inspiration, the breath is volume or flow limited, respectively. Some ventilators also have the capability to select an inspiratory flow pattern (constant, sinusoidal, accelerating, or decelerating). Despite a number of studies, data fails to demonstrate any advantage of one gas flow pattern over the others in all circumstances.

Cycling refers to the manner by which a ventilator transitions from inspiration to exhalation. If inspiration ceases after a preset time, the breath is said to be time cycled. Likewise, if inspiration ceases after a preset volume or inspiratory pressure is reached, the breath is volume or pressure cycled, respectively.

Exhalation proceeds after a valve is opened within the exhalatory limb of the ventilator circuit. As with normal respiration, exhalation is a passive process. During mechanical ventilation, the patient will remain in the exhalation phase until another breath is triggered.

Ventilators are described by the manner in which they operate during the first three phases of respiration. For example, an infant ventilator may be described as providing time-triggered, pressure-limited, and time-cycled breaths. Most clinicians, however, do not routinely refer to ventilator function in this manner. Rather, they refer to a particular mode of ventilation. A mode of ventilation is a shorthand method for describing how a ventilator performs the phases of the respiration. Modes of ventilation are selected based on the clinical situation.

Control Mode Ventilation

Control mode ventilation (CMV) is time triggered. Each breath is initiated at a preset time interval. By definition, the ventilator will not respond to the patient's spontaneous respiratory efforts. CMV should be reserved for patients who are apneic. A patient who is breathing spontaneously would be uncomfortable on this mode of ventilation because it would not be responsive to his or her needs and would give the alert patient breaths asynchronously with the patient's spontaneous respiration.

Assist Mode Ventilation

In assist mode ventilation, mechanical breaths are initiated by the patient's spontaneous respiratory effort. The ventilator accomplishes this by sensing a change in circuit pressure or gas flow (pressure or flow triggered). This mode allows the patient to "interact" with the ventilator. That is, the ventilator is responsive to the patient's needs on a synchronous fashion. The assist mode is rarely used by itself because no respiratory support would be afforded to a patient who became apneic.

Assist/Control Mode Ventilation

Assist/control mode breaths are initiated in response to the patient's spontaneous respiratory efforts. If a breath is not initiated during a preset time interval, however, the ventilator will deliver a controlled breath. This combination of assisted and controlled breaths offers the advantages of both modes. It allows the patient to interact with the ventilator, thereby serving the patient's respiratory needs. Should the patient become apneic or too weak to initiate a mechanical breath, the ventilator would continue to provide support in the form of controlled breaths triggered by a period of apnea.

Intermittent Mandatory Ventilation

Intermittent mandatory ventilation (IMV) was initially developed as a method for weaning patients from CMV back to total independent spontaneous respiration. During IMV, mechanical breaths are delivered at a preset frequency (time triggered). In between mechanical breaths, the patient is allowed to breathe spontaneously. Spontaneous breaths are permitted by one of two mechanisms. The ventilator will either have a continuous flow of gas in the circuit or an intermittent flow of fresh gas which is accessed by the patient's spontaneous effort opening a demand valve.

IMV is thought to have a number of benefits. First, it decreases the amount of positive pressure to which the lung is subjected. It has been suggested that this will decrease the impedance of venous return to the right heart associated with positive pressure ventilation. Spontaneous respiration also is associated with improved ventilation to the dependent areas of the lung, which theoretically should result in less ventilation-perfusion ($\dot{V}/\dot{Q}$) mismatching. In addition, allowing spontaneous breathing will assist in preserving the patient's respiratory muscular tone.

Synchronized Intermittent Mandatory Ventilation

Synchronized intermittent mandatory ventilation (SIMV) is similar to IMV except that mechanical breaths are triggered by the patient's respiratory effort instead of being time triggered. If no effort is detected during a preset time interval, a controlled breath is delivered. Like IMV, the patient breathes spontaneously between ventilator breaths. The advantage of SIMV is that it allows the patient to interact with the ventilator to a greater degree, and thus allows the patient to be more comfortable while on the ventilator. If a high enough rate is selected, this mode is similar to the assist/control mode.

Mandatory Minute Ventilation

Mandatory minute ventilation (MMV) is used during the process of weaning a patient from the ventilator. The patient breathes spontaneously while the ventilator measures his or her minute ventilation (frequency $\times$ tidal volume). A mechanical breath is delivered when the patient's cumulative minute ventilation falls below a preset amount. As the patient's spontaneous respiration improves, the amount of mechanical respiratory support decreases. MMV is not commonly used in the United States because no clear advantage over more frequently used modes has been demonstrated in the literature.

Pressure Support Ventilation

Pressure support ventilation (PSV) is pressure triggered, pressure limited, and flow cycled. This means that mechanical breaths are initiated by the patient's spontaneous effort. The ventilator then delivers a preset pressure into the circuit. This pressure can be set to provide any fraction of the total respiratory support needed by the patient. The ventilator cycles to exhalation when the flow in the circuit decreases below some preset level. This allows the patient to determine the length and volume of the delivered breath. Pressure support can be used solely or to assist sponta-neous respiration between mandatory breaths as a method of weaning.

Continuous Positive Airway Pressure/Positive End-Expiratory Pressure

The application of a continuous airway distending pressure in the absence of mechanical breaths is referred to as continuous positive airway pressure (CPAP). When mechanical breaths are present, this baseline airway pressure is termed positive end-expiratory pressure (PEEP). The advantage of CPAP/PEEP is that it increases FRC by reexpanding atelectatic areas of the lung, which improves respiratory compliance and ultimately decreases the patient's work of breathing. The recruitment of atelectatic areas of the lung also decreases $\dot{V}/\dot{Q}$ mismatch, improving oxygenation. A lower, less toxic concentration of oxygen can then be used.

CPAP and PEEP must be used with caution. It should never be used in respiratory diseases associated with overinflation, such as asthma. When used in these settings, CPAP/PEEP is associated with a number of complications related to increased alveolar distending pressures. Higher distending pressures can result in decreased venous return to the right heart, and thus will decrease cardiac output and impair oxygen delivery to the tissues. Intravascular volume expansion may minimize this effect. Increased distending pressures also translate into higher mean airway pressures, which increase the likelihood of complications from pulmonary barotrauma. Additionally, overdistention of alveoli can cause increased $\dot{V}/\dot{Q}$ mismatching, resulting in decreased oxygen delivery to peripheral tissues.

CPAP/PEEP also is associated with an increase in intracranial pressure. Consequently, elevated levels of CPAP/PEEP should be avoided in patients with intracranial hypertension.

PROCEDURE

Initiation of mechanical ventilation begins with selecting an appropriate ventilator. In most situations, choices are limited to either a volume controller or a pressure controller. Volume controllers are used most commonly in children weighing greater than 10 kg. They offer the advantage of being able to track changing respiratory compliance. When a patient's compliance decreases, pulmonary pressures increase as the delivered tidal volume remains constant. Ventilators of this type are equipped with an alarm to indicate increasing airway pressures, which assists in more effective ventilator management. Most volume controllers, however, cannot deliver the small tidal volumes required for patients weighing less than 10 kg.

Pressure controllers are most commonly used in smaller children and neonates. In contrast to volume controllers, delivered tidal volumes depend on the patient's respiratory compliance and resistance. A decrease in compliance will result in a smaller tidal volume as peak inspiratory pressure is constant. Because no procedure exists to directly measure tidal volume when using these ventilators, adequacy of ventilation is assessed clinically (i.e., chest excursion and auscultation of breath sounds) and by blood gas determination.

As with most procedures, using a systematic approach helps to avoid errors and omissions. The following information provides a starting point for initiating mechanical ventilation. It is not meant to imply that a "cook book approach" to mechanical ventilation is available that will work in all situations. The method in which a patient is ventilated is largely determined by the underlying disease process present.

Volume Controlled Ventilation

The first step in initiating volume controlled ventilation (Table 84.2) is selecting a mode. The most commonly used modes are SIMV and assist/control. They allow the most patient-ventilator interaction and will ensure adequate ventilation should the patient become apneic or too weak to initiate a breath. SIMV offers a number of advantages over the assist/control mode and is often the first choice. When initiating mechanical ventilation, a higher ventilator respiratory rate can be selected, and the ventilator will perform in a manner similar to the assist/control mode. As the patient's respiratory status improves, the ventilator rate can be decreased, allowing the patient to take a larger number of unassisted breaths which will provide a means for weaning the patient from the ventilator. In the assist/control mode, both spontaneous and time-triggered breaths are assisted. This exposes the patient to more positive airway pressure and its associated risks.

Regardless of the type of mode selected, it is important to ensure adequate alveolar ventilation and tissue oxygenation. Alveolar ventilation is determined by tidal volume and frequency of ventilation (rate). As previously stated, tidal volume of a normal patient is ap-

Table 84.2.
Initial Ventilator Setup

	Volume Controller	Pressure Controller
1. Select a ventilatory mode	Usually SIMV, but assist/control may be used	Infant ventilators usually have only one mode (time triggered, pressure limited, time cycled)
2. Provide adequate inspiration	Tidal volume of 10 mL/kg (Range is usually 8–15 mL/kg)	PIP to cause adequate inspiration to rise and fall of chest with good breath sounds Newborn well 15 cm H_2O RDS 25 cm H_2O 1 year 20–30 cm H_2O
3. Set the ventilator frequency	Physiologic norm for age (Table 84.3)	Physiologic norm for age (Table 84.3)
4. Set the inspiratory time (I time)	Calculated to keep I : E ratio of 1 : 2, unless clinically contraindicated	Calculated to keep I : E ratio of 1 : 2, unless clinically contraindicated
5. Set the F_iO_2	100% initially, then wean to maintain adequate O_2 saturation	100% initially, then wean to maintain adequate O_2 saturation
6. Set the PEEP	3–5 cm H_2O pressure, unless clinically contraindicated	3–5 cm H_2O pressure, unless clinically contraindicated
7. Assess the patient	Clinically and by blood gas determination, to ensure adequate oxygenation and ventilation	Clinically and by blood gas determination, to ensure adequate oxygenation and ventilation

proximately 6 to 8 mL/kg. The tidal volume set on the ventilator, however, should range from 8 to 15 mL/kg. Tidal volume at 10 mL/kg is a reasonable starting point. One reason for the difference is that the ventilator circuit is compressible and some of the delivered tidal volume will remain within it. Ventilator rate is usually set at the age-specific norm (Table 84.3).

Next the operator must select an inspiratory time. Inspiratory time is calculated after determining the desired respiratory rate. Under normal circumstances, one-third of a normal respiratory cycle is spent in inspiration (I:E ratio of 1:2). If a respiratory rate of 20 is desired, for example, each breath will take 3 seconds. The inspiratory time should be set at one-third this value or 1 second.

Oxygenation is determined by F_iO_2 and mean airway pressure. Initially the ventilator should be set to deliver 100% oxygen. This setting should be weaned provided oxygenation is adequate (SaO_2 greater than 95%). Mean airway pressure is most commonly augmented by the application of PEEP, which is usually set at 3 to 5 cm H_2O, unless clinically contraindicated. If the F_iO_2 can be weaned to less than 60%, this level of PEEP should be maintained. Under certain clinical situations, it will be necessary to further increase the PEEP so the F_iO_2 can be weaned to less toxic levels.

Assessment of Settings

After selecting these parameters, it is important for the clinician to assess the adequacy of mechanical ventilation, which is accomplished by observing the rise and fall of the chest and auscultating breath sounds. If ventilation appears to be inadequate, the tidal volume should be increased. In contrast, the tidal volume should be decreased if the observed chest movement is hyperdynamic. Adequate oxygenation should be assessed both clinically (i.e., color, heart rate) and by measurement of the oxygen saturation. After the patient has been stabilized, these observations should be verified by arterial blood gas determination.

If concerns exist over the patient's oxygenation or ventilation, use of the ventilator should be discontinued and the patient ventilated with a bag-valve device with 100% oxygen. If the patient can be adequately ventilated with a bag-valve device but deteriorates when placed on the ventilator, either a mechanical problem exists or inadequate ventilation parameters were selected. The ventilator should be checked to ensure proper setup. Respiratory therapy staff can be an excellent resource for this problem. If the patient's clinical condition does not improve with manual ventilation, a problem with the patient may exist. The position and patency of the endotracheal tube should be assessed. The patient also should be evaluated for any possible complications of positive pressure ventilation such as pneumothorax. When the specific problem is identified and corrected, the patient can then be reconnected to the ventilator and another assessment performed. Afterward a blood gas determination should be made to ensure adequate CO_2 elimination and oxygenation. Adjustments in the ventilation parameters are made on the basis of these observations. Table 84.2 summarizes the steps for initiating volume controlled ventilation.

Most conscious patients who are being mechanically ventilated will have some degree of pain and/or anxiety. Clinically, the patient will appear to be fighting the ventilator, which can result in difficulties with oxygenation and ventilation. When this occurs, it is important for the clinician to exclude any problems with patient condition or ventilator function. Sedatives and/or analgesics can then be used to make the patient more comfortable and thereby enhance patient-ventilator interaction.

Pressure Controlled Ventilation

The major difference between pressure controlled and volume controlled ventilation is that a peak inspiratory pressure (PIP) is selected instead of a tidal volume. An easy method to determine the initial PIP is to use a manometer attached to the endotracheal tube through a bag-valve device. While manually ventilating, the clinician notes the peak pressure required to demonstrate an adequate rise of the chest. This pressure should then serve as the PIP when initiating mechanical ventilation. If a manometer is not available, clinical experience will help dictate the initial PIP setting. In general, a neonate with no lung disease will require a PIP of about 15 cm

Table 84.3.
Suggested Ventilator
Rates Based On Age

Age	Rate (per min)
<2 mo	40
2 mo–6 mo	35
6 mo–12 mo	30
12 mo–6 yr	25
>6 yr	20

H_2O, whereas a neonate with RDS will need about 25 cm H_2O. In children weighing closer to 10 kg, a PIP of 20 to 30 is commonly needed to provide an adequate tidal volume. An even higher PIP may be necessary depending on the severity of the lung disease. Ventilatory frequency and inspiratory time should be set at the age-appropriate physiologic norm. As with volume controlled ventilation, the F_iO_2 should be initially set at 100% and the PEEP at 3 to 5 cm H_2O pressure.

After the patient is connected to the ventilator, a clinical assessment of the adequacy of ventilation should be performed as described after setup of volume ventilation. It is important to remember that no direct measurement of tidal volume is available while using pressure controlled ventilation. Therefore, more frequent blood gas determinations are often necessary, at least initially, to help gauge the patient's clinical condition. Noninvasive monitoring with pulse oximetry (Chapter 77) and end-tidal capnometry (Chapter 78) also can be helpful. As described earlier, sedatives and/or analgesics (Chapter 35) should be used to maintain patient comfort while on the ventilator. Table 84.2 summarizes the steps for initiating pressure controlled ventilation.

When determining the best strategy for ventilating a patient, the pathophysiology of the underlying disease process must be considered. This is not only important for providing effective ventilation, but also for avoiding complications. Ventilator management as it pertains to specific pathophysiologic processes will be discussed next.

Parenchymal Lung Disease

The hallmark of most parenchymal lung diseases is the formation of pulmonary edema. The decrease in FRC and the increase in closing capacity that results leads to subsegmental atelectasis. Ultimately, difficulties in maintaining adequate oxygenation ensue because of ventilation-perfusion mismatch. Therapy should be directed at increasing FRC above closing capacity which can be accomplished through the application of increased levels of PEEP. The amount of PEEP needed will directly correlate with the sever-

ity of the pulmonary insult. PEEP should be further increased in a stepwise fashion by 2 to 3 cm H_2O pressure until adequate oxygenation is achieved with nontoxic levels of oxygen (an F_iO_2 of less than 60%). As discussed, increased PEEP can have adverse effects on venous return to the right heart and cardiac output. These adverse effects can be lessened by intravascular volume loading. Care must be taken to select the amount of PEEP that will optimize oxygenation and cardiac output.

Worsening parenchymal lung disease is associated with a decrease in respiratory compliance. If the tidal volume is held constant, peak inflating pressures will increase. High inflating pressures are associated with pressure-induced lung injuries. One ventilation strategy used to avoid these complications is pressure controlled ventilation with permissive hypercapnia. The goals of this strategy are to maintain adequate oxygenation while limiting maximal lung inflation pressures. This goal is accomplished by restricting the PIP to less than 35 to 40 cm H_2O pressure, PEEP to less than 15 cm H_2O pressure, and F_iO_2 to less than 60%. If oxygenation is still marginal (below 85% SaO_2), further increases in mean airway pressure are achieved by increasing the inspiratory time (shortening the I:E ratio). In addition, careful attention to fever control and appropriate use of sedation will help decrease the end organ oxygen demands.

This combination of decreased peak inspiratory pressure, increased PEEP, and longer inspiratory time will reduce minute ventilation. The resultant increase in pCO_2 is termed permissive hypercapnia because this is the desired effect. Under these conditions, attempts to normalize the pCO_2 would require an increase in the ventilatory frequency. Unfortunately, using a longer inspiratory time and increased ventilatory rate will result in the delivery of a mechanical breath before the preceding exhalation is complete. This "stacking of breaths" will lead to alveolar overdistention and higher airway pressures. The patient should, therefore, be managed in a hypercapnic state. In their review, Feihl and Perret (2) have reported that patients can be safely managed with a pCO_2 of up to 80 mm Hg. Hypercarbia is well tolerated when developed chronically, due to a compensatory metabolic alkalosis. In the acute situation, sodium bicarbonate or THAM, an amine buffer that does not generate CO_2, may be administered to correct a respiratory acidosis when the pH falls below 7.15. Permissive hypercapnia is contraindicated in patients with increased intracranial pressure, because carbon dioxide is a potent cerebral vasodilator and, under these conditions, intracranial pressure may worsen.

Lower Airway Obstruction

Diseases such as asthma and bronchiolitis produce varying degrees of lower airway obstruction. Lower airway obstruction causes pulmonary hyperinflation due to mucous plugging and smooth muscle constriction. When positive pressure is applied, further hyperinflation occurs which may produce a profound decrease in venous return and, therefore, cardiac output. The end result will be a decrease in peripheral tissue oxygenation. A strategy exists, however, to minimize this effect. First, mean airway pressure should be kept to a minimum. In general, this means providing no PEEP or limiting it to a maximum of 2 to 3 cm of H_2O pressure. Another method of decreasing pulmonary hyperinflation is by avoiding "inadvertent" or "auto-PEEP." When lower airway obstruction is present, more time is required to fully empty the lung. If the exhalatory time allowed by the ventilator is too short, another breath will be initiated before the lung has emptied back to the baseline FRC. Again, this stacking of breaths results in worsening hyperinflation and increased mean airway pressure, a phenomenon called inadvertent or auto-PEEP. The amount of time required for exhalation should directly correlate with disease severity. In these situations the I:E ratio should be at least 1:2. It may be necessary to increase the I:E ratio to 1:3 or longer in children requiring ventilation with asthma.

Lower airway obstruction also results in increased work of breathing by increasing respiratory resistance. As discussed earlier, this can contribute to respiratory failure. Providing mechanical ventilation will decrease the oxygen demands of the respiratory musculature and prevent further respiratory mus-

cle fatigue, which should improve oxygen delivery to other peripheral tissues.

Cardiac Disease

Declining cardiac function places a number of stresses on the pulmonary system. The resultant pulmonary vascular congestion leads to the formation of interstitial edema. Interstitial edema can lead to alveolar collapse and to further $\dot{V}/\dot{Q}$ mismatch.

In addition, cardiac output falls as cardiac function worsens, and thus impairs oxygen delivery to the peripheral tissues. Oxygen delivery is determined by cardiac output and the concentration of oxygen in the blood. When cardiac output falls, the body must increase the concentration of oxygen in the blood to maintain oxygen delivery. The body accomplishes this by increasing respiratory rate and effort. The increased work of breathing required to accomplish this, however, places increased oxygen demands on the body. As discussed, this may ultimately result in respiratory failure.

Goals of mechanical ventilation in patients with cardiac dysfunction are therefore aimed toward reexpanding areas of atelectasis and decreasing the work of breathing. Areas of collapse are reexpanded by the application of PEEP. It is important to be cautious in using PEEP. Excessive PEEP will cause hyperinflation of the alveoli which may result in increased pulmonary vascular resistance. Increased pulmonary vascular resistance has a negative effect on cardiac output due to a decrease in left ventricular filling. In the setting of heart disease, cardiac output is highly dependent on left ventricular filling. Therefore, higher mean airway pressures can significantly affect cardiac output. It is reasonable to start with a PEEP of 3 to 5 cm H_2O. The amount of PEEP can then be titrated to improve oxygenation while maintaining venous return.

Mechanical ventilation in patients with cardiac disease also will decrease the total work of breathing. When the work of breathing is decreased, the oxygen demand by the respiratory musculature also is decreased. Oxygen that would have been used by the respiratory musculature can be used by other peripheral tissues. In this way, the total oxygen demands placed on the cardiopulmonary circulation are reduced.

SUMMARY
1. Select a ventilator—volume or pressure controller
2. Select a mode of ventilation
3. Provide adequate ventilation
   a. Set tidal volume or peak inspiratory pressure (PIP)
   b. Set the rate (Table 84.3)
4. Provide adequate oxygenation
   a. Set F_iO_2
   b. Set positive end-expiratory pressure (PEEP)
5. Set inspiratory time
6. Assess patient for adequate ventilation
   a. Adequate rise and fall of chest
   b. Adequate breath sounds
   c. Arterial blood gas determination (adequate pCO_2)
7. Assess patient for adequate oxygenation
   a. Adequate heart rate and color
   b. Adequate oxygen saturation (SaO_2)
   c. Arterial blood gas determination (adequate P_AO_2)
8. Make changes as necessary and reassess

COMPLICATIONS

A number of complications are associated with using mechanical ventilation. In general, these complications are the result of endotracheal tube placement, positive airway pressure, or ventilator failure. Careful attention to specific details of ventilator management will assist in avoiding these complications.

Injuries resulting from the presence of an endotracheal tube are primarily the result of pressure placed on the airway mucosa. These injuries may range from mild swelling to severe ulceration, and may occur at any point the airway is in contact with an endotracheal tube. A more comprehensive discussion of these complications appears in Chapter 16. To avoid endotracheal tube related injuries, a proper size tube should be used. It is best if the air leak occurs around the tube beginning at no more than 20 cm H_2O pressure. To check for an air leak, the endotracheal tube should be connected to an anesthesia bag attached to a manometer. The airway pressure is slowly increased by carefully closing the pop-off valve. While watching the airway pressure rise on the manometer, the clinician should listen for an air leak. An air leak can be heard by listening at the patient's mouth or by placing a stethoscope over the cricothyroid membrane. Cuffed endotracheal tubes should not be used in prepubertal patients. If a cuffed tube is used, it should be inflated with air to less than 20 cm H_2O pressure.

Using excessive positive airway pressure can result in alveolar overdistention and possibly rupture. Overdistention of alveoli may reduce cardiac output as described in the Procedure section. Alveolar rupture results in the accumulation of air into sites outside the pulmonary tree. Clinical significance of these extrapulmonary air accumulations depends on their location and size. Pneumothorax, pulmonary interstitial emphysema, pneumomediastinum, pneumopericardium, pneumoperitoneum, and subcutaneous emphysema are possible complications that may result from alveolar rupture. Incidence of these complications can be reduced by using the smallest lung volumes and lowest airway pressures that will maintain adequate oxygenation and ventilation.

When a patient's clinical status deteriorates, it is important to assess whether a ventilator malfunction has occurred. As discussed, this is most easily accomplished by hand ventilating the patient with a bag and 100% oxygen. If the patient's condition improves, a problem most likely exists with the ventilator. Once the malfunction is identified and corrected, the patient can then be placed back on the ventilator. The patient should then be reassessed to ensure the malfunction has been remedied. Ventilator malfunctions can be kept to a minimum by frequently evaluating the patient's condition and the operation of the ventilator. All health care providers involved in the care of mechanically ventilated patients should have a thorough understanding of the ventilators used at their institutions.

SUMMARY

Mechanical ventilation can be a life saving procedure in many clinical settings. Decisions regarding ventilator setup and management are based on the patient's physiology and underlying pathophysiology. Carefully repeated clinical assessments of patient condition and ventilator function will aid in the effective use of this treatment and help to avoid complications. The importance of this cannot be overstated, as the success of mechanical ventilation largely depends on the knowledge and expertise of the operator.

REFERENCES

1. Chatburn RL. Assisted ventilation. In: Blummer J, ed. A practical guide to pediatric intensive care. 2nd ed. St. Louis: CV Mosby, 1990, pp. 943–955.
2. Feihl F, Perret C. Permissive hypercapnia: how permissive should we be? Am J Respir Crit Care Med 1994;150:1722–1737.
3. Hubmayr RD, Abel MD, Rehder K. Physiologic approach to mechanical ventilation. Crit Care Med 1990;18:103–113.
4. Martin LD, Rafferty JF, Walker K, Gioia FR. Principles of respiratory support and mechanical ventilation. In: Rogers M, ed. Text book of pediatric intensive care. 2nd ed. Baltimore: Williams & Wilkins, 1992; pp. 134–193.
5. Pfaff JK, Morgan WJ. Pulmonary function in infants and children. In: Wilmott R, ed. Respiratory medicine I. Pediatr Clin North Am 1994;41:401–423.
6. Reynolds AM, Ryan DP, Doody DP. Permissive hypercapnia and pressure-controlled ventilation as

treatment of severe adult respiratory distress syndrome in a pediatric burn patient. Crit Care Med 1993;21:468–471.

7. Ring JC, Stidham GL. Novel therapies for acute respiratory failure. In: Orlowski JP, ed. Pediatric critical care. Pediatr Clin North Am 1994;41: 1325–1362.

8. Rusconi F, Castagneto M, Gagliardi L, Leo G, et al. Reference values for respiratory rate in the first 3 years of life. Pediatrics 1994;94:350–355.

9. Schuster DP. A physiologic approach to initiating, maintaining, and withdrawing mechanical ventila-tory support during acute respiratory failure. Am J Med 1990;88:268–278.

10. Shapiro BA. A historical perspective on ventilator management. New Horizons 1994;2:8–18.

11. Tobin MJ. Mechanical ventilation. N Engl J Med 1994;330:1056–1061.

12. Venkataraman ST, Orr RA. Mechanical ventilation and respiratory care. In: Furhman B, ed. Pediatric critical care. St. Louis: CV Mosby, 1992, pp. 519–543.

13. Rogers, MC, ed. Textbook of pediatric intensive care. Baltimore: Williams & Wilkins, 1987; p. 115.

GASTROINTESTINAL PROCEDURES

Section Editor: James F. Wiley II

CHAPTER 85

MANAGEMENT OF ESOPHAGEAL FOREIGN BODIES

Jeff E. Schunk and Nanette C. Kunkel

INTRODUCTION

Children often swallow foreign bodies because of their inquisitive nature and propensity for pica (1). Esophageal impaction of these objects occurs frequently and removal is often necessary to avoid serious complications (2–7). Most esophageal foreign bodies are blunt or smooth, and coins are the most common (1, 8–10). Other esophageal foreign bodies include bones, meat, toys, and less commonly, sharp objects. Esophageal foreign bodies may occur at any age, although they are found more commonly in children aged 6 months to 6 years.

A variety of techniques and settings may be used for esophageal foreign body removal, depending on the type of physician specialist who performs the procedure. Local referral patterns, the nature of the foreign body, the duration and extent of symptoms, and familiarity with various techniques will determine the method of choice. Frequently used removal methods include endoscopy in the operating room (8, 9, 11), flexible endoscopy in the outpatient setting (12), the Foley catheter technique (13–15), and advancement with a Bougie dilator (16, 17).

ANATOMY AND PHYSIOLOGY

Esophageal foreign bodies occur most commonly in children without underlying disease at predictable sites of normal anatomic narrowing (8, 9). These sites include the thoracic inlet (cricopharyngeus), the right mainstem ronchus-aortic arch, and the gastroesophageal junction (lower esophageal sphincter) (Fig. 85.1) (8, 9, 18, 19). Children with underlying esophageal pathology are predisposed to foreign body impaction at sites of pathologic narrowing that may not correspond to the typical sites.

It is generally recommended that all esophageal foreign bodies should be removed. Local reaction, both inflammatory and muscular, may adversely affect esophageal motility and can lead to adjacent airway narrowing. Although esophageal perforation is most likely to occur from an impacted sharp object (21), complications also have been reported from impacted blunt objects. These include esophageal perforation (4), tracheo-esophageal fistula (6), esophageal-aortic fistula (5), and upper airway compromise from local reaction (22). No serious complications have been reported from blunt esophageal foreign bodies impacted for less than a few days. Removal of an esophageal foreign body typically results in rapid return to normal esophageal function and relief of any symptomatology.

INDICATIONS

Patients with esophageal foreign bodies often present with a foreign body sensation, pain, or symptoms of impaired esophageal function such as vomiting, drooling, or dysphagia. Airway compromise with stridor or wheezing also may occur. However, many children

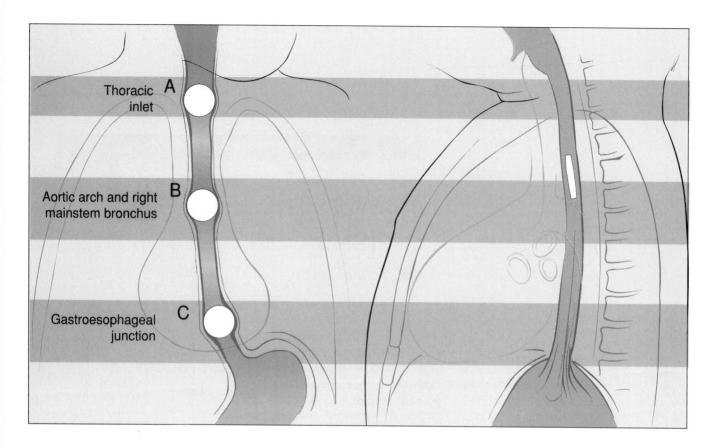

Figure 85.1.
Common sites of
esophageal impaction of
smooth foreign bodies.

with esophageal foreign bodies have no symptoms. In two studies performed in the emergency department (ED), 30% (18) and 44% (20) of the children with esophageal foreign bodies were asymptomatic.

Patients with coins at the lower esophageal sphincter for less than 24 hours may be observed for passage into the stomach. Patients with coins at the thoracic inlet or with symptoms should undergo emergent removal. Operative endoscopic removal is the traditional method of choice. It requires operating room personnel, an anesthesiologist and/or anesthetist, and an experienced surgeon. It is safe and efficacious in essentially all cases, and it allows for airway control and visualization of the esophagus (8, 11, 19). This method can be used for all esophageal foreign bodies and only rarely is thoracic surgery required due to mediastinal complications resulting from esophageal foreign bodies (perforation, mediastinitis, mediastinal mass).

Flexible, nonoperative endoscopy is usually performed by the gastroenterologist. It is efficacious in selected cases (blunt object im-pacted less than 1 to 2 weeks), although it does require pediatric equipment (12). Sedation may be necessary. This method affords advantages similar to operative endoscopy except that airway control is not guaranteed.

The Foley catheter technique is typically performed by a radiologist in the radiology suite. It is used successfully (67 to 98%) (13, 17, 23–25) for uncomplicated blunt esophageal foreign bodies with impaction duration less than 3 to 5 days. It also has been used in patients with underlying esophageal conditions (15). This technique offers the main advantages of reduced cost, no risk of general anesthesia, and no requirement for hospitalization.

Advancement of an esophageal foreign body into the stomach with a Bougie dilator is typically performed by the pediatric surgeon in the ED or under fluoroscopy. This technique is reserved for patients who have no respiratory symptoms, no underlying esophageal conditions, and who have esophageal impaction with blunt objects (coins) of short duration (usually less than 24 hours) (7, 16, 18). This method offers the advantage of avoiding the cost and risk of general anesthesia and hospitalization. In addition, it may be performed without fluoroscopy. Conversely, patients are at the theoretical risk of later impaction of the foreign body at another site in the gastrointestinal tract such as the pylorus or cecum.

Patients with respiratory symptoms, recent esophageal procedures, sharp foreign objects, or objects impacted for a long duration should only be considered for operative endoscopic removal. Patients with blunt foreign bodies of shorter duration (less than 3 to 5 days) can be considered for flexible endoscopy or the Foley catheter technique. Bougie advancement is generally reserved for single coins impacted less than 24 hours in children without esophageal disease (7, 17).

EQUIPMENT

Any esophageal foreign body removal attempt should be done with resuscitation equipment readily available, along with personnel experienced in its use. Specific techniques previously discussed require special equipment appropriately sized for the pediatric patient.

PROCEDURE

The emergency physician is most often concerned with proper diagnostic evaluation to identify the location and nature of an ingested foreign object. This is followed by appropriate preparation for the expected procedure. Diagnosis is usually straightforward with the typical radioopaque esophageal foreign body (coin) visible on plain radiograph. Less frequently a barium swallow is needed to outline a nonopaque esophageal foreign body. Recently, some authorities have reported success with using a handheld metal detector for localization of ingested coins (26–28).

In preparation for operative endoscopy, the patient should have nothing orally, have intravenous access, and undergo preoperative lab evaluation. The same preparation is needed if the patient is to undergo flexible endoscopy, although preparation for outpatient conscious sedation and monitoring also is required.

The Foley catheter technique is usually done without sedation. The patient is placed in the prone oblique or prone Trendelenburg position. Under fluoroscopic guidance, a Foley catheter (8 to 12 French) is passed distal to the foreign body and the balloon inflated with 3 to 5 cc barium. Gentle traction is applied to pull the esophageal foreign body out to the mouth where the foreign body is grasped or expectorated. Alternatively, the esophageal foreign body may be pushed into the stomach (13, 15, 17, 23–25).

Appropriately selected patients eligible for Bougie advancement are placed in the upright or prone position. A well-lubricated (proper size for the expected esophageal lumen diameter) dilator is gently advanced through the mouth and into the stomach. This technique has been used with and without fluoroscopy (16, 17).

Noninvasive Techniques

Several authorities have noted that some esophageal foreign bodies will pass spontaneously (9, 18, 20). Such spontaneous passage seems to be more common with esophageal foreign bodies impacted at the gastroesophageal junction (9). For this reason, expectant observation of short duration (24 hours) in the asymptomatic individual who has a blunt

---

SUMMARY
1. Identify location of foreign body by plain radiography, barium swallow, or metal detector
2. Determine duration of esophageal impaction (if possible) and any patient history of esophageal abnormality or surgery
3. If object is at lower esophageal sphincter and is not sharp or potentially harmful to patient, observe for 24 hours to allow for spontaneous passage
4. If object is not causing respiratory distress and has been impacted for a short period of time, consider Foley catheter removal, advancement with a Bougie dilator, or nonoperative endoscopy
5. If object is sharp, causes respiratory distress, has a long duration of impaction, or if patient has underlying esophageal abnormality, then prepare patient for removal by operative endoscopy

foreign body impacted for less than 1 day in this location may offer a reasonable alternative to active removal or advancement of the esophageal foreign body (8, 18, 29).

Although some have advocated pharmacologic means to promote passage of an esophageal foreign body (diazepam, glucagon, etc.), these agents have not been adequately studied in pediatric patients and routine use cannot be recommended.

COMPLICATIONS

Potential complications may vary with the removal method. Reported complications of operative esophagoscopy include dislodgment of the endotracheal tube; coughing at extubation; arrhythmia, vomiting, or laryngospasm during endoscopy; and stridor and laryngospasm after endoscopy (8, 11). Complications from the Foley catheter technique include vomiting, epistaxis, transient respiratory distress, and (rarely) esophageal injury (14, 24). Foreign body aspiration into the airway has not been reported with the Foley catheter technique. Significant complications from Bougie advancement in selected cases have not been reported (16, 17). Any technique that involves manipulating the esophagus carries a risk of esophageal injury, perforation and mediastinitis.

SUMMARY

Esophageal foreign bodies are common in children. They are usually blunt and lodge at sites of anatomic narrowing. The nature of the foreign body, duration of impaction, clinical condition, past medical history, hospital practice, and local referral patterns may determine the method used. All techniques should be attempted only by those clinicians familiar with their use and capable of managing any potential complications.

REFERENCES

1. Binder L, Anderson WA. Pediatric gastrointestinal foreign body ingestions. Ann Emerg Med 1984;13:112–117.
2. Byard RW, Moore L, Bourne AJ. Sudden and unexpected death—a late effect of occult intraesophageal foreign body. Pediatr Pathol 1990;10:837–841.
3. Katz KR, Emmens RW, Wood BP. Esophageal obstruction and abscess formation secondary to impacted, eroding tiddlywink. Am J Dis Child 1989;143:961–962.
4. Nahmah BJ, Mueller CF. Asymptomatic esophageal perforation by a coin in a child. Ann Emerg Med 1984;13:627–629.
5. Vella EE, Booth PJ. Foreign body in the oesophagus. BMJ 1965;2:1042.
6. Obiako MN. Tracheoesophageal fistula. a complication of foreign body. Ann Otol Rhinol Laryngol 1982; 91:325–327.
7. Jona JZ, Glicklich M, Cohen RD. The contraindications for blind esophageal bougienage for coin ingestion in children. J Pediatr Surg 1988;23:328–330.
8. Crysdale WS, Sendi KS, Yoo J. Esophageal foreign bodies in children, 15-year review of 484 cases. Ann Otol Rhinol Laryngol 1991;100:320–324.
9. Spitz L. Management of ingested foreign bodies in childhood. BMJ 1971;20:469–472.
10. Baraka A, Bikhazi G. Oesophageal foreign bodies. Br J Med 1975;1:561–563.
11. Hawkins DB. Removal of blunt foreign bodies from the esophagus. Ann Otol Rhinol Laryngol 1990;99: 935–939.
12. Bendig DW. Removal of blunt esophageal foreign bodies by flexible endoscopy without general anesthesia. Am J Dis Child 1986;140:789–790.
13. Campbell JB, Quattromani FL, Foley LC. Foley catheter removal of blunt esophageal foreign bodies. Experience with 100 consecutive children. Pediatr Radiol 1983;13:116–119.
14. Campbell JB, Condon VR. Catheter removal of blunt esophageal foreign bodies in children. Pediatr Radiol 1989;19:361–365.
15. Nixon GW. Foley catheter method of esophageal foreign body removal: extension of applications. AJR 1979;132:441–442.
16. Bonadio WA, Jona JZ, Glicklich M, Cohen R. Esophageal Bougienage technique for coin ingestion in children. J Pediatr Surg 1988;23:917–918.
17. Kelley JE, Leech MH, Carr MG. A safe and cost-effective protocol for the management of esophageal coins in children. J Pediatr Surg 1993;28:898–900.
18. Schunk JE, Corneli H, Bolte R. Pediatric coin ingestions, a prospective study of coin location and symptoms. Am J Dis Child 1989;143:546–548.

19. Chaikhouni A, Kratz J, Crawford F. Foreign Bodies of the esophagus. Am Surg 1985;51:173–179.
20. Hodge D, Tecklenburg F, Fleisher G. Coin ingestion: does every child need a radiograph? Ann Emerg Med 1985;14:443–446.
21. Nandi P, Ong GB. Foreign body in the oesophagus: review of 2394 cases. Br J Surg 1978;65:5–9.
22. Pasquariello PS, Kean H. Cyanosis from a foreign body in the esophagus. Clin Pediatr 1975;14: 223–225.
23. Towbin R, Lederman HM, Dunbar JS, Ball WS, Strife JL. Esophageal edema as a predictor of unsuccessful balloon extraction of esophageal foreign body. Pediatr Radiol 1989;19:359–360.
24. Schunk JE, Harrison AM, Corneli HM, Nixon GW. Fluoroscopic Foley catheter removal of esophageal foreign bodies in children: experience with 415 episodes. Pediatrics 1994;94:709–714.
25. Campbell JB, Foley LC. A safe alternative to endoscopic removal of blunt esophageal foreign bodies. Arch Otolaryngol 1983;109:323–325.
26. Biehler JL, Tuggle D, Stacey T. Use of a transmitter-receiver metal detector in the evaluation of pediatric coin ingestions. Pediatr Emerg Care 1993;9: 208–210.
27. Ros SP, Cetta F. Successful use of a metal detector in locating coins ingested by children. J Pediatr 1992;120:752–3.
28. Ros SP, Cetta F. Metal detectors: an alternative approach to the evaluation of coin ingestions in children? Pediatr Emerg Care 1992;8:134–136.
29. Schunk JE. Foreign body—ingestion/aspiration. In: Fleisher GR, Ludwig S, eds. Textbook of pediatric emergency medicine. 3rd ed. Baltimore: Williams & Wilkins, 1993, p. 210.

CHAPTER 86

GASTRIC INTUBATION

Harold K. Simon and William Lewander

INTRODUCTION

Inserting a gastrointestinal tube for medical purposes dates back to Boerhave (1668–1738), who first suggested their use, and John Hunter, who reported conveying food and medicine in 1790 for a case of "paralysis of the muscles of deglutition" (1). Occasional case reports followed but it was not until 1921, when Levin introduced the smooth catheter-tipped tube, that gastric intubation became a routine medical procedure (2, 3).

Intoxication, trauma, abdominal obstruction, and upper gastrointestinal bleeding require emergent gastric intubation. The procedure is commonly performed by physicians and nurses in both the emergency department (ED) and intensive care settings. The placement of a gastric tube is straightforward, but requires close attention to technique to avoid serious complications.

ANATOMY AND PHYSIOLOGY

The approach to gastric intubation in children is similar to the adult patient. Major anatomic obstacles to gastric tube placement are the nares, choanae, adenoids, tonsils, tongue, and epiglottis (Fig. 86.1). Unlike adults, however, children have increased tonsillar and adenoidal tissue size that may predispose them to traumatic bleeding during gastric intubation, especially if excessive force is used. In addition, the relative macroglosia in young children and the smaller nostril diameter may impede nasogastric intubation. In some pediatric patients, orogastric intubation will be required if it becomes evident that nasogastric intubation will result in excessive trauma.

The cribriform plate, an anatomic site deserving special emphasis, is a thin bone located in the superior aspect of the nasal cavity. It separates the intracranial cavity from the nasal cavity. This bone may be fractured following severe facial or head trauma, which would allow potential access into the intracranial cavity. Placement of a nasogastric tube in the presence of such an injury has resulted in introduction of the tube into the cranial vault, an obviously catastrophic result (4). Care must be taken before nasogastric intubation to ensure that a cribriform plate disruption is not present.

Physiologically, the gag reflex impedes gastric tube placement by closing the nasopharynx via the levator veli palatini and tensor veli palatini muscles (cranial nerve X) and constricting the pharyngeal musculature (cranial nerve IX and X). Impairment of the gag reflex often occurs in patients with altered mental status. In such patients, passage of the tube may actually be easier because the patient does not struggle. However, the risk of aspiration of gastric contents into the lungs increases greatly because the tracheal protection afforded by an intact gag reflex is diminished or absent. In addition, the gastric tube may be inadvertently passed into the trachea because the warning signs of cough or lack of phonation would not be present. Finally, children can have congenital anomalies that may make their anatomy unique from adults and which may also act as an impediment to gastric intubation such as choanal atresia, esoph-

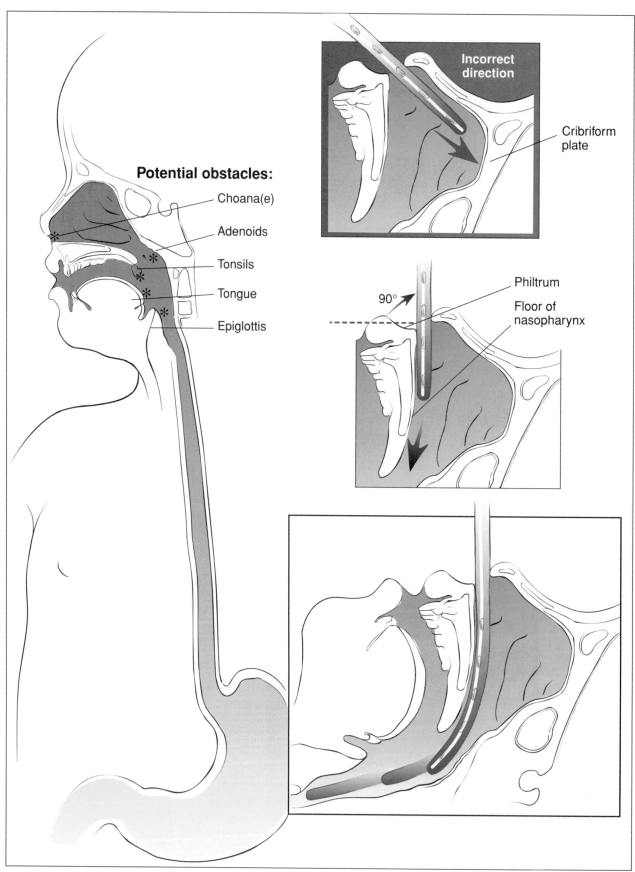

Potential obstacles:

Choana(e)

Adenoids

Tonsils

Tongue

Epiglottis

Incorrect direction

Cribriform plate

Philtrum

Floor of nasopharynx

90°

Figure 86.1.
Anatomy of the oropharynx with potential sites of impedance during nasogastric intubation.
Note the correct path for nasogastric tube insertion and the proximity to the cribriform plate.

ageal atresia, esophageal strictures, and tracheoesophageal fistula.

INDICATIONS

Gastric intubation is widespread in the daily
practice of pediatric emergency medicine.
Emergent indications include gastric decontamination of toxins, gastric lavage, gastrointestinal decompression (as in cases of obstruction), evaluation of gastrointestinal
hemorrhage, introduction of radiographic
contrast for imaging studies, and the administration of activated charcoal or medications
(see also Chapters 93 and 126). Nutritional
alimentation is a common nonemergent indication for gastric intubation.

Gastric intubation can be accomplished
by either the nasogastric or orogastric approaches. The nasogastric route allows for
easier gastric tube taping and is better tolerated by the conscious patient. However, the
position of the cribriform plate in the roof of
the nasal cavity must be considered when
placing a nasogastric tube. The possibility of
inadvertent intracranial placement can occur
if any cribriform disruption takes place (4, 5).
Other disadvantages of nasogastric intubation include the potential for adenoidal and
tonsillar bleeding, and the size limitation of
the nares.

The clinician should perform orogastric
intubation rather than nasogastric intubation
in the settings of head or facial trauma with
potential cribriform plate injury suggested by
copious nasal bleeding or clear nasal secretions. Coagulopathy, epistaxis, nasal obstruction, difficult nasal passage, and small nares
for the required gastric tube size (see Chapter
127) are other common indications for orogastric intubation.

Blind gastric intubation should not be
performed in patients with a poor gag reflex
before securing an airway because of the risk
of aspiration. Blind gastric intubation also
should be avoided in patients with high-lying
esophageal foreign bodies or in cases of caustic ingestions because of the risk of
esophageal perforation. Of note, esophageal
varices are not a contraindication for gastric
intubation. Blind nasogastric intubation has
been shown to be safe in patients with suspected, or even proven, varices (6, 7, 8).

EQUIPMENT

Airway equipment (oxygen, bag-valve-
mask)
Suction
Tape
Gastric tube (size appropriate to pass with
minimal resistance through the nares)
Surgical lubricant
Nasal decongestant spray such as phenyle-
pherine (optional)
Syringe (30 to 60 mL)
Tincture of benzoin
Lidocaine jelly 2% (optional)
Anesthetic spray such as cetacaine (optional)
Magill forceps
Tongue blade
Laryngoscope

The Levin tube and the Salem sump are
the two most common types of gastrointestinal tubes. The Levin tube is a single lumen,
nonradiopaque design and the Salem sump is
a double lumen, radiopaque tube. The major
advantage of the double lumen tube is that the
smaller vent lumen allows for outside air to
be drawn into the stomach enabling continuous flow. The single lumen design of the
Levin tube increases the likelihood that it will
become obstructed by the gastric mucosa
when suction is applied. This features limits
the usefulness of the Levin tube in gastric decompression and lavage. Conversely, the
constant flow of the double lumen Salem
sump facilitates controlled suction forces and
makes it less likely to adhere to the gastric
wall. This feature makes the Salem sump
more effective for suctioning of stomach contents (6).

PROCEDURE

The procedure should be explained to the
family and the patient (when appropriate) before tube insertion. Adequate airway control
must be guaranteed before attempting gastric
intubation. Monitoring of the patient during
the procedure should include heart rate, respiratory rate, and pulse oximetry for the unconscious patient. The clinician also should
stabilize the neck if cervical spine injury is
suspected. In the case of the comatose patient
with an intact gag reflex, the child is placed in
a decubitus position with the head down

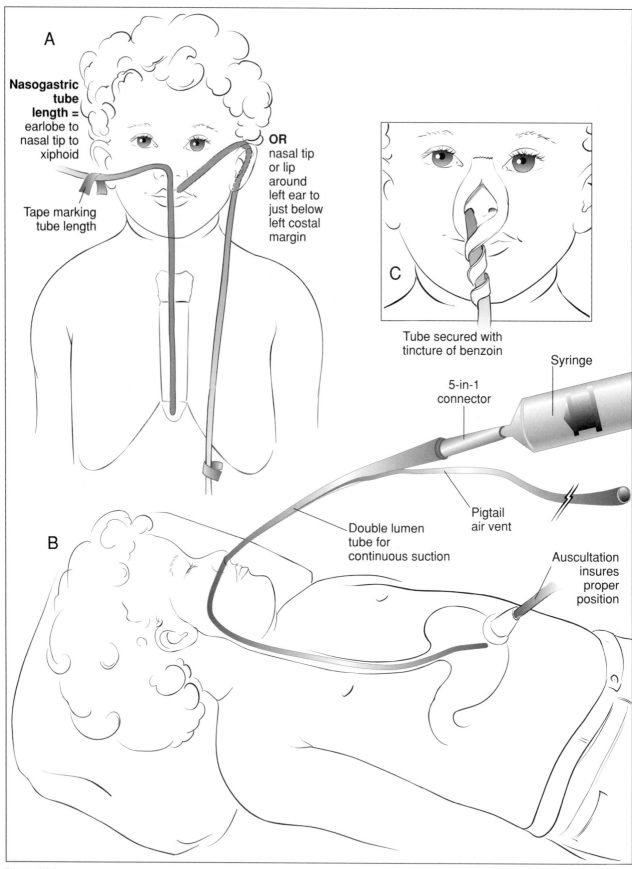

Figure 86.2.

A. External landmarks for determining proper gastric tube length.

B. Confirmation of nasogastric placement.

C. Taping of nasogastric tube.

(when cervical spine injury is not suspected) to minimize the risk of aspiration. A comatose patient with a poor gag reflex should be endotracheally intubated before proceeding with gastric intubation (see Chapter 16). All necessary equipment must be readily available along with any assistants. Suction equipment and oxygen should be immediately available and operating properly.

The oropharynx is next suctioned clear of secretions. For nasogastric intubation, the length of the desired tube is estimated by adding the distance from the tip of the nares to the earlobe, and the distance from the nose to the xiphoid (Fig. 86.2) (9, 10). Alternatively, the length of the tube can be measured by externally placing it from the tip of the nose or the lip (depending on the approach used) back to the ear and down to the left upper quadrant just below the left costal margin. The tubing length can be marked with a piece of tape. In small children or in the case of uncooperative patients, an assistant can help secure the child's head in place.

Nasal decongestant such as phenylephrine is sprayed into the nares to shrink the nasal mucosa before nasogastric intubation. A small amount of lidocaine 2% jelly is placed in the naris before introducing the tube to partially limit the discomfort of the procedure. A well-lubricated tube should then be gently passed through the naris, perpendicular to the philtrum (not angled superiorly) with pressure directed caudally toward the hypopharynx to avoid the cribriform plate and the nasal mucosa. If the clinician encounters difficulty, he or she can attempt to use the contralateral naris or a smaller tube. Difficult passage caused by curling of the tube may be lessened by stiffening the tube in ice, but excessive force should never be used. In cases when cervical injury is not suspected, flexion of the neck also may facilitate placement. If the relative macroglossia in young children and infants proves to be an impediment to placement, the tongue can be gently depressed with a tongue blade. The site of impedance often can be palpated in the neck and help guide further efforts.

As a last resort, direct visualization with a laryngoscope (see Chapter 16) is performed using appropriate sedation. The esophagus is visualized inferior to the larynx. The gastric tube is then passed directly into the esopha-

gus. Guidance using McGill forceps may be necessary when passing a nasogastric tube in this manner (6).

Once the tube reaches the hypopharynx, insertion should be rapid and continuous as the patient swallows. The clinician can overcome esophageal resistance by having the older, cooperative patients sip water, therefore improving esophageal peristalsis. If coughing, choking, or changes in phonation occur (indicating tracheal insertion) or if significant gagging occurs (indicating coiling in the esophagus) the clinician should remove the tube and reattempt insertion. If the patient is crying or talking during the procedure, this is a good indication that the gastric tube has not been inadvertently placed in the trachea.

Tube placement is checked by aspirating stomach contents and then introducing 3 to 10 mL of air (depending on the size of the child) via a catheter-tipped syringe placed at the end of the tube. Auscultation over the epigastric region should reveal a rush of air (rumbling sound) as evidence of proper placement. If correct placement is questioned, the tube should be repositioned or removed. Placement should be confirmed with a radiograph in unconscious patients or whenever uncertainty about positioning exists. Although several methods of securing the tube have been described (11), the basic approach includes securing a small piece of tape with tincture of benzoin to the nasal bridge or cheek. The distal end of the horizontally cut tape is wrapped around the segment of tube extending from the nostril. Orogastric tubes can be secured in a similar manner to the lateral cheek.

COMPLICATIONS

While gastric tube placement is generally well tolerated, several complications exist. The primary method for avoiding most significant complications of gastric intubation is never to use excessive force during the procedure. This point cannot be overemphasized. If the tube does not pass relatively easy, then another route should be used, or the tube should be passed under direct visualization using a laryngoscope. Creation of a false passage may occur when the tube is inserted into a natural cul-de-sac (such as a py-

SUMMARY
General Considerations
1. Fully discuss procedure with patient and family to limit anxiety
2. Have necessary equipment and assistants available
3. Position patient and protect airway when indicated
4. Stabilize neck if any question of cervical spine injury
5. Suction patient clear of secretions
6. Use well lubricated, size appropriate tube
7. Apply topical anesthetic for nasogastric placement
8. Estimate desired length—tip of nares to earlobe and nose to xiphoid, or nostril back around ear and down just below left costal margin
9. Gently pass tube into desired position in caudally directed manner, going straight into the nostril, not up
10. Check placement with infusion of air; confirm placement with radiograph as needed

Specific Considerations in the Unconscious Patient
1. Consider head down, decubitus positioning and endotracheal intubation before gastric intubation in comatose patients to reduce risk of aspiration
2. All unconscious patients should have radiographic confirmation of positioning.

riform sinus) and persistent and inappropriate force is applied. Forced passage of a gastric tube also may result in avulsion of tonsillar and adenoidal tissue, which may cause significant bleeding or airway obstruction if the dislodged segment of tissue is large enough to occlude the trachea (3, 12–14). Accidental intracranial passage of a gastric tube may be prevented by avoiding the nasogastric approach in patients with facial or head trauma who have possible cribriform plate disruption. Finally, prevention of endotracheal tube dislodgment when passing a gastric tube requires careful securing of the endotracheal tube (see Chapter 16) before gastric tube placement.

SUMMARY

Gastric intubation is a commonly used procedure in the ED and in the inpatient setting. Physicians and nurses should be knowledge-able regarding the use, placement, and potential complications of gastric intubation. If done with care and proper technique, this procedure can be performed successfully with minimal difficulty in most cases.

REFERENCES

1. Paine JR. The history of the invention and development of the stomach and duodenal tubes. Ann Intern Med 1934;8:752–763.
2. Levin AL. A new gastroduodenal catheter. JAMA 1921;76:1007.
3. Hafner CD, Wylie JH, Brush BE. Complications of gastrointestinal intubation. Arch Surg 1961;83:147–160.
4. Young RF. Cerebrospinal fluid rhinorrhea following nasogastric intubation. J Trauma 1979;19:789–791.
5. Wyler AR, Reynolds AF. An intracranial complication of nasogastric intubation. J Neurosurg 1977;47:297–298.
6. Glauser JM. Nasogastic intubation. In: Roberts JR, Hedges JR, eds. Clinical procedures in emergency medicine. 2nd ed. Philadelphia: WB Saunders, 1991, p. 640–648.
7. Lopez-Torres A, Waye JD. The safety of intubation in patients with esophageal varices. Am J Dig Dis 1973;18:1032.
8. Ritter DM, Rettke SR, Hughes RW, Burritt MF, Sterioff S, Illstrup DM. Placement of nasogastric tubes and esophageal stethoscopes in patients with documented esophageal varices. Anaesth Analg 1988;67:283.
9. Abdominal procedures. In: Simon R, Brenner BE, eds. Emergency procedures and techniques. Baltimore: Williams & Wilkins, 1987, pp. 1–7.
10. Gastointestinal intubation. In: Van Way III. The pocket manual of basic surgical skills. St. Louis: CV Mosby, 1986, pp. 179–185.
11. Sader AA. New way to stabilize nasogastric tubes. Am J Surg 1975;130:102.
12. Wald P, Stern J, Weiner B, Goldfrank L. Esophageal tear following forceful removal of an impacted orogastric lavage tube. Ann Emerg Med 1986;15:80–82.
13. Lind LJ, Wallace DH. Submucosal passage of a nasogastric tube complicating attempted intubation during anesthesia. Anesthesiology 1978;49:145–147.
14. Weiner BC. Management of oral gastric lavage tube impaction of the esophagus. Am J Gastroenterol 1986;81:1202–1204.

CLINICAL TIPS

1. Topical anesthetic jelly (nasogastric tube) or topical anesthetic spray (orogastric tube) limits the discomfort of the procedure.
2. If excessive choking or gagging occurs, the tube should be removed.
3. Talking or crying during the procedure is a good indication that the gastric tube has not been inadvertently placed in the trachea.
4. If difficulty is encountered, palpation of the neck may reveal the site of impedance.
5. Gentle downward displacement of the tongue with a tongue blade may facilitate passage of a nasogastric tube in the young child or infant.
6. If unable to advance the tube, congenital malformations such as choanal atresia, esophageal atresia, and esophageal strictures should be considered.
7. Excess force must never be used in passing a nasogastric tube.

Gastrostomy Tube Replacement

John W. Graneto

Introduction

In 1980 percutaneous endoscopic gastrostomy (PEG) was introduced for children who require long-term nutritional support (1). The endoscopic PEG was found to be simpler and safer than surgical gastrostomy (2). Its use quickly became a popular method of providing enteral access for children suffering from chronic illnesses that lead to impaired and insufficient oral intake, the most common being anoxic brain injury (2). Nutritional support and medication administration—either long term or for brief periods postoperatively—are easily achieved in these patients with a PEG tube. The increasing frequency with which these tubes are being used in pediatric patients, combined with the tendency of the tubes to dislodge or malfunction, make replacement of gastrostomy tubes a common procedure for the emergency physician.

Anatomy and Physiology

Children can have impaired swallowing function for a variety of reasons including anoxic brain injury, gastroesophageal reflux, esophageal injury from lye ingestion, congenital esophageal anomalies (e.g., stenosis, stricture, duplication, or tracheoesophageal fistula), achalasia, familial dysautonomia, and any disease that interferes with oropharyngeal muscle tone and coordination (e.g., muscular dystrophy, Werdnig-Hoffmann disease,

or myasthenia gravis). These children may be unable to ingest sufficient oral intake to prevent eventual dehydration, or they may have such uncoordinated swallowing reflexes that they are highly prone to aspirate orally ingested substances into the lungs. Using a PEG tube avoids these problems by allowing direct access to the stomach which obviates the need for oral administration of medications and feedings.

The anterior or anterolateral surface of the stomach wall is the usual site of insertion of a PEG tube. The PEG tube stoma traverses the stomach wall beginning at the internal mucosa extending outward to the visceral lining and approximating these layers to the parietal peritoneal lining of the abdominal wall. After several weeks, a fistulous tract forms and adherence of these layers to each other becomes permanent.

Indications

Gastrostomy tubes require replacement for several reasons. Tubes can deteriorate over time and become dysfunctional during the natural course of their use (3). PEG tubes also can become blocked, which is normally caused by formula accumulations that dry and solidify. One study has shown certain formulas to be more prone to clogging than others when exposed to acidic stomach contents. These include Ensure®, Pulmocare® and Osmolite® (4). Tubes also can become blocked due to mechanical twisting, kinking, and undissolved medications. In general, attempts to unstop these types of blockages should not be made with stylets or other probing devices because these efforts can potentially rupture the feeding tubes below the skin surface leading to intraabdominal leakages. Blocked tubes that cannot be made functional should be removed and replaced.

Active children can cause their PEG tubes to become accidentally dislodged from the stomach. Although the specific incidence of this event is not well known, some authorities suggest that this occurs relatively frequently. Inadvertent removal of the PEG tube is an important indication for timely tube replacement. Because the stoma site will begin to close over in a short time (usually within hours) after gastrostomy tube removal, prompt catheter replacement is of prime importance. Delays in tube replacement will increase the difficulty of passing a temporizing device, such as a Foley catheter (5). If a Foley catheter is placed promptly after the PEG tube is removed, the procedure can usually be accomplished in the emergency department (ED) or office setting without requiring anesthesia or intervention by a subspecialist. No attempt to remove a well-positioned yet malfunctional tube should be made without assurance that the replacement equipment and personnel to perform the replacement are readily available.

Although PEG tube replacement is most commonly a simple procedure, spontaneous expulsion of a tube that was recently placed (within 1 to 2 weeks of the initial operative procedure) is a special case. In such situations, the stomach wall may not have had time to adhere to the peritoneal lining and overlying skin. Attempts at reestablishing a PEG tube or temporizing with a Foley catheter can disrupt the fistula tract with the formation of a false lumen into the peritoneum. Instillation of formula through the improperly positioned tube can cause a chemical and bacterial peritonitis with potentially life-threatening consequences. Therefore, patients requiring PEG tube replacement in the immediate postoperative period should have consultation from the ED with the surgeon or gastroenterologist who originally placed the tube.

EQUIPMENT

Replacement tube
Lubricant (e.g., K-Y Jelly®)
10 mL syringe
30 to 60 mL syringe
Stethoscope
Tape
Benzoin
Absorbent dressing

Figure 87.1.
Types of gastrostomy tubes.

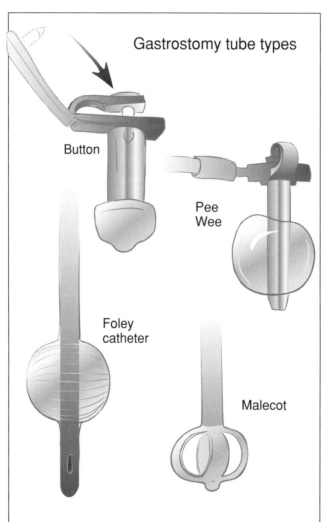

Gastrostomy tube types

Button

Pee Wee

Foley catheter

Malecot

Replacing a nutritional feeding tube in the ED does not necessarily mean that the dislodged tube must be replaced with the same type of tube. If the original type of equipment is available, however, this should be the preferred replacement equipment used. A wide variety of PEG tubes are currently available on the market, most of which are made of silicone, rubber, or polyurethane. Many tubes are similar, with only minor differences in their design, connectors, and lengths. The more common types are (a) balloon ended, such as a Foley catheter, (b) mushroom shaped (dePezzer), such as the Button® made by BARD and the MIC-KEY, or (c) collapsible wings, such as the Malecot (Fig. 87.1).

The Button® manufactured by BARD Interventional Products, was first developed in 1984. Its advantages over conventional gastrostomy tubes include less skin irritation, fewer problems with migration and dislodgment, and no awkward lengthy tube exposed externally. The Button® tube does not have to be changed as frequently as conventional products (6, 7). The Button® has gained popularity and is favored by both patients and families.

Attempts to use the same size replacement tube as the original also should be a goal. Usual catheter sizes range from 18 to 28 French.

PROCEDURE

Clogged Tube

If a blockage has occurred, the clinician should gently instill warm water into the tube and allow it to flow back out repeatedly until patency is established. Whether carbonated soda is more effective than other liquids is debatable; specifically, diet cola has been reported anecdotally as the most effective medium for clearing the tubes. Parents should be advised that the best way to avoid these occurrences is with proper flushing of the tube before and after each use.

Open Stoma

Foley catheter insertion is the most common temporizing measure for replacing gastrostomy feeding devices. This is especially important for emergency physicians practicing in a community setting, as Foley catheters would be the most readily available equipment for such a temporizing measure (Fig. 87.2).

Assessment of the child should rule out intraabdominal pathology. Using sedation and/or analgesia may assist in keeping the child calm during the procedure (see Chapter 35). A replacement tube the same size as the malfunctioning or dislodged tube, or a temporizing balloon-tipped Foley catheter, should be obtained and checked. For tubes with inflatable balloons, balloon integrity should always be checked. For collapsible wing or mushroom-tipped catheters, the clinician must make sure the stylet or obturator properly distends the distal tip so that it is narrowed before passage through the stoma site.

Before removing the malfunctioning tube, the clinician detaches any clamps or external sources of stabilization. If the dysfunctional catheter is balloon tipped, a Luer-Lok™ syringe or other adaptable syringe is connected to the balloon port of the old gastrostomy tube and balloon contents are withdrawn. If the tube requires a stylet or obturator for removal, it is inserted to extend the distal tip within the stomach wall.

If the child can follow commands, the clinician should instruct him or her to take a deep breath and hold it while the old tube is gently pulled out. If removal of the current but malfunctional tube is not possible by gentle traction, the tube may be cut at the abdominal wall surface and the internal components allowed to pass through the gastrointestinal tract. The distal portion will normally pass spontaneously through the gastrointestinal tract or it may be removed later endoscopically (8). The stoma site is covered liberally with water soluble lubricant or topical anesthetic. The stoma site is approached with the new catheter held perpendicular to the skin. The new catheter is gently inserted with continuous pressure into the stoma site and advanced steadily until well inside the stomach (Fig. 87.2).

At this point, the balloon is filled with saline or water to ensure stability (if a balloon-type tube is used) or the obturator or stylet is removed (if a mushroom or collapsible wing tube is used). To check for proper functioning and placement, the operator

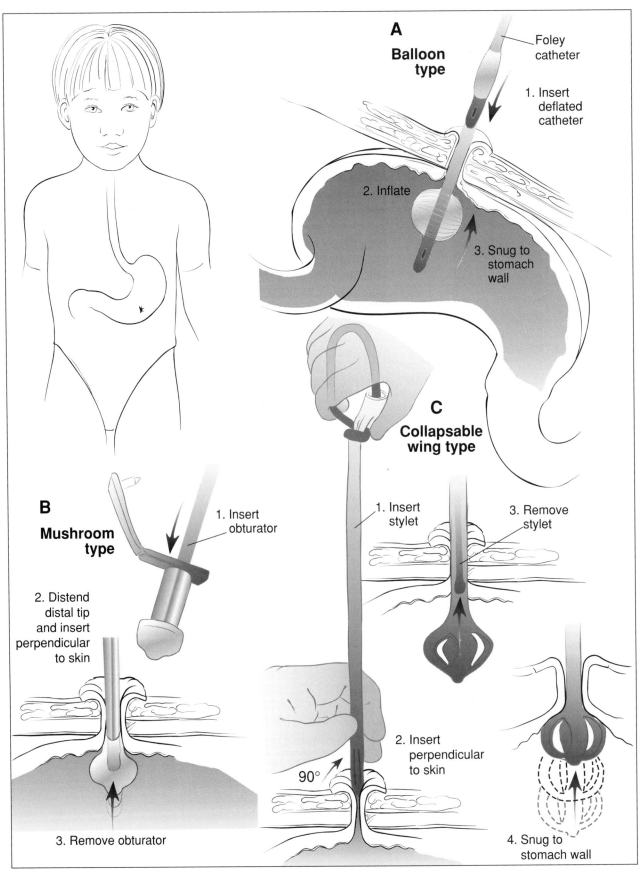

A
Balloon type

Foley catheter

1. Insert deflated catheter

2. Inflate

3. Snug to stomach wall

C
Collapsable wing type

1. Insert stylet

3. Remove stylet

2. Insert perpendicular to skin

90°

4. Snug to stomach wall

B
Mushroom type

1. Insert obturator

2. Distend distal tip and insert perpendicular to skin

3. Remove obturator

Figure 87.2.
Gastrostomy tube replacement.
A. Foley catheter.
B. Mushroom tube with obturator.
C. Collapsible wing tube with stylet.

should first attempt to aspirate stomach contents using a syringe attached to the tube, and second, to listen over the stomach when instilling 10 to 15 mL of air. Hearing borborygmi will confirm the proper location. The tube should be secured and covered or the distal end port closed. Tape or sutures are used to secure the tube in place. A dressing may be applied or the tube may be freely exposed to the air.

Using gastrograffin or other contrast media to confirm proper position radiographically is not necessary provided the previous two methods of placement confirmation are successful. If any question arises about the actual site of placement, radiographic studies are indicated. Likewise, if the clinician is suspicious of a perforated viscous, a noncontrast upright abdominal-chest radiograph is indicated to rule out free air in the peritoneum.

Closed Stoma

Using a guide wire or stylet in a Malincott tube replacement for a recently closed stoma is an option that should be reserved for the surgeon or gastroenterologist. In most instances, intravenous access can be obtained should the appropriate consultant not be immediately available. Improper technique can result in establishing a "false lumen" with the potential serious complications of a ruptured viscous or separation of the gastric wall from the stoma site.

Jejunostomy Tube Replacement

Malfunctioning or dislodged jejunostomy tubes should be replaced by the subspecialist who initially performed the jejunostomy. Nasoduodenal tubes may be placed under fluoroscopy by an experienced radiologist as a temporary measure. Blind passage of a weighted nasoduodenal tube (Dubhoff) is difficult in children and should not be performed.

COMPLICATIONS

Excessive force combined with using a tube that is too large may lead to accidental insertion into the peritoneal cavity through a false lumen, separation of the stomach wall from the peritoneal wall resulting in peritoneal insertion of the distal tube, or lysis of adhesions of the stomach wall away from the abdominal wall causing pneumoperitoneum. If a false lumen is formed and is not recognized, formula may be instilled into the space, resulting in chemical peritonitis (9). These complications can be avoided by appropriately sizing the replacement tube and using continuous firm pressure when replacing the gastrostomy tube. Furthermore, a gastrostomy tube should not be used for instillation of feedings unless correct positioning is confirmed as previously described.

Insufficient advancement of the replacement tube, which leaves the distal tip in the fistula rather than in the stomach lumen, can lead also to disruption of the fistula and pain when the stylet is withdrawn or the balloon is filled. Continued patient discomfort after tube placement is an indication of this problem. In most instances, the replacement tube should be advanced several centimeters through the stoma before anchoring it.

As mentioned, delay in replacement may result in closure of the gastrostomy fistula. Other complications include wound infections at the skin site or bleeding at the site of insertion caused by trauma to the area. Use of adequate lubrication and avoidance of excessive force can minimize the potential for bleeding and infection. Finally, a replacement Foley catheter tube not secured properly may migrate farther into the gastrointestinal tract (potentially causing obstruction), or it may migrate up into the esophagus (10, 11). Esophageal migration has been associated with perforation (12, 13).

SUMMARY

1. Assess child's condition. Restrain if necessary. Consider using sedation and/or analgesia
2. Obtain replacement tube and check for proper functioning
3. Remove any clamps from malfunctional tube and
   a. Withdraw liquid balloon contents
   —OR—
   b. Insert stylet or obturator
4. Have child take a deep breath and gently pull out old tube
5. Lubricate replacement tube and stoma site generously
6. Insert replacement tube perpendicularly into stoma site
7. Advance with continuous steady pressure
8. Fill balloon with saline/water
   —OR—
   Remove obturator/ stylet
9. Aspirate stomach contents and listen over stomach while injecting air through replacement tube
10. Secure tube and cover distal end

CLINICAL TIPS

1. Water or saline is best for inflating catheter balloons.
2. Prompt opening of fistulous tract of a recently dislodged tube is the most effective way to maintain patency.
3. When inserting the tube, continuous and steady pressure rather than intermittent poking or jabbing will generally be more helpful.
4. Fluid-filled replacement tubes may have more stability during replacement.

Chapter 87
Gastrostomy Tube
Replacement

This problem is easily avoided by pulling the Foley tube back against the stomach wall after the balloon has been inflated and properly securing the excess tubing extending from the gastrostomy site.

SUMMARY

Whether replacing a spontaneously expelled gastrostomy tube or fixing one that is malfunctional, various options exist for the emergency physician. The procedures performed vary somewhat depending on the type of equipment used. Key points include timely intervention before the fistulous tract has time to close over and avoidance of using excessive force at all times. Proper postplacement evaluation is essential to ensure proper functioning and prevent complications.

REFERENCES

1. Gauderer MWL, Ponsky JL, Izant RJ. Gastrostomy without laparotomy: a percutaneous endoscopic technique. J Pediatr Surg 1980;15:872–875.
2. Gauderer MW. Percutaneous endoscopic gastrostomy. A 10-year experience with 220 children. J Pediatr Surg 1991;26(3):288–294.
3. Kadakia SC, Cassaday M, Shaffer RT. Prospective evaluation of Foley catheter as a replacement gastrostomy tube. Am J Gastroenterol 1992;87(11): 1594–1597.
4. Marcuard SP, Perkins AM. Clogging of feeding tubes. J Parenteral Enter Nutr 1988;12:403.
5. Ruddy RM. Illustrated techniques of pediatric emergency procedures. In: Fleisher GR, Ludwig S, eds. Textbook of pediatric emergency medicine. Baltimore: Williams & Wilkins, 1993, pp. 1638–1639.
6. Steele NF. The Button: replacement gastrostomy device. J Pediatr Nurs 1991;6(6):421–424.
7. Townsend LC. Practical considerations of the gastrostomy button. Society of Gastroenterology Nurses and Associates, 1991 August 18–26.
8. Korula J, Harma C. A simple and inexpensive method of removal or replacement of gastrostomy tubes. JAMA 1991;265:1426–1428.
9. Marshall JB, Bodnarchuk G, Barthel JS. Early accidental dislodgment of PEG tubes. J Clin Gastroenterol 1994;18:210–212.
10. Cassaday M, Kadakia SC, Yamamoto K, Parker A. Foley feeding catheter migration into the small bowel. J Clin Gastroenterol 1992;15:242–244.
11. Browne BJ, Kaufman B, Brown C. Internal displacement of a gastrostomy button: an unusual case of gastric outlet obstruction. J Pediatr Surg 1993;28:1575–1576.
12. Whiteley S, Liu PH, Tellez DW, McGill LC. Esophageal rupture in an infant secondary to esophageal placement of a Foley catheter gastrostomy tube. Pediatr Emerg Care 1989;5:113–116.
13. Konigsberg K, Levenbrown J. Esophageal perforation secondary to gastrostomy tube replacement. J Pediatr Surg 1986;21:946–947.

CHAPTER 88

PARACENTESIS

Natalie E. Lane and Ronald I. Paul

INTRODUCTION

Paracentesis, or a peritoneal tap, is the procedure of entering the peritoneal cavity through the abdominal wall and aspirating a collection of fluid with a finely gauged needle. The peritoneum is normally bathed in a small amount of fluid. Ascites, derived from the Greek word "askites" meaning bag or bladder, is a collection of fluid in the peritoneal cavity whose volume is in excess of the normal amount. Paracentesis may be used as a diagnostic tool in the evaluation of ascites or a therapeutic procedure for the relief of respiratory distress secondary to large accumulations of ascites. An understanding of the patient's anatomy and the pathophysiology of ascites is essential to the correct performance of this procedure. Treatment rooms in the hospital, office, or clinic are appropriate settings for a diagnostic tap. For the relief of respiratory distress, paracentesis should be performed in an emergency department (ED) or in an intensive care unit. Both sites should be equipped with monitoring and resuscitative equipment.

ANATOMY AND PHYSIOLOGY

No one pediatric age group is predisposed to the development of ascites. Unlike adults, who often develop ascites secondary to acquired diseases, ascites in children is more often the result of congenital defects. Obstructive urinary tract anomalies are the most common cause of neonatal ascites (1). Other forms of ascites can be seen with a diverse group of diseases including hydrops fetalis, occult perforations of the gastrointestinal tract, cardiac abnormalities with associated congestive heart failure, portal hypertension, postoperative Fontan procedures, peritonitis, metabolic diseases, malnutrition, neoplasias, lymphatic obstruction, and obstructed ventriculoperitoneal shunts. The basic pathologic mechanisms resulting in ascites include (*a*) high venous hydrostatic pressure (i.e., congestive heart failure, portal hypertension), (*b*) decreased plasma colloid oncotic pressure, (i.e., hypoproteinemia), (*c*) lymphatic obstruction, (*d*) genitourinary obstruction, (*e*) inflammation (i.e., peritonitis), and (*f*) ruptured viscus (2, 3).

Marked ascites is clinically noted by a protuberant abdomen and bulging flanks in the supine position. Shifting areas of dullness may be noted by percussion of the abdomen as the patient moves from a supine to a decubitus position. The clinician can appreciate fluid waves by placing the hands on a supine patient's opposing flanks (4). Regardless of the etiology of ascites, infants and small children may develop clinical symptoms by both direct and indirect effects on respiratory function. With marked ascitic fluid collections, restriction of diaphragmatic movement and compression of lower lung fields occur resulting in decreased functional residual capacity, increased ventilation-perfusion mismatch, and eventual respiratory compromise.

In adult patients with cirrhosis and ascites, rapid removal of peritoneal fluid (8 L, or approximately 120 mL/kg, over one hour)

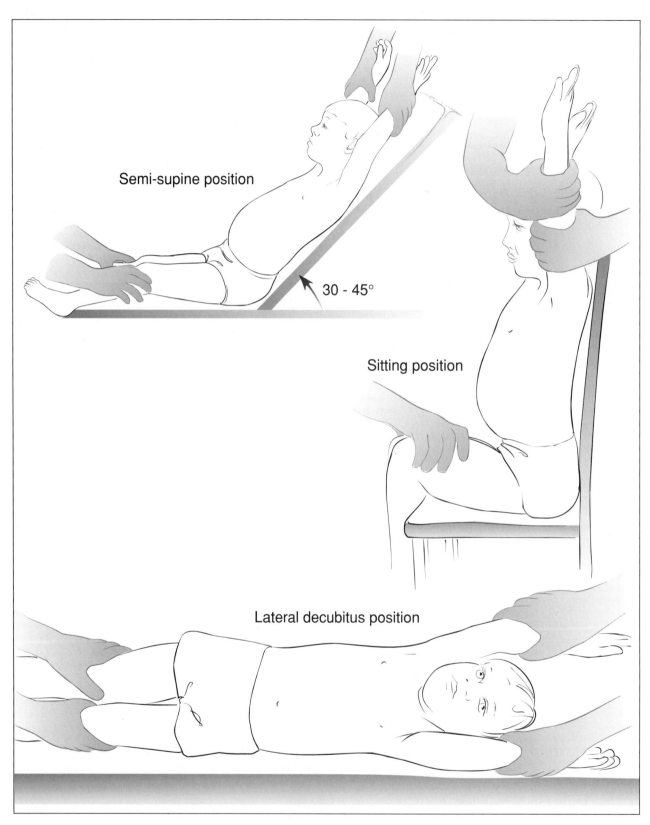

Semi-supine position

30 - 45°

Sitting position

Lateral decubitus position

Figure 88.1.
Patient positions for paracentesis.

has been associated with increased cardiac output 1 hour after paracentesis (5). However, prerenal azotemia, hyponatremia, decreased central venous pressure, decreased pulmonary capillary wedge pressure and decreased cardiac output subsequently developed 24 hours later in these patients. Albumin replacement (8 g albumin for every 1 L of peritoneal fluid removed) prevented these effects.

INDICATIONS

Paracentesis for therapeutic purposes is often temporizing until the etiology is determined and treated. In some situations, ascitic fluid is difficult to locate and a radiologist should be consulted. Ultrasound may detect as little as 10 mL in an optimal setting and can discern loculated areas of fluid (6, 7). Radiographic films of the abdomen reflect indirect findings and only are helpful if a large amount of fluid is present.

Paracentesis should never be performed through an area of cellulitis. In addition, relative contraindications include patients with prior abdominal surgeries, due to the possibility of perforation of adhered bowel loops. In these patients, paracentesis should be performed in consultation with a pediatric surgeon. Patients with abnormal coagulation studies are at risk of developing an expanding abdominal wall hematoma (8). Coagulopathy, however, is not a contraindication to performing paracentesis. Pregnant patients also can undergo paracentesis with selection of the proper puncture site (see Procedure).

EQUIPMENT

Antiseptic solution
Intravenous catheter—16 to 22 gauge
20 mL syringe
1% lidocaine with or without epinephrine
5 to 10 mL syringe with 25- to 30-gauge needle

Sterile specimen vials
Sterile gauze dressings

Monitoring equipment should be used and intravenous access should be obtained in cases of large volume removal. These patients should be monitored for heart rate, respirations, blood pressure, and oxygen saturation.

PROCEDURE

Once ascites is identified either by physical examination or radiography, the child should be placed in one of three positions: sitting, semi-supine, or lateral decubitus. The patient is secured by assistants or restraints. The bladder should be emptied by catheterization (Chapter 98). Gastric distension should be remedied by gastric intubation (Chapter 86). The site of aspiration is prepped with an antiseptic solution and sterile drapes are applied.

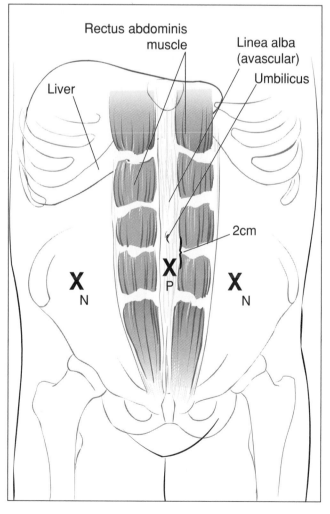

Figure 88.2.
Neonatal insertion site (N) below the umbilicus, lateral to the rectus abdominis muscle. Pediatric insertion site (P) along the midline at the avascular linea alba, 2 cm below the umbilicus.

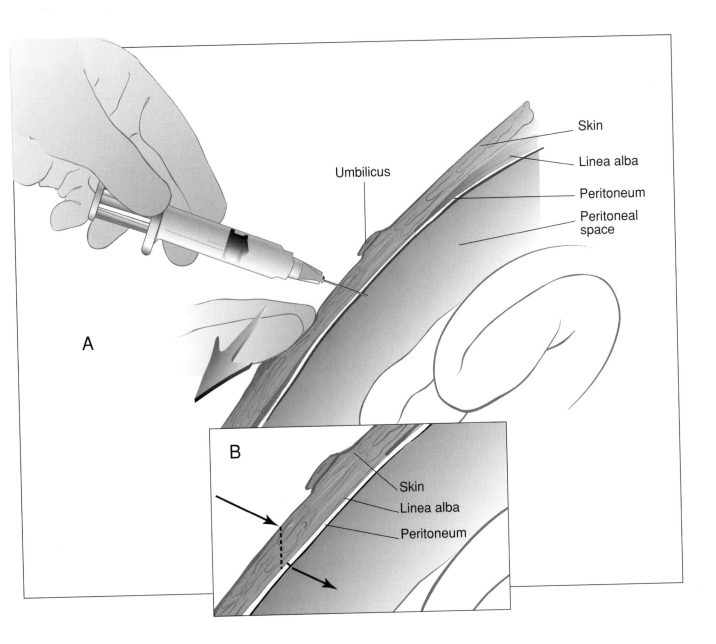

Umbilicus

Skin

Linea alba

Peritoneum

Peritoneal
space

A

B

Skin
Linea alba
Peritoneum

Figure 88.3.
Z-track formation and
controlled removal of
ascitic fluid.
A. Needle insertion with
caudal traction on
overlying skin.
B. Z-track formation after
release of skin and removal
of needle.

Needle insertion can be performed in various sites. In neonates an area lateral to the rectus abdominis muscle and below the umbilicus is chosen to avoid the liver and spleen (9) (Fig. 88.2). The most common site in children is the midline at the avascular linea alba, 2 cm below the umbilicus (1) (Fig. 88.2). Needle insertion in pregnant patients should be above the umbilicus and lateral to the midline. Care should be taken not to pierce the rectus abdominis muscle and risk puncturing the superior or inferior epigastric artery.

Once the site is chosen, several milliliters of 1% lidocaine, with or without epi-

nephrine (maximum infiltration: 4 mL/kg lidocaine without epinephrine, 7 mL/kg lidocaine with epinephrine) are infiltrated subcutaneously down to the peritoneum using a small gauge needle. The clinician then inserts an intravenous catheter at a 30 to 45° angle through the wheal of anesthesia while one hand pulls the skin caudally (Fig. 88.3). The clinician advances the needle and syringe with negative pressure applied until he or she feels a "pop" as the catheter passes through the peritoneum and fluid is visible in the syringe. While holding the needle, the plastic sheath is advanced into the peritoneal cavity. The needle is removed and the syringe reapplied to the catheter with subsequent collection and removal of fluid. Overly rapid removal of fluid can cause adverse effects as described, if intravenous albumin replacement is not provided (see Anatomy and Physiology). On removing the catheter and syringe, the oblique angle and formation of a Z-track will allow for sealing and prevention of a leak (Fig. 88.3) (8).

Fluid (20 to 50 mL) should be sent for diagnostic evaluation including cell count and differential, Gram stain, cultures (bacterial, viral, fungal), acid-fast bacillus smear, cytology, total protein, albumin, glucose, lactic dehydrogenase, amylase, blood urea nitrogen, creatinine, potassium, ammonia, and specific gravity. Interpretation of peritoneal fluid studies is well described elsewhere (2).

SUMMARY

1. Prepare patient under sterile conditions after placing in restrained sitting, semisupine, or lateral decubitus position (Fig. 88.1)
2. Catheterize the bladder and consider nasogastric intubation to relieve gastric distension
3. Anesthetize area of choice with 1% lidocaine (Fig. 86.2)
4. Insert intravenous catheter with syringe attached while retracting the skin overlying the site caudally (Fig. 86.3)
5. Advance intravenous catheter with negative pressure applied to syringe until "pop" is felt and fluid fills syringe. Advance catheter, remove needle and reattach syringe.
6. Remove enough fluid for therapeutic results and/or diagnostic tests
7. Remove catheter when finished and apply clean gauze dressing

---

COMPLICATIONS

Complications occur in 1 to 3% of patients following paracentesis (10). Persistent peritoneal leak, abdominal wall hematoma, and scrotal swelling are most common. Persistent fluid leaks can be prevented by creating a Z-track during the initial puncture. If a leak occurs, it can be stopped by a pressure dressing or suturing of the puncture site. Abdominal wall hematomas are usually self-limiting. Rarely, patients with preexisting clotting abnormalities may develop expanding hematomas and hemorrhage. Correction of the underlying clotting disorder and blood transfusion should adequately treat this complication. Scrotal swelling results from dissection of ascites fluid through tissue layers and does not require specific treatment in most cases.

More serious complications include intraperitoneal hemorrhage, bowel or bladder puncture, and bacterial peritonitis. Nasogastric tube placement, bladder catheterization, and attention to proper technique decreases the risk of viscous perforation and the potential sequelae of hemorrhage and bowel or bladder perforation. Bacteria can be introduced into the peritoneal cavity if sterile precautions are not followed. Strict adherence to sterile technique during the procedure and avoidance of areas of infection prevent seeding of the puncture site and bacterial peritonitis.

SUMMARY

Ascites occurs uncommonly in neonates and children. When present and causing respiratory distress or when fluid is needed for diagnostic consideration, paracentesis is indicated. The procedure is safe when performed in an appropriate setting by pediatric or emergency physicians familiar with the procedure and its potential complications.

REFERENCES

1. Rice TB, Pontus SP. Abdominal paracentesis. In: Fuhrman BP, Bradley JJ, eds. Pediatric critical care. St. Louis: CV Mosby, 1992, pp. 147–51.
2. Cochran WJ. Ascites. In: Oski FA, ed. Principles and practice of pediatrics. 2nd ed. Philadelphia: JB Lippincott Co., 1994, pp. 1902–1907.
3. Dudley FJ. Pathophysiology of ascites formation. Gastroenterol Clin North Am 1992;21:215–235.
4. Williams JW, Simel DL. Does this patient have ascites? How to divine fluid in the abdomen. JAMA 1992;267:2645–2648.
5. Arroyo V, Gines P, Planas R. Treatment of ascites in cirrhosis: diuretics, peritoneovenous shunt, and large volume paracentesis. Gastroenterol Clin North Am 1992;21:237–255.
6. Dinkel E, Lehnart R, Troger J, et al. Sonographic ev-

CLINICAL TIPS

1. The sitting or semisupine position is more comfortable for patients in respiratory distress.
2. Formation of the Z-track with caudal traction of overlying skin while placing the needle will seal the defect in the peritoneum and prevent leakage when the catheter is removed.
3. Repositioning the patient may improve flow of ascitic fluid through the catheter.
4. Controlled flow of ascitic fluid may be accomplished by a three-way stopcock or intravenous tubing with a flow gauge.
5. Large amounts of ascites fluid may be safely removed if albumin replacement is given intravenously (8 g albumin/1 L peritoneal fluid removed).

idence of intraperitoneal fluid—an experimental study and its clinical implications. Pediatr Radiol 1984;14:299–303.

7. Wyllie R, Fitzgerald D, Arasu T, Joseph F. Ascites: pathophysiology and management. J Pediatr 1980; 97:167–176.

8. Runyon BA. Paracentesis of ascitic fluid—a safe procedure. Arch Int Med 1986;146:2259–2261.

9. Valaes T. Neonatal ascites. In: Gellis S, Kagan B, eds. Current pediatric therapy. Philadelphia: WB Saunders Co., 1990, pp. 701–703.

10. Mallory A, Schaefer JW. Complications of diagnostic paracentesis in patients with liver disease. JAMA 1978;239:628–630.

CHAPTER 89

HERNIA REDUCTION

Mark C. Clark

INTRODUCTION

Hernia is defined as a protrusion of an organ or structure through the wall of the cavity normally containing it. This chapter will focus on abdominal hernias, primarily indirect inguinal hernias. This type of hernia is the most common congenital anomaly requiring surgery, accounting for 37% of all surgeries in a large pediatric hospital (1, 2). Femoral hernias are a rare occurrence at any age but are exceedingly rare in the pediatric population. In a 10-year survey of pediatric hernias, only 6 femoral hernias presented as compared with 1134 inguinal hernias, representing only 0.5% of the hernias (3, 4). Direct inguinal hernias are also rare in the pediatric population and often occur after an indirect inguinal hernia repair (1). The umbilical hernia is common, particularly in African-American infants. It rarely incarcerates and usually resolves by the time the child is 5 years of age (1, 2).

Incarcerated inguinal hernia occurs when the contents of the sac cannot be easily reduced into the intraabdominal cavity. Strangulation produces vascular compromise that leads to necrosis of the viscera (1). Prompt reduction of the inguinal hernia before ischemia develops is the main goal of management. The primary problem facing the physician is not the management of the inguinal hernia, which is relatively straightforward, but the diagnosis. The aim of this chapter is to provide a better understanding of the clinical presentation of the inguinal hernia and its expeditious management to prevent complications when incarceration occurs.

ANATOMY AND PHYSIOLOGY

The processus vaginalis, a protrusion of the anterior abdominal wall peritoneum, appears at approximately 12 weeks gestation when it invaginates into the internal ring of the inguinal canal. From here the processus vaginalis begins its descent down the inguinal canal into the scrotum or the labia. In males, the testes, which are intraabdominal organs following the processus, enter the scrotum between 32 and 40 weeks of gestation (1, 2, 5). The right testicle arrives last in the scrotum possibly explaining why inguinal hernias are more frequent on the right side. The processus vaginalis in females travels alone, ending in the labia majora, the remnants of its descent being the canal of Nuck. The processus vaginalis begins to close before birth, and although the exact time is controversial, it is estimated at birth that an 80 to 94% patency of the processus is evident, which decreases to 20 to 30% patency in adulthood (1). From this data, it can be deduced that the processus vaginalis closes slowly, and furthermore that a hernia is not inevitable when the processus vaginalis remains patent.

The partial or complete failure of the obliteration of the processus vaginalis predisposes to the formation of indirect inguinal hernias and different types of hydroceles (Fig. 89.1). The processus vaginalis may remain widely patent resulting in a scrotal hernia (complete inguinal hernia). A communicating hydrocele may develop when the proximal processus vaginalis remains patent, but the neck of the communication is quite narrow. This allows peritoneal fluid to enter

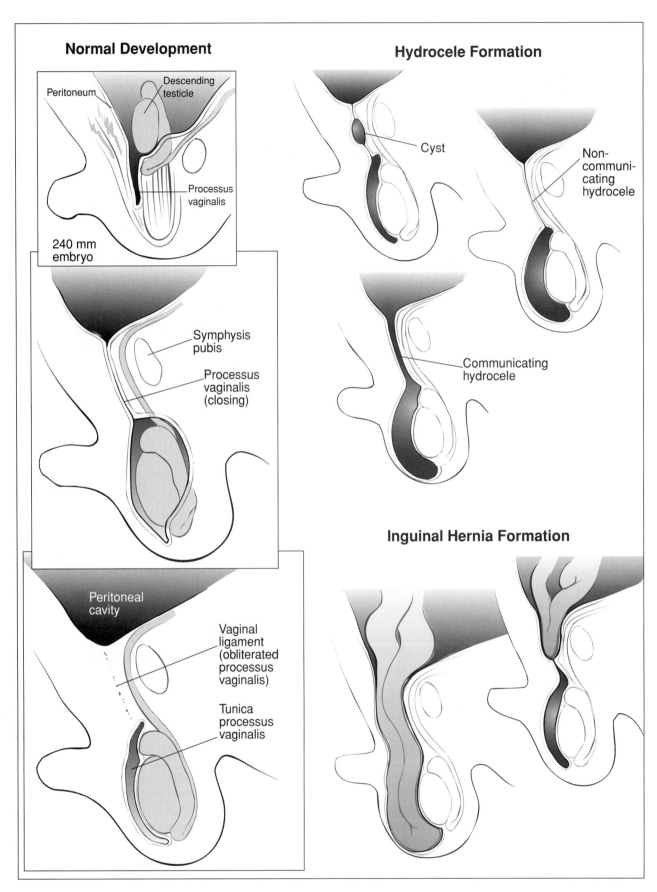

Figure 89.1.
Common anomalies of the inguinal canal.

and exit the scrotal sac, but the patent neck is not large enough to allow entry of abdominal viscera. The processus may obliterate distally leaving a patent proximal sac and the potential for an inguinal hernia. A commonly observed type of isolated hydrocele of the tunica vaginalis (noncommunicating hydrocele) occurs when fluid collects within the tunica vaginalis and the inguinal processus obliterates proximally. A hydrocele of the cord occurs when the processus closes irregularly leaving a patency and fluid collection isolated to the cord (6).

Most indirect inguinal hernias occur in healthy children, but some predisposing diseases increase the incidence of indirect inguinal hernias (Table 89.1) (1, 5, 6). Most of these conditions increase intra-abdominal pressure or fluid, cause abdominal wall defects, or otherwise prevent the processus vaginalis from closing normally.

INDICATIONS

Inguinal hernias occur in approximately 1 to 5% of the general pediatric population, but increase to 9 to 11% in premature infants (1, 2, 5). Most inguinal hernias present in the first year of life, with a peak incidence during the first 3 months of life. Overall, 60% of inguinal hernias are diagnosed on the right, 10% are bilateral, and 30% are solitary on the left (7). Bilateral hernias are much more common in premature infants. In a composite of numerous studies, boys outnumber girls for inguinal hernias 8.5 to 1 (1, 8, 9).

Incarcerations of inguinal hernias occur more frequently in girls, in premature infants, and during the first year of life. Incarceration is believed to be more common in girls because the hernia often contains an ovary (1, 8, 10–14).

Diagnosis of indirect inguinal hernia is made by observing a reducible inguinal or scrotal mass that occurs with crying or straining. In many patients inguinal hernias can be highly suspected when the parents give a reliable history of an inguinal bulge that either spontaneously or manually reduces (15, 16). When a child presents with such a history, the clinician must then search for certain corroborative physical findings. Spermatic cord thickening can be detected by rolling the

proximal cord between the thumb and the index finger. The thickening is caused by the hernia sac. The silk glove sign is positive if the clinician rubs the index finger over the spermatic cord at the pubic tubercle and feels two layers rubbing together like silk cloth. The silky sensation is produced by the two opposing sides of the hernia sac rubbing against each other. Neither of these signs is pathognomonic for a hernia, but may be helpful in arriving at the diagnosis (17). A quiet infant can be made to strain the abdominal muscles by stretching supine with the legs extended and the arms held straight above the head. Most infants will struggle to get free and thus will increase intraabdominal pressure, often causing the inguinal hernia to protrude. In the older child, the same can be accomplished by asking the child to blow up a balloon, perform the Valsalva maneuver, or cough while standing.

Incarcerated inguinal hernias present with crying, irritability, and vomiting, which can progress to abdominal distention and bowel obstruction if not reduced quickly. If the child is known to have an inguinal hernia, the incarcerated inguinal hernia may appear to the parents to be more tense and tender than before. Strangulated hernia occurs when an incarcerated bowel or solid organ infarcts and becomes necrotic. Strangulation should be suspected when the child has a fever, bloody stools, testicular swelling in addition to scrotal swelling, leukocytosis, or an inflamed scrotum or inguinal canal. Most pediatric surgeons believe the total time of incarceration to be an unreliable predictor of bowel strangulation (18).

Differentiating a hydrocele from an inguinal hernia is a diagnostic challenge in clinical practice. First, the clinician should clearly remember that bowel can transilluminate like a hydrocele, but the hydrocele is noted for its brilliant transillumination (2). Another important finding is that the hydrocele usually has a definite upper limit and never extends into the internal ring of the inguinal canal. A hydrocele is generally movable, smooth, nontender, and feels cystic. In addition, a rectal examination can sometimes help confirm an inguinal hernia by palpation of the bowel as it enters the internal ring of the inguinal canal internally. Listening for bowel sounds over the scrotum may also be

Table 89.1.
Conditions Associated with Inguinal Hernia

Abdominal wall defects
Ascites
Connective tissue disorders
Continuous ambulatory peritoneal dialysis
Cryptorchidism
Cystic fibrosis
Genitourinary anomalies
Intersex syndromes
Mucopolysaccharidoses
Myelomeningocele
Prematurity
Positive family history
Ventriculoperitoneal shunt

Table 89.2.
Differential Diagnosis
of Inguinal and Scrotal
Swelling

TESTICULAR SWELLING
   Testicular torsion
   Testicular tumor
   Epididymitis
   Epididymoorchitis
   Testicular trauma
   Torsion of the appendage of
      epididymis or testicle
   Hydrocele of the tunica vaginalis
   Communicating hydrocele
   Varicocele
INGUINAL SWELLING
   Retractable testicle
   Undescended testicle
   Hydrocele of the cord
   Incarcerated ovary
   Incarcerated dermoid cyst
   Appendicial abscess
   Groin abscess
   Inguinal lymphadenitis
SCROTAL SWELLING
   Idiopathic scrotal edema
   Allergic scrotal edema
   Henoch-Schönlein purpura
   Kawasaki disease
   Insect bite

helpful. When a hydrocele of the cord is present it can be clinically indistinguishable from an incarcerated inguinal hernia (7).

Acute scrotal and inguinal swelling includes a myriad of diagnostic possibilities (Table 89.2). Testicular torsion is another diagnosis that should not be missed. In testicular torsion the testicle is usually exquisitely tender, high riding, and the cremasteric reflex will be lost. In inguinal hernias the cremasteric reflex also may be absent, but with testicular torsion the swelling should not extend into the external ring of the inguinal canal (19, 20).

Unless the child is extremely ill appearing with signs of toxicity from gangrenous bowel, manual reduction should be attempted (6). In a survey of 40 senior pediatric surgeons, all replied that they would attempt manual reduction in clinically stable patients without signs of peritoneal irritation (18). Goals of early reduction of an incarcerated inguinal hernia are to prevent strangulation from occurring, decrease the risk of testicular atrophy, and stabilize the child before surgery (5). Pediatric surgeons have an increased complication rate when operating on an incarcerated inguinal hernia and, consequently, prefer to avoid doing it if possible (2, 10).

In the past, evidence of bowel obstruction has been considered a contraindication for manual reduction of a hernia. Obtaining radiographs showing evidence of bowel obstruction is not uncommon with these patients. In one study in which 12 of 14 infants 2 years old and younger showed radiographic evidence of bowel obstruction, the success of manual reduction was not affected by this finding. It was previously a pediatric surgery policy at the involved hospital to order such radiographs with all incarcerated hernias, but the practice was discontinued after this study (11). In the previously mentioned survey, 75% of pediatric surgeons replied they would still attempt manual reduction for incarcerated inguinal hernias even if the child had abdominal distention and radiographic evidence of intestinal obstruction (18).

Manual reduction should not be attempted by the emergency physician in a child who appears toxic or febrile, has bloody diarrhea, entrapped viscera that are black or blue, peritoneal signs, or leukocytosis greater than 15,000/mm^3 (6, 18). Even though it is considered virtually impossible to reduce necrotic bowel, cases have been reported (21).

EQUIPMENT

Ice pack
Necessary equipment for proposed route of
   sedation and/or analgesia (see Chapter 35).

PROCEDURE

Recent years have shown a gradual improvement in the published figures for manual reduction of incarcerated inguinal hernias. Most recently two studies have had 95.5% (151 of 158) and 100% (30 of 30) success rates in reduction of incarcerated inguinal hernia in children less than 2 years old (the age group in which incarceration occurs most commonly) (22, 23). Earlier studies had reported successful reductions in the 70 to 80% range (10, 11).

No prospective study has examined the success rate using different techniques of manual reduction. Instead most authorities report using some combination of sedation, ice packs, elevation, and gentle taxis (manual reduction). When pediatric surgeons were surveyed, they were quoted to use gentle manipulation 95% of the time, sedation 75%, elevation 55%, and ice packs only 18% of the time (18). The technique behind manual reduction is to apply bimanual pressure along the inguinal canal and use the hand most distal to "milk out" the gas or contents of the incarcerated bowel (Fig. 89.2). After reducing the contents of the incarcerated bowel, pressure should be slightly increased over the distal hernia as compared with the proximal aspect to reduce the bowel. The pressure should be held constant up to 5 minutes (24). If this fails, most authorities would recommend sedation, Trendelenburg positioning, and a covered ice pack or cold pack to the groin. Many clinicians favor these measures on the first attempt. Morphine sulfate (0.1 mg/kg) intramuscularly is a good choice for parenteral sedation and pain relief. When the child relaxes or falls asleep, gentle taxis as previously described should be reattempted.

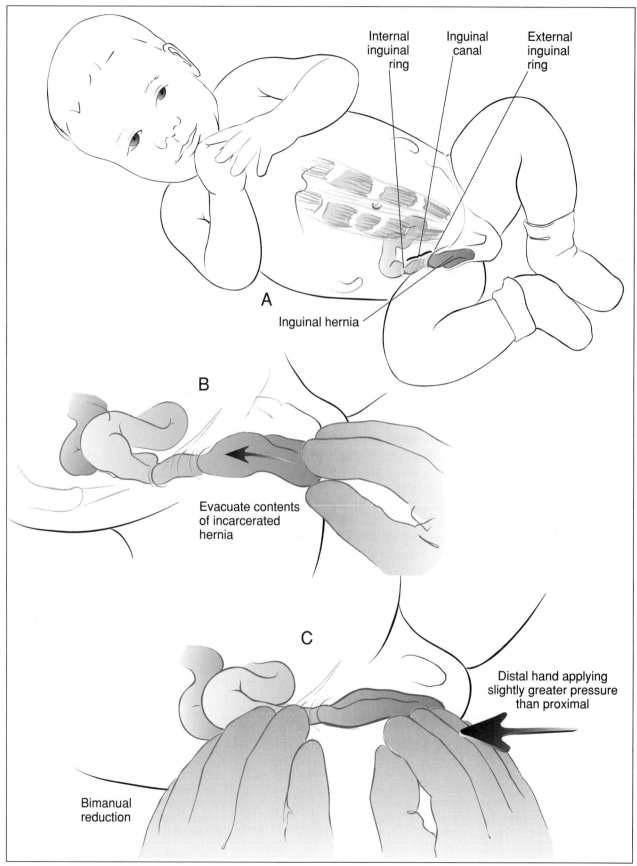

Figure 89.2.
Bimanual reduction of an inguinal hernia.
A. Anatomy of an inguinal hernia.
B. Gas and stool are first "milked out" of the bowel to reduce its size.
C. Constant pressure is applied for up to 5 minutes (distal to proximal) to reduce the bowel itself.

SUMMARY
1. Confirm the presence of a true hernia before attempting reduction.
2. Ensure that peritoneal signs are not present, and, to the extent possible, that the bowel is not ischemic. If either finding is questionable, seek immediate surgical consultation.
3. Consider sedation
4. Warm hands before contacting patient
5. Apply gentle, firm bimanual pressure along entire inguinal canal, using hand most distal to "milk out" contents or gas within incarcerated bowel
6. After reducing contents of incarcerated bowel, apply increased pressure over distal as compared with proximal inguinal canal
7. If bowel fails to reduce after 5 minutes of continuous pressure, try sedation if not used on first attempt, Trendelenburg positioning, and ice pack to groin and repeat procedure
8. Contact surgeon for all incarcerated hernias to arrange admission and semielective or emergent surgery

COMPLICATIONS

Reduction of necrotic or strangulated bowel is the most feared complication. As reviewed by Rowe and Lloyd, however, the incidence of intestinal infarction is extremely low. Between 1960 and 1965 the intestinal resection rate among 351 patients with incarcerated inguinal hernias was 1.4%. A review of three series published since 1978 indicate no resection of bowel in 221 patients with incarcerated inguinal hernias (2). Although no cases have been reported of necrotic bowel being reduced, careful examination before reduction should avoid this potential complication (21).

After reducing an inguinal hernia, the physician should ensure that the inguinal canal is empty, especially the internal ring. Cases of incompletely reduced bowel (one wall of the bowel still incarcerated), have been reported that result in necrotic bowel (Richter's hernia) (1). Most experts recommend that children with reduced incarcerated inguinal hernia be admitted to the hospital to observe for such complications and to schedule for semielective repair of the hernia. It is known that recurrent incarceration occurs frequently and often soon after the previous incarceration (13, 25).

In a female, an irreducible incarcerated inguinal hernia should suggest the possibility of ovarian herniation (11). It was previously thought that an asymptomatic, irreducible herniated ovary could be managed by elective surgical reduction. It is now known that a relatively high incidence of future torsion with strangulation occurs in this situation. For this reason, females with incarcerated ovaries should normally have urgent surgical correction (11, 12).

The vascular supply to the testis can be compromised by the incarcerated inguinal hernia resulting in ischemic necrosis and atrophy of the testis. From the available data, ischemic changes in the testes are relatively common with incarcerated inguinal hernias, but the rate of infarction is actually low. Children most at risk for this complication are premature infants, infants less than 6 months of age, and those who have unsuccessful manual reduction and require emergency herniorrhaphy (11, 14).

Two factors influence the success of an attempted hernia reduction. The longer the duration of symptoms at the time of presentation and the younger the child, the higher the incidence of nonreduction (11). The complication rate for irreducible inguinal hernias is 22 to 33% with emergency surgery as opposed to 1.7 to 4.5% for manually reduced hernias with elective repair (9, 10). Children with irreducible incarcerated inguinal hernias need emergent pediatric surgery consultation and also require similar care as any child with a surgical abdomen, including intravenous antibiotics, correction of fluid and electrolyte abnormalities, and nasogastric suctioning with the assumption that emergency herniotomy will have to be performed (2, 7). The primary reason pediatric surgeons now admit children with reduced incarcerated inguinal hernia for early semielective repair is to prevent the future possibility of recurrent incarceration and irreducibility with their associated complications (8, 9, 10, 11, 13, 15, 18, 22, 25).

CLINICAL TIPS
1. Femoral hernias and direct inguinal hernias are rare in children.
2. An indirect inguinal hernia presents with a mass at the internal ring of the inguinal canal.
3. A hydrocele is usually smooth, nontender and mobile, has brilliant transillumination (bowel can also transilluminate), and does not extend into internal ring of the inguinal canal.
4. Communicating hydrocele often has a history of shrinking during the night.
5. When parents give a reliable history for an inguinal hernia, provocative maneuvers may cause the inguinal hernia to protrude.
6. Even with irreducible incarcerated inguinal hernias, strangulation is rare.
7. Most attempts at reduction of an incarcerated inguinal hernia are successful.
8. Irreducible inguinal hernias in girls are more likely to be an incarcerated ovary.
9. Evidence of bowel obstruction is not a contraindication to manual reduction of an inguinal hernia.

Summary

Correct performance of hernia reduction requires recognition of the presence of an incarcerated hernia, proper manual technique, and appropriate observation after hernia reduction. In most cases, reduction can be successfully performed by an emergency physician. Patients with hernias that are irreducible or with signs of peritonitis need emergent surgical consultation and surgical repair.

References

1. Bronsther B, Abrams MW, Elboim C. Inguinal hernias in children—a study of 1000 cases and a review of the literature. JAMA 1972;27:522–584.
2. Rowe MI, Lloyd DA. Inguinal hernia. In: Welch KJ, Randolph JG, Ravitch MM, O'Neill JA, Rowe MI, eds. Pediatric surgery. 4th ed. Chicago: Year Book Medical Publishers, 1986, pp. 779–793.
3. Chapman WHH. Femoral hernia in children: an infrequent problem revisited. Military Medicine 1991;156:631–633.
4. Nayeem N. Femoral hernia in children. Br J Clin Pract 1990;44:383–384.
5. Weber TR, Tracy TF. Groin hernias and hydroceles. In: Ashcraft KW, Holder TM, eds. Pediatric surgery. 2nd ed. Philadelphia: WB Saunders, 1993, pp. 562–570.
6. Grosfeld JL. Current concepts in inguinal hernia in infants and children. World J Surg 1989;13: 506–515.
7. Blumberg NA. Infantile umbilical hernia. Surg Gynecol Obstet 1980;150:187–192.
8. Moss RL, Hatch EI. Inguinal hernia repair in early infancy. Am J Surg 1991;161:596–599.
9. Rescorla FJ, Grosfeld JL. Inguinal hernia repair in the perinatal period and early infancy: clinical considerations. J Pediatr Surg 1984;19:832–837.
10. Rowe MI, Clatworthy HW. Incarcerated and strangulated hernias in children. Arch Surg 1970;101: 136–137.
11. Davies N, Najmaldin A, Burge DM. Irreducible inguinal hernia in children below 2 years of age. Br J Surg 1990;77:1291–1292.
12. Boley SJ, Cahn D, Lauer T, Weinberg G, Kleinhaus S. The irreducible ovary: a true emergency. J Pediatr Surg 1991; 26:1035–1038.
13. Stylianos S, Jacir NN, Harris BH. Incarceration of inguinal hernia in infants prior to elective repair. J Pediatr 1993;28:582–583.
14. Friedman D, Schwartzbard A, Velcek FT, Klotz DH, Kottmeier PK. The government and the inguinal hernia. J Pediatr Surg 1979;14:356–359.
15. Skinner MA, Grosfeld JL. Inguinal and umbilical hernia repair in infants and children. Surg Clin North Am 1993;73:439–449.
16. Dennis C, Enquist IF. Strangulating external hernia. In: Nyhus LM, Condon RE, eds. Hernia. Philadelphia: JB Lippincott Co., 1978, pp. 279–299.
17. Gilbert M, Clatworthy HW. Bilateral operations for inguinal hernia and hydrocele in infancy and childhood. Am J Surg 1959;97:255–259.
18. Rowe MI, Marchildon MB. Inguinal hernia and hydrocele in infants and children. Surg Clin North Am 1981;61:1137–1145.
19. Lassaletta L, Fonkalsrund EW, Tovar JA, Dudgeion D, Asch M. The umbilical hernias in infancy and childhood. J Pediatr Surg 1975;10:405–409.
20. Rabinowitz R. The importance of the cremasteric reflex in acute scrotal swelling in children. J Urol 1984;132:89–90.
21. Klein BL, Ochsenschlager DW. Scrotal masses in children and adolescents: a review for the emergency physician. Pediatr Emerg Care 1993;9: 351–361.
22. Puri P, Guiney EJ, O'Donnell L. Inguinal hernia in infants: the fate of the testis following incarceration. J Pediatr Surg 1984;19:44–46.
23. Stringer MD, Higgins M, Capps ANJ, Holmes SJK. Irreducible inguinal hernia. Br J Surg 1991;78: 504–505.
24. Schnaufer L, Mahboubi S. Abdominal emergencies. In: Fleisher GR, Ludwig S, eds. Textbook of pediatric emergency medicine. 3rd ed. Baltimore: Williams & Wilkins, 1993, pp. 1307–1335.
25. Sparnon AL, Kiely EM, Spitz L. Incarcerated inguinal hernia in infants. Br Med J 1986; 293:376–377.

CHAPTER 90

TREATMENT OF UMBILICAL GRANULOMA

Angela C. Anderson and Seema Sachdeva

INTRODUCTION

An umbilical granuloma results from chronic local infection of the umbilical cord. Prevention of umbilical granuloma formation is usually accomplished by keeping the umbilical cord dry and by applying a topical antimicrobial agent daily (e.g., isopropyl alcohol or bacitracin) (1). Removal of an umbilical granuloma is a simple procedure, usually performed in the office setting or a low acuity area of the ED.

ANATOMY AND PHYSIOLOGY

The umbilical cord is normally comprised of the umbilical vein and two umbilical arteries embedded in a gelatinous substance called Wharton's jelly. Persistence of the embryologic connection between the umbilicus and the ileum is known as a vitelline or omphalomesenteric duct. A patent urachus (allantois) describes a continued connection between the umbilicus and the bladder. These latter two anomalies can mimic an umbilical granuloma.

Umbilical cord separation usually occurs 1 to 2 weeks after birth. The remaining umbilical stump is covered by a thin layer of skin. Scar tissue with wound healing occurs within 12 to 15 days after separation. Delayed cord separation beyond 3 weeks of age is associated with defects in cellular immunity (2, 3).

Blood vessels in the stump remain anatomically patent during this time although they are functionally closed. Eventually the umbilical arteries become the lateral umbilical ligaments and the umbilical vein transforms into the ligamentum teres. While patent, the blood vessels are potential portals of entry for invasive pathogens such as *Staphylococcus aureus*, group B *Streptococcus*, and *Clostridium tetani*. Chronic local infection leads to migration of moist granulation tissue at the base of the cord. The resulting granuloma is soft and vascular with pink coloration. It may be associated with small amounts of bleeding or drainage.

INDICATIONS

Small umbilical granulomas often regress with continued application of isopropyl alcohol. However, large or pedunculated umbilical granulomas frequently bleed and may lead to umbilical disfigurement. In general, large or bleeding granulomas deserve removal.

Several umbilical abnormalities must be differentiated from an umbilical granuloma before any attempt is made at removal (Table 90.1 and Fig. 90.1). Omphalitis, characterized by periumbilical erythema and cord drainage, is caused by bacterial infection of the umbilical stump. Pathogens include group A *Streptococcus*, group B *Streptococcus*, or *Staphylococcus aureus*. This condi-

Table 90.1.
Differentiating Features of Umbilical Abnormalities

	Umbilical Granuloma	Patient Omphalomesenteric Duct	Patient Urachus	Omphalitis	Umbilical Polyp	Omphalocele
Appearance	Reddish to pink mass	Pale pink orifice	Like the surrounding navel skin	Periumbilical erythema, discharge may be present	Red nodule	Protruding sac with glistening surface
Palpation	Dry, velvety feel	Moist, velvety feel	Wet due to presence of urine	Indurated feel	Moist with some excoriation of surrounding skin	Usually soft, may feel firm if liver is a part of herniated contents
Presentation	Serous-Serosanguinous foul smelling discharge or mass after cord separates off	Discharge (mucus, gas, meconium and fecal matter) present at birth or delayed until second week of life	Urinelike discharge at birth or soon after, sometimes delayed for several months	Mild local erythema, sometimes frank purulent discharge with extensive periumbilical involvement may be present	Mucous discharge and mass visible after cord separates	Protruding sac through umbilical area at birth
Orifice and tract	Absent	Present	Present	Absent	Absent	Absent
Diagnosis	Probe test is negative	Probe test is positive Injection of contrast material into the orifice demonstrates the tract and its communication with the gastrointestinal tract	Cystography and injection of contrast material into the orifice outlines the tract	Gram stain and culture	Biopsy confirms the presence of mucous membrane of small intestine	Physical examination
Treatment	Silver nitrate cauterization. If persistent, electrodesiccation, cryotherapy, or surgical treatment may be used	Surgical repair	Surgical repair	Oral or parental antibiotics	Cauterize if sure no tract present	Immediate surgical repair

tion represents a true cellulitis of the abdominal wall which may extend internally via the still patent umbilical vessels to cause liver abscess, portal vein thrombosis, and umbilical arteritis. Abscess formation within the cord may cause a red umbilical mass that could be mistaken for an umbilical granuloma. However, the presence of periumbilical erythema and fever should lead to the correct diagnosis.

Umbilical polyps are remnants of the vitelline or omphalomesenteric duct. An umbilical polyp appears bright red and nodular. It may be associated with mucoid discharge and is comprised of intestinal mucosa. A patent vitelline or omphalomesenteric duct appears as a pale pink orifice with flatus or feculent discharge and is often adjacent to an umbilical polyp. Typically, this duct extends from the ileum to the base of the umbilicus.

A patent urachus occurs when the allantoic duct fails to close and is associated with bladder outlet or urethral obstruction. Diagnosis is made by careful observation for intermittent urine flow from the umbilicus. The urachus appears as an opening at the base of the umbilicus occasionally associated with reddened surrounding mucosa.

An omphalocele is a protrusion of abdominal contents into the base of the umbilical cord. The abdominal organs within the omphalocele are visible through the transparent peritoneum. Although large omphaloceles will not be confused with an umbilical granuloma, small omphaloceles may appear as yellow-white protrusions within the cord.

EQUIPMENT

75% silver nitrate on a wooden applicator stick

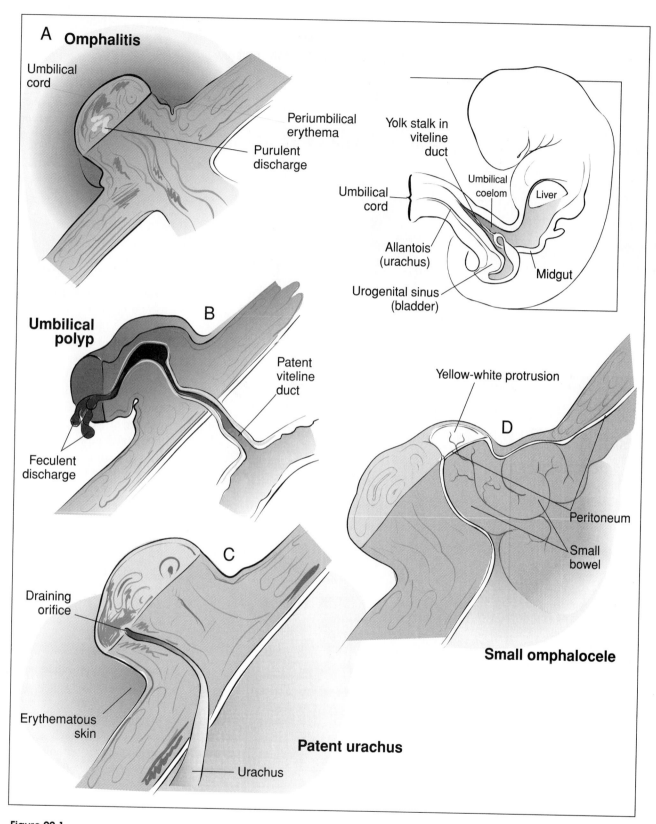

Figure 90.1.
Anomalies of the umbilical cord that must be differentiated from umbilical granuloma.

Clean gauze or cotton
Sterile suture
Sterile scissors

Silver nitrate is an antiseptic cauterizing agent. Effective cautery requires aqueous activation of the silver nitrate. The depth of silver nitrate cautery is limited by coagulation necrosis.

PROCEDURE

The desired site for silver nitrate application is carefully inspected for evidence of infection or other anomaly as described previously (Fig. 90.2). The tip of the silver nitrate stick is applied for 2 to 3 seconds to the umbilical granuloma, avoiding surrounding tissue. Cautery is signaled by a change in color from red to grey or black. If the surface of the lesion is dry, the tip of the applicator should be moistened with tap water before the procedure. Multiple applications with a single stick may be necessary with some large granulomas. Caution must be exercised to prevent contact of the silver nitrate with adjacent skin. Any excess silver nitrate or umbilical drainage should be wiped with gauze or cotton at the end of the procedure. Applications may be repeated every 3 to 5 days until the umbilical granuloma has resolved. Alternatively, large, pedunculated granulomas may be tightly ligated at the base. Subsequently, the granuloma may fall off or be cut off approximately 1 week after ligation. The base is then cauterized with silver nitrate as previously described.

SUMMARY
Large Nonpedunculated Granuloma
1. If granuloma appears dry, wet silver nitrate applicator with water
2. Apply silver nitrate to granuloma for 2 to 3 seconds until mucosa turns grey or black
3. Apply repeatedly with single stick, taking care to avoid healthy skin or spillage of silver nitrate.
4. Blot excess silver nitrate off the granuloma and surrounding skin
5. Repeat application in 3 to 5 days as needed

Large Pedunculated Granuloma
1. Tie off base of granuloma using thick (1.0 to 3.0) silk or nylon surgical tie
2. In 1 week, remove remnant of granuloma, if necessary, and cauterize base of granuloma using technique described.

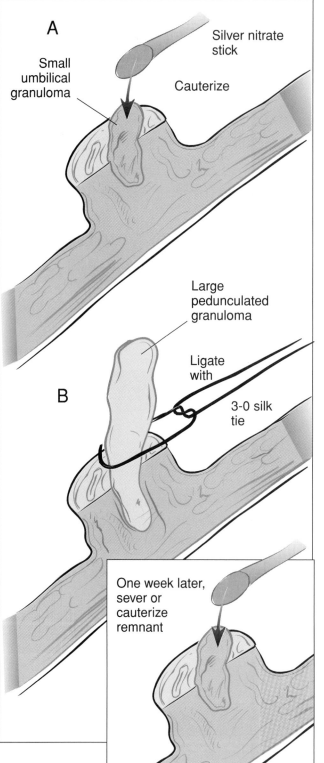

Figure 90.2.
Umbilical granuloma removal
A. Cautery with silver nitrate stick
B. Ligation using thick silk or nylon tie

COMPLICATIONS

Silver nitrate can cause chemical burns if applied to the skin, mucous membranes, or cornea (4, 5). Careless application with spillage of silver nitrate-containing fluid onto the abdomen has caused significant burns. This problem can be avoided by limiting cautery to one silver nitrate stick per procedure and carefully drying the treated area with gauze or cotton at the end of the procedure (6).

Cautery of vitelline duct remnants, a patent urachus or omphalocele makes subsequent diagnosis and surgical treatment difficult. In the case of an omphalocele, cautery may risk peritonitis and underlying organ injury. Cautery of an omphalitis risks further spread of infection and creates a poorly healing, infected abdominal wound.

SUMMARY

Umbilical granuloma removal is a simple procedure that is commonly performed in the outpatient pediatric setting. Care must be taken to differentiate an umbilical granuloma from other umbilical anomalies and to avoid damage to normal skin when performing this procedure.

REFERENCES

1. Kennedy JL. Disorders of the umbilicus. In: Gellis SS, Kagan BM, eds. Current pediatric therapy. Philadelphia: WB Saunders Co, 1991, p. 700.
2. Davies EG, Issacs D, and Levinsky RJ. A lethal syndrome of delayed umbilical cord separation, defective neutrophil mobility and absent natural killer cell activity. Abstr Br Pediatr Assoc 1982:46.
3. Hayward AR, Leonar, J, Wood CBS, et al. Delayed separation of umbilical cord, widespread infections and defective neutrophil mobility. Lancet 1979; 1:1099.
4. Laughrea PA, Arentsen JJ, Laibson PR. Iatrogenic ocular silver nitrate burn. Cornea 1985;4:47–50.
5. Fletcher PD, Wyman BS, Scopp IW. Acute necrotizing ulcerative gingivitis: sequelae following treatment with silver nitrate. J Dent 1976; 46:122–124.
6. Chamberlain JM, Gorman RL, Young GM. Silver nitrate burns following treatment for umbilical granuloma. Pediatr Emerg Care 1992;8:29–30.

CLINICAL TIPS

1. If the umbilical mass is bright red, flesh-colored, or excessively moist, cautery should not be performed until further evaluation for an orifice by probe test is performed.
2. Fever and periumbilical redness suggest omphalitis and should preclude any attempts at umbilical cautery.
3. No more than one applicator stick should be used when performing umbilical granuloma cautery.

CHAPTER 91

ORAL REHYDRATION

Julius G. Goepp

INTRODUCTION

Children with acute gastroenteritis and dehydration are commonly treated in the emergency department (ED) (1). Morbidity and mortality are related to the acute loss of circulating fluid volume, ultimately resulting in diminished tissue perfusion, metabolic acidosis, and shock. Goals of therapy in this instance are (*a*) rapid restoration of circulating intravascular volume (water and electrolytes), (*b*) correction of acid-base disturbances, and (*c*) reduction in stool output and vomiting. Of great importance to successful therapy is the recognition that parents often identify the gastrointestinal symptoms, not the threat of dehydration, as the primary concern. This conception must be addressed for any therapy to be effective.

Although oral rehydration therapy has been demonstrated to meet the goals previously described even in severely dehydrated children, its use in the United States has been limited. The most frequent obstacles to successful oral rehydration in the ED are false perceptions that oral rehydration is too slow or is not a definitive procedure. These beliefs are held as frequently by physicians and nurses as by parents. Generally, 5 minutes spent preparing for and describing oral rehydration therapy to family and staff will reduce or eliminate these obstacles. Particularly helpful is introducing the concept of one teaspoon (5 mL) per minute. In addition, oral rehydration therapy spares the child the pain of an intravenous line and promotes more direct parental involvement in the management of the child's dehydration.

ANATOMY AND PHYSIOLOGY

Acute gastroenteritis is caused by a variety of viral and bacterial pathogens. Regardless of the etiology, however, diarrhea always results when gastrointestinal fluid secretion exceeds fluid absorption. Once fluid losses begin, various physiologic processes follow. Metabolic acidosis from decreased tissue perfusion causes further decline in end-organ function, such as decreased myocardial contractility, which may exacerbate the effects of shock. Reduced renal perfusion triggers the renin-aldosterone system, resulting in sodium and water retention at the expense of increased urinary potassium losses. Ultimately, hypokalemia results in decreased bowel motility with the potential for further third space fluid losses (2).

Oral rehydration therapy can safely and rapidly restore circulating volume. Oral rehydration solutions consist of balanced mixtures of simple or complex carbohydrates and sodium. Small carbohydrate molecules promote absorption of sodium by "facilitated cotransport" (3) which in turn promotes water absorption. Oral rehydration therapy has been demonstrated to provide rehydration as rapidly as intravenous solutions and with equally good correction of electrolyte and acid-base disturbances.

INDICATIONS

Oral rehydration therapy may be used in any conscious infant, child, or adolescent with acute gastroenteritis, including the patient

Table 91.1.
Fluid Therapy Chart

Degree of Dehydration	Signs	Rehydration Phase (First 4 hours, repeat until no signs of dehydration remain)[1,2]	Maintenance Phase (Until illness resolves)
Mild	Slightly dry mucous membranes, increased thirst	ORS* 50–60 mL/kg	Breast feeding, undiluted lactose-free formula, ½-strength cow's milk or lactose-containing formula
Moderate	Sunken eyes, sunken fontanel, loss of skin turgor, dry mucous membranes	ORS 80–100 mL/kg	Same as above
Severe	Signs of moderate dehydration plus one or more of the following: rapid thready pulse, cyanosis, rapid breathing, delayed capillary refill, lethargy, coma	I.v. or i.o.** isotonic fluids (0.9% saline or Ringer's lactate), 40 mL/kg/hr until pulse and state of consciousness return to normal, then 50–100 mL/kg of ORS based on remaining degree of dehydration[3]	Same as above

[1] If no signs of dehydration are present, rehydration phase may be omitted. Proceed with maintenance therapy and replacement of ongoing losses.
[2] Replace ongoing stool losses and vomitus with ORS, 10 mL/kg for each diarrheal stool and 5 mL/kg for each episode of vomitus.
[3] While parenteral access is being sought, nasogastric infusion of ORS may be started at 30 cc/kg/hr, provided airway protective reflexes remain intact.
* ORS = oral rehydration solution
** i.o. = intraosseous

with mild, moderate, or severe dehydration. Patients with signs of shock also should receive intravascular fluid replacement in the early stages. Table 91.1 shows the degrees of dehydration, the associated signs and symptoms, and the recommended fluid therapy. The fluid deficit indicated in Table 91.1 should be replaced in the ED over the first 4 hours. The maintenance phase consists of the remaining time the child is symptomatic from acute gastroenteritis and is being managed with feeding and fluids at home.

Vomiting is not a contraindication to oral rehydration therapy, but requires some modification of the technique (see Procedure). Vomiting children or those refusing to drink may receive fluid via a nasogastric tube (Chapter 86), provided they have intact airway protective reflexes. Contraindications to oral rehydration therapy include the suspicion of an acute surgical abdomen, obtundation, or loss of airway protective reflexes.

EQUIPMENT

Specific equipment used depends on the child's age:
Cup
5 mL syringe
Small infant bottle (2 oz Volutrol) with nipple
Clock or watch with sweep second hand

Physiologically appropriate oral rehydration solution (Pedialyte®, Rehydralyte®, Ricelyte®, World Health Organization oral rehydration solution (Jianas Bros. Packing Co., Kansas City, MO, (812) 421-2880).

Optional:
Flexible 5-French or 8-French silastic feeding tube and Kangaroo Pump

Fluids with high concentrations of sugars such as soft drinks, fruit juices, and fruit punch will actually exacerbate diarrhea by an osmotic effect. For purposes of discussion, the terms physiologically appropriate solution and oral rehydration solution refer to solutions containing glucose not more than 3%, sodium from 50 to 90 mEq/L, and potassium and base to correct losses. Although Pedialyte® and Ricelyte® are generally referred to as oral maintenance solutions, some authorities do not commonly differentiate between the so-called oral maintenance solutions and oral rehydration solutions. For practical purposes in the industrialized world, solutions containing sodium in the above-mentioned range provide adequate restoration of circulating volume in children with mild to moderate dehydration. Children with severe dehydration (more than 9%) should be given a true rehydration solution containing sodium concentration of 70 to 90 mEq/L (Rehydralyte® or WHO solution).

The compositions of various solutions

Table 91.2.
Composition of Various Solutions used for Oral Rehydration

Solution	Glucose/CHO g/L	Sodium mEq/L	HCO$_3$ mEq/L	Potassium mEq/L	Osmolality mmol/L
Pedialyte®	25	45	30	20	250
Ricelyte®	30*	50	30	25	200
Rehydralyte®	25	75	30	20	310
WHO packet	20	90	30	20	330
Cola#	700	2	13	0.1	750
Apple juice#	690	3	–	32	730
Gatorade#	255	20	3	3	330

* Rice Syrup Solids
\# Soft drinks, full-strength fruit juices, and sports drinks are physiologically inappropriate fluids for children with diarrhea because of their high osmotic load. They should not be used for rehydration.

commonly used in children with acute gastroenteritis are given in Table 91.2. Note the high osmolality and low sodium content of the physiologically inappropriate solutions (cola, apple juice, and sports drinks).

PROCEDURE

Oral rehydration therapy works best when the clinician incorporates the child's parents into the process. The specific procedure undertaken will depend on parents' and clinicians' preferences. The overriding principle is that continuous small quantities of oral rehydration solution must be provided. Giving an 8 kg infant 8 oz of fluid ad lib usually results in a messy and discouraging episode of vomiting. Most parents will not be able to restrict a thirsty infant to an ounce every few minutes, unless they are given careful and explicit procedural instructions. Most importantly, giving 5 mL (1 tsp) of fluid per minute results in 300 mL per hour, or 30 mL per kg in a 10 kg baby. This rate is sufficient to rehydrate almost any infant or small child over a 2- to 4-hour period. The goal of oral rehydration therapy is to replace the entire deficit in 4 hours or less.

The child's fluid deficit should be calculated from his or her present weight and degree of dehydration. This volume of fluid should be replaced during the ED visit. The child and parent should be placed in a relatively quiet place (but where they can be observed), and the parent should be instructed to feed the child 5 mL of oral rehydration solution from a syringe every minute. A clock with a second hand should be provided. If the child vomits, the emesis should be collected

in a basin for quantification, but the 5 mL per minute of fluid should continue to be given. The child will swallow more fluid than he or she vomits. Children almost never really "throw up everything."

After 15 minutes, the physician should check that 60 to 75 mL of oral rehydration solution has been consumed. Parents may need frequent encouragement in the first 15 to 30 minutes. Periodically, emesis should be measured and compared with fluid intake. Almost uniformly, intake will greatly exceed output, but output must be measured to convince parents of this fact. Most infants and young children will readily absorb 300 mL per hour by this mechanism, and will meet or exceed the calculated replacement volume in 2 to 4 hours.

Toddlers present a special challenge. Generally, their degree of dehydration is less severe than infants. An active toddler with diarrhea and vomiting who vigorously refuses to drink oral rehydration solution can be sent home without formal rehydration in the ED in most instances. Such children may be given saltine crackers and half-strength apple juice. Consumption of 10 saltines along with 8 oz (240 mL) of half-strength juice provides approximately 70 mEq/L of sodium and 88 g/L of complex carbohydrates, comparable with oral rehydration solutions. Dilution of juice is important to reduce the osmotic load presented to the gut. Complex carbohydrates are well tolerated with diarrhea because of their low osmotic contribution (4).

For the truly dehydrated infant or toddler who refuses oral rehydration therapy, who has painful oral lesions, or who is simply too tired to drink, nasogastric feeding is appropriate. A soft, flexible feeding tube should be

SUMMARY
1. Calculate fluid deficit from physical examination (Table 91.1)
2. Begin fluid replacement with physiologically appropriate solution (Table 91.2)
3. Use cup and spoon or cup and syringe to provide 5 mL (1 tsp) per minute (rate=300 mL/hr)
4. Replace calculated deficit plus ongoing losses over 4 hours
5. When child is clinically rehydrated, discharge to home on alternating oral rehydration solution and regular feedings from a variety of high complex carbohydrate, low simple sugar feedings
6. Be certain to remind parents that:
   a. Oral rehydration therapy alone does not reduce stool output. Full feedings will reduce both output and duration of symptoms.
   b. In general an episode of acute gastroenteritis lasts 5 to 7 days. As long as good hydration is maintained, diarrheal stools alone are not harmful.
7. If the child refuses oral rehydration solutions:
   a. Give saltine crackers and half-strength apple juice
   b. Discharge patient when he or she eats 10 crackers and drinks 8 oz (240 mL) of half-strength juice with instructions as indicated

placed and secured (Chapter 86). A Kangaroo pump can be used to infuse oral rehydration solution at 20 to 30 mL/kg/hr. This technique is often useful in severely dehydrated children as an initial approach when intravascular access is being sought, particularly in children in whom intraosseous access is inappropriate. The nasogastric approach must not be used in an obtunded or comatose child.

After successful rehydration, as determined by disappearance of clinical signs of dehydration, home care instructions are critical. Parents must understand that oral rehydration solution alone replaces fluid but does not reduce diarrheal symptoms. Symptomatic improvement will depend in large part on proper feeding practices (5). Appropriate feedings (selected from the entire range of foods normally taken by the child, which contain large proportions of complex carbohydrates and small quantities of simple sugars) should begin immediately following rehydration. Continuing clear liquids or dilute formulas are not necessary.

COMPLICATIONS

Complications rarely occur with oral rehydration therapy. Overhydration (2 to 3%) may occur but is of no clinical relevance. However, the clinician must be certain that the diagnosis of acute gastroenteritis is correct, and that appropriate efforts are made to identify acute abdominal or infectious processes presenting as vomiting and diarrhea. In well-nourished infants, hyper- or hyponatremia is not a risk provided that appropriate and properly mixed solutions are used. Pre-existing electrolyte disturbances are usually corrected by proper oral therapy (5). A small proportion (approximately 1%) of infants may have acute glucose intolerance resulting in explosive watery stools within hours of taking oral rehydration solution (ORS). These infants must receive intravenous hydration with nothing by mouth until improved. Prevention of complications related to technique depends on recognition of di-

Figure 91.1.
Rehydration Orders

Mild Dehydration:			Moderate Dehydration:		
60 mL ORS/kg x _____ kg = _____ mL ORS			80 mL ORS/kg x _____ kg = _____ mL ORS		
Deliver calculated volume over 2 – 4 hours by administering 5 mL/minute as tolerated					

Treatment Record

Hours After Rx Start	Time	T	P	R	BP	Volume ORS* Calculated to be Given	ORS* Ingested	Other Ingested	Volume IV given	Stool Loss (mL)	Vomit (mL)	Assessment of Dehydration	Init.
Start													
1													
2													
3													
4													

Discharge instructions: _____

*ORS = oral rehydration solution

minished airway protective reflexes and proper placement of nasogastric tubes if used.

Frequent observation and reevaluation of patients undergoing oral rehydration therapy will permit prevention or detection of complications. Ongoing intake and output calculations allow the clinician to identify the occasional child who cannot keep up with losses and who requires parenteral therapy; using the oral rehydration flow chart will simplify the calculations (Fig. 91.1).

SUMMARY

Oral rehydration therapy is a simple and effective technique for rapid restoration of circulating volume when losses are due to acute gastroenteritis. Oral rehydration therapy may be used for mild, moderate, or severe dehydration and can be used in vomiting children. Careful attention to teaching parents and staff, and the delivery of 5 mL (1 tsp) per minute, results in the most successful therapy. After rehydration, appropriate feeding should commence.

REFERENCES

1. Glass RI, Lew JF, Gangarosa RE, LeBaron CW, Ho MS. Estimates of morbidity and mortality rates for diarrheal diseases in American children. J Pediatr 1991;118(4):S27–S33.
2. Hirschhorn N. The treatment of acute diarrhea in children. An historical and physiological perspective. Am J Clin Nutr 1980;33:637–663.
3. Hirschhorn N, Greenough WB. Progress in oral rehydration therapy. Sci Am 1991;264(5):50–56.
4. Khin-Maung-U, Greenough WB. III. Cereal-based oral rehydration therapy. I. Clinical Studies. J Pediatr 1991;118:S72–S79.
5. Goepp J, Santosham M. Oral rehydration therapy." In: Oski FA, McMillan J, eds. Principles and practice of pediatrics supplement. 2nd edition. Philadelphia: JB Lippincott Company, 1994.

CLINICAL TIPS

1. Oral rehydration therapy is less invasive and takes no more time than intravenous rehydration.
2. Parents should receive specific instructions to give no more than 1 teaspoon (5 mL) of oral rehydration solution per minute.
3. The child should be checked approximately every 15 to 30 minutes and the volume of fluid consumed compared with the amount of emesis.
4. In most cases, the amount of fluid consumed will greatly exceed the amount of fluid vomited.

REDUCING A RECTAL PROLAPSE

Gary Schwartz

INTRODUCTION

Rectal prolapse, a relatively uncommon clinical entity, refers to the prolapse of the rectal mucosa through the anus. In some instances, the rectal mucosa must be manually reduced if spontaneous reduction does not occur. Reduction can be easily performed by the pediatrician, emergency physician, or parent after adequate instruction. Although the procedure itself is not difficult, the presence of rectal prolapse in a young child should prompt the clinician to consider underlying causes for the condition.

ANATOMY AND PHYSIOLOGY

Rectal prolapse begins with an internal prolapse of the upper rectum into the lower rectum. Further extension of the upper rectal mucosa through the anus creates a partial prolapse, the most common form seen in children. Continuation of this process results in a complete rectal prolapse (Fig. 92.1). Anatomic predisposing factors that may explain the predilection for rectal prolapse in certain children include vertical course of the rectum, flat sacrum and coccyx, and a lack of levator ani support (1).

Conditions that cause increased intraabdominal pressure, hardening of the stools, or muscle weakness are also commonly associated with rectal prolapse (Table 92.1). Children under 3 years of age seem most susceptible to rectal prolapse with the highest incidence found under 1 year of age. The elderly comprise another high-risk group predisposed to rectal prolapse (2–4). Malnutrition most commonly causes rectal prolapse in underdeveloped countries, whereas in the United States, most patients with rectal prolapse have stool abnormalities such as chronic constipation or diarrhea (1, 2). Cystic fibrosis is the most serious of the potential etiologies for rectal prolapse in an otherwise well patient. Patients with cystic fibrosis have an 18% overall incidence of rectal prolapse (5). For this reason, children with noninfectious diarrhea and no other etiology for rectal prolapse or with recurrent idiopathic prolapse should be considered for a sweat chloride determination or other diagnostic tests for cystic fibrosis.

INDICATIONS

Children with rectal prolapse appear well. Rectal prolapse may even come to attention as an incidental finding by a clinician who notices a mass protruding from the anus. Often spontaneous reduction will occur before the patient is examined by medical personnel. In this instance, the physician's examination may only reveal laxity of rectal tone. For these patients, consideration should be given to the possibility that the mass described by parents represented a rectal prolapse.

Any patient with a visible rectal prolapse should have it reduced. Before reduction other conditions that can mimic rectal pro-

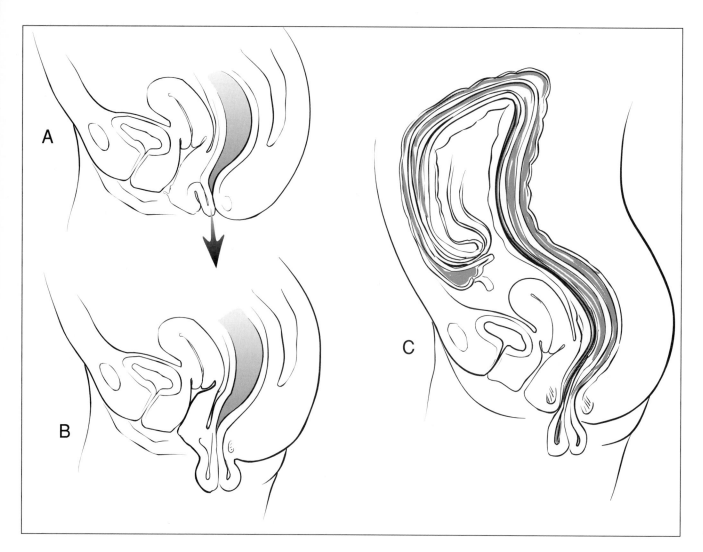

Figure 92.1.
Anatomy of a rectal
prolapse.
A. Partial prolapse.
B. Complete prolapse.
C. Prolapsed
intussusception.

Table 92.1.
Causes of Rectal Prolapse

Constipation
Diarrhea
Cystic fibrosis
Malnutrition
Excessive straining
Meningomyelocele
Idiopathic

**Chapter 92
Reducing a Rectal
Prolapse**

lapse, such as rectal hemorrhoids, a prolapsed rectal polyp, or an ileocecal intussusception protruding through the anus should be considered. Of these, intussusception requires emergent diagnosis and treatment. Differentiating features of intussusception include ill appearance of the child and inability to pass a finger between the prolapsed bowel and the anal sphincter. Hemorrhoids and rectal polyps should be easily identified because they do not involve the entire rectal mucosa.

Before reduction, sedation may be given, depending on the size of the rectal prolapse and the discomfort of the patient (see Chapters 34 and 35). Many small prolapses can be reduced with local comfort measures only. Patients who have undergone an unsuccessful attempt at reduction should receive sedation before renewed efforts.

EQUIPMENT

Gloves
Lubricant
Gauze
Tape
Sedation (as needed)

PROCEDURE

As mentioned, this procedure may require sedation for the child who is crying or fighting, as this will increase intraabdominal pressure and make reduction more difficult. The child is placed prone in the knee-chest position on the parent's lap or on the examination table. With gloved hands, the clinician should place gentle but firm pressure on the prolapsed mucosa (Fig. 92.2). A finger may be placed in the rectum to guide reversal of the prolapse.

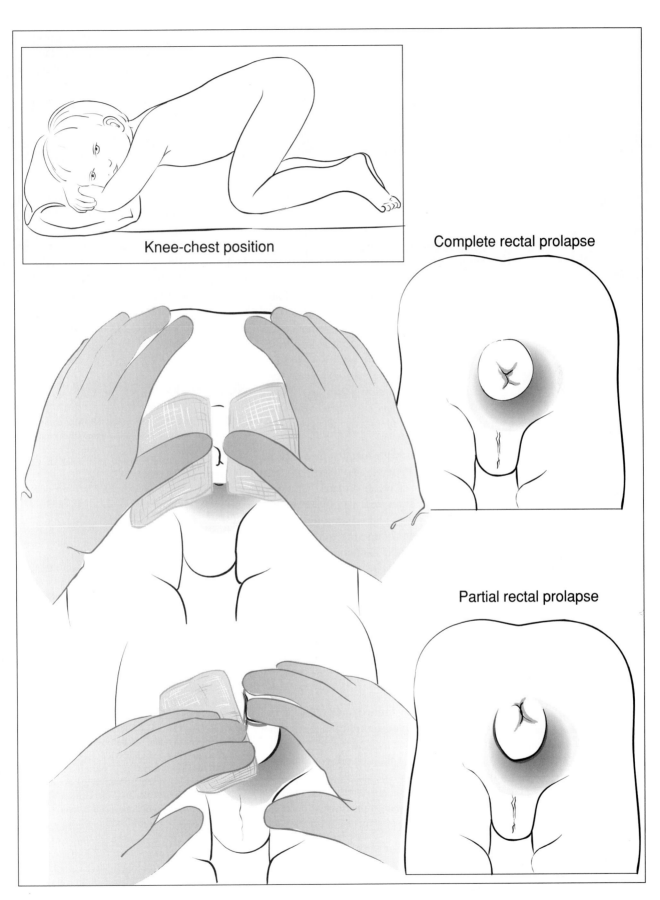

Knee-chest position

Complete rectal prolapse

Partial rectal prolapse

Figure 92.2.
Rectal prolapse reduction.

SUMMARY
1. Sedate child as needed
2. Position child prone in knee-chest position
3. Generously lubricate prolapsed mucosa with water-soluble lubricant
4. With gloved hands apply circumferential pressure on prolapsed mucosa while guiding rectum internally with finger placed in central orifice
5. Apply a pressure dressing with Vaseline-impregnated gauze, dry gauze, and tape

CLINICAL TIPS
1. The protruding rectal mass should be carefully examined to ensure that the patient does not have hemorrhoids, a prolapsed polyp or a prolapsed intussusception before attempting reduction.
2. The diagnosis of cystic fibrosis should be considered in an otherwise well child with noninfectious diarrhea and rectal prolapse.
3. Sedation and careful manual compression of the mucosa to decrease edema may help when reduction of the rectal prolapse is difficult.
4. Parents should be informed that the rectal prolapse is likely to recur and prophylactic treatment should be provided for potential underlying causes.

If the prolapsed mucosa has been out for a prolonged period of time, swelling may require manual compression of the prolapse before successful reduction. After reduction, a pressure dressing may be used between bowel movements. Parents must be warned that this reduction may be temporary and rectal prolapse may recur for several months. If this becomes a problem, retaping with a Vaseline gauze over the anus and bulky dressing may be helpful. As the child grows, the condition should resolve. Unlike inguinal hernias, rectal prolapses rarely become incarcerated in children. However, emergent surgical consultation is indicated if the prolapse cannot be reduced.

After reduction, a prophylactic regimen should be started to prevent recurrences. This regimen is directed at the precipitating cause of the prolapse. If constipation is the cause, this should be treated with laxatives and stool softeners. Diarrhea is treated as indicated depending on the underlying etiology. When cystic fibrosis patients are treated with pancreatic enzyme supplements, their symptoms should improve (5).

Few patients with rectal prolapse need surgical repair. Patients who have recurrent severe episodes of rectal prolapse requiring physician reduction and have no treatable underlying etiology should be referred to a pediatric surgeon. Numerous surgical procedures are available including anal encirclement with suture (a modified Theirsch procedure), sclerosing solution injections, linear cauterization of the anorectum, and posterior suspension with levator repair (6–10).

COMPLICATIONS

Local pain and self-limited mucosal bleeding are the most common complications encountered when reducing a rectal prolapse. Inability to reduce the rectal prolapse could potentially lead to local edema with bowel wall ischemia. In almost all cases, however, the described technique combined with appropriate sedation results in a successful reduction.

Finally, mistaking a prolapsed ileocecal intussusception for a rectal prolapse could result in delayed treatment of intussusception with significant morbidity. This possibility dictates a close examination of any mass protruding through the anus.

SUMMARY

Rectal prolapse through the anus, a condition most common in young children, can usually be reduced by the emergency physician or primary care provider. All patients with rectal prolapse deserve careful consideration of underlying etiologies, especially cystic fibrosis. Pediatric surgical consultation should be considered for patients with severe, recurrent prolapse unresponsive to conservative medical management.

REFERENCES

1. Ramanujam PS, Venkatesh KS. Management of acute incarcerated rectal prolapse. Dis Colon Rectum 1992;35:1154–1156.
2. Corman ML. Rectal prolapse in children. Dis Colon Rectum 1985;28:535–539.
3. Zempsky WT, Rosenstein BJ. The cause of rectal prolapse in children. Am J Dis Child 1988:142:338–339.
4. Armstrong AL, Bivins BA, Sachatello CR. Rectal prolapse: a brief review. J Ky Med Assoc 1978;XXX:329–332.
5. Stern RC, Izant RJ, Boat TF, Wood RE, Mathews LW, Doershuk CF. Treatment and prognosis of rectal prolapse in cystic fibrosis. Gastroenterology 1982;82:707–710.
6. Krasna IR. A simple purse string suture technique for treatment of colostomy prolapse and intussusception. J. Pediatr Surg 1979;14:801–802.
7. Wyllie GG. The injection treatment of rectal prolapse. J Pediatr Surg 1979;14:62–64.
8. Kay NRM, Zachary RB. The treatment of rectal prolapse in children with injections of 30% saline solutions. J Pediatr Surg 1970;5:334–337.
9. Hight DW, Hertzler JH, Philippart AI, Benson CD. Linear cauterization for the treatment of rectal prolapse in infants and children. Surg Gynecol Obstet 1982;154:400–402.
10. Ashcraft KW, Garred JL, Holder TM, Amoury RA, Sharp RJ, Murphy JP. Rectal prolapse: 17-year experience with the posterior repair and suspension. J Pediatr Surg 1990;25:992–995.

MANAGEMENT OF UPPER GASTROINTESTINAL BLEEDING

James G. Linakis and James F. Wiley II

INTRODUCTION

Severe upper gastrointestinal bleeding occurs uncommonly in children. However, in pediatric patients with underlying predisposition to portal hypertension and esophageal varices, bleeding can be life-threatening and difficult to control. Gastric lavage is the initial technique used to confirm upper gastrointestinal bleeding, regardless of the amount of blood loss or the etiology. Lavage is useful in estimating the rate of hemorrhage and aids in endoscopic evaluation by evacuating the stomach before the examination. Emergency physicians and, in certain cases, advanced prehospital personnel should be able to perform this procedure in a child of any age.

If the bleeding causes hemodynamic instability, vasopressin may be used to decrease blood flow through the portal circulation. Vasopressin has a 50 to 70% success rate in controlling upper gastrointestinal bleeding (1). It may be used in a child of any age and should be administered in the emergency department (ED) or intensive care unit setting.

Gastroesophageal tamponade with a Sengstaken-Blakemore (S-B) tube is rarely required in the pediatric patient for temporary control of bleeding from ruptured gastroesophageal varices. Most studies report that the S-B tube provides hemostasis in 50 to 90% of patients who are bleeding from esophageal varices (2, 3). Gastroesophageal tamponade is a high-risk procedure and should be performed only by a physician skilled in its use.

ANATOMY AND PHYSIOLOGY

Upper gastrointestinal bleeding may arise from the esophagus or stomach. In children, varices, gastritis, esophagitis, and peptic ulcer disease account for the majority of bleeding etiologies (4). Varices develop as a result of portal hypertension. Most serious upper gastrointestinal bleeding in pediatric patients results from ruptured varices.

The portal venous system includes the portal vein, the superior mesenteric vein, and the splenic vein which direct venous drainage from the stomach, small intestines, large intestines, spleen, and pancreas through the liver sinusoids. Portal hypertension results from relative obstruction of portal venous blood flow, which leads to the development of portal to systemic collateral veins, or varices. These varices develop close to veins draining into the caval systems. Esophageal and gastric varices, resulting from dilation of the anastomosis between the left gastric vein and the esophageal vein, are the most likely to bleed spontaneously because they are under the highest amount of pressure. Other communications occur between the superior rectal vein from the portal system and the middle and inferior rectal veins of the caval system or between the left branch of the portal vein and the paraumbilical veins. Although the anatomy is the same regardless of age, children with portal hypertension more commonly have congenital anomalies whereas adults with varices typically have cirrhotic liver disease caused by chronic ethanol abuse.

Chapter 93
Management
of Upper
Gastrointestinal
Bleeding

951

Mallory-Weiss esophageal tears, esophagitis, gastritis, and peptic ulcer disease are the most frequent mucosal causes of upper gastrointestinal bleeding in children. Mallory-Weiss tears are disruptions at the posterior gastroesophageal junction which occur from frequent forceful emesis. The amount of bleeding associated with Mallory-Weiss tears is usually small. Esophagitis usually complicates gastroesophageal reflux or follows from esophageal candidiasis. Gastritis may be infectious or toxic and reflects diffuse involvement of the stomach mucosa. Large amounts of bleeding may occur with a diffuse gastritis. Peptic ulcer disease is underappreciated in children and can lead to life-threatening bleeding or perforation as in adult patients (5).

INDICATIONS

The most common cause of severe upper gastrointestinal bleeding in children is from esophageal varices due to increased portal hypertension. Congenital malformations such as biliary atresia or polycystic disease, acquired mechanisms, such as cavernous transformation of the hepatic vein following umbilical vein catheterization in the neonatal period, or idiopathic causes are the major categories of portal hypertension in children (6).

Children with significant upper gastrointestinal bleeding may have tachycardia, pallor, poor skin perfusion, tachypnea, orthostatic hypotension, or frank hypovolemic shock. The quality of the emesis (coffee ground or bright red) does not indicate the amount or the seriousness of emesis. The volume of emesis may help quantify the amount of blood loss that has occurred but does not help determine if blood loss is ongoing. Significant upper gastrointestinal bleeding can occur without any hematemesis (5). For this reason, any child suspected of having significant bleeding based on history or physical examination should undergo gastric lavage to determine if hemorrhage continues.

When available, a pediatric gastroenterologist should be involved early in the management of patients with persistent hemorrhage, because endoscopy will be required to help localize the site of bleeding and to control the hemorrhage via sclerotherapy, cauterization, or esophageal banding. Angiography with infusion of vasopressin or injection of embolic material directly into the artery perfusing the bleeding site may be performed by invasive radiologists if the usual measures to control bleeding fail (7).

Vasopressin infusion is indicated for continued, hemodynamically significant hemorrhage. It should be carried out only after fluid and blood products have been given and should be considered a temporizing measure only until endoscopy can be performed.

The Sengstaken-Blakemore tube may be used for severe variceal bleeding that cannot be controlled with vasopressin infusion, sclerotherapy, or esophageal banding. Given the high morbidity and mortality associated with this procedure, however, it is preferable for it to be placed by a pediatric gastroenterologist or invasive radiologist skilled in its use.

EQUIPMENT

Gastric lavage—refer to Chapters 86 and 126
Vasopressin administration:
  Large bore intravenous line, preferably a central line
  5% dextrose in water
Sengstaken-Blakemore tube:
  Pediatric S-B tube for children less than 12 years of age or adult S-B tube for adolescents
Lubricating jelly
0.1% intranasal cocaine, 2% lidocaine jelly or a nasal spray containing ephedrine or pseudoephedrine
Normal saline
60 mL syringe
Y-connector
Manometer
Surgical clamps
Stethoscope
Tape
Scissors

The S-B tube is a triple-lumen rubber tube with a proximal esophageal balloon and a distal gastric balloon (Figs. 93.1, 93.2). Two of the three lumina inflate these balloons, and the third lumen is used for nasogastric suction. Alternatively, the Linton-Nachlas tube has two lumina for suction of

Chapter 93
Management of
Upper
Gastrointestinal
Bleeding

952

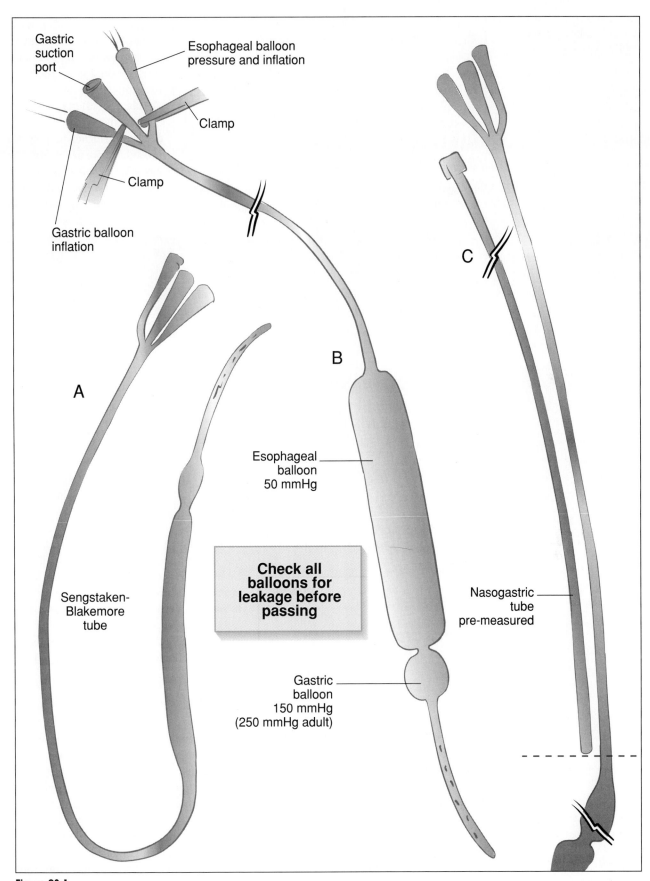

Figure 93.1.
A. Uninflated Sengstaken–Blakemore tube.
B. Inflated Sengstaken–Blakemore tube showing correct position of clamps.
C. Length of nasogastric tube to a point just above the esophageal balloon should be premeasured.

953

Figure 93.2.
Correct positioning of
Sengstaken–Blakemore
tube.

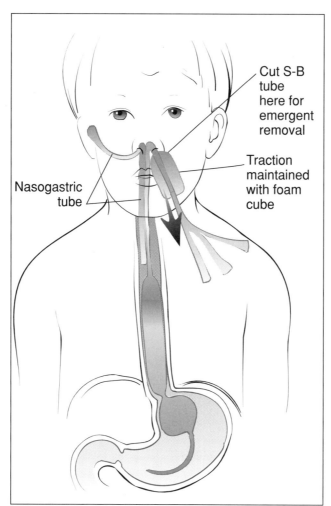

Nasogastric tube

Cut S-B tube here for emergent removal

Traction maintained with foam cube

the stomach and esophagus respectively, and has a single gastric balloon for tamponade.

PROCEDURE

Gastric Lavage

A nasogastric tube is first inserted to the proper position. A complete discussion of this procedure is given in Chapter 86. To perform lavage, 10 mL/kg of normal saline is infused into the stomach. Iced saline lavage offers no advantage over room temperature saline and may predispose to hypothermia, especially in small children. The saline is allowed to remain in the stomach for 2 to 3 minutes and then is withdrawn by gentle suction. Lavage is continued until the fluid return is clear. Returned volume of fluid should approximate the volume of fluid infused. If the

lavage fluid cannot be withdrawn, the tube is repositioned, the patient is repositioned, or more fluid is instilled into the stomach. If the return is not clearing after 10 minutes, continued lavage is of no benefit and further diagnostic procedures are necessary. The nasogastric tube should be kept in place and left to low suction, which is helpful in diagnosing intermittent bleeding and estimating the rate of blood loss.

Vasopressin Administration

A large bore intravenous line, preferably a central line, should be inserted for administrating vasopressin. The infusion is begun at 0.1 U/min and the dose is increased hourly by 0.05 U/min up to a maximum of 0.2 U/min in children under 5 years of age, 0.3 U/min in children over 5 years and under 12 years of age, and 0.4 U/min in children over 12 years of age. The patient should undergo continuous cardiac and blood pressure monitoring. Serial electrocardiograms (ECG) are also recommended. Blood products should continue to be transfused concomitantly. Once bleeding has stopped, the infusion is continued for at least 12 to 24 hours at the lowest effective dose to avoid recurrence of bleeding (7).

Sengstaken-Blakemore Tube

All balloons should be checked for leakage by inflating them underwater—the esophageal balloon should be tested to a pressure of 50 mm Hg and the gastric balloon should be tested with 150 mL of air in a pediatric tube and 250 mL of air in an adult tube (Fig. 93.1).

Before passage of the S-B tube, a nasogastric tube is placed alongside it to premeasure the distance for subsequent insertion.

Chapter 93
Management of
Upper
Gastrointestinal
Bleeding

954

The tip of the nasogastric tube should lie just above the proximal portion of the esophageal balloon. Alternatively, a nasogastric tube can be tied to the S-B tube, passing both tubes as a single unit (Boyce adaptation).

The stomach is emptied before the procedure to decrease the risk of aspiration. The balloons should then be evacuated of all air and twisted around the S-B tube to facilitate passage of the tube. The tube is lubricated and the head of the patient's bed is raised to 30°. Local anesthesia with intranasal cocaine or lidocaine jelly and a decongestant spray containing ephedrine or pseudoephedrine may be used in the nose, but not in the pharynx so as to preserve the patient's gag reflex. The tube should then be passed into one nostril, through the nasopharynx, and into the esophagus. Flexion of the neck may facilitate passage. It may be necessary to pass the tube through the mouth in small children.

The tube is passed into the stomach and any remaining gastric contents are removed. Placement of the tube in the stomach is confirmed radiographically after injecting a small amount of air into the gastric balloon (20 to 50 mL, depending on the age of the child). The gastric balloon should then be inflated with up to 150 mL of air in a pediatric balloon and 250 mL of air in an adult balloon. Only air should be used to inflate the balloons. The intake lumen should be double clamped with a surgical clamp.

Gentle traction is then applied until the gastric balloon is felt to be lodged at the gastroesophageal junction. To continue to provide traction, the tube can be taped to the mouthpiece of a football helmet. Traction also can be maintained with a split cube of foam rubber (Fig. 93.2). The tube is inserted between the two halves, and the cube is placed against the nose and strapped to the tube. Alternatively, the tube simply can be taped to the patient's nose.

Once the tube is in place, the stomach is lavaged with saline until the aspirate is clear. In many cases, the inflated gastric balloon alone will be sufficient to control bleeding by preventing flow of blood from the stomach into the esophagus and/or by directly occluding the gastric varices and submucosal vessels near the cardioesophageal junction. If the bleeding cannot be controlled, the esophageal balloon is inflated with air to 30 to 40 mm Hg.

To inflate the esophageal balloon, one end of a Y-connector is inserted into the lumen opening. A mercury manometer is attached to the other end of the Y-connector, and the balloon is inflated until a pressure of 30 to 40 mm Hg is attained. The esophageal tubing is then clamped.

At this point, if a nasogastric tube has not already been attached to the S-B tube, an appropriate size nasogastric tube is passed through the contralateral nare into the esophagus until the clinician feels it abut the upper portion of the esophageal balloon. This tube is then attached to intermittent suction, which is necessary to prevent aspiration of oral, nasal, and pharyngeal secretions. The nasogastric tube should be passed even if the esophageal balloon is not inflated, because the inflated gastric balloon does not allow the patient to swallow secretions. A radiograph is mandatory to verify tube positioning.

Once passed, the tube is left in place for 24 hours, unless a complication occurs. Patients often need to be sedated to tolerate the S-B tube and restraints also may be required. If bleeding is controlled, the esophageal balloon is deflated first, and then the gastric balloon approximately 1 hour later. The gastric tube is then irrigated for 1 to 2 more hours, and then removed.

Airway obstruction can occur with dislodgment of an esophageal balloon or an underinflated gastric balloon into the pharynx. Slow deflation or rupture of the gastric balloon may enable the esophageal balloon to migrate proximally and obstruct the airway at the oropharynx or larynx. If this happens, the tube should be grasped at the mouth and cut just below the entrance of the three channel inlets of the S-B tube thereby deflating the balloons (Fig. 93.2). The tube is then removed immediately.

COMPLICATIONS

Gastric Lavage

The complications of gastric lavage are similar to those of gastric intubation, as described in Chapter 86. In addition, use of iced saline

**Chapter 93
Management
of Upper
Gastrointestinal
Bleeding**

955

SUMMARY

Gastric Lavage
1. Place gastric tube (Chapter 86)
2. Instill 10 mL/kg room temperature normal saline
3. Withdraw saline after 2 to 3 minutes.
4. Continue until return is clear
5. If return is not clearing after 10 minutes, stop lavage and put nasogastric tube to low intermittent suction

Vasopressin Administration
1. Insert large bore intravenous line (Chapter 75) or central line (Chapter 18)
2. Infuse vasopressin at 0.1 U/min and increase by 0.05 U/min up to the maximum by age
3. Continue infusion at minimum dose that controls bleeding for 12 to 24 hours after bleeding ceases

Sengstaken-Blakemore Tube Insertion
1. Sedate or restrain patient
2. Inflate all balloons of S-B tube underwater to check for leaks
3. Prepare also to pass a regular nasogastric tube so that it rests above proximal portion of esophageal balloon
4. Empty stomach
5. Remove all air from S-B tube balloons and heavily lubricate tube
6. Apply nasal vasoconstrictors and topical lidocaine gel to tube
7. Pass tube through nostril or mouth using a bite block into stomach
8. Inflate gastric balloon with 20 to 50 mL of air and confirm appropriate position radiographically
9. Once good position is confirmed, inflate gastric balloon with 150 mL of air in a pediatric balloon or 250 mL of air in an adult balloon
10. Double clamp gastric intake lumen
11. Apply traction until gastric balloon abuts gastroesophageal junction, and secure tube to nose
12. Lavage stomach through S-B tube
13. If bleeding continues, inflate esophageal balloon until bleeding stops or to a maximum measured pressure (using a Y-connector and mercury manometer) of 30 to 40 mm Hg
14. Pass nasogastric tube through contralateral nares to a distance that places lumen just proximal to inflated esophageal balloon
15. Confirm nasogastric tube placement with radiograph

solution for lavage can lead to hypothermia in younger patients.

Vasopressin Administration

Vasopressin is a vasoconstrictor that can cause tissue ischemia in the heart, kidneys, extremities and gastrointestinal tract. These side effects are dose dependent. Water intoxication from excess antidiuretic hormone effect is a possible consequence of a high dose, prolonged vasopressin infusion (1).

Sengstaken-Blakemore Tube

Sengstaken-Blakemore tube placement carries a high risk of morbidity and mortality. Major complications such as airway obstruction, pulmonary aspiration, and esophageal injury occur in up to 35% of patients, and mortality as a direct result of tube use is reportedly in 5 to 20% or patients (2, 7–9).

Upper airway obstruction, as mentioned, can occur if the gastric balloon becomes deflated, allowing the esophageal balloon to move cephalad and occlude the trachea. Aspiration and even sudden death may occur if secretions collecting in the proximal esophagus are not cleared promptly by the nasogastric tube or if copious regurgitation of gastric contents occurs (2). Ensuring appropriate placement and patency of the nasogastric tube and emptying the stomach before S-B tube placement help lower the risk of aspiration.

Esophageal laceration, necrosis, or rupture can occur if either the esophageal or gastric balloon is malpositioned or overinflated. Injuries to the esophagus are more likely after 24 hours of tamponade, although necrosis may be prevented by deflating the balloons intermittently at 6-hour intervals (2, 8, 9). Great care must be taken to position the S-B tube correctly and to avoid overinflation of the esophageal and gastric balloons to prevent major complications.

Chest discomfort and small amounts of bleeding from local mucosal irritation in the nose, esophagus, and stomach frequently follow S-B tube placement. Rare complications include hemothorax, innominate vein ob-

Chapter 93
Management of
Upper
Gastrointestinal
Bleeding

956

struction, and tracheoesophageal fistula (10, 11). Lastly, improper S-B tube placement or inappropriate use of the S-B tube for nonvariceal upper gastrointestinal bleeding can lead to further hemorrhage while risking all of the potential complications of the procedure.

SUMMARY

Correct management of severe upper gastrointestinal hemorrhage in children requires an understanding of the correct procedures and the proper indications for each. Gastric lavage is indicated for initial management of upper gastrointestinal bleeding in children and adults, regardless of etiology. Vasopressin is infused when a hemodynamically significant hemorrhage is evident and after fluid and blood products have been administered in patients with esophageal varices and portal hypertension. Gastroesophageal balloon tamponade, although rarely used in the pediatric age group, can be an effective way to temporarily control bleeding from gastric or esophageal varices. Because of the high risk for serious complications, this procedure should only be performed by a physician skilled in its use and only when more conservative methods to control bleeding have failed.

REFERENCES

1. Johnson WC, Widrich WC, Ansell JE, et al. Control of bleeding varices by vasopressin: a prospective randomized study. Ann Surg 1977;186:369–374.
2. Bauer JJ, Kreel I, Kark AE. The use of the Sengstaken-Blakemore tube for immediate control of bleeding esophageal varices. Ann Surg 1974;179:273.
3. Feneyrou B, Hanana J, Daures JP, et al. Initial control of bleeding from esophageal varices with the Sengstaken-Blakemore tube. Am J Surg 1988;155:509.
4. Ament ME, Berquist WE, Vargas J, Perisic V. Fiberoptic upper intestinal endoscopy in infants and children. Pediatr Clin North Am 1988;35:141–155.
5. Ament M. Diagnosis and management of upper gastrointestinal tract bleeding in the pediatric patient. Pediatr Rev 1990;12:107–116.
6. Alvarez F, Bernard O, Brunelle F, et al. Portal obstruction in children. I. Clinical investigation and hemorrhage risk. J Pediatr 1983;103;696–702.
7. Boyle JT. Gastrointestinal emergencies. In: Fleisher GR, Ludwig S, eds. Textbook of pediatric emergency medicine. 3rd ed. Baltimore: Williams & Wilkins, 1993, pp. 896–901.
8. Conn HO, Simpson JA. Excessive mortality associated with balloon tamponade of bleeding varices: a critical reappraisal. JAMA 1967;202:587.
9. Chojkier M, Conn HO. Esophageal tamponade in the treatment of bleeding varices: a decadal progress report. Dig Dis Sci 1980;25:267.
10. Juffe A, Tellez G, Eguaras MG, et al. Unusual complication of the Sengstaken-Blakemore tube. Gastroenterology 1977;72:724.
11. Akgun S, Lee DW, Weissman PS, et al. Hemoptysis and tracheosophageal fistula in a patient with esophageal varices. Am J Med 1988;85:450.

CLINICAL TIPS

1. The amount of bleeding cannot be estimated by what the patient vomits.
2. Signs of hemorrhagic shock require aggressive measures and early consultation of a gastroenterologist in a patient suspected of upper gastrointestinal bleeding.
3. Gastric lavage should be performed with room temperature saline.
4. Vasopressin infusion and Sengstaken-Blakemore tube insertion are only helpful in patients with upper gastrointestinal bleeding from varices.
5. Vasopressin infusion should be administered through a central line if possible.
6. A Sengstaken-Blakemore tube should only be inserted by a person with experience in its use.
7. Great care must be taken to ensure appropriate placement of a Sengstaken-Blakemore tube.
8. To remove the S-B tube, the esophageal balloon is deflated first, and the gastric balloon is deflated 1 to 2 hours later.
9. Airway obstruction may be life threatening and requires immediate cutting and removal of the S-B tube.

Chapter 93
Management
of Upper
Gastrointestinal
Bleeding

957

GENITOURINARY PROCEDURES

Section Editor: Mark D. Joffe

PREPUBERTAL GENITAL EXAMINATION

Cindy Christian and Joanne M. Decker

INTRODUCTION

Examination of the prepubertal genitalia should be part of a complete physical examination during well-child care visits. Although the performance of this examination is not routine in an acute care setting, under certain circumstances it is essential. The purpose is either to ensure normal anatomy during routine checkups or to evaluate for pathology in children who present with complaints specific to the genital area. The examination is generally done by physicians or specially trained nurses in a variety of outpatient and inpatient settings. Until recently, the physician has paid little attention to normal and abnormal prepubertal genital anatomy, particularly in girls. Although the technique of examining young patients is relatively simple, the interpretation of findings can be difficult. This chapter will discuss the approach to performing a proper genital examination in the prepubertal child, basic genital anatomy, and common abnormalities and problems encountered. Specific indications for performing the examination also will be discussed. If, by history or examination, sexual abuse is suspected, Chapter 97 may be used as a reference for the proper method of collecting forensic evidence. Examination of the genitalia in the adolescent patient is reviewed in Chapter 96.

ANATOMY AND PHYSIOLOGY

Genital anatomy and physiology are largely influenced by hormonal changes throughout childhood, so that individual patients will have significant variation in the appearance of the genitalia depending on the child's age.

The normal, full-term infant male should have a clearly identifiable penis, with an average length of 3 to 4 cm. Any newborn boy with a penis measuring less than 2.5 cm should be referred to an endocrinologist (1). The examining physician should note if the urethral opening is in the normal position at the apex of the glans, or displaced ventrally (hypospadias) or dorsally (epispadias). Infants with either of these abnormalities require urologic evaluation. In the uncircumcised newborn boy, the foreskin is rarely retractable and should not be forced. The scrotum should be fused. A bifid (partitioned) scrotum is abnormal and requires evaluation for ambiguous genitalia. Hydroceles are common in the newborn period and, in isolation, require only follow-up examinations. The testicles should be palpable in the scrotum or easily located in the distal inguinal canal. The child with a true undescended testicle should be referred to a surgeon.

Occasionally, a prepubertal boy can present with a painful, swollen penis. In the absence of a known trauma, this swelling may be due to inflammation of the glans (balanitis) or the foreskin and the glans (balanoposthitis). The inflammation will usually resolve if treated with warm soaks and an oral antibiotic such as cephalexin. In uncircumcised boys, a painful swollen penis could be caused by an unretractable foreskin (phimosis) or a foreskin that is retracted over the glans and now cannot be reduced to the normal position (paraphimosis). Procedures for paraphimosis reduction are described in Chapter 101. The clinician should remember, however, that it is normal to be unable to retract the foreskin back from the normal position in an uncircumcised boy until he is about 3 years of age. Essentially no other changes are apparent in the male external genitalia until the onset of puberty. The first genital change to occur is the enlargement of testicular diameter to greater than 2.5 cm. The average age of onset of testicular enlargement is 11.6 years, with a standard deviation of approximately 1 year (2). A boy younger than age 9 with testicular enlargement should be referred to an endocrinologist for evaluation of precocious puberty.

In a newborn girl, it is important to identify all normal genital structures (Fig. 94.1). In term infants, maternal estrogen causes the labia majora to appear well developed and plump. The labia generally cover the rest of the genitalia and must be separated to visualize the other structures. In preterm infants, the labia majora are thinner and separated, and may actually make the clitoral prepuce appear unusually prominent. The labia majora should never be fused posteriorly nor demonstrate rugae. Either finding would indicate ambiguous genitalia. The clitoris is located ventrally at the anterior fusion of the labia minora. If any prepubertal girl is found to have a clitoris that measures greater than 3 mm in length and 2 mm in width, she should be referred to an endocrinologist for clitoromegaly. In the supine position, the urethral meatus should be located just inferior to the clitoris, between the labia minora. The vaginal orifice is located inferior to, and separate from, the urethra. The hymenal membrane should be seen just inside the entrance to the vagina, partially obscuring visualization of the vagina. It is present in all girls with otherwise normally formed genitalia. Effects of maternal estrogen on the newborn hymen cause it to appear thickened and opaque. The newborn girl may have some white or blood-tinged vaginal discharge (also secondary to maternal hormone effect), which should resolve by 2 weeks of age. Finally, the inguinal areas should contain no palpable gonads or hernias.

In the prepubertal girl, the physician should pay more attention to the anatomy of the vulva. The appearance of the vulva changes dramatically in the first years of life, as maternal estrogen effects wane. In the prepubertal girl, the vulvar mucosa may appear quite erythematous due to the normal appearance of the vasculature in the relatively thin tissue. The labia majora are less prominent than in an adolescent or an adult, exposing the vulvar structures to some extent, which leaves these structures more vulnerable to injury from straddle-type falls. Likewise, the labia minora in the prepubertal child are thin. They meet posteriorly to form the posterior fourchette, which may exhibit some friability in young girls. This friability does not necessarily indicate a pathology. Occasionally the epithelium of the labia minora are fused, as a result of nonspecific irritation. Fused labia minora may impede visualization of the hymen and vagina. In most cases, this is functionally insignificant and will eventually lyse with estrogen at puberty. Some children are symptomatic, however, with urinary dribbling and secondary vulvovaginitis. These children require a short course (no more than 2 weeks) of topical estrogen. Manual lysis of the adhesions is not recommended as an initial therapy.

Some experts have devoted much attention in recent years to the hymenal anatomy in prepubertal children. Great variation exists in the appearance of the hymenal tissue and configuration of the hymenal orifice in young girls. Generally, the hymen is thin and may be translucent, with a lacy vascular pattern. In other children, a normal hymen may appear redundant and more opaque. Hymenal types are generally classified by both shape of the tissue and appearance of the opening (Fig 94.2). Findings are described based on their location in relation to a clock face with 12 o'clock at the ventral position. A crescentic hymen is probably the most common. The tissue is U shaped and appears slung between the 11-o'clock and 1-o'clock positions. An-

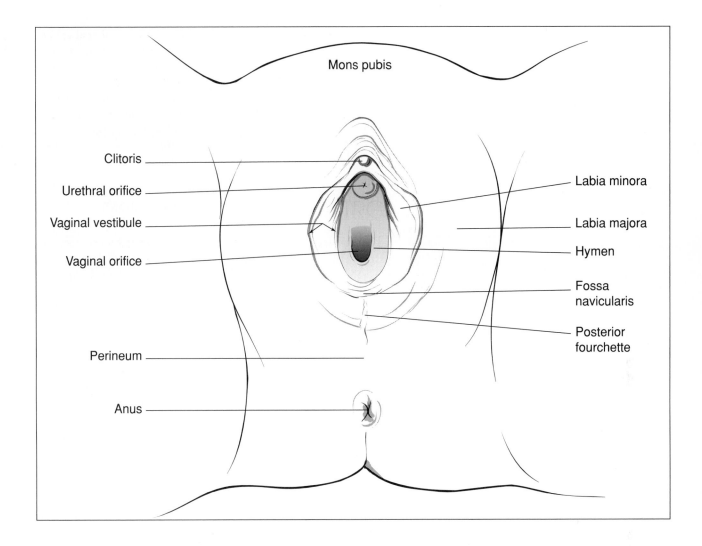

Clitoris

Urethral orifice

Vaginal vestibule

Vaginal orifice

Perineum

Anus

Mons pubis

Labia minora

Labia majora

Hymen

Fossa
navicularis

Posterior
fourchette

nular hymens are ring shaped with a central orifice. A septated hymen is identified by a midline septum of tissue that creates two hymenal openings. The examiner should ensure that the septum is isolated to the hymen and does not continue internally. This can be done visually and/or with a small curved probe placed to encircle the septum if possible. A cribriform hymen contains multiple small openings and is an unusual variation. Microperforate hymens contain one small opening, which can be found anywhere on the hymenal surface. Unlike any of the discussed configurations, an imperforate hymen is abnormal and requires surgical correction.

Genitalia of prepubertal girls are susceptible to vulvovaginal irritation for several reasons. The prepubertal vagina lacks labial fat pads and pubic hair, which in the adolescent and adult serve to protect the vulva and vagina. The pH of the prepubertal vagina is neutral, providing a favorable milieu for bacterial overgrowth. Finally, prepubertal girls may not be meticulous about their hygiene, predisposing to fecal contamination of the vulvar and urethral areas. Unlike adolescent or adult patients, in whom a specific microbiologic cause of vulvovaginitis is usually identified, the majority of symptomatic prepubertal girls have nonspecific vulvovaginitis.

The anal anatomy of infants and young children is similar in both boys and girls. The anus should appear as a separate opening on the perineum, with symmetric, thin radiating rugae. Anal tags in the midline position are common and are not necessarily pathologic. In infants, small anal fissures can develop as a consequence of straining or constipation. Small, superficial anal fissures should not be confused with larger tears extending deeper

Figure 94.1.
Anatomy of the female
external genitalia.

Chapter 94
Prepubertal Genital
Examination

Figure 94.2.
Normal variants in hymenal
structure.

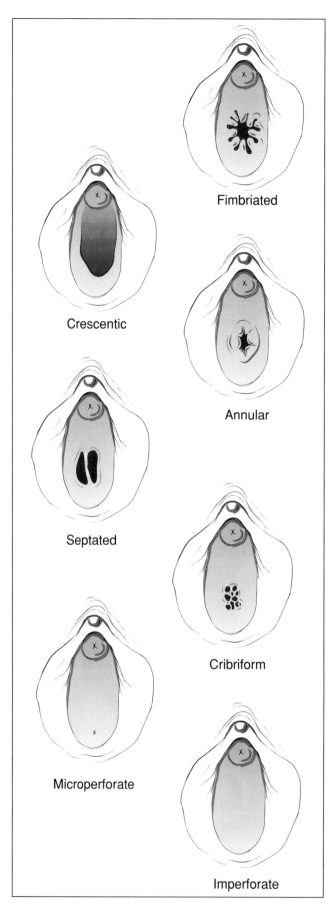

Crescentic

Fimbriated

Annular

Septated

Cribriform

Microperforate

Imperforate

into the external anal sphincter as a result of anal trauma. The anus should have a brisk wink reflex and normal tone. Children with stool in the rectal vault may exhibit anal dilation during examination. This should not be considered abnormal.

INDICATIONS

In the well-child care setting, inspection of the genitalia should routinely be done as part of the physical examination. This practice will help the child become accustomed to it as part of a normal physical examination. In addition, the physician will be able to assess for any abnormalities and become familiar with the normal variability of the prepubertal anatomy. In the acute care setting, examination of the genitalia is mandatory for any child with the following complaints: vaginal or penile discharge and/or bleeding, dysuria, genital rash, pruritus or pain, a history of genital or perineal trauma, rectal pruritus or pain, or a history of possible sexual abuse.

In general, the examination can be successfully performed with a gentle approach and patience. However, examination under sedation or general anesthesia has certain specific indications. Patients with irretrievable vaginal (Chapter 95) or rectal foreign bodies or with vaginal bleeding of uncertain etiology require a more extensive examination under general anesthesia. In children with genital and/or anal trauma, thorough evaluation and optimal repair of lacerations is best achieved under general anesthesia. Finally, young victims of sexual assault occasionally require immediate forensic evidence collection (Chapter 97). For those children who cannot cooperate with the forensic examination, sedation may be necessary. It is important to stress that most children can be examined without the need for pharmacologic agents. Physical restraint is not optimal and seldom necessary in the examination of the infant or toddler. It is contraindicated in examination of the school-aged child.

Referrals to specialists are guided by examination findings. For example, discovery of a genital mass would require consultation by an oncologist or gynecologist. Endocrinologists should be involved when the examining physician discovers ambiguous genitalia or precocious puberty. Patients with hypospadias, imperforate hymen, significant genital trauma, undescended testicles, hernias (Chapter 89), or other operatively correctable diagnoses should be referred to the proper surgical subspecialist. Children with unexplained genital injuries or sexually transmitted diseases should be referred not only to a child protective service and the police, but also, if possible, to a physician with expertise in the evaluation and follow-up of sexually abused children.

EQUIPMENT

Examining gloves
Patient gown
Light source (e.g., goose-neck lamp)
Colposcope or otoscope
Several calcium alginate swabs (calgiswabs)
    if cultures are indicated (Table 97.1)
Standard size culture swab
Sterile nonbacteriostatic saline
Microscopic slides
Culture and/or transport media for gonorrhea
    and chlamydia
Viscous lidocaine (optional)

PROCEDURE

The patient should be informed before starting that a full physical examination including an evaluation of the genitalia will be done. To ensure that the child understands the precise nature of the examination, it is wise to use terms for anatomic parts with which the child is familiar. Parents of young children can relate the names for genitalia used in their household. The child may be given the choice of having the parent present during the examination. Most young children want a parent in the examining room during the evaluation, whereas older children often opt to be alone. If a parent is not going to be in the room, another member of the health care team should be present to chaperone during the procedure. After the examination is explained, the child should disrobe without the physician present. Examining gowns are typically used, except for very young patients who either do not know the difference or want to be able to see everything that is happening. Before starting the examination, the physician should be sure all necessary equipment is easily accessible.

Genital examination of the young child should be preceded by a general physical examination to evaluate for evidence of systemic illness, which also allows the child to become familiar with the examiner and places the genital examination in a medical context. For children who are uncooperative, examination can be limited to the heart, lungs, and abdomen. The abdomen is auscultated and palpated for organomegaly, masses, and tenderness. The clinician should feel for inguinal adenopathy, which may indicate infection. Genital examination begins with assessment of Tanner staging of pubic hair for all patients and of the breasts in girls.

Boys

Examination of the penis and scrotum is straightforward. With the patient in the supine position, the clinician should lift the penis off the scrotum. The penis should be evaluated for any abnormalities including skin lesions such as warts, vesicles, or chancres. In an uncircumcised boy, the foreskin area should be examined for inflammation (balanoposthitis) or other abnormalities. In a boy under age 3 years, the foreskin may not yet be retractable and should not be forcibly retracted. An erection of the penis during the examination is not uncommon. If it occurs, it may be ignored or explained as a normal body response during a genital examination.

The scrotum is evaluated for any swelling, skin lesions, or bruising. Testicles should be palpable in the scrotum or in the in-

SUMMARY
1. Explain how examination will be performed before patient disrobes; answer any questions
2. Begin with general physical examination and Tanner staging
3. Have child assume supine frog-leg position—parent may sit on the examining table at child's head for support
4. Examine labia majora, perineum, and buttocks for abnormalities.
5. Grasp labia majora between thumbs and index fingers and pull laterally, downward, and outward; inspect vulva
6. Identify clitoris, urethra, and hymen and assess hymenal patency
7. If necessary, examine child further in knee-chest position.
8. If indicated, obtain specimens for culture by separating labia majora, pausing so hymenal orifice widens, and passing small swab into vaginal vault
9. Perform bimanual examination using recto-abdominal approach to locate uterus and assess for any abnormal masses
10. Allow patient to dress privately and then discuss findings of examination and any necessary follow-up

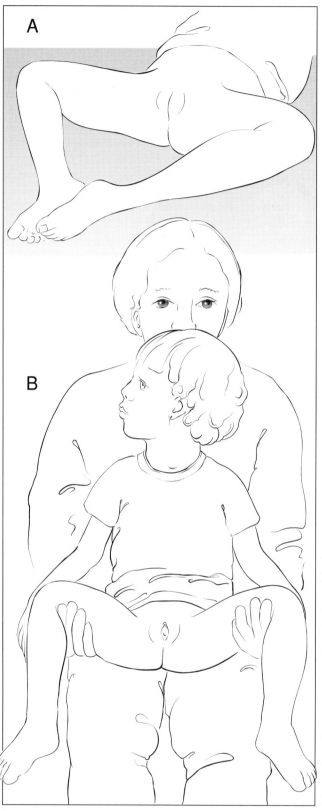

Figure 94.3.
Supine frog-leg position.

guinal canal. If a testicle is not obviously apparent, the clinician should press the index finger of one hand over the center of the ipsilateral inguinal canal, which should prevent the testicle from retracting proximally into the canal. The thumb and index finger of the opposite hand should palpate for the testicle beginning at the inguinal area and working gently down the canal to the scrotum. If the testicle is still not found, the patient should be examined in a standing position or sitting with his legs crossed. This technique uses gravity to assist in bringing down a retractile testicle. Inability to locate a testicle using any of these methods should prompt a referral to a urologist for presumed undescended testicle.

Girls

In contrast to the three stages of the adolescent pelvic examination (Chapter 96), a careful external examination is all that is generally required for the prepubertal patient. Few prepubertal girls can tolerate a speculum examination while awake, especially if they have complaints related to the genitals. If a bimanual examination is necessary, it is generally done rectoabdominally and not via the vagina. Importantly, the thin, nonestrogenized hymen of the prepubertal child is sensitive to even minimal contact with the clinician's examining finger or a swab. This discomfort can often result in the patient becoming fearful and uncooperative. For this reason, it is best to manipulate the hymen as little as possible during the examination. As mentioned previously, an unhurried, careful approach generally yields the best results.

The external examination can be done on an examining table, on a gynecologic table with stirrups, or with the patient sitting in the parent's lap. Because the examination is difficult to perform if the parent and child are sitting in a chair, the clinician should instead suggest that the parent sit on the examining table near the patient's head during the examination. Only children who are very uncooperative require examination in their parent's lap. The genital examination is done either in the supine frog-leg position (Fig. 94.3) and/or in the knee-chest position (Fig. 94.4). Most examinations begin with the child in the supine frog-leg position, as this position is usually less intimidating for the patient. Using the knee-chest position subsequently provides the physician with better visualization of the vaginal vault, because the anterior hymenal tissue falls forward in this position. The knee-chest position also may be used for better evaluation for a vaginal foreign body, or when the edges of the hymen need to be carefully assessed (as in cases of suspected sexual abuse) and cannot be seen well in the supine position. It should be emphasized that the knee-chest position is often perceived as a vulnerable position for the child because she cannot see what is happening. Therefore, the supine frog-leg position should always be used initially for the prepubertal genital examination.

To place the child in the frog-leg position, the clinician should ask the child to lie on her back, bend her knees and "flop her legs out like a frog" or "open them like a book" (Fig. 94.3). The child should be encouraged to place the bottoms of her feet together and to abduct her knees completely (2).

To place the child in the knee-chest position (Fig. 94.4), the clinician should ask the child to lie on her belly, with her buttocks in

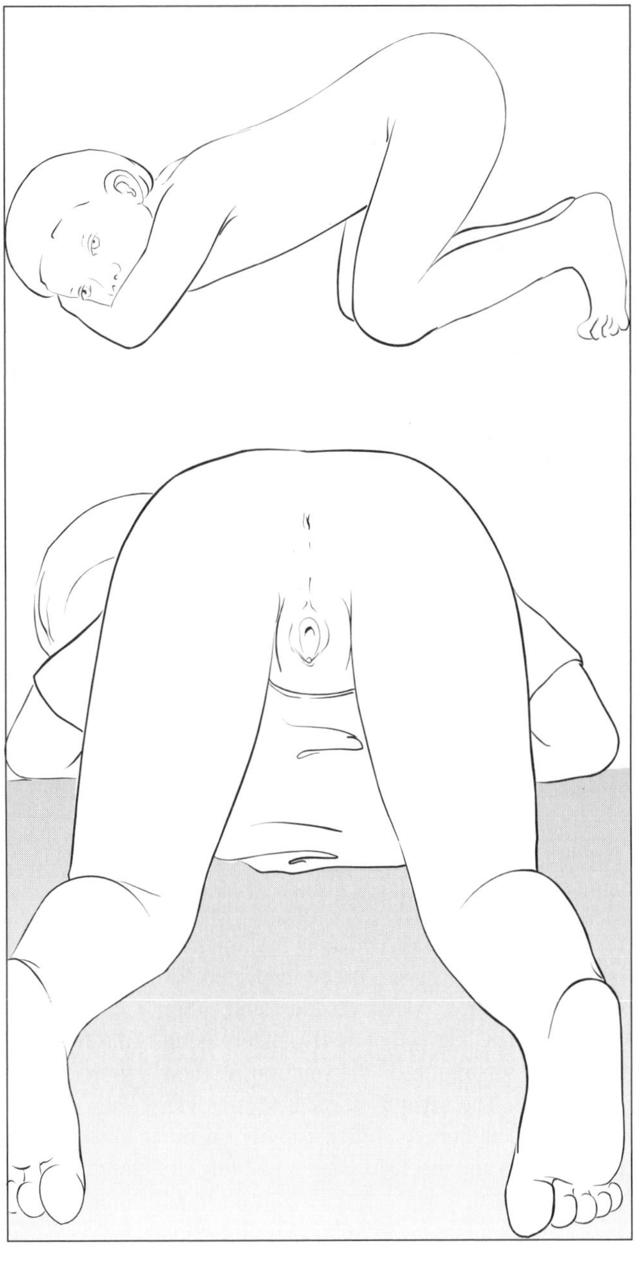

Figure 94.4.
Knee-chest position.

the air. Her head and chest should rest on the examining table. Most of her weight should rest on her bent knees, which should be 6 to 12 inches apart to allow for the best visualization of the genitalia (3). An assistant (or the child's mother) should spread the buttocks by gently pulling them laterally and slightly upward.

At the beginning of the genital examination, the light source is turned on and directed toward the child's perineum. Talking casually to her throughout the examination often relaxes the patient and facilitates the evaluation. The child should be told when she will feel the gloved hand of the clinician on her

**Chapter 94
Prepubertal Genital
Examination**

967

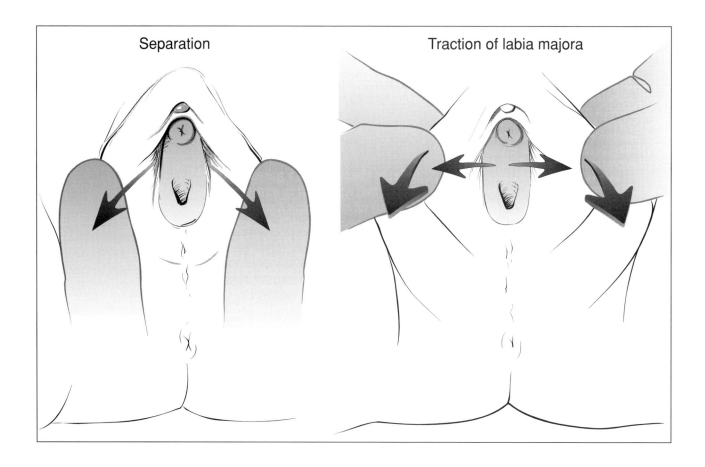

Separation

Traction of labia majora

Figure 94.5.
Techniques for inspection of the vulva.
Left: labial separation.
Right: labial traction—the labia majora are grasped between the thumbs and index fingers and gently pulled laterally, downward, and outward.

thighs or genital areas. The labia majora, perineum, and buttocks should be inspected for discharge, rashes, warts, vesicles, and other abnormalities. The vulva is visualized using either the separation or the traction method (Fig. 94.5). The separation method involves placing the thumbs or index fingers on the labia majora and displacing them laterally. In the labial traction method, the lower portions of the labia majora are held between the clinician's thumbs and index fingers, and the labia are pulled laterally, downward, and outward. This procedure should not hurt the patient and generally allows for better visualization of the vulvar structures than simply separating the labia.

The vulvar structures are examined for clitoromegaly, warts, vesicles, discharge, or signs of trauma. The clinician should identify the labia minora, the urethral meatus, and the hymen. The hymen should be assessed for patency and the configuration noted (Fig. 94.2). Some young girls have redundant hymenal tissue, which makes visualization of the vaginal orifice difficult. For these chil-

dren, the knee-chest position may be preferable. Alternatively, a small moistened calgiswab can be used to carefully manipulate the hymen and locate the opening. The calgiswab may be bent to encircle a septated hymen and to ensure that the septum does not extend internally. The clinician must remember, however, that the hymen is sensitive and manipulation usually causes discomfort. If the hymenal tissue must be manipulated, the clinician can apply a small amount of viscous lidocaine. The posterior fourchette and perineum are then examined for any abnormalities.

Patients with a history of sexual abuse or with vaginal discharge identified during the examination may require laboratory or forensic evaluation (Chapter 97). Most sexually transmitted diseases in prepubertal girls cause vaginitis and not upper tract disease. Specimens for culture, therefore, can be obtained from the vaginal vault rather than the cervix. For children with copious discharge, a swab of the discharge handled correctly will usually lead to identification of the pathogen.

For children with minimal discharge, intravaginal swabs are necessary. Calgiswabs are the appropriate swabs for obtaining vaginal cultures in a young girl. The swab should be premoistened with nonbacteriostatic saline. Labial traction should be performed with the nondominant, gloved hand. The clinician should pause for a few seconds to allow the child to relax. As the child relaxes, the hymenal orifice will enlarge, allowing for painless insertion of the swab past the hymenal tissue. The swab is inserted approximately 2 to 3 cm and kept there for 10 to 15 seconds (or less if the patient cannot tolerate the procedure) to absorb secretions. Gonorrhea, chlamydia, and general vaginal cultures are prepared in accordance with laboratory protocol. Rapid immunofluorescent tests for chlamydia are contraindicated in the evaluation of the prepubertal child with vaginitis due to high false-positive rates. Wet mounted and potassium hydroxide (KOH) preparations are prepared in the standard manner. Any vesicles noted should be unroofed and swabbed for herpes culture using a swab premoistened with special transport medium (see also Chapters 123 and 124).

The bimanual examination of the prepubertal child is done with a finger in the rectum as opposed to the vagina (Fig. 94.6). Lubrication of the gloved finger is essential. The smallest finger possible should be used for the rectal examination in an infant. Gentle pressure on the abdomen and palpation with the finger that is inserted in the rectum is usually sufficient to locate the uterus. The adnexae are generally not palpable in the prepubertal child, and the detection of any mass in these areas should be further investigated.

Once the examination is complete, the patient should be allowed to dress in privacy. After the patient is clothed, examination findings are reviewed with the patient (as appropriate) and the parent, and any necessary follow-up is discussed.

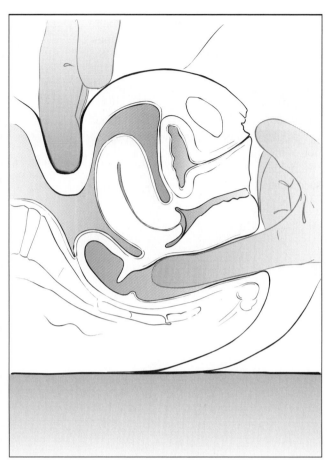

Figure 94.6.
Rectoabdominal bimanual examination allows palpation of the uterus and adnexal areas in the prepubertal child.

CLINICAL TIPS
1. An unhurried and sensitive approach will save time and make the examination more pleasant for both the clinician and the patient.
2. Talking to the child during the examination helps the patient relax.
3. Having a third person in the room can provide support to the patient and can protect the clinician from allegations of impropriety.
4. Labial traction, accomplished by gently pulling the labia majora laterally, downward, and outward (Fig. 94.5) allows for better visualization.
5. Pausing before inserting a swab lets the hymenal orifice enlarge to allow passage of the swab without touching the hymen.

COMPLICATIONS

The most significant complication that can occur is psychological trauma to a child who is forcibly restrained during the examination. As previously discussed, most children will cooperate with the examination if the clinician provides a careful explanation and uses a calm, unhurried approach. If the clinician is still unable to gain cooperation, the examination should be stopped. At this point either sedation should be considered or the examination should be deferred.

SUMMARY

Genital examination of the prepubertal girl should be part of routine well-child care. This allows the physician to appreciate the range of normal hymenal variation and assess for abnormalities. Indications for performing a genitoanal examination in other settings are based on complaints or symptoms related to the genitalia. The examining physician must be familiar with prepubertal anatomy. The examination should be brief and painless, allowing the child the opportunity to watch (if desired) and ask questions. Specimens for culture or forensic evaluation can be obtained in a painless manner to preserve the cooperation of the child. Any abnormalities or uncertain findings should be referred to the proper subspecialist.

REFERENCES

1. Hoekelman R. The physical examination of infants and children. In: Bates B, ed. A guide to physical examination and history taking. Philadelphia: JB Lippincott Co., 1987.
2. Giardino AP, Finkel MA, Giardino ER, Seidl T, Ludwig S. A practical guide to the evaluation of sexual abuse in the prepubertal child. Newbury Park, CA: Sage Publications, 1992.
3. Emans SJ, Goldstein DP. Pediatric and adolescent gynecology. 3rd ed. Boston: Little, Brown & Co., 1990.

CHAPTER 95

VAGINAL FOREIGN BODY REMOVAL

Angelo P. Giardino and Cindy W. Christian

INTRODUCTION

Vaginal foreign bodies in the prepubertal child frequently lead to vaginitis, vulvovaginitis, nonspecific genitourinary symptoms, and friability of the vaginal tissues with or without frank vaginal bleeding (1, 2). Patients with vaginal foreign bodies commonly are symptomatic and present with either bright red vaginal bleeding or purulent, foul-smelling, sometimes bloody vaginal discharge (3). Asymptomatic foreign bodies have also been described. Once diagnosed, the object must be removed from the vagina to avoid a progression of genitourinary symptoms and superinfection of the vaginal area. Serious complications may occur as sequelae of long-standing vaginal foreign bodies, including traumatic lesions to the vagina, bladder, rectum, and urethra, as well as fistula formation (4).

Early reports described a "veritable museum of curiosities" removed from the vagina, including batteries, beads, bits of toys, folded paper, cherries, cotton, corks, crayons, hairpins, insects, marbles, marker tips, nuts, paper clips, pencil erasers, pins, plum pits, safety pins, sand, shells, splinters of wood, stones, tampons, toilet tissue, and twigs (1–3, 5, 6). The most common material recovered is toilet tissue, which may be fecally contaminated (2, 5). Owing to natural curiosity, body exploration, and hygienic habits, toddlers and school-age girls are the most likely to present with vaginal foreign bodies.

In the prepubertal child irrigation of the vagina with normal saline may be sufficient to dislodge the foreign body. If unsuccessful, removal under general anesthesia may be required. In the adult patient, using forceps, vacuum suction, and other gynecologic and/or obstetrical instruments have been advocated (4, 6–8). These are unlikely to be tolerated in the prepubertal child and are generally not appropriate for this age group. Occasionally, a moistened cotton swab can be used to retrieve toilet tissue visible in the vaginal vault. Examination for a foreign body should be done in accordance with the techniques described in Chapter 94. The knee-chest position allows for good visualization into the vaginal vault and is recommended for cases of a possible foreign body. If a foreign body is suspected, saline irrigation should be performed by the examining physician or nurse practitioner. This procedure can be easily accomplished with equipment generally available in the ambulatory setting, including clinics, EDs, and primary care offices. It is a simple procedure in which success depends primarily on the cooperation of the child and the patience of the provider.

ANATOMY AND PHYSIOLOGY

A full discussion of the anatomy and physiology of the prepubertal genitalia is included in

SUMMARY
1. Explain procedure to child
2. Set up equipment—fill 60 cc syringe with saline and firmly attach to 8-French feeding tube; prime feeding tube with saline
3. Visualize hymenal orifice using labial traction; allow child to relax before inserting feeding tube
4. Apply viscous lidocaine to hymen with cotton swab if needed
5. Gently pass distal end of catheter through hymenal orifice into vagina until slight resistance is felt
6. Tell child she may feel cold water "at her bottom"
7. Irrigate vagina until effluent is clear.

Chapter 94. The foreign body, frequently fecally contaminated toilet tissue, causes an inflammatory reaction that leads to vaginitis with vaginal wall irritation, friability, vaginal bleeding, and/or discharge. Symptoms generally resolve promptly after removal.

Just as the hymen is not an obstacle to inserting foreign material, it also is not an obstacle to removing soft or solid foreign bodies in the vagina. The clinician frequently may encounter variations in hymenal configuration, but should not change the basic approach to foreign body removal. It must be remembered, however, that the periurethral and hymenal tissues are highly innervated and sensitive to touch.

INDICATIONS

The differential diagnosis in a prepubertal female who presents with vaginal bleeding with or without discharge should include vaginal foreign body. Additionally, nonspecific genitourinary symptoms with or without abdominal pain should raise the suspicion of a vaginal foreign body. Classically, the vaginal foreign body is associated with a purulent, foul-smelling, bloody vaginal discharge. Although vaginal bleeding is probably the most common presentation, routine vaginal inspection during a well-child examination may lead to visualization of a foreign body (3). Irrigation of the vagina is indicated if a foreign body is seen or strongly suspected based on the signs and symptoms.

If a foreign body is strongly suspected but is not visualized and irrigation fails to dislodge the object, or if symptoms persist, a surgical and/or gynecologic consult is necessary. Frank, uncontrolled bleeding requires more aggressive action than irrigation, but rarely occurs with foreign bodies in young children. In cases of significant bleeding, a search for the source of the bleeding is warranted, with the goal of repairing a possible laceration or identifying a mass and/or oncologic process.

Foreign body removal from the vagina cannot be accomplished without some degree of cooperation by the patient. Some children may benefit from mild sedation. Forced removal in the uncooperative child is contraindicated.

EQUIPMENT

Examination table
8-French feeding tube
60-mL syringe
Normal saline (warmed and tested for temperature or at room temperature)
Viscous lidocaine
Cotton swabs
Emesis basin
Absorbent underpads
Light source

PROCEDURE

Early reports advocated instrumentation of the sedated or anesthetized child to visualize and remove the object (1, 5). Recent experience suggests that irrigating the vagina is the initial procedure of choice for the prepubertal child (2, 3). If the object is visualized and accessible, a premoistened cotton swab can be used to "roll" the object out. Vigorous manipulation of the vagina with rigid instruments is contraindicated. Irrigation is less likely to cause discomfort than manipulation with rigid instruments. Verbal consent should be obtained.

Vaginal Irrigation of the Prepubertal Vagina

As mentioned previously, the child with a suspected vaginal foreign body should first be examined using the techniques described in Chapter 94. Examination in the knee-chest position may allow visualization of the foreign body in the vagina. Before irrigating the vagina, the procedure should be explained to the child. It is helpful to show the patient that the tubing used is flexible, soft, and thin in diameter.

The equipment is prepared by attaching a 60-mL syringe filled with saline (warmed and tested following standard protocol for warming crystalloid (9, 10) or at room temperature) to an 8-French feeding tube (Fig. 95.1). Saline is run through the feeding tube.

The child is placed in the supine position on absorbent underpads. An emesis basin may be pressed against the buttocks to collect

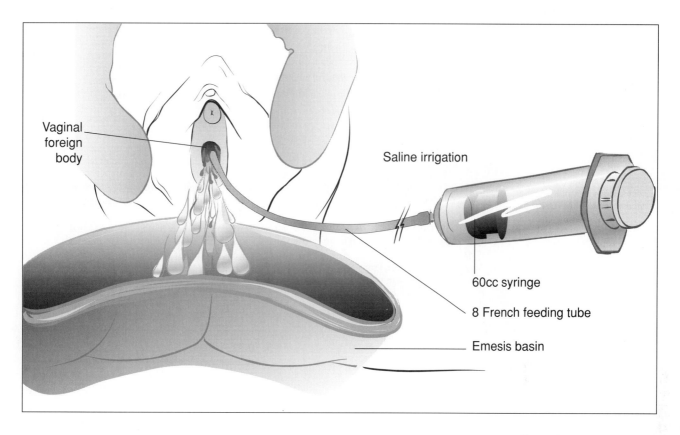

Vaginal foreign body

Saline irrigation

60cc syringe

8 French feeding tube

Emesis basin

Figure 95.1.
Vaginal irrigation with a feeding tube can remove some foreign bodies from the vagina.

saline that runs out of the vagina during irrigation. The labia majora are separated with "down and out" traction. A small amount of viscous lidocaine may be applied with a cotton swab to the hymenal tissue to decrease discomfort. Because the feeding tube is flexible and thin, many children can cooperate without receiving a topical anesthetic. After separating the labia, the child is given time to relax so the hymenal orifice will open. The clinician gently inserts the distal end of the feeding tube past the hymenal orifice into the vagina until he or she encounters some resistance. The child is then informed that she will feel cool water "at her bottom." The tube is held in place and irrigation is begun.

If irrigation results in recovering small bits of toilet paper, it should continue until the effluent is clear. It is unlikely that continued irrigation will successfully remove a foreign body after 2 or 3 unsuccessful attempts. After irrigating the vagina, the child is given a towel to dry herself and is allowed to dress. It is important to discuss the findings and further plans after the patient is dressed.

COMPLICATIONS

Few complications are associated with this procedure if performed in an unhurried, careful manner. Inserting the feeding tube should not injure the tissues in any way. The pressure generated from the setup described is not great and should not cause injury to the vagina. Forceful restraint and irrigation of the vagina in an uncooperative child poses a risk for traumatic injury and should be avoided. In such situations, examination under anesthesia is the safer option. The most common problem is failure to successfully remove a foreign body that is lodged in the proximal vagina.

SUMMARY

Vaginal foreign body should be in the differential diagnosis of prepubertal girls who present with vaginal bleeding or malodorous discharge. Toilet paper is the most common foreign body found in the prepubertal vagina. Foreign bodies can occasionally be removed

CLINICAL TIPS
1. An unhurried approach will ultimately save time.
2. Examination in the knee chest position improves the vision into the vagina.
3. Allowing the child to relax after separating the labia will enlarge the hymenal orifice. Avoiding contact with the hymenal tissue will decrease discomfort.
4. Application of viscous lidocaine to the hymen may improve cooperation.
5. Warmed saline is more comfortable for the child.

**Chapter 95
Vaginal Foreign Body
Removal**

with a moistened cotton swab or with vaginal irrigation. Vaginal irrigation is a simple procedure that should be attempted before referring the child to a specialist. Many children, however, will ultimately require an examination under anesthesia.

References

1. Ambuel JP. Foreign bodies in the vagina of children. J Peds. 1959;54:113–114.
2. Emans SJH, Goldstein DP. Pediatric and adolescent gynecology. 3rd ed. Boston: Little, Brown & Co., 1990.
3. Paradise JE, Willis ED. Probability of vaginal foreign body in girls with genital complaints. AJDC 1985;139:472–476.
4. Wittich AC, Murray JE. Intravaginal foreign body of long duration: a case report. Am J Obstet Gynecol 1983;169:211—212.
5. Henderson PA, Scott RB. Foreign body vaginitis caused by toilet tissue. AJDC. 1966;111:529–532.
6. Emge KR. Vaginal foreign body extraction by forceps: a case report. Am J Obstet Gynecol 1992;167:514–515.
7. Pelosi MA, Giblin S, Pelosi MA. Vaginal foreign body extraction by obstetric soft vacuum cup: an alternative to forceps. Am J Obstet Gynecol 1993;168:1891–1892.
8. Escamilla JO. Vaginal foreign body extraction by forceps: case report. Am J Obstet Gynecol 1993;169:233–234.
9. Werwath DL, Schwab CW, Scholten JR, Robinett W. Microwave ovens: a safe new method of warming crystalloids. Am Surg 1984;50:656–659.
10. Leaman PL and Martyak GG. Microwave warming of resuscitation fluids. Ann Emerg Med 1985;14:876–879.

ADOLESCENT PELVIC EXAMINATION

Angelo P. Giardino and Cindy W. Christian

INTRODUCTION

The adolescent pelvic examination allows thorough examination of the female external and internal genital structures and anus. A pelvic examination in the emergency setting is indicated for an adolescent female presenting with vaginal discharge, abnormal uterine or vaginal bleeding, amenorrhea, lower abdominal pain, severe dysmenorrhea, exposure to a sexually transmitted disease (STD), suspected pregnancy, genital or anal pruritus, suspected foreign body, pelvic inflammatory disease, and suspected sexual assault (1–4). Pelvic examinations are routinely indicated in the ambulatory setting for all sexually active teens, for patients seeking birth control, for STD surveillance, and for routine health assessment in all women over approximately 17 years of age (1, 5, 6).

Properly trained pediatricians, emergency physicians, and other health care providers can perform pelvic examinations with skill and accuracy. Consultation with specialists is sometimes required. Patients with possible oncologic problems or those who are pregnant should be referred to an obstetrician and/or gynecologist (OB/GYN). Consultation with an endocrinologist may be necessary for hormonal aberrations such as virilization or delayed puberty.

Despite its value, the pelvic examination is often associated with dread by both patent and physician (7). Patient anxiety is especially great at the time of the first pelvic examination, and may reach an anxiety level similar to that seen in patients before surgery (8). The most common patient concern is of pain from the procedure and this fear is directly related to the information peers have passed on to the patient (8). Additional sources of anxiety include embarrassment over having breasts and genitals exposed and examined, feelings of vulnerability during the examination, perception of losing control of one's body, concern that a gynecologic disorder will be discovered, and concerns about personal cleanliness and hygiene (8, 9). Positioning, presence of a support person, and gender of the clinician have all been associated with the adolescent's perception of the discomfort and the level of anxiety associated with the procedure (9, 10, 11).

Reproductive and sexual functions are obviously sensitive subjects, and examinations of the genital and anal area require a thoughtful approach. Using force or restraint is always contraindicated. Sedation or anesthesia are acceptable only in the most extreme cases when examination cannot be deferred, such as patients with severe, uncontrollable vaginal bleeding. Patient requests regarding gender of clinician should be accommodated whenever possible (7, 12).

Pelvic examination of the adolescent differs from the genital examination in the prepubertal child (Chapter 94) in its inclusion of an internal speculum and bimanual examination. Pelvic examinations are typically performed on adolescent patients between 12 and 18 years of age, with Tanner stages of 2 through 5. Tanner stages are analogous to sexual maturity ratings and reflect the presence of secondary sexual characteristics (13).

Although few would argue that a pelvic examination is an important part of a comprehensive physical examination in the adolescent patient, it remains a procedure viewed as technically difficult. With adequate training, the correct equipment, an unhurried approach, and a sensitive demeanor the procedure can be accomplished with a minimum of discomfort to the patient.

ANATOMY AND PHYSIOLOGY

The external and internal structures of the adolescent female genital and anal anatomy are similar to those described in the prepubertal child. They differ, however, in terms of size and estrogen effect. The length of the vagina grows from approximately 3 to 4 cm in the infant to approximately 10 to 12 cm in the sexually mature adolescent female (14). The translucent hymenal membrane in the prepubertal child changes under the influence of estrogen and appears pink, thickened, and opaque on examination. With puberty, the labia majora, mons pubis, and perineal area increase in pigmentation and develop pubic hair. The vaginal pH becomes acidic, normal vaginal flora changes, and a physiologic leukorrhea composed of desquamated epithelial cells and cervical mucus develops (15).

EQUIPMENT

Pelvic examination table with stirrups
Light source
Running water
Water-soluble lubricant
Culture materials—gonorrhea, chlamydia (in the adolescent patient rapid slides may be appropriate)
Microscopic slides
Fixative and Ayre wooden spatulas for Pap smears (if performed)
Normal saline
KOH and Gram stain materials
Plastic test tubes

Sample swabs
Specula of different sizes
Hand mirror for patient use
Examining gloves, gowns, and sheets

Different specula exist and are recommended for different ages and sizes of patients; Huffman (½ × 4¼ inches) used for nonsexually active adolescents, Pederson (⅞ × 4½ inches) for sexually active, nulliparous adolescents, Graves (1⅜ × 3 inches) for the parous female (16). Infant specula are not recommended.

PROCEDURE

Before the procedure, the clinician should discuss the pelvic examination with the patient, specifically addressing issues related to discomfort during the examination and the presence of a support person in the room during the examination. A chaperone should be in the room regardless of the gender of the clinician.

During the examination, the clinician should inform the patient about what is happening and what sensations to expect. After the pelvic examination, the patient should be given the opportunity to dress in private and, finally, the clinician should discuss findings and explain follow-up procedures.

Written consent for the pelvic examination is not necessary. Verbal consent should be obtained from the patient. Parental consent is not necessary in most situations although institutional protocols should be consulted.

Pelvic examination of the adolescent patient contains the following basic steps: (*a*) the external examination, (*b*) the speculum examination, and (*c*) the bimanual examination, generally done in that order. The patient should empty her bladder before beginning the examination. She should be asked to disrobe, including her panties, and cover herself with a sheet provided while the clinician waits outside the room.

The external examination begins by having the patient lie on the examining table. Placing a pillow under the patient's head makes the examination more comfortable and demonstrates concern for the patient's comfort. The abdomen is examined by first inspecting its shape and contour. Auscultation for bowel and/or fetal heart sounds and percussion for liver size and tenderness should follow. Tenderness of the liver may be present with Fitz-Hugh and Curtis syndrome. The remainder of the abdomen is palpated for masses, tenderness, guarding, or rebound. The inguinal area is palpated for adenopathy, which may indicate pelvic infection.

The patient is instructed in how to assume the lithotomy position, at which time the stirrups are adjusted for comfort. The patient should abduct her knees and relax her thighs into a frog-leg position. Phrases such as "separate your knees" are preferable to "spread your legs." This position will relax the pelvic musculature. First, a visual inspection of the external genitalia should note the Tanner stage as evidenced by pubic hair (and breasts). Before touching the patient the clinician should inspect for lesions, bleeding, or discharge. If the patient complains of pruritus, the pubic hair is inspected for signs of pubic lice (pediculosis pubis). A gloved hand is then placed on the patient's thigh and, while maintaining a running dialogue with the patient, the labia and mons pubis are palpated.

The labia majora are separated (Fig. 96.1.) and the vulva is inspected for signs of infection or injury. Warts, vesicles, or signs of inflammation are identified. The perianal area is checked for condyloma. Palpation of the periurethral, Skene's, and Bartholin's glands for masses or discharge follows. Clitoromegaly, estrogen status of the mucosa, and the configuration of the hymen are noted. Assessing for hymenal patency is necessary to determine if a speculum examination should proceed. The majority of adolescents with normal anatomy can tolerate a speculum examination if appropriate equipment and technique are used. A Huffman speculum is narrow, but long enough to allow for viewing the cervix. Sexually active adolescents are comfortably examined with a Pederson speculum. Obese or parous patients are best examined with the larger Graves speculum.

The speculum examination begins by first running the speculum under warm water, which both warms and lubricates the speculum allowing for a more comfortable examination. Lubricant gel is not necessary and may interfere with some specimen collections. The clinician inserts a gloved index finger of the dominant hand into the vagina, applying gentle pressure posteriorly, which will

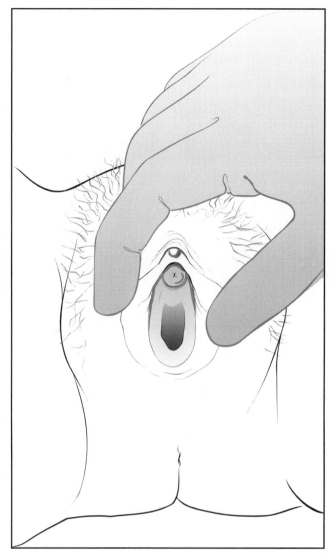

help relax the pubococcygeal muscle. In addition, identifying the location of the cervix at this time will help guide the speculum into proper position. The speculum is introduced into the vagina at a 45° angle in a downward direction, with the blades oriented vertically. (Fig. 96.2). This can be done before removing the finger from the vagina. After the speculum is inserted and rotated to the horizontal position, the blades are opened slowly to expose the cervix. Initially inserting the speculum with the blades oriented vertically minimizes patient discomfort caused when the blade edges impinge on the lateral vaginal walls. It should also be remembered that pressure applied anteriorly will compress the urethra between the speculum blade and the pubic symphysis and cause pain. If the cervix is

Figure 96.1.
Labia majora are separated with thumb and index finger for inspection of the vulva.

Chapter 96
Adolescent Pelvic Examination

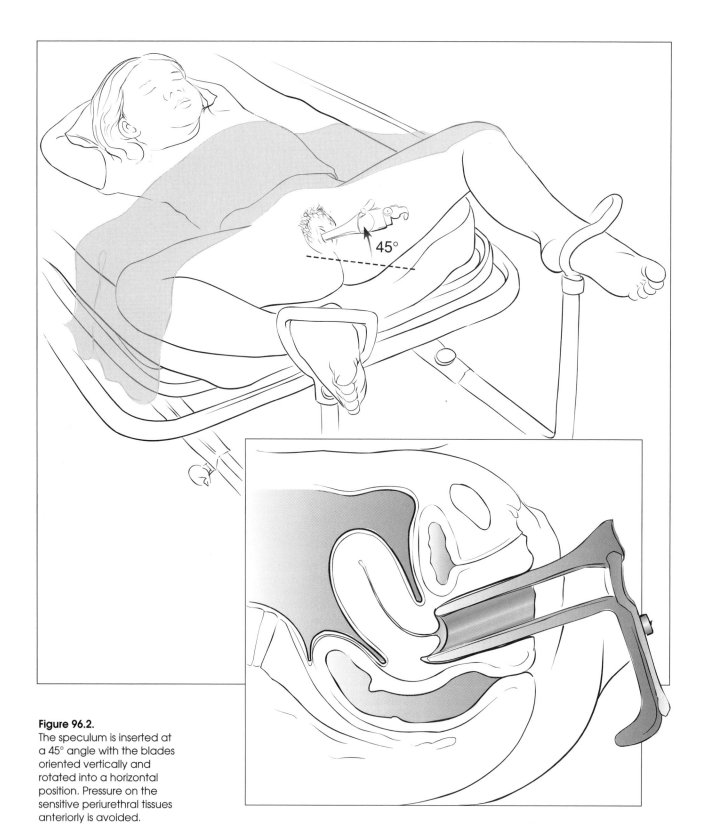

Figure 96.2.
The speculum is inserted at a 45° angle with the blades oriented vertically and rotated into a horizontal position. Pressure on the sensitive periurethral tissues anteriorly is avoided.

not visualized, the blades should be closed, repositioned, and reopened.

The surface of the cervix generally is smooth and pink. Many adolescents have columnar epithelium from the internal os ex-tending onto the external cervix. This ever-sion of the mucosa is known as ectropion, and may be normal or indicate infection.

If indicated, a Pap smear should be obtained first, before the cervical cells are

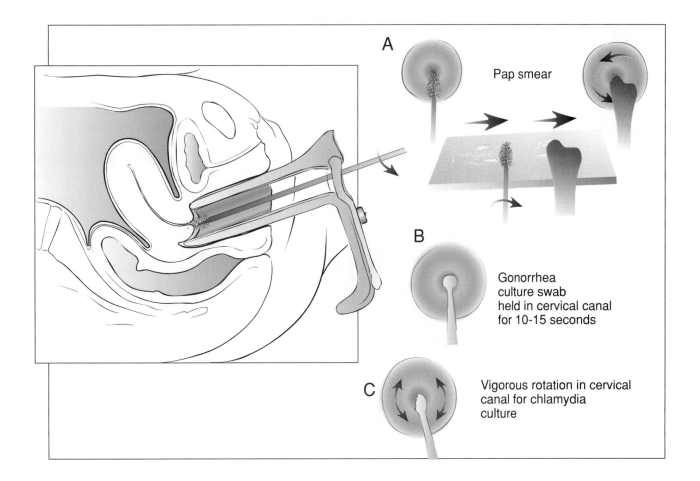

A. Pap smear

B. Gonorrhea culture swab held in cervical canal for 10-15 seconds

C. Vigorous rotation in cervical canal for chlamydia culture

disturbed. Cells from the endocervix and the cervical os are sampled (Fig. 96.3). A cotton-tipped swab or cytobrush is rotated in the endocervical os in one direction. The swab is removed and rotated in the opposite direction on one-half of a glass slide. Next, an Ayre wooden spatula is used to scrape the cervix. The spatula is rotated 360° to sample the entire surface of the cervix and smeared on the second half of the glass slide. Fixative is immediately applied to preserve the sample. Air drying of the sample will render the Pap smear unreliable.

Cultures for gonorrhea are obtained by inserting a swab 1 to 2 cm into the cervical canal for 10 to 15 seconds (to allow the swab to absorb secretions). The specimen is applied to a culture plate with medium specific for identification of *Neisseria gonorrhoeae*. Plates just taken from a refrigerator are too cold and can result in falsely negative culture results. The sample is transported to the laboratory in a sealed container with a carbon dioxide tablet. A sample obtained in the same manner can be placed on a slide for Gram stain.

Chlamydia cultures are obtained by inserting a swab with either a plastic or metal stick (wood inhibits chlamydia growth) into the cervical canal and rotating the swab vigorously to pick up endocervical cells. The swab is removed and placed in culture medium. The swab is rotated onto a test slide if a rapid test is being used.

Sampling of the vaginal secretions is necessary to diagnose trichomonas, bacterial vaginosis, or candida. A wet prep or potassium hydroxide (KOH) prep is performed by collecting a sample of vaginal secretions from the posterior fornix using a swab. The swab is then mixed with a few drops of normal saline, or slides are prepared directly.

Once all specimens are obtained, the speculum is slowly removed while the vaginal walls are inspected. After the cervix is released, the blades of the speculum are closed and the instrument withdrawn from the vagina maintaining gentle pressure posteriorly.

The last part of the pelvic examination is the bimanual palpation (Fig. 96.4). This allows for assessment of the size, position, and configuration of the internal pelvic organs.

Figure 96.3.
Specimen collection.
A. Sample for Pap smear is obtained with cytobrush or swab and rotated onto slide. Spatula is rotated 360° on cervix and smeared on glass slide.
B. Swab of cervical discharge is inoculated onto medium for gonorrhea culture.
C. Cervical cells are obtained for chlamydia culture or rapid test.

Figure 96.4.
Bimanual examination.
A. The uterus is squeezed between the fingers on the cervix and the hand on the lower abdomen.
B. The adnexa on both sides are palpated.

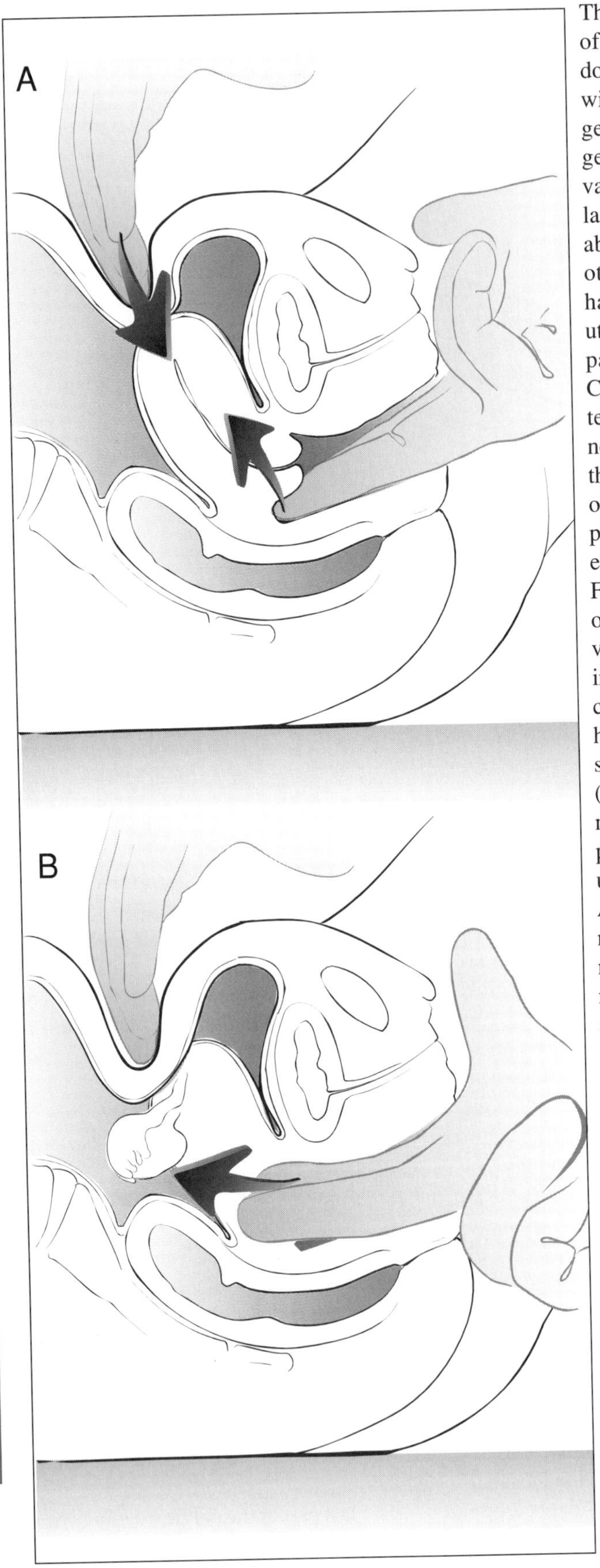

SUMMARY
1. Tell patient what will be done and what she will feel
2. Respect patient's modesty—use drapes and gown
3. Begin with abdominal examination and Tanner staging
4. Separate labia majora and inspect vulva
5. Use speculum warmed and lubricated with water
6. Insert gloved finger to determine location of cervix and relax posterior musculature
7. Be careful not to apply pressure anteriorly as speculum is inserted
8. Insert speculum at 45° angle with blades oriented vertically; then rotate speculum to horizontal position
9. If cervix is not seen, close blades and reposition speculum
10. Obtain specimens for Pap smear; fix immediately
11. Obtain culture specimens for sexually transmitted infections
12. Use gloved, lubricated finger(s) for bimanual examination
13. Rectoabdominal examination may be useful if bimanual examination is not tolerated
14. Discuss findings and arrange for follow-up

**Chapter 96
Adolescent Pelvic Examination**

The index and middle fingers of the clinician's gloved, dominant hand are lubricated with a water-soluble lubricant gel. One or two fingers are gently inserted into the vagina. When the patient is relaxed, external pressure to the abdomen is applied with the other hand. As the internal hand lifts and supports the uterus, the external hand palpates for size and position. Cervical motion or uterine tenderness is noted. The adnexa are palpated by placing the internal fingers laterally to one side of the fornix and pressing deeply on the ipsilateral lower abdominal wall. Finding the pulsations of the ovarian artery in the lateral vaginal recess and then sliding the fingers medially to locate the adnexa are sometimes helpful (2). The adnexa is a smooth, walnut-size mass (normal ovary size is approximately 3 cm in diameter). Palpation of the adnexa can be uncomfortable for the patient. Any extreme tenderness, mass, enlargement, or asymmetry of the adnexa is abnormal. Both sides must be examined.

The rectoabdominal examination is especially helpful when the vaginal bimanual examination cannot be tolerated, when the uterus is retroverted and/or retroflexed, or when the patient has complaints specific to the rectum or anus (17). It is not mandatory in the adolescent patient. The rectal examination should follow the vaginal bimanual examination and is performed with one lubricated gloved finger.

After the examination is complete, the patient is offered tissues to wipe away lubricant, and left alone to dress. When the patient is clothed, the clinician then discusses the findings and arranges any necessary follow-up.

COMPLICATIONS

Even with the most sensitive approach some discomfort from the pelvic examination is unavoidable. Complications due to technique include pain and anxiety, which may lead to avoidance of future health care interactions. Patient discomfort can be minimized by discussing the expected sensations associated with the examination before its performance and listening to the patient's concerns. Paying attention to techniques such as warming the speculum, avoiding pressure on the urethra, having patient void before examination, using the appropriate speculum, using water to lubricate the speculum before insertion, and using drapes and gowns to ensure modesty can further reduce discomfort from pelvic examination (18). Allowing the patient to assume a semirecumbent position and to use a handheld mirror to permit viewing of the examination also may decrease anxiety and discomfort (11). Pelvic examination should never cause physical injury.

SUMMARY

The pelvic examination is part of routine care for all sexually active adolescents and all adolescents older than 17 or 18 years. Pelvic examinations should be done on all female patients with complaints specific to the genital or rectal area and for those with unexplained abdominal pain. Proper training in the technical and interpersonal aspects of pelvic examination can improve the diagnostic accuracy and reduce patient discomfort.

REFERENCES

1. Beach RK. The adolescent pelvic examination: an office guide. Adolescent Health Update 1991;4:3–7.
2. Wilson MD, Joffe A. Step-by-step through the pelvic exam. Contemp Pediatr 1988;5:92–104.
3. Kreutner AK. Examination of the adolescent female. In: Kreutner AKK, Hollingsworth DR. Adolescent obstetrics and gynecology. Chicago: Year Book Medical Publishers, Inc., 1978, pp. 47–65.
4. Vandeven AM, Emans SJ. Vulvovaginitis in the child and adolescent. Pediatr Rev 1993;14:141–147.
5. Talbot CW. The gynecologic examination of the pediatric patient. Pediatr Ann 1986;15:501–508.
6. Biro FM. Reproductive care in the office: screening methods. In: McAnarney ER, Kreipe RE, Orr DP, and Comerci GD. Textbook of adolescent medicine, 1992, pp. 654–665.
7. Braverman PK, Stasburger VC. Why adolescent gynecology? Pediatricians and pelvic examinations. Pediatr Clin North Am 1989;36:471–487.
8. Millstein SG, Adler NE, Irwin CE. Sources of anxiety about pelvic examinations among adolescent females. J Adol Health Care 1984;5:105–111.
9. Seymore C, DuRant RH, Jay MS, Freeman D, Gomez L, Sharp C, and Linder CW. Influence of position during examination, and sex of examiner on patient anxiety during pelvic examination. J Pediatr 1986;108:312–317.
10. Phillips S, Friedman SB, Seidenberg M, Heald FP. Teenagers' preferences regarding the presence of family members, peers, and chaperones during examination of genitalia. Pediatrics 1981;68:665–669.
11. Swartz WH. The semisitting position for pelvic examination. JAMA 1984;251:1163.
12. Cowell CA. The gynecologic examination of infants, children, and young adolescents. Pediatr Clin North Am 1981;28:247–266.
13. Slap GB. Normal physiologic and psychosocial growth in the adolescent. J Adol Health Care 1986;7:13s–23s.
14. Muram D. Anatomy: anatomic and physiologic changes. In: Heger A, Emans SJ. Evaluation of the sexually abused child. New York: Oxford University Press, 1992, pp. 71–73.
15. Wheeler MD. Physical changes of puberty. Endocrinol Metabol Clin North Am 1991;20:1–14.
16. Emans SJH, Goldstein DP. Pediatric and adolescent gynecology. 3rd ed. Boston: Little, Brown & Co., 1990.
17. Greydanus DE, Shearin RB. Adolescent sexuality and gynecology. Philadelphia: Lea & Febiger, 1990, pp. 17–42.
18. Primose RB. Taking the tension out of pelvic exams. Am J Nurs 1984;84:72–74.

CLINICAL TIPS
1. An unhurried and sensitive approach, and talking the patient through the procedure, will save time and make the examination more pleasant for both the clinician and the patient.
2. A chaperone ahould always be present during a pelvic exam (regardelss of the sex of the clinician) in addition to the patient's support person to protect the clinician from allegations of impropriety.
3. A speculum appropriate for the age and size of the patient should be selected.
4. When inserting and removing the speculum, the clinician should be careful to both avoid putting pressure anteriorly (against the urethra) and not to trap pubic hairs.

FORENSIC EXAMINATION OF THE SEXUAL ASSAULT VICTIM

Robert Allan Shapiro and Charles J. Schubert

INTRODUCTION

Physicians are often called on to evaluate children who may have been victims of sexual abuse. It is estimated that 20% of American women and 5 to 10% of American men will experience some form of sexual abuse as children (1). Evaluation for sexual abuse includes a history from the alleged victim and/or guardian and a physical examination. When indicated, laboratory tests for sexually transmitted diseases and forensic specimens for the police are obtained. In this chapter, the term "forensic specimens" refers to samples collected for a police investigation, not for medical treatment. The procedure must be performed with precision and documentation must be complete because the evaluation may later be scrutinized in a court of law. Procedures presented in this chapter will satisfy legal requirements when performed properly.

ANATOMY AND PHYSIOLOGY

Before conducting an evaluation, the anatomy of the genitalia and examination techniques in Chapters 94 and 96 should be reviewed. The appearance of the normal genitalia changes dramatically from infancy to childhood to adolescence. Many "normal" variants of the prepubertal and adolescent hymen are encountered, as well as great variation in the normal color and skin appearance

of the anus. Errors in clinical judgment may occur if the physician is unfamiliar with the normal range of anatomic findings and the changes that occur with age.

Physical examination of many victims of sexual abuse will be normal (2, 3) (Fig. 94.2). Abuse by fondling and oral contact, for example, usually cause no identifying physical signs. Penetration of a young child's vagina often will result in injury and recognizable findings on examination. Penetration of the vulva without vaginal penetration in the young child, or vaginal penetration in the pubertal female, most often causes no injury. Rectal and penile injuries are unusual. The amount of force used, the frequency of abuse, the use of lubricants, the size of the object penetrating the child, and the child's age are factors that will determine the likelihood of injury and an abnormal examination. Furthermore, when injuries heal findings of trauma are often absent. Approximately 30% of sexually abused children will have completely normal examinations, 50% will have nonspecific findings, and the remaining 20% will have findings indicative or suspicious of sexual abuse (2).

The most specific indicators of vaginal penetration are injuries to the hymenal ring. Acute trauma is indicated by bleeding, fresh tears, abrasions, or bruising to the hymen or to one of the structures immediately adjacent to the hymen (Fig. 97.1). Healed trauma from vaginal penetration may result in hymenal

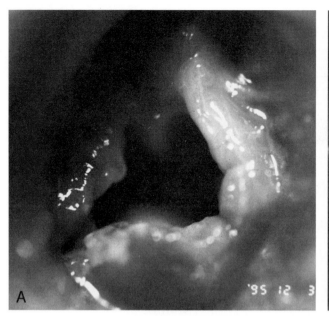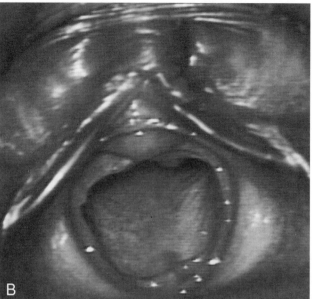

Figure 97.1.
Traumatic vaginal injuries from sexual abuse.
A. Laceration of the hymen results in a deep notch at 8 o'clock.
B. Attenuation (thinning) of the hymen.

scars, transections (a deep notch extending through the entire width of the hymen), significant thinning, attenuation or deep notching of the inferior hymen between 5 and 7 o'clock, or complete absence of the hymen. Small notches, bumps, minor irregularities, absence of hymen between 10 and 2 o'clock, redundant hymenal tissue, labial adhesions, and erythema are not specific for abuse (4).

Penetration of the rectum in sexual abuse may cause lacerations, perianal bruising, or decreased rectal tone. Except during infancy, constipation rarely causes rectal fissures and sexual abuse should be considered in all children with this finding. Digital examination of the rectum usually is not necessary. Rectal tone should be assessed by observation of the anal diameter as the buttocks are spread apart. However, stool in the rectal vault also may cause a decrease in rectal tone and should be ruled out by digital examination if decreased tone is observed.

Straddle injuries are a common etiology of genital trauma. These injuries commonly result in bruising and lacerations to the skin overlying the pubic symphysis or of the labia majora. Straddle injuries are frequently asymmetric. Sexual abuse should be considered if the trauma is midline or involves the hymen.

INDICATIONS

Evaluation for sexual abuse or assault is needed whenever illegal sexual activity has been disclosed or discovered. The definition of illegal sexual activity varies from state to state. When in doubt about whether a crime has been committed, police in that jurisdiction should be consulted. In most states, any sexual activity with a child under 13 years of age is illegal and requires an evaluation. Teenagers between the ages of 13 and 15 who have sexual activity with a partner 4 or more years older may be engaging in illegal activity. Again, local law enforcement should be consulted to determine if a reportable crime has been committed. Incest and any sexual activity that is forced on a minor against his or her will must be evaluated and reported.

Children who are victims of sexual abuse frequently report fondling of their genitalia or rectum, oral sex, attempted intercourse, sodomy, or demands to masturbate the perpetrator. Most often the perpetrator is a male who has access to the child, such as a member of the child's family, a close family friend, or one of the child's caretakers. Sexual abuse occurs in children of all ages. Of the victims, 80% are female. The child may dis-

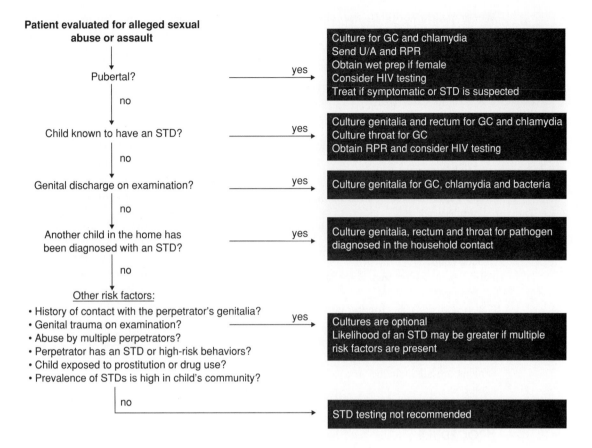

Patient evaluated for alleged sexual abuse or assault

Pubertal? — yes → Culture for GC and chlamydia
Send U/A and RPR
Obtain wet prep if female
Consider HIV testing
Treat if symptomatic or STD is suspected

no ↓

Child known to have an STD? — yes → Culture genitalia and rectum for GC and chlamydia
Culture throat for GC
Obtain RPR and consider HIV testing

no ↓

Genital discharge on examination? — yes → Culture genitalia for GC, chlamydia and bacteria

no ↓

Another child in the home has been diagnosed with an STD? — yes → Culture genitalia, rectum and throat for pathogen diagnosed in the household contact

no ↓

Other risk factors:
• History of contact with the perpetrator's genitalia?
• Genital trauma on examination?
• Abuse by multiple perpetrators?
• Perpetrator has an STD or high-risk behaviors?
• Child exposed to prostitution or drug use?
• Prevalence of STDs is high in child's community?
— yes → Cultures are optional
Likelihood of an STD may be greater if multiple risk factors are present

no ↓

STD testing not recommended

Figure 97.2
Indications for STD testing.

close the abuse, or it may be discovered by others. The last incident of abuse before evaluation may have been years ago or within hours of presentation.

Indications for STD testing in cases of sexual abuse vary among experts. A suggested approach is presented in Fig. 97.2. Testing all adolescent victims is warranted given the high incidence of STDs in this population. If the victim is an asymptomatic prepubertal child, testing is recommended if the prevalence of STDs is high in the community in which the child lives or if the history suggests an increased risk of infection. Symptomatic prepubertal children should have infections documented by culture and children diagnosed with one STD should be tested appropriately for others.

Forensic specimens must be collected if the last abuse and/or assault occurred within 72 hours of the evaluation and the history suggests that semen, saliva, blood, or hair of the alleged perpetrator may be found on the victim's body or clothing. (5, 6)

Conscious sedation or examination under general anesthesia may be indicated for the uncooperative or combative patient whose ex-

amination cannot be deferred. This includes victims with acute genital or rectal trauma and victims for whom police evidence must be collected. Patients older than 2 or 3 years should not be restrained against their will because forced rectal and genital examinations may be psychologically harmful to them. Most patients, however, will cooperate if their fears are addressed by the physician and they are reassured that the evaluation will not be painful. Young children will cooperate more often with the evaluation if they are allowed to sit on a parent's lap.

EQUIPMENT

If culturing for STDs:
Thayer-Martin plates (rapid testing methods not acceptable)
Chlamydia culture media
Calgiswabs (do not use swabs with wooden sticks)
Approximately 5 mL sterile saline (do not use bacteriostatic saline)
Pelvic examination tray (for adolescent patients)

Wet prep materials (glass test tube and slide, swab, saline)

If collecting forensic specimens:

Letter size envelopes

2×2 piece of filter paper (or equivalent)

2×2 sterile gauze pads

Large cotton swabs

Sheets of paper towel

Sterile saline (5-mL respiratory vials work well)

Sterile test tube

Small paper bag for storage of the victim's underwear

Large paper bag for storage of the victim's larger clothing items

Woods lamp

Pelvic examination tray (for the adolescent patient)

Comb and scissors (for the adolescent patient)

Large paper envelope to store all of the above

(Note: items for collecting forensic specimens are all included in a self contained rape kit)

PROCEDURE

A series of procedures are described in this section. These procedures should be performed in the order listed. Steps accompanied by (**ALL**) should be done for every patient; steps accompanied by (**STD**) should be done for patients requiring STD cultures; and steps accompanied by (**FORENSIC**) should be done only for patients requiring forensic specimen collection. Patients receiving a forensic examination should undergo the standard steps of STD testing as indicated.

A history of the abuse and/or assault is obtained (**ALL**). The physician may not have the time or the expertise needed to obtain a complete history of the alleged abuse and/or assault. It is sufficient to limit the history to a description of the sexual abuse and/or assault, the identity of the alleged perpetrator, the time, date, and place of last episode, the last menstrual period (if applicable), the date and time of last consensual intercourse (if any), and the method of birth control (if any). This information should reveal any indications for STD testing and forensic evidence collection, and will be helpful in deciding the disposition of the victim. A more complete interview

should be done by a trained medical social worker. Trained personnel also will offer anticipatory guidance to the family and assess the safety of the home.

The patient is prepared for the examination (**ALL**). The procedure is explained to the victim and family. If possible, the patient should not bathe, void, or defecate before forensic specimen collection. The patient is allowed to choose who he or she would like to be present during the examination. (The alleged perpetrator should not be allowed to stay with the patient.) The patient is reassured that the examination will not be painful. Young children should be allowed to sit on a parent's lap. A general examination is performed, documenting any signs of injury (**ALL**). All injuries are photographed.

Clothing of the patient that is stained with blood, semen, or saliva is placed into the large paper bag (**FORENSIC**). The bag is sealed with tape and labeled with the date, the patient's name, and a description of the bag's contents. The patient's underwear is placed into the small paper bag and the bag is sealed with tape. The underwear is collected even if the patient has changed underwear since the assault. The bag is sealed and labeled as described.

A sample of the patient's saliva is collected (**FORENSIC**). The saliva sample will be used to determine the patient's secretor status of blood group antigens and should be obtained in all cases when forensic specimens are collected. The filter paper is handled with gloved hands. The patient is asked to moisten part of the paper with the tongue and a circle is drawn around the dampened area (Fig. 97.3). The filter paper is then placed into an envelope, sealed with tape, and labeled as described.

Oral specimens for semen are collected (**FORENSIC**). Using two cotton-tipped swabs, saliva from the victim's upper and lower gum lines is collected. These two swabs are placed into an envelope, sealed with tape, and labeled as described.

A pharyngeal culture for gonorrhea is collected (**STD**). A pharyngeal specimen is collected using a fresh cotton-tipped swab, culture media is inoculated and labeled as described.

The skin is examined for seminal stains and bite marks, particularly around the genitalia, thighs, and buttocks (**FORENSIC**). Stains are swabbed with a piece of 2 × 2 gauze that has been lightly moistened with sterile saline. The center of bite marks are swabbed for saliva. The room is then darkened and the victim's body is scanned with the Woods lamp. A green fluorescence indicates other possible seminal stains. The gauze is placed into an envelope, sealed, and labeled as described. If more than one stain is found, each stain is collected separately and placed into separate envelopes.

The genitalia and rectum are inspected for signs of injury and infection (**ALL**). Documentation of findings includes the estimated age of any injuries (fresh, healing, old) and whether the findings are consistent with sexual abuse or assault.

A rectal specimen for semen is collected (**FORENSIC**). Two cotton swabs are lightly moistened with sterile saline and inserted into the victim's rectum. After 5 to 10 seconds, the swabs are withdrawn and placed into an envelope. The envelope is sealed and labeled as described.

Rectal and vaginal cultures for gonorrhea and chlamydia are obtained (**STD**). In prepubertal females, the vaginal mucosa is cultured just proximal to the hymen using a calcium alginate swab moistened with sterile saline. In adolescent females, cervical specimens are obtained. Urethral cultures are obtained in males. Swabs with plastic or aluminum handles should be used for all chlamydia cultures, because the wood handles of other swabs are toxic to the organisms. Chlamydia specimens must be sent for culture (*not* immunoassay or other rapid methods) to avoid false-positive results and meet the legal standard.

Any loose pubic hairs are collected (**FORENSIC**). If the victim has pubic hair, a paper towel is placed under his or her buttocks and the pubic hair is combed. Any loose hair that falls onto the towel is wrapped, along with the comb, in the paper towel and placed into an envelope. The envelope is sealed and labeled as described.

If the victim is a preadolescent and has no pubic hair, the skin near the child's genitalia and rectum is inspected carefully for stray hairs. If found, they are collected and wrapped in a paper towel. The folded towel is placed into an envelope, sealed, and labeled

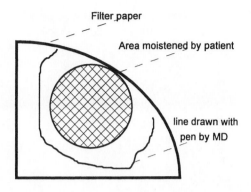

as described. If the victim has pubic hair, 5 to 10 pubic hairs are cut with the scissors as close to the skin as possible. The cut hairs are wrapped in a clean paper towel and placed into an envelope. The envelope is sealed and labeled as described. The scissors can be discarded.

A genital specimen for semen is collected (**FORENSIC**). If the patient is an adolescent female, two cotton swabs are used to collect vaginal secretions. If the patient is a male or a prepubertal female, a 2 × 2 gauze is lightly moistened with sterile saline and the external genitalia is swabbed. The swabs or gauze are placed into an envelope, and the envelope is sealed and labeled as described.

Wet mounted preparations for sperm and Trichomonas are obtained from the mouth, genitalia, and rectum (**FORENSIC**). In prepubertal females, small calcium alginate swabs are used to collect vaginal secretions so that trauma and discomfort are minimized. To prevent the wet mounted preparations from drying before microscopic analysis is complete, the swabs are placed into individual sterile test tubes which have been filled with a small amount of sterile saline. Each tube is labeled as described.

Each envelope is examined to make certain that the outside surface contains a clear description of the specimen, the victim's name, and the current date (**FORENSIC**). Envelopes are sealed with tape. All forensic specimens are placed into a large envelope, and the envelope is labeled as described. The chain of custody—a legal term referring to the need to identify at all times the person possessing the evidence and to whom and at what time it was passed to another—is thus secured. Until the evidence is locked in a secure location or is given to the police, it must

Figure 97.3.
A sample of the victim's saliva is collected. The saliva sample will be used to determine the victim's secretor status of blood group antigens, and should be obtained in all cases when forensic specimens are collected. The filter paper is handled with gloved hands. The victim is asked to moisten an area of the paper with the tongue and a circle is drawn around the damped area as illustrated. The filter paper is then placed into an envelope, sealed with tape, and labeled appropriately.

Figure 97.4.
Microscopic view of
immotile sperm.

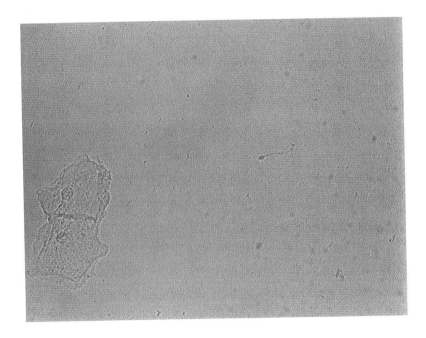

remain in the hands of the physician or nurse to secure the chain of custody. If the chain of custody includes periods of time when the evidence was not accounted for, such as a time when it was left on a counter unattended, an opportunity would have existed for tampering. This break in the chain might compromise the validity of the evidence during a legal proceeding. The chain of custody should be thoroughly documented.

The wet mounted preparations are examined for sperm and Trichomonas (**FOREN-SIC**). If they are to be examined in the hospital laboratory, they must be taken by the physician or nurse to maintain the chain of custody. If sperm are found, motility should be documented. The microscopic appearance of sperm is shown in Figure 97.4. Any slides prepared from the wet mounted preparations are placed into cardboard slide holders, labeled, and placed into the large evidence envelope. The envelope is then sealed with tape. The completed evidence envelope is placed into a locked and secure closet or drawer until it is given to the investigating police officer (**FORENSIC**). Written documentation is completed (**ALL**).

Prophylaxis against STDs and pregnancy should be considered for the adolescent (**STD**). The prevalence of sexually transmitted infections in sexually abused prepubertal children is low and STD prophylaxis is generally not needed. Serum for HIV and syphilis testing is obtained (**STD**). Test-ing should be repeated in 3 to 6 months after the last episode of abuse.

The county children's protective service (CPS) should be called to report suspected child sexual abuse (**ALL**). The police are called to report alleged assault. Discharge planning must be discussed with the CPS social worker in cases of abuse. In most instances, the child can be safely discharged to home if he or she will not be in contact with the alleged perpetrator. Situations will arise when emergency placement into foster care or admission to the hospital will be required to ensure the child's safety. CPS has the legal authority to make this decision.

The victim and/or family should be told that the examination is complete and reassured that tests for any physical complications or problems resulting from the abuse have been done (**ALL**). The family's questions should be answered, and examination findings and the reporting process should be explained.

COMPLICATIONS

The alleged victim, whether in fact abused or not, has gone through an emotional ordeal and is asked to tolerate a sometimes uncomfortable and embarrassing evaluation. The physician can help the victim deal with the evaluation and begin the psychological healing by remaining sensitive and unhurried

SUMMARY

Procedure	*ALL	*STD	*FORENSIC
1. History and examination	✓		
2. Outer clothing specimen			✓
3. Underwear specimen			✓
4. Saliva specimen			✓
5. Oral semen specimen			✓
6. Pharyngeal culture		✓	
7. Skin stains specimen			✓
8. Genital-rectal examination	✓		
9. Rectal semen specimen			✓
10. Genital-rectal cultures		✓	
11. Loose pubic hair specimen			✓
12. Cut pubic hair specimen			✓
13. Genital semen specimen			✓
14. Wet prep collection			✓
15. Wet prep examination			✓
16. Chain of custody			✓
17. Documentation	✓		
18. HIV and syphilis testing	✓		
19. Reporting	✓	✓	
20. Discharge	✓		

*ALL denotes procedures that should be performed for all potential victims of sexual abuse or assault. STD denotes procedures that should be performed for patients requiring testing for sexually transmitted diseases. FORENSIC denotes procedures that should only be performed for patients requiring collection of forensic specimens. Patients receiving a forensic examination should undergo routine STD testing as indicated.

CLINICAL TIPS

1. Commercial rape kits will save time and increase the precision of forensic evidence collection.
2. Examination and collection of specimens should not be rushed. Careful attention to details, labeling of specimens, and documentation are critical.
3. Swabs moistened with sterile saline will be less painful.
4. The number of persons handling specimens should be limited and the chain of custody must be maintained.
5. If the patient is unco-operative, the need for an emergency evaluation should be reassessed. If forensic specimens and emergency examination are not needed, the examination may be less stressful if completed at a later date.

throughout the evaluation. Forcing an unco-operative victim to undergo an examination adds to the emotional trauma. Referral for evaluation in a setting more conducive to co-operation or sedation occasionally needs to be considered.

As mentioned previously, forensic evidence should not be left unattended. The chain of custody must be documented and maintained to prevent legal invalidation of the collected evidence. All forensic specimens must be stored in paper envelopes. Specimens stored in plastic bags will not dry properly and will be of less use to the forensic laboratory.

SUMMARY

Physicians are required to evaluate and report all cases of suspected sexual abuse and/or assault. A report by telephone should be followed by a written report. Clear documentation and attention to details are required. Evaluation will vary depending on the details of the specific case. A sensitive and unhurried approach can minimize any additional distress caused by evaluation procedures. The

physician is an important advocate for the victim of sexual abuse and should be available and willing to testify in court if needed.

REFERENCES

1. Finkelhor D, Hotaling G, Lewis IA, Smith C. Sexual abuse in a national survey of adult men and women: prevalence, characteristics, and risk factors. Child Abuse and Neglect 1990;14:19–28.
2. Adams JA, Harper K, Knudson S, Revilla J. Examination findings in legally confirmed child sexual abuse: it's normal to be normal. Pediatrics 1994;94: 310–317.
3. Berenson AB. The prepubertal genital exam: what is normal and abnormal. Current Opinion in Obstetrics and Gynecology 1994;6:526–530.
4. Giardino AP, Finkel MA, et al. A practical guide to the evaluation of sexual abuse in the prepubertal child. Newbury Park, CA: Sage Publications, Inc., 1992, pp. 75–79.
5. Jenny C. Forensic examination: the role of the physician as "medical detective." In: Heger A, Emans SJ. Evaluation of the sexually abused child: a medical textbook and photographic atlas. New York: Oxford University Press, 1992, pp. 51–61.
6. Kanda MB, Orr LA. Specimen collection in sexual abuse. In: Ludwig S, Kornbert AE, eds. Child abuse: a medical reference. 2nd ed. New York: Churchill Livingstone, 1992, pp. 265–279.

Chapter 97
Forensic Examination
of the Sexual Assault
Victim

CHAPTER 98

BLADDER CATHETERIZATION

Douglas A. Boenning and Fred M. Henretig

INTRODUCTION

Bladder catheterization is performed most often in children to obtain urine in a sterile manner for culture and urinalysis (1). The procedure allows for relatively easy and timely access to urine, particularly in the young child who cannot void on command. A bladder catheter also may be placed for monitoring urine output and relieving obstruction. Both bladder catheterization and suprapubic aspiration of urine may be used to obtain sterile urine (1), the latter procedure most typically in young infants (Chapters 99 and 134). Nurses and nurse extenders are most likely to perform catheterization in emergency department or inpatient settings. In general, the physician may be called on to perform more challenging catheterizations, especially when abnormal anatomy is present. A urologist might be consulted for particularly difficult catheterizations, when an experienced pediatrician or emergency physician is unable to pass a catheter. The procedure is usually straightforward and impacts on all pediatric age groups, although it is performed most frequently in children under age 3 years to obtain urine for culture. Some obvious psychosocial issues impact on children of all age groups (and parents) regarding exposed genitalia and perceived violation of this sensitive area. Some cultural groups may even fear that a daughter's virginity will be compromised by urinary catheterization (2). All patients and/or parents thus deserve a brief but careful explanation of the relevant anatomy and details of the procedure. Respect for modesty and privacy is critical and will be highly appreciated by the older child and all parents.

ANATOMY AND PHYSIOLOGY

The relevant anatomy of the prepubertal child is generally similar to the adult, except for the obvious differences in size and lack of secondary sexual characteristics. In boys, the urethral meatus is usually easy to locate, but the long course of the urethra and its relative fixation at the level of the symphysis pubis can make passage of the catheter trying (3). Holding the penis straight with slight traction at 90° vertical to the abdominal wall straightens the urethral course as much as possible (Fig. 98.1).

In the uncircumcised neonate or infant boy, a tight foreskin can make the task of locating the urethral meatus an even greater challenge. Usually gentle retraction of the foreskin will expose enough of the glans to visualize the meatus. Some infant boys with chronic ammoniacal diaper dermatitis may acquire meatal stenosis and thus require a smaller catheter than might otherwise be typical for their age. Whereas difficult catheterization in the adult male may result from prostatic hypertrophy, urethral obstruction in a young boy may indicate the presence of posttraumatic urethral stricture or congenital anomalies.

In the young female child, the urethra is short and generally easy to catheterize once the orifice is visualized. However, the opening is in close proximity to the vaginal introi-

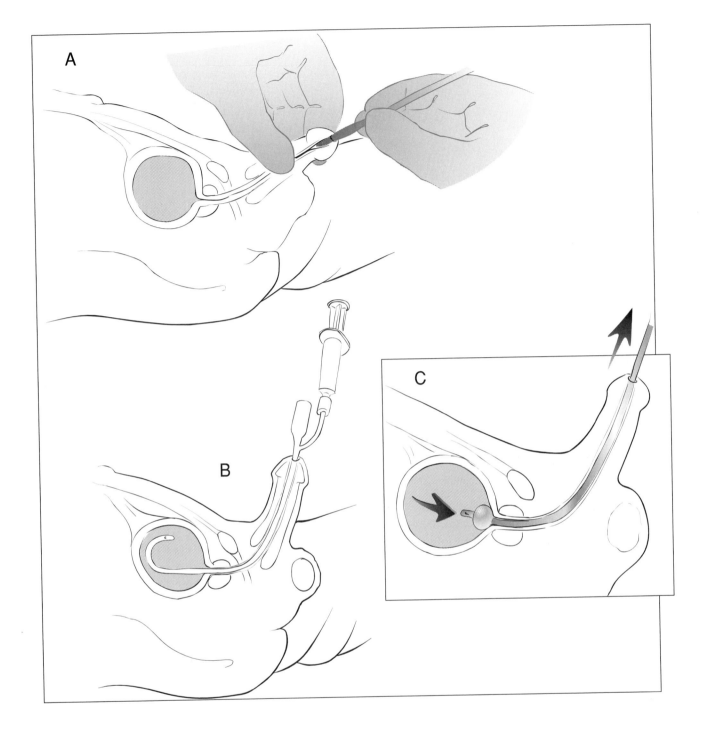

Figure 98.1.
Bladder catheterization for boys.
A. The catheter is advanced gently with the penis held perpendicularly to the suprapubic abdominal wall.
B. The catheter is fully advanced before an attempt is made to inflate the balloon.
C. The catheter is withdrawn slowly after balloon inflation until it lodges against the trigone.

tus, and the mucosa of the introitus may cover the urethral meatus, making it difficult to locate (4) (Fig. 98.2). It may be noted that gentle lateral traction of the labia and gentle downward pressure on the cephalad aspect of the vaginal introital fold with a sterile cotton-tipped applicator allows visualization of the infantile female urethral meatus more readily (4) (Fig. 98.3). Alternatively, gently grasping the labia between thumb and forefinger and

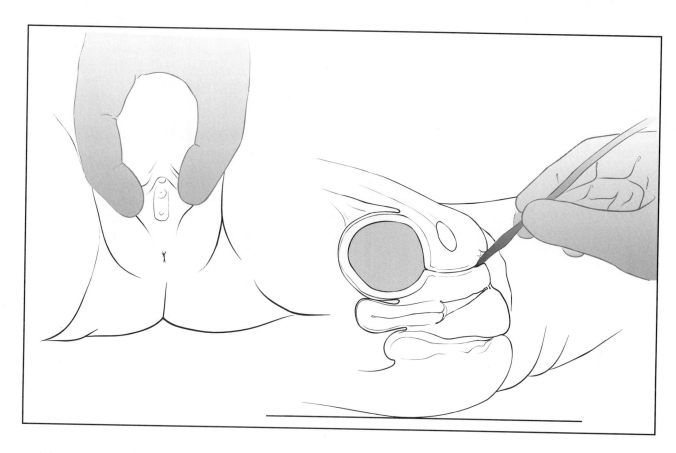

Figure 98.2.
With girls, the urethra is
short and generally easily
catheterized with
adequate visualization of
the urethral meatus.

applying gentle lateral and outward traction (toward the clinician) also may expose the urethral meatus (Fig. 98.4). Two additional considerations may complicate urethral visualization in girls. Female hypospadias results when the meatus opens into the distal anterior wall of the vagina. A catheter with a curved tip (coudé) may allow catheterization, usually just inside the introitus on the roof of the vagina. Additionally, labial adhesions may be present in infant girls. In this context, another technique such as suprapubic aspiration is generally preferred for simple collection of urine.

INDICATIONS

The most common indication for catheterizing a young child in the ED or ambulatory setting is to obtain a sterile urine specimen for laboratory analysis (1). Other indications generally include preventing or relieving urinary obstruction, the need for cystourethrography, and close monitoring of urine output. In infants and small children with suspected urinary tract infection or nonlocalizing signs of fever or possible sepsis, a cleanly obtained

urine specimen is paramount to reaching a diagnosis. Commonly, either bladder catheterization or suprapubic aspiration is used. The latter procedure is considered by many authorities to be the gold standard for obtaining bacteriologically uncontaminated specimens; however, it is frequently unsuccessful with small bladder volumes of urine which are common in ill or dehydrated infants (1) (see also Chapter 99). The most common indication for placement of an indwelling urinary catheter in children is to monitor urine output in the critically ill or injured child. Other situations that may indicate catheterization on occasion include (a) the need to perform urgent cystourethrography, (b) children suffering contusions or burns (scald, flame, or chemical) to the perineum and thus at risk of meatal swelling and obstruction to urine outflow, (c) as a temporizing measure to relieve lower urinary tract obstruction (e.g., in a male neonate with posterior urethral valves), (d) in children with neurogenic bladder due to spinal dysfunction as a result of trauma or congenital anomalies such as spina bifida, and (e) following general anesthesia and/or surgery-induced urinary retention.

Figure 98.3.
The female urethral meatus
may be better exposed by
applying gentle lateral
traction to the labia with
simultaneous downward
traction applied to the
introital mucosa.

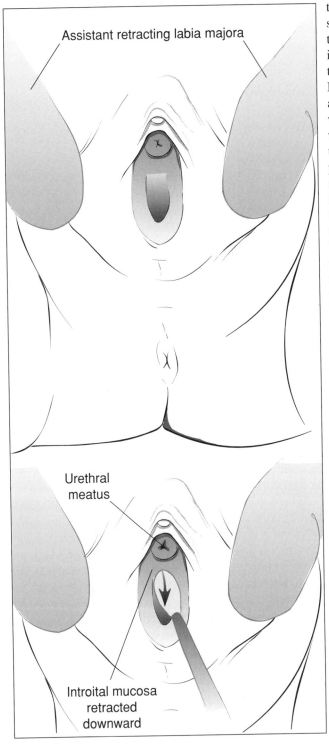

Assistant retracting labia majora

Urethral
meatus

Introital mucosa
retracted
downward

tion of hematuria, glycosuria, specific gravity), and is certainly adequate for establishing gross patency and function of the urinary system. Many children aged 2 years and older are able to provide a voided specimen. For the child who can voluntarily void, the urethral meatus may be prepped and urine caught in a sterile container. In addition infants under 6 months may at times be induced into voiding urine using one of two tricks. The Perez reflex consists of ventrally suspending the infant in one hand and stroking the para-spinal region with the other hand (5). An assistant or urine bag is needed to catch the resultant urine flow. The second method is wetting the abdomen with an alcohol pad. The resultant cooling effect from evaporation has been reported to induce spontaneous voiding (6). This latter phenomenon may explain why many infants spontaneously urinate when they are being prepared for catheterization. If only urinalysis is needed, clean catch specimens are usually adequate. Documentation of physiologic urine production (e.g., after intravenous hydration) can be accomplished in many patients by simply placing an adherent plastic urine bag on the child after adequately prepping the perineum. In the dehydrated child, invasive methods of obtaining urine should be postponed for 60 to 90 minutes after initiating intravenous hydration to allow for some bladder filling. Otherwise, a highly concentrated few milliliters of "sludge" will be obtained rendering a urinalysis difficult to interpret and often necessitating a subsequent, additional attempt at catheterization.

Relative contraindications to bladder catheterization begin primarily with careful consideration of whether less invasive methods would suffice in a given clinical context (3). Voided urine may be sufficient to use for urinalysis in some circumstances (e.g., detec-

The primary absolute contraindication to

placement of a catheter is the trauma patient with possible urethral injury (7). This is typically suspected with the findings of blood at the urethral meatus, displaced or high-riding prostate gland on rectal examination, or perineal hematoma.

EQUIPMENT

Sterile gloves and drapes
Cotton balls or cotton sponges
Povidone-iodine solution
Forceps
Lubricant
Catheter
Specimen collection cup
Connectible drainage bag and tubing (if desired)

Most hospitals today use preassembled catheterization equipment trays (Fig. 98.5). Appropriate urinary catheter sizes are age and size dependent (see Table 6.2). The neonate can usually be catheterized with a 5-French feeding tube. Pediatric urinary catheter sizes are typically: infants—8 French, young children—10 French, and older children—12 French.

It may be helpful to ensure the availability of an extra pair of gloves and an extra catheter should contamination occur during the procedure.

An extra specimen cup may allow the discarding of the first few drops of collected

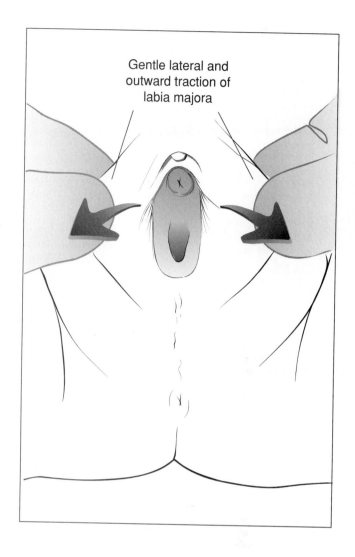

Gentle lateral and outward traction of labia majora

Figure 98.4.
The female urethral meatus also may be exposed in some girls by gentle simultaneous lateral, outward, and upward traction on the labia majora.

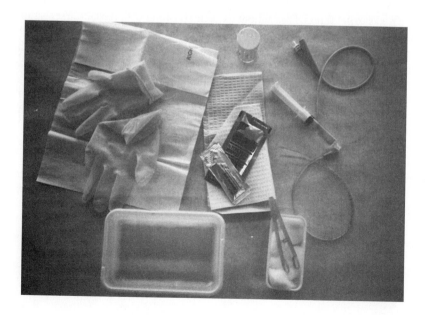

Figure 98.5.
Many hospitals use catheterization trays that include all the necessary equipment other than the urethral catheter. Photo shows an added pediatric balloon and a straight catheter.

SUMMARY

1. Provide careful explanation of relevant anatomy and procedural technique to patients and families, and seek history of latex or iodine allergy
2. Maintain strict adherence to sterile technique
3. Inspect and test catheter tip (and balloon) before insertion
4. In boys, gently retract the foreskin as necessary and pull back over glans after completing procedure
5. In boys, hold penis with gentle traction away from and perpendicular to lower abdomen while advancing catheter
6. In girls, achieve visualization of urethral meatus with gentle traction on labia and/or downward displacement of cephalad aspect of vaginal introital fold with cotton-tipped applicator
7. With an indwelling catheter, it is important to advance catheter well into bladder before balloon inflation to avoid urethral injury if balloon were inadvertently placed in proximal urethra

urine, if sufficient quantity is present, so as to get the most uncontaminated specimen possible for microbiologic testing.

Latex allergy is common in spina bifida patients, and thus latex-free equipment should be available particularly for this population

An assistant, preferably other than the parent, is usually necessary with female infants and young children of either gender.

PROCEDURE

Verbal consent should be obtained and the procedure explained carefully to the caretaker and child, in age-appropriate language, avoiding medical jargon and anatomic terms (Chapter 9). Intermittent catheterization should be a quick procedure with rare complications given adequate assistance, proper equipment, and appropriate restraint and/or cooperation from the patient. A history of any previous difficulties with catheterization suggesting aberrant anatomy should be sought, and a history of latex or iodine allergy.

Sterile technique is used throughout (Chapter 7). The catheterization tray is opened and inspected for appropriate contents, and any necessary equipment and assistance are gathered. Curtains are drawn and privacy maintained as much as possible. Before establishing a sterile field, the perineum is inspected and the urethral opening identified. Many babies in diapers will have powder, ointments, or medicated creams on the perineum that will need to be removed with soap and water before establishing a sterile field. The patient is placed supine, with girls in a frog-leg position, and an absorbent pad underneath the buttocks. The equipment is placed on a drape between the patient's legs or below the feet. The lubricant is opened and cotton balls are saturated with povidone-iodine solution, reserving one or two dry cotton balls. Sterile drapes are placed on the perineum with the cutout area exposing the genitalia. Direct over-the-shoulder lighting, similar to that for a gynecologic examination, is particularly helpful for identifying the urethra in girls.

Catheterization of Boys

Intermittent catherization is performed with a single-lumen (straight) catheter. Insertion of an indwelling catheter is described later in this section. For circumcised patients, the clinician holds the penis using the nondominant hand and swabs the glans and urethral meatus with a povidone-iodine saturated cotton held in tweezers or forceps. The dominant hand is maintained in sterile condition. In the uncircumcised patient, the foreskin is gently retracted, if possible, for cleaning and visualization of the meatus. If the foreskin is tight, the clinician should aim for the center of the glans. After sterile preparation, the catheter tip is inspected for any defects or sharp edges. The catheter is held approximately 20 cm proximal to the tip to form a loop. This loop will help to minimize inadvertent contamination of the proximal part of the catheter via inadvertent contact with nonsterile areas. The lubricated catheter tip is inserted into the meatal opening and advanced while holding the shaft 90° from the body, applying gentle traction to the penis (Fig. 98.1. A, B). The catheter tip may meet some resistance at the level of the prostatic urethra due to external bladder sphincter contraction. Advancement may be aided by maintaining gentle pressure with the catheter, awaiting sphincter relaxation. Bladder sphincter relaxation may be enhanced in the older, cooperative child by plantar flexing the toes and by slow, deep breathing to further relax the abdominal wall and pelvic floor musculature. During inhalation the sphincter is most relaxed, allowing the best opportunity for advancing the catheter. The catheter should never be forced, to avoid creating a traumatic fistula or false tract. Along with the tactile sensation of bladder entry, urine should appear in the catheter tubing. The proximal end of the catheter is then positioned in the sterile collection container if it has not been already.

Some clinicians discard the first few drops of urine to obtain a sample with the least possible periurethral contamination; however, in an infant the clinician generally takes what he or she can get. The catheter is withdrawn after an adequate volume is obtained. If a scant volume is produced, the catheter can be slightly withdrawn while massaging the lower abdomen to coax some additional residual volume from the bladder. In the uncircumcised patient, it is important to pull the foreskin forward over the glans on completion of the procedure to avoid paraphimosis.

Catheterization of Girls

Aside from locating the female urethral meatus, as previously noted, catheterization of the female patient is often easier than that of the male patient. If the vagina is unintentionally catheterized, despite efforts at visualizing the urethral meatus (see Anatomy and Physiology), leaving the catheter in place might serve as a useful landmark during further attempts at locating the urethra. As with the male patient, the female patient is positioned supine in a private location, while necessary equipment and assistance are arranged. The perineum is prepared with sequential swabbing using a cotton ball and antiseptic from anterior to posterior, then dried with a sterile cotton ball. If an assistant is not available, the clinician uses the nondominant hand to keep the labia separated while inserting the lubricated catheter tip until urine is obtained (Fig. 98.2.A,B).

Indwelling Catheters

Indwelling bladder catheters have a double or triple lumen tube with an expandable balloon near the distal tip to help secure them in the bladder. General preparation for catheterization is the same as for the intermittent procedure. The catheter balloon should be tested for competence before insertion by sequential filling with the recommended volume of sterile saline, observing for leakage, and then withdrawing saline to ensure complete emptying of the balloon. When inserting the catheter into the bladder, the balloon should be expanded only when urine flow is established and the catheter has been further advanced its full length to the Y connector. The clinician thereby avoids inadvertent injury to the proximal urethra by an improperly positioned balloon (Fig. 98.1.B). After balloon expansion, the catheter should be withdrawn until gentle resistance denotes that the balloon is lodged at the bladder neck (Fig. 98.1.C). The catheter is then taped securely to the patient's leg and connected to a closed collecting system. In the combative child or adolescent, manual restraints and/or temporary sedation may be required to prevent urethral trauma.

COMPLICATIONS

Unfavorable outcomes that are generally avoidable include inflicting de novo urethral or bladder injury due to forcing a catheter, exacerbating urethral injury in the trauma patient, causing paraphimosis by failing to restore a retracted foreskin to its normal position, introducing infection by failure to adhere to sterile procedure, and failing to deflate a balloon catheter (3). Each of these complications may be anticipated and can be largely avoided by adherence to the methods described in this chapter. For most intermittent diagnostic catheterizations, the catheter is inserted for such a short time that infection is a rarely seen complication. Retained indwelling catheters may be due to intravesical knotting or balloon failure (3, 8). A knotted catheter may be due to the introduction of an excessive length of straight catheter, particularly a highly flexible feeding tube, into the bladder, allowing loops of catheter to intertwine. A knotted catheter may be removed by untying it using a guide wire passed through the main lumen, or by more invasive urologic techniques such as urethral dilation with urethral sounds or, if necessary, suprapubic removal (8). Failure of a balloon to deflate is usually due to a flap valve defect in the inflating lumen or syringe adaptor malfunction (3). A reasonable first course of action is to remove the adaptor plug, which may allow the saline from the balloon to flow out. If that is unsuccessful, a fine vascular access guide wire is gently passed, with rotation, through the inflating channel in an effort to disrupt the presumed flap valve defect. If this fails, the next step would be to cut the catheter off a few centimeters from the urethra, in hope that the defect was external (distal) to the cut. If the balloon does not immediately deflate, it is then necessary to carefully attach a new, sterile, closed collecting system, while pursuing further options. Additional approaches might include attempts to rupture the balloon by overexpansion, installation of an erosive substance, or direct piercing with a needle introduced suprapubically. The optimal approach among these techniques is controversial and, therefore, is best determined after consultation with a urologist.

Summary

For the nontoilet-trained young child, diagnostic bladder catheterization is often an important technique for obtaining a sterile urine sample for microscopic analysis and culture. The same procedural principles apply as for initiating continuous monitoring of urine flow in critically ill or injured children. Pediatric patients and families, particularly parents of young girls, need a careful explanation of the relevant anatomy and procedural methods. Anatomic considerations in children include tight foreskin in uncircumcised male infants and difficult visualization of the urethral meatus, female hypospadias, and labial adhesions in girls. Appropriate size catheters are age and size dependent. Several simple guidelines exist to ease visualization of the urethral meatus. A urinary catheter should never be forced because this is the most likely cause of complications related to local trauma. Indwelling catheters pose additional concerns including increased risk of infection and the potential for the complication of a retained catheter. Nevertheless, both intermittent and indwelling urinary catheterizations of children have proven to be safe procedures and should be integral components of every emergency department's routine pediatric protocols.

References

1. Pollack CV, Pollack ES, Andrew ME. Suprapubic bladder aspiration versus urethral catheterization in ill infants: success, efficiency, and complication rates. Ann Emerg Med 1994;23:225–230.
2. Wong DL. The child who is hospitalized. Nursing care of infants and children, 5th ed. St. Louis: CV Mosby, 1995, pp. 1176–1177.
3. Zbaraschuk I, Berger RE, Hedges JR. Emergency urologic procedures. In: Roberts JR, Hedges JR, eds. Clinical procedures in emergency medicine. Philadelphia: WB Saunders, 1991, pp. 867–874.
4. Redman JF, Bissada NK. Direct bladder catheterization in infant females and young girls. Clin Pediatr 1976;15:1060–1061.
5. Whaley LF, Wong DL. The child who is hospitalized. Nursing care of infants and children. 4th ed. St. Louis: CV Mosby, 1991, pp. 1220–1222.
6. Ellis R. Once more into the void. Contemp Pediatr 1989;6(8):164.
7. Feeman S, Chapman J. Urologic procedures. Emerg Med Clin North Am 1986;4:543–560.
8. Kanengiser S, Juster F, Kogan S, Ruddy R. Knotting of a bladder catheter. Pediatr Emerg Care 1989; 5:37–39.

SUPRAPUBIC BLADDER ASPIRATION

Michael F. Altieri

INTRODUCTION

Suprapubic bladder aspiration refers to the introduction of a sterile needle through the abdominal wall into the bladder of a young child to obtain a urine specimen. This technique allows for the sterile collection of urine from incontinent children in sepsis evaluations when isolating an organism from the urinary tract may be of paramount importance. This procedure also avoids any passage of urine through a potentially contaminated urethral conduit and exposure to bacterial flora of the perineal skin.

Aspiration of the bladder was first described by Huze and Beeson (1) in 1956 as a method to collect sterile urine. The safety and efficiency of suprapubic bladder aspiration have been established in several studies (2–6). Alternatives to suprapubic bladder aspiration are midstream clean catch collection and urethral catheterization. In obtaining a clean catch specimen, the urine passes through the urethra, which may lead to contamination. It is also extremely difficult to obtain a clean catch urine specimen in a female patient because the short urethra usually causes urine to flow over the perineal skin (7). The timing has to be right—the clinician must be ready when the incontinent child decides to void.

Suprapubic bladder aspiration is a safe and relatively simple procedure. It is usually performed by physicians, and can be accomplished in most inpatient and outpatient settings.

ANATOMY AND PHYSIOLOGY

Urinary tract infections are common in children. During early infancy they are more likely in boys and are often secondary to anomalies of the urinary tract. Beyond the age of 3 to 4 months, urinary tract infections are much more common in girls, probably as a result of the diminished protection against bacteria prvided by a short urethra.

The precise pathogenesis of urinary tract infections has not been determined, but several factors have been shown to play a role in their etiology. In infancy many infections are the result of bacteremia. Beyond infancy most infections result from bacteria ascending the urethra to the bladder. The majority of the organisms causing these infections are colonic flora. Thus *Escherichia coli* is by far the most common cause of urinary tract infection in children. Other urinary pathogens include *Klebsiella, Proteus,* group D streptococcus (enterococcus), and staphylococcal species.

Suprapubic bladder aspiration may be performed in newborns, infants, and children under 2 years of age. In this age group the bladder is an abdominal rather than a pelvic organ, making it accessible to needle aspiration. Few anatomic structures have to be identified before performing the procedure. The clinician merely locates the umbilicus and the symphysis pubis prior to inserting the needle. The needle passes through skin, rectus muscle, and peritoneum and into the anterior superior wall of the bladder.

INDICATIONS

Suprapubic bladder aspiration may be indicated in incontinent children under 2 years of age, when collection of sterile urine is necessary and urethral contamination must be avoided. One common clinical situation when suprapubic bladder aspiration is used would be the septic workup of a febrile infant, in whom a urinary tract infection will often be found. In these cases, obtaining uncontaminated urine that allows identification of a true pathogen is imperative. In addition, suprapubic bladder aspiration is an option in a young child who will receive antibiotic therapy for presumed bacteremia or other major infections to rule out involvement of the urinary tract. Aspiration of the bladder may also be used when uncontaminated urine must be obtained from the incontinent child who has gastroenteritis and frequent diarrheal stools.

Urethral catheterization is widely used in lieu of suprapubic bladder aspiration, and it is the procedure of choice in many facilities. However, drawbacks include catheter contamination during insertion and potential difficulty in finding the urethral orifice in the infant female. The urethral meatus also can be difficult to find in the uncircumcised male with a minimally retractable foreskin.

Using a urine bag to collect a specimen is the least desirable way of obtaining urine, especially when the urine is to be used for culture. Urine obtained in this fashion makes contact with the skin in the genital area and has a high contamination rate. Urine bags are also known to leak and to be contaminated by diarrheal stool.

EQUIPMENT

Sterile procedure gloves
Antiseptic solution (10% Betadine)
Sterile 4 × 4 gauge sponges
Sterile 10-mL syringe
22- or 23-gauge 0.5″ needle
Sterile specimen container
Adhesive bandage

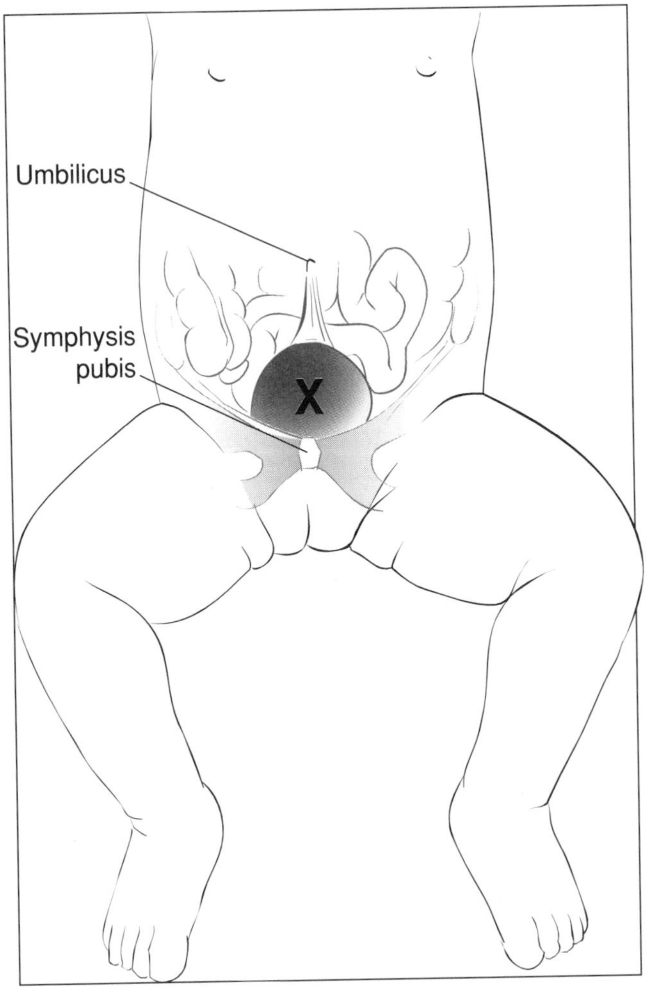

PROCEDURE

The child is securely restrained on his or her back in the frog-leg position, which facilitates stabilization of the pelvis (Fig. 99.1) (8). The skin from the umbilicus to the urethra is prepared with a 10% Betadine solution and the insertion site is identified. The insertion site is in the midline 1 to 2 cm above the pubic symphysis on the abdominal wall. The site can be draped with a sterile cloth and, if desired, local anesthetic such as 1% lidocaine may be infiltrated at the site. This is an optional part of the procedure because needle insertion for the procedure is probably less painful than lo-

Figure 99.1.
Frog-leg position and identification of the insertion site.

**Chapter 99
Suprapubic Bladder
Aspiration**

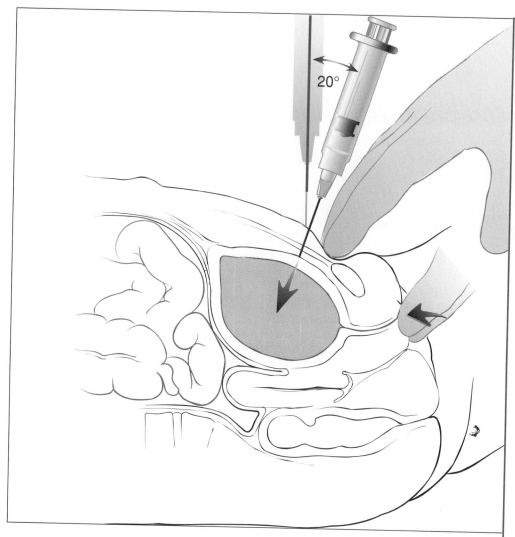

Figure 99.2.
The skin is punctured and the needle is advanced in a cephalad direction angled approximately 20° from the vertical while applying mild negative pressure to the syringe. If this is unsuccessful, the needle is withdrawn and a second attempt is made at the same site with the needle oriented vertically.

SUMMARY
1. Securely restrain child on his or her back in the frog-leg position
2. Prepare skin from the urethra to the umbilicus with betadine solution
3. Identify insertion site 1 to 2 cm superior to pubic symphysis in the midline and drape site.
4. Infiltrate lidocaine locally at insertion site (optional)
5. To prevent patient from urinating during the procedure, occlude urethral opening by squeezing the penile urethra in boys or applying pressure to the urethral meatus in girls
6. Insert needle through the abdominal wall in a slightly cephalad direction approximately 20° from vertical and apply negative pressure to syringe as needle is advanced
7. If unsuccessful, withdraw needle and reinsert it at the same site oriented perfectly upright (vertical)
8. If still unsuccessful, hydrate the child for at least 1 hour before reattempting procedure. Alternatively, use ultrasound after hydration to identify a full bladder (see Chapter 134)
9. When urine is obtained, place it in a sterile container for transport to the laboratory
10. Clean remaining betadine from the site and place an adhesive bandage over puncture wound

cal infiltration anesthesia. Next the urethral opening should be occluded by squeezing the penile urethra in the boy or applying pressure to the urethral meatus in the girl. Many infants will urinate when they feel pressure on the lower abdomen, making occlusion of the urethra necessary to avoid losing the specimen.

The skin is punctured and the needle is advanced in a cephalad direction angled approximately 20° from the vertical while applying mild negative pressure to the syringe (Fig. 99.2). In this way, the needle will puncture the center of a full bladder. When the needle enters the bladder cavity, urine will be aspirated. If the bladder is partially empty, however, this angle of entry may result in passing the needle over the top of the bladder and unsuccessful aspiration. In such cases, the needle is withdrawn to the skin and reoriented vertically (so that a lower part of the abdominal cavity will be entered) and the procedure is repeated. If still unsuccessful the clinician should delay at least 1 hour before a repeated attempt. During this time the child is hydrated with fluids to attempt filling the bladder. Ultrasonography may also be used to identify an adequately filled bladder prior to aspiration (see Chapter 134). When successful, the urine is placed in a sterile container to

**Chapter 99
Suprapubic Bladder
Aspiration**

be transported promptly to the laboratory. Betadine around the insertion site is then cleaned from the skin and a small adhesive bandage is placed over the puncture wound.

COMPLICATIONS

The complication rate from this procedure is low, but a few adverse effects have been described after suprapubic bladder aspiration (9). Hematuria, usually mild and transient, can occur secondary to needle perforation of the bladder wall. Intestinal penetration may occur when a loop of bowel overlies the bladder, but the small hole rarely leads to peritonitis (10). Infection of the needle track also has been reported.

These complications of suprapubic bladder aspiration are not common but are difficult to avoid. The best way to ensure the lowest complication rate is to carefully identify the landmarks for insertion and introduce the needle only 1 to 2 cm above the pubic symphysis on the abdominal wall. The needle should initially be aimed in a slightly cephalad direction toward the center of the bladder. Complications related to needle insertion may also be reduced by using ultrasound guidance, since the clinician is more likely to puncture a full bladder rather than a loop of bowel. Infection is best prevented by strict adherence to aseptic technique (see Chapter 7). The insertion site should be carefully prepared with betadine before the procedure and then cleaned and dressed after the needle has been removed.

SUMMARY

Although largely supplanted by urethral catheterization in recent years, suprapubic bladder aspiration remains a safe and effective procedure for obtaining sterile urine from an incontinent child. Complications from this procedure are rare. In addition, suprapubic bladder aspiration offers the advantage of being easily and quickly performed while avoiding contamination during insertion of a catheter, as often occurs when urethral catheterization is attempted with a struggling child. Suprapubic aspiration is a valuable but underutilized technique which is most useful for obtaining an uncontaminated urine specimen from the infant undergoing a sepsis evaluation.

REFERENCES

1. Huze LB, Beeson PB. Observations of the reliability and safety of bladder catheterization for bacteriologist study of urine. N Engl J Med 1956;255:474.
2. Stamey T.A. Pathogenesis and treatment of urinary tract infections. Baltimore: Williams & Wilkins, 1980.
3. Simon G. Suprapubic bladder puncture in a private pediatric practice. Part Grad Med 1982 July;72(1); 63–64.
4. Mustonen A, Vhari M. Is there bacteremia after suprapubic aspiration in children with urinary tract infection? J Vrol 1978 June;119(6):822–823.
5. Walker D, Richard G. Suprapubic bladder aspiration in infants and children. J Fam Pract 1979;8:1047–8.
6. Burkemeyer BM. Suprapubic aspiration of urine in very low birth weight infants. Pediatrics 1993;92: 457–459.
7. Roberts JR, Hedges JR. Clinical procedures in emergency medicine. Philadelphia: WB Saunders Co., 1985.
8. Cole HS. GU infections. Drug therapy 1978 May;64.
9. Fleisher G, Ludwig S. Textbook of pediatric emergency medicine. Baltimore: Williams & Wilkins, 1983.
10. Polnay L, Fraser AM, Lewis JM. Arch Dis Child, 1975 Jan;50(1):80–86.

MANUAL DETORSION OF THE TESTES

Kate M. Cronan and Stephen A. Zderic

INTRODUCTION

Testicular torsion occurs when the testes rotate on the vascular pedicle producing sharp pain secondary to ischemia. A final diagnosis of testicular torsion will be made in 20 to 25% of children presenting with acute scrotal pain. The differential diagnosis includes torsion of the testicular appendage, epididymitis, incarcerated inguinal hernia, and trauma. Clinicians should not be misled by a history of testicular trauma, which is often obtained in children with testicular torsion.

Time is of the essence because many patients present after enduring ischemic pain for 12 or more hours. Studies suggest that the gonadal salvage rate is lower in the adolescent patient, which is felt to be secondary to patient delay in seeking medical attention (1). It is for this reason that manual detorsion of the testes can be quite useful as a temporizing therapeutic maneuver until an operating room is available for definitive open surgical reduction and orchiopexy.

ANATOMY AND PHYSIOLOGY

Torsion of the testes occurs in children with testes that are not adequately fixed by the tunica vaginalis to the intrascrotal soft tissues. This "bell-clapper" deformity enables the testicle and spermatic cord to twist, which obstructs both venous outflow and arterial inflow through the spermatic vessels. Vascular obstruction can be partial or complete. After 8 hours of warm ischemia, the odds increase that testicular atrophy will result, but gonadal salvage may still be possible after prolonged symptoms if the obstruction is incomplete.

Torsion of the testes results in the triad of acute diffuse scrotal pain, high-riding gonad, and absent cremasteric reflex. This triad comes about because twisting of the spermatic cord results in a retraction of the testes back toward the pubic tubercle. The twisting action leaves the cremasteric muscle fibers unable to exert their normal pulling action, which forms the basis for the valuable cremasteric reflex test. Stroking the inner thigh causes the cremasteric reflex to result in a sudden brisk upward deflection of the testicle (Fig. 100.1). This sign, if present, excludes spermatic cord torsion (2). It must be stressed, however, that many normal male patients will not have a positive cremasteric reflex; hence this sign is helpful only if present. The deflection must be upward, and it must be significant (1 to 2 cm) to have the optimal reliability. Stroking the thigh produces a wrinkling of the scrotal skin, and the inexperienced observer may mistake this for a cremasteric reflex. When a torsion is present, examination of the testicle will reveal a tense and extremely tender gonad with no ability to discriminate between the epididymis and the testes.

Testicular torsion is a clinical diagnosis, and the patient should be seen as quickly as possible by a urologist. Ordering scans and

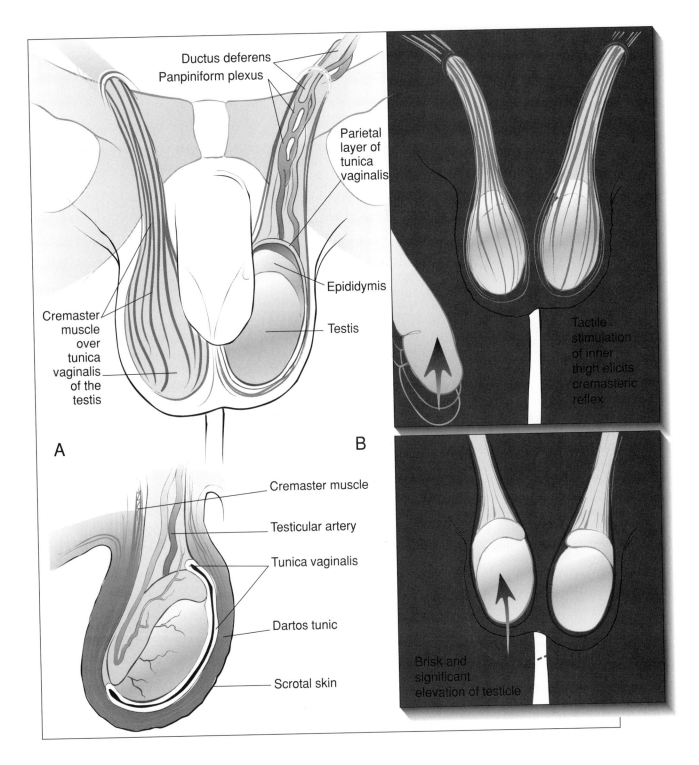

Figure 100.1.
Normal scrotal anatomy and the cremasteric reflex.
A. The testes and epididymis are enveloped within the tunica vaginalis. Attached to the testes and epididymis are the gonadal artery and vein within the cremaster muscle fibers.
B. Stroking the inner thigh produces shortening of the cremaster muscle with upward excursion of the gonad. This shortening should be significant (1 to 2 cm) so as to not be confused with simple wrinkling of the dartos muscle.

Chapter 100
Manual Detorsion of
the Testes

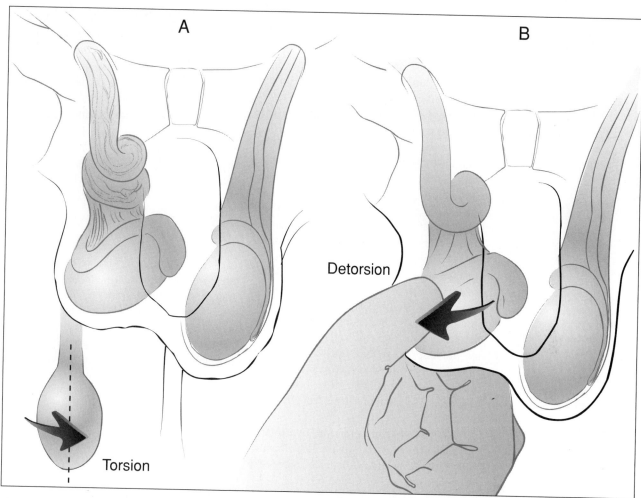

Detorsion

Torsion

ultrasounds by telephone without examining the patient can waste valuable time. In only 5% of the cases of acute scrotal pain are these tests indicated.

INDICATIONS

Manual detorsion of the testes may be used to acutely relieve the ischemic pain in patients with testicular torsion. It is highly effective if used early in the course (before 8 hours of symptoms). Manual detorsion is almost never successful after prolonged ischemia because the swelling and edema become so marked. If urologic consultation is unavailable or will be significantly delayed, the emergency physician, pediatrician, or family physician may attempt this maneuver. If the urologist will be arriving within a short period, he or she should be allowed to examine the patient before manual detorsion.

A urologist should be consulted regarding any case of acute scrotal pain in a child, but as mentioned, detorsion may be attempted if the urologist is going to be significantly delayed in arrival or if the child must be transferred to another facility. Detorsion is indicated only if the etiology of the acute scrotum is torsion of the spermatic cord. Although attempting this maneuver in the presence of epididymitis or a torsed appendix testis will probably not produce any harm, it will be extremely painful and yield no benefit to the patient.

EQUIPMENT (OPTIONAL)

Doppler stethoscope
Lidocaine 1% for spermatic cord block
Intravenous catheter
Morphine and/or midazolam

PROCEDURE

Testes twist with inward rotation in 90% of all cases of testicular torsion. The average

Figure 100.2.
Manual detorsion.
A. Torsion of the testes with two inward twists has resulted in a new high-lying position.
B. The testis is grasped with the fingers and rotated outwardly with two full 360° twists.

SUMMARY

1. Triad of acute scrotal pain, high-riding testis, and absent cremasteric reflex suggest testicular torsion
2. Always seek urologic consultation for initial assessment and follow-up
3. Manual detorsion may be successful and of value in first 8 to 12 hours of symptoms
4. Administer intravenous conscious sedation and/or perform spermatic cord block as indicated
5. Torsion almost always occurs with inward or internal rotation—rotate testis within scrotum in outward direction one or two 360° turns
6. Prompt relief of pain and return to normal position in scrotum suggest successful detorsion
7. Following successful detorsion, surgical exploration and orchiopexy should proceed as soon as possible

CLINICAL TIPS

1. Torsion involves an average of two 360° inward twists.
2. A positive cremasteric reflex excludes testicular torsion. An absent cremasteric reflex does not rule it in.
3. Detorsion results in relief of pain and a normal configuration of the scrotum.
4. Urologic consultation is vital and urgent for patients with testicular torsion. Scrotal exploration is always indicated after manual detorsion.

number of twists in the cord is two (720°) (3). Thus a successful detorsion must involve gently grasping and rotating the testicle within the scrotum in an outward direction, in a series of 360° twists (Fig. 100.2). A dose of intravenous morphine and/or midazolam to blunt the discomfort of detorsion may help the child cooperate and minimize the pain from the procedure. This practice is unlikely to confuse the clinical presentation in cases when the pain is severe. Alternatively, using a local block of the spermatic cord can alleviate the pain of the procedure. Manual detorsion without either of these ancillary procedures often produces brief discomfort, followed by relief of pain that is almost instantaneous. Often, after initiating the detorsion maneuver, the testicle flips over into the normal configuration. The successful detorsion is marked by the sudden onset of pain relief that is quite dramatic and gratifying. Using the Doppler stethoscope in diagnosing spermatic cord torsion has been shown to have minimal predictive ability; however, it may be useful in monitoring effects of detorsion (4).

After successful detorsion, orchiopexy should not be delayed despite relief of symptoms. Often, even after a clinically successful detorsion, exploratory surgery reveals a 180° twist with persistent venous congestion. When considering the likelihood that a patient who suddenly feels better will not return for follow-up and the potential consequences, the urologist should proceed with scrotal exploration as soon as an operating room is available. Admission to the hospital for observation while waiting 2 to 4 hours for operating room time is certainly preferable to gonadal loss.

COMPLICATIONS

Other than discomfort, no complications to the detorsion procedure occur. Failure does not worsen the ischemia of the gonad. It is imperative, however, that manual detorsion be viewed as only a temporizing measure before surgical intervention. If the physician or patient does not fully understand this, the patient may be lost to follow-up and suffer a subsequent torsion of the testicle.

SUMMARY

In most large metropolitan areas, prompt urologic consultation is available to assess children with acute scrotal pain. In other areas, transfer of the child to another facility may be necessary. Testicular torsion is an emergency in which duration of symptoms before treatment is related to success in gonadal salvage. Manual detorsion can temporarily reestablish perfusion to the testes and may be safely used in the emergency setting when rapid consultation is unavailable. Definitive surgical therapy is always indicated in children with testicular torsion.

REFERENCES

1. Barada JH, Weingarten JL, Cromie WJ. Testicular salvage and age-related delay in the presentation of testicular torsion. J Urol 1989;142:746.
2. Rabinowitz R. The importance of the cremasteric reflex in acute scrotal swelling in children. J Urol 1984; 132:89.
3. Cattolica EV. Preoperative manual detorsion of the torsed spermatic cord. J Urol 1985;133:803.
4. Betts JM, Norris M, Cromie WJ, Duckett JW. Testicular detorsion using Doppler ultrasound monitoring. J Ped Surg 1983;18:607.

CHAPTER 101

PARAPHIMOSIS REDUCTION

Michael Green and Gary R. Strange

INTRODUCTION

Phimosis is a condition in which tightness of the foreskin prevents it from being retracted with gentle manipulation. Paraphimosis occurs when a tight foreskin is retracted and cannot easily be reduced. The constricting band of foreskin tissue can lead to venous obstruction, swelling of the glans and potentially ulceration and penile gangrene. Reduction of paraphimosis is often done by physicians in the emergency department (ED) and occasionally in other clinical settings.

The foreskins becomes increasingly retractile over the first few years of life as the tissue separates from the glans penis, promoted by nighttime erections (1–3). Physicians should counsel parents not to forcibly retract the foreskin for cleansing. When it retracts easily, children can be taught to wash the glans and return the foreskin to its anatomic position. Many children presenting to the ED with paraphimosis have had their foreskins forcibly retracted by uninformed caretakers. In addition, medical professionals may forcibly retract a tight foreskin for bladder catheterization and fail to immediately reduce it. Paraphimosis is most common in infants and small children.

Several procedures have been suggested for reducing paraphimosis. Reduction may be straightforward, especially if performed before the development of significant edema. In more long-standing cases, however, reduction can be difficult and, occasionally can require surgical intervention.

ANATOMY AND PHYSIOLOGY

Separation of the glans from the foreskin typically begins about the time of birth. Gairdner found that the foreskin was retractable in only 4% of neonates, 20% of 6 month olds, 50% of 1-year-olds, 80% of 2-year-olds, and 90% of 3-year-olds (2). Although a fully retractable foreskin can become entrapped producing paraphimosis, this problem is much more likely to develop in the tight, partially retractable foreskin of young patients. Paraphimosis can also occur in circumcised boys who have some residual foreskin.

The pathophysiology of paraphimosis involves constriction proximal to the glans penis by a tight ring of retracted foreskin tissue. As the duration of paraphimosis increases, distal accumulation of blood, lymph, and edema fluid lead to swelling which further impedes spontaneous reduction. Reduction by a medical professional is necessary to prevent eventual strangulation and tissue necrosis. Once the constriction is resolved, normal blood flow into and out of the foreskin and glans penis will return.

INDICATIONS

Paraphimosis in younger pediatric patients is most often identified by parents during diaper changes. The retracted foreskin becomes progressively more edematous proximal to the exposed glans penis. Previously unrecognized paraphimosis may be found in the infant who presents with intractable crying.

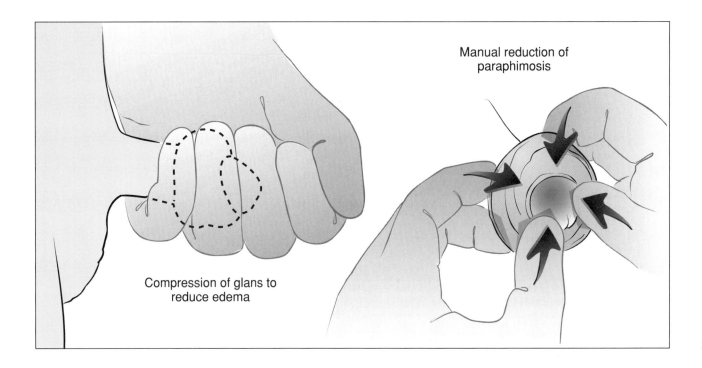

Figure 101.1.
With the thumbs on the glans penis and fingertips on the tight band of foreskin, the glans is pushed as the foreskin is pulled over the glans.

Manual reduction of paraphimosis

Compression of glans to reduce edema

Older boys typically complain of pain as swelling causes increasing constriction and eventually ischemia of the glans. Manual reduction by one of the techniques described in this chapter is indicated whenever spontaneous reduction of the foreskin does not occur. This should be performed as early as possible to eliminate pain and to prevent complications. If initial attempts at reduction are unsuccessful, urgent consultation with a urologist should be obtained.

EQUIPMENT

Ice packs
Gloves
Anesthetic lubricant
Needles, syringes, local anesthetic for dorsal
    nerve block
Babcock clamps
Scalpel

PROCEDURE

Sedation and analgesia (Chapters 34 and 35) may be required for selected patients, particularly if aggressive manipulation is necessary. A block of the dorsal nerve of the penis (Chapter 37) also is effective for eliminating the pain of the procedure.

If a Foley catheter is in place, it should be removed. Reduction may then occur spontaneously or, in mild cases, may be easily performed with manual manipulation. Nonsurgical techniques should be attempted before surgical approaches, but long delays must be avoided. Currently accepted approaches include compression and manual manipulation, Babcock clamp reduction, puncture procedure, dorsal slit reduction, and immediate circumcision.

Nonsurgical Reduction

Nonsurgical reduction of a paraphinosis can be performed or facilitated using several techniques (4–6). Simple compression of the glans penis with the tips of the operator's thumbs, while pulling distally on the retracted foreskin with the fingertips, will often draw the constricting band over the glans penis, thereby reducing the paraphimosis (Fig. 101.1). This technique should be attempted initially and is successful in a majority of cases. Failure is usually related to prolonged paraphimosis and resultant swelling of the foreskin and glans penis.

If simple reduction is initially unsuccessful, it may be necessary to decrease the swelling before reduction can be achieved. This is accomplished with gentle compres-

Chapter 101
Paraphimosis
Reduction

sion by the clinician's hand for 5 minutes, or applying a compression dressing. Ice is a safe and often effective alternative method for decreasing edema. A mixture of ice and water sealed in a rubber glove is applied to the foreskin and glans penis for 3 minutes at a time. Careful monitoring is required to prevent cold or pressure injury. The reduction technique previously described can be attempted again, which is often successful once the swelling has diminished.

If reduction fails despite attempts at decreasing swelling, reduction using noncrushing (Babcock) clamps may be attempted (7). Clamps are placed on the constricting ring in each quadrant, followed by continuous, gentle, and equal traction pulling the foreskin over the glans. This method also has a high success rate (Fig. 101.2).

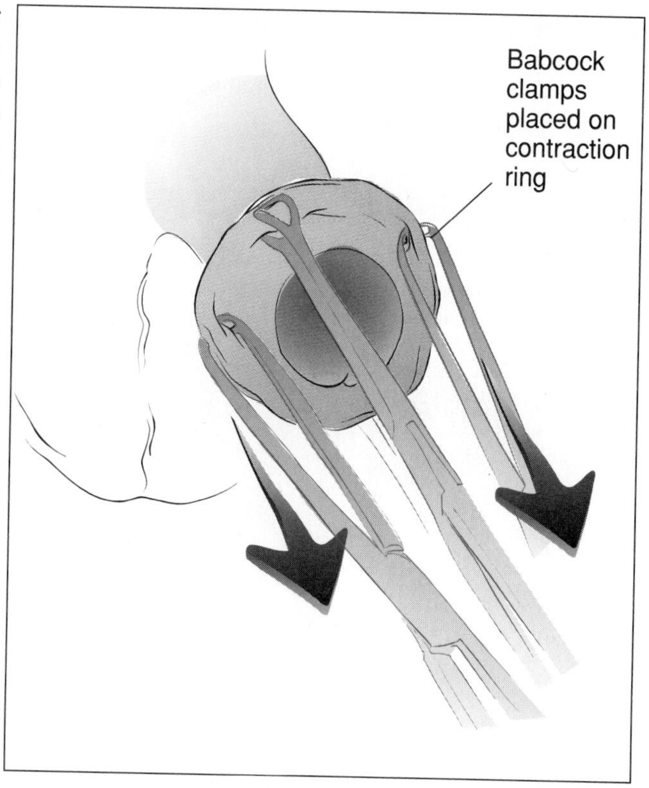

Urologic consultation is indicated for all cases not reducible with simple techniques and for possible postreduction consideration of circumcision.

Surgical Reduction

If noninvasive techniques prove unsuccessful, a surgical approach such as puncture, dorsal slit, or immediate circumcision should be used (8). Urologic consultation should precede any type of surgical intervention whenever feasible. The puncture technique uses a needle to remove fluid from the edematous foreskin. The swollen foreskin tissue is punctured, after which fluid is expressed with gentle compression thereby facilitating reduction. A dorsal slit procedure or an emergency circumcision are occasionally necessary. These procedures should be performed by a urologist or experienced surgeon.

Successful reduction after any of the described techniques will be obvious as the foreskin returns to position over the glans penis. Residual edema will take hours or days to fully resolve. Follow-up with a urologist is

Babcock clamps placed on contraction ring

Figure 101.2.
Noncrushing (Babcock) clamps are placed on the constricting portion of the foreskin in each quadrant. Gentle, continuous, equal traction is applied until reduction is achieved.

advisable—especially in cases that are difficult to reduce—to assess the healing of the penis and to consider elective circumcision.

COMPLICATIONS

Complications are rare from paraphimosis reduction. Overaggressive manual reduction or compression can injure the glans penis and foreskin. Ice can cause a cold injury if not monitored properly. In inexperienced hands the surgical techniques can lead to injury of the penis, especially if the child is not adequately sedated, locally anesthetized, and/or restrained.

SUMMARY

Early reduction of paraphimosis is indicated to avoid skin ulceration and necrosis of the distal penis. Gentle, continuous compression followed by manual manipulation is often a successful technique, as is the use of noncrushing clamps. Application of these procedures, after removal of a Foley catheter if present, and careful, monitored application of ice packs is successful in most cases. Surgical approaches such as dorsal slit incision and immediate circumcision may occasionally be necessary. Urologic consultation should precede any surgical procedures.

REFERENCES

1. Herzog LW, Alvarez ST. The frequency of foreskin problems in uncircumcised children. Am J Dis Child 1986;140:254.
2. Gairdner D. Fate of the foreskin: a study of circumcision. Brit Med J 1949;2:1433.
3. Oster J. Further fate of the foreskin: incidence of preputial adhesions, phimosis, and smegma among Danish schoolboys. Arch Dis Child 1968;43:200.
4. Barry CN. A simple method for reduction of paraphimosis. J Urol 1954;71:450.
5. Cletsoway RW, Lewis EL. Treatment of paraphimosis. US Armed Forces Med J 1957;8:361.
6. Zbaraschuk I, Berger RE, Hedges JR. Emergency urologic procedures. In: Roberts JR, Hedges JR, eds. Clinical procedures in emergency medicine. Philadelphia: WB Saunders, 1991.
7. Skoglund RW, Chapman WH. Reduction of paraphimosis. J Urol 1970;104:137.
8. Schenck GF. The treatment of paraphimosis. Am J Surg 1930;8:329.

CHAPTER 102

MANAGEMENT OF ZIPPER INJURIES

Joel A. Fein and Stephen Zderic

INTRODUCTION

Injury to the skin and soft tissues of the penis and scrotum commonly results among pediatric patients from entrapment inside a zipper mechanism. Most of these injuries occur in school-age boys during opening or closing of the zipper, when tissue may be caught in the tracks or become entangled within the fastener mechanism (1). The goal of therapy is to provide a relatively painless and rapid extrication of the involved area without inflicting further injury. The techniques are straightforward and may be performed by physicians at any level of training. If local or regional anesthesia is not required, non-physician health care providers also may perform the procedures outlined in this chapter.

ANATOMY AND PHYSIOLOGY

The school-aged boy who is dressing himself without using protective undergarments is at highest risk for zipper injuries. For this reason, parents should be wary of pajamas that contain such mechanisms. Although any loose tissue can become caught inside a zipper, the majority of zipper injuries involve uncircumcised penile foreskin. The redundant tissue located on the ventral aspect of the circumcised penis also is at risk for this type of injury. Once the tissue is caught inside the zipper, swelling may occur and may complicate the extrication procedure.

A zipper is composed of two opposing rows of teeth that interlock inside a sliding zipper fastener mechanism. The sliding portion consists of two face plates that are bridged by a "diamond" or median bar. As the fastener mechanism draws the two rows of teeth together on either side of the median bar, it aligns them such that the teeth interlock. Unless this alignment is maintained in a two-dimensional plane, the teeth edges fall apart. This relationship is the basis for the following techniques, which work equally well for both metal and plastic zippers.

INDICATIONS

Whenever tissue is entangled inside a zipper fastener or between the teeth of a zipper, the clinician should attempt to extricate the tissue. Using excessive force is not warranted and may cause further damage to the tissue. No absolute contraindications exist to these techniques, but if the extraction proves difficult, urologic referral is most appropriate. A urologist should be consulted for cases that involve the urethra or fail to respond to the following procedures. Any blood at the meatus or hematuria should alert the clinician to the possibility of an underlying urethral injury.

EQUIPMENT

Betadine solution or alcohol pad
Mineral oil

Figure 102.1.
Cutting the median bar of the zipper with a wire cutter or bone cutter will allow the side plates to separate and the tissue to be freed.

SUMMARY
1. Restrain child and prepare entrapped tissues with antiseptic solution
2. Use local or regional anesthesia if extrication is difficult.
3. Place mineral oil on involved area and apply gentle traction
4. Cut median bar with wire or bone cutters if traction fails
5. Separate rows of teeth and free entrapped tissue
6. Provide local wound care
7. Instruct parents to observe at home for complications of wound infection or urethral obstruction

CLINICAL TIPS
1. Conscious sedation may be necessary with an anxious patient.
2. Ice may reduce the swelling and facilitate the extrication of the entrapped skin.
3. Cutting the zipper out of the pants or pajamas makes it easier to cut the median bar.
4. If the above-described techniques are unsuccessful, a urologist may need to perform a circumcision under general anesthesia.

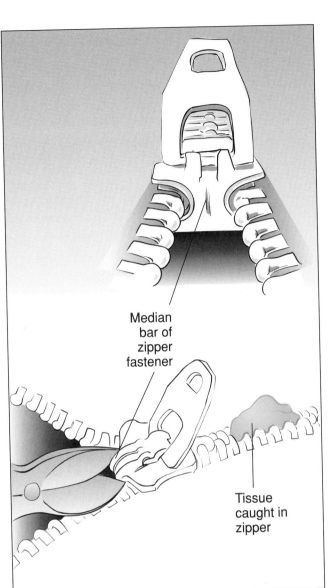

Median bar of zipper fastener

Tissue caught in zipper

Bone cutter or wire cutter (Fig. 102.1)
Bandage scissors

PROCEDURE

The clinician can approach the extraction of tissue from a zipper mechanism using one of the following techniques: (*a*) mineral oil extraction, (*b*) cutting the median bar, or (*c*) cutting the zipper cloth.

Oral or intranasal sedation (Chapter 35) should be considered before starting the procedure. Ice should be applied through a moist cloth to minimize swelling while setting up the sedation and anesthesia. Most children will require local or regional anesthesia after a superficial disinfectant is applied. A direct injection to the affected site may increase edema and complicate the extraction; so that regional anesthesia techniques such as dorsal penile block (Chapter 37) or circumferential penile block should therefore be considered.

After appropriate anesthesia is undertaken and the child is restrained appropriately for age (Chapter 3), mineral oil may be applied liberally to the surface of the involved tissue and gentle traction applied to the zipper (2). At this point, the tissue may slide out of the zipper mechanism without further injury.

If gentle traction does not free the tissue, then the median bar of the zipper fastener should be cut with the wire cutters or bone cutter (3, 4) (Fig. 102.1). With the median bar cut, the side plates of the zipper fastener separate and the zipper teeth fall apart.

A similar result can be accomplished by cutting the zipper cloth around the area of injury (Fig. 102.2). A bandage scissors is used to make several cuts completely through the cloth on both sides of the zipper, above and below the entrapped skin. The side plates will easily separate freeing the tissues that had been trapped. In general, assuming the appropriate tools are available, the median bar method is easier.

After the tissue is freed from the zipper mechanism, any open wounds should be cleaned and dressed with a sterile, dry gauze. Discharge instructions should address the possible complications of skin infections and urethral obstruction. Attempts to prevent recurrent injury should include a discussion of the protection afforded by undergarments and avoiding pajamas with zippers.

COMPLICATIONS

Some complications of the recommended procedures occur as a result of the initial injury; however, subsequent damage to the skin can be avoided by using only gentle traction during extrication. To avoid lacerating underlying skin when cutting the median bar the child must be properly restrained, and wire cutters or bone cutters with the smallest possible mouth should be used. Urethral obstruction with urinary retention may result from posttraumatic edema, and can occur up to 8 hours after the procedure. This may require temporary placement of a Foley catheter. Urologic consultation is indicated if complications occur.

SUMMARY

Zipper injuries occur most commonly among school-aged boys who dress themselves without wearing protective undergarments. Boys who wear pajamas that have a zipper mechanism are especially prone to these injuries. Usually the penile foreskin of an uncircumcised boy is entrapped in the tracks or the fastener of a zipper, although any loose tissue of the penis or scrotum may be caught. The goal of the clinician is to extricate the entrapped tissue while minimizing pain and without causing further injury. Measures to reduce pain include sedation, applying ice to the affected site, and local or regional anesthesia. For uncomplicated injuries, liberal application of mineral oil followed by gentle traction may be the only measures required for removal. When this is inneffective or when larger segments of tissue are entrapped, it is usually necessary to cut the median bar of the zipper with a wire cutter or to cut the zipper cloth around the area of injury with scissors. Although complications are infrequent, the clinician must take great care to avoid injuring the urethra during extrication and to carefully inspect the penis for signs of preexisting urethral trauma caused by the zipper. Suspicion of urethral injury warrants consultation with a urologist before performing any procedures.

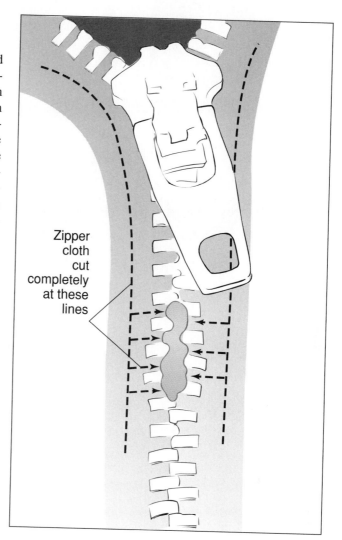

Zipper cloth cut completely at these lines

Figure 102.2.
Cutting completely through the zipper cloth on both sides will enable the side plates to be separated.

REFERENCES

1. Saraf PS, Rabinowitz R. Zipper injury of the foreskin. Am J Dis Child 1982;136:557–558.
2. Kanegaye JT, Schonfeld N. Penile zipper entrapment. A simple and less threatening approach using mineral oil. Pediatr Emerg Care 1993;9:90–91.
3. Nolan JF, Stillwell TJ, Sands JP. Acute management of zipper-entrapped penis. J Emerg Med 1990;8:305–307.
4. Oosterlinck W. Unbloody management of penile zipper injury. Eur Urol 1981;7:365–366.

Obstetrical Procedures for Adolescents

Vidya T. Chande

Introduction

Emergency physicians and prehospital care providers must be familiar with the procedure for delivering a newborn, as transfer to a labor suite before delivery is not always possible. Even physicians who work solely in a pediatric emergency department (ED) need a working knowledge of the steps involved. This chapter will focus on normal spontaneous vaginal delivery and the needs of the adolescent mother. A more extensive discussion of newborn delivery can be found in other textbooks (1, 2).

The majority of women delivering babies today do so under the guidance of a health care professional who has special training in obstetrics. Women are encouraged to seek prenatal care and to contact their health care provider at the first signs of labor. Occasionally, however, young women unexpectedly present to the ED or clinic in active labor. It is the physician's job to decide if the pregnant adolescent can be transferred to a labor and delivery suite or if preparation on site for an imminent delivery is necessary.

Pregnant adolescents are less likely to seek prenatal care and may be at greater risk of delivering in the ED because of their complex social situations (3). In fact, the pregnant adolescent may deny being pregnant even as the baby is about to be born. Therefore, providers of emergency care must assess the pregnant adolescent carefully because her first medical contact for pregnancy may be at the time of delivery.

An adolescent patient presenting in labor is likely to be extremely anxious and complaining of severe abdominal pain. The patient may be screaming hysterically and may be unable to answer medical questions. The physician may have to rely solely on the findings on physical examination, such as the size of the uterus and observed uterine contractions, to determine that the patient is pregnant and about to deliver.

Anatomy and Physiology

Labor is defined as progressive dilatation of the uterine cervix in association with repetitive uterine contractions. Normal labor is a continuous process that leads to delivery of the products of conception, including the baby and the placenta. The progress and outcome of labor are influenced by four factors: the bony and soft tissues of the maternal pelvis, the contractions of the uterus, the fetus, and the placenta (4).

Just before the beginning of labor, a small amount of blood-tinged mucus is discharged from the vagina. This "bloody show" is a plug of cervical mucus mixed with blood and is evidence of cervical dilatation.

Rupture of the fetal membranes occurs before onset of labor in approximately 10% of women. The majority of women whose membranes rupture first go into labor within 24 hours. If labor does not begin within 24 hours, the pregnancy is considered to be complicated by prolonged rupture of the membranes, a risk factor for neonatal sepsis.

Diagnosis of true labor can be made when the following features exist: (*a*) contractions occur at regular intervals, (*b*) intervals between contractions gradually shorten, (*c*) intensity of contractions gradually increases, (*d*) discomfort localizes in the back and abdomen, (*e*) cervix dilates, and (*f*) discomfort does not stop with sedation.

Labor is usually divided into three stages. The first stage begins with the onset of labor and ends when dilatation of the cervix is complete. The average duration of the first stage of labor is 8 to 12 hours in the primiparous patient and 6 to 8 hours in the multiparous patient. The progress of the first stage of labor can be monitored by assessing the cervix for effacement and dilatation, and determining the fetal station. Effacement of the cervix is a process of thinning out of the cervix. Effacement is expressed in terms of the length of the cervical canal compared with an uneffaced cervix. For example, 0% indicates no effacement whereas 100% indicates the cervix is very thin (less than 0.25 cm thick).

Dilatation of the cervical os is expressed by estimating the diameter of the cervical opening by direct palpation with the sterile-gloved fingers. Complete dilatation occurs at 10 cm.

Fetal station refers to the position of the presenting part in relation to the level of the ischial spines. If the presenting part is at the spines, it is at "zero station." If the presenting part is above the spines, the distance is reported in minus figures (e.g., −1 to −3 cm or "floating"); if below the spines, the distance is reported in plus figures (e.g., +1 to +3 cm or "on the perineum").

The second stage of labor extends from full dilatation of the cervix to complete birth of the infant. This stage varies from a few minutes to 1 to 2 hours. The third stage of labor is the period from birth of the infant until delivery of the placenta is complete. Many adolescents presenting in labor will be primiparous and therefore should be expected to labor for 8 to 12 hours before delivering the infant. The second stage of labor also may be longer in the primiparous patient.

The vertex (head) is the presenting part in 95% of deliveries. As shown in Figure 103.1, the sequence of events in vertex presentations is:

A. Engagement: Engagement refers to the passage of the head through the pelvic inlet. This usually occurs in the last two weeks of pregnancy in the primiparous patient and at the onset of labor in the multiparous patient.

B. Flexion and descent: Flexion is necessary for passage of the smallest diameter of the head through the smallest diameter of the bony pelvis. Descent is gradual and is affected by the previously mentioned forces that influence labor.

C. Internal rotation: Internal rotation occurs with descent of the head and is necessary for the presenting part to traverse the ischial spines.

D. Extension: Extension occurs after the head has begun to pass through the introitus.

E. External rotation: External rotation occurs after delivery of the head as it rotates to the position it occupied at engagement. The shoulders then descend along the same pathway as the head, and the remainder of the fetus is delivered.

Vertex vaginal delivery usually occurs spontaneously. The primary role of the clinician is to help control the process to avoid sudden expulsion of the fetus, which could lead to injuries to the mother and infant.

INDICATIONS

When a patient presents in labor, the clinician must assess the fetus and mother rapidly. If delivery is imminent, the infant should be delivered before transfer; if not, the mother should be transferred to a delivery suite where personnel are more accustomed to obstetrical procedures.

If complete cervical effacement and dilatation are evident, immediate delivery may be necessary. Delivery is imminent when the contractions last 1 to 2 minutes and occur at intervals of 2 to 3 minutes, and the infant's head is at the perineum. An obstetrician should be contacted immediately while the physician prepares for the delivery.

Every effort should be made for compli-

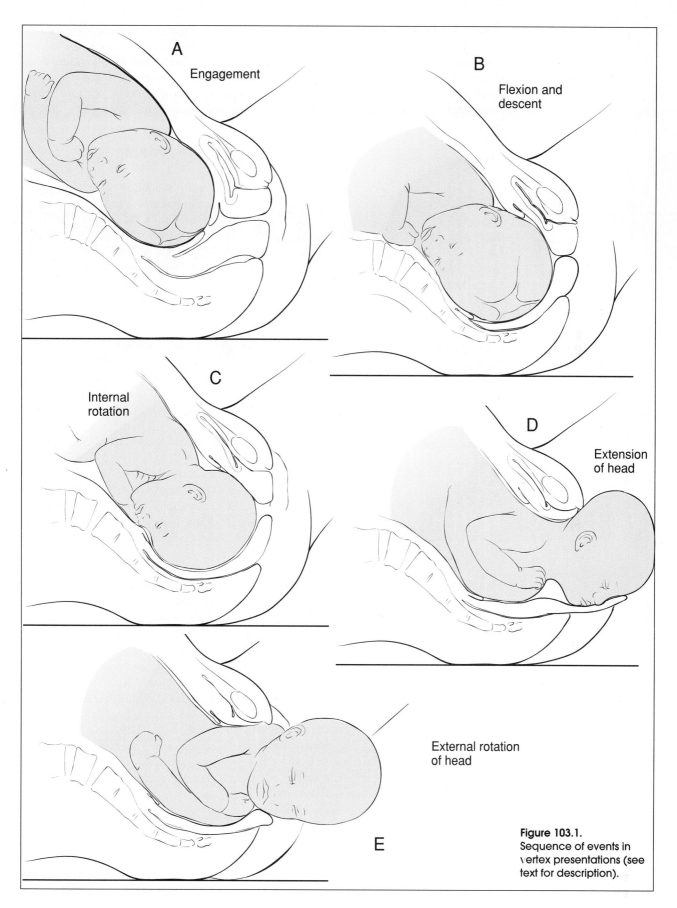

A **Engagement**

B **Flexion and descent**

C **Internal rotation**

D **Extension of head**

E **External rotation of head**

Figure 103.1.
Sequence of events in vertex presentations (see text for description).

cated deliveries to occur in a delivery suite. Heavy maternal bleeding and fetal distress are obstetrical emergencies requiring immediate involvement of an obstetrician, and should not be managed by ED or clinic staff alone. Breech presentations also are more difficult to manage and have a higher risk of morbidity and mortality for the mother and fetus.

EQUIPMENT

Mask, cap, gown
Goggles
Sterile gloves
Large basin (for placenta)
Scissors
2 Kelly clamps or umbilical tape
Bulb syringe
Cord clamp
Povidone-iodine solution
Sterile towels
Sterile drapes
Warm blankets
Heated isolette or overhead warming lights
Infant resuscitation tray
Name bands

PROCEDURE

At least two clinicians should be present at the delivery. One person should attend to the mother while the other attends to the newborn. A support person for the mother, either a family member or another health care provider, also should be present. A social worker may be included as part of the team if the mother is particularly upset and difficult to manage.

The procedure should be explained to the mother (and father, if present). The mother's support person should be seated by the mother's head. Adolescent mothers especially need to be encouraged to remain calm and to work with the clinician to deliver the baby as smoothly as possible. The mother is often frightened by the process of labor and benefits from a calm, soothing voice. A primiparous adolescent is especially likely to have little understanding of what is happening and to be extremely anxious. The presence of a support person for the adolescent mother during labor and delivery is important because it

helps calm the mother and improves the outcome for both mother and infant (5).

All personnel should follow universal precautions by wearing a gown, gloves, mask, cap, and goggles before proceeding with the delivery (see Chapter 7).

Initial Assessment

A brief history should be obtained to determine (a) onset and frequency of contractions, (b) gestational age of the fetus, (c) presence of bleeding, (d) possible rupture of membranes, (e) prenatal care, (f) intercurrent illnesses, and (g) fetal activity (2). A brief physical examination should be performed and fetal heart tones should be recorded.

Vaginal Examination

If no vaginal bleeding is present, a manual vaginal examination should be performed to determine the position of the fetus and to determine if delivery is imminent. This evaluation should assess cervical effacement, dilatation, and fetal station (1). A vaginal examination should never be performed by anyone other than an obstetrician for a third-trimester gestation with vaginal bleeding. Inadvertent manipulation of a placenta previa may cause profuse and uncontrollable vaginal bleeding.

The mother should be positioned on a bedpan with her legs widely separated (1). The perineum should be cleansed with an antiseptic solution before beginning the examination. Scrubbing should be anterior to posterior, away from the vaginal introitus. The clinician should use the thumb and index finger of a sterile-gloved hand to separate the labia. The index and third finger of the second hand (also sterile-gloved) should be used to perform the vaginal examination. If complete dilatation and effacement of the cervix are evident and the infant's head is at the perineum, preparation for delivery should begin immediately.

Delivery of the Infant

The mother should be positioned supine on the stretcher, with legs bent at the knees and flexed and abducted at the hips (2). The clinician should stand or sit between the mother's legs. The mother's perineum should again be cleansed with povidone-iodine solution, wiping anterior to posterior, and the legs and abdomen covered with sterile drapes. The adolescent mother should be encouraged to remain calm so that the delivery will proceed smoothly.

Spontaneous vaginal delivery of the infant presenting by vertex is divided into three phases (1): delivery of the head, delivery of the shoulders, and delivery of the body. Delivery is about to occur when the presenting part distends the vulva (crowning). Speed of delivery should be controlled to avoid forceful expulsion of the infant.

Delivery of an infant presenting breech (feet first) is more difficult and the infant and the mother are at greater risk of injury. An obstetrician should be called immediately to manage breech deliveries.

Delivery of the Head

A gentle, gradual delivery is best for the mother and the infant. As the head advances, the clinician places one hand over the occiput to control delivery. The second hand, draped with a sterile towel to avoid fecal contamination, may apply gentle pressure on the perineum from the coccygeal region upward (modified Ritgen maneuver) (Fig 103.2). This maneuver will help extend the head at the proper time, thus protecting the maternal perineal musculature.

In vertex presentations, the forehead is followed by the face, chin, and neck. After the head has been delivered, a finger should palpate the infant's neck to check for a loop of umbilical cord encircling the neck (nuchal cord). The umbilical cord encircles the neck in 20 to 25% of deliveries. If a nuchal cord is present, it should be palpated to check for pulsation and then gently slipped over the infant's head. If the cord is tight, it should be clamped in two places and cut between the clamps, and the remainder of the delivery should proceed.

Once the head has been delivered, the infant's face should be wiped and the mouth and nose should be suctioned with a bulb syringe. Special maneuvers are necessary if thick meconium is present (Chapter 39).

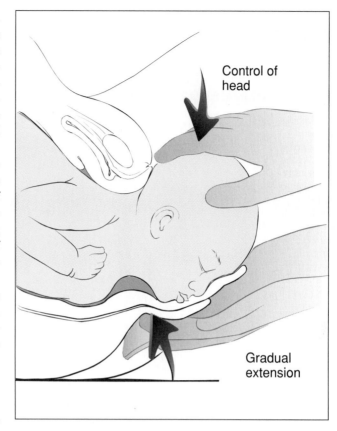

Delivery of the Shoulders

Delivery of the shoulders also should proceed gradually. Gentle downward traction on the head will help deliver the anterior shoulder, followed by gentle upward traction which delivers the posterior shoulder (Fig. 103.3). Forceful traction, especially with rotation, can cause injury to the infant's brachial plexus and great vessels.

Shoulder dystocia (shoulders unable to pass through the birth canal after delivery of the head) complicates 0.15 to 0.6% of all deliveries (2). This is an obstetrical emergency because the umbilical cord may become occluded, leading to fetal hypoxia. An obstetrician should be notified of shoulder dystocia immediately at the first suspicion that the shoulders may not pass. Exaggerated flexion and abduction of the maternal hips often resolves the problem in mild dystocia. Downward traction at the pubic symphysis also may dislodge the impacted anterior shoulder. Other maneuvers are occasionally necessary for more severe dystocia but are beyond the scope of this chapter.

Figure 103.2.
Gentle, upward pressure on the perineum protects the perineal musculature from injury.

Figure 103.3.
Delivery of the anterior and
posterior shoulders.

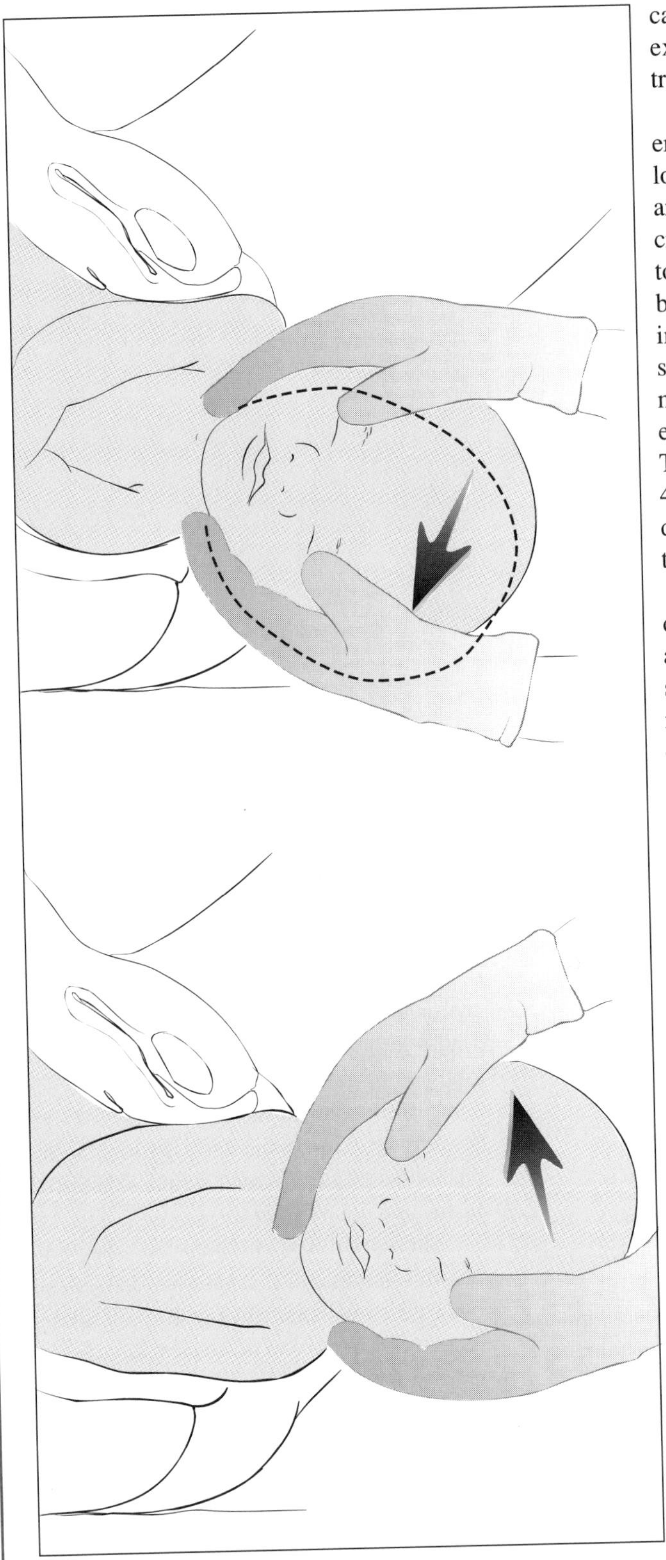

Summary
1. Perform brief assess-
   ment of mother in-
   cluding vital signs
   and fetal heart tones
2. If mother is in early
   labor, transfer her to
   delivery suite
3. If contractions are 2
   to 3 minutes apart and
   infant's head is dis-
   tending perineum,
   prepare for emer-
   gency delivery
4. Notify obstetrician
   that assistance is
   needed immediately
5. Assign one person for
   mother and one for
   infant; set up equip-
   ment for delivery and
   newborn resuscitation
6. Position mother on
   her back with hips
   flexed and abducted
   and knees flexed;
   mother's support per-
   son should be at head
   of bed
7. Clean perineum with
   povidone-iodine solu-
   tion and drape ab-
   domen and legs
8. As head emerges, ap-
   ply one hand to head
   to control speed of
   delivery; other hand
   exerts upward pres-
   sure on perineum
   (Fig. 103.2)
9. Check neck for loop
   of umbilical cord—if
   present, slip over in-
   fant's head; if cord is
   tight, clamp in two
   places and cut be-
   tween clamps
10. After head is deliv-
    ered, wipe face and
    suction nose and
    mouth

Delivery of the Body and Extremities

The body and extremities should deliver easily after the head and shoulders have been delivered. The clinician must be prepared to
control the remainder of the delivery and
catch the newborn should it be
expelled forcefully. Gentle
traction may be necessary.

After the infant is delivered, the head should be held
lower than the body at a 15°
angle to allow drainage of secretions from the airway and
to allow a small transfusion of
blood from the placenta to the
infant. The umbilical cord
should be clamped within 1
minute of delivery to avoid
excess transfusion of blood.
Two Kelly clamps are placed
4 to 5 cm from the infant's abdomen and the cord is cut between the clamps.

The infant should then be
dried and placed under a radiant warmer to prevent cold
stress. The nose and mouth
may be suctioned again if necessary and the infant should be
assessed by the second clinician at the delivery (6). This
person should evaluate the infant's respiratory effort and
heart rate, and provide additional resuscitative measures
as needed (see Chapter 38).

Delivery of the Placenta

After delivery of the infant,
the uterus will continue to
contract to allow the placenta
to deliver. Placental separation from the uterine wall usually occurs within 5 minutes
after delivery of the infant.
Signs of placental separation
include: (*a*) the uterus becomes globular, (*b*) a small
gush of blood occurs, (*c*) the
umbilical cord protrudes further from the vagina, and (*d*)
the uterus rises in the abdomen (1,7).

The mother should then be asked to bear
down to expel the placenta. The placenta
should not be delivered by pulling on the cord
because this may lead to uterine injury or

tearing of the placenta causing retained parts. Delivery of the placenta may be assisted by applying pressure to the abdomen just above the pubic symphysis. This will elevate the uterus into the abdomen and push the placenta into the vagina. The placenta may then be guided out of the vagina. The placenta should be kept in a basin for further inspection to ensure that no missing pieces have been retained in the uterus.

The uterus should be palpated after delivery of the placenta to stimulate contraction and reduce blood loss. Oxytocin (10 i.u.) may be given intravenously to aid in the contraction of the uterus (4).

Postpartum Care

The perineum, vagina, and cervix should be inspected for lacerations. If any lacerations are noted, they should be repaired in a sterile manner by a clinician familiar with the techniques. This procedure can take place after transfer. After determining that the mother and infant are in stable condition a maternity service is contacted, detailed information about the emergency delivery is provided, and the mother and infant are transferred for complete evaluation and admission.

COMPLICATIONS

Excessive traction on the head and neck can cause injury to the brachial plexus and/or great vessels. Brachial plexus injury (Erb's palsy) usually resolves over time. Shoulder dystocia can result in fractures of the clavicle, which are not uncommon after delivery of large infants. Brachial plexus injury and clavicle fracture should be suspected when a newborn does not move one arm or if asymmetry of the Moro or startle reflex is observed.

Postpartum hemorrhage is the most common cause of obstetric hemorrhage and is an obstetrical emergency (2, 8). An obstetrician should be notified while initial management is begun by the emergency physician. Intravascular volume should be replaced with crystalloid and blood products as needed. The most common causes of immediate postpartum hemorrhage are uterine atony, lacera-

tions of the vagina and cervix, and retained placental fragments. Uterine atony may be treated with uterine massage and oxytocin (20 to 40 i.u. in 1 L crystalloid). If the uterus remains boggy, an ergot preparation may be given to stimulate uterine contraction. Ergots may cause hypertension and should be avoided in women with preeclampsia or preexisting hypertension. Any lacerations should be repaired and the uterus should be inspected manually for fragments of placental tissue.

Infant distress is another complication that providers must be prepared to address (6). Clinicians must be prepared to treat an asphyxiated newborn, even if delivery is progressing without apparent complications (Chapter 38). An infant resuscitation tray should be available for all deliveries and a provider should be assigned to the evaluation and treatment of the infant.

SUMMARY

Delivery of a newborn is a procedure best done by the patient's obstetrical care provider. Whenever possible, the expectant mother should be transferred to a delivery suite or an obstetrician should be called to the scene of emergency delivery. Occasionally in emergency situations other clinicians may be called on to manage a delivery. The majority of vaginal vertex deliveries occur spontaneously and the primary role of the clinician is to control the speed of delivery to avoid injury to the mother and the infant. Two clinicians should be available to attend the delivery—one for the mother and one for the infant. Equipment for resuscitation of the infant should be available and universal precautions should be observed during the delivery.

REFERENCES

1. Cunningham FG, MacDonald PC, Gant NF, Levenok KJ, Gilstrap LC, eds. Williams obstetrics. 19th ed. Norwalk, CT: Appleton & Lange, 1993.
2. Doan-Wiggins LA. Emergency childbirth. In: Roberts JR, Hedges JR, eds. Clinical procedures in emergency medicine. 2nd ed. Philadelphia: WB Saunders, 1993, pp. 903–907.

11. Deliver shoulders (Fig. 103.3) and rest of body
12. Clamp umbilical cord in two places and cut between clamps within 1 minute
13. Assess infant and provide resuscitation as needed
14. Wait for placenta to separate. Assist mother in delivering placenta with downward pressure on abdomen—do not pull on umbilical cord. Save placenta for inspection
15. Massage uterus to stimulate contractions and prevent further bleeding; oxytocin (10 i.u.) can be given intravenously
16. Check cervix and perineum for lacerations

CLINICAL TIPS
1. The clinician should remain calm, even though this procedure is not commonly performed. Most deliveries proceed spontaneously without difficulty.
2. Universal precautions should be observed.
3. Neonatal resuscitation equipment should be ready to use.
4. An isolette should be turned on before delivering the baby.
5. A support person who can help the mother focus on the delivery should be included.

Chapter 103
Obstetrical
Procedures for
Adolescents

3. Wegman ME. Annual summary of vital statistics—1993. Pediatrics 1994; 94:792–803.

4. Benson RC, ed. Current obstetric and gynecologic diagnosis and treatment. 5th ed. Los Altos, CA: Lange Medical Publications, 1984.

5. Kennell J, Klaus M, McGrath S, Robertson S, Hinkley C. Continuous emotional support during labor in a US hospital. JAMA 1991; 265:2197–2201.

6. Chameides L, Hazinski MF, eds. Textbook of pediatric advanced life support. 2nd ed. Dallas, TX: American Heart Association, 1994.

7. Scherger JE. Management of normal labor and birth. Primary Care 1993; 20(3):713–9.

8. Gianopoulos JG. Emergency complications of labor and delivery. Emerg Med Clin North Am 1994; 12(1):239–256.

ORTHOPAEDIC PROCEDURES

Section Editor: Brent R. King

CHAPTER 104

SPLINTING PROCEDURES

Jean E. Klig

INTRODUCTION

Orthopaedic immobilization methods represent a continuum of external support for musculoskeletal injuries. Splints are part of this spectrum and are vital tools for the initial management of many injuries in children. The goal of splinting is to provide support at key points around an injury to allow for (*a*) decreased pain, (*b*) mechanical stabilization of bones, soft tissues, and neurovascular structures, (*c*) decreased risk of further injury to the affected area, and (*d*) decreased risk of swelling-related injuries such as a compartment syndrome. In contrast to the circumferential limits of a cast, a splint allows for minor fluctuations in extremity size without a risk to neurovascular structures of the immobilized limb.

Splints can be used both for initial injury care and for definitive treatment in certain cases. They are often used for the acute management of nondisplaced closed fractures in children for a minimum of 24 to 48 hours after initial injury because they allow for extremity swelling without external compression. Although extremity swelling is minimal beyond 48 hours after a fracture, splints can be used for up to 2 weeks before a cast must be applied. Splints also offer a valuable temporizing measure in children with equivocal injuries such as joint sprains. In a child, painful injury to a joint with an open epiphysis must initially be assumed to be a nondisplaced Salter-Harris type I fracture even if radiographs are unremarkable. Sprains in children are therefore considered fractures,

and are optimally treated with a splint. For older adolescents, splints may be used as definitive treatment for more severe joint sprains. Overall, the rule of "when in doubt, splint" is key to the treatment of pediatric musculoskeletal injuries (1).

Splinting methods in this chapter can be used in children of all ages, and are used in prehospital, emergency, and ambulatory settings. Splint techniques can be performed by many skilled medical personnel.

ANATOMY AND PHYSIOLOGY

Pediatric and adult fractures are different because children's bones are continually in the process of growth. A growing long bone has four anatomical parts: physis, epiphysis, metaphysis, and diaphysis (Fig. 104.1). Growth occurs in two regions. The bone increases in length at the growth plate (physis) by endochondral ossification. Increase in width occurs at the periosteum by membranous ossification. As a result, the strongest part of a child's bone is the periosteum and adjacent joint capsules and ligaments—the growth plate is the weakest area (2). Given the strength of the periosteum, capsule, and ligaments of a child's bone, dislocation and sprain and/or strain injuries are rare. Fractures are common.

Certain fractures are unique to children. The great tensile strength of pediatric bones often results in buckling (torus), bending (greenstick), or compression fractures. Physeal or growth plate fractures are character-

Figure 104.1.
Pediatric long bone.
Children's bones have
extensive tensile strength
and are weakest in areas
of growth. Fractures of the
shaft often manifest as
buckling (torus) or bending
or fraying (greenstick), but
injuries to the growth plate
region can vary.

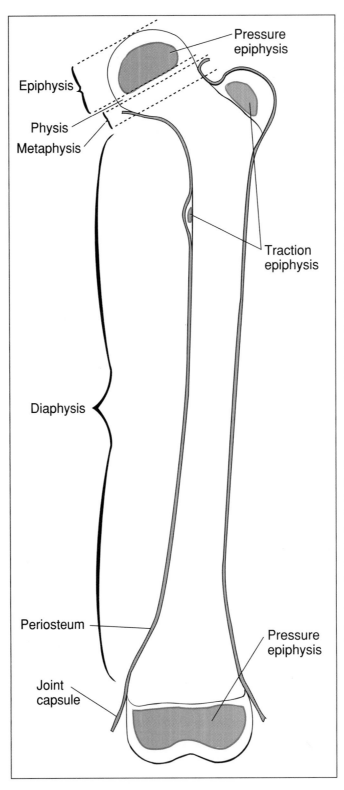

the epiphyseal plate, which fractures into the articular surface; type IV entails a fracture through the epiphyseal plate and metaphysis; type V is a compression fracture of the growth plate.

Differences in the pediatric anatomy impact on splinting practices in two key ways. First, the dynamics of bone growth allow for remodeling of angulated fractures. Fractures with up to 30° of angulation in the plane of joint motion can be splinted without reduction. Second, children tend to not suffer muscle stiffness or spasm. Splints can therefore be used liberally without significant risk of musculoskeletal rigidity.

INDICATIONS

Given the rate at which children's bones grow and remodel, early diagnosis and treatment is vital to fracture care. Splints can be applied for most pediatric fractures, except for those requiring orthopaedic consultation (detailed later in this section). Clinical findings include: inability and/or reluctance to use the affected limb; pain with limb movement; swelling, discoloration, deformity at the fracture site; crepitus; and reproducible bone point tenderness to palpation (3). Radiographs should always be obtained to support positive or abnormal clinical findings. Negative radiographs do not rule out a Salter I fracture. Reproducible bone tenderness near a joint with an open epiphysis is sufficient indication for a splint. Sprains are rare in children and are usually presumed to be Salter I fractures (4,5).

ized by the Salter-Harris classification (Fig. 104.2): type 1 injures the zone of provisional calcification without fracture; type II is a slip of the epiphyseal plate with a fracture through the metaphysis; type III is a slip of

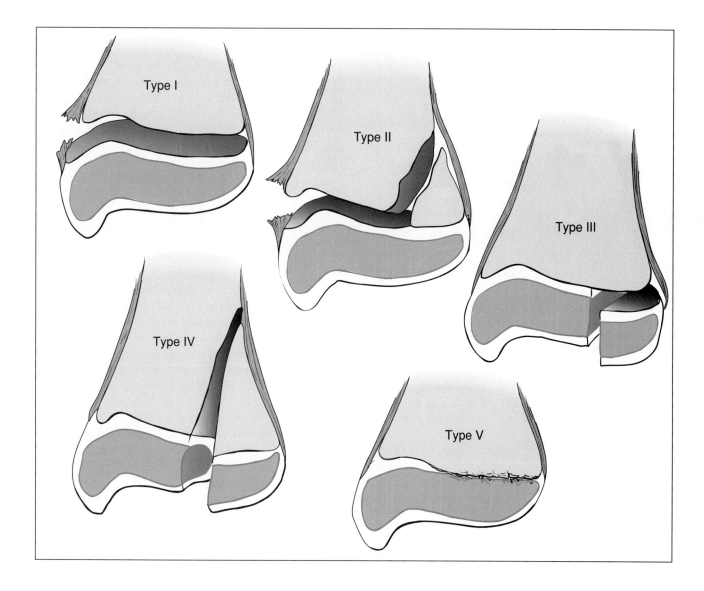

Radiographs should be reviewed for fracture type, growth plate involvement, and degree of bone angulation. Injuries that are splinted based on clinical suspicion of a fracture (negative radiographs) should be re-examined with follow-up films in 5 to 10 days.

Orthopaedic consultation should be sought immediately for any extremity fracture with evidence of neurovascular compromise (Chapter 109), including extreme pain at rest, pain with passive movement, pallor, paralysis, or paresthesias. Consultation also is required for open fractures, elbow and femur fractures, fractures angulated greater than 30°, or fractures involving the growth plate (Salter III to V). If follow-up fracture care is uncertain, orthopaedics should be consulted for definitive treatment.

Beyond fracture care, splints are sometimes used in children to immobilize areas where wound healing may be impaired by motion. This includes areas with extensive sutures, sutures over joint areas, burns, or infected and/or dirty wounds.

EQUIPMENT

Although preformed splints are available, many do not fit children. This section lists essential pediatric splint materials. Splints can be formed with either plaster or fiberglass material. Fiberglass is stronger, more durable, lightweight, and easier to apply. Prefabricated splint roll is commercially available and incorporates padding, plaster or fiberglass, and cotton stocking into one unit

Figure 104.2.
Salter-Harris classification for fractures in growth plate region.

for ease of application. Padded aluminum splints also are available in a variety of sizes for children.

Cotton stocking material (stockinette)
Elastic (Ace®) bandage*
Soft cotton roll (Webril®)
Commercial splint roll*
Plaster roll or sheets, or fiberglass roll
Prefabricated splint*
*Optional

PROCEDURES

General Splint Principles

Most splints incorporate four layers (Fig. 104.3). A stockinette is placed against the skin to provide protection. This is optional, but is often used for comfort. Webril® is placed around the stockinette to provide padding, especially at bony prominences. Plaster or fiberglass is placed over the Webril® to maintain the position of immobilization. An Ace® bandage or stockinette is rolled around the plaster or fiberglass to secure the splint to the limb and protect the firm layer. The Ace® bandage or stockinette can be used as a measuring tape to gauge the length of splint needed.

Steps to general application of a splint are:

1. Cut dry plaster or fiberglass and stockinette to fit area to be splinted. Try to use the opposite, unaffected extremity to measure these materials. Dimensions are provided for each splint. Areas where the splint will bend around joints can have notches cut laterally to minimize folding of the plaster or fiberglass.
2. Slide stockinette on extremity.
3. Roll webril around stockinette.
4. Position the child's extremity for optimal plaster or fiberglass application.
5. Wet plaster or fiberglass material and apply. Avoid using overly warm water because the splint will release further heat as it hardens on the child's extremity.
6. Perform initial splint shaping at large joints.
7. Overwrap plaster or fiberglass with Ace wrap or cotton roll.
8. Shape splint contours to final form.
9. Maintain splint positioning of joint until plaster or fiberglass has completely hardened.

Splinting in children requires both adequate preparation and patience. Three elements for successful application of a pediatric splint are positioning, molding, and adequate hardening. Always ensure that the child is properly positioned for the splint and has sufficient support or restraint to maintain that position. After the splint is molded for proper joint positioning, have an assistant or parent hold that position until the splint has fully hardened. It is best to advise the parent or assistant to hold the splint in position until 15 minutes is counted on a time clock.

Pediatric splints involve some general pitfalls. To make an effective splint, the clinician must use appropriate size and shape splint materials, adequately pad all bony prominences, and avoid bunching of the Ace bandage at joint sites. The clinician should not wrap the splint too tightly around the limb or allow plaster to fully encircle injury site. When premeasuring dry plaster sheets, the clinician needs to allow an extra 1 inch for shrinkage. Because hardening plaster releases heat, wet the plaster with cool to tepid water, and beware of excessive heat retention if elastic bandage overwrap is used (6). Splints for young children should have an extra overwrap layer applied for protection. Without an added wrapping layer, a splint will end up removed by the curious toddler!

All patients with splints should receive discharge instructions, with the following points: (a) the patient should elevate the injured limb and apply ice to injury often for

Figure 104.3.
Basic splint assembly. Sugar tong splint.
A. Measure and prepare all required materials. Position child as indicated for the splint.
B. Apply stockinette, then overwrap with webril.
C. Moisten plaster or fiberglass, apply as indicated providing initial shaping.
D. Overwrap with Ace wrap or stockinette and provide final shaping. Parent must hold child 15 minutes for splint to harden.

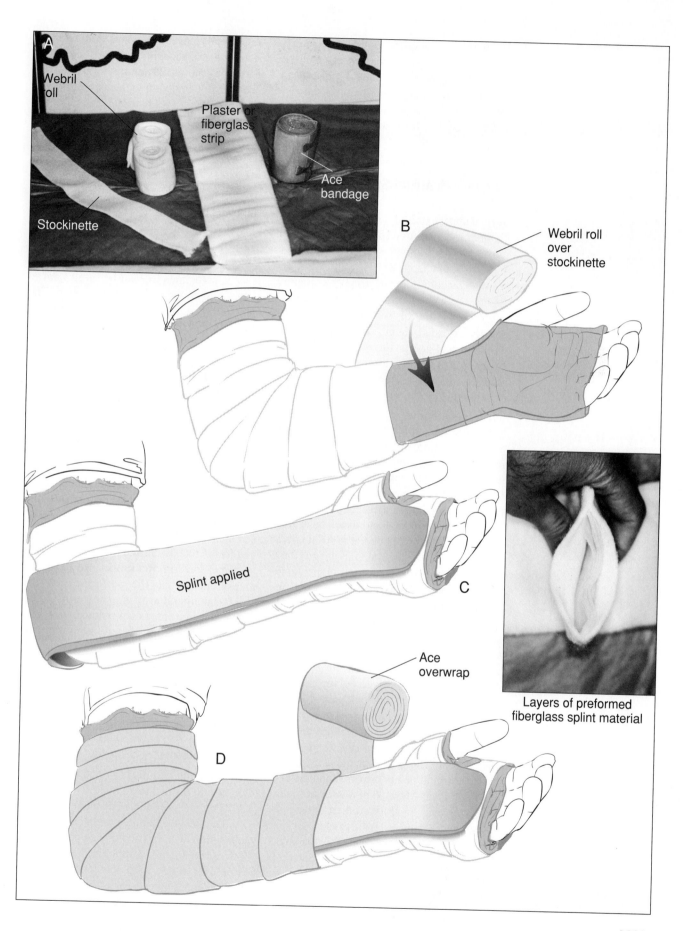

A
Webril roll
Stockinette
Plaster or fiberglass strip
Ace bandage

B
Webril roll over stockinette

Splint applied

C

D
Ace overwrap

Layers of preformed fiberglass splint material

36 hours, (b) the splint should be kept dry, (c) guidelines for pain management should be provided, (d) the patient must be instructed to return immediately for pain or sensory changes distal to the splint, or for pain underneath the splint, (e) orthopaedic follow-up should be provided.

Upper Extremity Splints

Several upper extremity splints can be used in children. A sugar tong splint can be used for most pediatric upper extremity fractures. When in doubt about which splint to use, apply a sugar tong. For most upper extremity splints, the wrist and hand are placed in the neutral position of function, with wrist slightly extended, thumb abducted, metacarpophalangeal joints flexed, and interphalangeal joints slightly flexed, as if grasping a softball.

Sugar Tong Splint
The sugar tong splint has a broad range of uses. Applied proximally, it can be used for stable humerus fractures. It is most frequently used distally for stable forearm and wrist fractures, and provides the most effective immobilization of these areas. A double sugar tong—both a proximal and distal sugar tong splint combination applied at a 90° angle at the elbow—can be used to immobilize elbow injuries. Note that a sugar tong splint should not be used for displaced fractures that require reduction.

A distal sugar tong splint is demonstrated in Figure 104.3. The *width* of the distal splint should slightly overlap the radial and ulnar edges of the arm. The *length* should extend from the dorsal aspect of the knuckles, around the elbow, to the volar palmar flexion crease. Position the child on his or her stomach with the injured arm at the edge, the forearm hanging down toward the floor (elbow flexed 90°). The parent or assistant should hold the arm at points proximal and distal to the splint area. After the plaster or fiberglass and overwrap layer is applied, shape the splint and keep the elbow flexed at 90° and the wrist in neutral position. Provide three-point fixation at the fracture site, as shown in Figure 104.3. This position should be held until the splint has dried completely.

The width of the proximal sugar tong should fully cover the dorsal and volar aspects of the upper arm. Its length should extend from the axilla medially, around the elbow, and laterally up to the acromioclavicular joint. Remember that the splint measurements can be performed on the child's uninjured arm. A proximal splint is most easily applied with the child positioned on the back and the arm resting on the chest, flexed 90° at the elbow. Shape the splint to follow the contours of the arm held at 90° of flexion at the elbow, and internally rotated at the shoulder.

Provide extra padding at bony prominences for comfort before applying the plaster or fiberglass layer. A second outer wrap layer is recommended, but be careful not to overly tighten the splint with this wrap. The splinted arm must be placed in a sling to support the sugar tong at the elbow.

Radial and Ulnar Gutter Splints
Gutter splints are indicated for metacarpal and/or proximal phalangeal fractures. An ulnar gutter splint immobilizes the plane of the fourth and fifth digits. A radial gutter splint immobilizes the plane of the second and third digits, with a hole cut for the thumb to pass through the splint.

The application of a gutter splint is shown in Figure 104.4. Dimensions of the splint should be: *width* to wrap to the midline of the hand on the dorsal and volar surfaces, and *length* to extend from the nail base to the proximal forearm. Remember that the splint measurements can be performed on the child's uninjured arm. As shown in Figure 104.4, position the patient with the forearm vertically erect. This is easily accomplished by seating a child in a parent's lap and having the parent hold the extremity at the elbow and by the uninjured fingers. After the plaster or fiberglass and overwrap layer is applied, shape the splint as follows: wrist in neutral position, metacarpophalangeal joints in 70° flexion, and proximal interphalangeal joints in 20 to 30° flexion. Have the parent hold this position until the splint has dried completely. It is best to instruct them to hold the position for 15 minutes as counted on a clock.

To make the gutter splint more comfortable, a thin layer of padding can be placed in between the fingers to minimize irritation. An extra layer of overwrap is recommended for children under 4 years (or active children) to keep the splint dry and protected. Using a sling is optional to keep the injury elevated, but is not feasible for infants and toddlers.

Thumb Spica Splint

A thumb spica splint is essentially a gutter splint adapted for the thumb. It is indicated for nondisplaced fractures of the first metacarpal bone and proximal phalanx of the thumb, and for fracture of the scaphoid bone.

The thumb spica is shown in Figure 104.5. Dimensions of the splint are the same as for the gutter splints, as is the position in which the child is held. Remember that the splint measurements can be performed on the child's uninjured arm. After the plaster or fiberglass and overwrap layer is applied, shape the splint as follows: wrist in neutral position, and thumb abducted and in slight flexion at the metacarpophalangeal and interphalangeal joints ("wine glass" position of the thumb). Have the parent hold this position until the splint has dried completely, approximately 15 minutes.

Colles' Splint

A Colles' splint provides volar support and can be used for distal forearm and wrist fractures as an alternative to the distal sugar tong splint. The sugar tong is more often used in young children because it provides dorsal and volar stability. As seen in Figure 104.6, the Colles' splint covers the following dimensions: *width* to fully cover the volar aspect of the forearm, and *length* to extend from the proximal fingers to the proximal forearm along the volar side of the forearm. Remember that the splint measurements can be performed on the child's uninjured arm. Posi-

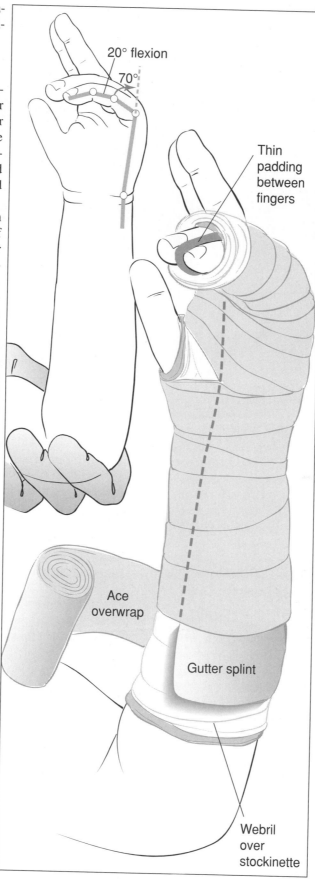

20° flexion

70°

Thin padding between fingers

Ace overwrap

Gutter splint

Webril over stockinette

Figure 104.4.
Ulnar gutter splint. For radial gutter splint, apply to opposite (radial) side with hole cut for thumb to pass through.

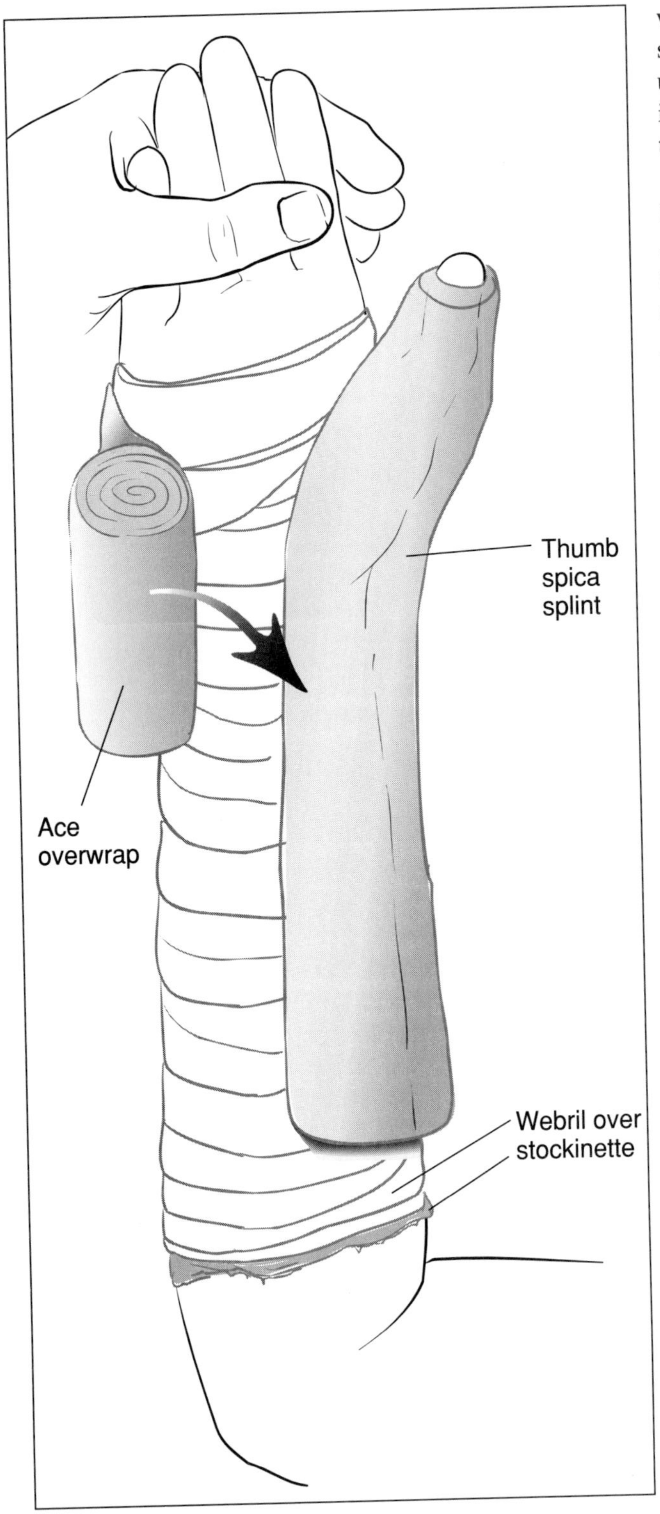
Thumb
spica
splint
Ace
overwrap
Webril over
stockinette

Figure 104.5.
Thumb spica splint.

tion the child lying on his or her side, with the dorsal side of the affected forearm against the stretcher, and held at the elbow and fingers as tolerated. After the plaster or fiberglass and overwrap layer is applied, shape the splint with the wrist in neutral position, and digits slightly flexed at all joints. Hold this position until the splint has dried completely. A sling is optional, but is not feasible for infants and toddlers.

Long Arm Splint

A long arm splint is used for stable injuries in the elbow area. Note that a double sugar tong splint also can be used for stable elbow injuries (see Sugar Tong Splint). It is imperative to obtain orthopaedic consultation for any supracondylar fracture, or injuries that may involve joint compromise.

The long arm splint is shown in Figure 104.7. Dimensions are *width* to cover one-half of the arm circumference, and *length* to extend from the dorsal aspect of the mid-upper arm, over the olecranon, and down the ulnar aspect of the forearm to the distal palmar flexion crease. Remember that the splint measurements can be performed on the child's uninjured arm. Position the child on the stomach with the injured arm at the edge, the forearm hanging down toward the floor (elbow flexed 90°). After the plaster or fiberglass and overwrap layer is applied, shape the splint with the elbow flexed 90° and the forearm in neutral position (Fig. 104.5). The parent or assistant should hold this position until the splint has dried completely, or time 15 minutes on the clock.

To ensure comfort, provide extra padding to bony prominences before applying plaster or fiberglass layer. Many casting materials cannot maintain the right angle shape of the long arm splint, so a sling must be worn to support the splint.

Digit Splints

Dynamic splinting is provided for interphalangeal joint sprains of fingers and/or for phalangeal toe fractures. For this splint method, place cotton padding between the injured digit and an adjacent uninjured digit. Securely tape the two digits together. Change the tape every few days for up to 3 weeks.

Padded metal finger splints are commercially available. These are indicated for mid-

Figure 104.6.
Colles' splint.
Not recommended for young children.

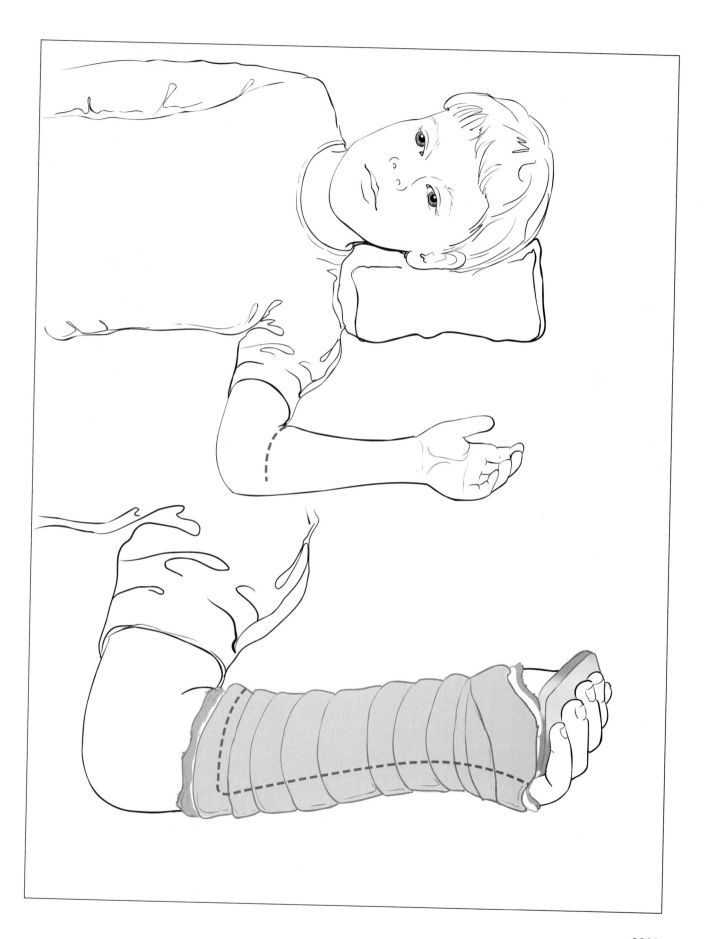

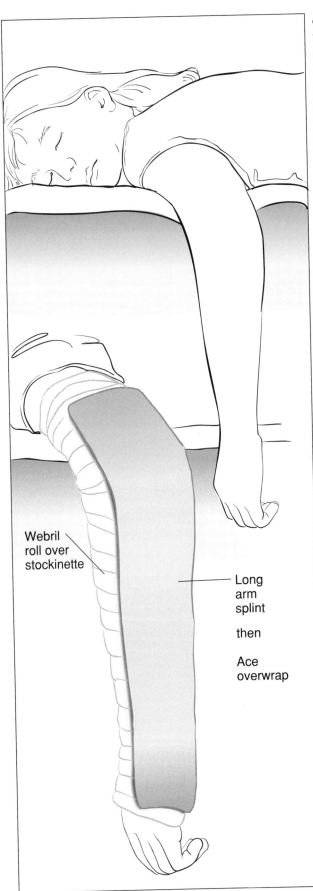

Figure 104.7.
Long arm splint.

Webril
roll over
stockinette

Long
arm
splint

then

Ace
overwrap

dle and distal phalangeal fractures of the hand. Several types of splints are available (Fig. 104.8). The splint should be shaped to hold the metacarpophalangeal joint flexed 50°, and the interphalangeal joint flexed 15 to 20°. Always provide extra tape so that a finger splint can be changed. For younger children, protect the finger splint by overwrapping with gauze roll.

Lower Extremity Splints

Knee Immobilizer—Long Leg Splint

Commercially made knee immobilizers are frequently used for soft tissue and/or ligament injuries of the knee. The long leg splint provides more extensive knee immobilization and can be used for fractures of the distal femur and proximal tibia and/or fibula. Sizing for younger children is often a problem with commercial knee immobilizers, and instead the long leg splint can be adapted for the knee.

Dimensions of the long leg splint are *width* to cover at least one-half of the leg diameter, and *length* to extend posteriorly from below the buttock to the heel of the foot. For knee immobilization only, the splint length should extend posteriorly from the midthigh to 3 inches above the malleoli. Position the patient prone—across a parent's lap or on an examination table—to apply the splint. After the plaster or fiberglass and overwrap layer is applied, shape the splint as follows: for fractures, place the knee in slight flexion and the ankle in neutral position; for knee injuries, place the knee in full extension. Maintain the required position until the splint has dried completely.

For comfort, provide extra padding at bony prominences before applying the plaster or fiberglass layer. Crutches are recommended for ease of ambulation, but should not be given to children under 6 years old. Unfortunately, children under 6 years must be transported by wheelchair or carried by a parent if they are unable to ambulate with the long leg splint or knee immobilizer. Careful patient and parent education is advised when crutches are provided to young children over 6 years; without proper guidance, they are often misused and therefore unsafe.

Posterior (Short Leg) Splint

A posterior leg splint provides support for injuries of the distal tibia and/or fibula, the ankle, and the foot. The stirrup splint (see next section) is often combined with a posterior splint to stabilize ankle injuries.

An assembled posterior splint (with stirrup) is shown in Figure 104.9. The splint *width* should cover at least one-half of the leg circumference. The *length* should extend posteriorly from the level of the fibular neck, over the heel of the foot, to the base of the digits. Remember that the splint measurements can be performed on the child's uninjured leg. To apply the splint, position the child prone on a stretcher or a parent's lap. After the plaster or fiberglass and overwrap layer is applied, shape the splint with the foot in neutral position at 90° to the leg. This position can be held by an assistant, or the child can be repositioned in a chair with the foot flat on the floor until the splint has dried completely.

For comfort, provide extra padding at bony prominences before applying the plaster or fiberglass layer. Avoid placing pressure at the region of the fibular neck to prevent compression of the peroneal nerve. A second outer wrap layer is recommended for young children to protect the splint. Be careful to not tighten the splint when applying this second overwrap. Crutches are recommended for ease of ambulation, but should not be given to children under 6 years old. Unfortunately, children under 6 years must be transported by wheelchair or carried by a parent after the splint is applied. Careful patient and parent education is advised when crutches are provided to young children over 6 years; without proper guidance, they are often misused and therefore unsafe.

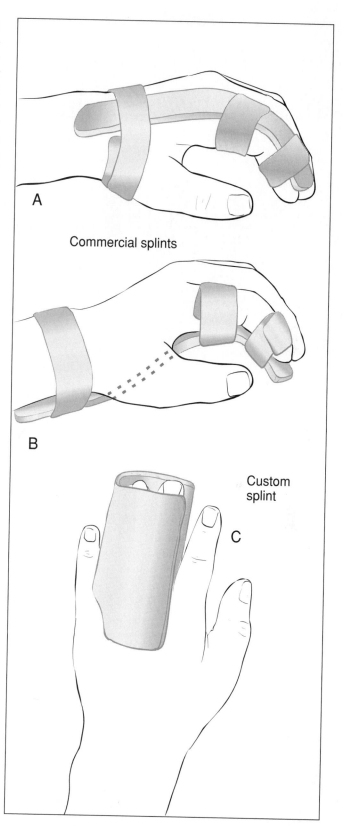

Figure 104.8.
Finger splints.
A, B. Commercial splints are available.
C. A custom splint.

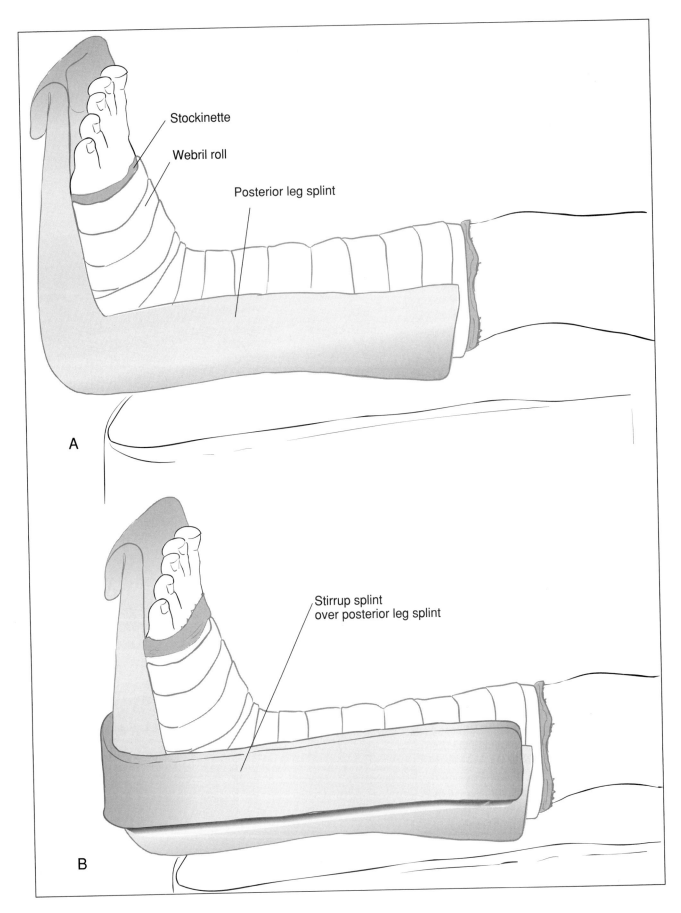

Stockinette

Webril roll

Posterior leg splint

A

Stirrup splint
over posterior leg splint

B

	Splint	Fracture Indications	Comments
Upper Extremity Splints	Colles'*	Distal forearm Wrist	Alternative to sugar tong. Not for young children.
	Digits*	Phalanx	
	Long arm	Elbow	MUST USE SLING
	Gutter	Metacarpal and/or proximal phalanx	RADIAL for 2nd/3rd digits ULNAR for 4th/5th digits
	Sugar tong	Humerus = proximal Forearm and wrist = distal	Useful for most upper extremity fractures. MUST USE SLING
	Thumb spica	1st metacarpal Proximal phalanx Scaphoid	
Lower Extremity Splints	Long leg	Distal femur Proximal tibia/fibula	CRUTCHES FOR CHILDREN OVER 6 YEARS
	Posterior (short leg)	Distal tibia/fibula Ankle Foot	CRUTCHES FOR CHILDREN OVER 6 YEARS
	Stirrup	Ankle (including soft tissue injuries)	Allows for weight bearing. Fits in a shoe.

*Prefabricated splints are commercially available

This type of splint has an important weakness. The area at the heel, where the splint bends at 90° can be broken by forceful dorsiflexion or plantar flexion of the foot and/or ankle. Parents and older children should be warned of this possiblity and older children should be encouraged to use crutches. In younger children this problem may be avoided by using fiberglass material, which is stronger or by combining the posterior splint with a stirrup or sugar tong splint.

Stirrup Splint (Sugar Tong)

Stirrup splints provide lateral support for ankle fractures or soft tissue injuries. Commercially made stirrup splints are available to provide dynamic splinting of the ankle, but cannot be used to manage fractures. As noted, stirrup splints often are used in addition to posterior splints to stabilize ankle fractures.

As seen in Fig. 104.9, the stirrup splint covers the following areas: *width* to cover at least one-half of the leg circumference, and *length* to extend mediolaterally from just below the fibular head, around the heel, and

ending just below the medial aspect of the knee. Position the patient as described for a posterior splint.

Stirrup splints conveniently fit in a loose shoe and allow for weight bearing to be initiated. Fiberglass material is recommended for this splint given that it may endure weight bearing. Crutches should be provided if full weight-bearing is contraindicated. These features benefit older children, but can be risky for the young. For children under 6 years, a stirrup splint is recommended only in combination with a posterior splint; crutches cannot be used.

COMPLICATIONS

Splints that are properly used are rarely associated with complications. Two well-established sequelae can be avoided through careful splint practices. Swelling commonly occurs around fracture areas. To avoid compromise of neurovascular structures, never fully encircle the injury, do not overwrap the splint tightly, and ensure that aftercare instructions include limb elevation. Prolonged immobilization often causes limb stiffness. Follow-up care for further injury manage-

CLINICAL TIPS

1. If in doubt as to whether a fracture is present in a child, place a splint until a follow-up radiograph is obtained.
2. Measure splint materials carefully using the child's opposite, unaffected limb.
3. Plan ahead! Proper positioning of the patient, molding of the plaster or fiberglass, and adequate drying time for hardening of the plaster or fiberglass are key for a functional and durable splint.
4. Always provide the patient and/or parents with discharge instructions and plans for follow-up care.

Figure 104.9.
A. Posterior leg splint.
B. A stirrup applied for added lateral stability.

ment is vital to ensure proper timing of splint and/or cast removal.

SUMMARY

Splints are essential for treating acute fractures and sprains not requiring immediate surgical intervention, and can offer definitive treatment for certain injuries. A knowledge of proper splint use and techniques of application is important for many medical personnel in the ambulatory setting. After a splint is applied, detailed discharge instructions and follow-up arrangements are vital to the success of treatment.

REFERENCES

1. Shaw D. Principles and techniques of splint musculo-cutaneous injuries. Emerg Med Clin North Am 1984; 2(2): 391–407.
2. Simon R. Emergency orthopaedics. 2nd ed. Norwalk CT: Appleton & Lange, 1987.
3. Chung S. Handbook of pediatric orthopaedics. New York: Van Nostrand Rheinhold Co., 1986.
4. Hodge D. Injury management principles. In: Barkin R, eds. Pediatric emergency medicine. St. Louis: Mosby, 1992.
5. Howes D. Plaster splints: techniques and indications. Ann Family Practice 1984; 30(3), 215–221.
6. Kaplan S. Burns following application of plaster splint dressings. J Bone Joint Surg 1981; 63A: 670–672.

CHAPTER 105

SHORT ARM AND SHORT LEG CASTS

David T. Bachman

INTRODUCTION

The use of emergency casting as a treatment for orthopaedic injuries can be traced to Antonius Mathysen, a Dutch military surgeon, who in 1851 used dressings impregnated with dehydrated gypsum in the management of fractures (1). Today, casting, whether with plaster or synthetic materials, remains the most common method of immobilizing and stabilizing fractures so that healing can occur. In most instances, casting is the definitive treatment. It must be remembered, however, that even the best applied cast is no substitute for a proper reduction. Applying a short arm or short leg cast is well within the scope of practice of pediatricians and emergency physicians. The only prerequisite is a solid understanding of acute orthopaedic injuries in the pediatric age group, such as provided in other textbooks (1, 2). With proper training and supervision, personnel working in the ambulatory setting including physician assistants, nurse practitioners, registered nurses, and technicians can apply simple casts. Notably, a properly applied splint (Chapter 104) can provide immobilization comparable to that afforded by a cast. Indeed, in the acute setting splinting is generally the treatment of choice, especially in the hands of those whose experience with casting is limited.

ANATOMY AND PHYSIOLOGY

Distinct differences exist between children and adults in the nature of skeletal injuries that occur and the management of those injuries. Most differences reflect the fact that unlike the bones of an adult (i.e., anyone who has reached skeletal maturity), those of a child are growing. The periosteum of the bones of a child is physiologically quite active. As a result, the potential for healing and, in many instances, for significant remodeling, is high. Nonunion essentially never occurs. Conversely, fractures in children frequently involve the growth plate, posing a risk to ongoing bone growth should management be improper. Many of those growth plate injuries result from mechanisms of injury that in adults would cause a ligamentous injury. For example, a severe valgus injury to the knee will result in a fracture through the distal femoral physis in a child rather than in a strain of the medical collateral ligament as would be the case in an adult. Overall, then, with any extremity injury in a child, the clinician must be highly suspicious of the possibility of a fracture.

Clearly, the most common indication for applying a cast is for the treatment of a fracture. In all instances, it must first be determined that the position of the fracture is satisfactory. Despite the potential for fracture remodeling in children, it is hardly safe to assume that remodeling can correct all deformities. Bowing and rotational deformities in particular have limited potential for remodeling.

Instances also occur in which clinical findings suggest a fracture but radiographic studies are negative. When this occurs, it is recommended that the involved extremity be immobilized until a definitive diagnosis can be established. Splinting is generally adequate in this setting, although in some cases, such as a suspected toddler's fracture in a young child, a cast will prove advantageous. Similarly, it may be preferable to cast rather than to splint certain soft tissue injuries, for example severe ankle sprains.

INDICATIONS

Specific settings in which it is appropriate for a nonorthopaedist to consider applying a short arm and short leg cast are outlined in this section. Once again, proper splinting will provide equally satisfactory treatment on a temporary basis for the injuries listed. The decision to cast rather than to splint should be made only after the nature of any accompanying soft tissue injuries (e.g., abrasions that require dressing changes) and the potential for ongoing swelling are considered. Certain fractures merit urgent orthopaedic consultation including complete fractures of the radius, ulna, and tibia, and fractures with significant displacement or growth plate involvement. Open and pathologic fractures by definition also require prompt referral. Even when the nonorthopaedist does choose to provide the initial treatment and apply a cast, he or she should always consider referral to an orthopaedic specialist for follow-up care.

The following are indications for a short arm cast:

1. torus fractures of the radius and ulna;
2. nondisplaced Salter-Harris type I fractures of the distal radius (may be clinical rather than radiographic diagnosis);
3. clinically suspected scaphoid (navicular) fractures (thumb spica) (discuss with hand specialist first if overt fracture); and

4. nondisplaced, stable metacarpal fractures.

The following are indications for a short leg cast:

1. minor fibula fractures (including suspected Salter-Harris type I of distal fibula);
2. toddler's fractures;
3. severe ankle sprains;
4. stable fractures of metatarsals; and
5. fractures of mid and hind foot.

EQUIPMENT

Stockinette—2, 3, and 4" widths
Cast padding—2, 3, and 4" widths
Plaster or fiberglass rolls—2, 3, 4, and 6" widths
Plaster strips (splints)—3 x 15", 4 x 15", and 5 x 30" sizes
Felt padding
Bucket
Gloves, gowns, shoe covers, drapes (towels)
Cast knife
Cast bender
Cast saw
Cast spreader
Cast shoes (canvas overboots)

For the most part, successful application of a cast depends more on proper technique than on the specific brand of materials used. Certain types of cast padding are easier to work with than others, but all are satisfactory. The biggest decision for the clinician is whether to use plaster or synthetic (fiberglass) casting material. Of the two, plaster is the least expensive, has the longest shelf life, and is the easiest to apply. Conversely, fiberglass is lighter, provides superior strength, dries and cures more rapidly, resists water much better, and is unlikely to cause thermal burns. The material chosen generally reflects availability and clinician experience and preference.

PROCEDURE

Certain steps must first be taken in applying all casts (1, 3–8). Before applying any cast, it is important to assemble all the necessary materials. To run short of casting material midway through the procedure is problematic indeed. The amount and width of stockinette, cast padding, and casting material needed will obviously reflect the size of the patient. Next, the patient should be prepared for the procedure. Proper positioning is important. Help of an assistant is often necessary, especially with younger children. With adequate explanation and reassurance—and if a parent is allowed to remain—most children will cooperate fully. Draping is also essential, both to protect patient clothing and modesty. The clinician, too, should take steps to protect his or her clothing. Gowns and shoe covers are recommended. Gloves are essential when working with fiberglass, as anyone who has worked with that material bare-handed can attest.

Before the actual cast is applied, the skin of the involved extremity should be washed with soap and water and thoroughly dried. All superficial wounds should be carefully cleansed and then covered with a thin, sterile dressing. If the wounds are more than minor, the clinician must consider initial splinting rather than casting until satisfactory wound healing has begun. Once cleansed, the extremity should be placed in the position in which it is to be cast. This positioning must be maintained throughout the duration of the procedure if ridging of the casting materials and pressure points are to be avoided. Next, stockinette can be applied (Fig. 105.1.A). Its use, although favored by many, is not an essential step. It does allow for smoother trimming at the ends of the cast. When used, it can be applied as one continuous piece overlying the whole portion of the extremity to be cast or as two segments at the upper and lower ends of the cast only (7). When it is applied in two segments, stretching and tension over bony prominences are avoided. If it is applied as a single piece, care should be taken to cut off any folds or wrinkles that result.

The cast padding is the next layer to be applied. The padding should be rolled on to the extremity from distally to proximally, each turn overlapping the previous one by half (Fig. 105.1.B, C). Overpadding is to be avoided, as it will result in a loose cast. Extra padding should be applied over bony prominences such as the ulnar styloid, the malleoli, and the heel. Small pieces of felt can be used if needed. Smooth application of the cast padding is essential; wrinkles should be cut or torn away.

If plaster is to be used, all the rolls needed to cast the extremity in question should then be set on end in water deep enough to cover them completely. Using cold or perhaps lukewarm water is recommended; the drying time when hot water is used is too fast to permit successful application. The end of the roll will be easier to find if it is folded back before immersion. Once the air bubbles cease, the rolls should be removed, then squeezed but not wrung to remove water. The more water removed, the faster the drying time. By pinching the end together somewhat, inconvenient telescoping of the roll during application will be prevented.

Beginning distally, the plaster rolls should be applied in the same direction as the padding, overlapping again by 50% (Fig. 105.1.D). The rolls must be held close to the extremity, using the thenar eminence to push the roll around the limb under moderate tension. The free hand should be used to take pleats as needed to guide the roll and to accommodate the changing diameter of the limb. When one roll is finished, the next should begin at the same point. Two turns should not be taken at the same point other than at the upper and lower ends of the cast. After 1 to 2 rolls of plaster have been applied, and when the plaster is the consistency of wet cardboard, smoothing and shaping should begin using the flat of the hand and the thenar eminence (Fig. 105.1.E)(1). Additional rolls can then be applied until a cast of uniform thickness (0.25") has been achieved. No more than 6 to 7 layers of plaster are generally needed. The cast should not be any thicker at the fracture site than elsewhere. Rubbing and smoothing should continue so as to guarantee that all layers of the cast fuse together into one strong unit. Notably, too much rubbing too late in the drying phase will cause the plaster to crumble. At all times during the smoothing, extreme care must be taken to avoid any focal indentations or pressure points. Before applying the final roll of plaster, the ends of the stockinette should be folded over and then covered with cast material so as to provide smooth ends for the cast (Fig. 105.1.F, G). Alternatively, the ends of the stockinette can be folded over and held in place using single, shorter strips of cast material.

When using fiberglass casting materials,

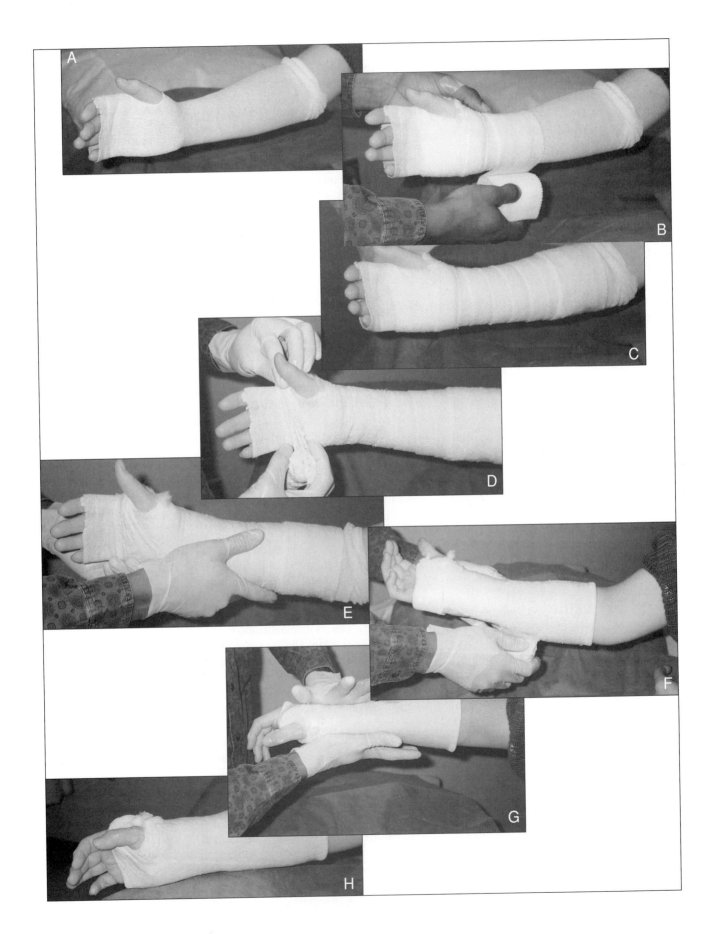

Summary

Short Arm Cast

1. Assemble materials (2 rolls plaster generally adequate, 2 to 3" size child, 4" adult; with fiberglass, use narrower rolls)
2. Position patient and extremity: supine, should be abducted 90°, elbow flexed 90°
3. Apply stockinette (optional): thumbhole necessary, avoid wrinkles (Fig. 105.1.A)
4. Apply cast padding: wrap from proximal palmar crease to about 1" below flexion crease of elbow. Make transverse tear in padding before wrapping around thumb webspace. Apply additional padding over ulnar styloid (Fig. 105.1.B, C)
5. Apply cast material rolls: roll from distal to proximal. Twist 180° when wrapping through thumb webspace. Before second roll, fold over ends of stockinette. Total of four to six layers of plaster, three of fiberglass, sufficient. Do not begin too distally. Allow for 90° flexion at metacarpal-phalangeal joints, for fanning of fingers, and for opposition of thumb to index and little fingers (Fig. 105.1.D, F)
6. Smooth and shape: begin rubbing when plaster consistency of wet cardboard. Mold to shape of forearm using palms and thenar eminence, not digits. Shape should be cylindrical, not round (Fig. 105.1.G)
7. Maintain immobilization during drying. Reassess for pressure points, pain relief, neurovascular compromise. Trim ends of cast as needed to allow for adequate finger and thumb motion (Fig. 105.1.H).
8. For thumb spica, use same approach except need to include thumb in extension in cast. Cut 2" cast padding to 1" size for use around thumb itself (Fig. 105.2)

Short Leg Cast

1. Assemble materials (3 rolls plaster generally adequate, 3 to 4" size child, 6" adult; with fiberglass, use narrower rolls)
2. Position patient and extremity—alternatives: (*a*) patient sitting, knee flexed to 90°, (*b*) patient supine, hip and knee flexed to 90°, assistant supporting leg, (*c*) patient prone, knee flexed to 90°
3. Apply stockinette (optional): if single piece, cut away transverse fold in front of ankle—better to apply two short segments at proximal and distal ends of cast (Fig. 105.3.A, B)
4. Apply cast padding: wrap from level of distal metatarsals to one fingerbreadth below tibial tubercle; apply additional padding over malleoli and heel
5. Apply cast material rolls: roll from distal to proximal. Total of five to seven layers of plaster, three of fiberglass, sufficient. If larger child weight bearing intended, will need to add reinforcing splints when using plaster. Can incorporate two plaster splints posteriorly, folding back last 1 to 2" at level of distal metatarsals (Fig 105.3.C). Alternatively, fold 4" plaster splints in half longitudinally, placing one posteriorly and in a stirrup (U-shape from medial to lateral). Do not begin too distally
6. Smooth and shape: begin rubbing when plaster consistency of wet cardboard. Mold to shape of lower leg using palms and thenar eminence, not digits (Fig. 105.3.D). Allow for flexion, fanning of all the toes (Fig. 105.3.E)
7. Maintain immobilization during drying. Reassess for pressure points, pain relief, neurovascular compromise. Fit for cast boot, crutches as needed. No weight bearing for minimum of 24 hours.

essentially the same considerations apply with a few exceptions. First, cold water must always be used to wet the rolls. Secondly, as it is not possible to make tucks as readily as with plaster, it is recommended that rolls of narrower width be used (i.e., 2" fiberglass rolls are generally adequate given its superior strength).

Once the cast is complete, positioning of the extremity must be maintained until adequate hardening occurs (Fig. 105.1.H). Any movement during this time—when the inter-

Figure 105.1.
Applying a short arm cast.
A. Maintain casting position and apply stockinette.
B, C. Apply cast padding on to the extremity distally to proximally, overlapping each turn.
D. Beginning distally, apply plaster rolls.
E. Smooth plaster and
F, G. fold over ends of stockinette to provide smooth ends for the cast.
H. Maintain positioning of the extremity until cast is hardened.

Figure 105.2.
Thumb spica cast.
Use the same approach as
short arm cast, except
need to include thumb in
an extension of the cast.
Cut 2″ cast padding to 1″
size for use around thumb
itself.

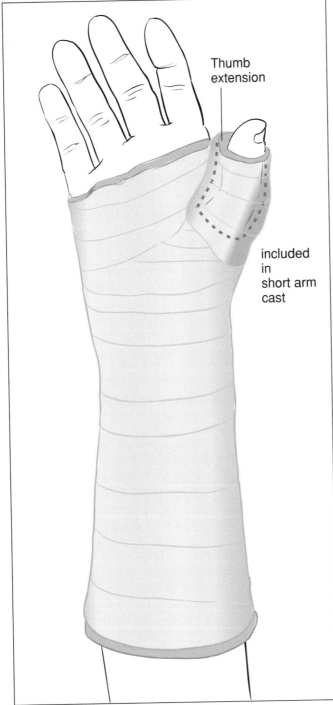

Thumb
extension

included
in
short arm
cast

locking of the plaster crystals is occurring—causes considerable loss of strength. (It takes 48 hours for a plaster cast to cure completely.) Once the cast hardens, the patient should be reexamined and questioned about pain relief, pressure points, and circulatory compromise. Written instructions regarding cast care and signs of complications should be provided and reviewed. A return for a formal cast check at 12 to 24 hours is suggested. Prescriptions for appropriate analgesics should be written and follow-up appointments planned.

COMPLICATIONS

Essentially all complications that can occur after the application of a cast can be prevented by careful adherence to technique. One complication—fracture displacement—occurs either when a cast is applied too loosely or improperly molded or when the wrong type of cast altogether is chosen. For complete midshaft fractures of the radius and ulna to displace in a short arm cast would hardly be surprising; a well-applied long arm cast is needed for such fractures, assuming initial alignment was satisfactory.

Another complication—pressure sores and skin necrosis—also can be prevented if adequate padding is provided and care is taken to avoid creating pressure points during the molding and smoothing steps. Once again, a cast that is too loose can prove problematic by allowing excessive movement between the cast and the underlying skin (5). Clinicians must remember that patients often first complain of burning pain or discomfort as a pressure sore develops. A window should be cut in the cast—or the cast removed and replaced—when such complaints arise.

A third complication, that of a thermal burn as the plaster sets, is completely avoid-

Figure 105.3.
Short leg cast.
A. Apply stockinette in either continuous piece or
B. Two short segments at proximal and distal ends of cast.
C. Apply cast material rolls.
D. Smooth and shape plaster.
E. Allow for flexion and fanning of all the toes.

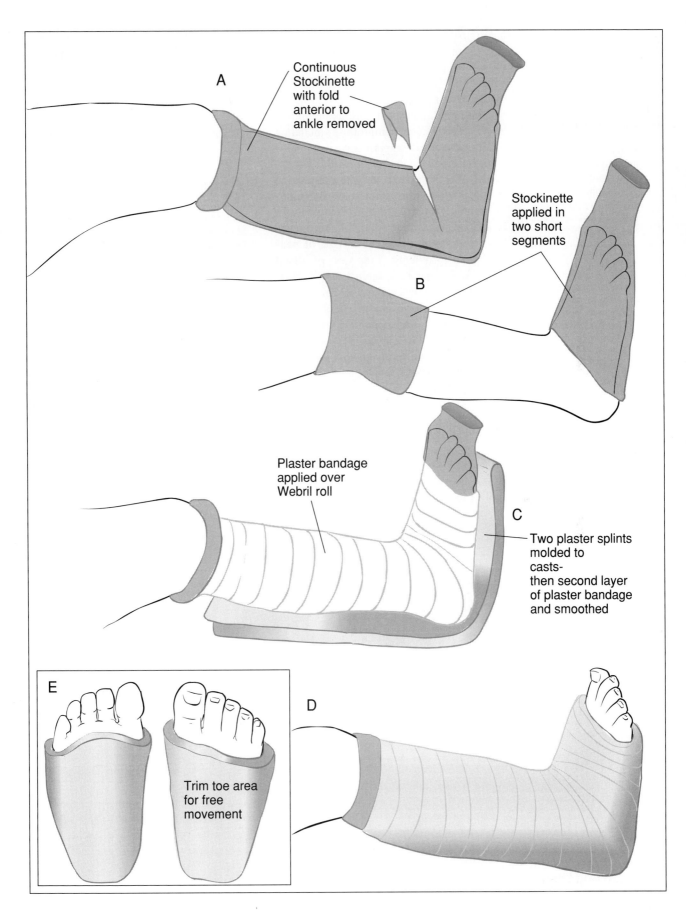

A — Continuous Stockinette with fold anterior to ankle removed

B — Stockinette applied in two short segments

C — Plaster bandage applied over Webril roll

Two plaster splints molded to casts- then second layer of plaster bandage and smoothed

D

E — Trim toe area for free movement

able if cold water is used and overly thick casts (more than 8 layers) are not applied. Care should be taken not to cover the cast with a pillow or other insulating material during the drying phase.

The final, and most serious complication—neurovascular compromise, including a fully developed compartment syndrome—is likewise preventable. As previously mentioned, a splint, which better allows for tissue swelling, is generally preferable to a cast in the setting of an acute fracture. Should a cast be applied, it is wise to split it *and* the underlying padding at the earliest signs of neurovascular problems. Presence of distal pulses is no guarantee against the development of compartment syndrome. Pain, particularly pain with the passive stretching of muscle, is the earliest sign of compartment syndrome and should never be ignored. Immediate orthopaedic consultation should be sought with the least suspicion of this complication (Chapter 109).

SUMMARY

Armed with an understanding of the principles of both pediatric orthopaedics and cast application, the pediatrician or emergency department physician should be able to provide the initial, if not definitive, casting for a number of simple fractures of the lower arm and leg. Complications can occur, but are avoidable if proper technique is followed and early symptoms and signs are not ignored.

REFERENCES

1. Rang M. Children's fractures. 2nd ed. Philadelphia: JB Lippincott Co., 1983, pp. 30–36.
2. Bachman DT, Santora SD. Orthopaedic Trauma. In: Fleisher GR, Ludwig S, eds. Textbook of pediatric emergency medicine. 3rd ed. Baltimore: Williams & Wilkins, 1992, pp. 1236–1287.
3. Browner BD, Jupiter JB, Levine AM, Trafton PG, eds. Skeletal trauma. Philadelphia: WB Saunders Co., 1992, pp. 222–225.
4. Iversen LD, Clawson DK. Manual of acute orthopaedic therapeutics. 3rd ed. Boston: Little, Brown, & Co., 1987, pp. 66–83.
5. Lewis RC. Handbook of traction, casting, and splinting techniques. Philadelphia: JB Lippincott Co., 1977, pp. 56–81.
6. Mercier LR. Practical orthopedics. 3rd ed. St. Louis: CV Mosby, 1991, pp. 15–22.
7. Rockwood CA, Green DP, Bucholz RW, eds. Rockwood and Green's fractures in adults. 3rd ed. Philadelphia: JB Lippincott Co., 1991, pp. 30–56.
8. Wr KK. Techniques in surgical casting and splinting. Philadelphia: Lea & Febiger, 1987, pp. 1–129.

HAND AND FINGER INJURIES

Robert Eberlein

INTRODUCTION

Fingertip and hand injuries occur frequently in children and may have significant functional or cosmetic morbidity associated with them. These injuries can occur in any mobile child and although they can usually be treated in an outpatient setting, they can be painful and are almost always frightening to the child.

This chapter discusses the outpatient management of common injuries to the hand and fingertips, including subungual hematomas, subungual foreign bodies, nailbed lacerations and avulsions, the mallet finger deformity, and boxer's fractures.

ANATOMY AND PHYSIOLOGY

The nailbed itself is a thin layer of epithelial tissue overlying the cortex of the distal phalanx (Fig. 106.1). The germinal matrix is the portion of tissue proximally which is responsible for most of the nail formation (1), and the lunula marks its distal end. This is the paler area seen to extend just beyond the eponychium, the fold of skin that covers the proximal nail. The sterile matrix is the more distal tissue of the nailbed and is responsible for a small amount of nail growth. The nail is tightly adherent to the sterile matrix but loosely held to the germinal matrix. The lateral margins of the nail are held in place by the lateral skin folds. The extensor tendon inserts onto the epiphysis of the distal phalanx whereas the flexor profundus tendon attaches distal to the epiphyseal plate. Blood supply to the fingertip is from the many branches of the two digital arteries. The pad of the fingertip is composed of fatty and soft tissues in which a multitude of exquisitely sensitive nerve endings exist.

Basic Examination of the Digits

Before initiation of therapy for a significant finger injury, it is important to perform and to document a careful examination of the involved finger (Fig. 106.2). This examination should focus on evaluation of motor function, sensory function, and vascular structures.

Motor function of the fingers should be assessed by testing both muscular strength and tendon function. In the cooperative child, these should be tested by asking the child to place his or her hand on the examination table with the palm up. The clinician then places two fingers on the involved finger just proximal to the distal interphalangeal (DIP) joint, holding the finger firmly against the table (Fig. 106.2.A). The patient is asked to bend the tip of the finger. If function is normal then the maneuver can be repeated against resistance. This tests both muscular strength and the function of the flexor digitorum profundus tendon. Next the child's noninjured fingers are held against the examination table and the child is again asked to bend his or her finger first without resistance and then against resistance (Fig. 106.2.B). This

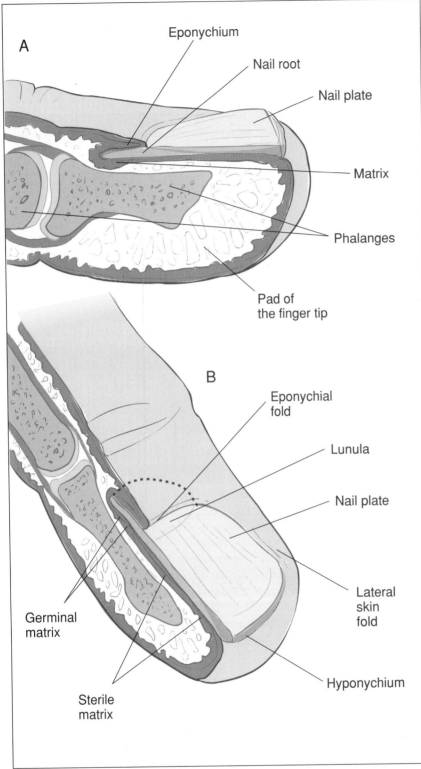

Figure 106.1.
Anatomy of the finger and nail bed.

manuever tests both proximal muscular strength and the function of the flexor digitorum superficialis tendon.

Pain associated with these maneuvers in the presence of a laceration on the palmar or lateral portion of the finger may indicate a tendon injury. In younger children who are less likely to cooperate, the mere act of holding the child's hand against the examination table may cause the child to flex the appropriate fingers. It may, however, be impossible to know whether associated pain is present so lacerations of the palmar side of young children's fingers should be thoroughly explored. Extensor tendon injury is less serious but should be identified. Cooperative children can be asked to close and open their hand or to curl and uncurl the affected finger. As suggested, exploration of finger lacerations is vital in young children.

Sensory function also is vitally important. Fingers that have normal motor function but impaired sensation may significantly limit the overall function of the individual digit and may affect the function of the hand itself. In older children, two-point discrimination can be tested using a paper clip opened and bent into a caliper with the points spread apart at least 10 mm (Fig. 106.2.C). The paper clip points are placed against the skin along the long axis of the finger and the child is asked to close his or her eyes and then to say whether he or she was touched by one or two points. The touch should be relatively light so as to minimize the stimulation of pressure receptors. The points of the paper clip are gradually brought closer together and the test is repeated until the child reports feeling only one point. Most normal children will sense two distinct points until the arms of the caliper are less than 6 mm apart. Because the finger has excellent invervation it is important to check sensation on both the medial and lateral sides and along the dorsal and palmar sides. In cooperative younger children it may only be possible to test gross sensation by simply asking the child whether he or she feels the touch of a finger. Once again, sensation should be checked in all areas of the finger. Finally, in young children, clinicians may have no good way to acertain the presence or absence of nerve injury. Some objective evidence can be obtained by placing the finger in a bowl of warm water for a few minutes. Injured fingers with areas of skin that have an interrupted nerve supply will not wrinkle.

Vascular supply to the fingers should be checked by testing capillary refill of the fingertip. Unless injury to the nail has occurred, refill is best tested by applying pressure to the tip of the finger until the skin beneath the nail is seen to blanch. Pressure is released and the time that it takes for pink color to return to the nail is noted. Normal capillary refilling time is less than 2 seconds.

SUBUNGUAL HEMATOMAS

A subungual hematoma (SUH) is an acute, painful collection of blood between the fingernail and the nailbed itself. It arises when the highly vascular nailbed is transiently crushed and the resultant extravasation of blood collects between the nail and the nailbed, creating a blue-black discoloration beneath the nail. The nail and its margins remain intact. As the hematoma enlarges, the pressure beneath the nail increases, compressing the highly sensitive nerve fibers within the fingertip. The result is a painful fingertip. Blunt trauma directed against the fingertip (or occasionally the toe) is the typical mechanism for developing an SUH. These can occur in any child capable of inducing such mechanisms (catching the fingertip in a closing door, striking it with a hammer, dropping a weight on it, etc.). This condition is best treated by timely decompression. Nail trephination affords rapid and complete relief and is easily accomplished in an office or emergency setting.

In cases of SUH with disruption of the nail or its margins, the nail itself should be removed and the nailbed explored for lacerations requiring repair (2). An underlying distal phalanx fracture may be present but hematoma size bears no direct correlation to the presence or absence of a fracture beneath (3). Any injury suspicious for fracture should be radiographically evaluated because these would require splinting and a displaced fracture of the distal phalanx can significantly disrupt the nail bed (see Nailbed Injury and

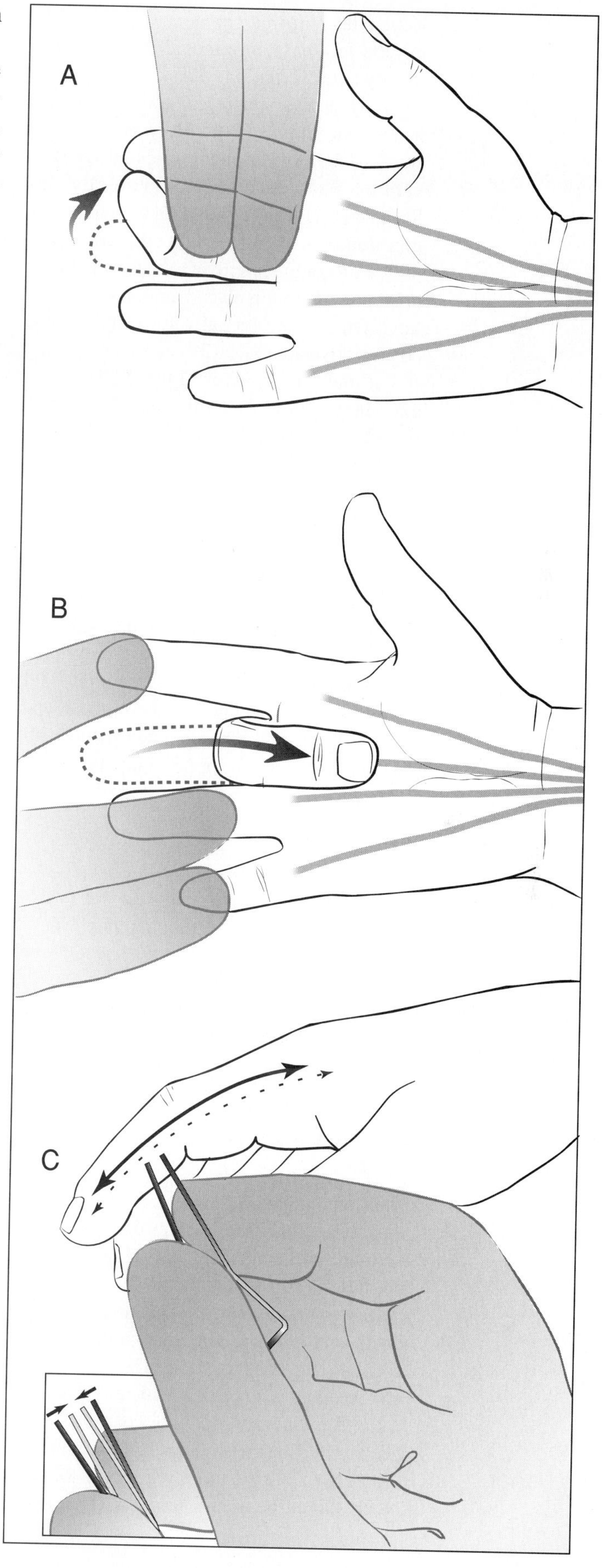

Figure 106.2.
Basic examination of the digits.

Repair later in this chapter). Traditionally, experts felt that nail removal was necessary for any large SUH (25 to 50% or larger) to adequately assess and repair any underlying nailbed lacerations (4–6). However, a recent study of otherwise uncomplicated SUH of various sizes demonstrated virtually any SUH can be adequately treated with trephination alone (3). No subsequent cosmetic deformities or complications existed even in the presence of nondisplaced underlying fractures. Other authorities also support this more conservative approach (2).

It must be emphasized that SUH can be extremely painful. Narcotics may be ineffective (2) and the child is likely to be frightened by the visual aspects of the wound. This fear is likely to increase the child's apparent distress. Relief of pain occurs rapidly once the hematoma is drained and this should be performed as expeditiously as possible. The blood usually remains liquid for 24 to 36 hours (7) or longer; therefore, drainage will still afford pain relief even if presentation is delayed somewhat. Beyond 48 hours it is felt that trephination will not release liquid blood. Radiographs should be obtained if the clinician has any concern for bony involvement.

Equipment

Syringe with 27-gauge needle
Bupivacaine (0.25%) without epinephrine
Antiseptic prep solution
Restraints (as needed)
Electrocautery device or, alternatively, a paper clip, butane lighter, and hemostats
Protective dressing

Procedure

Nail trephination involves creating a hole in the nail over the hematoma, allowing drainage of the blood beneath (Fig. 106.3). If the hole is too small, blood can clot in the hole preventing complete drainage and adequate pain relief. A hole 3 or 4 mm is usually adequate and one large hole is better than several small ones, each of which may clot (2).

After age-appropriate restraints have been used (Chapter 1), anesthesia can be provided by a digital block (Chapter 4). This block should be used for any anxious child,

any child with underlying fractures whose pain will persist, and children who will be drained with the paper clip method. Many children, however, complain the pain associated with digital block is worse than the brief, if any, pain associated with electrocautery trephination (8). For most children on whom the electrocautery device will be used, no anesthesia is necessary (9).

Gently clean the overlying nail with antiseptic solution. If alcohol is used it must be allowed to dry as it can ignite when heated. The electrocautery device is held perpendicular to the nail over the SUH, heated, and then gentle downward pressure is used to create the hole. Blood will rapidly exit through the hole and the remainder may be extruded by gentle pressure on the nailbed. A high speed nail drill also is available and is used in a similar fashion to trephinate the nail.

Alternatively, a paper clip held by hemostats may be heated with a butane lighter and used to create the drainage hole using gentle downward pressure perpendicular to the nail. If performed well, the heated clip rapidly penetrates the nail and cools as it hits the underlying blood with minimal discomfort to the patient. If several attempts are needed to penetrate the nail the resultant pressure on the nailbed can increase the child's discomfort unless the digit is adequately anesthetized.

After drainage a protective dressing can be applied and the patient instructed to soak the digit in warm water 3 times daily for 2 days, redressing after each soak. Any underlying fracture will require splinting for at least 14 days and may require evaluation by a hand specialist.

Complications

Complications of nail trephination are rare. Some authorities believe trephination converts an underlying fracture to a potentially more serious open fracture (10) and they routinely prescribe 48 hours of antibiotics. In a recent study, however, no infectious complications were noted in patients trephinated with underlying fractures and in whom antibiotics were withheld (3). Many authorities feel antibiotics are unnecessary unless the child is immunocompromised or the vascular supply to the area is marginal (7). The parents and child should be warned that the discoloration beneath the nail often persists, that blood may continue to ooze for a day or two, and that the nail may fall off. If so, the nail will take 3 to 4 months to grow in again (7). Carbon deposits may persist at the site of trephination but are benign (2).

Summary

Subungual hematomas are common minor injuries typically treated in an outpatient setting by emergency physicians, pediatricians, or family practitioners. They can be painful and nail trephination provides immediate relief.

SUBUNGUAL FOREIGN BODIES

Subungual foreign bodies may occur in the fingers or toes of any mobile child. Removal of the foreign body offers relief from pain, minimizes risk of infection, and can be performed in most outpatient settings.

Subungual foreign bodies are typically wedged between the nail and the nailbed although penetration of either can occur. Mixed bacteria accompany the foreign body beneath the nail and can cause infection. This is especially true of wooden foreign bodies. When a wooden foreign body is allowed to remain beneath the nail resultant infection is virtually guaranteed.

Because the nailbed is so pain sensitive, rapid removal of subungual foreign bodies relieves some pain although the irritated tissues will generally have some persistent discomfort even after removing the offending agent. Timely removal primarily limits the risk of infection. Radiographs should be obtained in any injury suspicious for bony involvement or to document the presence of a radiopaque foreign body. Telephone consultation with a hand surgeon is advised for foreign bodies that are already clearly infected, foreign bodies that cannot be removed, or if concern exists for bony involvement and possible subsequent osteomyelitis due to deep nailbed penetration.

Figure 106.3.
Nail trephination.

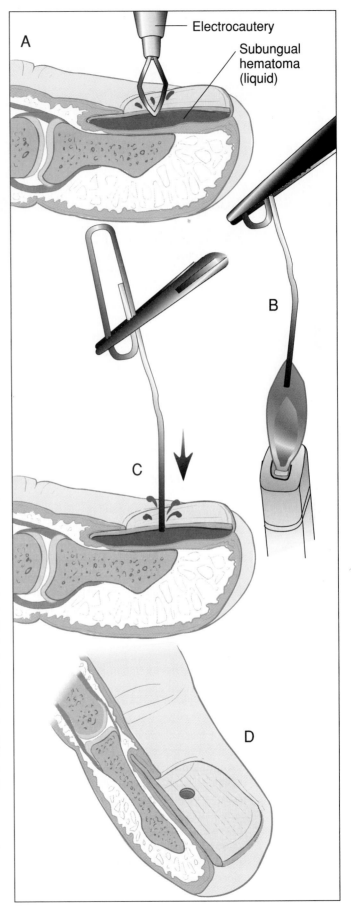

Equipment

Syringe with 27-gauge needle
Bupivacaine (0.25%) without epinephrine
Restraints as needed
Hemostats or forceps
Scissors
No. 11 scalpel
Sterile protective dressing

Procedure

Age-appropriate restraints (Chapter 3) should be instituted before removing the foreign body in any anxious child or for those who will need local anesthesia. Fingers can be immobilized by taping the involved digit and its neighbor to a small pediatric arm board. The technique for removing the foreign body depends on the position of the foreign body beneath the nail (Fig. 106.4).

If the foreign body protrudes beyond the end of the nail it may be grasped with a hemostat or a small pair of forceps and gently removed. A small protruding stump of foreign body can be pinned against the nail using a scissor tip, needle, or scalpel blade and gently drawn forward until it is out from beneath the nail.

Distal foreign bodies that cannot be grasped can be removed by several other methods. A 25- to 27-gauge needle can be bent at its tip to a 90° angle using a hemostat, then rotated slightly to snag the object and then gently withdraw it (11). Alternatively, a No. 11 blade can be held horizontally, perpendicular to the nail and scraped proximally to distally across the nail overlying the foreign body. This procedure will shave down the nail until the foreign body is exposed and can be grasped and removed (9). Most children can tolerate these methods without anesthesia.

Deeper or firmly embedded foreign bodies and any procedures resulting in nailbed manipulation will require a digital block (Chapter 37). After adequate anesthesia, the nail may be lifted on either side of the foreign body using the sharp point of a pair of scissors to separate the nail from the nailbed. The scissor is held so that the point is angled slightly dorsally and the point is run along the undersurface of the nail to avoid damaging the nailbed. Two or three tracts parallel to the long axis of the finger should release enough of the nail from the nailbed to allow the foreign body to be grasped with forceps and removed (9). For objects that cannot be removed by release of the fingernail as previously described, a V-shaped wedge may be cut out of the elevated nail overlying the foreign body to allow access for removal (7).

Heavily contaminated or large wooden foreign bodies that have fragmented are best dealt with by removing the entire nail. This procedure always requires a digital block, which allows full access to the site for any necessary debridement and cleaning. Debridement of the nailbed tissue itself should be kept to a minimum (see Nailbed Injury and Repair). A thorough cleaning and irrigation with several hundred milliliters of sterile saline using a large syringe and an 18-gauge plastic catheter minimizes residual bacteria and foreign body particles. The entire nail can be removed using the technique just mentioned, extending scissor tracts to the proximal and lateral limits of the nail. The dorsal eponychial fold must similarly be released from the proximal nail and the lateral skin folds freed from the nail. The scissor tracts must be kept parallel to the long axis of the finger. Once the foreign debris has been removed and the finger irrigated and gently scrubbed, the nail should be replaced. A hole should be placed into the nail in the center with either an electrocautery device, scissor tip, or similar device and the nail should be slid back beneath the eponychial fold to maintain this space. Two 5.0 nylon sutures should be placed through the nail at its mid-lateral positions and through the lateral skin folds to hold it in place. These sutures should be removed in 3 weeks. The new nail will grow from proximal to distal and will take 3 to 4 months to regenerate.

A sterile, nonadherent dressing with antibiotic ointment beneath will serve to protect the underlying tissue, promote healing, and prevent infection. This dressing may be removed in 12 to 24 hours and the finger soaked in warm water 2 to 3 times daily, redressing after each soak. Antibiotics are unnecessary unless the wound is already infected, the foreign body was heavily contaminated, or deep penetration of the nailbed with possible bony inoculation has occurred. In such cases, a 5- to 7-day course of appropriate antibiotics (e.g., cephalexin) should be prescribed.

Complications

Complications are rare and are mainly infectious. Retained wooden foreign bodies are likely to cause infection but can be minimized by ensuring that the entire foreign body has been removed. Wood, which has been soaked with blood or water, splits and fragments easily and small pieces may remain after the main portion has been withdrawn. Removal of the overlying nail with direct visual inspection is the surest means of limiting this problem.

Because the nailbed and the underlying bone are in close proximity, foreign bodies which deeply penetrate the nailbed itself can inoculate the distal phalynx and cause subsequent osteomyelitis (7). Thorough cleansing and irrigation of the wound site after nail removal and 5 days of an appropriate antibiotic are recommended. The child and the parents also should be warned to return immediately for increasing pain, tenderness, redness, swelling, or fever over the next several weeks.

Summary

Subungual foreign bodies are painful and carry a significant risk for infection, especially if wooden. Prompt removal minimizes the risk of infection and helps to alleviate the associated discomfort.

NAILBED INJURY AND REPAIR

Significant trauma to the fingertip often results in avulsion of the fingernail and laceration of the underlying nailbed. Appropriate repair of these wounds at the time of injury yields the best results (Fig. 106.5).

Normal nail growth following a nailbed laceration requires the presence of a smooth nailbed. Irregular nailbeds heal with scar formation, as do nailbeds with avulsed tissue

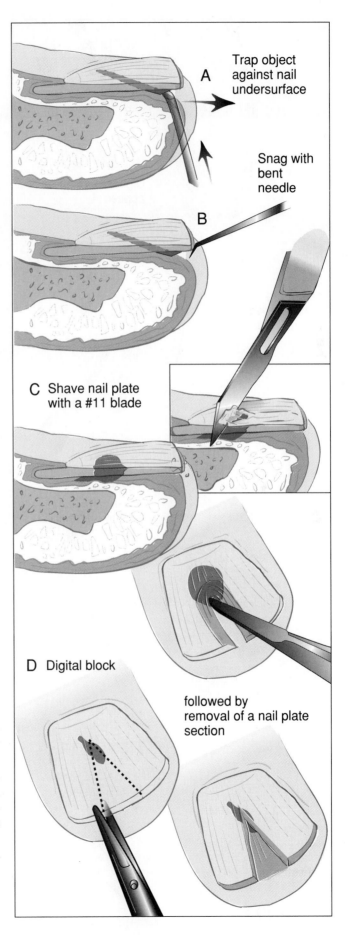

Figure 106.4.
Removing subungual foreign bodies.

A Trap object against nail undersurface

Snag with bent needle

B

C Shave nail plate with a #11 blade

D Digital block

followed by removal of a nail plate section

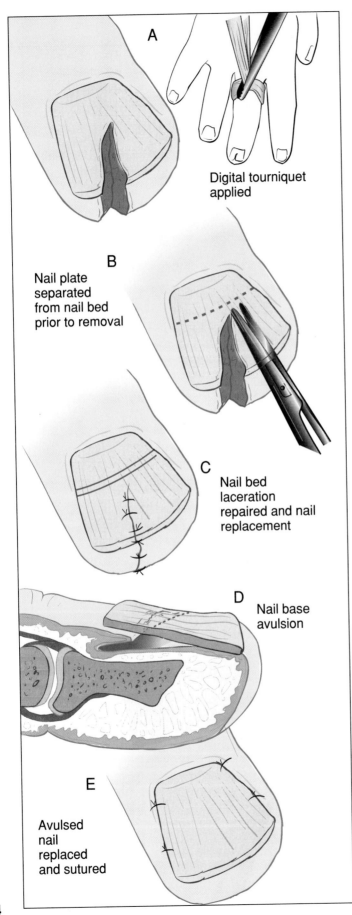

A
Digital tourniquet applied

B
Nail plate separated from nail bed prior to removal

C
Nail bed laceration repaired and nail replacement

D
Nail base avulsion

E
Avulsed nail replaced and sutured

which are allowed to heal by secondary intention. Scar tissue will not produce new nail tissue or bind to the new nail (1, 12, 13) perhaps resulting in an abnormally formed or split fingernail, or in a nail that fails to adhere to the underlying nailbed Likewise, the eponychial and lateral skin folds must remain open to prevent scarring between the skin folds and the underlying nailbed. This scarring makes it difficult for the new fingernail to grow. In most cases the new fingernail either forces its way through the scar tissue, resulting in a painful, inflamed fingertip or splits at the point where the skin is adherent to the nailbed, resulting in a split fingernail (1).

It is important to remember that many injuries to the fingertip do not require extensive exploration or repair. For example, uncomplicated subungual hematomas are usually associated with small nailbed lacerations but these are best treated with nail trephination alone (see Subungual Hematomas earlier in this chapter). However, in cases of nail disruption, partial nail avulsion, or skin margin laceration, the nail must be removed completely for adequate examination and repair (6, 12).

The clinician should remember a few basic principles when dealing with nailbed injuries. Final outcome often depends on the initial care of the wound. Meticulous repair of the nailbed will minimize problems of scar formation with subsequent splitting or nonadherence of the fingernail. Minimal debridement of the fingernail or the nailbed should be attempted as the nailbed tissue heals well when sutured back into place and even small scars due to absent tissue can result in bothersome splitting or nonadherence of the nail. Every attempt should be made to replace avulsed nailbed tissue.

Significant fingertip injuries should be evaluated radiographically for evidence of underlying fractures. Any displacement must be corrected and if the fracture is unstable a hand surgeon should be consulted. Stability of all underlying fractures must be ensured to prevent recurrent damage to the nailbed caused by the movement of unstable bone

Figure 106.5.
Repairing the nailbed injury.

fragments. This may require Kirschner wiring (4, 6). Finally, a thorough examination of the tendon function must be performed as tendon injuries can be overlooked when concentrating on the wound. Skin and nailbed lacerations may be of any form. Nail avulsions can occur distally if the nail tip itself is forced dorsally. Crushing forces to the nail from the dorsal surface can pull the less adherent proximal nail out from beneath the eponychium. Careful inspection of the avulsed nail may show fragments of nailbed adherent to the nail. The hand surgeon to whom the child is being referred may appreciate a call describing the nature of the wound even if his or her help is not immediately required.

Equipment

Syringe with 27-gauge needle
Bupivacaine (0.25%) without epinephrine
Restraints as needed
Antiseptic prep solution
Tourniquet
Suture set
Fine absorbable suture (6.0 or 7.0, preferably chromic)
Magnifying eyewear
No. 15 scalpel
Dressing and splint
Electrocautery device

Procedure

Initial care of any nailbed injury includes age-appropriate restraints, used as needed (Chapter 3), and adequate anesthesia for the digit, typically as a digital block (Chapter 37). If the child is unable to tolerate the procedure with local anesthesia alone then conscious sedation or general anesthesia will be required.

The fingernail should be removed to allow full access to the nailbed (Fig. 106.5.A, B). The nail is gently separated from the underlying adherent nailbed with the sharp end of a scissors tip. The tip should be held parallel to the finger, angled slightly dorsally, then inserted between the nail and nailbed and advanced slowly keeping the tip pressed against the nail to avoid damaging the nailbed. The scissor tip is moved proximally in several

tracts until the nail is freed from the underlying nailbed (Fig. 106.5.B). Then, similarly, the eponychial and lateral folds are freed from the nail by inserting the scissor tip between the skin folds and the fingernail itself. The fingernail may have some avulsed nailbed attached to it, which must be saved for reimplantation into its space in the nailbed. Once the nail is removed, the nailbed may be gently irrigated with several hundred milliliters of sterile saline using a large syringe and an 18-gauge plastic catheter.

A bloodless field is required and a digital tourniquet should be used for this purpose. Attempts at repair will be futile if the wounds are constantly oozing blood. After sterile preparation of the entire finger a sterile penrose drain may be wrapped snugly around the base of the finger, stretched slightly, and clamped with a hemostat (Fig. 106.5.A). Alternatively a sterile glove of the patient's size can be used. The rubber tip of the involved digit is cut off the glove and the glove is placed on the hand. The cut rubber finger is rolled back proximally until it reaches the hand, which will provide an even, compressive tourniquet to help maintain a bloodless field (12). A pneumatic tourniquet also can be used. The upper arm is wrapped with several layers of padding such as webril, the tourniquet is then applied and inflated above the systolic pressure. A blood pressure cuff may similarly be used but these devices are not designed for prolonged inflation and therefore tend to loose pressure during use. Regardless of the method chosen, tourniquet time and pressure should be minimized as much as possible. If the pneumatic cuff is used, the patient should be warned that the involved arm will become numb once inflated and will be uncomfortable when the tourniquet is released but that these sensations will resolve. The arm will become painful beneath the cuff after approximately 20 minutes which limits the actual amount of time for repair while the cuff is inflated. Actual repair of the lacerations is facilitated by using magnifying eyewear. Adequate repair will be difficult otherwise.

Nailbed lacerations may be linear or stellate but results will be excellent if both approximation and suturing of the nailbed tissues are precise (Fig. 106.5.C). All lacerations should be repaired with fine absorbable suture on side-cutting needles (7.0

chromic is preferred by most but vicryl or 6.0 sutures also are acceptable) (4, 6). More proximal lacerations may extend beneath the eponychium and if this is suspected the germinal matrix must be exposed. The eponychium is cut back several millimeters, perpendicular to its edges, at the point it curves distally. Retraction of this eponychial skin fold then allows adequate access to the proximal germinal matrix for inspection and repair (4, 6, 13). Once the germinal matrix is repaired, the eponychial cuts may be closed with 5.0 nylon suture.

Nailbed avulsions often occur proximally when the fingertip is crushed, pulling the less adherent proximal nail out from beneath the eponychium so that it rests above the skin (Fig. 106.5.D). These nails must be removed and the nailbed examined for lacerations or tissue avulsions (12). Complete or distal nail avulsions also must be fully examined.

Nailbed tissue may adhere to the nail that has avulsed. Small fragments are best left attached to the nail and replaced as a unit with the nail. The nail with the attached nailbed fragments should be replaced, supported with adhesive wound closure tape, and sutured into place to provide adequate immobilization (14) (Fig. 106.5.E). Larger fragments can be gently trimmed off the nail with a No. 15 scalpel blade and sutured back into place with fine absorbable suture (13). Large injuries with absent, destroyed, or hopelessly contaminated tissues will require nailbed grafting and therefore a hand surgeon should be consulted (4, 6, 13). Occasionally a nail avulsion will tear the germinal matrix proximally and pull it out from beneath the eponychium while remaining attached distally. These wounds also are best handled by a hand surgeon (6).

Lacerations to the lateral or eponychial skin folds should be repaired with 5.0 or 6.0 nylon using the usual skin techniques being careful to maintain the eponychial fold while approximating the skin edges precisely.

All nailbeds require splinting, which is best accomplished with the original nail itself. The nail should be gently cleaned and a hole placed into the center of the nail to allow for drainage. The nail is replaced into position beneath the eponychium and sutured in place through the lateral skin folds with two 5.0 nylon sutures (4, 6, 12, 13). Another method is to use a nail stitch. This is similar to the two-stitch method, but leaves the suture intact and is tied back across the nail. This also provides self-tamponading pressure. This provides protection for the sensitive nail bed, keeps the eponychial skin fold open and acts as a splint (7). If unable to use the original nail, a nonadherent splint of silastic, mesh gauze, or the sterile foil from a suture packet may be secured beneath the eponychial fold and left in place for 3 weeks (12, 13). A protective dressing and splint may be applied and should be left in place until follow-up visit in 24 hours.

Complications

Failure to provide a smooth, well-approximated nailbed may result in a split or nonadherent nail (1, 4, 6, 7, 12, 13). Scar tissue formation may also be followed by a sensitive nailbed and fingertip (13). Allowing the eponychial fold to scar also results in a split nail or pain as the nail tries to grow through the adhesion (12). Lateral fold scarring can result in ingrown nails (12). Fractures must be anatomically reduced to prevent disfigurement and recurrent nailbed injury due to bony motion (4, 6). Infection is rare and usually occurs only in wounds heavily contaminated with organic matter. Five days of an appropriate antibiotic would be warranted in such cases (6, 12).

Summary

Nailbed injuries often can be repaired with good results if meticulous tissue reapproximation is achieved. Care must be taken to reduce all associated fractures and to avoid eponychial or lateral skin fold scarring.

FINGERTIP AVULSIONS

Fingertip avulsions can usually be managed in an outpatient setting by primary care providers. All ages of children can be affected—their wounds typically arising from having their finger caught in a closing door, although slicers, mowers, etc. also contribute to these injuries.

In contrast to adults, distal amputations or partial avulsions heal extremely well in children, especially before adolescence. Reports have been given of children less than 2 years old regenerating entire distal tips after amputation when managed conservatively (15).

Wounds involving only distal soft tissue or wounds with a small amount of exposed bone should be managed conservatively whereas amputations at or proximal to the distal interphalangeal (DIP) joint should be microsurgically reimplanted as the child's future occupation and hobbies cannot be predicted (4). In contrast to adults, exposed bone need not be shortened unless extensive soft tissue loss has occurred or the child is over 12 years of age (4, 9). Teenagers should have these wounds cared for similar to adults with bone shortening and the creation of a skin flap to cover the bone. All injuries should be evaluated radiographically. Any finger that is contaminated or requires a flap or shortening procedure requires consultation by a hand surgeon.

Equipment

Syringe with 27-gauge needle
Bupivacaine (0.25%) without epinephrine
Suture set
Rongeurs to shorten bone (if necessary)
Nylon suture
Irrigation supplies
Dressings and splints
Digital tourniquet
Restraints as needed
Antibiotics

Procedure

For all distal amputations or partial avulsions digital block should be performed. The child should be restrained and sedated as necessary and a bloodless field obtained with a digital tourniquet (see Nailbed Injury and Repair).

Wounds involving avulsion of the distal skin and pulp are best managed conservatively with thorough irrigation, debridement of devitalized tissues, and nonadherent sterile dressings that are changed often. This applies to all children regardless of age (4, 7, 9).

Wounds involving exposed distal bone also should be managed conservatively in all children less than 12 years of age (4) but older adolescents should probably have the bone trimmed with Rongeurs and a skin flap created to cover the bone. The skin should be closed with 5.0 nylon suture, creating a shortened but closed digit (7).

Partial tip avulsions with an intact volar skin bridge will frequently survive as a composite graft in children less than 2 years of age (7, 13). These should be cleaned, irrigated, debrided, and the skin approximated with 5.0 nylon suture. In older children and adolescents these should be debrided away as the survival of these flaps falls rapidly with age. A delayed free graft can be applied several days later if necessary (4, 10), and a conservative approach is the best initial care (irrigation, debridement, dressings). Contaminated wounds in adolescents should not be closed primarily but rather also closed or grafted in a delayed fashion (10).

Antibiotics should be given for all exposed fractures of the distal phalynx. A first parenteral dose should be given at the time of initial care followed by a 5- to 7-day oral course (7). Cleanliness and serial dressing changes must be stressed to the parents and adequate follow-up with a hand surgeon ensured.

Complications

Complications are primarily due to infections. They can be limited by thorough debridement, irrigation, delayed closure or grafting if heavily contaminated, frequently changed sterile occlusive dressings, and appropriate use of antibiotics.

Summary

Despite the gruesome appearance of distal fingertip amputations, young children regenerate these tissues well and have much better results than adults when managed conservatively.

MALLET FINGER

The mallet finger deformity typically occurs when the extended finger is hit head on by another object (e.g., a baseball). Lacerations to the dorsal finger at the level of the DIP also can produce a similar deformity. When the extensor tendon separates from the remainder of the distal phalanx a mallet finger deformity arises. The profundus flexor tendon pulls the distal fragment volarly. The fingertip cannot be straightened as the extensor tendon is no longer attached to the distal phalanx. In younger children the epiphyseal plate will separate and the proximal epiphysis remains attached to the extensor tendon. In adolescents whose epiphyseal plate has fused, the tendon pulls off the distal phalanx with or without a portion of the dorsal lip of the distal phalanx itself. Hand surgeon involvement is necessary if the extensor tendon is lacerated near its distal insertion (7). Consultation is advised if a dorsal lip or epiphysis has avulsed off the proximal aspect of the distal phalanx as these injuries occasionally require open repair (9).

Equipment

Radiographs
Splinting materials
0.25% bupivacaine
Syringe with 27-gauge needle
Alcohol prep swab

Procedure

The closed mallet finger injury without fracture heals well with splinting (Fig. 106.6). A dorsal foam finger splint should be applied which holds the DIP fully extended and brings the extensor tendon and the distal phalynx into juxtaposition. Full flexion should be allowed at the PIP. This splint must be maintained for 6 to 8 weeks. If the DIP falls into flexion at any time the tenuous healing of tendon to bone may be lost and the healing process must begin anew. The splint may be carefully removed when wet or dirty but the parents and child must be warned to ensure constant extension at the DIP joint until the new splint is applied (7).

Mallet finger deformities associated with fractures or epiphyseal separations may need operative repair. A splint should be applied (as previously described) until the patient can be seen by the hand surgeon (9).

Mallet finger deformities due to tendon laceration need suture fixation of the tendon, which should be performed by a hand surgeon (7). The wound should be thoroughly cleansed and irrigated, the skin loosely closed with 5.0 nylon suture, and a splint applied. A 5-day course of oral antibiotics is appropriate.

All mallet fingers, once splinted, should be elevated and analgesics given for 48 hours. Delaying treatment or inadequate splinting of a mallet finger can lead to permanent disability. The fingertip will never fully extend and can effectively destroy the career of a budding musician or athlete.

Mallet finger deformities are easy to identify with a careful examination. Splinting in extension will yield good results but the patient must be warned to maintain extension at all times.

FRACTURES

Fractures of the fifth metacarpal head, or boxer's fractures, occur when the closed fist hits another solid object with the striking point centered over the fifth metacarpal head. The metacarpal neck fractures and the fragments often impact securely (4). Midshaft phalangeal fractures may be associated with displacement, angulation, or rotation. Angulation of up to 40 to 50° at the fifth metacarpal neck in a boxer's fracture is tolerated and heals well if no rotational deformity occurs and if the fragments are stable (4).

Midshaft phalanx fractures should be thoroughly evaluated for rotational deformity, angulation, or displacement and any abnormalities must be corrected. To assess for rotational deformity, have the child slowly make a fist. As the fingertips approach the palm they should all point toward the radial syloid. If the tip of the fractured finger points elsewhere then a rotational deformity is present in the fracture (Fig. 106.7). Referral to a hand surgeon is advised as these fractures may be unstable and can result in permanent disability if they do not heal accurately. Radiographs, both prereduction and postreduction, should be obtained in all suspected fractures.

After ensuring the lack of rotational deformity in a boxer's fracture, radiographs should be reviewed to assess the angulation

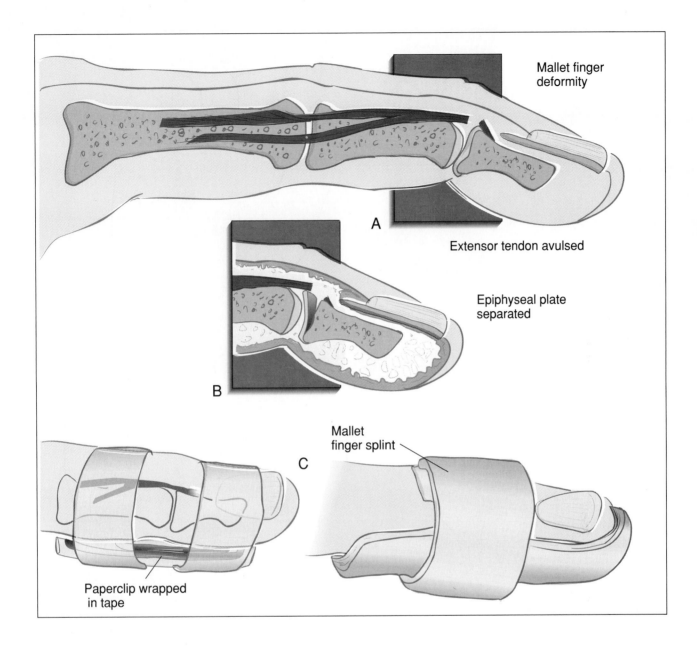

Mallet finger deformity

Extensor tendon avulsed

A

Epiphyseal plate separated

B

Mallet finger splint

C

Paperclip wrapped in tape

Figure 106.6.
Closed mallet finger injury repair.

of the fracture. No reduction is needed if the angulation is less than 50°. If over 50°, the metacarpal head must be reduced. After cleaning the skin with alcohol, inject a weight-appropriate volume of 0.25% bupivacaine into the soft tissue surrounding the fracture. Once the area is anesthetized, reduce the fracture using both hands. Place the thumbs on the dorsal surface of the fifth metacarpal, one over the head and one over the midshaft with the index fingers below to provide a sufficient grasp of the two fragments of bone. Using a slowly increasing force reduce the fracture by pushing the thumbs toward each other in a volarly directed fashion. This may be difficult or even impossible if the frag-

ments are tightly impacted. Place the child in an ulnar gutter splint (Fig. 104.4) and provide a sling for elevation with adequate analgesics for 48 hours.

Midshaft phalangeal fractures without rotation or displacement can be splinted using a dorsal foam splint, immobilizing the joints on either side of the fracture. Keep the wrist extended at 30°, the MP joints at 40° flexion, and IP joints at 15° flexion (4).

Proximal and middle phalanx fractures may be angulated and should be reduced if angulation is prominent. Use a digital block and reduction techniques as described. Always assess for rotation. Any fracture that cannot be reduced is rotated, and any fracture

**Chapter 106
Hand and Finger
Injuries**

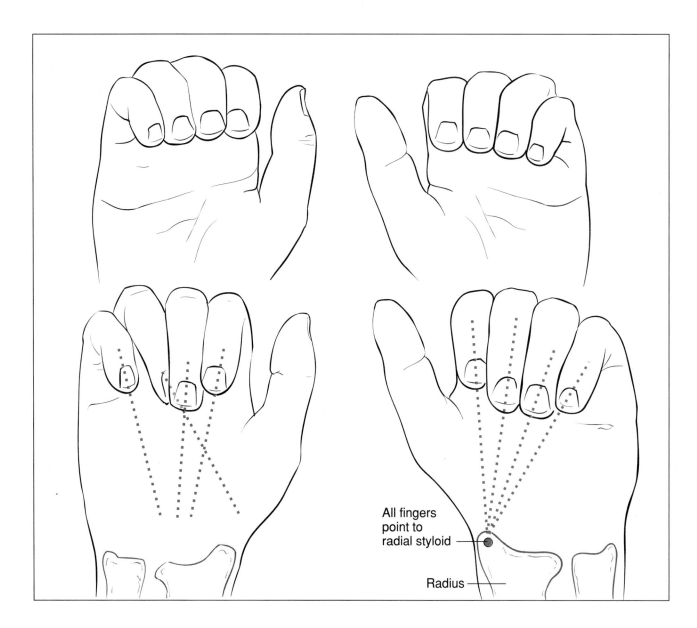

All fingers
point to
radial styloid

Radius —

Figure 106.7.
Upper row depicts normal
fingers. Lower row depicts
rotational deformities in
fingers of right hand.

that involves the joint should be splinted and referred to a hand surgeon.

Complications

Boxer's fractures are rarely disabling but rotational deformities can occur and can interfere with the power aspect of the child's grasp. Midshaft phalangeal fractures also can rotate or angulate and if untreated can interfere with functional use of the hand. This is especially true of proximal phalangeal fractures which may require open reduction or have contractures of the PIP (4). Splinting must always adequately immobilize the joints above and below the fracture to prevent mo-

tion at the fracture site with delayed healing or nonunion.

Summary

Most simple fractures of the fingers and hand can be managed in an outpatient setting but care must be taken to look for the mallet finger deformity. Be sure to fully assess for rotational or joint involvement as these will necessitate a hand surgeon.

REFERENCES

1. Zook E. Anatomy and physiology of the periony-
   chium. Hand Clinics 1990;6:1.

2. Roberts J. Evaluation and treatment of subungual hematoma. Emerg Med News 1993 Feb.;15:2.

3. Seaburg D, Angelos W, Paris P. Treatment of subungual hematomas with nail trephination: a prospective study. Am J Emerg Med 1991;9(3):209.

4. Tintinalli J, Krome R, Ruiz E. Emergency medicine—a comprehensive study guide. 3rd ed. New York: McGraw-Hill, 1992.

5. Simon R, Wolgin M. Subungual hematoma: association with occult laceration requiring repair. Am J Emerg Med 1987;5:302.

6. Van Beek A, Kassen M, Adson M, Dale V. Management of acute fingernail injuries. Hand Clinics 1990;6:23.

7. Roberts J, Hedges J. Clinical procedures in emergency medicine. 2nd ed. Philadelphia: WB Saunders, 1991.

8. Milstein D, Milstein S. Letter to the editor. Emerg Med News 1993;15:5.

9. Fleisher G, Ludwig S. Textbook of pediatric emergency medicine. 2nd ed. Baltimore: Williams & Wilkins, 1988.

10. Carter P. Common hand injuries and infections. Philadelphia: WB Saunders, 1983.

11. Davis L. Letter to the editor. J Fam Prac, 1980;11:5.

12. Roberts J. Fingernail avulsion and injury to the nail bed. Emerg Med News 1993;15:3.

13. Shepard G. Management of acute nail bed avulsions. Hand Clinics 1990;6:39.

14. Zook E. Discussion of "Management of acute nail bed avulsions," Hand Clinics 1990;6:57.

15. Rosenthal L, Reiner M, Bleicher M. Nonoperative management of distal fingertip amputations in children. Pediatrics 1979;64:1.

ARTHROCENTESIS

Mark C. Clark and Steven G. Rothrock

INTRODUCTION

Arthrocentesis involves using a needle and a syringe to aspirate synovial fluid from a joint. In evaluating the child with a warm, tender, swollen joint—an acute monoarticular arthritis—it is often impossible to diagnose or exclude septic arthritis without arthrocentesis. Children can present with a wide range of inflammatory arthropathies (Table 107.1). Clinical presentation of any of these may resemble septic arthritis.

Arthrocentesis is a relatively simple and safe procedure that can easily be performed by a physician in an emergency department (1). Many physicians, however, are reluctant to perform arthrocentesis (2–6). This reluctance is unwarranted. As this chapter demonstrates, the emergency physician can safely and appropriately aspirate all extremity joints except for the hip (2–4, 7, 8).

INDICATIONS

Acute pain and swelling in a joint always requires immediate evaluation. Although many less serious causes of monarthritis exist, inadequately treated infectious arthritis carries a risk of prolonged morbidity and even mortality. Arthrocentesis should be performed in virtually every patient with monarthritis, especially if infection is suspected (7). No other sufficient diagnostic method is available for discriminating septic arthritis from other monarthritides than arthrocentesis (5).

Decompression of traumatic hemarthro-

sis is controversial in hemophiliacs and nonhemophiliacs. Most experts, however, believe arthrocentesis is indicated in painful tense effusions (2–6). In patients with hemophilia, arthrocentesis should not be done until coagulation factor replacement has been completed. The physician may want to consult with the hematologist or orthopaedist who cares for the child before performing arthrocentesis for hemarthrosis. Other indications and the few contraindications for arthrocentesis are listed in Tables 107.2 and 107.3.

PROCEDURE

If the few basic principles for arthrocentesis are followed, most sites for aspiration are intuitive. Miller, an anatomist, published two landmark articles describing optimal sites for arthrocentesis (9). His criteria for selecting sites for arthrocentesis are as follows:

1. The site should be as far removed as possible from tendons, large nerves, or blood vessels.
2. A palpable bony landmark should be available in the immediate vicinity of the insertion site.
3. If the landmark is not easily palpable when the joint is in the best position for insertion, the joint may be palpated in one position and subsequently moved to the position for insertion.
4. Methods such as distraction or positioning which will enlarge the target area (the joint cavity) should be used.

Table 107.1.
Common Causes of Arthritis in Children

Septic arthritis
Traumatic hemarthrosis
Postinfectious reactive arthritis
Juvenile rheumatoid arthritis
Serum sickness
Systemic lupus erythematosus
Henoch-Schönlein purpura
Lyme arthritis

5. Positioning should be such as to stretch the part of the capsule and any supporting ligaments that might be penetrated by the needle tip.
6. The direction of penetration should be such as to minimize the danger of scoring the articular cartilages (9).

General Approach

In the young or uncooperative child, judicious use of sedation may be indicated (Chapter 35). The joint needs to remain completely immobile during arthrocentesis to prevent scoring the articular cartilage with the needle. A papoose and an assistant may be required to accomplish this goal.

Sterile technique is followed with first using alcohol to wipe away dirt and skin oils. Then povidone-iodine solution should be painted three successive times over the aspiration site. Finally, only a small area of povidone-iodine is wiped from the entry site with alcohol to avoid the introduction of any antiseptic into the joint and risk sterilizing septic joint fluid. Using drapes and even gloves has not been universally recommended (2, 3, 10, 11). However, in light of universal precautions and the behavior of children, sterile drapes and gloves should be used (4, 12).

Equipment needed for arthrocentesis is readily available in all emergency departments (Table 107.4). As a rule, the physician should use the largest needle that can atraumatically aspirate a joint because synovial fluid can be difficult to withdraw secondary to its viscosity. In general, this would be an 18- to 20-gauge needle for the knee and a 20- to 23-gauge needle for small joints. Choice of syringe size should be based on the estimated volume of the joint effusion.

Local anesthesia may be used but none should be allowed to enter the joint because it

Table 107.2.
Indications for Arthrocentesis

1. Rule out the possibility of septic arthritis
2. Diagnosis of other inflammatory effusions
3. Relief of pain from a tense effusion
4. Confirm the diagnosis of a suspected traumatic hemarthrosis caused by occult fracture or internal derangement
5. Follow the progress of treatment of a septic arthritis
6. Irrigation, decompression, and culture of septic joint

Table 107.3.
Contraindications for Arthrocentesis

Absolute:
1. Cellulitis overlying site of aspiration
Relative:
2. Coagulopathy—hemophilia or warfarin therapy
3. Joint prosthesis
4. Septicemia

may sterilize infected joint fluid and may affect synovial fluid analysis (4, 5). An alternative method is using a vapocoolant, like ethyl chloride, that can be sprayed on the skin to frost it and produce anesthesia (13, 14). This may be ideal in children because it forgoes using local anesthetic which can in itself be painful. Another (albeit unproven) method by which anesthesia of the skin may be accomplished is by applying lidocaine-prilocaine paste. This paste must be applied to the skin over the intended site of needle entry then covered with an occlusive dressing for 30 minutes to 1 hour before the procedure. The paste is then wiped away before skin preparation.

The needle insertion site can easily be lost after the joint becomes sterilely prepared and draped, as these can obscure visual and tactile landmarks. To overcome this hindrance, the joint should be palpated for bony landmarks before preparing and draping so that tactile reference points will be available for guidance during arthrocentesis. The insertion site can be marked on the skin with a closed retractable pen. Placing the joint in the recommended position (see Specific Joints in this chapter) will stretch the joint capsule at the entry site and allow for maximum joint space in which to insert a needle. Distraction

Table 107.4.
Equipment

Alcohol sponges
Povidone-iodine solution
Sterile gauze dressings (2'' × 2'')
Sterile disposable 2 mL, 10 mL,
    20 mL syringes
18-, 20-, 22-gauge, 1.5'' needles
Test tubes (red top and lavender top)
Ethyl chloride
1% lidocaine solution
Sterile drapes
Sterile gloves
Adhesive bandage

on the joint may be necessary at times to increase the joint space even further. The recommended direction of needle insertion (see Specific Joints) offers the best method to avoid scoring the cartilage.

Often a distinct "pop" can be felt when the needle passes the joint capsule and enters the joint cavity. As the needle advances toward the joint space, the clinician should draw back on the plunger of the syringe. Generally, entry into the joint cavity will be confirmed by the aspiration of synovial fluid. If synovial fluid stops flowing into the syringe, and joint fluid still remains, flow will often be reestablished by repositioning the needle or by reinjecting a small amount of joint fluid.

Specific Joints

Knee/Superolateral Approach (Fig. 107.1)

Position: Patient's knee should be extended as much as tolerated. (Full extension facilitates entry into the joint.)

Insertion: The needle is inserted slightly lateral to the superolateral border of the patella.

Direction: The needle is directed slightly inferiorly and slightly posteriorly to pass underneath the patella, aiming for the intercondylar fossa.

Comments: Relaxation of the quadriceps greatly facilitates needle placement.

Knee/Medial Approach (Fig. 107.2)

Position: The knee may be fully extended or flexed to 45°.

Insertion: The needle is inserted at the midpoint of the patella or the superomedial border of the patella.

Direction: The needle is directed underneath the patella aiming for the intercondylar fossa.

Comments: Experts are divided on which method is easier. It may be easier to use this method if the joint effusion is small, whereas others believe the superolateral approach to be easier if joint effusion is large with bulging at the superolateral pouch.

Ankle/Tibiotalar Joint (Fig. 107.3)

Position: The ankle should be slightly plantar flexed as the joint space will be widened

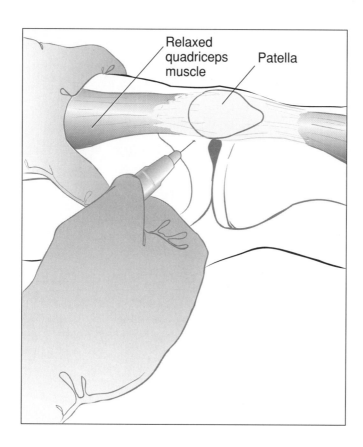

Figure 107.1.
Arthrocentesis of knee via superolateral approach.

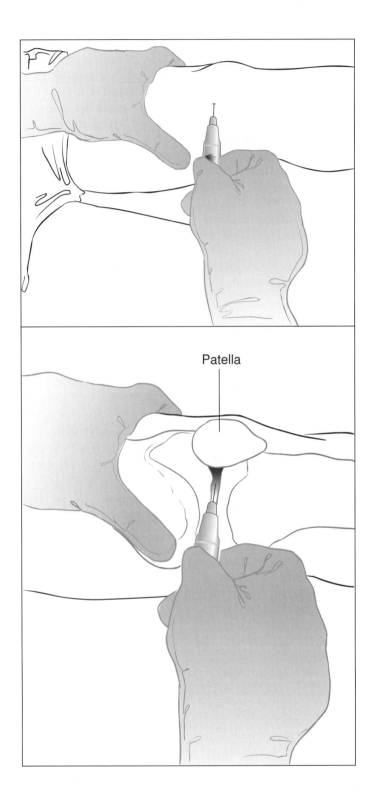

Patella

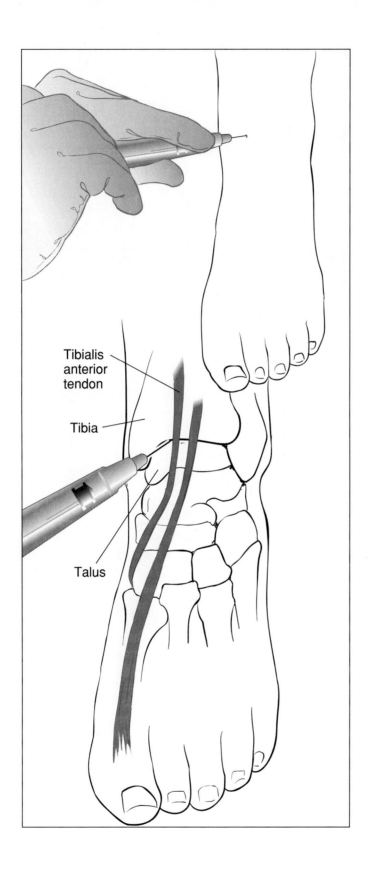

Figure 107.3.
Arthrocentesis of ankle at
tibiotalar joint.

Tibialis
anterior
tendon

Tibia

Talus

Figure 107.4.
Arthrocentesis of ankle at
subtalar joint.

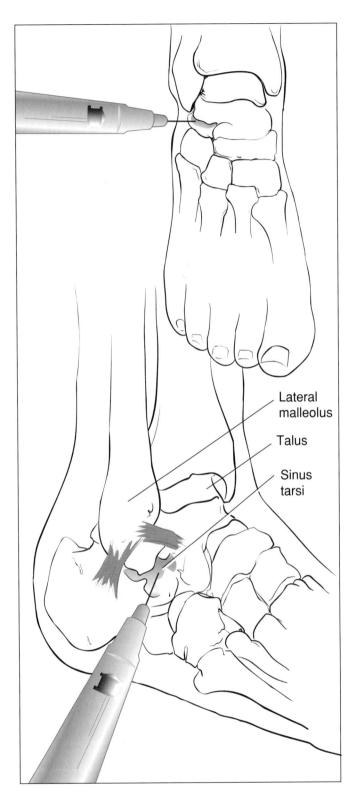

Lateral
malleolus

Talus

Sinus
tarsi

for arthrocentesis and will be in a position
of comfort for a patient with a joint effusion.

Insertion: The needle is inserted anterior to
medial malleolus, in a sulcus just medial
to the tibialis anterior tendon.

Direction: The needle is directed posterolat-
erally.

Ankle/Subtalar Joint (Fig. 107.4)
Position: The ankle is at 90° and slightly inverted.

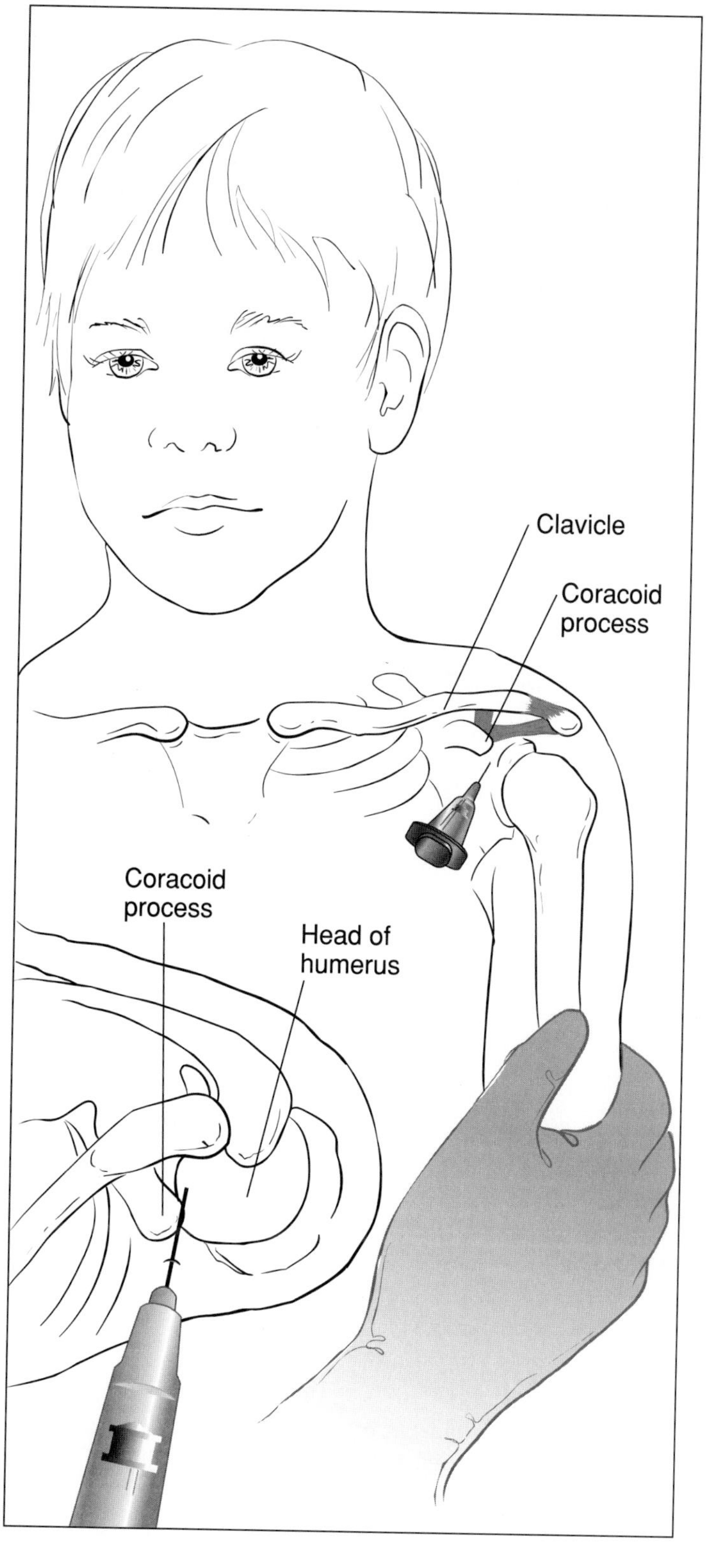

Figure 107.5.
Arthrocentesis of shoulder.

Clavicle

Coracoid
process

Coracoid
process

Head of
humerus

Insertion: The needle is inserted just distal to tip of the lateral malleolus.

Direction: The needle is held horizontal to the subtalar joint and directed medially.

Comments: This can be a difficult joint space to enter.

Shoulder (Fig. 107.5)

Position: The patient is allowed to sit upright with the arm at rest and the hand in the lap.

Insertion: The needle is inserted just inferior and lateral to the coracoid process.

Direction: The needle should be directed

**Chapter 107
Arthrocentesis**

Figure 107.6.
Arthrocentesis of elbow.

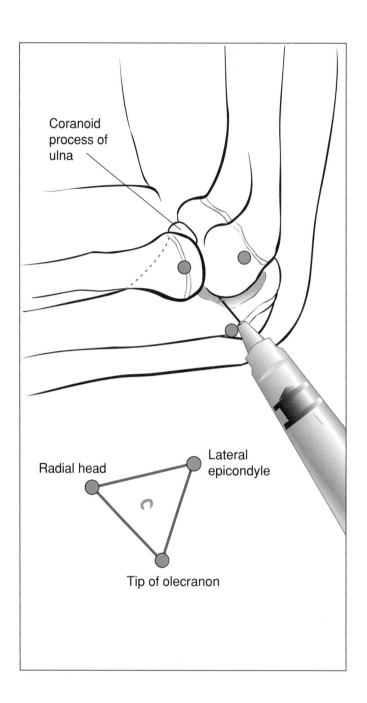

Coranoid
process of
ulna

Radial head

Lateral
epicondyle

Tip of olecranon

posteriorly or posteriorly and slightly superiorly and laterally.

Comments: Arthrocentesis of this joint can be
difficult. In an uncooperative child, sedation is encouraged. Consultation may be
required.

Elbow (Fig. 107.6)

Position: The patient's elbow is held at
90°, preferably resting on a table or a
bed.

Insertion: The needle is inserted in the center of the anconeus triangle, a space between the lateral epicondyle of the

humerus, the radial head, and the olecranon process.

Direction: The needle should be directed medially and slightly anteriorly toward the
coronoid process of the ulna.

Comments: If a significant effusion is present, this space will often bulge outward.

Wrist (Fig. 107.7)

Position: The wrist is flexed 30° and ulnarly
deviated.

Insertion: The needle is inserted just distal to
the dorsal radial tubercle (of Lister) and in

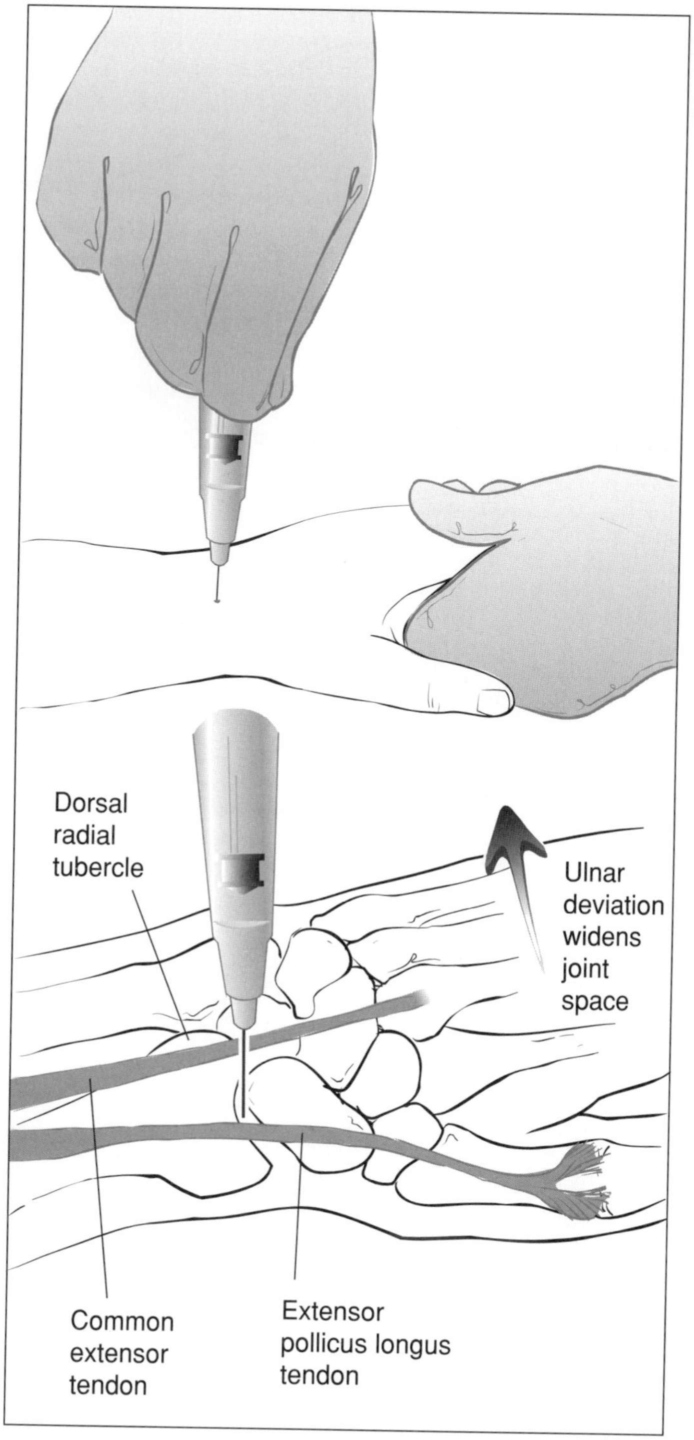

Figure 107.7.
Arthrocentesis of wrist.

Dorsal
radial
tubercle

Ulnar
deviation
widens
joint
space

Common
extensor
tendon

Extensor
pollicus longus
tendon

the sulcus between the extensor pollicis longus tendon and the common extensor tendon to index finger.

Direction: The needle is inserted perpendicular to the skin.

Comments: Application of traction to the hand may facilitate the procedure by widening the joint space.

**Metacarpophalangeal and
Interphalangeal Joints (Fig. 107.8)**

Position: The fingers are flexed 15 to 20°

Insertion: The needle is inserted dorsally, just medial or lateral to the extensor tendon.

Direction: The needle is directed perpendicular to the skin.

Comments: The needle does not have to enter

Chapter 107
Arthrocentesis

SUMMARY

1. Discuss procedure with parents and child and obtain informed consent
2. Review technique for arthrocentesis of specific joint by studying corresponding text and figure—remember to note joint positioning, insertion sites based on bony landmarks, and direction needle should be inserted
3. Gather necessary equipment
4. Consider sedation, immobilization, and need for an assistant
5. Palpate bony landmarks to find reference points in locating insertion site—may want to mark skin with closed retractable pen
6. Prepare joint entry site for sterile technique
7. Anesthetize entry site with local anesthetic or vapocoolant
8. Place joint in correct position and consider joint distraction
9. Direct needle as recommended in specific approaches to lessen chance of scoring cartilage
10. Remember to send synovial fluid for analysis (listed in order of importance): culture and sensitivity, Gram stain, and cell count with differential
11. Send synovial fluid to lab in sterile glass or plastic tube without additives for immediate culture and Gram stain, and ideally a heparinized tube for cell count and differential (50 U heparin/mL synovial fluid)
12. Examine synovial fluid in clear test tube for color and clarity

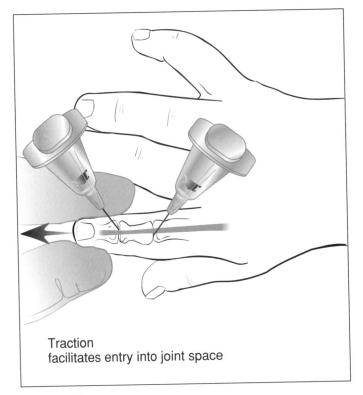

Traction
facilitates entry into joint space

Figure 107.8.
Arthrocentesis of metacarpophalangeal and interphalangeal joints.

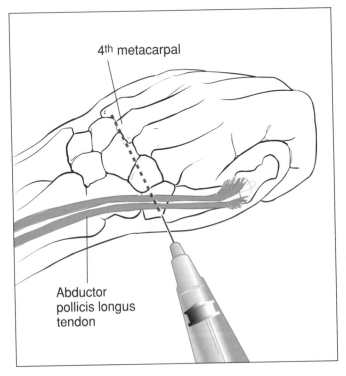

4th metacarpal

Abductor
pollicis longus
tendon

Figure 107.9.
Arthrocentesis of thumb at carpometacarpal joint.

between the joint surfaces. Applying traction facilitates entry into the joint space.

Thumb/First Carpometacarpal Joint (Fig. 107.9)

Position: The thumb should be opposed with the little finger or placed in the palm of the hand with a closed fist.

Insertion: The needle is inserted proximal to the prominence at the base of the first metacarpal on the palmar side of the abductor pollicis longus tendon.

Direction: The needle should be directed toward the base of the fourth metacarpal.

Comments: The abductor pollicis longus tendon is easiest to palpate when the thumb is extended.

COMPLICATIONS

Complications with arthrocentesis can occur, but with careful technique, should be rare. Infection can be prevented by observing sterile technique and avoiding sites with cellulitis or skin lesions. Articular cartilage does not repair itself; therefore, diligence should be maintained to avoid scoring the cartilage with the needle. Needle entry should be only deep enough to allow aspiration, and joint position and entry sites should be chosen that allow for the maximum space. A small amount of traumatic capsular bleeding usually occurs, but bleeding is rarely significant, unless a coagulopathy is present (2, 5, 10). Patients with hemophilia should have clotting factor replacement performed beforehand. Finally, hypersensitivity reaction can occur with local anesthetics, as with any procedure involving these agents. A careful history of medical allergies should be taken before the procedure and resuscitative equipment should be readily available in case such a complication does occur (Table 107.5)

SYNOVIAL FLUID ANALYSIS

Examination of synovial fluid is often said to be the most useful test in rheumatology, constituting a liquid biopsy of the joint. The primary purpose of synovial fluid analysis is to determine the cause of the arthritis and to differentiate inflammatory from noninflammatory

arthritis. No other sufficiently reliable method is available for differentiating septic arthritis from severe inflammatory arthritis (6).

Many synovial tests used for this purpose in the past have now been found to add little diagnostic information. Virtually all important information from synovial fluid analysis that influences diagnosis and treatment can be obtained by a cell count and differential, culture, and Gram stain (15, 16). Some authorities have recommended a long list of chemical, immunologic, and microbiologic studies borrowed from routine tests of other body fluids. However, the application of these tests to synovial fluids is unproven. In some cases routine tests such as synovial fluid protein and glucose have been found to not offer any additional diagnostic information to that already obtained by synovial cell count and differential (16). Viscosity has been found to be less useful than previously thought, because synovial fluid viscosity can be decreased by inflammatory diseases and edematous conditions. The mucin clot test offers a subjective and an inexact measurement of hyaluronate which decreases in inflammatory joint effusions. More objective and accurate ways to measure inflammation are available, such as cell count and differential (6, 15). Crystal analysis by polarized light microscopy is not necessary because gouty arthritis is not seen in children. Controversy exists regarding synovial assays for protein, glucose, enzymes, immune complexes, rheumatoid factor, Lyme titers, and antinuclear antibody in children. In some cases and in some geographic locations these tests may be indicated. One strategy that can be used by the emergency physician is to set aside some of the recovered fluid. Then, if the child proves to not have a straightforward infectious or traumatic arthritis, fluid is available for further testing.

The absolute cell count is the major factor that discriminates inflammatory from noninflammatory arthritis. The white blood cell count indicates the degree of inflammation, suggests the likelihood of infection, and estimates the rate of potential joint destruction. Synovial fluid can be classified into four groups: normal, noninflammatory, inflammatory, and septic. Classification has limited diagnostic usefulness because fluid from a single joint may fall into any group (Table 107.6) (5). A wide spectrum of leukocytosis exists in both sterile and septic joint effusions

Table 107.5. Complications

Joint infection
Articular cartilage injury
Joint bleeding
Hypersensitivity reactions

CLINICAL TIPS

1. Joints may have more than one route of entry. The preferred route is usually the shortest distance from the point of entry to the joint space and avoids skin lesions or superficial infections, major vessels, tendons, and nerves. An approach on the extensor side of the joint usually accomplishes this goal.

2. The skin over the aspiration site can be marked with a closed retractable pen while manually examining the unprepared joint.

3. Local anesthetic should not be injected into joint cavity because it may cause artifact and sterilize septic synovial fluid.

4. Discomfort of arthrocentesis can be decreased sufficiently by a local vapocoolant, such as ethyl chloride.

5. Because joint fluid is so viscous, use the largest needle that can atraumatically enter the joint cavity.

6. Size of the syringe should correspond with the estimated volume of the joint effusion.

7. Remember to loosen the seal on the syringe before aspirating the joint to prevent trauma from undue struggling with the syringe.

Table 107.6.
Synovial Fluid Analysis[a]

	Normal	Noninflammatory	Inflammatory	Septic
Cell count (per mm^3)	<200	200–2000	2000–75,000	often >100,000†
PMNs (%)	<25%	<50%	>50% often	>75%†
Color	colorless to straw	straw to yellow	cloudy yellow	cloudy, yellow, green
Clarity	transparent	transparent	translucent	opaque

† WBC and % of PMN leukocytes will be less if organism is less virulent, or if patient is partially treated or immunocompromised.
[a] Compiled from references 19 and 20.

and strict classification is imprudent (7, 17, 18).

Perhaps the most urgent reason for performing synovial fluid analysis is to identify septic arthritis. If arthrocentesis obtains limited amounts of fluid, the order of importance for synovial studies are bacterial culture, Gram stain, and finally cell count and differential. As a rough guideline, if newsprint can be read through the synovial fluid in a glass tube, the effusion is probably noninflammatory (5).

SUMMARY

Arthrocentesis in children is a straightforward procedure whose primary role in the emergency department is to identify septic arthritis. An understanding of the anatomical reasons for selection of the needle entry site into the joint cavity and familiarity with this aseptic technique should lead to successful arthrocentesis and further prevention of the already rare complications. Evaluation of the synovial fluid is now less complicated in light of recent recommendations to omit redundant and misleading tests.

REFERENCES

1. Gatter RA, Schmacher Jr. HR. Joint aspiration: indications and technique. In: Gatter RA, Schumacher Jr HR, eds. A practical handbook of synovial fluid analysis. Philadelphia: Lea & Febiger, 1991, pp. 14–23.
2. Samuelson CO, Cannon GW, Ward JR. Arthrocentesis. J Fam Pract 1985;20:169–184.
3. Ezell SL, Kobernick ME, Benjamin GC. Arthrocentesis. In: Roberts JR, Hedges JR, eds. Clinical procedures in emergency medicine. 2nd ed. Philadelphia: WB Saunders, 1991, pp. 847–859.
4. Carlson W, DiGiulio GA, Gewitz MH, et al. Illustrated techniques of pediatric emergency procedures. In: Fleisher GR, Ludwig S, eds. 3rd ed. Baltimore: Williams & Wilkins, 1993, pp. 1663–1667.
5. Hasselbacher P. Arthrocentesis and synovial fluid analysis. In: Schumacher Jr. HR, ed. Primer on the rheumatic diseases. 9th ed. Atlanta: Arthritis Foundation, 1988, pp. 55–60.
6. Cohen AR. Hematologic emergencies. In: Fleisher GR, Ludwig S, eds. 3rd ed. Baltimore: Williams & Wilkins, 1993, pp. 718–744.
7. Baker DG, Schumacher Jr. HR. Acute monarthritis. N Engl J Med 1993;329:1013–1020.
8. Leversee JH. Aspiration of joints and soft tissue injections. Primary Care 1986;13:579–599.
9. Miller JA. Joint paracentesis from an anatomic point of view. II. Hip, knee, ankle and foot. Surgery 1957; 41:999-1011.
10. Gatter RA. Arthrocentesis technique and intrasynovial therapy. In: McCarty DG, Koopman WJ, eds. Arthritis and allied conditions. 12th ed. Philadelphia: Lea & Febiger, 1993, pp. 711–720.
11. Owen DS. Aspiration and injection of joints and soft tissues. In: Kelley WN, Harris ED, Ruddy S, Sledge CB, eds. Textbook of rheumatology. Vol 1. 3rd ed. Philadelphia: WB Saunders, 1989, pp. 621–636.
12. Kasser JR. Bone and joint infections. In: Canale ST, Beaty JH, eds. Operative pediatric orthopaedics. St. Louis: CV Mosby, 1991, pp. 1047–1067.
13. Gatter RA, Schumacher HR. A practical handbook of joint fluid analysis. 2nd ed. Philadelphia: Lea & Febiger, 1993, pp. 7–14.
14. Abeles M, Garjian P. (letter) Do spray coolant anesthetics contaminate an aseptic field? Arth Rheum 1986;29:576.
15. Eisenberg JM, Schumacher HR, Davidson PK, Kaufmann L. Usefulness of synovial fluid analysis in the evaluation of joint effusions: use of threshold analysis and likelihood ratios to assess a diagnostic test. Arch Intern Med 1984;144:715–719.
16. Schmerling RH, Delbanco Tl, Toteson ANA, Trentham DE. Synovial fluid tests—what should be ordered? JAMA 1990;264:1009–1014.
17. McCutchan HJ, Fisher RC. Synovial leukocytosis in infectious arthritis. Clin Orthop 1990;257:226–230.
18. Singleton JD, West SG, Nordstrom DM. "Pseudoseptic" arthritis complicating rheumatoid arthritis: a report of six cases. J Rheumatol 1991;18: 1319–1322.
19. Doughty RA, Rose C. Pain-joints. In: Fleisher GR, Ludwig S, eds. Textbook of pediatric emergency medicine. 3rd ed. Baltimore, Williams & Wilkins, 1993, pp. 377–381.
20. Schumacher Jr. HR. Synovial fluid analysis and synovial biopsy. In: Kelly WN, Harris ED, Ruddy S, Sledge CB, eds. Textbook of rheumatology. 3rd ed. Philadelphia: WB Saunders, 1989, pp. 637–649.

REDUCTION OF COMMON JOINT DISLOCATIONS AND SUBLUXATIONS

Grace M. Young

INTRODUCTION

Dislocation is the complete disruption of the normal articulation of a joint. Subluxation is partial dislocation in which the integrity of the joint is disrupted but the articulating surfaces maintain some degree of apposition. Disruption is identified by the position of the distal articulating surface relative to the proximal articulating surface.

Axial and rotatory forces that cause dislocations in the adult more often cause epiphyseal fractures in the child or adolescent. Although the immature skeleton usually has generalized joint laxity, ligaments and capsular structures around joints in a child are strong relative to the physis. For these reasons, ligamentous and joint injuries occur infrequently in the younger child and increase in incidence in the adolescent whose growth plates are closing or closed. The exception is the child whose joints are inherently lax due to a congenital disorder such as Ehlers-Danlos, Down's, or Marfan's syndromes; these children are at increased risk for joint dislocations.

More common traumatic joint injuries in children and adolescents include subluxation of the radial head and dislocations of the finger, shoulder, patella, and hip joints. Discussions in this chapter will be limited to isolated dislocation or subluxation that is not associated with a fracture and that can be managed by the emergency physician in the acute setting. Dislocations of the elbow and knee joints have significant potential for neurovascular compromise, will occur rarely in the child, and should be primarily managed by the pediatric orthopaedist.

Most reduction maneuvers for dislocations discussed in this chapter are based on traction and countertraction applied to the muscles and ligaments of the joint. Traction is the use of continuous mechanical force to overcome muscle spasm that is caused by injury during dislocation. Traction produces muscle fatigue and eventual muscle relaxation. The joint then distracts slightly and allows reduction of the dislocation. Traction also relieves impaction or entrapment of bone, tendon, or ligament caused by the dislocation.

Successful reductions require adequate analgesia and anesthesia, an accurate knowledge of joint anatomy, and a slow deliberate technique. Early reduction prevents joint dysfunction. Radiographs generally should be obtained before and after the reduction maneuver to delineate the joint structure and articulation; an associated fracture that may be obscured by the dislocation must be excluded. Immobilization of the joint after reduction prevents redislocation. Ice, elevation, and nonsteroidal antiinflammatory medication promote healing. Exercise restores full range of motion (ROM) and strength.

Before receiving treatment of any joint injury, the child must be managed using the guidelines of pediatric trauma resuscitation. Life-threatening trauma, especially any compromise of the airway, breathing, or circulation (oxygenation, ventilation, or perfusion), must first be excluded and multiple organ injury appropriately treated. In addition, the child or adolescent whose injured limb shows any signs or symptoms of acute neurovascular compromise or compartment syndrome (pain, pallor, painful passive motion, pulselessness, paresthesia, paresis) requires immediate reduction and orthopaedic consultation.

RADIAL HEAD SUBLUXATION

Introduction

Radial head subluxation (RHS) is partial dislocation of the head of the proximal radius from its articulation with the proximal ulna and the capitellum of the distal humerus in the radiohumeral joint. Its synonyms include nursemaid's elbow, pulled elbow, and temper tantrum elbow (1, 2). Pure complete elbow dislocations are rare in children. Whereas, in contrast to adults, dislocation of the elbow is the second most common joint dislocation after that of the shoulder (3).

Radial head subluxation is the most common joint injury in the pediatric age group. It occurs in toddlers between the ages of 1 and 4 years, but rarely before age 1 year or after age 8 years. The presenting history usually recalls an abrupt pull or lift on the arm that subsequently results in the child's refusal to use the arm. This force is imparted by either the caretaker, by the child, or less commonly by a fall (2–5). The most common scenario originated the term nursemaid's elbow: a nursemaid caretaker yanks abruptly on the outstretched arm of a recalcitrant toddler while trying to cross a busy intersection or to prevent his or her stumble. The child's left arm is more commonly affected perhaps because a right-handed adult is more likely to hold the child's left hand. Circumstances that may induce bilateral RHS include the child who falls while grasping onto a bar or side rail, or swinging the child whose arms are both extended (1–5).

The reduction maneuver is quick and straightforward. It can be done in the ED or outpatient setting by a skilled physician, it requires little strength, and it usually is successful (3–5).

Anatomy and Physiology

The radial head is attached to the proximal ulna and capitellum of the distal humerus, primarily by the annular ligament. The annular ligament acts as a sling to guide supination and pronation. When the forearm is in supination, the oval-shaped radial head sits prominently at the radioulnar joint and maintains the annular ligament distal to its epiphysis. As the forearm is pronated, the contour of the radial head flattens, which allows the annular ligament to slide proximally over the radial head. RHS usually occurs after any sudden longitudinal traction force on the wrist or hand when the elbow is in extension and the forearm in pronation. These forces may stretch and tear the annular ligament at its distal attachment to the radial neck. Without this distal tether, the annular ligament slips and becomes entrapped proximally in the radiocapitellar joint to cause subluxation of the radial head. The forearm locks in pronation because supination becomes quite painful. Forced supination mechanically loops the annular ligament into its appropriate position over the radial head by using the radius as a lever. Because of this unique anatomy, reduction may be easily achieved by simple forced supination of the forearm (2, 3).

Radiographs of the elbow joint in RHS reveal normal bone and anatomic relationships. On occasion, a child's RHS may be reduced in the radiology suite when the technician supinates the forearm to obtain a true AP projection of the elbow (2, 4). The presence of a "posterior fat pad sign," an abnormal lucency at the posterior distal humerus, or a displaced "radiocapitellar line" (the radial head and neck normally intersects the capitellum) or anterior humeral line (line along the anterior distal humerus that intersects middle third of the capitellum) is indicative of intraarticular hematoma, fracture, or other injury (Fig. 108.1). These signs exclude the diagnosis of RHS and suggest the need for orthopaedic evaluation. Although several authorities (6, 7) report the association of RHS with displacement of the radiocapitellar line,

Chapter 108
Reduction of
Common Joint
Dislocations and
Subluxations

1076

it is difficult to assess its validity because radiographs of their patients' arms were in the position of comfort and not true lateral projections. Gross dislocation or fracture, such as condylar fracture of the distal humerus or ulnar fracture with radial head dislocation (Monteggia fracture-dislocation), exclude simple subluxation and require immediate orthopaedic consultation.

Indications

Clinical diagnosis of RHS as suggested by a typical history and physical examination is usually sufficient to perform the reduction maneuver without first obtaining radiographs. The usual presenting complaint is refusal to use the affected arm and the history offers a plausible mechanism. The classic clinical presentation for RHS is that of a quiet, nondistressed child who holds the affected arm at his or her side, refusing to use or supinate it, and possibly supporting the affected hand with the other. The affected forearm is in pronation and the elbow in extension (Fig. 108.2.A) (1–5). A brief physical examination reveals no soft tissue swelling or ecchymosis, rare isolated radial head tenderness, intact distal neurovascular function, no gross bony deformities, and no obvious evidence of trauma. Examination also should include palpation of the clavicles. Supination is strongly resisted; otherwise, full ROM is exhibited at the elbow (4, 5).

The presence of any significant swelling, tenderness, suspicion of fracture, complete dislocation, or neurovascular compromise requires radiographic evaluation and precludes immediate use of this reduction maneuver. A pediatric orthopaedist also should be consulted.

Equipment

For reduction: none

Procedure

The child should sit comfortably in the parent's lap. The clinician, using the nondominant hand, supports the affected elbow gently with the palm and applies moderate pressure

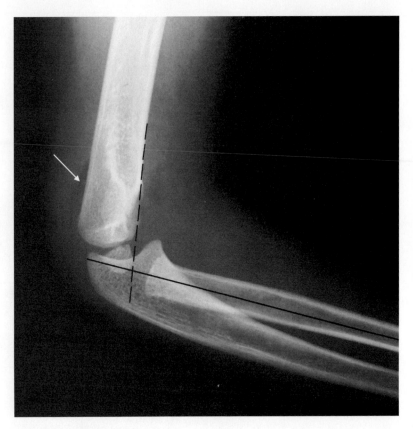

Figure 108.1.
Lateral view radiograph of elbow reveals posterior fat pad sign (*arrow*) and slight posterior displacement of capitellum relative to anterior humeral line (*dashed line*) indicative of supracondylar fracture. The radiocapitellar line (*solid line*) in this patient is normal.

on the radial head with either the thumb or fingers. With the dominant hand, the clinician grasps the wrist of the affected arm by placing the fingers on the volar aspect of the wrist and the thumb on the dorsal aspect (Fig. 108.2.B–D). In one quick, deliberate motion while applying gentle longitudinal traction, the forearm is forcefully and fully supinated, and the elbow flexed. In 80 to 90% of maneuvers, a palpable or audible "click" or "clunk" at the radial head area accompanies and is predictive of a successful reduction (1, 2, 4, 5). Pain and much distress is usually elicited during supination but subsides quickly after reduction and with consoling (4). In greater than 90% of children with RHS, return to use occurs within 10 to 15 minutes or earlier after reduction. Voluntary use of the affected arm within 30 minutes after the maneuver confirms the clinical diagnosis and successful reduction of RHS (4, 5).

After a successful reduction, no treatment, immobilization, or radiography is required except education for prevention. A second attempt or more may be needed if the child does not use the arm within 15 to 30 minutes despite encouragement. If no im-

Chapter 108
Reduction of
Common Joint
Dislocations and
Subluxations

1077

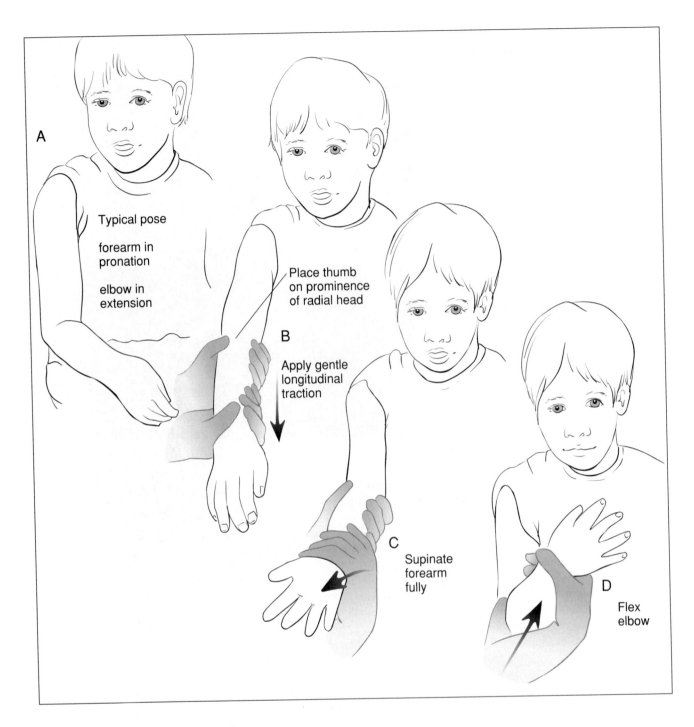

Labels within figure:

A

Typical pose

forearm in pronation

elbow in extension

Place thumb on prominence of radial head

B

Apply gentle longitudinal traction

C

Supinate forearm fully

D

Flex elbow

Figure 108.2.
Procedure for reduction of radial head subluxation.

provement is seen after several appropriate reduction attempts and the injury is associated with a fall or trauma, further evaluation and diagnostic radiography is needed (4, 5).

If reduction is delayed more than 8 to 12 hours, full recovery may take up to 1 to 2 days. Immobilization with a posterior splint may be applied with reevaluation in 24 hours. Spontaneous return of arm use at home may occur. If the child persistently refuses to use the arm, he or she should be evaluated for other pathology and referred to a pediatric orthopaedist (4, 5).

Complications

No complications other than recurrence have been reported with this maneuver (3). Recurrence of RHS ranges between 5 and 40%; recurrence decreases as the child's joint structures strengthen (4, 5). Chronic mild subluxation may be a sequelae after RHS, but no long-term studies are available. The older child who has recurrent RHS may require surgical repair of the annular ligament. An irreducible subluxation is rare and may require an open reduction (3, 5).

In the child with persistent nonuse of the arm, subtle avulsion or condylar fractures may not be initially evident. Septic joint, osteomyelitis, fracture of the clavicle, or a traumatic radial head dislocation also must be considered. Rarely, the median or ulnar nerves are stretched or entrapped (3, 5).

DIGIT DISLOCATIONS

Introduction

Interphalangeal (IP) joint dislocations of the fingers and toes are common. Dislocation of the proximal interphalangeal (PIP) joint occurs more frequently than that of the distal interphalangeal (DIP) joint in the child or adolescent. Dorsal PIP dislocation occurs most commonly (8–10). Forced hyperextension with axial compression causes a dorsal PIP (or DIP) joint dislocation, when the middle (or distal) phalanx is dislocated dorsal to the proximal (middle) phalanx. Volar IP joint dislocations, when the distal phalanx is dislocated volar to the middle phalanx for example, are relatively uncommon (8, 9, 11). Forced hyperflexion results in a volar IP dislocation. An IP dislocation usually results from an athletic injury or the finger being entrapped between objects. Typically, the finger was jammed or bent backward while playing football, basketball, or baseball (8, 9, 11). Most dislocations are managed easily with a closed reduction maneuver in the ED. After reduction, the IP joint is usually stable and the ligaments in the child usually heal without complication. All finger dislocations should have subsequent reevaluation by a hand specialist to manage potential subtle ligamentous, cartilaginous, or bony injury (8, 9).

Anatomy and Physiology

The interphalangeal joint is a hinge joint that allows only flexion and extension and con-

sists of several ligamentous complexes (Fig. 108.3). The volar plate provides stability against hyperextension injury and dorsal dislocation of the phalanx. It often ruptures during a dorsal dislocation and may be associated with an avulsion fracture at the base of the phalanx. The strong collateral ligament complex resists hyperextension and lateral dislocation injury. The extensor hood complex stabilizes against hyperflexion injury and volar displacement of the phalanx (8, 11). Phalanges act mechanically as lever arms during forced hyperextension or hyperflexion. The longer lever arm of the PIP joints accounts for the higher frequency of PIP dislocations, whereas the shorter lever arm of the DIP joints results in fewer DIP dislocations (12). Once reduced, the IP joint is usually stable (8).

Although determination of specific ligamentous injury is important, the degree of joint function and stability after an injury is clinically more significant. An accurate and detailed examination is crucial and requires digital block anesthesia. Passive hyperextension tests the integrity of the volar plate; radial and ulnar stress, the collateral ligaments. Limitation of active flexion and extension, especially against resistance, may suggest tendinous or ligamentous rupture or intraarticular osteochondral fragment. An external skin laceration after a blunt hyperextension injury suggests a volar plate rupture (8, 9, 11).

Radiographs of the affected digit before and after reduction reveal the alignment of the phalanges, the nature of dislocation, and the presence of any bony fracture (Fig. 108.3.A,B). Optimal diagnosis requires three views: AP, true lateral, and oblique. A physeal, avulsion, or distal tuft fracture, or an osteochondral fragment can be subtle and may be present only on one or two views (8, 9).

Indications

An IP joint dislocation is typically associated with forced hyperextension or hyperflexion of the digit. It presents with gross deformity, diffuse pain, tenderness, and swelling, and is confirmed by radiographs and requires immediate reduction.

Any digit that has neurovascular compromise, an open joint dislocation, ligamen-

Chapter 108
Reduction of
Common Joint
Dislocations and
Subluxations

1079

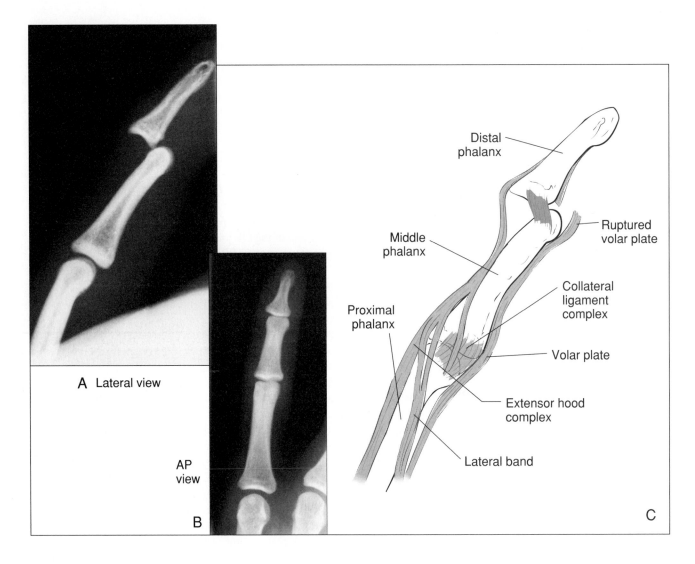

A Lateral view

AP view

B

Distal phalanx

Ruptured volar plate

Middle phalanx

Collateral ligament complex

Proximal phalanx

Volar plate

Extensor hood complex

Lateral band

C

Figure 108.3.
Radiographic (**A, B**) and schematic (**C**) representation of an interphalangeal joint dislocation.

tous or volar plate rupture, joint instability, or an associated fracture also should have immediate orthopaedic consultation. A lateral or volar PIP joint dislocation, although rare, requires an orthopaedist for possible open reduction with internal fixation (8, 11, 12). Dislocation of the metacarpophalangeal (MCP) joint, although rare in adults, may be more common in children. MCP dislocation usually requires open reduction and should be managed primarily by a pediatric orthopaedist (9).

Equipment

For digital block anesthesia:
Antiseptic solution (povidone-iodine or alcohol swabs)
Lidocaine 1% without epinephrine
25- or 27-gauge, 0.63" needle

For reduction:
Gauze, 4" × 4"
For immobilization:
Foam-padded malleable splint, appropriately sized
Tape

Procedure

Before performing the reduction maneuver, all rings should be removed from the affected finger. Digital block anesthesia (Chapter 37) requires 10 to 15 minutes for optimal anesthetic affect.

With the patient's hand or foot securely braced, the clinician firmly grasps the dislocated phalanx; dry gauze loosely wrapped around the phalanx may improve the grip. The joint is hyperextended with gentle longitudinal traction for a dorsal dislocation, or hy-

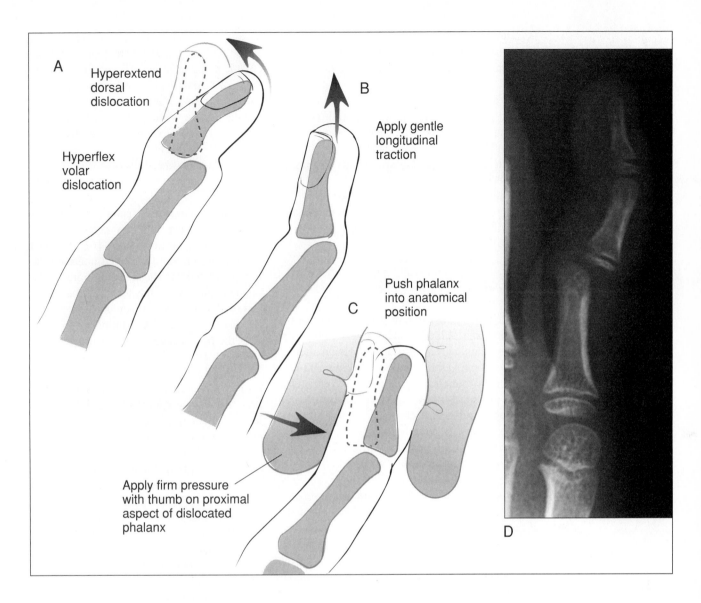

A. Hyperextend dorsal dislocation / Hyperflex volar dislocation

B. Apply gentle longitudinal traction

C. Push phalanx into anatomical position / Apply firm pressure with thumb on proximal aspect of dislocated phalanx

D.

Figure 108.4.
Procedure for reduction of dorsal DIP joint dislocation (**A–C**). Radiograph of PIP joint dislocation (**D**).

perflexed for a volar dislocation. The dislocated phalanx is then pushed gradually into its normal anatomic position. Traction should not be vigorously applied in a child because it may interpose soft tissue or an osteochondral fragment into the distracted joint space and prevent reduction (Figure 108.4) (9, 10).

After reduction, the affected joint must be examined for flexor-extensor tendon function, active ROM, localized tenderness, and instability in the medial-lateral and dorsal-volar directions. Comparison of these motions with the other digits is helpful in a child who has inherently lax joints. Any joint instability or neurovascular compromise after reduction requires immediate pediatric orthopaedic consultation (9–11).

The joint should be immobilized with a foam-padded splint immediately after reduc-tion to prevent redislocation or instability. For a dorsal PIP dislocation, the splint is applied dorsally with the joint in 20 to 30° of flexion. For a volar DIP dislocation, the splint is applied only to the DIP joint on the volar aspect; the DIP should be in full extension and the PIP joint be allowed to have full ROM. Immobilization should continue 14 to 21 days for a PIP joint dislocation and 10 to 14 days for a DIP joint dislocation. Buddy taping to an adjacent digit, thereafter for 3 to 6 weeks, allows active ROM and prevents hyperextension. In the younger child whose cause of dislocation was more likely liga-mentous laxity rather than rupture, immobilization by buddy taping for 10 to 14 days is an acceptable alternative treatment (8–11).

Postreduction radiographs confirm correct joint alignment and identify subtle frac-

Chapter 108
Reduction of
Common Joint
Dislocations and
Subluxations

1081

tures, especially chip or avulsion fractures. Stress views may further assess functional stability with active ROM and joint congruity (9, 11).

Despite appropriate management with rest, ice, and elevation, pain and swelling may persist for 6 to 12 months. Nonsteroidal antiinflammatory medication is helpful. Because joint instability or dysfunction may be obscured by extensive swelling, all finger joint dislocations should be referred for orthopaedic or hand specialist evaluation within 2 to 3 weeks following reduction (8, 10, 11).

Complications

Complications are rare with early reduction, although persistent pain and swelling are common. Inadequate immobilization after reduction may result in redislocation, and prolonged immobilization in muscle contracture. Volar plate injury may lead to recurrent dislocation with chronic laxity, hyperextensibility (swan neck deformity on active extension), or flexion contracture (pseudo-boutonniere deformity without DIP hyperextension). Late or delayed reduction commonly results in loss of joint motion, joint instability, and limitation of function of the hand (8, 9, 11, 12).

Unsuccessful reduction is typically caused by intraarticular entrapment of the volar plate, extensor hood ligaments, or osteochondral fragment from an associated avulsion fracture; or a buttonhole dislocation of the phalangeal neck through the joint capsule. Failure to diagnose an unstable joint, open joint injury, or associated epiphyseal or avulsion fracture should be avoided (8–12).

SHOULDER DISLOCATION

Introduction

Shoulder dislocation is the displacement of the proximal humerus from its normal articulation in the glenoid fossa. In the adolescent, anterior dislocation of the shoulder is the most common joint dislocation (13, 14). The usual mechanism is a forced abduction and external rotation of the arm about the shoulder. Shoulder dislocations in the adolescent usually result from a direct blow to the shoulder or a fall on an outstretched arm during an athletic injury or a fight (15). A child younger than 12 years of age rarely dislocates the shoulder joint. Forces that dislocate the shoulder in the mature skeleton fracture the physis of the proximal humerus in the immature skeleton of a child.

The humeral head dislocates in an anterior and inferior direction in more than 90 to 96% of glenohumeral dislocations (13). Posterior dislocations of the shoulder are rare in pediatric patients, but may occur during a convulsion or cardioversion (16). Posterior dislocations present with fixed internal rotation of the humeral head. Even more rarely, the humeral head dislocates in a superior direction, known as luxatio erecta humeri (17). Recurrent shoulder dislocations are frequent after the first because the anterior capsule is stretched.

Although many methods have been described for reduction of a shoulder dislocation, few are appropriate for the child or adolescent. Maneuvers using leverage (Kocher) (13), overhead traction (Milch, Cooper) (18, 19), external rotation (14, 20), or lateral traction (Eskimo) (13) should not be used in the child or adolescent. Reduction by these techniques is associated with the most complications, especially in the child and adolescent. Complications include further neuromuscular, vascular, and periarticular soft tissue injury; fracture of the humeral neck and glenoid rim; spiral fracture of the humeral shaft; and more significant pain (13, 14, 21). These maneuvers will not be discussed in this section.

For the pediatric patient, reduction by forward flexion with gravity (Stimson) (19, 22–24), scapular manipulation (21, 25–27) and abduction (Hippocrates) (13, 28) are best. These reduction techniques are 70 to 90% effective with the first attempt (13, 21) and are commonly performed by emergency physicians in the ED setting.

Anatomy and Physiology

In the shoulder joint, the relatively large humeral head articulates with a shallow glenoid fossa of the scapula. A thin and inelastic joint capsule envelops the two bony structures and its attachments (Fig. 108.5). The joint capsule, glenohumeral ligament,

Chapter 108
Reduction of
Common Joint
Dislocations and
Subluxations

1082

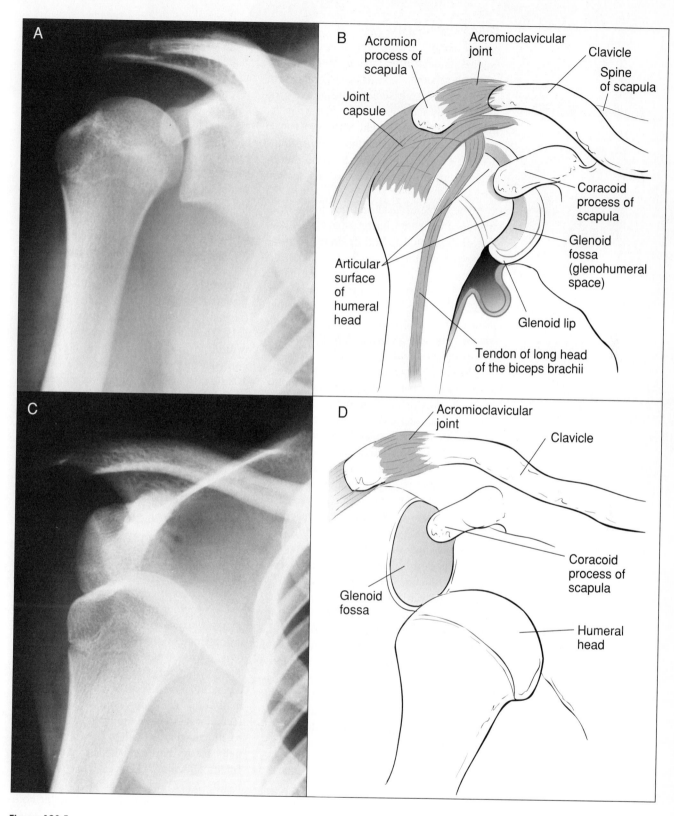

Figure 108.5.
A, B. Normal shoulder joint.
C, D. Anterior dislocation of the shoulder.

Chapter 108
**Reduction of
Common Joint
Dislocations and
Subluxations**

1083

subscapularis muscle, long head of the biceps brachii tendon, and the rotator cuff muscles (supraspinatus, infraspinatus, teres minor) function together to restrain glenohumeral dislocation. Successive failure of each of these fibrous and muscular structures results in a dislocation, during which 10 to 15% tear. An acute force directed at the anterior shoulder can easily disrupt this tenuous glenohumeral articulation and cause dislocation (16).

The humeral head and the glenoid rim fracture frequently during anterior dislocation of the shoulder. Both fracture when the humeral head impacts against the anterior-inferior rim of the glenoid. Fracture of the humeral head appears as a smoothly margined bony defect, called a Hill-Sachs lesion, at its posterior-lateral cortex. Fracture of the glenoid rim, also known as a Bankart lesion, occurs less commonly (15, 16, 29).

In the child or adolescent, vascular or nerve injury occurs rarely after an uncomplicated shoulder dislocation. In the adolescent, however, the rotator cuff muscles commonly tear during dislocation, and concurrent fracture of the proximal humerus is common in the child (29). The brachial plexus and circumflex nerves are injured infrequently. Axillary nerve dysfunction results in decreased deltoid muscle contraction and decreased light touch sensation over the deltoid. The axillary artery may sustain traction or compression injury during dislocation or secondary to forceful reduction (14, 16, 30).

The forward flexion and abduction maneuvers use the traction-countertraction principle to lever the humeral head into the glenoid fossa. Both maneuvers fatigue the shoulder girdle muscles, relax the biceps muscle and neurovascular structure, and distract possible humeral head impaction on the glenoid. The forward flexion-gravity technique allows a spontaneous reduction by gravity, time, and muscle relaxation; the abduction technique applies active opposing forces.

Scapular manipulation maneuvers the glenoid to release humeral head impaction and to affect reduction. When the humeral head dislocates from forced abduction and external rotation, the glenoid fossa is forced medially and the inferior tip of the scapula abducted. Although scapular manipulation

has not been studied in patients younger than 17 years (21, 25), this technique is atraumatic, uses minimal force, causes little pain, and has no reported complications in adults.

Radiographs of the shoulder should be obtained before and after the reduction maneuver. The combination of AP, axillary, and scapular Y views accurately identifies dislocation, position of the humeral head, and associated fracture. The AP projection demonstrates the normally symmetric glenohumeral space (Fig. 108.5.A,B). The axillary projection delineates the coracoid, acromion process, and humeral head, and identifies impaction fracture (14). The scapular Y view (Fig. 108.6) best shows the position of the humeral head in relation to the Y-shaped projection of the scapula, that neither the AP nor the axillary views demonstrate as clearly (31). The humeral head normally overlies a central position on the glenoid between the coracoid and acromion processes (see Fig. 108.6.A,B); in a dislocation, it is shifted to an abnormally anterior (see Fig. 108.7.C,D), posterior, inferior, or rarely, superior position (14, 31). An additional apical oblique view may better identify a fracture of the humeral head or glenoid rim (29, 32, 33). More obscure fracture or abnormality is demonstrated by CT or MRI scans.

Indications

Dislocation of the shoulder confirmed by radiographs requires immediate reduction. Typically the adolescent presents with an anterior shoulder dislocation after a fight or sports injury. The patient is leaning forward in moderate to severe pain and has a characteristic loss of the normal shoulder contour. This asymmetry is due to an unoccupied subacromial space where the humeral head normally sits. The elbow is in flexion; the affected arm is held in abduction and external rotation, and is difficult to internally or externally rotate. Peripheral pulses, capillary refill, motor strength, and sensation are usually intact distal to the dislocation (13).

In the presence of neurovascular com-

Figure 108.6.
Scapular Y view of shoulder.
A, B. Normal.
C, D. Anterior dislocation.

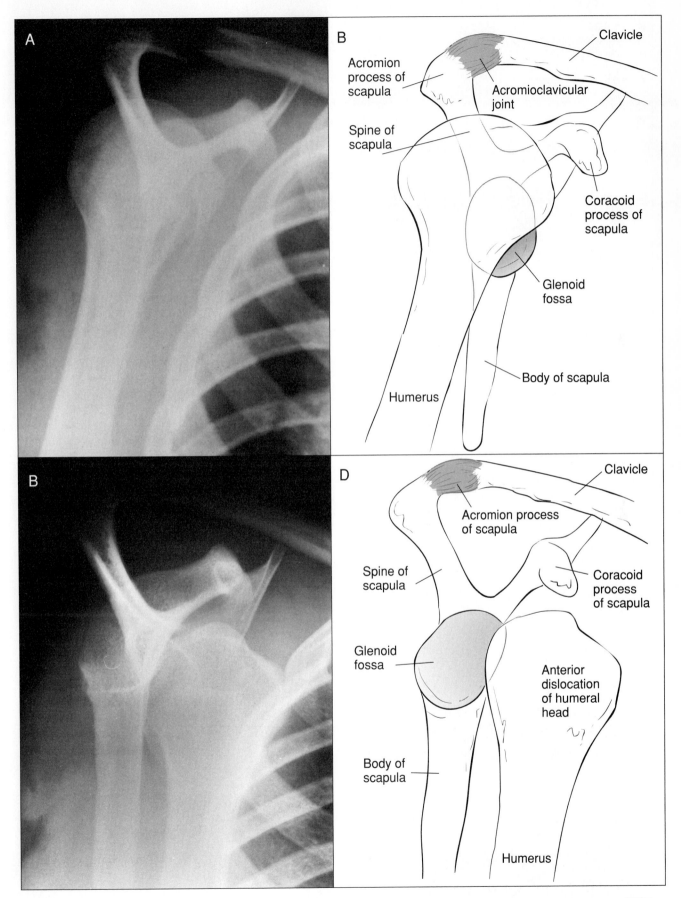

A

B

B

D

Clavicle

Acromion
process of
scapula

Acromioclavicular
joint

Spine of
scapula

Coracoid
process of
scapula

Glenoid
fossa

Body of scapula

Humerus

Clavicle

Acromion process
of scapula

Spine of
scapula

Coracoid
process
of scapula

Glenoid
fossa

Anterior
dislocation
of humeral
head

Body of
scapula

Humerus

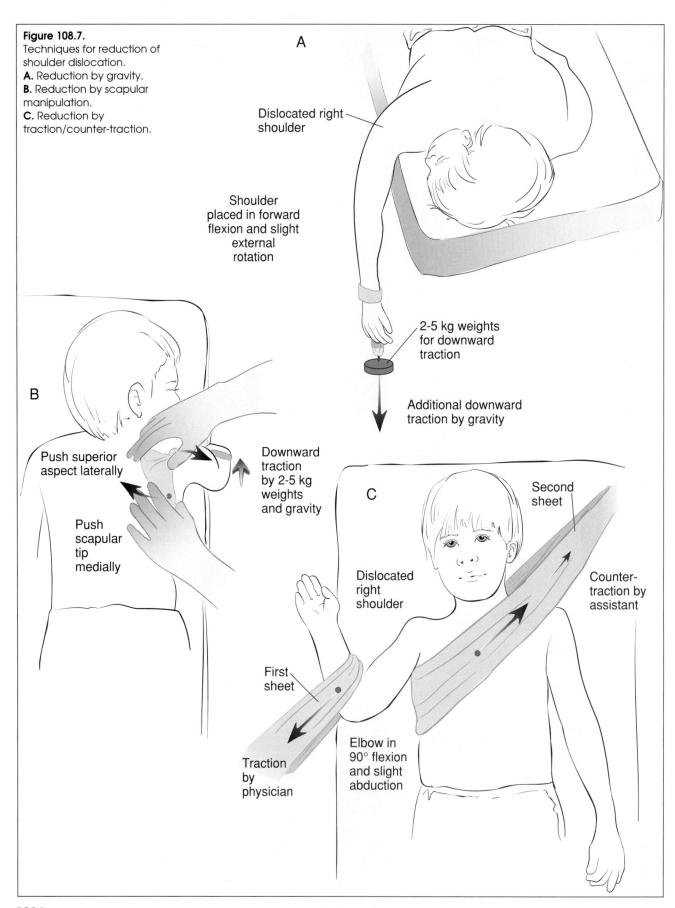

Figure 108.7.
Techniques for reduction of shoulder dislocation.
A. Reduction by gravity.
B. Reduction by scapular manipulation.
C. Reduction by traction/counter-traction.

A

Dislocated right shoulder

Shoulder placed in forward flexion and slight external rotation

2-5 kg weights for downward traction

Additional downward traction by gravity

B

Push superior aspect laterally

Push scapular tip medially

Downward traction by 2-5 kg weights and gravity

C

Second sheet

Dislocated right shoulder

Counter-traction by assistant

First sheet

Traction by physician

Elbow in 90° flexion and slight abduction

promise, humeral neck fracture, intraarticular bony fragments, or a posterior or superior (luxatio erecta humeri) dislocation, an immediate orthopaedic consultation also should be obtained. An associated humeral head fracture does not preclude reduction of a shoulder dislocation in the ED (13, 16).

Equipment

Medications for conscious sedation
Monitoring equipment
For reduction:
  Weights—2-5 kg
  or two sheets
For immobilization:
  Sling and swathe
  Shoulder immobilizer

Procedure

After interposed intraarticular fragments are excluded, the following reduction maneuvers are appropriate for the child and adolescent. Reduction may be achieved by the forward flexion-gravity maneuver and, if unsuccessful, followed by scapular manipulation or traction-countertraction techniques.

Reduction by Forward Flexion-Gravity (Fig. 108.7.A)

The patient is placed in a prone position with the affected arm hanging vertically over the edge of the stretcher. The shoulder is in forward flexion and slight external rotation. In this position, gravity offers downward traction. Additional traction is applied to the arm with 2 to 5 kg weights strapped on the wrist. With sufficient time (20 to 30 minutes), muscle relaxation and analgesia, the shoulder muscles fatigue and the humeral head gradually relocates into the glenoid fossa. When reduction occurs, the affected arm swings freely and painlessly in the forward position. Reduction requires minimal exertion or strength, even in the most muscular adolescents; no other assistance generally is needed. Although patience and a hemodynamically stable patient are required, this maneuver is atraumatic, simple, and safe. The major disadvantage of this procedure is that, while prone, the patient is less accessible if he or she requires acute resuscitation (13, 22, 23).

Reduction by Scapular Manipulation (Fig. 108.7.B)

Similar to reduction by gravity technique, the patient is placed in a prone position with the affected arm hanging vertically over the edge of the stretcher. Downward traction using 2 to 5 kg weights for 5 minutes produces muscle fatigue and relaxation of the shoulder muscles. To achieve reduction, the scapula is rotated gently by simultaneously pushing its tip medially and its superior aspect laterally. A palpable or audible "clunk" occurs with a successful reduction. This technique has similar advantages and disadvantages to reduction by gravity.

This technique also may be performed with the patient seated. When this approach is used, the patient is seated facing the back of a stable chair. The patient rests his or her chest against the back of the chair and an assistant applies traction to the affected arm. Manipulation of the scapula is performed as previously described. When shoulder reduction is accomplished by scapular manipulation, less sedation and analgesia may be required. (21, 25, 27).

Reduction by Traction-countertraction (Fig. 108.7.C)

The patient is placed in a supine position. The elbow of the affected side is in slight abduction and 90° flexion. With the physician next to the patient's hip on the side of the affected shoulder, one sheet is looped around the flexed forearm just distal to the elbow and around the physician. A second sheet is wrapped around the patient's chest under the axilla of the affected side and around the assistant; using this sheet, the assistant provides countertraction. Continuous and gradually increasing longitudinal traction on the abducted arm with countertraction across the chest gradually achieves reduction. Both the physician and the assistant may gain mechanical advantage by leaning back on the sheets. As the shoulder muscles fatigue, reduction may be assisted with gentle internal and external rotation of the shoulder. Reduction of the humeral head into the glenoid fossa often is clearly observed and occasionally may be accompanied by a palpable or audible "clunk." This technique requires more physical

Chapter 108
Reduction of
Common Joint
Dislocations and
Subluxations

1087

strength. It also may cause significant pain, and always requires a minimum of two people for reduction. (13, 28, 29).

After a successful reduction, active motion and a normal contour at the shoulder is usually restored immediately. Assessment of distal neurovascular status after reduction is crucial because of possible concurrent brachial plexus or vascular injury. Radiographs of the shoulder after reduction, including the AP and scapular Y views, confirm a successful reduction. An apical oblique view may improve diagnosis of subtle fractures of the humeral head, glenoid lip, or humeral neck (29). A sling and swathe or shoulder immobilizer applied for 1 to 3 weeks usually offers adequate immobilization (13, 14, 16, 34). Restriction of the affected arm from abduction, external rotation, and excessive use allows healing of the anterior capsule and glenoid ligaments without laxity. Immobilization may be removed for bathing (16). The patient should then be referred for orthopaedic evaluation and physical rehabilitation within 1 to 2 weeks and further restricted from sports activities for 3 to 6 weeks (15, 16, 32).

Complications

The most common complication is recurrent dislocation of the shoulder which is due to a stretched subscapular tendon and capsular laxity. The most significant factor for recurrence is age; the younger the patient, the more likely is redislocation (14-16). In patients younger than 20 years, 80 to 90% have recurrent shoulder dislocation, rising to 64% in patients younger than 30 years. Higher recurrence rates may be associated with a glenoid rim fracture or a humeral head impaction fracture of the greater tuberosity. Operative procedures may decrease recurrence rates (13, 15, 34).

Irreducible dislocations of the shoulder occur because of interposition of soft tissue, long head of the biceps tendon, or bony fragments of the greater tuberosity into the joint capsule; or bony instability from a glenoid lip fracture. Posterior dislocations should not be missed. These patients usually require an open reduction and stabilization of the shoulder joint (13).

Neural injury involves the brachial plexus in 10 to 25% of cases, and most commonly, involves the axillary nerve. Rarely in the younger child, avascular necrosis of the humeral head, vascular injury including that of the axillary artery, or degenerative arthritis occur. Muscle contracture from immobilization is unlikely in the child (15, 30). Complications of the reduction technique, although infrequent, result from excessively forceful traction and compression on neurovascular structures in the axilla. Humeral neck and spiral humeral shaft fractures occur rarely from an overly forceful attempt at reduction (14, 30).

PATELLA DISLOCATION

Introduction

In a dislocation, the patella is displaced from its normal anterior and central position on the knee joint. It is often associated with disruption of its ligamentous or tendinous attachments. Patellar dislocation most commonly occurs in the 14- to 18-year-old athletic adolescent. The injury affects predominantly adolescent girls (35, 36), the left patella (37), and participants of team sports, such as football, basketball, and baseball (37). The recurrence rate also is higher in girls than in boys. Typical mechanisms include the twisting motion of hitting a baseball or when figure iceskating, valgus stress, or a direct blow to the knee (35, 37, 38). A closed reduction maneuver usually is rapid and nearly effortless; it is commonly performed by the emergency physician in the ED (35).

Anatomy and Physiology

The patella, a triangular sesamoid bone, forms the anterior roof of the knee joint. It is embedded in the distal tendon of the quadriceps extensor femoris muscle, which inserts at the tibial tuberosity on the proximal tibia. The patella is normally located anterior and central to the knee joint (Figure 108.8).

Lateral dislocation of the patella is most common (37, 39). Sudden internal rotation of the femur on a fixed foot imparts a valgus stress (knock-knee) on the knee. Abrupt forceful contraction of the quadriceps directs

Chapter 108
Reduction of
Common Joint
Dislocations and
Subluxations

1088

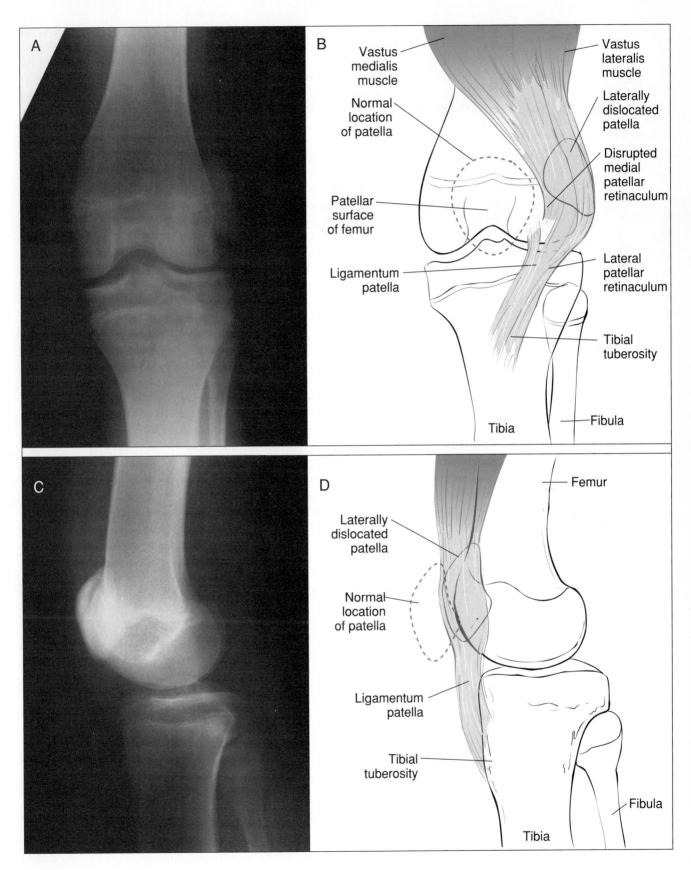

Figure 108.8.
Patella dislocation.

1089

strong lateral forces on the patella and causes the lateral displacement of the patella. A weak vastus medialis muscle is unable to oppose lateral forces on the patella imposed by the other quadriceps muscle groups (37, 39, 40). The vastus medialis muscle may tear when the knee is suddenly forced to internally rotate (38). In addition, a blow laterally directed to the medial aspect of the patella, or medially directed to the lateral knee posterior to the patella, also cause patellar dislocation (37). Dislocation of the patella causes disruption of its medial ligamentous and tendinous attachments, avulsion fracture of its medial margin, or rupture of the medial retinaculum (36, 40). A joint effusion or hemarthrosis often occurs concurrently (36, 39). A palpable defect of the vastus medialis oblique suggests muscular or ligamentous rupture (37, 39).

Individuals who are more predisposed to patellar dislocations have genu valgus (knock-knees), lateral position of the tibial tuberosity, flattened lateral femoral condyles, and weak quadriceps muscles (37, 38). In patients who are more likely to have recurrent dislocation, passive lateral hypermobility of the patella, dysplastic distal one-third of the vastus medialis oblique, high or lateral position of the patella, and history of previous dislocation or subluxation of the patella are characteristic (37). Children with Down's syndrome, neuromuscular disorders, and nail-patella syndrome have congenital ligamentous laxity and are particularly prone to patellar dislocation (37–40).

Radiographic examination of the patella requires three views of the knee joint. A standard AP and lateral view best show dislocation of the patella (Fig. 108.8). An infrapatellar or "sunrise" projection of the patella with the knee in 20° flexion offers an evaluation of the isolated patella and its integrity (38, 40). Because the patella ossifies after about age 5 years (37), the infrapatellar view is more helpful in the older child or adolescent. In a clinically apparent patellar dislocation, radiographs often are obtained after reduction (39).

Indications

An acute patellar dislocation is usually obvious by the presenting history and on clinical presentation. On examination, the knee is held in slight flexion and the patella is observed or palpated lateral to the knee. Radiographs of the knee confirm the patella's lateral location. Reduction of the clinically apparent patellar dislocation may precede obtaining radiographs.

Most often the patella reduces spontaneously before medical attention and is in its normal position on presentation to the ED. A typical history and physical examination should confirm a spontaneously reduced acute dislocation of the patella. The alert adolescent ably describes the malposition of the kneecap. A positive "apprehension sign," pain and anxiety elicited on passive lateral motion of the patella, is characteristic for an acute patellar dislocation that spontaneously reduced (37, 38). Other signs include tenderness of the medial retinaculum or excessive mobility of the patella (36, 37, 39, 40). The adolescent with spontaneous reduction must receive similar postreduction management despite the patella's apparently normal anatomic position (38, 40).

Suspicion of fracture, intraarticular pathology, osteochondral fracture, ligamentous disruption, or atypical dislocation of the patella require immediate pediatric orthopaedic consultation and possible open reduction (37, 39–42)

Equipment

For reduction: None
For immobilization:
   Standard knee immobilizer, appropriately
      sized
   or plaster splints

Procedure

Gradual full extension at the knee generally achieves reduction without complications. The patient is placed in a supine position with the hips in flexion to relax the quadriceps muscles. The knee is brought slowly to full extension; slight pressure on the laterally displaced patella applied in a medial direction facilitates reduction (Fig. 108.9). The knee joint is then evaluated for tenderness, effusion, ligamentous laxity and passive hypermobility. In a clinically apparent patellar dislocation, prompt reduction before radiog-

Chapter 108
Reduction of
Common Joint
Dislocations and
Subluxations

1090

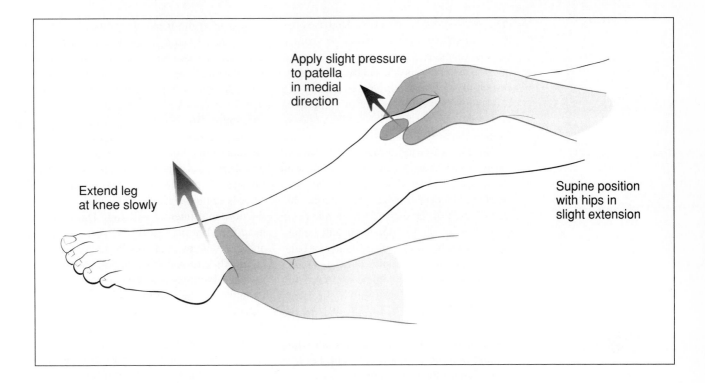

Apply slight pressure to patella in medial direction

Extend leg at knee slowly

Supine position with hips in slight extension

Figure 108.9.
Technique for reduction of patellar dislocation.

raphy quickly relieves acute severe pain and restores normal patellofemoral anatomy (35, 38, 39).

After reduction, radiographs of the knee should be obtained to exclude any fracture or avulsion. A complete series includes three views: AP, lateral, and infrapatellar. The knee should be immobilized in extension with either a standard knee immobilizer or plaster splints. Immobilization continues for up to 6 weeks with full weight bearing as tolerated. Aggressive physical therapy to strengthen the quadriceps muscles (37, 38) and evaluation by a pediatric orthopaedist at 1- to 2-week intervals are recommended (37).

Complications

Recurrent patellar dislocation is common after initial dislocation. Although 33% of adolescents of ages 15 to 18 years have recurrence, 60% of those ages 11 to 14 years recur (37). Early surgical intervention to prevent recurrence is controversial (35, 37).

Medial retinaculum rupture and osteochondral, patellar, and lateral femoral condyle fractures commonly accompany patellar dislocations and should not be missed. Degenerative changes and osteoarthritis of the patellofemoral joint may result from damage to the articular surface of the patella by intraarticular fracture or fragments (35, 36, 39, 42). Rare late complications include patellar instability due to abnormal anatomy, quadriceps atrophy, infrapatellar nerve injury, and loss of flexion and extension (38). Postreduction radiographs and orthopaedic consultation for evaluation and follow-up are crucial to the exclusion and management of these potential complications (36, 38, 40).

An irreducible dislocation of the patella may result from significant joint effusion; aspiration may aid reduction (37, 40). Rarely, an atypical dislocation occurs when the patella is rotated, intraarticular, or entrapped by the femoral condyles. Successful reduction requires an immediate pediatric orthopaedic consultation and open reduction (35, 36, 39, 42).

HIP DISLOCATION

Introduction

Dislocation of the hip joint is a true orthopaedic emergency and requires immediate orthopaedic consultation. Less than 5 to 10% of all traumatic hip dislocations occur in chil-

Chapter 108
Reduction of
Common Joint
Dislocations and
Subluxations

1091

dren (43, 44). Early reduction decreases risk of complications, such as avascular necrosis of the femoral head. Occasionally, diagnosis of a hip dislocation is delayed because of concurrent multiple organ injury, especially in a child with a severe closed head or neck injury, or an ipsilateral fracture of the pelvis or femoral shaft (43–46).

In the older child or adolescent, violent forces are necessary to cause hip dislocation and the patient should be managed first as a victim of multiple trauma. Stabilization and management of the patient's respiratory and hemodynamic status should precede reduction of a limb with no distal neurovascular compromise (47). Examples of high velocity trauma include motor vehicle collision, fall from a great height, and sports injury from football or skiing (43, 44, 47, 48). In the younger child, hip dislocation also may result from low energy forces, such as a fall while running or a fall from a low height, because of their generalized ligamentous laxity (43, 44, 47, 49). Hip dislocation appears to be more common than hip fracture in the younger child (45, 46, 50).

Posterior hip dislocations are more commonly seen than anterior hip dislocations in both children and adults (43, 44, 47–52). Very rarely, central dislocations occur through a ruptured triradiate cartilage (44). More boys sustain hip dislocations than girls (43, 44, 48–55). Associated acetabular injury and ipsilateral long bone fracture are common in the older child or adolescent (43, 45, 46, 54).

After treatment of hemodynamic instability and life-threatening injury, closed reduction of traumatic posterior dislocation of the hip without associated fracture may be performed in the acute setting by the emergency physician or with an orthopaedic surgeon. Anterior hip dislocations are usually reduced in the operating suite with general anesthesia.

Anatomy and Physiology

The femoral head articulates with the acetabulum of the pelvis to form the hip joint (Fig. 108.10). The acetabulum is formed by the confluence of the ilium, ischium, and pubis; its physis is the triradiate cartilage. Growth of the acetabulum progresses in a centrifugal direction until the triradiate cartilage fuses at age 15 to 18 years. Trauma to the triradiate cartilage or a central dislocation through the triradiate cartilage may present with acetabular dysplasia during adulthood. Such injury may be overlooked during initial trauma resuscitation (56–58).

Dislocation of the hip joint results from an acute force that thrusts the femoral head and shaft against the acetabulum. A posterior dislocation of the femoral head occurs if the force is applied when the hip is in flexion, adduction, and internal rotation. The femoral head then lies posteriorly between the ilium and the ischium. A child who falls onto both knees while running or tripping, and an adolescent who impacts a knee against the car's dashboard while a passenger in a motor vehicle collision are typical examples of when the disruptive force is directed posteriorly and results in a posterior dislocation. The sciatic nerve which traverses posterior to the femoral head may be injured from a posteriorly dislocated hip (49, 51, 57). Rarely, traumatic posterior hip dislocation is associated with concurrent separation of the femoral capital epiphysis (50).

An anterior dislocation of the femoral head results if force is applied on the hip when it is in abduction, external rotation, and extension. In an anterior dislocation, the femoral head lies anteriorly between the ilium and the pubis and is more frequently associated with neurovascular compression or injury of structures in the inguinal canal. A child who rides a sled into a tree and an adolescent who is the victim of a football tackle are examples of inflicted forces that cause anterior dislocation of the hip from excessive abduction and extension. Compression of the femoral vessels or other inguinal structures may result from an anterior hip dislocation (47, 49, 52, 57).

The metaphyseal and epiphyseal vascular supply to the femoral head remain functionally separate until physeal closure at puberty. Branches of the lateral and medial femoral circumflex artery provide the major vascular supply to the femoral head. Until ages 5 or 6 years, the lateral femoral circumflex artery is the major supplier; thereafter, the terminal lateral epiphyseal branches of the medial femoral circumflex artery predominate. Although the artery of the ligamentum teres, a branch of the obturator

Chapter 108
Reduction of
Common Joint
Dislocations and
Subluxations

1092

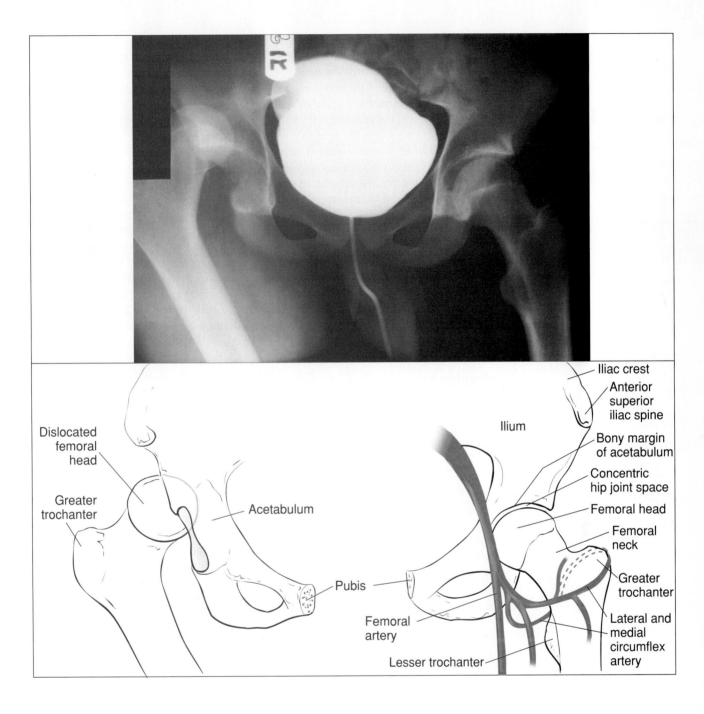

Labels on figure:

Dislocated femoral head

Greater trochanter

Acetabulum

Pubis

Iliac crest

Anterior superior iliac spine

Ilium

Bony margin of acetabulum

Concentric hip joint space

Femoral head

Femoral neck

Greater trochanter

Lateral and medial circumflex artery

Femoral artery

Lesser trochanter

Figure 108.10.
Normal (*left*) and dislocated (*right*) hip.

artery, is a lessor contributor to the femoral head, it is most often torn in a hip dislocation (44, 60). A dislocated femoral head frequently compresses or injures these vessels. Slow progressive ischemia, intracapsular hematoma, and avascular necrosis of the femoral head result. Reduction within 6 hours of dislocation appears to decrease risk of avascular necrosis of the femoral head in the adult. Factors that increase risk for avascular necrosis include more severe trauma, delayed reduction, older age, and concomitant injury

to the hip and pelvis (43, 44, 47, 51, 59, 61, 62).

In the older adolescent or adult, dislocations are often associated with fracture of the acetabular rim, femoral neck, greater trochanter, pelvic ring, or sacroiliac joint (49, 54). These fractures result from impaction forces directed through the ipsilateral femoral head or through the foot with leg extended. Examples include a flexed knee against the dashboard or a vertical fall onto a fully extended leg (43, 47, 58). Blunt trauma to the hip and pelvis also may injure adjacent pelvic and intraabdominal organs, particularly the bladder, urethra, and pelvic vasculature.

A true AP projection of the pelvis is crucial for accurate radiographic diagnosis; the hips must be in neutral position (Fig. 108.10). Inlet and outlet views assess the integrity of the hip joint and an AP posterior oblique view at 45° (LeTour-Judet view) defines the acetabulum (58). Normally, the contour of the femoral head is concentric with respect to the acetabulum. Deviation from this concentric relationship implies a hip dislocation. Imaging by CT and MRI scan best delineates fracture of the acetabulum, acetabular rim, and posterior articular surface, intra-articular fracture or fragments, and associated pelvic fracture. Radiographic diagnosis is further enhanced by angiography and arthrography (58, 63).

Indications

Dislocation of the hip requires immediate reduction to avoid further potential injury to the femoral head and to relieve patient discomfort. In a posterior hip dislocation, the hip appears to be in fixed adduction, internal rotation, and flexion, with some degree of thigh shortening. In an anterior hip dislocation, the hip presents in excessive abduction, external rotation, and extension, without leg length shortening. In both posterior and anterior dislocations, the hip is markedly tender but usually without swelling or ecchymosis. Radiograph of the AP hip confirms dislocation (44, 45, 47).

Suspicion of any of the following requires immediate pediatric orthopaedic consultation and open reduction: open dislocation, neurovascular injury, acetabular fracture, ipsilateral femur or pelvic fracture, a nonconcentric or loss of joint cavity space, or central dislocation with triradiate cartilage disruption (44, 46, 56). If the patient is expected to receive general anesthesia for other surgical procedures, reduction of the hip dislocation should be done intraoperatively.

Equipment

Medications for conscious sedation; consider general anesthesia
Monitoring equipment

For reduction:
Minimum of two assistants
For immobilization:
Leg traction device or materials for spica cast

Procedure

Reduction of a hip dislocation follows initial trauma resuscitation in the patient with multiple trauma. A successful reduction requires adequate analgesia and muscle relaxation for the patient, in addition to optimal mechanical advantage for the physician. The reduction maneuver or the side effects of parenteral sedation may compromise the hemodynamically unstable patient. In the younger child, administration of general anesthesia is preferred over outpatient sedation techniques.

To achieve reduction, the femoral head must be maneuvered laterally and anteriorly from its dislocated position posterior and medial to the acetabular rim. The patient is positioned with the affected hip and knee each in 90° flexion; the hip in slight internal rotation and adduction (Fig. 108.11). An assistant stabilizes the pelvis with downward immobilization on both anterior iliac crests. Continuous traction to the distal femur in line with the deformity fatigues and overcomes muscle spasm. The femoral head, aided by gentle rotatory motion of the femur, is gradually brought over the posterior acetabular rim and into the acetabulum (45, 46, 52, 64, 65).

The patient may be placed in a prone position (Fig. 108.11.A) with the thigh hanging vertically from the stretcher and downward vertical traction applied on the femur (45). In this position, gravity offers an additional mechanical advantage during downward traction. Excessive force is generally not needed. Or, the patient may be supine and upward traction applied (Fig. 108.11.B). The physician then frequently mounts the stretcher to gain mechanical advantage.

With a successful reduction, the hip and knee should extend easily with minimal soft tissue resistance (45). To maintain reduction, the hip is maintained in anatomic position, slight abduction and external rotation, using longitudinal traction in the older child or a spica cast in the younger child. An isolated hip dislocation requires a minimum of 7 to 10 days of hospitalization with bed rest. Al-

Chapter 108
Reduction of
Common Joint
Dislocations and
Subluxations

1094

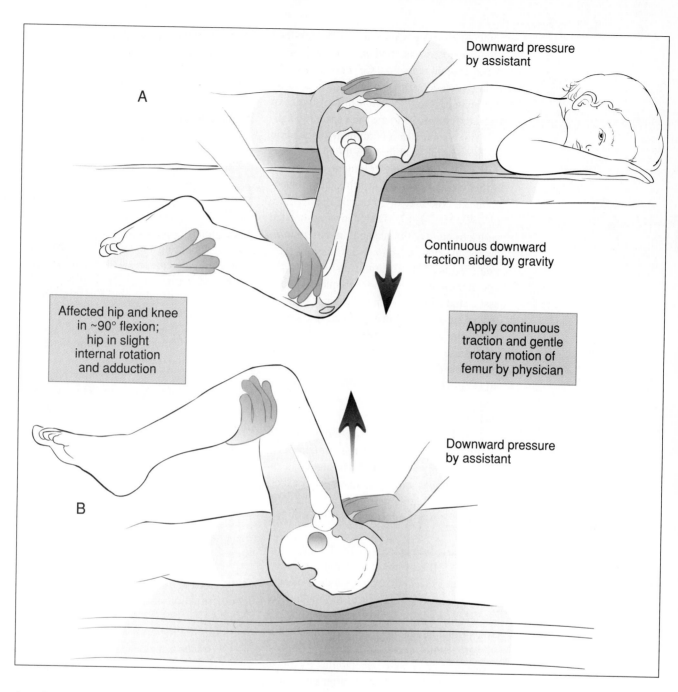

A

Downward pressure
by assistant

Continuous downward
traction aided by gravity

Affected hip and knee
in ~90° flexion;
hip in slight
internal rotation
and adduction

Apply continuous
traction and gentle
rotary motion of
femur by physician

Downward pressure
by assistant

B

though specific recommendations vary, a 4- to 6-week period of nonweight bearing and immobilization allows for soft tissue healing after dislocation (45, 46). Weight bearing on the hip generally begins 6 to 8 weeks after dislocation if CT or MRI scan is normal. This may begin earlier for the younger child and later for the adolescent (44, 49, 51, 52, 61).

A concentric hip joint space on postreduction radiographs confirms a successful reduction after the initial maneuver and during hospitalization. Early use of CT, MRI, angiography, or bone scan detects interposed

tissue, impaired perfusion, or ischemic changes of the femoral head. The child or adolescent with hip dislocation should be followed until skeletal maturity with interval radiographic imaging (44, 45, 50, 63).

Complications

Unsuccessful reduction by a closed maneuver is the most frequent complication and usually presents as nonconcentric reduction or loss of

Figure 108.11.
Techniques for reduction of hip joint dislocation.

Chapter 108
Reduction of
Common Joint
Dislocations and
Subluxations

1095

joint cavity space. Concentric reduction then requires closed reduction under general anesthesia or open reduction. Common causes for failure include inadequate muscle relaxation and analgesia, interposition of soft tissue or fracture fragment into the joint space, acetabular rim fracture, or a buttonhole dislocation of the femoral head through the hip capsule. Soft tissue or fracture fragment may result from avulsion fracture, torn ligament, osteochondral fracture, or intraarticular fracture (44, 49, 50, 54, 57). Dislocation associated with a fracture of the acetabulum or femur requires an open reduction with internal fixation (51, 54, 57). Recurrent dislocations are uncommon and occur more frequently when associated with severe initial trauma, delayed reduction, a concurrent acetabular fracture, or a capsular tear (49, 57, 58).

Missed diagnosis of dislocation of the hip occurs frequently in the presence of an ipsilateral femur fracture, separation of femoral capital epiphysis, young age (younger than 8 years), and central dislocations (52, 54, 57, 59, 63). Unrecognized dislocation or vascular injury increases the child's risk for complications. Complications of the reduction technique, although rare, may result from excessive force; ligamentous injury to the knee occurs if it was used as a fulcrum for reduction.

Avascular necrosis of the femoral head occurs in 10% of hip dislocations. The incidence of avascular necrosis increases with delayed reduction, injury to the medial circumflex artery, or persistent or enlarging intracapsular hematoma. A child should be followed until skeletal maturity because avascular necrosis or acetabular dysplasia may present 2 or more years after dislocation (43, 44, 49, 51, 52, 54, 57, 59, 66).

Limited ROM, pain, weakness, fatigue, and limp are common after a dislocation of the hip. These symptoms generally resolve with strengthening and ROM exercises. Late complications are unusual in children, including residual symptoms, narrowing of the joint space, thigh atrophy, osteoarthritis, femoral head deformity, acetabular dysplasia, or ectopic bone formation. An adduction deformity may result from physeal injury or avascular necrosis of the femoral head (43, 47, 48, 50–52, 54, 57, 60, 66).

REDUCTION OF JOINT DISLOCATIONS WITH NEUROVASCULAR COMPROMISE

Introduction

Isolated dislocation of the elbow, knee, or ankle are rare in children, but have the greatest association with neurovascular compromise. These dislocations are therefore true orthopaedic emergencies. The elbow, knee, and ankle joints dislocate only after violent forces such as that from motor vehicle related injuries, and often present with significant neurovascular compromise. Dislocations of this nature do not usually occur before adolescence. The forces necessary to dislocate these joints usually fracture the bones. Reduction of these dislocations should be immediately managed by the orthopaedist.

Reduction by the emergency physician may be reasonable, however, in the event that an orthopaedist is not immediately available *and* the injured limb shows signs or symptoms of acute neurovascular compromise. As in any child or adolescent with injuries caused by excessive forces, concurrent stabilization and management of the patient's respiratory and hemodynamic status are imperative. If the patient is expected to receive general anesthesia for other surgical procedures, reduction of dislocation should be done intraoperatively.

Reduction methods using traction and countertraction are generally successful for joint dislocations with neurovascular compromise. Radiographs after reduction reveal likely fracture, persistent malalignment, or other bony abnormality. Emergent evaluation by arteriography reveals arterial damage such as intimal tears, not otherwise clinically apparent. Exploration under general anesthesia best enables anatomic reduction and vascular or ligamentous repair of the affected joint. Reduction methods for dislocation of the elbow, knee, and ankle are described in this section.

Indications
Complete dislocation of the elbow, knee, and ankle show gross deformity which may be confirmed by diagnostic radiography. Dislocations with neurovascular compromise re-

Chapter 108
Reduction of
Common Joint
Dislocations and
Subluxations

1096

quire immediate reduction and do not absolutely require radiographs before reduction. Any joint dislocation that has persistent neurovascular deficits, or that cannot attain or maintain anatomical reduction, must be managed intraoperatively.

Equipment

Medications for conscious sedation; consider general anesthesia
Monitoring equipment
For reduction: None or assistant(s)
For immobilization: Splinting and strapping materials

Complications

Associated fractures, which occur commonly, must be excluded by radiographs after reduction. Irreducible dislocation, open dislocation, or dislocation with associated intraarticular fracture requires exploration and open reduction. Observation for neurovascular deficits, ischemia, or compartment syndrome should be continuous, aggressive, and is best initially as an inpatient.

Elbow Dislocation

Elbow dislocation is the displacement of both the proximal radius and the ulna from their respective articulation with the distal humerus. A posterior dislocation is most common and affects the nondominant elbow, occurs mostly in adolescent males, and is associated with forceful impact onto the hyperextended arm. Isolated dislocation without associated fracture is unusual—50 to 60% of children have associated fracture of the distal humerus, radial head, or coronoid process (3, 67–69).

Stretch injury to the ulnar nerve occurs frequently from elbow dislocation. Although neurovascular injury is uncommon in isolated elbow dislocations in children, early recognition is imperative. Careful examination of the hand and forearm should include capillary refill, radial and ulnar pulses for potential brachial artery injury; and motor and sensory components of the radial, median, and ulnar nerves for possible injury. Reduction optimally should occur in less than 2 hours after dislocation. If greater than 4 hours, the incidence of complications increase (3, 67, 69).

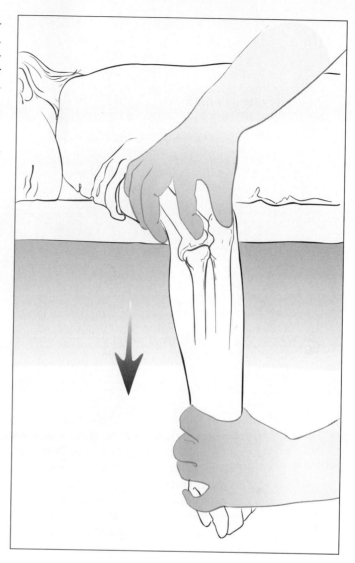

Procedure

With the patient in prone position, either the entire arm or only the forearm is allowed to hang over the side of the stretcher (Fig. 108.12). Traction is applied to the proximal forearm with the elbow in slight (70 to 80°) flexion, either by the physician or with weights for 15 to 20 minutes. Gentle countertraction on the humerus may be applied by an assistant. Forward and downward force applied to the olecranon with the physician's thumbs with simultaneous gentle elbow flexion usually affects reduction. Immobilization with a posterior splint with the elbow in 90° flexion remains for 2 to 3 weeks (3, 70, 71).

Complications

Hyperextension or pronation of the elbow during dislocation or reduction may cause en-

Figure 108.12.
Technique for reduction of elbow joint dislocation.

Chapter 108
Reduction of
Common Joint
Dislocations and
Subluxations

1097

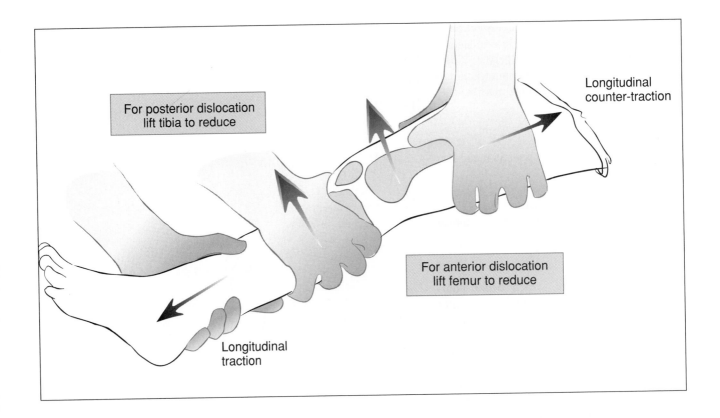

For posterior dislocation
lift tibia to reduce

Longitudinal
counter-traction

For anterior dislocation
lift femur to reduce

Longitudinal
traction

Figure 108.13.
Technique for reduction of
knee joint dislocation.

trapment or injury of the median or ulnar nerve, brachial artery, or brachialis muscle. Failure to recognize associated fracture of medical epicondyle, proximal radius, or coronoid process should be avoided. Long-term complications include flexion contracture, valgus instability, or heterotopic bone formation (3, 69, 72–75).

Knee Dislocation

Knee dislocation is the displacement of the tibiofemoral articulation. It is associated commonly with popliteal artery tear (30 to 40%) and peroneal nerve injury (10 to 15%). Knee dislocation involves the rupture of both anterior and posterior cruciate ligaments and disruption of the collateral ligaments. Anterior dislocation is most common and usually occurs with popliteal artery injury. Acute hyperextension of the knee causes rupture of the anterior cruciate ligament and posterior capsule, which allows anterior tibiofemoral displacement. Posterolateral dislocation is associated with peroneal nerve damage. Typically, knee dislocation occurs after a motor vehicle crash; significant dislocations are often reduced at the scene (76–80).

The popliteal artery is at particular risk of intimal tears because it is anchored and vulnerable in the popliteal fossa. Popliteal artery disruption causes distal ischemia, vascular occlusion, and limb loss if reduction is delayed or left undiagnosed. The peroneal (tibial and common peroneal) nerve usually sustains traction injury although less frequently. Careful distal examination of the lower leg and foot should include capillary refill, dorsalis pedis pulse, posterior tibial pulse, and peroneal nerve function. Presence of distal peripheral pulses and capillary refill does not preclude arterial injury. Arteriography best defines vascular integrity. Knee dislocation also is associated with tibial spine fracture, osteochondral fractures of the femur or tibia, and meniscal injuries; these injuries represent avulsion fractures secondary to an anterior cruciate ligament tear. Reduction optimally should occur in less than 6 hours after dislocation. If greater than 6 to 8 hours, the incidence of limb loss is greater than 85% (79–83).

Procedure
With the patient in prone position, gentle longitudinal traction is applied to the lower leg (Fig. 108.13). To reduce an anterior disloca-

tion, the femur is lifted anteriorly or the proximal tibia pushed posteriorly into anatomic position. For a posterior dislocation, extension at the knee and lifting the proximal tibia into the reduced position follows longitudinal traction. After reduction, poor distal pulses or perfusion requires immediate surgical exploration. Arteriography should be obtained after reduction of any knee dislocation and when performed for abnormal circulation should not delay vascular repair. Reconstruction of ligaments occurs after reduction in a timely fashion but need not be immediate. Immobilization with a posterior splint of the knee in 15° flexion occurs for 4 to 6 weeks (77–79).

Complications
Pressure to the popliteal area or hyperextension at the knee must be avoided to prevent further popliteal artery or peroneal nerve damage. Popliteal artery injury or associated fracture should not be missed. Irreducible dislocation may be secondary to interposed soft tissue, entrapment of the medial femoral condyle, buttonhole tear in the medial capsule, or ligamentous instability. Popliteal artery thrombosis or peroneal nerve deficits may present after reduction and lead to significant neurologic deficits or limb loss (77, 78, 81–84).

Ankle Dislocation

Ankle dislocation is the displacement of the distal tibia and fibula from their articulation with the talus bone of the foot. All ligamentous and capsular attachments from the tibia and fibula to the talus are usually torn. Posterior dislocation occurs most commonly and results from forced plantar flexion. Anterior dislocation results from forced dorsiflexion of the foot or a direct blow to the heel when

Figure 108.14.
Technique for reduction of ankle joint dislocation.

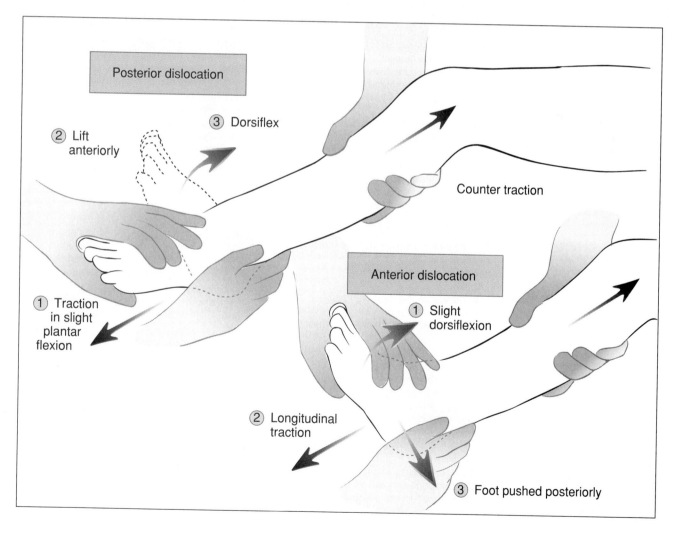

the foot is in dorsiflexion. Ankle dislocations usually have concurrent fracture of the malleoli (85–88).

Procedure

The patient is placed in a supine position with the knee in slight (30° to 45°) flexion (Fig. 108.14). Traction is applied to the foot by the physician while countertraction in the long axis of the limb is applied to the calf and proximal lower leg by an assistant. The physician's dominant hand holds the heel and the other hand grasps the forefoot. Traction and countertraction is applied with the foot in slight plantar flexion for a posterior dislocation, or in slight dorsiflexion for an anterior dislocation. To reduce a posterior dislocation, the foot is then lifted anteriorly and dorsiflexed gently. For an anterior dislocation, the foot is brought into further dorsiflexion. The foot is then pushed posteriorly and plantar flexed gently. A second assistant may apply additional force on the distal tibia: posteriorly directed in a posterior dislocation, or anteriorly directed in an anterior dislocation. Successful reduction is evident by the position of the talus in the mortise, a joint line that is parallel to the ground. Immobilization with a posterior splint followed by cast with the ankle in neutral position occurs for at least 4 to 6 weeks (87).

SUMMARY

Radial Head Subluxation
1. Have child sit comfortably in caretaker's lap
2. Support child's arm in nondominant hand, applying moderate pressure on radial head with thumb or fingers
3. Hold child's wrist in dominant hand, placing fingers on volar aspect of wrist and thumb on dorsal aspect
4. Apply gentle longitudinal traction to arm
5. While maintaining traction, in one motion supinate arm then fully flex it
6. An audible reduction click may be heard
7. If procedure is successful, child should be using arm within 20 to 30 minutes
8. If several appropriate attempts fail, radiographs should be obtained
9. If radiographs are normal, child should be placed in a sling and referred to an orthopedist; spontaneous reduction may occur in a day or two

Digit Dislocation
1. Remove all rings from affected finger and achieve anesthesia with a digital block.
2. Securely brace affected hand or foot
3. Apply gentle traction to affected digit.
4. For dorsal dislocation joint is gently hyperextended; for volar dislocation, hyperflexed
5. Push dislocated phalanx into its proper position
6. Obtain radiographs after reduction and splint digit

Shoulder Dislocation
A. Reduction by gravity
1. Use appropriate analgesia and sedation and monitor patient
2. Have patient lie on stretcher in prone position with affected arm dangling over side
3. Attach 2 to 5 kg weight to arm
4. Allow arm to hang for 20 to 40 minutes
5. After reduction arm will swing freely and painlessly in forward position

B-1. Reduction by scapular manipulation—prone position
1. Use appropriate analgesia and sedation and monitor patient
2. Have patient lie on stretcher in prone position with affected arm hanging over side
3. Attach 2 to 5 kg weight to arm or have assistant apply downward traction to arm
4. Gently rotate scapula by simultaneously pushing its tip medially and its superior aspect laterally
5. An audible or palpable "clunk" occurs with successful reduction.

B-2. Reduction by scapular manipulation—seated position
1. Use appropriate analgesia and sedation, if needed
2. Have patient sit in chair facing back of chair
3. While assistant applies forward traction to affected arm, scapula is rotated as described in B-1

C. Reduction by traction-countertraction
1. Use appropriate analgesia and sedation and monitor patient
2. Patient is placed in supine position with elbow of affected side in slight abduction and 90° of flexion.
3. Sheet is looped around flexed forearm distal to elbow, then around clinician (clinician should be standing next to hip on affected side)
4. Have assistant loop second sheet about himself or herself and then around patient's chest under axilla on affected side.
5. Exert continuous longitudinal traction on affected arm, gradually increasing force until the reduction is achieved—it may be necessary to lean back against sheets to gain mechanical advantage

Chapter 108
Reduction of
Common Joint
Dislocations and
Subluxations

1100

Patella Dislocation

1. Use appropriate analgesia and sedation and monitor patient
2. Place patient in supine position with hips in flexion
3. Bring knee joint to full extension while gradually applying medial pressure on patella to achieve reduction
4. Appropriately immobilize knee after examination

Hip Dislocation

A. Supine position
1. Use appropriate analgesia and sedation and monitor patient
2. Place patient in supine position with both hip and knee in 90° flexion and hip in slightly internal rotation and adduction
3. Have assistant stabilize pelvis with downward pressure applied to both iliac crests
4. Apply continuous traction to distal femur in line with deformity
5. Use gentle rotary motion of femur to gradually bring femoral head over posterior acetabular rim and into the acetabulum
B. Prone Position
1. Use appropriate analgesia and sedation and monitor patient
2. Place patient in prone position with thigh hanging vertically from stretcher
3. Apply downward vertical traction on distal femur until reduction is achieved

For both techniques, postreduction radiographs should be obtained. Casting may be needed for appropriate immobilization.

Posterior Elbow Dislocation

1. Use appropriate analgesia and sedation and monitor patient
2. Apply traction to proximal forearm with elbow slightly flexed.
3. Apply forward and downward pressure to olecranon while flexing elbow.
4. Apply appropriate immobilization.

Knee Dislocation

1. Use appropriate analgesia and sedation as needed and monitor patient
2. Place patient in prone position
3-A. For anterior dislocation lift femur anteriorly or push proximal tibia posteriorly.
3-B. For posterior dislocation, apply longitudinal traction then extend knee while lifting proximal tibia into reduced position
4. Angiography should be performed after reduction.
5. If no vascular injury is present, immobilize appropriately.

Ankle Dislocation

1. Use appropriate analgesia and sedation as needed and monitor patient
2. Place patient in supine position
3. Apply traction to foot while assistant applies countertraction to lower leg; dominant hand should hold heel and nondominant hand the forefoot
4. For posterior dislocation, apply traction with foot in a slight plantar flexion
5. For posterior dislocation, lift foot anteriorly while gently dorsiflexing it
6. For anterior dislocation, apply the traction with foot in slight dorsiflexion
7. For anterior dislocation, further dorsiflex foot then push it posteriorly while plantar flexing it gently
8. Immobilize ankle appropriately

Complications

Anterior or posterior tibial vessel injury or avascular necrosis of the talus are common after ankle dislocation. Other complications include posttraumatic arthritis, recurrent subluxation of the peroneal tendons, talar instability, or sympathetic dystrophy. Nonunion or malunion with deformity may occur if there is concurrent fracture (85, 87, 88).

REFERENCES

1. Boyette DP, Ahoskie NC, London AH. Subluxation of the head of the radius "nursemaid's elbow." J Pediatr 1948;32:278–281.
2. Salter RB, Zaltz C. Anatomic investigations of the mechanism of injury and pathologic anatomy of "pulled elbow" in young children. Clin Orthop 1971;77:134–143.
3. Ogden JA. Elbow. In: Ogden JA, ed. Skeletal injury in the child. 2nd ed. Philadelphia: WB Saunders, 1990, pp. 425–449.
4. Quan L, Marcuse EK. The epidemiology and treatment of radial head subluxation. Am J Dis Child 1985;139:1194–1197.
5. Schunk JE. Radial head subluxation: epidemiology and treatment of 87 episodes. Ann Emerg Med 1990; 19:1019–1023.
6. Frumkin K. Nursemaid's elbow: a radiographic demonstration. Ann Emerg Med 1985;14:690–693.
7. Snyder HS. Radiographic changes with radial head subluxation in children. J Emerg Med 1990; 8:265–269.
8. Jobe MT. Fracture and dislocations of the hand. In: Gustilo RB, Kyle RF, Templeman DC, eds. Fractures and dislocations. St. Louis: CV Mosby, 1993, pp. 611–644.
9. Beatty E, Light TR, Belsole RJ, Ogden JA. Wrist and hand skeletal injuries in children. Hand Clin 1990;6(4):723–738.
10. Thayer DT. Distal interphalangeal joint injuries. Hand Clin 1988;4(1):1–4.

CLINICAL TIPS

1. Use analgesia and sedation as needed.
2. Restraint may sometimes be required.
3. Monitor the patient well.
4. Consider the possibility of neurovascular compromise.
5. Seek orthopaedic consultation in dislocations with significant potential morbidity BUT if a consultant cannot be available in a timely fashion, attempt to reduce the dislocation.
6. After a successful reduction, immobilize the joint appropriately.

**Chapter 108
Reduction of
Common Joint
Dislocations and
Subluxations**

11. Vicar AJ. Proximal interphalangeal joint dislocations without fractures. Hand Clin 1988;4(1):5–13.

12. Khuri SM. Irreducible dorsal dislocation of the distal interphalangeal joint of the finger. J Trauma 1984;24(5):456–457.

13. Riebel GD, McCabe JB. Anterior shoulder dislocation: a review of reduction techniques. Am J Emerg Med 1991;9(2):180–188.

14. Plummer D, Clinton J. The external rotation method for reduction of acute anterior shoulder dislocation. Emerg Med Clin North Am 1989;7(1):165–175.

15. Hoelen MA, Burgers AMJ, Rozing PM. Prognosis of primary anterior shoulder dislocation in young adults. Arch Orthop Trauma Surg 1990;110(1):51–54.

16. Yu J. Anterior shoulder dislocations. J Fam Pract 1992;35(5):567–571,575–576.

17. Davids JR, Talbott RD. Luxatio erecta humeri. A case report. Clin Orthop 1990;(252):144–149.

18. Garnavos C. Technical note: modifications and improvements of the Milch technique for the reduction of the anterior dislocation of the shoulder without premedication. J Trauma 1992;32(6):801–803.

19. Janecki CJ, Shahcheragh GH. The forward elevation maneuver for reduction of anterior dislocations of the shoulder. Clin Orthop 1982;164:177–180.

20. Danzl DF, Vicario SJ, Gleis GL, Yates JR, Parks DL. Closed reduction of anterior subcoracoid shoulder dislocation. Evaluation of an external rotation method. Orthop Rev 1986;15(5):311–315.

21. Kothari RU, Dronen SC. Prospective evaluation of the scapular manipulation technique in reducing anterior shoulder dislocations. Ann Emerg Med 1992;21(11):1349–1352.

22. Stimson LA. An easy method of reducing dislocations of the shoulder and hip. Med Record 1900;57:356–357.

23. Lippert FG. A modification of the gravity method of reducing anterior shoulder dislocations. Clin Orthop 1982;165:259–260.

24. Waldron VD, Hazel D. Tips of the trade: 37. Technique for reduction of shoulder dislocation. Orthop Rev 1991;20(6):563,566.

25. Anderson D, Zvirbulis R, Ciullo J. Scapular manipulation for reduction of anterior shoulder dislocations. Clin Orthop 1982;164:181–183.

26. Kothari RU, Dronen SC. The scapular manipulation technique for the reduction of acute anterior shoulder dislocations. J Emerg Med 1990;8:625–628.

27. McNamara RM. Reduction of anterior shoulder dislocations by scapular manipulation. Ann Emerg Med 1993;22(7):1140–1144.

28. Hippocrates. Injuries of the shoulder. Dislocations. Clin Orthop 1989;246:4–7.

29. Harvey RA, Trabulsy ME, Roe L. Are postreduction anteroposterior and scapular Y views useful in anterior shoulder dislocations? Am J Emerg Med 1992;10(2):149–151.

30. Travlos J, Goldberg I, Boome RS. Brachial plexus lesions associated with dislocated shoulders. J Bone Joint Surg [Br] 1990;72B(1):68–71.

31. Silfverskiold JP, Straehley DJ, Jones WW. Roentgenographic evaluation of suspected shoulder dislocation: a prospective study comparing the axillary view and the scapular Y view. Orthopaedics 1990;13(1):63–69.

32. Garth WP, Slappey CE, Ochs CW. Roentgenographic demonstration of instability of the shoulder: the apical oblique projection. A technical note. J Bone Joint Surg [Am] 1984;66A(9):1450–1453.

33. Kornguth PJ, Salazar AM. The apical oblique view of the shoulder: its usefulness in acute trauma. AJR Am J Roentgenol 1987;149(1):113–116.

34. Marans HJ, Angel KR, Schemitsch EH, Wedge JH. The fate of traumatic anterior dislocation of the shoulder in children. J Bone Joint Surg [Am] 1992;74A(8):1242–1244.

35. Cofield RH, Bryan RS. Acute dislocation of the patella: results of conservative treatment. J Trauma 1977;17(7):526–531.

36. Vainionpaa S, Laasonen E, Silvennoinen T, Vasenius J, Rokkanen P. Acute dislocation of the patella. J Bone Joint Surg [Br] 1990;72B(3):366–369.

37. Cash J, Hughston JC. Treatment of acute patellar dislocation. Am J Sports Med 1988;16(3):244–249.

38. Kettelkamp DB. Management of patellar malalignment. J Bone Joint Surg [Am] 1981;63A(8):1344–1348.

39. Bassett FH. Acute dislocation of the patella, osteochondral fractures, and injuries to the extensor mechanism of the knee. Instr Course Lect 1976;25:40–49.

40. McManus F, Rang M, Heslin DJ. Acute dislocation of the patella in children. The natural history. Clin Orthop 1979;139:88–91.

41. Carragher AM, Todd A, Blake G. Acute traumatic lateral patellar dislocation. Ann Emerg Med 1989;18:1362–1363. 42. Corso SJ, Thal R, Forman D. Locked patellar dislocation with vertical axis rotation. A case report. Clin Orthop 1992;279:190–193.

43. Hougaard K, Thomsen PB. Traumatic hip dislocation in children. Follow up of 13 cases. Orthopaedics 1989;12(3):375–378.

44. Rieger H, Pennig D, Klein W, Grunert J. Traumatic dislocation of the hip in young children. Arch Orthop Trauma Surg 1991;110(2):114–117.

45. Ogden JA. Hip. In: Ogden JA, ed. Skeletal injury in the child. 2nd ed. Philadelphia: WB Saunders, 1990, pp. 661–682.

46. Canale ST, King RE. Fractures of the hip. Traumatic dislocations. In: Rockwood CA, Wilkins KE, King RE, eds. Fractures in children. Vol. 3. 3rd ed. Philadelphia: JB Lippincott, 1991, pp. 1093–1116.

47. McGoff JP, Ramoska EA. Traumatic hip dislocation in a child. Ann Emerg Med 1987;16(1):108–110.

48. Leenen LP, van der Werken C. Traumatic posterior luxation of the hip. Neth J Surg 1990;42(5):136–139.

49. Offierski CM. Traumatic dislocation of the hip in children. J Bone Joint Surg [Br] 1981;63B(2):194–197.

50. Bennett JT, Cash JD. Reduction of a non–concentrically relocated hip dislocation in a 7-year-old boy. Clin Orthop 1992;(280):208–213.

51. Schlonsky J, Miller PR. Traumatic hip dislocations in children. J Bone Joint Surg [Am] 1973;55A(5):1057–1063.

52. Barquet A. Traumatic anterior dislocation of the hip in childhood. Injury 1982;13(5):435–440.

53. Thompson VP, Epstein HC. Traumatic dislocation of the hip. A survey of 204 cases covering a period

Chapter 108
Reduction of
Common Joint
Dislocations and
Subluxations

1102

of 21 years. J Bone Joint Surg [Am] 1951; 33A:746–778.

54. Barquet A. Traumatic hip dislocation in childhood. A report of 26 cases and review of the literature. Acta Orthop Scand 1979;50(5):549–553.

55. Stueland D, Rothfusz RR. Posterior hip dislocation in a rural emergency department. Wis Med J 1992; 91(5):211–213.

56. Bucholz RW, Ezaki M, Ogden JA. Injury to the acetabular triradiate physeal cartilage. J Bone Joint Surg [Am] 1982;64A(4):600–609.

57. Moseley CF. Fractures and dislocations of the hip. Instr Course Lect 1992;41:397–401.

58. Pitt MJ, Ruth JT, Benjamin JB. Trauma to the pelvic ring and acetabulum. Semin Roentgenol 1992; 27(4):299–318.

59. Hougaard K, Thomsen PB. Traumatic posterior dislocation of the hip associated with separation of the capital epiphysis. Orthopaedics 1990;13(8): 891–894.

60. Ogden JA. Changing patterns of proximal femoral vascularity. J Bone Joint Surg [Am] 1974; 56A:941–950.

61. Barquet A. Avascular necrosis following traumatic hip dislocation in childhood: factors of influence. Acta Ortho Scand 1982;53(5):809–813.

62. Pai VS, Kumar B. Management of unreduced traumatic posterior dislocation of the hip: heavy traction and abduction method. Injury 1990;21(4):225–227.

63. Glynn TP, Kreipke DL, DeRosa GP. Computed tomography arthrography in traumatic hip dislocation. Intra–articular and capsular findings. Skeletal Radiol 1989;18(1):29–31.

64. DeLee JC. Dislocations and fracture–dislocations of the hip. In: Rockwood CA, Green DP, Bucholz RW, eds. Rockwood and Green's fractures in adults. Vol. 2. 3rd ed. Philadelphia: JB Lippincott, 1991, pp. 1574–1652.

65. Howard CB. A gentle method of reducing traumatic dislocation of the hip. Injury 1992;23(7):481–482.

66. Barquet A. Natural history of avascular necrosis following traumatic hip dislocation in childhood: a review of 145 cases. Acta Orthop Scand 1982; 53(5):815–820.

67. Josefsson PO, Nilsson BE. Incidence of elbow dislocation. Acta Orthop Scand 1986;57:537–538.

68. Mehlhoff TL, Noble PC, Bennett JB, Tullos HS. Simple dislocation of the elbow in the adult. J Bone Joint Surg [Am] 1988;70A:244–249.

69. Beaty JH. Fractures and dislocations about the elbow in children. Instr Course Lect 1992;41: 373–384.

70. Meyn MA, Quigley TB. Reduction of posterior dislocation of the elbow by traction on the dangling arm. Clin Orthop 1974;103:106–108.

71. Wilkins KE. Fractures and dislocations of the elbow region. Dislocation of the elbow joint. In: Rockwood CA, Wilkins KE, King RE, eds. Fractures in

children. Vol. 3. 3rd ed. Philadelphia: JB Lippincott, 1991, pp. 780–807.

72. Nevaiser JS, Wickstrom JK. Dislocation of the elbow: a retrospective study of 115 patients. South Med J 1977;70:172–173.

73. Josefsson PO, Johnell O, Gentz CF. Long–term sequelae of simple dislocation of the elbow. J Bone Joint Surg [Am] 1984;66A:927–930.

74. Josefsson PO, Gentz CF, Johnell O, Wendeberg BO. Surgical versus nonsurgical treatment of ligamentous injuries following dislocation of the elbow joint. J Bone Joint Surg [Am] 1987;69A:605–608.

75. Borris LC, Lassen MR, Christensen CS. Elbow dislocation in children and adults. A long–term follow–up of conservatively treated patients. Acta Orthop Scand 1987;58:649–651.

76. Gartland JJ, Benner JH. Traumatic dislocations in the lower extremity in children. Orthop Clin North Am 1976;7:687–700.

77. Beaty JH. Fractures and dislocations of the knee. Knee injuries. Knee dislocations. In: Rockwood CA, Wilkins KE, RE King, eds. Vol. 3. Fractures in children. 3rd ed. Philadelphia: JB Lippincott, 1991, pp. 1254–1255.

78. Schenck RC. The dislocated knee. Instr Course Lect 1994;43:127–136.

79. Gustilo RB, Cabatan DM. Traumatic dislocation of the knee. In: Gustilo RB, Kyle RF, Templeman DC, eds. Fractures and dislocations. St. Louis: CV Mosby, 1993, pp. 885–895.

80. Scott WN, Insall JN. Injuries of the knee. Traumatic dislocations of the knee. In: Rockwood CA, Green DP, Bucholz RW, eds. Rockwood and Green's fractures in adults. Vol. 2. 3rd ed. Philadelphia: JB Lippincott, 1991, pp. 1895–1914.

81. Ogden JA. Knee. In: Ogden JA, Skeletal injury in the child. 2nd ed. Philadelphia: WB Saunders, 1990, pp. 745–786.

82. Manaster BJ, Andrews CL. Fractures and dislocations of the knee and proximal tibia and fibula. Semin Roentgenol 1994;29(2):113–133.

83. Merrill KD. Knee dislocations with vascular injuries. Orthop Clin North Am 1994;25(4):707–713.

84. Dart Jr, CH, Braitman HE. Popliteal artery injury following fracture or dislocation at the knee: diagnosis and management. Arch Surg 1977;112: 969–973.

85. Moehring HD, Tan RT, Marder RA, Lian G. Ankle dislocation. J Orthop Trauma 1994;8(2):67–172.

86. Daffner RH. Ankle trauma. Semin Roentgenol 1994;29(2):134–151.

87. Vander Griend RA, Savoie FH, Hughes JL. Fractures of the ankle. Dislocations of the ankle. In: Rockwood CA, Green DP, Bucholz RW, eds. Rockwood and Green's fractures in adults. Vol. 2. 3rd ed. Philadelphia: JB Lippincott, 1991, p. 2030.

88. Wroble RR, Nepola JV, Malvitz TA. Ankle dislocation without fracture. Foot and Ankle 1988; 9(2):64–74.

Chapter 108
Reduction of
Common Joint
Dislocations and
Subluxations

1103

APPROACH TO FRACTURES WITH NEUROVASCULAR COMPROMISE

Scott H. Freedman and Brent R. King

INTRODUCTION

Neurovascular compromise should be considered whenever a child presents with an injured extremity. Although children with cool, pale, or cyanotic injured extremities are of obvious concern, serious injuries also can be subtle (1, 2). It is essential that individuals who care for children in either the prehospital setting or the emergency center be adept in the evaluation and initial management of the injured extremity. Depending on the circumstances, such as a lengthy prehospital extrication or transport, it may be several hours before the child receives definitive orthopaedic care. Emergency personnel therefore may be expected to perform limb-saving procedures including fracture reduction or limb manipulation in a neurovascularly impaired extremity. When the clinician is considering the rare but serious entity of compartment syndrome, expedient diagnosis and management are essential. The emergency physician must be able to measure intracompartmental pressures if an orthopaedic surgeon is not available to do so.

This chapter highlights specific orthopaedic injuries in children that may be limb threatening (3–7). All pediatric age groups may be affected, but due to the nature of certain injury patterns, school-age children and adolescents are the usual victims. Specific information about casting (Chapter 105), splinting (Chapter 104), and exsan-

guinating hemorrhage (Chapter 27) is provided elsewhere in this text and will not be discussed in detail in this chapter.

ANATOMY AND PHYSIOLOGY

Upper Extremity

The forearm is divided into an anterior (volar) and posterior (dorsal) compartment by a fascial sheath, interosseus membrane, and intermuscular septum. Each compartment contains its own muscle groups, innervation, and blood supply. An injury to the forearm that causes an elevation in compartmental pressures can result in the development of a compartment syndrome. A detailed discussion of compartment syndrome (8, 9) is provided later in this chapter. Table 109.1 lists the anatomic structures and their functions in the forearm and leg compartments.

The elbow joint is a complex synovial hinge joint between the distal humerus and the proximal radius and ulna. The spool-shaped trochlea and the rounded capitulum of the humerus articulate with the trochlear notch of the ulna and the cupped radial head, respectively. Flexion at the elbow is primarily provided by the brachialis muscle and is limited by apposition of the anterior surfaces of the arm and forearm, by tension of the posterior muscles, and by the radial and ulnar collateral ligaments. Extension at the elbow is primarily provided by contraction of the

Chapter 109
Approach to
Fractures with
Neurovascular
Compromise

1105

Table 109.1.
Compartment Structures of the Forearm and Leg

FOREARM
    Anterior (Volar) Compartment
    muscles: pronator teres, flexor carpi radialis, palmaris longus, flexor carpi ulnaris, flexor digitorum superficialis, flexor pollicis longus, flexor digitorum profundus, pronator quadratus
    blood supply: ulnar and radial arteries
    nerve supply: all muscles supplied by median nerve and its branches, except flexor carpi ulnaris and medial part of flexor digitorum profundus supplied by ulnar nerve. Principal action: flexion and pronation, intrinsic finger function (abduction, adduction), cutaneous sensation to palmar surface of hand.
    Posterior (Dorsal) Compartment
    muscles: extensor carpi radialis brevis, extensor digitorum, extensor digiti minimi, extensor carpi ulnaris, anconeus, supinator, abductor pollicis longus, extensor pollicis brevis and longus, extensor indicis
    blood supply: posterior and anterior interosseous arteries
    nerve supply: deep branch radial nerve. Principal function: wrist and finger extension; essentially no sensory function.
LEG
    Anterior Compartment
    muscles: tibialis anterior, extensor digitorum longus, peroneus tertius, extensor hallucis longus
    blood supply: anterior tibial artery
    nerve supply (principal): deep peroneal nerve. Principal function: cutaneous distribution of the anterior web space between the first and second toe, dorsiflexes foot and toes, inverts foot at ankle.
    Lateral Compartment
    muscles: peroneus longus and peroneus brevis
    blood supply: branches of the peroneal artery
    nerve supply: superficial peroneal nerve. Principal function: cutaneous distribution of the front of the leg and dorsum of the foot, foot and ankle eversion.
    Deep Posterior Compartment
    muscles: popliteus, tibialis posterior, flexor digitorum and hallucis longus
    blood supply: posterior tibial and peroneal arteries
    nerve supply: posterior tibial and peroneal nerves. Principal action: toe plantar flexion and assist in foot inversion, sensation to plantar aspect foot.
    Superficial Posterior Compartment
    muscles: gastrocnemius, soleus, plantaris longus.
    nerve supply: sural nerve. Principal function: sensation to dorsal lateral portion of foot and ankle. Gastroc-soleus complex is chief ankle and foot plantar flexor though supplied by tibial nerve (deep posterior compartment structure).

Table 109.2.
Ossification Centers of the Elbow

Ossification Center	Age of Appearance
Capitulum	1–2 yr
Radial head	5–7 yr
Internal (medial) humeral epicondyle	5–9 yr
Trochlea	9–10 yr
Olecranon	9–11 yr
External (lateral) humeral epicondyle	11–14 yr

the centers of ossification fuse at age 14 to 15 years whereas in boys fusion occurs at around 18 to 21 years of age.

An additional important feature of the bones of the elbow has to do with the actual structure of the supracondylar region of the humerus. In children the distal metaphysis of the humerus is flared and flat. Posteriorly it is indented due to the olecranon fossa and anteriorly it is thinned due to the coronoid fossa. The supracondylar region is a relatively weak section of bone that is somewhat susceptible to fracturing especially when the ossification centers are not fused. The brachial artery and its branches, the radial and ulnar arteries, and the median and radial nerves are the principal neurovascular structures that could be damaged in a complex supracondylar elbow fracture.

The median nerve arises from the medial and lateral cords of the brachial plexus. It descends along the lateral side of the axillary and brachial artery in the upper arm. At the midshaft of the humerus, it crosses the brachial artery to its medial side. It enters the forearm by passing between the two heads of the pronator teres muscle and descends on the deep surface of the flexor digitorum superficialis muscle. It innervates all the muscles of the forearm except the flexor carpi ulnaris and the medial half of the flexor digitorum profundus which are innervated by the ulnar nerve. At the wrist the median nerve gives rise to the palmar cutaneous branch which provides sensory innervation to the lateral half of the palm. It enters the palm by passing below the flexor retinaculum and through the carpal tunnel.

The ulnar nerve arises from the medial cord of the brachial plexus (C8 and T1). It descends along the medial side of the axillary and brachial arteries in the anterior compartment of the arm. Around the midshaft of the humerus the ulnar nerve dives posteriorly and

triceps muscle. Extension is limited by contact of the olecranon with the olecranon fossa of the humerus. In evaluating children, one must be knowledgeable of the age at which the ossification centers first appear and fuse so as to not misinterpret an ossification center with a fracture. This is particularly challenging when interpreting radiographs of the elbow. CRITOE is a commonly used mnemonic that can help the clinician remember the ossification centers and ages at which they appear and fuse (Table 109.2). In girls

**Chapter 109
Approach to
Fractures with
Neurovascular
Compromise**

1106

comes out behind the medial epicondyle of the humerus. It has no branches above the elbow. It enters the anterior compartment of the forearm by passing between the two heads of the flexor carpi ulnaris muscle and then descends deep to this muscle passing through the middle of the forearm medially to the ulnar artery. In the distal forearm the ulnar nerve becomes relatively superficial again passing above the flexor retinaculum before dividing into superficial and deep branches.

The radial nerve is the main continuation of the posterior cord of the brachial plexus. It passes from the axilla into the arm between the brachial artery and the long head of the triceps muscle. Accompanied by the brachial artery, the radial nerve takes a spiral course around the humerus in the radial groove. When it reaches the distal third of the arm, the nerve pierces the lateral intermuscular septum and passes between the brachialis and brachioradialis muscles to the lateral epicondyle of the humerus. There the radial nerve divides into its deep and superficial branches. The deep branch primarily innervates the extensor muscles in the arm, forearm, and wrist while the superficial branch provides cutaneous innervation to the dorsum of the hand and wrist. A significant injury to the radial nerve in or around the elbow could result in wrist drop characterized by the inability to extend the wrist. Table 109.3 summarizes the principal function and cutaneous sensation to the arm, forearm, and hand provided by the median, ulnar, and radial nerves.

Arterial circulation to the arm is primarily supplied by the brachial artery and its branches. The brachial artery is a continuation of the axillary artery and passes through the upper arm just medial to the humerus. It provides a number of muscular branches in the arm. In the inferior part of the cubital fossa just medial to the biceps brachii tendon and opposite the radial head, the brachial artery divides into the radial and ulnar arteries. The radial artery passes along the lateral side of the forearm, and the ulnar artery traverses the medial side.

Principal superficial venous drainage in the arm, forearm, and hand is provided by branches off the basilic and cephalic veins. In the cubital fossa, the median cubital vein is the largest vein and serves as the communicating vein between the basilic and cephalic veins. Extreme variation exists in the exact anatomic associations of the veins in the cubital fossa. Deep venous drainage of the arm is provided by the two brachial veins that begin in the elbow and traverse with the brachial artery to the axilla before ending in the axillary vein.

Lower Extremity

The lower limb consists of four parts: the pelvis, consisting of the hip bones (fusion of the ilium, the ischium, and the pubis) and

Table 109.3.
Major Nerves of Forearm: Function and Sensation

	Function	Cutaneous Sensation
WRIST AND HAND		
Median nerve	Flexes wrist; abducts hand	Palmar surface wrist; medial half of palmar surface (first 3½ digits)
Radial nerve	Extends and abducts hand at wrist joint	Dorsum of hand: lateral half
Ulnar nerve	Flexes wrist; adducts hand	Dorsum of hand: medial half; also medial half of fourth and all of fifth digit.
FINGERS		
Median nerve	Flexes middle phalanges of medial 4 digits; flexes distal phalanges of fingers. Abducts thumb; opposes thumb to little finger. First and second digits: flexes at MCP joints and extends IP joints	Palmar aspect thumb; both sides second, third, and lateral half fourth digit
Radial nerve	Extends IP and MCP joints of thumb; helps extend index finger. Abducts, extends thumb at carpometacarpal joint	Dorsal surface proximal phalanges first, second, and lateral half third digit
Ulnar nerve	Flexes little finger. Opposes little finger to thumb. Adducts and abducts fingers. Third and fourth digits: flexes at MCP joints, extends at IP joints.	Both sides fifth digit and medial half fourth digit. Dorsal surface proximal portion and lateral fourth and medial third digit

Chapter 109
Approach to
Fractures with
Neurovascular
Compromise

1107

their connections between the vertebral column and the femur; the thigh, containing the femur connecting the knee and the hip; the leg, containing the tibia and fibula connecting the ankle and the knee; and the foot, and the connection to the ankle. A full discussion of the entire lower limb is beyond the scope of this chapter and, as necessary, it is recommended to consult a comprehensive anatomy textbook (8,9). Because the greatest risk for neurovascular injuries in the lower extremity occur around the knee and in the compartments of the leg, much of the discussion will focus on these areas.

The Knee

As with the elbow, the knee is a synovial hinge joint. Articulation at the knee is between the large rounded condyles of the distal femur, the flattened condyles of the proximal tibia, and the facets of the patella. Principal movement of the knee is flexion and extension, but some lateral and medial rotation is present. Flexion is limited by contact of the posterior muscles in the calf and thigh, whereas full extension is usually limited by the knee ligaments to 0° although some individuals can hyperextend their knees by as much as 5 to 10°.

The popliteal fossa is the diamond-shaped region in the posterior aspect of the knee. It is bordered superolaterally by the biceps femoris muscle, superomedially by the semimembranosus and semitendinosus muscles, and inferolaterally and inferomedially by the lateral and medial heads of the gastrocnemius muscle, respectively.

Important neurovascular structures that traverse from the thigh to the calf lie deep within the popliteal fossa and are generally well protected from damage by a strong, thick fascial covering. However, in instances of a knee dislocation, displaced fractures through the physes of the proximal tibia or distal femur, or penetrating injuries to the fossa, a relatively high risk for concomitant neurovascular injuries to the leg and foot is evident. The popliteal artery and vein, the small saphenous vein, the tibial and common peroneal nerves, and the end branch of the posterior femoral cutaneous nerve all are contained in the fossa.

The popliteal artery is the direct continuation of the femoral artery beginning at the adductor hiatus in the thigh and ending by dividing into the anterior and posterior tibial arteries at the inferior border of the popliteus muscle. It provides numerous genicular tributaries to the knee, muscular branches to the thigh and leg, and cutaneous branches to the posterior leg. If the artery is damaged (severed, partially lacerated, or if it undergoes vasospasm), circulation to the leg could be profoundly compromised with resultant ischemic damage.

The popliteal vein connects the anterior and posterior tibial veins with the femoral vein. It commences in the distal border of the popliteus muscle and courses through the popliteal fossa superficial to the popliteal artery before ending at the adductor hiatus. The small saphenous vein runs between the heads of the gastrocnemius before draining into the popliteal vein.

The primary structures that innervate the leg and foot pass through the popliteal fossa. The sciatic nerve divides into the tibial and common peroneal nerves at the superior tip of the fossa. The tibial nerve is the larger branch and passes directly through the center of the fossa. It lies superficial and medial to the popliteal vessels. The nerve is just beneath the popliteal fascia and is covered by the two heads of the gastrocnemius muscle. The tibial nerve supplies articular branches to the knee, motor branches to the muscles of the posterior leg and the plantar flexors of the foot, and it joins a branch of the common peroneal nerve to form the sural nerve which innervates the lateral aspect of the ankle and sole of the foot.

The common peroneal nerve branches off the sciatic nerve and passes down the leg along the superolateral boundary of the popliteal fossa with the biceps femoris tendon. It passes superficial to the head of the gastrocnemius muscle out of the fossa before winding around the neck of the fibula. At this point it divides into the superficial and deep peroneal nerves and is susceptible to injury by its highly superficial location. The common peroneal nerve supplies articular branches to the knee and proximal tibiofibular joints, motor branches to the dorsiflexor and evertor muscles of the foot, and cutaneous sensory branches that innervate the skin of the calf.

Chapter 109
Approach to
Fractures with
Neurovascular
Compromise

1108

The Leg

A deep sheath of fascia encapsulates the leg by surrounding its contents and attaching to the medial and lateral borders of the tibia. Two intermuscular septa together with an interosseous membrane between the tibia and fibula divide the leg into three compartments: anterior, posterior, and lateral. The posterior compartment is further subdivided into a superficial and deep compartment by a transverse intermuscular septum passing between the tibia and fibula. Each compartment contains its own muscle group, blood supply, and nerve supply. Because the structures of the leg are well contained within these thick fascial septae, an injury that results in increased swelling may lead to increased compartmental pressures. This compartmentalization with the high propensity for injuries to the leg make it the most common site for the development of compartment syndrome. It is therefore important to be knowledgeable of the structures contained in the leg compartments (Table 109.1) (Fig. 109.1.A, B).

NEUROVASCULAR EXAMINATION OF THE INJURED EXTREMITY

Before obtaining radiographs and administering anesthesia, a methodical physical examination of an injured limb should be done and thoroughly documented. Examination of an injured child is often emotionally charged and difficult from the onset. Every effort must be made to establish rapport and to comfort the child. The examination never should be rushed. It may be helpful to have a family member present who will serve as a calming force for the fearful or uncooperative child. Assessment should be done with great care in an effort to be thorough and yet to cause no further pain or trauma.

Initial appropriate immobilization of the injured extremity is essential. A simple, padded splint should be applied to the suspected fracture taking care to include the joints above and below the injury. At first it is best to splint the injured limb in its deformed position to provide stability and comfort while minimizing the aggravation of any soft tissue or neurovascular damage. The splinted

extremity should then be elevated and ice applied in a manner not to interfere with the remainder of the examination (see Chapter 104).

At times the patient's injury is so painful that examination is near impossible. In such cases, analgesia should not be withheld and in fact will likely improve examination by localizing findings. It is recommended to titrate an intravenous narcotic (e.g., morphine sulfate 0.05 to 0.2 mg/kg or fentanyl 1 to 3 μg/kg) until adequate analgesia is obtained. The goal is to decrease pain and fear without inducing a state of deep sedation (see Chapter 34). It is obviously important to exclude other potentially life-threatening injuries (e.g., head, chest, abdomen) first.

Always inspect the injury before palpation or movement. Inspection is begun by first removing all clothing and jewelry that may interfere with complete visualization of both the injured limb and the contralateral limb. Dressings may need to be temporarily removed. If the injured extremity has already been immobilized, it is still imperative to perform a complete neurovascular examination. The splint or traction device may have been inadequately applied, and a long bone fracture may be improperly aligned and shortened or excessively stretched with resulting neurovascular compromise in either case. The appliance must be properly adjusted and the extremity fully reassessed.

Note the child undisturbed at rest. A child will always attempt to maintain the injured limb in a position of maximal comfort. Observe for active movement of the fingers and toes distal to the injury and compare findings to the contralateral limb. Note any gross bony or musculotendon deformities, swelling, and overlying ecchymoses. Lacerations, punctures, gunshot wounds (probable entry and exit sites), and degloving injuries may imply an open fracture. Active bleeding, arterial or venous in nature should be noted and controlled by applying direct pressure. The amount of blood loss from an open fracture is often grossly underestimated (1). Because major nerves nearly always run together with arteries, avoid blindly clamping a bleeding artery as this may cause injury to the accompanying nerve. Furthermore, applying a tight tourniquet proximal to the bleeding vessel may lead to irreversible ischemic dam-

Chapter 109
Approach to
Fractures with
Neurovascular
Compromise

1109

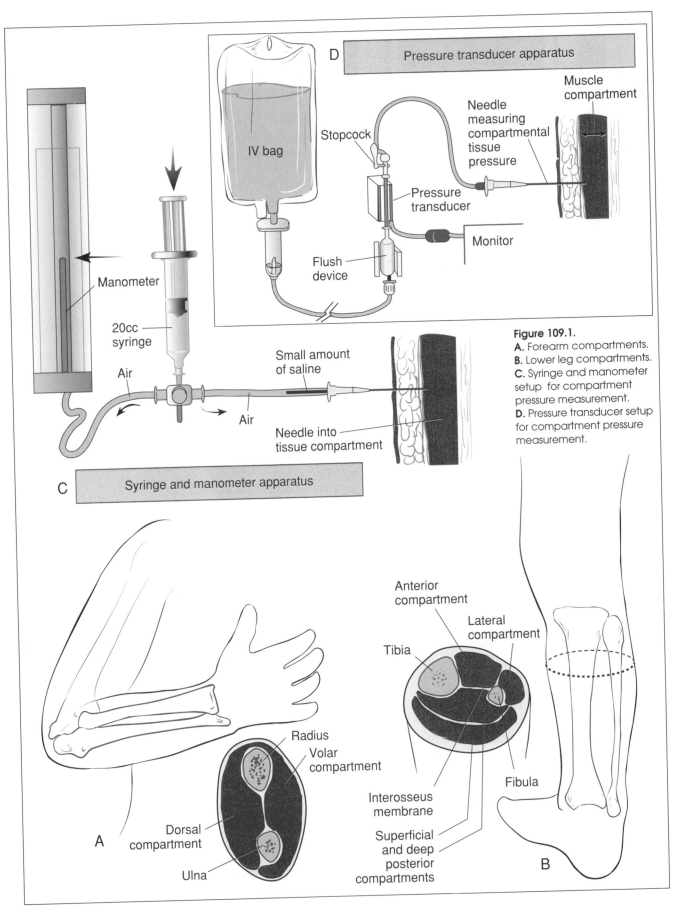

D Pressure transducer apparatus

Muscle compartment

Needle measuring compartmental tissue pressure

IV bag

Stopcock

Pressure transducer

Flush device

Monitor

Manometer

20cc syringe

Air

Air

Small amount of saline

Needle into tissue compartment

Figure 109.1.
A. Forearm compartments.
B. Lower leg compartments.
C. Syringe and manometer setup for compartment pressure measurement.
D. Pressure transducer setup for compartment pressure measurement.

C Syringe and manometer apparatus

Anterior compartment

Lateral compartment

Tibia

Radius

Volar compartment

Interosseus membrane

Dorsal compartment

Fibula

Superficial and deep posterior compartments

Ulna

A

B

1110

age to the distal part. This method to control a major hemorrhage should be reserved for an irreversibly damaged or crushed extremity for which applying direct pressure is ineffective (1) (see Chapter 27).

Circulation is next assessed. Pallor or cyanosis is noted distal to the injured part and color is compared with the uninvolved extremity. Temperature and perfusion also is compared with the uninjured limb. An expanding hematoma overlying the site of injury usually indicates significant arterial injury. In contrast, complete arterial transection or an intimal tear in a tight space may lead to minimal blood loss. The clinician must always examine for the presence and quality of bilateral peripheral pulses, but must exercise care in interpreting the findings. Pulses may remain palpable in the presence of arterial injury due to collateral flow or pulsatile fluid wave transmission. Conversely, absent pulses may reflect transient arterial spasm that by itself has little significance (2). However, the finding of diminished or absent pulses in the presence of an extremity injury never should be attributed to a spasm without a more complete evaluation. When necessary, emergency angiography should be performed. For upper extremity injuries, an Allen test can be done to assess arterial inflow to the hand. The child must cooperate by raising and clenching his or her hand. The clinician tightly compresses both the radial and ulnar arteries until the palmar surface is blanched. The hand is lowered and opened and then one vessel is released and reperfusion of the hand observed. The test is repeated, releasing the other artery and comparing the difference in reperfusion time. Normally both the radial and ulnar arteries should adequately reperfuse the palmar surface in less than 3 seconds. Again the Allen test also should be performed in the uninvolved limb for comparison.

Sensation should be assessed by localizing light touch using a cotton wisp. Two-point discrimination is done using the blunt ends of a paper clip, 1 cm apart. It may not be possible to reliably assess sensation by either of these methods in a nonverbal or uncooperative child. Still, the clinician should almost never use painful discrimination for the examination of the young child as it is itself painful and rarely provides useful informa-

tion (10, 11). It is still possible to assess sensation in the hand in the infant or fearful child. Because autonomic nerve fibers travel in nerve bundles, the wrinkle test can be done to assess sensation to the hand. The hand is first submerged in warm water for 5 to 10 minutes. The hand and fingers are then inspected for wrinkling. Those areas with impaired sensation will not wrinkle (10).

Motor function is next evaluated in both the injured and the uninjured extremity. Function and strength are carefully assessed and compared. In the evaluation for compartment syndrome, it is imperative to passively stretch and have the child actively flex the limb and the muscle group of concern. For example, the anterior compartment of the leg is the most common site for development of a compartment syndrome. The primary nerve supply is via the deep peroneal nerve that serves in foot dorsiflexion by innervating the tibialis anterior and extensor digitorum longus muscles. In the event of a compartment syndrome, these muscles are weakened and active foot dorsiflexion and toe extension are impaired. Furthermore, passively flexing the toes results in severe pain due to ischemia from pressure buildup in this compartment. Anesthesia (local, regional, or general) should then be provided as necessary, before obtaining radiographs or exploring the wound.

In the special case of the obtunded and/or comatose child, the physician must have a higher index of suspicion for neurovascular impairment and consequently a lower threshold for intervention (e.g., measuring intracompartmental pressures) (12). Any orthopaedic injury that leads to neurovascular compromise represents a potentially limb-threatening emergency. Insufficient arterial blood flow to a distal extremity can result from either vessel transection or laceration caused by a bony fragment or projectile missile (e.g., gunshot wound). Arterial spasm or compression caused by extrinsic pressure from the fractured bone or edematous tissue also may lead to ischemic damage. Venous obstruction is usually the result of tissue swelling from the injury or from tightly applied circumferential casts or dressings. If unrecognized or untreated, this could lead to the development of a compartment syndrome (12).

Chapter 109
Approach to
Fractures with
Neurovascular
Compromise

1111

Nerve injury may be temporary due to stretching, and nerve dysfunction generally resolves within 6 months. However, permanent dysfunction can result from ischemic necrosis in late compartment syndrome. Nerves, like vessels, also can be transected. It is therefore essential to make a rapid, accurate assessment and appropriate intervention to prevent permanent functional impairment or loss of the involved limb.

The proximity of the brachial artery to the elbow, the popliteal artery to the knee, and the pudendal artery to the pelvis make these three areas (elbow, knee, pelvis) particularly vulnerable to vascular compromise following a significant injury. The radial, median and ulnar nerves around the elbow and the tibial and common peroneal nerves at the knee are at relative high risk for nerve impairment. Therefore much attention will be focused on recognizing and treating supracondylar humeral fractures and severe knee injuries. It must be stressed, however, that any complicated fracture or dislocation may be unstable and lead to associated vascular ischemia or nerve damage. A brief overview of unstable pelvic, femoral shaft, and complex tibia-fibula and ankle fractures is included. Features that aid in the prompt recognition, diagnosis, and management of compartment syndrome are highlighted first.

COMPARTMENT SYNDROME

Pathophysiology

Generally speaking, insufficient blood flow to an extremity may lead to ischemic damage as early as 4 hours after an injury (3, 13, 14). Irreversible damage can occur 6 to 12 hours after onset of compromised vascular perfusion (4, 11, 15, 16).

Compartment syndrome represents any condition that leads to elevated tissue pressure within muscle groups enveloped by fascial sheaths. The actual incidence of compartment syndrome in children is unknown, but it is safe to say that it is a rare entity (12). Still, due to the potentially grave consequences if unrecognized and untreated, it is prudent to consider the diagnosis of compartment syndrome when faced with an extremity at risk.

The pathophysiology of compartment syndrome has been well studied (3, 4, 12–22). The increased pressure within the confined space leads to restriction of blood flow distally with subsequent ischemic insult to the extremity. It was previously believed that the ischemia leading to compartment syndrome was secondary solely to impaired arterial blood flow. Acute compartment syndrome, however, is known to occur in the presence of palpable distal arterial pulses. Current theory holds that it is narrowing of the arterial-venous pressure gradient either by increased venous pressure or decreased arterial pressure that causes hypoperfusion and ischemic injury. Subsequent reperfusion within the closed compartmental space leads directly to elevated pressure by increased flow in the restricted space and indirectly to increased pressure from local tissue edema. Further ischemia develops leading to necrosis and limb dysfunction.

A myriad of conditions may lead to compartment syndrome (3, 12). The basic principle again, is either the contents within the confined sheath unduly swell or the envelope surrounding the muscle group is overly constricting. Bleeding directly into the compartmental space secondary to blunt trauma (fractures, contusions), penetrating trauma (gunshot wounds) with arterial injury, primary limb surgery, or fracture reduction all may lead to the development of compartment syndrome. Excessively tight MAST suits, casts, air splints, or dressings may lead to compartment syndrome by excessive, external constricting pressure. Intraosseous infusions, snakebites, burns, and cardiac catheterizations may result in an increased compartmental volume from intravenous fluid infiltration or capillary leak and are known causes of compartment syndrome in children.

A chronic or recurrent form of compartment syndrome may develop from prolonged, excessive muscle use. Its pathogenesis is not well understood and the physician must have a high clinical suspicion for diagnosis. If considered, acute management is cessation of exercise and referral to an orthopaedic specialist (3, 4). Supracondylar fractures of the humerus, combined radius and ulnar fractures, femur fractures with skin traction, and tibia fractures are the most com-

Chapter 109
Approach to
Fractures with
Neurovascular
Compromise

1112

mon mechanisms of injury leading to compartment syndrome in children (12).

The clinician should always consider the diagnosis of compartment syndrome when a child presents with complaints of pain seemingly out of proportion to that expected from the nature of injury (12). A nonverbal or especially fretful, uncooperative child makes diagnosis more difficult and often requires more careful scrutiny. Discretion and care must be given to administering heavily sedating analgesia that may interfere with serial examinations. Severe pain elicited by actively flexing or passively stretching the suspected muscle groups is an especially sensitive sign and should heighten the clinician's concern. Paresthesias may be caused by ischemia to nerves traversing and innervating the suspected compartmental region. Decreased sensation to light touch or to two-point discrimination are reliable in defining distal sensory impairment. Swelling and palpable tenderness over the muscle group rather than the fracture site has been described by some as the earliest physical findings in compartment syndrome (14). As previously noted, palpable distal pulses and intact capillary perfusion do *not* rule out the diagnosis of compartment syndrome. Absent pulses and delayed perfusion are generally precarious signs of late presentation and heighten the likelihood that myonecrosis has already occurred.

Early recognition and diagnosis via tissue pressure measurement allow for timely therapeutic intervention, namely emergency fasciotomy and prevention of permanent limb dysfunction. A multiply injured child who is obtunded or comatose is especially difficult to evaluate because of the inability to perform a complete neurologic examination. An infant or highly uncooperative child may similarly be difficult to evaluate thoroughly. As noted, the only reliable signs on examination may be a tensely swollen, exquisitely tender extremity.

Because many patients will present in a cast, splint, or bandage, all appliances should be removed if the clinician suspects compartment syndrome. The involved limb is then iced and elevated. If improvement is not observed within 1 hour, an orthopaedic surgeon must be emergently consulted. If one is not readily available (within 4 hours of onset of

symptoms), the ED physician must consider measuring compartmental pressures.

Measurement of Intracompartmental Pressures

Normal intramuscular resting pressure approximates zero (3,16). As pressure within a compartment increases, perfusion decreases. No one standard recommendation represents the lowest accepted pressure, above which performing a fasciotomy is always warranted. Rather, abnormally high pressures range from 30 to 45 mm Hg. Some authorities recommend surgical decompression when the intracompartmental pressure approaches 10 to 30 mm Hg of the diastolic blood pressure (4). A general rule to follow would be to consult an orthopaedic surgeon when the diagnosis is suspected on clinical grounds. If tissue pressures are measured greater than 30 mm Hg, surgical decompression should likely be performed (3, 4, 12, 13).

In animal investigations, 6 hours of warm ischemia resulted in irreversible damage in 50% of the muscles studied. Eight to 12 hours of severe ischemia led to near complete and irreversible damage (16). It is thus imperative to act quickly in the face of a potentially devitalized compartment. When the orthopaedist is not available to measure compartment pressures, the emergency physician must be prepared to measure pressures so as to either expedite transfer to an available, nearby facility or assist the orthopaedist in diagnosis.

Whitesides et al. (3, 4, 16, 17, 21, 23) described a relatively straightforward technique for tissue pressure monitoring that can be done entirely with equipment and material found in the emergency room or office setting.

Equipment
Plastic extension tubes (2)
18-gauge needles (2)
20-mL syringe
Three-way stopcock
Vial bacteriostatic normal saline
Mercury manometer
Local anesthesia

The skin over the involved compartment is first prepared by cleansing with a povi-

Chapter 109
Approach to
Fractures with
Neurovascular
Compromise

1113

done-iodine solution. The site of needle insertion is anesthetized with local anesthetic. It is important to avoid injection into the suspected compartment as this may further raise the pressure and aggravate the situation.

The manometer measurement device is assembled as shown in Figure 109.1.C. First, intravenous extension tubing is connected to the front and rear ports of a three-way stopcock and a 20-mL syringe with the plunger at the 15-mL mark is connected to the upper port. A sterile 18 gauge needle is used to release the vacuum of a bottle of bacteriostatic normal saline. Once the vacuum has been released this needle is connected to the front port of the stopcock. The front port of the stopcock is opened and the plunger of the syringe slowly withdrawn until saline fills approximately half of the length of the tubing attached to the front port. It is important to withdraw the saline from the bottle slowly and smoothly so as to minimize bubble formation within the extension tubing and ensure that the saline only fills half of the extension tubing; the syringe should contain only air. The stopcock is then used to close the front port, and the needle is removed from the saline bottle. This needle is carefully removed and replaced with a new sterile needle. Keeping the front port stopcock closed during needle transfer will prevent loss of saline from the extension tubing. Next the extension tubing attached to the rear port is connected to the manometer. The needle is inserted into the desired muscle compartmental space and the stopcock is opened to both extension tubes and to the syringe. This produces a closed system whereby air is free to flow into both extension tubes as the pressure increases. Next the plunger is depressed slowly, forcing a rise in pressure within the system. As this is done, the mercury column within the manometer will slowly rise until the pressure within the system is equivalent to that within the tissue compartment. Then, as the pressure within the system surpasses tissue pressure, the saline contained within the extension tubing will be forced toward the needle, which will cause visible movement of the saline within the extension tubing. The reading on the mercury manometer at the time the saline begins to move represents the compartmental pressure. If more than one compartment pressure is to be measured, the system is reclosed and a new 18-gauge sterile needle is used each time.

Other techniques for measuring pressures include both the wick and the slit catheter methods (3, 4, 15–19). Both offer the advantage of continuous pressure monitoring but are cumbersome and not practical in either the emergency room or office setting.

The *Horizon PressureSense* intracompartmental pressure monitor is a portable, battery-operated, lightweight device the size of a penlight. It is relatively simple to use; requiring only the attachment of a needle and syringe apparatus and zeroing of the monitor before insertion in the injured limb. After injection of 0.5 mL of saline into the compartment, the pressure can be read directly off the monitor. Manufactured by Horizon Medical, Inc. (Santa Ana, CA), detailed directions are included in the package. Other brands (e.g., *Styker*) of portable pressure sensing devices also are available. Finally, certain types of electronic equipment commonly found in EDs can be used to measure intracompartmental pressures. The two most often used are intravenous pumps and monitors with arterial line capabilities.

To use an intravenous pump, the pump in question must have an internal electronic manometer that reports the pressure within the system. The procedure for this technique is as follows: First, a bag of normal saline is placed onto the pump apparatus using the same technique as would be used for intravenous infusion. Next a needle appropriate for measuring intracompartmental pressures (see previous section in this chapter) is attached to the distal end of the infusion tubing, occupying the location normally occupied by the intravenous catheter. If the intravenous pump can be moved up and down, then it should be placed level with the involved extremity. Then the pump should be set to infuse a small volume of fluid (e.g., 2 to 5 mL/hr). Next the baseline pressure within the system is recorded by pressing and holding the pressure button on the infusion pump. Ideally, of course, this baseline pressure should be zero but often, it is not. Notably, many pumps have a limit to the amount of negative pressure that they are able to report, and pressures below this are inaccurately reported. If the baseline pressure reported is negative, this should be taken into considera-

Chapter 109
Approach to
Fractures with
Neurovascular
Compromise

1114

tion. After the baseline pressure is recorded, then the needle is inserted into the compartment as previously described. The pressure button on the infusion pump is pressed and held, the pressure within the compartment is reported on the pump display. Positive baseline pressures and those negative baseline pressures that are within the limits of the machine's reporting ability can be added to or subtracted from the reported number as appropriate.

To use a monitor for recording intracompartmental pressures, the monitor and infusion system is set up for arterial line monitoring but with two exceptions (Fig. 109.1.D). First, the fluid to be infused need not be heparinized and second, it is not necessary for a bag of intravenous fluid to be placed into the pressure bag. As described, a needle is placed on the distal end of the infusion setup, instead of an intraarterial catheter. The system is then zeroed just as would occur before measuring an intraarterial pressure. When the needle is inserted into the compartment, the pressure reading obtained from the monitor is the intracompartmental pressure. This pressure reading is displayed in the area normally used to display the blood pressure from an arterial line.

Fasciotomy

Operative fasciotomies represent definitive treatment for an established compartment syndrome. The basic principle involves incising through the overlying skin and enveloping fascial sheaths of each involved compartment to release the constricted tissues and muscles. Suffice it to say the variety of fasciotomies requires extensive knowledge of local anatomic structures. Details of the operative techniques and fine anatomy are beyond the scope of this book, but are described in other text books (3, 4, 12, 13, 20).

Complications

Complications of neurovascular ischemia may be acute or delayed (13). When compartment syndrome develops and goes unrecognized or untreated, the consequences can be devastating. Volkmann's ischemia is defined as the neurologic sequelae of compartment syndrome; the pain from passively stretching the involved muscle groups and the sensory and motor deficits that result from the neurovascular compromise. Volkmann's ischemic contracture is the functionless limb that results from the untreated ischemia. It may occur following fractures of the elbow, forearm, wrist, tibia, and femur.

The claw hand deformity is Volkmann's contracture resulting from untreated forearm ischemia. In its most severe form, ischemic necrosis causes flexor contractures in the elbow, forearm, wrist, hand and fingers, and nerve damage causes intrinsic paralysis in the hand and wrist. This results in elbow flexion and forearm pronation. Characteristic findings in the hand and wrist are wrist flexion, hyperextension of the metacarpophalangeal joints, flexion of the interphalangeal joints and thumb contracture and thus the claw hand appearance (14).

When myonecrosis progresses, several consequences may occur (2, 13, 14). The necrotic limb is at risk for bacterial gangrene infection and the associated serious complications of overwhelming sepsis. One of the more common occurrences of muscle breakdown is myoglobinuria. If the patient's hydration status is not optimal, and myoglobin production exceeds kidney filtration capacity, renal failure may develop. Death can result from either of these serious complications.

FRACTURES AND DISLOCATIONS

Supracondylar Humeral Fractures

Pathophysiology
The most common mechanism of injury is a fall on the outstretched hand with the elbow in extension. Forces are transmitted proximally up the elbow fracturing the supracondylar region. If enough force is generated, the proximal fragment is driven posteriorly and the distal fragment displaced anteriorly. This type of extension injury represents 95 to 99% of all supracondylar humeral fractures. Due to the nature of this injury, it is always important to adequately evaluate the wrist and shoulder for an associated injury (5, 24–33).

Chapter 109
Approach to
Fractures with
Neurovascular
Compromise

1115

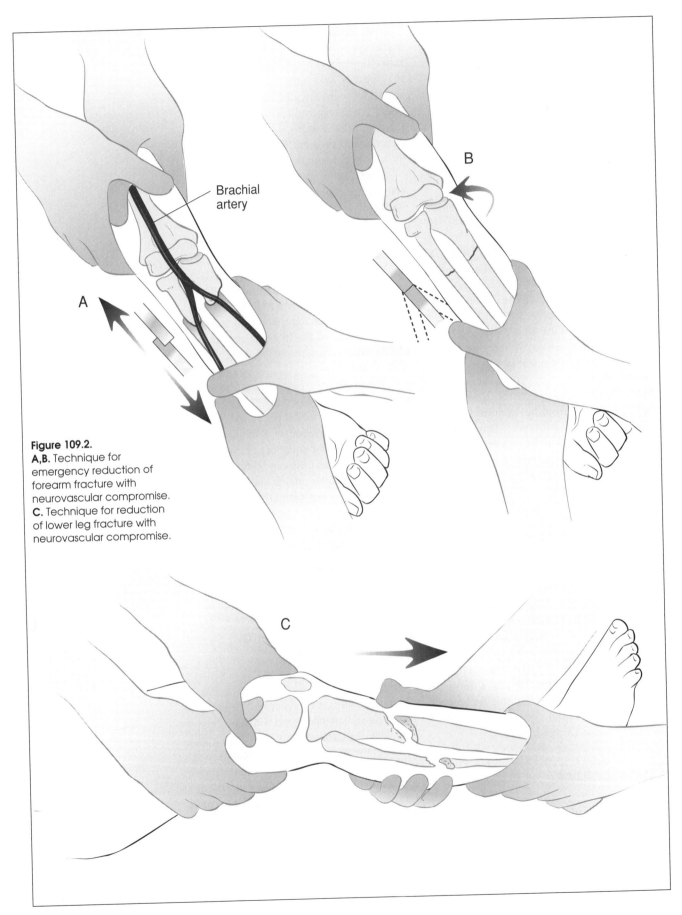

Figure 109.2.
A,B. Technique for emergency reduction of forearm fracture with neurovascular compromise.
C. Technique for reduction of lower leg fracture with neurovascular compromise.

Brachial artery

A

B

C

A direct blow to the flexed elbow with resultant fracture will cause anterior displacement of the proximal fragment of the humerus and posterior displacement of the distal fragment. This flexion injury is far less common than the extension type.

The elbow joint is traversed by the brachial artery and median, radial, and ulnar nerves. It is therefore not uncommon for neurovascular compromise to develop in the forearm or hand as a complication of this injury. In the extension injury, if the distal fragment is displaced medially, the radial nerve may be stretched and tented over the laterally displaced proximal fragment. If the distal fragment is displaced laterally as when the lateral periosteum remains intact, the median nerve is pulled tautly over the medially placed proximal fragment. The medial displacement pattern occurs more frequently, and thus radial nerve injuries develop more commonly. In the flexion-type injury, the ulnar nerve is more commonly stretched and injured because it is tightly bound to the medial intermuscular septum proximal to the fracture fragment and the cubital tunnel distal to the fracture. Overall in a review of 4520 fractures, 7% had concomitant nerve injuries, 45% were radial nerve injuries, 32% median nerve injuries, and 23% ulnar nerve injuries (25). Others report a 12% incidence of peripheral neuropathies developing after supracondylar humeral fractures (26). The anterior interosseus nerve was the most commonly injured branch of the median nerve resulting in loss of flexion of the distal phalanges of the thumb and index finger. Because nearly all nerve injury is from traction, full recovery can generally be expected within 6 months after injury.

Although the brachial artery may be completely transected, arterial spasm is far more common. In fact, neurovascular compromise commonly occurs after a fracture even when no displacement of the distal fragment has occurred. Swelling and hemarthrosis in the cubital fossa may lead to arterial spasm and/or occlusion. A compartment syndrome can develop if ischemia is prolonged (5, 20, 23–30).

Equipment and Procedures

Because it has a significant risk for neurovascular injury, reduction of the extension-type fracture with posterior displacement of the distal humeral fracture fragment will be detailed here. When a supracondylar humeral fracture of the elbow leads to neurovascular compromise in the forearm or hand, an orthopaedic surgeon must be emergently consulted. The arm should be immobilized, elevated, and iced. If the specialist is unavailable and the condition does not improve, it is the responsibility of the emergency room physician to reduce the fracture to restore flow and function to the distal arm.

Equipment
Appropriate sedative and/or hypnotic agents (Chapter 35)
Monitors and resuscitation equipment
Splinting material
Doppler transducer

Intravenous anesthesia should be administered to the child. The goal is to provide sufficient relief of pain and muscle relaxation so the child does not struggle and the muscles do not spasm during fracture reduction and immobilization.

Once ready, an assistant immobilizes the arm proximal to the fracture site. The physician exerts longitudinal traction at the wrist until the arm length is approximately normal. The elbow is slightly hyperextended to release any locked fracture fragments. This is done while pressure is applied in the anterior direction against the distal humeral fragment. At this point, medial and lateral angulation should be corrected. The assistant applies gentle posterior traction on the proximal humerus while this is being done. The elbow is then flexed to maintain proper alignment and posterior pressure is applied to the distal fragment. Distal pulses are assessed. If diminished or absent, the brachial artery may have spasmed due to tenting of the artery over the anteriorly displaced proximal bony fragment. If the fingers remain nonedematous, warm, pink, well perfused, and fully functional, these findings are far more significant than the presence or absence of a radial pulse. Slightly flexing the extremity to approximately 5 to 15° should restore circulation and the distal pulse. If pulse and perfusion remain abnormal, arteriography and/or surgical exploration are required (26, 27). Continuous pulse oximetry of an ipsilateral finger during

Chapter 109
Approach to
Fractures with
Neurovascular
Compromise

1117

SUMMARY
1. Stabilize patient; follow ABCs under ATLS protocol
2. Remove all clothing (including footwear) and jewelry covering and distal to injured extremity
3. Stop active bleeding with direct pressure dressing
4. Observe child and inspect injury: note position extremity maintained, note gross deformities, findings consistent with an open fracture, color. Always examine contralateral limb in same manner
5. Unless obvious neurovascular compromise is present, gently apply temporary, simple, padded splint to injured part initially leaving it in its deformed position. Include joints above and below suspected fracture to provide adequate stability. Elevate and ice injured limb (if neurovascular compromise is present, see 12 and 14, below)
6. Observe movements distal to injury. Have child move fingers and toes. Specifically, assess radial nerve function via finger, wrist extension, test median nerve with thumb to fingers apposition, and ulnar nerve can be assessed by spreading and adducting fingers. For lower extremity injuries, have child dorsiflex and plantarflex toes
7. Palpate extremity distal to injury by assessing temperature, capillary perfusion, and quality of distal pulses

the procedure is a quick way to ascertain whether perfusion is intact distally (28–30).

A long arm posterior splint is then applied (Chapter 104). If the distal fragment was displaced medially, the elbow should be slightly pronated for splinting. In contrast, if the distal fragment was laterally displaced, the forearm should be immobilized in supination. A sling is then applied and the patient is hospitalized for careful neurovascular checks. Postreduction radiographs are then obtained.

If reduction of fracture fails once, it should not be repeated due to risk of more substantial brachial artery damage with excessive manipulation. In this case an overhead olecranon reduction apparatus must be applied by an experienced orthopaedist. In fact, any nerve or vascular injury warrants overhead traction (27).

Assessing Effectiveness of Procedure

A postreduction radiograph is taken to document elbow position. Peripheral pulses, color, temperature, perfusion, and movement in the fingers and hand are repeatedly assessed and recorded. Emergent angiography is obtained should vascular injury be suspected. Inability to maintain a closed reduction or limb-threatening neurovascular damage may be an indication for an open, surgical reduction (27, 29).

Complications

Malunion is a complication that can result after any healed displaced fracture. In the supracondylar humeral fracture in children, cubitus varus ("gunstock" deformity), and valgus deformities are seen. The most frequent cause is malposition of the distal humeral fragment. Elbow stiffness and impaired function are complications from prolonged immobilization more often seen in adults. As noted previously, a clawhand deformity is a complication resulting from untreated compartment syndrome in the forearm (14, 24–31).

Distal Upper Extremity Injuries

Although potentially less serious than supracondylar fractures, injuries to the distal forearm are far more common. The mechanism of injury is similar to that previously described—a fall onto an outstretched arm. The resultant injuries usually involve the distal radius and ulna (e.g., Colle's fracture). In most cases this type of injury does not result in neurovascular compromise, but in cases of extreme angulation of the bones or significant local edema, the arterial and/or nerve supply to the hand may be compromised. Therefore all patients presenting to the ED with these types of injuries should have a careful examination of the hand as described previously (see Neurovascular Examination of the Injured Extremity).

If the examination demonstrates that either the blood supply or innervation to the hand is compromised, then emergency reduction is appropriate. After adequate analgesia has been administered, an assistant grasps the upper arm above the elbow to stabilize it. The physician then exerts gentle longitudinal traction on the arm distal to the fracture (Fig. 109.2.A,B). The procedure is successful if circulation to the hand is restored. Definitive reduction need not be accomplished until later.

LOWER EXTREMITY INJURIES

Injuries Around the Knee

Pathophysiology

In children, physis (growth plate) fractures (Salter type) occur with greater frequency than ligamentous injuries due to the relative weakness of the growth plate compared with the supporting ligaments. A frontal blow to a fixed thigh with the knee hyperextended may drive the lower leg forward. The result may be a fracture through the growth plate of the distal femur with anterior displacement of the distal epiphysis.

Occurring less frequently is a fracture-separation at the proximal tibial growth plate. The physis of the proximal tibia is well protected laterally by the fibula and anteriorly by the overhanging epiphyseal tubercle. Additionally the insertion of the surrounding knee ligaments and musculotendons offer further protective support to the growth plate. However, a violent, direct blow to the proximal tibial epiphysis (e.g., motor vehicle running over the lower leg) may cause a fracture through the physis with posterior displacement of the proximal metaphysis into the popliteal fossa. More common, though still rare, is an indirect mechanism whereby a blow occurs to the hyperextended lower leg with the knee fixed. This injury may occur in an adolescent after a sports injury or in a preadolescent after a fall or motor vehicle accident and result in fracture-separation through the tibial growth plate with similar posterior displacement of the proximal tibial metaphysis. For reasons stated, a knee dislocation without fracture is a rare event in children. All three types of injuries, however, are discussed due to their relatively high associated risk of vascular compromise (2, 20). The popliteal artery is tightly secured at the popliteal fossa by being anchored proximally at the adductor hiatus and distally at the soleus muscle. It provides primary circulation to the lower leg. Its tributaries provide poor collateral circulation at the popliteal fossa. Because the artery is firmly fixed in place, a fracture-separation around the hyperextended knee may posteriorly displace a fracture fragment to impinge on the popliteal artery. The nerve supply, principally composed of the tibial and common peroneal nerves, is more loosely attached than the artery, and therefore nerve injury is much less likely than vascular damage (7, 34).

A meticulous examination of the leg and foot is mandatory whenever any of these injuries is suspected. Evaluation should include assessment for associated femur and pelvic fractures which may not be immediately apparent. Both dorsalis pedis and posterior tibial pulses should be palpated or Doppler measured and compared with the uninjured side. The foot may be cold or pale. The lower leg may be cyanotic with delayed capillary refill if venous return is impaired. Muscle function and sensation in the lower leg, foot, and toes must be carefully assessed. If marked pain, muscle belly tenderness, and swelling are indicated, diagnosis of compartment syndrome should be seriously considered. Elevated compartment pressures in the lower leg will confirm the diagnosis.

Penetrating injuries around the knee also warrant special attention. Because late complications include development of arteriovenous fistulas and pseudoaneurysms, noninvasive duplex studies of the lower extremity are required even in the face of apparent vascular

competence. An emergency angiogram should be obtained in all cases of severe knee injuries that risk involving the popliteal artery. This is especially important because distal pulses may appear normal soon after the injury (3, 7, 34).

Chapter 108 details the procedure for reduction of a knee dislocation. The principles are generally the same when faced with a neurovascularly compromised leg from a fracture-separation through the physis of the distal femur or proximal tibia.

Unstable Pelvic Fractures

An unstable pelvic fracture is most commonly the result of a high impact force (e.g., motor vehicle accident or a fall) directly crushing the pelvis. Similarly by a fall from a great height, an indirect blow may be transmitted up through the femurs driving the femoral heads back into and fracturing the pelvic ring.

Any pelvic fracture has the potential for significant bleeding, which leads to hemodynamic compromise and shock. If a trauma victim is hemodynamically compromised due to blood loss from an unstable pelvic fracture, an immediately available, acceptable intervention is applying a pneumatic antishock garment until circulation is restored and operative intervention undertaken (Chapter 28). Serial hematocrits are obtained to assess blood loss. Evaluation for associated bladder and abdominal visceral injuries is always performed (1, 12).

Femoral Shaft Fractures

Fractures of the femoral shaft that impair circulation distally may be manifested by a cool, pale, pulseless foot. Alternatively, even in a grossly displaced fracture no neurovascular injury may be observed. However, gentle, longitudinal traction in line with the long axis should be attempted when circulation is impaired. As traction is being applied, the leg is turned gradually from the deformed position. As circulation is restored in the foot, the leg is immobilized in a traction splint. Splinting is always done after displaced femur fractures to minimize hemorrhage into the thigh

SUMMARY
(CONTINUED)

8. Carefully palpate injured part noting deformity pattern, hematoma, crepitus. Listen for bruits. In upper extremity pay careful attention to cubital fossa and in lower extremity injuries closely examine popliteal fossa. Evaluate for tenderness and swelling over associated compartments

9. Assess sensation distal to injury. In upper extremity, test on dorsum of hand (radial nerve), thumb or index finger (median nerve), and fifth finger (ulnar nerve). In the leg, always assess sensation in web space between first and second toes (deep peroneal nerve)

10. Passively stretch injured part to evaluate further for compartment syndrome

11. Administer anesthesia, if not already done and if child is in pain

12. Adequately splint injured part—if neurovascular impairment exists before splinting, an attempt should be made to reduce the fracture—see text for details of extremity manipulation and stabilization. Reassess neurovascular status after traction splint or appliance is in place to ensure that no new deficits are present

13. Obtain appropriate radiographs with comparison views as needed

14. Consult orthopaedic surgery—See text for management in event of concern of compartment syndrome

and prevent further neurovascular or soft tissue injury.

Doppler arterial pressures should be obtained in both the affected and uninvolved leg using a blood pressure cuff. A decrease in systolic arterial pressure of greater than or equal to 20 mm Hg in the involved extremity as compared with the uninjured limb may indicate significant arterial compromise. Many authorities recommend an intraoperative arteriogram at this point. In the case of obvious circulatory compromise, an emergency arteriogram must be obtained. Serial hematocrits also need to be obtained as significant and insidious hemorrhage may develop after a displaced femur fracture (1, 12).

Tibia and Fibula Shaft Fractures

The great majority of tibia and fibular shaft fractures are nondisplaced or incompletely displaced. A rare, but significant event is fracture through both the tibia and fibula with complete displacement. Should limb-threatening, vascular compromise occur, emergency reduction by gentle longitudinal traction is required (Fig. 109.2.C). As with the femoral shaft fracture, the leg may need to be turned from the plane of deformity while applying traction. When aligning a tibial fracture, the second toe should align with the tibial tubercle. This may need to be done even before radiographs are obtained (i.e., in a prehospital setting) as in the case of an obviously deformed lower leg with a pale, cool, pulseless foot.

Once a dorsalis pedis or posterior tibial pulse is obtained and perfusion restored to the foot, a posterior splint is applied (Chapter 104) and full orthopaedic consultation (including possible arteriography) obtained. These patients need close observation for signs of developing compartment syndrome (1, 10).

Ankle Fractures

Another rare but significant injury in the pediatric (usually adolescent) population is a severely displaced ankle fracture with associated dislocation. These injuries may result in neurovascular impairment around or distal to the ankle joint. If prompt orthopaedic care is unavailable and neurovascular impairment exists as evidenced by a cool, pale, or pulseless foot, fracture-dislocation reduction should be performed. An assistant should apply steady, gentle proximal countertraction and the injured ankle should be carefully rotated for proper alignment. As described, the second toe should be aligned with the tibial tubercle. A splint is applied taking care to avoid pressure over the bony prominences, and neurovascular status is reassessed (1, 10).

SUMMARY

Recognition and diagnosis of major arterial injury are relatively straightforward when pain, pulselessness, pallor, paralysis, and poikilothermia are present. In such cases immediate surgical intervention is mandatory in an attempt to restore vascular flow for limb salvage (2). In fact, by the time an injured extremity is cool and functionless, it is likely that irreversible damage has already occurred (16).

Often the presentation is more complex and even subtle. Signs of arterial injury include significant bleeding, an expanding hematoma, diminished or absent pulses, a bruit, distal ischemia, unremitting pain, or impaired distal sensation. Arterial intimal tears may initially have findings of normal pulses. Perfusion also may be normal distally unless small vessel collapse occurs. For these reasons, frequent neurovascular reassessments are required. Knowledge of regional anatomy, mechanism of injury, and a high index of suspicion are needed when evaluating for vascular injury. As detailed in this chapter, injuries around the elbow or knee should be carefully and serially evaluated for signs of neurovascular impairment. Unstable pelvic fractures and displaced femur fractures may lead to significant blood loss and require immediate orthopaedic evaluation. Evaluation of penetrating extremity trauma may include Doppler flow noninvasive studies and/or angiography.

All children who sustain a fracture or dislocation require a thorough neurovascular examination. A complete examination includes assessment of color, temperature, capillary refill, pulses, movement, and sensation. Neurovascular compromise in the face of an

Chapter 109
Approach to
Fractures with
Neurovascular
Compromise

1120

orthopaedic injury is defined as impairment in blood flow or motor function or sensation in a distal extremity. Lack of cooperation and equivocal findings due to the child's developmental stage, fear, and pain warrant serial examinations and more careful observation. A neurovascularly compromised limb provides a mandate for emergent orthopaedic consultation.

REFERENCES

1. Extremity trauma. In: American College of Surgeons, eds. Advanced trauma life support course. Chicago, 1989, pp. 181–200.
2. Chervu A, Quiñonez-Baldrich WJ. Vascular complications in orthopaedic surgery. Clin Orthop Rel Res 1988;235:275–288.
3. Mubarak SJ, Hargens AR. Compartment syndromes and Volkmann's contracture. Philadelphia: WB Saunders, 1981.
4. Van Ryn DE. Compartmental syndrome. In: Roberts JR, Hedges JR, eds. Clinical procedures in emergency medicine. Philadelphia: WB Saunders, 1991, pp. 859–866.
5. Niemann KMW, Gould JS, Simmons B, Bora FW. Injuries to and developmental deformities of the elbow in children. In: Bora FW, ed. The pediatric upper extremity: diagnosis and management. Philadelphia: WB Saunders, pp. 13–246.
6. Moore KL. Clinically oriented anatomy. 2nd ed. Baltimore: Williams & Wilkins, 1985, pp. 626–793.
7. Beaty JH, Roberts JM. Fractures and dislocations of the knee. In: Rockwood C, Wilkens K, King R, eds. Fractures in children. 3rd ed. Philadelphia: JB Lippincott, 1991, pp. 1171–1205.
8. Snell R, Smith M. Clinical anatomy for emergency medicine. CV Mosby, 1993, pp. 575–739.
9. Netter FH. The Ciba collection of medical illustrations. Vol. 8. Musculoskeletal system. Ciba-Geigy Corporation, 1987, pp. 30–108.
10. Bucknam CA. Vascular complications of fractures and dislocations. In Gossling HR, Pillbsbury SL, eds. Complications of fracture management. Philadelphia: JB Lippincott, 1984, pp. 123–140.
11. Dieckmann RA, Markison RE. Hand trauma. In: Grossman M, Dieckmann RA, eds. Pediatric emergency medicine. Philadelphia: JB Lippincott, 1991; pp. 300–304.
12. Simon R, Koenigsknecht S. Emergency orthopaedics. The extremities. 2nd ed. Appleton & Lange, 1987.
13. Willis RB, Rorabeck CH. Treatment of compartment syndrome in children. Orthop Clin North Am 1990; 21(2):401–412.
14. Moore RE, Friedman RJ. Current concepts in pathophysiology and diagnosis of compartment syndromes. Journal Emerg Med 1985;7:657–662.
15. Lapuk S, Woodbury D. Volkmann ischemic contrac-
ture: a case report. Orthop Rev 1988;17(6):618–624.
16. Allen MJ, Stirling AJ, Crawshaw CV, Barnes MR. Intracompartmental pressure monitoring of leg injuries. J Bone Joint Surg 1985;67-B(1):53–57.
17. Whitesides TE, Haney TC, Morimoto K, Harada H. Tissue pressure measurements as a determinant for the need of fasciotomy. Clin Orthop Rel Res 1975; 113:43–51.
18. Garrett WV, Thompson JE, Talkington CM, Smith BL. The role of fasciotomy in the acutely ischemic lower extremity. Chapter 33. In: Kempczinksi RF, ed. The ischemic leg. Chicago: Year Book Medical Publishers, 1985, pp. 483–493.
19. Matsen FA, Mayo KA, Sheridan GW, Krugmire RB. Monitoring of intramuscular pressure. Surgery 1976; 79(6):702–709.
20. Mubarak SJ, Hargens AR, Owen CA, Garetto LP, Akeson WH. The wick catheter technique for measurement of intramuscular pressure. J Bone Joint Surg 1976;58-A(7):1016–1020.
21. Nogi J. Common pediatric musculoskeletal emergencies. Emerg Med Clin North Am 1984;2(2):409–422.
22. Rang M. Fractures with vascular damage. In: Rang M, ed. Children's fractures. Philadelphia: JB Lippincott 1983, pp. 44–48.
23. Whitesides Jr TE, Haney TC, Hiranda H, et al. A simple method for tissue pressure determination. Arch Surg 1975;110:1311–1313.
24. Sherk H, Black JD. Orthopaedic emergencies. In: Fleisher GR, Ludwig S, eds. Pediatric emergency medicine. Baltimore: Williams & Wilkins, 1993, pp. 1397–1398.
25. Harris IE. Supracondylar fractures of the humerus. Orthopaedics 1992;15(7):811–817.
26. McGraw JJ, Akbarnia BA, Hnael DP, Keppler L, Burdge RE. Neurologic complications resulting from supracondylar fractures of the humerus in children. J Pediatr Orthop 1986;6(6):647–650.
27. Furrer M, Mark G, Ruedi T. Management of displaced supracondylar fractures of the humerus in children. Injury 1991;22(4):259–262.
28. Vasli LR. Diagnosis of vascular injury in children with supracondylar fractures of the humerus. Injury 1988;19(1):11–13.
29. Clement DA. Assessment of a treatment plan for managing acute vascular complications associated with supracondylar fractures of the humerus in children. J Pediatr Orthop 1990;10(1):97–100.
30. Ray SA, Ivory JP, Beavis JP. Use of pulse oximetry during manipulation of supracondylar fractures of the humerus. Injury 1991;22(2):103–104.
31. Klassen RA. Supracondylar fractures of the elbow in children. In: Morrey BF, ed. The elbow and its disorders. Philadelphia: WB Saunders, 1985; pp. 182–221.
32. Worlock PH, Colton C. Severely displaced fractures of the humerus in children: a simple method of treatment. J Pediatr Orthop. 1987;7:49–53.
33. Alburger PD, Weidner PL, Betz RR. Supracondylar fractures of the humerus in children. J Pediatr Orthop 1992;12(1):16–19.
34. Montgomery J. Dislocation of the knee. Orthop Clin North Am 1987;18(1):149–156.

Chapter 109
Approach to
Fractures with
Neurovascular
Compromise

1121

MINOR EMERGENCY PROCEDURES

Section Editor: John Loiselle

GENERAL WOUND MANAGEMENT

James M. Callahan and M. Douglas Baker

INTRODUCTION

Traumatic injuries are commonly encountered in pediatric patients. Ten million patients present to emergency departments (EDs) in the United States each year for treatment of traumatic wounds (1). A significant percentage of these patients will be children. Goals of therapy in dealing with cutaneous wounds include restoration of function and structural integrity, prevention of infection, and production of cosmetically acceptable healing. These goals are interrelated and adherence to sound principles of general wound management will lead to achieving them.

Effective wound management can be initiated by either EMS personnel or parents at the scene of an injury and is continued by nursing and medical personnel in the ED. The aim of therapy is to prevent secondary tissue damage or the development of infection, so that the majority of wounds can heal primarily. Adequate preparation of equipment and a well-established treatment plan is key to success.

General surgical principles including the adherence to standard aseptic techniques (Chapter 7) apply to all traumatic wounds. Appropriate restraint (Chapter 3), anesthesia, sedation, and pain control (Chapters 35 to 37) will lead to improved outcomes. Preparation of the wound is an important prelude to actual wound closure, which is discussed in Chapter 111.

ANATOMY AND PHYSIOLOGY

A working knowledge of both skin biomechanics and the mechanisms of soft tissue trauma is necessary to manage wounds effectively. In addition, many factors can modify the overall effect and outcome of a particular injury in a given patient. Knowledge of these factors also is important.

The skin is remarkably resistant to traumatic forces (2), and is highly elastic due to its high content of elastin fibers. It also has a large number of collagen fibers which give it added strength (2). A significant amount of force is required to cause tissue disruption.

The skin is constantly under static and dynamic tension. Static tension is caused by the force exerted on the skin by the underlying tissues at rest and the natural tension of the skin itself (3). Dynamic tension is caused by joint movement, muscle contraction, and gravity (3). Wounds under a large amount of tension tend to heal with wide, unattractive scars (3). Wound edges that retract more than 5 mm are thought be under strong, static tension (4). Wounds under low tension (edge retraction less than 5 mm) tend to heal with minimal scars. Those wounds that cross joints or are perpendicular to wrinkle lines often lead to unattractive scars regardless of the repairer's skill (4). Patients and their families should be warned about these issues before repairs are made.

The skin is inhabited by microorganisms

which can be a source of endogenous infection when trauma causes tissue disruption. Most of the bacteria in the skin reside in the horny layer of dead skin cells which are in the process of being sloughed off. The stratum corneum below this layer is composed of tightly packed, viable cells which act as a barrier to bacteria (1). Exogenous sources of bacteria also can lead to wound infections.

The amount of bacteria present on the skin varies by anatomic location. Three distinct zones are characterized by the density of residing microorganisms (1). Moist areas (i.e., axillae, perineum, web spaces, and intertriginous areas) have extremely high bacterial concentrations and therefore are prone to infection when disrupted traumatically. Dry areas (i.e., back, chest, abdomen, arms, and legs) have low bacterial concentrations. Exposed areas (i.e., face, head, hands, and feet) have high bacterial concentrations with the exception of the palms and dorsal surfaces of the hand where concentrations are low (1). Lacerations caused by contact with the oral cavity, especially the teeth (i.e., bite wounds) are highly contaminated and particularly prone to infection. Wounds that contact vaginal secretions or feces also will usually become infected.

It is important to consider the mechanism of injury in the management of soft tissue trauma. Wounds are caused by mechanical or thermal forces (Chapter 115). Mechanical forces are of three types: shearing, tension, or compression (2).

Shearing occurs when forces of equal magnitude are applied to the skin in opposite directions along parallel planes (Fig. 110.1.A) (2). A cut with a sharp edge (e.g., a knife or glass) is an example of a shearing force. Little energy is transmitted to surrounding tissues and, therefore, little devitalization of adjacent areas is seen. These wounds have a low potential for infection. Low velocity missile injuries (e.g., .22 caliber rimfire bullets and handguns other than the .44 magnum pistol) cause mostly a shear and compression injury which is confined to the actual missile tract (1). Direct injuries to internal organs or major vessels account for the morbidity and mortality associated with these wounds.

High velocity missile wounds (including rifled slugs from a shotgun at a range of less than 45 meters) cause not only a shearing injury along the wound tract but also devitalization of adjacent tissues secondary to compression and the entrainment of large amounts of skin bacteria and debris. These wounds are highly prone to infection. They should be managed by extensive and repeated debridement of the wound in the operating room to remove devitalized tissue (1).

Tension injuries occur when the skin is struck with a blunt or semiblunt object at an angle of less than 90° (Fig. 110.1.B). Avulsion injuries and flap lacerations are common (2). Usually these injuries are associated with a larger force applied to the skin than is seen with shearing injuries. Devitalized tissue is more often seen adjacent to the wound. In addition, the vascular supply to a flap may be compromised leading to necrosis. Tension wounds are more difficult to repair and more prone to infection.

Compression injuries, usually caused by blunt trauma directed at an angle of 90° against skin which often overlies bones cause the most tissue disruption (2) (Fig. 110.1.C). Stellate lacerations with adjacent hematomas and abrasions are commonly seen. Large areas of devitalized tissue can result, and infection rates 100 times as high as those seen with shearing injuries have been reported (1).

Tissue damage caused by an object is directly related to the amount of kinetic energy the object transmits to the tissues involved. The kinetic energy of an object is described by the equation

$$KE = \frac{1}{2}MV^2$$

where M equals the mass of the object and V equals the object's velocity. Increasing the velocity, therefore, has greater impact on the amount of tissue damage caused than increasing the mass of the object. Whether the material reacts with the biologic tissue or is relatively inert will determine if it will potentiate the development of infection. The configuration or shape of the object also will determine the nature of the wound it causes (2).

The environment in which the wounding event occurs will greatly modify the nature of the wound. Swamps, marshes, and other wet environments tend to have high bacterial loads. Wounds occurring on farms may be contaminated by animal feces. Soil and dirt also have been shown to inhibit the infection fighting capabilities of both the cellular and humoral immune systems (1). Organic components and inorganic clay components of soil inhibit white blood cell phagocytic and killing mechanisms and the bactericidal nature of human serum (1, 6–8). These same elements also inactivate many antibiotics (9). Soil from swamps and similar areas also have a high proportion of organic materials. Sand, a large-grained, inert component of soil, and the black dirt found on the surface of highways do not seem to lead to this same inhibition (1).

Finally, characteristics of the patient will influence both the type of wound caused by a particular insult and the healing process. Patient age, general health, and intercurrent illnesses or medication can affect skin integrity and the processes involved in wound healing. Malnutrition, shock states, severe anemia, and uremia promote delayed healing and increased infection rates (2). Chronic use of steroids can cause thinning of the skin analogous to the aging process leading to large, shallow avulsions or flap injuries (2). These drugs can also impair healing mechanisms and increase infection rates.

Knowledge of the mechanism of injury, characteristics of the wounding object, the environment in which the wound was sustained, and the health status of the patient are important to consider in the approach to general wound management. Developing an appropriate treatment plan based on the characteristics of the wound and the patient will improve outcome. Characteristics that lead to increased areas of devitalization, delayed healing, or increased infection rates require specialized approaches to wound management.

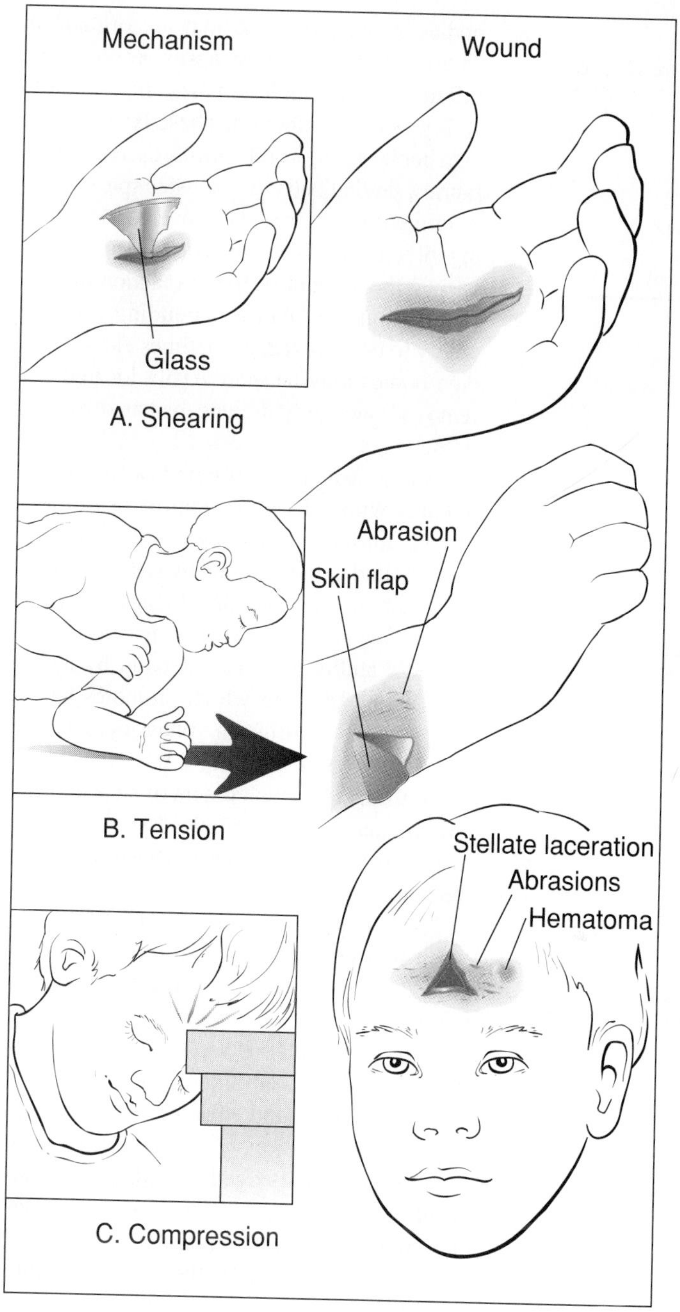

Figure 110.1.
Common mechanisms of injury and resulting wounds.
A. Shearing injury.
B. Tension injury.
C. Compression injury.

INDICATIONS

All wounds will benefit from some management. The level of care necessary for the particular injury must be determined by the clinician. Local cleansing and irrigation is important in almost all wounds, whereas additional interventions must be considered frequently but are only indicated in specific situations.

Certain situations indicate the removal of a foreign body within a wound (Chapter 113). In general, objects that are easily seen and grasped, objects likely to cause intense inflammation, objects in close proximity to vital structures, or objects that are detected due to the development of a soft tissue infection should be removed (10). Relatively inert foreign bodies that cause little tissue reaction and are not threatening because of their position or potential for migration may be left in place especially if exploration would lead to further tissue damage (2, 11). Other foreign

Chapter 110
General Wound
Management

Table 110.1.
Tetanus Prone Wounds

Wounds contaminated with soil,
feces, saliva
Bite wounds
Crush wounds
Puncture wounds
Avulsion wounds
Missile wounds
Burns and frostbite

bodies, especially those that are organic in nature, cause an intense tissue reaction and inflammation which impairs the wound's ability to resist infection. These types of foreign bodies (e.g., wood, thorns, cactus spines, fabrics, devitalized skin, rooster spurs) must be diligently sought and removed or devastating infections may result (10, 15, 16). Metals vary in the amount of tissue reaction and inflammation they cause depending on their ability to be oxidized. Sometimes elusive foreign bodies may be more easily located and removed once they are encapsulated by scar tissue.

In grossly contaminated wounds and wounds with a large amount of devitalized tissue, debridement can decrease wound infections and complications by removing bacteria, debris, and devitalized tissue. Devitalized tissue has been shown to impair the wound's ability to resist infection by acting as a culture medium which promotes bacterial growth, inhibiting phagocytosis by leukocytes, and limiting other leukocyte functions by the development of an anaerobic environment (31). Devitalized skin, fat, and muscle have been shown to cause comparable amounts of infection.

It is important to use debridement only when it is necessary so as to not "make the wound *your* wound." Jagged-edged, uneven wounds have a much longer wound edge than straight lacerations. If closed carefully, this leads to a decreased amount of tension per unit length of wound edge and better wound edge approximation (1). Converting such wounds to straight-edged wounds by debridement of skin and underlying tissue increases the amount of tension required to keep wound edges approximated and, therefore, the width of the scar (1). Debridement of facial fat should be avoided as unsightly depressions may result at the site of repair.

Fluid in a wound cavity, whether it is blood, pus, or serous fluid, will damage the defense mechanisms of the wound and lead to an increased risk of infection. Drains can be used to evacuate these fluids and improve healing. Drains should not be used prophylactically, however, as they actually may increase infection rates by damaging wound resistance to infection and permitting retrograde contamination of the wound by surface bacteria (43).

Wounds particularly prone to infection should be considered for delayed closure. These include markedly contaminated wounds, wounds with purulent material already present, wounds greater than 6 hours old, missile wounds, wounds secondary to severe crush injury, wounds caused by human or animal bites, and wounds that have come into contact with feces, saliva (bites), or vaginal fluids. Such wounds, if cleaned appropriately and managed in an open fashion for 4 to 5 days, will develop a marked resistance to infection and can undergo delayed closure at that time (38, 41).

All wounds carry the risk of tetanus as a potential complication. Contaminated wounds (especially involving soil or feces), wounds with devitalized tissue, and deep puncture wounds are particularly prone to contamination with *Clostridium tetani* (55). Patients who have not received at least three previous doses of tetanus toxoid or whose immunization status is unknown should receive tetanus immune globulin (TIG) 250 IU intramuscularly if the wound is tetanus prone (Table 110.1). Recommendations for using TIG and tetanus toxoid based on the number of previous doses of toxoid, the type of wound, and the length of time since the last toxoid are provided in Table 110.2.

Increasing numbers of rabies cases have been reported among wild animals in recent years (52, 53). Skunks, foxes, raccoons, and bats have a significant prevalence of rabies depending on their geographic location. Transmission of infection to stray and do-

Table 110.2.
Tetanus Prophylaxis

No. Doses of Tetanus Toxoid	Time Since Last Dose	Clean Wound		Tetanus Prone Wound	
		TIG	dT*	TIG	dT*
<3 or unknown	<5 yr	No	Yes	Yes	Yes
	5–10 yr	No	Yes	Yes	Yes
	≥10 yr	No	Yes	Yes	Yes
≥3	<5 yr	No	No	No	No
	5–10 yr	No	No	No	Yes
	≥10 yr	No	Yes	No	Yes

* In children under 7 years of age, DTP or pediatric DT (if pertussis vaccine is contraindicated) should be given.

Table 110.3.
Indications for Rabies Prophylaxis

1. Bites of wild carnivores (especially bats, foxes, raccoons, skunks, and woodchucks)
2. Bites of unknown or unavailable dogs and cats in rabies endemic areas
3. Bites of ill-appearing dogs and cats pending testing (may be discontinued if testing negative) or of animals who become ill during a 10-day observation period. Animals who are healthy and can be observed for 10 days do not need to be sacrificed and initial prophylaxis can wait until the animal develops symptoms
4. Individual cases of bites by cattle, rodents, and lagamorphs (rabbits and hares, although they almost never transmit rabies)

Immunoprophylaxis is indicated if the animal is acting strangely (very aggressive behavior or nocturnal animals out during daylight hours)

mestic dogs and cats, cattle, and even people have been reported. Bites by known, healthy, provoked domestic pets (dogs and cats) are unlikely to transmit rabies. Bites by unknown or unavailable animals or by skunks, foxes, raccoons, and bats should be treated as if the animal was rabid. Animals that can be observed and remain healthy for 10 days after biting a person could not have transmitted the virus. The virus has been transmitted in an aerosolized fashion in caves inhabited by bats (52, 53). Wounds for which rabies prophylaxis is indicated are listed in Table 110.3.

EQUIPMENT

Sterile gloves and mask
Manual sphygmomanometer to aid hemostasis
Hair clippers for scalp wounds
Iodophor or chlorhexidine-based solution for skin cleansing
Sterile saline solution for irrigation
Syringe—35 mL for irrigation
Splashshield device for irrigation (may use 19-gauge needle or angiocath)
High porosity sponge
Sterile drapes
Gauze sponges
Antibiotic ointment—water-based
Microporous polypropylene dressings
Microporous tape
Cotton tip applicators
Needle driver
Scissors and/or scalpel

Forceps and/or skin hooks (may be made from 25-gauge needle and applicators)
Wound closure and anesthetic materials as needed (Chapters 37 and 111)

It is important, especially with pediatric patients, to have all the equipment ready at the outset. Delays to get more equipment will only heighten the anxiety of the child as he or she waits for the procedure to begin. Instruments which may look threatening should be prepared out of the child's sight. The equipment should be appropriate for the degree of involvement and complexity of the procedure.

Protective equipment for health care personnel is extremely important (Chapter 8). Universal precautions should be followed by all personnel in dealing with wounds. Wound irrigation, hemostasis, and wound closure present opportunities for potentially contaminated blood to come into contact with the skin or mucous membranes of personnel involved in the procedure. A study in an adult ED population showed that 4% of patients who had blood drawn had unrecognized human immunodeficiency virus (HIV) infection. Patients with penetrating trauma had an increased seroprevalence rate independent of other known risk factors (5). Although the seroprevalence rate in children would be expected to be lower, it could approach 4% depending on the age of the child (increased rates in adolescents) and local incidence.

Splash guard devices can facilitate high pressure irrigation while providing protection for physicians, nurses, and ancillary personnel. They are disposable and easy to use. They also are less threatening in appearance to a toddler or young school-aged child than a needle or intravenous catheter. The Zerowet® splashshield (Zerowet, Inc., Los Angeles, CA) attaches to both Luer-Lok or slip-tip syringes and has a 19-gauge aperture producing an adequate flow of irrigating solution.

Skin hooks, which can be fashioned from 25-gauge needles bent with a needle driver or hemostat and attached to the end of a cotton-tipped applicator, cause much less tissue trauma than forceps when approximating skin edges. Forceps (rather than fingers) should be used to catch suture needles that have been driven through a wound. Disposable instrument trays can be custom ordered to include the equipment most often required at a particular institution. Disposable trays are usually less expensive than recleaning, resterilizing, and packing reusable instruments. Good quality, standard instruments are available in disposable packages. Particularly fine instruments or instruments for specialized procedures which will only be used occasionally are more readily available and usually of better quality when purchased as reusable, surgical quality instruments.

PROCEDURES

Hemostasis

As with any traumatic injury, the patient's overall status first should be assessed. Critical, life-threatening injuries should receive the highest priority. The airway and breathing should be assessed and stabilized. Vascular access should be obtained if the patient is hemodynamically unstable. Bleeding needs to be controlled. Even with minor wounds a thorough, secondary survey must be completed to ensure that concurrent injuries are not missed because the clinician's attention is drawn to the potentially disfiguring but not life-threatening laceration.

Control of bleeding, if it is significant, is an important part of the primary survey. Smaller wounds can wait until primary issues are addressed. Direct pressure followed by the application of a pressure dressing will lead to effective hemostasis in the vast majority of traumatic wounds (3, 4) (Fig. 27.1). EMS or ED personnel should ensure that all kinked or twisted flaps are returned to their original anatomic position to decrease the chance of vascular compromise.

Applying saline-soaked gauze pads will decrease heat loss from the wound while preventing desiccation of the wound edges, which in turn decreases amounts of devitalized tissue, lowers infection rates, and improves wound healing. If hemostasis cannot be achieved with direct pressure and the wound is on an extremity, the extremity should first be elevated for 1 minute. A sphygmomanometer placed proximal to the wound can then be inflated to a pressure just above the patient's systolic blood pressure

(Fig. 27.2). Tissue damage will not occur for approximately 2 hours following inflation (4).

Emergency Department Evaluation

The ED evaluation begins with taking an adequate history and performing a thorough physical examination using aseptic techniques (1) (Chapter 7). The mechanism and time of injury, characteristics of the wounding material, and location of the patient when the injury occurred should be noted. The possibility of a foreign body in the wound should be ascertained from the history. The patient's general health status, medication use, and immunization status, especially with regard to tetanus, should be determined.

A good physical examination of the injury requires hemostasis so that blood does not obscure the clinician's view. A sphygmomanometer can be used as previously noted. Distal function is tested first. Neurovascular integrity and the function of all tendons possibly involved in the injury must be examined cautiously before anesthesia is used. Bones underlying or near the wound should be carefully palpated to elicit crepitus, instability, or tenderness which could indicate the presence of a fracture. Radiographs should be obtained as indicated.

After the initial physical examination, the wound should be anesthetized (Chapter 37). When adequate anesthesia is obtained, *every* wound should be explored, even those that will not be sutured. The clinician should place the patient in a position that makes the wound easily accessible and use adequate lighting. Appropriate anesthesia and hemostasis should provide a nearly bloodless and painless environment in which the clinician can work.

Regarding extremities, exploration should be done through a full range of motion of the affected area. The examination also should be done in the position in which the injury occurred. Vascular structures, nerves, and tendons must be examined for incomplete injuries even if the distal examination seemed normal. The wound examination also should include a search for foreign bodies and devitalized tissues. Wound repair that will require the open reduction of fractures, reanastomosis of vascular structures, or nerve or tendon repair should be taken to the operating room where more controlled conditions allow for better wound healing (1). Extremely large wounds or wounds requiring extensive repairs in sensitive areas (e.g., perineum, medial canthus of the eye, extensive intraoral wounds) also should be considered for management in the operating room.

Foreign Bodies

The clinician must consider the possibility that a foreign body is contained in the wound based on history of the injury and the physical examination. Foreign bodies are rarely discovered unless they are anticipated by the person caring for the patient (10). Thorough exploration may reveal a foreign body in the wound but does not guarantee that one does not exist. Foreign bodies may be larger than the wound defect, especially if the wound extends into fatty tissue. Seeing the bottom of the wound decreases but does not eliminate the chance that a foreign body is present (13). Physical examination alone cannot exclude the presence of a foreign body in fatty tissues.

Wounds suspicious for the presence of foreign bodies should be radiographed. Multiple projections, surface markers, proper film exposure techniques (use of soft tissue penetration settings) and the use of fluoroscopy can increase the sensitivity of radiographs in the detection of foreign bodies (10). Most radiopaque objects, even if small, are easily demonstrated. All types of glass should be detectable on appropriately exposed radiographs regardless of their lead or heavy metal content (11). Glass fragments as small as 0.5 mm can be visualized on radiographs (12). Multiple projections will cast the shadow away from overlying bones and can result in alignment of the long axis of the foreign body with the long axis of the radiograph beam, increasing chances for detection. Using xeroradiographs, computed tomography scans, and ultrasound (Chapter 137) may increase the sensitivity in detecting less radiopaque foreign bodies (10). Nonradiopaque foreign bodies may present as filling defects, or air may be evident surrounding them on films (10).

Once a foreign body is detected, the decision must be made whether or not it will be removed based on its location and degree of reactivity. Removal of foreign bodies is discussed in Chapter 113.

Wound Cleansing and Irrigation

Using antiseptic solutions for wound cleansing is somewhat controversial. Certainly the intact skin surrounding a wound should be cleansed with an antiseptic solution (usually an iodophor, hexachlorophene, or chlorhexidine containing solution). Obvious dirt or other foreign materials should be removed from the wound by irrigation or gentle scrubbing (Fig. 110.2.A). Experimental evidence in laboratory animals suggests that using antiseptic solutions within the wound may damage tissue defenses and actually potentiate the development of infection (17, 18). In these studies the detergent component of scrub solutions seemed to be especially damaging to wound defenses. Povidone-iodine in the absence of detergents did not seem to increase infections but offered no therapeutic benefit over saline alone (18).

In contrast, a clinical trial showed that gently scrubbing wounds with a 1% povidone-iodine solution for 60 seconds reduced the incidence of wound infections when compared with saline irrigation alone (19). Most authorities recommend using only saline or nontoxic surfactants within wounds to effect cleansing (17, 18, 20–22). A good axiom to follow is "The only solution that should be placed in a wound is one that can be safely poured in the physician's eye" (23), although testing various solutions in this way is not recommended.

Saline irrigation of wounds has become a standard practice in treating contaminated or dirty wounds. High pressure irrigation of at least 8 lb/in^2 is required to remove most foreign material (20, 24) (Fig. 110.2.B). High pressure irrigation of this magnitude can be accomplished using a 35-ml syringe and a 19-gauge plastic vascular catheter. Usually 200 to 300 mL is the minimum volume desired for irrigation. It has been shown that irrigation fluid disseminates laterally through the sides of the wound but does not penetrate beneath

Figure 110.2.
A. Gentle mechanical scrubbing of contaminated wound.
B. High pressure irrigation using a Zerowet® splashshield.

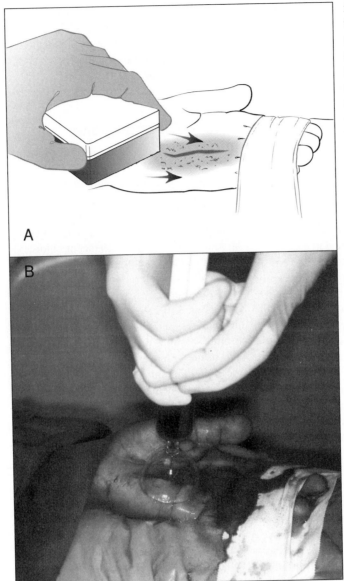

in urban, adult ED populations (2, 25). Using splash-shields has been shown to effectively decrease splatter onto the face and chest of the irrigator and correctly using the Zerowet® splashshield eliminated all facial splash (26).

Irrigation can effectively eliminate large particles, soil, and loose pieces of devitalized tissue but not bacteria and small particles. Mechanical scrubbing of wounds with sponges is effective in removing bacteria but can lead to tissue damage and decreased resistance to infection. Sponges with a low porosity are more damaging, and soaking the sponge in saline does not decrease the damage caused (27). Various surfactant compounds in the polyol family have been developed for use with sponges including Pluronic F-68® (Shur Medical Corp., Beaverton, OR) and Poloxamer 188® (Calgon Corp., St. Louis, MO) (20–22, 27). These compounds have been shown to be effective and safe and do not potentiate tissue damage. Scrubbing should be used in particularly contaminated wounds and when irrigation may distort the wound edges and compromise the cosmetic result obtained (e.g., in the periorbital area where the loose areolar tissue is easily distended by lateral dissemination of irrigation fluids) (20, 22).

the wound bed (24). Bacteria which contaminate wounds did not seem to be carried with the irrigating fluid in this model. Irrigation damaged tissue defenses in experimentally infected wounds. Therefore, this technique should only be used in contaminated wounds where the benefits of cleansing are more advantageous than the consequences of tissue damage (24).

Irrigation also can be hazardous for medical personnel irrigating the wound. The splash of blood and possibly infective agents into the eyes or mucous membranes of the irrigator may transmit HIV, hepatitis B, and other bloodborne infections. As mentioned previously, studies have shown surprisingly high seroprevalence rates for these infections

Hair Removal

Hair has long been regarded as a potential source of wound contamination, and data in the surgical literature support this view (1, 28). Hair also can make both the placement and removal of sutures difficult and, in the latter case, more painful. Razor removal of hair has resulted in increased rates of postoperative infections in surgical patients (29, 30). Removal of hair with electric clippers has led to decreased infection rates (29). The blade assemblies of electric clippers need to be adequately sterilized after each use (29) which can be difficult in a busy ED, especially if multiple scalp lacerations are being treated at the same time. Alternatively, petroleum jelly can be used to keep unruly hairs out of the wound while suturing takes place. Eyebrows should never be shaved or clipped, as they serve as important landmarks for wound alignment during repair and once shaved (or clipped), they may not grow back.

Debridement

Debridement can be an important step in wound management. It should be used to remove heavily contaminated tissue and also to remove devitalized tissue that will foster bacterial growth (Fig. 110.3) (31). However, debridement can also cause problems with wound healing. Excessive removal of tissue results in increased tension at the wound margins and subsequently increased scarring. If complete debridement of the wound is contraindicated because of the presence of vital structures or the probability of a poor cosmetic result, high pressure irrigation should be used. This should be followed by meticulous debridement of all clearly nonviable tissue (31).

Antibiotics

One major goal of wound care is preventing infection, which will lead to a decreased rate of complications and to a more aesthetically pleasing scar. The rate of infection in properly cleansed, nonbite wounds is generally quite low (less than 1%). Nevertheless, using prophylactic antibiotics has been advocated in many clinical situations involving minor soft tissue trauma. It is important to remember that many wound characteristics and the mechanism of injury greatly influence the rate at which infections develop.

The effect that soil contaminants have on host defenses has already been discussed. These same soil contaminants tend to inhibit the action of amphoteric and basic antibi-

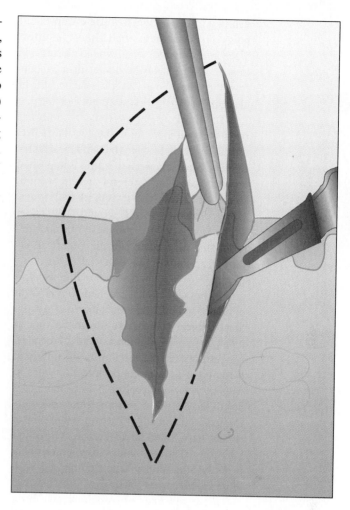

Figure 110.3
Wound debridement is performed to remove heavily contaminated or non-viable tissue.

otics. Acidic antibiotics such as penicillins and cephalosporins do not react with these contaminants and are not inactivated (32).

The size of the bacterial inoculum is extremely important in determining if infection develops. An inoculum of greater than or equal to 10^6 bacteria per gram of tissue is generally necessary to produce infection in otherwise healthy skin (33). Cleansing the wound (irrigation and scrubbing) and debridement, if necessary, are intended to decrease the bacterial load in the wound.

Investigators have attempted to determine the effectiveness of antibiotics in reducing wound infections. One study using experimental animals showed that to be successful, antibiotics must be given soon after the injury (34). In this study systemic antibiotics were effective in preventing infection in contaminated wounds if administered within 1 hour of the time the experimental wound was made. In wounds that were closed immediately after the injury, antibiotics were effective in preventing infection when initiated up to 24 hours later. Antibiotics had almost no effect (75% infection rate) when wound closure and treatment were delayed greater than 3 hours from the time of injury. Additional benefits of cleansing and irrigation were not evaluated.

This work also showed that wounds left open show an increase in their vascular permeability which leads to the buildup of a protein exudate in the wound. Fibrin is deposited and envelops the bacteria in the wound, shielding it from the effects of antibiotics. Using proteases in the wound (trypsin or Travase) will break down these fibrinous deposits and may potentiate the beneficial effects of antibiotics (32, 34).

By 3 to 6 hours the bacterial concentration within wounds has reached 10^6 per gram of tissue, and infection rates increase greatly. Some clinical studies have shown that time to repair has a marked impact on infection rates, suggesting that the institution of antibiotic therapy has little effect on infection rates in wounds not closed before 3 to 6 hours (35, 36). These studies support the work performed with animals. However, other clincal studies have found no difference in infection rates for pediatric wounds closed greater than 6 hours after injury when compared with those closed earlier (56).

Increased rates of infection have been found in wounds involving the hands and feet (36, 37). These seem more related to the types of injury seen in these regions and differences in the level of bacterial contamination than to a decreased biologic resistance to infection inherent in these sites (38). Despite this finding, randomized clinical trials have failed to show any benefit of prophylactic antibiotics in wounds involving the hand (39, 40). No studies have addressed the efficacy of prophylactic antibiotics in lower extremity wounds. Despite the lack of convincing data that prophylactic antibiotics are efficacious in treating minor soft tissue injuries, most experts suggest certain indications for using antibiotics in soft tissue injury (38) (Table 110.4).

If the choice is made to give an antibiotic, one with a broad spectrum which is effective against both staphylococci and streptococci, as well as facultative organisms, should be chosen. Cephalexin is an inexpensive, well-tolerated, and effective choice. Oxacillin, dicloxacillin, and amoxicillin-

Table 110.4.
Indications for Prophylactic Antibiotics

1. Patient prone to development of infective endocarditis
2. Immunosuppressed patients (relative indication)
3. Soft tissue lacerations occurring in previously lymphedematous tissue
4. Wounds judged to be contaminated or dirty by the clinician (especially in dependent areas)
5. Stellate lacerations with adjacent abrasions resulting from high impact
6. Delayed wound cleansing and repair (between 6 and 18 hours after injury, bacterial colony counts reach potentially infective concentrations, and therefore open management and delayed closure should be considered)
7. Wounds contaminated by saliva, feces, vaginal fluids (open management and delayed closure should be considered)
8. Missile wounds

clavulinic acid also are effective. Penicillin-sensitive patients can be cautiously treated with cephalosporins. If the patient also had a history of cephalosporin sensitivity, erythromycin or erythromycin-sulfisoxazole are acceptable alternatives. Antibiotics are not a substitute for meticulous wound care and aseptic techniques.

Drains

Drains should be placed to evacuate any fluid-filled wound cavities. Vented, closed suction drainage is the most efficacious system (42).

Animal and Human Bites

Bite wounds are especially prone to infection due to the high inoculum of bacteria that usually accompanies them and the fact that they are often either puncture wounds or crush-type injuries. Puncture wounds require specific wound management techniques which are described in Chapter 112. Bite wounds are common injuries. Over one million people are bitten by dogs each year in the United States, most of them children, and dog bites account for about 1% of ED visits (44, 45, 52). The incidence of cat, human, and other mammalian bites is lower but still significant.

Dog bites become infected somewhat more frequently than lacerations in general (45). However, with meticulous wound preparation, including high pressure irrigation and debridement of devitalized tissues, most can be safely sutured to effect primary closure. *Staphylococcus, Streptococcus, Bacteroides* species, anaerobic cocci, and *Pasteurella multocida* are the most common infecting organisms (45–47). Obviously infected wounds should be cultured and antibiotic therapy directed by sensitivities. Prophylactic antibiotics are probably indicated for dog bites of the hand, bites greater than 6 hours old, or bites that inflict a puncture wound.

Amoxicillin-clavulinic acid is an excellent choice for use in animal bite wounds. When appropriate per kilogram doses are used and given at least 6 hours apart (with food), gastrointestinal side effects can be minimized. Erythromycin is used in patients who are penicillin sensitive (48). Some practitioners prefer dicloxacillin or cephalexin because they cost less and produce fewer side effects. They argue that although the in vitro activity of dicloxacillin and cephalexin against *Pasteurella* is inadequate, the clinical outcome with these agents in dog and cat bites is good (49).

Cat bites have a higher incidence of infection (47, 50) and should not be closed if at all possible (48). These are usually small caliber puncture wounds which result in inoculation of bacteria relatively deep below the skin surface. The microbiology of infecting organisms is similar to that seen in dog bites, although *P. multocida* is implicated in up to 50% of infected cat bites (45, 47, 49). All cat bite wounds should receive meticulous irrigation and debridement and prophylactic antibiotics. Irrigation and debridement may be difficult to achieve due to the small size of the break in the skin.

Animal bites also raise the issue of rabies prophylaxis. Soap and water cleansing of wounds will decrease the transmission of rabies. Wounds at risk for rabies infection should not be sutured (53, 54). Bites that carry a risk of rabies (Table 110.3) require passive and active immunization. Human rabies immune globulin is administered in a dose of 20 IU/kg. The wound is infiltrated with one-half the dose and the remainder is given intramuscularly at a site distant from the site of active immunization. Injection in the gluteal area is recommended. In instances when local infiltration is either impractical or particularly painful, the entire dose may be given intramuscularly.

Human diploid cell vaccine (HDCV) should be given in a dose of 1 mL intramuscularly on the initial day of treatment and repeated on days 3, 7, 14, and 28 (53, 54). The deltoid area is the preferred injection site. Rabies vaccine adsorbed (RVA) is an alternative to HDCV. It is considered equivalent in terms of safety and efficacy and is given in the same dose and according to the same schedule as HDCV.

Human bites have traditionally been thought of as having a high infection rate (47, 51). Yet it has been argued that this is more related to the site and mechanism of injury and delays in seeking treatment than any unique characteristics of human bites or their microbiology (49). Human bites often involve a high impact mechanism of injury (i.e., fist fights, sports injuries) which results in tissue crushing and devitalization. This might partially explain why injuries to the dorsum of the hand (closed fist injuries) have a much higher infection rate than other bite wounds. Wounds to the dorsal metacarpal-phalangeal (MCP) joints should be considered bite wounds until proven otherwise, as the patient is often reluctant to admit involvement in an altercation. It is especially important to examine these wounds through a full range of motion, including full flexion, for penetration of the joint capsule or extensor tendons. A tendon injury that occurred when the fist was clenched may not be visible in the wound field when the fingers are extended.

Staphylococci, streptococci (including group A streptococcus), *Bacteroides* sp., anaerobic cocci, and *Eikenella corrodens* are organisms implicated in infections caused by human bites (45, 49, 50). Human bite wounds should not be closed unless on the face or on a well-vascularized area and then only if they are thoroughly irrigated and debrided (48). All persons with puncture wounds or lacerations resulting from human bites should be treated with prophylactic antibiotics. Most human bites in children result only in abrasions or contusions which require only surface cleansing. For human bite wounds requiring antibiotic treatment, amoxicillin-clavulinic acid is again an excellent choice (48). If dicloxacillin or cephalexin is used, penicillin must be added to cover *E. corrodens*. Giving a patient two medicines instead of one is likely to decrease patient compliance.

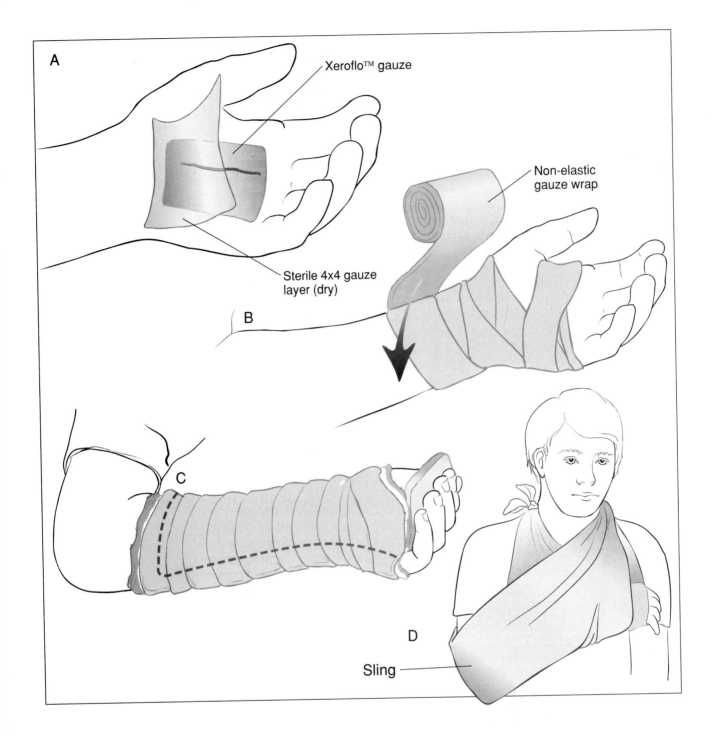

Figure 110.4.
Wound dressing.
A. Application of a moist nonadherent dressing followed by a dry covering.
B. Application of a nonelastic gauze wrap.
C. Application of a splint.
D. Wound elevation.

Tetanus Prophylaxis

All wounds should be assessed for the risks of tetanus as a potential complication, and the immunization status of all patients should be determined. Tetanus immune globulin (TIG) 250 IU should be administered intramuscularly when indicated for tetanus prone wounds (Table 110.1). When indicated, a single dose of tetanus toxoid should be administered intramuscularly as soon as possible after the injury (Table 110.2).

Postrepair Wound Care

Dressings are an important part of wound care. An effective dressing will prevent contamination of the wound by exogenous bacteria and promote epithelial migration and healing (1). As long as the outer surface of the dressing remains dry, it is an effective barrier to bacteria. By day 3 after primary closure, wounds are remarkably resistant to infection from external contamination.

Drying of the wound impairs healing. A dressing which prevents evaporation of water will keep the eschar and dermis at the wound site moist and promote rapid reepithelialization (Fig. 110.4.A) (1). Nonwoven, microporous polypropylene dressings are recommended and should be attached to the skin by side strips of microporous tape (1). Water-based antibiotic ointments under the dressings keep wound edges moist, which facilitates both healing and suture removal.

Facial wounds do not need to be dressed. To remove blood clots along the wound edge which will potentiate scar development, these wounds should be swabbed with half-strength hydrogen peroxide three to four times per day until suture removal (1). Abraded skin should be coated with water-soluble ointments. Wounds in cosmetically sensitive areas, especially abrasions, should be covered with sunblock with a protection factor of at least 15 for 6 months after injury to prevent development of hyperpigmented scars.

Pressure dressings with nonelastic gauze wrap can prevent fluid accumulation in wounds, thereby inhibiting the development of infection (Fig. 110.4.B). The amount of pressure applied proximal to extremity wounds is decreased to prevent edema development. Immobilization improves the ability of a wound to resist infection (1). Extremity wounds should be elevated and immobilized by slings and splints as needed (Fig. 110.4.C, D). Wounds that are closed primarily can be washed and gently patted dry after 48 hours.

SUMMARY
1. Obtain hemostasis with direct pressure to wound, or elevate extremity for 1 minute and then apply a sphygmomanometer.
2. Obtain adequate history including:
   Mechanism of injury
   Wounding object—mass, velocity, characteristics
   Environment in which injury occurred
   Time of injury
   General health of patient
   Medications
   Allergies
   Immunization status
3. Perform thorough physical examination including:
   Assessment of distal neurovascular function
   Assessment of tendon integrity
   Palpation of adjacent bony structures
4. Anesthetize wound
5. Explore every wound through full range of motion and in position of injury
6. Prepare all necessary equipment in advance
7. Evaluate for presence of foreign bodies
8. Remove all reactive foreign bodies (vegetable materials, wood, organic materials, clothing) and foreign bodies near vital structures or with potential to migrate
9. Cleanse wound using high pressure irrigation
10. Use mechanical scrubbing for particularly contaminated wounds
11. Debride obviously contaminated wounds and all devitalized tissue
12. Consider using antibiotics for:
    Contaminated wounds
    Bite wounds
    Crush wounds
    Foot wounds
    Other indications (Table 110.4)
13. Place drains if fluid is present
14. Administer appropriate tetanus and rabies prophylaxis
15. Apply dressing
16. Immobilize wound
17. Elevate wounded area when possible

Vigorous rubbing should be avoided as this can damage healing edges of the wound and lead to dehiscence and/or increased scarring.

COMPLICATIONS

Complications from general wound management techniques covered in this chapter should be minimal. Poor results including wound infections and less than optimal scars are more likely to result if these principles are not followed. Meticulous and thorough wound preparation, including a complete and detailed history and physical examination, is as important as the actual wound closure. As mentioned previously, antibiotics are never a substitute for thorough wound cleansing, debridement, and good aseptic technique. Overzealous debridement, especially in cosmetically important areas and areas under high amounts of static skin tension, will lead to scars that are wider than necessary and unsightly. Using antiseptic scrub solutions and other foreign substances in wounds may actually potentiate wound infections.

SUMMARY

General wound management techniques are often as important as actual wound closure in determining the eventual outcome in cases of soft tissue trauma. A working knowledge of skin biomechanics and wounding mechanisms will provide the basic information necessary for developing a rational treatment plan for each individual patient and injury. Adequate preparation and attention to detail throughout the process will minimize the risk of wound infection and maximize the chances of an optimal wound repair.

REFERENCES

1. Edlich RF, Rodeheaver GT, Morgan RF, Berman DE, Thacker JG. Principles of emergency wound management. Ann Emerg Med 1988;17:1284.
2. Trott A. Mechanisms of soft tissue trauma. Ann Emerg Med 1988;17:1279.
3. Thacker JG, Stolnecker MC, Allaire PE, Edgerton MT, Rodeheaver GT, Edlich RF. Practical applications of skin biomechanics. Clin Plast Surg 1977; 4:167.
4. Edlich RF, Rodeheaver GT, Thacker JG. The evalu-
ation of wounds in the emergency department. In: Tintinalli JE, Krome RL, Ruiz E, eds. Emergency Medicine: a comprehensive study guide. 3rd ed. New York: McGraw Hill, 1992; pp. 1027-1030.
5. Kelen GD, Fritz S, Qaqish B, Brookmeyer R, Baker JL, Cuddy RM, Goessel TK, Floccare D, Williams KA, Silvertson KT, Altman S, Quinn TC. Unrecognized human immunodeficiency virus infection in emergency department patients. N Engl J Med 1988; 318:1645.
6. Hauvy BB, Rodeheaver GT, Pettry D, Edgerton MT, Edlich RF. Inhibition of nonspecific defenses by soil infection potentiating factors. Surg Gynecol Obstet 1977;144:19.
7. Dougherty SH, Fiegel VO, Nelson RD, Edgerton MT, Edlich RF. Effects of soil potentiating factors on neutrophils in vitro. Am J Surg 1985;150:306.
8. Rodeheaver GT, Pettry D, Turnbull V, Edgerton MT, Edlich RF. Identification of wound potentiating factors in soil. Am J Surg 1974;128:8.
9. Roberts AH, Rye DG, Edgerton MT, Rodeheaver GT, Edlich RF. Activity of antibiotics in contaminated wounds containing clay soil. Am J Surg 1979; 137:381.
10. Lammers RL. Soft tissue foreign bodies. Ann Emerg Med 1988;17:1336.
11. Felman AH, Fisher MS. The radiographic detection of glass in soft tissue. Radiology 1969;92:1529.
12. Tandberg D. Glass in the hand and foot: will an x-ray film show it? JAMA 1982;248:1872.
13. Avner JR, Baker MD. Lacerations involving glass: the role of routine roentgenograms. AJDC 1992; 146:600.
14. Anderson MA, Newmeyer III WL, Kilgore Jr ES,. Diagnosis and treatment of retained foreign bodies in the hand. Am J Surg 1982;144:63.
15. Cooler JO, Kleiman MB, West K, Grosfeld J. Retained spur following a rooster attack. Pediatrics 1992;90:106.
16. Cracchiolo III A,. Wooden foreign bodies in the foot. Am J Surg 1980;140:585.
17. Custer J, Edlich RF, Prusak M, Madden J, Pauela P, Wangensteen OH. Studies in the management of the contaminated wound V. An assessment of the effectiveness of PhisoHex and betadine surgical scrub solutions. Am J Surg 1971;121:572.
18. Rodeheaver GT, Bellamy W, Kody M, Spatafora G, Fitton L, Leyden K, Edlich RF. Bactericidal activity and toxicity of iodine-containing solutions in wounds. Arch Surg 1982;117:181.
19. Gravett A, Sterner S, Clinton JE, Ruiz E. A trial of povidone-iodine in the prevention of infection in sutured lacerations. Ann Emerg Med 1987;16:167.
20. Edlich RF, Rodeheaver GT, Thacker JG. Wound preparation. In: Tintinalli JE, Krome RL, Ruiz E, eds. Emergency Medicine: a comprehensive study guide. 3rd ed. New York: McGraw Hill, 1992; pp. 1037–1039.
21. Rodeheaver GT, Kurtz L, Kircher BJ, Edlich RF. Pluronic F-68®: a promising new skin wound cleanser. Ann Emerg Med 1980;9:572.
22. Bryant CA, Rodeheaver GT, Reeum EM, Nichter LS, Kenney JG, Edlich RF. Search for a nontoxic surgical scrub solution for periorbital lacerations. Ann Emerg Med 1984;13:317.

Chapter 110
General Wound
Management

23. Branemark PI, Albrektsson B, Lindstrom J, Lundborg G. Local tissue effects of wound disinfectants. Acta Chir Scand 1966;357 (suppl.):166.

24. Wheeler CB, Rodeheaver GT, Thacker JG, Edgerton MT, Edlich RF. Side effects of high pressure irrigation. Surg Gynecol Obstet 1970;143:775.

25. Kelan GD, Green GB, Prucell RH, et al. Hepatitis B and hepatitis C in emergency department patients. N Engl J Med 1992;326:1399.

26. Pigman EC, Karch DB, Scott JL. Splatter during jet irrigation cleansing of a wound model: a comparison of three inexpensive devices. Ann Emerg Med 1993; 22:1563.

27. Rodeheaver GT, Smith SL, Thacker JG, Edgerton MT, Edlich RF. Mechanical cleansing of contaminated wounds with a surfactant. Am J Surg 1975; 129:241.

28. Dineen P, Druisin L. Epidemics of postoperative wound infections associated with hair carriers. Lancet 1973;2:1157.

29. Alexander JW, Fischer JE, Boyajian M, Palmquist J, Morris MJ. The influence of hair removal methods on wound infections. Arch Surg 1983;118:347.

30. Masterson TM, Rodeheaver GT, Morgan RF, Edlich RF. Bacteriologic evaluation of electric clippers for surgical hair removal. Am J Surg 1984;144:301.

31. Hauvy B, Rodeheaver G, Veusko J, Egerton MT, Edlich RF. Debridement: an essential component of traumatic wound care. Am J Surg 1978;135:238.

32. Edlich RF, Rodeheaver GT, Thacker JG. Antibiotics and drains in wound management. In: Tintinalli JE, Krome RL, Ruiz E, eds. Emergency medicine: a comprehensive study guide. 3rd ed. New York: McGraw Hill, 1992; pp.1040–1042.

33. Magee C, Hauvy B, Rodeheaver GT, Fox J, Edgerton MT, Edlich RF. A rapid slide technique for quantitating wound bacterial count. Am J Surg 1977;133:760.

34. Edlich RF, Smith QT, Edgerton MT. Resistance of the surgical wound to antimicrobial prophylaxis and its mechanism of development. Am J Surg 1973; 126:583.

35. Morgan WT, Hutchinson D, Johnson HM. The delayed treatment of wounds of the hand and forearm under antibiotic cover. Br J Surg 1980;67:140.

36. Thirlby RC, Blair III J, Thal ER. The value of prophylactic antibiotics for simple lacerations. Surg Gynecol Obstet 1983;156:212.

37. Rutherford WH, Spence RAJ. Infection in wounds sutured in the accident and emergency department. Ann Emerg Med 1980;9:350.

38. Edlich RF, Kenney JG, Morgan RF, et al. Antimicrobial treatment of minor soft tissue lacerations: a critical review. Emerg Med Clin North Am 1986; 4:561.

39. Grossman JAI, Adams JP, Kunec J. Prophylactic antibiotics in simple hand lacerations. JAMA 1981; 245:1055.

40. Haughey RE, Lammers RL, Wagner DK. Use of antibiotics in the initial management of soft tissue hand wounds. Ann Emerg Med 1981;10:187.

41. Edlich RF, Rogers W, Kasper G, Kaufman D, Tsung MS, Wangensteen OH. Studies in the management of the contaminated wound: I. Optimal time for closure of contaminated open wounds. II. Comparison of resistance to infection of open and closed wounds during healing. Am J Surg 1969;117:323.

42. Golden GT, Roberts TL, Rodeheaver GT, Edgerton MT, Edlich RF. A new filtered sump tube for wound drainage. Am J Surg 1975;129:716.

43. Magee C, Rodeheaver GT, Golden GT, Fox J, Edgerton MT, Edlich RF. Potentiation of wound infection by surgical drains. Am J Surg 1976;131:547.

44. Rest JG, Goldstein EJC. Management of human and animal bite wounds. Emerg Med Clin North Am 1985;3:117.

45. Brook I. Microbiology of human and animal bite wounds in children. Pediatr Infect Dis J 1987;6:29.

46. Callaham M. Dog bite wounds. JAMA 1980;244: 2327.

47. Aghababian RV, Conte Jr JE,. Mammalian bite wounds. Ann Emerg Med 1980;9:79.

48. Trott A. Care of mammalian bites. Pediatr Infect Dis J 1987;6:8.

49. Callaham M. Controversies in antibiotic choices for bite wounds. Ann Emerg Med 1988;17:1321.

50. Edlich RF, Spengler MD, Rodeheaver GT, Silloway KA, Morgan RF. Emergency department management of mammalian bites. Emerg Med Clin North Am 1986;4:595.

51. Baker MD, Moore SE. Human bites in children. AJDC 1987;141:1285.

52. Schmidt MJ, Olson JG, Krebs JW. Rabies goes wild. Contemp Pediatr 1993;10(8):36.

53. Fishbein DB, Robinson LE. Rabies. N Engl J Med 1993;329:1632.

54. American Academy of Pediatrics. Rabies. In: Peter G, ed. 1994 Red book: report of the committee on infectious diseases. 23rd ed. Elk Grove, IL: American Academy of Pediatrics, 1994; pp.388–395.

55. American Academy of Pediatrics. Tetanus. In: Peter G, ed. 1994 Red book: report of the committee on infectious diseases. 23rd ed. Elk Grove, IL: American Academy of Pediatrics, 1994; pp. 458–463.

56. Baker MD, Lanuti M. The management and outcome of lacerations in urban children. Ann Emerg Med 1990;19:1001–1005.

LACERATION REPAIR

Robert McNamara and John Loiselle

INTRODUCTION

Over one-third of injuries in children involve a laceration, making it the most common specific injury for which care is sought in a pediatric emergency department (1, 2). In addition, a significant number of these patients seek treatment in primary care clinics (3). Laceration repair accounts for one-half of all procedures performed on injured children (1, 2).

A laceration refers to a traumatic linear disruption of the dermis. Repair of such injuries serves several purposes. Early repair following appropriate wound management (Chapter 110) restores the skin's protective barrier and thereby reduces the risk of infection and fosters rapid healing. Suture placement also can assist in hemostasis by tamponading vessels involved in the laceration. Providing optimal cosmesis, particularly for wounds involving the face, is another important goal with laceration repair.

The incidence of lacerations in children is strongly correlated with the developmental level of the child. The initial rise in incidence occurs with the ability to ambulate. Lacerations peak at 2 years of age when the child has attained greatest mobility but lacks equivalent motor coordination. Half of childhood lacerations occur in children under 5 years of age, and frequently involve falls on broken glass bottles, wooden furniture, asphalt, or concrete (1). Lacerations resulting from assaults or altercations are more common in adolescents.

Animal bites also are a frequent source of lacerations in children. This is especially true in the preschool and early school years, when inadvertent provocation can result in an attack by the animal.

Common sites of lacerations in children are the head (60%), the upper extremities (23%), and the lower extremities (15%) (1, 4). Lacerations of the head or face are proportionately greater in children under 2 years of age, as older children are more likely to break a fall by extending an arm or leg.

The majority of childhood lacerations can be treated without subspecialty assistance (1, 2). Need for consultation depends on a number of factors, including the level of skill and experience of the clinician, the complexity of the laceration and involvement of underlying structures, the location of the laceration, and the ability of the child to cooperate.

In view of the frequency of lacerations during childhood, the importance of early repair, and the straightforward methods required for the majority of these injuries, every clinician treating acute injuries in children should be capable of suturing lacerations.

ANATOMY AND PHYSIOLOGY

Knowledge of the anatomy and regenerative properties of the skin is crucial to performing an optimal laceration repair. Layers of the skin are depicted in Figure 111.1. The epidermis is the most external layer and is composed of epithelial cells whose function is to protect deeper tissues from infection and desiccation.

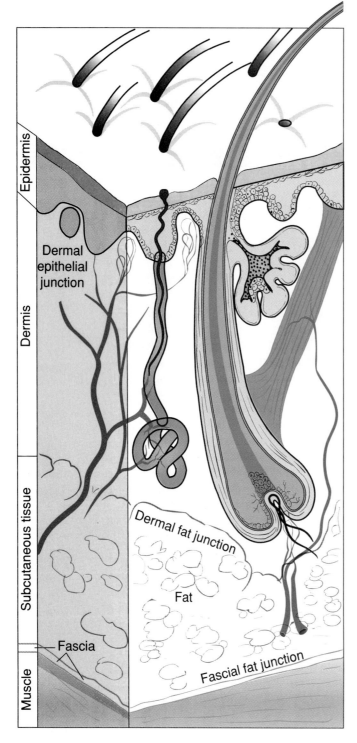

Figure 111.1
Anatomy of the skin layers.

tissue is bounded below by a sheet of connective tissue called the fascia.

The depth of the wound and the particular layers that have been disrupted are important factors in determining the best type of closure. Early contraction at the deeper levels following injury frequently results in an inaccurate estimate of wound depth. The wound must be explored thoroughly for this reason. The clinician must also carefully search for injuries to underlying structures, such as tendons which may have shifted with flexion or extension from below the visible external area of involvement. Certain layers retain sutures best: the fascial-fat junction, the dermal-fat junction, and the level just below the dermal-epithelial junction (Fig. 111.1). Adequate support of tissues is a prerequisite for an optimal closure and requires approximation of each involved layer. Improper alignment of layers results in an uneven surface which produces a shadow and obvious scarring.

Intact skin is under constant tension. This tension has both a static and a dynamic component. The skin in a particular location of the body possesses an intrinsic amount of tension which runs in a distribution depicted by Kraissel's lines, also known as the relaxed skin tension lines (RSTL) (11, 14) (Fig. 111.2). Tension along these lines determines the initial extent of separation that occurs along a laceration and the ultimate width of the scar. Sutures provide temporary support until the skin can regenerate tissue capable of overcoming this tension and maintaining closure of the wound. The extrinsic component of tension is produced by underlying muscles and joints. Skin overlying the knee, for example, is under varying amounts of tension depending on whether the knee is flexed or extended. Lacerations running perpendicular to these lines of tension subsequently gape more and require stronger sutures over a longer period to provide adequate support. These lacerations are consequently at an increased risk of scarring. Lacerations that run parallel to joints, normal skin folds, or Kraissel's lines can be expected to heal more rapidly and with better cosmetic results.

→

Figure 111.2.
Kraissel's lines or relaxed skin tension lines.

Immediately subjacent is the dermis which contains blood vessels, nerve endings, collagen, and fibroblasts. Below the dermis is subcutaneous tissue which is mainly composed of fat cells. Hair follicles, nerve fibers, and blood vessels also are located in this layer. The extent of subcutaneous tissue varies with the particular area of the body. The subcutaneous

**Chapter 111
Laceration Repair**

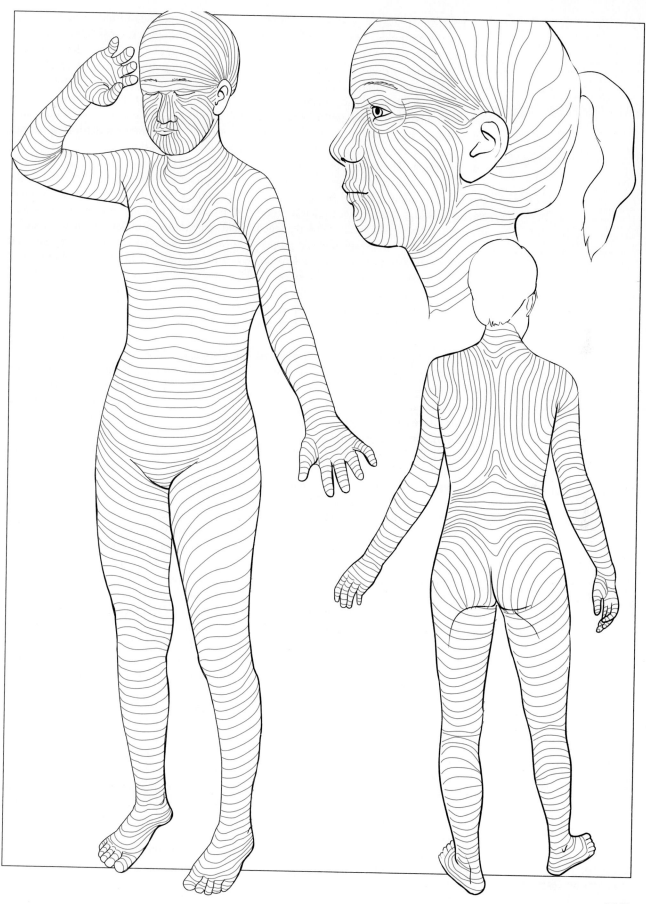

The normal healing process of skin occurs over a prolonged period and involves multiple, sometimes overlapping, stages. The process is typically divided into coagulation, inflammation, epithelialization, angiogenesis, collagen metabolism, and wound contraction. Coagulation occurs within the first hours following injury and involves vasospasm, platelet aggregation, and fibrous clot formation. The inflammatory phase is marked by increased capillary permeability and invasion of the wound by leukocytes. Neutrophils and macrophases release proteolytic enzymes which break down damaged tissue. Both cells possess phagocytic properties and ingest debris and bacteria. Chemotactic factors which stimulate fibroblast migration and replication are released during this phase. The inflammatory process peaks about 24 hours after the injury and lasts for several days.

The epidermis is the only layer with true regenerative capabilities. All other layers heal by laying down collagen or scar tissue. New epithelial cell growth occurs along the lacerated edges of the epidermis. In a sutured laceration complete bridging of the wound occurs within 48 hours. Epithelial cell growth is stimulated by the same factors that affect fibroblast proliferation (10). The placement of sutures creates a new wound through the epithelium and the new epithelial cells will migrate along the track of the suture. These cells frequently disappear once the suture is removed; however, when sutures are left in place for prolonged periods of time or are placed under excessive tension, these epithelial cells are more likely to remain and form punctate scars along the edge of the wound.

The various stages of wound healing depend on the delivery of substrates including nutrients, oxygen, and inflammatory cells to the site of injury. New vessel growth or angiogenesis is crucial in providing this means of delivery. Capillary production in the area of injury is stimulated by hypoxia, lactase production and stimulating factors produced by macrophages (10). Angiogenesis peaks 4 days following injury.

The formation of collagen, the principal structural protein, is essential in restoring the original tensile strength of the skin. Fibroblast deposition of collagen components begins within 48 hours of the injury. Various enzymatic processes result in the formation of fibrils. Subsequent cross-linking of these fibrils gives the collagen its maximal strength. Although the process of collagen synthesis reaches a peak in the first week, production and remodeling proceeds for up to 12 months. A new scar will reach only one-quarter of its ultimate strength by a month and less than two-thirds by 4 months (5).

Wound contraction is a poorly understood process in which the full wound thickness moves toward the center of the wound. This occurs 3 to 4 days following the injury and appears to be independent of collagen formation. Current research suggests that contractile cells called myofibroblasts may be involved in this process (10).

Various factors, both internal and external, will inhibit the normal process of healing. Underlying immune deficiencies or prolonged steroid use can affect the inflammatory stage. The presence of crushed tissue or debris surrounding the laceration, as frequently occurs with blunt trauma, will significantly impede epithelial cell replication. Epithelialization is optimized by meticulous attention to wound cleansing, debridement, and foreign body removal (Chapters 110 and 113). Collagen synthesis is a complex process that depends on the presence of a number of trace minerals, vitamins, and plasma proteins, as well as an adequate supply of oxygen. Poor nutrition, underlying illness, or vascular disease will adversely affect this process.

As the microscopic process of healing proceeds, the appearance of the wound also undergoes predictable stages of evolution and remodeling. The clinician must be cognizant of this transformation and prepare the patient who otherwise might be anxious to have an unsightly scar revised before it has reached its final state. What may initially appear to be a cosmetically appealing result following suture removal often will go through a stage in which it becomes increasingly thickened, reddened, and elevated. This occurs during the active period of fibrous tissue production and remolding which lasts approximately 3 months. Over the ensuing 3 months the scar can be expected to fade and recede as capillaries collapse and the cellular content is replaced by connective tissue, so that the appearance 6 months following the initial laceration is essentially the final scar.

Hypertrophic scarring and keloid formation are the result of abnormal healing that can occur despite proper wound management and suturing technique. Hypertrophic scars are composed of red, raised, pruritic tissue which is the result of excessive collagen deposition occurring within the original boundaries of the wound. Formation of such scars is related to the amount of time the wound spends in the inflammatory phase and the presence of excessive tension on the wound. Keloids are nodular masses of scar tissue which also contain increased amounts of immature collagen and migrate beyond the original extent of the wound. Keloids occur with greater incidence in dark-skinned individuals and have a higher propensity for certain areas of the body such as the sternum, deltoid, and mandible.

Children appear to have advantages in healing ability over adults. Studies suggest that in adults stages of healing begin later, occur at a slower rate, and do not reach the same level as in children. With increasing age collagen biosynthesis and cross-linking are decreased (5), the rate of epithelialization is reduced (6), and the proliferative capacity and contractility of fibroblasts are diminished (7). The underlying reason for these changes is difficult to determine due to the presence of multiple confounding factors. It is unclear whether these changes in wound healing are the result of prolonged environmental exposure, underlying disease, or simply the natural process of aging.

INDICATIONS

Basic goals of wound repair are to restore the integrity and the function of the injured tissues (11). To achieve these goals, preventing infection is important and minimizing scar formation is desirable. Wound closure ensures early restoration of the natural skin barrier, avoiding prolonged healing and protecting against subsequent infection. Wounds located on the face are of obvious concern regarding scar formation; however, excessive scar formation in any area can be a source of annoyance or embarrassment for the patient.

Minor soft tissue wounds are a common, unavoidable part of pediatric acute care. Anxiety of the patient and family surrounding the repair of these injuries, especially facial wounds, can be a source of much stress for the clinician. For these reasons, the ability to approach this situation in a clearly planned and confident manner is essential to the clinician's long-term survival in pediatric emergency care. Skilled minor wound care can be a source of great patient and personal satisfaction and should receive major consideration in the education of emergency care providers.

Reasons to Seek Consultation

Not every wound should be repaired by the emergency physician. Consultation should be considered in the following circumstances (11, 12):

1. Wounds with an underlying fracture;
2. Wounds requiring nerve repair, vascular repair, or tendon closure;
3. Wounds that would be better treated under general anesthesia due to their extent or location;
4. Situations in which the emergency physician has insufficient time to devote to proper care of the wound; and
5. Circumstances the emergency physician considers beyond his or her expertise.

The consulting service will vary with the injury and can range from general surgery (for a laceration complicated only by its extent) to plastic surgery, otorhinolaryngology, oral surgery, and orthopedics for more specialized circumstances.

A difficult situation arises when the family insists on a plastic surgeon for a relatively minor wound that is well within the capacity of the emergency physician. To readily consult plastic surgery in all such cases is a poor strategy (13). Often a simple closure yields a wholly acceptable result and the expense of a plastic surgeon and the time delay caused by such consultation is inappropriate for the situation (13). The clinician should reason with and inform the family that he or she is capable of handling the wound. The clinician also should inform the family that the need for revision will be unlikely but, if required, this can be performed without difficulty at a later date under more favorable conditions.

With complicated wounds, immediate repair even by an experienced plastic surgeon may not always be the best strategy (14). A complicated revision in the acute phase is considered less desirable by some authorities for the following reasons: (*a*) a higher risk of infection may necessitate suture removal and undermine the initial effort; (*b*) it is more difficult to make the proper cuts for Z-plasty, etc. in damaged tissue as opposed to the firm scar base that will be present at a later date; (*c*) less time is available to study the natural tendencies of the wound; and (*d*) the patient has no basis of comparison with which to judge the outcome of plastic surgery (14).

Some emergency physicians will feel comfortable with extensor tendon repair; however, the requirement for prolonged close follow-up and attention to patient compliance coupled with the potential for significant disability make referral a strong consideration in these cases. The emergency physician also must be aware that delayed repair of certain injuries, including nerve and tendon transection and complicated facial lacerations, is an acceptable response on the part of his or her consultant (13).

Infectious Considerations

The main reason not to close a soft tissue wound is to avoid a subsequent infection. The risk of infection in a wound depends on the interaction of patient factors, the wound environment, and the care provided by the physician (9, 11, 15–18). When wound evaluation indicates that primary repair would be associated with a high risk of infection, it is recommended to leave the wound open for delayed primary closure or to allow healing by secondary intention (11, 17).

Delayed primary closure is rarely used in the management of pediatric wounds, because the rate of wound infection in children is quite low. Studies examining all types of pediatric lacerations primarily repaired with sutures report infection rates of under 2% (19, 20). It also is important to realize that if primary repair fails due to wound infection, the subsequent management is similar to delayed primary closure (15).

Patient Factors
Patient factors associated with an increased rate of infection include the presence of dia-betes, immunosuppression, renal failure, liver failure, obesity, and malnutrition (9, 16, 18). Infection rates 5 to 8 times higher in surgical wounds have been demonstrated in the presence of diabetes, obesity, and malnutrition (18). Wound infection rates for pediatric patients with these conditions are unknown, as wound studies generally exclude such patients (19, 20). Presence of an underlying illness should not be the sole reason for avoiding wound closure, and the majority of wounds in these patients are amenable to primary repair. It is important, however, to pay close attention to wounds in such patients and to ensure adequate follow-up.

Local Factors
Local factors regarding the wound itself are the main source of wound problems in the ED (9). The clinician should always consider the following factors before wound closure.

Time Delay
Time is a variable factor in the closure of wounds as some, such as a highly contaminated puncture wound, should never be closed and others may be safely closed at almost any time after the injury (15). The golden period of wound repair is frequently mentioned but is a concept that varies depending on the evaluation of the individual wound. Primary determinants of an acceptable time period for primary wound closure are the degree of contamination of the tissue and the vascular supply of the area (9, 15).

Several studies have demonstrated that if a wound contains greater than 10^5 bacteria per gram of tissue the infection rate will be high (21–23). The mean time to achieve this level of contamination in one study was 5.17 hours, leading some authorities to consider the golden period to be quite short (21). Actual clinical studies, however, have produced results that support individual evaluation of wounds to determine if the time delay for closure is acceptable. No difference was found in infection rates for pediatric wounds sutured greater than 6 hours after injury as compared with those repaired earlier (20). A study of wounds in a third world setting found that it was safe to close general wounds for a period up to 19 hours whereas scalp wounds could be closed at any time

(24). Regarding hand wounds, time was not a factor in infection for a period up to 18 hours (23).

The primary determinant of the patient's ability to resist wound infection will be the local circulation to the wound site (25). For that reason injuries to well-vascularized areas such as the scalp, face, and tongue may be comfortably repaired many hours after presentation (9, 25). In the previously mentioned study, 97% of scalp wounds closed after 19 hours healed without complications (24).

Wound Contamination and Crush Injury

The degree of bacterial contamination is an important determinant of wound infection (21-23). Unfortunately, the method to perform quantitative bacterial analysis of a wound is somewhat cumbersome and time consuming, keeping this practice largely an item of research interest. The presence of devitalized tissue in a wound is considered a major risk factor for wound infection (11, 25, 27). Experimentally, inserting devitalized fat, muscle, or skin into a wound increases the infection rate (27). This occurs through inhibition of leukocyte function, creation of an anaerobic environment, and the support of bacterial growth by the "culture medium" nature of the devitalized tissue (27).

Crush injuries are generally considered at higher risk for infection due to the presence of devitalized tissue and, more importantly, disturbances of local blood flow (26). Although this makes intuitive sense, clinical series supporting this fact are limited. Separate studies on hand injuries demonstrated conflicting results when comparing infection rates in crush versus laceration type injuries (22, 28). In areas where the vascular supply is good such as the scalp, the overall infection rate will be low regardless of the mechanism of injury (24, 29).

The ability to sharply debride devitalized or heavily contaminated tissue will have a major impact on the decision to close a wound primarily (9, 17). Debridement can convert a crushed, dirty wound into a clean, sharply incised laceration suitable for primary repair. Similarly, adequate wound irrigation can be expected to reduce the bacterial contamination of a wound and decrease the rate of subsequent infection (Chapter 110).

Wound Location

Although wound location itself will usually not preclude primary repair, some general issues are pertinent to remember in evaluating wounds. Most studies demonstrate an increased rate of wound infection for injuries to the lower extremities (19, 20, 29). This is thought to be due to the relatively poor blood supply to the lower extremities (19, 25). The foot may be at a particularly high risk (11). Upper extremity wounds also are considered at higher risk for infection, particularly hand wounds, for reasons similar to the lower extremities (25, 29).

Areas with significant exposure to endogenous bacteria such as the mouth, vagina, and perianal area are theoretically at high risk for infection (11). These same areas, however, also have an excellent vascular supply, counterbalancing the increased bacterial exposure (25). Closure of wounds in the mouth is generally considered acceptable if no major time delay has occurred (30, 31). The low rate of infection of episiotomy incisions indicates some margin of safety for primary wound repair in the perineum. If in doubt about closure in special areas consultation should be considered.

Location of a wound also may influence where the repair is best undertaken. Wounds of the perineum may require closure in the operating room for the best result in terms of patient fear and anxiety. Wounds in inaccessible areas of the oral cavity also may require such management.

Bite Wounds

Considerable controversy exists surrounding the proper management of both human and animal bite wounds. The clinician's decision for closure in the case of a bite wound must weigh the various factors related to wound infection with the supposition that the wound is contaminated with bacteria before therapeutic intervention (9). The important considerations then become the vascular supply to the area and the ability of the clinician to clean the wound and decrease the bacterial contamination present (32).

In all types of bite wounds the hand is at especially high risk for infection (32-39) due to the relatively poor blood supply of many structures in the hand, as well as anatomical features which make cleaning a bite of the hand difficult if not impossible (33).

Human Bites

The notorious reputation of human bites is primarily based on one injury alone, the closed fist injury, when a laceration over the flexed metacarpal-phalangeal joint is sustained from the tooth of an opponent (32). Forces involved to create a skin break are generally sufficient to inoculate the tendon and its coverings which lie just under the skin in this area. Frequently, deeper injury occurs to the bone, cartilage, and joint space. When the hand is subsequently extended, the bacteria is carried into areas not accessible to routine cleansing in the ED (32, 33). In the pediatric age group these wounds are usually infected by the time of presentation (36, 37). Admission to the hospital is generally indicated for an infected closed fist injury (33, 37)

All patients presenting with a wound over the metacarpal head should be considered to have a human bite wound until proven otherwise. It is prudent to treat all such wounds in this location as a bite wound regardless of the history provided by the patient. If the wound is not infected at presentation it should be thoroughly evaluated by wound exploration and radiographic study to detect any underlying injury that would prompt hospitalization. Patients scheduled for outpatient treatment must have their wounds thoroughly cleansed, left open, and elevated. They are routinely treated with antibiotics and must be capable of early follow-up (33).

Human bites in other areas are of no greater risk than animal bites (32). Two studies of human bites in children indicate that the chance of infection in superficial abrasions is extremely low and that antibiotics are of no value. The literature on suturing human bite lacerations in children is limited; however, the placement of deep sutures was associated with an increased infection rate in a small series (36). Primary closure of wounds that can be adequately cleansed in well-vascularized areas should not present a problem. The typical small forehead laceration that is caused by a playmate's tooth is an example of a bite wound that should not be closed unless the wound is surgically extended for proper cleansing (36).

Dog Bites

Most animal bites that are considered for suturing in the ED are inflicted by canines. These wounds are assumed to be contaminated although it has been stated that meal-eating (as opposed to meat-eating) dogs do not have sufficient oral bacteria to create an inoculum at the level of 10^5 bacteria/g of tissue (9). As with human bites, dog bites to the hand are at higher risk for infection regardless of the use of antibiotics (35, 38, 39).

If coupled with excellent wound care and meticulous closing technique, suturing of facial dog bite wounds can safely be accomplished without using antibiotics (40). In a repair of 145 recent (less than 6 hours old) facial dog bites in 45 children after pressure irrigation with normal saline solution and wound edge excision, an infection rate of only 0.4% was reported even though no antibiotics were administered (40).

Regarding primary suturing of dog bite wounds in the face and other areas, the clinician must again consider the vascular supply and the ability to adequately clean the wound (32). Puncture type wounds can be expected to have a poor outcome if sutured, whereas large dog bite lacerations that can be adequately cleansed generally do well. Dog bite lacerations of the face, facial structures and scalp should generally be repaired primarily if cosmetically indicated (32, 39).

Other Animal Bites

Wounds caused by cats are generally not considered for suturing as they are usually puncture type wounds. Lacerations caused by monkeys have a notorious reputation based on anecdotal reports, whereas those caused by large herbivores such as horses will be associated with significant crush injury (32). Recommendations on primary closure of these wounds are lacking given their relative infrequency.

Foreign Bodies and Wound Closure

The presence of a nonirritant foreign body such as a small piece of metal or glass is not a contraindication to primary wound closure (41). Such wounds can be closed and managed expectantly if the foreign body is difficult to remove, is not in a critical area (e.g., a joint space or near a vital structure), and is not positioned so that it would be a likely source of ongoing irritation for the patient. Certainly, the patient and family should be informed of the presence of a foreign body and the rationale for the planned course of action.

Irritant foreign bodies such as wooden splinters or thorns should be removed at the time of presentation to avoid infectious complications (41) (see also Chapter 113). The presence of even minute amounts of soil in a wound invites infection, and wounds with suspected soil remaining should not be closed primarily (11).

Gunshot and Stab Wounds

Low velocity gunshot wounds that do not damage underlying structures can be managed on an outpatient basis. The traditional care of these wounds includes open treatment (no sutures) and basic wound care without using antibiotics (42). These wounds generally heal well without antibiotic therapy despite retained metallic fragments in the wound (42).

Stab wounds must be evaluated for depth and involvement or penetration of underlying structures before closure. This frequently necessitates surgical consultation. These wounds may be categorized as puncture wounds or simple, sharply incised lacerations. In the latter slashing type injury, such wounds may be closed as any other. Deeper puncture type injuries are traditionally managed in an open fashion (Chapter 112).

Dead Space

Eliminating any pocket in the depths of the wound that could collect blood or serum and thereby potentiate infection often is accepted as an essential step in wound management. This must be distinguished from the technique of a layered closure to decrease tension on the wound edge, which has cosmetic advantages (11, 12) Although theoretically useful, the suture closure of dead space to decrease infection has not been shown to be beneficial and may actually be detrimental (49–51). In a rabbit study using wounds inoculated with bacteria, it was demonstrated that, although dead space increased the rate of infection, suture closure of this dead space actually worsened the situation (50). It also is recommended to avoid sutures in the fat layer (12, 49, 51).

EQUIPMENT

The emergency physician frequently accepts the available equipment for wound repair in the ED as a *fait accompli*. Yet the frequent use of this equipment and the important nature of the task require that high quality instruments be available when needed. The clinician must accept nothing less. Basic surgical tool requirements useful for wound repair are listed below.

Needle holder—appropriately sized for suture needle. An excessively large needle holder will flatten a small needle after a few uses.

Nontraumatic tissue forceps—with no hooks to avoid crushing tissue. An alternative to using forceps is single- or double-pronged skin hooks (43).

Tissue scissors—a sharp, tightly cutting pair is essential for debridement.

Hemostats—these may be useful in situations when bleeding vessels will require ligation.

Scalpels—No. 10 or 15 blade may be necessary for sharp debridement.

Sterile drapes—an adequate amount to keep the wound area sterile. In the repair of facial wounds the hole in the drape should not be so small as to obscure useful landmarks (30). Facial drapes can be foregone if they cause excess anxiety in a child.

Sterile gauze—a ready supply of a sufficient number is frequently overlooked in setting up for laceration repair.

Sterile gloves and mask—important to reduce contamination of the wound by the clinician (11, 43). These items and a facial splashshield also should be considered necessary for protecting the clinician.

Light—an adequate light source is essential and will preferably be directed into the wound unobstructed from above.

Bed—the patient and bed should be positioned in a way to maximize comfort of both the patient and the clinician during the procedure. Using arm extensions and pillows should be considered and the height of the bed should be raised to a workable level.

Suture material (11, 43-46)—generally divided into absorbable and nonabsorbable based on the retention of tensile strength less than or greater than 60 days. Using catgut as an absorbable suture is no longer recommended. Two general types of synthetic absorbable sutures, Dexon® and Vicryl®, are both excellent choices for general wound repair.

Several types of nonabsorbable sutures are available for percutaneous suturing; however, the general choice for emergency physicians will be a nylon (Dermalon®, Ethilon®) or a polypropylene (Prolene®) suture. The monofilament sutures are preferred over braided or multifilament sutures which are thought to increase the risk of wound infection by providing interstices for bacteria to be shielded from leukocytes. A lower coefficient of friction allows a suture to smoothly pass through tissue. This same property, however, lessens the stability of the knot. Most synthetic sutures possess a low coefficient of friction and therefore the clinician should use at least four throws when tying knots with this material.

Silk is more reactive than synthetic suture material which limits its usefulness for general wound repair. The relatively soft feel of silk and its workability make it a consideration for repairs of the eyelid or mouth. In these areas silk sutures are usually removed in a few days thus lessening the reactivity problem.

Generally, the smallest size suture acceptable for the repair is recommended to reduce the amount of foreign material in the wound. The size of nonabsorbable sutures most commonly used in the ED run, in increasing order of diameter, from 6.0 to 3.0. Facial repairs will be conducted with 5.0 or 6.0 sutures, whereas 4.0 is commonly used for other areas. Use of 3.0 suture is usually limited to the scalp or areas of significant tension such as over joints. However, most scalp injuries and wounds over joints can be adequately managed with 4.0 suture. Absorbable sutures will remain in the wound for a long period and therefore using 5.0 is generally recommended although 4.0 may be advisable in areas with increased tension.

Needles—the reverse cutting needle is the best choice for general wound repair in the ED. This needle has the main cutting edge situated on the outside of the curve of the needle so that the cut is made away from the wound edge, which prevents the suture material from further cutting into the tissue along the path of the needle cut.

PROCEDURE

Wound Preparation

Anesthesia

Adequate anesthesia and a cooperative patient are essential for proper wound preparation (25). Principles of wound anesthesia and cleansing are covered extensively in Chapters 37 and 110. Using small gauge needles for the slow injection of a buffered anesthetic deep in the wound coupled with distraction by applying pressure around the wound will generally allow for reasonable cooperation by the patient (15). Complete anesthesia of the affected area must be accomplished before wound manipulation. It is the fault of the one providing anesthesia, and not the patient, if this is not satisfactory. If anesthesia is inadequate, the clinician must retreat and start over to ensure a wound repair that is the least distressing for both the patient and family. The repair of lacerations is perhaps the most common indication for using conscious sedation in the young child (Chapter 35).

Exploration

Exploration of all wounds with proper hemostasis to allow for complete visualization is mandatory to detect underlying injury or foreign bodies. Hemostasis usually can be achieved by local pressure or by using a blood pressure cuff inflated above systolic pressure in an extremity that has been elevated for 1 minute before cuff inflation (11). It is essential to explore wounds of the extremities through their full range of motion and to be particularly meticulous in examining them in the position of wounding. For example, the typical knee wound is approached with the patient's leg in full extension when most injuries occur in some degree of flexion. Exploration of injuries to the plantar surface of the foot may be facilitated by turning the (prone) patient around on the stretcher and elevating the foot into view with the head of the stretcher.

The clincian should have little hesitation to extend a wound using a scalpel if needed for proper wound exploration. The resultant added length of wound should heal in an acceptable fashion given the sharply incised nature of the wound extension. Once a foreign body is found within a wound this should be a signal to the clinician that more lies in wait for discovery. If the clinician is contemplating primary repair, he or she must continue to explore the wound until assured that no soil or irritant foreign bodies remain (11, 41).

Debridement

Removing devitalized or heavily contaminated tissue from a wound is a fundamental principle of wound care (9, 11, 25, 27). Sharp debridement of a contaminated wound may allow closure of a wound that would otherwise be treated with delayed primary closure (17). Debridement may be accomplished by excising the entire wound, sometimes referred to as wound ellipsing, or in a more selective fashion. Wounds that are amenable to excision are those in areas lacking vital underlying structures and where sufficient excess tissue is available to allow closing the wound without undue tension (11).

Although it decreases the likelihood of infection, excision can worsen the eventual cosmetic result. Excision should generally follow the RSTL as described previously (Fig. 111.2) (14, 47, 48). In fact, it is wise to excise only those wounds that can be easily done in a manner that will closely parallel the RSTL (11, 14). Excision performed on a jagged wound that is not parallel to the RSTL may produce a straight edge but will have a wide scar due to the tension on the wound. The same jagged laceration with multiple components running in different directions will be essentially a natural Z-plasty (14). Such a wound will have some segments following the RSTL and will likely heal in a more acceptable manner than the "clean" excision (11, 14).

Debridement of facial wounds should be conservative (14, 30). Given the excellent blood supply of the face, it is difficult to be sure tissue is truly devitalized. It is wiser to refrain from debridement rather than to sacrifice tissue that may live (14). Loss of tissue is the most significant limiting factor to the success of later plastic scar revision (47). An important cosmetic structure such as the philtrum should never be debrided (30).

If a wound is excised the effect of the natural contraction of the wound on surrounding structures must be anticipated. For example, a wide horizontal excision on the forehead may heal with a thin scar but cock the eyebrow on that side (30).

Certain areas are less amenable to excision and debridement. These areas include the nose, lip, hand, forearm, anterior lower leg, and the foot (12, 17, 27). When excising in a hairy region such as the eyebrow, all cuts must be angled parallel to the direction of the hair shafts and follicles to avoid excess follicle loss and a wide hairless scar (30, 47).

The technique of wound excision involves making a smooth, elliptical cut around the wound area to be excised (Fig. 111.3). This usually will, but does not necessarily, encompass the entire wound. It is recommended that the eventual length of the excision exceed the width by a factor of three (12). It is wise to mark the desired path of the skin cut. Two general methods are recommended for completing the excision. The skin can be scored with a scalpel and the cut completed with a pair of sharp tissue scissors (12)

Figure 111.3.
Elliptical incision of a jagged laceration.

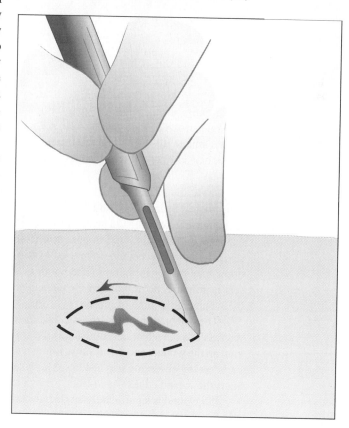

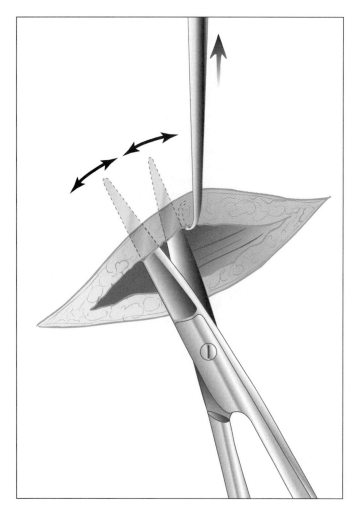

Figure 111.4.
Undermining a wound reduces the degree of tension present after the repair.

or the entire depth of the cut may be made with one stroke of the scalpel (48). With either technique it is important to obtain a perpendicular cut completely through the dermis.

Minimizing Scar Formation
Although at times even the best of efforts will result in an unsightly hypertrophic scar (56), several important techniques are used to minimize excess scar formation. The width of a scar is primarily determined by the tension on the wound at the time of closure (11, 46, 48, 57). The orientation of the wound related to the RSTL is the major determinant of the tension on the wound, and this is most simply ascertained by observing it at rest to see how far apart the wound edges gape (49).

If a wound is significantly angled or perpendicular in relation to the RSTL it will likely heal with a wide scar (11, 30, 48). As mentioned, this is a primary consideration

when contemplating wound excision. It is important to remember that the RSTL in the individual patient do not always follow the book (47, 49). The wrinkle lines which are so useful in adults to determine the orientation of the RSTL are not as evident in children. A practical technique to determine the orientation of skin tension is to simply pinch the skin and observe which direction has the longest furrows and, hence, the least tension (56).

When a wound is under tension certain methods are used to counteract this influence and reduce the eventual width of the scar. The primary method to counteract tension is to place subcutaneous sutures before percutaneous sutures (12). Techniques such as Z-plasty and W-plasty to reduce the tension on less favorably placed wounds are used by plastic surgeons and their performance is beyond the scope of this chapter (14, 30, 47). A relatively simple technique for reducing tension is to undermine the adjacent soft tissue to decrease the natural static tensions of the surrounding skin. A paucity of clinical studies on this technique exist; however, a wound study in a porcine model found that undermining generally decreased the forces required to close a wound (58).

Undermining is generally carried out in the plane of the subcutaneous fat for a distance of several millimeters or up to twice the width of the wound (Fig. 111.4) (12, 48). A pair of scissors or a scalpel is used to loosen the subdermal fatty tissue. The goal is to allow the skin edges to be brought together with very little tension. A note of caution has been raised about using undermining in contaminated wounds (11). The disruption in blood supply potentially caused by this largely unproven technique may lead to an increased risk of infection and offset any cosmetic improvement (11).

Simple scars that are most visible are characterized by abnormal color or an uneven surface which casts shadows (12). Good technique can help minimize the latter problem by producing a flatter scar through eversion of skin edges, matching skin heights, proper suture placement, and care in handling tissue.

Wound edges must be everted at the time of closure (12, 46, 48). Eversion is accomplished by placing the percutaneous suture so that its depth is greater than its width (Fig. 111.5) (12, 46). Alternatively, a mattress type suture can be used to produce eversion of the wound edge (12, 48). The difficulty with mattress sutures, however, is their tendency to cause ischemia of the wound edge (9). As discussed later in this chapter, using the lateral mattress suture for eversion may be preferable in this situation (48).

Absolute matching of the skin heights must be accomplished when the wound is sutured (12). Going in and out of each wound edge separately, using two passes with the suture needle, is the best strategy in wounds that are uneven (11). For precise approximation of the wound edges in jagged or stellate lacerations, meticulous placement of individual sutures is recommended (11, 46).

Most scar formation is a natural reaction to tissue injury and therefore the tissue to be repaired should be handled as gently as possible (17, 48). This can be ensured by using noncrushing clamps and by using only the fingers or skin hooks to handle the skin edges (17, 43, 48).

It is important for the clinician to be aware of circumstances when unsightly scarring is likely. For example, curved or U-shaped flap lacerations, often termed trap door lacerations, tend to yield poor results by virtue of the natural contraction of the wound to a point central in the flap (43, 47). When these are encountered in cosmetic areas, such as the forehead, it is wise to consider referral or to warn the parents of the likely need for revision.

Suturing Techniques

General Principles
Key principles to remember regarding the use of sutures include:
1. Every suture is a foreign body and the least amount of sutures should be used for the shortest time period that is sufficient. Corollaries to this include using deep sutures only when necessary, limiting the number of knots in a buried suture to three, and using the smallest size

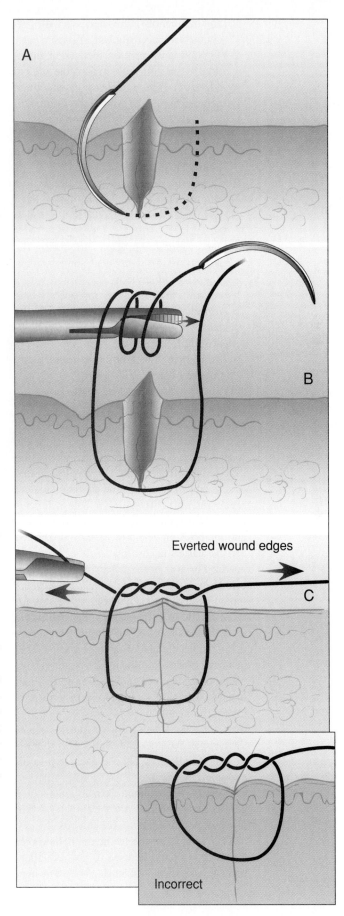

Figure 111.5.
The simple interrupted skin suture secured with an instrument tie.

and number of sutures necessary for percutaneous placement (44, 45, 49).

2. Tight sutures increase the risk of infection by causing ischemia of the wound edge (11). If the suture is tight enough to necrose tissue, the hold of the suture will be weakened (52). It is important to anticipate swelling in the wound area and to approximate the tissue rather than tightly close it.

3. Generally, wounds under greater tension should have more skin sutures placed and these should be closer to the wound edge (12).

4. Two general approaches to sewing the wound are recommended. Some authorities advocate dividing the wound with a central stitch because any extra tissue forming a "dog ear" will usually flatten out over time (48). Others insist on approaching the wound from one end and using special techniques to remove any dog ear (12).

Basic Use of Tools

Needle choice should be appropriately sized to allow desired penetration depth into the wound edge. For the novice practioner using the needle holder should be carefully studied because the majority of time wasted in wound repair relates to its use (53). The needle is best held perpendicular to the needle holder and the position where the needle is grasped can be varied according to the clinician's needs. For soft tissue repair it is generally best to grab the needle relatively close to the thread end (swage). This hold will allow for more needle to be passed through the tissue and will make it easier to retrieve the needle using the needle holder or forceps (53). This position, however, allows for greater risk of needle breakage and makes it more difficult to apply force. If the tissue to be penetrated is tough, the needle must be grasped closer to the point (53). When using the needle holder the clinician should make every effort to position the needle only once at each step to increase efficiency.

Wound edges should be manipulated in a gentle manner using only the fingers, a skin hook, or nontraumatic tissue forceps (17, 43, 48). To avoid damage to the epithelial layer the forceps should be used to grasp the dermal-fat junction when suturing (12). The nee-

dle should be retrieved only with the needle holder or a pair of forceps to avoid injury to the clinician. For similar reasons, the clinician should not use the fingers to help push the tissue over the needle.

Types of Stitches
Simple Interrupted Skin Sutures
Because the simple interrupted skin suture is most commonly used, this technique should be mastered first. As mentioned previously, it is essential to obtain eversion of the wound edges to minimize scar formation. Eversion means that the wound edges are rolled slightly outward with the two edges of the wound lined up exactly. To achieve wound edge eversion the path of the needle must be directly down or angled slightly away from the wound edge (12, 46) (Fig. 111.5.A). Additionally, the depth of the suture path must be greater than the width. The entire depth of the wound edge can be pulled perpendicular to the skin by grasping the fat-dermal junction with forceps and driving the needle straight down (12). The needle must trace an equal path through both sides of the wound to ensure accurate apposition of the wound. This is most easily achieved by pulling the needle though one side and out of the wound before reentering deep in the opposite side of the wound.

Another technique described for obtaining wound edge eversion is to pucker the wound edges in an everted manner with finger and thumb pressure before passing the needle completely through both sides of the wound (43).

Knot tying can be a source of frustration but is easily mastered with practice. The general technique most useful for knot tying in the ED is the instrument tie (Fig.111.5). This is best accomplished by pulling most of the suture through the wound so that only a few centimeters of thread are exposed at the first insertion site. At this stage, the remaining longer length of thread attached to the needle is grasped in the nondominant hand. The needle holder, grasped in the dominant hand, is placed across the longer (needle) length of thread, and the thread is then looped twice over the tip (Fig. 111.5.B). The needle holder then grasps the short (free) end of suture and pulls this away from the side of the wound initially entered, which will lay the double knot flat (Fig. 111.5.C). The knot is tightened so that the skin edges just come together. Further tightening beyond this point risks wound edge ischemia. The process is now reversed, with the needle holder again placed across the longer length of suture which is then looped once under the tip. The needle holder then grasps the free end of the suture, and returns it to the initial needle entry side of the wound, while the needle length of suture is carried back to the initial needle exit side of the wound. This alternating "over and under" method of tying results in a surgeon's knot. For monofilament sutures this should be repeated first in the over and then in the under manner for a total of four throws to secure the knot.

Most skin repair will be performed with monofilament sutures that, due to their low coefficient of friction, allow for further loosening or tightening of previously tied knots (45). This takes some pressure off the need for perfect wound edge approximation at placement of the first throw in tying. This same property, however, can cause knots to loosen excessively when attempting to secure them. To combat slippage of the first knot a locking technique may be used (53). In this technique, after the first double knot is laid flat, the pull of the hands is immediately reversed to lock the knot (53). To retain the lock, the next throw must be placed without tension on the segments.

Excess knots will actually weaken the suture and should be avoided (46). The ends of the suture should be cut long enough to allow easy handling for removal.

Subcutaneous Sutures

The primary reason to place subcutaneous sutures is to counteract tension on the wound and thus decrease the width of the subsequent scar. Using synthetic absorbable sutures to close the deep tissues will decrease the tension on the wound (11, 12, 48, 49). Placing such sutures in the dermal layer is especially important; however, the fascial junction surrounding muscle also is important to close (11, 12, 43, 49). It is essential in repairing injured muscle that the fascia is incorporated in the suture as the muscle itself will not hold a stitch (30, 43). When deep sutures are placed in the dermis in cosmetic areas it is generally recommended that the knot be buried (i.e.,

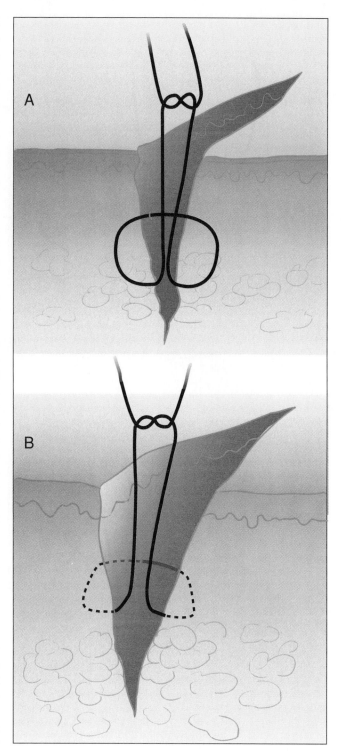

pointing downward toward the base of the wound) to keep as much foreign material as possible away from the healing wound edge (12, 46, 48). Using deep sutures in any wound at risk for infection must be undertaken cautiously or not at all (25, 54).

The fascial layer can be closed with sim-

Figure 111.6.
A. The buried subcutaneous suture.
B. The horizontal dermal stitch.

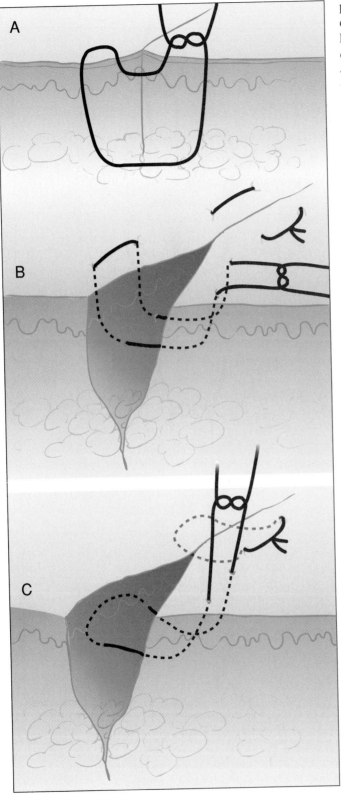

ple sutures, but subcutaneous sutures in the dermal layer will need to be inverted with the knot buried in areas where the skin is thin or cosmetic appearance is important (12, 46, 48). The initial insertion point of these subcutaneous sutures will be in the depths of the wound, typically at the fat-dermal junction (Fig. 111.6.A). Exposure of the correct entry point can be facilitated by using tissue forceps or a skin hook. The needle is rotated up through the tissue to exit in the dermis. At this point it is essential to pause and make sure that the second insertion point in the opposing dermis is at an equal vertical and horizontal level with the exit point of the first pass. Once this is ascertained the downward pass of the suture becomes a mirror image of the first pass, exiting at the same level as the original insertion. The needle end and free end of the suture should be on the same side of the loop. The knot is then tied, generally with only three throws to minimize suture material in the wound (45).

A simple but useful variation of the traditional subcutaneous suture is the horizontal dermal stitch (Fig. 111.6.B) (43). In this technique the dermis is aligned by placing a simple stitch in a horizontal plane. The loop and knot are at the same level in the subcutaneous tissue. This suture provides a nice approximation of the wound edge before skin closure but carries the disadvantage of an inability to bury the knot. This suture is most practical when nearing the end of a subcutaneous closure when room is limited to maneuver for an inverted suture.

Interrupted Mattress Sutures

Three basic types of mattress sutures are the vertical, the horizontal, and the half-buried horizontal (Fig. 111.7). These techniques are useful to provide eversion of the wound edges. The traditional vertical mattress suture involves taking a large deep course with the first pass of the needle and then taking a smaller stitch close to the wound edge. The knot is then tied on the side of the wound entered initially. It is important to avoid the tendency to apply excess tension when tying these knots. Notably, the vertical mattress suture may cause ischemia of the wound edge (9). The horizontal mattress suture closes a greater length of wound than the vertical mattress suture but usually results in less accurate

Figure 111.7.
Mattress sutures.
A. Vertical mattress suture.
B. Horizontal mattress suture.
C. Half-buried horizontal mattress suture.

approximation of the wound edges. The half-buried horizontal mattress stitch offers some advantages in that the number of skin punctures is halved and less tension is on the free edge of the wound opposite the knot (43).

Corner Stitch and V-Y Advancement Flap
The corner stitch is simply a variation on the half-buried mattress suture (Fig. 111.8). When applying this type of suture it is often wise to extend the apex of the V to form a Y, which will release some of the tension on this corner (43). The extension into a Y shape can be complimented with undermining as described previously to further decrease tension.

Continuous Skin Sutures
The sole reason to use a continuous stitch is to save time. This method poses some potential problems as breakage of one point may unravel the entire stitch (43). These sutures also may risk ischemia of the wound edge or early formation of stitch marks if they are pulled too tight (43, 54). Ischemia is more likely to be a problem if an interlocking method is used. Some authorities feel that continuous sutures are problematic if focal wound infection occurs; however, the suture can be cut and unwound from the infected area and secured with tape (54). This method is generally recommended for relatively straight clean wounds under little tension (43). Others prefer interrupted sutures for cosmetic areas. Careful placement of the individual sutures in a continuous stitch however, can yield an excellent result (12).

The most useful continuous stitch is the simple running stitch (Fig. 111.9.A), which is started by making a simple interrupted stitch and only cutting the end of thread not attached to the needle. The physician then performs sequential passes perpendicularly across the wound the same distance apart as normally placed interrupted sutures. Care is taken to take bites of equal depth from side to side. After each pass the length of thread should be pulled to close the wound and the placement evaluated before proceeding to the next pass. If the placement is unacceptable the needle can be backed out through the stitch site and the pass reattempted. Slight tension can be maintained on the thread that has already been used to suture so that the en-

tire wound does not have to be reapproximated after each suture. Once the desired length is closed the running stitch is most simply ended by reversing the direction of the needle pass using an entry site close to the previous exit site. This allows a narrow loop to be formed on one side that can be tied with the final pass to the opposite side (Fig. 111.9.A).

The continuous interlocking stitch is conducted in virtually the same manner as the simple running stitch except that the needle is

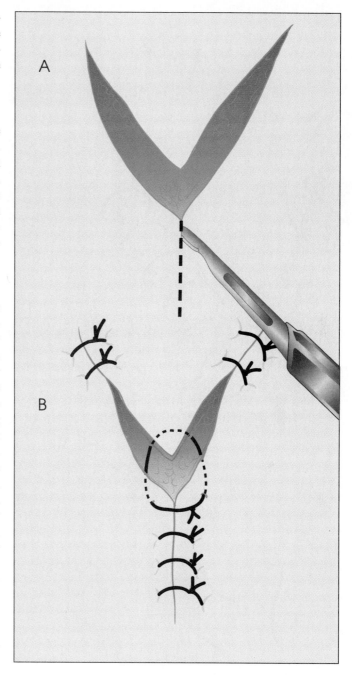

Figure 111.8.
Corner stitch and V-Y advancement flap.
A. Extension of the wound at the apex of the V.
B. Half-buried horizontal mattress stitch and simple interrupted stitches in the repair of a Y-shaped laceration.

Chapter 111
Laceration Repair

1157

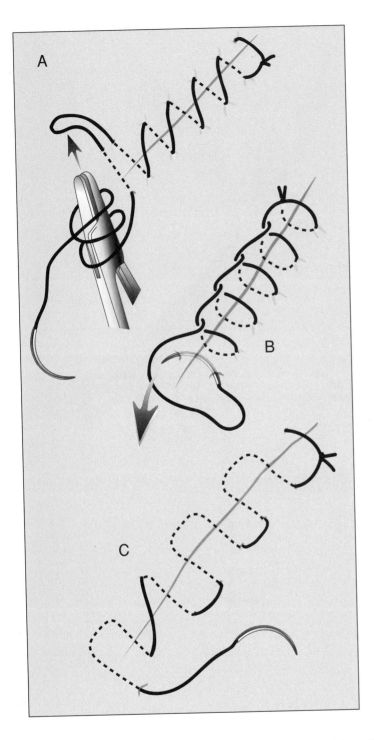

Figure 111.9.
Continuous skin sutures.
A. The simple continuous running skin stitch.
B. The continuous interlocking skin stitch.
C. The running lateral mattress stitch or continuous half-buried horizontal mattress stitch.

does not offer much time-saving advantage as it requires precise placement from side to side. However, it does prevent the occurrence of stitch marks and can be left in place for 2 to 3 weeks (47). These features make it a useful technique in patients prone to keloid formation and in situations such as young children when repeat trauma to the area is a concern (43, 48). It is generally not recommended to use a running subcuticular stitch in wounds at risk of infection (11, 55). This technique should generally not be used in a wound under significant tension before skin closure (43).

This technique is often used for cosmetic closures because of the lack of potential for stitch marks; however, exact alignment of the vertical heights of the wound is difficult (43). Furthermore, in cosmetic areas, sutures are generally removed in 3 to 4 days, well before the risk period for stitch marks (25, 46, 56).

This suture is usually begun by passing the suture through the skin at one end of the wound to exit in the dermis (Fig. 111.10). The wound is then closed by making small passes, usually less than 1 cm in width, in alternating sides of the wound in the dermal layer parallel to the skin surface. To ensure adequate alignment, each pass is usually begun slightly behind the exit point of the previous pass (43). Obviously, placement of each pass must be at the same level of dermis throughout the wound to ensure a good result. If the clinician must sew a long distance, it is advisable to bring the suture up to the surface on occasion to allow for easier removal (Fig. 111.10). Using skin tapes compliments this technique (11). The clinician can end the suture by bringing it out through the skin surface. The two ends of exposed suture can be taped in place using skin adhesive. If the clinician is worried about the security of the repair, he or she can initiate the process with an interrupted suture and end with a looping back placement as performed with the running skin suture (Fig. 111.9.A) to secure the free ends.

Alternatives to Suturing

Staples

The availability of relatively inexpensive disposable skin staplers has increased the use of this method of wound repair in the ED. Ex-

passed through a loop created by pulling the length of thread down in the direction the clinician is suturing (Fig. 111.9.B). A variation of the running stitch that uses the eversion advantage of a mattress suture is the running lateral mattress stitch (Fig. 111.9.C). It is recommended in this technique that a loop be intermittently run over the top to facilitate removal of this suture (48).

The running subcuticular stitch usually

perimentally, staples produce less inflammation in wounds than sutures while yielding a similar tensile strength (59). The major advantages in using staples are in time saved and in a decreased risk in exposure of the clinician to blood-borne diseases (60). Staples are particularly useful in long linear lacerations produced by slashing with a knife or razor edge. Some authorities recommend staples only for sharply incised wounds (61). Clinical reports, however, indicate their usefulness in other situations (60, 62).

Clinically, staples have been most commonly used for closing scalp lacerations (60, 62). Using staples is not recommended in the face for cosmetic reasons, in the hands and feet for comfort reasons, or in the scalp of a patient who will undergo complex cranial imaging (61, 62).

The wound is prepared for staple placement in the same manner as for traditional suture placement. This includes using subcutaneous sutures when needed to reduce tension (61). Placement of the staples is best achieved when an assistant everts the wound edges with tissue forceps or finger pressure.

A staple remover is a simple device that is often needed to correct inaccurate placement at the time of repair. This can then be given to the patient to bring to the follow-up visit for staple removal. Staples are generally left in place for a period similar to sutures in the same area.

Wound Tapes

Using wound tapes as the sole method of primary wound repair is acceptable for linear lacerations under minimal tension (11, 61). Their use in pediatric emergency care is common. One study reported that 20% of lacerations in children were closed with wound tapes (20). If the wound can be managed using only a topical anesthetic and does not require anesthesia by injection for cleansing or debridement, tapes can be applied painlessly (56). Wound tapes also are useful in reinforcing or refining other repairs including subcuticular methods (11). To avoid stitch marks in cosmetic areas, sutures can be removed in 2 to 3 days and replaced with skin tapes (48). If sutures are found to be under tension at any time it is recommended to remove them and apply skin tapes (48, 49).

Because wound tapes do not cause the

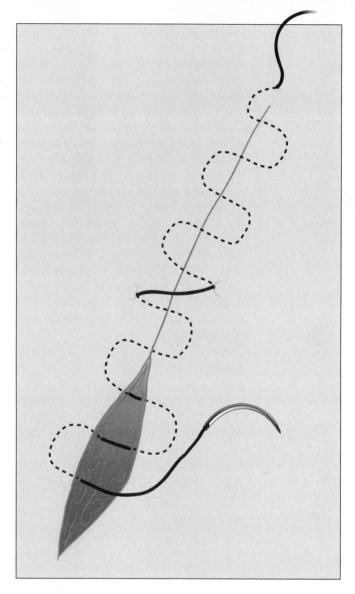

inflammatory process associated with suture placement it is not surprising that taped wounds are less likely to become infected than sutured wounds (16, 63). Skin tapes generally will not allow for the meticulous approximation required with stellate wounds and therefore such wounds generally require percutaneous sutures (11). Wound tapes are of no use in areas that are naturally moist or excessively hairy such as the scalp, axilla, palms, and soles (11, 61). Lacerations with surrounding abrasions present a problem if no sufficient uninjured skin is proximate to the wound to allow for application of an adhesive to the skin.

After wound preparation, the technique of tape application is simple. This requires cleansing, drying, and applying an adhesive

Figure 111.10.
Continuous subcuticular stitch.

(e.g., tincture of benzoin) to the surrounding skin before tape placement. The skin adhesive should not be allowed to spill into the wound as it is an irritant (11). The skin heights must be approximated carefully and equally to ensure a good result. The tapes are placed perpendicularly across the wound leaving some space for the wound to ooze. Extra tape parallel to the wound over the ends of the previously placed strips may help prevent skin blisters which occur from tension at the tape ends (61).

A study of the various available wound tapes recommended the Shur-Strip® brand over Steri-Strip® or Clearon® tapes (64). Although the strength of all three brands was sufficient for minor wound purposes, the Shur-Strip® possessed greater adhesiveness and had the capability to elongate in the presence of wound edema (64).

Hair Ties

A hair tying method for scalp lacerations may be useful for patients with longer hair who have no need for subcutaneous repair (65). In one study, the hair was tied in knots as with sutures and then cut out in a few days. Complaints were few; however, there was mild wound separation in 8% of the patients (64).

Tissue Adhesives

Using tissue adhesives for clean, pediatric facial lacerations less than 4 cm in length produced cosmetic results equal to suture repair (66). The tissue adhesive method also was faster and less painful than sutures (66). Currently, a preparation for this technique is not FDA approved for use in the United States.

Delayed Primary Closure

The technique of delayed primary closure is based on experimental studies of contaminated wounds. In one study, the infection rate of experimentally contaminated wounds was high if they were closed on the first day but became uncommon in these wounds if closure was delayed until after 4 days (69). This technique will not be used as often in pediatric wound care because heavily contaminated and crush wounds from street brawls, farming, and industrial accidents are infrequent in this population (19).

It was previously recommended that hand wounds undergo special consideration for delayed primary closure, but this is unnecessary for most civilian hand wounds (22). Additionally, this technique may lead to desiccation of vital hand structures.

The wound that is to undergo delayed primary closure is initially approached in a manner similar to other wounds. Adequate anesthesia is required for cleansing and debridement. The wound cavity is then filled with a sterile, fine mesh gauze and covered using a bulky dressing. The wound is then left completely undisturbed for 4 to 5 days unless pain, fever, or other signs indicate potential wound infection (17, 49, 70). At 4 to 5 days the wound, if uninfected and free of debris and devitalized tissue, can be approximated with sutures or skin tapes. These wounds will heal with excellent tensile strength as the injury will just be entering the active phase of regeneration (70).

To avoid the need for repeat anesthesia of the wound, sutures can be placed in healthy tissue away from the wound edge at the time of the first visit and then tied at the time of follow-up (17, 49). Alternatively, on day 4 or 5, rather than just apposing the wound edges, the clinician may opt to sharply incise both edges to create a freshly cut surface for approximation (17). This delayed wound excision is primarily used to improve the cosmetic result, as a direct closure should heal without problems.

Approach to Specific Areas

Scalp

Scalp wounds are common and generally heal in an uncomplicated manner due to the excellent vascular supply. Emergency physicians must not be cavalier in their approach to these wounds as significant underlying injury may be present. Additionally, a subgalea wound infection can cause serious morbidity (43). It is wise to explore all scalp wounds both visually and digitally to exclude the presence of a fracture or foreign body. Care should be taken to look under any flaps of tissue (30). Debridement of the scalp is generally not a high priority as the excellent vascularity will ensure the survival of even heavily contused tissue (30). The scalp is not as elastic in older children and excessive ellipsing may create tension in closure. Bleeding vessels usually respond to wound closure followed by pressure. It is usually not necessary to tie off individual bleeders (30).

Scalp wounds are generally prepared in the same manner as other wounds, with the obvious obstacle of the hair. Scalp wounds can usually be closed without prior hair removal. However, this may cause technical difficulties in suture placement and removal (67). Although the clinician is warned regarding unnecessary hair removal due to an increased risk of infection, this recommendation is based on studies of preoperative patients (25). It is unlikely that a scalp wound would become infected solely due to hair removal. Clipping the hair rather than shaving is a reasonable suggestion for scalp wounds (25).

Closure of the galea is recommended. Two general methods have been proposed for this. Some authorities feel that the galea should be closed together with the other skin structures by taking one large bite of tissue (43). This is recommended to decrease the amount of foreign body (suture) within the wound (43). Others advocate separate closure of the galea with absorbable sutures (60, 62, 67).

Scalp wounds often are amenable to repair by continuous skin sutures or staples. Suture size is usually 4.0 or larger and the highly visible blue coloring of Prolene® may offer advantages at the time of removal.

Forehead

The forehead is one of the easiest areas to predict the tension on the wound, as the RSTL run transversely. Lacerations that are vertically oriented will tend to heal with a wide scar (30). Lacerations angled greater than 35° from the RSTL will have a poor result (14). For anatomical reasons a vertical laceration situated in the midline is less likely to be problematic (30). Curved flap lacerations in this region may heal poorly due to the trap door effect caused by central contraction of the scar (43, 47). When the clinician is confronted with a large, unfavorably situated forehead wound, he or she should consider referral or warn the parents about the potential need for revision.

Forehead lacerations are common in children, and relatively few are referred to a plastic surgeon. However, the factor of skin tension must be appreciated even in small lacerations. The small vertical forehead laceration will be under tension and is therefore not suitable for primary closure by skin tapes. Efforts to counteract skin tension, including undermining and deep suture placement, should be considered. Using skin tapes to augment the repair initially and then for another 5 to 7 days after suture removal is recommended. Many people have small but unsightly forehead scars acquired as a result of an ED repair during youth. Extra care in the initial management and follow-up of these wounds will decrease the likelihood of such a result. Horizontally positioned lacerations, in contrast, heal well with skin tapes.

Windshield injuries unfortunately are common and typically present with multiple lacerations, abrasions, and some areas of tissue loss. Each individual laceration must be explored for the presence of glass (30). Multiple small wounds can be handled by a combination of loose single stitches, taping, or minor wound excision (30, 47). Subsequent dermabrasion or dermoplaning may be necessary for such injuries (47).

Eyebrows

Two essential points to remember in approaching lacerations of the eyebrow are that shaving the area must be avoided and that all excisional cuts must be angled parallel to the direction of hair follicle growth (30, 41, 47, 48). Regrowth of eyebrow hair is unpredictable; correct alignment of the eyebrow after it is shaved is difficult if not impossible; and perpendicularly placed excision cuts will damage an excessive number of hair follicles, leaving a wide hairless area. Debridement of the eyebrow, as with other facial structures, should be conservative (14, 30). Because the eyebrow is a major cosmetic landmark, approximation of this structure must be exact (47).

Eyelids

Simple lacerations of the eyelid are easily repaired but the following are indications for consultation with an ophthalmologist (30, 43, 68):

1. The presence of yellow fat indicates possible penetration of the orbital septum.
2. Lacerations of the free margin of the eyelids require meticulous repair to avoid subsequent deformity and disability.

3. The patient with a deep upper lid laceration should be evaluated for ptosis which indicates the need for repair of the levator palpebrae muscle.
4. Lacerations medial to the punctum on the lower lid can damage the lacrimal duct. The duct must be probed through the punctum with fine suture material and the wound examined for visualization of the suture indicating duct injury.
5. Medial eyelid injuries can disrupt the canthal ligament which will require special repair.

Nose

The superior aspect of the nose can be handled similar to other facial tissue whereas the inferior portion, due to the tight nature of the skin, is not amenable to significant excision (30). Fractures commonly accompany these lacerations; however, primary repair of the laceration may be undertaken in consultation with an otorhinolaryngologist. The presence of an underlying fracture will generally require the addition of antibiotic coverage. Facial blocks are useful when dealing with nasal lacerations. The free rim of the nose (around the nares) is an important cosmetic landmark and must be carefully closed.

Complete lacerations are closed in layers using absorbable sutures on the mucosal side (30, 68). The skin of the distal nose does not hold stitches well and the site is prone to forming stitch marks and abscesses. For this reason some authorities recommend a subcuticular suture for this area (43, 68). Alternatively, fine sutures can be used with early removal and subsequent skin taping. Skin taping, however, is difficult with adolescents, as the skin of the nose is quite oily (43).

Ears

Closure of ear wounds not involving the cartilage proceeds as with other wounds. If the cartilage has been violated it must be covered in some manner early in the care of the patient (30, 31, 43, 68). Small widths can be removed if needed for closure. If a large amount is exposed, early consultation should be sought for possible removal and preservation in a subcutaneous pocket.

If possible, the wound should be closed without suturing the cartilage to lessen the risk of infection (31). This is generally possible when the cartilage laceration is small and the cartilage edges are well apposed before suturing. If the cartilage is to be sutured, the perichondrium must be included as the cartilage will not hold a stitch. The posterior ear skin may be closed with absorbable sutures if the ear would need to be excessively bent to remove these sutures.

A conforming dressing should be applied by using moistened cotton balls to fill in the ear concavities and the space behind the ear (Chapter 58). A large compression wrap is then applied around the head. This is left in place for 2 days, and the wound is then examined for a subperichondrial hematoma which would require aspiration.

Lip

As described fully in Chapter 69, principles of lip closure are few and include conservative debridement with no debridement of the philtrum, a layered closure, and exact approximation of the vermillion border (30, 31, 43, 47, 68).

Tongue and Intraoral Lacerations

Fortunately most lacerations of the tongue in children will heal well without sutures. Those that are deep or involve a division of the free edge will need to be closed to avoid subsequent disability, prolonged healing, and later entrapment of food (43, 68). Other intraoral lacerations must be evaluated to ensure that no injury to the salivary ducts or facial nerves has occurred. Repair of these mucosal injuries is necessary only for deep lacerations to accelerate healing and to avoid complications (see Chapter 69).

Other Facial Areas

Evaluation of injuries to underlying structures, particularly the parotid duct and facial nerve, is essential for lacerations involving the lateral aspects of the face. Due to the underlying bony prominence, the cheek area is prone to a particular type of injury. The patient presents with a small laceration secondary to a blunt mechanism that may have significant muscle violation beneath the surface. If this is not recognized and repaired an unsightly depressed scar may result (47). Palpation of a soft tissue defect under the small laceration may be a clue to this injury. Extension of the skin wound is necessary to effect this type of repair and may be necessary to allow adequate visualization to determine if such complex repair is needed.

The chin is a common area for lacerations in children and the mechanism is virtually always blunt trauma from a fall. These wounds are tempting to debride but this is usually not necessary (30). If the wound is not under tension, as appreciated by visualizing the wound at rest, wound tapes can be used on the chin.

Extremity Lacerations

It is generally best to avoid deep sutures when possible in extremity lacerations where the baseline incidence of wound infection is higher (31). The high rate of infection of wounds in the lower extremities calls for careful evaluation of the need for any sutures at all in these wounds (19, 20, 29). This may be particularly pertinent to lacerations of the foot (11).

Lacerations over joints, especially the knee, will require prolonged immobilization of that joint if sutures are placed. Sutures may be foregone in some minor wounds in these areas rather than putting the patient through the inconvenience and expense of joint immobilization.

Lacerations through the tip of the finger are common in young children and are often caused by a closing door. These injuries can appear dramatic but usually heal well. Significant bony involvement should prompt consultation with an orthopedic surgeon, but most of these injuries can be handled by the emergency physician. Recommendations for handling these injuries are found in Chapter 106.

Continued Wound Care

Using antibiotics in the management of simple wounds is often an area of distinct disparity between the results of research and what is actually practiced. For routine lacerations, using antibiotics does not appreciably lower infection rates. In fact, some evidence indicates the opposite effect (71). Regarding hand lacerations, several studies indicate no benefit to using antibiotics (28, 72, 73). Some authorities suggest antibiotics for wounds when the predicted infection rate will be greater than 10% (1). This strategy, however, has not been proven in a clinical trial and the rate of infection in routine pediatric lacerations is well below this threshold (19, 20).

Human bite wounds of the hand are associated with a higher risk of infection, particularly for the closed fist injury (32). It is recommended that all such hand wounds receive antibiotics (32). Penicillin is a reasonable choice in noninfected wounds as it covers oral flora adequately. If a wound becomes infected, staphylococcal coverage must be added with continuation of the penicillin to cover *Eikenella corrodens,* a common organism in human bite wound infections (32). Bites in areas other than the hands generally heal well if they can be adequately cleansed and do not routinely require antibiotics. Facial dog bites, subject to excellent wound care, rarely become infected (40). Although many physicians feel the need to prescribe antibiotics for such wounds, little scientific basis for this practice exists.

Intraoral and perioral lacerations are considered to be contaminated wounds due to the high bacterial count of saliva (11, 68). Using antibiotics in such injuries is unproven and is an area of controversy (31, 48). If a clinician chooses to use an antibiotic, penicillin is adequate (68).

The need for a dressing on the sutured wound is quite limited. The purposes of wound dressings are to absorb secretions, to protect the wound surface, and to prevent infection from an external source (74). Most minor wounds do not ooze excessively and the wound edge is sealed to the outside within several hours (46, 74, 75). Clinical studies do not demonstrate an increased rate of infection in wounds that are not dressed (74).

Similar logic applies to the safety of early gentle cleansing with mild soap and water (75, 76). It is generally recommended to wait 8 to 24 hours before undressing or cleansing the wound. Wounds in certain areas such as the scalp are only dressed if a compression wrap is desired. If a dressing is applied to an extremity it is important to ensure that no pressure is applied proximal to the wound, risking edema (11).

Wound edges should be kept moist and free of scab in cosmetic areas (11). If scab is allowed to become interposed in the wound edges it will be replaced by scar tissue (11). Using both half-strength hydrogen peroxide and lubricating ointments within 6 hours of wound repair is recommended (11). Antibiotic ointments are commonly used for prophylactic purposes on wounds when in fact their main benefit is lubricating the edge rather than preventing infection (75).

Local heat application increases the perfusion to wounds and has a role in the prevention or management of wound infection (77). Other measures to consider include wound elevation and immobilization through bulky dressings or loosely fitted splints. A common oversight is failure to elevate hand injuries with the use of a simple sling. Likewise, prescribing crutches for lower extremity and foot lacerations often encourages the

SUMMARY
Wound Preparation
1. Provide conscious sedation as needed
2. Anesthetize wound
3. Provide hemostasis
4. Explore wound for foreign bodies or injuries to underlying structures
5. Remove contaminated or devitalized tissue through debridement and excision
6. Thoroughly cleanse wound
7. Undermine wound edges when necessary to reduce tension

Using Needle Holder
1. Grasp needle away from swage and closer to tip for tougher tissue
2. Hold needle perpendicular to needle holder
3. Enter skin perpendicular to surface
4. Stabilize or manipulate skin edges with skin hook or nontraumatic forceps
5. Retrieve needle after each pass with needle holder or forceps

Instrument Tie
1. Pull suture through wound, leaving a few centimeters at insertion site
2. Grasp longer (needle) length of suture in dominant hand
3. Loop suture twice *over* tip of needle holder
4. Grasp free end of suture with needle holder
5. Pull shorter (free) end through loops and away from side of wound initially entered
6. Tighten knot so that skin edges just come together
7. Loop needle end of suture once *under* tip of needle holder
8. Grasp free end of suture with needle holder
9. Pull free end through loop and back to initial needle entry side of wound

SUMMARY
(CONTINUED)
10. Repeat single loop tie, first in over and then in under manner, for a total of four throws
11. Cut both ends of suture allowing adequate length to retrieve suture at time of removal

Simple Interrupted Skin Sutures
1. Enter skin with needle directed downward or angled sightly away from wound edge
2. Drive needle to a depth greater than its width
3. Trace a symmetric path through both sides of wound
4. Secure suture with an instrument tie

Inverted Subcutaneous Sutures
1. Insert needle from within wound at fat-dermal junction
2. Rotate needle up through tissue and exit in dermis
3. Insert needle in opposing dermis at an equal vertical and horizontal level
4. Rotate needle down through tissue and exit at fat-dermal junction
5. Bring both ends of suture to same side of loop
6. Secure suture with a knot consisting of three throws

Interrupted Mattress Sutures
Vertical Mattress
1. Place a wide, deep stitch across wound—use two steps (retrieving needle from within wound) when necessary
2. Reverse directions from previous stitch, entering same side as recent exit but at a point closer to wound edge and in line with previous pass
3. Complete a smaller and shallower pass on same side as initial entry site and equidistant from wound edge as second entry site
4. Tie knot on side of wound that was initially entered

Horizontal Mattress
1. Place an initial stitch of same dimensions as a simple interrupted suture pass
2. Reenter skin lateral to exit point and equidistant from wound edge
3. Perform a second pass reversing directions from previous stitch and exiting at a point lateral to initial entry site and equidistant from wound edge, so that free and needle ends of suture remain on same side of wound
4. Tie knot on side of wound that was initially entered

Half-Buried Mattress or Corner Stitch
1. Enter skin below and just lateral to point of V
2. Exit within wound
3. Evert tip of flap with skin hooks or forceps

4. Pass needle through dermis of flap tip, parallel to skin surface
5. Enter wound on opposite side of point of V
6. Exit through skin at a point below and lateral to point of V, symmetrically across from initial insertion site
7. Secure suture with an instrument tie

Continuous Skin Sutures

Simple Running Stitch

1. Place a simple interrupted suture at one end of laceration without cutting needle end of suture
2. Travel length of laceration performing sequential passes perpendicular to laceration and equidistant from each other
3. Maintain tension on needle end of suture following each pass
4. Reverse direction of needle pass once end of laceration is reached
5. Enter skin close to previous exit site, and leave a narrow loop on that side by only partially pulling suture through
6. Secure end of suture with an instrument tie using narrow loop as free end of suture

Running Subcuticular Stitch

1. Pass suture through skin at one end of wound and exit in dermis
2. Travel length of wound making small passes (less than 1 cm in width) within dermis and parallel to skin surface
3. Alternate sides of wound with each entry site slightly behind previous exit point and at same vertical level of dermis
4. Complete suture by bringing needle out through skin surface at end of wound
5. Cut needle from suture
6. Tape free ends of suture to skin surface using skin adhesive

Wound Tapes

1. Clean and dry skin surrounding laceration
2. Apply adhesive to surrounding skin
3. Place tape strips perpendicularly across wound leaving some space for oozing
4. Place extra tape strips across ends of previous strips and parallel to wound

Delayed Primary Closure

1. Anesthetize wound
2. Explore wound
3. Debride and excise wound as needed
4. Thoroughly cleanse wound
5. Fill wound cavity with sterile, fine mesh gauze
6. Cover wound with a bulky dressing
7. Remove dressing in 4 to 5 days and approximate edges with sutures or skin tapes if no infection or devitalized tissue is evident

patient to remain in the erect position. Crutches should be accompanied by admonitions to limit their use to essential travel for meals and bodily functions.

Sutures should be removed early and replaced with tapes if wound edema creates significant tension on them (46, 48). Increased pull on the sutures will lead to earlier formation of stitch marks. Stitch marks occur because of epithelialization of the suture tracks and can be avoided by removing sutures within 7 days (25, 46). The general schedule for suture removal is 3 to 5 days for the face, 7 days for scalp and anterior trunk lacerations, and 10 to 14 days for the extremities and back (30, 31, 43, 44).

COMPLICATIONS

Any disruption of the skin involving the dermis will heal by the formation of scar tissue. A primary goal in suturing lacerations should be to minimize the size and visibility of the scar. Formation of keloids and hypertrophic scars are the unavoidable result of an abnormal healing process; however, a poorly or incorrectly performed step in suture closure will increase the likelihood of producing an unsightly scar.

An uneven skin surface resulting from an elevation or depression of scar tissue will cast a shadow across the skin making the defect more obvious. This may result from a failure to adequately align the skin layers or from inverting rather than everting the epithelial layer during the closure. Formation of a hematoma in the subcutaneous layers can result in a depression in the skin surface once the hematoma has been absorbed. This may be avoided through closure of all skin layers.

Failure to accurately align natural landmarks such as the eyebrow or the vermilion border of the lip will be noticeable no matter how invisible the actual scar.

So-called dog ears result from excess tissue on one edge of the wound which is gathered at the end of the laceration. This may be a consequence of inaccurate alignment of wound edges by the clinician or the inevitable result of a laceration with avulsed tissue leaving unequal lengths of opposing wound edges. The clinician can avoid malalignment by sewing inward from both ends or by

CLINICAL TIPS

1. Adequate immobilization, sedation, and anesthesia are key to successful laceration repair in children.
2. Natural landmarks should be used. Shaving eyebrows and using epinephrine in anesthetizing the vermilion border obscures two important landmarks
3. Shaving the hair is generally unnecessary in the repair of scalp wounds.
4. The intrinsic and extrinsic tension forces across a laceration must be considered when planning the repair.
5. Delayed closure of wounds should be decided based on the location and the degree of contamination of the wound.
6. Only skin hooks, nontraumatic forceps, or fingers, should be used in handling wound edges.
7. The fewest number of sutures should be used for the shortest time period that is sufficient.
8. Three layers support sutures best: the fascial-fat junction, the dermal-fat junction, and the level just below the dermal-epithelial junction. Fat and muscle will not hold a stitch.
9. Wounds under greater tension should have more skin sutures placed and these should be closer to the wound edge.

throwing an initial suture in the center of a long laceration dividing it into two smaller, more manageable lacerations. Additional corrective methods are possible in instances when the formation of a dog ear is unavoidable.

Optimal healing depends on the transport of oxygen and nutrients to the site of injury. Excessive undermining or rough handling of tissue can disrupt this process, resulting in the death of tissue and increased scar formation.

Sutures also can produce scars. Excessive tension placed on the sutures will result in strangulation and ischemia of the tissue. Sutures may actually tear through the wound margin. Healing will occur by formation of more scar tissue rather than the natural regeneration of the epithelium. Sutures that are left in place for excessive periods also will leave permanent stitch marks. Knots of subcutaneous sutures will increase tissue reaction at the skin surface and may even break through the surface if not buried.

Functional impairment can result from undue tension imposed by sutures placed across a laceration that occurs in a location requiring a significant degree of mobility, such as a joint. Contractures occur when inadequate tissue is available to allow full mobility following healing. They also can occur as a result of the abnormal continuation of the normal process of wound contraction. Contractures occasionally can be averted through using splints that allow the laceration to heal in the position of greatest extension. In certain instances it may be preferable to allow the wound to heal by secondary intention.

SUMMARY

Because lacerations occur commonly in children, laceration repair is a necessary skill for the clinician treating acute injuries in this patient population. Additional expertise is sometimes necessary, but the majority of wound closures do not require a subspecialist. Careful attention to the location and mechanism of the laceration, and an assessment of the risk of infection will help the clinician determine the best type of stitch, the size and type of suture material, and the need for prophylactic antibiotics. The clinician should possess a thorough knowledge of the

properties of the skin and the orientation of relaxed skin tension lines. Exploration of the wound, proper cleansing and preparation, and appropriate follow-up wound care are also essential in optimizing function and minimizing scar formation. The best results are obtained when adequate mobilization, sedation, and analgesia are used.

REFERENCES

1. Baker MD, Selbst SM, Lanuti M. Lacerations in urban children: a prospective 12 January study. AJDC 1990;144:87–92.

2. Krauss BS, Herakal T, Fleisher GR. General trauma in a pediatric emergency department: spectrum and consultation patterns. Ped Emerg Care 1993; 9(3):134–138.

3. Gofin R, Lison M, Morag C. Injuries in primary care practices. Arch Dis Child 1993;68:223–226.

4. Templeton JM, Ziegler MM. Minor trauma and minor lesions. In: Ludwig S, Fleisher GR, eds. Textbook of pediatric emergency medicine. 3rd ed Baltimore: Williams and Wilkins, 1993.

5. Traub AC, Quettlebaum FW. Cutaneous wound closure: early staple removal and replacement by skin tapes. Contemp Surg 1981;18:93–101.

6. Uitto J. Connective tissue biochemistry of the aging dermis. Age-related alterations in collagen and elastin. Dermatol Clin 1986;4(3):433–446.

7. Holt DR, Kirk SJ, Regan MC, Hurson M, Lindblad WJ, Barbul A. Effect of age on wound healing in healthy human beings. Surgery 1992;112(2): 293–297.

8. Kono T, Tanii T, Furukawa M, Mizuno N, Kitajima J, Ishii M, Hamada T. Correlation between aging and collagen gel contractility of human fibroblasts. Acta Derm Venerol 1990;70(3):241–244.

9. Robson MC. Disturbances of wound healing. Ann Emerg Med 1988;17:1274–1278.

10. Hunt TK. The physiology of wound healing. Ann Emerg Med 1988;17:1265–1273.

11. Edlich RF, Rodeheaver GT, Morgan RF, Berman DE, Thacker JG. Principles of emergency wound management. Ann Emerg Med 1988;17:1284–1302.

12. Dushoff IM. A stitch in time. Emerg Med 1973 January;1–16.

13. McDowell AJ. Extravagant treatment of garden variety lacerations. Plast Reconstr Surg 1979;63: 111–112.

14. Borges AF. Timing of scar revision techniques. Clin Plast Surg 1990;17:71–76.

15. Berk WA, Welch RD, Bock BF. Controversial issues in clinical management of the simple wound. Ann Emerg Med 1992;21:72–80.

16. Hunt TK. Disorders of repair and their management. In: Hunt TK, Dunphy JE, eds. Fundamentals of wound management. New York: Appleton-Century-Crofts, 1979, pp. 68–168.

17. Burke JF. Infection. In: Hunt TK, Dunphy JE, eds. Fundamentals of wound management. New York: Appleton-Century-Crofts, 1979, pp. 170–240.

18. Cruse PJE, Foord R. A 5-year prospective study of 23,649 surgical wounds. Arch Surg 1973;107: 206–210.

19. Rosenberg NM, DeBaker K. Incidence of infection in pediatric patients with laceration. Ped Emerg Care 1987;3:239–241.

20. Baker DM, Lanuti M. The management and outcome of lacerations in urban children. Ann Emerg Med 1990;19:1001–1005.

21. Robson MC, Duke WF, Krizek TJ. Rapid bacterial screening in the treatment of civilian wounds. J Surg Res 1973;14:426–430.

22. Marshall KA, Edgerton MT, Rodeheaver GT, Magee CM, Edlich RF. Quantitative microbiology: its application to hand injuries. Am J Surg 1976;131: 730–733.

23. Nylen S, Carlsson B. Time factor, infection frequency and quantitative microbiology in hand injuries. Scand J Plast Reconstr Surg 1980;14: 185–189.

24. Berk WA, Osbourne DD, Taylor DD. Evaluation of the "golden period" for wound repair: 204 cases from a third world emergency department. Ann Emerg Med 1988;17:496–500.

25. Edlich RF, Rodeheaver G, Thacker JG, Edgerton MT. Technical factors in wound management. In: Hunt TK, Dunphy JE, eds. Fundamentals of wound management. New York: Appleton-Century-Crofts, 1979, pp. 364–454.

26. Cardany CR, Rodeheaver G, Thacker J, Edgerton MT, Edlich RF. The crush injury: a high risk wound. JACEP 1976;5:965–970.

27. Haury B, Rodeheaver G, Vensko J, Edgerton MT, Edlich RF. Debridement: an essential component of traumatic wound care. Am J Surg 1978;135: 238–242.

28. Haughey RE, Lammers RL, Wagner DK. Use of antibiotics in the initial management of soft tissue hand wounds. Ann Emerg Med 1981;10:187–192.

29. Rutherford WH, Spence RAJ. Infection in wounds sutured in the accident and emergency department. Ann Emerg Med 1980;9:350–352.

30. Dushoff IM. About face. Emerg Med 1974 November;24–77.

31. Crow RW. Sports-related lacerations. Promoting healing and limiting scarring. Phys Sports Med 1993;21:143–147.

32. Callaham M. Controversies in antibiotic choices for bite wounds. Ann Emerg Med 1988;17:1321–1330.

33. Callaham ML. Human and animal bites. Topics Emerg Med 1982 April;1–13.

34. Lindsey D, Christopher M, Hollenbach J, Boyd JH, Lindsey WE. Natural course of the human bite wound: incidence of infection and complications in 434 bites and 803 lacerations in the same group of patients. J Trauma 1987;27:45–48.

35. Boenning DA, Fleisher GR, Campus JM. Dog bites in children: epidemiology, microbiology, and penicillin prophylactic therapy. Am J Emerg Med 1983; 1:17–21.

36. Baker DM, Moore SE. Human bites in children, a 6-year experience. Am J Dis Child 1987;141: 1285–1290.

37. Schweich P, Fleisher G. Human bites in children. Ped Emerg Care 1985;1:51–53.

38. Rosen RA. The use of antibiotics in initial management of recent dog bite wounds. Am J Emerg Med 1985;3:19–23.

39. Callaham M. Prophylactic antibiotics in common dog bite wounds: a controlled study. Ann Emerg Med 1980;9:410–414.

40. Guy RJ, Zook EJ. Successful treatment of acute head and neck dog bite wounds without antibiotics. Ann Plast Surg 1986;17:45–48.

41. Davies D, Smith R. The hand: II. Plast Reconstr Surg 1985;290:1729–1734.

42. Brunner RG, Fallon WF. A prospective, randomized clinical trial of wound debridement versus conservative wound care in soft tissue injury from civilian gunshot wounds. Am Surg 1990;56:104–107.

43. Lammers RL. Principles of wound management. In: Roberts JR, Hedges JR, eds. Clinical procedures in emergency medicine. Philadelphia: WB Saunders, 1991; pp. 515–565.

44. Swanson NA, Tromovitch TA. Suture materials, 1980s: properties, uses, and abuses. Int J Dermatol 1982;21:374–378.

45. Capperauld I. Sutures in wound repair. In: Westaby S, ed. Wound care. St. Louis: CV Mosby, 1986; pp. 47–57.

46. Macht SD, Krizek TJ. Sutures and suturing-current concepts. J Oral Surg 1978;36:710–712.

47. Borges AF. Scar analysis and objectives of revision procedures. Clin Plast Surg 1977;4:223–237.

48. Robinson DW. Simple revision of scars. Clin Plast Surg 1977;4:217–222.

49. Edlich RF. Technical considerations in closure of skin wounds. In: Sparkman RS, ed. The healing of surgical wounds. Pearl River, NY: Davis & Geck, 1985; pp. 2–19.

50. DeHoll D, Rodeheaver G, Edgerton MT, Edlich RF. Potentiation of infection by suture closure of dead space. Am J Surg 1974;127:716–720.

51. Milewski PJ, Thomson H. Is a fat stitch necessary? Br J Surg 1980;67:393–394.

52. Westaby S. Wound closure and drainage. In: Westaby S, ed. Wound care. St. Louis: CV Mosby, 1986; pp. 32–46.

53. Anderson RM, Romfh RF. Technique in the use of surgical tools. New York: Appleton-Century-Crofts, 1980.

54. McLean NR, Fyfe AHB, Flint EF, Irvine BH, Calvert MH. Comparison of skin closure using continuous and interrupted nylon sutures. Br J Surg 1980;67:633–635.

55. Irvin TT. Simple skin closure. Br J Hosp Med 1985; 33:325–333.

56. Davies DM. Scars, hypertrophic scars, and keloids. Br Med J 1985;190:1056–1058.

57. Wray RC. Force required for wound closure and scar appearance. Plast Reconstr Surg 1973;72:380–382.

58. McGuire MF. Studies of the excisional wound: I. Biomechanical effects of undermining and wound orientation on closing tension and work. Plast Reconstr Surg 1980;66:419–427.

59. Roth JH, Windle BH. Staple versus suture closure of skin incisions in a pig model. Can J Surg 1988;31: 19–20.

60. Ritchie AJ, Rocke LG. Staples versus sutures in the closure of scalp wounds: a prospective, double-blind, randomized trial. Injury 1989;20:217–218.

61. Trott A. Alternative methods of wound closure. In: Roberts JR, Hedges JR, eds. Clinical procedures in emergency medicine. Philadelphia: WB Saunders, 1991; pp. 565–573.

62. Brickman KR, Lambert RW. Evaluation of skin stapling for wound closure in the emergency department. Ann Emerg Med 1989;18:1122–1125.

63. Connolly WB, Hunt TK, Zederfelt B, Cafferata HT, Dunphy JE. Clinical comparison of surgical wounds closed by suture and adhesive tapes. Am J Surg 1969;117:318–322.

64. Rodeheaver GT, Halverson JM, Edlich RF. Mechanical performance of wound closure tapes. Ann Emerg Med 1983;12:203–206.

65. Davies MJ. Scalp wounds. An alternative to suture. Injury 1988;19:375–376.

66. Quinn JV, Drzewiecki A, Li MM, Stiell IG, Sutcliffe T, Elmslie TJ, Wood WE. A randomized, controlled trial comparing a tissue adhesive with suturing in the repair of pediatric facial lacerations. Ann Emerg Med 1993;22:1130–1135.

67. Howell JM, Morgan DO. Scalp laceration repair without prior hair removal. Am J Emerg Med 1988; 6:7–10.

68. Cantrill SV. Facial trauma. In: Rosen P, ed. Emergency medicine: concepts and clinical practice. St. Louis: CV Mosby, 1992; pp. 355–370.

69. Edlich RF, Rogers W, Kasper G, Kaufman D, Tsung MS, Wangensteen OH. Studies in the management of the contaminated wound. I. Optimal time for closure of contaminated open wounds. II. Comparison of resistance to infection of open and closed wounds during healing. Am J Surg 1969;117:323–329.

70. Dimick AR. Delayed wound closure: indications and techniques. Ann Emerg Med 1988;17: 1303–1304.

71. Day TK. Controlled trial of prophylactic antibiotics in minor wounds requiring suture. Lancet 1975; 2:1174–1176.

72. Roberts SHN, Teddy PJ. A prospective trial of prophylactic antibiotics in hand lacerations. Br J Surg 1977;64:394–396.

73. Grossman JAI, Adams JP, Kunec J. Prophylactic antibiotics in simple hand lacerations. JAMA 1981; 245:1055–1056.

74. Chrintz H, Vibits H, Cordtz TO, Harreby JS, Waaddegaard P, Larsen SO. Need for surgical wound dressing. Br J Surg 1989;76:204–205.

75. Goldberg HM, Rosenthal SAE, Nemetz JC. Effect of washing closed head and neck wounds on wound healing and infection. Am J Surg 1981;141: 358–359.

76. Noe JM, Keller M. Can stitches get wet? Plast Reconstr Surg 1988; 81:82–84.

77. Rabkin JM, Hunt TK. Local heat increases blood flow and oxygen tension in wounds. Arch Surg 1987;122:221–225.

Management of Plantar Puncture Wounds

Howard Dixon III

Introduction

Plantar puncture wounds are a common problem among children, accounting for 0.8% of emergency department (ED) visits (1), and have the potential of serious complications if treated incorrectly. The vast majority of plantar puncture wounds are caused by nails, and generally occur during the summer (1, 2). Coring or enlargement of the puncture site may be beneficial in contaminated wounds or those with a possible foreign body by allowing for improved visualization, irrigation, and drainage. This procedure is easily performed by physicians or other health care providers in office or ED settings.

Anatomy and Physiology

Because of the close proximity of the tarsal bones to the skin surface and the greater force exerted on this weight-bearing area, puncture wounds of the forefoot penetrate deeper and have the highest risk of infectious complications, followed by the arch and lastly the heel. Complications include cellulitis, soft tissue abscess, foreign body granuloma, pyarthrosis, and osteomyelitis. Infection occurring in the first few days following the puncture is most commonly due to *Staphylococcus aureus* or group A *Streptococcus*. Pyarthrosis and osteomyelitis secondary to puncture wounds are overwhelmingly due to *Pseudomonas aeruginosa* (1, 2). The incidence of infections is reportedly as high as 15% (1), with the incidence of osteomyelitis estimated to be 0.4 to 0.6% (3). It should be noted that such estimates are likely high, as a large percentage of patients do not seek medical attention for superficial puncture wounds. Patients presenting late (7 days or greater) are at an increased risk for infectious complications (1). In addition, children appear to be at greatest risk for permanent sequelae as a result of these infections (2). Most puncture wounds are considered to be tetanus prone and, thus, require tetanus prophylaxis (see Table 110.2).

Indications

Indications for coring include grossly contaminated wounds and those suspicious for foreign body. Minor or clean superficial wounds to the plantar surface do not require enlargement, which can be a painful procedure to the child (4, 5). If coring is undertaken, local anesthesia should be used along with consideration for a peroneal nerve block (see Chapter 37). Wounds that have obvious deep tissue infection such as osteomyelitis or pyarthrosis will require surgical consultation as will those wounds presenting with a retained foreign body that the primary physician is unable to remove (6).

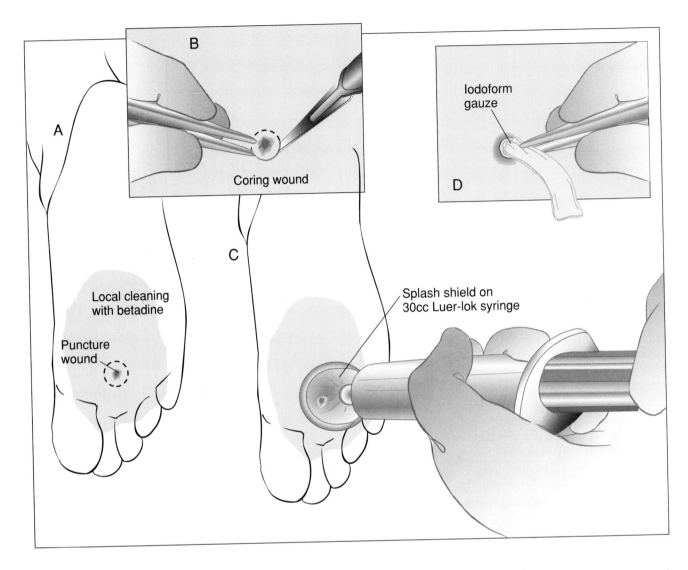

EQUIPMENT

Lidocaine—1 to 2% *without epinephrine*
Syringes—10 and 30 mL
Needle— 25 or 27 gauge, 1.5 inch
Scalpel blade (No. 11) or 4 mm disposable
  punch biopsy corer
Forceps
Normal saline
Povidone-iodine solution—10%
Angiocath or splashshield—18-gauge
Iodoform gauze—0.25 inch
Gauze dressing
Adhesive strips
Sterile gloves

PROCEDURE

Initially, most puncture wounds require evaluation for potential foreign bodies with plain radiographs. However, if a high degree of suspicion exists regarding the presence of radiolucent foreign bodies, a computerized tomography or ultrasound (Chapter 137) should be considered. Soaking the foot in an antiseptic solution has not been proven useful (7). Cleansing the external surface with povidone-iodine, however, is recommended (Fig. 112.1.A). Wounds that require coring should receive local or regional anesthetic (Chapter 37). Probing the wound is controversial, as this may result in a foreign object being pushed even deeper into the foot and also may cause damage to underlying nerves and vessels. With a No.11 scalpel blade (or 4 mm punch biopsy corer or cuticle scissors), a 2 mm circular rim of full-thickness skin is removed (Fig. 112.1.B). Irrigation into the wound tract with normal saline may be performed (Fig. 112.1.C) using a 30 mL syringe and an 18-gauge angiocath or splashshield.

Any debris or foreign objects should be removed with care. The physician may also opt to pack the tract with iodoform gauze (Fig. 112.1.D) before applying a bulky dressing.

Empiric antibiotics have not been shown to be effective and should be avoided unless evidence of infection is present (8). Patients should be instructed to avoid weight-bearing over the next 5 days and to keep the foot elevated when possible. Close follow-up within 48 hours is essential because even wounds that are properly managed may become infected. In addition, patients and/or parents should be warned about the possibility that osteomyelitis may be delayed in its manifestation. Innoculation of the bone with bacteria can sometimes take days or weeks before progressing to frank osteomyelitis. The initial skin wound may heal completely during this time. The patient complains of persistent pain with touch or weight-bearing, although the prior plantar puncture wound may be forgotten. This misleading course of events can lead to delayed diagnosis and more extensive damage to the bone. Consequently, when giving discharge instructions the clinician should carefully explain that delayed pain or tenderness around the site should prompt another evaluation of the patient, even if coring has been performed. It is also advisable to instruct the patient or parent that the phrase "possible infection in the bone" should be explicitly stated to the follow-up health care provider to trigger a heightened suspicion for osteomyelitis. Tetanus toxoid and tetanus immune globulin should be administered before discharge when indicated (Chapter 110).

COMPLICATIONS

Painful scarring may result from coring. Damage to underlying vessels, nerves, and fascia can occur with excessive debridement or coring. Limiting the amount of probing and depth of the tract will reduce damage to surrounding areas. Complications such as infections, cellulitis, pyarthrosis, and osteomyelitis are not as common to the procedure as they are to the puncture itself. Follow-up within 24 to 48 hours aids in early recognition of potential problems.

SUMMARY

Plantar puncture wounds are a common problem during childhood. Wounds that are grossly contaminated and those suspected of harboring a foreign body may benefit from coring or enlarging the wound site to effect improved irrigation and drainage. Close follow-up is mandatory to recognize the serious potential complications of pyarthrosis and osteomyelitis.

REFERENCES

1. Fitzgerald RH, Cowan DE. Puncture wounds of the foot. Orthop Clin North Am 1975;6:965.
2. Jarvis JG, Skipper MD. Pseudomonas osteochondritis complicating puncture wounds in children. J Ped Ortho 1994;14:755.
3. Chisolm CD, Schlesser JF. Plantar puncture wounds: Controversies and treatment recommendations. Ann Emerg Med 1989;18:1352.
4. Zukin DD, Inaba AS, Wuerker C. Soft tissue injuries. In: Barkin RM, ed. Pediatric emergency medicine: concepts and clinical practice. St. Louis: CV Mosby, 1992.
5. Resnick CD, Fallat SM. Puncture wounds: therapeutic considerations and a new classification. J Foot Surg 1990;29:147.
6. Inaba AS, Zukin DD, Pero M. An update on the evaluation and management of plantar puncture wounds and Pseudomonas osteomyelitis. Pediatr Emerg Care 1992;8:38.
7. Verdile VP, Freed HA, Gerard J. Puncture wounds to the foot. J Emerg Med 1989;7:193.
8. Joseph WS, LeFrock JL. Infections complicating puncture wounds of the foot. J Foot Surg 1987; 26:S30.

SUMMARY
1. Obtain radiographs to identify potential foreign body, fracture, or to evaluate for osteomyelitis if late presentation
2. Place patient in prone position
3. Prepare wound in an antiseptic fashion
4. Administer local or peroneal block
5. Coring—remove 2 mm rim of full-thickness skin from around puncture site
6. Remove any debris or foreign bodies
7. Irrigate wound with saline under high pressure
8. Pack wound with iodoform gauze
9. Apply bulky dressing
10. Administer tetanus toxoid and tetanus immune globulin when indicated
11. Encourage nonweight bearing for 5 days and elevation of extremity
12. Administer antistaphylococcal antibiotics if evidence of cellulitis
13. Refer for surgical management if retained foreign body or osteomyelitis is present
14. Follow-up in 24 to 48 hours

CLINICAL TIPS
1. Clean or superficial wounds need not undergo coring.
2. Wounds of the forefoot and those with late presentations are more likely to become infected.
3. A high index of suspicion must be maintained for a retained foreign body and for osteomyelitis in late presentations.

Chapter 112
Management of
Plantar
Puncture Wounds

SUBCUTANEOUS FOREIGN BODIES

Steven G. Rothrock

INTRODUCTION

Although most lacerations, puncture wounds, and abrasions that bring children to medical attention are minor in nature, physicians must be prepared to adequately care for those children whose wounds are complicated by foreign bodies. Studies have revealed that a significant percent of lacerations or puncture wounds in children presenting to pediatric emergency departments involve retained foreign bodies (1–3). Retained foreign bodies place these children at risk for infections, neurologic damage, scarring, and other serious complications while accounting for a significant number of malpractice claims against treating physicians. Considering that such a large number of children will present with this problem, physicians must have a complete understanding of foreign body management.

The most common types and locations of retained foreign bodies differ depending on the age of the patient. Infants who crawl can easily puncture their hands and knees with objects on the ground such as splinters, gravel, and glass. As children begin to walk, they are at risk for puncture wounds to the soles of their feet, most commonly from nails. Adolescents and teenagers are increasingly exposed to BBs, bullets, knives, and other forms of violence.

The complexity of the removal procedure, the optimal setting for removal, and the clinician involved vary depending on numerous factors. Superficial, easily visualized objects in benign locations can frequently be removed safely and completely in the office or emergency department (ED). Other foreign bodies require a surgical subspecialist and removal under the controlled conditions of an operating room.

ANATOMY AND PHYSIOLOGY

Polymorphonuclear neutrophils cause an initial tissue response by releasing a variety of hydrolytic enzymes, sometimes leading to pustules and rapid destruction, extrusion of the substance, or secondary infection with abscess formation. Alternately, subacute or chronic inflammation may follow or a foreign body granuloma may develop. The granuloma is formed by macrophages and giant cells which lay down collagen and fibrin and wall off foreign material from the rest of the body. Thus, foreign bodies may be present without symptoms if they are innocuous, or they may cause secondary localized infections or chronic inflammation if irritating material is present (10).

Glass, wood, and metal account for over 80% of all embedded foreign bodies (8). Although glass and metallic fragments often are innocuous to tissues, they also may migrate to, damage, and/or lacerate tendons and nerves and muscles, or lead to chronic inflammatory changes that may be mistaken for osteolytic lesions or pseudotumors on plain radiography. Wood and vegetable material such as thorns, spines of cacti, or wooden splinters are more toxic to tissues frequently causing inflammation and serving as a nidus for infection (5). Vegetable matter (including wood) can carry fungal organisms leading to phycomycoses (10). Particulate matter may produce cosmetic disfigurement or inflammatory papules and nodules. Subcutaneously embedded silica often causes no acute symptoms; however, granulomas can occur from 6 months to 60 years after traumatic implantation (10, 11). Graphite from pencils can lead to pigmented tattooing in soft tissues (12). Rubber is an excellent medium for growth of *Pseudomonas* organisms, placing children at risk for complications of perichondritis and osteomyelitis when the sole of a tennis shoe is penetrated (5).

The location of a foreign body is an important factor in the ease of its removal and its propensity to cause complications. The hand is one of the most common areas in which foreign bodies become lodged (4). Because of the abundance of overlapping tissue planes, foreign bodies frequently are missed on physical examination even when radiopaque (13, 14). Although the complexity of the anatomy makes the hand difficult to examine, it also places these patients at risk for nerve, tendon, vessel, and muscle injury as well as localized infections.

The foot also is a difficult area to evaluate for the presence of foreign bodies. Foreign bodies (usually a piece of sock or shoe) are important causative factors in patients who develop infections following puncture wounds of the foot (2).

Foreign bodies can lodge proximally in extremities causing tendon, muscular, neurologic, or vascular damage. Migration to or involvement of tendon sheaths, joints, or blood vessels should always be considered when evaluating pediatric patients with suspected extremity foreign bodies.

INDICATIONS

Determining the presence of a foreign body is often difficult. Several historical and physical examination clues, however, should heighten the clinician's suspicion of an embedded foreign body. In glass-induced wounds, glass fragments are more frequently retained if the head or the foot is involved, or if the wound occurred during a motor vehicle accident (4). Particulate matter, dirt, rust, or skin can be tracked into the wound if cloth or a shoe is penetrated by a sharp object (e.g., a nail), especially if the object is 4.5 mm or greater in diameter (5). Fragments often are left behind if prior attempts have been made to remove wood or vegetable matter (6). In fact, a foot infection that is not improving after treatment with antibiotics is highly suggestive of a retained foreign body.

The presence of a foreign body is not always obvious on gross inspection. Glass is notoriously difficult to visualize within a wound (4). Gross visualization often does not detect glass in children even when the bottom of the wound can be seen. However, lacerations that are less than 0.5 cm in depth have been shown to rarely contain glass (7). Other useful clues to the presence of a foreign body include inordinate wound pain, tenderness with deep palpation over the wound, pain with passive movement of that area (especially after local topical anesthesia), pain associated with a mass, or skin discoloration (5). Often, no history is available in the preverbal child. The only clue may be a slowly resolving cellulitis, draining sinus, culture-negative abscess, or radiographic abnormality consistent with a pseudotumor, joint destruction, periosteal thickening, or a lytic lesion (2, 8, 9).

Plain radiography identifies most glass and metallic foreign bodies (9). Although ingested aluminum often is not seen with plain radiography, embedded aluminum usually is visible on plain films (15). When glass or metal is less than 1 to 2 mm in diameter or overlies bone, it may not be visualized (16). Wood can be identified on plain films in only 15% of cases (8, 9). After 48 hours, air trapped within the wood is absorbed and tissue fluids saturate it, making wood almost impossible to identify on plain films (9). Plastic and vegetable matter have similar densities to wood and are not seen on most plain films (5).

Ultrasonography should be considered a first-line technique for identifying nonradiopaque foreign bodies (Chapter 137). Sensitivity and specificity in identifying foreign bodies such as plastic, wood, and vegetable matter exceed 90% (17–20). In fact, almost all foreign objects create a reflective surface by ultrasonography (17–20). However, air and gas do not conduct sound waves and bone impedes transmission of sound waves to deeper tissues. Therefore, identifying foreign bodies adjacent to bone, air, or gas with ultrasonography is difficult (17, 19).

Computerized tomography (CT) and magnetic resonance imaging (MRI) are used primarily (*a*) when foreign material is in a critical area, (*b*) when the surgical approach and exploration may be altered by better three-dimensional analysis of anatomy, or (*c*) when alternate techniques such as ultrasonography and plain radiography are inadequate or equivocal (21). MRI is superior to CT in visualizing foreign bodies with densities similar to surrounding tissue and also soft tissue reactions such as edema, hemorrhage, and infection (21). MRI should be avoided in patients with potential metallic foreign bodies including prior surgical hardware and vascular clips (22). Both imaging techniques take excess time, are expensive, and may require sedation (and monitoring) of the young or apprehensive child.

One of the most difficult decisions to make when caring for a child with a retained foreign body is whether to remove it. Unfortunately, no clear cut guidelines are available for removal. Foreign bodies that are highly inflammatory, potentially toxic or infectious, or those that might involve or migrate to tendons, nerves, vessels, joints, or open fractures should be removed. Foreign bodies that have the potential to cause an allergic reaction, persistent pain, or a cosmetic deformity also should be removed. If the object is small, innocuous, and does not involve important structures it often can be left in place (Table 113.1). However, the clinician should consider the fact that a child has a much longer potential life expectancy than an adult and thus has a greater lifetime risk of developing problems from a retained foreign body. Sequelae from joint, bone, muscle, and tendon injuries are potentially more serious to a growing child than to an adult. Thus, clinicians should be more reluctant to leave a foreign body in place in a child. If a foreign body is left in place, local care of the wound and referral to a surgical specialist for elective re-

Table 113.1.
Indications for Removing Foreign Bodies

Reactive materials likely to cause inflammation or infection (e.g., thorns, spines, wood, other vegetable material, and clothing)
Heavy bacterial contamination
Toxicity (e.g., spines with venom, heavy metals)
Impingement on or damage to tendons, vessels, or nerves
Impairment of mechanical function
Intraarticular location
Proximity to fractured bone
Potential for migration toward important anatomic structures
Intravascular location
Persistent pain
Established inflammation or infection
Allergic reaction
Cosmesis or psychological distress

Used with permission from Lammers RL, Magill T. Detection and management of foreign bodies in soft tissue. *Emerg Med Clin North Am* 1992;10:767–781.

moval at a future date are appropriate. The reason for leaving a foreign body in place should be explained completely to the patient and family if this treatment option is chosen.

Contraindications to foreign body removal in the ED include foreign bodies embedded in the chest, abdomen, or neck. If an object is embedded in the trunk or neck, it should be left in place so that adequate dissection of the wound tract (usually by a surgeon under general anesthesia) can be made with the object still in place. Removing such an object may cause a tamponaded vessel to bleed or inhibit the ability to identify the tract of the object throughout its length. The decision of whether to remove a foreign object also includes considering the amount of time and effort necessary and the potential damage of wound exploration. In general, attempts at exploration in the ED should not exceed 30 minutes. If more time is needed, if important structures are injured or at risk for injury, or if more than a short-acting sedating agent is needed, subspecialty consultation should be sought for removal of the foreign body under more controlled circumstances.

EQUIPMENT

Tourniquet or blood pressure cuff
Gauze pads
Needle (25-gauge needle or smaller) and syringe

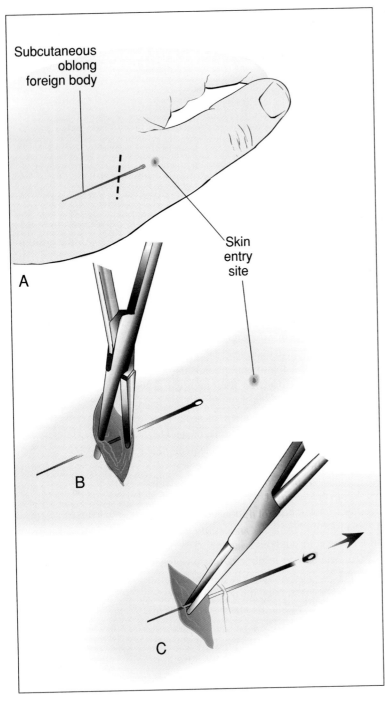

Figure 113.1.
Removal of foreign body oriented parallel to skin surface.

Forceps—with and without teeth for grasping object and skin

Hemostat—curved and straight for grasping object

Large syringe—with 18-gauge needle or angiocath for irrigation

Normal saline—sterile for irrigation

Salicylic acid—40% for superficial splinters

Elmer's® glue for small cactus spines

PROCEDURE

The first step to removing a foreign body is to identify and localize the object. Several radiologic techniques can assist in localizing foreign bodies that cannot be directly visualized. Paper clips or needles should be placed at 90° angles to each other over the surface of a wound before obtaining a plain radiograph. Several films can be taken to localize a foreign body in two or more planes. If the foreign body is radiopaque and not able to be localized using this technique, fluoroscopy or CT can often identify the site and aid in removal (23). If the foreign body is not radiopaque, ultrasonography and CT guidance can be used for localization and removal (23, 24). Finally, metal detectors have been used successfully to assist with metallic foreign body removal from extremities (25).

Before beginning any procedure, all equipment should be assembled. Before and after manipulation or application of anesthesia to a wound, the clinician should assess tendon function, nerve function, and the vascular status of the involved extremity. The wound is examined with the underlying tendons and muscles extended and flexed through their entire range of motion to reproduce all relationships of the wound to the underlying structures. To ensure proper visualization of the wound, anesthesia, complete immobilization, and proper lighting are critical (Chapters 3 and 37). Using local anesthetic agents that contain epinephrine should be avoided on digits and end organs. A tourniquet applied proximally to the wound or a blood pressure cuff inflated to 20 mm Hg above the systolic blood pressure will provide adequate hemostasis. Neither the tourniquet nor the inflated cuff should be used for more than 30 minutes at a time. Alternately, if a wound only involves a finger, a sterile glove (sized for the patient's hand) may be

Lidocaine—1% or 2% with or without epinephrine depending on wound location

Betadine—for preparation of sterile field around wound

Drapes—for sterile field

Sterile needles or paper clips—for localization during radiography

Scalpel—No. 15 blade for enlarging wound or en bloc removal of foreign body

applied to the involved hand. The fingertip of the glove covering the involved digit is cut and rolled to the base of the finger, which limits blood flow to the finger during examination of the wound and maintains a sterile field (26). Cleansing the area around the wound with betadine and placing sterile drapes around the wound will ensure no contamination from skin flora (Chapters 7 and 110).

If the foreign body is not readily visible, extending or enlarging the wound with a No. 15 scalpel blade should be considered. If only superficial dermis and epidermis are incised, the risk of damaging underlying structures will be minimized when enlarging the wound. If possible, the clinician should attempt to incise along natural skin folds and not perpendicular to skin creases (see Fig. 111.2). The wound can be carefully explored by spreading the soft tissue with a hemostat. Blind probing with any instrument should be avoided, especially in areas where vital structures are located such as the hand, foot, or face. In children, vital structures are much closer to the skin and to each other and have a higher risk of injury during manipulation of a wound.

Once the foreign body is located, examination of its entire length and identification of its exact anatomic location will ensure that important structures are not involved. The foreign body can be grasped with forceps or a hemostat and removed as one piece if it is metal or glass. Following removal, reexploration of the wound will ensure that no important structures were damaged during removal and that no pieces of the foreign body were left behind. If the wound is clean, does not contain particulate matter or devitalized tissue, and is less than 12 to 24 hours old, it should be thoroughly irrigated and sutured. Debridement of devitalized tissue, placement of a penrose drain, or delayed primary closure are indicated for older or contaminated wounds.

Difficult to find, relatively clean embedded objects that are parallel to the skin, such as a long thin needle or a piece of glass, are best approached by incising the skin perpendicular to the midpoint of the object's long axis (5). Gentle spreading of tissues with a hemostat will aid in locating the object. The object then can be grasped with the hemostat and removed via its original entrance site or

through the newly created incision (Fig. 113.1). The incision is then closed.

If the foreign body enters perpendicular to the skin and is difficult to find, attempted localization through a linear incision is not recommended. This will displace the foreign body to one side of the wound. Instead, a small elliptical incision (large enough to ensure that the foreign body can be removed)

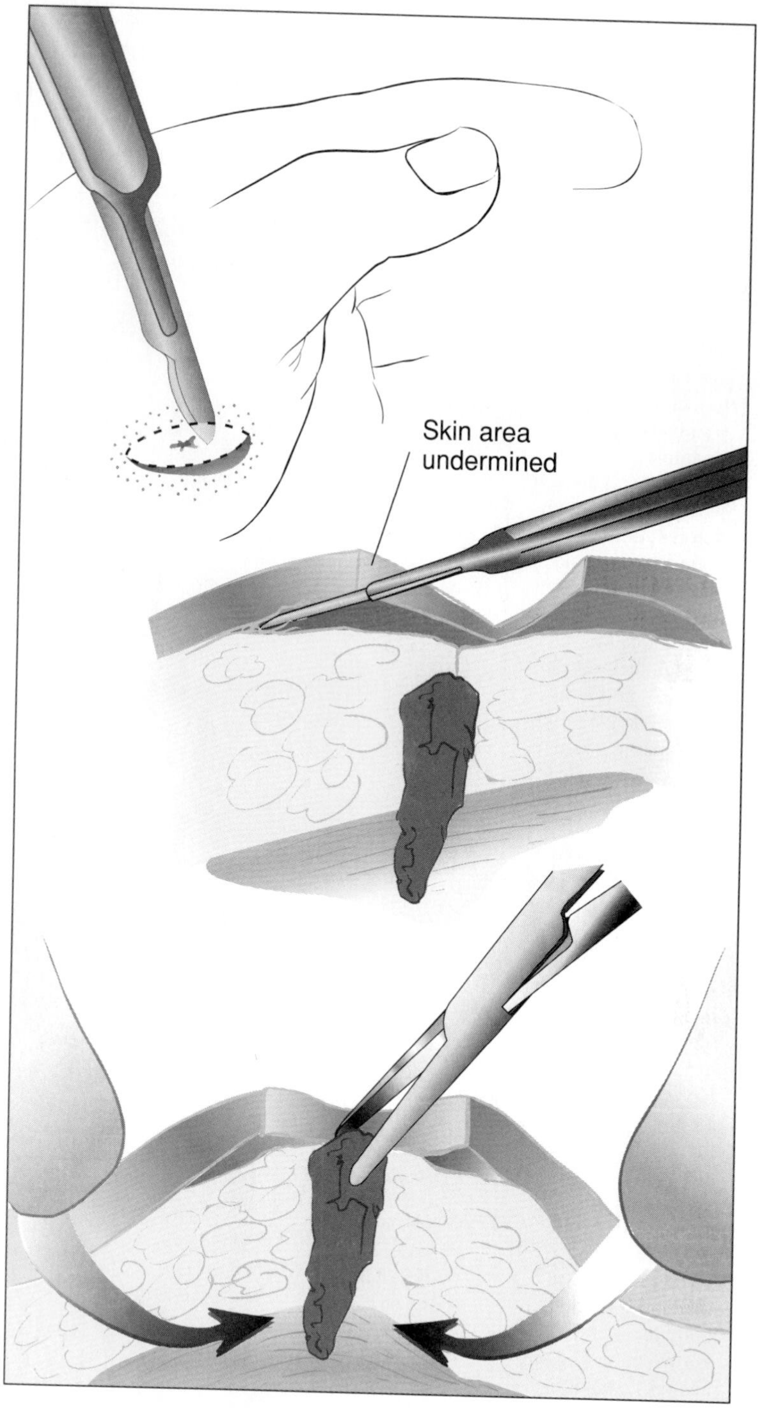

Skin area undermined

Figure 113.2.
Removal of foreign body oriented perpendicular to skin surface.

Figure 113.3.
En bloc removal of foreign
body and surrounding
contaminated tissue.

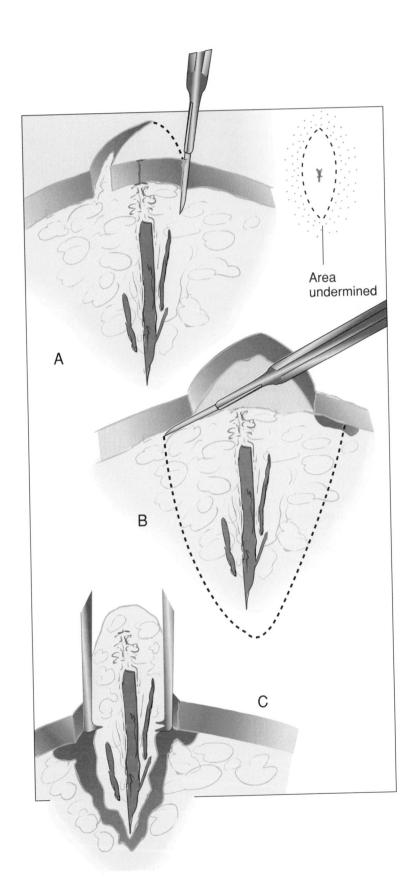

Area
undermined

A

B

C

SUMMARY

1. Use appropriate ra-
   diographic technique
   and surface markers
   to identify possible
   foreign body
2. Examine extremity
   proximal and distal to
   wound to ensure ten-
   don function, neuro-
   logic function, and
   vascular status are intact
3. Examine tendons
   through their entire
   range of motion to
   ensure that potential
   overlapping tissue
   planes present during
   injury are reproduced
4. Provide adequate lo-
   cal analgesia, con-
   sider conscious seda-
   tion, and immobilize
   patient and extremity
5. Control for hemosta-
   sis by applying proxi-
   mal tourniquet or
   blood pressure cuff
   expanded to 20 mm
   Hg above systolic
   blood pressure for no
   more than 30 minutes
   at a time
6. Set time limit of 30
   minutes for explo-
   ration of wound
7. Explore wound so
   that entire foreign
   body location is
   known including any
   anatomic relation-
   ships with important
   structures
8. Remove entire for-
   eign body including
   devitalized or in-
   fected tissue

should be made with the entrance site of the foreign body in its center (Fig. 113.2). The skin is then undermined 0.25 to 0.50 inch in all directions. The foreign body can be displaced into the middle of the wound by compressing the skin surface. It then can be grasped and removed with a hemostat. If no contamination is evident, thorough irrigation followed by wound closure should be performed.

Removing vegetable matter and wooden splinters requires special care. If the end of a splinter or piece of wood is grasped, it often fragments leaving multiple pieces in the wound. If the piece is already fragmented or cannot be removed without fragmentation, either an incision down the entire long axis of the foreign body should be made or en bloc removal of the material and surrounding tissue is performed. To cut down to the foreign body, an incision made over its entire long axis and removal via the new skin incision rather than through the entrance wound is indicated. Thorough irrigation of the entire tract and removal of all foreign debris should follow.

Before performing en bloc removal of a foreign body and surrounding tissue, the clinician must first ensure that no tendons, nerves, or vessels are present in the surgical field. An elliptical incision is then made around the wound (including the entire area to be removed to a depth below the foreign body). The surrounding skin is undermined 0.25 to 0.50 inch in all directions. The entire block of tissue then can be removed by grasping the piece of tissue and applying upward traction (Fig. 113.3). If performed properly, no fragments will be left behind and contaminated tissue will be excised. En bloc removal also should be considered for superficial objects that are difficult to visualize or have the potential to stain, infiltrate, damage, or irritate surrounding tissue.

Superficial splinters also can be removed using keratolytic agents. Salicylic acid hydrates the stratum corneum, loosens the cell margins of the dermis, and detaches the splinter fragment (27). Applying 40% salicylic acid with an occluding adhesive strip is 73% successful at 72 hours and 100% successful at 7 days in removing subcutaneous splinters parallel to the skin surface (27).

Cactus spines comprise another unique class of foreign bodies that present problems with removal. Large and medium spines (that do not have barbs on their tip) can be removed with the same technique as embedded long needles (28). Traction can be applied to the long axis of the spine, because cactus needles do not fracture easily. Small cactus spines are more difficult to remove. Patients with punctures due to small cactus spines can have over 1000 embedded spines. Several techniques can be used for removal. Toothless forceps alone, or in combination with the application of a thin layer of glue (Elmer's®), covered with a single layer of gauze which is lifted after drying will remove most spines (29). Less successful techniques include applying a facial peel, adhesive tape, cellophane sealing tape, or ostomy cement, waiting for it to dry, and then pulling most of the spines off at once (28, 29).

Although few prospective studies have addressed the utility of antibiotics in preventing infections in patients undergoing foreign body removal, it is generally recommended that patients with wounds that are devitalized (dusky appearing with a tenuous or poor blood supply), older than 12 to 24 hours, contaminated (with dirt, vegetable or particulate matter), or patients who are immunocompromised receive prophylactic antibiotics. Either a penicillinase resistant penicillin derivative, erythromycin, or a first generation cephalosporin are commonly used for this purpose (2, 12, 15). Because of the serious nature of hand infections, an antibiotic for most hand wounds that previously contained a foreign body is recommended. Until further studies are performed, physicians should consider these factors and individualize treatment decisions to each particular case.

A 1- or 2-day follow-up of all patients already infected or at risk for developing an infection will aid in detecting potential complications before any serious sequelae occur.

COMPLICATIONS

Complications of wound exploration and foreign body removal parallel those of retained foreign bodies. Prolonged manipulation of tissue can lead to superficial and deep wound infections including cellulitis, abscesses, lymphangitis, septic arthritis, and osteo-

Chapter 113
Subcutaneous Foreign
Bodies

myelitis by repeatedly damaging tissue. Conversely, infections can occur if foreign material is left behind (especially if the foreign material is irritating such as wood, vegetable matter, or graphite). Physicians must weigh the risk of introducing an infection against the risk of foreign material causing an infection.

Repeated wound handling can directly damage nearby structures including nerves, arteries, tendons, muscle, and bone. This is especially true of younger patients whose smaller size makes these consequences more likely. Scarring may occur if dermal or subcutaneous tissue is crushed or devitalized during exploration. To minimize this damage, a time limit for exploration should be set and tissue handled as little as possible during the procedure. Talc from surgical gloves also may be introduced into a wound during exploration and foreign body removal, causing a localized allergic reaction that may be confused with an early infection.

All techniques of limiting hemostasis can compromise arterial flow to the involved area. Vasoconstricting agents are contraindicated near end organs such as fingers, toes, nose, ears, penis, or for tissue that has a compromised arterial supply (e.g., partially devitalized skin). Application of tourniquets and blood pressure cuffs should not exceed 20 to 30 minutes at a time. Breaks of 1 to 2 minutes to limit pain and tissue hypoperfusion are recommended. Neuropraxia, intimal vascular damage, vascular thrombosis, and gangrene have been reported with prolonged use of tourniquets, primarily if left on for more than 2 continuous hours (30, 31). The technique of rolling the fingertip of a glove to the base of the involved finger can lead to pressures as high as 1000 mm Hg if too small a glove is used, whereas an appropriate size glove for the patient's hand provides adequate hemostasis with lower pressures and less risk of damage (32).

SUMMARY

The ability to remove subcutaneous foreign bodies is an important skill physicians must possess when dealing with injured pediatric patients. Although this procedure has many potential complications, knowledge of a vari-

ety of alternative techniques will increase the clinician's ability to successfully remove foreign bodies. Properly preparing the pediatric patient and the wound for exploration will save time, effort, and decrease potential complications from this procedure. Immobilization and anesthesia are two important factors that physicians must address in young and often apprehensive children before any attempt at foreign body removal. Finally, setting a time limit and handling tissue as little as possible will reduce the risk of injuring tissue and important adjacent structures.

REFERENCES

1. Baker MD, Lanuti M. The management and outcome of lacerations in urban children. Ann Emerg Med 1990;19:1001–1006.
2. Chisholm CD, Schlesser JF. Plantar puncture wounds: controversies and treatment recommendations. Ann Emerg Med 1989;18:1352–1357.
3. Fitzgerald RH, Cowan JD. Puncture wounds of the foot. Orthop Clin North Am 1975;6:965–972.
4. Montano JB, Steele MT, Watson WA. Foreign body retention in glass-caused wounds. Ann Emerg Med 1992;21:1360–1363.
5. Lammers RL, Magill T. Detection and management of foreign bodies in soft tissue. Emerg Med Clin North Am 1992;10:767–781.
6. Chow D, Cooke TD, Feltis T. Thorn-induced synovitis. Can Med Assoc J 1987;136:1057–1058.
7. Avner JR, Baker D. Lacerations involving glass. Am J Dis Child 1992; 146:600–602.
8. Brewer Jr TE, Leonard RB. Detection of retained wood following trauma. North Carolina Med J 1986; 47:575–577.
9. Flom LL, Ellis GL. Radiologic evaluation of foreign bodies. Emerg Med Clin North Am 1992;10: 163–177.
10. Epstein WL, Fukuyama K. Mechanisms of granulomatous inflammation. Immunology Series 1989;46: 687–721.
11. Mowry RG, Sams Jr. WM, Caulfield JB. Cutaneous silica granuloma. A rare entity or rarely diagnosed? Report of two cases with review of the literature. Arch Dermatol 1991;127:692–694.
12. Barnett RC. Soft tissue foreign body removal. In: Roberts JR, Hedges JR, eds. Clinical procedures in emergency medicine. 2nd ed. Philadelphia: WB Saunders, 1991, pp. 581–591.
13. Anderson A, Newmeyer WL, Kilgore ES. Diagnosis and treatment of retained foreign bodies of the hand. Am J Surg 1982;144:63.
14. Morgan WJ, Leopold T, Evans R. Foreign bodies in the hand. J Hand Surg 1984;9:194–196.
15. Langsam A. Solid foreign bodies in the soft tissue: diagnosis and management. Delaware Med J 1985; 57:701–702.

16. Courter BJ. Radiographic screening for glass foreign bodies—What does a "negative" foreign body series really mean? Ann Emerg Med 1990;19: 997–1000.

17. Banerjee B, Das RK. Sonographic detection of foreign bodies of the extremities. Br J Radiol 1991;64: 107–112.

18. Blyme PJH, Lind T, Schantz K, Lavard P. Ultrasonographic detection of foreign bodies in soft tissue: a human cadaver study. Arch Orthop Trauma Surg 1990;220:24–25.

19. Crawford R, Matheson AB. Clinical value of ultrasonography in the detection and removal of radiolucent foreign bodies. Injury Br J Accident Surg 1989; 20:341–343.

20. Gilbert FJ, Campbell RS, Bayliss AP. The role of ultrasound in the detection of nonradiopaque foreign bodies. Clin Radiol 1990;41:109–112.

21. Bodne D, Quinn SF, Cochran CF. Imaging foreign glass and wooden bodies of the extremities with CT and MR. J Comput Assist Tomogr 1988;12: 608–611.

22. Lewis TT, Case A, Troughton A, Bloom PA, Goddard P. Metallic foreign body localization with magnetic resonance imaging. Radiol Today 1991;57: 16–17.

23. Bissonnitte RT, Connell DG, Fitzpatrick DG. Preoperative localization of low-density foreign bodies under CT guidance. Can Assoc Radiol J 1988;39: 286–287.

24. Bradley M, Kadzombe E, Simms P, Eyes B. Percutaneous ultrasound guided extraction of nonpalpable soft tissue foreign bodies. Arch Emerg Med 1992; 9:181–184.

25. West A, Glucksman E. The use of a metal locator in an accident and emergency department. Arch Emerg Med 1987;4:57–61.

26. Barnett A, Pearl RM. Readily available, inexpensive finger tourniquet. Plast Reconstr Surg 1983;71: 134–135.

27. Copelan R. Chemical removal of splinters without epidermal toxic effects. J Am Acad Dermatol 1989; 20:697–698.

28. Lindsey D, Lindsey WE. Cactus spine injuries. Am J Emerg Med 1988;6:362–369.

29. Martinez TT, Jerome M, Barry BC, Jaeger R, Xander JG. Removal of cactus spines from the skin. A comparative evaluation of several methods. Am J Dis Child 1987;141:1291–1292.

30. Dove A, Clifford R. Ischemia after use of a finger tourniquet. Br Med J 1982;284:256.

31. Pedowitz RA. Limb tourniquets during surgery. Acta Orthop Scand 1991;62 (Suppl 245):17–33.

32. Brown CK, Wootsen SL, Fair LK. Retained foreign body: a fingernail fragment. J Emerg Med 1993;11: 259–264.

HAIR TOURNIQUET REMOVAL

John Loiselle and Richard T. Cook, Jr.

INTRODUCTION

Hair-thread tourniquet syndrome refers to conditions in which an appendage (e.g., finger, toe, or penis) is circumferentially constricted by a hair or thread, leading to impairment of lymphatic and eventually venous return (1, 2). Cases involving entrapment of other body parts such as the female genitalia (clitoris and labia), though unusual, have also been reported (3). Hair tourniquets most frequently occur in the first few months of life, although they occasionally occur in toddlers. Removal of a hair tourniquet involves cutting the constricting band, thereby eliminating the vascular compression and restoring perfusion. Principles that should be adhered to when releasing the constricting band include protecting entrapped soft tissue from harm while avoiding injury to the neurovascular and tendon structures of the appendage. The removal procedure in most cases can be performed in the ambulatory office or in the emergency department. This procedure is usually performed by the emergency physician, general pediatric practitioner, or family physician, but if significant edema has occurred with ensuing distortion of tissues, surgical consultation may be necessary.

ANATOMY AND PHYSIOLOGY

Anatomic structures involved in a digital hair tourniquet include the layers of the skin, as well as the nerves, blood vessels, and lymphatics (Fig. 114.1). The neurovascular bundles of the fingers and toes are located on the dorsal and palmar or plantar aspects of both the radial and ulnar margins. The major neurovascular structures of the penis and clitoris are located on the dorsal surface at the 12-o'-clock position. Deeper structures of the penis which may become involved include the dorsally located corpora cavernosum and also the corpus spongiosum, which is located on the ventral surface and surrounds the urethra (4).

Hair tourniquets have been associated with postpartum hair loss (telogen effluvium), mothers with long hair (particularly blonde in a caucasian child), use of mittens or booties in infants, and hair shed in the bathtub (2, 6, 12). Reports also have been made of tourniquets being placed intentionally (2, 11). It is postulated that the offending hair is often wet when it first becomes wrapped around the appendage, and as it dries it contracts, thus leading to the initial constriction (1, 5, 6, 7). Constriction of venous and lymphatic vessels with inhibition of venous return by a hair tourniquet leads to edema which further increases the swelling, compounds the compression of the vessels, and compromises distal perfusion in a vicious cycle. If the constricting agent has been in place long enough, it can cut through the skin layers. Epithelialization may then occur obscuring the hair beneath an overlying skin bridge. Injury may be caused by ischemia and by direct damage to structures through the cutting action of the tourniquet. Necrosis and gangrene of digits (5, 11) and erosion through the urethra with resulting fistula formation have been reported (8, 9).

Figure 114.1.
Neurovascular and
structural components of
the fingers and penis.

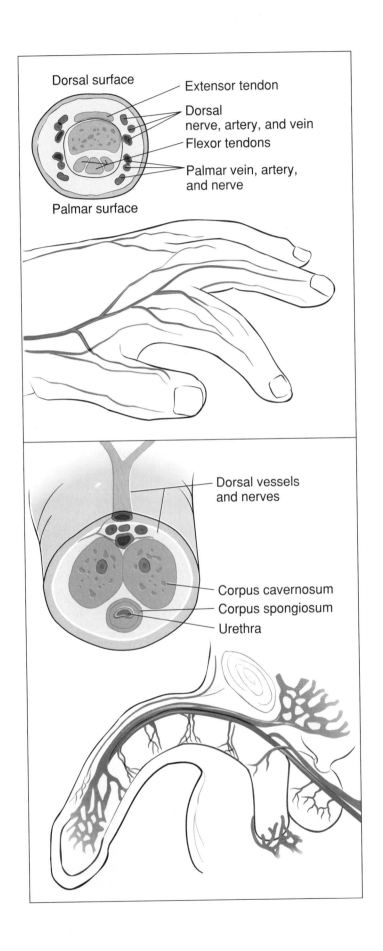

Dorsal surface

Extensor tendon

Dorsal
nerve, artery, and vein

Flexor tendons

Palmar vein, artery,
and nerve

Palmar surface

Dorsal vessels
and nerves

Corpus cavernosum

Corpus spongiosum

Urethra

INDICATIONS

The child with a constricting band of hair or thread may present in several ways. Most frequently the child has an erythematous, swollen, painful appendage. When inspected carefully, a sharp, circumferential demarcation is present beyond which the digit is affected. At the point of demarcation an extra crease or indentation is noted. Because of the difficulty in localizing a source of pain in the infant, it is important not to overlook this as a possible diagnosis when evaluating the presentation of irritability and crying (3).

A number of other processes may present in a similar fashion. Hair tourniquets involving the penis may initially be confused with a paraphimosis in the uncircumcised male (5), or balanitis, a localized infection of the glans penis. Similarly, a hair tourniquet on the digit may mimic infectious processes such as a cellulitis, felon, or paronychia. Rarely encountered entities resulting in band-like constrictions around the digits include congenital amnionic bands and ainhum, a rare condition of spontaneous bandlike constriction and ischemia occurring in toes of dark-skinned people (1, 2).

Frequently the hair or thread is visible and may simply be cut or unwrapped. When the strand is not visible or has eroded through the dermis and involves underlying structures, or if uncertainty exists regarding completeness of removal, a surgical or urologic consult may be necessary.

EQUIPMENT

Local or regional anesthesia materials (Chapter 37)
Scalpel blade—No. 11
Povidone-iodine solution
Fine-tipped forceps
Ear curette
Ophthalmic spud
Fine-tipped hemostat
Blunt probe
Fine-tipped scissors

PROCEDURE

The technique used for removing a hair tourniquet and the need for involving specialists depends on the perceived risk to the ap-

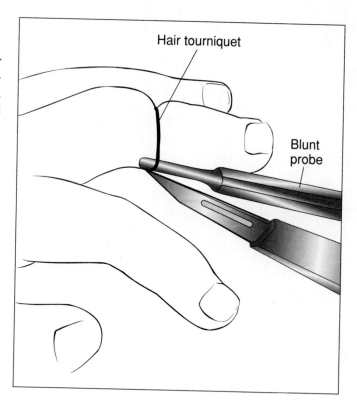

Hair tourniquet

Blunt probe

Figure 114.2.
Removal of a hair tourniquet with a blunt probe.

pendage, the involvement of underlying structures, the depth of the hair, and the appendage involved. If a loose end of the constricting hair can be located, it may be only necessary to grasp it firmly with gloved fingers, fine forceps, or a hemostat and gently unwind it. It should be noted that a single strand may have broken into several and this process may need to be repeated.

In cases when the constricting band does not seem too deeply imbedded in the soft tissue, a blunt probe or metal ear wax curette may be gently inserted beneath the constriction (Fig. 114.2). Insertion is facilitated when performed in a proximal to distal direction while applying traction to the skin. The hair generally penetrates less deeply and may be more accessible on the dorsal aspect of the fingers or toes. Once the strand is isolated with a metal object, it can be cut with fine-tipped scissors. Alternatively, a scalpel blade may be used to cut through the hair onto the probe or curette, which serves to protect the underlying skin.

In situations in which the degree of edema or depth of penetration of the hair makes this technique impossible, direct incision of the band to ensure release is necessary. Surgical consultation should be considered at this point.

Figure 114.3.
A. Incisional removal of a hair tourniquet from a digit.
B. Incisional removal of a hair tourniquet from a penis.

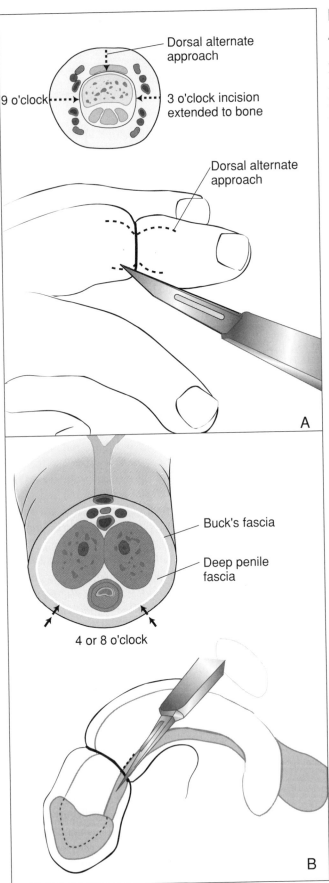

Dorsal alternate approach

9 o'clock

3 o'clock incision extended to bone

Dorsal alternate approach

A

Buck's fascia

Deep penile fascia

4 or 8 o'clock

B

SUMMARY
1. Grasp loose fibers and gently unwind
2. Insert blunt probe or curette beneath hair or thread
3. Isolate fiber from underlying soft tissue
4. Remove fiber
   a. Cut fiber with fine-tipped scissors
   or
   b. Cut through fiber and onto probe or curette with No. 11 scalpel blade
5. Explore for presence of additional strands
6. Evaluate neurovascular status and/or tendon function

Incisional approach
Digit
1. Perform digital nerve block on involved digit
2. Prepare and drape digit and surrounding area in sterile fashion
3. Incise along digit perpendicular to tourniquet to the depth of bone
   a. Incise laterally at 3-o'clock or 9-o'clock position
   or
   b. Incise dorsally at 12-o'clock position
Penis
1. Apply local or regional anesthesia
2. Prepare and drape penis and surrounding area in sterile fashion
3. Incise lateral inferior surface at either 4- or 8-o'clock position

---

Chapter 114
Hair Tourniquet
Removal

Incisional Approach

Digits

A digital nerve block is performed (Chapter 37), and the digit and surrounding area is prepped and draped in a sterile fashion. The major consideration when determining the best site for an incision in the removal of a hair tourniquet is the location of underlying structures. Because the neurovascular bundles lie at the dorsal and palmar aspects of the radial and ulnar portions of the digits, one recommended approach is to make the incision between the bundles using a No. 11 scalpel blade at either the 3-o'clock or 9-o'clock position (Fig. 114.3.A). The incision should be made longitudinally along the digit with the blade perpendicular to the strand and the skin surface. The incision is made in a proximal to distal direction, and should be extended to the bone to ensure incision of the fiber.

An incision on the dorsal surface provides an acceptable alternative approach (2) (Fig. 114.3.A). Although this may result in an incision into the extensor tendon, a longitudinal incision parallel to the direction of the tendon fibers should heal well with splinting and general wound care. This incision has the advantage of avoiding the neurovascular bundles entirely.

Penis

Following the application of a topical anesthetic or a penile nerve block (Chapter 37), the penis and surrounding area is prepped and draped in a sterile fashion. In the penis the main neurovascular structures reside on the dorsal surface and the urethra on the ventral surface. The recommended site for an incision is on the lateral inferior surface at the 4- or 8-o'clock position (Fig. 114.3.B.). Attempts should be made to stay in the deep penile fascia at the junction of the corpus cavernosum and spongiosum (11). Given that the fascia is a relatively tough layer, the clinician may elect to make light incisions of the skin cutting slightly deeper with successive strokes through the same initial incision, with the goal of cutting the constricting band without penetrating the fascial layer into the lumen of the corpora. Urologic assistance should generally be obtained before embarking on such an incision, unless the penis is deemed to be at immediate risk.

Evidence of reperfusion usually occurs within several minutes after release of the constricting band; however, depending on the tissue insult caused by the constriction, it may be days before normal perfusion has returned completely. When any question remains as to whether the circumferential constriction has been completely removed, surgical consultation should be obtained.

Neurovascular status and/or tendon function should be documented following the procedure. The need for tetanus prophylaxis should be addressed. An extremity should be placed in an elevated position to allow for passive drainage. Reevaluation in 24 hours will help to ensure that all constricting bands have been removed and that the soft tissue is adequately perfused and free from infection.

COMPLICATIONS

Damage to neurovascular structures may be the result of prolonged ischemia, the cutting action of the tourniquet, or the incision. Similarly, injuries to the corpus collosum, corpus spongiosum, or urethra are possible with incisional removal of hair tourniquets involving the penis. Dorsal incisions in the fingers and toes generally do not cause functional damage to tendons, however, tenosynovitis may result from injury to the tendon sheath.

Once penetration of the superficial layers of the skin has occurred, whether by the hair or the incision, infection is a risk.

SUMMARY

Diagnosis of a hair or thread wrapped around an appendage such as a finger, toe, or penis may be obvious or may test the diagnostic skills of an astute clinician. In the uncomplicated case, removal is a simple matter of unwinding the offending hair. If the hair has been present for a prolonged period, progressive edema and penetration into deeper layers of skin may necessitate an incisional approach to ensure complete removal. A consultant is frequently necessary at this point. Although serious consequences have been reported with delay in recognizing and removing such objects, successful removal generally results in reperfusion with few if any complications.

REFERENCES

1. Alpert JJ, Filler R, Glaser HH. Strangulation of an appendage by hair wrapping. N Engl J Med 1965; 273:866–867.
2. Barton DJ, Sloan GM, Nichter LS, Reinisch JF. Hair-thread tourniquet syndrome. Pediatrics 1988; 82(6):926–929.
3. Henretig R. In: Fleisher G, Ludwig S, eds. textbook of pediatric emergency medicine. 3rd ed. Baltimore: Williams & Wilkins, 1993, p. 144.
4. Gross, CM (ed.) Grey's anatomy. 28th ed. Philadelphia: Lea & Ferbiger, 1966.
5. Haddad FS. Penile strangulation by human hair— Report of three cases and review of the literature. Urol Int 1982;37:375–388.
6. Mariani PJ, Wagner DK. Topical cocaine prior to treatment of penile tourniquet syndrome. J Emerg Med 1986;4(3):205–208.
7. Summers JL, Guira AC. Hair strangulation of the external genitalia. Ohio ST Med J 1973;69:672–673.
8. Toguri AG, Light RA, Warren MW. Penile tourniquet syndrome caused by hair. So Med J 1979; 72(5):627–628.
9. Harrow BR. Strangulation of penis by a hidden thread (letter). JAMA 1967;199(2):171.
10. Press S, Schnachner I, Paul P. Clitoris tourniquet syndrome. Pediatrics 1980;66:781.
11. Kerry RL, Chapman DD. Strangulation of appendages by hair and thread. J Pediatr Surg 1973; 8(1):23–27.
12. Quinn NJ. Toe tourniquet syndrome. Pediatrics 1971;48:145.

BURN MANAGEMENT

Kathy N. Shaw and Marc H. Gorelick

INTRODUCTION

In 1985, over 400,000 children were treated in an emergency department (ED), clinic, or physician's office for burn injuries (1). Most of these burns occurred in the home and the majority were preventable. Young children less than 4 years of age have the highest incidence of injury from burns. They are most at risk for scald burns requiring hospitalization and for death in house fires. Overall, burn injuries are the third leading cause of accidental death in children (1–3). Burns also are a significant mechanism of child abuse (4–5).

Four different types of burns may occur depending on the source of injury. Thermal burns are the most common type of burn injury seen in children (1, 2). They occur as a result of scalds, contact burns, or flame injuries. Chemical burns in children usually involve ingestion or contamination with acids or alkalis found in household products. Electrical burns are usually low voltage injuries that occur in toddlers mouthing electrical cords or playing with sockets. Although rare, high voltage injuries may be seen, typically in older children or adolescents. Radiation burns in children are usually due to sunburn (6).

Most burns are minor and can be treated in an outpatient setting. In order to make decisions regarding management, the physician must be able to determine the depth or degree of the burn, the percentage of body surface area involved, whether the pattern of injury is typical of abuse, and whether deformity or loss of function may occur. Once a burn is de-

termined to be minor, trained nursing or EMS personnel can often provide local care. The care the minor burn patient receives is crucial to ultimate outcome. Many of the same principles apply to burns as those discussed under basic wound care (Chapter 110). Goals are to relieve pain, prevent infection and additional trauma, and minimize scarring and contracture. Treatment of the major burn victim should be performed by physicians trained in burn management. The initial care of the major burn victim is critical to both immediate survival and ultimate outcome (7). Expert pediatric respiratory management is often needed for major burn victims with smoke inhalation. Mortality for these children is much higher than for those children with comparable burns but no smoke inhalation (8).

ANATOMY AND PHYSIOLOGY

The skin is the largest organ in the body and has many important functions. It acts as a barrier to infection and loss of body water, a thermal regulator, a sensory organ, and an excretory organ. Of the skin's three layers (Fig. 115.1), the dermis contains the blood vessels, nerves, and epithelial appendages (e.g., hair) as well as sebaceous and sweat glands that are necessary for most of the skin's primary functions and for self-repair. The depth of the burn injury therefore determines the extent of the damage to this organ and its ability to heal (Table 115.1). Superficial or first degree burns affect only the epidermis or tough protective barrier. A mild sunburn is a typical ex-

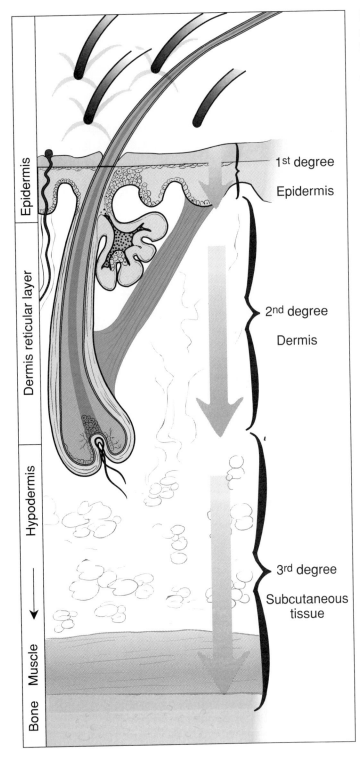

Figure 115.1.
Skin layers and
corresponding classification
of burn depths.

Chapter 115
Burn Management

burns involve the entire dermis including neurovascular structures. Fourth degree burns extend into the muscle, fascia, or bone.

Both the depth or degree of the burn and the extent of skin involvement determine the severity of the injury and affect the skin's ability to maintain its physiologic functions. First degree burns are not included in calculations of the extent of involvement unless the area exceeds 25 to 30% of the body surface area. Estimates of body surface area (BSA) involvement in babies and young children cannot be done using the "rule of 9's" because they have a proportionately larger head and smaller lower extremities (Fig. 115.2). Emergency departments should have access to tables listing BSA by body part and age of the child such as the Lund and Browder charts (9). For smaller burns, the area can be estimated by comparing the child's palm size, which is 1% of BSA, with the burned area.

INDICATIONS

Treatment of burns depends on the severity of injury, location, characteristics of the child, and mechanism of injury (Table 115.2). A first degree burn is identified by pain, erythema, and subsequent peeling, but healing occurs without scarring. A typical second degree burn is painful, red, blanches with pressure, has weeping blisters, and usually heals with minimal or no scarring. Deep second degree burns may appear white and be anesthetic but often will blanch with pressure. Third degree burns are dry, leathery, white or charred in appearance, painless, and require grafting because the dermis has been destroyed. The depth of the burn sometimes can be difficult to determine in the first few hours and may require repeated examinations.

Minor burns are usually treated in the ED or office by trained personnel including nurses and EMTs under the supervision of a physician. A minor burn is defined as a second degree burn that covers less than 10% of BSA in children under 6 years of age, and less than 15% in older children and adults, or a third degree burn covering less than 2% of the BSA. Exceptions include burns which may cause loss of function, severe deformity, or are associated with a higher risk of infection

ample. Partial thickness or second degree burns extend into the dermis. Deep second degree burns may mimic third degree burns, as most of the skin elements are destroyed. Healing is prolonged and hypertrophic scarring may occur. Full thickness or third degree

Table 115.1.
Characteristics of Burns by Degree

Degree	Symptoms/Physical Examination	Healing	Causes
First (superficial)	Pain 48–72 hr Erythema Mild edema Blanches	Epithelium may peel in 5–10 days No scarring	Ultraviolet light
Second (partial thickness)	*Superficial* Painful Bright red Weeping blisters	*Superficial* 10–14 days Minimal or no scarring	*Superficial* Short flash Brief scald
	Deep White/yellow or mottled +/− anesthetic	*Deep* 25–35 days Hypertrophic scarring Requires grafting	*Deep* Scalds Short flash
Third (full thickness)	Dry, leathery Anesthetic Pearly white → charred Thrombosed veins visible		Flame Scald Electrical

such as burns of the hands, face, eyes, ears, feet, perineum, or genitalia. In addition, burns should not be classified as minor if the child has an underlying disease which may affect the healing process, if the burn is suspected to have occurred from child abuse or neglect, if the caretaker is unable to care for the burn, or if the burn is circumferential and may require escharotomy or crosses a flexion crease indicating a more severe injury.

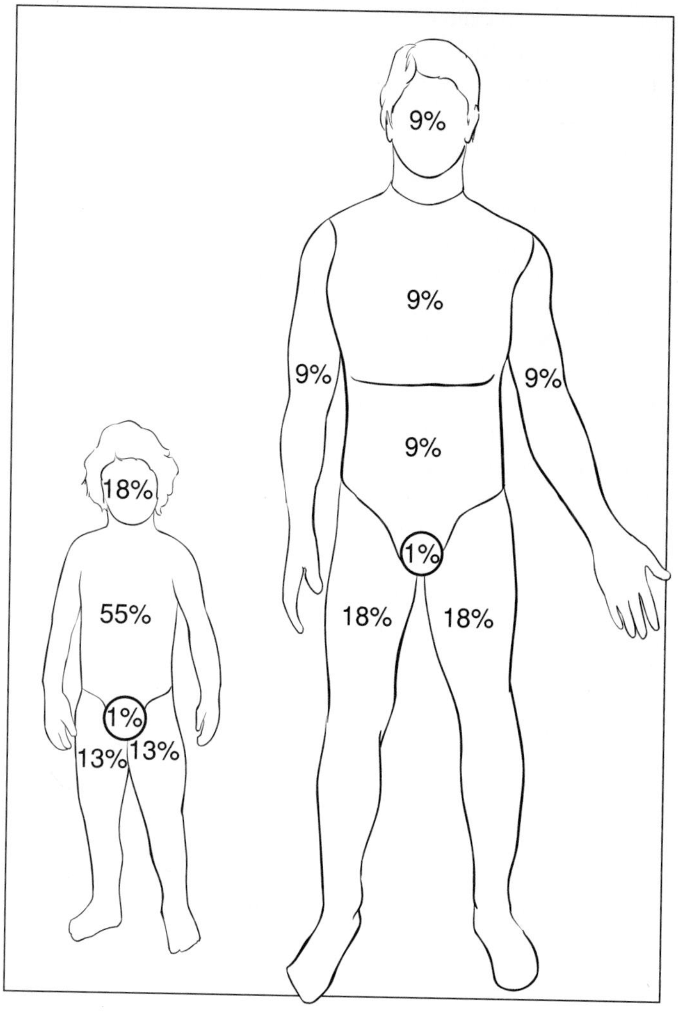

Figure 115.2.
Differences in the percent of body surface area distribution between a child and an adult.

Table 115.2.
Classification of Burns in Children

Classification	Burn		Associated Factors	Disposition
Major	2°: >20% BSA 3°: >10% BSA Circumferential Crosses flexion crease	or	Potential loss of function Increased risk of infection Severe deformity e.g., burns of hands, face, ears, nose, feet, perineum, genitalia e.g., immunosuppressed child High voltage injury Smoke inhalation	Burn center Pediatric intensive care
		or		
Moderate	2°: 10–20% 3°: 2–10%	+ or or	None of above Parental inability to care for burn Child abuse suspected	Hospitalization or close follow-up by specialist
Minor	2°: <10% BSA 3°: <2% BSA	+	None of above	Outpatient treatment

Major burns include second degree burns of greater than 20% and third degree burns of more than 10% of the BSA in children. In addition, burns associated with smoke inhalation, major trauma, or high voltage electrical burns, should be considered major burns. When concern arises about the healing process, the clinician also should consider it a major burn. These should be treated by a physician knowledgeable in burn care. General or plastic surgeons should be consulted as needed and when available, especially for procedures such as escharotomy and treatment of burns which may cause disability or disfigurement. Most major burns require the special facilities and personnel of a burn center. Transfer to a center with pediatric intensive care should be considered for children with inhalational or high voltage electrical injuries regardless of the extent of the burns. Most burns of moderate extent also require hospitalization or close follow-up by a physician knowledgeable in burn management.

EQUIPMENT

Standard resuscitation equipment—includes airway equipment, supplemental oxygen, intravenous access, and isotonic intravenous fluids such as lactated Ringer's. A cardiorespiratory monitor and pulse oximeter also should be available.

Cleaning and debridement
  Sterile saline or water
  Syringes—30 to 60 mL
  Gauze pads
  Povidone-iodine solution—one quarter strength
  Forceps
  Scissors
Dressing
  Sterile sheet (for major burns)
  Tongue depressor (to apply topical agents)
  Topical antimicrobial agent—most commonly used is 1% silver sulfadiazine (Silvadene®, Thermazine®) cream. This has the advantages of broad spectrum of activity, ease and comfort of application, and lack of absorption. Its use, however, is not recommended on the face (6). Other broad spectrum preparations such as bacitracin/polymixin B (Polysporin®) may be used for small burns, particularly those involving the face. Mafenide acetate (Sulfamylon®) is another topical antimicrobial cream which is occasionally used, but should be avoided in the outpatient setting due to the potential for serious systemic side effects (6).
  Inner dressing—generally divided into conventional and synthetic (10, 11). Conventional dressings are those made from cotton gauze. The gauze may be plain, or impregnated with a greasy material such as petrolatum to render it nonadherent; examples include Aquaphor®, Vaseline®, and Adaptic®. Xero-

form® gauze also incorporates 3% bismuth tribromophenate as an antibacterial agent.

A wide variety of synthetic materials also is available. These have been designed to render frequent dressing changes unnecessary. Some dressings commonly available in the United States include semipermeable polyurethane films such as OpSite® and Tegaderm® (adhesive) and Epi-Lock® (nonadhesive), and hydrocolloid dressings such as DuoDerm®, and composites including Biobrane® and Epigard®.

A number of investigators have failed to demonstrate clear superiority of any of the various types of dressings—all provide satisfactory results when properly used (29–36). Conventional dressings continue to be the most widely used, and have the advantages of being readily available and simple to apply. Moreover, most health care providers are familiar with their use. Synthetic dressings, by obviating the need for frequent dressing changes, may make home care easier and may minimize patient discomfort. Several studies comparing different dressings have found total costs to be similar (29, 33). Thus the choice of dressing method is largely a matter of patient and physician preference.

Outer dressing
    Cotton gauze rolls
    Stockinette or burn netting
    Tape
Miscellaneous
    Scalpel—No. 10 or 15 for escharotomy
    Splinting materials (Chapter 104)

PROCEDURE

Major Burns

Initial Resuscitation Measures

Treatment of major burns begins with appropriate prehospital care. The clinician should focus primary attention on management of the airway, breathing, and circulation. The cervical spine should be immobilized if concomitant trauma is suspected. The burn wound may initially be immersed in cool water to provide rapid return to normal temperature. Ice, however, should be avoided as ex-

cessive cold leads to potentiation of ischemic damage (12). Chemical burns should be vigorously irrigated with water. Appropriate dressings include a dry sterile sheet or saline-soaked gauze; both provide immediate pain relief and some degree of protection of the wound. Home remedies such as butter or other ointments are not indicated.

In the ED, sterile technique must be meticulously practiced from the outset in the care of patients with major burns, including masks and gowns for medical personnel (Chapters 7 and 8). Resuscitation continues, with particular attention to fluid management. Large-bore intravenous access is mandatory, preferably through unburned skin. Isotonic crystalloid, such as normal saline or lactated Ringer's, is administered in boluses of 20 mL/kg as needed to restore circulatory stability. A number of formulas for estimating fluid needs of burned children over the first 24 hours have been developed, the details of which are beyond the scope of this book (13–19). Children with electrical burns must be monitored for cardiac dysrhythmias. Importantly, such patients frequently have internal injuries more extensive than those suggested by the external appearance of the burn.

Emergent Escharotomy

A problem unique to the burn victim is compromised ventilation or regional circulation due to restrictive eschar in circumferential full thickness burns of the chest or extremities, respectively. In such cases, incisional decompression or escharotomy is performed emergently as a palliative measure (7, 20, 21). A single incision is made with a No. 10 or 15 scalpel, extending the full length of the burn, and carried down through the eschar to the layer of the subcutaneous fat; occasionally, extension down to the deep fascia is necessary. Anesthesia or analgesia is not required, as the nerve fibers have been destroyed, and bleeding is typically minimal. The preferred site of the escharotomy incision is along the lateral or medial aspect of the limb, or bilaterally in the anterior axillary line on the chest (Fig. 115.3). Extension along the costal margins also may be necessary. Following decompression, rapid improvement in chest excursion or limb perfusion should be observed. If not, the incision should be checked for adequacy of length and depth.

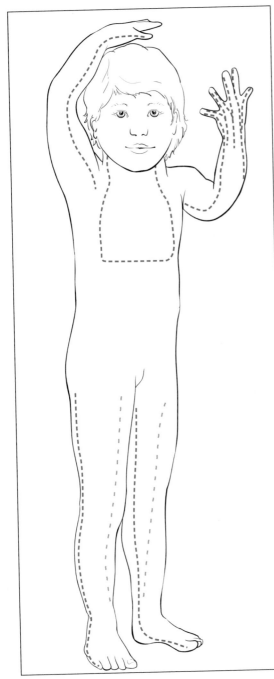

Figure 115.3.
Escharotomy incision sites in a child.

Burn Preparation

Care of the burn itself in the ED is similar to that described for the prehospital setting. Because the burned child is typically in a great deal of pain, analgesia must be provided as early as possible (22). All clothing is removed from burned areas. Adherent molten material such as tar should be cooled with water but left in place. The burns are then irrigated and protected with dry sterile sheets or saline-soaked gauze. It should be noted that prolonged use of saline-soaked gauze can cause discomfort for the patient from cooling. In addition, small infants may need to be placed under an overhead warmer to prevent hypothermia due to evaporative heat loss. Further wound care, such as debridement or application of any topical agents, should be left to the discretion of the surgeon who will assume further care of the child with major burns (23). Supportive measures in the ED include any necessary ongoing resuscitative interventions, maintenance of analgesia, and tetanus immunoprophylaxis as needed.

Minor Burns

The treatment of minor partial thickness burns is directed toward providing an optimal environment for wound healing to occur (21).

A number of approaches that meet this goal are possible. While considerable debate exists in the literature on various points of burn care, most burns can be managed successfully using one of several methods. The choice of approach in a specific case depends on a number of factors including characteristics of the burn and the patient, and physician preference.

Burn Preparation and Debridement

In all cases the wound must be prepared. Clothing should be removed from the burned area. Chemical burns are irrigated with large amounts of water or saline; a small child may be placed in a sink for this purpose. As with major burns, if adherent tar is present it should be left in place. Applying a solvent ointment such as petrolatum or Aquaphor® allows easy removal of the tar after 24 to 48 hours (7).

The process of preparing and dressing a partial thickness burn can be quite painful. Adequate pain control, which usually requires narcotics, must be provided before proceeding (Chapter 34). For larger burns, conscious sedation may be necessary (Chapter 35).

First degree burns require no debridement, and the eschar of a full thickness burn also should be left undisturbed at the initial ED encounter. Any loose, necrotic, or clearly nonviable tissue should be debrided from partial thickness burns using a forceps and scissors (Fig. 115.4.A). Topical application of an anesthetic (e.g., viscous lidocaine) over small burns may help limit pain. The toxic dose of anesthetic must not be exceeded. Overzealous debridement at the initial visit should be avoided. Great controversy exists over the management of intact blisters, but firm evidence in support of the various approaches is scarce (6, 7, 23, 25–27). Generally, blisters should be left intact in fresh (less than 24 hours old) burns. Large (greater than 5 cm) bullae, especially those crossing joints, are best opened and debrided at the time of the first dressing change, whereas small blisters are left intact. Ruptured blisters are generally unroofed, particularly if the wound appears dirty, to prevent bacterial infection beneath the open epithelium, although some evidence exists that debridement is unnecessary (27). Aspiration of blisters is to be avoided.

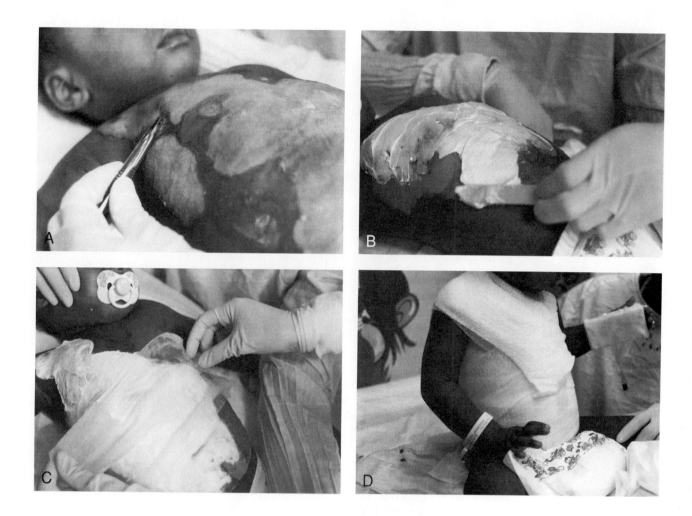

After the burn is debrided, it is gently but thoroughly cleansed with a bland soap or dilute (quarter-strength) solution of povidone-iodine, using 4 × 4 cm gauze pads. Gentle saline irrigation is followed by pat drying with sterile sponges before applying a dressing. Sterile technique must be adhered to during all stages of burn care.

Burn Dressings

The simplest method of burn treatment is the open or exposure method, in which the exposed wound itself provides a natural dressing—blister, crust, or eschar. Because of the difficulty in keeping open wounds clean in children, the open method is usually reserved for burns less than 1 cm, or burns of the face or neck, where dressing application is problematic (23). Following preparation of the burn as previously described, a topical antibacterial ointment such as bacitracin/polymixin B is applied. This ointment is more cosmetically acceptable for an undressed burn than silver sulfadiazine. The patient or parent is then instructed to clean the burn and reapply ointment one or two times a day until healed.

Most burns in children are treated with some type of closed dressing. Two basic approaches are described here. In the first approach, the clinician uses a conventional gauze-type dressing. Antibacterial cream such as silver sulfadiazine is applied to the cleansed and debrided wound to a thickness of approximately 2 to 3 mm (0.063 inch) using a sterile tongue blade, covering the entire surface (Fig. 115.4.B). The burn is then covered with a layer of gauze sponges. Alternatively, the antibiotic cream may be applied first to the gauze, or a nonadherent type of gauze dressing may be used, with or without an antibacterial agent (Fig. 115.4.C). This first layer is then wrapped in several layers of roller gauze to create a bulky, absorbent outer dressing (Fig. 115.4.D). In burns of the hand,

Figure 115.4.
Conventional burn dressing.
A. Debridement.
B. Application of topical antimicrobial agent.
C. Nonadherent inner dressing.
D. Absorbent outer dressing.

wads of gauze can be placed between the fingers and in the palm to create a protective bulky dressing. Finally, the entire dressing is covered with stockinette, elastic bandage, or burn netting to keep the child from unwrapping it. A glove or shirt can be fashioned from these materials for burns of the extremities or trunk.

Conventional dressings are usually changed once or twice daily. It should be noted that silver sulfadiazine becomes inactivated by tissue secretions and loses effectiveness after 12 hours (28). Some authorities prefer to have most patients return in 24 hours for the first dressing change. Home care consists of removing the dressing, removing all antibacterial cream, cleansing with a mild soap and water, and reapplying the dressing as previously outlined. Outpatient analgesics such as acetaminophen with codeine should be supplied for the first few dressing changes. Follow-up visits with a primary care provider at 3 and 7 days are recommended, with more frequent visits for supervised dressing changes if compliance is a problem. The parent is instructed to return if signs of infection develop.

As an alternative to conventional dressing materials, a variety of synthetic dressings are available, intended to serve as a temporary skin substitute. The burn is prepared in the manner described. The dressing material is cut to fit the burn, overlapping the adjacent healthy skin by 1 to 2 cm. The dressing is placed over the wound under moderate tension, smoothing out any wrinkles and pressing out any air or fluid from beneath. Dressings without adhesive (e.g., Biobrane®, Epi-Lock®) are secured with paper tape or adhesive strips along the margins. The inner dressing is then covered with roller gauze and stockinette as with the conventional dressings.

Synthetic dressings should be reexamined in 24 hours. If the dressing is not adhering to the skin it must be removed. If the wound has remained clean, it may be redressed in the same manner. Failure to adhere after 48 to 72 hours (two or three attempts) requires a change in management. If the synthetic dressing is adhering properly, only the outer dressing is changed. The inner dressing is kept in place until healing is complete (approximately 14 days for a partial thickness burn). The outer dressing can be changed daily at home, with less frequent changes needed as the quantity of exudate decreases. As in the case of a conventional dressing, twice weekly follow-up visits should be made with the primary care provider.

SUMMARY

Major Burns
1. Initiate necessary resuscitation measures
2. Provide adequate analgesia
3. Remove clothing
4. Perform emergent escharotomy if indicated
   A. Incise full length of burn down to subcutaneous fat
   B. Incise along lateral or medial aspect of limb, or bilaterally in anterior axillary line for chest
5. Irrigate burns with saline
6. Cover burns with sterile dry sheets or saline-soaked gauze
7. Maintain body temperature with overhead warmers as needed
8. Administer tetanus immunoprophylaxis when indicated
9. Contact burn center as necessary

Minor Burns
1. Provide adequate analgesia
2. Prepare wound
   A. Irrigate burns with saline
   B. Debride necrotic or clearly nonviable tissue using forceps and scissors
   C. Gently clean burns with mild soap or quarter-strength povidone-iodine
   D. Pat dry with sterile sponges
3. Apply wound dressing
   A. Open
      1. Apply antibiotic ointment (e.g., bacitracin/polymixin B) to face, neck, or small (less than 1 cm) extremity burns
   B. Closed
      1. Apply inner dressing
         a. Conventional
            i. Coat burn with a layer of silver sulfadiazine
            ii. Cover area with sterile gauze
         b. Synthetic
            i. Cut material to fit burn with a slight overlap of adjoining healthy skin
            ii. Apply material without wrinkles or trapped air
            iii. Secure material with tape
      2. Apply outer dressing
         a. Wrap inner dressing in several layers of roller gauze
         b. Cover dressing with a stockinette or elastic bandage
4. Splint extremities with partial or full thickness burns that extend across joints
5. Administer tetanus immunoprophylaxis when indicated

Splinting

Joints crossed by extensive partial or full thickness burns should be splinted in the position of function, using standard splinting techniques (Chapter 104). This is particularly important when synthetic dressings are used, to minimize motion and increase the chance of successful adherence. Patients with such burns should be referred to a surgeon for follow-up.

COMPLICATIONS

With the loss of the epidermal barrier, burn wounds are commonly colonized with microorganisms, which may lead to local or even systemic infection. The rate of burn wound infection is greatest in children and the elderly. Certain burns are more prone to infection: deep partial thickness and full thickness burns, burns of the lower extremities and perineum, and those involving greater than 30% of body surface area (37). When infection occurs, healing is delayed and extension of the depth of injury is possible. Preventing infection is therefore paramount, which is best accomplished by careful attention to appropriate technique. Prophylactic systemic antibiotics are not indicated (38).

The risk of hypothermia in children with extensive burns may be increased with the application of saline-soaked gauze if efforts to maintain body heat are not followed. This is especially critical in young infants who have a larger ratio of BSA to volume.

Extensive fluid and blood loss with resulting cardiovascular instability may be triggered by overaggressive early debridement of extensive burns. Debridement of major burns should be performed under controlled conditions and in consultation with specialists in burn management.

SUMMARY

The vast majority of burns can be effectively managed in the outpatient setting; however, the physician must be capable of categorizing and classifying burns to provide optimal burn care for children. Recognition of child abuse, risk factors for poor burn healing, and associated injuries are important when deciding care and disposition. The focus for minor burns is on relief of pain, prevention of infection and additional trauma, and minimization of scarring and contracture. ED care for the major burn patient may affect survival and ultimate prognosis. Knowledge of when to seek consultation and transfer to tertiary care facilities is crucial. Finally, the ED personnel should consider burn prevention counseling as an important aspect of burn care of young children.

REFERENCES

1. McLoughlin E, McGuire A. The causes, cost, and prevention of childhood burn injuries. AJDC 1990; 144:677–683.
2. Centers for Disease Control. Childhood injuries in the United States. AJDC 1990;144:627–646.
3. Malek M, Chang B. The cost of medical care for injuries to children. Ann Emerg Med 1991; 20(9):997–1005.
4. Purdue G, Hunt J, Prescott P. Child abuse by burning. An index of suspicion. J Trauma 1988; 28(2):221–224.
5. Hyden PW, Gallagher TA. Child abuse intervention in the emergency room. Pediatr Clin North Am 1992;39(5):1053–1081.
6. Schonfeld N. Outpatient management of burns in children. Pediatr Emerg Care 1990;6(3):249–253.
7. Baxter CR, Waeckerle J. Emergency treatment of burn injury. Ann Emerg Med 1988;17(12): 1305–1315.
8. Thompson PB, Herndon DN, Traber DL, Abston S. Effect on mortality of inhalation injury. J Trauma 1986;26(2):163–165.
9. Lund CC, Browder NC. The estimation of areas of burns. Surg Gynecol Obstet 1944;79:352–358.
10. Quinn KJ, Courtney JM, Evans JH, Gaylor JDS. Principles of burn dressings. Biomaterials 1985; 6:369–377.
11. Queen D, Evans JH, Gaylor JDS, Courtney JM, Reid WH. Burn wound dressings. A review. Burns 1987; 13(3):218–228.
12. Purdue GF, Layton TR, Copeland CE. Cold injury complicating burn therapy. J Trauma 1985; 25(2):167–168.
13. Finkelstein JL, Schwartz SB, Madden MR, Marano MA, Goodwin CW. Pediatric burns. An overview. Pediatr Clin North Am 1992;39(5):1145–1163.
14. Carvajal HF. A physiologic approach to fluid therapy in severely burned children. Surg Gynecol Obstet 1980;150:379–384.
15. Graves TA, Cioffi WG, McManus WF, Mason AD, Pruitt BA. Fluid resuscitation of infants and children with massive thermal injury. J Trauma 1988; 28(12):1656–1659.
16. Pruitt B. Advances in fluid therapy and the early care of the burn patient. World J Surg 1978; 2:139–150.

CLINICAL TIPS

1. Appropriate burn management depends on the depth and extent of the burns.
2. Burns in children may be a manifestation of abuse.
3. Most major burns in children require the expertise of a burn center.
4. Initial resuscitation measures should be addressed before definitive burn care.
5. Analgesia should be provided as early as possible.
6. Aspiration of blisters should be avoided.
7. A final covering of stockinette or burn netting limits the ability of the young child to remove the dressing.
8. The young burn victim is at significant risk of heat loss due to the relatively high ratio of BSA to volume.

17. O'Neill JA. Fluid resuscitation in the burned child. A reappraisal. J Pediatr Surg 1982;17(5):604–607.
18. Demling RH. Fluid replacement in burned patients. Surg Clin North Am 1987;67(1):15–30.
19. Merrell SW, Saffle JR, Sullivan JJ, Navar PD, Kravitz M, Warden GD. Fluid resuscitation in thermally injured children. Am J Surg 1986;152: 664–669.
20. Bennett JE, Lewis E. Operative decompression of constricting burns. Surgery 1958;43(6):949–955.
21. Pruitt BA, Dowling JA, Moncrief JA. Escharotomy in early burn care. Arch Surg 1968;96:502–507.
22. Osgood PF, Szyfelbein SK. Management of burn pain in children. Pediatr Clin North Am 1989; 36(4):1001–1013.
23. Griglak MJ. Thermal injury. Emerg Med Clin North Am 1992;10(2):369–383.
24. Zawacki BE. Reversal of capillary stasis and prevention of necrosis in burns. Ann Surg 1974; 180(1):98–102.
25. Forage AV. The effects of removing the epidermis from burnt skin. Lancet 1962;690–693.
26. Rockwell WB, Ehrlich HP. Should burn blister fluid be evacuated? J Burn Car Rehab 1990;11(1):93–95.
27. Andrejak M, Davion T, Gineston JL, Capron JP. Management of blisters in minor burns. Brit Med J 1987;295:181.
28. Warden GD. Outpatient care of thermal injuries. Surg Clin North Am 1987;67:147–157.
29. Stair TO, D'Orta J, Altieri MF, Lippe MS. Polyurethane and silver sulfadiazene dressings in treatment of partial thickness burns and abrasions. Am J Emerg Med 1986;4(3):214–217.
30. Afilalo M, Dankoff J, Guttman A, Lloyd J. Duoderm hydroactive dressing versus silver sulfadiazine/ bactigras in the emergency treatment of partial skin thickness burns. Burns 1992;18(4):313–316.
31. Lobe TE, Anderson GF, King DR, Boles ET. An improved method of wound management for pediatric patients. J Pediatr Surg 1980;15(6):886–889.
32. Cockington RA. Ambulatory management of burns in children. Burns 1989;15(4):271–273.
33. Gerding RL, Emerman CL, Effron D, Lukens T, Imbembo AL, Fratianne RB. Outpatient management of partial thickness burns: Biobrane® versus 1% silver sulfadiazine. Ann Emerg Med 1990; 19(2):121–124.
34. Gerding RL, Imbembo AL, Fratianne RB. Biosynthetic skin substitute versus 1% sulfadiazine for treatment of inpatient partial thickness thermal burns. J Trauma 1988;28(8):1265–1269.
35. Waffle C, Simon RR, Joslin C. Moisture-vapour-permeable film as an outpatient burn dressing. Burns 1988;14(1):66–70.
36. Wyatt D, McGowan DN, Najarian MP. Comparison of a hydrocolloid dressing and silver sulfadiazine cream in the outpatient management of second degree burns. J Trauma 1990;30(7):857–865.
37. Dodd D, Stutman HR. Current issues in burn wound infections. Advan Pediatr Infect Dis 1991; 6:137–162.
38. Boss WK, Brand DA, Acampora D, Barese S, Frazier WH. Effectiveness of prophylactic antibiotics in the outpatient treatment of burns. J Trauma 1985; 25(3):224–227.

INCISION AND DRAINAGE OF A CUTANEOUS ABSCESS

Grace M. Young

INTRODUCTION

A cutaneous abscess is a localized cavity of purulent material in the superficial skin and soft tissue. It causes a fluctuant swelling or mass, with inflammatory changes in the surrounding soft tissue. The abscess may progress to a spontaneous discharge of its contents through its external or internal surface. (1–3)

The preferred treatment for the cutaneous abscess is surgical incision and drainage (1–5). Percutaneous needle aspiration alone inadequately drains an abscess cavity and often results in persistent or recurrent abscess formation. Incision and drainage of an abscess prevents potential bacteremic dissemination or extension into important adjacent tissues (e.g., vascular structures). The procedure is simple, may be done quickly, and is usually curative for all age groups. It is commonly performed by physician and physician extenders in the emergency or outpatient setting.

Evaluation and treatment of superficial abscesses accounts for 1 to 2% of all emergency and outpatient visits (1–5). Although it is one of the most common soft tissue infections, only a few controlled studies are found on the treatment of cutaneous abscesses in adults and children.

ANATOMY AND PHYSIOLOGY

A cutaneous abscess occurs after disruption of the normal barriers of the skin which pre-vent natural bacterial colonization from becoming an infection. Localized cellulitis first develops when bacteria proliferate within the skin and subcutaneous tissues. As bacterial enzymatic activity produces necrosis, liquefaction, and a leukocytic response, pus forms and an abscess results. Cellulitis generally resolves with antibiotic therapy, whereas an abscess usually does not respond to antibiotics alone without open drainage of the pus.

Common causes for the disruption of the normal skin barriers to infection include direct trauma to, or a foreign body in, the skin or soft tissues; injection or accumulation of bacterial inoculum (e.g., injury from cat bite or rusty nail); decreased or inadequate blood or lymphatic circulation (e.g., necrosis, hemorrhage); or poor host systemic immunity (e.g., debilitating disease, immunocompromised host). Proliferation of bacteria subsequently occurs which may progress to a folliculitis or abscess. Often a keratin plug may sufficiently obstruct the normal outflow of a secretory gland and prevent the normal clearance of bacterial colonization. Areas prone to such obstruction are the axilla, groin, perineum, and breast (4). In the infant or younger child, common sites also include the perianal area from mucocutaneous infection or enterocutaneous fistula (3), and the digits from finger sucking or biting (8).

The causative organism usually reflects that of the indigenous flora of the specific site. Overall, *Staphylococcus aureus* is the predominant organism isolated from most abscesses, especially as a single isolate. Aerobic organisms indigenous to the skin and secretory gland typically cause abscesses distant from the oral or anogenital areas in the general population; they include *S. aureus,* coagulase-negative staphylococcus, and α-hemolytic and β-hemolytic streptococcus. Oral flora are found in abscesses that result from prolonged or repeated contact with the mouth, as in the fingers or toes of infants (see Chapters 117 and 118), as well as in dental abscesses (Chapter 66). Fecal flora are usually isolated from abscesses of the anogenital, vulvovaginal, inguinal, and perirectal areas. These bacteria are most commonly mixed aerobic and anaerobic organisms: *Escherichia coli,* group D streptococcus, *Neisseria gonorrhoeae, Peptostreptococcus, Enterobacter,* or *Bacteroides* species. Abscesses of the axilla are commonly caused by Gram-negative aerobic organisms, *E. coli* or *Enterobacter* species (4–6, 8).

Organisms which cause abscesses in the child have a similar distribution as that in adults except that *Haemophilus influenzae* and group B streptococcus are more commonly isolated from abscesses in children younger than 2 years (6, 8). In general, mixed aerobic and anaerobic flora predominate in the abscesses of the head and fingers in children. The organisms commonly isolated include *E. coli* and anaerobic organisms, such as *Peptostreptococcus, Bacteroides, Fusobacterium,* and *Clostridium* species, because these abscesses are typically associated with oral or perianal flora (4–6, 8).

INDICATIONS

Clinically, both cellulitis and an abscess may appear as a localized area of pain (dolor), erythema (rubor), warmth (calor), edema (tumor), or induration; the patient usually complains of localized pain and swelling without fever. Fluctuance on physical examination with or without spontaneous drainage usually indicates the presence of an abscess (2, 5). A definitive diagnosis of an abscess can be made with the successful percutaneous needle (18 gauge) aspiration of pus from the site (2).

The treatment for a cutaneous abscess is surgical incision and drainage (1–4). Optimal management of cutaneous abscesses in the emergency or outpatient setting requires the following appropriate conditions: (*a*) the inflammatory mass is an acute, superficial and localized cutaneous abscess without extension to deeper structures; (*b*) the child will be adequately cooperative when the procedure is performed under local or regional anesthesia; and (*c*) the child has no other apparent medical condition that precludes outpatient management, such as airway or anatomical anomalies. If these conditions are not met, or if the depth, extent, or cosmetic implications of the abscess are questionable, a pediatric surgical consultation and treatment under general anesthesia may be more appropriate.

Cellulitis without abscess and other causes for inflammatory masses are contraindications to incision and drainage. Congenital remnants of embryonic structures in the neck often present in the younger child as persistent or recurrent anterior neck masses. Congenital neck masses which often become infected include branchial cleft cyst, thyroglossal duct cyst, or cystic hygroma. Tinea capitis infrequently produces an inflammatory response called a kerion which presents as a tender, boggy, erythematous scalp mass. Tuberculous cervical adenitis (scrofula) and mycotic aneurysm occur rarely in the child. Other causes include viral (herpetic whitlow or zoster), chemical (insect or arachnid toxins), or idiopathic inflammation (autoimmune disorders). These masses should not be incised in the outpatient setting without further diagnostic evaluation.

Chronic or recurrent abscesses with fibrotic walls are difficult to drain adequately in the outpatient setting and may require intraoperative excision under general anesthesia. Further, abscesses within the central triangle of the face, which may drain into the cavernous sinus, have high potential for morbidity and require surgical consultation.

EQUIPMENT

For sterile preparation and dressing of abscess cavity:
    Antiseptic solution (povidone-iodine)
    Gauze (4 × 4)
    Sterile drapes
    Gauze packing strips (plain, iodoform)
    Cloth tape
For local or regional anesthesia:
    Lidocaine 1% without epinephrine

Needle—27 or 25 gauge, 1″
Syringe, 3 or 5 mL
For incision of abscess cavity, probing the
cavity, clearing loculations, grasping skin
edges, and manipulating gauze packing
strip and dressing:
Scalpel blades—No. 11 for small stab inci-
sion; No. 15 for larger cutaneous inci-
sion or elliptical excision
Hemostat clamps, small
Forceps, toothed
Scissors
For irrigation of abscess cavity:
Syringe—20 mL with 18-gauge intra-
venous catheter
Irrigation solution (normal saline, sterile
water, or hydrogen peroxide)
Monitoring equipment if parenteral sedation
is used

PROCEDURE

To increase the success of adequate drainage,
direct visualization and access to the abscess
site must be optimized by careful positioning
and selective immobilization. An assistant
may be helpful with patient restraint. The site
is cleansed with antiseptic solution and
draped using sterile technique (Chapter 7).
The surrounding noninfected skin and subcutaneous tissue is first anesthetized using 1%
lidocaine without epinephrine by local infiltration (Fig. 116.1) or regional block (Chapter 37). The roof of the abscess is then anesthetized by intradermal injection along the
linear course of the proposed incision (Fig.
116.2). For the larger abscess or one in a
more difficult location, the child may benefit
from parenteral sedation and analgesia. Nitrous oxide is often an excellent choice in this
situation (Chapter 36). Unfortunately, pain
often is unavoidable despite adequate anesthesia, especially during the spreading and
breaking of loculations. For most children,
pain diminishes with the drainage of pus and
relief of pressure from the abscess. Using
ethyl chloride alone is usually ineffective for
this procedure (2).

Organisms for culture and identification
should be obtained by percutaneous needle
aspiration from the abscess after sterile
preparation (2). Pus obtained from an open
incision may preclude the isolation of anaerobic bacteria. Gram stain of the pus may be
helpful in the choice of antibiotics if pre-

scribed. Routine Gram stain and culture are
generally not indicated in the uncomplicated
cutaneous abscess.

The abscess cavity is incised with the
scalpel blade; a linear incision parallel to the
skin folds (Fig. 116.2) minimizes subsequent
scarring. The incision should extend the entire length of the cavity to permit optimal
drainage. For a smaller (less than 1 cm) abscess, the No. 11 scalpel blade is used to
make a stab opening at the point of maximal

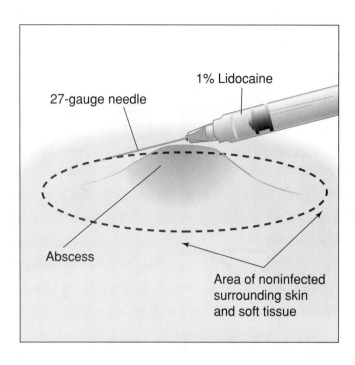

Figure 116.1.
Administration of local
anesthesia to a
subcutaneous abscess.

Figure 116.2.
Anesthetic administration
along proposed incision
site.

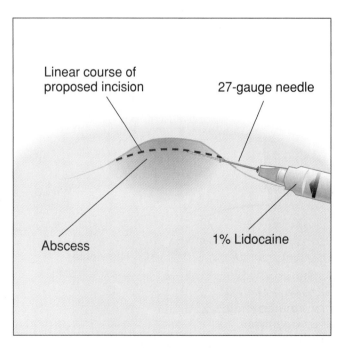

Figure 116.3.
Linear incision of a
cutaneous abscess.

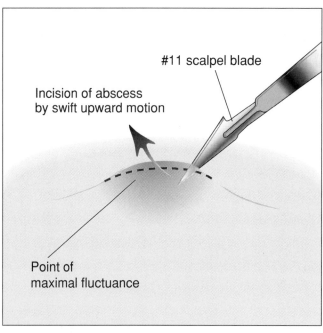

After the abscess is incised, the cavity is probed; any loculations of pus and necrotic debris are cleared by blunt spreading with a hemostat clamp (Fig. 116.5), or with the clinician's fingers if the size of the cavity permits. Copious irrigation of the abscess follows with normal saline, sterile water, or peroxide solution to remove all the pus and necrotic tissue (Fig. 116.5). Retained blood, plasma, and cellular debris sustain continued infection and should be continuously drained after this initial procedure. Many superficial abscesses empty completely after incision and irrigation, and have no remaining cavity. These require warm soaks to keep the incision open until healing commences. If a cavity remains, it is filled loosely with a gauze packing strip to ensure continued drainage of blood and coagulum (Fig. 116.6). A 1 cm end is left external to the wound edges to act as a wick and aid subsequent removal of the packing strip. The choice of packing material, plain or iodine-laden (iodoform) gauze, is not based on scientific evidence but rather on the mechanical process of a wick. Layers of dry gauze and tape complete the external wound dressing.

fluctuance, followed by one swift upward motion of the blade to complete the incision (Fig. 116.3). For a larger (more than 1 cm) abscess, the No. 15 scalpel blade is preferred to make an elliptical excision (Fig. 116.4) of the thin, nonviable or necrotic overlying skin and to facilitate drainage. An opening sufficiently wide to allow complete drainage of pus is crucial to the successful treatment of the abscess cavity.

Using antibiotics is controversial. Host defense and the depth and extent of the abscess determine the use of adjunctive antibiotic therapy. Although a cutaneous abscess usually resolves with open surgical drainage, transient bacteremia does accompany the incision and drainage procedure (6, 8). Oral antibiotics may be effective for those with surrounding areas of mild cellulitis or lymphangitis. Parenteral antibiotic therapy is warranted for the abscess that is associated with sys-

Figure 116.4.
Elliptical incision of a
cutaneous abscess.

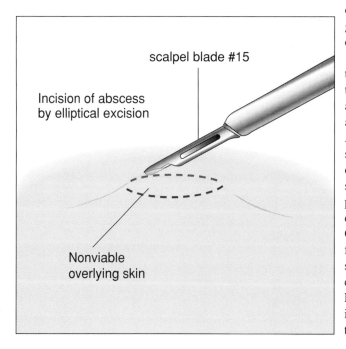

temic symptoms and signs of toxicity; that involves deeper tissue structures (tenosynovitis, fascitis, pyomyositis); or that occurs in the person predisposed to infection (immunocompromised, insulin-dependent diabetes, autoimmune disease, immunosuppressed by high dose steroid therapy or chemotherapy) (1, 4, 5).

The choice of antibiotics varies with the site of the abscess and the identification of the bacterial organism. Broad spectrum antibiotics may be administered empirically for typical organisms while awaiting culture results. For outpatient therapy, a 5- to 10-day course of cephalexin, erythromycin, or amoxicillin-clavulinic acid is effective, because penicillin resistance is common (6). However, the presence of a low pH, inactivating enzymes, and a fibrotic capsule in the abscess may render the penicillins and cephalosporins ineffective (8). Alternatively, clindamycin, metronidazole, or cefoxitin are effective parenteral antibiotics with better penetration of the abscess cavity and excellent coverage of anaerobic bacteria (2, 4, 8).

The gauze packing strip is removed within 24 to 48 hours and the wound irrigated. If the cavity continues to drain pus or necrotic debris, it should be repacked and rechecked in the next 24 hours. For abscesses in facial or other cosmetic areas, earlier removal of packing and reevaluation of the wound is best. After the packing is removed, warm soaks for 15 to 20 minutes several times daily for the next 4 to 5 days should be sufficient to maintain open wound edges and allow for continued drainage. Healing usually occurs in 7 to 10 days, with or without antibiotics (2). An inade-

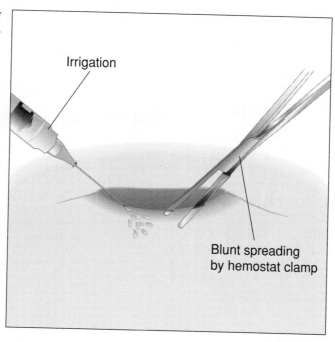

Irrigation

Blunt spreading by hemostat clamp

Figure 116.5.
Removal of loculations and irrigation of an abscess.

quate tetanus immune status requires appropriate immunization (see Table 110.2). Finally, close follow-up care ensures optimal management and decreases complications after incision and drainage of an abscess.

COMPLICATIONS

Few complications arise from this procedure and those that do occur are most commonly from inadequate drainage. Misdiagnosis oc-

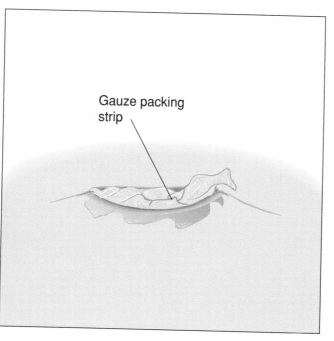

Gauze packing strip

Summary
1. Optimize approach to and visualization of abscess site
2. Anesthetize around abscess site and along proposed incision course by intradermal infiltration with 1% lidocaine without epinephrine
3. Perform percutaneous needle aspiration for Gram stain and culture when indicated
4. Incise entire length of abscess cavity
5. Spread open abscess cavity bluntly with hemostat clamp or fingers. Clear all loculations of purulent material. Irrigate copiously and evacuate cavity completely
6. Pack remaining cavity loosely with gauze packing strip and cover with dry gauze dressing
7. Consider need for antibiotics (cephalexin, amoxicillin-clavulinate, or erythromycin)
8. Provide tetanus toxoid immunization when indicated
9. Change gauze packing strip and check wound within 24–48 hours or earlier
10. Encourage warm soaks 15 to 20 minutes several times daily after gauze packing strip is removed
11. Reevaluate frequently

Figure 116.6.
Packing the abscess cavity with a gauze packing strip.

Chapter 116
Incision and Drainage
of a Cutaneous
Abscess

curs if an inflamed mass mimics an acute abscess, or if an abscess involves vital structures. Inflamed masses that occur within the neck of a child may be infected congenital cysts as described previously. Abscesses in the cervical, axillary, or inguinal areas may be closely adjacent to neurovascular structures. These lesions may worsen after inappropriately proceeding with an incision and drainage in the outpatient setting without further diagnostic evaluation.

Other complications may arise from failure to recognize the child who may be predisposed to endocarditis or bacteremia (e.g., valvular heart disease, immunocompromise, or immunosuppression). As with any wound healing process, scar and keloid formation may follow (Chapter 110).

SUMMARY

Surgical incision and drainage of the uncomplicated cutaneous abscess generally prevents progression or bacteremic dissemination. After optimal anesthesia and analgesia, the abscess cavity is incised with a scalpel over its entire length, probed with forceps and hemostat clamp to clear all loculations, and irrigated to ensure adequate drainage. Gauze packing strips and antibiotics are used if indicated. Optimal management includes close follow-up care.

REFERENCES

1. Llera JL, Levy RC. Treatment of cutaneous abscess: a double-blind clinical study. Ann Emerg Med 1985; 14(1):15–19.

2. Halvorson GD, Halvorson JE, Iserson KV. Abscess incision and drainage in the emergency department. Part I. J Emerg Med 1985;3(3):227–232.

3. Meislin HW. Pathogen identification of abscesses and cellulitis. Ann Emerg Med 1986;15(3):329–332.

4. Meislin HW, Lerner SA, Graves MH, et al. Cutaneous abscesses: Anaerobic and aerobic bacteriology and outpatient management. Ann Intern Med 1977; 87(2):145–149.

5. Llera JL, Levy RC, Staneck JL. Cutaneous abscesses: natural history and management in an outpatient facility. J Emerg Med 1984;1(6):489–493.

6. Brook I, Finegold SM. Aerobic and anaerobic bacteriology of cutaneous abscesses in children. Pediatrics 1981;67(6):891–895.

7. Fine BC, Sheckman PR, Bartlett JC. Incision and drainage of soft tissue abscesses and bacteremia [letter]. Ann Intern Med 1985;103(4):645.

8. Brook I, Frazier EH. Aerobic and anaerobic bacteriology of wounds and cutaneous abscesses. Arch Surg 1990;125(11):1445–1451.

Chapter 116
Incision and Drainage
of a Cutaneous
Abscess

INCISION AND DRAINAGE OF A PARONYCHIA

Fred M. Henretig

INTRODUCTION

A paronychia is an infection of the soft tissue structure in the space surrounding the nails. It occurs commonly in all age groups, and is located on the fingers and occasionally on the toes. When a paronychia evolves to a closed pocket of pus, proper treatment involves adequate drainage. Several techniques are commonly recommended for treating the varying stages of this process. Recent overviews of paronychia have appeared (1–4), though no controlled studies comparing various treatment approaches are found. Management of the common acute paronychia in children of any age should be well within the repertoire of emergency physicians and pediatricians, and is typically performed in the ambulatory setting.

ANATOMY AND PHYSIOLOGY

The structure of the nail complex is illustrated in Figure 117.1.A. When the seal between the proximal nail fold and the nail plate is disrupted, bacteria gain entry and infection ensues (Fig. 117.1.B). The bacterial etiology of both pediatric and adult paronychias have been studied, and reflect both skin (staphylococcal and streptococcal species) and typical oral flora. Most infections are mixed and more than 70% include oral anaerobes (6, 7). In children, typical insults during infancy include tight-fitting sleeper outfits causing toe

paronychias and overzealous nail trimming causing involvement of both fingers and toes, as well as digital sucking and nail-biting in toddlers, preschool, and school-age children. Hangnails and minor trauma related to work account for many acute paronychias in adolescents and adults.

As infection evolves, pus may accumulate under the eponychium (cuticle) and under the nail fold along the sides of the nail plate (Fig. 117.2). With further extension, pus may dissect under the nail plate, potentially compromising the ventral floor of the germinal matrix which is primarily responsible for nail growth (5). Ultimately, the infection may spread to contiguous structures causing osteomyelitis, tenosynovitis, or pyarthrosis (4). Adequate drainage of enclosed purulence will relieve pain, hasten resolution, and usually obviate such complications.

INDICATIONS

A paronychia may begin as cellulitis with redness, swelling, and tenderness along the edge of the nail, without frank pus accumulation. At this stage treatment may be nonsurgical, utilizing warm soaks, elevation, splinting, and appropriate antibiotics (cephalosporin or amoxicillin-clavulinate). Any appearance of frank pus or fluctuance warrants a drainage procedure, and little is lost by erring on the side of early drainage in uncer-

Figure 117.1.
A. Structure of the nail.
B. Course of bacterial infection.

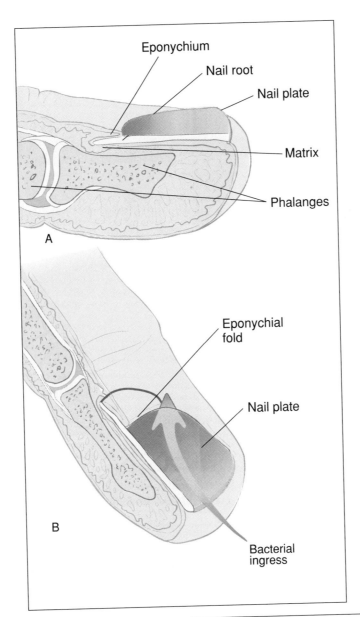

Eponychium

Nail root

Nail plate

Matrix

Phalanges

A

Eponychial fold

Nail plate

B

Bacterial ingress

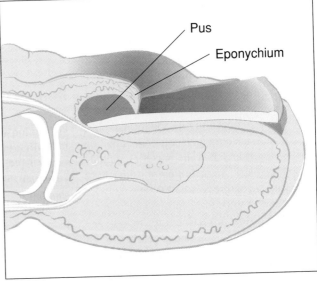

Pus

Eponychium

Chapter 117
Incision and Drainage
of a Paronychia

Figure 117.2.
Pus accumulation under the eponychium.

tain cases. For small pockets of pus at the base of the nail (the most common pediatric situation), simple lifting of the eponychium off the base of the nail is sufficient. When pus accumulates below the base or side of the nail plate, additional drainage is afforded by removing of proximal or lateral strips of nail, respectively. It is not necessary or desirable to incise periungual skin as part of the initial approach to acute paronychias. By contrast, failure of a paronychia to resolve appropriately after treatment or chronic-recurrent paronychia usually necessitates referral to a hand specialist for consideration of more aggressive surgery (e.g., eponychial marsupialization and nail plate removal) (5).

EQUIPMENT

Ethyl chloride spray
Lidocaine 1 to 2% *without epinephrine*
Syringe and needle—25 to 27 gauge
Antiseptic prep solution (e.g., Betadine)
Scalpel blade—No. 11
Small hemostat or clamp
Gauze strip packing
Scissors, small
Gauze pads

PROCEDURE

For most patients who require only the lifting of a small area of eponychium, anesthesia beyond patient distraction and possibly ethyl chloride spray is usually unnecessary. Children who require extensive drainage and/or nail plate incision will need digital block anesthesia (Chapter 37). Brief soaking of the digit may soften the eponychium and facilitate the procedure. After superficial disinfectant is applied, and anesthesia as appropriate is undertaken, the child should be restrained momentarily as appropriate for age (Chapter 3). A No. 11 scalpel blade or the tip of a small hemostat is introduced under the eponychial fold, parallel to the surface of the nail plate, and extended into the depth of the enclosed pocket of pus (Fig. 117.3.A). Since the overlying tissue involved is usually thin and devitalized, this can often be done with one quick pass of the scalpel blade or hemostat, causing a minimal amount of pain. For larger parony-

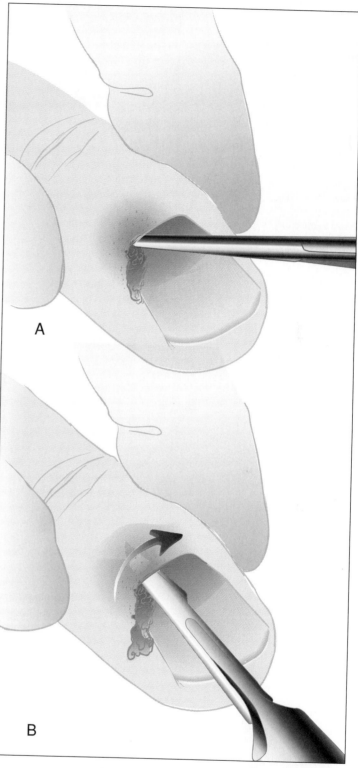

Figure 117.3.
Drainage of the paronychia.

chias involving most of the nail base, the blade or hemostat tips may be fanned through the range of the pocket (Fig. 117.3.B). When pus is encountered below the lateral edge of the nail, the nail fold skin should be gently

Figure 117.4.
Involvement below the
lateral nail edge and
removal of the lateral nail.

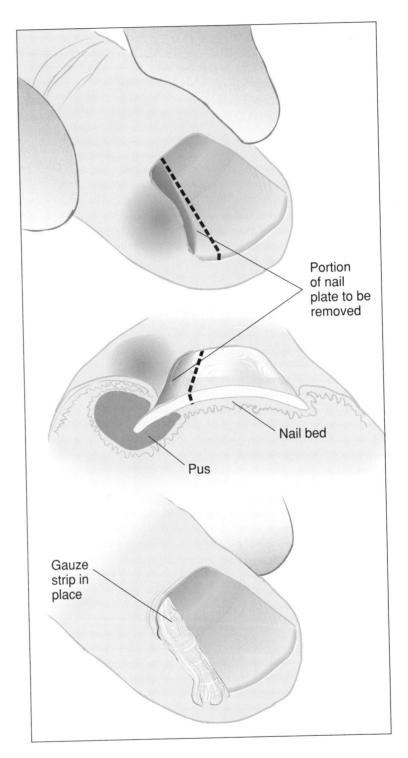

Portion
of nail
plate to be
removed

Nail bed

Pus

Gauze
strip in
place

SUMMARY
1. Restrain child when
   necessary
2. Prepare antiseptic
   field
3. Apply ethyl chlo-
   ride/digital block
   anesthesia
4. For proximal, superfi-
   cial involvement; lift
   eponychium and use
   packing as needed.
   Minimal anesthesia
   may be necessary in
   this setting
5. For subungual puru-
   lence; lift epony-
   chium and remove
   part of nail-plate
6. Cover site with outer,
   bulky gauze dressing
7. Consider local and/or
   oral antibiotics
8. Encourage warm
   soaks (when packing
   removed)
9. Follow-up in 24 to 48
   hours for more com-
   plex procedures to
   evaluate site and re-
   move packing, and/or
   5 to 7 days for resolution
10. Refer to subspecialist
    for persistence be-
    yond 10 days or con-
    tinued recurrence

lifted, and a thin longitudinal strip of nail is incised and removed (Fig. 117.4). If the pus has dissected below the proximal base of the nail, then the proximal one-third of the nail is removed in a strip perpendicular to the long axis of the nail. A small superficial incision in the eponychium in the longitudinal plane at the corner of the nail may facilitate lifting the nail plate (Fig. 117.5).

When the nail plate is so incised, or if a deep pocket remains after simple lifting of a large proximal paronychia, a small strip of gauze packing should be left in place to ensure continued drainage. The wound should

**Chapter 117
Incision and Drainage
of a Paronychia**

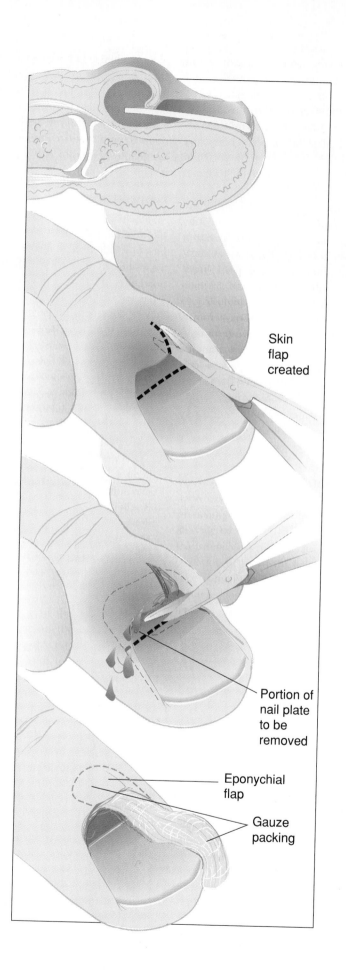

Skin flap created

Portion of nail plate to be removed

Eponychial flap

Gauze packing

Chapter 117
Incision and Drainage
of a Paronychia

1209

then be dressed with sterile, dry gauze. Warm soaks also will promote drainage, and should be initiated the same day if no packing is used, or after the packing is removed, typically in 24 hours after simple eponychia elevation, or at 48 hours when both eponychial lifting and partial nail plate removal have been used. Some authorities prefer to begin warm soaks the same day regardless of whether packing is used. Local antibiotic ointments are unproven in efficacy, but may facilitate compliance with soaks. Systemic antibiotics are likewise of uncertain additional benefit, but often are prescribed. Amoxicillin-clavulinate for 5 to 7 days would be a logical choice given the typical mixed flora (6). Follow-up evaluation generally is warranted at 24 to 48 hours for any paronychia treatment with an extended drainage procedure and/or packing. Most patients will have resolution in 5 to 7 days; persistence beyond 10 days or continued recurrence should prompt consideration of evaluation for osteomyelitis and subspecialty referral.

Complications

Complications of the recommended procedures are few. Removal of the proximal nail plate may potentially damage the germinal matrix, and thus should be done gently. The nail plate will lift easily if significant subungual pus is present. Previously recommended approaches that involved extensive incision of periungual skin have been associated with chronic scarring and nail deformity (1). Complications related to contiguous spread of infection generally are related to delayed or inadequate drainage, but may rarely develop despite appropriate treatment; hence the need for good follow-up.

Conclusion

Paronychia is the most common hand infection in children. Management usually can be accomplished entirely within the ambulatory setting by emergency physicians or pediatricians familiar with the procedure. The mainstay of treatment is the timely provision of adequate drainage and close attention to follow-up.

REFERENCES

1. Canales FL, Newmeyer WL 3d, Kilgore ES Jr. The treatment of felons and paronychias. Hand Clin 1989; 5:515.
2. Silverman RA. Diseases of the nail in infants and children. Adv Dermatol 1990;5:153.
3. Hausman L. Hand infections. Orthop Clin North Am 1992;23:171.
4. Mack GR. Common problems of the hand. Adv Dermatol 1992;7:315.
5. Bednar MS, Lane LB. Eponychial marsupialization and nail removal for surgical treatment of chronic paronychia. J Hand Surg 1991;16A:314.
6. Brook I. Bacteriologic study of paronychia in children. Am J Surg 1981;141:703.
7. Brook I. Aerobic and anaerobic microbiology of paronychia. Ann Emerg Med 1990;19:991.

INCISION AND DRAINAGE OF A FELON

Courtney A. Bethel

INTRODUCTION

A felon is an infection of the distal fat pad of the digit. Unlike a paronychia, a felon is a deep soft tissue infection involving the distal pulp of a finger or thumb that may not communicate with skin until late in the course. Incision and drainage are often required to prevent the spread of infection to bone and to relieve pain. Several techniques have been advocated, all of which involve surgical drainage with as little interruption of vascular, neurologic, and structural components as possible. No technique has been definitively shown to be best.

A felon may occur in any age group. The emergency or primary care physician with experience in minor surgical procedures may perform the procedure on the cooperative patient with regional anesthesia alone. For uncooperative patients, conscious sedation may be necessary (see Chapter 35).

ANATOMY AND PHYSIOLOGY

The distal finger consists of a relatively closed compartment bounded by the nail and skin on the dorsal and distal aspects, by skin on the palmar surface, and by the flexion crease of the distal interphalangeal joint proximally (Fig. 118.1). The fingertip is composed of tough, fibrous tissue which is anchored to the periosteum by strands of tissue called septae. These septae are most dense at the flexor crease, fingertip, and on each side at the dorsal-palmar junction. The septae are least dense at the center of the touch pad. The flexor digitorum profundus tendon inserts at the proximal one-third to middle of the distal phalanx. Blood is supplied by digital arteries which lie parallel and lateral to the phalanx. The digital nerves lie palmar and superficial to the arteries. Both arteries and nerves begin to arborize just beyond the distal phalangeal epiphysis.

A felon may arise from a minor puncture wound, splinter, or fissure and can go unnoticed by the patient until the severe throbbing pain and localized swelling begin. Cases have also been reported of iatrogenic felon formation as the result of repeated fingersticks (1). Young children and diabetic patients, who commonly undergo finger sticks to obtain blood, are therefore at increased risk for developing a felon.

Infection in this closed compartment may progress in several ways. Inflammation and edema cause increased pressure and a compartment syndrome develops. As pressure rises, the arteries collapse and tissue necrosis including the periosteum and cancellous bone (osteitis) may ensue (2). The epiphysis is spared as its blood supply is outside the closed space, which allows regeneration of eroded bone in children. The extent of regeneration depends on the virulence of the organism and patient age (2). Conversely, the fibrous septae, being least dense in the central area of the fingerpad, may allow abscess ex-

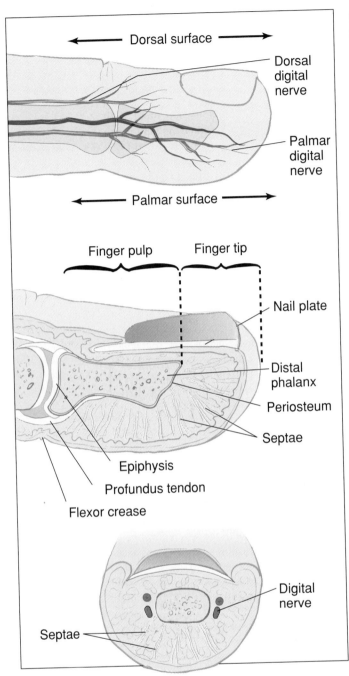

Figure 118.1.
Anatomy of the fingertip.

suckers. Complications of an untreated felon include tenosynovitis, flexion contracture, septic arthritis, and osteomyelitis (3).

INDICATIONS

Felons are characterized by intense throbbing pain made worse by dependent position, and localized distal pulp swelling with erythema. Differential diagnosis includes herpetic whitlow (distinguished by the presence of vesicles and a history of recurrence), osseous metastasis, and superficial abscess extension from a paronychia.

Early in the infection, before frank pus formation, the need for incision and drainage may be obviated with immobilization, strict elevation, and broad spectrum antibiotics (4, 5). The patient with a tense fingertip should be surgically decompressed even when no frank pus drainage or fluctuance is present, as ischemic necrosis may precede skin necrosis and pus drainage (5, 6). Once pus and abscess formation have occurred, treatment of this deep space infection involves early incision and drainage, appropriate antibiotic therapy, elevation and immobilization, and close follow-up. Incisions that injure the digital nerves or uninvolved tissue must be avoided. These include the fishmouth and through-and-through techniques (3, 7).

Significant lymphangitis, tenosynovitis, or suspicion of osteomyelitis should prompt hand surgery referral for admission and intravenous antibiotic therapy with operative incision and drainage.

EQUIPMENT

Sterile gloves
Digital tourniquet—sterile penrose drain with hemostat
Scalpel blade—No. 11
Fine hemostat
Iodophor gauze or sterile umbilical tape—0.25 inch
Syringe—20 mL with sterile saline for irrigation
Bandage material—adaptic, gauze fluffs, kerlix
Digital splint—plaster or preformed
Sling
Catheter—18-gauge, intravenous

tension to overlying skin. In this case a draining sinus may result. Rarely, the abscess located deep in the pulp may dissect around the side of the phalanx and cause an associated paronychia.

Although the bacteriology in children has not been extensively studied, the primary pathogens consist of skin flora, especially Staphylococcus aureus. Oral flora also are common in children who are finger and thumb

PROCEDURE

A comfortable, well-lit area with an assistant and fine sterile instruments are required for the procedure. Adolescent and teenage patients may cooperate with metacarpal or digital nerve block placement (Chapter 37) using lidocaine or bupivacaine. Conscious sedation and age-appropriate restraint are recommended for younger children (Chapters 3 and 35). The digit may be secured to a sterile tongue depressor at the level of the middle phalanx and again more proximally on the hand to minimize movement of the tip (Fig. 118.2). The involved digit, after the nerve block, is sterilely prepared and draped. A bloodless field is achieved with a digital tourniquet such as a penrose drain clamped at the base of the finger, or simple manual pressure along the radial and ulnar digital arteries. The tourniquet should be released briefly every 20 to 30 minutes to avoid prolonged ischemia of the finger.

The incision is made in the area of greatest tenderness or closest to the region where the abscess is "pointing," which may be identified with a blunt probe. A felon with maximal tenderness at the center of the terminal pulp is incised longitudinally using a No. 11 scalpel blade (Fig. 118.3). The incision does not cross the distal interphalangeal joint flexor crease. Any loculations are gently disrupted using a small hemostat. A small amount of pus may be expressed. Dissecting proximally may extend the process to the tendon sheath of the flexor digitorum profundus and should be avoided. The wound is irrigated with saline through an 18-gauge intravenous catheter. A sterile gauze wick (plain or antibiotic impregnated umbilical tape or 0.25 inch iodophor gauze) is loosely placed in the depth of the wound. The digital tourniquet is removed and a sterile gauze bulky dressing and sling for elevation are applied.

A felon with maximal fluctuance located on the radial or ulnar aspect of the distal pulp is incised along the lateral surface using a No. 11 scalpel blade with the bevel facing distally (Fig. 118.3.A). The incision is made midway between the fingertip and the distal flexor crease and just below the nail. The scalpel blade is advanced into the pulp space, where pus is most likely to be found. The incision may be carried in a J-shaped fashion along the involved side of the digit. In general, the length will be approximately 0.5 to 1.0 cm. Using a small hemostat, the loculations are gently disrupted to adequately drain all pus (Fig. 118.3.B). The wound is then irrigated with sterile saline. An antibiotic impregnated gauze wick is fashioned and inserted into the incision with the hemostat (Fig. 118.3.C), and the tourniquet removed. A sterile, nonstick gauze bulky dressing is applied, with a sling for elevation.

Follow-up evaluation in 24 to 48 hours for wick removal and inspection is mandatory. Strict elevation, splinting, systemic antibiotics, and warm soaks beginning the following day will speed healing and reduce discomfort. Antistaphylococcal antibiotics are recommended (3–5, 8, 9). Prolonged healing or persistent drainage and/or pain necessitate hand surgery consultation.

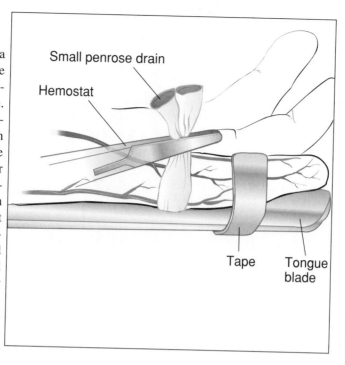

Figure 118.2.
Immobilization and hemostasis of the finger.

Labels: Small penrose drain; Hemostat; Tape; Tongue blade

SUMMARY
1. Immobilize involved digit
2. Administer conscious sedation as needed
3. Perform digital or metacarpal nerve block of affected digit
4. Sterilely prepare and drape digit
5. Apply tourniquet to provide hemostasis
6. Incise area of maximal tenderness with No. 11 scalpel blade
   A. Use longitudinal incision of anterior surface if fluctuance is located at center of terminal pulp
   B. Use lateral incision in a plane parallel to fingernail when fluctuance is along radial or ulnar aspect of distal pulp
7. Disrupt loculations at base of abscess gently with small hemostat
8. Irrigate wound with sterile saline through 18-gauge intravenous catheter
9. Place loose gauze wick in wound
10. Remove tourniquet
11. Apply nonstick dressing, splint, and sling

Chapter 118
Incision and Drainage
of a Felon

Figure 118.3.
A. J-shaped lateral incision of a felon.
B. Disruption of loculations within a felon.
C. Wick placement.
D. Longitudinal incision on the palmar surface of the distal finger.

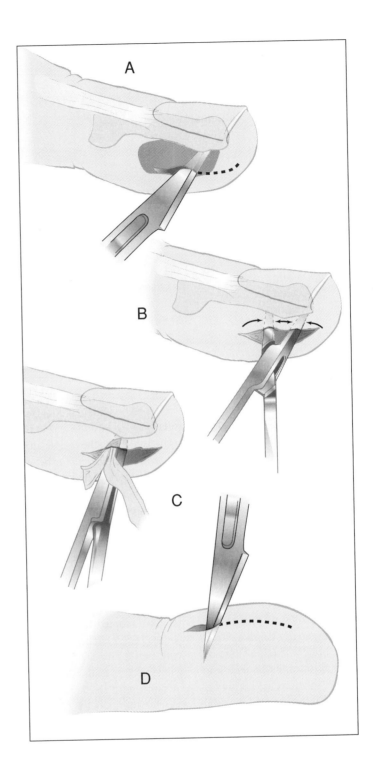

CLINICAL TIPS
1. A tense fingertip or pointing abscess requires incision and drainage.
2. Excessive disruption of septae as caused by a fishmouth incision may result in an unstable touch pad.
3. Lateral incisions should be made on one side only and just below the fingernail and phalanx to avoid injury to the digital nerves.
4. Incision type and location are determined by the point of maximum fluctuance.

COMPLICATIONS

Flexor tenosynovitis may arise as a direct result of felon formation but more commonly from iatrogenic injury to the tendon or sheath. An unstable touch pad may result from complete disruption of the septae as oc- curs in the fishmouth incision, which extends from the ulnar to radial side of the digit pass- ing through the fingertip. For this reason, many authorities recommend avoiding this approach. A painful scar occurs when the dig- ital nerve is injured. This may be prevented by making the incision just beneath the nail and dissecting carefully along the periosteum of the tuft. Anesthesia of the tip has occurred with damage to both digital nerves as a result of through-and-through incisions. To minimize the risk of iatrogenic complications, care is taken to review the relevant anatomy, use sterile technique and appropriate antibiotic coverage, and provide close follow-up with prompt referral for complications.

SUMMARY

Felons usually require incision and drainage with antistaphylococcal antibiotic coverage. The incision should be located at the point of maximal fluctuance and should allow adequate drainage while avoiding injury to vascular, neurologic, and structural components of the finger. Close follow-up is essential. Hand surgery referral should be sought for any complications of a felon or the incision and drainage procedure.

REFERENCES

1. Perry A, Gottlieb L, Zachary L. Fingerstick felons. Ann Plastic Surg 1988; 20:249–251.
2. Flatt AE. Infections. The care of minor hand injuries. 3rd ed. St. Louis: CV Mosby, 1972; pp. 247–250.
3. Leddy JP. Infections of the upper extremity. In: Bora FW, ed. Pediatric upper extremity diagnosis and management. Philadelphia: WB Saunders, 1986, pp. 362–363,
4. Kilgore ES, Brown LG, Newmeyer WL, Graham WP, Davis TS. Treatment of felons. Am J Surg 1975; 130: 194–198.
5. Bolton H, Fowler P, Jepson R. Natural history of pulp space infection and osteomyelitis of the distal phalanx. J Bone Joint Surg 1949; 31B:499–504.
6. Carter PR. Common hand injuries and infections: a practical approach to early treatment. Philadelphia: WB Saunders, 1983; pp. 216–219.
7. Lewis RC. Infections of the hand. Emerg Med Clin North Am 1985; pp. 3(2):263–275,
8. Canales FL, Newmeyer WL, Kilgor ES. Treatment of felons and paronychias. Hand Clin 1989; 5(4):515–523.
9. Hausman L. Common bacterial Infections. Orthop Clin North Am 1992; 23(1):174–176.

CHAPTER 119

INGROWN TOENAIL REPAIR

Shari L. Platt and George L. Foltin

INTRODUCTION

Ingrown toenail is a commonly seen, yet infrequently described, ailment in the pediatric population. It occurs when the lateral edge of the nail plate penetrates the adjacent soft tissue of the nail fold, usually on the great toe. Therapy is aimed at relieving pain, treating associated infection, and preventing recurrence and the development of a chronic condition.

Predisposing factors toward the development of an ingrown toenail include a severely incurvated or hypertrophic nail, an axially rotated digit, and the wearing of tight-fitting footwear or feet pajamas. In the pediatric ED, the adolescent male is the patient most at risk (1, 2).

Ingrown toenail in the infant is rare. It is commonly due to congenital hypertrophy of the lateral nail folds of the hallux, congenital malalignment of the great toenail, or distal embedding with a normally directed nail. Conservative treatment with local care and symptomatic relief is recommended. Surgical intervention is never indicated, as these conditions usually resolve spontaneously as the infant grows (3).

Commonly thought of as a problem seen by podiatrists and surgeons, many ingrown toenails can be managed by emergency medicine and primary care practitioners in the ambulatory setting. In most cases, proper treatment and follow-up care is curative. More severe cases, however, may have recurrences.

ANATOMY AND PHYSIOLOGY

The term ingrown toenail is actually a misnomer, because it is rarely caused by growth of the nail into the groove. It is actually due, in most cases, to primary hyperplasia of the epithelium within the nail groove in response to external pressure and irritation on the toe from poorly fitting footwear. A minority of cases are additionally due to primary nail plate deformity such as a congenitally thick lateral nail margin or an increased curvature into the nail groove. This may predispose the patient to an increase in external irritation and reactive tissue hypertrophy in the nail groove region, which results in exquisite pain with erythema and edema at the nail fold. If left untreated, hyperkeratosis and purulent granulation formation develop (1, 2, 4, 5) (Fig. 119.1).

Prevention involves conscientious nail hygiene with frequent nail trimming. Toenails should be trimmed in a horizontal cut creating a squared edge, rather than a curved edge. A curved edge may result in the formation of a sharp spicule of nail remaining in the nail groove. This spicule will create a nidus for hyperkeratosis and ingrown toenail symptomatology (1).

INDICATIONS

Ingrown toenail can be categorized by severity and chronicity. These categories help to guide the clinician toward an appropriate

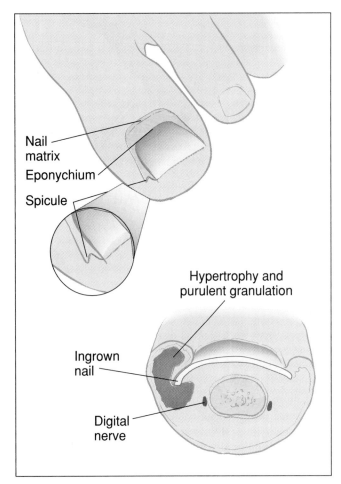

Figure 119.1.
Anatomy of ingrown toenail.

Nail matrix
Eponychium
Spicule
Hypertrophy and purulent granulation
Ingrown nail
Digital nerve

Table 119.1. Treatment Algorithm for Ingrown Toenail

Stage	Treatment
I	Conservative management
II (mild)	Angular nail resection with debridement
II (severe)	Partial nail resection
III	Partial nail resection with: a. Plastic nail tip reduction b. Germinal matrix ablation or Total nail avulsion

ment modality in the patient presenting with an ingrown toenail.

EQUIPMENT

Digital block anesthesia
1 or 2% lidocaine *without epinephrine*
Syringe with 25- or 27-gauge needle
Digital tourniquet
Betadine/antiseptic cleanser
Sterile gauze 4 × 4
Sterile cotton or petrolatum gauze
Alcohol or collodion
Scalpel blade—No. 11
Nail cutter or splitter
Hemostat, small
Antibacterial ointment
Nail file, small
Suture material for wedge resection
Silver nitrate sticks
Minicuret

PROCEDURES

Conservative

Conservative management begins with cleansing of the nail groove with an alcohol swab. An exquisitely tender and possibly infected nail edge may require digital block anesthesia (Chapter 37) before manipulation, even for the most conservative therapies. Bleeding may be minimized by applying of a digital tourniquet before any procedure. A minicuret can then be used to remove any visible debris or nail spurs. If the nail is curved to form a central peak, the central portion of

treatment modality. It should be stressed, however, that the pediatric population presenting with symptoms of an ingrown toenail are most commonly at the mildest end of the spectrum, and although a surgical method of treatment is described in detail, conservative measures are generally the more appropriate first line of therapy.

According to the staging by Heifetz, the mildest cases are classified as stage I. This stage presents as focal pain, erythema, and swelling at the lateral margin of the nail bed. Stage II progresses with worsening inflammation and may result in infection and formation of purulent granulomatous tissue. Stage III is a chronic and severe disease state. It involves the development of granulation tissue with hyperkeratosis and hypertrophy of the nail wall (5, 6). The algorithm in Table 119.1 is recommended for determining treat-the nail surface may be filed down until the nail bed matrix is visible through the thinned nail, which allows for release of the curvature pressure. The affected nail edge is then lifted out of the nail groove with a hemostat, rotating away from the nail fold (Fig. 119.2). Debris is again removed by curettage, and granulation tissue may be ablated via application of a silver nitrate stick for no longer than 1 minute. A small piece of cotton soaked in alcohol or petrolatum gauze is then firmly packed under the nail edge. The patient may replace the alcohol-soaked swab daily. Another similar approach is to pack a wisp of cotton under the nail edge, and soak it with collodion. This may remain for 3 to 6 weeks, and then should be replaced until the nail grows beyond the distal aspect of the nail fold. The patient must be instructed to follow strict foot hygiene habits consisting of warm water soaks of the affected toe, trimming of the nail transversely as it grows, and wearing loose-fitting footwear. This procedure, if followed with good patient compliance, is associated with a success rate as high as 96% in patients with stage I and mild stage II disease (1, 2, 4–8).

Angular Nail Resection with Debridement

In more severely affected stage II patients, or in mildly affected stage II patients who fail to perform the rigorous postprocedural footcare required in the conservative management, a slightly more aggressive mode of therapy may be required.

The least invasive surgical procedure is a wedge resection of the distal portion of the affected nail including removal of the nail spicule. A digital block is required for anesthesia before this procedure. A digital tourniquet may be applied proximally to minimize bleeding. The nail is cleansed and a triangular wedge of nail is excised to a point one-third to two-thirds the distance from the eponychium as shown in Fig. 119.3. The nail wedge and the nail spicule must be completely removed. The remaining nail edge should be filed down so that it may grow smoothly along the nail groove. The exposed nail matrix should be debrided and cleansed.

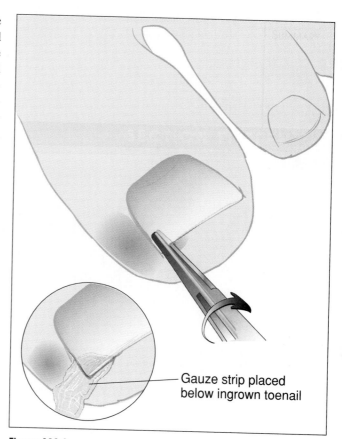

Figure 119.2.
Conservative management of ingrown toenail.

Gauze strip placed below ingrown toenail

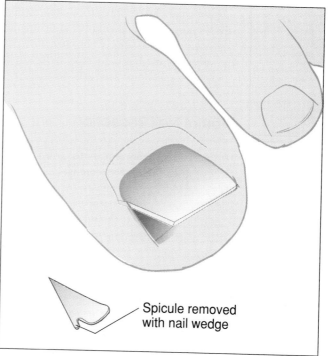

Figure 119.3.
Angular nail resection.

Spicule removed with nail wedge

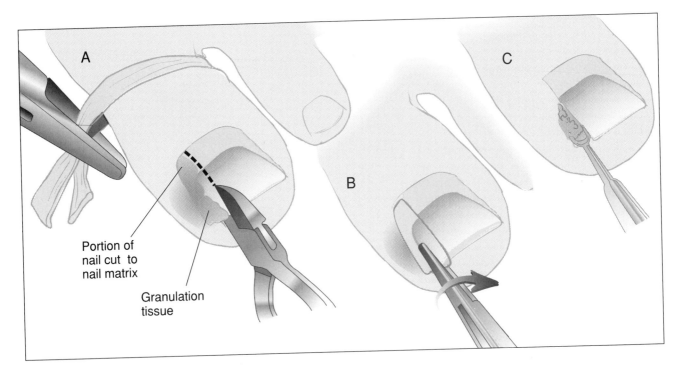

Trauma to the nail groove must be avoided, as this can lead to scarring and obliteration. All keratotic material must be removed with a sharp blade. The nailbed should be dressed with antibacterial ointment and gauze. Close follow-up within 48 hours should be arranged for a wound check. This procedure is palliative in most cases and curative in many mild stage II cases. A significant chance exists, however, for the tissue to again hypertrophy and nail ingrowth to recur (1).

Partial Nail Resection

In the patient who suffers recurrence after wedge resection, or for more advanced stage II cases with hyperkeratosis and granulation development, a more definitive surgical procedure is required. It should again be emphasized that this procedure is rarely necessary in younger children and should be performed only when indicated. A partial nail resection without nail matrix ablation is the most widely recommended treatment for the more severe case of ingrown toenail.

Following a digital block, the nail is cleansed and prepared with a bacteriostatic solution. A digital tourniquet is placed for hemostasis. The affected nail edge is cleansed and debrided, allowing for loosening of the imbedded nail edge. The nail is cut longitudinally, approximately one-third the distance from the lateral edge, using a nail cutter or splitter (Fig. 119.4.A). The incision must advance toward and continue through the eponychium, so that the entire nail portion inclusive of the nail root may be resected as shown. The resected nail is then removed using a hemostat, via a slow, steady rotating motion toward the intact nail edge to minimize damage to the nailbed (Fig. 119.4.B). The exposed nailbed is then gently debrided and cleansed to remove all the keratotic and granulation tissue (Fig. 119.4.C). Additional pressure may be applied during this procedure to ensure hemostasis (1, 5, 9).

This surgical method is often quite successful if it is followed with rigorous nail hygiene and appropriate trimming. In most cases, the nail will regrow in a normal manner leaving little or no deformity. Recurrence is common but less likely with further nail care, and usage of loose-fitting footwear. Oral antibiotics are recommended only for those patients who present with additional signs of infection, such as a purulent exudate or cellulitis, or in the immunocompromised patient. Wound follow-up is essential after 24 to 48 hours (5).

Approaches to Stage III

In recurrent cases, a partial nail resection may be followed by a plastic nail lip reduction, after resolution of the initial infection. Surgical consultation is advisable in such cases. The procedure involves a soft tissue wedge resection of a triangular segment just lateral to the affected nail groove (Fig. 119.5). Suture closure of the wedge results in drawing the nail lip and groove lateral and downward (Fig. 119.5). This reduction is usually effective in preventing the recurrence of nail ingrowth into the nail groove (4, 5).

In more severe and chronic cases of ingrown toenail, a partial nail resection procedure is performed in conjunction with nailbed and matrix ablation, using either surgical technique or phenol application. The recurrence rate is significantly reduced after the ablation; however, the risks of this procedure include nail growth deformity and significant soft tissue damage due to phenol leakage along the nail groove (1, 4, 5, 7, 9, 10). In severe cases, total nail resection has been per-

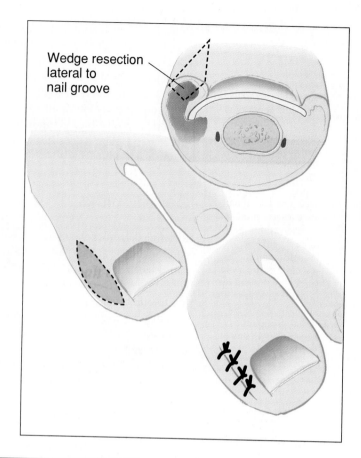

Figure 119.5.
Nail lip reduction.

SUMMARY

Conservative
1. Administer digital nerve block anesthesia
2. Clean nail groove with alcohol pad
3. File central nail peak as needed
4. Elevate nail edge from groove
5. Remove debris from nail groove with curettage and debridement
6. Apply silver nitrate to granulation tissue as needed
7. Pack cotton or gauze beneath nail edge
8. Apply bulky dressing
9. Emphasize follow-up home care
   A. Change packing as needed until nail extends beyond distal aspect of nail fold
   B. Initiate warm water soaks after 24 hours
   C. Trim nail transversely
   D. Wear loose-fitting shoes
10. Follow-up with physician for wound evaluations at 24 to 48 hours and again after 1 to 2 weeks

Angular Nail Resection
1. Administer digital nerve block anesthesia
2. Clean nail groove with alcohol pad
3. Cut triangular wedge from distal nail
4. Remove nail wedge and spicule
5. File remaining nail edge
6. Remove debris from nail groove with curettage and debridement
7. Apply antibacterial ointment
8. Apply bulky dressing

SUMMARY (CONTINUED)
9. Emphasize follow-up home care as for conservative method
10. Follow-up with physician for wound evaluations at 24 to 48 hours and again after 1 to 2 weeks

Partial Nail Resection
1. Administer digital nerve block anesthesia
2. Clean nail groove with alcohol pad
3. Place digital tourniquet for hemostasis
4. Cut the nail longitudinally through eponychium
5. Remove resected nail edge with a hemostat ensuring total nail root removal
6. Remove debris from nail groove with curettage and debridement
7. Apply antibacterial ointment
8. Apply bulky dressing
9. Consider oral antibiotics
10. Emphasize follow-up home care as previously discussed
11. Follow-up with physician for wound evaluations at 24 to 48 hours and again after 1 to 2 weeks

Plastic Lip Reduction
1. Make elliptical incision through granulation tissue lateral to affected nail groove
2. Extend incision in wedge-shaped fashion
3. Remove resulting triangular-shaped segment of tissue
4. Bring together opposing sides of wound with sutures

formed. This intervention, however, is associated with a high rate of recurrence and is not a recommended mode of treatment (1, 5). As stated, a child with stage III disease requiring any of these more aggressive surgical interventions normally should be referred for podiatric consultation and follow-up, as these procedures require a significant level of experience and skill.

COMPLICATIONS

Bleeding is frequently associated with procedures involving full or partial removal of the nail. Placement of a digital tourniquet will generally provide adequate hemostasis during the procedure. Additional applied pressure may be required once the tourniquet is removed. Infection may be a complication of the disease process itself or may result from performing the procedure. As mentioned previously, recurrence of ingrowth is often unavoidable especially in the more severe cases. Any surgical intervention or overaggressive debridement may result in abnormal or absent nail regrowth due to damage to the nail groove or matrix.

SUMMARY

Ingrown toenails are commonly seen in the ambulatory setting. The physician should be familiar with the various treatment options outlined in this chapter. Treatment must be individualized for each patient based on severity and chronicity of the condition. In children, a conservative approach is encouraged, and good foot hygiene and footwear usage must always be stressed.

REFERENCES

1. Malusky LP. Podiatric procedures. In: Roberts JR, Hedges JR, eds. Clinical procedures in emergency medicine. Philadelphia: WB Saunders, 1991, pp. 819–824.
2. Jackson JL, Linakis JG. Ankle and foot injuries. In: Barkin RM, ed. Pediatric emergency medicine concepts and clinical practice. St. Louis: CV Mosby, 1992, p. 374.
3. Rufli T, von Schulthess A, Itin P. Congenital hypertrophy of the lateral nail folds of the hallux. Dermatology. 1992;184:296–297.
4. Seibert JS, Mann RA. Dermatology and dfisorders of the toenails. In: Mann RA ed. DuVries' surgery of the foot. St. Louis, The CV Mosby, 1978, pp. 498–504.
5. Coughlin MJ. Toenail abnormalities. In: Mann RA, Coughlin MJ, ed. Surgery of the foot and ankle. St. Louis, CV Mosby, 1993, pp. 1049–1071.
6. Reijnen JAM, Goris RJA. Conservative treatment of ingrowing toenails. Br J Surg 1989;76:955.
7. Murray WR. Management of ingrowing toenail. Br J Surg 1989;76:883.
8. Ilfeld FW. Ingrown toenail treated with cotton collodion insert. Foot Ankle 1991;11:312.
9. Wee GC. Atlas of improved surgical procedures for common foot disorders. Springfield: Charles C. Thomas, 1972, pp. 5–32.
10. Leahy AL, Timon CI, Craig A, Stephens RB. Ingrowing toenail: improving treatment. Surgery 1990;107:566–567.

FISHHOOK REMOVAL

Douglas S. Diekema and Linda Quan

INTRODUCTION

Removal of a fishhook can pose a challenge to those working in the emergency department (ED). Most frequently the hook will find its way into a finger or foot. The barb on the end of the hook prevents easy removal, but several time-honored techniques provide effective means of extraction. No clinical trial has compared the most common methods, although all have been the subject of colorful discussion in letters to the editor of various medical journals. The string technique of fish hook removal has been used in the field by fishermen for years, a testimony to its reliability and straightforward nature. But other methods, as described in this chapter, have their ardent supporters as well.

ANATOMY AND PHYSIOLOGY

Because most fishhooks embed in skin and subcutaneous tissue, understanding the anatomy of the skin and of the hook facilitates successful removal. Important anatomic and physiologic characteristics of the skin are described in detail in Chapters 110, 111, and 115. Most fishhooks consist of an eyelet at the end of a straight shank and a curved belly which ends in a barb (Fig. 120.1). The barb is usually located on the inner curve of the hook, pointed away from the hook's tip. When the sharp point of the hook enters tissue, the barb engages and prevents the hook from being pulled back through the entrance site. Atraumatic removal of the hook requires that the barb be disengaged from the surrounding tissue.

INDICATIONS

The location of the fishhook may determine which of the three methods described in this chapter will best accomplish removal. The push-through method is most effective when the point of the hook is near the surface of the skin, allowing it to be pushed through easily. This method is less useful when the tip is buried deep, as pushing it through would cause additional significant tissue damage. The rapidity, painlessness, and lack of dependence on special tools make the string technique ideal for use in the field or when local anesthesia is not available or desirable. It may also be the best technique for deeply embedded hooks. To be performed successfully, however, the body part containing the hook must be immobilized during the removal procedure. Therefore, the string technique should not be used on body parts that cannot be fully immobilized, such as ears. This technique also may be contraindicated for fishhooks located near the eye, as the airborne hook might injure the patient's eye. Finally, the needle technique can be used in the ED for those hooks embedded superficially. The more deeply embedded the hook, however, the more difficult it may be to find the barb with the needle tip.

Although the vast majority of fishhooks can be easily removed in the field or in the office or ED, fishhooks that have penetrated the globe require immediate consultation with an ophthalmologist. Likewise, consultation with a surgeon may be judicious for those hooks that have embedded near vital structures. This may apply to fishhooks in the neck, near the radial artery, and in the genitals.

Figure 120.1.
Structure of a fishhook.

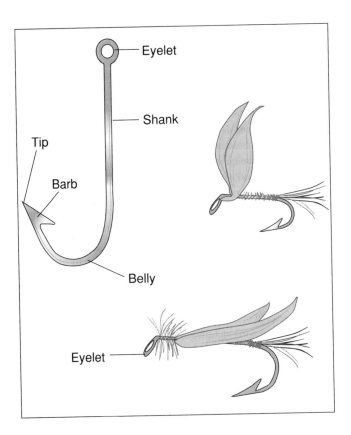

EQUIPMENT

Gloves
Wire cutter
Antiseptic prep solution (e.g., Betadine)
Lidocaine 1 to 2% without epinephrine (for push-through and needle techniques)
Syringe or needle for local anesthesia (27-gauge)
Safety goggles (for string technique)
String, fishing line, or 1.0 silk (for string technique)
Needle, 18-gauge (for needle technique)

PROCEDURE

Before removing the embedded barb, the clinician should remove multiple hooks or attached lures if present. Often, lures and additional hooks can be unscrewed while grasping the embedded hook with a hemostat. A wire cutter can be used to isolate the embedded hook from other hooks attached to the same shaft. Once the embedded hook has been disconnected from any attachments, the skin and fishhook should be prepared with betadine and the barbed hook can be removed from the skin using one of the following techniques.

Push-Through Method

The push-through method of removal requires a digital block or local infiltration of the skin overlying the point of the hook with 1% lidocaine (Fig.120.2.A). The point of the hook is then advanced and pushed through the skin (Fig.120.2.B), the barb clipped off with a wire cutter (Fig. 120.2.C), and the remainder of the shank and belly backed out of the wound (Fig120.2.D). The exit site is usually small and therefore suturing is not indicated.

String Technique

The string technique begins by securing the body part containing the fishhook firmly against a table or flat surface to prevent movement during the procedure. A piece of string (e.g., silk suture) about 3 feet long

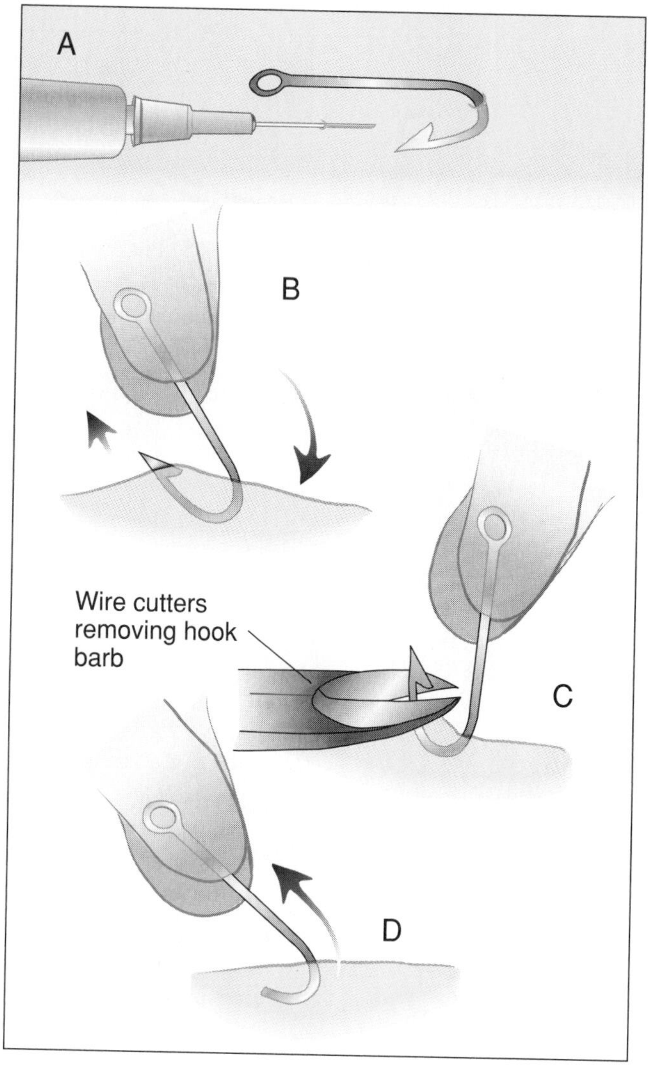

Figure 120.2.
Push-through method of
fishhook removal.

A

B

Wire cutters
removing hook
barb

C

D

should be looped around the belly of the fish-hook (Fig.120.3.A). If the shank has been cut, the remaining portion of the shank can be grasped with a strong hemostat which then will act as a substitute shank. The ends of the string should be wrapped securely around the clinician's right index finger (or left finger if the clinician is left handed). The eye and shank of the fishhook should be firmly grasped between the clinician's left index fin-ger and thumb, and then depressed, disengag-ing the barb from surrounding tissue (Fig. 120.3.B). The left middle finger applies slight pressure downward on the shank toward the patient's skin. The loop is then pulled slowly away from the hook, horizontally in the plane of the shank's long axis until just taut. Using

the right index finger, the loop is allowed to relax slightly and then, reversing direction, jerked suddenly away from the fishhook, flicking the hook from the skin (Figure 120.3.C). When done properly, this technique does not require local anesthesia (1). Because the hook often flies out of the wound, protec-tive goggles should be worn by both patient and clinician, and bystanders should be cleared from the expected flight path (2).

Needle Technique

A third technique uses a needle to cover the hook's barb, allowing the clinician to back the fishhook out of the skin. After local infil-

Figure 120.3.
String technique of
fishhook removal.

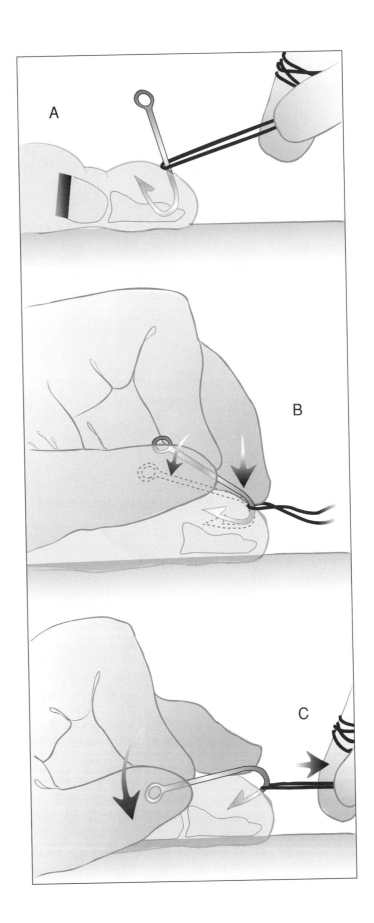

SUMMARY

1. Remove attached lures and additional hooks from embedded hook
2. Prepare field in antiseptic fashion
3. Inject local anesthesia or perform a digital block
4. Push-through method
    A. Push tip of hook through anesthetized skin
    B. Clip barb
    C. Back shank and belly of fishhook out of wound
5. String technique
    A. Secure body part involved
    B. Loop string around belly of fishhook
    C. Wrap ends of string around index finger
    D. Depress shank of hook with opposite index finger and thumb
    E. Forcefully jerk string to remove hook
6. Needle technique
    A. Insert 18-gauge needle along inside of fishhook belly
    B. Engage barb with needle opening
    C. Back needle and hook out of skin together
7. Administer tetanus booster if indicated

tration with 1% lidocaine using a 27-gauge needle, an 18- or 20-gauge needle is inserted through the wound along the shaft of the hook (Fig. 120.4.A). With the bevel of the needle facing the inside of the hook's belly, the needle is advanced along the hook's belly until the needle opening slides over (engages) the barb of the hook (Fig.120.4.B). Once the barb has been covered, the needle and hook are held firmly together while backing the hook and needle out of the wound as a unit (Fig. 120.4.C).

Following removal of the fishhook, routine wound care should prove adequate. The wound should be cleansed and a tetanus booster given if necessary. Antibiotics are not generally indicated (1, 3).

COMPLICATIONS

Complications are rare when these procedures are performed properly. As with any wound, infection is a rare complication (4). The wound should be thoroughly irrigated and cleansed, and the patient instructed to return if any signs of infection arise. The push-through technique may cause additional tissue damage as it is advanced through intact skin. The deeper the needle, the higher the risk of causing significant damage. The string technique is effective and safe when done properly. If the body part containing the fishhook is not properly secured, however, movement when the hook is jerked can result in tissue damage and pain. Most failures of this technique are thought to be due to the lack of a quick and confident yank on the string. As mentioned, the patient and clinician should both wear protective goggles to prevent eye injury. Finally, the needle technique becomes more difficult to perform without causing excessive local trauma when the fishhook is deeply embedded.

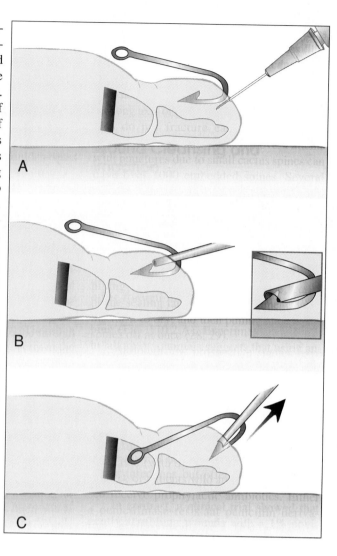

Figure 120.4.
Needle technique of fishhook removal.

CLINICAL TIPS
1. The push-through method works best when the point of the hook is near the skin surface, minimizing additional tissue damage as the barb is advanced through the skin.
2. The needle technique works best when the hook is superficially embedded.
3. The string technique is simple enough to be done in the field and, when performed correctly, requires no anesthesia.

SUMMARY

Removal of the embedded fishhook can be easily accomplished in the field, in the office, or in the ED by personnel familiar with the procedures outlined in this chapter. After removal of the hook, cleansing the wound and follow-up care should suffice.

REFERENCES

1. Friedenberg S. How to remove an imbedded fishhook in five seconds without really trying. New Eng J Med 1971;284:733–734.
2. David SS. Fish hook removal. Lancet 1991; 338: 1463–1464.
3. Cooke T. How to remove fish hooks with a bit of string. Med J Aust 1961;48:815–16.
4. Barnett, RC. Removal of fish hooks. J Hosp Med 1980;70:56–57.

Chapter 120
Fishhook Removal

CHAPTER 121

RING REMOVAL

Susan M. Fuchs

INTRODUCTION

Occasionally children try on a parent's ring or toy jewelry, only to realize that the ring cannot be removed. By the time the child arrives in the emergency department or office, several attempts to remove the ring have often been made, resulting in increased swelling of the affected finger. Another scenario is an adolescent who injures a finger distal to a ring. In these cases, the injury (possibly a fracture) results in swelling which does not allow removal of the ring. With continued swelling, ring removal is often necessary to avoid vascular compromise to a digit. Although this chapter focuses on rings, other round objects (washers, metal nuts) can be treated in a similar manner.

ANATOMY AND PHYSIOLOGY

The degree of vascular compromise of the finger depends on the magnitude and duration of swelling. Initial swelling is usually due to injury or attempts at ring removal and does not compromise circulation. Further swelling of the finger can result in obstruction of venous and lymphatic drainage, which in turn exacerbates the swelling. The risk of complete obstruction of circulation and gangrene can occur in 10 to 12 hours (1).

Acute swelling of a finger also can result from an allergic reaction, insect bite, or burn to the finger, in which case edema is the primary problem. When a finger is injured due to a fracture or dislocation, the deformity can itself prevent ring removal with or without significant swelling. Compared to those of an adult, the fingers of a young child tend to be chubby, which may further exaggerate the effects of swelling. The time to presentation also will affect the amount of swelling, but does not necessarily correlate directly.

INDICATIONS

A child often will present with a complaint about a painful finger, whereas an adolescent may be more stoic. Conversely, finger injury may be the initial presentation, only to have ring removal discovered as a secondary problem.

Several methods can be attempted to save the ring; however if the digit is already ischemic or if a displaced fracture or a dislocation occurs distal to the ring, the ring should be cut off immediately.

Perfusion of the finger is in doubt when it is pale, mottled, and has diminished or absent capillary refill. If perfusion is questioned, a pulse oximeter lead can be attached to the fingertip (Chapter 77). If a reading is obtained (a pulse wave form), perfusion is still present (2).

Assuming there is no circulatory compromise to the finger, one factor in determining the best removal method is the type of ring, i.e., plastic versus metal, narrow band versus wide band, inexpensive versus expensive or irreplaceable. It may be easier to cut a plastic ring with a ring cutter than attempt another technique, whereas if the ring is a broad, strong metal band, the string methods may be a better starting point, assuming no vascular compromise has occurred.

EQUIPMENT

Water-soluble lubricant (e.g., KY jelly)
2.0 or 3.0 silk suture, string, or umbilical tape—20″ piece
Hemostats or mosquito clamps
Ring cutter
Elastic tape, 1″ wide (intravenous tourniquet or penrose drain)
Blood pressure cuff
Monitoring equipment if conscious sedation has been administered

It is beneficial to have all equipment available for the various methods, rather than to begin searching for the ring cutter after other methods fail.

PROCEDURE

Because some of these methods may be upsetting and painful for an infant or child, consideration should be given to (a) letting the parent hold the child during the procedure (Chapter 2), (b) pain relief by administering a digital block (Chapter 37), and/or (c) possibly using conscious sedation (Chapter 35).

Before beginning any of the methods described in this chapter, the procedure should be explained to the child and parents, and the equipment demonstrated. Any needles should be shielded from the child's view. The parent can assist the child in elevating the affected hand. While preparing the equipment, the parent or child should apply ice to the finger for 5 minutes to limit further swelling. The hand and finger are then cleansed with sterile water, keeping the hand elevated as much as possible during the procedure.

Depending on the methods attempted at home or en route to the hospital, the degree of swelling, duration of swelling, and the desire to preserve the ring, one or more of the following techniques can be performed (see Indications).

String Pull

With the string pull, one end of the suture (string) is slipped beneath the ring and pulled through until both ends are of equal length. A hemostat may be used to grasp the suture under the ring. The ring and distal finger are then lubricated. The suture is grasped with the clinician's fingers or a hemostat, and pulled in a circular motion. The suture should be rotated around to different sections of the ring and pulled along the axis of the finger to gradually advance the ring off (3) (Fig. 121.1).

If this method is not successful, a digital block should be administered before the next maneuver. If the block is performed with medication deposited into the web space, or via a volar metacarpal approach, no significant additional swelling of the finger should occur.

String Wrap

With the string wrap, one end of thick silk suture (string or umbilical tape) is passed under the ring so that 5 inches remains on the proximal side of

Figure 121.1.
String pull method of ring removal.

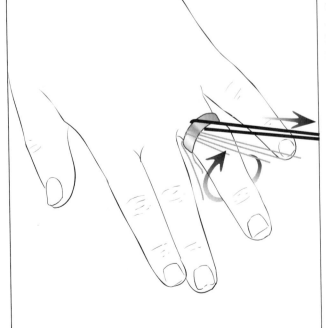

the finger. A hemostat may be used to slide the suture under the ring. The remaining suture is wrapped tightly around the swollen finger beginning just distal to the ring. Each loop of the suture should touch so that no tissue bulges between loops. The wrap should be continued beyond the proximal interphalangeal joint (PIP) (1, 2, 4) (Fig. 121.2). When the wrap is complete, the proximal piece of string (under the ring) is pulled toward the fingertip with the clinician's fingers or a hemostat. As the string gradually unwinds, it should ease the ring over the PIP joint and off the finger. If the string was not long enough, or the wrapping not tight or close enough, this procedure may have to be repeated.

Ring Cutter

The ring cutter has a guard over the wheel to prevent cutting the skin, and this characteristic should be explained to the child and parent. The ring cutter should be examined to ensure that the saw-tooth wheel of the ring cutter is sharp, approximates the cutter guard, and turns easily. It should then be cleaned with alcohol and dried with gauze. Next the cutter guard is placed under the ring. Due to swelling of the tissue this frequently causes pain. The easiest place to cut is the thinnest portion of the ring, but the best position to perform this procedure is usually on the palmar surface. If possible, the ring should be turned until the thinnest section is on the pal-

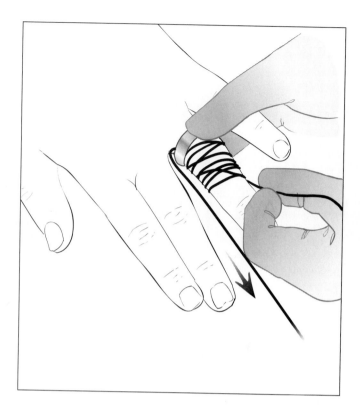

mar surface. The wheel is placed on the ring, the handle of the ring cutter is grasped and pressure applied while the wheel is turned (5) (Fig. 121.3). If the ring begins to heat up, the procedure should be stopped until the metal cools. Occasionally the ring cutter wheel is too dull to cut the ring, and another ring cutter must be used.

Once the ring is cut, the ends should be manually pulled apart or spread using a hemostat or clamp, before removing the ring.

Figure 121.2.
String wrap method of ring removal.

Figure 121.3.
Ring cutter method of ring removal.

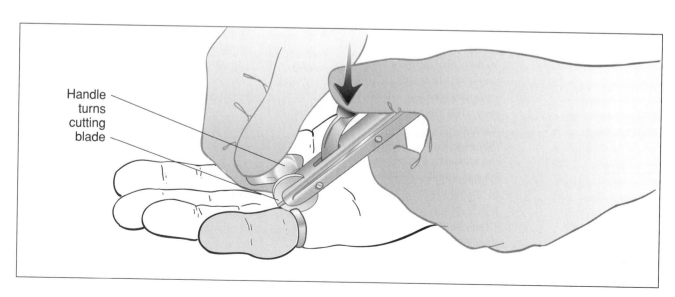

Handle turns cutting blade

Occasionally a second cut will be needed to remove the ring. This cut should be made 0.5 to 1.0 cm from the first cut. It should be noted that the pressure of the ring cutter can bend one cut side into the finger. To protect the finger from the sharp edges of the first cut, a thin piece of gauze or a Band-Aid should be placed underneath the ring. Once the second cut is complete the free piece can be removed and the ends of the ring pulled apart using a hemostat. The parents should be informed that most rings removed in this way can be taken to a jeweler for repair.

Elastic Tape Method

The elastic tape method was recently described and used successfully on an adult (6). Its use has not been reported in children or adolescents, but may prove beneficial when severe swelling occurs, and the ring cannot be cut. The procedure actually exsanguinates the finger as a way to reduce the edema. It is similar to the string wrap method, but uses elastic tape and a blood pressure cuff. Before attempting this method, sedation will probably be necessary.

Either 1-inch wide elastic tape, an intravenous tourniquet, or a 1 inch penrose drain is wrapped tightly around the finger from the tip of the finger to the ring, i.e., in a distal to proximal direction. The hand is then elevated above the head, and the finger wrapped in an ice pack. After 15 minutes, a blood pressure cuff is applied to the patient's forearm and inflated to 250 mm Hg. The tape is then removed. If the edema is reduced sufficiently to remove the ring, one of the previously discussed methods can be used. If the finger is still too swollen, this procedure can be repeated until the swelling is reduced enough to permit ring removal.

Following ring removal using any of these techniques, the patient should be reminded to not place a ring on the affected finger until all swelling has resolved. The digit should be cleaned and perfusion reassessed (color, capillary refill). If flow does not appear to be restored after ring removal, it should be checked using a pulse oximeter. If no flow is evident after 5 to 10 minutes or all efforts at removal have failed, a hand or vascular surgeon should be consulted.

CLINICAL TIPS

1. The ring cutter should be tested before beginning the procedure, including a visual inspection of the ring cutter or a test on a piece of plastic.
2. The patient and/or parents should be informed before the procedure that one of the options includes cutting the ring. Some will prefer that this be tried first.
3. The decision to use a digital block should be based on the patient's degree of discomfort, level of cooperation, and the likelihood of ring removal by the first method chosen. In some cases with young children, the use of string and ring cutters far outweighs the threat of a needle.

SUMMARY

1. Explain procedure to child and parents
2. Elevate hand
3. Apply ice to finger for 5 minutes to see if swelling will diminish
4. Cleanse area with sterile water and keep hand elevated as much as possible during procedure

String Pull

5. Slip one end of suture or string beneath ring and pull through until both ends are of equal length. A hemostat may be used to grasp suture under ring
6. Lubricate ring and distal finger
7. Grasp suture with fingers or a hemostat
8. Pull in a circular motion. Slip suture around to different sections of ring, and pull as ring gradually moves off of finger
9. Clean digit and reassess perfusion (color, capillary refill)

String Wrap

5. Administer a digital block
6. Pass end of suture or string under ring so 5 inches remains on proximal side of finger. A hemostat may be used to slide suture under ring
7. Tightly wrap remaining suture around swollen finger beginning just distal to ring
8. Continue wrap beyond proximal interphalangeal (PIP) joint
9. Pull proximal end of string toward fingertip with fingers or a hemostat. As it gradually unwinds, it should ease ring over PIP joint and off of finger
10. Remove suture from finger
11. Repeat procedure as needed
12. Clean digit and assess perfusion (color, capillary refill)

Ring Cutter

5. Administer a digital block
6. Examine ring cutter to ensure that sawtooth wheel is sharp, approximates cutter guard, and turns easily
7. Clean ring cutter with alcohol and then dry with gauze
8. Turn ring, if possible, until thinnest section is on palmar surface of finger
9. Place cutter guard under ring
10. Place wheel on ring, grasp handle of ring cutter and apply pressure while turning wheel. If ring begins to heat up, stop until metal cools
11. When ring is cut, manually pull apart ring, or spread ends using a hemostat or clamp, and remove ring
12. When necessary, make a second cut 0.5 to 1.0 cm from first cut. Protect finger from sharp edges of first cut with a thin piece of gauze or a Band-Aid slipped underneath ring. Once second cut is complete remove free piece and pull ends of ring apart using hemostats
13. Examine finger for cuts, clean finger, and check perfusion
14. Take ring to jeweler for repair

COMPLICATIONS

Trauma to the digit in the form of a cut or bruise can occur during ring removal. Cleansing and a dressing (Band-Aid) are all that is needed. If a digital block was used, the patient may experience a throbbing pain as the anesthetic wears off.

SUMMARY

Although the order in which ring removal has been outlined takes into account the desire to save the ring, if this is not a priority, using the ring cutter is the most reliable method. Obviously the decision regarding which method to use depends on the patient, the degree of swelling, the presence or absence of vascular compromise, the presence of an injury distal to the ring, and the type of ring.

REFERENCES

1. Young JR. Unring a finger. Emerg Med 1982 Sept; 15:107–108.
2. Jastremski MS. Ring removal. In: Jastremski MS, Dumas MS eds. Emergency procedures. Philadelphia: WB Saunders, 1992, pp. 141–143.
3. Mizrahi S, Lunski I. A simplified method for ring removal from an edematous finger. Am J Surg 1986; 151:412–413.
4. Barnett RC. Soft tissue foreign body removal. In: Roberts JR, Hedges JR, eds. Clinical procedures in emergency medicine. 2nd ed. Philadelphia: WB Saunders, 1991, p. 588.
5. Carlson DW, DiGiulio GA, Gewitz MH, Givens T, Handler SD, Hodge D, et al. Illustrated techniques of pediatric emergency medicine. In: Fleisher GR, Ludwig S, eds. Textbook of pediatric emergency medicine. 3rd ed. Baltimore: Williams & Wilkins, 1993, pp. 1658–1659.
6. Cresap CR. Removal of a hardened steel ring from an extremely swollen finger. Am J Emerg Med 1995;13: 318–320.

INTRAMUSCULAR AND SUBCUTANEOUS INJECTIONS

A. Felipe Blanco and James F. Wiley II

INTRODUCTION

Since its introduction in the second half of the 19th century, intramuscular injection has been a main route of drug delivery for the prophylaxis and treatment of disease (1). This mode of drug administration is most useful when the patient's disease and/or the pharmacokinetic properties of the drug preclude oral dosing, and an intravenous route is unavailable or unnecessary. The technique is straightforward and may be used for patients of all ages. New drugs and new applications for current drugs have increased the variety and frequency of agents delivered by this route.

Subcutaneous injection predates intramuscular injection in medical history. One of its first uses was for the prophylactic injection of cow pox to provide immunity against small pox in the mid-18th century (1). Subcutaneous injection serves a more limited but still important role in drug delivery for pediatric care.

ANATOMY AND PHYSIOLOGY

Site selection for intramuscular injection involves several considerations. The site should avoid major nerves and blood vessels. The muscle mass should be large enough to allow retention and absorption of the injected drug, and anatomic landmarks used for injection should remain consistent from patient to patient. In children, the four sites for intra-

muscular injection are the anterolateral thigh (vastus lateralis muscle), the ventrogluteal area (gluteus medius muscle), the upper arm (deltoid muscle), and the buttock (gluteus maximus muscle) (Fig. 122.1). Site preference depends on age and nutrition status of the child as shown in Table 122.1 (2). Malnourished children may have decreased muscle mass at one or more injection sites and therefore require special consideration.

Intramuscular injection creates a depot for drug absorption from the muscle into the systemic circulation. However, this route does not always ensure rapid or complete bioavailability. Absorption depends on the lipophilicity and concentration of the drug, on the total surface area available, and on blood flow at the injection site. Absorption varies by injection site—most rapid from the deltoid muscle, slowest from the gluteal muscles, and intermediate from the vastus lateralis muscle (3). Injected drug absorption increases with exercise and decreases or stops with circulatory disturbances such as shock, hypotension, congestive heart failure, and myxedema.

Intramuscular injection presents the delivered drug as a potential antigen to macrophages and T cells within the muscle. Furthermore, intramuscular injection causes tissue injury which leads to a migration of many inflammatory cells of different types to the area. As a result, an amnestic response may occur within T lymphocytes, leading to a type IV immunologic response after reex-

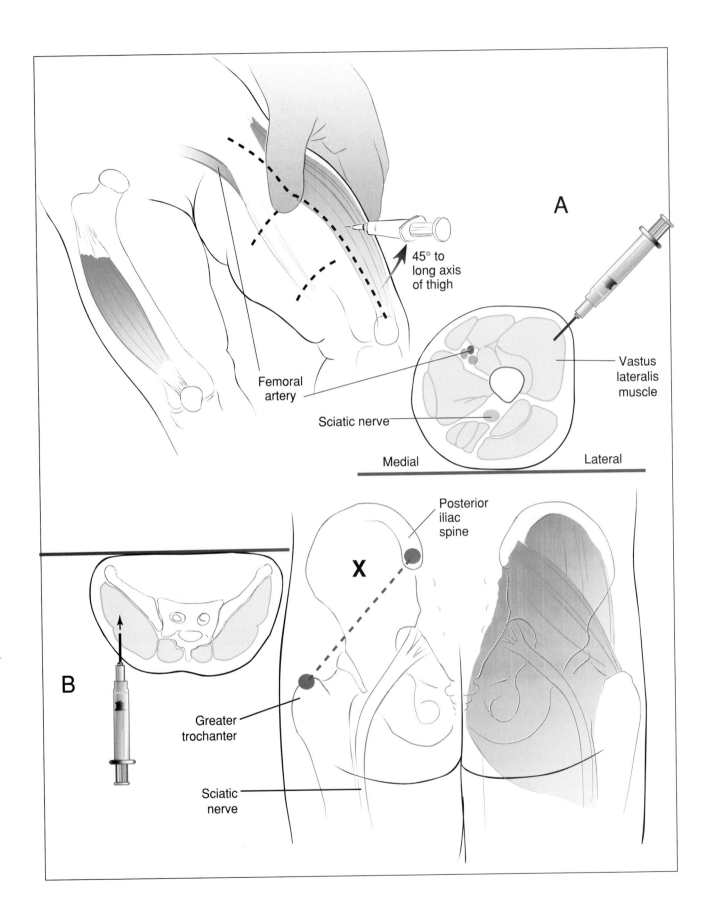

45° to
long axis
of thigh

A

Femoral
artery

Sciatic nerve

Vastus
lateralis
muscle

Medial

Lateral

Posterior
iliac
spine

X

B

Greater
trochanter

Sciatic
nerve

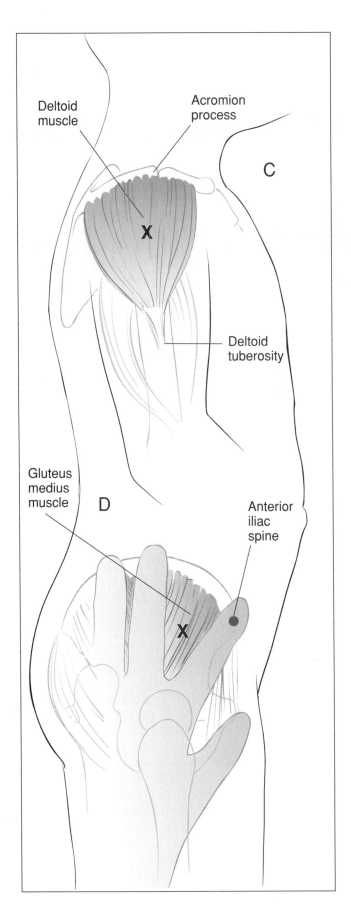

Figure 122.1.
Intramuscular injection sites.
A. Anterolateral thigh (vastus lateralis muscle). Technique: Pinch the muscle with free hand, to stabilize and expose more muscular mass. Insert the needle in the anterolateral aspect of the thigh, at the junction of the middle and distal thirds, at an angle of 45° to the long axis of the thigh.
B. Dorsogluteal (maximus, medium, minimus gluteal muscles). Technique: With the patient prone, locate the head of the greater trochanter of the femur and the posterior iliac spine. The line between these two points divides the gluteal area into upper outer and lower inner portions. Insert the needle superior and lateral to this line, at approximately halfway between the two anatomical points mentioned. The needle must go perpendicular to the stretcher, not to the patient's skin.
C. Upper lateral arm (deltoid muscle). Technique: Expose the arm from the shoulder to the elbow. Pinch the deltoid muscle with free hand to stabilize and expose more muscular mass. Insert the needle perpendicular to the skin at a point halfway from the acromion process of scapula to the deltoid tuberosity of the humerus.
D. Ventrogluteal (gluteus medius, tensor fasciae latae muscle) (Von Hochstetter's site). Technique: Locate the anterior iliac tubercle with left index finger on the right side of the patient, or vice versa. Extend the middle finger of the same hand to the most superior point of the iliac crest forming a triangle between these two fingers and the iliac crest. Insert the needle in the center of the triangle and perpendicular to the skin.

Table 122.1.
Preferred Injection Sites

Age (yr) or Clinical Status	Sites (Muscle)*
<2	Anterior lateral thigh (vastus lateralis)
	Ventral gluteal (gluteus medius)
2–10	Anterior lateral thigh
	Ventral gluteal
	Upper arm (deltoid)
>10	Upper arm
	Anterior lateral thigh
	Ventral gluteal
	Dorsal gluteal (gluteus maximus)
Malnourished	Anterior lateral thigh
	Ventral gluteal

* Sites listed in descending order of preference

posure to the drug. Thus intramuscular injection may predispose an individual to hypersensitivity and allergic reactions to the drugs received.

Intramuscular injection causes direct tissue injury and pain. Muscle enzymes (aspartate transaminase, creatinine phosphokinase) are elevated by injection. This is especially true when large volumes are used, when the drug is intrinsically irritating or when the pH of the injectate is far from physiologic range (3). Inadvertent injection into an artery or vein compounds the potential for tissue injury. Arterial injection may cause subsequent vasospasm and potential drug toxicity in the distal tissues. Arterial or venous injection

Table 122.2.
Drugs Frequently Used for Intramuscular or Subcutaneous Injection

Agent	Pain	Potential Complications
Intramuscular Administration		
Vaccine		
DPT	+ + +	+ + +
Hepatitis B	+	+
HiB	+	+
Antibiotics		
Penicillin G procaine	+ + +	+
Penicillin G benzathin	+ + +	+
Ceftriaxone	+ + + +	+ +
Ampicillin sodium	+ +	+
Analgesics		
Morphine sulfate	+	+
Meperdine HCL	+	+
Other		
Phenobarbital sodium	+	+
Diphenhydramine HCL	+	+
Naloxone HCL	+	+
Subcutaneous Administration		
Epinephrine 1:1000	+ + +	+
Insulin	+	+
MMR	+ +	+ +

also carries the risk of untoward systemic effects with certain agents, such as lidocaine. Table 122.2 lists drugs commonly injected via the intramuscular route and their potential for tissue injury.

The goal of subcutaneous injection is to deliver the drug into the adipose tissue, which lies below the dermis layer of the skin and above the muscle layer. The optimal sites for this task are the upper lateral shoulder, the anterior thighs, and the abdomen, because they have a relative abundance of fat with few surface veins. The adipose layer has a smaller blood supply relative to the muscle layer; therefore, drug absorption after subcutaneous injection is less consistent and slower than intramuscular injection. Drugs given subcutaneously, such as growth hormone and insulin, are best absorbed from the abdomen followed by the arms, thighs, and buttocks (4, 5). The potential for allergic reactions and tissue injury discussed for intramuscular injections also applies, although to a lesser extent, to subcutaneous injections. Table 122.3 lists the agents commonly delivered by subcutaneous injections.

INDICATIONS

Intramuscular Injection

Common reasons for using intramuscular injections in the ambulatory setting include immunization, infectious prophylaxis, treatment of existing infection, pain management, and sedation (Table 122.3). This route of drug delivery ensures compliance and avoids first-pass metabolism. With some infectious diseases (e.g., streptococcal pharyngitis, and certain gonococcal infections) a single intramuscular shot of antibiotic has proven as efficacious as a multiple-day, orally administered drug regimen (6, 7). Potential advantages of intramuscular drug administration, however, should be weighed against the pain of the procedure and potential risks of local injury and allergic reaction when used in the outpatient setting. Intramuscular injections should be avoided in patients with bleeding dyscrasias and circulatory instability. Hematoma formation and hemorrhage can cause extensive local tissue damage in patients with hemophilia, thrombocytopenia, von Willebrand's disease, disseminated intravascular coagulation, and other clotting disorders. In addition, patients in shock do not absorb drugs well from intramuscular injections and may suffer complications from erratic drug delivery.

Intramuscular injections should not be given near cutaneous vascular malformations because these sites increase the risk of inadvertent intravascular injection. Injection through denuded skin or near a skin infection (impetigo, cellulitis) risks internal spread of a local infection. Drugs that have a high likelihood of precipitation at the site and incomplete bioavailability should not be administered. Phenytoin and digoxin, for example, are not recommended for injection for this reason. Other drugs that precipitate to varying degrees at the injection site include ampicillin, diazepam, and quinidine (3).

Subcutaneous Injection

Subcutaneous injections are most useful for delivering certain immunizations (measles, mumps, rubella) and specific drugs (epinephrine, naloxone, insulin). The clinician can quickly give epinephrine subcutaneously and expect a response within 3 to 5 minutes in a patient with adequate circulation who presents with status asthmaticus or who requires treatment for a severe allergic reaction. Subcutaneous administration of insulin remains the primary route of treatment for many patients with diabetes mellitus. Continuous subcutaneous infusions are becoming more common in the treatment of a variety of conditions including diabetes mellitus, growth hormone deficiency, and chronic cancer pain.

Clinicians should avoid subcutaneous injections in patients with inadequate circulation, as little to no drug delivery will occur. Bleeding dyscrasias are a relative contraindication to subcutaneous injection, although some hematologists recommend the subcutaneous administration of the diphtheria/pertussis/tetanus (DPT) immunization in hemophiliacs to avoid the greater risk of intramuscular injection. Subcutaneous injections should not be given through areas of cellulitis, impetigo, or denuded skin.

PROCEDURE

Intramuscular Injection

Equipment
Antiseptic solution—usually isopropyl alcohol 70%
Sterile syringe and needle—20- to 25-gauge, 1″ (2.54 cm)
Sterile dry cotton ball or gauze
Injectant

Four sites are suitable for injection in children (2) (Fig. 122.1). The maximum volume of injection varies according to muscle mass and age (Table 122.3.) The patient should not be informed of the injection until it is time to perform the procedure. The injectant is drawn up, out of view of the patient, using a large needle (18 to 21 gauge). The large needle is removed and an injecting needle (23 to 25 gauge) is attached to the syringe. The injecting needle is tightly connected to the syringe hub to avoid leakage of the drug during injection. The need for the shot should be explained in an age-appropriate fashion. The patient is restrained (Chapter 3) and the skin cleansed with an antiseptic solution, which is allowed to dry.

The needle is quickly inserted down to the muscle (the hub of the syringe should be at the skin surface) and aspirated to ensure that the needle is not in a blood vessel. The solution is injected slowly and the needle removed. A cotton ball or gauze is then applied over the site with moderate pressure.

Subcutanous Injections

Equipment
Antiseptic solution—usually isopropyl alcohol 70%
Sterile tuberculin or insulin syringe with 27-gauge, 0.5″ needle
Sterile dry cotton ball or gauze
Injectant

The shot should not be discussed with the child until just before it is administered. The needle should be tightly connected to the syringe. The injectant is drawn up in the syringe out of view of the patient. Next the need for the injection is explained in an age-appro-

Table 122.3.
Maximum Recommended Volumes for Intramuscular Injection

Age (mo)	Volume (mL)
0–3	0.5–1.0
3–24	1.0
24–60	1.0–1.5
>60	1.0–2.0

priate fashion. A site is selected (upper outer arm, lateral thigh, or abdomen) that has no visible superficial veins or cutaneous vascular malformations (Fig. 122.2). The skin is cleansed with an antiseptic solution, which is allowed to dry. The needle is quickly inserted into the subcutaneous layer at a 45° angle to the skin. The drug is injected and the needle withdrawn. A gauze or cotton ball is applied to the site until bleeding stops.

COMPLICATIONS

Complications following intramuscular injection arise from the needle wound, incorrect technique, and the substance delivered to the tissue. In one multihospital study of 12,123 patients who received intramuscular injections, the local complication rate was 0.4%, with abscess formation being most frequent (8). Most information derives from case reports which highlight the serious potential for injury but provide no incidence data for each complication. Main complications arising from the needle wound are infection and inadvertent puncture of vital structures. Reports exist of cellulitis with abscess formation (staphylococcal, clostridial, and sterile), clostridial myositis, and frank gangrene associated with intramuscular injections (9–11). Using sterile disposable needles, giving attention to site cleansing before the procedure, and avoiding sites with adjacent infection usually will prevent such complications.

Repetitive injections can cause muscle contracture, permanent muscle fibrosis, and intramuscular hemorrhage with hematoma formation despite correct technique. Rotating injection sites in children who receive multiple injections and avoiding obviously traumatized areas prevent these complications (12, 13).

Permanent nerve injury and intraarterial injection with vascular damage necessitating skin grafting or limb amputation have occurred from incorrect needle positioning before injection. Premature or small infants and malnourished children are at particular risk for these dreaded complications. Needle aspiration before injection and adherence to suggested injection sites, needle length and injectant volumes will prevent these rare but potentially disastrous outcomes.

Of the four intramuscular sites, the dorsal gluteal area most often is associated with significant nerve or vascular injury. The most frequent complication at this site is sciatic nerve injury, but superior gluteal nerve, posterior femoral cutaneous nerve, and pudendal nerve damage have been reported from injections at this site (8). In the upper arm, radial nerve injuries result from injections to the lower portion of the proximal third of the arm and axillary nerve damage has followed deltoid injection with excessively long needles (14). The lateral thigh and ventral gluteal regions appear to be safer for injection than the upper arm and dorsal gluteal area. However, femoral artery thrombosis in an infant has been reported after an intramuscular injection in the anterolateral thigh with a longer needle than recommended (11). No neuromuscular complications have yet been reported from the ventral gluteal area.

Inadvertent subcutaneous injection can cause a large red site of inflammation as the injected drug spreads through the subcutaneous layer. Differentiation between subcutaneous injection and cellulitis may be difficult. Subsequent lipodystrophy and skin pigmentation can occur depending on the irritative characteristics of the injectant (15). This complication often follows injection with a short needle, drug delivery during the initial skin puncture, or early withdrawal of the needle while drug is still being injected.

Intramuscular drug injection can also create a significant immunologic response that predisposes patients to severe allergic reactions and anaphylaxis. Allergic reactions to drugs are unpredictable. For this reason, *all children receiving intramuscular injections on an outpatient basis should be observed for a minimum of 30 minutes following injection to ensure no signs of an acute allergic response before being discharged.*

Pain is an unavoidable adverse effect of an intramuscular injection. Immediate pain, however, can be minimized by preparing the child psychologically, cooling the skin site, and by rapid skin puncture. Delayed pain is due to (*a*) aseptic irritation and neurosis, which varies in degree with the different substances given, (*b*) an immune response to the injectate, (*c*) infection, or (*d*) muscle spasm.

Intramuscluar Injection
1. The drug should be appropriate for the intramuscular route.
2. The patient should be assessed for contra-indications to the procedure (bleeding dyscrasia, cellulitis).
3. Techniques should be used to reduce psy-chological stress.
4. A safe age-appropriate site should be cho-sen (Table 122.1).
5. Needles should be switched after drawing up injectant.
6. The smallest diameter needle that will permit free flow of the injectate should be used (not less than 25-gauge to ensure aspiration of blood if a vein or artery is inadvertently entered).
7. Appropriate needle length should be used (usually 1″, although longer for obese or adolescent patients).
8. The antiseptic should be dry before the skin is penetrated.
9. The injection solution should be warmed to room temperature.
10. The needle should be inserted quickly through the skin to minimize pain.
11. The plunger of the syringe should not be depressed during needle insertion.
12. Aspiration for blood before injection en-sures the needle is not in a blood vessel.
13. Slow and steady injection reduces pain.
14. Irritating injectants (ceftriaxone) may be mixed with 1 mL of 1% lidocaine before injection.
15. Alternating sites for subsequent injections reduces the risk of muscle contractures.
16. Premature infants, young infants, or mal-nourished infants or children deserve extra caution.

Subcutaneous Injection
1. Psychological stress may be avoided with a variety of distraction techniques.
2. Overlying blood vessels must be avoided.
3. Quick needle insertion reduces pain.
4. Rotating injection sites prevents lipodys-trophy, lipoatrophy, and subcutaneous nodules or scarring.

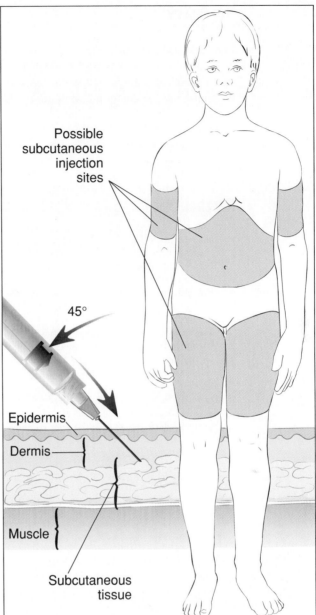

Possible subcutaneous injection sites

45°

Epidermis

Dermis

Muscle

Subcutaneous tissue

Figure 122.2
Subcutaneous injection.

Of these, only avoidance of infection is within control of the shot giver. Pretreatment with acetaminophen or a nonsteroidal antiin-flammatory drug 30 minutes before injection may blunt the delayed pain due to tissue reac-tion.

Compared with intramuscular injection, complications of subcutaneous injection are less severe. Local infection, allergic reaction, and abscess may occur, but muscle contrac-ture, intraarterial injection, and nerve injury are highly unlikely due to the shorter needle used and the recommended sites of injection. Untoward systemic effects may follow inad-vertent intravenous injection. Care should be taken to avoid superficial veins when per-forming a subcutaneous injection. Finally, subcutaneous nodules and scarring may form after repetitive subcutaneous injections to a particular site. These nodules may alter the absorption of the drug. This problem is most frequent in diabetics who do not carefully ro-tate sites. In these patients, insulin injection into subcutaneous nodules hampers insulin delivery to the circulation, thereby resulting in poor glucose homeostasis. Rotating injec-tion sites and avoiding preexisting scars pre-vent this complication.

Chapter 122
Intramuscular and
Subcutaneous
Injections

SUMMARY

Intramuscular and subcutaneous injection of substances are commonly performed in a variety of clinical settings. With knowledge of technique, the procedures are straightforward and cause minimal complications. Small infants and malnourished children are more prone to adverse effects and require special care when receiving injections.

REFERENCES

1. Howard-Jones N. The origin of hypodermic medication. Sci Am 1971 January;224:96–102.
2. Bergson P, Standford S, Kaplan A. Intramuscular injections in children. Pediatrics 1982;70:944–948.
3. Greenblatt DJ, Koch-Weser J. Drug therapy: intramuscular injection of drug. N Engl J Med 1976;295: 542–546.
4. Beshyah SA, Anyaoku V, Niththyananthan R, Sharp P, Johnston DG. The effect of subcutaneous injection site on absorption of human growth hormone: abdomen versus thigh. Clin Endocrinol 1991;35: 409–412.
5. Bantle JP, Weber MS, Rao S, Chattopadhyay MK, Robertson RP. Rotation of the anatomic regions used for insulin injections and day-to-day variability of plasma glucose in type I diabetic subjects. JAMA 1990;263:1802–1806.
6. Rajan VS, Sng EH, Thirumorthy T, Goh CL. Ceftriaxone in the treatment of ordinary and penicillinase-producing strains of Neisseria Gonorrhoeae. Br J Vener Dis 1982;58:314–316.
7. Report of the committee on infectious diseases. 22nd ed. Elk Grove Village, Il; American Academy of Pediatrics, 1991, p. 443
8. Greenblatt D, Allen M. Intramuscular injection site complications. JAMA 1978;240:542–544.
9. Beecroft P, Redick S. Possible complications of intramuscular injections on the pediatric unit. Pediatr Nurs 1989;15:333–336.
10. Berggren RB, Batterton TD, McArdle G, et al. Clostridial myositis after parenteral injections. JAMA 1964; 188:1044.
11. Talbert JL, Haslam RHA, Haller JA. Gangrene of the foot following intramuscular injection in the lateral thigh: a case report with recommendations for prevention. J Pediatr 1967;70:110.
12. McCloskey JR, Chung SMK: Quadriceps contracture as a result of multiple intramuscular injections. Am J Dis Child 1970;131:416.
13. Alvarez EV, Munters M, Lavine LS, et al. Quadriceps myofibrosis: a complication of intramuscular injections. J Bone Joint Surg 1980;62A:58.
14. Broadbent TR, Odom GL, Woodhall B. Peripheral nerve injuries from administration of penicillin: report of four clinical cases. JAMA 1948;140:1008.
15. Buchta RM. Atrophy after parenteral injection. Am J Dis Child 1976;130:900.

LABORATORY SKILLS

Section Editor: James F. Wiley II

Obtaining Biologic Specimens

Louis M. Bell and Nicholas Tsarouhas

General Introduction

Biologic specimens can be an important adjunct to the history and physical examination. Poorly obtained specimens not only may lead to erroneous diagnoses, but also may cause undue morbidity. This chapter will discuss the indications, materials, procedures, and complications involved with the collection of biologic specimens. The interpretation of these results also will be addressed.

Blood Cultures

Introduction

Blood cultures are the cornerstone to the diagnosis of bacteremia and sepsis. The Gram stain is of controversial benefit (1) and may have no value unless bacteremia is overwhelming (2). Consequently, most institutions do not routinely Gram stain blood specimens. For this reason, it is important to optimize the procedure for obtaining a proper blood culture. Isolation of the offending microorganism is crucial to diagnosis and management of patients with blood-borne bacterial disease.

Anatomy and Physiology

Peripheral veins are the most common vessels from which blood cultures are drawn. The veins used most often in pediatric blood draws are those in the antecubital fossa. However, because of the occasional difficulty in obtaining blood specimens from young children and infants, other sites also are frequently used (Chapter 75). Using the femoral vein, located medial to the femoral arterial pulsation and below the inguinal ligament, is sometimes discouraged because of the possible difficulty in appropriately cleaning the site. This difficulty is more of a problem in the adult patient and therefore need not be excluded as a potential site in the child.

Arteries are equally acceptable sites for blood cultures. The radial artery is most commonly used, but the ulnar, dorsalis pedis, posterior tibial, and even temporal arteries are occasionally used (Chapter 74). In the newborn, the umbilical artery or vein is often used as a site from which to draw blood cultures. These are most helpful if drawn at placement of the line (Chapter 40). Capillary collections are not acceptable as blood culture specimens.

Indications

The obvious indication for drawing a blood culture is in the toxic-appearing child. This child should always have a blood culture drawn to rule out sepsis. Many additional scenarios, however, deserve special note.

Children with immunodeficiencies obviously are more susceptible to develop serious bacterial infections. Examples include children with oncologic disease, acquired immunodeficiency syndrome, chronic renal failure, and sickle-cell anemia. Patients on immunosuppressive medication also are at higher risk for sepsis. Antirejection drugs in patients status after organ transplants, and chronic steroids for asthma or kidney disease, make these children more vulnerable. Neonates are immunocompromised by virtue of the immaturity of their immune systems. All febrile infants less than 2 months of age warrant a full sepsis evaluation. Additionally, other signs of illness such as irritability, lethargy, poor feeding, or apnea may indicate sepsis. Although fever often is the presenting symptom, note that some of these children may not have the ability to mount a febrile response. All of these scenarios require increased vigilance with respect to possible sepsis.

Much has been written in the pediatric literature regarding occult bacteremia. Strictly speaking, it is defined as bacteremia confirmed microbiologically despite no clinical signs of sepsis. Considerable disagreement exists regarding who is at risk. Most agree that children less than 2 years old are at greatest risk, but some expand this range to 3 years old. Temperature is another source of contention. Most sources place the high risk cutoff at above 39.0 to 39.4 °C. The incidence of occult bacteremia in this setting is usually stated to be 3 to 5%. The usual offending microorganism is *Streptococcus pneumoniae*. A far less common culprit, *Haemophilus influenzae* type b, is becoming even more rare since routine immunization was instituted against this pathogen.

A crucial aspect of the diagnosis of endocarditis deals with the isolation of the offending microorganism. It had previously been accepted that the highest yield for the blood culture was that done at the time of the fever spike. Most agree now, however, that the bacteremia is continuous and the timing is not so important. More important is doing serial cultures to increase the yield. Microorganisms usually implicated include *Streptococcus viridans*, *Staphylococcus aureus*, *Staphylococcus epidermidis,* and *enterococci*. Children with congenital heart disease, prosthetic valves, or history of rheumatic fever are at highest risk. A high degree of suspicion should be maintained in any child with

a prolonged fever. A new heart murmur also is highly suspicious. Supportive evidence may include a low hemoglobin, high white blood cell count, or high erythrocyte sedimentation rate.

Children with long-term venous access catheters (Broviac® or Hickman®) who develop fever are commonly admitted to the hospital to rule out line infection. Because of the potential seriousness of a line infection, these children have central and peripheral blood cultures drawn and then are started on presumptive antibiotic therapy until culture results are known. The most common microorganisms implicated in these infections are the Gram-positives *S. aureus* and *S. epidermidis*. Occasionally, also seen are Gram-negative infections. Any febrile child with a central line presenting with chills, change in mental status, or hypotension should be presumed to have line sepsis. Oncology patients receiving long-term chemotherapy and children with gastrointestinal or nutritional disorders comprise a large part of this population.

Immunocompetent children rarely develop pure anaerobic infections. When anaerobes are involved, the infection often is polymicrobial. Examples include dental infections, human bites, and abscesses. Some authorities believe that if an anaerobic infection is strongly suspected, a separate anaerobic blood culture should be obtained.

Fungi often are difficult to grow in routine blood cultures. Other than sometimes taking several weeks to grow, special media and techniques often are required. For instance, *Malassizia furfur,* a lipid-dependent yeast, grows poorly in standard culture, but well in media overlaid with olive oil (3). This species is known to cause systemic infection in babies with central venous catheters in neonatal intensive care units. The laboratory should be consulted when fungi are suspected.

Equipment

Peripheral Blood Culture
Iodine swabs
Alcohol swabs
Blood culture tube or bottle
Tourniquet
Butterfly needle
Syringe—3 to 5 mL

Gauze
Band-Aid
Sterile gloves
If vacutainer system is used:
  Vacutainer needle and holder, or
  Vacutainer butterfly and holder
If newly placed intravenous catheter is used:
  Peripheral intravenous catheter
  T-connector

Central Line Blood Culture
Steel clamp
Iodine swabs
Blood culture tube or bottle
Syringes—5 mL
Sterile transfer needle
Heparin or saline flush
Sterile gloves
Sterile drape

Needleless Central Line Blood Culture
Steel clamp
Iodine swabs
Vacutainer tube (for discarded blood)
Vacutainer needle and holder
Needleless cannula
Vacutainer tube (for blood culture)
Heparin or saline flush
Sterile gloves
Sterile drape

**Totally Implanted Venous Access System
Blood Culture**
Huber needle with a 90 ° bend
Extension tubing with side clamp
Gauze to stabilize needle
Equipment as listed for central line blood culture

The most commonly used disinfectants are iodine and alcohol. Most institutions use disposable swabs of povidone-iodine (Betadine®). This preparation yields 1% available iodine. One adult study compared these 1% iodine pads with iodine tincture pads (2% iodine/47% ethanol) and found less contamination with the latter (4). Disposable alcohol swabs most commonly used contain 70% isopropyl alcohol.

Tubes and bottles are the two main types of receptacles used for blood cultures (Fig. 123.1). Tubes are used with media systems, whereas bottles are used with broth techniques. A common media system uses the

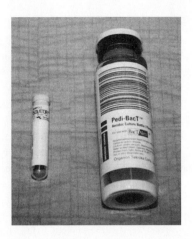

Figure 123.1.
Blood culture tube and bottle.

Isolator 1.5® microbial tubes. This system basically involves extracting the collected blood from the tube and then directly plating the collected blood onto media. With this technique, independent colonies can be counted and identified, which is one advantage of media systems over broth systems.

With broth systems (BACTEC® or Pedi-BacT®), the blood is inoculated into the bottle and this culture is not disturbed unless bacterial growth is sensed by automated systems. The broths are enriched with mixtures to enhance bacterial growth (soybean-casein digest, brain heart infusion, etc.). Additionally, antibiotic-binding resins often are added. Sodium polyanethol sulfonate (SPS) usually is added for its anticoagulant properties and its ability to counteract antibacterial factors in the blood (1).

Many authorities believe that the broth system is superior for a variety of reasons. Most importantly is the fewer contaminated specimens. The media system involves several processing steps which expose the culture, whereas the broth system is closed until a microorganism is detected. Additionally, the broth system is more sensitive and more rapid to detect a potential pathogen. Finally, the broth system, because it is automated, involves far less labor and therefore cost.

Procedures

Peripheral Blood Culture
As with all pediatric procedures, the first step involves establishing a relationship with the child and parent. Once the procedure is explained to both, the appropriate restraint technique is chosen (Chapter 3). Once the desired

site is selected, the tourniquet is applied. The next step is to sterilize the site. Most prefer to start with a betadine swab, wiping the site in concentric circles outward from the anticipated point of venipuncture. This is repeated with two more betadine swabs. The clinician must now allow the betadine to dry for 1 minute. The most common breach of technique is not to wait these 60 seconds for this important step (5). After the betadine has dried, the site is wiped with an alcohol swab. It is important to not contaminate the area by repalpating the vein once the site has been sterilized.

With the site now prepared, the vein is punctured and the blood is withdrawn (Chapter 75). The appropriate volume for blood culture depends on the institution's culture system. Generally, 0.5 mL of blood is the minimum necessary for a good result. Note that blood is inherently bactericidal, so "the more the better" is not always true. Many broth systems recommend up to 5 mL of blood. Only one blood culture tube or bottle is sufficient for the vast majority of pediatric situations. Notable exceptions may include endocarditis, central line infections, and strong suspicion for anaerobic infections.

The unclotted blood should be inoculated into the tube or bottle as quickly as possible after the draw. Studies done in children (5) and adults (6, 7) have shown no benefit to changing needles between the one used for the blood draw and the one used to inoculate the tube or bottle. This former practice of changing needles is now agreed to be a "no-benefit, high-risk procedure" (8). Similarly, needles should not be recapped; they should be discarded immediately into a sharps container. It is estimated that one-third of all needlestick injuries occur during recapping (9).

A common practice in many institutions involves drawing blood specimens through a newly placed, peripheral intravenous catheter. This also is acceptable for blood cultures, provided that strict attention is paid toward the sterility of the culture. Using the same technique to sterilize the site with three Betadine® pads and one alcohol pad, the intravenous catheter is inserted (Chapter 75). An assistant attaches a T-connector with syringe, and then withdraws the blood. The T-connector is removed and a sterile needle is inserted onto the blood-filled syringe. It is important to dispense the first inoculum of blood into the blood culture receptacle.

Central Line Blood Culture

The most important step, again, is sterilizing the site (Chapter 76). Betadine® swabs are used to disinfect the connection between the extension tubing or cap and the hub. The tubing or cap is then disconnected, and the hub itself again is disinfected. A sterile syringe is attached, and 0.5 mL (infant) to 1 mL (child) is withdrawn for discard. Another syringe is attached and the blood culture specimen (0.5 to 1 mL) is collected. A sterile needle is attached to the syringe, and the blood is inoculated into the receptacle. Note that the catheter should be flushed with heparin or saline when the blood draw is completed.

Needleless Central Line Blood Culture

As per other cultures, the actual technique is discussed elsewhere (Chapter 76), and only the blood culture aspects are reviewed. The key point is, again, disinfection. The rubber cap of the central line is swabbed well with Betadine®, as are the tops of the vacutainer tubes. The needleless cannula, which is attached to the vacutainer needle, is then pushed into the rubber cap of the central line. The vacutainer tube for discard is now attached, and approximately 1 mL is withdrawn and discarded. The vacutainer blood culture tube is now attached and 1 to 2 mL of blood is collected. When the needleless cannula is removed, the rubber cap is swabbed with Betadine®, and then the line is flushed with heparin or saline.

Totally Implanted Venous Access System Blood Culture

Blood cultures are just as easily performed with implanted systems as with standard central lines. The complete technique is described in Chapter 76. Once the subcutaneous cylinder is palpated, it is disinfected with three Betadine® swabs, followed by an alcohol swab. After connecting the Huber needle to tubing and a syringe, it is inserted through the diaphragm to the back of the reservoir. Again, the first 1 to 2 mL of blood is discarded, and then the blood culture specimen is collected in a separate syringe. After the blood has been collected, the system is flushed with heparin or saline.

Interpretation of Results

A great deal has been written on the interpretation of blood culture results. Certain clues are useful to distinguish between infection and contamination. The most important factor is the clinical status of the patient. Recovery of a virulent microorganism in a well child supports contamination. Growth factors that support contamination include an organism that takes several days to grow out, one that grows in only one of several collections, one that grows in the enrichment broth only, and one with multiple species present. Finally, certain microorganisms (diphtheroids, coagulase-negative staphylococci, micrococcus, and ba-cillus) are common contaminants in immunocompetent hosts with no "hardware".

Another area of difficulty lies with determining central line infections. It often is problematic to determine if the cultured microorganism (usually a staphylococcus or a Gram-negative rod) is a primary line pathogen. This key distinction has great import on the therapeutic regimen. If the line is the source of infection—(and not merely colonization)—the clinician needs to consider line removal.

Many authorities believe that quantitative blood cultures are important in interpreting blood culture results. Yagupsky and Nolte (10), in an extensive review on quantitative studies, note a clear trend toward low colony counts in contaminated blood cultures compared with true positive cultures. Diagnosis of coagulase-negative staphylococcal sepsis in young infants may be aided through these techniques (11). Quantitative studies also may prove useful in monitoring antibiotic efficacy and predicting the severity of clinical disease (10, 12). Several authorities believe that quantitative methods are important in diagnosing central line infections (13–15). Others note that this information has not been shown to be necessary to management, or to correlate with outcome (16).

Quantitative blood cultures hold promise in resolving many of these issues of contamination, colonization, and infection. However, all clinicians and investigators agree that the most important information is gained from the history and physical examination of the patient. The clinical picture is always the crucial variable that dictates the therapeutic plan.

Complications

Complications related to the procurement of blood cultures are divided into two groups: those causing potential adverse effects on the patient and those causing potential adverse effects on the results. The latter refers mainly to contaminated specimens. The blood culture may become contaminated from the patient's own normal skin flora, the blood drawer's hands, or the laboratory technician's respiratory droplets. If the clinician strictly adheres to the above-mentioned procedure, the contamination rate should generally not exceed 2 to 3% (4). Complications related to phlebotomy or interruption of an implanted line are discussed in Chapters 75 and 76.

RESPIRATORY SPECIMENS

Introduction

Respiratory infections are one of the most common reasons pediatric patients are brought to medical attention. Furthermore, despite the advances of critical care pediatrics, these infections still cause a significant number of pediatric deaths each year. It is therefore of utmost importance to know which study is indicated, how to properly and safely collect the specimen, and how to interpret the results. An accurate diagnosis is the cornerstone of a sound therapeutic plan.

Anatomy and Physiology

It is important to understand the anatomy of the respiratory system to know where to search for a pathogen, what normal flora and cells can be expected to be found, and what structures can be damaged by the procedure. A good nasopharyngeal sample yields a specimen with ciliated, columnar epithelial cells. The majority of respiratory viruses, *Chlamydia trachomatis* and *Bordetella pertussis,* are best recovered from here. The oropharynx is the area where group A β-hemolytic streptococcus (GABHS) is detected. Although the palatine tonsils regress by puberty, any inflamed areas of the posterior pharyngeal wall may harbor this causative pathogen of tonsillitis.

The trachea, because of its position inferior to the pharynx, is not an ideal location to recover potential bacterial pathogens. Procedures to recover tracheal microorganisms are invariably contaminated by pharyngeal flora. Furthermore, it usually is unclear if the recovered tracheal microorganisms accurately reflect the etiology of the suspected pneumonia. The bronchoalveolar lavage (BAL) and protected respiratory brush (PRB) procedures attempt to sample as close as possible to the area of pulmonary pathology. Both techniques ideally sample secondary or tertiary bronchi. The PRB has the added advantage of eliminating much of the upper airway contamination.

Indications

The most common indication for the throat swab is to detect GABHS. "Strep throat" is a common cause of pharyngitis in the school-aged child. Although usually seen in children 2 years of age and older, it can occur at any age. It commonly presents as sore throat with fever, and often is associated with headache and abdominal pain. Physical examination usually reveals pharyngeal erythema, often accompanied by tonsillar enlargement and exudate.

An important reason to culture even those with classic disease is for management of acute and postinfectious sequelae. Untreated patients may develop suppurative complications (otitis media, cervical adenitis, peritonsillar abscess) and nonsuppurative complications (rheumatic fever, glomerulonephritis). Scarlet fever, which can be recognized by its characteristic sandpaper-like erythematous rash, commonly occurs with pharyngitis and is caused by a group A streptococcal exotoxin.

Another reason for culturing patients is to appropriately manage contacts of the index patient who subsequently develop illness. Symptomatic family members should probably be cultured. Posttreatment cultures are indicated only in patients who are at high risk for rheumatic fever or who are persistently symptomatic (17).

Throat swabs also are commonly used to detect gonococcal pharyngitis. Gram stain and culture of an exudative pharyngitis are indicated in the appropriate clinical setting.

Patients at risk include those sexually active, and children who are suspected victims of abuse.

Another use of the swab culture is to screen the anterior nares (and other body sites) for *Staphylococcus aureus* and its associated toxins. For example, some strains of *S. aureus* elaborate a toxic shock syndrome toxin (TSST-1). Demonstration of *S. aureus* carriage also is important for infection control purposes in newborn nurseries, hospital outbreaks, and interhospital transfers.

Indications for using the nasopharyngeal swab (NPS) are becoming less common. To improve the yield, many of the previous indications are being replaced by recommendations for the nasopharyngeal aspirate (NPA). For example, detection of *B. pertussis* was previously done from an NPS, but now is being replaced by the NPA. The NPS is still being used, however, in the detection of *C. trachomatis* and measles virus.

As mentioned, most authorities now recommend an NPA to maximize the yield for the diagnosis of pertussis. Additionally, using the NPA obviates the need for special transport media. Notably, the best time to recover the microorganism is early in the illness, such as before the paroxysmal phase. Respiratory syncytial virus (RSV) is another circumstance when the NPA delivers a much greater yield than NPS. NPA is the collection method of choice for adenovirus, influenza virus, and parainfluenza virus.

Tracheal aspiration is probably more useful as a therapeutic rather than a diagnostic procedure. It usually is done through an endotracheal tube (ETT) to remove airway secretions and debris in order to optimize gas exchange, and to prevent atelectasis and infection. Diagnostically, the aspirate occasionally may be helpful in the investigation of infectious respiratory disease. Bacterial tracheitis is one such example.

A useful technique in diagnosing severe or unusual lower respiratory disease is BAL. One disease in which it has proven especially useful is *Pneumocystis carinii* pneumonia (PCP). This disease of immunocompromised patients is readily diagnosed by staining BAL washings. This early diagnosis avoids empiric therapy and leads to early treatment and improved outcome. Other common diseases of the immunocompromised also may be diagnosed with BAL; these include cytomegalovirus, *Aspergillus fumigatus*, *Candida albicans*, and *Legionella pneumophila*. Additionally, other bacterial, mycobacterial, and viral diseases can be diagnosed by BAL. Most agree that BAL is indicated before open lung biopsy to diagnose many of these diseases.

Protected respiratory brush (PRB) technique has become popular in many intensive care settings. This procedure is touted as a sensitive and specific approach to ventilated patients to determine the cause of pneumonia and to differentiate between infection and colonization (18). This technique is widely agreed to be useful in diagnosing many types of acute pneumonia. It also may have a role in routine surveillance culturing of stable, mechanically ventilated patients (19).

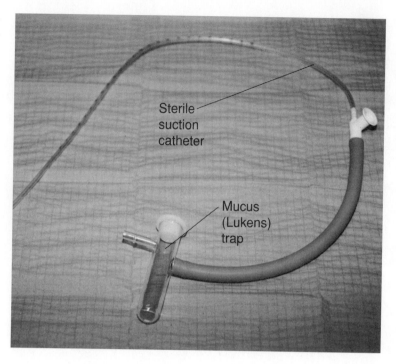

Figure 123.2.
Mucus (Lukens) trap with sterile suction catheter attached.

Equipment

Throat Swab
Sterile Dacron or rayon-tipped swabs with self-contained medium for transport, or
Sterile Dacron or rayon-tipped swabs
Sheep blood agar for direct inoculation

Nasopharyngeal Swab (NPS)
Calcium alginate or Dacron swab (aluminum shaft for *C. trachomatis*)
Regan-Lowe or Bordet-Gengou medium for *B. pertussis*
Tryptose phosphate broth with 5% bovine albumin, Hanks balanced salt solution with 5% gelatin or 10% albumin or buffered sucrose phosphate for *C. trachomatis* (20)

Nasopharyngeal Aspirate (NPA)
Lukens or mucus trap (Fig. 123.2)
Sterile suction catheter (Table 123.1)
Sterile nonbacteriostatic saline
Suction source (Table 123.1)

Tracheal Aspirate
Same as for nasopharyngeal aspirate, with oxygen source and catheter with side holes in addition to end holes.

Bronchoalveolar Lavage (BAL)
Same as for nasopharyngeal aspirate and tracheal aspirate. May be performed through a bronchoscope.

Protected Respiratory Brush
Telescoping, double-lumen brush catheter (Fig. 123.3)
Sterile scissors
Sterile, specimen collection container
Betadine®

Procedures

Throat Swab
In a cooperative child, the clinician first asks the patient to open the mouth, stick out the tongue, and say "ah." In a crying child, the clinician must coordinate the attempt with the patient's screaming. Either way, the goal is to swab the posterior pharynx, tonsils, and any areas of exudate or erythema. Care should be taken to avoid contact with the tongue or an-

Table 123.1.
Suction Catheters and Pressures

Age	Catheter Size*	Suction Pressure**
Premature infant	6	80–100
Infant	8	80–100
Preschool age	10	100–120
School age	12	100–120
Adolescent	14	120–150

* Catheter sizes given use French system
** Pressures in mm mercury

Chapter 123
Obtaining Biologic
Specimens

terior oral cavity. If a self-contained transport medium is used, usually the base must be broken to saturate the swab that has been reinserted into its container. These must be transported to the laboratory for processing within 4 hours. If plates are used, the specimen is gently swabbed onto the appropriate medium at bedside.

The same swabs may be used to culture and then inoculate Thayer-Martin chocolate agar in the detection of *Neisseria gonorrhoeae*. This agar inhibits growth of normal flora and nonpathogenic *Neisseria* species found on mucosal surfaces. Additionally, a carbon dioxide pellet or vial is included with these plates to enhance growth. After the plate has been swabbed with the specimen, the carbon dioxide is dispensed by either adding the pellet or shattering the vial. The system should be sealed to prevent the release of the carbon dioxide.

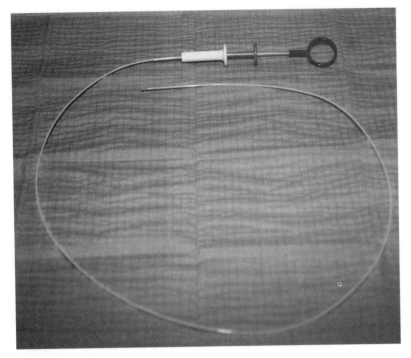

Figure 123.3.
Protected respiratory brush.

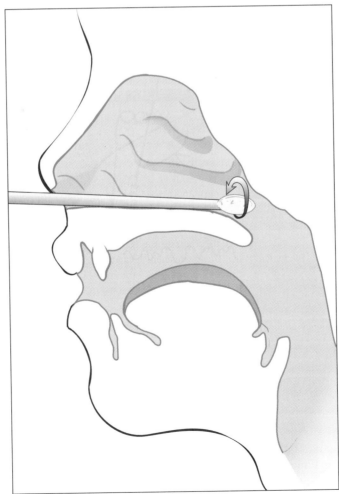

Figure 123.4.
Nasopharyngeal swab in nasopharynx.

Nasopharyngeal Swab

The nasopharyngeal swab (NPS) is obtained by inserting the swab a few centimeters into the nasopharynx (Fig. 123.4) and then rotating it gently to maximize the number of ciliated columnar epithelial cells. The specimen is then placed in the appropriate transport medium or streaked onto a plate at bedside.

Nasopharyngeal Aspirate

The nasopharyngeal aspirate (NPA) is set up by attaching the mucus trap to the suction source, and then to the sterile suction catheter. The wrapper is then removed from the catheter which is now gently inserted into the nasopharynx (Fig. 123.5). An approximate measurement of the appropriate distance is that from the tip of the nose to the tragus. Once the catheter is in the desired location, suction is applied. Using a slow, twirling mo-

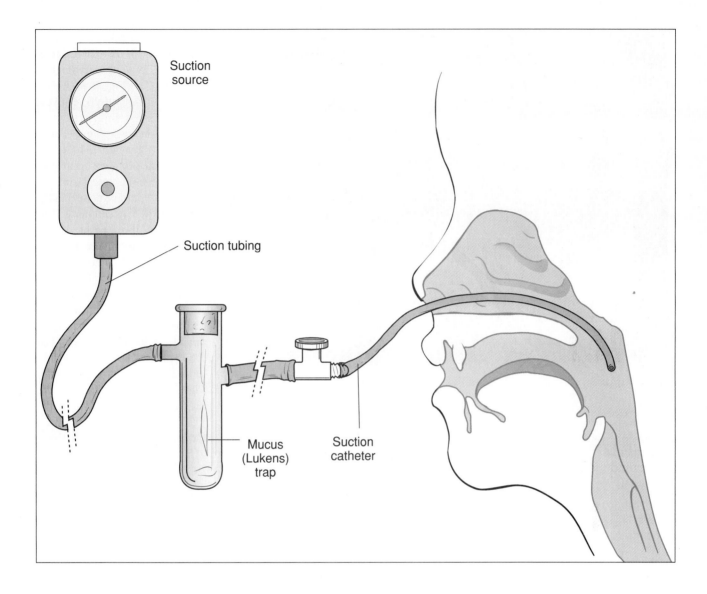

Figure 123.5.
Nasopharyngeal aspirate in
nasopharynx.

tion, the catheter is now withdrawn. Retained secretions in the catheter may be collected into the trap by suctioning a few milliliters of sterile, nonbacteriostatic saline. The original rubber tubing of the trap is now disconnected from the catheter and attached to the trap to seal and close the system.

It is important to transport these specimens to the laboratory as quickly as possible. Viral specimens should not be frozen. If laboratory processing is to be delayed, the specimens should be stored (no longer than a few days) at 4°C. Note also that viruses are inactivated by ultraviolet light, therefore specimens should be shielded appropriately.

Tracheal Aspirate

The tracheal aspirate procedure (Fig. 123.6) is similar to the NPA. The endotracheally in- tubated patient is first preoxygenated with 100% oxygen for 1 minute. The oxygen source is then removed. The sterile suction catheter, which is attached to the mucus trap and suction source as described, is quickly guided into the ETT with a sterile, gloved hand. The catheter is advanced until mild re- sistance is encountered (the carina), and is then withdrawn 1 to 2 cm. Suction is now ap- plied and the specimen is collected using a slow, twirling motion. The catheter is now withdrawn and removed.

The patient is immediately reoxygenated with 100% oxygen, and then placed on the previous ventilator settings. Note that if the aspirate is difficult to collect because of thick secretions, a few milliliters of sterile, nonbac- teriostatic saline are instilled into the ETT, the patient is given a few hand-ventilated

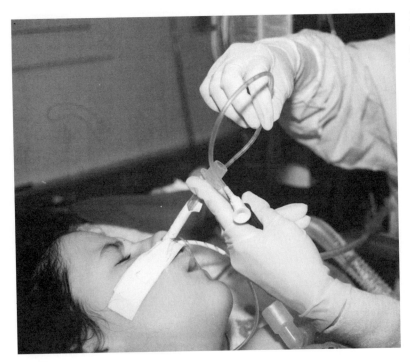

Figure 123.6.
Tracheal aspirate
performed by nurse.

Protected Respiratory Brush

The protected respiratory brush (PRB) specimens are obtained using a telescoping, double-lumen brush catheter (Fig. 123.7). This apparatus has a distal, polyethylene glycol occlusion to minimize contamination. Also needed are sterile scissors, a sterile specimen collection container, and betadine.

The PRB procedure also can be done either with bronchoscopic assistance or blindly. If the procedure is to be done blindly, the distance that the PRB apparatus will be advanced must first be premeasured. One method uses the patient's most recent anteroposterior chest radiograph (19). From this radiograph, the distance from the end of the ETT to midpoint of the right mainstem bronchus is recorded. The PRB is ultimately advanced based on this measurement and on the child's weight—if the child weighs less than 10 kg, the PRB is advanced 1 cm additionally; if 10 to 20 kg, 2 cm; and if greater than 20 kg, 3 cm further.

After measurement, the patient is preoxygenated. The PRB apparatus is then advanced into the ETT. At the desired distance, the inner catheter is advanced out of the outer catheter by squeezing the inner and outer handles together, which jettisons the protective polyethylene glycol plug. The clinician, using back and forth motion of the thumb ring, now brushes this bronchus several times with the previously protected brush. When completed, the brush is retracted back into the catheters, and the unit is withdrawn. The brush must now be sterilely recovered. The outer catheter and then the inner catheter are sterilized with Betadine®. The brush is then exposed, and is cut with sterile scissors into a sterile container for transport to the laboratory. This procedure is illustrated in Figure 123.7.

breaths, and the above mentioned procedure is repeated. The aspirate is transported as described.

Bronchoalveolar Lavage

The bronchoalveaolar lavage (BAL) procedure is similar to the tracheal aspirate. The patient is preoxygenated as previously described, and the suction catheter is advanced. The key difference is that the catheter is passed beyond the carina until firm resistance is met (ideally into a second or third generation bronchus). Sterile, nonbacteriostatic saline is now instilled by sterile syringe through the catheter. The volume instilled is approximately 1 to 2 cc/kg to a maximum of 20 cc. The saline is allowed to dwell for several seconds and then is suctioned into a mucus trap as described. Ideally, 80% of the volume instilled should be withdrawn. This lavage may be repeated, providing the patient tolerates the procedure. Note that catheter placement is greatly improved if this procedure is aided by a fiberoptic bronchoscope.

Interpretation of Results

Many institutions routinely perform a throat swab for rapid GABHS antigen detection, with the culture. This is usually a latex agglu-

Figure 123.7.
Protected respiratory brush procedure.
A. Catheter inserted into bronchus.
B. Brush advanced out of catheter to collect specimen.
C. Brush withdrawn back into catheter for removal.
D. Brush tip sterilely cut with scissors into specimen cup for transport.

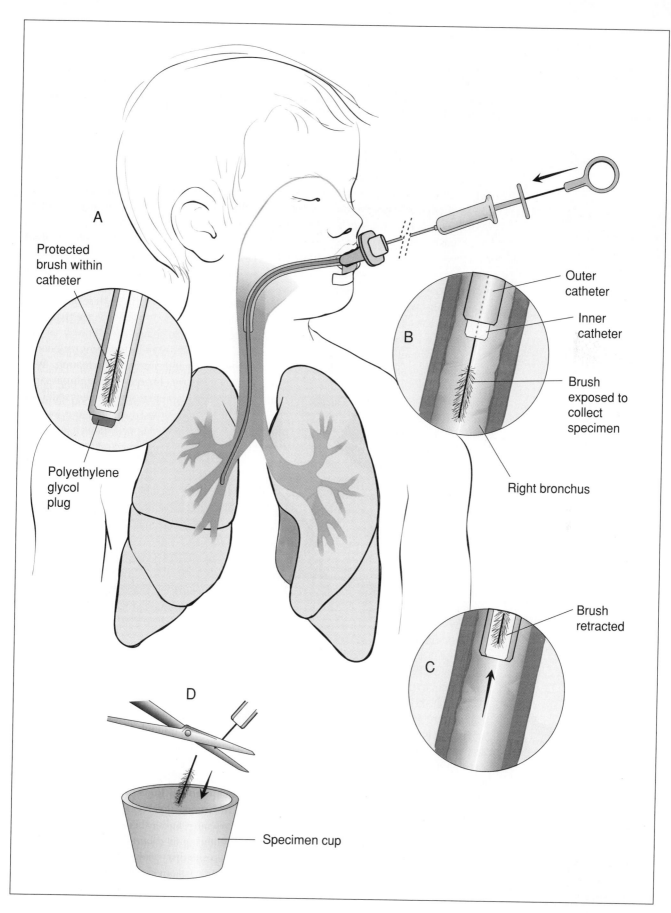

A

Protected brush within catheter

Polyethylene glycol plug

B

Outer catheter

Inner catheter

Brush exposed to collect specimen

Right bronchus

C

Brush retracted

D

Specimen cup

tination or an enzyme-linked immunosorbent assay (ELISA). The sensitivity of these rapid studies is reported at 70 to 90% (20), and the specificity is better than 98% (2). It is recommended that cultures be performed on rapid tests that are negative. The culture is the gold standard, and takes 24 to 48 hours to incubate. Proper technique is key to an accurate result. The 10% false-negative rate reported on properly performed cultures (21) is most likely due to antibiotic pretreatment and overgrowth of other microorganisms. Carriers of GABHS account for most of the false positives. Considerable variation exists on how physicians manage presumed streptococcal pharyngitis. On patients with negative rapid studies, some initiate treatment pending the culture results, whereas others opt to wait until the culture results are known. Some physicians do only cultures, whereas others do no studies and treat all patients fitting the appropriate clinical picture of GABHS infection.

Interpreting the throat swab for *N. gonorrhoeae* is less confusing. Though a Gram stain with Gram-negative diplococci associated with leukocytes may be helpful, most generally follow the results of the culture. The *S. aureus* screen of the anterior nares, however, must be interpreted with caution. Ten to 30% are colonized with *S. aureus,* and 10% of the normal *S. aureus* strains which colonize the nares can produce TSST-1 (17).

Chlamydia and measles virus both may be detected by rapid antigen studies done on the nasopharyngeal swab. Fluorescent antibody (FAB) and ELISA are the two most common techniques used. Note that it is difficult to culture both organisms.

As mentioned, *B. pertussis* should be probed with nasopharyngeal aspirate, rather than nasopharyngeal swab. Interestingly, the rapid method (usually the FAB), though relatively insensitive, still may be more sensitive than culture. *B. pertussis* is a fastidious bacterium that is difficult to recover. For this reason, many laboratories perform both FAB and culture to enhance detection. The rapid detection of RSV is reported to have sensitivities of 80 to 90% (17) and a specificity of greater than 96% (22). The ELISA (which is easily automated) is preferred over the FAB as the latter requires high-quality antisera, fluoresceinated conjugants, a fluorescent microscope, and an experienced microscopist (20). RSV culture generally takes 5 to 7 days.

Adenovirus, influenza virus, and parainfluenza virus may be detected by the rapid methods previously mentioned. The key is for the NPA to collect a sufficient number of cells. Culture of these viruses may take several days to 2 weeks.

The difficulty with interpreting tracheal aspirates is due to contamination and colonization. A pure growth of one microorganism with many neutrophils is highly suggestive, but unfortunately rare. The patient's clinical status must be carefully considered when interpreting these results.

The excellent sensitivity and specificity of BAL has made it the diagnostic procedure of choice in diagnosing PCP. Most research, however, has centered on the bronchoscope-assisted BAL. It remains to be seen if the procedure, when performed blindly, is equally effective.

The PRB may offer the clinician the most easily interpreted information. When done properly, little contamination should occur. Again, more research needs to be done on blind collections.

Complications

Throat swab, nasopharyngeal swab, and nasopharyngeal aspirate have similar, minor complications. Gagging is probably the most common complication. Occasionally, emesis occurs. Supine infants who vomit should immediately be turned to one side to prevent aspiration. Traumatic bleeding may occur with the throat swab, and epistaxis is not uncommon with the nasopharyngeal procedures. These are nearly always mild and self-limited. Occasionally, the NPA catheter is difficult to pass into the nasopharynx. The clinician needs to recall that the nasal "tunnel" goes back (in the direction of the occiput) and not up toward the eyes. Minor discomfort is common to all procedures.

Complications associated with tracheal aspirate, bronchoalveolar lavage, and protected respiratory brush are understandably more serious. These are obviously sicker patients, and all three techniques necessitate temporary airway compromise. Continuous monitoring of vital signs and pulse oximetry is mandatory. Hypoxemia is the foremost complication. It is crucial to minimize the duration of the procedure. Pre- and postoxygenation with 100% oxygen is important for adequate reserve and rapid recovery, respectively. Bradycardia, secondary to vagal stimulation, may occur. Other dysrhythmias, presumably secondary to hypoxia, may rarely be seen. The procedure should be stopped immediately if these rhythm disturbances are encountered. Bronchoconstriction may occur, especially in those with reactive airways. Atelectasis may result if the catheter diameter is excessively large or if the procedure takes too long. Increased intracranial pressure is a consideration in a small population of patients. This most likely results from gagging, and may be prevented by lidocaine (intravenous or tracheal spray).

Traumatic mucosal injury to the airways may occur with any of these procedures. It is therefore important to use soft catheters, minimal necessary suction pressures, and gentle technique. Bleeding is especially possible with the PRB. Despite the seemingly harsh brushing, however, significant bleeding is rare. Pneumothorax, fortunately, is rare with the PRB procedure.

DERMATOLOGIC SPECIMENS

Introduction

In pediatrics, the majority of children with a new onset of cutaneous lesions (and fever) have an infectious disease whether viral, bacterial, or fungal. In most instances, characterization of the lesions on physical examination will lead to the correct diagnosis without need for specimen collection. However, because the skin is accessible, it is a good source from which specimens can be obtained for microscopic examination, isolation, identification, and susceptibility testing of pathogenic microorganisms.

Anatomy and Physiology

Impetigo is a common infection of the epidermis usually caused by group A streptococci or *Staphylococcus aureus* (23). Infections start with thin-walled vesicles or pustules which easily rupture and release a cloudy yellow exudate. When dried, the fluid forms honey-colored crusts. The exudate may inoculate other areas of the body and spread the infection. In addition, *S. aureus* causes a bullous form of impetigo which begins with a flaccid pustule sometimes quite large in diameter (3 to 4 cm). Lesions often can be seen in opposing skin surfaces, referred to as kissing lesions. In cases of extensive or atypical impetigo, wiping away the crusted exudate or unroofing the bullae to culture the fluid will help confirm the diagnosis (see Procedures in this section).

Cellulitis is a deeper inflammation of the skin involving the subcutaneous tissues. Hallmarks of this infection are erythema with ill-defined borders, swelling, and pain. Cellulitis may develop secondary to trauma, or following a superficial skin eruption such as primary varicella. *S. aureas,* group A streptococci, *Streptococcus pneumoniae,* and *Haemophilus influenzae* type b are possible etiologies of cellulitis (23, 24).

Fever, rigors, and vomiting may be the initial symptoms of meningococcemia. The majority of children will develop cutaneous lesions. The lesions are usually petechial, but blanching macular, papular, or even urticarial lesions may be noted initially (23). As the disease progresses, the petechiae may enlarge and develop a vesicular center or even necrosis. The lesions are most prominent on the extremities and trunk. The etiology is *Neisseria meningitidis* and is isolated from the blood in virtually all patients. If a child has been pretreated with antibiotics, demonstrating organisms on Gram stain obtained by scraping the cutaneous lesions is occasionally helpful. Although reports vary, organisms are seen on Gram stain or culture in approximately 50 to 70% of cases (25, 26).

Finally, it is important to remember that despite signs and symptoms of shock, and petechial lesions that initially suggest meningococcemia, other pathogens such as *S. pneumoniae, Neisseria gonorrhoeae,* and *H. influenzae* type b also may cause a similar illness and presentation. In adolescents with disseminated gonococcal infections due to *N. gonorrhoeae,* migratory arthritis and skin lesions are hallmarks of the disease and have been called the arthritis-dermatitis syndrome. The skin lesions are usually few in number and thorough physical examination is required to not overlook them. They can be found most commonly on the distal extremities. The lesions may start as papules but evolve into pustules on an erythematous base.

Although skin lesions should be cultured (with joint effusions and blood), they are frequently negative.

Only *S. aureus*, which belongs to phage group II (types 3A, 3B, 3C, 55, 71), can cause staphylococcal scalded-skin syndrome (SSSS) (23, 24). An exfoliative exotoxin, often originating at a distant site not on the skin, causes generalized bulla formation and exfoliation. Initially, the child may present with fever and erythroderma, which progresses shortly to large flaccid bullae filled with clear fluid. The upper layer of the epidermis appears wrinkled, and may be removed with only light pressure (Nikolsky's sign). The organism usually is not recovered from the areas of exfoliation. Instead, a primary cellulitis, the nares, conjunctiva, stool, or blood should be cultured.

Occurring most frequently with *Pseudomonas* or fungal septicemia, ecthyma gangrenosa is characterized by a rounded, indurated, painless mass with a central necrotic black center. Notably, the border, which can be irregular, is usually red and nonblanching or purpuric. Gram-stained smear of the exudate, or scraping of the lesions, will show either the Gram-negative rods of *Pseudomonas* or the large Gram-positive cocci of a fungal infection.

Herpes simplex virus is one of the most common viral infections of man. Herpes simplex virus (HSV) infection is unique to humans, who serve as the only natural host of the virus. Herpesvirus hominis has two major groups, type 1 and type 2 (23). Children often exhibit the results of primary infection including herpes gingivostomatitis, herpes keratoconjunctivitis, herpes vulvovaginitis and progenitalis (in sexually active adolescents), neonatal herpes, Kaposi's varicelliform eruption (eczema herpeticum), and herpetic whitlow (primary cutaneous inoculation). Except for herpetic whitlow, the cutaneous and mucous membrane involvement is characterized by grouped or clustered vesicular lesions on an erythematous base. In the mouth, the lesions may coalesce into yellowish, painful plaques. In general, fever and pain accompany the primary infection. Herpetic whitlow is more commonly pustular in appearance, and forms deep bullous swellings on the fingers. It often appears as deep, painful bubbles under the skin sur-

rounded by erythema (23). Mucous membrane vesicle or conjunctival cultures can be collected to confirm the diagnosis (see Procedures in this section).

Another member of the herpes virus family, varicella-zoster virus (VZV) causes a common childhood disease, chicken pox. This primary infection is widespread, with attack rates of 85% among susceptible siblings, and less among day care attendees. Although common and easily recognized, it can be lethal in the immunocompromised host, and can spread quite easily among susceptible hospitalized children. The incubation period following exposure is 10 to 21 days, with most children developing symptoms at 14 to 16 days. The infection begins with a prodrome of low grade fever, headache, and malaise. The onset of rash begins as papules, which progress to vesicles, pustules, and finally crusted lesions. Two hallmarks of the disease are the characteristic appearance of the delicate vesicle described as a "dewdrop on a rose petal," and the lesions are present in various forms (papules, vesicles, umbilicated pustules) simultaneously. Umbilicated vesicles and pustules also are common. The lesions involve the scalp, face, trunk, and extremities, and come in crops usually over the first 3 days after onset. The child is no longer infectious when the lesions crust.

Herpes zoster or shingles occurs as VZV reactivates following the primary chicken pox illness. Factors that lead to reactivation of the latent VZV and the characteristic grouped vesicles on an erythematous base in a dermatomal distribution, are currently being intensely researched. Although zoster is thought of as occurring only in adults, children also may present with shingles. These children usually have a history of chicken pox in the first year of life. The rash resolves in 7 to 14 days in 90% of children (23). In an otherwise healthy child with shingles, an immunologic evaluation is not indicated. Occasionally, depending on the circumstances, diagnosis may be confirmed with a culture and/or fluorescent monoclonal antibody test.

Superficial fungal skin infections are common in children. Their young age and normally close play predispose them to three common types of fungal infections: the dermatophytoses (tinea or ringworm), tinea versicolor, and candidiasis (thrush and diaper dermatitis). Tinea infections usually are caused by strains of *Microsporum* and *Trichophyton* (23, 27).

Tinea capitus is the most common dermatophytosis of childhood (23). Characteristically, hair loss occurs with the hair shafts broken off close to the scalp in a circular pattern. Slight redness and scaling also may be noted. Diagnosis by Wood's lamp is less likely than in times past. *Microsporum audonine* infection, once the most common cause of tinea capitus, causes the hair to fluoresce a brilliant green color. Currently, however, *Trichophyton tonsurans* causes the majority of cases and does not fluoresce under a Wood's lamp (23).

Tinea corporis, because of its round or oval appearance with a raised scaling border, is often referred to as ringworm. Lesions may present in many forms, however, including eczematous, vesicular, and pustular. Scrapings of the lesions for culture will confirm diagnosis.

Onychomycosis (tinea unguium) is a common, chronic fungal infection of the fingernails and toenails. It occurs primarily in adolescents and adults and is difficult to cure. However, mucocutaneous candidiasis, associated with congenital immunodeficiency and endocrinopathy (e.g., hypoparathyroidism), can present in childhood with recurrent superficial *Candida* infections—especially onychomycosis.

Scabies is a contagious pruritic disease caused by the arachnid mite, *Sarcoptes scabiei,* which is less than 0.5 mm in length. The mite burrows underneath the skin in the stratum corneum and deposits eggs. History reveals intense pruritus, especially at night, usually with multiple family members affected. The rash is characterized by pruritic papules, vesicles, pustules, and occasionally (only 10% of cases) linear burrows associated with scaling (32). Importantly, the distribution of the rash is different between infants and young children versus older children, adolescents, and adults. In infants and toddlers, the axilla, lumbosacrum, groin, trunk, head, neck, palms, and soles can be affected. In older children and adults, the head is almost never involved and the rash is limited more to the extremities, interdigital webs, and flexures of the wrists and arms; however, the breasts, areolae, genitalia, and waist also can be involved. Diagnosis occasionally can be confirmed by a skin scraping which reveals the eggs or a mite. The yield of the skin scraping is frustratingly low in children, and often diagnosis is based purely on the history and physical examination (32).

Indications

As previously stated, in many cases obtaining specimens from the skin is not necessary, as the diagnosis is established during the history and physical examination. As referenced in Table 123.2, obtaining dermatologic specimens in children includes four general indications. First is the immunocompetent child in which the presentation is atypical, and the culture or rapid diagnostic test is helpful in confirming the suspected diagnosis. Second is the immunocompromised child who, in most cases, should have the diagnosis confirmed with specimen collection. These children are at risk for more extensive and/or atypical infections with opportunistic microorganisms. Special treatments may be needed in these cases. Third, any child who is severely ill (sepsis or shock) should have cutaneous specimens sent to the microbiology and/or virology laboratories for Gram stain or rapid diagnostic tests. Obviously, resuscitation and antimicrobial therapy should be instituted before specimen collection. Fourth is any infection in which the spread among hospitalized children is possible. For example, the use of a negative pressure isolation room (which are often few in number) usually justifies confirming the diagnosis of chicken pox. Virtually no contraindications exist for these procedures.

Equipment

Unroofing pustules and crusts
Isopropyl alcohol
Needle—18 to 23 gauge
Tuberculin syringe
Sterile swab with self-contained transport medium

Petechiae, ecthyma gangrenosa
Isopropyl alcohol
Scalpel—No. 11 blade

Table 123.2.
Indications for Dermatologic Procedures

Infection	Lesion Type	Procedure	Procedure Indicated	Comments*	Tests
BACTERIAL Impetigo	Pustules Crusted lesions	Unroofing	Rarely	2, 4	Gram stain and culture
Meningococcemia	Petechiae** Purpura**	Scraping	Always	3	Gram stain and culture
Staphylococcal scalded-skin syndrome	Bullae Pustules Exfoliation	Unroofing	Always	3; search for the primary site of infection	Gram stain and culture
Pseudomonal (or fungal) sepsis	Ecthyma Gangrenosa	Scraping	Always	3	Gram stain and culture
VIRAL Herpes simplex virus	Vesicles Pustules	Unroofing	Occasionally	1, 2; in neonates always obtain specimen	Rapid diagnostic slide; culture
Varicella	Vesicles Pustules	Unroofing	Rarely	1, 2	Rapid diagnostic slide; culture
Zoster	Vesicles Pustules	Unroofing	Rarely	1, 2	Rapid diagnostic slide; culture
FUNGAL Tinea corpous Tinea capitus Onychomycosis	Scaling papules Alopecia Vesicle, pustules	Scraping	Occasionally	2, 4	Oricult
SCABIES	Papules Pustules Vesicles	Scraping	Occasionally	1, 2, 4	Microscopic evaluation

* Comments
1. Obtain a specimen if child is admitted to the hospital for infection control purposes; the child should be placed in isolation pending results.
2. If diagnosis is unclear or if the child is immunocompromised, then obtain specimen.
3. Always obtain a specimen; the results of the culture may be important in treatment.
4. With extensive infection requiring hospitalization, culture may be helpful in determining appropriate treatment.

** Other cause of petechiae and purpura include *H. influenzae* type b, *N. gonorrhoeae*, *S. pneumoniae*. Rocky Mountain spotted fever, purpura fulminans.

Glass slide
Sterile swab with self-contained transport medium

Unroofing vesicles
Isopropyl alcohol
Needle—23 gauge sterile
Sterile mini-tip Dacron or rayon-tipped swab on a metal or plastic shaft
Glass slide
Viral transport media

For conjunctival lesions
same as above and
Chlamydia collection kit
Viral/*Chlamydia* collection media

It is important to note that calcium alginate tipped or wooden shaft swabs should not be used for collecting these specimens, because they inhibit growth of some viruses, *Chlamydia,* and bacteria (28, 29). These specimens should be transported in viral transport medium. The medium includes gentamicin to inhibit bacterial overgrowth, and nutrients (sucrose, L-glutamic acid, bovine albumin, etc.) to support viral and chlamydial growth (30).

Fungal skin and nail scraping
Adhesive tape
Scalpel—No. 11 blade (for nails)
Toothbrush (for skin and scalp)
Sterile swab (for weeping lesions)
Wood's lamp
Oricult-DTM® (Orion Diagnostica; Espoo, Finland; Fig. 123.10)

Scraping for scabies
Isopropyl alcohol
Scalpel—No. 11 blade
Mineral oil
Glass slide

Procedures

Unroofing Pustules and Crusted Lesions
An intact pustule should be chosen. Alcohol

should be lightly applied and allowed to dry completely. The pustule is unroofed with a 23-gauge needle. The fluid and the basal cells are collected by rotating the swab vigorously in the pustule. If *N. gonorrhoeae* is suspected, inoculate Thayer-Martin agar. The agar, with carbon dioxide pellet or vial in an airtight pouch, will enhance the growth (31).

If the pustule is large, an 18-gauge needle on a tuberculin syringe can be used to puncture the pustule. The pustule fluid can be sent for Gram stain and culture. Crusted lesions will require crust removal. The moist base of the lesion should be vigorously swabbed with a premoistened sterile swab and sent to the microbiology laboratory for Gram stain and culture (Fig. 123.8).

Petechiae, Purpura, Ecthyma Gangrenosa
Lesions should be carefully scrutinized. Vesicles, pustules, or bullae are preferable. If none are present, a new petechial or purpuric lesion is selected. Enough specimen for Gram stain and culture will be obtained only by scraping vigorously into the skin to cause an abrasion and weeping. The material should be collected from the margin of the larger lesion. The material can then be transferred to a glass slide for Gram stain, and the swab is sent for Gram stain and culture (Figure 123.9). Gram-stained smears from petechial skin lesions have been reported to show Gram-negative, bean-shaped diplococci, consistent with meningococci, in 50 to 70% of cases. Organisms can be demonstrated in endothelial cells and neutrophils. Although cultures from these scrapings are frequently negative, blood and/or CSF cultures are frequently positive.

Unroofing Vesicles and Conjunctival Sampling
A new skin vesicle should be chosen and alcohol applied lightly. Vigorous wiping is avoided so as to not disrupt the vesicle integrity. The alcohol is allowed to dry completely. With a 23-gauge sterile needle, the vesicle is carefully unroofed, taking care to not cause bleeding. After unroofing, the mini-tipped rayon or Dacron swab is rolled vigorously in the base of the lesion. The collection of cells from the vesicle base are then transferred to the glass slide by rolling the swab onto the glass, spreading the cells over

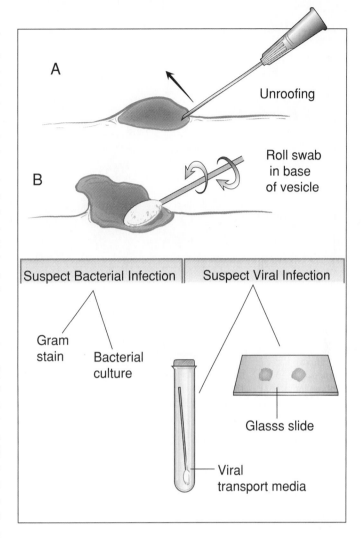

Figure 123.8.
Procedure for unroofing a vesicle or pustule.

a small circular area (diameter of a pencil eraser) in each of two locations on the slide (one for a control). The slide is allowed to air dry, and submit to the clinical virology laboratory. To test for both HSV and VZV, a separate slide should be prepared for each virus. The slides are air dried and labelled appropriately with the patient's name and collection date. The used swab should be placed in viral transport media and sent for routine viral culture. This procedure is illustrated in Figure 123.8.

A fluorescent monoclonal antibody test can be performed on the slides. When adequate cells are present on the slides, the sensitivity and specificity are approximately 95% (29, 32). These tests can be performed in 1 to 2 hours. It is important to remember that HSV grows in tissue culture as quickly as bacteria—usually within 72 hours. VZV take much longer to be isolated in tissue culture (7 to 14 days).

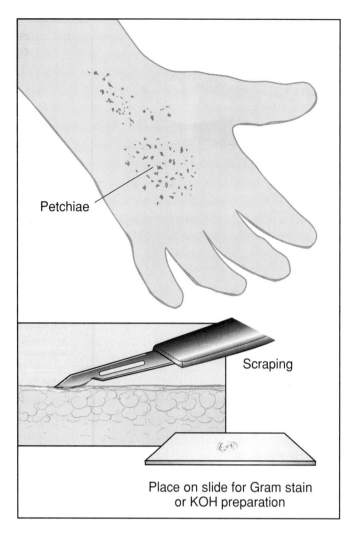

Petchiae

Scraping

Place on slide for Gram stain
or KOH preparation

Figure 123.9.
Procedure for scraping
petechiae and superficial
fungal infections (tinea
corporis, tinea capitus,
onychomycosis).

cells, will render the slide uninterpretable. Chlamydial culture remains the more sensitive procedure, and a specimen should be sent for routine culture when submitting a slide for rapid antigen detection (30).

Fungal Skin and Nail Scraping
A scraping is collected from the edge of a dry lesion with two glass slides or toothbrush and placed directly onto Oricult-DTM® or other suitable fungal detection system. Wet or weeping skin lesions should be swabbed with a Dacron swab. The swab is inoculated by rolling over the agar surface. Forceps also can be used to collect hairs. Those that resist the pull should be left in place; those that are loose should be selected. The medium is inoculated by pressing the hairs gently against the agar surface. For onychomycosis, a scalpel should be inserted under the protruding nail and scraped. The scrapings are collected on the Oricult-DTM® agar (Fig. 123.10). Inoculate the agar at 30°C, or at room temperature, with the lid on loosely to allow free passage of air.

Scraping for Scabies
The most likely lesions to yield evidence of mite infestation (e.g., mite, ova, larval, or fecal material) are fresh papules or burrows. A bright light is helpful. Areas of excoriation are not suitable. Once the lesion is identified, alcohol is applied lightly to the skin and allowed to dry completely. A single drop of mineral oil is applied to the papule. The epidermis is superficially abraded with a scalpel blade and the material is transferred to a slide and examined under a microscope with 10 × power to identify signs of *Sarcoptes scabiei* (33).

Interpretation of Results

Proper specimen collection and handling are vital components of any good diagnostic laboratory. Each laboratory has slightly different requirements for handling specimens. The time and expense of performing these procedures for the diagnosis of bacterial, viral, and fungal infections necessitate an understanding of those requirements. Most diagnostic laboratories have specimen collection and transport guidelines which should be reviewed by those clinicians collecting the specimens.

Conjunctival swabs should be taken by stroking the lower conjunctival space of the eye five or six times with a cotton swab to obtain epithelial cells. To diagnose HSV or adenovirus, the swab is used to spread the cells over a small circular area (diameter of a pencil eraser) in each of two separate areas of a glass microscope slide. The slides are air dried. A fluorescent monoclonal antibody test should be performed. The swab should be sent in viral transport medium for viral isolation (30).

If *Chlamydia* is suspected, the swab is dropped into viral/chlamydial transport medium. Specimens are inoculated onto tissue culture cells and stained with *Chlamydia*-specific monoclonal antibodies after 48 hours of incubation. Using a rapid antigen detection kit (e.g., Syva Microtrak®) also is an option. Specimen collection is critical, and the kit instructions for collection and slide preparation should be strictly followed. Gross contamination of pus or discharge, or a lack of epithelial

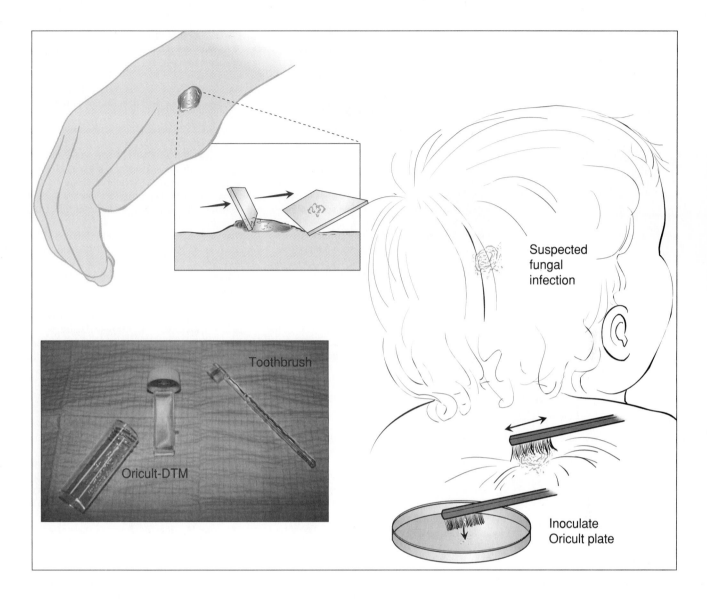

Growth in the Oricult-DTM® system for superficial fungal infection usually occurs in 2 to 7 days. A change in the color of the agar slide from translucent yellow to red, beneath white colonies, indicates the presence of dermatophytes. The sample is considered negative if no growth has appeared within 14 days. False-positive results are sometimes seen with certain saprophytic molds which are contaminants. Although a red color change may occur, it usually occurs only when molds have formed well-developed colonies, often with darkened aerial hyphae.

Complications

Minimal complications are associated with these procedures. They are, therefore, rarely contraindicated. Possible complications include bleeding, pain, or subsequent infection at the site of the procedure. For the vast majority of patients, however, the complications are well tolerated.

REFERENCES

1. Ackerman VP, Pritchard RC. Blood culture techniques. A survey in Australasian Laboratories. Pathology 1987;19:265–273.
2. Jui J, Brancato, FP. Blood cultures and anaerobic culture techniques. In: Roberts JR, Hedges JR, eds. Clinical procedures in emergency medicine. 2nd ed. Philadelphia: WB Saunders, 1991, pp. 1093–1099.
3. Aschner JL, Punsalang A, Maniscalco WM, Menegus MA. Percutaneous central venous catheter colonization with malessezia furfur: incidence and clinical significance. Pediatrics 1987;80:535–539.
4. Strand CL, Wajsbort RR, Sturmann K. Effect of

Figure 123.10.
Collection of specimen from presumed fungal lesions.

Chapter 123
Obtaining Biologic
Specimens

iodophor vs iodine tincture skin preparation on blood culture contamination rate. JAMA 1993;269:1004–1006.

5. Isaacman DJ, Karasic RB. Lack of effect of changing needles on contamination of blood cultures. Pediatr Infect Dis J 1990;9:274–278.

6. Krumholz HM, Cummings S, York M. Blood culture phlebotomy: switching needles does not prevent contamination. Ann Intern Med 1990;113:290–292.

7. Thamlikitkul V, Chokloikaew S, Tangtrakul T, Siripoonkiat P, Wongpreedee N, Danchaivijitr S. Blood culture: comparison of outcomes between switch-needle and no-switch techniques. Am J Infect Control 1992;20:122–125.

8. Leisure MK, Moore DM, Schwartzman JD, Hayden GF, Donowitz LG. Changing the needle when inoculating blood cultures: a no-benefit and high-risk procedure. JAMA 1990;264:2111–2112.

9. Jagger J, Hunt EH, Brand-Elnaggar J, Pearson R. Rates of needle-stick injury caused by various devices in a university hospital. N Engl J Med 1988;319:284–288.

10. Yagupsky P, Nolte FS. Quantitative aspects of septicemia. Clin Microbiol Rev 1990;3:269–279.

11. St. Geme JW, Bell LM, Baumgart S, D'Angio CT, Harris MC. Distinguishing sepsis from blood culture contamination in young infants with blood cultures growing coagulase-negative Staphylococci. Pediatrics 1990;86:157–162.

12. Marshall GS, Bell LM. Correlates of high grade and low grade Haemophilus influenzae bacteremia. Pediatr Infect Dis J 1988;7:86–90.

13. Flynn PM, Shenep JL, Stokes DC, Barrett FF. In-situ management of confirmed central venous catheter-related bacteremia. Pediatr Infect Dis J 1987;6:729–734.

14. Raucher HS, Hyatt AC, Barzilai A, et al. Quantitative blood cultures in the evaluation of septicemia in children with broviac catheters. J Pediatr 1984;104:29–33.

15. Wing WJ, Norden CW, Shadduck RK, Winkelstein A. Use of quantitative bacteriologic techniques to diagnose catheter-related sepsis. Arch Intern Med 1979;139:482–483.

16. Decker ND, Edwards KM. Central venous catheter infections. Pediatr Clin North Am 1988;35:579–612.

17. Peter G, Lepow M, McCracken GH, Phillips CF, eds. Report of the committee on infectious diseases. 22nd ed. Elk Grove Village, IL: American Academy of Pediatrics, 1991.

18. Chastre J, Viau F, Brun P, et al. Prospective evaluation of the protected specimen brush for the diagnosis of pulmonary infections in ventilated patients. Am Rev Resp Dis 1984;130:924–929.

19. Clarke WR, Bell LM, Conte VH, McGowan KL. Blind endobronchial cultures: an alternative respiratory culturing method in children with chronic respiratory failure. J Crit Care 1992;7:230–235.

20. Feigen RD, Cherry JD, eds. Textbook of pediatric infectious diseases. 3rd ed. Philadelphia: WB Saunders, 1992.

21. Bisno AL. The rise and fall of rheumatic fever. JAMA 1985;254:538–541.

22. Ahluwalia GS, Hammond GW. Comparison of cell cultures and three enzyme-linked immunosorbent assays for the rapid diagnosis of respiratory syncytial virus from nasopharyngeal aspirate and tracheal secretion specimens. Diagn Microbiol Infect Dis 1988;9:187–192.

23. Hurwitz S. Bacterial and protozoal infection of the skin (Chapter 10, pp. 275–310); Viral diseases of the skin (Chapter 11, pp. 318–341); Skin disorders due to fungi (Chapter 13, pp. 372–400). In: Clinical pediatric dermatology. 2nd ed. Philadelphia: WB Saunders, 1993.

24. Swartz MN, Weinberg AN. Infections due to Gram-positive bacteria (Chapter 176). In: Fitzpatrick TB, Eisen AZ, Walff K, et al., eds. Dermatology in general medicine. 3rd ed. New York: McGraw-Hill, 1987, pp. 2100–2121.

25. Schachner LA, Hansen RC, eds. Pediatric dermatology. New York: Churchill Livingstone, 1988, p. 1320.

26. Demis DJ. Bacterial infections. In: Clinical cermatology. Vol. 3. Philadelphia: JB Lippincott Company, 1990, p. 2.

27. Goslen JB, Kobayashi GS. Fungal diseases with cutaneous involvement (Section 27, Chapter 181). In: Fitzpatrick TB, Eisen AZ, Wolff K, et al., eds. Dermatology in general medicine. 3rd ed. New York: McGraw-Hill, 1987.

28. Chernesky MA, Ray CG, Smith TF. Laboratory diagnosis of viral infections. Cumitech 1982;15:1–17.

29. Greenberg SB, Krilov LR. Laboratory dagnosis of viral respiratory disease. Cumitech 1986;21:1–16.

30. Lennette DA, Schmidt NJ. Diagnostic procedures for viral, rickiettsial, and chlamydial Infections. 5th ed. New York: American Public Health Association, 1979.

31. Isenberg HD, Schoenkrecht FD, Graevenitz A. Collection and processing of bacteriological specimens. Cumitech 1979;9:1–22.

32. McIntosh K, Pierik L. Immunofluorescence in viral diagnostics. In: Coonrod JD, Kunv LJ, Ferroro MJ, eds. The direct detection of microorganisms in clinical samples. Orlando: Academic Press, 1983.

33. Hurwitz S. Insect bites and parasitic infestations (Chapter 14). In: Clinical pediatric dermatology. 2nd ed. Philadelphia: WB Saunders. 1993, pp. 405–413.

CHAPTER 124

CLINICAL LABORATORY PROCEDURES

Meta Podrazek and James F. Wiley II

INTRODUCTION

This chapter deals with laboratory tests that may be commonly performed by a physician or other health care provider during the emergent care of a child. The format for this discussion concentrates on the scientific background of the test, the equipment required, the procedure, and the interpretation of results. As of January 1995, significant federal oversight governs the performance of all clinical laboratory tests.

Recent regulations under the Clinical Laboratory Improvement Act (CLIA) of 1988 require that all sites of laboratory testing register with the Health Care Financing Administration (HCFA) and obtain a provider number. According to CLIA, tests are classified as waived, physician-performed microscopy, moderate complexity, and high complexity. Waived tests require certification only, without any further requirement except to agree to random inspection which ensures that only waived tests are being performed. Laboratories performing physician-performed microscopy are subject to quality control and assurance regulations but are exempt from routine laboratory inspections. All other tests are classified as moderate complexity or high complexity and require external proficiency testing, establishment of written quality control and quality assurance procedures, special personnel requirements, and laboratory inspections every 2 years (1). In some instances, satellite laboratory activities in the emergency department (ED) can be administrated by the hospital clinical laboratory which may have the resources to comply with CLIA regulations. The most current CLIA designation (as of June 1995) is indicated for each test discussed.

INFECTIOUS DISEASE

Gram Stain

Background

The Gram stain, named for Hans Christian Gram, differentiates two large groups of bacterial species: Gram-positive and Gram-negative organisms. The procedure requires applying crystal violet, a dye taken up by the bacterial cell wall, then Gram's iodine, which aids in bonding dye to the cell wall. Next, decolorization with an acetone-alcohol agent and counterstaining with safranin solution are performed. The Gram-positive organisms retain the crystal violet dye and resist decolorization, thus appearing purple in color. Gram-negative organisms, however, take up the dye and are then susceptible to decolorization, and on microscopic examination appear pink. The ability to resist decolorization is due to the cell wall composition of each organism. The Gram-positive cell wall contains a thick peptidoglycan layer with numerous teichoic acid cross-linkages. These cross-links contribute to cell wall resistance to alcohol decolorization. In contrast, the cell wall of the Gram-negative organism has a thin layer of peptidoglycan and a thick external coat of lipoplysaccharides and protein islands (2, 3).

Other cells in a Gram-stained specimen include erythrocytes and leukocytes, which initially stain with application of crystal violet; the stain then washes out with an application of decolorizer. Subsequent safranin counterstain results in a cell appearance of pink or red. Yeast cells, resisting decolorization and staining purple, are Gram-positive in their Gram reaction, but fungal mycelia are Gram variable (2). This procedure is designated as moderately complex by the FDA and thus requires proficiency testing, designated personnel, written quality control and assurance measures and laboratory inspection every 2 years.

Equipment

Glass slide and coverslip
Crystal violet solution
Ethyl alcohol 95% (optional: acetone-ethyl alcohol mixture)
Gram's iodine
Safranin solution
Heat source (optional: 95% methanol)

Procedure

Gram staining requires specimen collection, preparation of the smear, staining, decolorization, counterstain application, drying, and microscopic examination. The primary goal of specimen collection is obtaining the body fluid or exudate material with minimal contamination. For example, careful cleaning of the surrounding skin before obtaining a wound exudate specimen helps to eliminate skin bacterial contaminants. Material collected in a syringe or plastic container is preferable to using cotton swabs, which can absorb components of the specimen. The specimen is thinly applied on a clean glass slide and air dried. Most specimens will adhere to the slide and do not require heat fixing. To heat fix, the slide is passed over a gentle flame several times. The slide should feel warm to the touch and should not be overheated, thus damaging the specimen. Alternatively, fixation can be performed with 95% methanol. The methanol is applied to the slide, allow it to run off for 1 minute, then air dried before staining. One then proceeds in the following fashion (3, 4).

The slide is flooded with crystal violet solution for 30 to 60 seconds and rinsed with tap water. Then the slide is flooded with Gram's iodine solution for 30 to 60 seconds and rinsed with tap water. Next, the decolorizer (95% ethyl alcohol or acetone-ethyl alcohol mixture) agent is used to rinse the slide for 5 to 30 seconds, until the drops running off the slide are no longer blue. For decolorizing agents that have higher acetone content, the decolorization is much more rapid (5 to 10 seconds). The agent used will dictate the rinsing time required for adequate decolorization. Thicker smears also may require more time for decolorization. Finally, the slide is flooded with safranin solution for 30 to 60 seconds, rinsed with tap water, and air dried. If using a paper towel or filter paper to facilitate drying the slide, it is important to ensure that the slide is blotted, as wiping may damage the specimen. The specimen is examined under a low then high power objective. Using an oil immersion lens allows better visualization of leukocytes, erythrocytes, and bacteria.

A more rapid method of Gram staining can be used. First, crystal violet is applied for a few seconds, followed by Gram's iodine solution for a few seconds. The slide is rinsed with decolorizing agent, and safranin solution (counterstain) is applied for a few seconds. The slide is then rinsed with tap water and dried.

Interpretation

Using the Gram stain technique serves many purposes. First, the Gram stain provides identification of bacteria on the basis of the Gram reaction; and second, numbers and morphology of bacteria can be seen on Gram stain. These two factors are valuable clues to the cause of disease and may help guide early treatment. Appropriate antibiotic therapy should not be dictated by Gram stain alone, but should be chosen based on all available clinical information. Gram staining, as it provides an opportunity for direct examination of the specimen, also determines the adequacy of the specimen for culture. For example, a sputum sample with more than 10 epithelial cells per low power field indicates contamination of the sample with oropharyngeal flora and is thus inadequate for culture.

The Gram stain is useful in many clinical settings including infections of the lower respiratory tract, genitourinary tract, skin and soft tissues, and joint spaces. Gram stains of cerebrospinal fluid and the buffy coat of peripheral blood (in the setting of meningitis and septicemia, respectively) are generally performed in the hospital laboratory, rather than in the ED. Gram stain findings for respiratory and gynecological pathogens are summarized in Table 124.1 (5, 6). Although not elucidated in this table, bacterial morphology and Gram reaction may help guide therapy in cases of septic arthritis, cystitis, and skin infections.

The decolorizing step, as previously described, distinguishes Gram-positive from Gram-negative organisms. Failure to perform this step correctly yields erroneous results. Underdecolorization occurs when rinsing with the decolorizing agent is not performed an adequate length of time. Thus cellular elements retain the crystal violet dye even in the absence of the thick peptidoglycan layer of Gram-positive organisms. Overdecolorization also may occur. The specimen that is decolorized for too long a period (especially when using the rapid-acting, high acetone content decolorizer) may remove crystal violet dye and lead to the erroneous interpretation of Gram-negative staining. Of note, any loss in cell wall integrity of Gram-positive organisms may allow the crystal violet to rinse away with the decolorizing step. The Gram-positive's teichoic acid cross-links may be affected by such factors as antibiotic treatment, the action of autolytic enzymes, or the age of the organism itself (2, 4). In light of the potential for misinterpretation, and the frequent difficulty in obtaining an adequate, contaminant-free specimen, the Gram stain is recommended as a diagnostic adjunct, not the sole determinant, in guiding appropriate presumptive antibiotic therapy.

Potassium Hydroxide Preparation

Background
The potassium hydroxide (KOH) preparation provides direct microscopic examination of clinical specimens in suspected fungal infections. Fungi have a polysaccharide-containing cell wall. The KOH solution is an alkali that digests proteinaceous material, such as host cellular material, while leaving the fungal cell wall intact (2). Thus using the KOH preparation can help confirm the diagnosis in clinically suspected fungal infections. The KOH preparation is designated as a physician-performed microscopy procedure and requires proficiency testing, test management, and quality control and assurance policies.

Equipment
Glass slide and coverslip
Scalpel—No. 15 blade
KOH solution (10%)
Heat source (optional)

Table 124.1.
Gram Stain Findings

Specimen Source	Organism	Gram Stain
Lower respiratory tract	• Contaminated specimen • Good quality specimen • *Streptococcus pneumoniae* • *Staphylococcus aureus* • *Haemophilus influenzae* • Viral pathogen • *Mycoplasma*	• >10 epithelial cells/LPF, <25 neutrophils/LPF • <10 epithelial cells/LPF, >25 neutrophils/LPF • GP* cocci in pairs and chains; inflammatory cells • GP cocci singly, in pairs, chains, clusters; inflammatory cells • GN* coccobacilli; inflammatory cells • No predominant bacterial organism • No predominant bacterial organism; mononuclear cells
Genital tract	• Normal flora (lactobacillus, gardnerella) • *Neisseria gonorrhoeae* • *Chlamydia trachomatis* • *Candida* sp. • *Gardnerella vaginalis*	• Large GP rods with smaller Gram-variable rods • GN intracellular diplococci, leukocytes • Many leukocytes • Branched hyphae, budding yeast • Mixed flora, Gram-variable rods, large GP rods in small numbers (0–5/HPF), clue cells, leukocytes

* GP = Gram-positive
* GN = Gram-negative

Procedure

The specimen is obtained and placed on a glass slide. For cutaneous infections, the site is cleaned with an alcohol swab and the active edge of the lesion is scraped with the edge of a microscope slide or scalpel blade. If the infection involves scalp and hair, one may select a short broken hair and remove using a hemostat, or gently scrape the scalp using the slide or scalpel. For vaginal infection, the specimen is collected using a cotton swab. Care must be used in viewing such specimens, as the cotton strands may resemble fungal hyphae on microscopic examination (7).

The specimen is covered with 1 to 2 drops of KOH solution and topped with the coverslip. Alternatively, the coverslip may be placed on the specimen and one drop of KOH solution placed at the edge of the preparation, allowing the solution to flow under the coverslip (7). One should wait at least 5 minutes before proceeding with the microscopic examination. If proteinaceous debris remains, potentially obscuring fungal elements, 5–10 minutes longer is allowed before reexamining microscopically. Alternatively, the clinician can pass the specimen quickly over a flame, which may speed the alkali digestion. One ought to be careful to not overheat or boil the material, as this will damage the specimen. The specimen is examined using a low (10×), then high power objective to identify fungal elements.

Interpretation

Fungi are separated into two groups, yeasts and molds, which differ in macroscopic appearance of colonies formed on culture media, microscopic morphologic features, and the mode of sporulation and characteristics of spores produced. Most of the clinically significant fungi reproduce by asexual sporulation. Three types of spores—arthroconidia, chlamydospore, and blastoconidia—may be identified by microscopic examination (Table 124.2) (Fig. 124.1) (2, 7).

As previously mentioned, care must be taken in preparing the specimen and interpreting microscopic findings. Overheating may damage the specimen and obliterate fungal elements. Foreign material such as the cotton fibers from a swab may masquerade as hyphae. Inadequate time allowed for the KOH preparation may impair fungi visualization as cellular debris obscure fungal elements. Such debris also may resemble fungal elements, further impeding accurate identification.

Cellophane Tape Preparation

Background

The adult pinworm, Enterobius vermicularis, lives in the cecum, colon, appendix, and rectum. The female adult migrates to the perianal area and deposits her eggs on the skin at nighttime. Thus perianal pruritus that interferes with sleep characterizes Enterobius infection. Cellophane (or cellulose) tape applied to the perianal skin in the morning, before the patient washes or defecates, will pick up the deposited eggs thus demonstrating infection. The pinworm examination is designated as a physician-performed microscopy procedure and requires proficiency testing, test management, and quality control and assurance policies.

Table 124.2.
Microscopic Examination of Fungi

Fungi	Site	Microscopic Appearance
Dermatophytoses *Microsporum* spp. *Trichophyton* spp. *Epidermophyton* spp.	Skin Hair/scalp Nails	Colorless, branched, septate hyphae (3–5 μm in diameter). Arthroconidia appear as square, rectangular, or barrel-shaped thick-walled cells: - within the hair shaft - on the hair shaft periphery - in chains in skin and nails
Tinea versicolor *Malassezia furfur*	Skin	Round yeast cells (3–8 μm in diameter). Dark, short, curved hyphae elements (2.5–4 μm in diameter)
Candidiasis *Candida albicans* *Candida* spp.	Skin Nails Mucous membranes Blood Urine	Branched, septate hyphae Blastoconidia • Individual round or oval budding yeast cells (3–4 μm in diameter) • Pseudohyphae, i.e., budding structures that are elongated and remain attached to mother cells (5–10 μm in diameter)

Equipment
Cellulose tape
Glass slide
Small paper label (approx. 1×2 cm)
Wooden tongue depressor
Glass test tube (optional)
Toluene (for use with frosted tape)

Procedure
A small paper label is placed at one end of a 1×8 cm length of tape (Figure 124.2). Then the tape strip is placed, adhesive side down, onto a microscope slide with the free end of the tape wrapped over the opposite edge of the slide. Next, the slide and tape are placed on a wooden tongue depressor. The tape is peeled back holding the paper label end, and wrapped (adhesive side out) over the end of the tongue depressor. While holding the slide against the tongue depressor, the tape is placed on the perianal area, pressing firmly with the tongue depressor.

The tongue depressor is removed, then the tape is brought back over the slide edge, adhesive side down again, and placed back onto the slide pressing firmly. The slide is examined under the low-power objective. When frosted tape is used, the tape is lifted, one drop of toluene is applied, the tape is pressed onto the slide, and examined microscopically to view eggs (8).

Alternatively, using a 1×8 cm strip of tape, each end of the tape is folded over (with the adhesive side folded on itself) about 1 cm at each end. The tape is stretched, adhesive side out, over the butt end of a test tube holding each end firmly with thumb and forefinger (Fig. 124.3). The tape is applied to perianal area, rocking the tube back and forth to cover more skin area. The tape is removed, applied to slide (adhesive side down) and viewed under the microscope (8). Toluene again, may be required to delineate eggs. Occasionally, adult worms also can be demonstrated by tape preparation.

Interpretation
When the adult female lays eggs, the eggs are partially embryonated. Within a few hours (by the time the cellophane tape preparation is performed) the eggs may be fully embryonated and are infective. Characteristic eggs are 50 to 60 μm in length and 20 to 30 μm in breadth. They are flattened on one side and

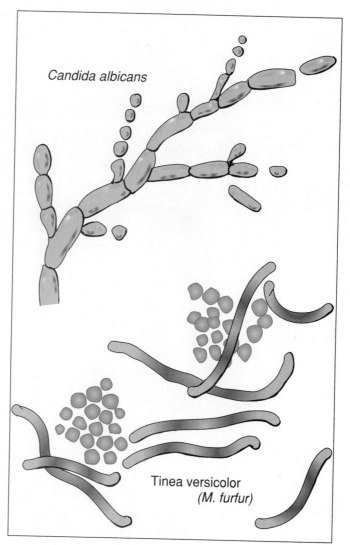

Candida albicans

Tinea versicolor
(M. furfur)

Figure 124.1.
Identification of fungal elements (40× magnification).

have a translucent, thick shell (8). Direct smears of fecal material may be prepared; tape preparations, however, better demonstrate the embryonated eggs. After treatment, follow-up tape preparations are obtained to demonstrate that the patient is free of infection. Tape preparations may be required for 3 to 4 consecutive days to confirm cure (9).

GYNECOLOGY

Wet Mount/Wet Preparation

Background
The wet preparation, useful in evaluating the patient with presumed vaginitis, cervicitis, or pelvic inflammatory disease, entails suspending a specimen in saline solution and subsequent microscopic examination for the identi-

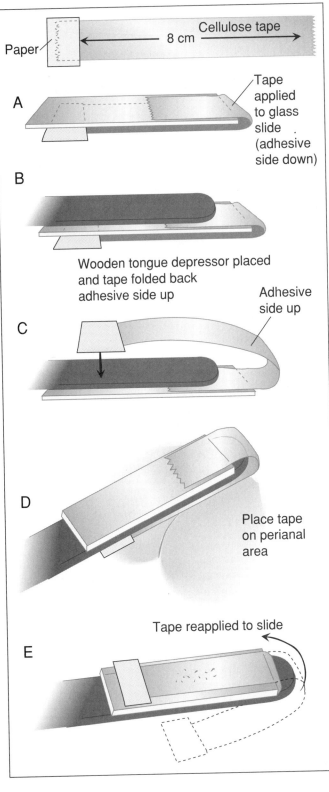

Paper

Cellulose tape

← 8 cm →

A
Tape applied to glass slide (adhesive side down)

B
Wooden tongue depressor placed and tape folded back adhesive side up

Adhesive side up

C

D
Place tape on perianal area

E
Tape reapplied to slide

quality control and assurance policies.

Equipment
Glass test tube with 1 mL sterile saline solution
Cotton-tipped swab
Glass slide and coverslip

Procedure
The vaginal fluid specimen is obtained using a cotton-tipped swab. The swab is placed in the tube containing saline. After agitating the swab in the tube, the swab is touched to the center of the glass slide and a coverslip applied. The slide is then examined under a low power objective to identify areas of visible cellular material or organisms, and then examined under high power.

Interpretation
The most common and diagnostically useful information obtained using the wet mount technique includes identification of leukocytes, clue cells, fungal elements, and trichomonads (Table 124.3) (Fig. 124.4). Frequently in a patient with vaginitis, the clinician will see many leukocytes on the wet preparation. These cells, 12 to 15 μm in diameter, are likely to have the multilobed, segmented nuclei consistent with polymorphonuclear leukocytes. This finding, although neither sensitive nor specific, may help to confirm a clinical impression of infectious vaginitis or cervicitis. Important to note, however, is the presence of white cells on wet preparation in cases of non-infectious leukorrhea.

Clue cells, a characteristic feature of *Gardnerella vaginalis* (or bacterial vagino-

fication of inflammatory cells and organisms. The wet preparation of vaginal or cervical specimens is designated as a physician-performed microscopy procedure and requires proficiency testing, test management, and

sis), also can be identified on wet preparation. The clue cell is a vaginal epithelial cell with adherent bacterial organisms. The cytoplasm and cell border are distorted by the bacteria giving the cytoplasm a lacy, granular appearance with a surrounding irregular border (10). Although clue cells have a high specificity for bacterial vaginosis, other bacterial organisms (including lactobacilli and streptococci) may adhere to epithelial cells and be confused with true clue cells. Sensitivity, reported in one study as more than 90%, has been shown in other studies to be lower and clearly dependent on clinician expertise in identifying the cells (11–13).

Trichomonads are the protozoa identified on wet preparation as small (5 to 15 μm in length), flagellated organisms that have jerky, nondirectional motility (8). Identification of the organism is specific and therefore diagnostic for trichomoniasis. In one study, however, protozoa were identified on wet preparations in only 60% of patients with culture-positive trichomoniasis (14). The low sensitivity may be related to several factors, most important of which include the rapid loss of protozoan motility (within 30 to 60 minutes of specimen preparation) and other specimen material (epithelial cells, leukocytes, and fungal elements) obscuring the organisms. Thus culture, Papanicolaou test, or monoclonal antibody techniques may be necessary for definitive diagnosis (the latter two of which are not routinely performed in the ED setting).

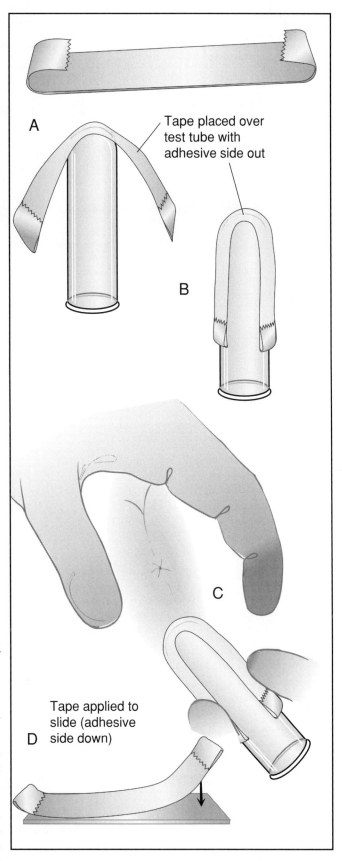

Figure 124.3. Collection of *Enterobius vermicularis* using test tube and cellophane tape.

Tape placed over test tube with adhesive side out

A

B

C

Tape applied to slide (adhesive side down)

D

Table 124.3.
Sexually Transmitted Infections in the Pediatric Patient

Organisms	Syndrome(s)	Clinical Findings	Laboratory Findings
Candida albicans	Vaginitis	• Erythema of vagina	• Branched and budding hyphae on KOH and wet preparation
Trichomonas	Vaginitis Cervicitis	• Copious discharge • Petechiae of cervix (''strawberry cervix'') and upper vaginal vault	• Trichomonads and leukocytes on wet preparation
Gardnerella vaginalis	Vaginitis	• Watery, malodorous discharge	• ''Fishy'' odor of specimen with addition of KOH due to release of amines • Clue cells on wet preparation • Vaginal pH greater than 4.5
Chlamydia trachomatis	Cervicitis PID*	• Patient may be asymptomatic • Purulent discharge • Erythematous, friable cervix (although cervical examination may be completely normal)	• Wet preparation with many leukocytes
Neisseria gonorrhoeae	Vaginitis Cervicitis PID*	• Patient may be asymptomatic • Mucopurulent discharge • Erythematous cervix	• Wet preparation with many leukocytes • Gram stain with Gram-negative intracellular diplococci and leukocytes

Figure 124.4.
Wet preparation of vaginal secretions: microscopic findings (100× magnification).

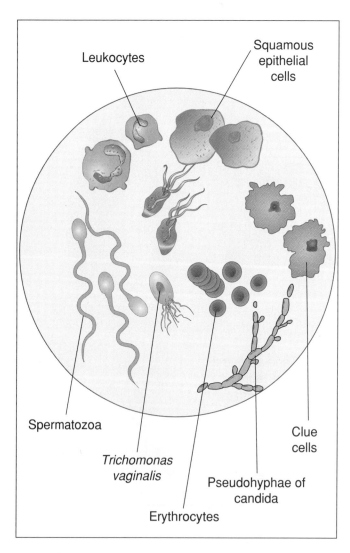

Leukocytes

Squamous epithelial cells

Spermatozoa

Trichomonas vaginalis

Erythrocytes

Pseudohyphae of candida

Clue cells

Urine Pregnancy Test

Background

Rapid urine pregnancy tests most commonly use immunosorbent assays with monoclonal antibodies to the β-subunit of human chorionic gonadotropin (HCG). The fertilized ovum at time of implantation, approximately 8 to 9 days after ovulation, secrets HCG. This glycoprotein, composed of α- and β-subunits, reflects the presence of placental trophoblast tissue, but also is secreted in abnormal pregnancies (including ectopic pregnancy, blighted ova, and fetal demise) and in association with certain malignancies. The α-subunit of HCG is similar to that of LH, TSH, and FSH. The β-subunit, in contrast, is the biologically active, immunospecific chain not found in pituitary hormones (15, 16).

Table 124.4.
Urine Pregnancy Tests: Test Procedures and Results

Test	Test Procedure	Approximate Test Time (minutes)	Positive test indicator	Additional information
Clearview HCG (19)	Place five drops of urine in sample window	5	Horizontal blue line in Result Window (with blue line in Control Window)	Semiquantitative; faint blue line in result window indicates HCG <50 (retest in 48–72 hrs)
Duoclon (20)	Add one drop of urine reagent on slide and stir	3	Agglutination (granular pattern on slide)	Agglutination occurs within 1–3 minutes
HCG-nostick (21)	Place buffer in vial, add 0.2 mL of urine, mix and place dipstick in vial	30	Rose-red color on reactive area of dipstick	Reaction time is 30 minutes at room temp. or 5 minutes using a rotator (170 rpm)
Icon II HCG (urine) (22)	Place five drops of urine at center of membrane and add reagents	5	Circular blue spot in Test Zone (with blue spot in Reference Zone)	Semiquantitative; color intensity indicates approx. HCG level
Pregnospia II (23)	Add 0.1 mL of urine to reagents and distilled water in vial	30	Change in color from original reddish-purple	Color change often occurs within 2–3 minutes (may require 30 minutes)
Pregnosticon Dri-Dot (24)	Add one drop each of urine and water to dried reagents on slide, then stir	4	No agglutination; green homogenous appearance to specimen	Positive result occurs within 2–3 minutes
QuickVue HCG-Urine (25)	Place three drops of urine in round Sample Well	3	Any pink to purple line next to the letter T in Results Window (with blue Control Line)	Positive result may occur as early as 1 minute
TestPack Plus HCG-Urine (26)	Place three drops of urine in Sample Well.	5	Positive sign (+) or any part of the vertical bar in the Result Window	Read only after appearance of red color in end of Assay Window; positive result may occur as early as three minutes

During the first trimester of pregnancy, serum HCG concentrations double approximately every 48 hours (doubling time is 29 to 43 hours during the first 35 days after conception, then slows to 48 to 65 hours between days 35 to 47) (17–19). Serum HCG levels peak during the third gestational month, reaching levels of 1,000,000 mIU/mL or more. Subsequently, serum and urine levels decline, then plateau to a level that is maintained throughout the normal gestation (15).

Many types of assays are used to identify β-HCG in the urine. Two of the most commonly used are the two-site immunometric ("sandwich") assay and agglutination inhibition assay (19). The first of these, immunometric assay, entails using antibody on a solid support surface that binds HCG; addition of a second, labeled antibody binds HCG at a different site and is thus captured by the solid-phase matrix. Because the monoclonal antibodies used have highly specific epitopes (the antigenic region of the molecule), each antibody binds selectively to the appropriate subunit of HCG. For example, one method uses an antibody in the solid-phase matrix which binds the α-subunit, thereby trapping

not only HCG but also LH, FSH, and TSH. Using a second labeled antibody recognizes the carboxyl-terminal part of the HCG β-subunit. The marker, usually an enzyme, results in a positive color reaction in the solid-phase matrix identifying the presence of HCG. The immunometric assay is the method for the most current and sensitive urine pregnancy tests. This is particularly useful in the ED setting because testing is easy to perform and results are rapidly obtained (14).

Agglutination inhibition assays, using sol particles or latex particles, also make use of antibodies against HCG. The particles used are coated with HCG; urine from the patient is mixed with anti-HCG antibodies, then the mixture is added to the HCG-coated particles. In the case of pregnancy, HCG in the urine binds to all available anti-HCG antibodies; thus, virtually no antibodies are available for binding with the HCG-coated particles resulting in no agglutination. Conversely, in the nonpregnant patient with no urine HCG, added anti-HCG antibodies bind with the particles and agglutination results. Slide or tube tests use agglutination inhibition method (14). Urine pregnancy tests are waived tests under CLIA.

Table 124.5.
Urine Pregnancy Tests: Test Methods and Sensitivities

Test	Manufacturer	Method	Sensitivity Threshold (mIU/mL)	Earliest (+) Result Relative to First Missed Menses (mm)
Clearview HCG	Wampole	IA	50	At or shortly after mm
Duoclon	Organon Teknika	LAI (slide)	500	Within 1 week of mm
HCG-Nostick	Organon Teknika	SPIA (slide)	50	At or shortly after mm
Icon II HCG	Hybritech	IA	50	At or shortly after mm
Pregnospia II	Organon Teknika	SPIA (tube)	150	Shortly after mm
Pregnosticon Dri-Dot	Organon Diagnostic	LAI (slide)	1000	4–12 days after mm
Quick Vue	Quidel	IA	25	Before 1st mm
TestPack Plus (HCG urine)	Abbott	IA	50	At or shortly after mm
TestPack Plus (HCG combo)	Abbott	IA	25	Before 1st mm

Equipment

Urine specimen (optimal: first-morning void)
Pregnancy test kit (Some test kits use either serum or urine specimens for qualitative HCG determination. All kits should include necessary slides or tubes, pipettes, reagents, and product information inserts.)

Procedure

Table 124.4 summarizes the procedure required using any one of eight commercially available pregnancy test kits (20–27). (See appropriate manufacturer's product insert for detailed procedure description.)

Interpretation

Table 124.5 summarizes test methods and sensitivity levels for some of the commer-cially available pregnancy test kits (20–27). When using rapid, qualitative urine pregnancy tests it is important to understand test limitations. Although these manufacturers report high sensitivities and specificities, the test result must be put in context with clinical information. False-negative or false-positive urine HCG results occur in a variety of clinical situations (Table 124.6).

Motile Sperm Microscopy

Background

Microscopic examination of vaginal secretions to identify motile sperm is an important and rapidly performed laboratory procedure in the ED. This procedure often is used in

Table 124.6.
Urine Pregnancy Tests: False-Positive and False-Negative Results

False Positives	Reason	Recommendation
Trophoblastic disease	Production of HCG	Close follow-up with serial quantitative HCG levels
Natural termination of pregnancy or therapeutic abortion (within 4 weeks)	Falling but still detectable levels of HCG	Serial quantitative HCG levels
Concomitant medication use	Interfering substance with assay	Review product information concerning interference testing
Hematuria or proteinuria	Interference with assay	Review product information concerning interference testing; repeat test

False Negatives	Reason	Recommendation
Dilute urine	Urine does not contain truly representative HCG levels	Use first-morning void for testing
Low urine pH (<3)	Interference with assay	Add no preservatives to urine specimen
Early pregnancy	Urine HCG level below sensitivity threshold of assay	Attempt accurate dating of last menses; review product information concerning sensitivity threshold; repeat test within 2 weeks
Ectopic pregnancy	Urine HCG level below sensitivity threshold of assay	Close follow-up with serial quantitative HCG levels, ultrasonic examination, and rapid consultation and intervention as appropriate

cases of alleged sexual assault and abuse. Sperm may remain motile in the vagina for 6 to 12 hours, and for an even longer period in the cervix. In controlled studies, 50% of sperm lost motility by 2 to 3 hours, providing the ED physician with a narrow window of opportunity for visualizing motile sperm (28). In contrast, nonmotile sperm can be seen on microscopic examination of a specimen days after intercourse, a confounding factor in evaluating a sexual assault victim who may have had recent voluntary intercourse. Thus, this important microscopic finding is only identified by the initial examining physician; the forensic pathologist involved in a sexual assault case will likely first evaluate specimens many hours after collection, precluding identification of motile sperm (28, 29). Motile sperm microscopy is designated as a physician-performed microscopy procedure and requires proficiency testing, test management, and quality control and assurance policies.

Equipment

Sterile container (e.g., glass test tube)
Small syringe or dropper
Sterile, nonbacteriostatic saline solution
Cotton-tipped swab
Glass slide and coverslip
Supravital stain (optional)
Glacial acetic acid (optional)

Procedure

The clinician may obtain the specimen in the older pediatric patient by aspirating secretions pooled in the posterior fornix using a small syringe or dropper. Optionally, the clinician may wash the vagina with 5 to 10 mL of saline, aspirate the fluid, and place it in a sterile container. A third option, especially in the small child, is placing a cotton-tipped swab in the vaginal orifice that is then placed in 2 to 3 mL of saline in a glass test tube.

Using a dropper or small syringe, a few drops of the specimen are placed on a clean glass slide and the coverslip applied. One examines the specimen under low and high power objective to identify motile sperm. Of-

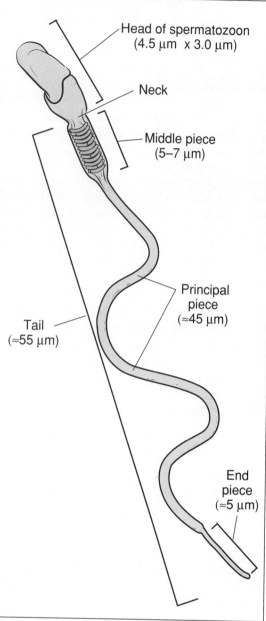

Head of spermatozoon
(4.5 μm x 3.0 μm)

Neck

Middle piece
(5–7 μm)

Principal
piece
(≈45 μm)

Tail
(≈55 μm)

End
piece
(≈5 μm)

Figure 124.5.
Spermatozoon anatomy (100× magnification).

ten sperm may be obscured by cellular material, especially red blood cells. Using glacial acetic acid provides lysis of red blood cells. Of note, however, is that the acid will leave sperm immotile. Another option is using supravital stain which lyses red blood cells and stains sperm blue for easier visualization. Supravital staining results in little loss of sperm motility (28, 29).

Interpretation

The mature human spermatozoon is about 60 μm long with two major components, the head (composed of acrosome and nucleus) and the tail (composed of neck, middle piece, principal piece, and end piece). The head is approximately 4.5 μm by 3.0 μm (in contrast to a polymorphonuclear neutrophil, approximately 12 to 15 μm in diameter). The principal piece is so named because it comprises the main portion of the flagellum or tail structure that propels the sperm (Fig. 124.5) (30).

False-negative interpretation of specimen occurs when inadequate sampling, specimen preparation, and/or interpretation occurs. For example, cellular material such as red blood cells may obscure sperm. Using glacial acetic acid, as previously described, results in immotile sperm. A motile protozoan that can be identified in vaginal secretions, *Trichomonas vaginalis*, may be confused with spermatozoa, yielding a false-positive result. This flagellated parasite is significantly smaller (5 to 15 μm in length) than the spermatozoon and is therefore distinguishable.

STOOL TESTS

Fecal Occult Blood Test

Background

The presence of occult blood in fecal material can be identified using many different commercial tests. Two of the most common are the Hemoccult® (SmithKline Diagnostics, Inc.) and Hematest® (Ames). These tests rely on the ability of hemoglobin to act as a peroxidase, catalyzing the reaction between peroxide and a chromogenic, organic compound.

The chromogenic substances are orthotolidine (impregnated in the Hematest® filter paper) and guaiac (impregnated in the Hemoccult® card's filter paper). Peroxide in the form of a solution or tablet is applied to the specimen and filter paper. If hemoglobin is present in the specimen, the chromogenic compound is oxidized and a color change to blue occurs (31). This test is waived under CLIA.

Equipment

For Hematest® method:
Filter paper and reagent table (provided in kit)

Cotton-tipped swab
Glass slide
Distilled water

For Hemoccult® method:
Hemoccult® card
Developer (stabilized aqueous solution of hydrogen peroxide and denatured ethanol)
Cotton-tipped swab

Procedure

For the Hematest® method (32), one obtains a sample of fecal material using a cotton-tipped swab or during the course of a routine rectal examination. After placing Hematest® filter paper on a glass slide, a thin streak of fecal material is smeared on the filter paper. Then, a Hematest® reagent tablet is placed on the smear, and one drop of distilled water on the Hematest® tablet. After waiting 5 to 10 seconds for the water to penetrate the tablet, one adds a second drop of water so that water runs down the side of the tablet and onto the specimen. A gentle tap of the slide may be required to allow the water droplets to reach the specimen. Any color change in the filter paper is noted. One observes for up to 2 minutes to detect a blue color.

For the Hemoccult® method (33), a sample of fecal material is obtained as described for the previous method. The examiner should open the Hemoccult® card front tab and apply a thin smear of the stool to the filter paper in the box designated "A." A second smear (sampled from a different part of the stool) can be applied to box "B." The tab cover is closed. Next, the flap on the reverse of the card is opened. Two drops of Hemoccult® developer are applied to the filter paper over each smear. After waiting 20 seconds, the filter paper is observed to detect a color change to blue. If uncertain, the specimen is directly examined by opening the obverse flap. Just below this area is an orange rectangle designated "Performance Monitor®" area. A drop of developer is applied here to provide a blue color with which the test area can be compared to confirm a positive result.

Interpretation

A blue color noted on the filter paper indicates the presence of hemoglobin in the stool specimen. The healthy person loses 2.0 to 2.5 mL of blood into the gastrointestinal tract daily. More than 2.8 mL of blood in a 24-hour period may indicate gastrointestinal disease. The chromogenic substances used in commercial kits vary in sensitivity. The Hemoccult® test, which uses guaiac, turns positive at a level of 5.0 mg of hemoglobin per gram of stool. This is considered the upper limit of normal stool peroxidase activity (34). Ostrow et al. demonstrated that in 90% of observations, 6.0 mg of added hemoglobin per gram of feces was detected using Hemoccult® testing, but at low levels of hemoglobin (1.5 mg per gram of feces) 80% resulted in negative tests. By contrast, Hematest®, which uses orthotolidine, was shown to be more sensitive (35). Christensen et al. (31) compared five commercial kits by collecting stool from healthy children and adding designated quantities of whole blood, such that 0 to 6 mL of hemoglobin were added per 100 grams of feces. Five kits were used to test 270 stool samples which revealed Hematest® was a significantly more sensitive test than Hemoccult®. The ability of the Hematest® to detect minute volumes of blood in stool also led to a greater percentage of false-positive results. For this reason, these authorities concluded that a slightly less sensitive test (i.e., Hemoccult®) was advantageous (31). False-negative test results can occur if (a) stool has a highly liquid content, (b) the aliquot sampled is not from the center portion of a formed stool, (c) ascorbic acid was recently ingested, (d) inadequate time is allowed for the peroxidase-catalyzed reactions, or (e) the specimen smear is too thick (34). Delay in applying developer solution and in reading the color change on the filter paper also can result in false negatives. Interfering factors that cause false-pos-

itive test results are summarized in Table 124.7.

HEMATOLOGY

Microhematocrit

Background

The hematocrit is the volume of packed red blood cells in a volume of whole blood and is expressed as a percentage. The test requires centrifugation to separate the blood cells from plasma. It is a test that is applicable and may be useful in evaluating patients who are polycythemic, but more commonly it is used in cases of suspected anemia.

The hematocrit (or packed cell volume) can be measured using the Wintrobe method which entails using a graduated tube 11.5 cm in height, filled with anticoagulant (EDTA) and specimen (patient's venous blood), that requires centrifugation for 30 minutes. A faster, less cumbersome method is the more commonly used microhematocrit test. The microcapillary hematocrit tubes, also filled with anticoagulant and blood specimen, when centrifuged reveal the separation of packed cells and a buffy coat. The height of the packed cells in the capillary tube corresponds to the hematocrit (36). The microhematocrit is waived under CLIA regulations.

Equipment
Microhematocrit centrifuge
Microhematocrit capillary tubes
Tube sealant
Microhematocrit reader card
Purple top tube (optional)

Procedure
A capillary blood specimen is obtained using the fingerstick or heelstick method (Chapter 42). A venous blood sample also may be used. The capillary tube is filled at least two-thirds full. This procedure is repeated so that two capillary tubes are filled. The second tube serves as an internal control and as a backup in case of breakage.

If the test is not to be performed immediately, a venous blood sample can be placed in a purple top tube which contains EDTA anticoagulant. The specimen must be well mixed

Table 124.7.
Fecal Occult Blood Testing: False-Positive Results

Peroxidase activity	Beef, mutton, salmon, sardines, yellow turnips, horseradish, apples, bananas, oranges, soups with dark meats
Gastrointestinal irritants	Alcohol, iron, salicylates, coumarin, Rauwolfia derivatives, colchicine, steroids, indomethacin, and other antiinflammatory medications
Concomitant conditions	Menstruation, bleeding hemorrhoids, anal fissure(s)

with anticoagulant and the test should be run within 24 hours. When ready for centrifugation, the examiner should remove the purple cap, place the capillary tube into the test tube, turn both horizontally without spilling blood and the capillary tube should fill. Then the end of each capillary tube is sealed and the tubes are placed in the centrifuge opposite each other, with the sealant ends on the outside, and the lid is closed.

Centrifugation may vary depending on the machine used. One option is centrifugation at 10,000 rpm for 3 minutes; however, more time may be required. After the centrifuge has come to a complete stop, the capillary tubes are removed. Two layers, the packed cell and plasma layers, should be visible. One should place the tube on the microhematocrit reader card, correctly position the tube on the card and, using the scale provided, read the hematocrit that corresponds to the height of the red cell column (36). This process is repeated for the second capillary tube and record the microhematocrits.

Interpretation

Hematocrit levels and the microhematocrit readings depend on many factors including age, sex, hydration status, and the altitude at which the patient lives. Inaccurate readings, either falsely low or high, can occur using the microhematocrit method described. Falsely low levels occur with improper reading of the microhematocrit reader card, significant delay between centrifugation and reading, and hemolysis or clotting of the blood sample being tested. A falsely elevated level occurs if the buffy coat (the gray layer above the red cell column) is included in the packed cell volume, and in patients with sickle-cell disease or other cases of unusually shaped red blood cells that result in plasma trapping in the red cell column. A falsely elevated level also occurs with incorrect use of the microhematocrit reader card, and in cases of inadequate centrifugation which causes incomplete packing of red blood cells (36).

A venous specimen collected in a EDTA-anticoagulated tube may present problems and lead to inaccurate hematocrit readings. The specimen must be adequately mixed with the EDTA. Inadequate mixing and withdrawal of specimen from the plasma-rich area result in falsely low hematocrit values; if specimen is drawn from the red cell-rich area, readings are falsely elevated. Too small a blood sample, with resultant EDTA overdilution of the blood leads to lower hematocrit readings. Finally, samples stored for longer than 24 hours before testing lead to falsely elevated levels (36).

Using the microhematocrit method for rapid hematocrit determination in adults in the ED setting was tested by Bartfield et al. (37). Two blood specimens per patient were collected and compared with laboratory CBC results. The ED hematocrits were slightly lower than the laboratory hematocrit (a difference of 0.539 ± 1.64 standard deviations) with 93% of all ED-measured hematocrits within three percentage points of the laboratory hematocrit results. The average of the two ED-measured hematocrits had excellent correlation with the laboratory result. These authors concluded that the microhematocrit method is rapid, easy to perform, and reliable, but that a formal CBC should be considered if the measured hematocrit is abnormally low.

HemoCue® Method of Hemoglobin Determination

Background

The HemoCue® hemoglobinometer is a portable and easy to use device that measures hemoglobin by spectrophotometry. The method requires a microburette, a small disposable receptacle for the blood sample that collects 10 μL of blood by capillary action. Dry reagents are deposited on the inner walls of the microburette cavity. The reagents include sodium deoxycholate, which lyses the red blood cells; sodium nitrate, which converts the hemoglobin iron from the ferrous to the ferric state to form methemoglobin; and sodium azide, which combines to form azide methemoglobin. The microburette is then placed in the HemoCue® photometer, which measures absorbance at two wavelengths, 565 nm and 880 nm. Within 15 to 45 seconds, the hemoglobin concentration is calculated and is digitally displayed in grams per deciliter (g/dL). The machine is programmed to disregard results when absorption figures from the two different wavelengths differ widely (38, 39). This test is waived by CLIA.

Equipment

Microburette and HemoCue® photometer

For capillary blood sample:
Lancet device
Alcohol swab

For venous or arterial sample:
Needle, 22 gauge, and small syringe
Alcohol swab
Purple top (EDTA-containing) tube

Procedure

A blood sample is obtained and placed in the microburette. If the fingerstick method is used, the drops of capillary blood are directly drawn into the microburette. If a venous or arterial sample is obtained, sample is placed in the EDTA tube, mixed by inverting the tube several times, then instilled into the microburette. The microburette must be completely filled, without the presence of air bubbles, for an accurate reading. Next, the microburette is placed into the HemoCue® photometer. The microburette sits easily onto a small shelflike receptacle that slides into the machine. After waiting 15 to 45 seconds, one reads the display.

Interpretation

The HemoCue® provides fast and accurate hemoglobin determinations. Multiple studies have been performed to test its accuracy, particularly in the ambulatory care setting. One investigation compared hemoglobin results obtained by the HemoCue® method with the standard laboratory coulter counter method (40). The capillary and venous blood samples were obtained from 200 pediatric patients who were noted to be anemic, nonanemic, or with a sickling disorder. Comparison of hemoglobin levels measured by HemoCue® with coulter methods revealed a mean difference between the two instruments of 0.35 g/dL in nonanemic patients, 0.33 g/dL in the anemic group, and 0.42 g/dL in patients with sickling disorders. In small proportions of patients, the difference in hemoglobin measurements exceeded 1.0 g/dL (8% for nonanemic patients and those with sickling disorders, and 4% for anemic patients). With such differences, the hemoglobin measured by HemoCue® was lower in each instance. Also confirmed was that the accuracy of HemoCue® hemoglobin estimates are not markedly affected by sickle cells.

Concern about the accuracy of Hemo Cue® using capillary, venous, and arterial samples prompted a study of 42 intensive care unit patients (39). The HemoCue® values were compared with coulter counter results, which revealed that sequential capillary samples were significantly more variable than venous or arterial samples, with 16% of the paired capillary hemoglobin estimates varying by more than 1.0 g/dL. Peripheral skin temperature did not influence the repeatable accuracy of capillary samples. Such variable estimates may be related to errors in obtaining specimen, especially inadequate filling of the microburette and the presence of air bubbles in the sample. When using fingerstick to obtain specimen, rouleaux formation and hemodilution at the fingertip may cause such variable hemoglobin readings. These authors (39) therefore advocate using a "bottle" method (i.e., placing the capillary specimen in an EDTA tube and after agitation, instilling the blood in the microburette) to improve HemoCue® accuracy. In doing so, Cohen et al. noted a sensitivity of 85% and specificity of 94% when HemoCue® was used to detect anemia (40).

Finally, false elevation of hemoglobin levels due to hyperlipemia was addressed by von Schenck et al. (38). Measurements of hemoglobin by the HemoCue® method in a nonanemic patient are not affected by lipemic blood specimens. Slight false increases in hemoglobin due to hyperlipemia were detected when hemoglobin values were in the lower range of anemia. However, comparison of HemoCue® with Hemalog 8/90 (a filter photometer commonly used for laboratory hemoglobin measurement) revealed more accurate results when hemoglobin was measured using the HemoCue® for anemic patients with hyperlipemic specimens.

URINE TESTING

Multiple Reagent Strip or Urine Dipstick

Background

Multiple reagent strips, or urine dipsticks, provide rapid chemical examination of urine specimens. The chemicals measure or detect urinary pH, protein, glucose, ketones, blood,

Table 124.8.
Urine Chemistry Testing by Dipstick: Reagents

Test	Reagent Multistix®	Chemstrip®
Ph	Methyl red	Methyl red
	Bromthymol blue	Bromthymol blue
		Phenolphthalein
Protein	Tetrabromphenol blue	3′,3″,5′,5″-tetrachlorophenol-3,4,5,6-tetrabromosulfophthalein
Blood	Dumeme hydroperoxide	Tetramethylbenzidine
	Tetramethylbenzidine	2,5-Dimethyl-2,5-dihyodroperoxyhexane
Glucose	Glucose oxidase	Glucose oxidase
	Peroxidase	Peroxidase
	Potassium iodide	Tetramethylbenzidine
Urobilinogen	Para-dimethylamine-benzaldehyde	4-methozbenzene-diazonium-tetrafluoroborate
Bilirubin	2,4-Dichloroaniline	2,6-Dichlorobenzene-diazonium
	Diazonium salt	Tetrafluoroborate
Nitrite	Para-arsanilic acid	3-Hydroxy-1,2,3,4-tetrahydro-7,8-benzoquinoline
	1,2,3,4-Tetrahydrobenzo(h)-quinoline-3-ol	Sulfanilamide
Leukocytes	Pyrrole amino acid ester	Indoxylcarbonic acid ester
	Diazonium salt	Diazonium salt
Specific	Poly(methylvinyl ether maleic anhydride)	EGTA
gravity	Bromthymol blue	Bromthymol blue
Ketone	Sodium nitroprusside	Sodium nitroferricyanide
		Glycine

bilirubin, urobilinogen, nitrite, specific gravity, and leukocytes. Two commercially available urine dipsticks are commonly used, the Chemstrip® and Multistix®. Each contain chemical-impregnated absorbent pads arranged on plastic strips. When the pad comes in contact with urine, a color-producing chemical reaction occurs which is then interpreted relative to a color chart supplied by the test manufacturer. The results may be quantitative (e.g., an estimate of milligrams per deciliter or pH) or semiquantitative (e.g., 1^+, 2^+, 3^+, 4^+) depending on the reagent used. The reagents impregnated in the dipstick pads are summarized in Table 124.8 (41, 42). The urine dipstick test is waived under CLIA regulations.

Equipment
Reagent strip
Color reference charts (provided on container)
Urine specimen in clean plastic or glass container (obtained via midstream clean catch, Foley catheterization, or suprapubic aspiration)

Procedure
The reagent strip is dipped in the urine specimen, allowing all reagent pads to contact urine. After 10 to 15 seconds, the strip is removed from urine. One should touch the edge of the strip on the container's rim as the strip is withdrawn or on an absorbent paper towel to remove excess urine. A specified time is allowed for the reaction for each reagent pad to occur. Appropriate times are indicated on the color chart. The strip is kept horizontally oriented while waiting so that no excess urine produces a runover of chemicals from one pad to an adjacent pad, distorting color results. Finally, under good light, the color of the strip's reagent pads is compared with the color chart, again keeping the strip horizontal. Color results should be identified within 2 minutes.

Interpretation
Normal urine pH ranges from 4.5 to 8.0; most often urine is slightly acidic, about 6.0. Urinary pH depends on the acid-base content of the bloodstream, the renal function of the patient, the patient's dietary intake, the presence of infection in the urinary tract, and the age of the urine specimen. A patient with high vegetable intake will have more alkaline urine due to bicarbonate formation by many fruits and vegetables, whereas high protein and meat diets produce acidic urine. Urinary tract infections caused by urea-splitting organisms tend to alkalinize urine. Urine specimens that sit for long periods before testing is performed may prove to be highly alkaline for this very reason, necessitating retesting a freshly voided specimen. Patients also may be prescribed medications that alter urinary

pH. Of note, one important interfering substance with urine pH testing is the adjacent reagent pad which contains acidic compounds for protein testing. This runover phenomenon may produce a falsely acidic pH test result in an alkaline urine specimen. The range of measurable pH levels by reagent strip testing is 5 to 9 for the most commonly used commercial tests (41, 42).

Proteinuria, as detected by reagent strip testing, may occur with glomerular membrane damage, tubular disorders that impair protein reabsorption, hematuria, infection, and increased serum levels of protein. Contamination of the specimen container with detergents and quaternary ammonium compounds may result in a false-positive reaction. An acid buffer is used in the reagent pad; however, a highly alkaline urine (too alkaline for the acid buffer to be effective) produces a false-positive result. Buffer removal, as occurs when urine sits on the reagent pad for too long, also may produce false-positive results. The lowest sensitivity threshold for reagent strips is approximately 6 to 7 mg/dL of protein (41, 42).

Glycosuria may indicate a high glucose content meal recently ingested by a healthy patient, glucose intolerance in a diabetic, or impaired tubular reabsorption of glucose as seen in thyroid and central nervous system disorders. False positives can result when urine containers contaminated with peroxide or oxidizing detergents simulate the glucose oxidase reaction. Substances that prevent oxidation of the chromogen or interfere with the enzymatic reaction may produce false-negative results. These include ascorbic acid, levodopa, aspirin, homogentisic acid, and 5-hydroxyindoleacetic acid. The sensitivity threshold for glucosuria testing via reagent strip is 100 mg/dL for Multistix® and 40 mg/dL for Chemstrip® tests.

Testing of blood in the urine is performed in suspected urinary tract infection, traumatic injury to the urinary tract, renal calculi, tumors, glomerulonephritis, and injury due to toxic chemicals or drugs. The most common interfering substance producing a false-positive result is urinary myoglobin which produces a grossly red-appearing urine and reacts positively with the previously described reagents. Contamination of urine with povidone-iodine or blood from menstrual flow also may produce a false-positive

result (43). Contaminating detergents, bacterial enzymes (e.g., E. coli peroxidase) and dietary peroxidase can produce positive reactions in the absence of hematuria. False negatives result with high ascorbic acid levels, elevated urine specific gravity and protein, and increased levels of urinary nitrite. A highly acidic urine specimen (especially below a pH of 5) may inhibit cellular hemolysis on the reagent pad with a resultant false-negative reading. Reagent strip testing detects approximately 5 to 10 red blood cells per microliter with increased sensitivity noted in detection of free hemoglobin compared with measurement of intact red blood cells (41, 42).

Urinary ketone detection is most commonly used in the diagnosis and management of patients with diabetes mellitus. Interfering substances include phthalein dyes (which produce a red color) and large concentrations of levodopa. A specimen that is improperly preserved before testing may result in bacterial breakdown of acetoacetic acid and falsely low ketone levels. Levels of acetoacetate as low as 5 to 10 mg/dL may be detected by reagent strips (41, 42).

Bilirubin, a degradation product of hemoglobin, can appear in the urine when the normal degradation process is disrupted with bile duct obstruction or hepatic damage. When exposed to light, bilirubin is rapidly destroyed and accurate urinary bilirubin testing becomes difficult. Oxidation of bilirubin to biliverdin (as occurs with exposure to room air) also impairs the diazo reaction. Thus rapid testing of fresh specimens is important in accurate detection of urinary bilirubin. As with identification of hematuria, high concentrations of nitrite and ascorbic acid lower test sensitivity. Detection of as little as 0.2 to 0.5 mg/dL is possible with reagent strips (41, 42).

Urobilinogen, another degradation product of hemoglobin, can be detected in urine in patients with liver disease or with hemolytic disorders. Reagent strips that use Erlich's reagent (p-dimethylamino-benzaldehyde) may result in false-positive tests if such interfering substances as sulfonamides, porphobilinogens, indican, and p-aminosalicylic acid are present. Chemstrip® uses a different reagent, as previously described, that results in a more specific test. Large concentrations of nitrite may result in false-negative results.

Results are described in Erlich units (with Multistix®) or as mg/dL (with Chemstrip®). The Chemstrip® sensitivity level is 0.4 mg/dL (41, 42).

The urinary nitrite test provides clinicians with a rapid screening test for urinary tract infection. Multiple studies have examined the clinical use and predictive value of testing urine for nitrite to detect urinary tract infections. Goldsmith and Campos analyzed 1010 urine specimens from infants and children and found low sensitivity levels (29% sensitive for urine culture results with or greater than 10^5 colony forming units/mL and 21% sensitive for cultures with or greater than 10^4 cfu/mL) and excellent specificity (99%). This study also found that the negative predictive value was 95% (44). False-negative results can be explained by lack of dietary nitrate, the organism Staphylococcus saprophyticus (a nonnitrate-reducing) bacterium, large concentrations of ascorbic acid in the specimen, and antibiotic inhibition of bacterial metabolism. Also with large numbers of bacteria, reduction of nitrite to nitrogen results in nondetectable levels by reagent strip testing. A urine sample that is allowed to sit for a prolonged period can result in proliferation of contaminant bacteria and false-positive test results, again emphasizing the requirement for testing a freshly voided specimen.

Leukocytes in the urine may indicate the presence of urinary tract infection (UTI). Urine testing and comparison with culture results reveal that the urine reagent strip that detects leukocyte esterase activity is 76% sensitive in urine specimens when subsequent cultures grow at or above 10^5 cfu/mL and 64% sensitive with or greater than 10^4 cfu/mL. Specificities are 81% and 82%, respectively, in the same study (44). Another investigation of this rapid screening test for detecting urinary tract infections in children reveals that a dipstick test of small (+1) or moderate (+2) leukocyte concentration was equivalent to approximately 10 leukocytes/hpf. Combining leukocyte and nitrite reagent strip testing was as sensitive as the laboratory urinalysis in detecting UTI, with fewer false-positive results. The authors caution, however, that in children under 2 years of age, the reagent strips that combined nitrite and leukocyte testing had only a 71% sensitivity (compared with the 87% detection for older children). Combining these two tests also revealed 98% negative predictive value (45). Specific interference of oxidizing agents (e.g., detergents) may result in false-positive results; however, this occurrence is uncommon. False-negative results may result with elevated urinary protein, glucose, or specific gravity.

The reagent pad that quantifies specific gravity provides readings in the 1.001 to 1.035 range. Specific gravity may be inaccurately measured by reagent strips in alkaline specimens due to the reagent bromthymol blue, which becomes active above a pH of 6.5, and thus requires adding a correction factor (0.005) to the results when alkaline urine is tested. Urinary protein may artificially elevate the specific gravity reading (42, 43).

Urine Glucose or Clinitest®

Background
The Clinitest® tablet is used for detecting urinary glucose and other sugars, such as galactose, fructose, lactose, and pentose (46). This is a copper reduction test that serves as a screening tool for the presence of metabolic disorders such as galactosemia. The tablet contains copper sulfate, sodium carbonate, sodium citrate, and sodium hydroxide. Addition of water and urine to the table results in the following reaction in the presence of urinary reducing substance (47):

Cupric ions + reducing substance → cuprous ions + oxidized substance

At the end of the reaction, the color change from blue, when compared with the manufacturer's color chart, approximates the amount of glucose or reducing substance present in the urine. Clinitest®, used in conjunction with the urine dipstick, confirms the presence of glucose (if the dipstick is positive), or detects other reducing sugars (if the dipstick is negative). The Clinitest® is waived under CLIA regulations.

Equipment
Fresh urine sample
Dropper
Test tube
Clinitest® tablet and manufacturer's color chart
Distilled water

Procedure

Two drops of urine are placed in the test tube. The dropper is rinsed and ten drops of distilled water are placed in the test tube with urine. Next, the Clinitest® tablet is placed in the test tube and the completion of the reaction is awaited. The solution should bubble and the test tube will feel hot to the touch. After the bubbling has ceased for 15 seconds, one should gently agitate the test tube, note color change, and compare with the manufacturer's color chart.

Interpretation

The color change in the presence of reducing substances progresses from a negative blue to brick red with increasing urinary sugar concentration (see test package insert). At high glucose levels, the color change may pass through the orange and red stage to return to a dark color (blue, blue-green, or green-brown) appearing negative for reducing substances, unless the preceding color change was noted.

The sensitivity level of the Clinitest® tablet is a minimum level of 200 mg/dL of glucose. A positive Clinitest® reaction, in addition to indicating the presence of glucose or other reducing sugars, may indicate the presence of ascorbic acid, salicylates, streptomycin, tetracycline, nalidixic acid, penicillin, methyldopa, probenecid, chloramphenicol, or cephalosporins in the urine. Thus a positive Clinitest® reaction may require confirmatory testing in the laboratory to rule out the presence of an interfering substance and to identify the specific sugar (46).

Urine Specific Gravity

Background

Specific gravity reflects the density of the dissolved chemicals in the urine specimen and thus the kidneys' ability to selectively reabsorb essential compounds and water from the glomerular filtrate. Although specific gravity can be determined chemically using a dipstick as previously discussed, an alternative approach is using a urinometer or refractometer.

The urinometer is a weighted float that, placed in a liquid, displaces a volume equal to its weight. Additional mass due to dissolved substances in the urine results in the float displacing a volume of urine smaller than that of distilled water. Thus the specimen's specific gravity determines the level to which the urinometer sinks. The urinometer is calibrated (1.000 to 1.040) in terms of urine specific gravity. The refractometer measures the refractive index of the solution (urine), which is the comparison of the velocity of light in air with the light in a solution. The concentration of compounds in solution determines both the velocity of and the angle at which light passes through the solution. The refractometer measures this angle and converts the refractive index to a specific gravity (42). Both tests are waived under CLIA regulations.

Equipment

If using urinometer:
  10 to 15 mL of urine
  Large container

If using refractometer:
  1 to 2 mL of urine
  Glass dropper or plastic syringe

Procedure

When using the urinometer, 10 to 15 mL of urine specimen is poured into a large container. The urinometer is placed in the specimen with a spinning motion. The urinometer must be in a large enough volume of urine that it does not rest on the bottom or touch the sides of the container. Finally, one reads the scale printed on the urinometer at the bottom of the urine meniscus.

When using the refractometer, one drop of urine is placed on the prism. The instrument is focused at a good light source. Then the specific gravity scale is read.

Interpretation

Specific gravity levels may fall between 1.001 and 1.035 which, in large part, depend on the patient's hydration status, specimen temperature, and presence of urinary glucose and/or protein. However, patients receiving high molecular weight intravenous fluids or radiograph contrast media may have abnormally high specific gravity levels detected (42).

Glucose and protein as high molecular weight substances increase the density of the urine specimen. Their contribution to the specific gravity is subtracted from the measured reading. The amount subtracted is based on the following: A gram of protein per deciliter of urine raises the specific gravity by 0.003; a gram of glucose per deciliter of urine raises the specific gravity 0.004.

The urinometer is calibrated for a particular temperature (approximately 20°C). A cold temperature artificially elevates specific gravity. Therefore, for every 3° that the specimen temperature is below urinometer calibration temperature, 0.001 must be subtracted from the specific gravity reading. This method is applicable especially if a specimen has been refrigerated before the reading, generally not the case in the ED setting.

Microscopic Examination of Urine Sediment

Background
Urine sediment refers to the multiple constituents of a urinary specimen that may include erythrocytes, leukocytes, epithelial cells, or casts composed of these cells. Also included are bacteria, yeast, or parasites, and spermatozoa, mucus, and crystals. Supravital staining of urine sediment may more clearly delineate these sediment constituents. This test is classified as physician-performed microscopy by CLIA.

Equipment
Urine specimen, freshly voided
Centrifuge tube and centrifuge
Glass slide and coverslip
Supravital stain (crystal violet and safranin)

Procedure
A clean catch or catheterized urine specimen is obtained. A freshly-voided specimen is examined. If a delay in examination is anticipated, the specimen is refrigerated and examined within 48 hours. At examination, the specimen is mixed well, placed in the centrifuge tube, and centrifuged at 1500 rpm for 5 minutes. Next, supernatant fluid is removed by aspiration with dropper or syringe. The centrifuge tube is tapped to resuspend the sediment. Then, 1 to 2 mL of the resuspended sediment is removed, a drop placed on the slide, and a coverslip applied.

The specimen is examined under low power to identify epithelial cells, crystals, mucus, bacteria, yeast, sperm, and artifacts. At least 10 low power fields are reviewed. Under high power, one seeks to identify casts, erythrocytes, and leukocytes. Another option to help delineate cellular components is to apply a drop of supravital stain to the specimen and reexamine under low and high power.

Interpretation
Erythrocytes in the urine are colorless disks on microscopic examination (Fig. 124.6). The cells shrink in concentrated urine, and swell and lyse in alkaline dilute urine. Smaller than leukocytes, erythrocytes are approximately 7 mm in diameter and may be confused with oil droplets or yeast. Red blood cells cannot enter the filtrate of an intact nephron; thus the presence of erythrocytes in the urine is abnormal and may be associated with injury to the glomerular membrane, or result from renal calculi, urinary tract infection, malignancies, damaged renal capillaries or vascular injury, and toxic- or allergy-mediated reactions. The appearance of erythrocytes in urine may indicate contamination due to vaginal bleeding or menstruation.

No visible erythrocytes on microscopic examination of sediment may indicate absence of bleeding, infection, or glomerular damage, but may represent a false-negative result. Red blood cells may be disrupted or lysed and only the hemoglobin is detectable by urine dipstick (chemical analysis) or by macroscopic appearance (red urine) in the presence of a negative microscopic examination. More than three red blood cells per high power field is considered abnormal (47).

Pyuria, a condition of white blood cells in the urine, occurs in the presence of infection, inflammation, or malignancy within the genitourinary system. Less than five white blood cells per high power field can be found in a normal urine specimen. Leukocytes are easier to identify than erythrocytes due to their larger size (diameter approximately 12 μm) and cellular components (visible cytoplasm and nuclei). Nuclear details, especially the multilobed nucleus of the polymorphonuclear leukocyte, can be enhanced with supravital staining. Renal tubular epithelial cells may be confused with leukocytes, again necessitating staining techniques.

Table 124.9.
Examination of Urinary Sediment: Casts and Associated Conditions

Cast	Associated Conditions
Hyaline	Glomerulonephris, pyelonephritis, stress, exercise, chronic renal disease, congestive heart failure
Red blood cell	Glomerulonephritis, exercise
White blood cell	Pyelonephritis
Epithelial cell	Renal tubular damage
Granular	Urinary stasis, urinary tract infection, stress, exercise
Fatty	Nephrotic syndrome

Casts are formed within the renal tubular lumen or collecting ducts and are generally cylindrical, with parallel sides and rounded ends. Casts form when urinary stasis, stress or exercise, pyelonephritis, glomerulonephritis, urinary tract infection, nephrotic syndrome, renal tubular damage, or chronic renal disease are present. A summary of the conditions associated with urinary casts is provided in Table 124.9.

Epithelial cells, sloughed from the cellular lining of the genitourinary system, are often found in normal urine specimens. Epithelial cells originate from the vagina and lower urethra (squamous epithelial cells), the renal pelvis, bladder, and upper urethra (transitional epithelial cells); and renal tubules (renal tubular epithelial cells). Squamous cells are irregularly shaped, large cells, easily identified under low power, with a central nucleus (about the size of erythrocyte) and abundant cytoplasm. They are frequently seen in a specimen that is obtained without adequate preparation, such as without using the clean catch technique. Transitional epithelial cells are smaller than squamous cells, round, and contain a central nucleus. In the absence of unusual morphology, these cells seldom indicate pathology. When large numbers of unusually shaped transitional epithelial cells are seen on microscopic examination of urine, renal carcinoma (and therefore cytologic examination) should be considered. Renal tubular cells are round, larger than

Figure 124.6.
Urine sediment: microscopic findings (100× magnification).

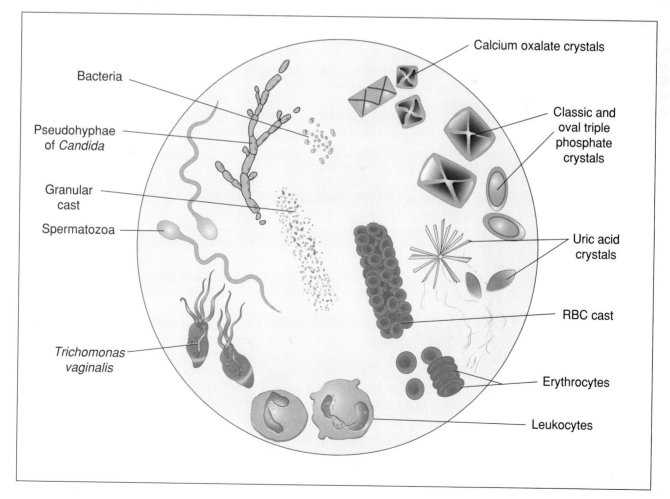

1285

leukocytes, with a single round nucleus. These cells, present in large numbers, indicate tubular injury as can be seen in infectious, inflammatory, toxin-mediated, and allergic processes. Tubular damage also occurs in renal transplant rejection. Staining techniques help distinguish leukocytes from renal tubular cells, particularly regarding nuclear detail and morphology.

Bacteria in the urine are identified in cases of pyelonephritis, urinary tract infection, and in contaminated urine specimens. The Gram-negative organisms are the most common pathogens and are most easily seen under high power using Gram-staining techniques. Specimens that remain at room temperature must be examined shortly after collection. With delay in microscopic examination, bacteria may represent multiplication of contaminant organisms rather than an acute infectious process.

Yeast cells, most commonly the *Candida albicans* species, seen in patients with vaginal candidiasis and/or diabetes may be confused with erythrocytes on microscopic examination of urine sediment. Another organism, *Trichomonas vaginalis*, the most commonly encountered parasite identified in urine, may resemble a leukocyte. Because of its flagellated structure and movement in urine, however, it is usually easily distinguished. Finally, spermatozoa can be seen in urine (please refer to the Gynecology section of the chapter for further discussion).

Mucous threads seen on examination of urine sediment are composed of protein material produced by cells of the genitourinary system. The threads are irregular in shape and better visualized under low light. Clumps of mucus can be similar in appearance to hyaline casts.

Crystals commonly seen in urine are present in healthy patients and in pathologic conditions. In acidic urine, urate crystals are reddish-brown or yellow. These different shaped crystals (rhomboid, wedge, needle, or rosette) can appear in urine specimens in the absence of disease, in patients with leukemia, and in some cases of arthritis. Calcium oxalate crystals, colorless prism shapes or octahedral shapes that resemble envelopes, may suggest ethylene glycol poisoning, but also appear in normal acidic urine specimens. In alkaline urine, the triple phosphate crystal is a colorless prism resembling a coffin lid. Calcium phosphate crystals, also colorless, can appear as plates, needles, or thin prisms. Abnormal crystals in urine include cystine, cholesterol, leucine, tyrosine, sulfonomides, radiographic dyes, bilirubin, and ampicillin. These crystals are depicted in Figure 124.6.

Finally, artifactual material often is found in urine specimens, including oil droplets, hair, fibers, or talcum powder, reinforcing the need for proper specimen collection and using clean containers, droppers, syringes, slides, and coverslips (42, 47).

BLOOD CHEMISTRY TESTING

Dextrostick®/Chemstrip®

Background
Reagent strip test for rapid determination of blood sugar contains color indicators and the enzymes glucose oxidase and peroxidase. Blood is placed on the reagent pad, and glucose oxidase catalyzes the D-glucose oxidation. Hydrogen peroxide that results from this reaction oxidizes the color indicators in the presence of peroxidase. The glucose concentration is a semiquantitative glucose measurement, completed by comparing the reagent pad with the color chart provided on the reagent strip container label (41). This test is classified waived by CLIA (when done with apparatus approved by FDA for home use).

Equipment
Reagent strip
Container label with color chart
Alcohol swab
Lancet or needle, sterile
Cotton ball
Clock or timer

Procedure
The reagent strip pads are compared with the unused color block on the color chart. The pads should not appear darker in color than the reference colors on the chart. A blood specimen is obtained using alcohol-swabbed fingertip and lancet or sterile needle. The finger is squeezed until one large blood droplet forms, then the droplet is touched to the reagent pad without smearing the blood sample or touching the pad with the fingers. After waiting 60 seconds, any excess blood is

wiped from test pad using a cotton ball. After waiting another 60 seconds, so that the total time elapsed (with blood in contact with the reagent pad) is 2 minutes, the reagent pad colors are matched with the color chart and the estimated glucose level is recorded (41).

Interpretation

Blood glucose level depends on a person's age, dietary intake, timing of test in relation to food intake, and presence of disease (e.g., diabetes, infection, alcohol intoxication). Chemstrip bG® provides a range of detectable glucose levels between 20 mg/dL and 800 mg/dL. Normal fasting glucose levels in an adult may range from 70 to 110 mg/dL and after meals, 110 to 180 mg/dL. The neonate's blood sugar, however, ranges from 35 to 90 mg/dL (41).

In a study of chemstrip glucose determination with glucose levels below 80 mg/dL, Chemstrip bG® has a 61% positive predictive value. When the Chemstrip bG® reading was negative (at or less than 40 mg/dL), the test always predicted the absence of hypoglycemia (48). Another study comparing Chemstrip bG® with Dextrostix® revealed Chemstrip bG® glucose levels were closer to true values and sometimes lower than measured glucose concentrations. Correlation between measured and actual glucose values proved better with Chemstrip bG® at all glucose levels tested (i.e., less than 60 mg/dL, 60 to 200 mg/dL, and 200 to 600 mg/dL (49).

Certain factors may interfere with glucose values as determined by the dextrostick method. Hyperlipidemic patients may have inaccurate glucose readings. In samples with glucose concentration above 200 mg/dL, elevated hematocrits (above 55%) may also artificially lower measured glucose levels (as much as 15%). Very low hemotocrits (below 35%) may artificially raise glucose values (up to 10%). In the hyperglycemic, hyperosmolar, and ketotic state, blood values may be underestimated by the dextrostick method. Certain drugs will interfere with the Chemstrip bG® reaction—dopamine or methyldopa, at concentrations of 10 mg/dL (much higher than the therapeutic concentration of either) will inhibit the reagent pad reaction (41). Care must also be taken in interpretating the neonate's blood sugar measured below 50 mg/dL by the dextrostick method and should be confirmed by the hospital laboratory.

EMERGENCY DEPARTMENT LABORATORIES

The type of clinical testing required in the ED depends on the volume of patients and severity of illness encountered. At minimum, an ED should have the capacity for rapid determination of hematocrit or hemoglobin, fecal occult blood testing, rapid determination of serum glucose, urine pregnancy testing, and urine dipstick testing. These tests are inexpensive, easy to perform, and valuable in assisting with diagnosis and treatment.

Other useful tests include KOH preparation, wet preparation of vaginal and cervical secretions, motile sperm microscopy, urine sediment microscopy, and Gram stain. However, these tests require a dedicated microscope, appropriate training, and, in the case of Gram stain, a high degree of laboratory oversight. Emergency departments with high patient volume may be best served by a stat laboratory within the department which has a dedicated laboratory technician who can perform a variety of tests including complete blood count, erythrocyte sedimentation rate, microscopic urinalysis, and Gram stain. An onsite stat laboratory has the advantages of test performance by a highly trained technician, rapid test turnaround, and the ability of the clinician to review test results easily with the technician. The principal drawback to an onsite stat laboratory is cost and space.

REFERENCES

1. Schuman AJ. Office labs: still worth it under CLIA? Contemp Pediatr 1993;10:50–74.
2. Baron EJ, Finegold SM, eds. Bailey and Scott's diagnostic microbiology. 8th ed. St. Louis: CV Mosby, 1990.
3. Murray PR. Microscopy. In: Wentworth BB, ed. Diagnostic procedures for bacterial infections. Washington, DC: American Public Health Association, 1987, pp. 681–683.
4. Quintiliani R, Bartlett RC. Examination of the Gram-stained smear (essay). Hoffman-LaRoche Inc., 1985.
5. Farmer MY, Hook EW, Heald FP. Laboratory evaluation of sexually transmitted disease. Pediatr Ann 1986;15(10):715–724.
6. Walsh RD, Cunha BA. Diagnostic significance of the sputum Gram stain in pneumonia. Hosp Physician 1992 October:37–44.
7. Larone DH. Medically important fungi: a guide to identification. 2nd ed. New York: Elsevier, 1987, pp. 173–177.

SUMMARY	
ED Test	**CLIA Status**
Blood glucose	W*
Fecal occult blood	W
Microhematocrit	W
Urine Clinitest®	W
Urine dipstick	W
Urine specific gravity	W
Urine pregnancy	W
Cellophane tape	PPM
KOH	PPM
Motile sperm	PPM
Urine sediment	PPM
Gram stain	MC

Key: W = waived;
PPM = physician-performed microscopy
MC = moderate complexity

*Waived when done by apparatus approved by FDA for home use.

8. Markell EK, Voge M, John DT, eds. Medical parasitology. 7th ed. Philadelphia: WB Saunders, 1992, pp. 72–74, 268–269, 421–422.

9. Garcia LS, Bruckner DA, Brewer TC, Shimizu RY. Techniques for the recovery and identification of cryptosporidium oocysts from stool specimens. J Clin Microbiol 1993;18(1):185–190.

10. Farmer MY, Hook EW, Heald FP. Laboratory evaluation of sexually transmitted diseases. Pediatr Ann 1986; 15(10):716–724.

11. Spiegel CA, Amsel R, Holmes KK. Diagnosis of bacterial vaginosis by direct Gram stain of vaginal fluid. J Clin Microbiol 1983;18(1):170–177.

12. Spiegel CA. Vaginitis. In: Wentworth BB, Judson FN, eds. Laboratory methods for the diagnosis of sexually transmitted diseases. Washington, DC: American Public Health Association, 1984, pp. 151–168.

13. Johnson J, Shew ML. Screening and diagnostic tests for sexually transmitted diseases in adolescents. Sem Pediatr Infect Dis 1993;4(3):142–150.

14. Krieger JN, Tam MR, Stevens CE, Nielsen IO, Hale J, Kiviat NB, Holmes KK. Diagnosis of Trichomoniasis. JAMA 1988;259(8):1223–1227.

15. Stephenson JN. Pregnancy testing and counseling. Pediatr Clin North Am 1989;36(3):681–696.

16. Braunstein GD. HCG testing. Vol. I. A clinical guide for the testing of human chorionic gonadotropin (monograph). Abbott Park, IL: Abbott Diagnostics Educational Services, 1993, pp. 3–23.

17. Braunstien GD. HCG testing. Vol. 2. Answers to frequently asked questions about HCG testing (monograph). Abbott Park, IL: Abbott Diagnostics Educational Services, 1991, pp. 4–17.

18. Pittaway DE, Reish RL, Wentz AC. Doubling times of human chorionic gonadotropin increase in early viable intrauterine pregnancies. Am J Obstet Gynecol 1985;152:299–302.

19. Fritz MA, Guo S. Doubling time of human chorionic gonadotropin (HCG) in early normal pregnancy: relationship to HCG concentration and gestational age. Fertil Steril 1987;47:584–589.

20. Product insert. Clearview HCG. Cranbury, NJ: Wampole Laboratories, Division of Carter-Wallace, Inc.

21. Product insert. Neo-planotest Duoclon slide. Durham, NC: Organon Teknika Corporation.

22. Product insert. HCG-Nostick. Durham, NC: Organon Teknika Corporation.

23. Product insert. Icon II HCG (urine). San Diego: Hybritech Inc.

24. Product insert. Pregnospia II. Durham, NC: Organon Teknika Corporation.

25. Product insert: Pregnosticon Dri-Dot. Durham, NC: Organon Teknika Corporation.

26. Product insert. Quidel Quick Vue One-Step HCG-Urine. Abbott Park, IL: Abbott Laboratories, Diagnostics Division.

27. Product insert. Abbott Park, IL: Abbott TestPack Plus HCG-Urine. Abbott Laboratories, Diagnostics Division.

28. Hoelzer M. Sexual assault. In: Tintinalli JE, ed. Emergency medicine: a comprehensive study guide. New York: McGraw-Hill, 1992, pp. 398–402.

29. Braen GR. Sexual assault. In: Rosen P, Barkin RM, eds. Emergency medicine concepts and clinical practice. St. Louis: CV Mosby, 1992, pp. 2003–2012.

30. Dym M. The male reproductive system. In: Weiss L, ed. Histology cell and tissue biology. New York: Elsevier Biomedical, 1983, pp. 1014–1017.

31. Christensen F, Anker N, Mondrup M. Blood in faeces. A comparison of the sensitivity and reproducibility of five chemical methods. Clin Che Acta 1974;57:23–27.

32. Product insert. Hemoccult. San Jose: SmithKline Diagnostics, Inc.

33. Product insert. Hematest. Elkhart, IN: Ames Company.

34. Jacobs DS, Kasten BL, Demott WR, Wolfson WL. Laboratory test handbook. Cleveland: Lexi-Comp/Mosby, 1988, pp. 621–622.

35. Ostrow JD, Mulvaney CA, Hansell JR, et al. Sensitivity and reproducibility of chemical tests for fecal occult blood with an emphasis on false-positive reactions. Am J Digest Dis 1973;18:930–940.

36. Fisher PM, Addison LA, Curtis P, Mitchell JM. The office laboratory. Norwalk, CT: Appleton-Century-Crofts, 1983, pp. 78–84.

37. Bartfield JM, Robinson D, Lekas J. Accuracy of microcentrifuged hematocrits in the emergency department. J Emerg Med 1993;11:673–676.

38. von Schenck H, Falkensson M, Lundberg B. Evaluation of "HemoCue," a new device for determining hemoglobin. Clin Chem 1986;32(3):526–529.

39. Chen PP, Short TG, Leung DHY, Oh TE. A clinical evaluation of the HemoCue haemoglobinometer using capillary, venous, and arterial samples. Anaesth Intensive Car 1992;20(4):497–503.

40. Cohen AR, Seidl-Friedman J. HemoCue system for hemoglobin measurement. Am J Clin Pathol 1988; 90:302–305.

41. Product insert. Chemstrip bG. Indianapolis: BioDynamics/bmc.

42. Strasinger SK. Urinalysis and body fluids. A self-instructional text. 2nd ed. Philadelphia: FA Davis, 1989, pp. 46–50, 54–86.

43. Litwin MS, Graham SD. False-positive hematuria (edit). JAMA 1985;254(13):1724.

44. Goldsmith BM, Campos JM. Comparison of urine dipstick, microscopy, and culture for the detection of bacteruria in children. Clin Pediatr 1989;29(4): 214–218.

45. Shaw KN, Hexter D, McGowan KL, Schwartz JS. Clinical evaluation of a rapid screening test for urinary tract infections in children. J Pediatir 1991; 118(5):733–736.

46. Product insert. Clinitest. Elkhart, IN: Ames Division, Miles Laboratories.

47. Free HM, ed. Modern urine chemistry. Elkhart, IN: Miles Laboratories, 1986, p. 44.

48. Maisels MJ, Lee CA. Chemstrip glucose test strips: correlation with true glucose values less than 80 mg/dL. Crit Care Med 1983;11(4):293–295.

49. Chernow B, Diaz M, Cruess D, Balestrieri F, Uddin D, Rainey TG, O'Brian JT. Bedside glucose determinations in critical care medicine: a comparative analysis of two techniques. Crit Care Med 1982; 10(7):463–465.

CHAPTER 125

Skin Testing

Zach Kassutto

Introduction

Intradermal injections can be used for the diagnosis of tuberculosis, allergy testing, or local anesthesia. The rationale for injecting into the dermis, as opposed to the subcutaneous layer of the skin or the muscle, is to elicit localized effects while limiting the systemic dispersion of the injected substances. Injecting into the dermis also can elicit specific immune responses that are easily detected by inspection and palpation. The procedure is quickly learned and is performed by a physician, nurse, or physician's assistant. Intradermal injections can be used with children in any age group. This chapter will focus primarily on using intradermal injections as related to tuberculosis.

The classic and most common application of this procedure is the intradermal injection of mycobacterium derivatives to diagnose previous mycobacterium infection. This procedure, first described by Mantoux in 1908 (1), is currently the most widely used and cost-effective tool for diagnosing tuberculosis. Given the recent resurgence of tuberculosis in the United States, this diagnostic procedure often is used in the emergency department (ED) setting.

Anatomy and Physiology

The skin is composed of three basic layers (see Fig. 129.1)—the epidermis, the dermis, and the subcutaneous tissue. The epidermis is a thin, superficial layer composed of an outer layer of dead, keratinized epithelial cells and an inner cellular layer. The dermis lies just beneath the epidermis and contains blood vessels, connective tissue, hair follicles, and sebaceous glands. The deeper subcutaneous layer contains mostly fat. This layer supports the blood vessels, nerves, and lymphatics that supply the more superficial layers. Sweat glands and roots of hair follicles also are found in the subcutaneous layer.

The tuberculin tests (tine and Mantoux) are the prototypes of a cell-mediated immune response (type IV hypersensitivity reaction). In the nonimmunocompromised patient, exposure to an antigen (e.g., *Mycobacterium tuberculosis*) results in the development of sensitized lymphocytes. Reexposure to the antigen (as in intradermal injection) causes these cells to release mediators at the site of reexposure, which results in induration and erythema (a positive test). If no reaction occurs, the patient was not exposed to a significant load of the antigen previously, or the patient is anergic. This type of reaction, called a delayed hypersensitivity skin test, usually manifests within 48 to 72 hours. Table 125.1 lists other potential antigens available for intradermal skin testing.

Other antigens such as antibiotics result in an immediate hypersensitivity reaction mediated by IgE on presensitized mast cells in the dermis (type I hypersensitivity reaction). This type of reaction can detect sensitivity to a host of other antigens including other drugs, microorganisms, pollens, animal dander, and helminths. A positive response is manifested by the triple response of Lewis et

Table 125.1.
Examples of Substances Injected Intradermally

Tests for *Mycobacterium* infection
  Old tuberculin (OT)
  Purified protein derivative (PPD)
Antigens for anergy testing
  Tetanus toxoid antigen
  Diphtheria toxoid antigen
  Streptococcus antigen
  Candida antigen
  Trichophyton antigen
  Proteus antigen
Negative controls for hypersensitivity
   testing
  Normal saline solution
  Glycerine
Tests for evidence of infection
  Leprosy
  Lymphogranuloma venereum
  Mumps
  Cat scratch disease
  Chancroid
  Brucellosis
  Tularemia
  Glanders
  Toxoplasmosis
  Blastomycosis
  Histoplasmosis
  Coccidioidomycosis
  Trichonosis
  Filariasis
Allergy testing
  Horse serum based antivenin
  Drugs (including antibiotics)
  Pollens
  Animal dander
  Bee venoms
Local anesthesia
  Lidocaine or other local anesthetic

al. (2). Initially the skin becomes pale, followed by an erythematous flare, and then a slight swelling or induration described as a wheal. This dermal reaction to histamine usually begins within 5 minutes of allergen exposure and peaks at approximately 30 minutes. Occasionally, a late phase reaction occurs 3 to 24 hours later which manifests as ill-defined edema.

INDICATIONS

When tuberculin is introduced into the dermis with a syringe, the test is called the Mantoux test. This test is the current gold standard for detecting tuberculosis. It is indicated acutely in suspected mycobacterial infection, or in patients with a significant tuberculosis exposure (Table 125.2). This diagnosis should be considered in children with chronic cough, pneumonia (especially of the upper lobes), adenopathy (particularly of the hilum) or adenitis (especially of the head or neck), or meningitis. Tuberculosis can involve virtually any body system including the lungs, central nervous system, gastrointestinal system, cardiovascular system, bones, joints, skin, and eyes. Children at high risk for tuberculous infection should be tested annually (Table 125.2). The screening multiple puncture tests are no longer recommended for the diagnosis of tuberculosis due to a high rate of false-positive (approximately 20%) and false-negative (up to approximately 10%) responses (3). The only absolute contraindication for intradermal tuberculin placement is a

Table 125.2.
Patients at Risk for Tuberculosis Infection

1. Contacts of adults with infectious tuberculosis
2. Patient or parents from country with high prevalence of tuberculosis
3. Frequent exposure to high risk adults (HIV-infected patients, homeless persons, drug abusers, poor and medically indigent city dwellers, nursing home residents, migrant farm workers)
4. Chest radiograph abnormalities suggestive of tuberculosis
5. Clinical evidence of tuberculosis
6. HIV seropositivity
7. Immunosuppressive disorders
8. Corticosteroids at immunosuppressive doses
9. Other medical risk factors (Hodgkin's disease, lymphoma, diabetes, chronic renal failure, malnutrition)
10. Incarcerated adolescents

Adapted from Lewis T, Grant RT. Vascular reactions of the skin to injury. Part II. Heart 1924;11:209.

severe skin reaction with prior testing. The patient will give a history of a bullous or necrotic type reaction. On examining the patient, it is also likely that a residual scarring from such a reaction will occur.

The Mantoux test using purified protein derivative (PPD) is also useful for the diagnosis of diseases due to nontuberculous mycobacterium (cervical adenitis is the most common example in children). These organisms share a number of common antigens with *M. tuberculosis* and account for many false-positive reactions when *M. tuberculosis* is being ruled out.

Skin testing also is used to test for allergic and anergic reactions. Tests other than intradermal injection are used by allergists to test for immediate hypersensitivity. These include the scratch test and the prick-puncture test. In the scratch test, a superficial scratch is made through the outer cornified layer of the skin. The allergen is then applied to the area. Nonspecific reactions can occur at the site in response to the local trauma alone, resulting in false-positive testing. This test is not recommended for routine use. In the prick-puncture test, allergen is applied to the skin surface and then a needle is passed through the substance into the epidermis. The needle tip is then elevated to lift a small portion of the epidermis. Clinicians feel the intradermal test is more sensitive and is therefore the test of choice in the ED. Skin tests for hypersensitivity to drugs or other substances are rarely, if ever, carried out in the emergency setting. In the rare event that a potential antigen needs to be given to a patient, an allergist can be consulted. In most cases, such as suspected antibiotic allergy, an alternative drug can be selected. If no alternative is available, and the situation is life threatening or the allergy history is vague, the drug is given with appropriate precautions in the event of anaphylaxis.

Intradermal injection also can be used for local anesthesia (Chapter 37), and for antitoxin allergy testing in cases of envenomations (Chapter 130).

EQUIPMENT

Alcohol swab
Sterile, disposable tuberculin syringe

Intradermal needle—small gauge (26 or 27), short (0.25 to 0.50"), beveled
Purified protein derivative (PPD)

Two commercial tuberculin preparations are currently available—purified protein derivative, and old tuberculin. Old tuberculin (OT), a heat-sterilized preparation of tubercle bacilli, was first produced by Robert Koch in the late 19th century. Koch proposed OT as a possible therapy for tuberculosis, but it proved to be ineffective. It is currently used primarily for tuberculosis screening. In the tine test (so called for the sharp prongs or tines which are used to puncture the skin), OT or PPD is introduced into the skin by a multiple puncture device (commercial brands include MonoVacc®, Aplitest®, and Tine®).

PPD also can be introduced into the skin with a so-called tuberculin syringe. The same size and type of equipment is used regardless of the patient's age (see Procedure).

If multiple antigens are to be injected for anergy testing, an anergy panel is available (Multitest CMI). This device consists of a plastic applicator with multiple sterile test heads preloaded with skin antigens and a negative control. As with the injection of any chemical or biologic product, monitoring and resuscitative equipment should be available in the event of an adverse reaction such as anaphylaxis.

PROCEDURE

This procedure is considered routine, and written consent is not required. The substance to be injected should not be outdated. The active fraction of all tuberculins are easily absorbed onto plastic or glass. These substances therefore need to be kept in a cool, dark place and should not be transferred from one container to another. To avoid reduced potency, tuberculin should be injected as soon as possible after it is drawn into the syringe.

A site for injection needs to be selected. Preferably it should be free of hair, obvious superficial blood vessels, pigmented lesions, and infected or other skin lesions. If scarred by the procedure, the location should have minimal cosmetic ramifications. The volar aspect of the forearm several inches distal to the elbow is the most frequently used area.

Infrequently, the patient's back can be used. The diaphragm of the vial stopper is wiped with 70% alcohol and then the substance to be injected is drawn into a tuberculin syringe. For PPD, use 0.1 mL or 5 TU (tuberculin units), because no current indications suggest otherwise. Air bubbles are removed from both the syringe and the lumen of the needle. Using circular motions, a 3 cm region of skin is cleansed with an alcohol swab. After the alcohol dries completely, the skin is stretched by placing thumb and forefingers at either side of the injection site. Alternatively, the forearm may be grasped from the posterior aspect which secures the arm and stretches the skin at the same time.

The syringe is held nearly parallel to the skin, with the bevel of the needle directed up. The angle of the needle to the skin should be less than 15° relative to the skin surface. The clinician then inserts the needle into the skin just past the opening in the bevel of the needle. The clinician pulls the plunger back to ensure that a blood vessel has not been entered. If blood is aspirated, the clinician should withdraw the needle and reattempt the procedure with a new syringe at a different location. The substance is injected while the skin is observed for the appearance of a wheal or a pale bleb (Fig. 125.1). Waiting several seconds after injecting the substance before removing the needle will minimize the amount of liquid that may seep through the injection site upon withdrawal of the needle. The needle is then removed slowly. The presence of a wheal confirms injection into the dermal layer. Absence of a wheal, or more than a small amount of bleeding at the injection site, indicates probable injection into the subcutaneous tissue (4).

The exact time and site of the injection is documented. The intradermal PPD test is standardized regarding the dose of tuberculin injected and the definition of the diameter of a positive response. PPD that seeps out of the skin may falsely decrease the amount of a dermal response in a patient who is sensitized.

After the injection, the perimeter of the injection site may be marked with a waterproof pen or skin marker so that the site of injection is easily located when the patient returns for follow-up. For the injection of allergens, the patient should be observed for 30 minutes for possible allergic reaction.

SUMMARY

1. Select site for injection, usually volar aspect of forearm
2. Draw up substance to be injected using sterile technique
3. Cleanse skin with 70% alcohol swab, allow to dry
4. Secure arm, and stretch skin at injection site
5. Hold syringe with bevel up and nearly parallel to skin; insert needle into superficial layers of skin just past tip of needle
6. Aspirate to ensure that a blood vessel has not been entered, then slowly inject substance
7. Slowly withdraw needle and confirm intradermal placement by presence of a wheal
8. Document site of injection and consider circling site with waterproof marker
9. Guarantee follow-up with physician in 48 to 72 hours for interpretation

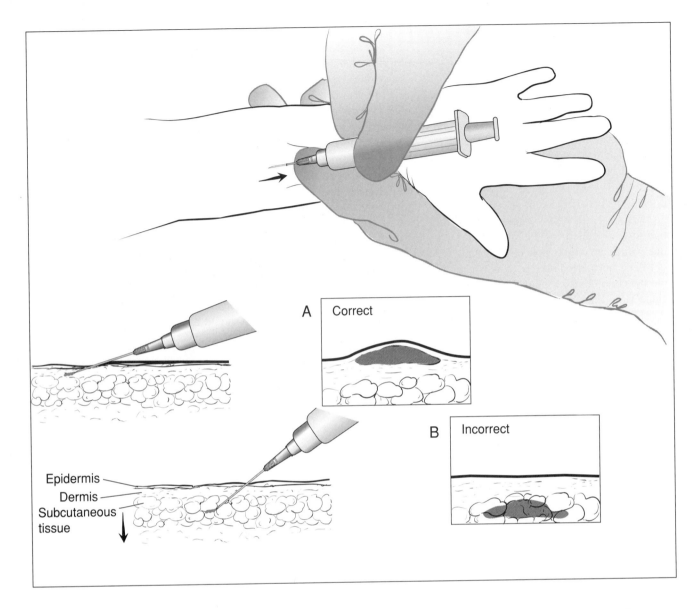

Figure 125.1.
Correct positioning of syringe and hands for intradermal injection. *Insets:* Intradermal placement of injectant.

A Correct

B Incorrect

Epidermis
Dermis
Subcutaneous
tissue

Some authorities advocate using a control injection with sterile normal saline on the opposite forearm. Isopropyl alcohol, for example, can cause a reaction that may be misinterpreted as a response to antigen. This technique is often used when testing for immediate hypersensitivity, but is not common for tuberculin testing.

Appropriate follow-up must occur (48- to 72-hour recheck in the case of a Mantoux test). All results should be interpreted by qualified medical personnel, and not by the patient or family member. Induration of greater than or equal to 15 mm is a positive test. A reaction that is less than 5 mm is negative. Reactions between 5 and 15 mm are interpreted based on the patient's age and risk factors (Table 125.3). Repeat testing may be

indicated 8 to 10 weeks after the first test. Many patients with tuberculosis demonstrate anergy early in the course of illness. Patients also may be anergic due to coinfections, young age, and immunosuppression. Other patients may have an increased response to skin testing. These include patients who have received BCG (bacillus calmette guerin) vaccination, or patients exposed to mycobacterium (including nontuberculous mycobacterium) who have had repetitive skin testing. This so-called booster phenomenon cannot be differentiated from the response to natural infection, and therefore has no bearing on the interpretation of the skin test.

The family should receive instructions to call or return at once if skin breakdown occurs, or if the patient develops evidence of a

Table 125.3.
Definition of Positive Mantoux Skin Test in Children

Reaction ≥5 mm
1. Close contact with known or suspected case of tuberculosis
2. Clinical or radiographic evidence of disease
3. Host factors increasing risk for tuberculosis (e.g., HIV, immunosuppressive disorders)

Reaction ≥10 mm
1. Age ≤4 years
2. Medical risk factors (see item 9 in Table 125.2)
3. Increased environmental exposure (see items 2 and 3 in Table 125.2)

Reaction ≥15 mm
All children, even without risk factors

Adapted from Committee on Infectious Diseases, American Academy of Pediatrics. Screening for tuberculosis in infants and children. Pediatrics 1994;93:131–134.

systemic allergic reaction (e.g., hives or respiratory distress). Other family members also may require testing for tuberculosis if exposure was significant.

COMPLICATIONS

Some hypersensitive patients may develop a severe reaction at the injection site which may range from vesiculation to ulceration and necrosis. Such strongly positive tests can result in scarring. For this reason, areas of lesser cosmetic importance are chosen for this test. All patients receiving PPD need to be questioned regarding such a reaction, as it is a contraindication to standard PPD testing. Other less significant reactions include transient bleeding or immediate erythema at the puncture site. Some patients develop pain or pruritus at the test site which may be relieved by cold packs or topical steroid preparations.

Anaphylaxis is rare with PPD, but can occur with the intradermal injection of allergens. This type of reaction is more likely with injections to the skin layers deeper than the dermis. A patient should be observed for approximately 30 minutes after receiving intradermal allergen. Complications can be minimized by taking a careful history and by using proper technique.

SUMMARY

A recent resurgence of tuberculosis is evident in this country. The Mantoux test is easy to perform, relatively inexpensive, and effective in diagnosing tuberculosis. The procedure is learned quickly, and has an important role in the ED setting.

REFERENCES

1. Mantoux C. Intradermoreation de la tuberculose. CR Acad Sci 1908;147:355.
2. Lewis T, Grant RT. Vascular reactions of the skin to injury. Part II. The liberation of a histaminelike substance in the injured skin, the underlying cause of factitious urticaria and of wheals produced by burning: and observations upon the nervous control of certain skin reactions. Heart 1924;11:209.
3. Committee on Infectious Diseases, American Academy of Pediatrics. Screening for tuberculosis in infants and children. Pediatrics 1994; 93:131–134.
4. McConnell EA. Giving intradermal injections. Nursing 1990 March;20(3):70.

CLINICAL TIPS
1. The substance to be injected should not be outdated.
2. Proper storage of the injected substance must be ensured.
3. The active component of PPD is easily absorbed onto plastic so it should be promptly injected after being drawn out of the vial.

TOXICOLOGIC AND ENVIRONMENTAL PROCEDURES

Section Editor: James F. Wiley II

GASTRIC EMPTYING

Mary A. Hegenbarth and Gary S. Wasserman

INTRODUCTION

Commonly used methods for gastrointestinal decontamination in children include induced emesis with syrup of ipecac, gastric lavage, activated charcoal, cathartics, and whole-bowel irrigation. Although many authorities attempt to compare the relative efficacies of ipecac-induced emesis, gastric lavage, and activated charcoal, it is difficult to conduct and interpret clinical studies of gastric emptying because of multiple variables including the substance(s) ingested, time since ingestion, unreliability of history, and differences in technique (1–16). Generally, ipecac or lavage—if indicated, performed soon after ingestion, and done properly—is probably of approximately equal effectiveness (30 to 80% of ingested toxin removed). However, despite the extensive use of both ipecac and gastric lavage, few reports have demonstrated improvement in patient outcomes. In recent years, the advisability of any gastric emptying procedure for most patients has been questioned, with many experts recommending activated charcoal as the primary treatment for patients with most nonlife-threatening ingestions (3, 4, 6, 13, 15, 17). Consultation with a clinical toxicologist or poison center is highly recommended if the clinician is unsure about the best method of gastrointestinal decontamination for a particular patient. Treatment should be individualized and should consider such factors as the severity of symptoms and expected toxicity, time elapsed, absorption characteristics, effectiveness of activated charcoal, and availability of antidotes.

Gastric lavage has a long history of use for evacuating the stomach after oral ingestion of toxins. In 1812, Physick used a hollow tube to lavage twin infants with laudanum (tincture of opium) overdose (18). Most pediatric patients requiring treatment for toxic ingestions are either young children less than 6 years of age with accidental poisoning, or adolescents with intentional ingestions due to suicide attempts or illicit drug use. The procedure is similar to gastric intubation described in Chapter 86, and is done in the hospital setting (primarily ED) by physicians and/or nurses. Gastric lavage is moderately difficult to perform and requires attention to detail for optimal effectiveness and avoidance of complications.

ANATOMY AND PHYSIOLOGY

Syrup of Ipecac

Syrup of ipecac (Ipecacuanha) is the most effective, safe emetic agent available for use in toxic ingestions. It contains two natural alkaloids, emetine and cephaeline. Emetine stimulates the vomiting center in the medulla while cephaeline locally irritates enteric mucosa. Ipecac-induced vomiting begins within 5 to 30 minutes (average 20), and occurs two to four times over the next 20 to 60 minutes.

Gastric Lavage

Small children obviously have smaller nasal and oral passageways, a shorter esophagus, and a smaller stomach than adults. Factors that may make lavage relatively difficult in young children include a large tongue, loose primary teeth, and an uncooperative attitude regarding the procedure. Lavage tubes are easily inserted too far into children, which may cause serious malposition despite clinical signs of adequate placement (19). Proper insertion length has been found to correlate with patient height (19, 20).

Gastric lavage aims to remove toxin from the stomach before absorption occurs; its effectiveness diminishes with increasing time since ingestion. Effectiveness also depends on the physical characteristics of the substance(s) ingested. Liquids are rapidly absorbed and are unlikely to be significantly recovered given the typical delay preceding lavage. Solid preparations are absorbed more slowly; absorption is further delayed with enteric-coated forms, substances that retard gastrointestinal motility, and those that tend to form concretions. Gastric lavage may have the undesired effect of accelerating absorption by enhancing pyloric emptying into the duodenum (9). This outcome is more likely if the patient is lying on the right side or if large aliquots of cold fluids are used (21–23). The left lateral decubitus position is preferred to maximize access of the tube to stomach contents and minimize pyloric emptying (Fig. 126.1). Young children are more susceptible to electrolyte changes than adults. Normal saline or 0.45 normal saline are recommended rather than water. Using warmed or at least room temperature fluid will prevent iatrogenic hypothermia and may aid in slowing pyloric transit time (21).

INDICATIONS

Syrup of Ipecac

Recent guidelines for ipecac limit its use to the immediate postingestion period (about 5 to 10 minutes). It is therefore primarily used in the home rather than in health care facilities and only for specific indications. It may be especially useful in recent, potentially toxic ingestions of substances that are not bound by charcoal (e.g., iron), and for those with large tablets, capsules, or plant/mushroom fragments that are difficult to remove with lavage.

Because of the delay in onset and continued emesis, ipecac is contraindicated for (*a*) ingestions that are not discovered immediately, (*b*) poisoning with substances that may cause rapid onset of altered mental status, respiratory depression, seizures, or dysrhythmias (e.g., tricyclic antidepressants, camphor, or clonidine), and (*c*) other substances for which emesis is contraindicated. Other contraindications to ipecac-induced emesis are dictated by special patient considerations such as previous esophageal surgery or the presence of a bleeding disorder (Table 126.1). Administration of activated charcoal is significantly delayed when ipecac has been given. With many poisons, the benefit of immediate activated charcoal administration outweighs the benefit of syrup of ipecac administration (Chapter 127).

Gastric Lavage

Gastric lavage is indicated for life-threatening toxic ingestions in which the benefit of the procedure is felt to outweigh the risk. Obtunded patients in one study who underwent gastric lavage within 1 hour of their ingestions had improved outcome compared with those who received only activated charcoal (12). For the majority of toxins, lavage is most effective if performed within the first 2 hours after ingestion, although drugs whose absorption is prolonged (aspirin, anticholinergics, etc.) may sometimes be recovered in significant amounts even after many hours. Specific indications for gastric lavage include (*a*) the unconscious poisoned patient, (*b*) ingestion of a highly toxic substance, especially one with rapid onset of central nervous system depression or seizures for which ipecac is contraindicated (cyclic antidepressants, clonidine, cyanide, camphor, etc.), and (*c*) large ingestions of strong acid (using a narrow, soft tube). Table 126.2 summarizes the contraindications to gastric lavage.

Consultation is recommended if the physician is unsure about the best method(s)

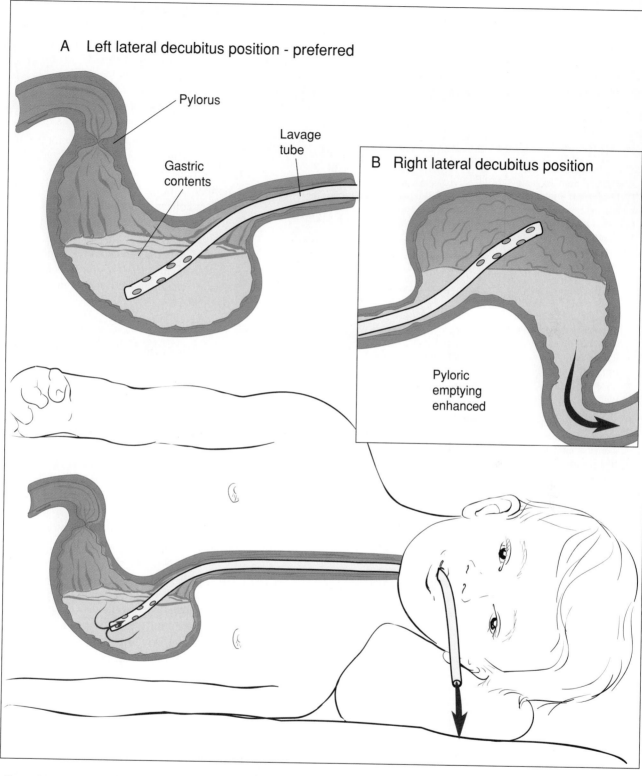

Figure 126.1.
Effect of patient position on pyloric emptying and availability of gastric contents to lavage (modified from Burke M. Gastric lavage and emesis in the treatment of ingested poisons: a review and a clinical study of lavage in 10 adults. Resuscitation 1972;1:91–105).
A. Left lateral decubitus (preferred). Access to gastric contents enhanced, pyloric emptying discouraged.
B. Right lateral decubitus. Pyloric emptying enhanced (undesirable).

Syrup of Ipecac
1. Administer syrup of ipecac:
   Age 6–12 mo—10 mL (one dose only)
   1–5 yr, 15 mL
   >5 yr, 30 mL
2. Give 4 to 8 oz of fluid
3. Expect vomiting within 20 to 30 minutes
4. Repeat dose once (except children less than 12 months) if no vomiting

Gastric Lavage
1. Ensure airway protection. Restrain and position patient in left lateral decubitus, head down position. Have suction on at bedside
2. Measure tube insertion distance and mark tube (Fig. 126.3)
3. Lubricate tube and insert gently through mouth to predetermined distance
4. Confirm tube placement by auscultation of insufflated air over stomach and by eventual return of gastric contents
5. Lavage patient using 10 mL/kg aliquots of saline (up to 150 mL) until return is clear
6. Instill activated charcoal/cathartic before withdrawing tube

Table 126.1.
Contraindications to Syrup of Ipecac

Absolute Contraindications
1. CNS depression present or impending
2. Convulsions present or impending
3. Cardiovascular instability present or impending
4. Absent gag reflex
5. Caustic-corrosive
6. Diaphragmatic hernia, unrepaired
7. Pulmonary edema
8. Hemorrhagic diathesis
9. Infants less than 6 months old
10. Most fundoplication procedures

Relative Contraindications
1. Most hydrocarbon ingestions (unless toxicity outweighs risk of aspiration)
2. Phenothiazines (potential dystonic reaction)
3. History of cardiovascular disorder
4. Hypertension
5. Cerebral vascular anomalies
6. Pregnancy, especially last trimester
7. Activated charcoal to be given

of gastrointestinal decontamination. For the majority of children with mild to moderate potential toxicity, activated charcoal alone may be the safest, most effective treatment; observation is often adequate for asymptomatic patients (14). Whole-bowel irrigation may be preferred for iron poisoning or sustained-release drugs (24, 25) (Chapter 128).

EQUIPMENT

Syrup of Ipecac

Syrup of ipecac, USP
Emesis basin
Protective clothing for patient and clinician

Table 126.2.
Contraindications to Gastric Lavage

1. Alkaline caustic ingestion
2. Most hydrocarbon ingestions, unless unusually large volume or containing a highly toxic component (e.g., insecticide)
3. Plant or mushroom ingestions, if fragments too large to pass
4. Previous esophageal or gastric injury, surgery, or anomaly (stricture, tracheo-esophageal fistula, gastric stapling, etc.), although children with gastric fundoplication can be safely lavaged
5. Ingestions likely to cause only mild symptoms (risks outweigh benefit)
6. Time since ingestion exceeds a few hours (see text for exceptions)
7. Airway compromise without prior endotracheal intubation

Gastric Lavage

Orogastric lavage tube with side holes or closed system (Fig. 126.2)
Tape measure
Lubricant for tube
Oral airway/bite block
Rigid suction device for emesis
Funnel and/or wide-tipped syringe for instilling and withdrawing fluid
Lavage fluid—warmed or room temperature normal saline, at least 1 to 2 L
Basin for collecting drainage
Sterile specimen container for toxicologic analysis
Activated charcoal and cathartic, if indicated
Restraint devices (e.g., papoose board, extremity restraints) for young or uncooperative patients
Protective clothing, eyewear, gloves for personnel
Resuscitative equipment including oxygen, bag-valve-mask device, and airway equipment
Monitoring of vital signs, cardiac rhythm, and oxygen saturation if unstable, intubated, or depressed level of consciousness

Large lavage tubes (24 to 50 French) are most effective for recovering solid fragments. The tube should be fairly rigid to prevent collapse and should have side holes. Tubes especially designed for gastric lavage (Lavacuator®, Edlich®, Ethox®) are preferred rather than soft rubber (Ewald®) or small Salem sump tubes. A 24-French tube is commonly used for young children; 34- to 42-French tubes are recommended for adolescents and adults. The syringe used for infusing and draining fluid should have a large bore opening or it will impede drainage. Commercially available kits for gastric lavage include appropriate tubes packaged with special wide-tipped syringes (e.g., Edlich® Gastric Lavage Kit, Monojet®). More elaborate closed system sets also are available. Their contents vary and may include special bags for fluid infusion and/or drainage collection, and adapters for direct charcoal administration (Code-Blue Easi-Lav®, Ballard Medical Products; No-Mes®, Ethox Corp.). The Code-Blue Easi-Lav® disposable closed system has unique one-way valves and dual plungers which have simplified gastric lavage while making it clean, efficient, and almost error-free. The closed system kits are more expensive than simple kits but are convenient for performing large volume lavages (Fig. 126.2).

PROCEDURES

Syrup of Ipecac

The dose of ipecac is 10 mL for infants 6 to 11 months, 15 mL for children 1 to 12 years, and 30 mL for adolescents and adults. Oral fluid, 4 to 8 oz, is recommended after administration. The dose of ipecac may be repeated once if emesis has not occurred within 20 to 30 minutes.

Gastric Lavage

The oral approach is preferred in almost all instances, as it allows passage of a larger tube without trauma to the nasal mucosa and turbinates. The main disadvantages of the oral route are that gagging is increased and that the patient may bite on the tube. A bite block may be helpful but often causes gingival and oral trauma. Formal consent is not generally obtained before gastric lavage, but the indications, technique, and potential complications should be discussed with the parents and child (as appropriate for age).

Next, the patient's ability to protect the airway is assessed by checking the gag reflex and the level of consciousness. If the airway reflexes are significantly depressed, the airway is protected by endotracheal intubation (Chapter 16). Intubation is rarely necessary in view of some authorities' experience. Many children who appear somewhat sleepy are promptly awakened upon tube insertion and are able to fully protect their airway. If any question arises about the adequacy of airway protection, however, the patient should be intubated before attempting lavage.

Adequate restraint is essential—at least two persons are usually necessary to perform lavage in an uncooperative child. Suctioning equipment should be working and at hand. Distance for tube insertion is measured by placing the tube on the child and measuring from the teeth to the epigastrium, allowing

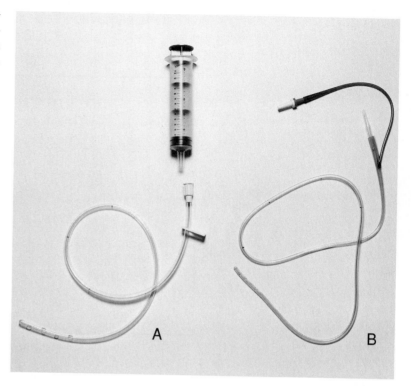

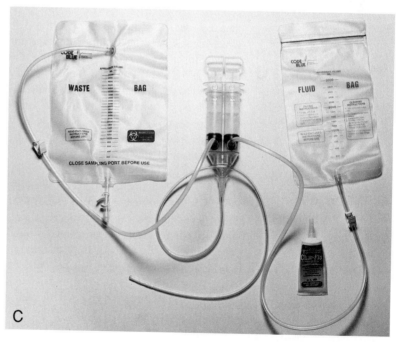

for curvature of the tube along the tongue and oropharynx. Proper tube insertion length also can be determined using the patient's height (Fig. 126.3). Marking the distance for tube insertion with tape or ink is suggested. The patient is positioned in the left lateral decubitus position to minimize pyloric emptying; mild Trendelenburg positioning (head lower

Figure 126.2.
A. Orgastric tube with syringe.
B. Salem sump tube (not recommended).
C. Closed system for gastric lavage.

Chapter 126
Gastric Emptying

Estimated Lavage Tube Insertion Depth for Gastric Emptying
Child's Height (inches)

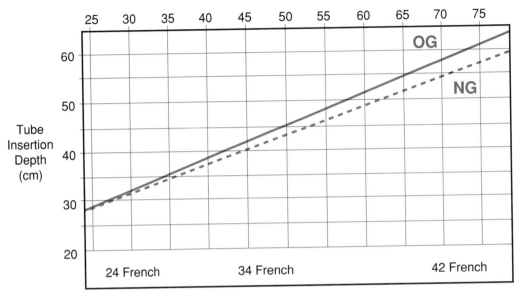

Figure 126.3.
Estimation of gastric tube insertion depth based on patient height. OG, Oro-gastric tube length; NG, Nasogastric tube length. (Modified from Scalzo AJ, Tominack RL, Thompson MW. Malposition of pediatric gastric lavage tubes demonstrated radiographically. J Emerg Med 1992;10:586. Used with permission of AJ Scalzo.)

than feet) decreases the risk of aspiration. The distal tube is generously lubricated and inserted into the oropharynx. If cooperative, the child is asked to swallow as the tube is gently advanced to the premarked length. Some authorities do not advise using topical anesthetic sprays or gels to ease passage, as they may interfere with the protective gag reflex. Flexing the neck may help pass the tube into the esophagus. In intubated patients brief deflation of the endotracheal tube cuff is advisable. The lavage tube should be removed if the patient develops respiratory distress, continual coughing, inability to phonate, or if the tube meets resistance or coils back through the mouth. Once the tube appears to have passed successfully, its position is determined by insufflating 5 to 20 cc of air with a syringe while listening for a rush of air over the stomach. If equivocal, air insufflation is repeated while listening in the axillary lung fields. Gastric contents usually drain if the tube is properly positioned. If gastric contents do not return, try advancing the tube a few centimeters as it may be in the distal esophagus. Although rarely needed, tests to exclude inadvertent tracheal position of the tube may be performed if difficulty arises in confirming proper tube placement. One such test is to instill a few milliliters of saline into the tube,

with coughing indicative of tracheal misplacement. Another method is to place the free end of the tube under water during expiration; if air bubbles are seen the tube is in the trachea. Although seldom needed, radiographs may be helpful to ensure proper placement if tube position is still uncertain.

The stomach should be drained of its contents before beginning lavage, and the initial gastric aspirate saved for toxicologic analysis in a sterile specimen container. Aliquots of 10 mL/kg (about 100 mL in children, up to 150 mL in adolescents) of saline are used for lavage. The fluid may be infused by gravity or with a syringe, but rapid, forceful fluid injection should be avoided which may force stomach contents out the pylorus. Next, the lavage fluid is drained by gravity (by holding the end of the tube below the level of the stomach) or removed by syringe aspiration; the amount returned should approximate the amount infused. The procedure is continued until the return fluid is clear (usually at least 1 L). In some patients significant amounts of toxin can be recovered by further lavage after visual clearing (5). If concretions are suspected (e.g., aspirin), it may be helpful to flex the child's hips and gently massage the stomach (26). When lavage has been completed, the tube may be used for installing activated charcoal and/or cathartics before withdrawal. Retching or vomiting commonly occurs when removing the tube. After lavage, the patient should be observed for any respiratory symptoms that might indicate pulmonary aspiration.

COMPLICATIONS

Syrup of Ipecac

Persistent emesis (over 1 hour), drowsiness, and diarrhea are the most common adverse effects of ipecac use. Aspiration may be a hazard in patients who develop significant CNS depression or seizures. More than two doses of syrup of ipecac may be toxic, producing cardiac depression, dysrhythmias, vascular collapse, excessive vomiting, abdominal cramping, and diarrhea.

Gastric Lavage

Although rare, gastric lavage is associated with potentially serious complications. The most common serious complication is pulmonary aspiration, which may occur despite the presence of a gag reflex or a cuffed endotracheal tube (14). Inadvertent lavage of the lungs may be catastrophic, particularly if charcoal is instilled (27). Additional respiratory complications include laryngospasm and respiratory insufficiency or hypoxia.

Trauma to the oral mucosa is common and may include dislodging of loose teeth. More serious esophageal or gastric lacerations and perforations are rare. Petechiae of the head, neck, and chest are sometimes produced. Mechanical problems with the tube such as kinking, curling back on itself, or knotting may make removal difficult. Esophageal spasm causing difficult tube insertion or removal has been reported. Esophageal spasm may occur after ingestion of any drug that interacts to disturb the dynamic equilibrium of smooth muscle innervation of the esophagus and lower esophageal sphincter. Overdose of β-adrenergic antagonists (beta-blockers) or anticholinergic drugs and irritant effects from the ingestion of large numbers of pills (secobarbital and meprobamate) have caused esophageal spasm. Treatment with sedatives, glucagon, or nitroglycerin has been anecdotally effective (28, 29). Electrolyte imbalance and hypothermia are potential problems in young children lavaged with cold or inappropriate lavage solutions.

Respiratory complications can be minimized by giving careful attention to the airway and respiratory status, patient position, and accurate tube placement. Gentle technique with careful positioning of bite blocks and good lubrication minimizes trauma. Hypothermia and hyponatremia are prevented by using warmed saline for lavage.

SUMMARY

Ipecac-induced emesis has limited usefulness for gastric emptying in a health care facility, but can easily be used at home. Strict attention must be paid to contraindications to its use (Table 126.1). Gastric lavage may be useful in the child with a recent, life-threatening ingestion. Airway protection must be ensured, and the child should be adequately restrained in the proper position, with working suction at hand. A large bore orogastric tube should be used; tube insertion length should be premeasured and position confirmed after placement. Pulmonary aspiration is the most common among several serious complications. For this reason, careful consideration of the risk versus benefit of gastric lavage should occur before its performance.

REFERENCES

1. Auerbach PS, Osterloh J, Braun O, et al. Efficacy of gastric emptying: gastric lavage versus emesis induced with ipecac. Ann Emerg Med 1986;15:692–698.
2. Tandberg D, Diven BG, McLeod JW. Ipecac-induced emesis versus gastric lavage: a controlled study in normal adults. Am J Emerg Med 1986;4:205–209.
3. Tenenbein M, Cohen S, Sitar DS. Efficacy of ipecac-induced emesis, orogastric lavage, and activated charcoal for acute drug overdose. Ann Emerg Med 1987;16:838–841.
4. Underhill TJ, Greene MK, Dove AF. A comparison of the efficacy of gastric lavage, Ipecacuanha and activated charcoal in the emergency management of paracetamol overdose. Arch Emerg Med 1990;7:148–154.
5. Young WF, Bivens HG. Evaluation of gastric emptying using radionuclides: gastric lavage versus

Chapter 126
Gastric Emptying

ipecac-induced emesis. Ann Emerg Med 1993;22:1423–1427.

6. Greensher J, Mofenson HC, Caraccio TR. Ascendancy of the black bottle (activated charcoal). Pediatrics 1987;80:949–951.

7. Vale JA, Meredith TJ, Proudfoot AT. Syrup of Ipecacuanha: is it really useful? Br Med J 1986;293:1321–1322.

8. Curtis RA, Barone J, Giacona N. Efficacy of ipecac and activated charcoal/cathartic: prevention of salicylate absorption in a simulated overdose. Arch Intern Med 1984;144:48–52.

9. Saetta JP, March S, Gaunt ME, Quinton DN. Gastric emptying procedures in the self-poisoned patient: are we forcing gastric content beyond the pylorus? J Royal Soc Med 1991;84:274–276.

10. Tenenbein M. Inefficacy of gastric emptying procedures. J Emerg Med 1985;3:133–136.

11. Saetta JP, Quinton DN. Residual gastric content after gastric lavage and Ipecacuanha-induced emesis in self-poisoned patients: an endoscopic study. J Royal Soc Med 1991;84:35–38.

12. Kulig K, Bar-Or D, Cantrill SV, Rosen P, Rumack BH. Management of acutely poisoned patients without gastric emptying. Ann Emerg Med 1985;14:562–567.

13. Albertson TE, Derlet RW, Foulke GE, Minguillon MC, Tharratt SR. Superiority of activated charcoal alone compared with ipecac and activated charcoal in the treatment of acute toxic ingestions. Ann Emerg Med 1989;18:56–59.

14. Merigian KS, Woodard M, Hedges JR, Roberts JR, Stuebing R, Rashkin MC. Prospective evaluation of gastric emptying in the self-poisoned patient. Am J Emerg Med 1990;8:479–483.

15. Kulig K. Initial management of ingestions of toxic substances. NEJM 1992;326:1677–1681.

16. Phillips S, Gomez H, Brent J. Pediatric gastrointestinal decontamination in acute toxin ingestion. J Clin Pharmacol 1993;33:497–507.

17. Hodgkinson DW, Jellet LB, Ashby RH. A review of the management of oral drug overdose in the Accident and Emergency Department of the Royal Brisbane Hospital. Arch Emerg Med 1991;8:8–16.

18. Major RH. History of the stomach tube. Ann Med History 1934;6:500–509.

19. Scalzo AJ, Tominack RL, Thompson MW. Malposition of pediatric gastric lavage tubes demonstrated radiographically. J Emerg Med 1992;10:581–586.

20. Strobel CT, Byrne WJ, Ament ME, Euler AR. Correlation of esophageal lengths in children with height: application to the Tuttle test without prior esophageal manometry. J Pediatr 1979;94:81–84.

21. Ritschel WA, Erni W. The influence of temperature of ingested fluid on stomach emptying time. Int J Clin Pharmacol 1977;15:172–175.

22. Burke M. Gastric lavage and emesis in the treatment of ingested poisons: a review and a clinical study of lavage in 10 adults. Resuscitation 1972;1:91–105.

23. Vance MV, Selden BS, Clark RF. Optimal patient position for transport and initial management of toxic ingestions. Ann Emerg Med 1992;21:243–246.

24. Tenenbein M. Whole bowel irrigation in iron poisoning. J Pediatr 1987;111:142–145.

25. Fleisher GR, Kearney TE, Henretig F, Tenenbein M. Gastric decontamination in the poisoned patient. Ped Emerg Care 1991;7:378–381.

26. Bartecchi CE. A modification of gastric lavage technique. JACEP 1974;3:304–305.

27. Harris CR, Filandrinos D. Accidental administration of activated charcoal into the lung: aspiration by proxy. Ann Emerg Med 1993;22:1470–1473.

28. Rinder HM, Murphy JW, Higgins GL. Impact of unusual gastrointestinal problems on the treatment of tricyclic antidepressant overdose. Ann Emerg Med 1988;17:1079–1081.

29. Panos RJ, Tso E, Barish RA, Browne BJ. Esophageal spasm following propranolol overdose relieved by glucagon. Am J Emerg Med 1986;4:227–228.

ACTIVATED CHARCOAL ADMINISTRATION

Michael Shannon

INTRODUCTION

The efficacy of activated charcoal in the treatment of poisoning was first described in the 1700s, although it was Tovery's survival after ingesting a strychnine and charcoal slurry before the French Academy of Medicine in 1831 that dramatized its lifesaving effects (1).

Activated charcoal is created from the exposure of carbon-containing materials (usually low ash wood) to steam and acids, producing a finely granular substance with a surface area of approximately 1000 m^2/g.

ANATOMY AND PHYSIOLOGY

The microscopic pores of activated charcoal permit adsorption of drugs and other large molecular weight substances. Activated charcoal, in fact, effectively adsorbs all toxins with the exception of alcohol, metals and minerals, hydrocarbons, and cyanide. Maximal adsorption of charcoal to toxin occurs when the charcoal:drug ratio is 10:1.

Because of its effectiveness both in preventing systemic absorption of an ingested toxin (i.e., enhancement of preabsorptive elimination) and in accelerating the elimination of already absorbed toxins (i.e., postabsorptive elimination enhancement), charcoal has become the most important single intervention in the treatment of toxic exposures.

Because gastric emptying and cathartic administration provide only modest benefit after toxic ingestion, increasing data support the administration of activated charcoal alone (2–3).

INDICATIONS

Activated charcoal is indicated in two distinct circumstances. First is after the ingestion of any toxin known to be adsorbed by activated charcoal. Second is to enhance the elimination of drugs that can be removed by gastrointestinal dialysis (e.g., theophylline, phenobarbital, salicylates) or drugs that are known to have substantial elimination of parent compound and/or pharmacologically active metabolite through the bile (e.g., tricyclic antidepressants, carbamazepine). In the case of theophylline and phenobarbital, oral charcoal will enhance the elimination of drug that has been administered intravenously (4).

The window of opportunity for clinical effectiveness depends on the absorption characteristics of the drug. With drugs in which gut absorption is complete within 2 to 4 hours, activated charcoal has a clear role. In contrast, for drugs with delayed gut absorption, for example, drugs with anticholinergic activity, activated charcoal is potentially effective in preventing drug absorption for up to 12 hours postingestion.

Contraindications to activated charcoal

SUMMARY
1. Prepare activated charcoal by mixing aqueous solution (1 mg/kg up to 50 to 60 g) with ice and add flavoring (cola or cherry syrup), if desired
2. Place mixture in cup with lid and offer to child through a straw
3. If child is too young to use straw, mixture may be placed in baby bottle with some enhancement of nipple
4. If child will not drink activated charcoal, then it should be instilled through an orogastric tube (Chapter 126) or via a small (10 to 14 French) nasogastric tube (Chapter 86)

CLINICAL TIPS
1. Most children will drink the charcoal if it is prepared properly.
2. Activated charcoal should not be administered to a child with an altered level of consciousness until the airway is protected.
3. Multiple doses of activated charcoal require special attention to cathartic administration: sorbitol should be given with the first dose and then after every third dose only if the patient passes no charcoal-laden stool.

are loss of airway control, ingestion of a caustic agent (because such victims should be NPO and because thorough endoscopic evaluation cannot be easily performed after charcoal administration), and gastrointestinal obstruction or perforation.

EQUIPMENT

Activated charcoal
Flavoring (cola or cherry syrup)
Cup with a lid
Straw
Ice
If patient is uncooperative:
    Nasogastric intubation (Chapter 86)

Activated charcoal is available in many forms. The simplest preparation is desiccated charcoal, which is reconstituted as needed for administration. The most common form of activated charcoal currently available consists of either charcoal suspended in water (with an added sweetener) or a cathartic, most commonly sorbitol. These preparations avoid the mess produced by the preparation of a charcoal slurry from powder. Less commonly used but also available are charcoal capsules or tablets. These forms are difficult with children because they require taking many tablets to achieve the minimally effective charcoal dose.

Activated charcoal is administered in a dose of 1 g/kg. Although many authorities advocate strict attention to the 10:1 activated charcoal:toxin ratio with no ceiling dose, the maximal dose is customarily 50 to 60 g. In circumstances when repetitive oral charcoal is administered, the typical dose is 1 g/kg body weight (maximum 50 to 60 g) every 4 hours. Alternatives to this include 0.5 g/kg every 2 hours.

PROCEDURE

Administration of activated charcoal to a child or adult is usually accomplished easily by having the patient slowly drink a charcoal slurry, prepared in a vehicle of water or cathartic (Fig. 127.1). Flavoring agents have little effect on adsorptive characteristics and

may be added. Placing the slurry in a covered cup and using a straw often makes the mixture more palatable. In the case of an infant or toddler, activated charcoal is rarely taken voluntarily (although this may be initially attempted), requiring that it be administered via an orogastric tube (if gastric lavage is being first performed) (Chapter 126) or by a small, nasogastric tube (if it is simple charcoal instillation).

Activated charcoal administration to the small child requires a 10- to 14-French nasogastric tube, sterile lubricant, a catheter tip syringe, and a restraining papoose. After the child is restrained and with the help of an assistant, the clinician inserts the nasogastric tube (Chapter 86). Tube placement should be confirmed either through the return of gastric contents or by air insufflation which is heard after placing a stethoscope over the stomach. With the patient's head restrained, the activated charcoal is infused slowly. After infusion is complete, the nasogastric tube is removed and the child released from restraints.

COMPLICATIONS

Complications from the administration of activated charcoal are rare. The primary complication is vomiting and aspiration of charcoal. This typically occurs in the setting of depressed consciousness or some other condition that reduces the ability to protect the airway. With patients who have potential airway compromise, protective endotracheal intubation should be considered before activated charcoal administration. The administration of repetitive oral charcoal also has been associated with charcoal inspissation, creating a mechanical obstruction. Finally, the repetitive administration of activated charcoal suspended in a cathartic may produce excessive fluid losses, particularly in young children. For this reason, charcoal and sorbitol mixtures should never be administered repetitively.

As with any procedure that has potential complications, a procedure note should be written which documents gastric intubation with confirmation of tube placement and instillation of activated charcoal without clinical evidence of aspiration.

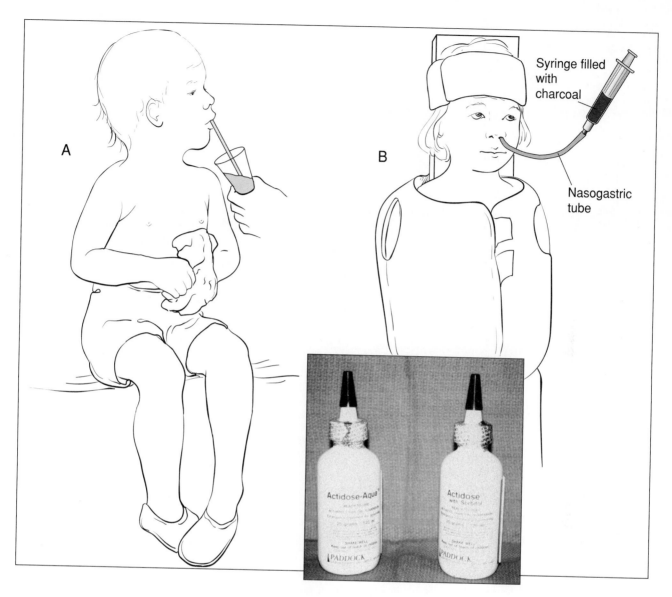

Figure 127.1.
Activated charcoal
administration.
A. Child voluntarily drinking
an activated charcoal
slurry.
B. Nasogastric
administration.

SUMMARY

Activated charcoal administration is commonly performed when treating poisoned patients. With proper preparation, many children will drink activated charcoal thus avoiding a nasogastric tube. Care must be taken with this procedure in patients who have impaired consciousness or who require multiple doses of charcoal.

REFERENCES

1. Derlet DW, Albertson TE. Activated charcoal—past, present and future. West J Med 1986;145:493–496.
2. Palatnick W, Tenenbein M. Activated charocal—an update. Drug Safety 1992;7:3–7.
3. Greensher J, Mofenson HC, Caraccio TR. Ascendancy of the black bottle (activated charcoal). Pediatrics 1987;80:949-950.
4. Pond SM. Role of repeated oral doses of activated charcoal in clinical toxicology. Med Toxicol 1986; 1:3–11.

Chapter 127
Activated Charcoal
Administration

WHOLE-BOWEL IRRIGATION

Milton Tenenbein

INTRODUCTION

Whole-bowel irrigation (WBI) is a procedure intended to prevent the absorption of poisons by removing them from the gastrointestinal tract. It consists of the rapid enteral administration of large amounts of the special irrigation fluid polyethylene glycol electrolyte lavage solution (PEG-ELS) over several hours (1). It is routinely used in patients of all ages as a colonoscopy preparative procedure. It differs from the other gastrointestinal decontamination procedures, syrup of ipecac-induced emesis, gastric lavage, and single-dose activated charcoal administration, in that it has the potential to decontaminate the intestines and the stomach. Although WBI has been shown to decrease the bioavailability of selected ingestants to a greater extent than these other procedures, because it is both labor intensive and time consuming, it should be restricted to specific indications.

Prevention of absorption is a cardinal tenet of treating the acute overdose patient. The traditional approach was either ipecac-induced emesis or gastric lavage as a primary intervention followed by activated charcoal as an adjunctive procedure. However, opinion has shifted to charcoal monotherapy (2–5) and current practice reflects this change.

Situations arise, however, when charcoal would be expected to be of limited benefit. These include ingestion of substances not adsorbed by charcoal, with iron being the most important, and presentation of a patient several hours after the ingestion of sustained release pharmaceuticals. These drugs can persist for prolonged periods within the intestines beyond the reach of ipecac, gastric lavage, and charcoal.

ANATOMY AND PHYSIOLOGY

Toxin absorption depends on such factors as digestion of the substance into small particles, dissolution of the substance, ionization state of the toxin (ionized form is poorly absorbed), location of the substance within the gastrointestinal tract (more surface area and blood flow to the proximal small intestine), and the transit time for the toxin through the gastrointestinal tract. Most toxins are absorbed in the proximal small intestine. The scientific basis for WBI is to increase the transit of poison past the area of absorption and thus decrease its bioavailability (1).

Human bioavailability studies in patients receiving whole-bowel irrigation have consistently shown decreases in drug absorption of 67 to 73%, exceeding the performances of syrup of ipecac, gastric lavage, and a single dose of activated charcoal when performed at comparable times after ingestion (6-8). Only 3500 MW polyethylene glycol electrolyte solution should be used for whole-bowel irrigation, because it was specifically designed to prevent fluid or electrolyte flux across the gastrointestinal epithelium (9).

SUMMARY

1. Pass 12-French nasogastric tube into stomach (Chapter 86)
2. Ensure gastric location by auscultation after air injection
3. Radiologically confirm that tip of tube is in midportion of stomach
4. Attach proximal end of tube to nasogastric tube feeding bag
5. Hang bag on intravenous pole
6. Seat patient or elevate head of bed to at least 45°
7. Place polyethylene glycol electrolyte lavage solution into feeding bag and allow it to flow into patient by gravity
8. Desired rates of flow:
   <6 yr—500 mL/hr
   6-12 yr—1000 mL/hr
   >12 yr—1500–2000 mL/hr
9. Endpoint is clear rectal effluent which can take many hours
10. Use commode or other receptacle to collect rectal effluent

CLINICAL TIPS

1. Nasogastric administration of irrigation solution is required because even the most cooperative patient will not consume a sufficient amount at the required rate.
2. Emesis is usually controlled by decreasing the rate of infusion for brief periods of time.
3. Positioning the patient upright promotes a more efficient whole-bowel irrigation.
4. A commode or similar receptacle is strongly recommended to collect the effluent.

Chapter 128
Whole-Bowel
Irrigation

INDICATIONS

Two primary indications for using whole-bowel irrigation are the ingestion of substances not adsorbed by charcoal and the ingestion of delayed release pharmaceuticals (Table 128.1) (7, 8, 14) which can persist within the gut for many hours beyond the reach of the other decontaminating procedures. Of the toxins not absorbed to activated charcoal, iron is most commonly ingested and consistently shown to be removed by WBI (10, 11). Whole-bowel irrigation also has been efficacious in treating ingestions of lithium (8), lead (12), and zinc (13). Ingestion of very large amounts of toxic substances and delayed presentation after ingestion are potential indications (11); however, these specific situations are difficult to identify in the clinical setting. Whole bowel-irrigation is also of potential benefit for the cocaine body stuffer (15), although this is an unlikely presentation in the pediatric age group.

Contraindications for WBI are ileus, gastrointestinal hemorrhage, obstruction, or perforation. Compromised circulation also is a contraindication because of the need to elevate the head of the bed. An absent gag reflex is a relative contraindication because of the risk for pulmonary aspiration.

EQUIPMENT

Polyethylene glycol electrolyte lavage solution
Nasogastric tube (10 to 12 French)
Intravenous pole
Reservoir bag used for tube feedings
Commode
Irrigation solution—available as a powder requiring reconstitution with tap water or as a ready-to-use product

Table 128.1.
Indications for Whole-Bowel Irrigation

I Strongly recommended . . .
Iron
Lithium
Modified (sustained) release pharmaceuticals
II Consider for . . .
Heavy metals
Lead salts
Zinc salts
Packets of illicit drugs

PROCEDURE

The nasogastric tube is passed into the stomach and gastric location is ensured by auscultation during air injection (Chapter 86). It is preferable to radiologically confirm that the tip of the tube is in the midportion of the stomach. The tube is then attached to a reservoir bag of irrigation solution which is hung from an intravenous pole (Fig. 128.1). Mechanical infusion pumps are not recommended because most cannot achieve the high flow rates required for adequate WBI. The patient should be seated or the head of the bed elevated to at least 45°. The desired rates of flow are 500 mL/hr for children less than 6 years, 1000 mL/hr for 6 to 12 years, and 1500 to 2000 mL/hr for above 12 years. The end point is a clear rectal effluent which takes many hours. A commode or similar receptacle is useful to collect the effluent.

A nasogastric tube is required because patients will not consume the irrigation fluid at the required rate. Only a small bore tube is needed for this procedure, although such a tube would not be suitable for gastric lavage or even gastric aspiration. Pretreatment with syrup of ipecac is undesirable because this tends to cause vomiting of the irrigating solution. Placing the patient in an upright position promotes the settling of the ingestant into the distal portion of the stomach, decreases the likelihood of vomiting, and establishes a dependent relationship of the intestines to the stomach. These measures favor a more efficient irrigation.

Although not frequent, emesis may complicate this procedure. When it occurs, it is usually a consequence of the ingestant itself, for example, theophylline or salicylates. Ingestant-induced emesis is best managed by antiemetics which must be given parenterally as WBI interferes with absorption of orally administered medications. Metoclopramide (initial dose 0.1 mg/kg every 6 hours, intravenously) is favored both for its antiemetic and gastric emptying properties. The likelihood of emesis also is decreased by keeping the patient's upper half of the body upright. If emesis occurs despite the discussed measures, the infusion rate may be decreased by 50% for 30 to 60 minutes with the intent of returning to the previous rate. These interventions control emesis in most situations.

A single dose of activated charcoal can be given before initiating WBI, but multiple doses of charcoal should not be given during the procedure. Charcoal adsorption of ingestant is blocked by the polyethylene glycol of the irrigating solution which occupies the binding sites. This has been shown to occur with the lower charcoal doses used in multiple-dose charcoal therapy to promote drug excretion but not with the larger initial dose that is used to prevent drug absorption (16).

Monitoring of WBI requires the usual nursing supervision for intravenous therapy; however, monitoring the patient's fluid or electrolyte status during the procedure is not necessary. The endpoint is a clear rectal effluent which takes many hours. If WBI is being used to remove foreign bodies from the gastrointestinal tract, then the appearance of a clear rectal effluent may not be a valid endpoint. In such instances, endpoints to consider are abdominal radiographs showing no radiopaque foreign bodies or passage of the expected number of foreign bodies in the rectal effluent (17). After completion of WBI, two to three liquid bowel movements are expected.

COMPLICATIONS

To date, no major complications from properly performed WBI have been reported. Theoretical concerns exist for pulmonary aspiration after emesis or perforation of a viscus if WBI is given in the presence of an ileus or gastrointestinal hemorrhage. However, relative to the other forms of gastrointestinal decontamination, WBI should be regarded as having a low risk to benefit ratio.

SUMMARY

Whole bowel irrigation is an effective but labor intensive gastrointestinal decontamination procedure for poisoned patients. It is not a panacea for all overdose patients and should be reserved for its specific indications.

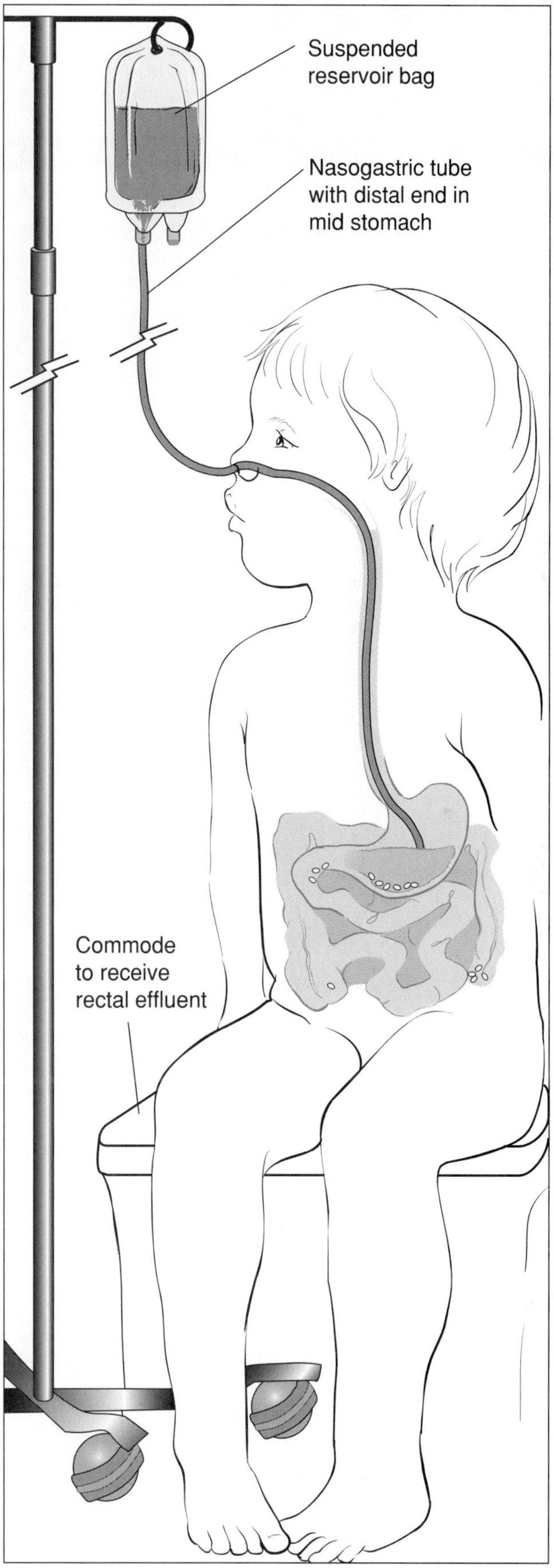

Figure 128.1.
Whole-bowel irrigation.

Suspended reservoir bag

Nasogastric tube with distal end in mid stomach

Commode to receive rectal effluent

REFERENCES

1. Tenenbein M. Whole-bowel irrigation as a gastrointestinal decontamination procedure after acute poisoning. Med Toxicol 1988;3:77–84.
2. Kulig K, Bar-Or D, Cantrill SV, Rosen P, Rumack BH. Management of acutely poisoned patients without gastric emptying. Ann Emerg Med 1985;14:562–567.
3. Albertson TE, Derlet RW, Foulke GE, Minguillon MC, Tharratt SR. Superiority of activated charcoal alone compared with ipecac and activated charcoal in the treatment of acute toxic ingestions. Ann Emerg Med 1989;18:56–59.
4. Merigian KS, Woodard M, Hedges JR, Roberts JR, Stuebing R, Rushkin MC. Prospective evaluation of gastric emptying in the self-poisoned patient. Am J Emerg Med 1990;8:479–483.
5. Kulig K. Initial management of ingestions of toxic substances. New Engl J Med 1992;326:1677–1681.
6. Tenenbein M, Cohen S, Sitar DS. Whole-bowel irrigation as a decontamination procedure after acute drug overdose. Arch Int Med 1987;147:905–907.
7. Kirshenbaum LA, Mathews SC, Sitar DS, Tenenbein M. Whole-bowel irrigation versus activated charcoal in sorbitol for the ingestion of modified release pharmaceuticals. Clin Pharmacol Ther 1989;46:264–271.
8. Smith SW, Ling LJ, Halstenson CE. Whole-bowel irrigation as a treatment for acute lithium overdose. Ann Emerg Med 1991;20:536–539.
9. Davis GR, Santa Ana CA, Morawski SG, Fordtran JS. Development of a lavage solution associated with minimal water and electrolyte absorption or secretion. Gastroenterology 1980;78:991–995.
10. Tenenbein M. Whole-bowel irrigation in iron poisoning. J Pediatr 1987;111:142–145.
11. Tenenbein M. Whole-bowel irrigation as a gastrointestinal decontamination procedure after acute poisoning. Med Toxicol 1988; 3:77–84.
12. Roberge RJ, Martin TG. Whole-bowel irrigation in an acute oral lead intoxication. Am J Emerg Med 1992;10:577-583.
13. Burkhart KK, Kulig KK, Rumack B. Whole-bowel irrigation as treatment for zinc sulfate overdose. Ann Emerg Med 1990;19:1167–1170.
14. Shenfield GM. Slow-release overdose. Med J Austral 1993;158:150–151.
15. Hoffman RS, Smilkstein MJ, Goldfrank LR. Whole-bowel irrigation and the cocaine body packer, a new approach to a common problem. Am J Emerg Med 1990;8:523–527.
16. Kirshenbaum LA, Sitar DS, Tenenbein M. Interaction between whole-bowel irrigation solution and activated charcoal, implications for the treatment of toxic ingestions. Ann Emerg Med 1990;19:1129–1132.
17. Scharman EJ, Lembersky R, Krenzelok EP. Efficacy of whole-bowel irrigation with and without metoclopramide pretreatment. Am J Emerg Med 1994;12:302–305.

SKIN DECONTAMINATION

David C. Lee

INTRODUCTION

The presentation of a child brought to the emergency department with a life-threatening dermal exposure can be dramatic. Similar to the sensational trauma patient, the health care provider must not solely concentrate on the exposure and forget the fundamentals of resuscitation. However, unlike the trauma patient, the health care provider also must address hazardous materials (HAZMAT) procedures policies of the health care team. Fortunately, with nearly all dermal exposures, the aphorism "the solution to the pollution is dilution" is valid.

ANATOMY AND PHYSIOLOGY

The skin is an extremely effective barrier to potentially toxic compounds. The ability for the skin to act as a barrier depends on the relative maturity and thickness of the epidermis, dermis, subcutaneous fat, and appendices (Fig. 129.1.A) (1–4).

The epidermis is composed of four layers which form a tough, water-insoluble covering. The rate-limiting step in the penetration of the skin for most substances is diffusion through the outer most layer (stratum corneum) (5). The thickness of the stratum corneum varies with age and location on the body (Fig. 129.1.B). The preterm infant does not have a fully formed stratum corneum and becomes more susceptible for dermal absorption (1, 6–7). Plantin et al. (8)

noted that dermal permeability is increased in premature infants, which falls steadily until approximately the age of 10 days. Epidermal and dermal thickness also differs in various areas of the body (8). Rates of absorption correlate proportionately with these variations. Vanrooij et al. showed a 69% difference on absorption of polyaromatic hydrocarbons from the groin as compared with the palm (Fig. 129.2) (9).

The dermis and subcutaneous fat, the two deeper layers of the skin, mainly act as a fibrous envelope and as an insulator. These layers and the deeper layers of the epidermis are rich in enzymes and can modify chemicals that penetrate through the stratum corneum. The skin is capable of phase I oxidative, phase II conjugation, reduction, and hydrolytic reaction (9–11).

Sweat gland ducts and hair follicle orifices may enable toxins to penetrate the skin. Their concentration also varies with age and anatomical site. The adult forehead has approximately 900 follicles per square centimeter as compared with none at the palms and soles.

The pediatric patient is more susceptible than the adult patient to suffer injury from dermal exposures, not only because of the differences in the structure of the skin, but also because of the higher rate of body surface area to body weight. Wester et al. has shown that the neonate exhibits roughly 3 times greater absorption rates as compared with the adult for an equal amount of exposure (12). Table 129.1 summarizes important factors that may enhance toxin absorption.

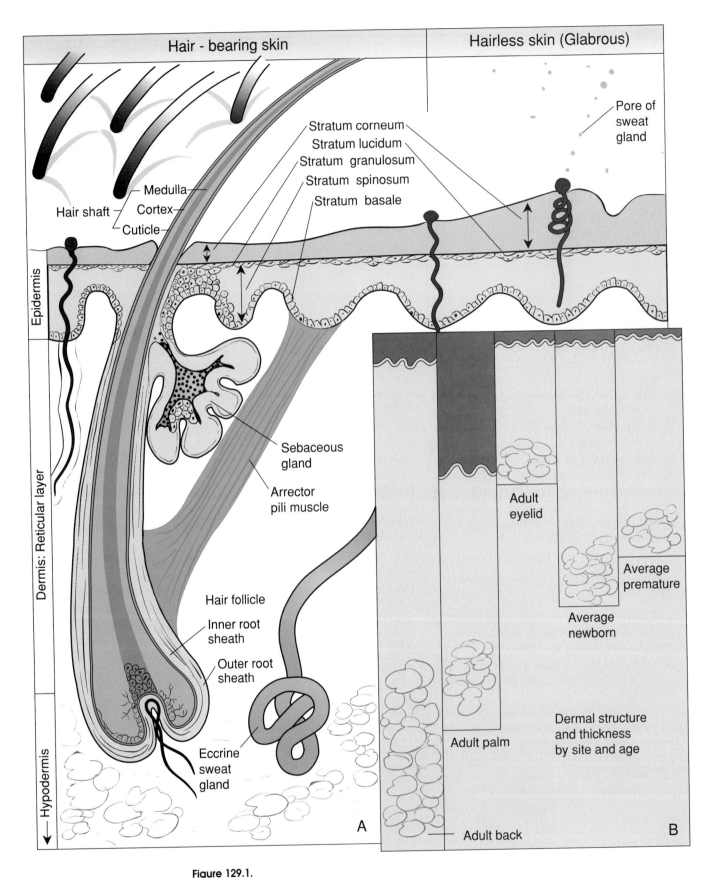

Hair - bearing skin

Hairless skin (Glabrous)

Pore of sweat gland

Stratum corneum
Stratum lucidum
Stratum granulosum
Stratum spinosum
Stratum basale

Medulla
Cortex
Cuticle
Hair shaft

Epidermis

Sebaceous gland

Arrector pili muscle

Dermis: Reticular layer

Hair follicle

Inner root sheath

Outer root sheath

Eccrine sweat gland

Hypodermis

Adult eyelid

Average premature

Average newborn

Adult palm

Dermal structure and thickness by site and age

Adult back

A

B

Chapter 129
Skin Decontamination

Figure 129.1.
A. Anatomy of the skin.
B. Variation in dermal structure and thickness (15).

INDICATIONS

Goals of decontamination are to prevent both absorption and systemic toxicity. No absolute contraindications exist for dermal decontamination. Lifesaving procedures, however, should not be delayed by the need for skin decontamination.

EQUIPMENT

Established area for decontamination in the ED as per HAZMAT protocols (13)

Green soap or other mild soap

Lukewarm normal saline irrigant (Table 129.2 lists alternative irrigants for rare exposures)

PROCEDURE

Before skin decontamination, health care personnel must ensure their safety by donning gloves, gowns, masks, and eye protection (13, 14). Resuscitative efforts aimed at addressing respiratory or circulatory compromise should not be delayed by skin decontamination. The patient should be placed in an area specifically designed for decontamination with establishment of special procedures to prevent contamination of other areas of the hospital with the exposure. Such areas should have a self-contained water drainage system (gurney with collection bottle or floor drain with a containment tank) and air ventilation that is filtered and goes to the outside.

Once stabilization procedures have been initiated, skin decontamination begins with removing all clothes and jewelry. These items should be handled carefully and placed in double plastic bags. Any solid or particulate matter is brushed off before washing to

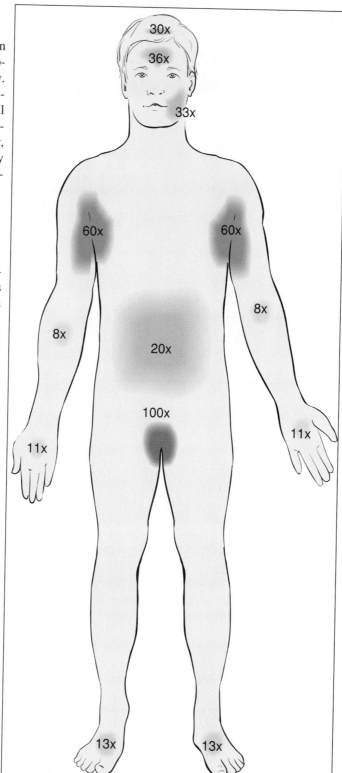

Figure 129.2.
Absorption rates of parathion in male adults (16).

Table 129.1.
Factors Enhancing Absorption

Host Properties
  Maturity of the dermis
  Integrity of the dermis
  Anatomical site
  Skin hydrations
Chemical Properties
  High lipid solubility
  Low molecular weight
  High chemical concentration
Physical Factors
  Occlusion or wrapping of the area
  Prolonged exposure
  Amount of surface area exposed
  Vehicle which toxin is dissolved in

SUMMARY

1. Place patient in proper area for decontamination—ensure adequate protection of health care personnel based on toxic exposure
2. Perform appropriate stabilization procedures and remove all clothing and jewelry
3. Brush off solid matter and blot any viscous liquid on skin
4. Starting at face and moving distally, rinse skin with cool, normal saline irrigant at low pressure (Table 129.2 lists exceptions)
5. Gently wash patient with mild soap (tincture of green soap) with special attention to hair, nails, intertriginous areas, face
6. Monitor temperature throughout procedure to avoid hypothermia

Table 129.2.
Chemicals Requiring Specific Decontamination*

Toxin	Classification	Treatment
Bitumen	Caustic without systemic toxicity	Copious irrigation with cold water until bitumen cools and hardens. Bitumen that is adherent to blistered skin should be removed with blister epithelium. Bitumen adherent to unblistered skin should be covered liberally with a hydrocarbon solvent (e.g., mineral oil) (17).
Chromic acid	Caustic with systemic toxicity	Standard decontamination with 10% ascorbic acid added to irrigant (18).
Hydrofluoric acid	Caustic with systemic toxicity	Standard decontamination followed by application of 10% calcium gluconate gel. Parenteral calcium administration by injection, venous or arterial infusion may be required. Patient at risk for hypocalcemia (19–21).
Lithium (elemental)	Caustic	Standard decontamination with removal of large particles and application of mineral oil to exposed areas.
Methyl mercury	Caustic with systemic toxicity	Standard decontamination with blister debridement and blister fluid removal (22).
Phenol	Caustic with systemic toxicity	Irrigate with polyethylene glycol mixture (2 parts PG to 1 part water) (23).
Phosphorus (elemental yellow phosphorus)	Caustic	Avoid exposure to air. Irrigate with 1 to 2% cupric sulfate solution and keep covered with water (24).
Radiation	Acute radiation syndrome	Obtain radiation monitoring device. Protect personnel if patient is radioactive. Decontaminate from periphery to center of area of exposure. Avoid creating new breaks in the skin. Allow wounds to bleed freely. Collect urine and feces for signs of internal decontamination (25–27).
Sodium (elemental)	Caustic	Standard decontamination with removal of large particles and application of mineral oil to exposed areas (28).

* These are theoretically optimal treatment protocols. Decontamination efforts should not be delayed for a significant time to institute these recommendations.

CLINICAL TIPS

1. Hazardous materials protocols should be developed for any hospital area likely to receive contaminated patients.
2. Airway, breathing, and circulation must be addressed before attempts at skin decontamination.
3. Early facial decontamination avoids further exposure by ingestion or inhalation.

prevent dissolution of solid matter and increased toxin absorption. Similarly, viscous liquid contaminants are blotted off. Room temperature saline is used at low pressures to rinse the patient. Forceful irrigation with warm water could theoretically cause dissolution of fine particles and vasodilatation. With large exposures, decontamination efforts should begin around the face and move distally.

After rinsing the patient, tincture of green soap or other mild soap is used to wash off further residue. Exposed skin should be handled gently to avoid accidentally abrading the skin and thereby further increasing toxin exposure. Special attention should be paid to areas where contaminants may collect—hair, nails, orifices, intertriginous areas, and areas of high dermal absorption such as the face and genitalia.

Certain rare exposures require special irrigants and procedures different from that just described as discussed in Table 129.2.

COMPLICATIONS

Hypothermia is the major potential complication of skin irrigation, requiring that temperature be monitored closely and warming be instituted as needed following decontamination (Chapter 132). Other problems associated with skin decontamination are failure to stabilize the patient before instituting irrigation and failure to protect health care personnel properly during decontamination.

SUMMARY

As compared with the adult patient, the pediatric patient is more susceptible to injury from a toxic dermal exposure. Fortunately, the basics of decontamination are technically simple to perform and easy to remember.

Chapter 129
Skin Decontamination

REFERENCES

1. Holbrook KA. Structure and biochemical properties of the skin of adults, children, and newborn infants. In: Schachner LA, Hansen RC, eds. Pediatric dermatology. New York: Churchill Livingstone, 1988, pp. 30–76.
2. Weston WL. Practical pediatric dermatology. 2nd ed., Boston: Little, Brown & Co., 1985, pp. 1–13, 365–367.
3. Tucker SB, Key MM. Occupational skin disease. In Rom WW, ed. Environmental and occupational medicine. 2nd ed. Boston: Little, Brown & Co., 1992, pp. 551–561.
4. Weinberg S, Hoekelman RA. Pediatric dermatology for the primary care practitioner. New York: McGraw-Hill, 1978, pp. 1–10.
5. McAuliffe DJ, Blank IH. Effects of UVA (320–400 nm) on the barrier characteristics of the skin. J Invest Dermatol 1991;96(5):758–762.
6. Freeman S, Maibach HI. Dermatologic toxicity. In: Haddad LM, Winchester JW, eds. Clinical management of poisoning and drug overdose. 2nd ed. Philadelphia: WB Saunders, 1990, pp. 355–369.
7. Ebling FJ. The normal skin. In: Rook A, Wilkinson DS, Ebling FJ, eds. Textbook of dermatology. 4th ed. Boston: Blackwell Scientific Publications, 1986, pp. 5–8.
8. Plantin P, Jouan N, Karangwa A, et al: Variations of the skin permeability in premature newborn infants. Value of the skin vasoconstriction test with neosynephrine. Arch Francaises De Pediatr 1992; 49(7):623–625.
9. Vanrooij JG, DeRoos JH, Bodelier-Bade MM. Absorption of polycyclic aromatic hydrocarbons through the human skin: differences between anatomic sites and individuals. J Toxicol Environ Health 1993;38(4):355–368.
10. Sanchez MR. Dermatologic principles. In: Goldfrank LR, Flomenbaum NE, Lewin NA, eds. Goldfrank's toxicologic Emergencies. 4th ed. Norwalk, CT: Appleton & Lange, 1990, pp. 187–208.
11. Guy RH, Hadgraft J. Principles of skin permeability relevant to chemical exposure. In: Hobson DW, ed. Dermal and ocular toxicity, fundamentals and methods. Boston: CRC Press, 1991, pp. 221–246.
12. Wester RL, Noonan PK, Cole MP, et al. Percutaneous absorption of testosterone in the newborn rhesus monkey: comparison to the adult. Pediatr Res 1977;11:737–739.
13. Bronstein AC, Currnace PL. Emergency care for hazardous materials exposure. St. Louis: CV Mosby, 1988, pp. 265–266.
14. Olson KR. Comprehensive evaluation and treatment of poisoning and overdose. In: Olson KR, ed. Poisoning and drug overdose. Norwalk, CT: Appleton & Lange, 1990, pp. 1–55.
15. Maibach HI, Feldman RJ, Milby TH, et al. Regional variations in percutaneous penetration in man. Arch Environ Health 1971;23:208–211.
16. Feldman RJ, Maibach HI. Percutaneous penetration of some pesticides and herbicides in man. Toxicol Appl Pharmacol 1974;28:126–132.
17. Pruitt BA, Edlich RF. Treatment of bitumen burns. JAMA 1982;247(11):1565.
18. Samitz MH, Scheiner DM, Katz SA. Ascorbic acid in the prevention of chrome dermatitis. Arch Environ Health 1968;17:44–45.
19. Shewmake SW, Anderson BG. Hydrofluoric acid burns: a report of a case and review of the literature. Arch Dermatol 1979;115:595–596.
20. Caravati E. Acute hydrofluoric acid exposure. Ann Emerg Med 1988;6:143–149.
21. Bracken WM, Cuppage F, McLaury RL, et al. Comparative effectiveness of topical treatments for hydrofluoric acid burns. J Occup Med 1985;27: 733–739.
22. Berkhart PG. Treatment of skin burns due to alkyl mercury compounds. Arch Environ Health 1961; 3:106–107.
23. Brown VK, Box VL, Simpson BJ. Decontamination procedures for skin exposed to phenolic substances. Arch Environ Health 1975;30:1–6.
24. Curreri PW, Asch MJ, Pruitt BA. The treatment of chemical burns: specialized diagnostic, therapeutic and prognostic considerations. J Trauma 1970; 10(8):634–642.
25. Miller EW, Miller RM. Environmental hazards: radioactive materials and wastes. Santa Barbara, CA: Contemporary World Issues ABC-CLIO, 1990, pp. 64–65.
26. Upton AC. Ionizing radiation. In: Rom WW, ed. Environmental and occupational medicine. 2nd ed. Boston: Little, Brown & Co, 1992, pp. 1071–1085.
27. Yow RB, Anderson BG. Radiation poisoning. In: Haddad LM, Winchester JW, eds. Clinical management of poisoning and drug overdose. 2nd ed. Philadelphia: WB Saunders, 1990, pp. 624–635.
28. Ellenhorn MJ, Barceloux DG. Medical toxicology: diagnosis and treatment of human poisoning. New York: Elsevier, 1988, pp. 8–9.

CHAPTER 130

ENVENOMATION MANAGEMENT AND TICK REMOVAL

G. Randall Bond

INTRODUCTION

Procedures used to treat envenomation and to remove ticks may be described in three categories: inactivation of venom, removal of envenomation apparatus or body parts, and local wound management. Procedures for treating envenomations vary greatly based on the offending organism. This chapter deals with the procedures involved with managing North American snakebites, North American scorpion stings, black widow spider bites, jellyfish envenomation, marine vertebrate envenomation, and tick infestation.

NORTH AMERICAN SNAKE BITES

Anatomy and Physiology

In North America, bites by poisonous snakes are overwhelmingly caused by members of the Crotalidae (pit vipers) family, which include rattlesnakes, and the Agkistrodon family, which includes water moccasins or cotton mouths and copperheads. These reptiles have hollow, hinged front fangs connected to venom glands which allow injection of venom subcutaneously much like a syringe and needle. Rattlesnakes are the largest North American snake and have the longest fangs, reaching a length of 3 to 4 cm.

Coral snakes have been found in the southeastern United States and the Sonoran Desert of Arizona. They can be identified by circumferential red and yellow rings that touch each other ("red on yellow, kill a fellow"). These snakes are relatively shy, and no human bites have been reported in Arizona in several years. Coral snakebites have a notable, neurotoxic venom that causes less wound swelling and tenderness than the North American pit vipers.

Although the potency and exact composition of venom varies significantly among species, all have the ability to cause local swelling, direct cellular injury, and shock (1). Some species such as the eastern diamondback rattlesnake primarily have hemorrhagic toxins, which cause aggregation of platelets or degradation of fibrinogen that can result in disseminated intravascular coagulation. Others such as the Mojave rattlesnake have neurotoxins which may cause weakness or muscle fasciculation.

Because a snake will deliver the same amount of venom whether biting an adult or a child, the degree of envenomation by weight is greater for children, and therefore pediatric patients are likely to present with the more severe symptoms for a given envenomation (2). In addition, a deeper bite into the muscle is theoretically more likely in children, although as in adults, bites through the fascia leading to elevated compartment pressures are rare. Two fang marks are typically seen after envenomation, although single or multiple marks are possible. Distance between fang marks indicates possible snake size.

Copperheads may have fangs as small as 3 to 4 mm making it difficult to detect the bite wound in this type envenomation.

Indications

The severity and need for intervention varies dramatically depending on the species and quantity of venom injected (1–20). Although toxicity may be delayed, most victims present with symptoms or show signs within the first 4 to 6 hours. All symptomatic patients should have frequent vital signs, fluid support, and adequate analgesia. Affected extremities should be elevated and, in the case of the hand, wrist, and forearm, a volar splint should be placed to allow comfort and adequate lymphatic drainage of venom (Chapter 104). A complete blood count with platelet count, prothrombin time (PT), partial thromboplastin time (PTT), fibrinogen, and urinalysis should be obtained in all patients. As mentioned, children are at particular risk following a snakebite because the venom dose per kilogram is higher; in addition, snakes can reach more vital areas (neck, torso) in the toddler or infant.

Administration of antivenin often is decided by close evaluation and continued assessment of the bite site. It is necessary to closely follow distal perfusion in a bitten extremity (4, 5). The most useful parameters include color and capillary refill. These should be assessed at least hourly and more frequently if compromise is suspected. Based on studies done with digital subtraction angiography, if color and capillary refill are questionable but the digit remains warm, it is likely that perfusion remains (6). Alternatively, a pulse oximeter placed on the distal portion of the finger may be used. The ability to record the pulse documents perfusion. Pain from wrapping or squeezing the fingertip of a bitten digit makes this technique poorly tolerated by patients. When tissue perfusion to the distal extremity is good and perfusion is only questioned in the area immediately surrounding a more proximal bite, surgical intervention is not required. Significant tissue loss is uncommon particularly with antivenin therapy (4, 7, 8). A nonperfused distal extremity requires surgical consultation (6, 9).

The extent of tissue edema and rapidity of its proximal spread following Crotalidae envenomation may be dramatic. At time of presentation to the ED three sites on the affected extremity should be marked. Sequential (every 30 minutes), circumferential measurements should be taken at these sites. If one site is increasing at a rate greater than 0.5 cm/hour, progression is considered to be rapid and antivenin administration should be strongly considered. Because of the extent of swelling and tenderness with direct pressure or motion, the question of compartment syndrome involving the calf or forearm frequently arises. Fortunately, a true compartment syndrome following rattlesnake envenomation is uncommon, particularly when antivenin is used (3, 4). Studies in animals have indicated that compartment syndrome occurs only when envenomation is directly into the compartment. Envenomation into the subcutaneous tissue over a compartment or into structures distal to the compartment will not result in a compartment syndrome (10). Because of the infrequent occurrence of a true compartment syndrome, direct measurements of compartment pressures should be obtained any time this complication is suspected before performing any type of surgical release or fasciotomy (Chapter 109).

Coral snake bites may not evoke a significant local reaction. Other than bite injury itself, minimum or no swelling or pain may be noted. Patients may experience nausea, vomiting, excess salvation, euphoria, and dizziness. Neurologic findings include paresthesia of the bitten extremity, weakness, ptosis, diplopia, dyspnea, fasciculation, and respiratory muscle paralysis (21).

The initial decision to give antivenin and how much to give has traditionally been based on the severity of envenomation. Mild envenomation describes swelling and tissue changes limited to the local bite site. Moderate envenomation includes significant local swelling with rapid proximal spread to affect half of the extremity. Severe envenomation is present when the entire extremity is affected or systemic signs of envenomation, coagulopathy, weakness, muscle fasciculation, or hypotension are present.

Systemic reaction is a clear indication for antivenin therapy. Conversely, mild envenomation does not necessarily require antivenin therapy. Controversy exists regarding the management of moderate to severe swelling alone, particularly following a copperhead bite (3, 4, 7, 8, 11, 12). Systemic reactions and local tissue necrosis are uncommon even in untreated patients with significant swelling following copperhead envenomation (7), which has led to less frequent use of antivenin in such cases.

Following envenomation by other species of Crotalidae, antivenin is probably indicated for anything other than mild local reaction (3, 4, 8, 11, 12). Some authorities recommend a small initial dose (5 vials of antivenin) to treat mild envenomation (3, 4, 11). Usually 10 vials of antivenin is the minimum dose once the clinician decides to give antivenin. Pediatric dosage is the same as the adult because the critical factor in antivenin efficacy is inactivating venom and the amount of venom inoculated into the patient is independent of the patient's size. Because the ultimate swelling cannot be predicted and optimal benefit is gained by early administration of antivenin, patients with rapid proximal progression of swelling should be considered moderate and receive antivenin. Patients with only local swelling but with evidence of distal vascular compromise also are candidates for antivenin (8). Before administering antivenin, consultation with a medical toxicologist is advised.

No early findings predict which victims of coral snake envenomation will have severe neurologic symptoms. All such patients should receive antivenin as soon as possible following the bite (21). Antivenin is available for the eastern and Texas coral snakes. This product also should be used following bites of the Sonoran coral snake.

Early administration has the potential to reduce ultimate tissue injury. Delayed administration may reverse coagulopathy or neurotoxicity but has less effect on local tissue injury. Unfortunately antivenin administration is associated with a 9 to 25% rate of acute hypersensitivity reaction and an almost universal experience of delayed reaction (serum sickness) (4, 11, 13-16). The decision to administer antivenin represents a risk and/or benefit choice.

Previous exposure to horse serum based products or an acute reaction to skin testing with antivenin are relative contraindications to administering antivenin. When definitely indicated, antivenin may still be given but administration should be modified (see Procedure) (4, 11, 17). Concurrent use of beta-blockers also is a contraindication. Beta-blockade reduces the efficacy of intervention should anaphylaxis occur. Because acute phase reactions are likely, antivenin should not be given to a patient concurrently taking beta-blockers unless the envenomation is presently life threatening. Massive edema and tissue destruction of coagulopathy are not adequate indications for antivenin in the presence of beta-blockade. Because 25% or more of coral snake bites may be nonenvenoming bites, positive skin test in an asymptomatic patient is considered a relative contraindication to antivenin administration (21).

Equipment

Antivenin Skin Testing
Horse serum from antivenin kit
Sterile normal saline
Tuberculin syringe with small gauge needle
Isopropyl alcohol disinfectant
Patent intravenous access

Antivenin Preparation and Administration
Polyvalent Crotalidae antivenin or coral snake specific horse serum antivenin
Diluent (10 mL)
250 mL bag of 5% dextrose in water or normal saline 0.9%
Intravenous infusion pump
Patent intravenous access
Monitoring and ancillary equipment and medications as for skin testing

Wyeth polyvalent antivenin is a partially purified protein precipitate from serum of horses which have been hyperimmunized with the venom from four species of pit viper: *Crotalus adamanteus* (eastern diamondback), *Crotalus atrox* (western diamondback), *Crotalus durissus terrificus* (tropical rattlesnake), and *Bothrops atrox* (fer-delance). Cross reactivity with the venom components of other crotalids allows this antivenin to be used in the management of envenomation by all North American and South American Crotalidae species.

Procedure

Skin Testing

Skin testing is performed to assess the relative risk that an individual has prior hypersensitization to horse serum and may experience an IgE mediated reaction. Using antivenin carries a 0 to 33% risk of an acute hypersensitivity reaction (itch, hives, wheezing, anaphylaxis) (13–16). When the skin test is positive, reaction to the antivenin occurs 50 to 100% of the time. When skin test is negative, reaction still occurs 10 to 28% of the time, because many of the reactions are not IgE mediated but are anaphylactoid, for example, the result of direct activation of complement by polymerized immunoglobulin (4, 13, 14).

Only those patients who will receive antivenin should have skin testing, because the test can sensitize patients for future antivenin administration. The cardiorespiratory status of the patient should be continuously monitored throughout the procedure, and appropriate drugs (epinephrine, diphenhydramine, ranitidine, intravenous steroids) and equipment (suction, oxygen, airway materials) for treating allergic reactions and anaphylaxis must be readily available. Adequate intravenous access should be ensured before skin testing. The horse serum provided with each vial of antivenin should be diluted to a concentration of 1 part horse serum to 10 parts sterile normal saline. A 0.02 mL volume of the diluted horse serum is injected intradermally on the volar aspect of the forearm, avoiding any veins or vascular malformations (Chapter 125 and Fig. 125.1). A control of 0.02 mL sterile normal saline may be placed in a similar manner adjacent to the horse serum site to aid in interpretation. The clinician then observes the skin site, vital signs, respiration, and general patient condition for 15 to 20 minutes. A positive reaction consists of a wheal, erythema, urticaria, or systemic reaction.

Antivenin Preparation and Administration

Antivenin administration is a relatively dangerous procedure that requires continuous cardiorespiratory monitoring, frequent patient assessments, and the capability for immediate intervention and treatment for anaphylaxis. The ED or the ICU is the most appropriate location for performing this procedure.

The Crotalidae antivenin is reconstituted with the 10 mL of diluent provided. Adequate dissolution of the lyophilized antivenin should be ensured by rolling each vial vigorously between the palms for several minutes until no particles or powder are observed when the vial is held up to a light. (Small globules of lipid may be seen, but no powder should be undissolved.) Next, 100 mL of the volume of a 250 mL bag of normal saline or 5% dextrose water (10 mL for each vial of antivenin administered) is removed from the bag. Ten vials (100 mL) of antivenin are then added to the bag for a total reconstituted volume of 250 mL. The fully flushed intravenous tubing containing antivenin should be passed through an infusion pump and inserted as close as possible to the patient's intravenous site to avoid lag time during the initial administration of antivenin. Infusion of antivenin is started at a rate of 2 mL/hour. The rate is doubled every 2 minutes to a maximum of 250 mL/hour (achieved at 15 minutes after initiation of infusion). Before each increase, the patient should be assessed for any signs of an acute allergic reaction.

Coral snake specific horse serum antivenin should be administered in the same manner as described for Crotalidae antivenin (21). Asymptomatic patients receive 5 vials and symptomatic patients receive 10 vials.

If an acute reaction occurs (itching, hives, hypotension, respiratory compromise), antivenin administration should stop immediately. Epinephrine (1:1000) at a dose of 0.01 mL/kg (maximum dose 0.3 mL) is given subcutaneously and indications for antivenin administration should be reevaluated. Consultation with a medical toxicologist is advised.

If the clinician determines that the patient should receive antivenin after an allergic reaction occurs, a second intravenous line should be inserted and the patient should receive diphenhydramine, ranitidine, and methylprednisolone intravenously. Epinephrine infusion is initiated at 0.05 ug/kg/minute. The antivenin should be further diluted to half the original concentration. Antivenin infusion is then administered at 2 mL/hour, doubling every 3 to 5 minutes to a maximum rate of 250 mL/hour as long as no reaction occurs. Dilution, reduction of infusion rate, and pretreatment with antihistamines and low dose epinephrine usually allow the infusion of antivenin without further complication (4, 17).

If coagulopathy is present, the patient's PT, PTT, fibrinogen, and platelet count should be checked 30 to 90 minutes following the completion of antivenin administration. If the abnormalities have significantly corrected and the rate of swelling has slowed, no further antivenin is needed. Coagulation parameters should then be rechecked in another 1 to 2 hours. If correction is not adequate or was only temporary, more antivenin is needed. Most significant envenomations require 15 to 30 vials to correct the abnormalities. These should be given in 5 to 10 vial aliquots in the same manner that the patient has previously tolerated. Resolution of swelling is not an endpoint for antivenin administration. Once swelling has occurred, it will continue to progress proximally at a slow rate over 24 to 36 hours. Resolution of swelling may take days to weeks.

The patient's tetanus status should be ascertained and tetanus toxoid administered as necessary. Prophylactic antibiotics (amoxicillin/clavulinic acid, a penicillinase resistant penicillin or a first generation cephalosporin) have frequently been recommended on theoretic grounds. No benefit to antibiotic administration has ever been objectively demonstrated and the only study to examine the issue found no benefit (18). Blebs and small areas of tissue necrosis usually require debridement.

Complications

Immediate hypersensitivity occurs in up to one-third of patients receiving antivenin. Patients who have received horse serum preparations before or have positive skin test are at particular risk. The decision to give antivenin in these patients requires an assessment of the risk the snakebite poses for the patient and the ability to prevent or control the expected allergic reaction. In most cases, only severe envenomations justify antivenin administration in patients at high risk for an allergic reaction.

Most patients who receive at least 5 to 10 vials of antivenin will experience a delayed serum sickness reaction. Serum sickness usually occurs 3 to 23 days following envenomation (17). Anticipatory therapy is not indicated. When it occurs, serum sickness should be treated with antihistamines and corticosteroids.

Complications associated with coral snake horse serum derived antivenin are similar to those outlined for Crotalidae antivenin. Coral snake antivenin may not reverse existing neurologic symptoms. The clinician should be prepared to provide respiratory support to patients with existing weakness at the time of antivenin administration.

SCORPION STINGS

Anatomy and Physiology

Although several species of scorpions are known to exist in the southwestern United States, only one has significant medical importance, the bark scorpion (*Centruroides sculpturatus*) (22). This scorpion makes its home primarily in the desert Southwest, almost exclusively in Arizona. Rare reports of envenomation have occurred in other parts of the United States when the scorpion has traveled from Arizona as a "hitchhiker" in luggage or in the trunk of a car (22).

Clinical Manifestations

When a scorpion sting occurs the most frequent symptom manifested, particularly in an older child or adult victim, is local pain. Local effects such as erythema, swelling, or blanching are absent. Often, tapping one finger over the sting site will elicit pain (the tap test). More severely affected individuals will experience pain and paresthesia of the affected extremity. When relatively more venom per kilogram body weight is injected (small children), peripheral motor neuron and cranial nerve manifestations may occur. These include uncontrolled jerking movements of the extremities, peripheral muscle fasciculation, tongue fasciculation, and facial twitching. The patient also may have opsoclonus, which consists of rapid disconjugate eye movements. When victims are experiencing a severe reaction, they will also frequently demonstrate agitation, extreme tachycardia, salivation, and respiratory distress (22–26). Given this constellation of symptoms, severely affected infants often are misperceived as experiencing seizures. Respiratory distress is most likely due to a combination of excess salivation, loss of pharyngeal tone, and uncoordinated contraction of the diaphragm and intercostal muscles. Rarely, respiratory compromise of infants and toddlers will progress to a point that endotracheal intubation and mechanical ventilation are required.

Indications

Although any victim of a scorpion bite can normally be managed solely with supportive care (analgesia, sedation, and adequate airway support), symptom resolution for scorpion stings in small children may occur more rapidly with *Centruroides* antivenin therapy (23). Antivenin therapy also may obviate or reduce the need for airway and ventilatory support (22, 23). Symptom severity in older children and adults rarely justifies the risk of antivenin administration.

Equipment

Skin testing equipment (listed on p. 1321)
Tuberculin syringe with small gauge needle
Diluent (10 mL)
Sterile normal saline
Isopropyl alcohol disinfectant
100 mL bag of 5% dextrose in water or normal saline 0.9%
Patent intravenous access
Intravenous infusion pump
Goat serum derived anti-*Centruroides* antivenin (This product is supplied by the Antibody Production Laboratory at Arizona State University and is available at most hospitals in the state of Arizona. This antivenin has been approved by the Arizona Board of Pharmacy but has never been tested by the Food and Drug Administration. Transportation across state lines is therefore illegal and it is not available outside of Arizona.)

Procedure

Skin testing should be performed only if anti-*Centruroides* antivenin is definitely to be ad-

ministered. As stated previously, antivenin administration is a hazardous procedure that requires continuous cardiorespiratory monitoring, frequent patient assessments, and the capability for immediate intervention and treatment for anaphylaxis. The ED or the ICU is the best site for this procedure.

One vial of goat serum anti-*Centruroides* antivenin is reconstituted with 10 mL normal saline and diluted in 100 mL of normal saline. The fully flushed intravenous tubing which contains antivenin is passed through an infusion pump and inserted as close as possible to the patient's intravenous site to avoid lag time during the initial administration of antivenin. The infusion of antivenin is started at a rate of 2 mL/hour and then doubled every 2 minutes to a maximum of 250 mL/hour (achieved at 15 minutes after initiation of infusion). Before each increase, the patient should be assessed for signs of an acute allergic reaction. If one vial does not completely treat signs and symptoms of envenomation within 30 minutes, a second vial should be administered. Antivenin administration must be stopped immediately if an allergic reaction occurs. Continuation of anti-*Centruroides* antivenin administration is not justified in the presence of an acute allergic reaction, and the patient should be provided appropriate medications to treat the allergic reaction and supportive care to treat the scorpion sting.

Complications

Complications that may occur with administration of *Centruroides* antivenin are similar to those associated with Crotalidae antivenin.

LATRODECTUS ENVENOMATION

Anatomy and Physiology

Black widow spiders are found in all states but Alaska. They prefer warm, dark, dry places outdoors or in basements and garages. Despite their wide distribution, however, these spiders avoid humans and their bites are relatively infrequent. About half of black widow spider bites are below the waist. Bites are characterized by an initial prick sensation such as that of a needle followed in 1 to 2 hours by regional lymph node tenderness. Symptoms are variable in time course and severity. Pain may start as early as 20 minutes following a bite but often does not start for 2 to 3 hours and frequently waxes and wanes. The bite site may be surrounded by a white area with a thin ring of erythema less than a centimeter from the bite (halo sign). This lesion rapidly fades and no tissue injury occurs. Muscle cramping in the affected extremity may be severe. Depending on the location of the bite, cramping also may affect the abdomen, chest, and/or back muscles. At times, the presentation of a black widow spider bite may be confused with an acute abdomen. Associated autonomic symptoms include nausea, vomiting, sweating, hypertension, and tachycardia. Significant symptoms often last for 36 to 72 hours. Following this period, milder symptoms or a feeling of being "not quite right" may persist for 1 to 2 weeks.

Indications

Today, with adequate supportive care, symptoms of black widow spider bites are rarely life threatening, even in small children. The cornerstone of management is adequate analgesia and hydration. Meperidine or morphine should be given in sufficient quantity. Calcium gluconate and muscle relaxants have been advocated as adjuvants, but relief is transient and inconsistent; partial or full relief occurs in only 4 to 50% of those patients treated (27, 28). *Latrodectus* antivenin has the advantage of offering rapid, complete relief of pain and the possibility of discharge from the ED, and may be considered in the treatment of severe envenomations.

Procedure

Instructions for reconstitution, skin testing, dilution, and administration of *Latrodectus* antivenin are as for Crotalidae envenomation. One vial is usually adequate for relief of symptoms. Allergic reaction is an absolute indication to stop antivenin administration and a contraindication to continued *Latrodectus* antivenin administration. Further care should be directed at treatment of the allergic reaction and supportive care.

Complications

Although frequently used in the past, antivenin use has declined with improvements in supportive care and reports of severe reaction including death. Recently in a review of 163 patients, acute reaction occurred in 5 of 58 receiving antivenin, one of which resulted in death (27). Only patients with life-threatening reactions which are uncontrolled with supportive care and who are without allergic contraindications should be considered candidates for antivenin.

JELLYFISH STINGS

Anatomy and Physiology

Jellyfish tentacles contain thousands of stinging cells called nematocysts, which are triggered by contact. When stimulated, nematocysts forcefully extrude a thin, threadlike appendage which penetrates human skin and injects a toxic venom. Several species are found in North American and Hawaiian waters, including the cabbage head jellyfish (*Stomolophus meleagris*), the Chesapeake Bay sea nettle (*Crysaora quinquecirrha*), and the Atlantic and Pacific Portuguese man-of-war (*Physalia physalis* and *Physalia utroculus*). The most dangerous species, the box jellyfish (*Chironex fleckeri*), is found only in Indian and South Pacific waters (29).

When jellyfish envenomation occurs, symptoms are almost immediate. Mild symptoms include itching, burning, urticaria, and local paresthesia. With more severe envenomation, significant pain radiates centrally. The contact point may demonstrate a whip-like tentacle print with subepithelial ecchymosis. Hemorrhagic vesicles may develop. Systemic symptoms vary from headache, vomiting, and malaise to syncope, delirium, coma, paralysis, renal failure, pulmonary edema, and cardiovascular collapse (29–32). Anaphylaxis has been reported (33). Only one death has been documented from the Atlantic Portuguese man-of-war (32). Severity of symptomatology depends on species, season, extent of contact, prior sensitization, and underlying health of the victim (29–32).

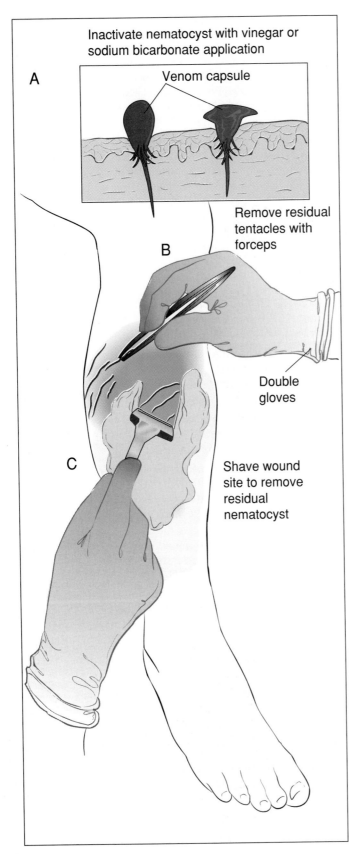

Figure 130.1.
Management of jellyfish
stings.

Indications

Suspected jellyfish stings may be treated as
described in Procedures in this section without significant concern about complications.

Equipment

Gloves—two pairs
5% acetic acid (vinegar) or bicarbonate of
    soda paste (Chesapeake Bay sea nettle)
Forceps
Shaving cream
Razor

Procedure

For jellyfish stings, supportive cardiorespiratory care should be provided and significant
allergic reaction treated before focusing on
wound treatment. In addition to supportive
care and analgesia, intervention is directed at
deactivation of the nematocysts, removal of
retained tentacle fragments, and skin care.
The clinician should don two pairs of surgical
gloves before handling the wound to avoid
accidental envenomation from residual nematocysts. The sting site should not be
washed, rubbed, or wiped. When providing
first aid at the scene, rinsing with sea water
may help remove some nematocysts. Lesions
from North American species, except the
Chesapeake Bay sea nettle, should be soaked
in a 5% acetic acid solution (vinegar) for 30
minutes to deactivate nematocysts (Fig.
130.1.A) (34). Stings from the Chesapeake
Bay sea nettle, which is found only in bays on
the Atlantic coast, should be treated with a
paste of sodium bicarbonate (baking soda)
(30, 31). Wounds should not be washed with
fresh water, as this may cause more nematocysts to discharge. Alternative first aid measures such as isopropyl alcohol and meat tenderizer are not as effective as acetic acid or
sodium bicarbonate (baking soda) and may
cause further nematocyst discharge (29, 30).
Tentacle fragments should be removed with
forceps (Fig. 130.1.B). Additionally, shaving
cream may be applied and the wound shaved
to remove residual nematocysts (Fig. 130.1.C).
Local wound care includes daily application
of Burrow's solution.

The role of allergic reaction in the slow resolution of skin lesions is unclear (29, 35). Many undischarged nematocysts have been found on a patient even after correct treatment as previously outlined (32). Therapy with topical corticosteroids is frequently recommended (29, 30). Prophylactic antibiotics are not indicated.

Complications

The main concerns in managing patients with jellyfish stings are to prevent inadvertent discharge of nematocysts which cause further symptoms and to avoid self-envenomation when treating these patients. Attention to proper pretreatment of the wound site before manipulation will prevent exacerbation of the sting. Double gloving and using forceps will prevent self-inoculation.

MARINE VERTEBRATE ENVENOMATION

Anatomy and Physiology

Another potential danger to swimmers is injury from marine vertebrates. Although the exact components of the toxin differ, the mechanism of venom delivery, systemic effects, and management of envenomation by various types of marine vertebrates are similar.

Stingray envenomation typically occurs when a person wading in shallow water accidentally steps on the ray. Reflexively, the tail "whips" to thrust the spine into the lower extremity of the victim. The spine has a serrated edge causing direct tissue injury. As the sheath over the spine is ruptured, venom is released into the wound. Envenomation results in severe pain, wound edema, and bleeding. Systemic manifestations include nausea, vomiting, diarrhea, headache, dizziness, muscle cramps, syncope, tachycardia, and hypotension. Stingrays have also caused deep, mortal wounds to the chest and abdomen in divers.

Scorpionfish (including lionfish, zebrafish, and stonefish) and catfish release venom into the victim when their spines are stepped on or mishandled. The spines cause local tissue injury. Because the spines are narrow, the wound is more often a puncture wound than the gash of a stingray. Venom is released when the overlying sheath is torn. Severity of symptoms varies by species of fish. Pain is intense and immediate. The wound initially may be ischemic and then becomes erythematous and edematous. Areas of anesthesia and hyperesthesia may be juxtaposed. Systemic reactions include those described for stingray venom as well as heart block, congestive heart failure, delirium, seizures, and limb paralysis. The most intense systemic symptoms follow envenomation by scorpionfish native to the South Pacific (36). Death has occurred in divers who become panicked after envenomations by stonefish during coral reef exploration. Catfish envenomation causes few systemic reactions (37).

Equipment

Cold saline
Warm water (42 to 43°C maximum temperature)
Same as for subcutaneous foreign body, puncture wounds, and laceration repair (Chapters 111 through 113)

Procedure

After envenomation by marine vertebrates, the wound should be irrigated as soon as possible with cold saline to remove residual venom and to inhibit venom absorption by vasoconstriction. Adequate analgesia should be provided. A local anesthetic or regional nerve block may be necessary (Chapter 37). Any obvious spine or sheath should be removed from the wound. The affected area (usually an extremity) should be immersed in water as warm as can be tolerated by the victim (42 to 43°C or 110°F, maximum temperature) for 30 to 90 minutes. After treating with warm water and achieving adequate pain control, the wound should be definitively explored and debrided. Radiographs are necessary following marine vertebrate envenomation to detect retained spines in wounds that may be difficult to adequately explore. Large wounds may require loose primary or delayed secondary closure (Chapters 111, 113).

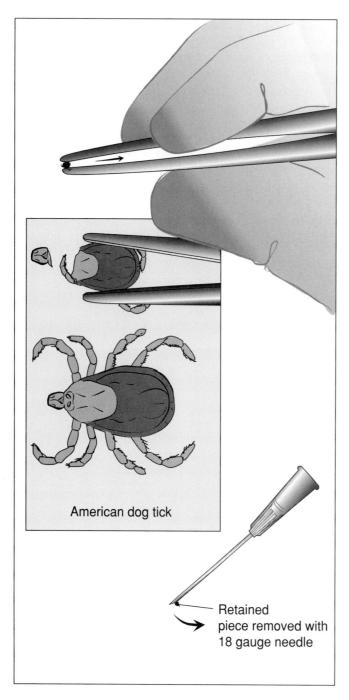

Figure 130.2.
Tick removal.

American dog tick

Retained piece removed with 18 gauge needle

2 days will identify patients in need of antibiotic treatment. Prophylactic antibiotics at time of first visit may be considered, but no evidence indicates that prophylactic antibiotics prevent subsequent wound infection after marine vertebrate envenomation.

TICK REMOVAL

Anatomy and Physiology

Children also frequently receive tick bites and may present in the ED for removal of the tick. Ticks are a common summertime finding on the skin of persons who live in rural areas or have recently visited the country. Ticks are most often found in moist or covered areas such as the scalp, axillae, groin, or genitalia. They usually fall off spontaneously after finishing their meal, but meals can last days.

Indications

Because the likelihood of transmission of tick-borne diseases such as Lyme disease, Rocky Mountain spotted fever, and ascending tick paralysis has been related to the duration of tick exposure, all ticks should be removed when discovered. Care must be taken in the removal of the tick to ensure that no body parts or attachment cement is left.

Equipment

Gloves
Forceps
Large needle (18 gauge)

Procedure

Several techniques for tick removal have been described, many of which come from American folklore (38). These include covering the tick with petroleum jelly, coating with fingernail polish, applying rubbing alcohol, or touching a hot object (e.g., a just extinguished match) to the hind part. When objectively examined none of these techniques resulted in successful removal, even after several hours (38). Mechanical removal is the only recommended technique (38, 39).

Complications

For patients with marine vertebrate injuries, the clinician must use caution during warm water immersion to avoid contact burns. Secondary infection (with or without retained foreign body) occurs frequently. Careful attention to wound management and early identification of a retained foreign body help reduce the likelihood of infection (Chapters 112, 113). Close patient follow-up in 1 to

To accomplish this, the tick should be grasped as close to the skin as possible using blunt, curved forceps held in a gloved hand (Fig. 130.2). The tick is then pulled out of the skin using a firm, steady motion directed perpendicular to the body. The skin should be closely examined to ensure that all tick parts have been removed. Any remaining material should be removed with forceps, or the site should be excised with an 18-gauge needle using a method similar to removing a splinter (Chapter 113). Finally, the site should be thoroughly cleansed with soap and water.

Complications

During the procedure, care should be taken to keep from crushing the tick to avoid exposing the host to more tick fluids and leaving tick parts in the skin. Because both human blood and tick secretions are potentially infectious, universal precautions should be observed.

SUMMARY

Antivenin Skin Testing
1. Perform skin testing only after deciding to administer antivenin
2. Perform skin testing only in a monitored environment
3. Be prepared to treat an immediate hypersensitivity reaction
4. Dilute provided horse serum 1:10 with normal saline or sterile water*
5. Inject 0.02 mL of the antivenin serum intradermally in the volar aspect of the forearm**
6. Consider placing 0.02 mL of a normal saline control adjacent to the antivenin site for comparison
7. Observe skin test site(s) for 15 to 20 minutes
8. A positive reaction is any wheal, erythema, urticaria, or systemic reaction

Antivenin Preparation and Administration
1. Only administer antivenin in a monitored environment (ED, ICU) with physician intervention immediately available
2. Reconstitute each vial of lyophilized Wyeth polyvalent Crotalidae antivenin with 10 mL of diluent provided†
3. Once diluent is added, roll each vial vigorously between palms for several minutes until no particles of powder can be observed when the vial is held up to the light. Small globules of lipid may be apparent but no powder should be undissolved.

SUMMARY
(CONTINUED)
4. Remove 100 mL (or 10 mL for each vial to be given) from a 250 mL bag of normal saline or D5W†
5. Add 10 vials of antivenin to bag making a reconstituted volume of 250 mL†
6. Use infusion pump for antivenin delivery ensuring that the antivenin is administered as close to intravenous site as possible
7. Start infusion of antivenin at 2 mL/hour; double rate of infusion every 2 minutes for next 15 minutes (maximum rate: 250 mL/hour)
8. Monitor patient closely for signs of allergic reaction

Continuation of Crotalidae Antivenin Administration in a Patient with an Allergic Reaction
1. Consultation with medical toxicologist is advised
2. Start second intravenous line
3. Administer diphenhydramine 1 mg/kg intravenously and ranitidine 2 mg/kg intravenously
4. Give methylprednisolone 2 mg/kg intravenously to minimize delayed hypersensitivity reaction
5. Start epinephrine infusion at 0.05 ug/kg/min; adjust infusion as necessary to control allergic signs and symptoms during further antivenin administration
6. Further dilute antivenin to one-half its original concentration
7. Resume antivenin infusion at 2 mL/hour and double every 3 to 5 minutes as tolerated

***Centruroides sculpturatus* Antivenin Administration**
1. Perform skin testing only if antivenin is to be used (see Summary—Antivenin Skin Testing)
2. Only administer antivenin in a monitored environment such as an ED or ICU where immediate management of anaphylaxis can occur
3. Reconstitute one vial of goat serum antivenin with 10 mL normal saline and dilute in 100 to 250 mL normal saline
4. Start infusion of antivenin at 2 mL/hour; double rate of infusion every 2 minutes for next 15 minutes (maximum rate: 250 mL/hour)
5. Monitor patient closely for signs of allergic reaction‡
6. If one vial does not result in resolution of symptoms within 30 minutes of completing administration, give second vial (22)

Nematocyst Deactivation and Removal after Jellyfish Stings
1. Wear double gloves before handling wound to avoid accidental envenomation
2. Do not wipe or rub wound

Summary

(Continued)

3. Soak lesions from all species except Chesapeake Bay sea nettle in 5% acetic acid solution (vinegar) for 30 minutes to deactivate nematocysts (33)
4. Treat Chesapeake Bay sea nettle wounds with paste of bicarbonate of soda (29, 30)
5. Remove tentacle fragments with forceps
6. Apply shaving cream and shave wound to remove residual nematocysts

Treating Marine Vertebrate Envenomation

1. Irrigate wound as soon as possible with cold saline
2. Provide analgesia—often local anesthetic or regional nerve block is necessary (Chapter 37)
3. Explore and debride wound to remove residual elements of sheath or spine
4. Place affected extremity in water as warm as can be tolerated by victim (42 to 43°C or 110°F, maximum temperature) for 30 to 90 minutes
5. Definitively explore and debride wound after adequate pain control and detoxification
6. Radiographs are necessary to detect retained spines (36)
7. Loose primary closure may be performed on large wounds

Tick Removal

1. Grasp tick as close to skin as possible using blunt, curved forceps held in gloved hand
2. Steadily pull firmly and directly away from skin
3. Examine skin to be sure all tick parts have been removed
4. Remove residual material with forceps or excise it with large gauge needle
5. Thoroughly clean skin with soap and water

* For *Centruroides sculpturatus* antivenin, reconstitute one vial with 10 mL of normal saline and skin test with 0.01 mL intradermally.
** For *Latrodectus* antivenin, reconstitute one vial with 2.5 mL of sterile water and test as for crotalid antivenin.
† Reconstitute Latrodectus antivenin in the same manner using 2.5 mL of diluent provided. Remove 2.5 mL from 100 mL of normal saline or D5W and add one vial of *Lactrodectus* antivenin for a total volume of 100 mL.
‡ If an allergic reaction occurs, stop infusion, administer epinephrine, diphenhydramine, ranitidine, and methylprednisolone as needed and provide supportive care.

Summary

Snake envenomations are infrequent but potentially life threatening in children. Assessment of the wound, administration of antivenin as indicated, and treatment of systemic effects provide the best approach to these injuries. With spider bites and scorpion stings, symptomatic treatment is usually the best approach. Jellyfish stings can be alleviated by simple measures which can be administered on the beach although victims should be watched carefully for signs of anaphylaxis. Marine vertebrate stings require appropriate wound management and warm water immersion. Tick attachment is a common pediatric problem requiring rapid removal that avoids further infectious exposure.

Clinical Tips

Antivenin Administration

1. Antivenin administration is most strongly indicated for persons who have suffered envenomation by rattlesnakes or neurotoxic snakes.
2. Close assessment of the patient's physical findings and response to supportive measures helps to determine the need for antivenin except after neurotoxic snakebite.
3. Patients on β-adrenergic blockers should not receive antivenin unless their envenomation is life threatening.
4. Patients with positive skin reaction to *Latrodectus* and *Centruroides* antivenin should not undergo antivenin administration. Crotalidae antivenin administration after positive skin test must be decided based on the severity of symptoms.
5. The majority of patients will develop serum sickness 2 to 3 weeks after antivenin administration.

Jellyfish Stings

1. Fresh water or isopropyl alcohol increases nematocyst discharge and should not be used.
2. Meat tenderizer is commonly used but also may promote nematocyst discharge.
3. Life-threatening anaphylactic reactions rarely occur from jellyfish stings in the United States.
4. Delayed pruritus and hives localized to the sting site are common.

Marine Vertebrate Envenomations

1. Adequate analgesia should be a high priority in the management of marine envenomations.
2. Care should be taken to avoid contact burns during warm water immersion.
3. Careful wound management is essential to a good outcome.
4. Secondary infection occurs frequently necessitating close patient follow-up.

Tick Removal

1. Crushing the tick increases the potential exposure to the patient and clinician.
2. All material must be carefully removed from the skin.
3. Universal precautions should be observed to avoid contamination by human or tick secretions.

REFERENCES

1. Russell FE, Carlson RW, Wainschel J, et al. Snake venom poisoning in the United States. JAMA 1975; 233:341–344.
2. White RR, Weber RA. Poisonous snakebite in central Texas. Ann Surg 1991;213:466–472.
3. Hurlbut KM, Dart RC, Spaite D, McNally J. Reliability of clinical presentation for predicting significant pit viper envenomation (abstract). Ann Emerg Med 1988;17:438.
4. Swindle GM, Seaman KG, Arthur DC, Almquist TD. The six-hour observation rule for grade I crotalid envenomation: is it sufficient? Case report of delayed envenomation. J Wilderness Med 1992; 3:168–172.
5. Wingert WA, Chan L. Rattlesnake bites in southern California and rationale for recommended treatment. West J Med 1988;148:37–44.
6. Curry SC, Kraner JC, Kunkel DB, et al. Noninvasive vascular studies in management of rattlesnake envenomation to extremities. Ann Emerg Med 1985; 14:1081–1084.
7. Burch JM, Agarwal R, Mattox KL, et al. The treatment of crotalid envenomation without antivenin. J Trauma 1988;28:35–43.
8. Downey DJ, Omer GE, Moneim MS. New Mexico rattlesnake bites: demographic review and guidelines for treatment. J Trauma 1991;31:1380–1386.
9. Roberts RS, Csencsitz TA, Heard Jr. CW. Upper extremity compartment syndromes following pit viper envenomation. Clin Orthop Related Research 1985; 193:184–188.
10. Garfin SR, Mubarak SJ, Akeson WH. Role of surgical decompression in treatment of rattlesnake bites. Surg Forum 1979;30:502–504.
11. Wingert WA, Sullivan JB, Sinkinson CA. Snakebite management: which approach to use. Emerg Med Report 1984;5:37–44.
12. Kunkel DB, Curry SC, Vance MV, et al. Reptile envenomation. J Toxicol—Clin Toxicol 1984;21: 503–526.
13. Spaite DW, Dart RC, Hurlbut K, et al. Skin testing: implications in the management of pit viper envenomation (abstract). Ann Emerg Med 1988;17:389.
14. Jurkovich GJ, Luterman A, McCullar K, et al. Complications of Crotalidae antivenin therapy. J Trauma 1988;28:1032–1037.
15. Jamieson R, Pearn J. An epidemiologic and clinical study of snakebites in childhood. Med J Aust 1989; 150:698–701.
16. Curro V, Stabile A, Michetti V. Antivenom treatment in snake bites (letter). Acta Pediatr Scand 1988;77:597–597.
17. Burgess JL, Dart RC. Snake venom coagulopathy: use and abuse of blood products in the treatment of pit viper envenomation. Ann Emerg Med 1991;20: 795–801.
18. Clark RF, Selden BS, Furbee B. The incidence of wound infection following Crotalid envenomation. J Emerg Med 1993;11:583–586.
19. Karlson-Stiber C, Persson H, Heath A, et al. Clinical experiences with specific sheep Fab fragments in the treatment of Vipera berus bites: a preliminary report (abstract). Vet Hum Toxicol 1993;35:333.
20. Smilkstein MJ. Therapy for toxicologic emergencies. Acad Emerg Med 1994;1:126–129.
21. Craig S, Kitchens MD, Van Mierop LHS. Envenomation by the eastern Coral snake. JAMA 1987; 258(12):1615–1618.
22. Curry SC, Vance MV, Ryan PJ, et al. Envenomation by the scorpion Centruroides sculpturatus. J Toxicol—Clin Toxicol 1984;21:417–449.
23. Bond GR. Antivenin administration for Centruroides scorpion sting: risks and benefits. Ann Emerg Med 1992;21:788–791.
24. Rachesky IJ, Banner W, Dansky J, et al. Treatment for Centuroides elixicauda envenomation. Am J Dis Child 1984;138:1136–1139.
25. Rimsza ME, Zimmerman DR, Bergeson PS. Scorpion envenomation. Pediatrics 1980;66:298–302.
26. Berg RA, Tarantino MD. Envenomation by the scorpion Centruroides elixicauda (C sculpturatus): severe and unusual manifestations. Pediatrics 1991; 87:930–933.
27. Clark RF, Kestner SW, Vance MV. Clinical presentation and treatment of black widow spider envenomation: a review of 163 cases. Ann Emerg Med 1992;21;782–787.
28. Key GF. A comparison of calcium gluconate and methocarbamol (Robaxin®) in the treatment of latrodectism (black widow spider envenomation). Am J Trop Med Hyg 1981:30(1)273–277.
29. Auerbach PS. Marine envenomation. New Engl J Med 1991;325(7):486–493.
30. Roson CL, Tolle SW. Management of marine stings and scrapes. West J Med 1989;150:97–100.
31. Burnett JW, Calton GJ. Jellyfish envenomation syndromes updated. Ann Emerg Med 1987;16: 1000–1005.
32. Stein MR, Marraccini JV, Rothschild NE, et al. Fatal Portuguese man-of-war (Physalia physalis) envenomation. Ann Emerg Med 1989;18:312–315.
33. Togias AG, Burnett JW, Kagey-Sobotka A, et al. Anaphylaxis after contact with a jellyfish. J Allergy Clin Immunol 1985;75:672–675.
34. Turner B, Sullivan P, Pennefather J. Disarming the bluebottle, treatment of Physalia envenomation. Med J Aust 1980;2:394–395.
35. Fisher AA. Toxic versus allergic reactions to jellyfish. Cutis 1984;34:450–454.
36. Lehmann DF, Hardy JC. Stonefish envenomation. New Engl J Med 1993;329(7):510–511.
37. Zeman MG. Catfish stings. A report of three cases. Ann Emerg Med 1989;18:211.
38. Needham GR. Evaluation of five popular methods for tick removal. Pediatrics 1985;75:997–1002.
39. Bowles DE, McHugh CP, Spradling SL. Evaluation of devices for removing attached Rhipicephalus sangueneus (Acari: Ixoididae). J Med Entomol 1992;29:901–902.

CHAPTER 131

COOLING PROCEDURES

John J. Kelly

INTRODUCTION

The spectrum of heat-related illness includes heat edema, heat tetany, and heat cramps, which are relatively benign and self-limiting maladies. The more perilous side of the spectrum of heat illness includes heat exhaustion and heat stroke. These entities have common prodromal symptoms of progressive lethargy, headache, nausea, vomiting, lightheadedness, and myalgias. The clinical hallmark of heat stroke is acute neurologic disability. This may manifest as ataxia, psychosis or irrational behavior, and seizures, with high body temperature (above 39°C, 102° F) and a history of heat stress (1).

Rapid cooling is an emergency procedure that reduces morbidity and mortality in the pediatric patient with heat stroke. This procedure must be done quickly in the prehospital phase of care and in the emergency department. These procedures are for the most part simple to perform and can be done by any health care worker.

ANATOMY AND PHYSIOLOGY

All humans produce heat as a by-product of metabolism and muscle activity. Recognition of hyperthermia requires rectal measurement of the temperature. Oral and axillary temperatures consistently underestimate core body temperature. Recently, otic measurement of temperature using infrared sensors has shown promise for providing a reading that more closely approximates hypothalamic tempera-

ture and thereby closer monitoring of change than rectal measurement. At this time, however, continuous measurement of otic temperature is not widely available and standardization of otic temperature measurement is undergoing further study (2–5).

Under normal circumstances, body heat is transferred from the core to the skin via cutaneous blood flow, where heat can be lost through radiation, evaporation, convection, and conduction. Radiation, the transfer of heat by nonparticulate means, accounts for 55 to 65% of heat loss depending on the gradient between core and ambient temperatures and the amount of exposed body surface area. Often, heat-related illness occurs when the ambient temperature approaches or exceeds the core body temperature. Children have a greater body surface area to mass than adults which allows for quicker cooling; however, children may lack the understanding or ability to remove themselves from an overheated environment. Evaporation of water from the dermal and pulmonary surfaces provides an additional 30% of heat loss. When the surrounding environmental temperature nears body temperature, evaporation becomes the only functioning mechanism for heat loss. When the insult of high relative humidity is added, evaporative heat loss is rendered ineffective and results in rising core temperature. Neonates and infants have a limited ability to perspire and therefore are significantly hampered in their ability to lose heat in hot, humid weather (6). Evaporation can provide a large heat exchange with the environment while preserving skin blood flow and is one of the major routes for heat reduction in the hyperthermic patient.

Together, convection and conduction, account for 15% of the body's heat loss under normal circumstances. Convection, the transfer of heat by particles of air or water having contact with the patient, is used therapeutically with evaporation. Evaporation of water requires more loss of heat than conduction, the direct transfer of heat from one object to another, which is the principle operative in ice water immersion. Human studies have shown evaporation techniques to be more effective in lowering core body surface temperature than ice water immersion (7).

Dehydration often occurs in conjunction with hyperthermia due to preceding strenuous exercise with sweating in the older child or adolescent or due to poor feeding in infants. Electrolyte abnormalities such as hypernatremia or hyponatremia may occur, particularly if the patient has a preexisting condition such as cystic fibrosis (hypernatremic sweat leads to hyponatremic, hypochloremic metabolic alkalosis). Other diseases that predispose patients to heat illness include congenital absence of sweat glands, congenital heart disease (impaired cardiac output under stress), diabetes mellitus/diabetes insipidus (increased water loss), familial dysautonomia (temperature instability), cerebral palsy (central hyperthermia and impaired thirst), and malnutrition or obesity (6, 8).

The body responds to an increase in core temperature as excessively warm blood reaches the preoptic area of the anterior hypothalamus. Initially, cholinergic stimulation of sweating increases, which is also enhanced by circulating catecholamines. At low rates of sweat production, sodium and chloride are reabsorbed within the sweat gland. At high rates of sweat production, sodium and chloride losses occur. With acclimatization over several days, salt losses are countered by increased aldosterone secretion with reabsorption of sodium and chloride in the sweat glands and kidneys (9). As mentioned, young children have a limited number of sweat glands and also are limited in their ability to regulate their body temperature through this mechanism. In addition, the posterior hypothalamus increases blood flow to the skin surface in response to overheating. Flow through the skin can comprise up to 30% of cardiac output and effectively transfer heat from the body core to the skin surface. Finally, feelings of being hot or thirsty prompt a person to seek a cooler ambient environment and replenish fluids lost through sweating. Often, children lack the developmental capabilities to tend to these needs on their own. It should be emphasized that drugs with antipyretic effects are not beneficial in treating hyperthermia because they alter the set point of the hypothalamus, and the basic pathophysiology of hyperthermia involves the overwhelming of hypothalamic temperature regulation (10).

INDICATIONS

Common settings for heat illness vary by age. In infants, the possibility of heat illness increases when the environmental setting is hot and humid and the infant is overdressed, left in a closed automobile, exposed to direct sunlight, bundled in blankets, or placed by a hot radiator (8). Children and adolescents who are subjected to strenuous activity in a hot and humid environment increase their risk for heat illness. The obese, young, underconditioned candidates for summer football camp, cross-country running, and marching commonly succumb to heat disorders (11). The athletic preadolescent's ability to transport muscle-generated heat and to produce sweat are both less than the ability of the older athlete. The preadolescent, however, possesses a remarkable facility for psychologically adapting to exercise in high temperature. This creates a combination of traits that places the young sports participant at unique risk to heat illness (8, 12).

Any patient with heat-related illness needs to be cooled down. The extent of the illness determines the extent of treatment. Considerable overlap occurs between heat exhaustion and heat stroke; therefore in patients with severe presenting signs of heat illness, aggressive treatment for heat stroke should be instituted. Because the critical clinical difference in heat stroke is the presence of acute neurologic disability, rapid aggressive cooling measures must be initiated before obtaining lab studies or entertaining a differential diagnosis (1). *If heat stroke is suspected, treat*

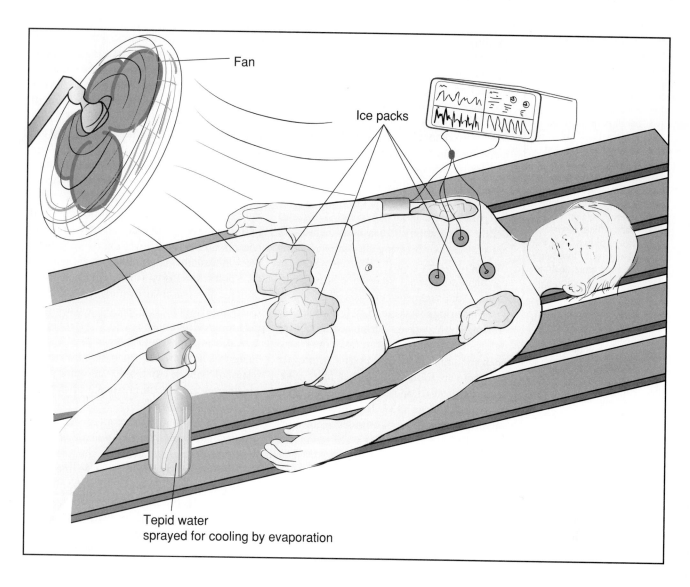

Fan

Ice packs

Tepid water
sprayed for cooling by evaporation

immediately. Cooling will not harm patients who are hyperthermic from other causes and will be lifesaving for the patient.

EQUIPMENT

Industrial size floor fan
Modified litter with a grated bottom or a net hammock
Ice packs
Spray bottle
Water-resistant monitor leads

PROCEDURE

When a heat stroke victim presents to the ED, the clinician should begin treatment with at-tention to airway, breathing, and circulation. At a minimum, a hyperthermic patient should receive supplemental oxygen, two large bore intravenous catheters, and an infusion of 5% dextrose in either 0.50 normal saline (school-age children or adolescents) or 0.25 normal saline (children less than 5 years of age) at 1.50 maintenance requirement. The patient's clothing should be stripped and a high rectal probe should be placed for continuous core temperature monitoring. A glass thermome-ter is not appropriate because it may break and injure the patient. Aggressive cooling measures should begin with using a powerful, industrial size floor fan placed at the foot of the bed and aimed directly at the patient (Fig. 131.1). Using tepid (60° F) water in a spray bottle, the patient's skin is kept moist by misting whenever the skin begins to dry.

Figure 131.1.
Cooling procedure in the hyperthermic patient.

SUMMARY

1. Remove all clothing and place high rectal temperature probe for continuous core temperature monitoring
2. Place patient on slotted gurney or suspend in hammock to maximize heat dissipation
3. Liberally spray patient with tepid (room temperature) water
4. Place patient in air stream of two large industrial size floor fans
5. If temperature decline is not satisfactory, apply ice packs to axilla, groin, and neck
6. Control shivering, seizures, and agitation with appropriate doses of benzodiazepines
7. Hypotensive patients require central venous pressure monitoring and careful administration of fluids to avoid pulmonary edema as core body temperature falls
8. Stop cooling measures when core body temperature falls to 39°C (102°F).

Cooling by evaporation provides heat exchange comparable to ice water immersion without shivering. Because evaporation and convection are more efficient modes of heat exchange as compared with conduction (and skin blood flow is preserved), some authorities have compelling arguments for recommending this technique (1). Furthermore, cooling by evaporation is more comfortable for the patient and allows for easier monitoring, stabilization, and treatment. Massaging the patient with ice to keep the skin moist during evaporation (9) has been mentioned, but may cause shivering. If further cooling treatment is necessary, then ice packs (or chemical cold packs) may be applied to the axilla, groin, and neck (Fig. 131.1).

Shivering, shaking, fasciculations, or convulsions may occur during cooling. Using chlorpromazine 50 mg intravenously has been recommended as a means to prevent shivering in adult patients but may lower seizure threshold and cause dystonia, especially in children (13). For these reasons, small doses of benzodiazepines seem more appropriate to control both shivering and seizures. Patients with agitation or acute psychosis as part of the spectrum of heat stroke also may be treated with benzodiazepines. Keeping the patient relaxed reduces the risk of the patient hurting self or members of the medical team. Haloperidol appears to be implicated in some cases of death from heat stroke and therefore should be avoided (13).

Hypotension is common in heat stroke and does not usually reflect dehydration. It is the result of high output failure due to shunting of blood through dilated skin vessels. This hypotension usually responds well to cooling, and it is unwise to give large fluid boluses. If hypotension persists after core temperature has decreased, then aggressive fluid challenge can be instituted with ongoing measurement of vital signs, urine output, and central venous pressure (or Swan-Ganz measurements). As peripheral vasodilatation resolves and blood volume returns to the central circulation, pulmonary edema or fluid overload is a real threat in those patients who were more than judiciously hydrated. If hypotension persists in the presence of cooling and fluid challenge, pressor agents may be required. In this instance, dopamine is preferred because, at low doses, it preserves renal and splanchnic circulation. Predominantly α-agents promote peripheral vasoconstriction and should be avoided (1, 13, 14).

Cooling measures should continue until the core temperature falls to 102°F (39°C). At this temperature, cooling techniques are stopped to avoid overcooling and resultant hypothermia, which may occur up to 6 hours after initial cooling. Core temperature should be monitored continuously during this time. Patients with heat stroke should be admitted to a monitored setting and observed for late complications such as irreversible central nervous system abnormalities, rhabdomyolysis, adult respiratory distress syndrome, liver injury, cardiovascular dysfunction, disseminated intravascular coagulation, and acute renal failure. Heat stroke is a multisystem insult that affects almost every organ (1, 13). Because true heat stroke is uncommon, a written protocol, which can guide the emergency medicine team's acute treatment of the victim, can be very helpful.

It appears that the evaporation technique is safer and more effective when compared with other common cooling techniques that use ice water (14). Evaporative methods carry no contraindications and can be quickly used when the ED has a written protocol and equipment standing by. Ice water immersion is more difficult to use especially in the uncooperative, agitated, psychotic, comatose patient who may need active airway management when in the bath. Ice water baths have had proponents, but currently few authorities recommend this modality as the treatment of choice. Theoretically, contact with ice water causes skin and subcutaneous vasoconstriction. This blocks heat exchange, is uncomfortable for the patient, and promotes skin shivering, all of which limit its effectiveness. The most critical drawback of ice water immersion is attempting to monitor and stabilize a very ill patient with possible hypotension and altered sensorium including psychosis, seizures, or coma.

Other techniques are reported in the literature but do not have proven efficacy such as iced gastric lavage (15), cold intravenous fluids, iced peritoneal lavage (16), or cold humidified oxygen. Infusion of chilled intravenous fluids and inhalation of cold humidified oxygen do not provide effective heat exchange. Iced gastric or peritoneal lavage has not undergone extensive study in humans. Finally, cardiopulmonary bypass is an effective means of lowering body temperature rapidly but is not routinely available for treating hyperthermia.

COMPLICATIONS

Complications which may occur as a direct result of acute cooling methods are minimal using the evaporation method described. However, "vigilance for the unexpected" should be the theme when treating heat illness. Patients may present with only mild confusion and progress quite rapidly to acute psychosis with agitation, seizures, or coma. Early institution of basic stabilization procedures, continuous monitoring, and cooling methods will help prevent difficult situations from turning into clinical disasters. Overshoot hypothermia must be avoided by constant monitoring of core body temperature with a target of 102° F (39° C) as the signal to stop cooling measures.

SUMMARY

Heat stroke requires immediate, aggressive treatment if suspected. While cooling measures are in progress, the clinician must keep a broad differential diagnosis for the etiology of the hyperthermia and perform a thorough clinical evaluation to find the true cause of the patient's malady. Rapid cooling by the evaporation method is the most simple and noninvasive technique to treat hyperthermia. Further, it is technically easier to monitor and treat the victim of heat illness while using evaporative cooling. Ice water immersion adds no additional benefit to the hyperthermic patient and makes supportive care more difficult. Pharmacologic interventions are limited to control of seizures, shivering, and agitation with the judicious use of benzodiazepines.

REFERENCES

1. Tek D, Olshaker JS. Heat illness. Emerg Med Clin North Am 1992;10(2):299.
2. Shinozaki T, Deane R, Perkins FM. Infrared tympanic thermometer: evaluation of a new clinical thermometer. Crit Care Med 1988;16:148–150.
3. Erickson RS, Kirklin SK. Comparison of ear-based, bladder, oral, and axillary methods for core temperature measurement. Crit Care Med 1993;21:1528–1534.
4. Milewski A, Ferguson KL, Terndrup TE. Comparison of pulmonary artery, rectal, and tympanic membrane temperatures in adult intensive care unit patients. Clin Pediatr 1991;(suppl)13–17.
5. Chamberlain JM, Terndrup TE, Alexander DT, Silverstone FA, Wolf-Klein G, O'Donnell R, Grandner J. Determination of normal ear temperature with an infrared emission detection thermometer. Ann Emerg Med 1995;25:15–20.
6. Avery ME. Heat-induced illness. In: Avery ME, First LR, eds. Pediatric medicine. Baltimore: Williams & Wilkins, 1989.
7. Weiner J, Khogali M. A physiologic body cooling unit for treatment of heat stroke. Lancet 1980;2:276–278.
8. Smith NJ. The prevention of heat disorders in sports. Am J Dis Child 1984;138:786.
9. Thompson AE, Mettler FA, Rozal HD. Environmental emergencies. In: Fleisher GR, Ludwig S, Henretig FM, et al., eds. Textbook of pediatric emergency medicine. Baltimore: Williams & Wilkins, 1988.
10. Simon HB. Hyperthermia. N Engl J Med 1993;329(7):483-487.
11. Dankes DM, Webb DW, Allen J. Heat illness in infants and young children: a study of 47 cases. Br Med J 1962;2:287.
12. Bar-Or O. Thermoregulation and fluid electrolyte needs. In: Smith NJ, ed. Sports medicine: health care for young athletes. Evanston, IL: American Academy of Pediatrics, 1983.
13. Knochel JP. Heat illness. In: Callahan ML, ed. Current practice of emergency medicine. Philadelphia: BC Decker, 1991.
14. Callahan M. Heat illness. In: Rosen P, et al., eds. Emergency Medicine. St. Louis: CV Mosby, 1988.
15. Syverud SA, Barker WJ, Amsterdam JT, et al. Iced gastric lavage for treatment of heat stroke: efficacy in a canine model. Ann Emerg Med 1985;14:424–432.
16. White JD, Kawath R, Nucci R, et al. Evaporation versus iced peritoneal lavage treatment of heat stroke: comparative efficacy in a canine model. Am J Emerg Med 1993;11(1):1.

CLINICAL TIPS
1. Antipyretics do not lower hyperthermia caused by environmental exposure.
2. Agents used for drug-induced hyperthermia (dantrolene, bromocriptine, L-dopa, carbidopa) are not effective for heat stroke.
3. Ice water immersion makes supportive care more difficult and may not be more effective than using evaporation measures.
4. Hypotensive shock from heat illness is caused by cardiogenic and hypovolemic mechanisms. Treat fluid losses judiciously with the aid of central venous pressure monitoring.

CHAPTER 132

WARMING PROCEDURES

Julie Lange Varga

INTRODUCTION

Children with profound accidental hypothermia, and even apparent clinical death, have been successfully resuscitated with good neurologic outcomes (1, 2). Patients with rectal temperatures as low as 16.0°C have survived with little or no demonstrable morbidity (3–6). More commonly, however, hypothermia presents less dramatically and yet must still be considered a life-threatening condition. Although persons of any age can be affected, the very young are particularly susceptible to hypothermia from cold exposure.

Warming techniques range from simple passive methods which any caregiver can perform, to highly complex procedures requiring special training, equipment, and personnel. Most techniques involve procedures described elsewhere in this text. The choice of technique rests on the clinical assessment and the recording of an accurate core temperature. The critical task for the clinician is distinguishing those patients requiring active rewarming from those for whom passive rewarming will suffice.

ANATOMY AND PHYSIOLOGY

For the purposes of this discussion, hypothermia is defined as a core body temperature of less than 35°C rectally (95°F). Fahrenheit can be converted to Celsius by the formula:

$$°C = (°F - 32)(5/9) \qquad (7).$$

Recently, otic measurement of temperature using infrared sensors has shown promise for providing a reading that more closely approximates hypothalamic temperature and thereby closer monitoring of change in core temperature than rectal measurement. At this time, however, continuous measurement of otic temperature is not widely available and standardization of otic temperature measurement is undergoing further study (8–11). Hypothermia can be classified into two categories: accidental hypothermia due to cold exposure in the presence or absence of an underlying disease, and hypothermia due to a primary disease such as trauma, hypoglycemia, sepsis, hypothyroidism and other endocrinopathies, metabolic disorders, or toxicologic exposures. Children's high body surface area to mass ratio and relatively low amount of subcutaneous fat make them especially susceptible to accidental hypothermia (7, 12). Neonates have further increased vulnerability to hypothermia due to their inability to produce heat by shivering (6). Children cool more quickly than adults when submerged in cold water which may provide some protection from the cardiovascular effects of cold exposure (2). Neonates and infants are unable to use behavioral adjustments to accommodate to extreme cold conditions. Adolescents are less likely to protect themselves from cold for social reasons and may succumb quickly to hypothermia during outdoor activities (13).

Four physical laws govern heat loss from the body. Radiation, the transfer of heat by nonparticulate means, accounts for 55 to 65% of heat loss, emanating mostly from the un-

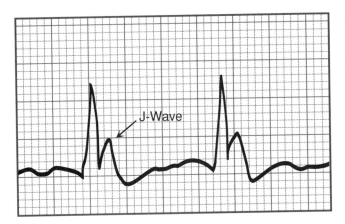

Figure 132.1.
ECG change with
hypothermia, J wave.

protected head. The degree of heat loss by radiation is directly related to the gradient between the core and ambient temperatures and the exposed body surface area. Evaporation of water from the skin and lungs accounts for approximately 30% of heat loss and is increased as wind speed increases. Convection is the transfer of heat by particles of air or water having contact with the heat source. Convective losses increase with shivering and with windy conditions. Conduction, the transfer of heat by direct contact, increases 5 times if the subject is wet and up to 30 times in cold water immersion. Fifteen percent of normal heat loss occurs by a combination of conduction and convection (7, 14).

As heat is lost and blood cools, the preoptic anterior hypothalamus stimulates superficial vasoconstriction which shunts blood away from the skin, and increased muscle tone which causes increased metabolism and heat production. When a critical muscle tone is reached, shivering begins which can increase heat production up to 4 times that of basal production. With progressive cooling, these homeostatic mechanisms fail, leading to decreased core temperature (7).

Certain generalizations can be made concerning clinical condition as correlated with core temperature (7). From 35°C to 32°C, general excitation characterized by vasoconstriction, shivering, and nonshivering thermogenesis occurs. At 32°C and below, homeostatic mechanisms fail. The progressive decline in metabolic rate results in decreased O_2 consumption and CO_2 production, and a shift of the oxyhemoglobin dissociation curve to the left. Slowing of the heart rate results in decreased cardiac output and, ultimately, hypotension. Progressive depres-

sion of central nervous system function is seen. When the core temperature reaches below 30°C the risk of cardiac arrhythmias increases; by 28°C increased myocardial irritability can result in ventricular fibrillation. The potential for ventricular fibrillation is increased when the electrocardiogram exhibits a J wave (Fig. 132.1). Coma, areflexia, severe hypotension, and asystole develop with progressively lower core temperatures.

The degree of hemodynamic instability, cardiac instability, and central nervous system depression will guide the selection of appropriate warming techniques to be used. Generally, passive rewarming or active core rewarming is chosen (see Indications in this chapter). Active external rewarming, meaning the use of overhead warmers or the application of heat directly to body surfaces using hot water mattresses, hot water bottles, or immersion in hot water causes early warming of the skin without reversing core hypothermia. In the setting of severe hypothermia, skin warming causes peripheral vasodilation with shunting of cold, acidemic blood from the periphery to the core. This process may initially cause a further decrease in core body temperature, a phenomenon known as core afterdrop. In addition, increased venous capacitance as a result of vasodilation may lower the effective preload and lead to decreased cardiac output and shock. The negative effects of active external rewarming may be lessened by application of heat to the head and trunk only (13).

INDICATIONS

Passive rewarming, which means removing the patient from the cold exposure and maximizing basal heat production using blankets or plastic bags on the extremities, is a generally safe and adequate approach for most patients with mild (35° to 34°C) or moderate (34° to 30°C) hypothermia who are clinically stable (7, 14–17). Active external rewarming with the application of heated materials to the body surface such as hot water bottles, heating blankets, overhead warmers, or hot water immersion is generally not recommended because it may lead to a lowering of core temperature, as peripheral vasoconstriction is reversed and cooler blood is shunted to central areas (7, 15–17). External rewarming, however, may have a role in treating otherwise healthy patients with mild hypothermia. If used, active external rewarming should be applied only to head and truncal areas to minimize peripheral vasodilatation (7, 14, 17, 18). Preterm infants with body temperatures between 30°C and 36°C have been successfully warmed on heated, water-filled mattresses (19).

For severe hypothermia (core temperature below 30°C), active core rewarming techniques may be indicated depending on the stability of the patient. Active core rewarming includes warm mist inhalation by mask or endotracheal tube ventilation, warm intravenous fluids, gastric irrigation, and bladder irrigation. Using more invasive methods such as peritoneal or thoracic irrigation should be considered for extremely hypothermic or unstable patients. Severely hypothermic patients may be extremely susceptible to ventricular fibrillation and care should be taken to avoid excessive stimulation of the patient. However, tracheal intubation has been performed without incident in many cases and should be initiated whenever necessary (12, 16).

In cardiac arrest, cardiopulmonary resuscitation should be initiated and a trial of defibrillation for a total of three shocks given. If the core temperature is below 30°C, further defibrillation and medication should be withheld and closed chest massage continued until the patient is warmed to a core temperature greater than 30°C, because the hypothermic heart is unresponsive to cardioactive drugs, pacing, and defibrillation (20). Cardiac arrest or instability requires rapid rewarming which is best accomplished with extracorporeal warming methods (2, 3, 7, 12, 21).

EQUIPMENT

Cardiac monitor
Core temperature monitor
Warm blankets or insulating blankets
Warm room
Fluid warmer
Face mask
Heated cascade nebulizer
Endotracheal tubes
Ventilator with heating cascade
Nasogastric tube or orogastric tube
Urethral catheters
Thoracostomy tubes
High flow fluid infuser
Thoracostomy drainage set with autotransfuser
Peritoneal lavage set
Cardiac bypass equipment
Hemodialysis equipment

PROCEDURE

All hypothermic patients should be placed on a cardiac monitor and have continuous core temperature monitoring, which is most easily accomplished with an electronic rectal probe. Passive rewarming involves preventing further exposure, removing wet clothing, providing a warm environment, and warm blanket exchanges or an insulating blanket. This process allows the patient's own thermogenic mechanisms to safely raise body temperature at a rate of 0.5°C to 2.0°C per hour (Fig. 132.2.A) (16). Active external rewarming is appropriate for infants and small children, and may raise temperature more quickly than passive rewarming in these patients (Fig. 132.2.B).

Active core rewarming can be accomplished by the successive application of techniques. Rates of rewarming range from 1°C to 3°C per hour with these techniques (Figs. 132.2.C, 132.2.D) (8, 16, 22). All patients may benefit from inspired warm oxygen, especially because hypothermia shifts the oxyhemoglobin dissociation curve to the left. The inspired air should be kept at approximately 45°C for patient comfort (7). Temperatures lower than this do not significantly increase core warming rates over passive techniques. Inspired air warmer than 50°C has been shown to cause thermal airway burns (14). Warm oxygen may be given by face mask via a heated cascade nebulizer (23) or by endotracheal tube and ventilator.

Intravenous fluids, warmed 40° to 41°C in a blood warming coil, should be infused to prevent further inadvertent cooling of the older child (school age and adolescent). Many hypothermic patients require volume resuscitation due to cold-induced diuresis. However, due to the relatively low rates of intravenous fluid infusion required for younger children

Figure 132.2.
A. Passive rewarming.
B. Active external rewarming.
C. Active core rewarming: Mild CNS and cardiovascular changes.
D. Active core rewarming: Severe CNS and cardiovascular changes.

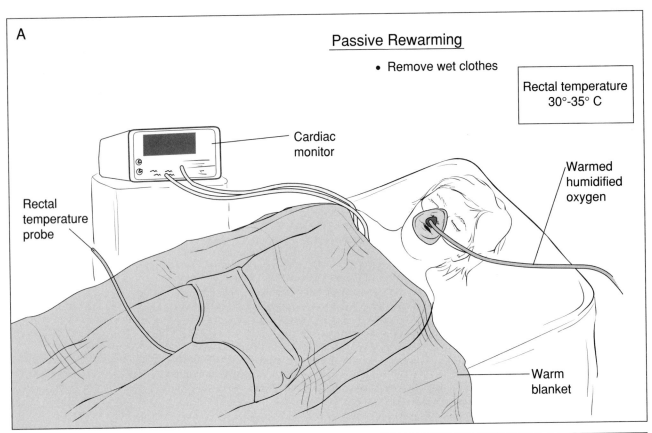

A

Passive Rewarming

- Remove wet clothes

Rectal temperature
30°-35° C

Cardiac
monitor

Warmed
humidified
oxygen

Rectal
temperature
probe

Warm
blanket

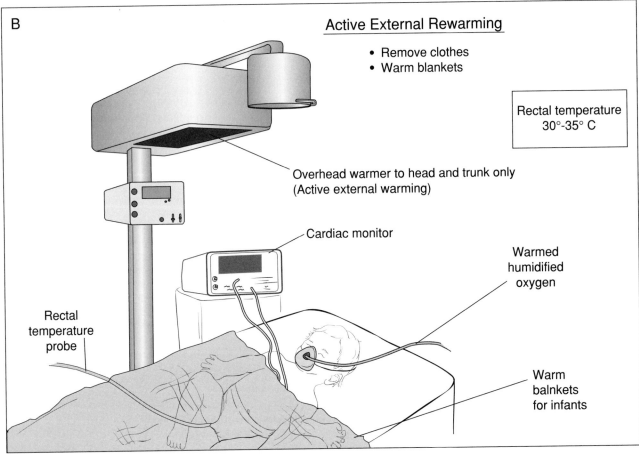

B

Active External Rewarming

- Remove clothes
- Warm blankets

Rectal temperature
30°-35° C

Overhead warmer to head and trunk only
(Active external warming)

Cardiac monitor

Warmed
humidified
oxygen

Rectal
temperature
probe

Warm
balnkets
for infants

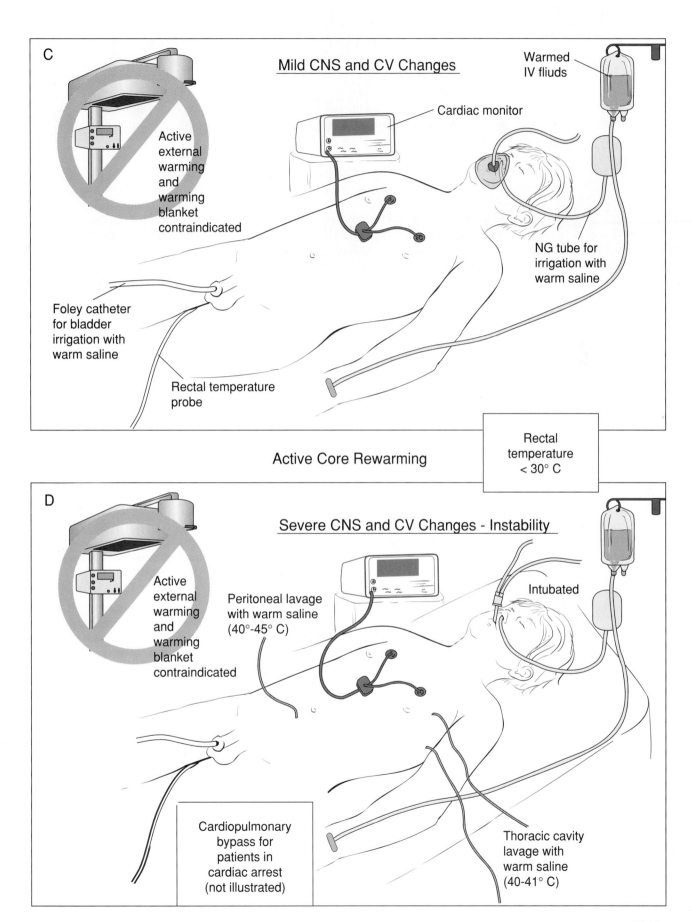

C

Mild CNS and CV Changes

Warmed IV fliuds

Cardiac monitor

Active external warming and warming blanket contraindicated

NG tube for irrigation with warm saline

Foley catheter for bladder irrigation with warm saline

Rectal temperature probe

Active Core Rewarming

Rectal temperature < 30° C

D

Severe CNS and CV Changes - Instability

Active external warming and warming blanket contraindicated

Peritoneal lavage with warm saline (40°-45° C)

Intubated

Cardiopulmonary bypass for patients in cardiac arrest (not illustrated)

Thoracic cavity lavage with warm saline (40-41° C)

(less than 5 years of age), radiant heat loss through the intravenous tubing eliminates the thermal benefit of warm IV fluids. Heat loss through intravenous tubing may be prevented by using short tubing of less than 25 cm from the warming source to the point of infusion. This technique, however, is not practical in most clinical settings (24).

Gastric and bladder irrigation with warmed fluids deliver heat to core structures in a relatively noninvasive fashion. Saline should be used in children to prevent electrolyte changes; adults safely tolerate infusion of warm tap water. Airway protection must be ensured. After placing a nasogastric or orogastric tube and/or a urethral catheter, aliquots of warmed fluid (40° to 45°C) are infused. Care should be taken to not distend the stomach or bladder. Rapid exchanges of fluid every 1 to 2 minutes will prevent cooling of the irrigant (17).

The peritoneal cavity provides a large surface area for heat exchange. Using techniques described elsewhere in this text, two peritoneal lavage catheters are placed and warmed saline (40° to 45°C) is infused at high flow rates via one catheter, while the other is drained to gravity or suction (Chapter 26). Alternatively, one catheter is used with frequent exchanges of warmed fluid (21). Warming rates to 4°C per hour can be achieved when peritoneal irrigation is combined with other less invasive warming methods (12, 22). Peritoneal irrigation should be considered for rapid rewarming of patients in cardiac arrest when extracorporeal methods are not available.

Thoracic cavity lavage can be achieved by two techniques. The closed technique involves placing two thoracostomy tubes in one side of the chest. One tube should be placed in the 4th intercostal space in the posterior axillary line and the other in the 3rd intercostal space in the midclavicular line (Chapter 30) (25). Warm saline (40° to 41°C) is infused in one tube with a highflow infuser while fluid is collected from the second tube using a thoracostomy autotransfuser drainage set. A one-tube system with a "Y-connector" also may be used by infusing aliquots of warm fluids and exchanging fluid every 1 to 2 minutes (17). The open technique for thoracic lavage is performed by left thoracotomy and direct instillation of warm saline (40° to 41°C) into the chest cavity (Chapter 32). Fluid is removed by continuous suction (17). Open thoracic lavage should be reserved for extreme cases with cardiac arrest or instability.

Extracorporeal warming via cardiopulmonary bypass or hemodialysis should be performed only by those personnel trained and experienced in these techniques. Application of extracorporeal warming is limited to patients in cardiac arrest or those who do not respond to less invasive techniques. Cardiac bypass is performed via the aorto-caval median sternotomy technique, or with femoral arterial and venous catheters (2, 21).

Warming procedures are continued until the patient is normothermic and hemodynamic stability is achieved. The patient

---

SUMMARY
Passive Rewarming
(Rectal temperature at or above 30°C)
1. Monitor core temperature continuously with electronic rectal probe and institute continuous cardiorespiratory monitoring
2. Remove wet clothing and place patient in warm environment
3. Rewarm using warm blanket or insulating blanket
4. Provide humidified inspired oxygen heated to 45°C
5. Instill intravenous fluids heated to 40° to 41°C
6. Active external rewarming, applied to head and trunk only, may be helpful for healthy patients with mild hypothermia

Active Rewarming
(Rectal temperature below 30°C)
1. Monitor core temperature continuously with electronic rectal probe and institute continuous cardiorespiratory monitoring
2. Intubate carefully as needed for airway control
3. Remove wet clothing and place patient in warm environment
4. Start passive rewarming as described. Do not institute active external rewarming
5. Begin bladder lavage in patients with mild cardiovascular and mental status changes using saline warmed to 40° to 41°C
6. Perform gastric, peritoneal, and thoracic lavage in patients with moderate to severe cardiovascular and mental status changes using saline warmed to 40 to 41°C
7. Consider cardiac bypass in patients with cardiac arrest or unresponsive dysrhythmias and rectal temperature below 30°C

should be continuously reassessed at each stage of warming and treatment of possible underlying conditions should be initiated simultaneously.

COMPLICATIONS

Passive warming and warm mist inhalation are associated with few problems and should be considered safe treatments for hypothermic patients. Overly aggressive, active external warming exposes patients to unnecessary risks by causing core temperature afterdrop, metabolic acidosis, and shock. Some evidence suggests a higher mortality rate in victims of prolonged hypothermia who receive active external rewarming (13). Complications of active core warming techniques are significant and particular to the procedures (thoracostomy, thoracotomy, peritoneal lavage) discussed elsewhere in the text. Therefore, active core rewarming should be reserved for patients with severe hypothermia marked by core temperature below 30°C. The most invasive active core warming techniques (i.e., open and closed thoracic lavage, peritoneal lavage, extracorporeal warming) should be reserved for patients with cardiovascular or central nervous system instability.

SUMMARY

Hypothermic patients who are stable may be safely warmed using passive techniques. Active core rewarming is necessary for severely hypothermic patients (core temperatures below 30°C, rectally) whose endogenous thermogenic mechanisms are depleted, and for patients with cardiovascular instability or severe central nervous system depression. Profoundly hypothermic patients may present with cardiac arrest. In such cases, particularly those involving children, aggressive warming using active core warming techniques may be associated with successful resuscitation and a good neurologic outcome.

REFERENCES

1. Letsou G, Kopf G, et al. Is cardiopulmonary bypass effective for treatment of hypothermic arrest due to drowning or exposure? Arch Surg 1992;127;525.
2. Antretter H, et al. Survival after prolonged hypothermia, N Engl J Med 1994;330:219.
3. DaVee T, Reineberg E. Extreme hypothermia and ventricular fibrillation. Ann Emerg Med 1980;9:100.
4. Nozaki R, et al. Accidental profound hypothermia. N Eng J Med 1986;315:1680.
5. Biggart M, Bohn D. Effect of hypothermia and cardiac arrest on outcome of near-drowning accidents in children. J Ped 1990;117:179.
6. Kemp A, Sibert J. Outcome in children who nearly drown: a British Isles study, British Med J 1991; 302(6782):931.
7. Reuler J. Hypothermia: pathophysiology, clinical settings, and managemen. Ann Inter Med 1978;89: 519.
8. Shinozaki T, Deane R, Perkins FM. Infrared tympanic thermometer: evaluation of a new clinical thermometer. Crit Care Med 1988;16:148-150.
9. Erickson RS, Kirklin SK. Comparison of ear-based, bladder, oral, and axillary methods for core temperature measurement. Crit Care Med 1993;21:1528-1534.
10. Milewski A, Ferguson KL, Terndrup TE. Comparison of pulmonary artery, rectal, and tympanic membrane temperatures in adult intensive care unit patients. Clin Pediatr 1991;(suppl):13-17.
11. Chamberlain JM, Terndrup TE, Alexander DT, Silverstone FA, Wolf-Klein G, O'Donnell R, Grandner J. Determination of normal ear temperature with an infrared emission detection thermometer. Ann Emerg Med 1995;25:15-20.
12. Danzl D, et al. Multicenter hypothermia survey, Ann Emerg Med 1987;16:1042.
13. Thompson A. Environmental emergencies. In: Fleisher G, Ludwig S, et al. eds. Textbook of pediatric emergency medicine. 3rd ed. Baltimore: Williams & Wilkins, 1993, pp. 815-818.
14. Danzl D. Accidental hypothermia. In: Rosen P, et al. eds. Emergency medicine: concepts and clinical practice. 3rd ed. St. Louis, CV Mosby, 1992, pp. 913–944.
15. Harnett R, Pruitt J, et al. A review of the literature concerning resuscitation from hypothermia. Part I.

CLINICAL TIPS

1. Active external rewarming in the severely hypothermic patient (core temperature below 30°C) may cause further drop of core temperature and lead to cardiac dysrhythmias.
2. Endotracheal and gastric intubation must be performed carefully in patients with severe hypothermia to avoid precipitation of cardiac dysrhythmias.
3. Open chest lavage or extracorporeal rewarming should be considered in the patient who has arrested from severe hypothermia.

The problem and general approaches. Aviat Space Environ Med 1983;54:425.

16. Miller J, Danzl D, et al. Urban accidental hypothermia: 135 cases. Ann Emerg Med 1980;9:456.

17. Sklar D, Doezema D. Procedures pertaining to hypothermia. In: Roberts J, Hedges J, eds. Clinical procedures in emergency medicine. 2nd ed. Philadelphia: WB Saunders, 1991, pp. 1100-1108.

18. Ledingham I, Mone J. Treatment of accidental hypothermia: a prospective clinical study. Br Med J 1980;280:1102.

19. Sarman I, et al. Rewarming preterm infants on a heated, water-filled mattress. Arch Dis Child 1989; 64:687.

20. Emergency Cardiac Care Committee and Subcommittees, American Heart Association. Guidelines for cardiopulmonary resuscitation and emergency cardiac care. Part IV: hypothermia. JAMA 1992;268: 2244-2246.

21. Harnett R, Pruitt J, et al. A review of the literature concerning resuscitation from hypothermia. Part II. Selected rewarming protocols. Aviat Space Environ Med 1983;54:487.

22. Otto R, Metzler M. Rewarming from experimental hypothermia: comparison of heated aerosol inhalation, peritoneal lavage, and pleural lavage. Crit Care Med 1988;16:869.

23. Shanks C, Sara C. Temperature monitoring of the humidifier during the treatment of hypothermia. Med J Aust 1972;2:1351.

24. Faries G, et al. Temperature relationship to distance and flow rate of warmed intravenous fluids. Ann Emerg Med 1991;20:1198.

25. Iversen R, Atkin S, et al. Successful CPR in a severely hypothermic patient using continuous thoracostomy lavage. Ann Emerg Med 1990;19: 1335.

ULTRASONOGRAPHIC TECHNIQUES

Section Editor: John Loiselle

GENERAL PRINCIPLES OF EMERGENCY DEPARTMENT ULTRASONOGRAPHY

John Loiselle

INTRODUCTION

The beginning of ultrasonography can be traced to the development of sonar in World War II. Applications in the field of medicine became apparent as early as the 1950s. Although initially considered a tool of radiologists, the use of ultrasonography spread to different subspecialties, notably cardiology and obstetrics, where it is now a routine and required skill. More recently its benefits have been demonstrated for specific applications within emergency medicine. In 1991 the American College of Emergency Physicians (ACEP) issued a position paper which endorsed the 24-hour availability of ultrasound technology within the emergency department (ED) and its use by appropriately trained, experienced, and credentialed emergency physicians (1). In addition, a report by the American Institute of Ultrasound in Medicine agreed that ultrasound examinations may be performed by appropriately trained emergency physicians in (*a*) certain immediate or life-threatening situations in which ultrasound examination is needed and other ultrasound physicians are not available, (*b*) certain urgent conditions in which ultrasound physicians cannot provide timely service on a 24-hour-a-day, 7-day-a-week basis, and (*c*) in situations in which ultrasound guidance may enhance the performance of certain procedures (2).

Many emergency medicine residency programs have already begun training residents in the emergent use of ultrasound (3, 4). It has been suggested that instruction in using of emergency ultrasonography be incorporated into the core curriculum of emergency medicine programs (5). Fellowships specializing in the use of ultrasound by emergency physicians already exist. It appears that using ultrasonography in the ED is rapidly becoming a useful and necessary skill.

The role of ultrasonography in the ED differs significantly from its previously recognized roles in other areas of medicine. For diagnostic purposes, ultrasound is generally used in the ED to answer a specific question, such as: Are products of conception clearly identifiable in the uterus? Its uses are limited to specific areas and cannot replace the more complete ultrasound studies typically performed by other specialists. Diagnostic ultrasonography has distinct advantages in the ED, where rapid, immediately available studies are crucial. It has been possible to obtain adequate examinations even during the performance of cardiopulmonary resuscitation (6).

Ultrasound functions not only as a diagnostic tool in the ED but also in providing guidance for performing various invasive procedures. It improves success rates and decreases complications in procedures commonly performed blindly (7–10). Ultrasound facilitates these procedures by allowing the clinician to follow the needle or other implement to the target, to mark the skin surface above the target, or to measure the distance from the skin surface to the target.

Chapter 133
General Principles of
Emergency
Department
Ultrasonography

1349

Although uses of ultrasound in the ED have been studied primarily in adults, a number of applications are useful for pediatric patients. Benefits have been demonstrated in all pediatric age groups, including neonates (11). Investigators have evaluated its usefulness in such cases involving pediatric trauma, removal of foreign bodies, adolescent pregnancies, and central line placement (12, 13).

The chapters in this section are not intended to serve as the only instructional aid in the use of ultrasound technology, but as an introduction to and review of the various techniques involved. As in the use and interpretation of any diagnostic procedure, routine standards must be applied. The individual must develop understanding and competency in the areas of application, visualization, and interpretation of ultrasound images. Specific indications must be developed to avoid overuse of this technique. Definitive expertise in using ultrasonography requires several years of subspecialty training. This is clearly not the goal for emergency physicians. However, training emergency physicians to use and interpret ultrasound for specific indications is possible in a reasonable period of time (14–17). ACEP has not proposed any standards for the training of emergency physicians, but authorities have suggested minimum hourly requirements in formal instruction, hands-on training, review of the literature, a number of successful studies, and formal review of studies with skilled sonographers (18, 19). These suggested requirements are consistent with those currently recommended in other nonradiologic specialties utilizing ultrasound (19). Chapters in this section address recommended numbers of studies to obtain competency in ED ultrasound utilization for particular applications. Ongoing review and quality assurance are a necessary part of maintaining proficiency in ED ultrasonography.

ANATOMY AND PHYSIOLOGY

Ultrasonography, like sonar, is based on the generation of sound waves, and relies on the ability of tissues within its path to propagate and reflect that wave to produce a two-dimensional image of objects in its field. The ultrasound transducer converts electrical energy to sound energy, which propagates through body tissues (Fig. 133.1.A). The denser the tissue, the better the sound wave is propagated. Sound waves propagate poorly through gas and do not reach structures separated from the transducer by a gas interface. This presents a problem for the unprepped patient with intestinal air who requires an abdominal scan. Wave propagation through bone is so rapid that ultrasound units are unable to accommodate it and therefore objects behind the bone cannot be detected.

Waves are reflected by interfaces of tissues of differing densities which produce echoes (Fig. 133.1.B). These echoes are detected by the transducer and converted back into electrical energy from which an image is constructed (Fig. 133.1.C). Echogenic or hyperechoic objects reflect most ultrasound waves and appear white on the ultrasound screen. Anechoic objects mainly transmit ultrasound waves and appear black on the screen. Objects of intermediate densities both transmit and reflect ultrasound waves and appear as varying shades of gray.

An acoustic window is an anechoic structure through which ultrasound waves can be transmitted to underlying structures of interest. A fluid-filled bladder is a commonly used acoustic window. Acoustic shadowing occurs when the ultrasound beam strikes a highly reflective surface, such as a renal stone or other calcified object, resulting in a dark shadow beyond the object. This may be helpful in identifying foreign bodies or a hindrance if distal objects become hidden within the shadow.

The resolution of ultrasound images depends on multiple factors. The strength of the echo, and therefore the image resolution, is proportional to the difference in density or acoustic impedance of adjacent tissues. Larger differences in tissue densities produce greater signal reflections and therefore greater resolution. Sound waves that strike perpendicular to the structure's surface rather than at an angle produce less scatter and a stronger echo and therefore provide greater resolution. Sound waves lose energy as they penetrate through a greater amount of tissue, and this beam attenuation results in lower resolution for distant objects.

Clinically relevant frequencies used in ultrasonography range from 2 to 9 megahertz (MHz). Transducers are available that produce specific frequencies within this range.

Chapter 133
General Principles of
Emergency
Department
Ultrasonography

1350

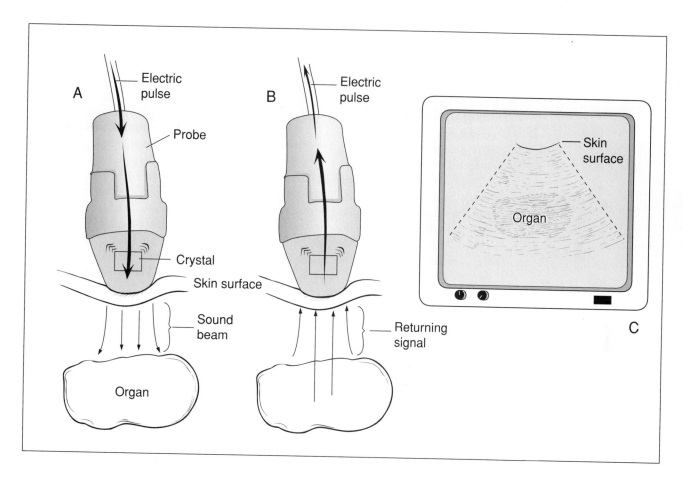

Figure 133.1.
A. Generation of an ultrasound beam by transducer.
B. Detection of a reflected ultrasound beam by transducer.
C. Corresponding image production on ultrasound screen

The focal zone of a transducer refers to the depth at which its image resolution is greatest and is determined by the frequency of the sound wave emitted. Higher frequencies produce greater resolution but penetrate less deeply below the body surface. A transducer that produces sound waves at a frequency of 2.25 MHz has optimal resolution capabilities at a depth of 8 to 12 cm. A 3.5 MHz transducer has a focal zone at 4 to 8 cm, and a 5 or 7.5 MHz transducer at 2 to 5 cm.

Ultrasonography is a noninvasive means of providing immediate bedside assessment of anatomy and function. The image on the screen is rapidly and continuously updated similar to the operation of a home television set, resulting in a real-time display which, to the clinician's eye, appears to move exactly as the body structures move.

As children and adults are susceptible to different disease processes, there are different indications and possibilities for the use of ED ultrasonography in different age groups. Using ultrasound in children offers both advantages and disadvantages. Children in general possess less adipose tissue and the depth to structures from the skin surface is not as great, which allows improved resolution of most structures in the body. Certain disease processes which are well known to complicate ultrasound studies (e.g., COPD, ascites) occur rarely in children. However, the smaller body of a child can make using a standard "adult" transducer impossible. Narrow rib interspaces limit the possible windows and transducer sizes that can be used. Morever, organs and structures are smaller and therefore harder to find and evaluate.

INDICATIONS

Ultrasound studies by emergency physicians are not intended to replace the physical examination, alternate studies, or ultrasound studies by a more experienced practitioner when available. Within the realm of the ED and the requirements of the emergency physician, several uses have been established for ultrasound. Its use in the ED is optimal for (*a*) relatively common conditions in which proficiency can be maintained, (*b*) conditions in

**Chapter 133
General Principles of
Emergency
Department
Ultrasonography**

1351

which emergent diagnosis is essential in dictating management, (c) situations in which no better diagnostic modality is available, (d) conditions in which ultrasound provides reasonable sensitivity and specificity in the hands of trained emergency physicians, and (e) conditions in which a rapid, focused study can be performed with findings that are readily detected and interpreted.

Currently a number of uses are established for pediatric ultrasonography by emergency physicians, several of which are discussed in detail in the remaining chapters of this section. In addition, certain ED ultrasound procedures which have been demonstrated as effective in adults are currently being explored for extrapolation to pediatric patients (15). A number of investigational uses also exist, although these will not be discussed.

The quality of the study in pediatric patients may be limited by a number of factors including agitation and lack of cooperation by the young child, tenderness with pressure from the transducer, inability to achieve proper positioning for the study, the small size of the child, and the size of the available equipment. It should be emphasized that ED ultrasonography must not interfere with procedures or evaluations of higher priority.

EQUIPMENT

The proper ultrasound machine and other specific equipment options will depend on the anticipated applications within the ED.

Ultrasound machine—optimally a unit capable of being upgraded and compatible with the different transducers necessary for anticipated uses. Many machines are equipped with standard features and numerous options, most of which are unnecessary for intended uses in the ED. The unit must be portable for rapid bedside deployment. A screen size of at least 5 inches diagonally is recommended for adequate visualization. The screen should be capable of displaying the image with a minimum of 64 shades of gray (20). Standard controls on an ultrasound machine include:

Overall gain—controls the power output or strength of the ultrasound signal and acts in a manner comparable to the brightness control on a television set.

Time gain compensation—accounts for beam attenuation by controlling beam strength at different levels to produce a consistent, uniform image. Near gain controls dampen the signals of superficial structures whereas far gain controls allow for enhancement of distant echoes. These are controlled automatically on some units. Others have multiple controls for different depths in a graphic equalizer format.

Zoom—provides image magnification.

Freeze frame—provides a still image for evaluation. This may be important when scanning structures in motion such as the heart, or when measurements or a hard copy are desired.

Electronic calipers—allows accurate measurements of objects being scanned.

Doppler—provides the capability to detect motion due to changes in wavelengths produced by an object moving toward or away from the transducer. Generally used to detect blood flow. Flow characteristics are depicted on-screen using color. Currently not considered cost efficient for most ED purposes (20).

Transducers—ultrasound waves are produced by a vibrating quartz crystal within the transducer by means of a piezoelectric effect. The alignment of these piezoelectric elements determines the focal length of the transducer. The higher the frequency of sound wave produced, the better the resolution, but the more superficial the soundwave penetration. The common frequencies available are 3.5 MHz for use in abdominal scanning, 5 MHz for cardiac examinations, and 7.5 MHz for superficial scanning such as foreign body detection. Varying sizes and shapes of transducers make them useful for particular types of scanning such as endovaginal, abdominal or transesophageal scans (Fig. 133.2). Some are the size of a fingertip for use in tight spaces. Transducers should be selected according to the likely uses of the machine in the ED.

Printer—essential in providing documentation of ultrasound findings both for the

Chapter 133
General Principles of
Emergency
Department
Ultrasonography

1352

medical record and for future quality review. Most units have the capability of labeling the print with identifying information.

Videotape recorder—useful in providing further documentation and for subsequent review of the study. It is a neccessary part of a quality assurance program.

Acoustic gel—provides interface between skin and transducer by conducting sound waves.

Acoustic standoff pads—act as an artificial acoustic window intended to provide additional distance to superficial structures so that structures remain within the transducer's focal zone. An intravenous fluid bag often provides an acceptable alternative.

PROCEDURE

The patient should be oriented regarding the procedure when maturational age and circumstances allow. Reassurance of the noninvasive, painless nature of the examination should lower anxiety and in most cases improve compliance of the child. This is especially important for procedures such as endovaginal scanning in the adolescent.

The position of the patient on the examining table will vary depending on the intended area to be scanned. Optimal positioning is discussed for each procedure in the relevant chapters. Correct positioning will provide the best and most accurate views of certain structures and will frequently determine the difference between an adequate and inadequate scan. Inability to position the patient properly due to lack of cooperation or contraindications to moving the patient may limit or exclude the use of scanning in particular cases.

The position of the clinician also is an important aspect of the examination. For each application the clinician should have a routine, comfortable position, an easily visible and accessible screen, and should also have the patient close enough so that the transducer can be readily manipulated to the desired position. The clinician must assume a position in which no interference occurs with the ongoing evaluation or management of the patient. In most cases the clinician will have

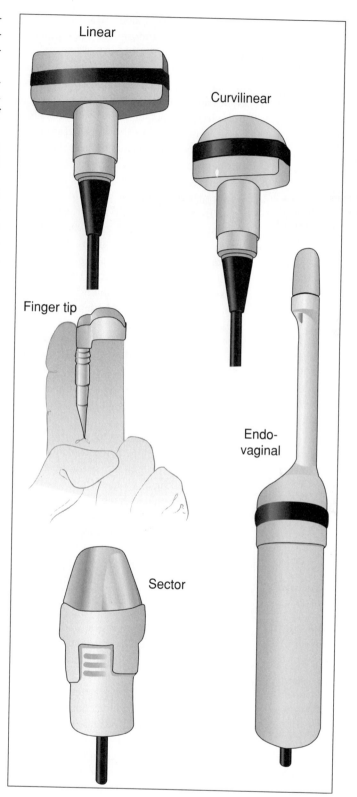

Figure 133.2.
Transducer types.

SUMMARY

1. Prepare patient for specific examination
2. Warm up ultrasound unit with proper initial knob settings
3. Position patient appropriately for desired examination
4. Apply gel to body surface overlying structure of interest
5. Grip transducer in a comfortable manner and orient marker dot
6. Image structure in multiple planes using angling and sweeping movements as necessary
7. Measure depth to structure and/or overall size as necessary
8. Record desired views with an appropriately labeled printout and videotape

CLINICAL TIPS

1. Preparing the patient for the examination often will reduce anxiety and result in a more useful scan.
2. Generous gel application reduces artifacts and improves the image.
3. Stabilizing the scanning hand improves the image and avoids motion artifact if the child shifts during the examination.
4. The appropriate frequency transducer must be chosen to produce the best image.
5. The best studies for the ED are those that can be performed rapidly, are easily interpreted, and are goal directed.

Chapter 133
General Principles of Emergency Department Ultrasonography

his or her dominant side toward the patient, with the area to be examined approximately at elbow level (Fig. 133.3.A).

The unit itself may require time to warm up and should be turned on as soon as it becomes apparent that ultrasonography may be used. Initial standard control settings should be determined for specific scans before actual use and the clinician should check that these settings are in place before proceeding. Fine tuning can then be performed as necessary. Common errors include not allowing adequate time for the unit to warm up and manipulating contrast and gain knobs excessively. Overuse of the gain to increase contrast will result in increasing artifacts and producing an inaccurate depiction of tissue densities (20). The gain should be adjusted using organs of known sonodensity for comparison.

The clinician should apply a generous amount of gel to either the body surface above the structure to be scanned or directly to the transducer. Inadequate amounts of gel result in poor transmission of sound waves known as contact artifact, as well as interference from bubbles within the gel.

Proper selection of the transducer frequency for the desired use is important. The focal zone of the transducer should be equivalent to the estimated depth of the structure of interest. As mentioned previously, acoustic standoff pads may be used to provide additional distance between the transducer and superficial target structures as needed (see Equipment). Several possible methods of gripping the transducer are used depending on the type of examination being performed and the clinician's preference. The pen grip is most commonly used as it provides good control and maneuverability for most examinations (Fig. 133.3.A). The hand holding the transducer should be supported against the patient's body to maintain contact and to provide a steady image if the patient shifts. Pressure should be adequate to maintain firm contact with the body surface and the gel, but not so firm as to cause discomfort to the patient. The transducer often can be moved closer to the target organ (e.g., to position the target within the focal zone of the transducer) by simply varying the pressure.

It is possible to view structures in a number of imaging planes. The two most frequently used are the sagittal and transverse planes (Fig. 133.3.B). Each view is gained by manipulating the transducer. This may include rotating in a 90 degree clockwise or counterclockwise direction, angling the probe against the body surface (Fig. 133.3 inset), or moving the transducer along the body surface.

Most transducers will produce a pie-shaped image on the ultrasound screen known as a sector scan. The point at the top of the screen corresponds to the tip of the transducer on the surface being scanned. The transducer contains a mark or indentation near its tip known as the marker dot. The orientation of the marker dot on the transducer determines the two-dimensional imaging plane that will be depicted on the screen. The marker dot, by convention, always points to the left side of the screen. In the standard transverse view the marker dot should face the patient's right-hand side, which will result in the patient's right-hand side being projected on the left side of the screen, in the same orientation as a CT scan image. A standard sagittal view is obtained with the marker dot facing the patient's head such that the cephalad part of the image appears on the left side of the screen. The ability to position the structure of interest within the screen is rapidly gained through experience. Angling the probe so that the marker dot points upward or moving the probe in the direction of the dot will move the object from left to right on the screen.

Measuring the depth to a structure or the length and width of a structure is performed by freezing an image on the screen and using the electronic calipers to mark the distance. Dimensions may be misinterpreted, however, if an oblique rather than a true transverse cut of the structure is obtained. Multiple cuts are necessary to provide the viewer with an accurate three-dimensional feel for the structure and to determine the optimal view. All photographed or recorded images should be labeled with the structure visualized and imaging plane used.

COMPLICATIONS

No harmful effects of ultrasound have been documented on patients or clinicians at en-

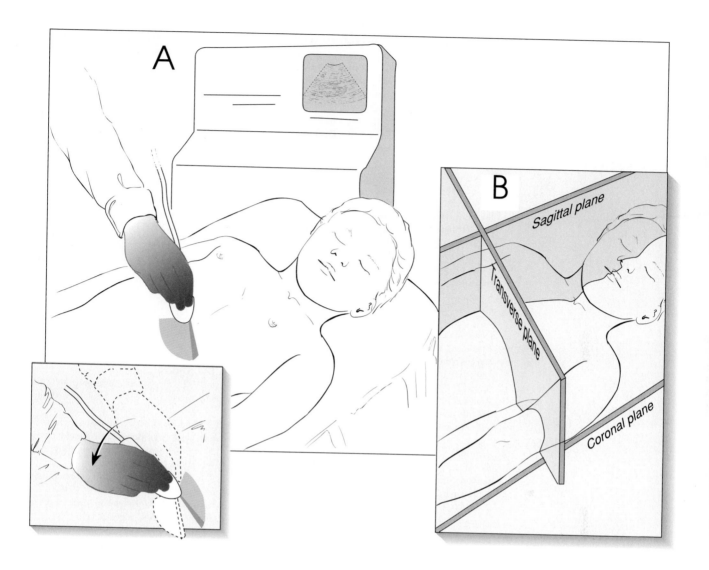

ergy levels that are used clinically (21). Current recommendations call for using the lowest energy level necessary to provide adequate visualization of objects, and minimizing the exposure to which individual patients are subjected.

Excessive force or pressure, as in any physical examination, has the possibility of inflicting soft tissue injury and the potential to precipitate injuries such as the rupture of intraabdominal abscesses or cysts.

SUMMARY

Emergency department bedside ultrasonography is a modality still in its early development, but is one which already shows evidence of being a useful adjunct to the physician's ability to accurately diagnose and

treat conditions in acutely ill and injured children. It can both avoid unnecessary invasive procedures and decrease the complications of others. It is not intended to replace a thorough history and physical examination or a more complete ultrasound study performed by other specialists. A number of studies have shown its accuracy for specific indications in the hands of properly trained emergency physicians. Structured training, credentialing, and quality assurance programs are important in acquiring and maintaining this skill.

REFERENCES

1. American College of Emergency Physicians. Position statement on the use of ultrasound for emergency department patients. January 24, 1991.

Figure 133.3.
A. Recommended position of clinician in relation to supine patient and ultrasound unit
B. Sagittal and transverse imaging planes. Alternating between the two planes is performed by rotating transducer 90°. Angling transducer changes transverse imaging plane (*inset*).

Chapter 133
General Principles of Emergency Department Ultrasonography

2. Initial report of AIUM Ad Hoc Committee on Ultrasound in Emergency Medicine.

3. Markham M, Hamilton GC. Objectives to direct the training of emergency medicine residents on off-service rotations; radiologic imaging 2: contrast and imaging techniques. J Emerg Med 1992;10(6): 767–774.

4. Cardenas E, Galli RL. Lower transabdominal endovaginal ultrasonography by emergency medicine residents. Ann Emerg Med 1993;22(5):920.

5. Heller MB, Verdile VP. Ultrasonography in emergency medicine. Emerg Med Clin 1992;10(1): 27–47.

6. Bocka JJ, Overton DT, Hauser A. Electromechanical dissociation in human beings: an echocardiographic study. Ann Emerg Med 1988;17:450–452.

7. Callahan JA, Seward JB, Tajik AJ, Holmes DR, Smith HC, Reeder GS, Miller FA. Pericardiocentesis assisted by two-dimensional echocardiography. J Thorac Cardiovasc Surg 1983;85:877–879.

8. Kuhn G, Burton J, Zelenka. Central venous access using portable ultrasound in the emergency department. Ann Emerg Med 1993;22(5):922.

9. Bradley M, Kadzombe E, Simms P, Eyes B. Percutaneous ultrasound guided extraction of nonpalpable soft tissue foreign bodies. Arch Emerg Med 1992; 9(2):181–184.

10. Alderson PJ, Burrows FA, Stemp LI, Holtby HM. The use of ultrasound to evaluate internal jugular vein anatomy and to facilitate central venous cannulation in pediatric patients. Br J Anaesth 1993;70: 145–148.

11. Gochman RF, Karasic RB, Heller MB. Use of portable ultrasound to assist urine collection by suprapubic aspiration. Ann Emerg Med 1991; 20(6):631–635.

12. Akgur FM, Kovanlikaya A, Kovalikaya I, Aktug T. Initial evaluation of children sustaining blunt abdominal trauma: ultrasonography vs diagnostic peritoneal lavage [Abstract]. In: Progress in pediatric trauma. Proceedings of the Fourth National Conference on Pediatric Trauma. Boston: Kiwanis Pediatric Trauma Institute, 1992:80.

13. Denys BG, Uretsky BF, Reddy PS, Ruffner RJ, Sandhu JS, Breishlatt WM. An ultrasound method for safe and rapid central venous access. N Engl J Med 1991;324:566.

14. Schlager D, Sanders AB, Wiggins D, Boren W. Ultrasound for the detection of foreign bodies. Ann Emerg Med 1991;20(2):189–191.

15. Ma OJ, Mateer JR, Ogata M, Kefer MP, Wittman D, Aprahamian C. Prospective analysis of a rapid trauma ultrasound examination performed by emergency physicians. J Trauma 1995;38(6):879–885.

16. Schlager D, Lazzareschi G, Whitten D, Sanders AB. A prospective study of ultrasonography in the ED by emergency physicians. Am J Emerg Med 1994; 12(2):185–189.

17. Jehle D, Davis E, Evans T, Harchelroad F, Martin M, Zaiser K, Lucid J. Emergency department sonography by emergency physicians. Am J Emerg Med 1989;7(6):605–611.

18. Olson DW. Gynecological applications of ultrasonography. In: Diagnostic ultrasonography for emergency medicine ACEP. St. Louis: CV Mosby, 1993.

19. Mateer J, Plummer D, Heller M, Olson D, Jehle D, Overton D, Gussow L. Model curriculum for physician training in emergency ultrasonography. Ann Emerg Med 1994;23:95–102.

20. Heller M, Jehle D. Ultrasound in emergency medicine. Philadelphia: WB Saunders, 1995.

21. American Institute of Ultrasound in Medicine. Official statement on clinical safety. March, 1988.

Chapter 133
General Principles of
Emergency
Department
Ultrasonography

Ultrasound-Assisted Suprapubic Bladder Aspiration

Robert F. Gochman

Introduction

Suprapubic bladder aspiration of urine is used to obtain urine in an aseptic fashion by passing a needle through the abdominal wall directly into the urinary bladder. This procedure is described fully in Chapter 99. Numerous studies have demonstrated the superiority of suprapubic bladder aspiration compared with other techniques of collecting urine for culture in infants and toddlers (1–7). Although the technique is inherently invasive, few serious complications have been reported with suprapubic bladder aspiration (8–10).

Reported rates of successfully obtaining urine by suprapubic bladder aspiration vary (1, 4, 6, 7, 11). Although many authorities emphasize the ease of collecting urine by this technique, suprapubic bladder aspiration performed in an emergency department (ED) setting is often unsuccessful. One primary factor affecting the success rate is the volume of urine in the bladder.

The development of relatively low-cost, portable ultrasound devices has expanded the availability of this noninvasive diagnostic technique to a variety of clinical settings. The value of portable ultrasonography in assisting suprapubic bladder aspiration in a pediatric ED has been demonstrated (12). This technique proved useful even when performed by physicians with no formal training in ultrasonography.

Ultrasound may be used as an adjunct in determining the presence of urine within the bladder before the standard suprapubic bladder aspiration procedure. In addition to the ED setting, this technique may prove valuable in neonatal intensive care units and other areas where suprapubic bladder aspiration is performed regularly. Although this technique has been described primarily by physicians, the relative ease of learning and performing the procedure should make it applicable to trained physician assistants, nurse practitioners, and nurses.

Anatomy and Physiology

The urinary bladder is an intraabdominal organ in infants and children less than 2 years of age, thus making it easily accessible by suprapubic bladder aspiration. In older children the bladder recedes into the pelvis and at that point enters the abdomen only when full. When suprapubic bladder aspiration is performed in the midline along the suprapubic crease, the needle passes through skin, rectus muscle and the anterior wall of the bladder. Using ultrasound, these tissues create a lighter background than the full bladder

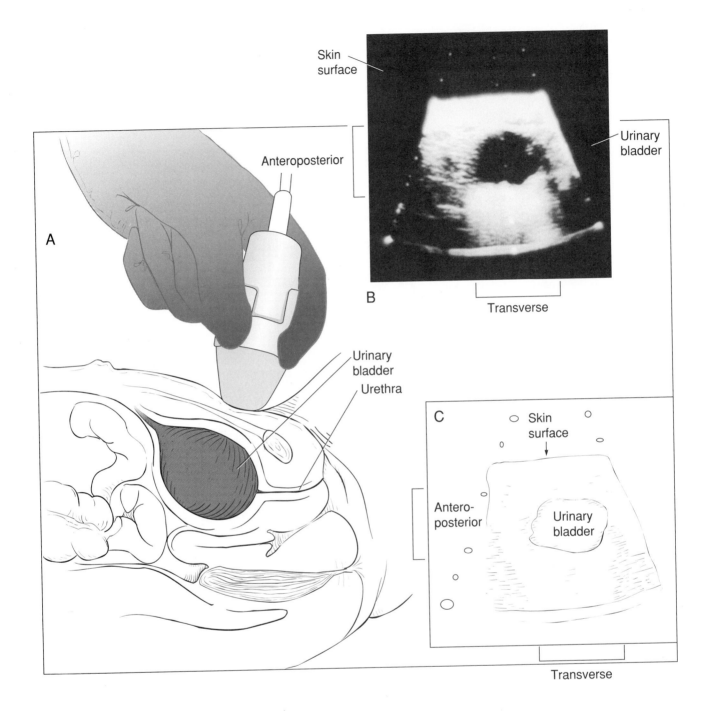

Figure 134.1.
A. Position of patient and ultrasound probe for scanning the bladder.
B. Ultrasound image of full urinary bladder in an infant.
C. Schematic depiction of ultrasound image.

**Chapter 134
Ultrasound-Assisted
Suprapubic Bladder
Aspiration**

which appears as a black ovoid structure. (Fig. 134.1).

Indications

Indications for suprapubic bladder aspiration are discussed in detail in Chapter 99. To sum-marize, this technique is indicated whenever a urine sample must be obtained in a sterile fashion from an incontinent patient to evaluate for a possible urinary tract infection. Using ultrasound as an adjunct to suprapubic bladder aspiration is indicated when the clinician is unsure whether the bladder is empty or full.

EQUIPMENT

Sterile gloves
Povidone-iodine solution
Sterile gauze
Sterile 5 mL syringe
Spinal needle—22 gauge, 1.5 (neonates)
Spinal needle—22 gauge, 1.5 (infants & todlers)
Sterile specimen container
Sterile bandage
Ultrasound device
Acoustic transmission gel

Many basic and enhanced ultrasound devices are presently available. Ideally, the machine would be portable with a standoff 7.5 MHz sector probe allowing for superficial scanning. The device should have the ability to measure the diameter of the bladder.

PROCEDURE

After obtaining the proper equipment needed for suprapubic aspiration, the clinician applies approximately 5 mL of ultrasound transmission gel to the infant's suprapubic region. For male patients, gentle pressure on the penile shaft should be maintained during the procedure to prevent spontaneous urination and loss of the specimen. The probe is gently applied to the suprapubic region in the midline and the area is scanned in the transverse plane, directing the probe caudad or cephalad as needed to maximize the size of the bladder image (Fig. 134.1.A). The anteroposterior (AP) and transverse internal bladder diameters are estimated to the nearest 0.5 cm. The bladder is considered to be full if both the maximum AP and transverse diameters are 2 cm or more, and empty if either diameter is less than 2 cm. These parameters have resulted in success rates greater than 75% (12). Greater success may be expected when larger bladder diameters are identified.

After ultrasonography, the probe and gel are removed from the patient's abdomen. If the bladder is full, suprapubic bladder aspiration should be attempted at once as described in Chapter 99. If empty, the bladder may be rescanned after a 30-minute waiting period allowing time for the bladder to fill. Thirty minutes allows for urine to accumulate while other procedures are completed; a longer waiting period may be impractical and imprudent in the ED setting.

COMPLICATIONS

Aside from the rare complications of suprapubic bladder aspiration (i.e., hematuria, infected needle tract, and bowel perforation) no additional risk of complication is expected with using ultrasound. In fact, by identifying an empty or full bladder before suprapubic bladder aspiration, the number of attempts and subsequent complications may be minimized.

SUMMARY

Portable ultrasonography is an easily learned technique for identifying the urinary bladder. Unlike other applications of ultrasonography, identifying a full bladder requires little expertise. Because the empty bladder is a potential space that only becomes visible as it fills, it is, quite simply, either there or not there. The value of ultrasound-assisted suprapubic bladder aspiration is therefore in confirming that a full or empty bladder exists, thus enhancing the success rate of suprapubic bladder aspiration and limiting the number of attempts.

REFERENCES

1. Aronson AS, Gustafson B, Svenningsen NW. Combined suprapubic bladder aspiration and clean-voided urine examination in infants and children. Acta Paediatr Scand 1973;62:396–400.
2. Bonadio WA. Urine culturing techniques in febrile infants. Pediatr Emerg Care 1987;3:75–78.
3. Edelmann Jr CM, Ogwo JE, Fine BP, Martinez AB. The prevalence of bacteriuria in full-term and premature newborn infants. J Pediatr 1973;82:126–132.
4. Nelson JD, Peters PC. Suprapubic aspiration of urine in premature and term infants. Pediatrics 1965;36:132–134.
5. Pryles CV. Percutaneous bladder aspiration and other methods of urine collection for bacteriologic study. Pediatrics 1965;36:128–131.

6. Pryles CV, Atkin MD, Morse TS, Welch KJ. Comparative bacteriologic study of urine obtained from children by percutaneous suprapubic bladder aspiration of the bladder and by catheter. Pediatrics 1959; 24:983–991.

7. Saccharow L, Pryles CV. Further experience with the use of percutaneous suprapubic bladder aspiration of the urinary bladder. Pediatrics 1969;43: 1018–1024.

8. Morrell RE, Duritz G, Oltorf C. Suprapubic aspiration associated with hematoma. Pediatrics 1982;69: 455–457.

9. Lanier B, Daeschner CW. Serious complication of suprapubic bladder aspiration of the urinary bladder. J Pediatr 1971;79:711.

10. Polnay L, Fraser AM, Lewis JM. Complication of suprapubic bladder aspiration. Arch Dis Child 1975; 50:80–81.

11. O'Callaghan C, McDougall PN. Successful suprapubic bladder aspiration of urine. Arch Dis Child 1987;62:1072–1073.

12. Gochman R, Karasic R, Heller M. Use of portable ultrasound to assist urine collection by suprapubic aspiration. Ann Emerg Med 1991;20:631–635.

CHAPTER 135

EMERGENT CARDIAC ULTRASONOGRAPHY

Kathleen A. Lillis and Dietrich Jehle

INTRODUCTION

Ultrasonography is a valuable recent addition to the diagnostic armamentarium of emergency physicians. Bedside sonography allows for more rapid diagnosis and treatment of patients with potentially life-threatening illnesses while using a noninvasive modality. Because of advances in the quality of imaging and portability of ultrasonography, trained emergency physicians can now obtain rapid access to information that greatly enhances the care of critically ill patients.

Limited emergent cardiac ultrasound performed at the bedside can provide valuable life-saving information in seconds. Studies have demonstrated that with little formal training, emergency physicians are capable of using ultrasound to diagnose specific emergent conditions (e.g., cardiac tamponade) (1). The optimal amount of training required to accurately detect such conditions, and the frequency of examinations necessary to maintain proficiency for emergency physicians has not yet been definitively determined. However, using recorded photographic images or hard copy, and videotaped examinations provides a means of quality assurance. Emergent echocardiography is most useful in pediatric patients to confirm the diagnoses of cardiac tamponade, pulseless electrical activity, and cardiac trauma.

ANATOMY AND PHYSIOLOGY

Cardiac tamponade results from the accumulation of fluid, pus, or blood within the pericardial sac. This restricts cardiac filling, limits stroke volume, and reduces blood pressure. If tamponade remains uncorrected it can result in cardiovascular insufficiency, shock, and eventually death.

Infection is the most common cause of pericarditis and the accumulation of pericardial fluid in children. Bacterial etiologies are more likely to result in cardiac tamponade. Up to 15% of patients develop pericardial effusions 1 to 3 weeks following cardiac surgery in a condition known as postpericardiotomy syndrome (2). Trauma, both penetrating and blunt, is increasingly seen as a cause of tamponade in older children and adolescents. Other causes include collagen vascular and oncologic disease.

Pulseless electrical activity (PEA) or electromechanical dissociation (EMD) is said to exist in the patient who displays electrical cardiac activity on a monitor, but has no detectable pulse. Pulseless electrical activity in children has multiple causes, including severe hypovolemia (including blood loss), cardiac tamponade, severe hypoxemia, tension pneumothorax, hypothermia, and ingestions. Detection of cardiac motility in the setting of PEA is crucial in determining the prognosis, underlying causes, and possible therapeutic interventions.

Impediments in adult echocardiography such as obesity, difficulty with positioning, and chronic obstructive pulmonary disease are less likely to pose limitations to ultrasound scanning in children.

For purposes of ultrasound evaluation, the heart can be categorized into two orthogonal planes: the long-axis plane and the short-axis plane. The long-axis plane transects the heart parallel to the long axis of the left ventricle. The short axis is obtained by transecting the heart perpendicular to the plane of the long axis. The four-chamber plane is a special long-axis plane that transects the heart parallel to the dorsal and ventral surfaces of the body (3). These planes are illustrated in Figure 135.1.

The pericardium is a dense tissue that forms a sac completely surrounding the heart and a small part of the aorta and pulmonary artery. This tissue is highly echogenic and is visualized as the outer border of the heart on ultrasound. The pericardium is composed of two layers: the visceral pericardium, and the parietal pericardium. Fluid between these layers is seen on ultrasound as an anechoic space between the two more reflective echoes. A small amount of fluid is normally present in this potential space and serves to lubricate the membranes. Generally, fluid is not visible anteriorly or in the nondependent areas of the supine patient. Any anterior displacement of the parietal pericardium represents an abnormal collection of fluid. Effusions tend to collect initially around the more dependent and mobile ventricles and later in the area of the less mobile atria.

Pericardial fat, pleural effusions, and subdiaphragmatic fluid may be confused with pericardial fluid. These anechoic stripes are not circumferential and do not demonstrate the normal variation in size between systole and diastole seen with pericardial fluid.

Hemopericardium is the most common feature of cardiac injury and is also seen as a circumferential echo-free space within the pericardium. An acute hemopericardium may present as a pericardial hematoma which has echogenic components. Any intrapericardial collection, either echo-free or echodense, in the setting of penetrating injury is presumed to represent penetrating cardiac injury.

Myocardial rupture is a rare complication of blunt chest trauma. Most patients die at the scene. In patients entering the EMS system alive, however, rapid diagnosis and treatment is essential for survival. Usually the pericardial sac contains the rupture and these patients present with hemopericardium and some degree of cardiac tamponade.

INDICATIONS

The role of pediatric cardiac ultrasound by the emergency physician is restricted to a few specific conditions in which it can provide immediate and unequivocal findings. It is in no way intended to supplant the role of a comprehensive echocardiographic examination. Currently this procedure has three main roles: (a) to detect a pericardial effusion in the appropriate clinical setting, (b) to detect a hemopericardium or cardiac rupture associated with chest trauma, and (c) to detect the presence of any cardiac motion associated with pulseless electrical activity.

Suspicion of cardiac tamponade must be acted upon within seconds. In an adolescent who has sustained a penetrating chest wound, an emergent echocardiographic examination can provide information regarding the extent of injury before a patient deteriorates. Emergent cardiac ultrasound gives the physician the ability to look inside the chest to confirm or refute the diagnosis at bedside.

Pericardial effusion in a child may present with a number of physical findings. Hypotension, especially when associated with evidence of increased central venous pressures, the presence of a pulsus paradoxus, chest pain, poor peripheral perfusion, or distended neck veins may all be signs of tamponade. However, no clinical findings associ-

Figure 135.1.
A. Imaging planes in emergent cardiac ultrasound.
B. Ultrasound image of short-axis plane of the heart.
C. Ultrasound image of four-chamber long-axis plane. (LV = left ventricle; RV = right ventricle; FO = foramen ovale; LA = left atrium; RA = right atrium; PVn = pulmonary veins.) (Ultrasound images reprinted with permission from Reed KL, Anderson CF, Shenker L. Fetal Echocardiography: An Atlas. New York: Alan A. Liss, 1988.)

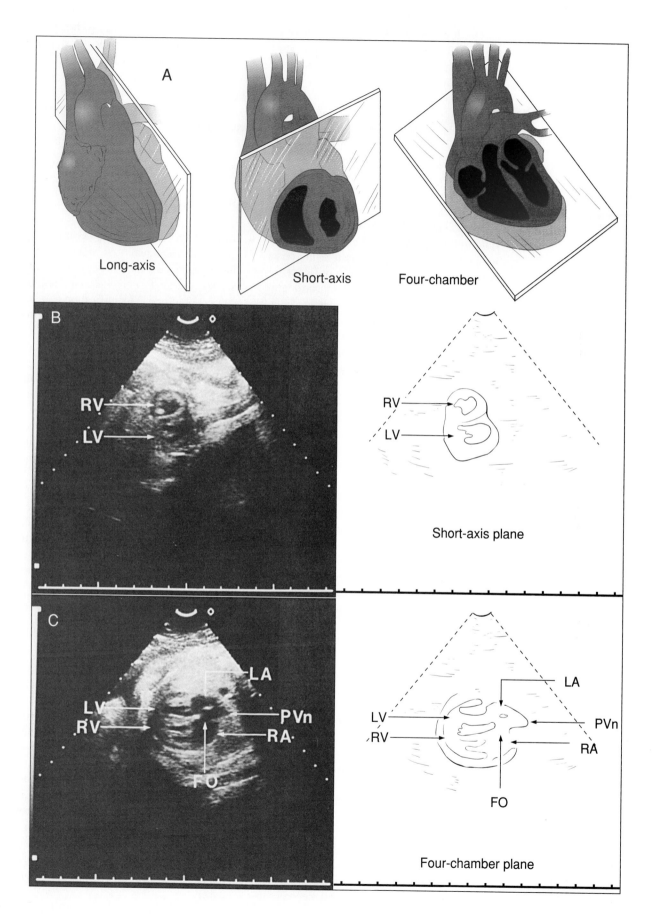

Long-axis

Short-axis

Four-chamber

RV
LV

RV
LV

Short-axis plane

LA
LV
RV
PVn
RA
FO

LA
LV
RV
PVn
RA
FO

Four-chamber plane

ated with tamponade are 100% sensitive or specific. The classic triad of distant heart sounds, hypotension, and elevated central venous pressure are rarely present in a child, making tamponade a difficult clinical diagnosis.

Standard available tests also are nonspecific in diagnosing cardiac tamponade. ECG changes or increased heart size on a chest radiograph may suggest pericardial fluid; however, normal results do not exclude its presence. The size of the cardiac silhouette on chest radiograph depends on the amount of fluid in the effusion and the distensibility of the pericardial sac. Effusions of acute onset generally do not result in a significant increase in the cardiac shadow. Echocardiography is therefore the procedure of choice in detecting the presence of a pericardial effusion (4). Limited ultrasound in the ED may provide important additional information, especially when time available before the need for intervention is limited.

Ultrasound also may be useful in the setting of blunt or penetrating chest trauma in cases of suspected hemopericardium or cardiac rupture. Its role may be limited to those patients with symptoms, or extended to those with a significant mechanism of injury in an attempt to anticipate potential deterioration.

Using ultrasound to diagnose cardiac trauma is not intended to replace other standard tests currently available. It should be used as a noninvasive, rapidly available modality to complement other clinical tools and to determine the presence of specific cardiac injury in a patient who has suffered chest trauma (5). Two-dimensional echocardiography performed in the ED for identifying penetrating cardiac injuries has decreased the time to diagnosis and has increased the survival rate and neurologic outcome of survivors (6).

In the setting of PEA, ultrasound may be used to determine whether cardiac function is truly absent or if the heart is pumping but unable to generate adequate stroke volume to register a blood pressure. In the former case the prognosis is essentially the same as for asystole, whereas in the latter instance a treatable cause may be determined and more aggressive interventions indicated (4).

Using cardiac ultrasonography for more advanced studies such as diagnosis of a particular congenital heart disease in neonates in the ED setting is not feasible. Although cardiac ultrasound by emergency physicians may demonstrate abnormal anatomy, it is unlikely to definitively diagnose the particular congenital lesion. The education and expertise necessary to make such a diagnosis is clearly attained only by the pediatric cardiologist.

EQUIPMENT

- Ultrasound machine—the scanner must have adequate image quality. It should be capable of displaying the image in at least 64 shades of gray. Fewer shades will significantly compromise identification and will impair the quality of a hard copy produced.
- The screen size must be at least 5 inches diagonally. Equipment with a small screen size is impractical for use in the ED and makes it difficult for more than one physician to view the screen at once.
- Measurement capabilities with an on-screen caliper system are necessary to make quantitative distinctions between normal and abnormal anatomy.
- Ultrasound machines used in the ED must be able to produce hard copies for permanent records. A free-standing printer which prints the screen image on specially treated paper is the most practical.
- Videotaping capabilities allow subsequent viewers to visualize ventricular wall or valvular motion that is not appreciated on a paper image.
- Any machine used in the ED must be portable and compact.
- Doppler ultrasound is an option that provides flow information simultaneously with the anatomic information displayed on the screen. This information is advantageous when scanning the heart, aorta, and other vascular structures, but is not required for basic scanning of children in the ED.
- Transducers with frequencies of 3.5 MHz and 5.0 MHz should be available. The 3.5 MHz transducer should have a narrow footplate to allow imaging between ribs in young children.
- Ultrasound gel is used to provide an acoustic interface between the chest wall and transducer.

Procedure

To perform a limited examination of the heart using ultrasound, four standard views are normally visualized. Each view is a two-dimensional image of the heart, in either the long- or short-axis plane, obtained through one of three windows (Fig 135.2). A window refers to a location on the body through which the transducer can image the heart. The four standard views for an ED study are the subcostal four-chamber view, the left parasternal short-axis view, the left parasternal long-axis view, and the apical four-chamber view.

The subcostal four-chamber view often provides the most important information for a single-view examination (7). To obtain this view, the patient should be in the supine position. Ultrasound gel is applied, and the transducer is placed at the left infracostal margin at the level of the xiphoid. The beam is aimed at the left shoulder and the marker dot pointed toward 9 o'clock. By rotating the transducer, the clinician can obtain the desired four-chambered view (Fig. 135.1.C). The structures closest to the transducer appear nearest the top of the display, and the marker points toward the left side of the screen. A small amount of hepatic parenchyma lies directly below the transducer. The right-sided chambers are posterior to the liver. The visceral and parietal pericardium are seen as single, bright reflecting surfaces. Fluid between these two pericardial layers can be seen as a separation of the bright echoes. The SC four-chamber view can provide essential information in a short period, and therefore should be used early in the ultrasound examination of the heart. The subcostal four-chamber view quickly screens for pericardial fluid while causing minimal interference with ongoing CPR. A limited, goal-directed examination may be performed within 1 minute (7).

The next two views are obtained by placing the transducer in the left parasternal window, which is immediately adjacent to the sternum between the second and fourth intercostal spaces (Fig. 135.2). Both left parasternal views may require positioning the patient in the left lateral decubitus position. These views may be difficult to obtain in poorly compliant or critically ill patients. The left parasternal long axis view is obtained by ro-

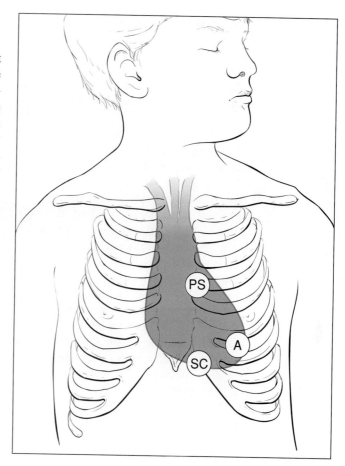

tating the transducer so the plane of the beam is parallel to a line drawn from the right shoulder to the left hip. The marker dot must therefore be pointed at approximately 4 o'-clock. This view allows visualization of the aortic valve and proximal ascending aorta, and provides a good assessment of left ventricular size. With pulseless electrical activity, CPR must be stopped momentarily while the examiner assesses for the presence or absence of wall and valve motion.

The left parasternal short-axis view is obtained by rotating the transducer so that the plane of the beam is perpendicular to the long axis of the heart (marker dot pointing at approximately 8 o'clock) (Fig. 135.1.B). By angling the transducer from the left hip to the right shoulder, the clinician can visualize sections extending from the apex through the mitral valve to the aortic valve.

The apical four-chamber view requires the patient to be in the supine or left lateral decubitus position. This view is obtained by placing the transducer directly over the point of maximum impulse with the beam directed

Figure 135.2.
Transducer locations for standard windows.
PS, parasternal;
A, apical;
SC, subcostal.

toward the right shoulder. The marker dot should be pointing at approximately 8 o'-clock. The transducer may need to be angled and/or rotated to obtain the desired view.

Although these standard views can provide essential information, it may be necessary to visualize other more useful planes by manipulating the transducer during the examination. The best view is the one that provides the desired information.

The subcostal four-chamber view is the best to visualize a pericardial effusion, followed by the left parasternal long-axis view. Once evidence of a pericardial effusion is demonstrated by ultrasound, clinical correlation is generally necessary to make the diagnosis of cardiac tamponade. A hyperdynamic heart, with diastolic collapse of the right atrium and ventricle, indicates that intrapericardial pressures from the effusion have exceeded intracardiac pressures, confirming the presence of cardiac tamponade. Respiratory variations of chamber diameters provide visual evidence of the mechanisms responsible for the paradoxical pulse. However, these observations require extensive ultrasound experience and are not easily demonstrated on ED studies.

The left parasternal long-axis view allows the physician visual access to the left ventricle, and is the preferred view to determine pulseless electrical activity. The apical four-chamber view and the subcostal four-chamber view provide good alternative views.

SUMMARY
(CONTINUED)
4. *Left parasternal long-axis view:* orient transducer so that marker dot is pointed to 4 o'clock
   Left parasternal short-axis view: rotate the transducer 90° from LPLA view so that marker dot is directed at 8 o'clock
   A. Angle transducer toward right shoulder to obtain view at aortic level
   B. Angle transducer perpendicular to chest wall to obtain view at mitral valve level
   C. Angle transducer toward left hip to obtain view at papillary muscle level
5. Stop CPR and assess ventricular wall motion
Apical Window
1. Place patient in supine or left lateral decubitus position
2. Place ultrasound gel and transducer at point of maximal impulse
3. Direct transducer at right shoulder
4. Point marker dot at 8 o'clock
5. Adjust image with slight angulation and/or rotation to obtain four-chamber view

COMPLICATIONS

No complications are associated with performing cardiac ultrasounds in children. However, limitations obviously exist. The accuracy of the procedure and subsequent decisions based on the results depend on the physician performing the examination. For example, to make the diagnosis of pulseless electrical activity, cardiac ultrasound will need to be performed on a child who is being resuscitated. It is unlikely that the brief cessation of CPR necessary to evaluate cardiac motion will have a significant detrimental effect on the patient. Pericardial fat, pleural effusions, and subdiaphragmatic fluid may be confused with pericardial fluid. Such a misinterpretation may lead to unnecessary pericardiocentesis. These anechoic stripes differ from effusions in that they are not circumferential. Previous experience has actually shown a decreased incidence of unnecessary pericardiocentesis and its associated risks (1). For limited studies such as these, the accu-

SUMMARY
Subcostal Window
1. Place patient in supine position
2. Place ultrasound gel and transducer at left infracostal margin at level of xiphoid
3. Aim transducer at left shoulder
4. Point marker dot at 9 o'clock
5. Adjust image by rotating transducer slightly to obtain four-chamber view
6. Identify echogenic visceral and parietal pericardial layers
7. Scan for echo-free space, representing fluid, separating pericardial layers
Parasternal Window
1. Place patient in supine or left lateral decubitus position
2. Place ultrasound gel and transducer at left parasternal area between second and fourth intercostal spaces
3. Aim transducer down at heart and slightly angled toward right shoulder

racy of trained emergency physicians has been excellent without significant misinterpretations (1).

SUMMARY

Echocardiography provides invaluable information to emergency physicians. Limited bedside cardiac ultrasound performed on children and adolescents is a noninvasive, immediately available method of examining the heart. Ultrasonography is most useful in this setting for diagnosing cardiac tamponade and pulseless electrical activity. The technique can be learned quickly and provides a high degree of accuracy for these indications. Early diagnosis and treatment of these conditions in the pediatric patient may be life saving.

REFERENCES

1. Mayron R, Gaudio FE, Plummer D, Asinger R, Elsperger J. Echocardiography performed by emergency physicians: impact on diagnosis and therapy. Ann Emerg Med 1988 Feb;17:150–154.
2. Cardiac emergencies. In: Ludwig S, Fleisher GR, eds. Textbook of pediatric emergency medicine. 3rd ed. Baltimore: Williams & Wilkins, 1993, pp. 559–564.
3. Hagan AD, DeMaria AN, eds. Clinical applications of 2D echocardiography and cardiac doppler. Boston: Little, Brown & Co., 1989, pp. 19–63.
4. Mazurek B, Jehle D, Martin M. Emergency department echocardiography in the diagnosis and therapy of cardiac tamponade. J Emerg Med 1991;9:27–31.
5. Beggs CW, Helling TS, Hays LV. Early evaluation of cardiac injury by two-dimensional echocardiography in patients suffering blunt chest trauma. Ann Emerg Med 1987 May;16:542–545.
6. Plummer D, Brunette D, Asinger R. Emergency department echocardiography improves outcome in penetrating cardiac injury. Ann Emerg Med 1992 June;21:709–712.
7. Heller M, Jehle D. Ultrasound in emergency medicine. Philadelphia: WB Saunders,1995, pp. 126–134, 184–194.

Ultrasound Evaluation of Potential Ectopic Pregnancy

Verena T. Valley and James R. Mateer

Introduction

The frequency of ectopic pregnancy is increasing, with an incidence of up to 1 in 64 pregnancies (1). Although the highest rate of ectopic pregnancy is reported to be in women over 30 years of age (2), the clinical suspicion for this diagnosis must remain high, even in patients as young as 11 years of age (the average age of menarche). In 1990 an estimated 1 million pregnancies occurred with over 500,000 births to teenagers (3). During the period from 1970 to 1987, teenagers had the highest mortality rates for ectopic pregnancy. Of these, black teenagers and other minority races had a mortality rate for ectopic pregnancy almost 5 times higher than that for white teenagers (4).

By definition, an ectopic pregnancy occurs when a fertilized ovum implants at a site other than the endometrial lining of the uterus. A heterotopic pregnancy is the combination of an ectopic and an intrauterine pregnancy. This is believed to occur in only 1/30,000 pregnancies (5), but may have a higher incidence in patients taking fertility drugs or patients with extensive tubal disease.

Current clinical evaluation methods used in the ED result in an alarming rate of misdiagnosis regarding ectopic pregnancy. Studies have show that over 40% of cases may be initially missed (6, 7). Improved methods of early diagnosis for ectopic pregnancy are needed to reduce the morbidity and mortality associated with this condition.

Ultrasound has proven to be a rapid and effective diagnostic tool in evaluating ectopic pregnancy. The main value of ultrasound is to determine the presence and viability of an intrauterine pregnancy (IUP). By proving the presence of an IUP, diagnosis of an ectopic pregnancy is essentially excluded. The lack of an IUP on ultrasound, however, suggests the possibility of an ectopic pregnancy, especially if associated with an adnexal mass or significant free pelvic fluid.

Ultrasonography using a portable unit can usually be performed without difficulty in standard ED pelvic examination rooms. The number of examinations required for clinical competence has not been extensively studied. Recent reports in the primary care literature, however, suggest that a physician can be trained to perform a limited obstetrical ultrasound examination with a program that includes 40 to 75 training scans (8, 9).

Anatomy and Physiology

Normal Pelvic Anatomy

Ultrasonographic characteristics of the postpubertal adolescent female are not significantly different from those of an adult female (10). For transabdominal scanning, the full bladder is used to displace bowel gas and serve as an acoustic window to the pelvis. The normal shape of the distended bladder is rectangular on transverse views and is teardrop shaped on longitudinal views.

In the immediate premenarcheal period, the ovaries and the uterus enlarge rapidly and attain a mean volume by menarche which approaches adult size (11). The maximum uterine size for nulliparous adults is 7 cm in length and approximately 4×5 cm in anteroposterior and transverse dimensions. For multiparous patients, these dimensions are increased by 1 to 2 cm in all planes. With an empty bladder the normal anteverted uterus lies at about 90° to the plane of the vagina, whereas a fully distended bladder can position the uterus almost parallel to the vagina. The cervix is usually midline; however, the fundus is commonly tilted slightly to the right or left of midline. The endometrium is visualized within the uterus as a central bright echo called the endometrial stripe. The sonographic size and appearance of the endometrial stripe vary during the menstrual cycle, with a normal width of 2 to 4 mm in the proliferative phase and 5 to 6 mm in the secretory phase. In addition, the endometrial stripe becomes more echogenic during the secretory phase. When searching for an early IUP the entire endometrial stripe must be visualized.

Uterine anomalies including a bicornuate or a septate uterus are occasionally seen. These often are first noted in early pregnancy when the gestational sac forms in one horn of the uterus.

The normal size of the ovary is $2 \times 2 \times 3$ cm in young adults. Identification is facili-

tated when the characteristic multiple follicles (0.5 to 1.0 cm diameter) are visualized around the periphery of the ovarian cortex (Fig. 136.1). When follicle size exceeds 2.5 cm, a physiologic cyst or other abnormality should be considered. The position of the ovaries is variable, but they are most commonly located near the posterior lateral pelvic wall just anterior to the internal iliac vessels and medial to the external iliac vessels.

The vagina is a hypoechoic tubular structure caudad to the cervix and immediately posterior to the bladder on a transabdominal scan. This structure is recognized by a central echogenic stripe which is formed by the opposing mucosal interface. The posterior fornix is closely related to the posterior cul-de-sac. The cul-de-sac is located posterior to the uterus and upper vagina. A small amount of fluid in the cul-de-sac is normal during midcycle.

Ultrasound Findings of Intrauterine Pregnancy

Recognizing an IUP is critical. The embryologic features of a normal IUP include (in chronological order of ultrasound appearance) the gestational sac, the yolk sac, the double decidual sac sign, the fetal pole, and fetal cardiac activity (Table 136.1).

In obstetrics, gestational age is traditionally defined based on the menstrual age—the time from the beginning of the last normal menses. Ultrasound imaging also follows this convention for references to gestational age. Gestational age can be determined by ultra-

Figure 136.1.
Longitudinal view of the left ovary demonstrating the characteristic follicular pattern. The ovary normally lies medial to the external iliac vein.

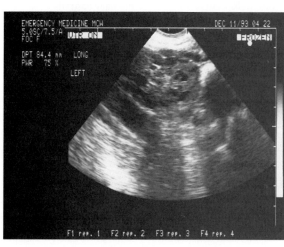
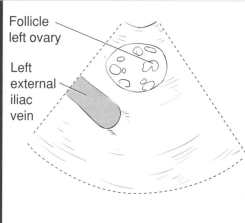

Follicle left ovary

Left external iliac vein

Table 136.1.
Ultrasonographic Gestational Markers
For Intrauterine Pregnancy

Structure	Transabdominal	Endovaginal
Gestational sac	5.5–6 wk	4.5–5 wk
Yolk sac (secondary)	6–6.5 wk	5–5.5 wk
Embryo (fetal pole)	7 wk	5.5–6 wk
Cardiac activity	7 wk	6 wk
Fetal parts	8+ wk	8 wk

sound as early as 5 weeks based on measurements of the internal diameter of the gestational sac. For more advanced early pregnancy (6 to 12 weeks' gestation), a crown-rump length can be determined by measuring the maximal length of the embryo excluding extremities and the yolk sac. The crown-rump length of the embryo during the first trimester is the most accurate measurement of gestational age that can be obtained by ultrasound during a pregnancy.

Gestational Sac

The gestational sac is the first developmental marker that can be imaged and has been reported to be 5 mm by the fifth gestational week (12). It can be seen at 4.5 to 5 weeks' gestation with endovaginal ultrasound and 5.5 to 6 weeks' gestation using the transabdominal approach. The ultrasonic appearance is that of a round, anechoic (echo-free or dark) sac measuring greater than 5 mm internal diameter surrounded by a thick concentric echogenic ring and located within the endometrial echo (Figs. 136.2 and 136.5).

Yolk Sac

The yolk sac has a characteristic appearance consisting of a bright, ringlike structure with an anechoic center. It is attached to the fetal umbilicus by a narrow stalk (Figs. 136.2 and 136.5). It is the first structure that can be accurately identified within the gestational sac. It also is the earliest reliable sign of an intrauterine pregnancy. Endovaginal ultrasound is the preferred method to evaluate an early or atypical intrauterine sac. The presence of a yolk sac is associated with a 62% incidence of a normal pregnancy (liveborn infant) (14). It can be seen at 5 to 5.5 weeks' gestation on endovaginal ultrasound and 6 to 6.5 weeks' gestation on transabdominal ultrasound. It usually is not seen after 12 weeks gestational age.

The presence of a yolk sac virtually eliminates the possibility that an intrauterine gestational sac represents a pseudogestational sac of ectopic pregnancy (13). A pseudogestational sac, or pseudo-sac of ectopic pregnancy, is a sac-like structure inside the uterus of a patient with an ectopic pregnancy. It is related to endometrial hormonal stimulation with edema fluid or blood accumulation. It can be differentiated from an early IUP by its lack of embryonic contents, absence of a double decidual sac, and lack of a definite thick, brightly echogenic decidual reaction.

Double Decidual Sac Sign

The double decidual sac sign consists of two concentric echogenic rings surrounding the gestational sac (Fig. 136.2). The inner ring represents the decidua capsularis, chorionic villi, and chorion surrounding an anechoic area. The outer ring represents the decidua

Figure 136.2.
Transverse view of the uterus demonstrating features of an early intrauterine pregnancy.

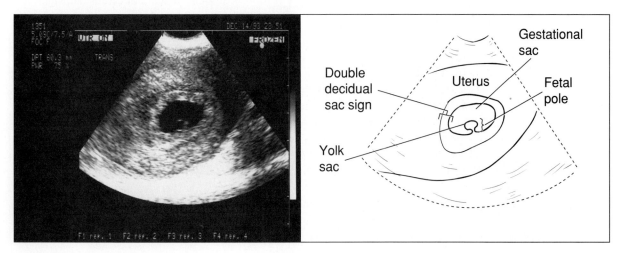

vera, or endometrium of the uterus. The ring between these layers is anechoic and is the remnant of the uterine cavity. Presence of the double decidual sac has been described as a sign of IUP; however, it is a less reliable sign for the diagnosis of a normally developing pregnancy (15). The presence of a double decidual sac sign is therefore suggestive of an IUP but is not by itself diagnostic.

Fetal Pole

The fetal or embryonic pole is recognized sonographically as a thickened area adjacent to the yolk sac and often can be seen when the embryo is 2 mm. It can be seen at 5.5 to 6 weeks' gestation on endovaginal ultrasound and 7 weeks' gestation on transabdominal ultrasound (Figs. 136.2 and 136.5).

Fetal Cardiac Activity

A fetal heart beat always should be present in a normally developing embryo at about 6.5 weeks' gestation and can generally be seen in a 2 or 3 mm fetus. Identification of cardiac activity is of particular importance as 97% of embryos with cardiac activity have a normal outcome (liveborn infant) (15–18). Cardiac activity is reliably seen at 6 to 6.5 weeks' gestation on endovaginal ultrasound and 7 weeks' gestation on transabdominal ultrasound but often can be identified as soon as an embryonic pole is visible.

Ultrasound Findings of Ectopic Pregnancy

Findings on an ultrasound examination that suggest an ectopic pregnancy include a definitive ectopic pregnancy and no definitive intrauterine pregnancy.

Definitive Ectopic Pregnancy

A definitive ectopic pregnancy is defined as the presence of a sac larger than 5 mm (maximum internal diameter) with a thick, concentric echogenic ring visualized outside the endometrial echo and containing a definite yolk sac or an obvious fetal pole (with or without fetal pulsations).

No Definitive Intrauterine Pregnancy

Diagnosis of an ectopic pregnancy must be

strongly considered when faced with a serum human chorionic gonadotropin (HCG) level above the discriminatory zone and no intrauterine pregnancy noted on the ultrasound examination. Serum HCG levels correlate with the size and gestational age of the embryo. The discriminatory zone of HCG (i.e., the level above which a normal intrauterine pregnancy is reliably visualized) was first described in 1981 (15). For transabdominal sonography this level has been most recently set at an HCG concentration of 3600 mIU/mL using the first international reference preparation (IRP) [equals 1800 mIU/mL via the second international standard (IS)] which correlates to a gestational age of approximately 6 weeks. With the advent of endovaginal sonography, the discriminatory zone of HCG is currently as low as 1025 mIU/mL IRP (approximately 500 mIU/mL second IS), consistent with 5 weeks' gestation. The absolute minimum value of HCG which identifies the discriminatory zone depends on the equipment used and the sonographer's technique. This value should ideally be established separately for each institution. The lack of an intrauterine pregnancy when the HCG is above the discriminatory zone, therefore, represents either an ectopic pregnancy or a recent abortion. This category accounts for the majority of ectopic cases diagnosed in an ED setting (19).

For patients with no IUP and an HCG below the discriminatory zone an early IUP is likely, but an early ectopic or a recent abortion with falling HCG levels cannot be excluded. For patients who lack an IUP, have no significant incidental findings, and have an HCG level below the discriminatory zone, the current standard of care is outpatient follow-up in 2 to 3 days for a repeat HCG level and ultrasound. Many patients in this category have an early IUP. This is confirmed by a 66% or greater increase in HCG level within 48 hours and identification of an IUP once the HCG is above the discriminatory zone.

Incidental Findings Suspicious for Ectopic Pregnancy

Certain ultrasound findings, although not the primary focus of a limited study in the ED, raise the index of suspicion for the presence of an ectopic pregnancy. Significant incidental findings on ultrasound include fluid in the cul-de-sac, adnexal masses, tubal rings, myomatous uterus, and an intrauterine device. Such findings require consultation with an obstetrician/gynecologist.

Fluid in the Cul-de-Sac
Moderate to large amounts of fluid which extend into the adnexa or the paracolic gutters suggest hemorrhage from a ruptured ectopic pregnancy or cyst.

Adnexal masses
Masses greater than 2.5 to 3.0 cm in diameter that are not simple cysts and are tender to palpation with the probe are suggestive of an ectopic pregnancy. Fetal heartbeats within masses have been observed in as many as 23% of cases (1). Additionally, these masses may contain amorphous material which is thought to represent blood, blood clots, and gestational material. This amorphic appearance was noted in 40% of tubal pregnancies (20).

Tubal Rings
Tubal rings are echogenic rings found outside the uterus which may indicate an early ectopic pregnancy. A tubal ring usually can be differentiated from a common corpus luteum cyst by its thick, round, brightly echogenic ring. A corpus luteum cyst is surrounded by less echogenic ovarian tissue which may contain characteristic follicles.

Myomatous Uterus
Fibroids can interfere with ultrasound examination due to acoustic shadowing. Findings in the ED may therefore be impossible to interpret.

Intrauterine Device
An intrauterine device (IUD) will cast a characteristic shadow on sonography and may interfere with imaging of the uterus.

INDICATIONS

Considerable overlap exists between the clinical presentation for an abortion versus an ectopic pregnancy. This is one reason why so many patients with ectopic pregnancy are initially misdiagnosed. It is therefore essential that the clinician first consider the possibility of ectopic pregnancy before a patient's condition is labeled as a spontaneous or threatened abortion. Bedside ultrasound can greatly facilitate differentiating these conditions in conjunction with other diagnostic tests and, as appropriate, close outpatient follow-up.

Indications for pelvic sonography include patients presenting with a positive urine pregnancy test and lower abdominal pain, an adnexal mass or tenderness, vaginal bleeding, orthostasis, or any other risk factors for ectopic pregnancy. A rule-out ectopic protocol integrating the use of bedside ultrasonography in the ED is currently being prospectively tested (Table 136.2) (19).

For the ED evaluation, the endovaginal approach is preferred over the transabdominal approach due to its higher image resolution in early pregnancy. In addition, the patient usually has an empty bladder, having recently submitted a urine sample for a pregnancy test. Advantages and disadvantages of each technique are listed in Table 136.3.

Endovaginal ultrasonography should not be performed if the diagnosis of vaginal bleeding due to a vaginal tear is suspected based on the history or physical examination. Physical examination should disclose the vaginal tear although bleeding may preclude it. An obstetrician-gynecologist should be consulted in this scenario.

EQUIPMENT

Ultrasound machine—a two-dimensional, real-time, black-and-white machine with hard copy (printer capabilities) is suggested.

Probes—a 3.5 to 5.0 MHz mechanical sector, annular array or curved array probe is necessary for transabdominal ultrasound. A 5.0 to 7.5 MHz mechanical sector, annular array or curved array endovaginal probe is necessary for endovaginal ultrasound.

Ultrasound gel

Disposable probe covers—required to avoid transmitting infection. Condoms are frequently used, although latex gloves also can be used to cover the endovaginal probe.

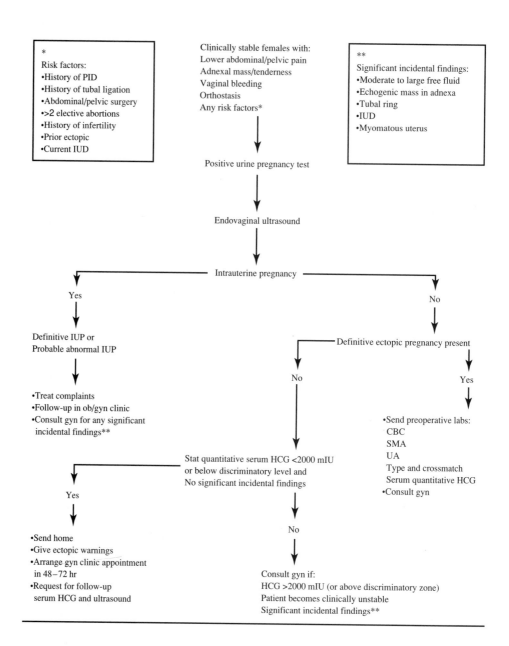

Table 136.2. Summary of Rule-Out Ectopic Protocol

*
Risk factors:
- History of PID
- History of tubal ligation
- Abdominal/pelvic surgery
- >2 elective abortions
- History of infertility
- Prior ectopic
- Current IUD

Clinically stable females with:
Lower abdominal/pelvic pain
Adnexal mass/tenderness
Vaginal bleeding
Orthostasis
Any risk factors*

**
Significant incidental findings:
- Moderate to large free fluid
- Echogenic mass in adnexa
- Tubal ring
- IUD
- Myomatous uterus

Positive urine pregnancy test

Endovaginal ultrasound

Intrauterine pregnancy

Yes

No

Definitive IUP or
Probable abnormal IUP

Definitive ectopic pregnancy present

No

Yes

- Treat complaints
- Follow-up in ob/gyn clinic
- Consult gyn for any significant
  incidental findings**

- Send preoperative labs:
  CBC
  SMA
  UA
  Type and crossmatch
  Serum quantitative HCG
- Consult gyn

Stat quantitative serum HCG <2000 mIU
or below discriminatory level and
No significant incidental findings

Yes

No

- Send home
- Give ectopic warnings
- Arrange gyn clinic appointment
  in 48–72 hr
- Request for follow-up
  serum HCG and ultrasound

Consult gyn if:
HCG >2000 mIU (or above discriminatory zone)
Patient becomes clinically unstable
Significant incidental findings**

Probe disinfectant—a number are available (21). Probe manufacturers provide information about safe and effective cleaning and disinfecting, as a particular disinfectant may be safe for some probes and destructive for others. Bleach wipes are acceptable for many probes.

Sterile gloves—necessary for the endovaginal examination.

Videotape recording capabilities—a highly recommended option for quality assurance and case review purposes.

PROCEDURE

The clinician should position the ultrasound machine next to the pelvic examination table such that the machine keyboard can be easily and comfortably accessed throughout the examination. Often the patient will want to see the screen; the machine can be easily adjusted in such a way to accommodate the patient's view.

The ultrasound equipment should be ready to go before the actual scanning. For

Table 136.3.
**Advantages and Disadvantages of
Transabdominal and Endovaginal Ultrasound**

Transabdominal	Endovaginal
Better overview	Better resolution
Less invasive	More comfortable than pelvic examination
Easier image orientation	Image orientation may be confusing
Requires full bladder	Best done with empty bladder

example, the patient's name (or medical record number) should be entered into the ultrasound machine and the videotape recorder should be on and ready to record. In addition, it is often helpful to label the initial screen as the longitudinal (or long) view as this is the first view in the scanning sequence. Placing the videotape recorder on both Record and Pause will allow the clinician to simply take the machine off of Pause to record the different anatomic views.

The clinician should avoid placing the patient in the Trendelenburg position, as any fluid present can help outline pelvic organs and tubes. Using a slightly reversed Trendelenburg position is recommended.

Transabdominal Imaging

A full bladder is necessary to displace bowel gas out of the pelvis and provide a homogenous sonographic window. It is possible for the bladder to be overfilled thus displacing

the uterus and ovaries beyond the focal zone of the probe. When this occurs, the patient should be asked to partially empty the bladder. If it is necessary to rapidly fill the bladder, this can be accomplished via retrograde introduction of sterile saline through a Foley catheter. Introduction of air bubbles should be avoided as this could interfere with imaging.

Imaging in transabdominal ultrasound is performed in the longitudinal (sagittal), transverse, and oblique planes. The image orientation in obstetrics and gynecology traditionally refers to the position of the probe with respect to the organ or structure of interest. Thus a true longitudinal view of the ovary or of a tilted uterus may be oblique to the long axis of the patient.

The ultrasound gel is applied to the patient's lower abdomen. A 3.5 to 5.0 MHz probe is placed in the midline immediately above the pubic symphysis. The orientation marker on the probe should be directed at the patient's head (Fig. 136.3.A). This position should provide a longitudinal view of the uterus directly below the anechoic bladder. The endometrial stripe is visualized using a side-to-side sweeping motion. In an anteverted uterus the cervix and cul-de-sac can be detected by angling the probe in a caudal direction.

From the midline longitudinal view, a slow sweeping motion laterally can be used to obtain longitudinal views of the ovaries (Fig. 136.3.B).

Figure 136.3.
A. Initial positioning of the transabdominal probe.
B. Transabdominal sweep of the right adnexa.

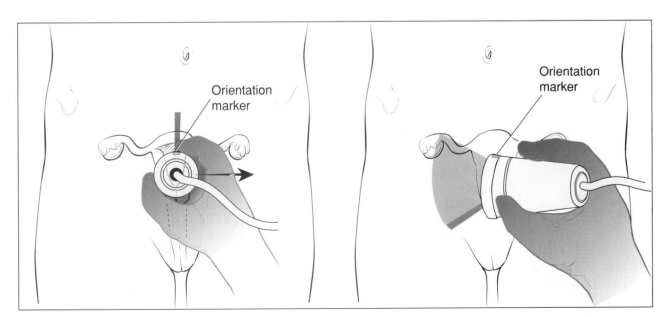

Orientation marker

Orientation marker

Beginning again from the midline longitudinal view, rotating the probe 90° counterclockwise will produce a transverse view of the uterus. The entire anteverted uterus from the fundus to the cervix can be viewed by angling the probe first cephalad and then caudad. A transverse view of the adnexa can be obtained by beginning with the transverse view of the uterus at the level of the fundus. The probe is angled laterally to aim at the adnexa. A slow sweep cephalad and then caudad will provide a view of the adnexa from top to bottom. The uterus and adnexa are carefully scanned for the presence of a gestational sac. The scan should be videotaped for further review.

Endovaginal Imaging

The patient should be given a short explanation of the procedure. Techniques that may facilitate the internal vaginal examination of an adolescent patient are described in Chapter 96. It is helpful to mention that the probe is smaller than most specula and is only inserted a short distance. Therefore, the endovaginal ultrasound examination may be more comfortable than the speculum examination. The option of having the patient place the tip of the probe into the vagina may make the patient less anxious.

Complete emptying of the urinary bladder is indicated to increase patient comfort with the procedure and to bring the uterus closer to the vaginal transducer.

The probe must be disinfected before each use with a commercially available preparation (Fig. 136.4.A). Ultrasound gel is applied to the tip of the probe. All air bubbles are removed as the probe is covered with a latex condom, probe cover, or a digit of a surgical latex glove (Figure 136.4.B). A small amount of gel applied to the outside of the probe cover facilitates insertion into the vagina. The examination is performed most easily with the patient on a pelvic examination table assuming a slightly reversed Trendelenburg position.

Standard imaging planes in an endovaginal scan are longitudinal and transverse to the uterus. The transverse plane is generally semicoronal to the body axis. Oblique planes are used as needed to visualize the adnexa. Pelvic structures can be guided toward the probe with the abdominal hand, and the probe

tip can be used to localize areas of tenderness detected by the bimanual pelvic examination.

The probe is held with the index finger on the probe orientation marker. The probe is slowly inserted approximately 3 to 4 inches into the vaginal vault with the orientation probe pointing up (Fig. 136.5.A). This orients the probe in the longitudinal position. The endometrial stripe is located on the ultrasound monitor and aligned by moving the probe either in the lateral or anterior-posterior planes to visualize its full extent. In a normally positioned or anteverted uterus, the fundus should appear on the left-hand side of the ultrasound monitor screen (Fig. 136.5.B). Often the uterus does not lie perfectly in the longitudinal plane and the probe must be rotated or angled until the endometrial stripe is seen. The endometrial stripe is then followed to the cervix. The entire endometrium is assessed for the presence of a gestational sac and contents (yolk sac, fetal pole, or fetal heart activity). The position of a gestational sac within the uterus is carefully noted with attention to the myometrial mantle.

Longitudinal sweeps of the adnexa are done from the midline position to either side (Fig. 136.6), which is accomplished by slowly angling the whole probe toward the lateral side wall of the pelvis while maintaining the orientation marker in the upright position. The longitudinal views of the adnexa are labeled left or right and videotaped for documentation and review.

The orientation marker and probe are then rotated 90° counterclockwise for the transverse views (Fig. 136.7). The endometrium again can be visualized from the fundus to the cervix. The probe is angled so that it is pointing toward the patient's anterior to view the fundus of the uterus, assuming an anteverted uterus. The probe is then gently angled posteriorly to visualize the body of the uterus and cervix. This maneuver ensures that the entire uterus is visualized. These views should be labeled transverse and videotaped for subsequent review.

The adnexa and posterior cul-de-sac are evaluated for the presence of significant incidental findings of fluid or masses. The adnexa are evaluated in the transverse plane by angling the probe toward the patient's right and left. As mentioned previously, ovaries often are found adjacent to the external iliac vein (Fig. 136.1). After locating the iliac

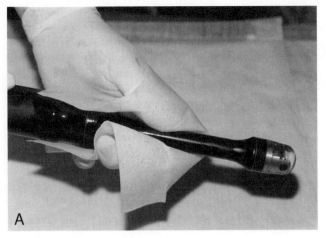

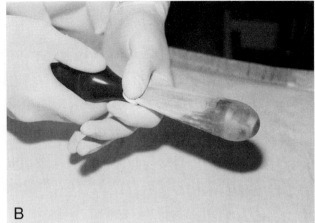

vein, the probe can be rotated or slightly angled anteriorly to image the ovary. The ovary has a characteristic follicular appearance which aids tremendously in its sonographic identification. Any masses should be assessed for tenderness with the probe tip.

The fallopian tubes may or may not be visualized. Normal tubes are difficult to image because of their small size. They are usu-

ally located lateral to the uterus behind the ovaries or in the cul-de-sac. The pathologic tube is more easily identified due to the accumulation of fluid, pus, or blood in the lumen or in the adjacent area.

The cul-de-sac should also be evaluated for the presence of fluid or blood clots. Using a high resolution probe may make a small amount of fluid in the cul-de-sac appear

Figure 136.4.
A. Disinfecting the endovaginal probe.
B. Application of the probe cover.

Figure 136.5.
Longitudinal view of the uterus and early intrauterine pregnancy with endovaginal ultrasound.
A. Endovaginal probe orientation and scanning field.
B. Ultrasound image.

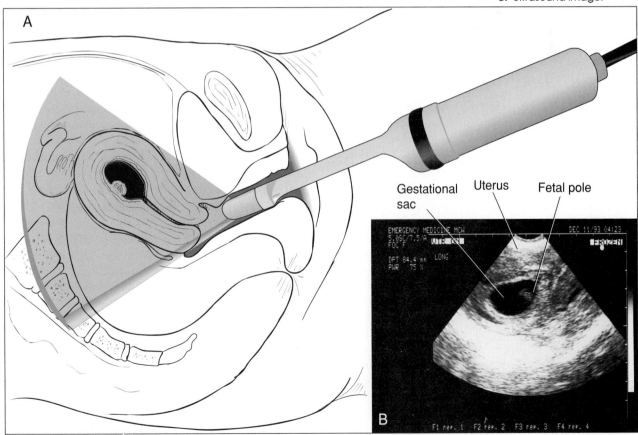

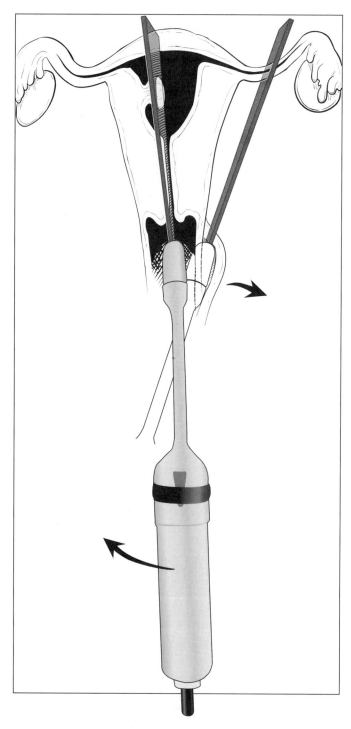

Magnification of the ultrasound images can help to identify structures and is a function found on the ultrasound keyboard. Zooming out (less image magnification) is often helpful when initially imaging the endometrial stripe and cervix or in determining the presence of fluid in the cul-de-sac. Zooming in (greater image magnification) provides better detail of intrauterine contents, especially fetal structures such as the fetal pole or yolk sac. The largest possible magnification that still enables orientation and recognition of the organs or pathology should be used.

PITFALLS

Many pitfalls are associated with ultrasound diagnosis of early pregnancy. For example, it is incorrect to assume that an HCG below the discriminatory zone excludes significant ultrasound findings. Many ectopics have been diagnosed with low HCG levels. The absolute level and rate of rise of HCG with an ectopic is variable and depends on the available vascular supply.

Fortunately a combined IUP and ectopic pregnancy, or heterotopic pregnancy, is rare (1/30,000); however, it is considered less rare in patients taking fertility drugs (up to 1/5000) and patients with tubal abnormalities. The significance is that the ultrasound examination is not completed when an IUP is identified. The clinician must routinely examine the adnexa and cul-de-sac for significant masses or fluid to exclude this possibility.

Interstitial pregnancies are a subset of ectopic pregnancies with implantation in the intrauterine portion of the fallopian tube or that portion of the tube which passes through the wall of the uterus. This subset is associated with a higher incidence of mortality due to the tendency to progress further before rupture and the increased likelihood of exsanguination due to this highly vascular and muscular site (23). This type of ectopic pregnancy is suspected when the gestational sac is not centrally located in the uterus. Diagnosis is confirmed by the lack of a complete, symmetric myometrial mantle around the entire gestational sac. In other words, with a normal intrauterine gestation, a uniform rim of solid tissue should represent the myometrial mantle around the gestational sac. Interstitial pregnancies

Figure 136.6.
Longitudinal sweep of the left adnexa with an endovaginal probe.

Chapter 136
Ultrasound Evaluation of Potential Ectopic Pregnancy

falsely large to the novice sonographer due to magnification. A small amount of free fluid is normally present especially in midcycle (22). Should the clinician find a large amount of fluid in the cul-de-sac, a transabdominal view of the pelvis may provide a more accurate estimation of fluid accumulation. Other intraperitoneal gutters where fluid may accumulate are also best investigated using the transabdominal approach.

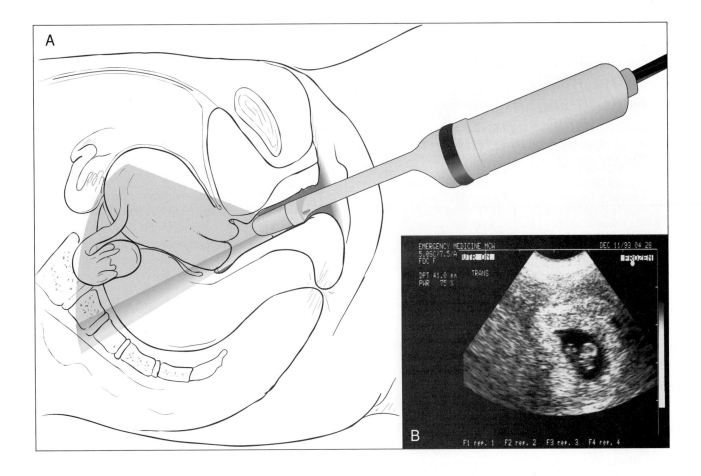

may appear intrauterine or extrauterine on the ultrasound study.

Advanced ectopics (8 or more weeks) have been misdiagnosed as an IUP when the gestational sac and contents appear normal. To avoid this pitfall it is important to routinely determine if the gestational sac lies within the endometrial echo with a complete myometrial mantle surrounding it.

Cervical ectopic pregnancy is rare, and it may be confused with the more common finding of an abortion in progress (with a low-lying gestational sac) or a large nabothian or cervical gland cyst. Endovaginal ultrasound and follow-up examinations are often needed to further evaluate this possible diagnosis.

Videotaping the ultrasound examination with careful image and orientation labeling may decrease the need for repeat ultrasound examinations. If the ultrasound is abnormal, the videotape can be reviewed with consultants and the need for a repeat ultrasound may be based on their recommendations.

Figure 136.7.
Transverse view of the uterus and early intrauterine pregnancy with endovaginal ultrasound.
A. Endovaginal probe orientation and scanning field.
B. Ultrasound image.

Chapter 136
Ultrasound Evaluation
of Potential Ectopic
Pregnancy

COMPLICATIONS

Currently no known risks to the patient or fetus are associated with the ultrasound energy used during the transabdominal or endovaginal ultrasound. Nevertheless, the power output of the machine should be maintained at the lowest possible level which produces a good image during ultrasound examination of the pregnant uterus.

SUMMARY

With the high rate of adolescent pregnancies, the possibility of ectopic pregnancy is a constant concern. The presence of an ectopic pregnancy is a difficult diagnosis to make based on the physical examination alone. Using bedside ultrasonography can enhance the emergency physician's diagnostic accuracy (19).

The recognition of an intrauterine pregnancy with careful examination of the adnexa can exclude the diagnosis of an ectopic pregnancy. The lack of an intrauterine pregnancy with an HCG above the discriminatory zone should be considered an ectopic pregnancy until proven otherwise. The possibility of an ectopic must be entertained before diagnosing a spontaneous or threatened abortion, as much overlap exists between these clinical presentations.

An understanding of the utility and limitations of ultrasonography with careful patient follow-up may ultimately decrease the morbidity and mortality associated with ectopic pregnancy.

REFERENCES

1. Mishell Jr. DR Ectopic pregnancy. In: Droegemuller W, Herbst AL, Mishell Jr DR, et al., eds. Comprehensive gynecology. St. Louis: CV Mosby, 1987, pp. 406–439.
2. Centers for Disease Control (CDC). Ectopic pregnancy—United States, 1987. MMWR 1990;39: 401–404.
3. NCHS. Advance report of final natality statistics, 1990. Hyattsville, Maryland: US Department of Health and Human Services, Public Health Service, CDC, 1993. (Monthly vital statistics report; vol 41, no. 9, suppl.)
4. CDC. Ectopic pregnancy surveillance—United States, 1970–1987. MMWR 1939 (SS-4):9–17.
5. DeVoe RW, Pratt JH. Simultaneous intrauterine and extrauterine pregnancy. Am J Obstet Gynecol 1948; 56:1119.
6. Stovall TG, Kellerman AL, Ling FW, Buster JE. Emergency department diagnosis of ectopic preg-

nancy. Ann Emerg Med 1990 October;19: 1098–1103.

7. Abbott J, Emmans LS, Lowenstein SR. Ectopic pregnancy: Ten common pitfalls in diagnosis. Am J Emerg Med 1990;8:515–522.

8. Hahn R, et al. Obstetric ultrasound training for family physicians: results from a multisite study. J Family Practice 1988;26(5):553–558.

9. Smith CB, Sakornbut EL, Dickinson LC, Bullock GL. Quantification of training in obstetrical ultrasound: a study of family practice residents. J Clin Ultrasound 1991;19:479–483.

10. Hayden CK, Swischuk LE. Pediatric ultrasonography. Baltimore: Williams & Wilkins, MD, 1987, p. 359.

11. Krantz KE, Atkinson JP. Gross anatomy. Ann NY Acad Sci 1967;142:551–575.

12. Bernaschek G, Rudelstorfer R, Csaicsich P. Vaginal sonography versus serum human chorionic gonadotropin in early detection of pregnancy. Am J Obstet Gynecol 1988;158:608.

13. Dodson MG. Transvaginal ultrasound. New York: Churchill Livingstone, 1991, pp. 173–175.

14. Nyberg DA, Mack LA, Harvey D, Wang K. Value of the yolk sac in evaluating early pregnancies. J Ultrasound Med 1988;7:129.

15. Kadar N, DeVore G, Romero R. Discriminatory hCG zone: its use in the sonographic evaluation for ectopic pregnancy. Obstet Gynecol 981; 58:156.

16. Stabile I, Campbell S, Brudzinskas JG. Ultrasonic assessment of complications during the first trimester of pregnancy. Lancet 1987; 2:1237.

17. Mantoni M. Ultrasound signs in threatened abortion and their prognostic significance. Obstet Gynecol 1985;65:471.

18. Cashner KA, Christopher CR, Dysert GA. Spontaneous fetal loss after demonstration of a live fetus in the first trimester. Obstet Gynecol 1987;70:827.

19. Mateer J, Aiman EJ, Brown M. Ultrasound evaluation of ectopic pregnancy by emergency physicians. Ann Emerg Med 1993 May;22:5, 921.

20. Rottem S, Thaler I, Levron J, Peretz BA, Itskovitz J, Brandes JM. Criteria for transvaginal sonographic diagnosis of ectopic pregnancy. J Clin Ultrasound 1990;18:274–279.

21. Odwin CS, Fleischer AC, Kepple DM, Chiang DT. Probe covers and disinfectants for transvaginal transducers. J Diagn Med Sonograph 1990; 6:130–135.

22. Davis FA, Gaines BB. Fluid in the female pelvis— cystic patterns. J Ultrasound Med 1986;5:75–80.

23. Telmus L, Pedowitz P. Intersitial pregnancy: a survey of 45 cases. Am J Obstet Gynecol 1953; 66: 1271.

ULTRASONOGRAPHIC FOREIGN BODY LOCALIZATION AND REMOVAL

Barbara J. Abrams

INTRODUCTION

Foreign body detection and removal are common problems in the pediatric ambulatory care setting. Although rarely life threatening, subcutaneous foreign bodies can be a source of frustration to patients, their parents, and physicians, as well as being associated with potentially significant complications (1–4). Furthermore, missed foreign bodies comprise the second most frequent basis for malpractice claims filed against emergency physicians (5).

Ultrasonography has been used effectively for detecting ocular foreign bodies; evaluating extremities by delineating muscle groups, tendons, and vascular structures; and preoperative localization of foreign bodies (6–13). It also has been used to localize and remove both radiopaque and nonradiopaque materials from extremities (1, 9, 13–15). Techniques for removing subcutaneous foreign bodies without the aid of ultrasound localization are discussed fully in Chapter 113.

Ultrasound offers the emergency physician a safe, painless means of (*a*) determining if a foreign body is present, particularly if nonradiopaque, (*b*) performing precise preoperative three-dimensional localization, and (*c*) maintaining visualization during foreign body removal (6, 8, 12, 15–17). It is particularly useful for confirming the presence of a foreign body in the pediatric population,

when the patient is often unable or unwilling to provide a thorough history. It also can be used to determine if the foreign body has been removed in its entirety, as wood, thorns and some cactus spines tend to fragment both with the initial skin puncture and during removal (4, 18).

Although it is not difficult to search for foreign bodies of the extremities with ultrasound, it does require patience, training, and the proper equipment. Definitive identification and removal of a foreign body with ultrasound requires practice. However, it has been demonstrated that physicians with no formal training background in ultrasonography can be highly effective in detecting foreign bodies in clinical simulations (16).

Due to the high initial start-up costs involved and the need to maintain proficiency, the technique is most useful in a high volume setting such as the emergency department.

ANATOMY AND PHYSIOLOGY

The response of the body to a foreign object depends, in part, on the type of material present in the wound. If the body is unable to expel the foreign material, macrophages will attempt to digest it. If these mechanisms fail, fibroblasts will form a collagen capsule around it, resulting in a granuloma. It is thought that subsequent capsular disruption

Chapter 137
Ultrasonographic
Foreign Body
Localization and
Removal

1383

secondary to trauma can result in delayed or recurrent inflammation (3, 19).

Over time, retained subcutaneous foreign bodies can have variable effects on the surrounding tissues. Foreign body type and location affect potential complications. Glass, metal, and plastics are relatively inert and may produce minimal sequelae in the body. Conversely, organic materials tend to cause a pronounced inflammatory response. In addition, foreign bodies can migrate and result in neuropraxia, delayed rupture of nerves and tendons, and vascular injury (20–23). They can also enter the circulation. Other complications are discussed in Chapter 113.

Basic Principles of Ultrasound

Whereas the visibility of objects on roentgenograms depends on their density compared with the surrounding tissues, ultrasonography detects differences in acoustic impedance between media. The density of a medium multiplied by the velocity of sound through that medium determines its acoustic impedance. The greater the difference in acoustic impedance between two media, the more sound waves are reflected back toward the transducer to produce an image. The difference in acoustic impedance at the air-tissue interface at the surface of the skin is so great that virtually 100% of the sound is reflected and no image is produced. Thus gel is used as a coupler to allow sound to enter into the tissues (3, 34, 37, 39).

Objects in the path of the beam either reflect, absorb, or transmit sound. The stronger the reflected sound (echoes) returning from an object, the brighter the image produced. When the beam of ultrasound is perpendicular to the foreign material, more sound is reflected back to the transducer and the dots comprising the image are brighter. Hence a better image or a better artifact is usually seen when the beam is perpendicular to the object. Furthermore, when the reflection of sound is strong secondary to large differences in acoustic impedance, some returning sound is repeatedly reflected between the transducer and the object, much like the repeating echo heard when a person shouts in a canyon. This recurring reflection of sound between the transducer and the object is a reverberation or comet tail artifact. Its appearance can be so striking that its presence can serve as a clear indication that a foreign body is present. This artifact, however, also can occur when air is present in the tissues as the air-tissue interface represents a significant difference in acoustic impedance (3, 8, 14, 34, 37, 38).

Small changes in beam orientation can have a great impact on the appearance of shadows, artifacts, or the imaging of the foreign object itself. For instance, tendons may appear echogenic if the beam is perpendicular, or hypoechoic if the beam is oblique to the tendon. The size, shape, orientation of the object in relationship to the surface of the skin, and whether the object is in the focal zone of the transducer also will affect its ultrasonographic visibility (4, 15, 26, 39, 40). Although vessels are visible with gray scale imaging, the addition of doppler makes their identification much easier (8, 10, 15, 30).

It cannot be overemphasized that the clinician needs to be familiar with the ultrasound equipment, the normal anatomy of the extremities, and the appearance of a variety of foreign bodies in longitudinal and transverse sections. The skin interface appears bright with the soft tissues represented as more hypoechoic. Practice on normal hands and feet will increase comfort with the appearance of tendons, vessels, muscles, and bones. Scanning should be performed both at rest and with active range of motion (8, 10, 12). Differences can be noted in the appearance of a tendon or object when the ultrasound beam is oblique versus perpendicular to the normal anatomy. Beef or chicken models may be used to observe the characteristic echo patterns produced by different materials. As mentioned previously, these patterns can alert the ultrasonographer that a foreign body is present and also may provide clues as to the composition of the object. For instance, metal and glass are often associated with reverberation artifacts and wood, pebbles, and sand can cause distal shadows .(4, 14–16, 26, 40) (Fig. 137.1). Organic materials can cause an intense inflammatory response which can highlight the echogenic object by creating a contrasting darker background around the object. These halos around objects also can represent abscesses and granulation tissue (1, 2, 4, 15). Further discussion of clinically important concepts in ultrasonography can be found in Chapter 133.

Chapter 137
Ultrasonographic
Foreign Body
Localization and
Removal

1384

INDICATIONS

In most cases, radiopaque materials are missed on initial examination because radiographs were never ordered (25). The history, such as injury involving a thin or breakable object, or physical examination consistent with retained foreign material, as well as the patient's subjective opinion that a foreign body is present, are the best means for determining if a diligent search including imaging studies is necessary. Clinical findings associated with retained objects include localized tenderness, sharp pain with palpation, pain associated with a mass, discoloration beneath the surface of the skin, a chronic draining sinus, a nonhealing wound, an abscess with sterile purulent cultures, or a persistent sterile monoarticular arthritis (2–4, 17, 22, 24).

A number of factors determine the need for foreign body removal. Foreign bodies that affect function or pose a risk of potential damage to underlying structures should be removed. In addition those causing, or likely to cause, toxic, inflammatory, or hypersensitivity reactions should be removed. A more complete discussion of indications to remove foreign bodies is provided in Chapter 113.

The modality most accessible to the emergency physician for foreign body detection is the plain radiograph. Although CT scanning, MRI, and xeroradiography are frequently mentioned in the literature as adjuncts to radiographs, these studies are generally not available on demand in many EDs.

Researchers in most large studies reported wood to be the most common foreign material found in the extremities, followed by either glass or metal (15, 25–27). Glass visualization on plain films depends on size and proximity to bone. Most glass fragments, regardless of lead content and pigmentation, and virtually all metal objects, can be visualized with plain radiographs (25, 28, 29). Wood, however, is only visualized from 5.5 to 15% of the time (2, 25, 30). Sometimes

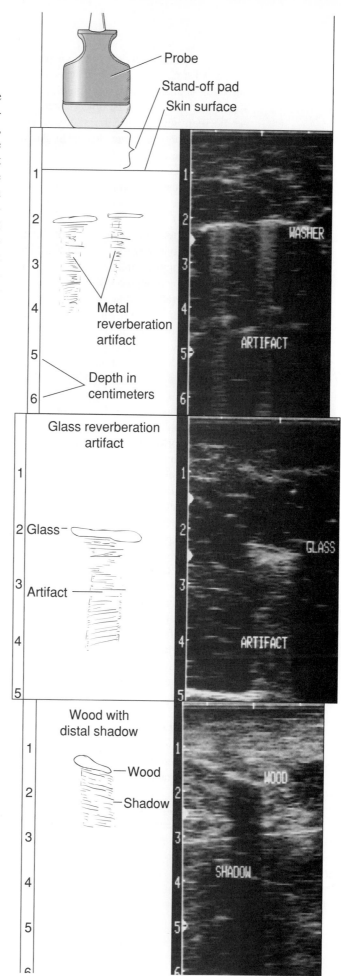

Figure 137.1.
Ultrasound images of various embedded materials.
A. Metal washer.
B. Glass.
C. Wood

secondary changes caused by foreign bodies, such as a filling defect, bony changes, or the introduction of air into the soft tissues, can be appreciated even when the object itself cannot be seen with plain films (22, 25, 31). Ultrasonography, however, has been shown to detect numerous nonradiopaque materials, including vegetable matter, sea urchin spines, thorns (rose, cactus, palm, blackthorns), sutures, fish bones, gauze, and plastic (1, 13, 14, 30, 32, 33, 35).

The effectiveness of plain films in the localization of foreign bodies is limited primarily by overlying bone and the size and density of a radiopaque foreign body. In addition, although radiographs outline the shape of a foreign body, they are not particularly useful for three-dimensional localization or visualization of nearby neurovascular structures and tendons (3, 4, 8, 12). By underpenetrating the film or using a soft-tissue technique, the resulting contrast between the foreign body and its surroundings can be enhanced and allow for better visualization. Plain radiographs are poor for demonstrating organic matter, especially if time has elapsed allowing for saturation of the object (4, 12, 17, 22, 25, 31).

Xeroradiography and fluoroscopy, although enhancing the likelihood of detection, are most effective for imaging radiopaque objects and expose the patient to higher doses of radiation.

CT can often detect foreign bodies not seen with other modalities; however, because of its cost and radiation dose, it is not recommended as a screening tool for foreign bodies. As with plain films and xeroradiography, small foreign bodies and saturated wood can be missed. MRI cannot be used for metallic objects or if a metal implant is nearby. Gravel also produces significant artifacts secondary to ferromagnetic particles and thus MRI is not recommended for wounds containing gravel. Both CT and MRI are expensive, require specialized personnel for their operation, and are generally impractical for foreign body detection in the ED. Furthermore, children may require sedation for these modalities. CT and MRI are therefore recommended only when other modalities fail (3, 4, 16, 30, 36).

Ultrasonography offers numerous advantages over other imaging techniques. It often can visualize radiopaque and organic foreign bodies with the use of portable equipment in the ED. It does not expose the patient to radiation and offers information for both three-dimensional localization of the object and its relationship to surrounding structures. Ultimately, this decreases operating time and incision size and allows the emergency physician to choose an optimal site for the incision.

EQUIPMENT

Ultrasound machine

Ultrasound transducer or probe—Image resolution in both the axial and lateral planes depends on the probe used. The higher the frequency of the probe (7.5 to 10 MHz), the better both the axial and lateral resolution and hence, the clearer the image produced. As frequency increases, however, the imaging depth decreases. This is not usually a problem, because the foreign bodies emergency physicians are generally interested in removing are relatively superficial. Smaller transducer heads are better for hard to image areas such as web spaces. Probe heads vary in size from a fingertip version to those measuring approximately 6 cm × 1.5 cm (see Fig. 133.2). The clinician must balance the asset of a smaller probe, which can be used in tight spaces, with a larger probe, which can provide a more adequate field of view.

Stand-off pad or gel pad—Not all probes are capable of imaging the first few millimeters beneath the surface of the skin, in which case a stand-off pad or bag of saline is useful. The stand-off or gel pad (Fig. 137.2) permits sound transmission and can be cut with a scalpel to the size and thickness necessary to allow the near zone on the monitor to include these first few millimeters beneath the skin's surface. They also are useful when scanning irregular surfaces or near bony prominences (41).

Ultrasound transmission gel

Standard equipment in removing a subcutaneous foreign body (Chapter 113)

Optional equipment:
  Printer or videotape connection—useful in documenting findings.
  Doppler capabilities—useful when working in highly vascular areas.

Chapter 137
Ultrasonographic
Foreign Body
Localization and
Removal

1386

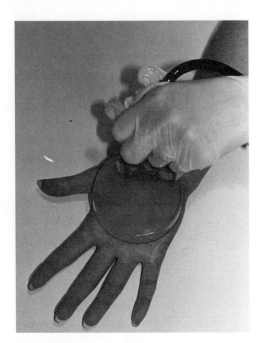

Figure 137.2.
Use of a stand-off or gel pad to scan for a shallow foreign body.

PROCEDURE

Identification

Ultrasound scanning for a foreign body generally does not require initial administration of anesthesia. A small amount of ultrasound transmission gel is applied to the skin surface above the location most likely to contain the foreign material. When scanning over broken skin or near secretions, the clinician can place a small amount of gel into the fingertip of a sterile glove or condom and place the transducer inside. The glove is smoothed against the transducer head to eliminate any air bubbles. Slow and methodical scanning is recommended, especially when the object is thought to be small. The search should be performed in a number of planes, as it is easy to miss an object such as a needle or toothpick when viewed only in transverse section (Fig. 137.3). A reasonable time limit should be set for detecting the object. Plain films should be obtained if a possibility exists that the object might be radiopaque. Plain radiographs often provide a larger field of view than can be easily scanned with ultrasound; they can therefore be used as a guide to focus the search. Plain films and ultrasound are

obviously not mutually exclusive and should be used together to detect objects that might be missed when using either modality alone (15–18). Foreign materials may appear as distinct objects or as one of numerous artifacts or shadows as previously described (see Anatomy and Physiology).

Localization

The image should correspond to the image expected in both longitudinal and transverse views. As shown in Figure 137.3, a typical sewing needle would appear to be approximately 3 to 5 cm in length with a comet tail artifact when viewed in longitudinal section. In transverse section, it would appear pinpoint with the same distal artifact. These artifacts may not be well visualized if the orientation of the beam is oblique to the object. Foreign bodies also may be more elusive when not perpendicular to the surface of the skin (4, 15).

Once the foreign object is located in at least two planes, the skin can be marked in a variety of ways. Using a marker, pen, or sterile tape, the skin is marked over the ends of an object, noting the depth listed on the ultrasound screen to the object at each point and the presence of any intervening structures. Alternatively, the skin over a foreign body is anesthetized and a localization needle is guided ultrasonographically to the object. When the needle contacts the foreign material, resistance or a grating sensation is frequently noted (6, 15, 17, 42). The skin surface may be marked using radiographic markers called Beekley spots, which are small metallic beads on an adhesive disc that can be easily repositioned (Fig. 137.4) (15).

Removal

Once the precise depth and orientation of the object are known, this information can be used to plan the site for incision. For instance, it may be advantageous to remove a foreign body from the lateral aspect of the heel, if feasible, as opposed to the weight-bearing plantar surface. Again, a time limit should be set for the procedure itself. An acceptable time limit is 15 to 30 minutes, considering that it is often necessary to maintain a bloodless field

Chapter 137
Ultrasonographic
Foreign Body
Localization and
Removal

1387

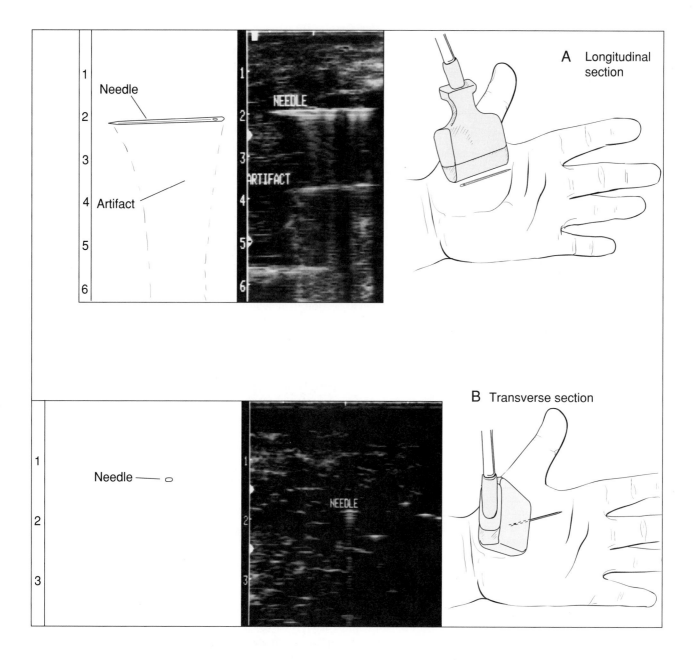

A Longitudinal section

B Transverse section

Figure 137.3.
Probe orientation and appearance of an embedded needle in different scanning planes.

**Chapter 137
Ultrasonographic
Foreign Body
Localization and
Removal**

(15, 17, 18). Prolonged attempts at removal in the ED are impractical and usually unsuccessful.

Anesthesia is applied to the area requiring manipulation (Chapter 37). By making a perpendicular incision adjacent to the end of a long thin object, the transducer can be held in the nondominant hand with the image of the object in a longitudinal projection (Fig. 137.5). Forceps or hemostats can then be observed while being guided to the proximal end of the foreign body through the incision. Traction applied along the longitudinal axis of the object will decrease the incidence of fragmentation. It is best to visualize both the

foreign body and the hemostat in the longitudinal plane (4, 15). Structures such as tendons can be evaluated by putting the extremity through a range of motion while visualizing the structure on the monitor.

The decision to remove a foreign body and the approach chosen must be based on the specifics of each situation. If removing material that is likely to break upon its removal, the ultrasound and/or the plain films should be repeated to ensure that it has been completely removed. After removal, standard wound care is administered (Chapter 110). If no remaining material is detected, patients should be advised to return to the ED if pain

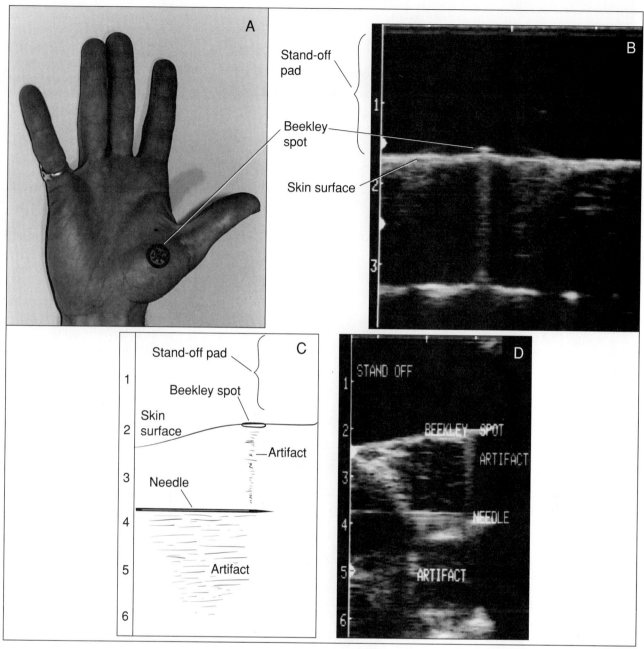

Figure 137.4.
Use of Beekley spots in localizing subcutaneous foreign bodies.

persists or infection develops, because a foreign body may still be present in the wound (3, 4, 17, 43).

COMPLICATIONS

The most frequently encountered problems with this procedure are generally the same for removal of any foreign body (Chapter 113). The addition of ultrasound to this common procedure poses no known additional biologic hazards at the intensities used for diagnostic purposes (34).

A few pitfalls, however, are associated with using ultrasound. Not all foreign bodies will be seen with ultrasound. It is important to take the time to perform a slow and careful examination. If one foreign body is detected, the possibility that a second or third foreign body may be present must be considered. A

Chapter 137
Ultrasonographic
Foreign Body
Localization and
Removal

1389

Identification

1. Apply ultrasound gel, transducer, and/or stand-off pad to area overlying most likely site of foreign body
2. Scan slowly and methodically
3. Scan area in a number of planes

Localization

1. Confirm object's size and shape by viewing in several planes
2. Evaluate depth of object at several points along its length
3. Mark skin surface at sites overlying object
4. Identify surrounding or overlying anatomic structures
5. Utilize adjuncts such as Beekley spots or a localization needle to further demarcate object

Removal

1. Determine optimal incision site based on previous information
2. Anesthetize area to be manipulated
3. Set reasonable time limit for attempted removal
4. Hold transducer in nondominant hand and scan object in longitudinal section
5. Direct hemostat or retrieval equipment to proximal end of object under ultrasound guidance
6. Repeat ultrasound scan to ensure complete removal of object
7. Administer standard wound care (Chapter 110)

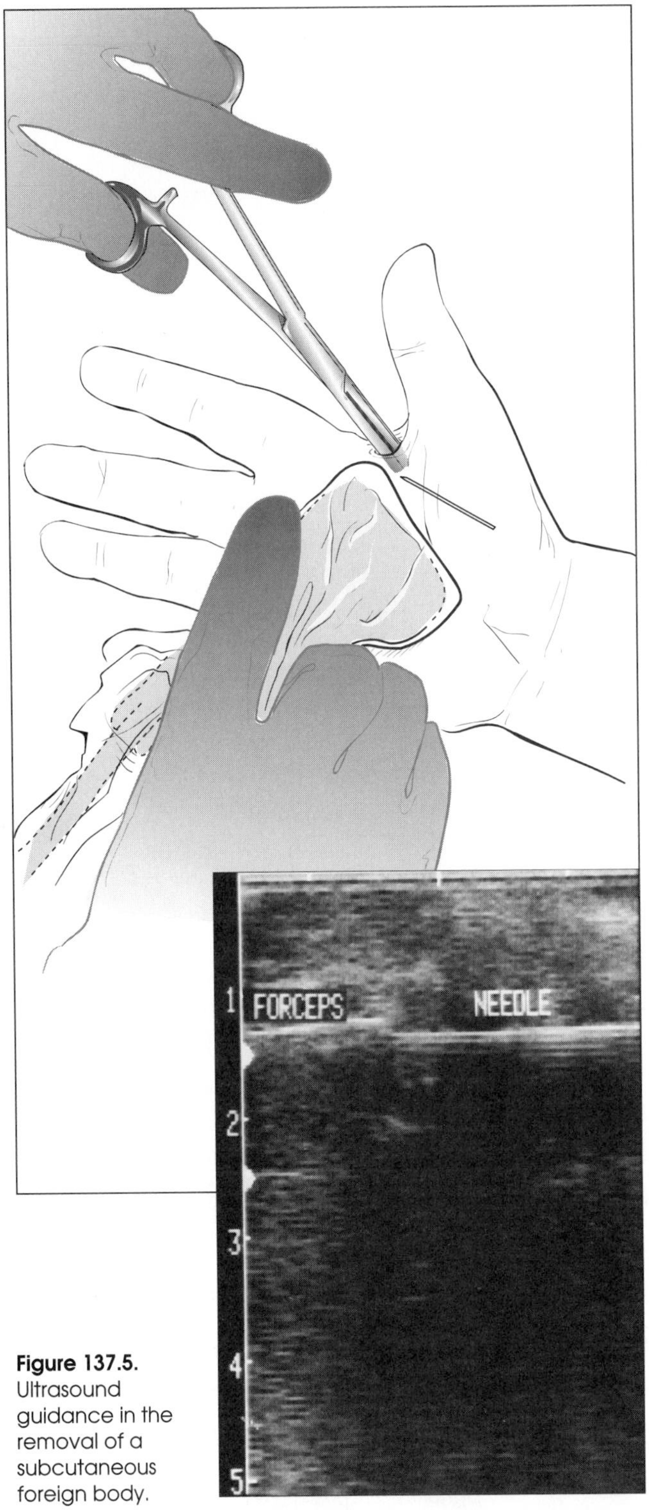

Figure 137.5. Ultrasound guidance in the removal of a subcutaneous foreign body.

result in time spent removing what appeared to be a foreign body but was not. This carries with it the possible surgical complications associated with removing any foreign object. False positives mentioned in the literature include fresh hematomas, calcifications, scars, cysts, keratin plugs, and atypical sesmoid or other small bones. Partially ossified cartilage in children can be mistaken for foreign bodies (1, 2, 4, 7, 8, 12, 15, 26, 30).

These errors can be minimized by careful scanning in multiple planes. The entire length of an echogenic structure should be scanned to ensure that it does not represent the head of a metacarpal bone. Similar structures in the same area or findings on plain films may suggest that ossified cartilage is being imaged. By using needle localization, the tissue can be incised to the suspicious site to visualize hematoma, scar tissue, or calcifications in soft tissue. With localization using a finder needle, bone hardness is useful in correctly identifying sesmoid and metacarpal bones. If it is not clear that a particular image represents a foreign body, comparative scanning of the opposite extremity can also be helpful (7, 15).

An oblique beam can change the appearance of a structure. Tendons may be mistaken for foreign bodies when scanned at a perpendicular angle. The same tendon may appear relatively hypoechoic and be mistaken for an area of inflammation when the beam is oblique to the tendon.

Air can be introduced into the tissue at the time of injury or surgical exploration. This can cause reverberation artifacts that

foreign body with a large shadow or artifact may obscure a more distal, smaller object. Objects also may be obscured by tendon, bone, or granulation tissue (3, 4, 40).

Another potential problem concerns misidentification of an image, which could

Chapter 137
Ultrasonographic
Foreign Body
Localization and
Removal

1390

may be incorrectly assumed to have been created by the presence of a foreign body; it can also make the ultrasound examination impossible. A wound recheck in 48 hours would allow time for air absorption, and a repeat ultrasound examination could be performed at that time. (1–4, 14, 26).

Using ultrasound may in fact reduce the complication rate. Because surrounding structures are visualized, complications associated with blind surgical exploration can be avoided. Furthermore, no ionizing radiation is used (2, 6, 8–12, 15, 30).

SUMMARY

As the natural curiosity of children often prompts exploration of their environment, pediatric patients commonly present with possible subcutaneous foreign body. Ultrasonography offers an advantage over plain films for the management of such cases, as it can visualize a number of nonradiopaque materials. In addition, because ultrasonography does not involve radiation, it often appeals to parents. Whereas the use of both plain radiographs and fluoroscopy often ends up necessitating blind surgical exploration, ultrasonography offers precise three-dimensional localization of the object and neighboring structures. This allows the physician to plan for an optimal incisional site and to remove the object under direct visualization. Considering that retained foreign materials may be associated with significant morbidity and liability, ultrasound can represent a valuable tool by providing the emergency physician with a simple, safe, noninvasive method of localizing and retrieving foreign objects.

REFERENCES

1. Banerjee B, Das RK. Sonographic detection of foreign bodies of the extremities. Br J Rad 1991;64:107–112.
2. Kobs JK, Hansen AR, Keefe B. A retained foreign body in the foot detected by ultrasonography. J Bone Joint Surg 1992;71:296–298.
3. Lammers RL. Soft tissue foreign bodies. Ann Emerg Med 1988;17:1336–1347.
4. Lammers RL, Magill T. Detection and management of foreign bodies in soft tissue. In: Chisholm CD, Howell JM, eds. Emerg Med Clini North Am. Philadelphia: WB Saunders, 1992:767–781.
5. Dunn JD. Risk management in emergency medicine. In: Emerg Med Clin North Am. Philadelphia: WB Saunders, 1987:51–69.
6. Coombs CJ, Mutimer KL, Slattery PG, Wise AG. Hide and seek preoperative ultrasonic localization of nonradiopaque foreign bodies. Aust NZ J Surg 1990;60:989–991.
7. Fornage BD, Rifkin MD, Touche DH, Segal PM. Sonography of the patellar tendon: preliminary observations. AJR 1984;143:179–182.
8. Fornage BD, Schernberg FL. Sonographic diagnosis of foreign bodies of the distal extremities. AJR 1986;147:567–569.
9. Fornage BD, Schernberg FL. Sonographic preoperative localization of a foreign body in the hand. J Ultrasound Med 1987;6:217–219.
10. Fornage BD, Schernberg FL, Rifkin MD. Ultrasound examination of the hand. Radiology 1985;155:785–788.
11. Fornage BD, Touche DH, Segal P, Rifkin MD. Ultrasonography in the evaluation of muscular trauma. J Ultrasound Med 1983;2:549–554.
12. Gooding GAW, Hardiman T, Sumers M, Stess R, Graf P, Grunfeld C. Sonography of the hand and foot in foreign body detection. J Ultrasound Med 1987;6:441–447.
13. Gordon D. Nonmetallic foreign bodies (letter). Br J Radiol 1985;58:574.
14. DeFlaviis L, Scaglione P, Del Bo P, Nessi R. Detection of foreign bodies in soft tissues: experimental comparison of ultrasonography and xeroradiography. J Trauma 1988;28:400–404.
15. Shiels WE, Babcock DS, Wilson JL, Burch RA. Localization and guided removal of soft tissue foreign bodies with sonography. AJR 1990;155:1277–1281.
16. Schlager D, Sanders AB, Wiggins D, Boren W. Ultrasound for the detection foreign bodies. Ann Emerg Med 1991;20:189–191.
17. Barnett RC. Soft tissue foreign body removal. In: Roberts JR, Hedges JR, eds. Clinical procedures in emergency medicine. Philadelphia: WB Saunders, 1991, pp. 581–591.
18. Lindsey D, Lindsey WE. Cactus spine injuries. Am J Emerg Med1988;6:362–369.
19. Peacock EE. Wound repair. 3rd ed. Philadelphia: WB Saunders, 1984, pp. 1–14.
20. Rachman R. Soft tissue injury by mercury from a broken thermometer. Am J Clin Path 1974;61:296–300.
21. Yu JC. Migration of broken sewing needle from left arm to heart. Chest 1975;67:626–627.
22. Cracchiolo A. Wooden foreign bodies in the foot. Am J Surg 1980;140:585–587.
23. Kleinman MB, Elfenbein DS, Wolf EL, Hemphill M, Kurlinski JP. Periosteal reaction due to foreign body-induced inflammation of soft tissue. Pediatrics 1977;60:638–641.
24. Swischuk LE, Jorgenson F, Jorgenson A, Capen D. Wooden splinter induced "pseudotumors" and "osteomyelitis-like lesions" of bone and soft tissue. AJR 1974;122:176–179.
25. Anderson MA, Newmeyer WL, Kilgore ES. Diagnosis and treatment of retained foreign bodies in the hand. Am J Surg 1982;144:63–65.
26. Gilbert FJ, Campbell RSD, Bayliss AP. The role of ultrasound in the detection of nonradiopaque foreign bodies. Clin Radiology 1990; 41:109–112.

CLINICAL TIPS

1. Scanning should always be performed in several planes.
2. Anatomic structures such as tendons can be detected with real-time scanning during motion of the extremity.
3. Practice in detecting foreign bodies can be obtained by scanning pieces of meat with imbedded objects.
4. Normal anatomic variants may be identified through comparative scanning of the uninvolved extremity.
5. Radiographs often provide a useful adjunct when scanning radiopaque objects.

Chapter 137
Ultrasonographic
Foreign Body
Localization and
Removal

1391

27. Morgan WJ, Leopold T, Evans R. Foreign bodies in the hand. J Hand Surg 1984;9-B:194–196.

28. Courter BJ. Radiographic screening for glass foreign bodies-what does a "negative" foreign body series really mean? Ann Emerg Med 1990;19: 997–1000.

29. Tandberg D. Glass in the hand and foot—will an x-ray film show it? JAMA 1982;248:1872–1874.

30. Crawford R, Matheson AB. Clinical value of ultrasonography in the detection and removal of radiolucent foreign bodies. Injury 1989;20:341–343.

31. Mucci B, Stenhouse G. Soft tissue radiography for wooden foreign bodies—a worthwhile exercise? Injury 1985;16:402–404.

32. Chau WK, Wu SSM, Wang JY. Ultrasonic detection of an intraabdominal foreign body. J Clin US 1985; 13:130–131.

33. Ginsburg MJ, Ellis GL, Flom LL. Detection of soft-tissue foreign bodies by plain radiography, xeroradiography, computed tomography, and ultrasonography. Ann of Emerg Med 1990;19:701–703.

34. Kremkau FW. Diagnostic ultrasound: principles, instruments and exercises. 3rd ed. Philadelphia: WB Saunders, 1989, pp. 10–56, and 226–230.

35. de Lacey G, Evans R, Sandin B. Penetrating injuries: how easy is it to see glass (and plastic) on radiographs? Br J Radiol 1985;58:27–30.

36. Russell RC, Williamson DA, Sullivan JW, Suchy H, Suliman O. Detection of foreign bodies in the hand. J Hand Surg 1991;16A:2–11.

37. Pinkney N. A review of the concepts of ultrasound—physics and instrumentation. 4th ed. Sonicor, Inc,. 1990, pp. 1–14.

38. Ziskin MC, Thickman DI, Goldenberg NJ, Lapayowkker MS, Becker JM. The comet tail artifact. J Ultrasound Med 1982;1:1–7.

39. Slasky BS, Lenkey JL, Skolnick ML, Campbell WL, Cover KL. Sonography of soft tissues of extremities and trunk. Seminars in Ultrasound 1982;3:288–330.

40. Suramo I, Pamilo M. Ultrasound examination of foreign bodies. Acta Radiol Diag 1986;27:463–466.

41. Nault P. Applying ultrasound to irregular surfaces. PT Mag 1993;94.

42. Bernardino ME, Jing BS, Thomas JL, Lindell MM, Zornoza J. The extremity soft-tissue lesion: a comparative study of ultrasound, computed tomography, and xeroradiography. Diag Radiol 1981;139:53–59.

43. Smoot EC, Robson MC. Acute management of foreign body injuries to the hand. Ann Emerg Med 1983;12:434–437.

44. Abrams BJ. Additional applications of ultrasonography. In: Diagnostic ultrasound for emergency medicine (handout), 1993;1–2.

45. Ellis GL. Are aluminum foreign bodies detectable radiographically? Am J Emerg Med 1993;11:12–13.

46. Green BF, Kraft SP, Carter KD, Buncic JR, Nerad JA, Armstrong D. Intraorbital wood: detection by magnetic resonance imaging. Ophthalmology 1990; 97:608–611.

47. Hansson G, Beebe AC, Carroll NC, Donaldson JS. A piece of wood in the hand diagnosed by ultrasonography. Acta Orthop Scand 1988;59:459–460.

48. Little CM, Parker MG, Callowich MC, Sartori JC. The ultrasonographic detection of soft tissue foreign bodies. Investigative Radiol 1986;21:275–277.

49. London PS. Wounds of deep significance: unsuspected foreign bodies in wounds (annotation). Injury 1972;3:179.

50. Matricardi L, Lovati R. Intestinal perforation by a foreign body: diagnostic usefulness of ultrasonography. J Clin Ultrasound 1992;20:194–196.

51. Pons PT. Foreign bodies. In: Rosen P, Baker FJ, Barkin RM, Braen GR, Dailey RH, Levy RC, eds. Emergency medicine: concepts and clinical practice. Washington, DC: CV Mosby, 1988, pp. 945–964.

52. Sanders RC. Clinical sonography: a practical guide. Boston: Little, Brown and Co., 1984, pp. 1–18.

53. Serrin DA, Eberhardt H, Hirsch JH. Ultrasonic localization of a wooden splinter in the foot. Med Ultrasound 1982;6:83–84.

54. Woesner ME, Sanders I. Xeroradiography: a significant modality in the detection of nonmetallic foreign bodies in soft tissues. AJR 1972;115:636–640.

55. Yeh HC, Rabinowitz JG. Ultrasonography of the extremities and pelvic girdle and correlation with computed tomography. Radiology 1982;143: 519–525.

Chapter 137
Ultrasonographic
Foreign Body
Localization and
Removal

1392

Ultrasound-Assisted Central Line Placement

Peter J. Alderson

Introduction

When indicated in the pediatric patient, access to the central circulation can be achieved from the internal and external jugular, subclavian, basilic, umbilical, and femoral veins. The site selected depends on the experience of the clinician and the indication for the catheter (1). As described in Chapter 18, attempting to cannulate the subclavian vein is fraught with potential problems in children. Furthermore, placement via the internal jugular vein may prove difficult to accomplish and is also associated with significant complications. Recent work suggests that the use of two-dimensional ultrasound scanning facilitates internal jugular vein cannulation and reduces the complication rate (2, 3). The technique may be equally applicable to femoral line placement.

Ultrasound-assisted central line placement should be regarded as a minor surgical procedure to be performed by an experienced physician. It should be done in an appropriate hospital setting such as the emergency department (ED), operating room, cardiac catheterization laboratory, or intensive care unit. The technique is quickly learned and has been shown to reduce both the time and number of needle insertions required to locate the internal jugular vein in children under 2 years of age (3). It is less useful in neonates and infants in whom the size of the ultrasound probe in comparison with the size of the patient tends to limit access.

Anatomy and Physiology

Although the internal jugular vein is typically described as running anterolaterally to the carotid artery, its location is subject to considerable variability. Ultrasound studies have demonstrated that in approximately 6% of patients the internal jugular vein may be thrombosed, absent, or unexpectedly small on one side (4, 5). The vein also may be located more laterally in the neck than expected, whereas in 10% of children it runs directly anterior to the carotid artery (3).

In children ranging in age from 3 days to 5.5 years the internal jugular vein at the level of the cricoid ring was reported to lie 4 to 10 mm below the surface of the skin and to vary in diameter from 2.5 to 12 mm. Vein depth and diameter tend to increase with age and weight (3).

Ultrasound scanning also has demonstrated that the cross-sectional area of the internal jugular vein is increased by placing the patient in Trendelenburg or by techniques such as the Valsalva maneuver which increase intrathoracic pressure (Fig. 138.1) (5). It would seem sensible to use this knowledge when possible during central line placement as it has been shown that palpation of the carotid artery or advancement of the venipuncture needle can obliterate the lumen of the internal jugular vein.

Comparable data concerning the subclavian vein are not currently available. In addition, the limited published information re-

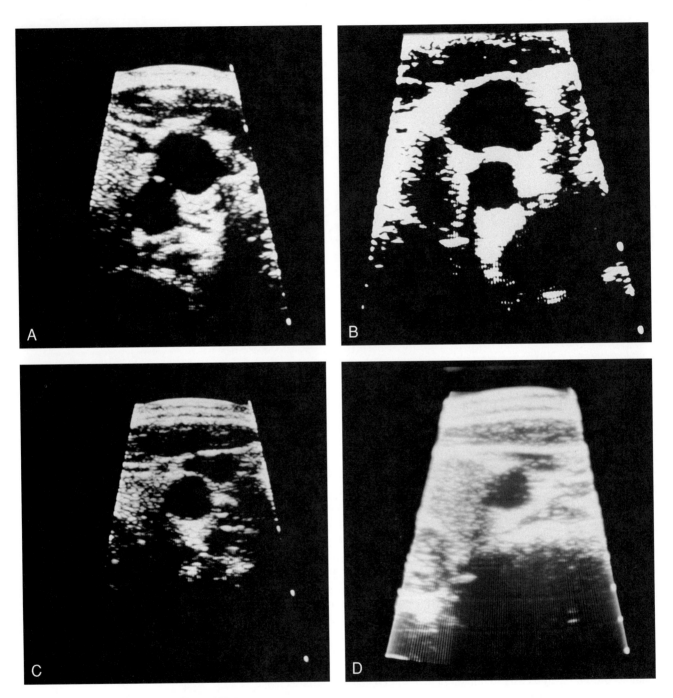

Figure 138.1.
Ultrasound appearance of neck vasculature.
A. Normal anatomy.
B. Increased internal jugular vein size with Valsalva maneuver.
C & D. Decreased internal jugular vein size with skin compression by transducer (C, gentle compression; D, more compression). (Reproduced with permission from Site~Rite® II, Dymax Corporation, Pittsburgh, PA.)

Chapter 138
Ultrasound-Assisted
Central Line
Placement

garding the femoral vein shows that it tends to be of smaller diameter (roughly 70%) in a given individual than the internal jugular vein but can be distended by approximately 20% with 15° head-up tilt (6). Considering the importance of femoral vein cannulation during pediatric resuscitation, further study of the use of ultrasound to facilitate this procedure is needed.

INDICATIONS

Central line placement can be complicated by the unfortunate selection of a small or thrombosed vessel. Such problems are clearly revealed by means of ultrasound scanning and thereby may be avoided.

If it is necessary to cannulate the internal jugular vein, it can be argued, based on the anatomic variation previously described, that a two-dimensional ultrasound scan should be obtained beforehand whenever possible.

Some evidence exists that in patients with a low central venous pressure the veins are exceptionally easy to compress (7). Visualization of the procedure may be useful in overcoming such problems during central line placement.

Finally, using ultrasound in demonstrating the relevant anatomy is a beneficial adjunct to teaching the techniques of central line placement.

EQUIPMENT

Ultrasound device—A lightweight and portable two-dimensional ultrasound scanner is preferred. The Site~Rite® machine produced by Dymax Corporation has controls optimized for visualizing the internal jugular vein and carotid artery. The 7.5 MHz transducer is fitted with an offset standardized to the expected depth of these vessels. Snap-on needle guides also are available. This machine has been cited in several studies using ultrasound guidance in central venous catheterization (2–4, 7, 9).

Transducer probe—The higher the operating frequency, the better both lateral and axial resolution of the scan become. Higher ultrasonic frequencies, however, are ab-

sorbed more strongly by human tissues so that deeper planes cannot be imaged without using inordinately high power levels. In practice a transducer with an operating frequency of 7.5 MHz appears satisfactory. Clearly the advance of technology may alter the choice of equipment.

It should be noted that Doppler ultrasound also can be used to locate patent arteries and veins. Although detailed information provided by a two-dimensional ultrasound scan concerning the depth, size, and anatomical relationships of the relevant vein is not available, the Doppler technique will allow the clinician to avoid absent or thrombosed vessels and to this extent provide guidance in central line placement.

Ultrasound gel
Needle guide
Sterile sheaths for the transducer probe
Skin marking pen
Sterile povidone-iodine ointment
Standard equipment for central venous line placement (Chapter 18)

PROCEDURE

The pediatric patient will have to remain still and inevitably some will require sedation and/or anesthesia (Chapter 35); however, most children requiring emergent central line placement will be severely compromised with a depressed sensorium. Positioning is of considerable importance, and it is recommended that the patient lie supine with a towel roll under the shoulders. The table is then tilted to 15° Trendelenburg and the child's head rotated away from the side to be cannulated.

The three levels of increasing sophistication in using ultrasound are localization, monitoring, and needle guidance.

Localization

At the simplest level the ultrasound scan is used to plan the procedure by visualizing the relevant vascular anatomy. Ultrasound gel is applied to likely venipuncture sites and the vessels are examined with the transducer probe. Initial placement of the probe should be above the clavicle and within the groove

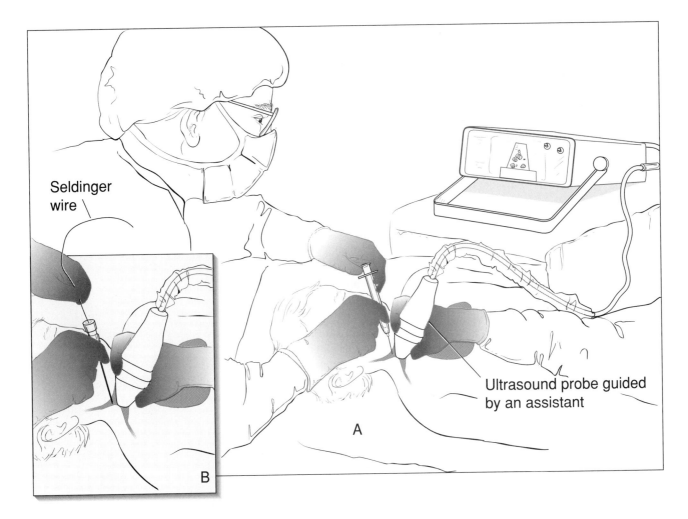

Seldinger wire

Ultrasound probe guided by an assistant

A

B

Figure 138.2.
A. Ultrasound-monitored internal jugular vein catheterization. Note the sterile sheath on the ultrasound probe and the role of the assistant.
B. Use of a needle guide in ultrasound-assisted internal jugular vein catheterization. Note the use of the Seldinger wire.

Chapter 138
Ultrasound-Assisted
Central Line
Placement

between the two heads of the sternocleidomastoid muscle. Scanning is performed in a transverse plane.

Several methods are useful in identifying the internal jugular vein by ultrasound. The internal jugular vein is generally located anterolaterally to the carotid artery. Differentiation of these vessels may be facilitated by performing a Valsalva maneuver in a cooperative patient or placing the patient in the Trendelenburg position. Both maneuvers should increase the diameter of the internal jugular vein without significantly affecting the size of the carotid artery. Pulsations within the carotid artery may also be useful in identifying that vessel. In addition, gentle compression with the transducer will partially collapse the internal jugular vein (Fig. 138.1). These techniques allow the physician to detect thrombosed or inappropriately small veins and to select the optimum route by which to access the central circulation. Verification of the precise anatomical relationship

between artery and vein will reduce the risk of accidental arterial puncture. In addition, the ultrasound scan gives guidance as to the approximate depth at which venipuncture should occur.

A suitable skin puncture site can be marked (or the course of the selected vein mapped) onto the overlying skin with a pen. The ultrasound gel and transducer probe are then removed and the standard procedure for central line cannulation is performed (Chapter 18).

Monitoring

At the next level of sophistication the ultrasound scan is used not only to plan the procedure but also to monitor the position of the venipuncture needle in real-time. The ultrasound probe needs to be positioned close to the chosen puncture site so that the venipuncture needle passes within the scan plane. This means that the probe impinges on the sterile field and must therefore be contained within a sterile sheath (Fig. 138.2.A). Sterile povidone-iodine ointment may be used as the ultrasound conductive medium, since it is easier to apply this to the skin than to maintain a pool of sterile ultrasound gel between the sheath and the transducer probe. The whole procedure actually requires three hands, so the presence of a suitably trained assistant will be required. The probe is again placed between the heads of the sternocleidomastoid muscle. Once the internal jugular vein has been identified, the probe is positioned so that the vessel image is centered on the ultrasound screen. The puncture site is anesthetized with 1% lidocaine, and the needle is inserted and advanced with continuous aspiration using ultrasound guidance.

This approach is more suitable for use in older children and is especially useful during procedure instruction when the trainee can assume the role of assistant. The advantage of this procedure is that the venipuncture needle is highly reflective of ultrasound and produces a white trace which can be observed advancing toward and then penetrating the lumen of the selected vessel. At the point of contact with the vessel the needle will be seen to indent the anterior surface of the vessel. Once access has been confirmed through the aspiration of blood into the syringe, the transducer is removed and the vessel is cannulated.

Needle Guidance

The third level of sophistication relies on the use of a suitable needle steering attachment or needle guide. Such a device is designed to restrict the movement of the venipuncture needle to a predetermined path in the image plane. The needle will therefore achieve venipuncture if inserted when the vein is visualized and transected by the electronically generated puncture line indicating the needle path. Either the probe and needle guide are both contained within the sterile sheath or it may be possible to sterilize the needle steering guide in glutaraldehyde and to clip it onto the ensheathed probe.

The initial approach is identical to the previously described monitoring procedure. Once the internal jugular vein has been identified and centered on the monitor, the needle

is held within the needle guide with the thumb (Fig. 138.2.B) and slowly advanced through the anesthetized skin. The progress of the needle is viewed on the ultrasound monitor while maintaining the internal jugular vein image within the electronically generated puncture line. Once penetration of the vessel lumen by the needle is visualized and blood aspirated, the transducer is removed and the procedure is completed in the standard fashion.

If the venipuncture is observed in real-time by means of ultrasound as in the latter

---

SUMMARY
1. Check equipment and ensure that child is appropriately monitored
2. Utilize sedation as needed
3. Place child in Trendelenburg position with a roll under shoulders and head turned away from side to be cannulated
4. Place ultrasound gel and transducer between two heads of sternocleidomastoid muscle and scan in transverse plane
5. Locate relative positions and depths of internal jugular vein and carotid artery
6. Modify position of child or route of access chosen depending on findings

Localization
a. Mark position of vein on skin surface
b. Remove ultrasound gel and transducer
c. Perform standard central venous catheterization using markings as a guide

Monitoring
a. Prep and drape patient before ultrasound scan
b. Place probe and ultrasound gel in sterile sheath or apply povidone-iodine ointment directly to skin as ultrasound conductive medium
c. Identify internal jugular vein and center image on ultrasound screen
d. Anesthetize the puncture site with 1% lidocaine as needed
e. Insert the needle and advance with continuous aspiration
f. Observe the needle penetrate the internal jugular vein on the ultrasound monitor
g. Remove transducer and complete central line cannulation in standard fashion

Needle Guidance
a. Connect needle guide to transducer
b. Center image of internal jugular vein on ultrasound screen and within electronically generated puncture line
c. Hold needle in needle guide with thumb
d. Advance needle while monitoring its progress on ultrasound screen
e. Remove transducer once penetration of vessel lumen has been visualized

two cases then it is possible to dispense with the usual syringe on the needle and instead use a Seldinger guide wire as a stylet. This prevents possible dislodgment of the needle from the vein when the syringe is discon-nected to thread the Seldinger wire, and also minimizes the risk of air embolism (8).

COMPLICATIONS

The incidence of complications during central line placement can be high and such complications may have serious consequences as discussed in Chapter 18. The most likely reason for complications such as arterial puncture and pneumothorax during internal jugular line placement is that the venipuncture is performed blindly. It is therefore expected that using two-dimensional ultrasound will reduce the complication rate associated with the placement of such central lines. Certainly the rate of carotid puncture during internal jugular venous cannulation in adults has been shown to be significantly reduced (9), but studies enrolling large numbers of pediatric patients are awaited. As yet no complications unique to ultrasound use have been reported during central line placement.

SUMMARY

If central line placement is indicated, then a two-dimensional ultrasound scan will clarify the vascular anatomy and help the clinician to both optimize the positioning of the patient and select a suitable puncture site. It is then possible to guide a finder needle into the chosen vein and to visualize threading of a guide wire in real-time. Using ultrasound will therefore reduce the time needed to achieve central line placement and increase the chance of a complication-free procedure.

REFERENCES

1. Steven JM, Cohen DE. In: Motoyama EK, ed. Smith's anesthesia for infants and children. 5th ed. St. Louis: CV Mosby, 1990.
2. Denys BG, Uretsky BF, Reddy PS. Ultrasound-as-sisted cannulation of the internal jugular vein: a prospective comparison to the external landmark guided technique. Circulation 1993;87:1557–1562.
3. Alderson PJ, Burrows FA, Stemp LI, Holtby HM. The use of ultrasound to evaluate internal jugular vein anatomy and to facilitate central venous cannulation in pediatric patients. Br J Anaesth 1993;70:145–148.
4. Denys BG, Uretsky BF. Anatomical variations of internal jugular vein location: impact on central venous access. Crit Care Med 1991;19:1516–1519.
5. Mallory DL, Shawker T, Evans RG, McGee WT, Brenner M, Parker M, Morrison G, Mohler P, Veremakis C, Parrillo JE. Effects of clinical maneuvers on sonographically determined internal jugular vein size during venous cannulation. Crit Care Med 1990;18:1269–1273.
6. Mortensen JD, Talbot S, Burkart JA. Cross-sectional internal diameters of human cervical and femoral blood vessels: relationship to subject's sex, age, body size. Anatomical Record 1990;225:115–124.
7. Armstrong PJ, Cullen M, Scott DHT. The Site~Rite® ultrasound machine—an aid to internal jugular vein cannulation. Anaesthesia 1993;48:319–323.
8. Nolsoe C, Nielsen L, Karlstrup S, Lauritsen L. Ultra-sonically guided subclavian vein catheterization. Acta Radiologica 1989;30:108–109.
9. Denys BG, Uretsky BF, Reddy PS, Ruffner RJ, Sandhu JS, Breishlatt WM. An ultrasound method for safe and rapid central venous access. N Engl J Med 1991;324:566.

TRANSPORT PROCEDURES

Section Editor: Brent R. King

CHAPTER 139

Preparing the Child for Interhospital Transport

Dennis R. Durbin

Introduction

Effective regionalized emergency care for children relies on the integration of several health care components into a continuum of pediatric care. Effective emergency care begins in the prehospital setting with immediate life-saving procedures, accurate triage, and rapid transport to the closest appropriate medical facility. Most critically ill or injured children are taken initially to a community hospital emergency department (ED) for primary stabilization. Many of these children, once properly stabilized, will require subsequent transport to a regional pediatric tertiary care center. Interhospital transport services are thus a critical link in the overall system of regionalized emergency care for children, bridging the patient's initial stabilization in the community hospital with definitive care in the tertiary care center.

The mode of transportation for a critically ill patient is an important factor in providing optimal comprehensive emergency care (1). Ground ambulances, helicopters, and fixed-wing aircraft may be available for pediatric interhospital transport. The correct mode of transport is the one that provides the most appropriate care to the child, while using scarce resources wisely. In addition, a variety of available personnel may compose the transport team (2–4). A team should be chosen to provide the skills and experience that best meet the needs of the patient during the transport. This chapter will highlight the most important factors to consider when arranging a pediatric interhospital transport, and will provide guidelines to help referring physicians choose the most appropriate vehicle and team type for a given transport.

Indications

Two general indications exist for the interhospital transport of children. First, the referring hospital may not have the inpatient resources necessary to care for the patient beyond initial stabilization in the ED. Second, the patient may have a diagnosis or severity of illness that would be best managed in a regional pediatric tertiary care center. Timely recognition of a child in need of interhospital transport is critically important. Delays are inherent in arranging an interhospital transfer, particularly when a specialized team from the receiving hospital is required. Therefore, clinical deterioration of the patient must be anticipated, and an appropriate transport team must be mobilized as early as possible during the patient's initial stabilization.

The transport of pediatric patients has no strict contraindications if, in the judgment of the referring physician, the child cannot be adequately cared for in the referring hospital. A relative contraindication to transfer is placing a patient in a mobile environment before ensuring adequate stabilization. It is the philosophy of most specialized pediatric transport teams to perform necessary procedures and critical interventions before placing the patient into a vehicle (5). This contrasts with the "scoop and run" philosophy of rapid transfer without regard for care delivered during transport. In only a minority of cases (e.g., expanding epidural hematomas, exsanguinating trauma) is speed of delivery to the tertiary care center the sole concern in pediatric interhospital transport. Just as important is the level of care delivered during transport. Therefore, every effort must be made to ensure that the vehicle type and team composition best meet the needs of the patient for the period during transport. Relative advantages and disadvantages of different vehicle and team types are discussed later in this chapter.

EQUIPMENT

To ensure a successful interhospital transport, the referring physician requires the most appropriate vehicle type and the best team composition. Availability of different vehicles and team types is highly variable in different regions of the country (1). Table 139.1 compares the relative advantages and disadvantages of ground ambulances, helicopters, and fixed-wing aircraft for pediatric transport. Ground ambulances are nearly universally available and, on average, are the most common mode of interhospital transport in the country. They are generally considered safer than either helicopters or fixed-wing aircraft, although accurate data directly comparing the safety of different vehicles are not available. Ground ambulances are the most cost-effective mode of transport over a limited range assuming normal road and traffic conditions.

The distinct advantage to helicopter transport is a rapid transport time over a wider range than with ground ambulances. When speed of delivery to the tertiary care center is the most critical factor to consider in the management of a patient, helicopter transport is frequently the optimal mode to use (6). However, the small space inside the helicopter cabin and constant noise and vibration from the rotors limit the ability of transport personnel to perform procedures during flight. In addition, helicopter transport is more costly than a comparable ground transport, and the availability of helicopters is always subject to weather conditions.

Fixed-wing aircraft are usually used for long distance transports (greater than 200 miles). Depending on the type of aircraft used, the cabin environment may allow for excellent patient monitoring and assessment. The major disadvantage of fixed-wing transport is the need to move the patient, typically by ground ambulance, from the referring hospital to a designated landing zone, transfer the patient into and then out of the aircraft at the destination site, and finally transport the patient again by ground ambulance to the receiving hospital. Multiple transfers pose risks of clinical deterioration of the patient, airway and intravenous catheter dislodgment, or equipment failure.

Referring physicians must ensure that the patient is not put at risk by any decrement in the level of care provided to the patient during transport. Therefore, careful attention to the qualifications and experience of transport personnel is mandatory. A number of choices in team composition are available. Table 139.2 highlights the relative advantages and disadvantages of the most common team compositions.

For some patients, the parents may function as adequate transport personnel. Clearly this should be reserved for those patients who

Table 139.1.
Comparison of Different Transport Vehicles

	Ground Ambulance	Fixed Wing	Helicopter
Availability	+ + +	+	+ +
Safety	+ +	+ +	+ +
Cabin environment (space, noise, vibration)	+	+ +	−
Transport time	+	+ +	+ + +
Range	<100 miles	200–2000 miles	100–150 miles
Cost	$500–1000	Varies	$2000–3500
Special issues	Road conditions	Multiple transfers	Weather conditions

Legend: + + +, Excellent; + +, Good; +, Fair; −, Poor.

are minimally ill with virtually no potential for deterioration and no need for ongoing monitoring. Transport via private car is generally the fastest and cheapest way to transfer a child between hospitals. Clinicians must recognize, however, that parents may not travel directly to the receiving hospital and that responsibility for the patient during the transport rests with the referring hospital. Despite these drawbacks, selected use of the parents' car helps reserve the more costly and scarce transport resources for those patients who most need them.

Local emergency medical services (EMS) ambulances are widely available and relatively cost effective for patients who are moderately ill with little risk of deterioration. Some patient monitoring and assessment can be performed, but the skills and experience of ambulance personnel for pediatric care may be limited. The addition of a nurse or physician from the referring hospital improves the level of skills and monitoring available to the patient, but may do so at the expense of scarce resources at the referring hospital. Moderately ill patients in need of continued noninvasive monitoring and at minimal risk of deterioration during transport may be adequately transported this way.

Broad-based transport teams are those that typically transport adult cardiac and trauma patients but can transport children when requested. Most helicopter transport teams would best be described this way. These personnel may have extensive training and experience in mobile intensive care, although their experience with critically ill children may be limited. When speed of transport is the primary factor to consider, these teams can generally be mobilized quickly and can deliver an appropriate level of care for a limited transport time.

Finally, specialized pediatric transport teams are becoming increasingly available in many parts of the country. These teams usually are based at the regional tertiary care center, and consist of nurses, physicians, respiratory therapists, or paramedics with specific training and experience in the transport of critically ill children. Because they must be mobilized from the tertiary care center, specialized teams are somewhat slower to arrive at the referring hospital, and are relatively costly compared with other forms of ground transport. The distinct advantage of the specialized pediatric transport team is the ability to deliver a high level of care and monitoring during transport. They are best used for moderately to severely ill children in need of continued monitoring or major interventions, or who are at risk of potential deterioration during transport.

Factors to consider in choosing the optimal method of interhospital transport for a child are (*a*) the diagnosis and severity of illness of the patient, (*b*) risk of deterioration during transport, (*c*) the urgency to arrive at the tertiary care center, (*d*) the distance between the two hospitals, (*e*) local geographic characteristics, (*f*) current weather and traffic conditions, (*g*) current availability of vehicles, and finally, when all other factors have been considered, (*h*) the relative cost (of both personnel and equipment) of the different options (1).

General guidelines to which referring physicians should adhere in arranging interhospital transport are that no decrement should occur in the level of care during all phases of stabilization and transport, and speed should not be overemphasized (6). It is often preferable to have a critically ill or potentially unstable patient wait for a dedicated pediatric transport team in a community hospital ED with access to life-saving equipment and personnel, rather than place that child in the care of personnel with limited pediatric experience, even though the latter mode of

Table 139.2.
Comparison of Different Transport Team Compositions

Type	Advantages	Disadvantages
Private car	Cost, speed, available	No care en route, unreliable
EMS/Ambulance	Cost, speed, some monitoring	Limited skills/interventions
+ RN and/or MD	Improved skills/monitoring	Uses scarce resources
Broad-based team	Cost, speed, improved monitoring and skills	Limited pediatric critical care
Specialized pediatric transport team	Highest level of care, monitoring	Limited availability, expensive

SUMMARY
1. Perform necessary interventions to stabilize patient
2. Contact transport personnel at receiving facility
3. Provide information to determine optimal mode of transport and team composition
4. Discuss transfer with patient and/or family and obtain consent
5. If possible, prepare all appropriate materials (copies of laboratory results, radiographs, etc.) prior to arrival of transport team
6. Update arriving transport team regarding any changes in clinical condition of patient
7. Assist in performing any necessary procedures to prevent potential clinical deterioration of patient en route (endotracheal intubation, paralysis and sedation, retaping lines and tubes, etc.)
8. Transfer patient only when sufficiently stabilized to allow safe transport

transport might be more rapidly available. Difficult decisions about optimal method of transport should always be made in consultation with the regional tertiary care center.

PROCEDURE

Perhaps the most important step in the interhospital transport of a critically ill child is the initial referral call. Likewise, the most important factor in determining the success of an interhospital transport is effective communication between the referring and receiving hospital staffs. The receiving hospital must determine the most appropriate bed assignment (ICU or regular ward) for the patient, and may need to prepare specialized diagnostic or therapeutic modalities for the patient's arrival. In addition, if a specialized pediatric transport team from the receiving hospital is employed, the optimal team composition must be determined. This degree of immediate preparation requires that key points of information on the patient's status be provided by the referring hospital in the initial referral call.

Figure 139.1 is a sample of the referral call log sheet used by the pediatric transport team at the Children's Hospital of Philadelphia. Specific identifying information about the patient and the referring physician are generally requested immediately in case the call is lost or disconnected. A brief summary of the patient's condition, including specific vital signs, and pertinent physical examination findings follow. Relevant laboratory and radiographic results should be provided. Finally, major interventions performed and the patient's response to them should be documented. If necessary, the physician at the receiving hospital may provide advice as to further evaluation or therapy for the patient. Disagreements about patient management should be openly discussed with the goal of rapidly reaching compromises that are in the patient's best interest. Follow-up phone calls during mobilization of the transport team may be necessary, and should allow for the provision of all requested information by either the referring or receiving hospital.

While awaiting the arrival of the transport team, referring hospital staff should ensure that the patient is optimally prepared for transport. Copies of radiographs and the patient's chart should be made, monitoring and assessment should be continued, and necessary procedures should be performed by the most experienced personnel. In addition, the patient's family should be prepared for the transport. They should understand the nature of their child's illness and the reason why transport is being arranged so that they may provide consent for the transport.

When the transport team arrives at the referring hospital, confusion frequently arises about responsibility for the patient and who is in charge. From a medical-legal standpoint, "shared responsibility" lies between both institutions. Specific roles and expectations of personnel should be discussed at the outset and agreement reached as amicably as possible. It is generally the responsibility of the transport team to decide when the patient is stable enough for transport.

An important part of successful pediatric interhospital transport is the advance preparation of the referring hospital before the need for transfer (5). A list of pediatric referral centers with phone numbers and a list of available regional transport services should be posted in the ED. Protocols for management of common pediatric life-threatening conditions can be developed and practiced in mock situations. A chart with dosing recommendations for the common pediatric code drugs should be readily available. The ED should be stocked with proper size endotracheal tubes, airway masks, laryngoscope blades, intravenous catheters, and blood pressure cuffs. The most convenient way to store pediatric equipment in a general ED is either to assemble a separate equipment pack or to reserve a drawer in the code cart for pediatric equipment.

Advance administrative preparation is increasingly required to ensure a smooth interhospital transfer. Predetermined referral patterns or payment agreements may exist, or insurance carriers may mandate referral to specific hospitals. Referring physicians should be aware of the administrative constraints to interhospital transport in their institution so that no unnecessary delays occur at the time of transport.

COMPLICATIONS

The interhospital transport of critically ill children is not a benign procedure. A number

CH The Children's Hospital of Philadelphia

TRANSPORT TEAM REFERRAL FORM

PATIENT PLATE IMPRINT

DATE: ___ / ___ / ___ TIME: ___ CALL RECEIVED BY: 080 377 ER 2160 ICU OTHER ___

NAME: AGE

REFERRING HOSPITAL:

WEIGHT ___ Kg

REFERRING M.D.: PHONE NUMBER: ( ) ___

REFERRING UNIT: DIAGNOSIS:

HISTORY AND INITIAL ASSESSMENT:

ALLERGIES: EXPOSURE TO COMMUNICABLE DISEASE:

RESPIRATORY

CYANOSIS Y N
RETRACTIONS Y N
APNEA Y N
SUPPLEMENTAL O_2 Y N
SaO_2: in RA ___ %
in O_2 ___ %
O_2 being delivered by:
Nasal Cannula face mask
Oxyhood blowby
INTUBATED Y N
IMV ___ PIP/PEEP ___

BLOOD GASES		
TIME		
SITE		
pH		
pCO_2		
pO_2		
BE		

CARDIOVASCULAR

COLOR:

CAPILLARY REFILL:

URINE OUTPUT:

MURMUR:

NEUROLOGIC

GLASGOW COMA SCALE		
Eye Opening	Spontaneous	4
	To Voice	3
	To Pain	2
	None	1
Verbal Response	Oriented	5
	Confused	4
	Inappropriate Words	3
	Incomprehensible Sounds	2
	None	1
Motor Response	Obeys Commands	6
	Localizes (Pain)	5
	Withdraw (Pain)	4
	Flexion (Pain)	3
	Extension (Pain)	2
	None	1
TOTAL		

PUPILS: Response to light: EQUAL UNEQUAL FIXED

SEIZURES Y N GENERALIZED FOCAL

VITAL SIGNS

	TIME	TEMP	HR	RR	BP
INITIAL					
@REFERRAL					
@UPDATE					

LAB RESULTS

CULTURES SENT:

CSF: WBC ___ RBC ___ PROT ___ GLUC ___

OTHER LABS:

XRAYS:

INTERVENTIONS	COMPLETED BY REFERRING HOSPITAL	RECOMMENDATIONS BY CHOP	RECOMMENDATION COMPLETED
MEDICATIONS			Y N
			Y N
IV FLUIDS / ACCESS			Y N
			Y N
VENTILATION			Y N
OTHER PROCEDURES			Y N

SIGNATURES:

RESIDENT ___ RN ___ ATTENDING ___

NUR-1032

Figure 139.1.
A referral log sheet used by the pediatric transport team at the Children's Hospital of Philadelphia.

of complications can occur either due to incomplete stabilization of the patient before transport or to the limitations of patient care and monitoring in a mobile environment (7–13). The patient's pretransport severity of illness and a lack of pediatric training and experience among team members are both related to the risk of morbidity during transport (7, 8). Recent reviews cite rates of adverse outcomes during transport between 5 and 20% (7–9). Chief among these are adverse events related to artificial airways and mechanical ventilation. Unrecognized need for tracheal intubation, airway dislodgment, and obstruction with secretions are among the most common serious morbidities incurred during transport (7–11). In addition, loss of intravenous access, physiologic deterioration of the patient (e.g., hypotension, bradycardia, hypoxemia), and equipment failure (e.g., exhausted O_2 supply, vehicular accident (14) all may occur during an interhospital transport.

The environment inside a transport vehicle is generally suboptimal for critical care. Limited space, noise, vibration, temperature, lighting, electrical interference (e.g., of helicopter navigational equipment), and constant motion impact on the function of monitoring equipment, the physiologic stability of the patient, and the ability of transport personnel to accurately assess patients and perform technical procedures (1, 15–17). In addition, transport personnel may be subject to motion sickness which may influence their judgment (18). Therefore, to minimize the risk of serious adverse events during transport, the clinician should perform interventions necessary to achieve stabilization prior to transport, and use transport personnel who are skilled and experienced in the mobile care of critically ill children whenever possible.

SUMMARY

Children requiring specialized or more intensive medical care must often be transported from one hospital to another to receive necessary treatment. Initial stabilization is performed in the transferring facility and definitive management is provided at the receiving facility. Although this would seem like a straightforward process, accomplishing a safe and successful transport of a critically ill child requires meticulous attention to detail. Once the decision has been made to transfer a patient, the medical personnel involved must select the appropriate mode of transportation and the optimal composition of the transport team. This selection is best made using information provided jointly by individuals from both facilities. In addition, the physician(s) caring for the patient at the transferring hospital must ensure that, to the extent possible, all the appropriate stabilization and preparation measures are performed prior to transport. Familiarity with these issues increases the likelihood that a transfer will occur smoothly and without incident.

REFERENCES

1. Schneider C, Gomez M, Lee R. Evaluation of ground ambulance, rotor-wing, and fixed-wing aircraft services. Crit Care Clin 1992;8(3):533.
2. Smith DF, Hackel A. Selection criteria for pediatric critical care transport teams. Crit Care Med 1983; 11(1):10.
3. McCloskey KA, Faries G, King WD, et al. Variables predicting the need for a pediatric critical care transport team. Pediatr Emerg Care 1992;8(1):1.
4. McCloskey KA, Johnston C. Pediatric critical care transport survey: team composition and training, mobilization time, and mode of transportation. Pediatr Emerg Care 1990;6(1):1.
5. McCloskey KA, Orr RA. Pediatric interhospital transport. In: Fleisher G, Ludwig S, eds. Textbook of pediatric emergency medicine. 3rd ed. Philadelphia: Williams & Wilkins, 1993.
6. McCloskey KA, Orr RA. Pediatric transport issues in emergency medicine. Emerg Med Clin North Am 1991;9(3):475.
7. Kanter RK, Tompkins JM. Adverse events during interhospital transport: Physiologic deterioration associated with pretransport severity of illness. Pediatrics 1989;84:43.
8. Kanter RK, Boeing NM, Hannan WP, Kanter DL. Excess morbidity associated with interhospital transport. Pediatrics 1992;90:893.
9. Macnab AJ. Optimal escort for interhospital transport of pediatric emergencies. J Trauma 1991;31: 205.
10. Gentleman D, Jennett B. Hazards of interhospital transfer of comatose head-injured patients. Lancet 1981;853.
11. Henning R, McNamarra V. Difficulties encountered in transport of the critically ill child. Pediatr Emerg Care 1991;7:133.
12. Fuller J, Frewen T, Lee R. Acute airway management in the critically ill child requiring transport. Can J Anaesth 1991;38:252.
13. Owen J, Duncan AW. Towards safer transport of sick and injured children. Anaesth Intens Care 1983; 11:113.
14. Auerbach PS, Morris JA, Phillips JB, et al. An analysis of ambulance accidents in Tennessee. JAMA 1987;258:1487.
15. Silbergleit R, Dedrick DK, Pape J, Burney RE. Forces acting during air and ground transport on patients stabilized by standard immobilization techniques. Ann Emerg Med 1991;20:875.
16. Shenai JP, Johnson GE, Varney RV. Mechanical vibration in neonatal transport. Pediatrics 1981;68:55.
17. Heiman HS. Safety and accuracy of an infant transport system. Pediatr Emerg Care 1993;9:324.
18. Wright MS, Bose CL. The transport environment: its effect on the function of medical attendants. Pediatr Emerg Care 1993;9:324.

CHAPTER 140

AEROMEDICAL TRANSPORT PROCEDURES

Scott H. Freedman and Brent R. King

INTRODUCTION

It has been well documented that morbidity and mortality related to the care of critically ill and injured children are decreased when care is provided in regionalized pediatric specialty hospitals. Documentation has been especially well demonstrated in neonatology, where facilities equipped with extracorporeal membrane oxygenation (ECMO) may save infants who would otherwise die (1, 2). In addition, providing care in a timely fashion dramatically improves outcome. The concept of the "golden hour" in trauma care is now sine qua non in emergency medical services systems (3). It is based on these principles that aeromedical transport has become instrumental in the process of caring for critically ill and injured children and neonates.

Air ambulances were first used during World War I to evacuate injured combat soldiers (4). The first commercial civilian air medical service was established in 1927 but this mode of transport did not gain widespread acceptance and use until the 1950s. The first documented use of aeromedical transport for a newborn occurred in 1967 when a premature neonate was transported from Zion, Illinois, to Peoria, Illinois, by helicopter. Using aircraft to transport children became routine in the early 1970s with the establishment of the first hospital-based helicopter program at St. Mary's Hospital in Denver in 1972 (5, 6). In 1986, the American Academy of Pediatrics (AAP) established guidelines for ground and air transport of children and neonates (7).

A discussion of some important ground transport procedures is provided in Chapter 139. Many of these concepts hold true for air transport. Issues such as the initiation of early interhospital communication, providing pertinent information including a comprehensive medical record, and timely on-site patient evaluation and stabilization are essential for a smooth, efficient turnaround. Table 140.1 summarizes the general responsibilities of the transferring and receiving facilities involved in a pediatric transport. Essential information required by air transport services is listed in Table 140.2. Additionally, many of the same supplies and medications are used for both ground and air transports.

Aeromedical transport, simply by its nature, has many unique characteristics. Medical team members should be familiar with aircraft cabin and safety features before departure. Table 140.3 lists safety instructions for helicopter travel. Noise and vibration have the greatest impact during helicopter transport affecting patient assessment and communication. Hypoxia, gas expansion, temperature, humidity, and gravitational forces are features unique to air travel (8–10). Each feature individually or in combination may adversely affect the care and condition of an ill or injured child transported in a helicopter or fixed-wing aircraft.

Table 140.1.
Transport Responsibilities

Transferring Facility
1. Stabilize patient
2. Early communication with accepting facility
3. Notify family—obtain consent
4. Copy pertinent record—include transfer summary, radiographs, medication list

Receiving Facility
1. Determine needs
2. Arrange for medical crew and vehicle
3. Provide ETA and offer further medical advice, when indicated
4. Prompt mobilization and arrival at bedside
5. Patient assessment and stabilization
6. Review record—most recent ABG, CXR's, dextrostix
7. Secure patient for transport—pay particular attention to airway, intravenous lines
8. Communicate with accepting facility—MD and nursing
9. Brief visit with family including additional consents
10. Intratransfer assessment, stabilization
11. Transfer care to receiving facility medical team
12. Follow-up with transferring facility

Table 140.2.
Information for Air Services

Information provided to helicopter service
1. Patient name, DOB, Weight, Sex
2. Patient location and destination—Address for both transferring and accepting hospital, including sending and receiving units
3. Name and contact telephone numbers for both sending and receiving physicians
4. Basic diagnosis
5. Nature of transport (neonatal-isolette, pediatric-stretcher)
6. Team composition (number of team members and weights)
7. Reason for transport (e.g., acuity of illness, traffic conditions)

Information provided to fixed-wing air service
1–7. Same as above
8. Responsible party/legal guardian (name, address, telephone number, when available)
9. Equipment required for transport (for commercial carriers, this includes any medications, oxygen, and feedings to be administered en route.)
10. Location of aircraft (provided by carrier service)

PHYSIOLOGY

Air flight physiology is governed by laws of physics dealing with pressure-volume changes at increasing altitudes. As a person ascends in an aircraft, the barometric (external) pressure decreases as the volume occupied by a gas increases (Boyle's law). The reverse is true during descent. Furthermore, at increasing altitudes as the barometric pressure decreases, the partial pressure of each gaseous component correspondingly decreases (Dalton's law). Therefore as an aircraft ascends, the partial pressure of oxygen decreases and the amount of available oxygen decreases as the gas molecules move apart. For example, at sea level the partial pressure of oxygen (PO_2) equals $21\% \times 760$ mm Hg = 160 mm Hg. At 8000 feet the percentage of oxygen remains 21%, but the barometric pressure has fallen to 565 mm Hg. The PO_2 at 8000 feet equals 119 mm Hg ($21\% \times 565$ mm Hg). Tables can be obtained that list the barometric pressure at increasing altitudes.

Hypoxia is the single greatest physiologic stressor encountered during air flight transport and it can adversely affect patients and crew members. In an unpressurized cabin, as altitude increases hypoxia develops. The initial compensatory sign of hypoxia is an increase in respiratory rate and effort.

When PO_2 falls to 50 to 60 mm Hg, CNS hypoxia often develops. The patient may become restless and agitated. Confusion, impaired memory, attention, judgment, and visual disturbances may develop. Neurologic symptomatology is directly related to the duration and severity of hypoxia. In the extreme case, sensory and cognitive dysfunction will progress to obtundation, coma, and death if not treated.

Recognizing the early, subtle signs of hypoxia will allow for timely intervention. All commercial fixed-wing aircraft and air ambulances are equipped with a compressor that is capable of partially pressurizing the cabin. The aircraft cabin is generally pressurized to a differential of approximately 8.6 psi. This means at a flight altitude of 35,000 feet where the atmospheric pressure is only 176 mm Hg (3.40 psi), the compressor adds another 445 mm Hg (8.6 psi) for a total pressure equal to 620 mm Hg (12.0 psi), which is equivalent to an approximate atmospheric pressure of 5000 feet. Alveolar PO_2 at a cabin pressure corresponding to an atmospheric pressure of 5000 feet is approximately 80 mm Hg. All air ambulances are pressurized in flights exceeding an altitude of 6000 feet.

Supplemental oxygen also should be provided when a child's pulmonary status may be compromised. The altitude oxygen requirement equation can be used to calculate oxygen percentage required at increasing al-

Table 140.3.
Safety Instructions for Helicopter Travel

1. All team members should be oriented to the aircraft and familiarized with the safety equipment on board before departure.
2. All team members should make sure they have no loose articles of clothing or accessories. Long hair should be tied back. Flat shoes should be worn.
3. The helicopter always should be approached from the front and from the downhill side.
4. Always wait for a signal from the pilot or crew member before approaching the aircraft.
5. Never allow anyone near the rear or tail of the helicopter (exception: rear-loading helicopters).
6. The flight crew is solely responsible for opening and closing the aircraft doors.
7. The flight crew is responsible for loading and unloading the patient and equipment. Assist the crew only when requested.

titudes. The formula is

$$F_iO_2 \text{ (required)} = F_iO_2 \text{ (present)} \times BP \text{ (present)/ } BP \text{ (alt)}$$

where F_iO_2 (present) is the patient's current fraction of inspired oxygen, BP (present) is the current barometric pressure, and BP (alt) is the barometric pressure at the expected cruising altitude. An example would be to calculate the required supplemental oxygen for a child on 50% O_2 at the referring hospital. The aircraft will be pressurized to a cabin altitude of 7000 feet. The barometric pressure at 7000 feet is 585 mm Hg. The supplemental oxygen the child would require is

$$F_iO_2 \text{ (required)} = 0.50 \times 760/585 = .65 \, O_2$$

If hypoxic effects develop, the crew members should first provide themselves with a supplemental oxygen mask and then attend to the patient. In such cases, the cabin pressure in the aircraft can usually be increased or the aircraft can fly at a lower altitude.

As previously mentioned, as altitude increases, gas volume proportionally increases. Gases expand in the body and exert pressure against surrounding tissues and organs. Physiologically, this explains yawning and ear popping on takeoff and landing. With patients who are transported, expanding air can result in a small pneumothorax becoming a clinically significant pneumothorax. Middle ear disease, dental caries or abscesses, and sinusitis are also exacerbated by gas expansion. Intestinal perforation could result from expansion of a gas bubble under pressure due to gastrointestinal obstruction. Nasogastric

tubes must be connected to a functioning portable or wall suction unit. Equipment that is under pressure may need adjustment under high altitude conditions. The pressure in a cuffed endotracheal tube should be slightly deflated before flying, and the cuff pressure must be periodically checked and adjusted as needed during the flight. A central line must be closely monitored, as a seemingly insignificant air bubble at atmospheric pressure can expand at high altitude with potentially serious consequences.

Temperature is also affected by increasing altitude. Air temperature decreases 1.5°C for every 1000-ft increase in altitude. All neonates should be transported in an enclosed isolette with a built-in heater and temperature gauge. All cabins should be equipped with heaters to prevent the infant or child from becoming hypothermic. The temperature of the child should be measured as frequently as other vital signs. The ambient temperature in the cabin should be monitored routinely. Warm intravenous fluids and humidified, warm oxygen should be used. The infant should be dressed with a cap and placed on a warming blanket, if needed, to prevent hypothermia. Effects of hypoxia are worsened under conditions of temperature extremes. A person's metabolic rate increases when exposed to marked changes in temperature thus increasing the oxygen requirement.

Humidity of the cabin environment is an additional consideration in air flight transport. As altitude increases, the humidity of the air drops substantially. Because the outside air serves as the source for air for pressurizing a cabin, the ambient conditions are dry. If not carefully considered, either the patient or the crew may experience signs of dehydration. During long transports, input and output of fluids by the patient must be carefully monitored and increased as necessary. Oxygen also should be humidified during lengthy transports for similar reasons.

Gravitational forces (G-forces) may be a factor when transporting children with head injury or vascular compromise (e.g., shock) as it causes peripheral pooling of blood. On takeoff or ascent, G-forces are directed toward the rear of an airplane. A child at risk for increased intracranial pressure should be loaded onto the plane with the head toward the front. During takeoff and ascent, blood would therefore pool in the lower part of the body preventing a sudden transient rise in intracranial pressure. Similar principles would dictate placing a child with hemodynamic instability with the head to the rear of the aircraft. In this case cerebral perfusion would be maintained even in a low output state. Alternatively, the stretcher could still be placed with the head to the front, and the foot of the bed could be elevated or fluid boluses could be given as needed.

Excessive noise and vibration are primarily results of the helicopter engine and rotor. An obvious disadvantage of a helicopter transport is that patient care may be compromised by the inability to fully assess and manage a patient when excessive noise or vibrations occur. Furthermore, stress from prolonged loud noise and vibration can cause hearing damage, headaches, and gastrointestinal or visual disturbances. Cotton should be placed in the infant's ears and children should be fitted with ear cups or ear plugs before takeoff. Medical team members must be provided helmets and headsets with an intercommunication system that does not interfere with the pilot's air traffic communication.

Although motion sickness is not unique to air travel, it does occur frequently. Steady rocking and vibrations during movement with visual loss of the horizon may disrupt a person's equilibrium. Nausea, vomiting, dizziness, blurred vision, or vertigo may result. Transdermal scopolamine can be applied prophylactically by team members known to be susceptible to motion sickness. For maximum benefit, the patch should be in place approximately 4 hours before travel and has lasting effect for up to 3 days. Drowsiness and blurred vision are side effects of scopolamine.

INDICATIONS

Many factors must be considered when choosing the optimal mode for transport. Patient acuity and distance to be traveled are the primary determinants when selecting the vehicle. Obviously, an unstable neonate or child with a life-threatening condition would benefit most from the shortest transport time possible (time actually spent in the vehicle, en route to the accepting facility). Transport time, however, is not solely dependent on miles traversed. In a congested inner city,

traffic (especially at peak rush hour periods), accidents, and construction detours may greatly prolong a ground transport. Similarly in a rural area, road and terrain conditions may make an outlying facility difficult to quickly access by ground.

Helicopter transport would seem to be a logical option when ground conditions or distance make ambulance transports impractical. Most civilian medical helicopters travel at speeds in excess of 150 mph with a range of up to 100 to 150 miles. A helicopter is generally used for transports covering more than 30 miles in one direction. However, an unstable child requiring urgent specialized care may be transported by helicopter at distances as short as 5 miles, whereas a ground ambulance at times may transport a stable child 100 to 150 miles. By virtue of their ability to make vertical takeoffs and landings, helicopters are able to reach patients in remote areas. Fixed-wing aircraft are generally used for transports in excess of 150 miles. Many additional variables also contribute to vehicle selection. Team and vehicle availability, proximity of landing zone or airport to referring hospital, prevailing weather conditions, and cost must also be considered.

Other factors may also have an impact on the decision to use air transport. Significant time delays in the availability of an aeromedical transport vehicle, flight crew, or medical team could impact vehicle selection. Inclement weather places great limitations on a helicopter's utility. Heavy fog or ice also would delay or prevent a fixed-wing aircraft from travel. Start-up, maintenance, and utilization costs are substantially higher for fixed-wing aircraft and helicopters than for ground ambulances.

Vehicle design and flying conditions should be considered. Cabin size is generally smaller in a helicopter than in an ambulance, and limitations for patient access and team size are greater. Although an ambulance is able to pull off the road or detour to a nearby hospital should a patient's condition deteriorate, a helicopter has no such luxury. If the medical crew wishes to directly communicate with a specialist at the receiving hospital while en route, this is easily accomplished via mobile telecommunications in an ambulance. In a helicopter or small fixed-wing aircraft, this is not always possible. Excessive noise and vibration may limit or prevent such communication. Additionally, because the helicopter cabin cannot be pressurized, hypoxic conditions may become clinically significant at altitudes exceeding 8000 feet. This is especially true in a child or neonate with pulmonary disease or profound anemia. Persistent pulmonary hypertension is markedly aggravated by hypoxic states. Children with sickle-cell disease and even sickle-cell trait may develop increased sickling of red blood cells and its associated complications (e.g., pain crises, acute chest syndrome) in hypoxic environments.

The obvious advantage of a fixed-wing aircraft is speed and range for long distance transports. The cabin in a fixed-wing aircraft can generally be pressurized to an altitude equivalent to at least 8000 feet. Hypoxia and risk of sudden decompression, however, still need to be recognized and managed. A fixed-wing transport requires moving the patient at least four times during a transport, transferring the patient from the hospital bed to a ground ambulance that travels to the airport and reloads the patient onto the airplane. Once the aircraft lands at its destination, reverse transfers must be done. A large distance between the hospital and the airport (at either end) may significantly add to the overall transport time.

EQUIPMENT

Tables 140.4 through 140.6 list recommended equipment, drugs, and supplies for a pediatric or neonatal transport. An equipment and medication bag should be prepared, organized, and labeled in advance. Before flying, all team members should have an orientation to the aircraft with an emphasis on location of all safety equipment. All units should have a cabin heater, an interior illuminator, and a voice communication system. Cabin heaters must be available to maintain ambient cabin temperature at least 24°C to preserve the physical properties of fluids and medications, as well as for the safety and comfort of the patient and crew. Voice communications systems cannot interfere with the aircraft communication system. Every unit must have an oxygen source and an electrical outlet invertor to supply AC/DC electric current. When choosing a specific unit, it must have adequate cabin space and configuration to allow for reasonable patient access. The transport team provides the information to the flight service regarding team size and type of transport (stretcher or isolette) when the actual unit is chosen.

Equipment for air transport is similar to that used for ground ambulance transport.

Table 140.4.
Transport Equipment List

Item	Model	Manufacturer(s)
1. ECG monitors	413, 413a	Tektronix Inc.*
	LIFEPAK5	Physio-control Inc.**
	506	Corometrics Medical System*
2. Pulse oximeter	N-10	Nellcor Inc.
	N-200	
3. Defibrillator—battery powered	LIFEPAK5	Physio-control Inc.**
4. Incubator, infant transport	ILSM-P	Airborne Life Systems
	20H	Ohio Medical Product
	AIRVAC	NARCO-Air Shields
	T167-1	
5. Ventilator, infant	BABYBIRD	Babybird
	MVP-10	Bio-Med Corp.
6. Oxygen analyzer	MINIOXG	Catalyst Research Corp.
	M25RAD	Oxy Med Inc.
7. Pumps, infusion syringe	AS20S	Travenol Labs
	AS-2F	
	MTP-100	
8. Blood pressure, noninvasive, indirect		Dinamap
		Ultrasonic Doppler
9. Portable suction unit		Laedral

* These neonatal models are capable of continuous monitoring of heart rate and rhythm, respiratory rate, skin temperature, and invasive or noninvasive blood pressure readings.
** Physio-Control Inc. manufactures a Lifepak monitor/defibrillator that provides continuous ECG monitoring/recording and DC defibrillation. The two instruments can be operated independently of each other.

Table 140.5.
Transport Nursing Bag

A. Medications
  1. Resuscitation: epinephrine, atropine, NaHCO$_3$, D50W, calcium (chloride, gluconate), dopamine, dobutamine, isoproterenol, digoxin, lidocaine, nitroprusside
  2. Paralytics: vecuronium, pancuronium, succinylcholine
  3. Sedatives/antiepileptics: diazepam, midazolam, lorazepam, phenobarbital, phenytoin
  4. Analgesics: morphine sulfate, fentanyl, meperidine
  5. Antibiotics: ampicillin, gentamicin, ceftriaxone, nafcillin, clindamycin, cefuroxime, vancomycin, amikacin.
  6. Miscellaneous: aminophylline, solumedrol, dexamethasone, diphenhydramine, nifedipine caps, neonatal tris-buffer, priscoline, furosemide, mannitol, NaCl and KCl concentrates, heparin flush, saline flush
  7. Intravenous fluid: normal saline, 5% albumin, D10W, D5 0.2NS, lactated Ringer's
B. Intravenous equipment
  Intravenous catheters (18-, 20-, 22-, 24-gauge angiocatheters) syringes, blood tubes, alcohol, Betadine, tape, armboards, tourniquets, intraosseous needles, tubing, butterflies and needles, Broviac caps, stopcocks, intravenous Y-connectors, cook catheter sets with 1% xylocaine, without epinephrine, Luer-Lok (adapters, T-connectors, and syringes)
C. Resuscitation/monitoring equipment
  Electrodes and leads, Dextrostix with lancets, nasogastric tubes (8, 5 French), urinary foley catheters (6, 8 French) and bags, BP cuffs (premie, child, adult), sphygmomanometer, Dinamap cuffs (#1, 2, 3, 4), temperature probes
D. Miscellaneous
  Spinal needles (22 gauge × 1.5″, 22 gauge × 3.5″), scalpels, restraints, cotton balls, premie hat and booties, pacifier

Table 140.6.
Transport Respiratory Supplies

1. Resuscitation bag (adult, child)
2. Face masks
  A. Resuscitation: adult, pediatric, infant, neonate
  B. Simple O$_2$: adult, child
  C. High concentration: adult, child
  D. Nasal cannulas: adult, pediatric, infant
3. Intubation equipment
  A. Laryngoscope blades: #0, 1, 1.5, 2, 3 Miller
  B. Laryngoscope handles: small, large
  C. Endotracheal tubes
    (Uncuffed (mm) 2.5, 3.0, 3.5, 4.0, 4.5)
    (Cuffed (mm) 3.0, 3.5, 4.0, 4.5, 5.0, 6.0, 7.0, 8.0)
  D. Suction equipment:
    Yankauer: small, large
    Catheters (French): 6, 8, 10, 12, 14
  E. Nasopharyngeal airways (French): 12 → 28
  F. Miscellaneous: spare batteries, spare bulbs, adaptors, scissors, tape, suture material and equipment, skin preparation, alcohol, gauze, blender/flowmeter, pulse oximeter probes.
4. Chest tubes
  A. Chest tubes: 10, 12 French
  B. Heimlich valves
  C. Tubing
5. Medications (nebulized)
  Albuterol, racemic epinephrine, atropine, isoproterenol, normal saline
6. Miscellaneous
  Stethoscope, ABG kits, CPAP bag setup with manometer

The transport team must bring all equipment and medications necessary for stabilization and transport. It must be assumed the referring hospital has no available pediatric drugs or resources to spare. All equipment must meet FAA regulations and be capable of providing pediatric life support in the transport setting. A transport isolette must be easily mobile, relatively lightweight, and durable.

The isolette ideally should have self-contained instrumentation with capabilities to monitor heart rate and rhythm, respiratory rate, central blood pressure, temperature (both patient and ambient), noninvasive blood pressure, and oxygen saturation. It should be equipped with a portable infant transport ventilator. The isolette must have a built-in power source and portable oxygen and air supply to serve both during transport in and out of the hospital and as an emergency backup should the vehicle supply fail. The power source should additionally be adaptable to the AC/DC current provided in the aircraft. The isolette should be compact to easily fit through standard hospital hallways and doorways and in and out the cabin door. Stretchers also must be easily mobile and

compact. Both the patient and the equipment should be easily and safely secured in the isolette or stretcher which is also well secured in the vehicle cabin.

All equipment used in air transport must meet FAA recommendations for use and safety. Equipment should be lightweight and portable to allow use during all stages of transport. Equipment must be durable to withstand repeated use under harsh weather conditions, vibrations, and changes in altitude and temperature. The equipment must be easy to maintain and operate. If necessary, both portable oxygen and battery power must be capable of supporting the patient for up to twice the expected transport time.

Basic equipment required for transport includes a monitor capable of measuring and recording heart rate and rhythm, respiratory rate, body temperature, and both invasive and noninvasive blood pressures. Pulse oximetry is now routinely monitored on nearly all pediatric transports. All monitors must be easy to read and operate in reduced lighting or in red tinted lights. A defibrillator, infusion pump, and suction units (portable and standard wall apparatus) also are essential equipment. The infusion pump should be battery powered and durable to prevent errors in the rate of infusion resulting from barometric pressure changes, vibration, altitude, and changes in position. The pump must be accurate to 0.1 mL per hr. Finally, all equipment should be checked frequently to ensure that it remains in optimum working order at all times.

PROCEDURE

Referring Hospital

When the referring physician has decided to transfer a patient, he or she must then attend to two important tasks. First, every effort should be made to ensure that the patient is both medically stable for the transport and that as many of the administrative tasks necessary to transport the patient as possible are completed. Medical stabilization begins with a recognition that the transport environment makes patient monitoring and care more difficult. Intravenous lines should be checked for patency and secured carefully. Tracheal and gastric tubes also should be checked and well secured. Whenever possible, medical interventions aimed at stabilizing the patient should be discussed with the receiving physicians and the transport crew. Regarding administrative procedures the most important of these is asking that at least one parent or legal guardian remain with the child at all times. This will ensure that necessary information and consent may be obtained before the actual transport.

The second task of the referring physician is to arrange for the transport. In most cases this will be a simple matter of calling a known transport service; however, rarely, the referring physician may be responsible for contacting the aeromedical provider directly. In this case the helicopter pilot will need certain information to ensure a safe landing and takeoff at the receiving facility (Fig. 140.1). This information should include the exact location of the helipad or landing area. Detailed information is usually appreciated unless the referring facility is well known to the aeromedical provider. Items such as cross streets, landmarks easily identified from the air, and the Keymap® location are helpful.

The pilot also should be notified of tall objects such as construction cranes, power lines, tall trees, or tall structures, which may interfere with the approach into the landing area. Even if the referring facility has a helipad, it is important to notify the pilot of any recent changes (e.g., construction) which might affect operations.

If the transferring facility does not have an acceptable landing area, then one must be established. Whenever possible, guidance should be sought from the aeromedical provider before establishing a landing zone because landing zones of different sizes are required for different aircraft, and a larger landing zone is required for night operations. In general, a small helicopter will require a 60×60 ft landing area for day operations and 100×100 ft for night operations. A medium-sized helicopter requires 75×75 ft for day operations and 125×125 ft at night. A large helicopter requires 120×125 ft for daytime and 200×200 ft at night. The ideal sight will be free of tall obstructing objects (e.g., phone wires) and debris which can be blown about by the aircraft's rotor wash. Additionally, it is best for the helipad to have a long open area on at least one side and preferably on two or more sides. Landing areas that are enclosed on all sides by trees or other tall objects force the aircraft to make direct vertical ascents and descents. This type of takeoff and landing places the greatest demands on the aircraft and leaves the least room for error. The landing zone should be as flat as possible—slopes of greater than 10° are unacceptable. If the landing area is not an established helipad, then the boundaries of the landing area should be marked by flares or other bright objects. If lights are used, these should not be directed into the pilot's eyes. Finally, smoke or other objects (e.g., a small flag) should be placed near the landing area so that the pilot can judge wind direction. Whenever possible the landing zone should be selected in concert with local EMS, fire department, or law enforcement. These agencies can be helpful with both selection of the landing area and crowd control near the landing area, which is particularly important when the sight chosen is a public roadway.

When the aircraft has landed, the referring personnel should in most cases wait un-

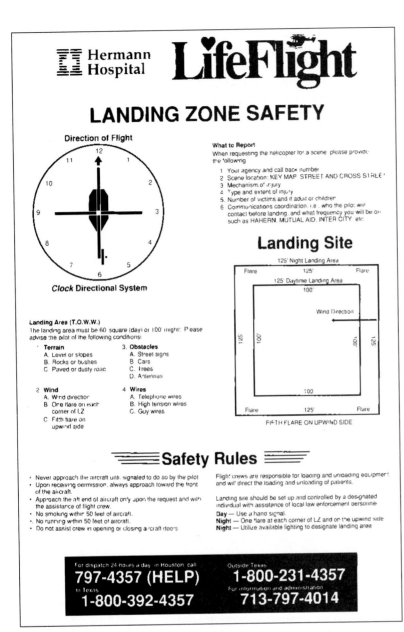

Figure 140.1.
Helicopter safety and landing zone information.

til the rotors have stopped turning before approaching the aircraft. It then should be approached from the front. Usually the pilot will wave ground personnel forward. Extra care must be taken when patient loading occurs with the rotor blades turning. The aircraft should not be approached until the pilot signals; then it should be approached from the front. If the aircraft has landed on a slope, it should be approached on the downhill side. Ground personnel should keep low because the rotor blades can dip in windy conditions. Extra care should be taken with rear loading helicopters. When patient loading occurs, personnel should not go beyond the midway point of the tail boom.

Receiving Hospital/ Transport Team

Once a transport call has been received and the decision made to provide aeromedical support, the team is mobilized. Information obtained from the transferring hospital includes not only diagnosis and status, but also specifics about intravenous access (number of lines and location), medications administered, and airway interventions. While waiting for the team to assemble, the equipment and supply bags are gathered and again checked to ensure that they are appropriately stocked. Backup batteries are brought as an additional power supply. Sufficient backup battery power and portable oxygen tanks must be available to provide care for the patient for 1.5 to 2 times the estimated transport time should the vehicle supply fail. Special drip infusions such as inotropes, prostaglandin, and fentanyl can be prepared in advance.

The medical team should be made familiar with the safety features, intercommunication system, and supply layout of the aircraft. This is ideally done at an orientation session but briefly reiterated before departure.

On arrival at the transferring hospital, the patient should be carefully assessed and stabilized before departure. Most complications that result during transport of a critically ill child are related to patient care rather than transport environmental factors.

It is imperative to ensure that the patient has a patent, stable airway before departure from the transferring facility. If the potential for respiratory embarrassment is relatively high, the child should undergo endotracheal intubation at the transferring hospital. If the child has already been intubated, proper airway placement of the endotracheal tube should be confirmed (recent chest radiograph and arterial blood gas, clinical assessment), and the tube should be securely taped in place. It is probably best to retape the endotracheal tube before transport, which allows for removal of any wet or loose tape and further decreases the potential risk of an accidental extubation during patient movement. The endotracheal tube should be thoroughly suctioned before transport. Either a nasogastric or an orogastric tube should be placed and mechanically suctioned to decompress the stomach of air, to reduce the risk of aspiration of gastric contents, and to improve respiratory compliance.

Similarly, all intravenous lines should be secured with clean, dry tape before transport. Each line should be clearly labeled. Whenever possible, fluids should be administered via syringe pumps to ensure accurate delivery en route. The rate of infusion of intravenous fluids may need to be increased to compensate for low humidity conditions or to treat transient hypotension resulting from the effect of gravitational forces during takeoff or rapid ascent. Intravenous lines not in use should be flushed with heparin and locked.

Because gas expands at high altitudes, small pneumothoraces may worsen; it is therefore often best to place a thoracotomy tube expectantly. Chest tubes are attached to either a Heimlich valve or portable suction. Colostomy and urinary bags should be drained of fluid and air.

If the patient is mechanically ventilated, he or she should be connected to the transport ventilator at bedside before movement. After the infant's airway has been deemed clinically stable, the patient is carefully moved to the transport isolette or stretcher. All intravenous lines should be untangled and easily accessible. Vital signs are rechecked. Attention must be given to maintaining euthermia as environmental conditions and temperature may change dramatically between the hospital room, the outside air, and the cabin during transport. The temperature inside the isolette should be preset and readied before arrival at the transferring hospital. Blankets are placed over the child. The child's wrists should be secured in place with Velcro or gauze restraints. The neonate or small infant transported in an isolette should have all extremities restrained to prevent sudden and potentially unsafe movement within the isolette. Safety belts are attached. In the airplane or helicopter cabin, the isolette or stretcher is locked in place with bars or chains to prevent movement during the flight. Cotton balls or ear cups should be placed to protect the patient's ears before helicopter takeoff. Consideration should be given to sedating and paralyzing the intubated patient before leaving the transferring hospital to prevent the child from attempting sudden movement or self-extubation during transit.

The neonate is especially susceptible to decompensation from stressors such as movement, touch, vibration, and noise, as well as changes in temperature, pressure, and altitude hypoxia. A higher concentration of oxygen will likely be needed as determined by the altitude oxygen requirement equation shown previously. Vital signs including a dextrostix should be again checked before departure. All electrode pads, monitor leads, intravenous lines, and tubes and drains are once again checked and secured. All monitors should have continuous LED displays placed in clear view of the transport nurse and physician.

During transport, vital signs are recorded at least every 15 minutes. It is possible to measure heart rate, systolic blood pressure, and oxygen saturation using the pulse oximeter. Blood pressure can be measured by placing the cuff on the same arm as the oximeter probe. The cuff is inflated until the oximeter readout disappears and then is deflated. The point at which the oximeter signal is reestablished represents the systolic pressure. Additionally, all intubated patients should have tracheal tube position confirmed, if not continuously using an end-tidal CO_2 detector, at least each time the patient is moved and then at regular intervals during the transport. Ideally, an end-tidal CO_2 monitor with a continuous digital readout is used. Colorometric means of measuring end-tidal CO_2 are less acceptable because the interpretation may be influenced by cabin lighting.

COMPLICATIONS

It is important to anticipate potential complications before any transport to be adequately prepared for intervention. For example, a sudden decrease in oxygen saturation on the pulse oximetry monitor can result from a mechanical or physiologic cause. The pulse oximeter leads and probe should be checked. The oxygen delivery source tank could be empty or the tubing kinked. The ventilator could be malfunctioning. The endotracheal tube itself could have dislodged or plugged, or the patient could possibly have developed a pneumothorax. Because assessment capabilities are limited by space, noise, and lighting, the transport team members must be prepared in advance to methodically evaluate the situation. Backup batteries and additional

SUMMARY
1. Perform necessary interventions to stabilize patient
2. Contact transport personnel at receiving facility
3. Provide information to determine optimal mode of transport and team composition
4. As necessary, provide additional information to aeromedical transport service to ensure safe landing and take-off (helipad location, potential obstructions, recent construction, etc.)
5. Establish landing zone if one does not already exist
6. Discuss transfer with patient and/or family and obtain consent
7. If possible, prepare all appropriate materials (copies of laboratory results, radiographs, etc.) prior to arrival of transport team
8. Update arriving transport team regarding any changes in clinical condition of patient
9. Assist in performing any necessary procedures to prevent potential clinical deterioration of patient en route (endotracheal intubation, paralysis and sedation, retaping lines and tubes, etc.)
10. Transfer patient only when sufficiently stabilized to allow safe transport

portable oxygen tanks should be readily available. A portable transilluminator and needle thoracostomy setup should be near the bedside. A team member should be prepared to manually ventilate the patient if a problem with the mechanical ventilator is suspected. The adage "If something can go wrong, it will" should be followed to anticipate and manage any real or apparent catastrophes. By being well prepared, a transport team can generally ensure a successful aeromedical transport.

SUMMARY

The goal of any transport is to provide competent and efficient pretransfer and intratransfer care. Many of the elements that lead to a successful ground transport (Chapter 139) are the same for aeromedical transport. For both, advanced preparation, communication, and teamwork are essential. Both air and ground transport have similar limitations in vehicle cabin size, patient access, and assessment capabilities. Noise, vibration, reduced lighting, and more difficult communication techniques (via intercommunication systems) make helicopter transports an even greater challenge. Altitude hypoxia, changes in barometric pressure, temperature, humidity, and gravitational forces are factors unique to air transport. A basic understanding of flight physiology is necessary to anticipate and plan for the potential impact on patient care.

Challenges and stressors of air medical transport generally can be alleviated by being well prepared for any complication that may arise. Early recognition of problems and prompt intervention often lead to a successful transport.

REFERENCES

1. Day SE, Chapman RA. Transport of critically ill patients in need of extracorpeal life support. Crit Care Clin 1992;8(3):581–596.
2. Yoder BA, Mull DM. Neonatal transport. Prob Crit Care 1990;4(4):581–598.
3. Pepe P. Prehospital and interhospital transport of the trauma patient. Prob Crit Care 1990;4(4):556–569.
4. Lam DM. Wings of life and hope. Prob Crit Care 1990;4(4):477–494.
5. Schneider C, Gomez M, Lee R. Evaluation of ground ambulance, rotor-wing, and fixed-wing aircraft services. Crit Care Clin 1992;8(3):533–564.
6. Brink LW, Neuman B, Wynn J. Air transport. Pediatr Clin North Am 1993;40(2):439–456.
7. Committee on hospital care, American Academy of Pediatrics. Guidelines for air and ground transportation of pediatric patients. Pediatrics 1986; 78(5):943–950.
8. Task force on interhospital transport. American Academy of Pediatrics. Guidelines for air and ground transport of neonatal and pediatric patients. Elk Grove Village, IL: American Academy of Pediatrics, 1993.
9. Blumen IJ, Abernethy MK, Dunne MJ. Flight physiology. Crit Care Clin 1992;8(3):597–618.
10. Fromm RE, Cronin LA. Issues in critical care transport. Prob Crit Care 1990;4(4):439–446.
11. Aoki BY, McCloskey K. Evaluation, Stabilization, and transport of the critically ill child. St. Louis: CV Mosby; 1992, pp. 321–341.
12. Pon S, Notterman D. The organization of a pediatric critical care transport program. Pediatr Clin North Am 1993;40(2):243–262.
13. Harris BH, Belcher JW. Equipment and planning for neonatal air transport. Med Instr 1982; 16(5):253–255.
14. Warren J, Guntupalli KK. Physiologic monitoring during prehospital and interhospital transport of critically ill patients. Prob Crit Care 1990; 4(4):459–469.
15. Talke P, Nichols RJ, Traber DL. Monitoring patients during helicopter flight. J Clin Monitor 1990; 6(2):139–140.
16. Klein K, Bills DM. Transport safety. In: McCloskey K, Orr R, eds. Pediatric transport medicine. St. Louis: CV Mosby 1995.

INDEX

References in italics denote figures; those followed by "t" denote tables.

equipment for, 1117
illustration of, *1116*
pathophysiology, 1115, 1117
Hydrocarbons, 61
Hydrocele
    clinical tips, 932
    formation, 929
    of inguinal canal
        illustration of, *928*
        inguinal hernia and, differential diagnosis,
            929–930
Hydrocephalus
    etiology of, 573
    shunts, 559
Hydrofluoric acid, skin decontamination of,
        1316t
Hydroxyzine, 450
Hymen
    prepubertal examination of, 962–963
    sensitivity of, 966
    sexual abuse indicators, 983–984, *984*
    structural variations, *964*
Hypercapnia, 896
Hypercarbia, 896
Hypersensitivity testing (*see also* Skin testing).
    antivenin formulations, 1322
    complications, 1292
    delayed, 1289
Hypertension, 28
Hyperthermia
    dehydration and, 1334
    symptoms of, 1333
Hypertrophy, electrocardiographic tracings
    left ventricular, *768, 769*
    right atrial, *767, 769*
    right ventricular, *767–768, 769*
Hyphema, 596
Hypnosis, 443
Hypospadia, female, catheterization in, 993
Hypotension, 1336
Hypothermia
    burns and, 1197
    classification of, 1339
    skin decontamination procedures and, 1316
Hypovolemia, 28
Hypovolemic shock, 88
Hypoxemia
    diffusion, 461
    nitrous oxide administration and, 461
    respiratory specimen techniques and,
            1256–1257
    thoracentesis and, 886
    tracheal suctioning and, 868
Hypoxia
    aeromedical transportation and, 1408
    clinical findings, 104
    pulse oximetry readings, 104

Immobilization
    of cervical spine
        anatomic and physiologic considerations,
            329–330
        assessment of, 338
        child vs. adult, 329, 330t, 344
        clinical tips, 340
        complications, 339t, 339–340

equipment
    car seats, *334*, 334–335
    cervical collar, 333–334, 336
    spine board, 333, *333*
indications for, 330–331
mechanisms of injuries, 329, 330t
procedure
    assessing prior immobilization, 335
    cervical collar application, 335–336, *336*
    in-line stabilization for airway control, 339
    manual stabilization, *338*
    radiographic options, *331–332*, 331–333
    semipermanent, 338–339
techniques for
    five-point restraint system, 20, *21*
    folded sheet, 17, 19, *19*
    papoose boards, 17, *18*
Immunometric assays, 1273
Impetigo
    culturing specimens, 1257
    description of, 1257
Implied parental consent, 67
IMV (*see* Intermittent mandatory ventilation).
Induction, rapid sequence
    anatomic and physiologic considerations
        airway reflexes, 142–143
        bradycardia, 143
        difficult intubations, conditions that predi-
            cate
            acquired, 143t
            congenital, 142t
            "full stomach" state, 143
            gag responses, 143
    ancillary agents
        atropine, 152–153
        lidocaine, 153
    clinical tips, 157–158
    complications, 156–157
    contraindications, 146
    definition of, 141
    equipment, 146, 146t
    indications, 145
        awake intubation, 145
        factors that influence decision, 144t,
            144–145
    modifications
        glaucoma, 156
        neurologic induction, 154–156
        neurologic intubation, 145
        situations that warrant, 141
    neuromuscular blockade
        depolarizing agents (*see* Succinylcholine).
        nondepolarizing agents, 152
    personnel for, 141–142
    pharmacologic agents
        desired effects, 143
        ideal properties, 143
    procedure
        cricoid pressure, 154
        factors that affect success, 153
        medications and dosages, 154t
        oxygenation and ventilation controls, 153
        preoxygenations, 153
    sedatives
        ketamine (*see* Ketamine).
        midazolam (*see* Midazolam).

direct
  with angled telescope, 706
  equipment, 703
  with flexible fiberoptic laryngoscope,
    706–709, *707*
  fiberoptic laryngoscopes, 703, 706–708
  indications, 701t, 701–702
  indirect
    equipment, 703
    illustration of, *705*
    patient positioning, 705, *706*
    procedure, 704–706
  physiologic effects, 171t
  in upper airway obstruction, 626
Laryngospasm, 709
Laryngotracheobronchitis
  aerosol therapy, 851
  characteristics of, 851
Larynx
  anatomy, *701*
  view with fiberoptic laryngoscopy, *708*
Lavage (*see also* Irrigation).
  bronchoalveolar
    complications, 1256–1257
    equipment, 1251
    indications, 1250–1251
    procedure, 1254
  diagnostic peritoneal
    anatomic landmarks, 357, *358*
    clinical tips, 364
    closed technique as alternative, 360
    complications, 363–364
    contraindications, 360
    description of, 357
    equipment, 360t, 360–361
    equivocal, criteria for, 363t
    indications
      criteria, 358–359, 360t
      penetrating trauma, 359–360
    positive, criteria for, 363t
    procedure
      anesthesia, 361
      fluid infusion, 363
      guide wire insertion, 361, *362*
      patient positioning, 361
    summary of, 363
  gastric
    anatomic characteristics, 1298
    clinical tips, 1303
    complications, 1303
    contraindications, 1300t
    effect on absorption, 1298
    equipment, 1300–1301
    factors that affect effectiveness, 1298
    indications, 1298–1299
    patient positioning, 1298, *1299*
    procedure
      inadvertent tube placement testing, 1302
      oral approach, 1301–1302
      patient restraint, 1301
      stomach drainage, 1302
      tube insertion length determinations,
        1301, *1302*
    summary of, 1300
    tubes, 1300–1301, *1301*

for upper gastrointestinal bleeding
  complications, 955–956
  procedure, 954
  summary, 956
Law of Poiseuille, 864
Left ventricular hypertrophy, electrocardio-
    graphic findings, *767, 769*
Leg
  compartment structures of, 1106t, 1109
  compartment syndrome, *1110*
Length, of patient
  for equipment selection, 42
  for weight estimation
    accuracy of, 39, 40
    Broselow system, 40, 41
    procedure, 41
Lens (*see* Contact lens).
Lidocaine
  administration, 153
  characteristics, 469t
  clinical uses
    dental abscess drainage, 727
    gastric intubation, 913
    intravenous regional anesthesia, 490
    orofacial anesthesia, 716, 721t
    paracentesis, 924
    regional auricular block, 653
    removal of vaginal foreign objects, 973
    suprapubic bladder aspiration, 1001
  dosage, 153
  properties of, 153
Lidocaine/adrenaline/tetracaine, as topical
    anesthetic, 472
Lids (*see* Eyelids).
Life support, basic
  airway passage, in infants
    adults and, comparison, 86
    anatomy and physiology, 86–87
  cardiopulmonary resuscitation (*see* Car-
    diopulmonary resuscitation).
  circulation
    checking the pulse, 93–94, *95*
    chest compressions, 95–97, *96–97*
    overview, 88–89
  clinical tips, 98
  complications, 97–98
  definition of, 85
  goals of, 85
  indications
    cardiopulmonary arrest, 91
    cardiopulmonary failure, 90–91
    overview, 89–90
    respiratory arrest, 90
    respiratory failure, 90
  procedure
    airway control, 91–92, *92*
    breathing, 92–93, *94*
    determining responsiveness, 91
    jaw thrust maneuver, 91–92, *93*
    "look, listen, feel" method, 92, *92*
    summary of, 95–96
Lighted stylet endotracheal intubation
  advantages, 211
  clinical tips, 211
  description of, 211
  procedure, 211, *214–215*
  summary of, 211

complications, 638
equipment, *635*, 635t
indications, 634–635
procedure
  hand position for pneumatic otoscopy, *637*
  patient restraint, 635–636, *636*
summary, 638–639
Ovarian herniation, 932
Ovaries, ultrasonographic imaging of, 1370, *1370*
Over-the-needle catheters
  description of, 802
  peripheral venous access use, 806–807
Oximetry (*see* Pulse oximetry).
Oxycellulose, in nasal packing, 666
Oxygen delivery
  complications, 108, 110
  equipment
    factors that affect, 104–105
    nasal cannula, 105, *105*
    nonrebreathing masks, 105–106, *106*
    oxygen hood, *107*, 107–108
    oxygen tent, 108, *109*
    partial rebreathing masks, 105–106
    simple oxygen mask, 105, *106*
  factors that affect, 103
  indications, 103–104
  oxyhemoglobin dissociation curve, *104*
  physiology of, 103
  procedure, 108
  to self-inflating resuscitation bags, 130–131
  utilization, 103
Oxygen hood
  description of, 107
  disadvantages, 108
  illustration of, *107*
Oxygen mask, for oxygen delivery, 105
Oxygen supplementation, during aeromedical transportation
  calculations to determine, 1408–1409
  for hypoxemia, 1408
Oxygen tent
  description of, 108
  illustration of, *109*
  maintenance, 108
Oxygen transport system
  illustration of, *824*
  pulse oximetry (*see* Pulse oximetry).
Oxyhemoglobin dissociation curve, *104, 125*
  description of, 824
  for emergent endotracheal intubation, *188*
  illustration of, *825*
Oxymetazoline, 206
Oxytocin, 1021

Pacing (*see* Cardiac pacing).
PAH preparation (*see* Potassium hydroxide preparation).
Pain
  anatomic and physiologic considerations, 437–439
  assessment of, 438
  definition of, 437

factors affecting, 438
in injection of local anesthetic, minimization of, 468
management (*see also* Analgesia).
  behavior therapy and, 442
  hypnosis, 443
  indications, 439–440
  medications
    complications, 443
    contraindications, 440
    description of use, 443
    narcotic, 441
    nonnarcotic, 440–441
    routes of administration, 439
  preparation and relaxation techniques, 441–442
  restraint, indications for, 442
  summary of, 442
in otitis media, 634
sedation for (*see* Conscious sedation).
understanding of, developmental sequence, 438t
undertreatment of, 439
Pancuronium
  administration, 152
  dosage, 152
  properties of, 152
Pap smear, 978, *979*
Papoose boards, 17, *18*
Paracentesis
  albumin replacement and, 923, 925
  anatomical and physiological considerations, 921, 923
  clinical tips, 925
  complications, 925
  contraindications, 923
  equipment, 923
  indications, 923
  procedure
    fluid collection, 924–925
    insertion sites, *923*
    patient positioning, *922*, 923
    procedure, 923–924
    "Z" track formation, *924*
  summary of, 925
Parallel margin infiltration
  description of, 468–469
  procedure, 470
  summary, 470
Paraphimosis
  pathophysiology of, 1007
  reduction
    anatomic and physiologic considerations, 1007
    with Babcock clamps, *1009*
    clinical tips, 1009
    complications, 1009
    description of, 1007
    equipment, 1008
    nonsurgical, *1008*, 1008–1009
    summary, 1008
    surgical, 1009
Parasympathetic nervous system, 848
Parasympatholytic agents
  anatomic effects, 848
  description of, 848

Index

1483

Two Great Companions to Textbook of Pediatric Emergency Procedures!

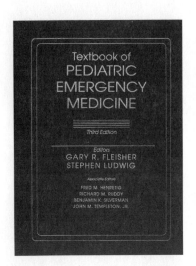

Textbook of Pediatric Emergency Medicine, Third Edition

Gary R. Fleisher, MD and Stephen Ludwig, MD

This is a valuable complement to Dr. Henretig and King's book. The expanded third edition includes new chapters on inter hospital/prehospital transport, HIV, sedation and analgesia, trauma and transplantation emergencies, plus new signs and symptoms for seizure, hypertension, hearing loss, dysphagia, and more.

1993/1844 pages/398 illustrations/#0-683-03255-0

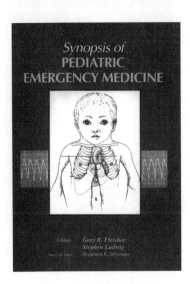

Synopsis of Pediatric Emergency Medicine

Gary R. Fleisher, MD, FAAP, FACEP and Stephen Ludwig, MD, FAAP

Here's the practical and portable answer to your busy, daily routine. Based on the authors' highly respected *Textbook of Pediatric Emergency Medicine*, the *Synopsis* has all the authority of the larger volume, yet presents the most clinically applicable basics in a succinct, easy-to-retrieve format. Perfect for bedside management, the text presents each aspect of pediatric emergency medicine in text keyed to both presenting complaint and disease entity. Valuable tables, algorithms, and current procedures are included.

1995/992 pages/205 illustrations/#0-683-03261-5

Preview these texts for a full month. If you're not completely satisfied, return them at no further obligation (US and Canada only).

Phone orders accepted 24 hours a day, 7 days a week (US only).

From the US, call: 1-800-638-0672
From Canada, call: 1-800-665-1148
From outside the US and Canada, call 410-528-4223
From the UK and Europe call 44 (171) 385-2357
From Southeast Asia call (852) 2610-2339

INTERNET
E-mail: custserv@wwilkins.com
Home page: http://www.wwilkins.com